This book is d

Rosen's Emergency Medicine

Volume 1

ROSEN'S
EMERGENCY MEDICINE
Concepts and Clinical Practice

sixth edition

Editor-in-Chief
John A. Marx, MD, FAAEM, FACEP
Chair and Chief
Department of Emergency Medicine
Carolinas Medical Center
Charlotte, North Carolina
Adjunct Professor
Department of Emergency
  Medicine
University of North Carolina
  School of Medicine
Chapel Hill, North Carolina

Senior Editors
Robert S. Hockberger, MD, FACEP, FAAEM
Chair
Department of Emergency
  Medicine
Harbor–UCLA Medical Center
Torrance, California
Professor of Clinical Medicine
David Geffen School of Medicine
  at UCLA
Westwood, Los Angeles, California

Ron M. Walls, MD, FAAEM, FACEP, FRCPC
Chair
Department of Emergency
  Medicine
Brigham and Women's Hospital
Associate Professor of Medicine
  (Emergency Medicine)
Harvard Medical School
Boston, Massachusetts

Editors
James G. Adams, MD, FACP, FACEP
Chair
Department of Emergency
  Medicine
Northwestern Memorial Hospital
Professor of Medicine
Northwestern University
  Feinberg School of Medicine
Chicago, Illinois

William G. Barsan, MD
Professor and Chair
Department of Emergency
  Medicine
University of Michigan
  Medical School
Ann Arbor, Michigan

Michelle H. Biros, MD, MS, FAAEM, FACEP
Research Director and Faculty
  Physician
Department of Emergency
  Medicine
Hennepin County Medical
  Center
Professor of Emergency Medicine
University of Minnesota
  Medical School
Minneapolis, Minnesota

Daniel F. Danzl, MD
Professor and Chair
Department of Emergency
  Medicine
University of Louisville School
  of Medicine
Louisville, Kentucky

Marianne Gausche-Hill, MD, FACEP, FAAP
Professor of Medicine
David Geffen School of Medicine
  at UCLA
Director of EMS and Pediatric
  Emergency Medicine Fellowship
Department of Emergency Medicine
Harbor–UCLA Medical Center
Torrance, California

Glenn C. Hamilton, MD, MSM
Professor and Chair
Department of Emergency Medicine
Wright State University School of
  Medicine
Dayton, Ohio

Louis J. Ling, MD, FACEP, FACMT
Professor of Emergency Medicine
  and Pharmacy
Associate Dean for Graduate
  Medical Education
University of Minnesota Medical
  School
Associate Medicine Director for
  Medical Education
Hennepin County Medical Center
Senior Associate Medical Director
Hennepin Regional Poison Center
Minneapolis, Minnesota

Edward J. Newton, MD, FACEP
Chair
Department of Emergency Medicine
Los Angeles County and University
  of Southern California Medical
  Center
Professor of Clinical Emergency
  Medicine
University of Southern California
  Keck School of Medicine
Los Angeles, California

MOSBY

ELSEVIER

MOSBY
ELSEVIER

1600 John F. Kennedy Boulevard, Suite 1800
Philadelphia, PA 19103-2899

ROSEN'S EMERGENCY MEDICINE: Concepts and Clinical Practice, 6th Edition
Three-Volume Set   0-323-02845-4
Online Edition   0-323-03686-4
E-dition   0-323-04302-X

NOTICE

Knowledge and best practice in this field are constantly changing. As new research and experience broaden our knowledge, changes in practice, treatment and drug therapy may become necessary or appropriate. Readers are advised to check the most current information provided (i) on procedures featured or (ii) by the manufacturer of each product to be administered, to verify the recommended dose or formula, the method and duration of administration, and contraindications. It is the responsibility of the practitioner, relying on their own experience and knowledge of the patient, to make diagnoses, to determine dosages and the best treatment for each individual patient, and to take all appropriate safey precautions. To the fullest extent of the law, neither the Publisher nor the Editors and Authors assume any liability for any injury and/or damage to persons or property arising out of or related to any use of the material contained in this book.

Library of Congress Cataloging-in-Publication Data

Rosen's emergency medicine : concepts and clinical practice.—6th ed. / editor-in-chief,
    John A. Marx ; senior editors, Robert S. Hockberger, Ron M. Walls ; editors, James Adams . . .
    [et al.]
       p. ; cm.
    Includes bibliographical references and index.
    ISBN-13: 978–0–323–02845–5   ISBN-10: 0–323–02845–4
    1. Emergency medicine. I. Title: Emergency medicine. II. Marx, John A. III.
Hockberger, Robert S. IV. Walls, Ron M. V. Adams, James VI. Rosen, Peter Emergency
medicine.
    [DNLM: 1. Emergencies. 2. Emergency Medicine. WB 105 E555 2006]
RC86.7.E5784 2006
616.02′5—dc22   2005041694

ISBN-13: 978–0–323–02845–5
ISBN-10: 0–323–02845–4

Acquisitions Editor: Todd Hummel
Developmental Editor: Kimberly Cox
Publishing Services Manager: Frank Polizzano
Project Manager: Robin E. Hayward
Cover Design Direction: Steven Stave
Text Designer: Jayne Jones
Marketing Manager: Dana Butler

Printed in China

Last digit is the print number: 9   8   7   6   5   4   3   2

Contributors

Cynthia K. Aaron, MD
Associate Professor of Emergency Medicine and
Pediatrics, Wayne State University School of
Medicine; Director, Medical and Clinical
Toxicology Education, Regional Poison Control
Center at Children's Hospital of Michigan, Detroit,
Michigan
161: Pesticides

Jean T. Abbott, MD, MH
Associate Professor, Division of Emergency
Medicine, Department of Surgery, University
of Colorado School of Medicine; Attending
Physician, Emergency Department, University
of Colorado Hospital, Denver, Colorado
177: Acute Complications of Pregnancy
206: End of Life

Norman S. Abramson, MD
Clinical Professor of Emergency Medicine,
University of Pittsburgh School of Medicine;
Attending Physician, Jefferson Regional Medical
Center, Pittsburgh, Pennsylvania
6: Brain Resuscitation

Riyad B. Abu-Laban, MD, MHSc, FRCPC
Assistant Professor, Division of Emergency
Medicine, Department of Surgery, University of
British Columbia Faculty of Medicine; Attending
Physician and Research Director, Department of
Emergency Medicine, Vancouver General Hospital,
Vancouver, British Columbia, Canada
55: Ankle and Foot

James G. Adams, MD
Chair, Department of Emergency Medicine,
Northwestern Memorial Hospital; Professor of
Medicine, Northwestern University Feinberg
School of Medicine, Chicago, Illinois

Stephen L. Adams, MD, FACP, FACEP
Professor of Medicine and Chief, Division of Sports
Medicine, Department of Medicine, Northwestern
University Feinberg School of Medicine; Medical
Director, Emergency Preparedness/Disaster
Services, Northwestern Memorial Hospital; Team
Physician, Chicago Cubs National League Baseball
Club, Chicago, Illinois
115: Tendinopathy and Bursitis

Kumar Alagappan, MD
Associate Professor of Clinical Emergency Medicine,
Department of Emergency Medicine, Albert
Einstein College of Medicine of Yeshiva
University, Bronx, New York; Associate Chair,
Department of Emergency Medicine, Long Island
Jewish Medical Center, New Hyde Park, New York
101: Headache

Brian Alverson, MD, FAAP
Staff Pediatrician, Sky Ridge Medical Center,
CarePoint, P.C., Lone Tree, Colorado
*168: Pediatric Respiratory Emergencies: Disease of the
Lungs*

**James T. Amsterdam, MD, DMD, MMM, FACEP,
FAAEM, FACPE**
Professor of Clinical Emergency Medicine,
Pennsylvania State University College of Medicine,
Hershey, Pennsylvania; Chair and Service Line
Director, Department of Emergency Medicine,
WellSpan/York Hospital, York, Pennsylvania
69: Oral Medicine

Christine Anderegg, MD
Medical Education Fellow and Clinical Instructor
of Medicine, David Geffen School of Medicine at
UCLA, Los Angeles, California
97: Sexually Transmitted Diseases

Deirdre Anglin, MD, MPH
Associate Professor of Emergency Medicine,
University of Southern California Keck School
of Medicine; Attending Physician, Los Angeles
County and University of Southern California
Medical Center, Los Angeles, California
67: Elder Abuse and Neglect

Felix Ankel, MD
Associate Professor of Emergency Medicine,
University of Minnesota Medical School,
Minneapolis, Minnesota; Residency Director,
Emergency Medicine, Regions Hospital, St. Paul,
Minnesota
84: Aortic Dissection

Robert E. Antosia, MD, MPH
Assistant Professor of Medicine, Harvard Medical
School; Attending Physician, Department of
Emergency Medicine, Beth Israel Deaconess
Medical Center, Boston, Massachusetts
47: Hand
54: Knee and Lower Leg

Chandra D. Aubin, MD
Assistant Professor of Emergency Medicine,
Washington University School of Medicine;
Attending Physician, Barnes-Jewish Hospital,
St. Louis, Missouri
10: Clinical Decision Making

Tom P. Aufderheide, MD, FACEP
Professor of Emergency Medicine, Medical College
of Wisconsin; Director of Research Services,
Department of Emergency Medicine, Froedtert
Memorial Lutheran Hospital, Milwaukee, Wisconsin
86: Peripheral Arteriovascular Disease

Adam Z. Barkin, MD
Attending Physician, Department of Emergency Medicine, Beth Israel Deaconess Medical Center; Instructor in Medicine, Harvard Medical School, Boston, Massachusetts
136: Sepsis Syndromes

Roger M. Barkin, MD, MPH, FAAP, FACEP
Clinical Professor of Pediatrics, University of Colorado Health Sciences Center; CarePoint, P.C., Denver, Colorado
165: Fever
171: Infectious Diarrheal Disease and Dehydration

Andrew R. Barnosky, DO, MPH
Assistant Professor, Department of Emergency Medicine, University of Michigan Medical School, Ann Arbor, Michigan
199: Occupational Medicine and Occupational Health in the Emergency Department

William G. Barsan, MD
Professor and Chair, Department of Emergency Medicine, University of Michigan Medical School, Ann Arbor, Michigan
99: Stroke

Bruce M. Becker, MD, MPH
Associate Professor, Departments of Community Health and Emergency Medicine, Brown Medical School; Attending Physician, Department of Emergency Medicine, Rhode Island Hospital and Hasbro Children's Hospital, Providence, Rhode Island
131: Parasites

Carol D. Berkowitz, MD
Professor of Clinical Pediatrics, David Geffen School of Medicine at UCLA, Westwood, Los Angeles, California; Executive Vice Chair, Department of Pediatrics, Harbor–UCLA Medical Center, Torrance, California
64: Child Maltreatment

Edward Bernstein, MD
Professor, Department of Emergency Medicine, Boston University School of Medicine; Professor of Social and Behavioral Sciences, Boston University School of Public Health; Vice Chair for Academic Affairs, Department of Emergency Medicine, Boston University Medical Center, Boston, Massachusetts
203: Multiculturalism and Care Delivery

Judith Bernstein, PhD, RNC
Associate Professor, Department of Emergency Medicine, Boston University School of Medicine; Associate Professor, Department of Maternal and Child Health, Boston University School of Public Health, Boston, Massachusetts
203: Multiculturalism and Care Delivery

Howard A. Bessen, MD
Professor of Medicine, David Geffen School of Medicine at UCLA, Westwood, Los Angeles, California and Harbor–UCLA Medical Center, Torrance, California
85: Abdominal Aortic Aneurysm

Elisabeth F. Bilden, MD, FACEP
Hennepin Regional Poison Center, Hennepin County Medical Center, Minneapolis, Minnesota; Department of Emergency Medicine, St. Luke's Hospital, Duluth, Minnesota
149: Antidepressants

Diane M. Birnbaumer, MD
Professor of Clinical Medicine, David Geffen School of Medicine at UCLA, Westwood, Los Angeles, California; Associate Program Director, Department of Emergency Medicine, Harbor–UCLA Medical Center, Torrance, California
37: Geriatric Trauma
97: Sexually Transmitted Diseases
181: The Elder Patient

Michelle H. Biros, MD
Research Director and Faculty Physician, Department of Emergency Medicine, Hennepin County Medical Center; Professor of Emergency Medicine, University of Minnesota Medical School, Minneapolis, Minnesota
38: Head

Robert A. Bitterman, MD, JD, FACEP
Department of Emergency Medicine, Carolinas Medical Center, Charlotte, North Carolina; Vice President, Emergency Physicians Insurance Company (EPIC), Auburn, California; Adjunct Associate Professor, Department of Emergency Medicine, University of North Carolina School of Medicine, Chapel Hill, North Carolina
93: Acute Gastroenteritis
207: Medicolegal and Risk Management

Kenneth E. Bizovi, MD
Assistant Professor of Emergency Medicine, Oregon Health and Science University; Staff Physician, Oregon Poison Center, Portland, Oregon
146: Acetaminophen

Thomas H. Blackwell, MD
Medical Director, Center for Prehospital Medicine, Department of Emergency Medicine, Carolinas Medical Center, Charlotte; Medical Director, Mecklenburg EMS Agency, Charlotte, North Carolina; Adjunct Associate Professor, Department of Emergency Medicine, University of North Carolina School of Medicine, Chapel Hill, North Carolina
191: Emergency Medical Service: Overview and Ground Transport

Frederick C. Blum, MD, FACEP, FAAP
Associate Professor of Emergency Medicine and Pediatrics, West Virginia University School of Medicine and West Virginia University Hospitals, Morgantown, West Virginia
11: Fever in the Adult Patient

Ira J. Blumen, MD
Professor, Section of Emergency Medicine, University of Chicago; Medical Director and Program Director, University of Chicago Hospitals, Chicago, Illinois
192: Air Medical Transport

Jennifer Bocock, MD
Assistant Professor and Education Coordinator, Wright State University School of Medicine, Dayton, Ohio; Attending Physician, Department of Emergency Medicine, Kettering Medical Center, Kettering, Ohio
30: Cyanosis

J. Stephen Bohan, MD, MS, FACP, FACEP
Executive Vice Chair and Clinical Director, Department of Emergency Medicine, Brigham and Women's Hospital; Assistant Professor, Harvard Medical School, Boston, Massachusetts
196: Guidelines in Emergency Medicine

Edward B. Bolgiano, MD, FACP, FACEP
Assistant Professor, Departments of Medicine and Surgery, University of Maryland School of Medicine; Chair, Department of Emergency Medicine, Bon Secours Hospital, Baltimore, Maryland
132: Tick-Borne Illnesses

Laura J. Bontempo, MD
Assistant Professor and Residency Program Director, Section of Emergency Medicine, Department of Surgery, Yale University School of Medicine, New Haven, Connecticut
125: Rhabdomyolysis

Marc Borenstein, MD
Chair, Department of Emergency Medicine; Program Director, Emergency Medicine Residency, Department of Emergency Medicine, Newark Beth Israel Medical Center, Newark, New Jersey
121: Selected Oncologic Emergencies

John C. Bradford, DO
Professor of Clinical Emergency Medicine, Department of Emergency Medicine, Northeastern Ohio Universities College of Medicine, Rootstown, Ohio; Attending Physician, Department of Emergency Medicine, Akron General Medical Center, Akron, Ohio
28: Vaginal Bleeding

William J. Brady, MD
Associate Professor, Department of Emergency Medicine, University of Virginia School of Medicine; Medical Director, Life Support Learning Center, University of Virginia Health System, Charlottesville, Virginia
14: Confusion
77: Acute Coronary Syndromes

Sabina Braithwaite, MD
Assistant Professor, Department of Emergency Medicine, University of Virginia School of Medicine; Medical Director, Paramedic Education, University of Virginia Health System, Charlottesville, Virginia
18: Dyspnea

David F. M. Brown, MD
Assistant Professor of Medicine, Harvard Medical School; Associate Chief, Department of Emergency Medicine, Massachusetts General Hospital, Boston, Massachusetts
15: Coma and Depressed Level of Consciousness
57: Foreign Bodies

James E. Brown, MD
Assistant Professor of Emergency Medicine; Program Director, Integrated Residency in Emergency Medicine, Wright State University School of Medicine, Dayton, Ohio
19: Chest Pain

Douglas D. Brunette, MD
Associate Professor, Department of Emergency Medicine, University of Minnesota Medical School; Program Director, Department of Emergency Medicine, Hennepin County Medical Center, Minneapolis, Minnesota
70: Ophthalmology

Keith K. Burkhart, MD
Professor of Clinical Emergency Medicine, Pennsylvania State University College of Medicine, Hershey, Pennsylvania
158: Lithium

Michael J. Burns, MD, FACP, FACEP
Clinical Professor, Departments of Medicine and Emergency Medicine, Division of Infectious Diseases, University of California, Irvine, School of Medicine, Irvine, California; Attending Physician, Emergency Medicine and Infectious Diseases, University of California, Irvine, Medical Center, Orange, California
182: The Immunocompromised Patient

John D. Cahill, MD, DTM&H
Assistant Professor and Lecturer, Department of International Health and Tropical Medicine, Royal College of Surgeons in Ireland; Attending Physician in Emergency Medicine and Infectious Disease, St. Luke's-Roosevelt Hospital Center, New York, New York
131: Parasites

Kirsten K. Calder, MD
Assistant Professor of Clinical Emergency Medicine, University of Southern California Keck School of Medicine; Department of Emergency Medicine, Los Angeles County and University of Southern California Medical Center, Los Angeles, California
178: Chronic Medical Illness During Pregnancy

Richard M. Cantor, MD, FAAP, FACEP
Associate Professor and Director, Pediatric Emergency Medicine, Department of Emergency Medicine; Medical Director, Central New York Regional Poison Control Center, State University of New York Upstate Medical University College of Medicine, Syracuse, New York
36: Pediatric Trauma

Stuart M. Caplen, MD
Chief, Department of Emergency Medicine, Englewood Hospital and Medical Center, Englewood, New Jersey
173: Neurologic Disorders

Andrea Carlson, MD
Department of Emergency Medicine; Director of Medical Toxicology, Advocate Christ Hospital and Medical Center, Oak Lawn, Illinois
163: Sedative Hypnotics

Dennis Chan, MD, FACEP
Chief of Emergency Services Sharp Memorial
  Hospital, San Diego, California
133: Tuberculosis

Theodore Chan, MD
Associate Professor, Department of Emergency
  Medicine, University of California, San Diego,
  School of Medicine, La Jolla, California
77: Acute Coronary Syndromes

Dane M. Chapman, MD, PhD
Director of Medical Simulation, Center for Clinical
  Reasoning and Procedural Competency, University
  of Colorado School of Medicine; Assistant Head
  and Director of Education, Division of Emergency
  Medicine, University of Colorado Health Sciences
  Center, Denver, Colorado
10: Clinical Decision Making

Daniel K. Chapman, MD, MPH
Assistant Professor, Division of Occupational
  Medicine, Department of Emergency Medicine,
  University of Michigan Medical School, Ann
  Arbor, Michigan
*199: Occupational Medicine and Occupational Health in
  the Emergency Department*

Douglas M. Char, MD, MA
Assistant Professor of Emergency Medicine,
  Washington University School of Medicine;
  Attending Physician, Barnes-Jewish Hospital and
  St. Louis Children's Hospital, St. Louis, Missouri
10: Clinical Decision Making

Carl R. Chudnofsky, MD
Associate Professor, Jefferson Medical College of
  Thomas Jefferson University; Chair, Department
  of Emergency Medicine, Albert Einstein Medical
  Center, Philadelphia, Pennsylvania
188: Procedural Sedation and Analgesia

Richard F. Clark, MD, FACMT
Professor of Medicine, University of California, San
  Diego, School of Medicine, La Jolla, California;
  Director, Division of Medical Toxicology,
  University of California, San Diego, Medical
  Center, San Diego, California
154: Hallucinogens

Phillip A. Clement, MD, FACEP
Clinical Assistant Professor, Department of
  Emergency Medicine, East Carolina University
  Brody School of Medicine; Attending Physician,
  Pitt County Memorial Hospital, Greenville, North
  Carolina
24: Diarrhea

Wendy C. Coates, MD
Associate Professor of Medicine and Chair, Acute
  Care College, David Geffen School of Medicine
  at UCLA, Westwood, Los Angeles, California;
  Director of Medical Education, Department of
  Emergency Medicine, Harbor–UCLA Medical
  Center, Torrance, California
95: Anorectum

Jamie L. Collings, MD
Assistant Professor, Northwestern University
  Feinberg School of Medicine; Residency Director,
  Department of Emergency Medicine, Northwestern
  Memorial Hospital, Chicago, Illinois
122: Acid-Base Disorders

Stephen A. Coluicciello, MD
Associate Chair, Department of Emergency
  Medicine, Carolinas Medical Center, Charlotte,
  North Carolina; Adjunct Professor of Emergency
  Medicine, University of North Carolina School of
  Medicine, Chapel Hill, North Carolina
113: Suicide
185: Substance Abuse

Edward E. Conway, Jr., MD, MS
Professor of Clinical Pediatrics, Albert Einstein
  College of Medicine of Yeshiva University, Bronx,
  New York; Chair, Department of Pediatrics, Beth
  Israel Medical Center, New York, New York
173: Neurologic Disorders

Mary Ann Cooper, MD
Professor, Departments of Bioengineering and
  Emergency Medicine, University of Illinois at
  Chicago, Chicago, Illinois
140: Electrical and Lightning Injuries

William H. Cordell, MD
Adjunct Clinical Professor in Emergency Medicine,
  Department of Emergency Medicine, Indiana
  University School of Medicine, Indianapolis,
  Indiana
202: Information Technology in Emergency Medicine

Todd J. Crocco, MD
Assistant Professor and Director of Clinical
  Research, West Virginia University School of
  Medicine, Morgantown, West Virginia
99: Stroke

Pat Croskerry, MD, PhD
Senior Research Scientist, Dalhousie University,
  Halifax, Nova Scotia, Canada; Attending
  Physician, Dartmouth General Hospital,
  Dartmouth, Nova Scotia, Canada
*204: Process Improvement and Patient Safety in the
  Emergency Department*

Natalie Cullen, MD
Assistant Clinical Professor, Wright State University
  School of Medicine, Dayton, Ohio; Attending
  Physician, Kettering Medical Center, Kettering, Ohio
25: Constipation

A. Adam Cwinn, MD, FRCPC
Associate Professor, Department of Emergency
  Medicine, University of Ottawa Faculty of
  Medicine; Head, Department of Emergency
  Medicine and Medical Director, Critical Care and
  Emergency Medicine, Ottawa Hospital, Ottawa,
  Ontario, Canada
52: Pelvis

Rita K. Cydulka, MD, MS
Associate Professor and Vice Chair, Department of Emergency Medicine, Case Western Reserve University School of Medicine; Attending Physician, Department of Emergency Medicine, MetroHealth Medical Center, Cleveland, Ohio
118: Dermatologic Presentations
124: Diabetes Mellitus and Disorders of Glucose Homeostasis

Daniel F. Danzl, MD
Professor and Chair, Department of Emergency Medicine, University of Louisville School of Medicine, Louisville, Kentucky
137: Frostbite
138: Accidental Hypothermia

Christine D. Darr, MD
Assistant Clinical Professor, University of Colorado School of Medicine; Medical Director, Pediatric Division, CarePoint, P.C., Denver, Colorado
167: Pediatric Respiratory Emergencies: Lower Airway Obstruction

Robert Dart, MD
Associate Professor and Vice Chair, Department of Emergency Medicine, Boston University School of Medicine, Boston, Massachusetts; Chief of Emergency Services, Quincy Medical Center, Quincy, Massachusetts
27: Acute Pelvic Pain

Mohamud Daya, MD, MS, FACEP, FACMT, DTM&H
Associate Professor, Department of Emergency Medicine, Oregon Health and Science University, Portland, Oregon
50: Shoulder

Kathleen A. Delaney, MD
Professor, Division of Emergency Medicine, University of Texas Southwestern Medical Center; Medical Director, Emergency Department, Parkland Memorial Hospital, Dallas, Texas
155: Heavy Metals

Theodore R. Delbridge, MD, MPH
Associate Professor of Emergency Medicine, University of Pittsburgh School of Medicine; Director of Emergency Services, University of Pittsburgh Medical Center Presbyterian, Pittsburgh, Pennsylvania
78: Dysrhythmias

Robert A. De Lorenzo, MD, FACEP
Associate Adjunct Professor, Uniformed Services University of the Health Sciences, Bethesda, Maryland; Program Director, Department of Emergency Medicine, Brooke Army Medical Center, Fort Sam Houston, San Antonio, Texas
20: Syncope

Susan M. Dunmire, MD
Associate Professor of Emergency Medicine and Academic Coordinator for Medical Student Education, Department of Emergency Medicine, University of Pittsburgh School of Medicine; Attending Physician, Emergency Department, University of Pittsburgh Medical Center Presbyterian, Pittsburgh, Pennsylvania
82: Infective Endocarditis and Valvular Heart Disease

Marc Eckstein, MD
Associate Professor of Emergency Medicine, University of Southern California Keck School of Medicine; Director of Prehospital Care, Los Angeles County and University of Southern California Medical Center; Medical Director, Los Angeles Fire Department, Los Angeles, California
42: Thoracic Trauma

Richard F. Edlich, MD, PhD
Professor Emeritus of Plastic Surgery and Biomedical Engineering; Founder, DeCamp Burn and Wound Healing Center, University of Virginia Health System, Charlottesville, Virginia; Director of Trauma Research, Education, and Prevention, Trauma Specialists, LLP, Legacy Emanuel Hospital, Portland, Oregon
60: Thermal Burns
61: Chemical Injuries

Mary A. Eisenhauer, MD, FRCPC
Associate Professor, Department of Medicine, University of Western Ontario Schulich School of Medicine; Emergency Physician, London Health Sciences Center, London, Ontario, Canada
48: Wrist and Forearm

Jay L. Falk, MD
Clinical Professor of Medicine and Emergency Medicine, University of Florida College of Medicine, Gainesville, Florida; Clinical Professor of Clinical Sciences, Florida State University College of Medicine, Orlando, Florida; Chief Academic Medical Officer, Orlando Regional Healthcare; Academic Chair, Department of Emergency Medicine, Orlando Regional Medical Center, Orlando, Florida
80: Heart Failure

Kim M. Feldhaus, MD
Staff Physician, Boulder Community Hospital, Boulder, Colorado
143: Submersion

Madonna Fernández-Frackelton, MD
Assistant Professor of Medicine, David Geffen School of Medicine at UCLA, Westwood, Los Angeles, California; Director, Adult Emergency Department, Harbor–UCLA Medical Center, Torrance, California
127: Bacteria

James F. Fiechtl, MD
Department of Emergency Medicine, Carolinas Medical Center, Charlotte, North Carolina
53: Femur and Hip

John T. Finnell, MD, MSc
Assistant Professor of Emergency Medicine, Department of Emergency Medicine, Indiana University School of Medicine, Indianapolis, Indiana
184: Alcohol-Related Disease

E. John Gallagher, MD
Professor and University Chair, Department of
Emergency Medicine, Albert Einstein College of
Medicine of Yeshiva University; Chief of Service,
Emergency Medicine, Montefiore Medical Center,
Bronx, New York
105: Peripheral Nerve Disorders

Marianne Gausche-Hill, MD, FACEP, FAAP
Professor of Medicine, David Geffen School of
Medicine at UCLA; Director of EMS and Pediatric
Emergency Medicine Fellowship, Department of
Emergency Medicine, Harbor–UCLA Medical
Center, Torrance, California
*175: Sudden Infant Death Syndrome and Apparent
Life-Threatening Events*

Mark E. Gebhart, MD, FAAEM
Assistant Professor of Emergency Medicine, Wright
State University School of Medicine; Staff
Physician, Emergency and Trauma Center, Good
Samaritan Hospital, Dayton, Ohio
31: Sore Throat

Joel M. Geiderman, MD
Co-Chair, Ruth and Harry Roman Emergency
Department, Burns and Allen Research Institute,
Cedars-Sinai Medical Center, Los Angeles,
California; Clinical Professor, Department of
Emergency Medicine, David Geffen School of
Medicine at UCLA, Westwood, Los Angeles,
California; Medical Director, Beverly Hills Fire
Department, Beverly Hills, California
46: General Principles of Orthopedic Injuries
49: Humerus and Elbow

Michael A. Gibbs, MD, FACEP
Clinical Professor of Emergency Medicine,
University of Vermont College of Medicine,
Burlington, Vermont; Attending Physician and
Chief, Department of Emergency Medicine, Maine
Medical Center, Portland, Maine
53: Femur and Hip
123: Electrolyte Disturbances

Brian P. Gilligan, MD
Attending Physician, Pediatric Emergency
Department, Wolfson Children's Hospital,
Jacksonville, Florida
8: Pediatric Resuscitation

Susan L. Gin-Shaw, MD
Department of Emergency Medicine, Mayo Clinic
Hospital Scottsdale, Scottsdale, Arizona; Staff
Physician, Arizona Heart Hospital, Phoenix,
Arizona
34: Multiple Trauma

Richard Goldberg, MD
Clinical Professor of Emergency Medicine,
Department of Emergency Medicine, Los Angeles
County and University of Southern California
Medical Center, Los Angeles, California; Staff
Physician, Providence Saint Joseph Medical
Center, Burbank, California
208: Wellness, Stress, and the Impaired Physician

James A. Gordon, MD, MPA
Assistant Professor of Medicine, Division of
Emergency Medicine; Director, Gilbert Program
in Medical Simulation, Harvard Medical School;
Attending Physician, Department of Emergency
Medicine, Massachusetts General Hospital,
Boston, Massachusetts
201: The Social Role of Emergency Medicine

John E. Gough, MD
Professor, Department of Emergency Medicine, East
Carolina University Brody School of Medicine;
Attending Physician, Pitt County Memorial
Hospital, Greenville, North Carolina
24: Diarrhea

Louis Graff, MD, FACP, FACEP
Professor of Traumatology and Emergency Medicine;
Professor of Clinical Medicine, University of
Connecticut School of Medicine, Farmington,
Connecticut; Assistant Clinical Professor, Division
of Emergency Medicine, Department of Surgery,
Yale University School of Medicine, New Haven,
Connecticut; Associate Chief of Emergency
Medicine, New Britain General Hospital, New
Britain, Connecticut
198: Observation Medicine and Clinical Decision Units

Timothy A. D. Graham, MD
Assistant Clinical Professor, Department of
Emergency Medicine, University of Alberta
Faculty of Medicine and Dentistry; Attending
Emergency Physician, University of Alberta
Hospital, Edmonton, Alberta, Canada
3: Monitoring the Emergency Patient

Richard O. Gray, MD
Assistant Professor of Emergency Medicine,
University of Minnesota Medical School;
Emergency Medicine Faculty Physician and
Director of Medical Student Education, Hennepin
County Medical Center, Minneapolis, Minnesota
83: Hypertension

John A. Guisto, MD, FACEP
Associate Professor, Department of Emergency
Medicine, University of Arizona Health Sciences
Center; Clinical Director, Emergency Department,
University Medical Center, Tucson, Arizona
135: Soft Tissue Infections

David A. Guss, MD, FACEP
Professor of Medicine and Surgery, University of
California, San Diego, School of Medicine, La
Jolla, California; Director, Department of
Emergency Medicine, University of California, San
Diego, Medical Center, San Diego, California
89: Liver and Biliary Tract

Leon Gussow, MD
Assistant Professor of Emergency Medicine, Rush
Medical College; Voluntary Attending Physician,
John H. Stroger, Jr. Hospital of Cook County,
Chicago, Illinois
163: Sedative Hypnotics

Rania Habal, MD, FACEP
Assistant Professor, New York Medical College, Valhalla, New York
179: Drug Therapy and Substance Abuse

Tenagne Haile-Mariam, MD
Assistant Professor, Department of Emergency Medicine, George Washington University Medical Center, Washington, DC
128: Viruses

Dina Halpern Kornblau, MD
Director, Division of Pediatric Neurology, St. Barnabas Hospital, Bronx, New York
173: Neurologic Disorders

Glenn C. Hamilton, MD, MSM
Professor and Chair, Department of Emergency Medicine, Wright State University School of Medicine, Dayton, Ohio
19: Chest Pain
33: Red and Painful Eye
119: Anemia, Polycythemia, and White Blood Cell Disorders
120: Disorders of Hemostasis

Mary Hancock, MD
Assistant Professor, Case Western Reserve University School of Medicine; Staff Physician, Department of Emergency Medicine, MetroHealth Medical Center, Cleveland, Ohio
118: Dermatologic Presentations

Christina E. Hantsch, MD
Associate Professor, Division of Emergency Medicine, Department of Surgery, Loyola University Chicago Stritch School of Medicine, Maywood, Illinois; Attending Physician, Emergency Medicine and Medical Toxicology, Loyola University Medical Center, Maywood, Illinois; Medical Director, Illinois Poison Center, Chicago, Illinois
160: Opioids

Stephen W. Hargarten, MD, MPH
Professor of Emergency Medicine, Medical College of Wisconsin, Milwaukee, Wisconsin
62: Injury Prevention and Control

Richard A. Harrigan, MD
Associate Professor, Department of Emergency Medicine, Temple University School of Medicine, Philadelphia, Pennsylvania
77: Acute Coronary Syndromes

David W. Harrison, MD, CCFP(EM), FRCPC
Clinical Associate Professor, University of British Columbia Faculty of Medicine; Medical Director, Hyperbaric Unit and Attending Physician, Division of Trauma Surgery, Vancouver General Hospital, Vancouver, British Columbia, Canada
190: The Difficult Patient

Ann L. Harwood-Nuss, MD, FACEP
Professor and Associate Dean for Educational Affairs, University of Florida Health Science Center Jacksonville, Jacksonville, Florida
98: Selected Urologic Problems

William G. Heegaard, MD
Associate Professor of Clinical Emergency Medicine, Department of Emergency Medicine, University of Minnesota Medical School; Faculty Physician, Department of Emergency Medicine, Hennepin County Medical Center, Minneapolis, Minnesota
38: Head

Katherine L. Heilpern, MD
Associate Professor and Vice Chair for Academic Affairs, Department of Emergency Medicine; Assistant Dean, Medical Education and Student Affairs, Emory University School of Medicine, Atlanta, Georgia
26: Jaundice

Robin R. Hemphill, MD, MPH
Associate Professor of Emergency Medicine, Vanderbilt University School of Medicine, Nashville, Tennessee
90: Pancreas

Sean Henderson, MD
Associate Professor of Emergency Medicine and Clinical Preventive Medicine, University of Southern California Keck School of Medicine, Los Angeles, California
42: Thoracic Trauma
180: Labor and Delivery and Their Complications

Robert Hendrickson, MD
Assistant Professor of Emergency Medicine, Oregon Health and Science University; Staff Physician and Clinical Toxicologist, Oregon Health and Science University and Oregon Poison Control Center, Portland, Oregon
146: Acetaminophen

Philip L. Henneman, MD
Professor and Chair, Department of Emergency Medicine, Tufts University School of Medicine, Boston, Massachusetts; Chair, Department of Emergency Medicine, Baystate Health System, Springfield, Massachusetts
23: Gastrointestinal Bleeding
91: Disorders of the Small Intestine
92: Acute Appendicitis

Gregory L. Henry, MD
Clinical Professor, Department of Emergency Medicine, University of Michigan Medical School; Emergency Physician, St. Joseph Mercy Hospital System, Ann Arbor, Michigan
17: Headache

H. Gene Hern, Jr., MD, MS
Assistant Clinical Professor of Medicine, University of California, San Francisco, School of Medicine, San Francisco, California; Associate Residency Director, Department of Emergency Medicine, Highland General Hospital of Alameda County Medical Center, Oakland, California
56: Wound Management Principles

Kendall Ho, MD, FRCPC
Assistant Professor, Department of Surgery; Associate Dean, Division of Continuing Professional Development and Knowledge Translation, University of British Columbia Faculty of Medicine; Attending Staff, Department of Emergency Medicine, Vancouver General Hospital, Vancouver, British Columbia, Canada
55: Ankle and Foot

Robert S. Hockberger, MD
Chair, Department of Emergency Medicine, Harbor–UCLA Medical Center, Torrance, California; Professor of Clinical Medicine, David Geffen School of Medicine at UCLA, Westwood, Los Angeles, California
40: Spinal Injuries
108: Thought Disorders

Gwendolyn L. Hoffman, MD, FACEP
Assistant Professor of Emergency Medicine, Michigan State University, East Lansing, Michigan; Chair, Emergency Services, Spectrum Health Blodgett and Butterworth Campuses, Grand Rapids, Michigan
5: Blood and Blood Components

Robert S. Hoffman, MD
Associate Professor of Emergency Medicine and Medicine (Clinical Pharmacology), New York University School of Medicine; Director, New York City Poison Control Center; Attending Physician, Bellevue Hospital, New York, New York
152: Cocaine and Other Sympathomimetics
157: Inhaled Toxins

Benjamin Honigman, MD
Professor and Head, Division of Emergency Medicine, Department of Surgery, University of Colorado School of Medicine, Denver, Colorado
142: High-Altitude Medicine

Mark A. Hostetler, MD, MPH
Assistant Professor, University of Chicago Pritzker School of Medicine; Chief, Section of Pediatric Emergency Medicine; Medical Director, Pediatric Emergency Department, University of Chicago Children's Hospital, Chicago, Illinois
170: Gastrointestinal Disorders

Debra E. Houry, MD, MPH
Assistant Professor, Department of Emergency Medicine, Emory University School of Medicine; Attending Physician, Emergency Department, Emory Healthcare, Atlanta, Georgia
177: Acute Complications of Pregnancy

Enoch T. Huang, MD
Assistant Clinical Professor of Emergency Medicine, University of California, Irvine, School of Medicine, Irvine, California; Fellowship Director, Undersea and Hyperbaric Medicine; Staff Physician, Departments of Emergency Medicine and Hyperbaric Medicine, Long Beach Memorial Hospital, Long Beach, California
200: Hyperbaric Medicine

J. Stephen Huff, MD
Associate Professor of Emergency Medicine and Neurology, Department of Emergency Medicine, University of Virginia Health System, Charlottesville, Virginia
14: Confusion
104: Spinal Cord Disorders

H. Range Hutson, MD
Assistant Professor of Emergency Medicine, Harvard Medical School; Department of Emergency Medicine, Massachusetts General Hospital, Boston, Massachusetts
68: Youth, Gangs, and Violence

Alson S. Inaba, MD, FAAP
Associate Professor of Pediatrics, University of Hawaii John A. Burns School of Medicine; Attending Physician, Pediatric Emergency Medicine, Kapiolani Medical Center for Women and Children; Pediatric Advanced Life Support National Faculty, American Heart Association Hawaii and Pacific Islands Region; Pediatric Advanced Life Support Course Director, The Queen's Medical Center, Honolulu, Hawaii
169: Cardiac Disorders

Jennifer Isenhour, MD
Adjunct Assistant Professor, Department of Emergency Medicine, University of North Carolina School of Medicine, Chapel Hill, North Carolina; Associate Residency Program Director, Department of Emergency Medicine, Carolinas Medical Center, Charlotte, North Carolina
43: Abdominal Trauma

Kenneth V. Iserson, MD, MBA, FACEP
Professor of Emergency Medicine, Department of Emergency Medicine; Director, Arizona Bioethics Program, University of Arizona College of Medicine; Emergency Physician; Chair, Bioethics Committee; Ethics Consultant, Institutional Review Board, University Medical Center, Tucson, Arizona
205: Bioethics

Kenneth Jackimczyk, MD
Attending Physician, Department of Emergency Medicine, Maricopa Medical Center, Phoenix, Arizona

Andy S. Jagoda, MD, FACEP
Professor and Vice Chair for Academic Affairs and Residency Director, Department of Emergency Medicine, Mount Sinai School of Medicine, New York, New York
106: Neuromuscular Disorders

Thea James, MD
Assistant Professor of Emergency Medicine, Boston University School of Medicine; Attending Physician, Boston University Medical Center, Boston, Massachusetts
203: Multiculturalism and Care Delivery

Timothy G. Janz, MD
Professor, Departments of Emergency Medicine and Internal Medicine, Wright State University School of Medicine, Dayton, Ohio
32: Hemoptysis
119: Anemia, Polycythemia, and White Blood Cell Disorders
120: Disorders of Hemostasis

Alan E. Jones, MD
Assistant Director of Research, Carolinas Medical
    Center, Charlotte, North Carolina; Adjunct
    Assistant Professor of Emergency Medicine,
    University of North Carolina School of Medicine,
    Chapel Hill, North Carolina
4: Shock

James B. Jones, PharmD, MD
Staff Physician, Mercy Hospital, Scranton,
    Pennsylvania
29: Back Pain

Robert C. Jorden, MD
Attending Physician, Penobscot Bay Medical Center,
    Rockport, Maine
34: Multiple Trauma

Nicholas J. Jouriles, MD
Professor of Emergency Medicine, Northeastern Ohio
    Universities College of Medicine, Rootstown, Ohio;
    Core Faculty, Emergency Medicine Residency,
    Akron General Medical Center, Akron, Ohio
81: Pericardial and Myocardial Disease

John Kahler, MD
Clinical Instructor, Department of Emergency
    Medicine, University of Michigan Medical School;
    Attending Physician, University of Michigan
    Health System, Ann Arbor, Michigan
98: Selected Urologic Problems

Amy H. Kaji, MD, MPH
Assistant Clinical Professor of Medicine, David
    Geffen School of Medicine at UCLA, Westwood,
    Los Angeles, California; Director, Disaster Resource
    Center, Department of Emergency Medicine,
    Harbor–UCLA Medical Center, Torrance, California
40: Spinal Injuries

Louise Kao, MD
Associate Director, Medical Toxicology Fellowship
    Program, Assistant Professor of Clinical
    Emergency Medicine, Indiana University School
    of Medicine; Department of Emergency Medicine,
    Methodist Hospital, Indianapolis, Indiana
189: The Combative Patient

Matthew T. Keadey, MD
Assistant Professor, Department of Emergency
    Medicine, Emory University School of Medicine;
    Chief of Service and Medical Director, Department
    of Emergency Medicine, Emory University
    Hospital, Atlanta, Georgia
183: The Solid-Organ Transplant Patient

Gabor D. Kelen, MD
Professor and Chair, Department of Emergency
    Medicine, Johns Hopkins University School of
    Medicine; Chief, Department of Emergency Medicine,
    Johns Hopkins Hospital, Baltimore, Maryland
130: AIDS and HIV

Eugene E. Kercher, MD
Associate Clinical Professor of Medicine, David
    Geffen School of Medicine at UCLA, Westwood,
    Los Angeles, California; Chair, Department of
    Emergency Medicine, Kern Medical Center,
    Bakersfield, California
110: Anxiety Disorders

Kelly E. King, MD
Medical Director, Casualty Care Research Center;
    Assistant Professor of Military and Emergency
    Medicine, Uniformed Services University of the
    Health Sciences, Bethesda, Maryland
22: Abdominal Pain

Susan Kirelik, MD
Medical Director, Pediatric Emergency Services;
    Chair, Department of Pediatrics, Sky Ridge
    Medical Center, Lone Tree, Colorado
*168: Pediatric Respiratory Emergencies: Disease of the
    Lungs*

Eileen Klein, MD, MPH
Associate Professor of Pediatrics, University of
    Washington School of Medicine; Attending
    Physician, Children's Hospital and Regional
    Medical Center, Seattle, Washington
9: Neonatal Resuscitation

Jeffrey A. Kline, MD
Director of Research, Carolinas Medical Center,
    Charlotte, North Carolina; Adjunct Associate
    Professor of Emergency Medicine, University of
    North Carolina School of Medicine, Chapel Hill,
    North Carolina
4: Shock
87: Pulmonary Embolism and Deep Venous Thrombosis

Andrew L. Knaut, MD, PhD
Assistant Professor, Department of Surgery, Division
    of Emergency Medicine, University of Colorado
    School of Medicine; Attending Physician, Denver
    Health Medical Center, Denver, Colorado
143: Submersion

Kristi L. Koenig, MD, FACEP
Professor of Clinical Emergency Medicine; Co-
    Director, Emergency Medical Services and Disaster
    Medical Sciences Fellowship, University of
    California, Irvine, School of Medicine, Irvine,
    California; Director of Public Health Preparedness,
    Department of Emergency Medicine, University of
    California, Irvine, Medical Center, Orange,
    California
194: Disaster Preparedness
195: Weapons of Mass Destruction

Joan Kolodzik, MD
Assistant Clinical Professor, Department of
    Emergency Medicine, Wright State University
    School of Medicine, Dayton, Ohio
30: Cyanosis

Joseph Kosnik, MD, FACEP, FAAEM
Adjunct Associate Professor, Department of
    Emergency Medicine, Wayne State University
    School of Medicine, Detroit, Michigan; Attending
    Physician, Department of Emergency Medicine,
    MidMichigan Medical Center, Midland, Michigan
153: Toxic Alcohols

Joshua M. Kosowsky, MD
Associate Clinical Director, Department of
    Emergency Medicine, Brigham and Women's
    Hospital; Instructor, Harvard Medical School,
    Boston, Massachusetts
76: Pleural Disease

Rashmi U. Kothari, MD
Associate Professor, Kalamazoo Center for Medical Studies, Michigan State University; Director of Emergency Medicine Research, Borgess Research Institute, Kalamazoo, Michigan
99: Stroke

Ted Koutouzis, MD
Clinical Instructor, Division of Emergency Medicine, Northwestern University Feinberg School of Medicine and Northwestern Memorial Hospital, Chicago, Illinois
115: Tendinopathy and Bursitis

Ken Kulig, MD
Associate Clinical Professor, Division of Emergency Medicine, Department of Surgery, University of Colorado School of Medicine; Toxicology Associate, University of Colorado–Affiliated Hospitals, Denver, Colorado
145: General Approach to the Poisoned Patient

Thomas Kwiatkowski, MD
Associate Professor of Emergency Medicine, Albert Einstein College of Medicine of Yeshiva University, Bronx, New York; Chair, Department of Emergency Medicine, Long Island Jewish Medical Center, New Hyde Park, New York
101: Headache

Christ G. Kyriakedes, DO
Associate Professor of Clinical Emergency Medicine, Department of Emergency Medicine, Northeastern Ohio Universities College of Medicine, Rootstown, Ohio; Program Director, Emergency Medicine Residency, Akron General Medical Center, Akron, Ohio
28: Vaginal Bleeding

Mark I. Langdorf, MD, MHPE, FACEP, FAAEM, RDMS
Chair and Medical Director; Associate Residency Director; and Professor of Clinical Emergency Medicine, Department of Emergency Medicine, University of California, Irvine, School of Medicine, Irvine, California and University of California, Irvine, Medical Center, Orange, California
182: The Immunocompromised Patient

Frank W. Lavoie, MD
Clinical Associate Professor, Department of Surgery, University of Vermont College of Medicine, Burlington, Vermont; Clinical Associate Professor, Department of Family Medicine, University of New England College of Medicine, Biddeford, Maine; Chief, Department of Emergency Medicine, Southern Maine Medical Center, Biddeford, Maine
107: Central Nervous System Infections

Eric J. Lavonas, MD
Director of Medical Toxicology Hospital Service, Carolinas Medical Center, Charlotte, North Carolina; Adjunct Assistant Professor of Emergency Medicine, University of North Carolina School of Medicine, Chapel Hill, North Carolina
159: Antipsychotics

David C. Lee, MD
Assistant Professor, New York University School of Medicine, New York, New York; Director of Research, Department of Emergency Medicine, North Shore University Hospital, Manhasset, New York
156: Hydrocarbons

Roger J. Lewis, MD, PhD, FACEP
Professor of Medicine, David Geffen School of Medicine at UCLA, Westwood, Los Angeles, California; Director of Research, Department of Emergency Medicine, Harbor–UCLA Medical Center, Torrance, California
197: Medical Literature and Evidence-Based Medicine

Michelle Lin, MD, FAAEM, FACEP
Assistant Clinical Professor of Medicine, University of California, San Francisco, School of Medicine; Attending Physician, Emergency Services, San Francisco General Hospital, San Francisco, California
51: Musculoskeletal Back Pain

Louis J. Ling, MD, FACEP, FACMT
Professor of Emergency Medicine and Pharmacy and Associate Dean for Graduate Medical Education, University of Minnesota Medical School; Associate Medicine Director for Medical Education, Hennepin County Medical Center; Senior Associate Medical Director, Hennepin Regional Poison Center, Minneapolis, Minnesota

William B. Long III, MD
Director of Trauma, Trauma Specialists, LLP, Legacy Emanuel Hospital, Portland, Oregon
60: Thermal Burns
61: Chemical Injuries

Mark J. Lowell, MD
Associate Professor, Department of Emergency Medicine, University of Michigan Medical School, Ann Arbor, Michigan
88: Esophagus, Stomach, and Duodenum

Douglas W. Lowery III, MD
Associate Professor of Emergency Medicine, Emory University School of Medicine; Vice Chair of Clinical Operations, Department of Emergency Medicine, Emory Healthcare, Atlanta, Georgia
114: Arthritis
183: The Solid-Organ Transplant Patient

Marie M. Lozon, MD
Associate Professor of Emergency Medicine and Pediatrics, University of Michigan Medical School; Director, Children's Emergency Services, University of Michigan Health System, Ann Arbor, Michigan
188: Procedural Sedation and Analgesia

Robert C. Luten, MD
Professor, Departments of Pediatrics and Emergency Medicine, University of Florida College of Medicine; Department of Emergency Medicine, Shands Jacksonville, Jacksonville, Florida
8: Pediatric Resuscitation

Binh T. Ly, MD
Assistant Clinical Professor, University of California, San Diego, School of Medicine, La Jolla, California; Associate Residency Director, Emergency Medicine; Associate Fellowship Director, Medical Toxicology, University of California, San Diego, Medical Center, San Diego, California
154: Hallucinogens

Everett Lyn, MD, MSc
Director of Education, Department of Emergency Medicine, Brigham and Women's Hospital; Assistant Professor, Harvard Medical School, Boston, Massachusetts
47: Hand
54: Knee and Lower Leg

Malcolm Mahadevan, MBBS, FRCSEd(A&E), MRCP(UK), FAMS
Clinical Senior Lecturer, National University of Singapore Faculty of Medicine; Consultant Emergency Physician and Director of Observation Services, National University Hospital, Singapore
198: Observation Medicine and Clinical Decision Units

William K. Mallon, MD
Associate Professor of Clinical Emergency Medicine, University of Southern California Keck School of Medicine, Los Angeles, California
180: Labor and Delivery and Their Complications

Diku P. Mandavia, MD, FACEP, FRCPC
Clinical Associate Professor of Emergency Medicine, University of Southern California Keck School of Medicine; Attending Staff Physician, Department of Emergency Medicine, Cedars-Sinai Medical Center, Los Angeles, California
73: Chronic Obstructive Pulmonary Disease

Mariann Manno, MD, FAAP
Associate Professor of Clinical Pediatrics, Department of Emergency Medicine, University of Massachusetts Medical School; Director of Pediatric Emergency Medicine, University of Massachusetts Memorial Health Care, Children's Medical Center, Worcester, Massachusetts
166: Pediatric Respiratory Emergencies: Upper Airway Obstruction and Infections

Catherine A. Marco, MD, FACEP
Clinical Professor of Surgery, Division of Emergency Medicine, Medical College of Ohio; Attending Physician, St. Vincent Mercy Medical Center, Toledo, Ohio
130: AIDS and HIV

Vincent Markovchick, MD
Professor of Surgery, Division of Emergency Medicine, University of Colorado School of Medicine; Director, Emergency Medical Services, Denver Health, Denver, Colorado
144: Radiation Injuries

Marcus L. Martin, MD
Professor and Chair, Department of Emergency Medicine, University of Virginia Health System, Charlottesville, Virginia
60: Thermal Burns
61: Chemical Injuries

John A. Marx, MD, FAAEM, FACEP
Chair and Chief, Department of Emergency Medicine, Carolinas Medical Center, Charlotte, North Carolina; Adjunct Professor, Department of Emergency Medicine, University of North Carolina School of Medicine, Chapel Hill, North Carolina
43: Abdominal Trauma

Maureen McCollough, MD, FACEP, FAAEM
Associate Professor of Clinical Emergency Medicine and Pediatrics, Keck School of Medicine of USC; Medical Director, Adult and Pediatric Emergency Departments, Los Angeles County University of Southern California Medical Center, Los Angeles, California
172: Renal and Genitourinary Tract Disorders

Mary Pat McKay, MD, MPH
Associate Professor of Emergency Medicine and Public Health, George Washington University Medical Center; Director, Center for Injury Prevention and Control, Ronald Reagan Institute of Emergency Medicine, Washington, DC
39: Facial Trauma

John G. McManus, MD
Assistant Professor, Oregon Health and Science University, Portland, Oregon; Researcher, U.S. Army Institute of Surgical Research, San Antonio, Texas
193: Tactical Emergency Medical Support and Urban Search and Rescue

David B. McMicken, MD, FACEP
Emergency Services, The Medical Center, Columbus Regional Healthcare System, Columbus, Georgia
184: Alcohol-Related Disease

Kemedy K. McQuillen, MD
Attending Physician, Advocate Christ Medical Center, Oak Lawn, Illinois
174: Musculoskeletal Disorders

Harvey W. Meislin, MD, FACEP
Professor and Head, Department of Emergency Medicine; Director, Arizona Emergency Medicine Research Center, University of Arizona Health Sciences Center, Tucson, Arizona
135: Soft Tissue Infections

Frantz R. Melio, MD, FACEP
Clinical Assistant Professor of Emergency Medicine, Department of Emergency Medicine, University of New Mexico School of Medicine, Albuquerque, New Mexico; Executive Director of Emergency Medicine, Trauma, and Sexual Assault Nurse Examiners (SANE); Attending Physician, Emergency Medicine, St. Vincent Hospital, Santa Fe, New Mexico; President, Northern New Mexico Emergency Medical Services, PC, Santa Fe, New Mexico
74: Upper Respiratory Tract Infections

Gregory P. Moore, MD, JD
Volunteer Clinical Faculty, Emergency Medicine Residency, University of California, Davis, Medical Center, Sacramento, California; Staff Physician, Kaiser Permanente, Sacramento, California
71: Otolaryngology
189: The Combative Patient

Gregory J. Moran, MD
Professor of Clinical Medicine, David Geffen School of Medicine at UCLA, Westwood, Los Angeles, California; Department of Emergency Medicine, Division of Infectious Diseases, Olive View–UCLA Medical Center, Sylmar, California
75: Pneumonia

Laurie J. Morrison, MD, MSc, FRCPC
Associate Professor and Director, Division of Emergency Medicine, Department of Medicine, University of Toronto Faculty of Medicine; Research Director, Prehospital and Transport Medicine Research Program, Department of Emergency Services, Sunnybrook and Women's College Health Sciences Centre, Toronto, Ontario, Canada
176: General Approach to the Pregnant Patient

Robert L. Muelleman, MD, FACEP
Chief of Emergency Medicine, University of Nebraska Medical Center, Omaha, Nebraska
117: Allergy, Hypersensitivity, and Anaphylaxis

Michael F. Murphy, MD
Clinical Associate Professor of Emergency Medicine, University of North Carolina School of Medicine, Chapel Hill, North Carolina; Clinical Chief of Anesthesiology, Lincoln Medical Center, Lincolnton, North Carolina; Attending Physician, Department of Emergency Medicine, Carolinas Medical Center, Charlotte, North Carolina
3: Monitoring the Emergency Patient

Lindsay Murray, MBBS, FACEM
Senior Lecturer in Emergency Medicine, University of Western Australia, Perth, Western Australia, Australia; Consultant Emergency Physician and Clinical Toxicologist, Sir Charles Gairdner Hospital, Nedlands, Perth, Western Australia, Australia; Medical Director, New South Wales Poison Centre, Children's Hospital at Westmead, Westmead, Sydney, New South Wales, Australia
147: Aspirin and Nonsteroidal Agents

Lewis S. Nelson, MD
Assistant Professor of Emergency Medicine, Department of Emergency Medicine, New York University School of Medicine; Associate Director, New York City Poison Control Center; Attending Physician, Bellevue Hospital, New York University Medical Center, New York, New York
157: Inhaled Toxins

John D. G. Neufeld, MD
Attending Physician, Department of Emergency Medicine, Calgary Health Region, Calgary, Alberta, Canada
35: Trauma in Pregnancy

Robert W. Neumar, MD, PhD
Assistant Professor, Department of Emergency Medicine, University of Pennsylvania School of Medicine, Philadelphia, Pennsylvania
7: Adult Resuscitation

Edward J. Newton, MD, FACEP
Chair, Department of Emergency Medicine, Los Angeles County and University of Southern California Medical Center; Professor of Clinical Emergency Medicine, University of Southern California Keck School of Medicine, Los Angeles, California
40: Spinal Injuries
45: Peripheral Vascular Injury
53: Femur and Hip
178: Chronic Medical Illness During Pregnancy

Kim Newton, MD
Assistant Professor of Emergency Medicine, University of Southern California Keck School of Medicine; Los Angeles County and University of Southern California Medical Center, Los Angeles, California
41: Neck

James T. Niemann, MD, FACEP, FACP
Professor of Medicine, David Geffen School of Medicine at UCLA, Westwood, Los Angeles, California; Department of Emergency Medicine, Harbor–UCLA Medical Center, Torrance, California
79: Implantable Cardiac Devices

Nnamdi Nkwuo, MD
Department of Emergency Medicine, Newark Beth Israel Medical Center, Newark, New Jersey
121: Selected Oncologic Emergencies

Eric K. Noji, MD, MPH
Senior Policy Advisor, Health and Homeland Security, Centers for Disease Control and Prevention, Atlanta, Georgia
194: Disaster Preparedness

Richard M. Nowak, MD, MBA
Clinical Associate Professor, Department of Emergency Medicine, University of Michigan Medical School, Ann Arbor, Michigan; Vice Chair, Department of Emergency Medicine, Henry Ford Health System, Detroit, Michigan
72: Asthma

John F. O'Brien, MD
Clinical Associate Professor of Emergency Medicine, University of Florida College of Medicine, Gainesville, Florida; Clinical Assistant Professor of Medicine, Department of Clinical Sciences, Florida State University College of Medicine, Orlando, Florida; Associate Program Director, Department of Emergency Medicine, Orlando Regional Medical Center, Orlando, Florida
80: Heart Failure

Jonathan S. Olshaker, MD
Professor and Chair, Department of Emergency Medicine, Boston University School of Medicine, Boston Medical Center, Boston, Massachusetts
13: Dizziness and Vertigo

Jeffrey Orledge, MD, MS
Assistant Professor, Medical College of Georgia and
Medical College of Georgia Health, Inc.; Medical
Director of Medical College of Georgia LifeNet Air
Medical Transportation Service, Augusta, Georgia
*193: Tactical Emergency Medical Support and Urban
Search and Rescue*

Edward J. Otten, MD, FACMT
Professor of Emergency Medicine and Pediatrics;
Director, Division of Toxicology, University of
Cincinnati College of Medicine, Cincinnati, Ohio
59: Venomous Animal Injuries

Daniel Pallin, MD, MPH
Associate Research Director, Brigham and Women's
Hospital; Instructor of Medicine (Emergency
Medicine), Harvard Medical School, Boston,
Massachusetts
54: Knee and Lower Leg

Arthur M. Pancioli, MD
Associate Professor, Department of Emergency
Medicine, University of Cincinnati College of
Medicine, Cincinnati, Ohio
103: Brain and Cranial Nerve Disorders

Paul M. Paris, MD, FACEP, LLD(Hon)
Professor and Chair, Department of Emergency
Medicine, University of Pittsburgh School of
Medicine; Chief Medical Officer, Center for
Emergency Medicine of Western Pennsylvania,
Pittsburgh, Pennsylvania
187: Pain Management

Jeffrey Pennington, MD
Residency Program Director and Senior Clinical
Instructor, Case Western Reserve University
School of Medicine; Residency Program Director,
MetroHealth Medical Center, Cleveland, Ohio
*124: Diabetes Mellitus and Disorders of Glucose
Homeostasis*

Debra Perina, MD
Associate Professor of Emergency Medicine and
Director, Prehospital Care Division, University of
Virginia Health System, Charlottesville, Virginia
18: Dyspnea

Andrew D. Perron, MD
Clinical Associate Professor, University of Vermont
School of Medicine, Burlington, Vermont;
Residency Program Director, Maine Medical
Center, Portland, Maine
104: Spinal Cord Disorders

Shawna J. Perry, MD
Assistant Professor, Department of Emergency
Medicine, University of Florida College of
Medicine; Director of Clinical Operations,
Department of Emergency Medicine, Shands
Medical Center, Jacksonville, Florida
*204: Process Improvement and Patient Safety in the
Emergency Department*

Michael A. Peterson, MD
Assistant Professor of Medicine, David Geffen
School of Medicine at UCLA, Westwood, Los
Angeles, California; Director of Emergency
Ultrasound Services and Emergency Ultrasound
Fellowship, Department of Emergency Medicine,
Harbor–UCLA Medical Center, Torrance, California
94: Large Intestine

James A. Pfaff, MD
Staff Physician, San Antonio Uniformed Services
Health Education Consortium, Brooke Army Medical
Center, Fort Sam Houston, San Antonio, Texas
71: Otolaryngology

Michael Alan Polis, MD, MPH
Chief, Collaborative Clinical Research Branch, Office
of Clinical Research (OCR), National Institute of
Allergy and Infectious Diseases (NIAID), National
Institutes of Health, Bethesda, Maryland; Clinical
Professor of Emergency Medicine, George
Washington University Medical Center,
Washington, DC
128: Viruses

Charles V. Pollack, Jr., MD, MA, FACEP
Associate Professor of Emergency Medicine,
University of Pennsylvania School of Medicine;
Chair, Department of Emergency Medicine,
Pennsylvania Hospital, Philadelphia, Pennsylvania
*2: Mechanical Ventilation and Noninvasive Ventilatory
Support*
16: Seizures
100: Seizures

Timothy G. Price, MD
Associate Professor, Department of Emergency
Medicine, University of Louisville School of
Medicine, Louisville, Kentucky
140: Electrical and Lightning Injuries

Thomas B. Purcell, MD
Adjunct Clinical Professor, David Geffen School of
Medicine at UCLA, Westwood, Los Angeles,
California; Attending Faculty, Department of
Emergency Medicine, Kern Medical Center,
Bakersfield, California
111: Somatoform Disorders
112: Factitious Disorders and Malingering

Linda Quan, MD
Professor of Pediatrics, University of Washington
School of Medicine; Attending Physician,
Children's Hospital and Regional Medical Center,
Seattle, Washington
9: Neonatal Resuscitation

Tammie E. Quest, MD
Assistant Professor, Department of Emergency
Medicine, Emory University School of Medicine,
Atlanta, Georgia
26: Jaundice

Rama B. Rao, MD
Assistant Clinical Professor of Emergency Medicine,
New York University School of Medicine;
Bellevue Hospital and New York University
Medical Center, New York, New York
152: Cocaine and Other Sympathomimetics

Robert C. Reiser, MD, MS, FACEP
Associate Professor, University of Virginia School of Medicine; Medical Director, Department of Emergency Medicine, University of Virginia Health System, Charlottesville, Virginia
12: Weakness

John R. Richards, MD
Associate Professor of Emergency Medicine, University of California, Davis, Medical Center, Sacramento, California
108: Thought Disorders

Wilfredo Rivera, MD
Assistant Professor, Department of Surgery, Division of Emergency Medicine, University of Texas Southwestern Medical School; Associate Medical Director, North Texas Poison Center, Dallas, Texas
148: Anticholinergics

David J. Roberts, MD
Adjunct Professor, University of Minnesota Medical School, Minneapolis, Minnesota; Consulting Toxicologist, North Memorial Medical Center, Robbinsdale, Minnesota; Medical Director, Hennepin Regional Poison Center, Minneapolis, Minnesota
150: Cardiovascular Drugs

Howard Rodenberg, MD, MPH
Director of the Division of Health and Environment and State Health Officer; Clinical Associate Professor, University of Kansas Medical School–Wichita, Kansas; Department of Health and Environment, Topeka, Kansas
192: Air Medical Transport

Kevin G. Rodgers, MD
Clinical Professor of Emergency Medicine and Co-Program Director, Emergency Medicine Residency, Indiana University School of Medicine, Indianapolis, Indiana
29: Back Pain

Victor S. Roth, MD, MPH
Assistant Professor, Division of Occupational Medicine, Department of Emergency Medicine, University of Michigan Medical School, Ann Arbor, Michigan
199: Occupational Medicine and Occupational Health in the Emergency Department

Richard E. Rothman, MD, PhD, FACEP
Associate Professor and Director, Fellowship and Residency Research Program, Department of Emergency Medicine, Johns Hopkins University, Baltimore, Maryland
130: AIDS and HIV

David H. Rubin, MD
Professor of Clinical Pediatrics, Weill Medical College of Cornell University, New York, New York; Chair and Program Director, Department of Pediatrics, St. Barnabas Hospital, Bronx, New York
173: Neurologic Disorders

Douglas A. Rund, MD
Professor and Chair, Department of Emergency Medicine; Associate Dean, College of Medicine and Public Health, Ohio State University, Columbus, Ohio
109: Mood Disorders

Jeffrey W. Runge, MD
Administrator, National Highway Traffic Safety Administration, Washington, DC; Adjunct Instructor of Emergency Medicine, University of North Caroline School of Medicine, Chapel Hill, North Carolina
62: Injury Prevention and Control

Michael S. Runyon, MD
Director of Medical Student Education, Department of Emergency Medicine, Carolinas Medical Center, Charlotte, North Carolina; Adjunct Professor of Emergency Medicine, University of North Carolina School of Medicine, Chapel Hill, North Carolina
87: Pulmonary Embolism and Deep Venous Thrombosis

Christopher S. Russi, DO
Assistant Professor of Emergency Medicine, Associate Residency Director and Director of Undergraduate Education, University of Iowa Carver College of Medicine, Iowa City, Iowa
17: Headache

Patricia R. Salber, MD, MBA, FACEP, FACP
Chief Medical Officer, Center for Practical Health Reform, Larkspur, California
66: Intimate Partner Violence and Abuse

Sally A. Santen, MD
Assistant Professor of Emergency Medicine, Vanderbilt University Medical Center, Nashville, Tennessee
90: Pancreas

John R. Saucier, MD
Clinical Assistant Professor of Surgery, University of Vermont College of Medicine, Burlington, Vermont; Attending Physician, Emergency Department, Maine Medical Center, Portland, Maine
107: Central Nervous System Infections

Diane Sauter, MD, FACEP
Clinical Assistant Professor of Emergency Medicine, Georgetown University; Attending Physician, Washington Hospital Medical Center, Washington D.C.
179: Drug Therapy and Substance Abuse

Neil Schamban, MD, FACEP
Vice Chair and Medical Director, Pediatric Emergency Department, Department of Emergency Medicine, Newark Beth Israel Medical Center, Newark, New Jersey
121: Selected Oncologic Emergencies

Diana C. Schneider, MD
Assistant Professor of Family Medicine and Internal Medicine, University of Southern California Keck School of Medicine; Medical Director, Adult Protection Team, Los Angeles County and University of Southern California Medical Center, Los Angeles, California
67: Elder Abuse and Neglect

Robert E. Schneider, MD
Clinical Associate Professor, Department of Emergency Medicine, University of North Carolina School of Medicine, Chapel Hill, North Carolina; Attending Physician, Department of Urology, Carolinas Medical Center, Charlotte, North Carolina
44: Genitourinary System

Sandra M. Schneider, MD, FACEP
Professor and Chair, Department of Emergency Medicine, University of Rochester Medical Center; Emergency Medicine Physician-in-Chief, Strong Memorial Hospital, Rochester, New York
151: Caustics

Carl H. Schultz, MD, FACEP
Professor of Clinical Emergency Medicine; Co-Director, Emergency Medical Services and Disaster Medical Sciences Fellowship, University of California, Irvine, School of Medicine, Irvine, California; Director, Disaster Medical Services, Department of Emergency Medicine, University of California, Irvine, Medical Center, Orange, California
194: Disaster Preparedness
195: Weapons of Mass Destruction

Richard Schwartz, MD, FACEP
Associate Professor and Chair, Department of Emergency Medicine, Medical College of Georgia and Medical College of Georgia Health, Inc., Augusta, Georgia
193: Tactical Emergency Medical Support and Urban Search and Rescue

Donna L. Seger, MD
Assistant Professor of Medicine and Emergency Medicine, Vanderbilt University Medical Center; Medical Director, Tennessee Poison Center, Vanderbilt University Medical Center, Nashville, Tennessee
147: Aspirin and Nonsteroidal Agents

Jennifer Seirafi, MD
Assistant Professor of Medicine (Voluntary Faculty), University of Miami School of Medicine; Attending Physician, Emergency Care Center, Jackson Memorial Hospital, Miami, Florida
102: Delirium and Dementia

Clare T. Sercombe, MD, FACEP
Staff Emergency Physician, North Memorial Medical Center, Robbinsdale, Minnesota
116: Systemic Lupus Erythematosus and the Vasculitides

Joseph Sexton, MD, FACEP
Attending Physician, Emergency Medicine, Bethlehem Emergency Care Specialists, St. Luke's Hospital, Bethlehem, Pennsylvania
132: Tick-Borne Illnesses

Marc J. Shapiro, MD
Assistant Professor, Brown University; Attending Physician, Department of Emergency Medicine, Rhode Island Hospital, Providence, Rhode Island
204: Process Improvement and Patient Safety in the Emergency Department

Nathan I. Shapiro, MD
Instructor of Medicine, Harvard Medical School; Research Director, Beth Israel Deaconess Medical Center, Boston, Massachusetts
136: Sepsis Syndromes

Ghazala Sharieff, MD, FACEP, FAAEM, FAAP
Associate Clinical Professor, Children's Hospital and Health Center/University of California at San Diego; Director of Pediatric Emergency Medicine, Palomar-Pomerado Hospitals/California Emergency Physicians, San Diego, California
172: Renal and Genitourinary Tract Disorders

Peter Shearer, MD
Assistant Professor and Assistant Residency Director, Department of Emergency Medicine, Mount Sinai School of Medicine; Attending Physician, Department of Emergency Medicine, Elmhurst Hospital Center; Attending Physician, Department of Emergency Medicine, Mount Sinai Hospital, New York, New York
106: Neuromuscular Disorders

Richard D. Shih, MD
Associate Professor of Surgery, New Jersey Medical School of the University of Medicine and Dentistry of New Jersey, Newark, New Jersey; Program Director, Emergency Medicine Residency Program, Morristown Memorial Hospital, Morristown, New Jersey
162: Plants, Mushrooms, and Herbal Medications

Lee W. Shockley, MD
Associate Professor, University of Colorado School of Medicine; Emergency Department Medical Director and Associate Residency Program Director, Denver Health Medical Center, Denver, Colorado
141: Scuba Diving and Dysbarism

Robert Silbergleit, MD
Assistant Professor, Department of Emergency Medicine, University of Michigan, Ann Arbor, Michigan
6: Brain Resuscitation

Barry Simon, MD
Associate Clinical Professor of Medicine, University of California, San Francisco, School of Medicine; Chair, Department of Emergency Medicine, Alameda County Medical Center, Oakland, California
56: Wound Management Principles

Jonathan I. Singer, MD, FAAP, FACEP
Professor of Emergency Medicine and Pediatrics, Wright State University School of Medicine; Staff Physician, Children's Medical Center, Dayton, Ohio
31: Sore Throat

Amardeep Singh, MD
Clinical Instructor, Rosalind Franklin University of Medicine and Science, North Chicago, Illinois; Emergency Physician, Mount Sinai Hospital, Chicago, Illinois
21: Nausea and Vomiting

Laura Slaughter, MD, FACP
Consultant, San Luis Obispo Sexual Assault Response Team (SART), San Luis Obispo, California; Consultant, Violence Intervention Program, Los Angeles County and University of Southern California Medical Center, Los Angeles, California
65: Sexual Assault

Jeffrey Smith, MD, MPH
Associate Professor of Emergency Medicine, George
Washington University School of Medicine and
Health Sciences; Director of Clinical Operations
and Trauma Services, Co-Director, Ronald Reagan
Institute of Emergency Medicine, Department of
Emergency Medicine, George Washington
University Hospital, Washington, DC
102: Delirium and Dementia

William S. Smock, MD, MS, FACEP
Professor, Department of Emergency Medicine,
University of Louisville School of Medicine,
Louisville, Kentucky
63: Forensic Emergency Medicine

Peter E. Sokolove, MD, FACEP
Associate Professor, Department of Emergency
Medicine, University of California, Davis, School
of Medicine, Davis, California; Vice Chair of
Education and Residency Program Director,
Department of Emergency Medicine, University of
California, Davis, Medical Center, Sacramento,
California
133: Tuberculosis

Brian Springer, MD
Assistant Professor, Department of Emergency
Medicine, Wright State University School of
Medicine, Dayton, Ohio
32: Hemoptysis

Maria Stephan, MD, FAAP
Associate Professor of Pediatrics, Department of
Pediatrics, Division of Emergency Medicine,
University of Texas Southwestern Medical School;
Attending Physician, Division of Emergency
Medicine, Children's Medical Center of Dallas,
Dallas, Texas
*186: Evaluation of the Developmentally and Physically
Disabled Child*

Jeffrey Sternlicht, MD
Attending Physician, Department of Emergency
Medicine, Greater Baltimore Medical Center,
Baltimore, Maryland
126: Thyroid and Adrenal Disorders

Brian Stettler, MD
Assistant Professor, Department of Emergency
Medicine, University of Cincinnati College of
Medicine, Cincinnati, Ohio
103: Brain and Cranial Nerve Disorders

Susan Stone, MD, MPH
Assistant Professor of Emergency Medicine and of
Anesthesiology and Pain Management, University
of Southern California Keck School of Medicine,
Los Angeles, California
206: End of Life

Stuart P. Swadron, MD, FACEP, FRCPC, FAAEM
Assistant Professor of Clinical Emergency Medicine,
University of Southern California Keck School of
Medicine; Program Director, Residency in
Emergency Medicine, Los Angeles County and
University of Southern California Medical Center,
Los Angeles, California
73: Chronic Obstructive Pulmonary Disease

David A. Talan, MD, FACEP, FIDSA
Professor of Medicine, David Geffen School of
Medicine at UCLA, Westwood, Los Angeles,
California; Chair, Department of Emergency
Medicine; Faculty, Division of Infectious Diseases,
Olive View–UCLA Medical Center, Sylmar,
California
75: Pneumonia

Vivek S. Tayal, MD, FAEP
Director of Ultrasound, Department of Emergency
Medicine, Carolinas Medical Center, Charlotte,
North Carolina; Adjunct Associate Professor of
Emergency Medicine, Department of Emergency
Medicine, University of North Carolina School of
Medicine, Chapel Hill, North Carolina
123: Electrolyte Disturbances

Jonathan M. Teich, MD, PhD
Attending Physician, Department of Emergency
Medicine, Brigham and Women's Hospital;
Assistant Professor of Medicine (Emergency
Medicine), Harvard Medical School, Boston,
Massachusetts
202: Information Technology in Emergency Medicine

Stephen R. Thom, MD, PhD
Professor, Department of Emergency Medicine,
University of Pennsylvania School of Medicine;
Chief, Hyperbaric Medicine, Institute for
Environmental Medicine, University of
Pennsylvania, Philadelphia, Pennsylvania
200: Hyperbaric Medicine

Stephen H. Thomas, MD, MPH
Assistant Professor of Surgery, Harvard Medical
School; Director, Undergraduate Emergency
Medicine Education, Massachusetts General
Hospital, Boston, Massachusetts
57: Foreign Bodies

Joshua L. Tobias, MD, FAAEM
Assistant Clinical Professor, David Geffen School
of Medicine at UCLA, Westwood, Los Angeles,
California; Director of Quality Assurance and
Assistant Program Director, Department of
Emergency Medicine, Kern Medical Center,
Bakersfield, California
110: Anxiety Disorders

Glenn Tokarski, MD
Senior Staff Physician, Emergency Medicine, Henry
Ford Health System, Detroit, Michigan
72: Asthma

Christian Tomaszewski, MD
Medical Director, HBO, Department of Emergency
Medicine, Carolinas Medical Center, Charlotte,
North Carolina; Adjunct Associate Professor
of Emergency Medicine, University of North
Carolina School of Medicine, Chapel Hill, North
Carolina
185: Substance Abuse

Susan P. Torrey, MD
Assistant Professor of Emergency Medicine, Tufts University School of Medicine, Boston, Massachusetts; Associate Residency Director, Department of Emergency Medicine, Baystate Medical Center, Springfield, Massachusetts
91: Disorders of the Small Intestine

T. Paul Tran, MD, MS, FACEP
Associate Professor and Research Director, University of Nebraska Medical Center, Omaha, Nebraska
117: Allergy, Hypersensitivity, and Anaphylaxis

Marshall G. Vary, MD
Assistant Professor of Clinical Psychiatry, Ohio State University; Chief Medical Officer and Senior Vice President, Riverside Methodist Hospital, Columbus, Ohio
109: Mood Disorders

Larissa I. Velez, MD
Assistant Professor of Emergency Medicine, University of Texas Southwestern Medical School; Associate Residency Director, Emergency Medicine; Staff Toxicologist, North Texas Poison Center, University of Texas Southwestern Medical Center and Parkland Health and Hospital System, Dallas, Texas
148: Anticholinergics
155: Heavy Metals

Salvator Vicario, MD, FACEP, FAAEM
Associate Professor of Emergency Medicine, University of Louisville School of Medicine, Louisville, Kentucky
139: Heat Illness

Robert J. Vissers, MD, FACEP, FRCPC
Adjunct Associate Professor, Oregon Health and Science University; Director, Department of Emergency Medicine, Legacy Emanuel Hospital, Portland, Oregon
190: The Difficult Patient

Ron M. Walls, MD, FAAEM, FACEP, FRCPC
Chair, Department of Emergency Medicine, Brigham and Women's Hospital; Associate Professor of Medicine (Emergency Medicine), Harvard Medical School, Boston, Massachusetts
1: Airway

Frank G. Walter, MD, FACEP, FACMT, FAACT
Chief, Division of Medical Toxicology; Associate Professor of Emergency Medicine, Department of Emergency Medicine, University of Arizona College of Medicine; Director of Clinical Toxicology, University Medical Center, Tucson, Arizona
149: Antidepressants

David G. Ward, MD, ABP
Staff Physician
Emergency Department
Heartland Regional Medical Center
St. Joseph, Missouri
171: Infectious Diarrheal Disease and Dehydration

Kevin R. Ward, MD
Associate Professor of Emergency Medicine and Physiology; Director of Research, Department of Emergency Medicine; Associate Director, Virginia Commonwealth University Reanimation Engineering Shock Center, Virginia Commonwealth University, Richmond, Virginia
7: Adult Resuscitation

Paul M. Wax, MD, FACMT
Professor of Clinical Emergency Medicine, University of Arizona; Banner-Good Samaritan Regional Medical Center, Phoenix, Arizona
151: Caustics

Robert L. Wears, MD, MS
Professor, Department of Emergency Medicine, University of Florida Health Science Center Jacksonville; Attending Physician, Shands Medical Center, Jacksonville, Florida; Visiting Professor, Clinical Safety Research Unit, Imperial College and St. Mary's Hospital, London, U.K.
204: Process Improvement and Patient Safety in the Emergency Department

Ellen J. Weber, MD, FACEP
Professor of Clinical Medicine, Division of Emergency Medicine, University of California, San Francisco, San Francisco, California
58: Mammalian Bites
129: Rabies

Suzanne R. White, MD, FACMT, FACEP
Professor and Clinician-Educator, Departments of Emergency Medicine and Pediatrics, Wayne State University School of Medicine; Medical Director, Children's Hospital of Michigan Regional Poison Control Center, Detroit, Michigan
153: Toxic Alcohols

Robert A. Wiebe, MD, FACEP, FAAP
Sarah M. and Charles E. Seay Distinguished Chair; Professor and Director, Division of Emergency Medicine, Department of Pediatrics, University of Texas Southwestern Medical Center; Director, Emergency Services, Children's Medical Center of Dallas, Dallas, Texas
164: General Approach to the Pediatric Patient

John M. Wightman, MD, MA
Associate Professor, Department of Emergency Medicine, Wright State University School of Medicine, Dayton, Ohio; Program Director (Military Component), Integrated Residency in Emergency Medicine, 88th Medical Group, Wright-Patterson Air Force Base, Ohio
22: Abdominal Pain
33: Red and Painful Eye

Saralyn R. Williams, MD
Associate Clinical Professor of Medicine, University of California, San Diego, School of Medicine, La Jolla, California; Assistant Medical Director, San Diego Division, California Poison Control System, San Diego, California
154: Hallucinogens

Mary A. Wittler, MD
Medical Toxicology Fellow, Department of
Emergency Medicine, Carolinas Medical Center,
Charlotte, North Carolina
159: Antipsychotics

John M. Wogan, MD
Chair, Department of Emergency Medicine, Greater
Baltimore Medical Center, Baltimore, Maryland
126: Thyroid and Adrenal Disorders

Jeannette M. Wolfe, MD
Assistant Professor of Emergency Medicine, Tufts
University School of Medicine and Baystate
Medical Center, Springfield, Massachusetts
92: Acute Appendicitis

Richard E. Wolfe, MD
Associate Professor, Harvard Medical School; Chief
of Emergency Medicine, Beth Israel Deaconess
Medical Center, Boston, Massachusetts
15: Coma and Depressed Level of Consciousness

Allan B. Wolfson, MD, FACEP, FACP
Professor of Emergency Medicine, University of
Pittsburgh School of Medicine; Program Director,
University of Pittsburgh Affiliated Residency in
Emergency Medicine, Pittsburgh, Pennsylvania
96: Renal Failure

Karen G. H. Woolfrey, MD, FRCPC, FACEP
Assistant Professor, Department of Medicine; Deputy
Director, Division of Emergency Medicine,
McMaster University; Research Coordinator and
Director of Residency Clinical Teaching Unit,
Emergency Department, St. Joseph's Hospital of St.
Joseph's Healthcare Hamilton, Hamilton, Ontario,
Canada
48: Wrist and Forearm

Samuel Yang, MD
Assistant Professor, Department of Emergency
Medicine, Johns Hopkins University School of
Medicine; Staff Physician, Department of
Emergency Medicine, Johns Hopkins Hospital,
Baltimore, Maryland
130: AIDS and HIV

Michael Yaron, MD
Associate Professor, Division of Emergency
Medicine, Department of Surgery, University of
Colorado School of Medicine, Denver, Colorado
142: High-Altitude Medicine

Donald M. Yealy, MD, FACEP
Professor of Emergency Medicine and Medicine,
University of Pittsburgh School of Medicine; Vice
Chair, Department of Emergency Medicine,
University of Pittsburgh Medical Center,
Pittsburgh, Pennsylvania
78: Dysrhythmias
187: Pain Management

Kelly D. Young, MD, MS
Associate Clinical Professor of Pediatrics, David
Geffen School of Medicine at UCLA, Westwood,
Los Angeles, California; Pediatric Emergency
Medicine Faculty, Harbor–UCLA Medical Center,
Torrance, California
197: Medical Literature and Evidence-Based Medicine

David K. Zich, MD
Assistant Professor of Medicine, Northwestern
University Feinberg School of Medicine;
Departments of Emergency Medicine and Internal
Medicine, Northwestern Memorial Hospital,
Chicago, Illinois
93: Acute Gastroenteritis

Gary D. Zimmer, MD, FAAEM
Assistant Professor, Department of Emergency
Medicine, Johns Hopkins University School of
Medicine; Director, Department of Emergency
Medicine, Harbor Hospital; Assistant Medical
Director for Baltimore Operations, Aeromedical
Transport Services Corporation, Baltimore,
Maryland
136: Sepsis Syndromes

Brian J. Zink, MD
Associate Professor and Associate Dean for Student
Programs, Department of Emergency Medicine,
University of Michigan Medical School, Ann
Arbor, Michigan
134: Bone and Joint Infections

D. Demetrios Zukin, MD, FAAP
Assistant Clinical Professor
Department of Pediatrics
University of California, San Francisco
San Francisco, California;
Attending Physician, Department of Emergency
Medicine
Children's Hospital Oakland
Oakland, California
165: Fever

Leslie S. Zun, MD, MBA
Professor and Chair, Department of Emergency
Medicine, Chicago Medical School of Rosalind
Franklin University of Medicine and Science,
North Chicago, Illinois; Chair, Department of
Emergency Medicine, Mount Sinai Hospital,
Chicago, Illinois
21: Nausea and Vomiting

Contributors

Preface to the Sixth Edition

Rosen's Emergency Medicine: Concepts and Clinical Practice culminates a 25-year tenure of what began as and remains the textbook for emergency physicians by emergency physicians. What remains in place? The editorial board is virtually intact save the fortunate acquisition of a stellar and experienced academician, Michelle Biros. The organization of the book still places Critical Management Principles at the forefront, in keeping with the mindset of the emergency physician, and then works its way through 7 parts, 32 sections, and 208 chapters, the last up from 201 in the prior edition. The annotations have been kept concise because of modern search capabilities but are thoroughly updated. This effects greater content within the same confines of space. The templates and formatting, which were reworked extensively for the previous edition, carry forward. Most significantly, hundreds of authors, authoritative in their field, have dedicated their skills and energy toward the foundation of this edition.

Yet this Sixth Edition demonstrates considerable change from its predecessor. This work is now in full color, a change intended to beautify but, more importantly, enhance the readability of the text. All figures and tables have been redrawn. The artwork has been updated. The bibliography now permits easier navigation. The complaint-based, algorithm-driven Cardinal Presentations section has been expanded. Finally, this text is now available as an Elsevier E-dition, wherein important changes in practice are posted to the website-based version. The postings are abstracted from recent peer-review journals, allowing the book and its diagnostic and management principles to be continually updated. This is critical given the ever increasing pace of change within our discipline.

This work ultimately reflects our contributors' expertise and reliance upon sound, evidence-based knowledge. We are grateful for their wisdom and willingness. Our editorial board has been exacting in wishing to ensure consistency and correctness. We are indebted to them for their perseverance. We are most appreciative of the efforts of Todd Hummel, Robin Hayward, and Judy Fletcher, our Publisher, Senior Project Manager, and Publishing Director, respectively, with Elsevier, and especially to those who support us on the home front, Tricia Wyatt and Gail Franklin (JAM), Maria Figueroa (RSH), and Diane Pugh and Janice Bingham (RMW), as it is they who continually pull us from the proverbial fire.

We will feel forever privileged for the honor of carrying forward this creation of Peter Rosen. It was his vision and courage that took this from fantasy to flight. And, borrowing from the Fifth Edition preface, it remains our "ongoing commitment to meet the dynamic and substantive needs of emergency medicine's academicians and clinicians alike."

JOHN A. MARX
ROBERT S. HOCKBERGER
RON M. WALLS

Preface to the First Edition

From the vision and foresight of a few physicians who perceived the need for a unique, disciplined, sensitive approach to the identification and stabilization of patients threatened with loss of life or limb, emergency medicine has rapidly developed into an exciting, academically recognized medical specialty. This textbook is dedicated to those who have accepted its responsibilities, challenges, and excitements.

We have attempted to define in depth the material on which our practice is based. There have been a number of efforts to write about emergencies, but we believe that this is the first to call solely on those people who themselves practice the specialty. In every chapter theory and knowledge pertinent to the practice of emergency medicine are presented.

This book is not an easy one; it was written based on published literature, not anecdote or prejudice. In many instances where the data are not available, both sides are presented with a suggested practice. The book is intended for all with a serious interest in or a need to know emergency medicine, including those who do not practice full-time emergency medicine, as well as the dedicated specialists who do.

The book is organized into two main sections—trauma and nontrauma. This division is artificial but does correspond to the first major decisions made in patient evaluations, because trauma usually affects individual anatomic structures whereas nontrauma is more likely to affect systems.

Despite this artificial separation, long and detailed discussion and instruction to authors concerning content and style ensued. We realize that we could not tap all available talent for contributions to the book, but we have made an effort to represent different schools of thought and regions of the country.

There are deliberate omissions; for example, we elected not to include any procedures. There was not enough room to create an atlas, but it was our desire to cover the chosen topics in detail. No effort has been made to address administration, management, disaster planning, or technical requirements of emergency medicine supplies or design. Prehospital care has been included only as it relates to individual topics, not as suggested protocol or from the vantage point of technician training programs.

It would be impossible to write a book this long and present nothing controversial. In fact we ourselves find sections we cannot totally accept, but in the process of working with multiple authors, we cannot with intellectual honesty put ideas into their material. We have, however, achieved our goal of presenting an in-depth vision of emergency medicine written by specialists in emergency medicine. We hope you will find the reading of this book as stimulating and enjoyable as we have found its creation.

PETER ROSEN
FRANK J. BAKER II
G. RICHARD BRAEN
ROBERT H. DAILEY
RICHARD C. LEVY

Acknowledgments

To our editors, for their enduring loyalty and dedication; to Karin, for her unwavering courage and grace; to my faculty and residents, who have given me so much; to Conner and Shelby, who have given me everything.

JAM

To Peter and the former editors for trusting us to continue their work; to the current authors and editors for the expertise, skill, and time they dedicated to this edition; to Ron for his critical thinking, enthusiasm, and much-needed sense of humor; to John for the few big things, the many small-but-important things, and the day-to-day leadership he provided as Editor-in-Chief; to my faculty, fellows, and residents for making each day an adventure; and to Patty, the love of my life.

RSH

With humble thanks to Peter, for his great vision in the creation of an extraordinary specialty and this compendium of its biology; to John and Bob, for their enduring friendship and collaboration; to the editors, for their sedulous attention to detail; and to Barb, Andrew, Blake, and Alexa, whose love defines me.

RMW

To my father, James J. Adams, whose strength will forever inspire me; to my mother Rita A. Adams, whose devotion to family will forever guide me; and to the many other members of my family: Cecelia, Joe, Jeff, Liz, Rob, David, Nicholas, Gregory, Leah, Katherine, and Sydney, whose support I rely on.

JGA

To all my former residents over the past 25 years from both Cincinnati and Michigan. I have been privileged to work with the best and I have learned a lot from all of you. I have to thank my children, David, Blake, and Anna, for keeping me thinking young and teaching me lots about life and family. My mom and dad have been a constant source of inspiration to me my entire life and they continue to be the role models I try to live up to. Most of all, I have to thank my wife and best friend, Mary, for her love and support over the past 30 years. She makes it all worthwhile.

WGB

To my family, friends, students, and teachers. I am continuously amazed, grateful, and humbled by your support and encouragement. Thank you.

MHB

To Joanna, Bags, Jules, and the Belties; and to our spry 91-year-old Floyds Knobs farmer neighbor, Odell Stiller, who quipped, "Doc, you'll never see my name or face in a book." Gotcha.

DFD

I dedicate this book to my husband David and our children, Sarah, Jeremiah, and Katie—for their patience, love, and support.

MGH

To Lynda, 35 years, a witnessed life, all because of a chance meeting in Ann Arbor just yesterday.

GCH

To emergency medicine residents and faculty everywhere, in their constant pursuit of knowledge but especially those at Hennepin County Medical Center for continuing to teach me. I am grateful to my parents, Rose and Joseph, for their commitment to education. Special thanks to Eric, Ali, Amanda, and, most of all, Beth for their love, patience, and understanding.

LJL

I would like to thank my teachers—my parents and my children, professors and patients, colleagues and students—who have patiently taught me about medicine and life; and my steadfast companion and wife Lynda, who has made the pursuit of wisdom possible.

EJN

Emeritus Editors
Peter Rosen
Roger M. Barkin

Past Editors
Frank J. Baker II (Editions 1 and 2)
G. Richard Braen (Editions 1, 2, and 3)
Robert H. Dailey (Editions 1, 2, and 3)
Jerris R. Hedges (Edition 3)
Richard C. Levy (Editions 1, 2, and 3)
Vincent Markovchick (Edition 4)
Mark Smith (Edition 3)

Contents

Volume 1

PART ONE
Fundamental Clinical Concepts

Section I
Critical Management Principles 2

Chapter 1
Airway 2
Ron M. Walls

Chapter 2
Mechanical Ventilation and Noninvasive
Ventilatory Support 26
Charles V. Pollack, Jr.

Chapter 3
Monitoring the Emergency Patient 35
Michael F. Murphy and Timothy A. D. Graham

Chapter 4
Shock...................................... 41
Alan E. Jones and Jeffrey A. Kline

Chapter 5
Blood and Blood Components 56
Gwendolyn L. Hoffman

Chapter 6
Brain Resuscitation 62
Robert Silbergleit and Norman S. Abramson

Chapter 7
Adult Resuscitation 75
Robert W. Neumar and Kevin R. Ward

Chapter 8
Pediatric Resuscitation 97
Brian P. Gilligan and Robert C. Luten

Chapter 9
Neonatal Resuscitation 118
Eileen Klein and Linda Quan

Section II
Cardinal Presentations 125

Chapter 10
Clinical Decision Making 125
Dane M. Chapman, Douglas M. Char,
and Chandra D. Aubin

Chapter 11
Fever in the Adult Patient 134
Frederick C. Blum

Chapter 12
Weakness 138
Robert C. Reiser

Chapter 13
Dizziness and Vertigo 142
Jonathan S. Olshaker

Chapter 14
Confusion 150
J. Stephen Huff and William J. Brady

Chapter 15
Coma and Depressed Level of
Consciousness 156
Richard E. Wolfe and David F. M. Brown

Chapter 16
Seizures 164
Charles V. Pollack, Jr.

Chapter 17
Headache 169
Gregory L. Henry and Christopher S. Russi

Chapter 18
Dyspnea 175
Sabina Braithwaite and Debra Perina

Chapter 19
Chest Pain 183
James E. Brown and Glenn C. Hamilton

Chapter 20
Syncope 193
Robert A. De Lorenzo

Chapter 21
Nausea and Vomiting 200
Leslie S. Zun and Amardeep Singh

Chapter 22
Abdominal Pain 209
Kelly E. King and John M. Wightman

Chapter 23
Gastrointestinal Bleeding 220
Philip L. Henneman

Chapter 24
Diarrhea 227
John E. Gough and Phillip A. Clement

Chapter 25
Constipation 237
Natalie Cullen

Chapter 26
Jaundice 243
Katherine L. Heilpern and Tammie E. Quest

Chapter 27
Acute Pelvic Pain 248
Robert Dart

Chapter 28
Vaginal Bleeding 254
John C. Bradford and Christ G. Kyriakedes

Chapter 29
Back Pain 260
Kevin G. Rodgers and James B. Jones

Chapter 30
Cyanosis 268
Jennifer Bocock and Joan Kolodzik

Chapter 31
Sore Throat 274
Jonathan I. Singer and Mark E. Gebhart

Chapter 32
Hemoptysis 279
Brian Springer and Timothy G. Janz

Chapter 33
Red and Painful Eye 283
John M. Wightman and Glenn C. Hamilton

PART TWO
Trauma

Section I
General Concepts 300

Chapter 34
Multiple Trauma 300
Susan L. Gin-Shaw and Robert C. Jorden

Chapter 35
Trauma in Pregnancy 316
John D. G. Neufeld

Chapter 36
Pediatric Trauma 328
Richard M. Cantor

Chapter 37
Geriatric Trauma 344
Diane M. Birnbaumer

Section II
System Injuries 349

Chapter 38
Head 349
William G. Heegaard and Michelle H. Biros

Chapter 39
Facial Trauma 382
Mary Pat McKay

Chapter 40
Spinal Injuries 398
Robert S. Hockberger, Amy H. Kaji,
and Edward J. Newton

Chapter 41
Neck 441
Kim Newton

Chapter 42
Thoracic Trauma 453
Marc Eckstein and Sean Henderson

Chapter 43
Abdominal Trauma 489
John A. Marx and Jennifer Isenhour

Chapter 44
Genitourinary System 514
Robert E. Schneider

Chapter 45
Peripheral Vascular Injury 536
Edward J. Newton

Section III
Orthopedic Lesions 549

Chapter 46
General Principles of Orthopedic
Injuries.................... 549
Joel M. Geiderman

Chapter 47
Hand 576
Everett Lyn and Robert E. Antosia

Chapter 48
Wrist and Forearm 622
Karen G. H. Woolfrey and Mary A. Eisenhauer

Chapter 49
Humerus and Elbow............ 647
Joel M. Geiderman

Chapter 50
Shoulder 670
Mohamud Daya

Chapter 51
Musculoskeletal Back Pain 701
Michelle Lin

Chapter 52
Pelvis **717**
A. Adam Cwinn

Chapter 53
Femur and Hip **735**
Michael A. Gibbs, Edward J. Newton,
and James F. Fiechtl

Chapter 54
Knee and Lower Leg **770**
Everett Lyn, Daniel Pallin, and Robert E. Antosia

Chapter 55
Ankle and Foot **808**
Kendall Ho and Riyad B. Abu-Laban

Section IV
Soft Tissue Injuries **842**

Chapter 56
Wound Management Principles **842**
Barry Simon and H. Gene Hern, Jr.

Chapter 57
Foreign Bodies **859**
Stephen H. Thomas and David F. M. Brown

Chapter 58
Mammalian Bites **882**
Ellen J. Weber

Chapter 59
Venomous Animal Injuries **894**
Edward J. Otten

Chapter 60
Thermal Burns **913**
Richard F. Edlich, Marcus L. Martin,
and William B. Long III

Chapter 61
Chemical Injuries **929**
Richard F. Edlich, Marcus L. Martin,
and William B. Long III

Section V
Violence and Abuse **940**

Chapter 62
Injury Prevention and Control **940**
Stephen W. Hargarten and Jeffrey W. Runge

Chapter 63
Forensic Emergency Medicine **952**
William S. Smock

Chapter 64
Child Maltreatment **968**
Carol D. Berkowitz

Chapter 65
Sexual Assault **977**
Laura Slaughter

Chapter 66
Intimate Partner Violence and Abuse **994**
Patricia R. Salber

Chapter 67
Elder Abuse and Neglect **1008**
Deirdre Anglin and Diana C. Schneider

Chapter 68
Youth, Gangs, and Violence **1017**
H. Range Hutson

Index .... **i**

Volume 2

PART THREE
Medicine and Surgery

Section I
Head and Neck Disorders **1026**

Chapter 69
Oral Medicine **1026**
James T. Amsterdam

Chapter 70
Ophthalmology **1044**
Douglas D. Brunette

Chapter 71
Otolaryngology **1066**
James A. Pfaff and Gregory P. Moore

Section II
Pulmonary System **1078**

Chapter 72
Asthma **1078**
Richard M. Nowak and Glenn Tokarski

Chapter 73
Chronic Obstructive Pulmonary
Disease **1097**
Stuart P. Swadron and Diku P. Mandavia

Chapter 74
Upper Respiratory Tract Infections **1109**
Frantz R. Melio

Chapter 75
Pneumonia **1128**
Gregory J. Moran and David A. Talan

Chapter 76
Pleural Disease **1143**
Joshua M. Kosowsky

Section III
Cardiac System **1154**

Chapter 77
Acute Coronary Syndromes **1154**
William J. Brady, Richard A. Harrigan,
and Theodore Chan

Chapter 78
Dysrhythmias 1199
Donald M. Yealy and Theodore R. Delbridge

Chapter 79
Implantable Cardiac Devices................. 1246
James T. Niemann

Chapter 80
Heart Failure 1258
John F. O'Brien and Jay L. Falk

Chapter 81
Pericardial and Myocardial Disease 1280
Nicholas J. Jouriles

Chapter 82
Infective Endocarditis and Valvular
Heart Disease 1300
Susan M. Dunmire

Section IV
Vascular System............................... 1310

Chapter 83
Hypertension 1310
Richard O. Gray

Chapter 84
Aortic Dissection 1324
Felix Ankel

Chapter 85
Abdominal Aortic Aneurysm 1330
Howard A. Bessen

Chapter 86
Peripheral Arteriovascular Disease 1342
Tom P. Aufderheide

Chapter 87
Pulmonary Embolism and Deep
Venous Thrombosis 1368
Jeffrey A. Kline and Michael S. Runyon

Section V
Gastrointestinal System 1382

Chapter 88
Esophagus, Stomach, and
Duodenum 1382
Mark J. Lowell

Chapter 89
Liver and Biliary Tract 1402
David A. Guss

Chapter 90
Pancreas 1426
Sally A. Santen and Robin R. Hemphill

Chapter 91
Disorders of the Small Intestine 1440
Susan P. Torrey and Philip L. Henneman

Chapter 92
Acute Appendicitis 1451
Jeannette M. Wolfe and Philip L. Henneman

Chapter 93
Acute Gastroenteritis 1460
Robert A. Bitterman and David K. Zich

Chapter 94
Large Intestine 1490
Michael A. Peterson

Chapter 95
Anorectum 1507
Wendy C. Coates

Section VI
Genitourinary System 1524

Chapter 96
Renal Failure 1524
Allan B. Wolfson

Chapter 97
Sexually Transmitted Diseases 1556
Diane M. Birnbaumer and Christine Anderegg

Chapter 98
Selected Urologic Problems 1572
John Kahler and Ann L. Harwood-Nuss

Section VII
Neurology...................................... 1606

Chapter 99
Stroke.. 1606
Rashmi U. Kothari, Todd J. Crocco,
and William G. Barsan

Chapter 100
Seizures.. 1619
Charles V. Pollack, Jr.

Chapter 101
Headache 1631
Thomas Kwiatkowski and Kumar Alagappan

Chapter 102
Delirium and Demetia 1645
Jeffrey Smith and Jennifer Seirafi

Chapter 103
Brain and Cranial Nerve Disorders 1664
Brian Stettler and Arthur M. Pancioli

Chapter 104
Spinal Cord Disorders 1675
Andrew D. Perron and J. Stephen Huff

Chapter 105
Peripheral Nerve Disorders.................. **1687**
E. John Gallagher

Chapter 106
Neuromuscular Disorders **1702**
Peter Shearer and Andrew Jagoda

Chapter 107
Central Nervous System Infections **1710**
Frank W. Lavoie and John R. Saucier

Section VIII
Psychiatric and Behavioral
Disorders.................................. **1726**

Chapter 108
Thought Disorders **1726**
Robert S. Hockberger and John R. Richards

Chapter 109
Mood Disorders **1734**
Douglas A. Rund and Marshall G. Vary

Chapter 110
Anxiety Disorders **1744**
Eugene E. Kercher and Joshua L. Tobias

Chapter 111
Somatoform Disorders........................ **1753**
Thomas B. Purcell

Chapter 112
Factitious Disorders and
Malingering.................................. **1761**
Thomas B. Purcell

Chapter 113
Suicide **1766**
Stephen A. Colucciello

Section IX
Immunologic and Inflammatory **1776**

Chapter 114
Arthritis **1776**
Douglas W. Lowery III

Chapter 115
Tendinopathy and Bursitis................... **1794**
Ted Koutouzis and Stephen L. Adams

Chapter 116
Systemic Lupus Erythematosus
and the Vasculitides **1805**
Clare T. Sercombe

Chapter 117
Allergy, Hypersensitivity, and
Anaphylaxis **1818**
T. Paul Tran and Robert L. Muelleman

Chapter 118
Dermatologic Presentations **1838**
Rita K. Cydulka and Mary Hancock

Section X
Hematology and Oncology **1867**

Chapter 119
Anemia, Polycythemia, and White
Blood Cell Disorders **1867**
Glenn C. Hamilton and Timothy G. Janz

Chapter 120
Disorders of Hemostasis **1892**
Timothy G. Janz and Glenn C. Hamilton

Chapter 121
Selected Oncologic Emergencies........... **1907**
Nnamdi Nkwuo, Neil Schamban,
and Marc Borenstein

Section XI
Metabolism and Endocrinology **1922**

Chapter 122
Acid-Base Disorders **1922**
Jamie L. Collings

Chapter 123
Electrolyte Disturbances **1933**
Michael A. Gibbs and Vivek S. Tayal

Chapter 124
Diabetes Mellitus and Disorders
of Glucose Homeostasis **1955**
Rita K. Cydulka and Jeffrey Pennington

Chapter 125
Rhabdomyolysis **1975**
Laura J. Bontempo

Chapter 126
Thyroid and Adrenal Disorders **1985**
Jeffrey Sternlicht and John M. Wogan

Section XII
Infectious Disease **2001**

Chapter 127
Bacteria...................................... **2001**
Madonna Fernández-Frackelton

Chapter 128
Viruses **2033**
Michael Alan Polis and Tenagne Haile-Mariam

Chapter 129
Rabies.. **2061**
Ellen J. Weber

Chapter 130
AIDS and HIV **2071**
Richard E. Rothman, Catherine A. Marco,
Samuel Yang, and Gabor D. Kelen

Chapter 131
Parasites **2096**
Bruce M. Becker and John D. Cahill

Chapter 132
Tick-Borne Illnesses **2116**
Edward B. Bolgiano and Joseph Sexton

Chapter 133
Tuberculosis **2145**
Peter E. Sokolove and Dennis Chan

Chapter 134
Bone and Joint Infections **2174**
Brian J. Zink

Chapter 135
Soft Tissue Infections **2195**
Harvey W. Meislin and John A. Guisto

Chapter 136
Sepsis Syndromes........................... **2211**
Nathan I. Shapiro, Gary D. Zimmer,
and Adam Z. Barkin

Index .... **i**

Volume 3

PART FOUR
Environment and Toxicology

Section I
Environment **2228**

Chapter 137
Frostbite **2228**
Daniel F. Danzl

Chapter 138
Accidental Hypothermia **2236**
Daniel F. Danzl

Chapter 139
Heat Illness **2254**
Salvator Vicario

Chapter 140
Electrical and Lightning Injuries.......... **2267**
Timothy G. Price and Mary Ann Cooper

Chapter 141
Scuba Diving and Dysbarism.............. **2279**
Lee W. Shockley

Chapter 142
High-Altitude Medicine...................... **2296**
Michael Yaron and Benjamin Honigman

Chapter 143
Submersion **2311**
Andrew L. Knaut and Kim M. Feldhaus

Chapter 144
Radiation Injuries............................. **2316**
Vincent Markovchick

Section II
Toxicology **2325**

Chapter 145
General Approach to the Poisoned
Patient **2325**
Ken Kulig

Chapter 146
Acetaminophen................................ **2331**
Kenneth E. Bizovi and Robert Hendrickson

Chapter 147
Aspirin and Nonsteroidal Agents........... **2339**
Donna L. Seger and Lindsay Murray

Chapter 148
Anticholinergics **2345**
Wilfredo Rivera and Larissa I. Velez

Chapter 149
Antidepressants **2352**
Elisabeth F. Bilden and Frank G. Walter

Chapter 150
Cardiovascular Drugs **2368**
David J. Roberts

Chapter 151
Caustics **2380**
Paul M. Wax and Sandra M. Schneider

Chapter 152
Cocaine and Other
Sympathomimetics **2386**
Rama B. Rao and Robert S. Hoffman

Chapter 153
Toxic Alchohols **2395**
Suzanne R. White and Joseph Kosnik

Chapter 154
Hallucinogens **2406**
Binh T. Ly, Richard F. Clark, and Saralyn R. Williams

Chapter 155
Heavy Metals **2418**
Larissa I. Velez and Kathleen A. Delaney

Chapter 156
Hydrocarbons **2428**
David C. Lee

Chapter 157
Inhaled Toxins **2432**
Lewis S. Nelson and Robert S. Hoffman

Chapter 158
Lithium 2442
Keith K. Burkhart

Chapter 159
Antipsychotics 2445
Mary A. Wittler and Eric J. Lavonas

Chapter 160
Opioids 2451
Christina E. Hantsch

Chapter 161
Pesticides 2457
Cynthia K. Aaron

Chapter 162
Plants, Mushrooms, and Herbal
Medications 2471
Richard D. Shih

Chapter 163
Sedative Hypnotics 2481
Leon Gussow and Andrea Carlson

PART FIVE
Special Populations

Section I
The Pediatric Patient 2494

Chapter 164
General Approach to the Pediatric
Patient 2494
Robert A. Wiebe

Chapter 165
Fever 2505
Roger M. Barkin and D. Demetrios Zukin

Chapter 166
Pediatric Respiratory Emergencies:
Upper Airway Obstruction and
Infections 2519
Mariann Manno

Chapter 167
Pediatric Respiratory Emergencies:
Lower Airway Obstruction 2532
Christine D. Darr

Chapter 168
Pediatric Respiratory Emergencies:
Disease of the Lungs 2554
Susan Kirelik and Brian Alverson

Chapter 169
Cardiac Disorders 2567
Alson S. Inaba

Chapter 170
Gastrointestinal Disorders 2601
Mark A. Hostetler

Chapter 171
Infectious Diarrheal Disease and
Dehydration 2623
Roger M. Barkin and David G. Ward

Chapter 172
Renal and Genitourinary Tract
Disorders 2635
Maureen McCollough and Ghazala Sharieff

Chapter 173
Neurologic Disorders 2657
David H. Rubin, Dina Halpern Kornblau,
Edward E. Conway, Jr., and Stuart M. Caplen

Chapter 174
Musculoskeletal Disorders 2689
Kemedy K. McQuillen

Chapter 175
Sudden Infant Death Syndrome and
Apparent Life-Threatening Events 2713
Marianne Gausche-Hill

Section II
The Pregnant Patient 2722

Chapter 176
General Approach to the Pregnant
Patient 2722
Laurie J. Morrison

Chapter 177
Acute Complications of Pregnancy 2739
Debra E. Houry and Jean T. Abbott

Chapter 178
Chronic Medical Illness During
Pregnancy 2761
Edward J. Newton and Kirsten K. Calder

Chapter 179
Drug Therapy and Substance Abuse 2779
Rania Habal and Diane Sauter

Chapter 180
Labor and Delivery and Their
Complications 2797
Sean Henderson and William K. Mallon

Section III
The Geriatric Patient 2824

Chapter 181
The Elder Patient 2824
Diane M. Birnbaumer

Section IV
The Patient with Compromised
Immune Function **2831**

Chapter 182
The Immunocompromised
Patient **2831**
Michael J. Burns and Mark I. Langdorf

Section V
The Patient with an Organ
Transplant..................................... **2846**

Chapter 183
The Solid-Organ Transplant
Patient **2846**
Matthew T. Keadey and Douglas W. Lowery III

Section VI
The Alcoholic or Substance Abuse
Patient **2858**

Chapter 184
Alcohol-Related Disease **2858**
David B. McMicken and John T. Finnell

Chapter 185
Substance Abuse **2882**
Stephen A. Colucciello and Christian Tomaszewski

Section VII
The Developmentally or Physically
Disabled Patient **2898**

Chapter 186
Evaluation of the Developmentally
and Physically Disabled Patient **2898**
Maria Stephan

Section VIII
The Patient in Pain **2913**

Chapter 187
Pain Management **2913**
Paul M. Paris and Donald M. Yealy

Chapter 188
Procedural Sedation and Analgesia **2938**
Carl R. Chudnofsky and Marie M. Lozon

Section IX
The Problem Patient **2956**

Chapter 189
The Combative Patient **2956**
Gregory P. Moore, Louise Kao, and Kenneth Jackimczyk

Chapter 190
The Difficult Patient **2972**
David W. Harrison and Robert J. Vissers

PART SIX
Emergency Medical Services

Chapter 191
Emergency Medical Service: Overview
and Ground Transport **2984**
Thomas H. Blackwell

Chapter 192
Air Medical Transport......................... **2994**
Howard Rodenberg and Ira J. Blumen

Chapter 193
Tactical Emergency Medical Support
and Urban Search and Rescue **3000**
Richard Schwartz, John G. McManus,
and Jeffrey Orledge

Chapter 194
Disaster Preparedness **3010**
Carl H. Schultz, Kristi L. Koenig, and Eric K. Noji

Chapter 195
Weapons of Mass Destruction **3021**
Carl H. Schultz and Kristi L. Koenig

PART SEVEN
The Practice of Emergency Medicine

Section I
Clinical Practice and
Administration **3034**

Chapter 196
Guidelines in Emergency Medicine **3034**
J. Stephen Bohan

Chapter 197
Medical Literature and
Evidence-Based Medicine **3046**
Kelly D. Young and Roger J. Lewis

Chapter 198
Observation Medicine and Clinical
Decision Units **3062**
Malcolm Mahadevan and Louis Graff

Chapter 199
Occupational Medicine and
Occupational Health in the
Emergency Department **3076**
Andrew R. Barnosky, Daniel K. Chapman,
and Victor S. Roth

Chapter 200
Hyperbaric Medicine **3088**
Enoch T. Huang and Stephen R. Thom

Chapter 201
The Social Role of Emergency
Medicine **3092**
James A. Gordon

Chapter 202
Information Technology in Emergency
Medicine **3097**
Jonathan M. Teich and William H. Cordell

Chapter 203
Multiculturalism and Care Delivery **3107**
Edward Bernstein, Judith Bernstein, and Thea James

Chapter 204
Process Improvement and
Patient Safety in the Emergency
Department **3119**
Pat Croskerry, Marc J. Shapiro, Shawna J. Perry,
and Robert L. Wears

Section II
Philosophical Issues of Practice **3127**

Chapter 205
Bioethics **3127**
Kenneth V. Iserson

Chapter 206
End of Life **3139**
Jean T. Abbott and Susan Stone

Chapter 207
Medicolegal and Risk Management **3156**
Robert A. Bitterman

Chapter 208
Wellness, Stress, and the Impaired
Physician **3174**
Richard Goldberg

Index .... **i**

PART ONE

Fundamental Clinical Concepts

CHAPTER

1 Airway

Ron M. Walls

PERSPECTIVE

Airway management is a defining element for the specialty of emergency medicine. Although practitioners from other specialties often have knowledge and skills that overlap those of the emergency physician, the ability to provide critical care and definitive airway management for all patients, regardless of the cause of their presentation, is unique to the specialty of emergency medicine. The emergency physician has primary responsibility for management of the airway. All techniques of airway management lie within the domain of emergency medicine. Rapid sequence intubation (RSI) is the cornerstone, but emergency airway management includes various intubation maneuvers, use of ancillary devices, approaches to the difficult airway, and rescue techniques when intubation fails.

Since the first reported use of neuromuscular blocking agents (NMBAs) in the emergency department by emergency personnel in 1971, there has been progressive sophistication of emergency airway techniques, pharmacologic agents, and special devices used to facilitate intubation.[1-3] The American College of Emergency Physicians stated in its policy on RSI that the use of NMBAs to facilitate tracheal intubation is within the domain of emergency medicine and that emergency physicians should possess the necessary knowledge, experience, and training to apply RSI in the clinical care of patients.[4] In the 1990s, widespread adoption of RSI as the method of choice for most emergency intubations in the emergency department occurred, and increasing attention has been focused on identification and management of patients with anticipated difficult intubation.[5,6]

PATHOPHYSIOLOGY

Decision to Intubate

A decision to intubate should be based on careful patient assessment with respect to three essential criteria: (1) failure to maintain or protect the airway, (2) failure of ventilation or oxygenation, and (3) the patient's anticipated clinical course and likelihood of deterioration.[7]

Failure to Maintain or Protect the Airway

A patent airway is essential for adequate ventilation and oxygenation. If the patient is unable to maintain the airway, patency must be established by artificial means, such as repositioning, chin lift, jaw thrust, or insertion of an oral or nasal airway. Likewise, the patient must be able to protect against aspiration of gastric contents, which carries significant morbidity and mortality. Traditionally, presence or absence of a gag reflex has been advocated as a reliable indicator of the patient's ability to protect the airway, but the gag reflex is absent in 12% to 25% of normal adults, and there is no evidence that its presence or absence corresponds to airway protective reflexes or the need for intubation.[8-11] A more reliable indicator may be the patient's ability to swallow or handle secretions, but this also remains to be tested. The recommended approach is to evaluate the patient's ability to phonate (which provides information about level of consciousness and voice quality), level of consciousness, and ability to manage his or her own secretions (e.g., pooling of secretions in the oropharynx, absence of swallowing spontaneously or to command.) In general, a patient who requires a maneuver to establish a patent airway or who easily tolerates an oral airway probably requires intubation for protection of that airway, unless a temporary or readily reversible condition, such as opioid overdose, is present.

Failure of Ventilation or Oxygenation

Ventilatory failure that is not reversible by clinical means or increasing hypoxemia that is not adequately responsive to supplemental oxygen is a primary indication for intubation. This assessment is clinical and includes evaluation of the patient's general status, oxygenation by pulse oximetry, and changes in the ventilatory pattern. Continuous capnography also can be helpful, but is not essential when oximetry readings are reliable. Arterial blood gases (ABGs) generally are not required to make a determination regarding the patient's need for intubation. In most circumstances, clinical assessment, including pulse oximetry, and observation of improvement or deterioration lead to a correct decision. ABGs are rarely helpful, and may be misleading, so, if obtained, they must be interpreted carefully in the context of the patient's clinical status.

Patients who are clinically stable or improving despite severe ABG alterations may not require intubation, whereas a rapidly tiring patient may require intubation when ABG values are only modestly disturbed or even improving.

Regardless of the underlying cause, the need for mechanical ventilation generally mandates intubation. External mask devices increasingly have been used to provide assisted mechanical ventilation without intubation (see Chapter 2), but despite these advances, most patients who need assisted ventilation or positive pressure to improve oxygenation require intubation.[12,13]

Anticipated Clinical Course

Certain conditions indicate the need for intubation even in the absence of frank airway, ventilatory, or oxygenation failure. These conditions are myriad and are characterized by a reasonable likelihood of predictable deterioration that would require airway intervention either to preserve the airway and ventilation or as part of the overall management of the patient. Intubation may be indicated relatively early in the course of severe cyclic antidepressant overdose. Although the patient is awake, protecting the airway, and exchanging gas well, intubation is advisable to guard against the strong likelihood of clinical deterioration, which can occur relatively abruptly and includes coma, seizure, cardiac dysrhythmia or arrest, and possible aspiration of activated charcoal or gastric contents.

Significant multiple trauma, with or without head injury, may be an indication for intubation.[14,15] Many of these patients are ventilating normally through a patent airway, and oxygen levels frequently are normal or supernormal with supplemental oxygen. Despite this, anticipated deterioration, loss of the ability to protect the airway, the need for invasive and painful procedures, or the need for studies outside the emergency department (e.g., computed tomography, angiography) may mandate intubation.[16] A patient with penetrating neck trauma may present with a patent airway and adequate gas exchange. Nevertheless, intubation is advisable with any evidence of vascular or direct airway injury because these patients tend to deteriorate and because increasing hemorrhage or swelling in the neck tends to both compromise the airway and confound later attempts at intubation.[17,18]

Although these indications for intubation may seem quite different and individualized, the common thread is the anticipated clinical course over time. In each circumstance, it can be anticipated that future events will compromise either the patient's ability to maintain and protect the airway or the patient's ability to oxygenate and ventilate. Knowledge of the natural history of the emergency condition is essential to determine whether intubation is necessary when airway compromise or gas exchange failure is not present on evaluation. A similar thought process is applied to any patient who will be leaving the emergency department for diagnostic studies (e.g., a computed tomography scan) or who may be transported to another facility. If it seems clinically likely that the patient may deteriorate, "prophylactic" or "preemptive" intubation is the prudent course.

CLINICAL FEATURES

Identification of the Difficult Airway

In most patients, even in the emergency department's precipitous and unpredictable environment, intubation is technically easy and straightforward. In large emergency department studies, overall intubation failure rates are about 1% for medical intubations and less than 3% in trauma patients.[1,19,20] Intubation failure occurs in approximately 1 in 200 to 1 in 2000 elective general anesthesia cases.[5,21,22] Bag/mask ventilation (BMV) is difficult in approximately one third of patients in whom intubation failure occurs, but combined failure of intubation and BMV is estimated to be exceedingly rare—1 in 5000 to 1 in 200,000 elective anesthesia patients.[22-24] These numbers cannot be applied directly to the emergency department situation but are reassuring in that they indicate a high degree of safety if a preintubation analysis of factors predicting difficult intubation is undertaken.[25]

The emergency nature of the patient's presentation often precludes postponement of the intubation, even for a short time, but knowledge of the difficulties presented by the patient's airway permits thoughtful planning and preparation for possible intubation failure. Preintubation assessment should evaluate the patient for difficult intubation, difficult BMV, and difficult cricothyrotomy. Knowledge of all three domains is crucial to successful planning.[5]

Neuromuscular paralysis should be avoided in patients for whom a high degree of intubation difficulty is predicted, unless the administration of NMBAs is part of a planned approach to the difficult airway. This approach may include use of a *double setup,* in which an alternative approach, such as cricothyrotomy, is simultaneously prepared.

Preintubation evaluation should be as comprehensive as clinical circumstances permit. A systematic approach to the patient is required. Most of the difficult airway markers discussed in the anesthesia and emergency medicine literature have not been scientifically validated.[25] Nevertheless, a methodical approach can be used to evaluate the patient, based on the accepted markers of difficult intubation. One such approach uses the mnemonic *LEMON* (Box 1-1).[5]

BOX 1-1. "LEMON" Approach for Evaluation of the Difficult Airway

Look externally, especially for signs of difficult intubation (by gestalt), difficult bag mask ventilation, and difficult cricothyrotomy
Evaluate the "3-3-2 rule"
Mallampati
Obstruction
Neck mobility

L—Look Externally

The patient first should be inspected for external markers of difficult intubation, simply by the gestalt of the intubator. Subjective clinical judgment can be highly specific (>90%), but severely insensitive (<20%) and so must be augmented by other evaluations.[23] Also at this time evaluation for difficult BMV and difficult cricothyrotomy occurs. Attributes of difficult BMV have largely been validated and can be summarized with the mnemonic *MOANS* (Box 1-2).[5,23] Difficulty with mask seal; obesity (because of redundant upper airway tissues, chest wall weight, and resistance of abdominal mass); advanced age (best judged by the physiologic appearance of the patient, but any age >55 years is at risk); edentulousness ("no teeth"), which independently interferes with mask seal; and stiffness or resistance to ventilation (e.g., asthma, chronic obstructive pulmonary disease, pulmonary edema, restrictive lung disease, term pregnancy) all cause or contribute to increased difficulty with BMV. The difficulty with BMV of the edentulous patient is the basis of the old, but wise, adage: "Remove dentures to intubate, leave them in to bag/mask ventilate."

Difficult cricothyrotomy can be anticipated whenever there is disturbance of the ability to locate and access the landmarks of the anterior airway via the neck. Prior surgery; the presence of hematoma, anatomic disruption, tumor, or abscess; scarring (as from radiation therapy or prior injury); or obesity, edema, or subcutaneous air each has the potential to make cricothyrotomy more difficult. The landmarks for cricothyrotomy are sought and identified as part of this first step in assessment of the difficult airway.

E—Evaluate 3-3-2

The second step in the evaluation of the difficult airway is to assess the patient's anatomy with respect to suitability for direct laryngoscopy. Direct laryngoscopy requires the ability to visualize the glottis by direct vision through the mouth, using alignment of the oral, pharyngeal, and laryngeal axes. Visualization requires that the mouth open adequately, that the submandibular space be adequate to accommodate the tongue, and that the larynx be positioned low enough in the neck to be accessible. These relationships have been explored in various studies by imaging and by external measurement of thyromental distance.[26] The "3-3-2 rule" is an effective summary of these geometric evaluations.[5] The 3-3-2 rule requires that the patient be able

to place 3 of his or her own fingers between the open incisors, 3 of his or her own fingers along the floor of the mandible beginning at the mentum, and 2 fingers from the laryngeal prominence to the floor of the mouth (Figure 1-1). A patient with a receding mandible and high-riding larynx is virtually impossible to intubate using direct laryngoscopy. Most patients are not sufficiently cooperative for such an evaluation, and the operator compares his or her fingers with the patient's fingers to estimate the sizes for the three tests.

M—Mallampati Score

Oral access is assessed using the Mallampati scale (Figure 1-2). Visibility of the oral pharynx ranges from complete visualization, including the tonsillar pillars (class I), to no visualization at all, with the tongue pressed against the hard palate (class IV). Class I and class II predict adequate oral access, class III predicts moderate difficulty, and class IV predicts a high degree of difficulty.[27]

O—Obstruction

Upper airway (supraglottic) obstruction may make visualization of the glottis, or intubation itself, mechanically impossible. Conditions such as epiglottitis, laryngeal tumor, Ludwig's angina, neck hematoma, or glottic polyps can compromise laryngoscopy, passage of the endotracheal tube (ETT), BMV, or all three. Physical examination for airway obstruction is combined with assessment of the patient's voice to satisfy this evaluation step.

N—Neck Mobility

Neck mobility is essential to allow the angled axes of the upper airway to be sufficiently repositioned to permit direct visualization of the glottis and is assessed by having the patient flex and extend the head and neck through a full range of motion. Neck extension is the most important motion, and simple extension may be as effective as the "sniffing" position in achieving an optimal laryngeal view.[28] Modest limitations of motion do not seriously impair laryngoscopy, but severe loss of motion may render laryngoscopy impossible. Cervical spine immobilization in trauma artificially reduces cervical spine mobility and predicts a more difficult laryngoscopy, but direct laryngoscopy is still highly successful in this group of patients.[14]

Identification of a difficult intubation does not preclude use of an RSI technique (see Figure 1-7). The crucial determination is whether the operator judges that the patient has a reasonable likelihood of intubation success, despite the difficulties identified, and that ventilation with a bag and mask will be successful in the event that intubation fails (hence the value of the MOANS assessment; see Box 1-2).

Measurement of Intubation Difficulty

The actual degree to which an intubation is "difficult" is highly subjective, and quantification is challenging.

BOX 1-2. MOANS Mnemonic for Evaluation of Difficult Bag/Mask Ventilation

Mask seal
Obesity
Aged
No teeth
Stiffness (resistance to ventilation)

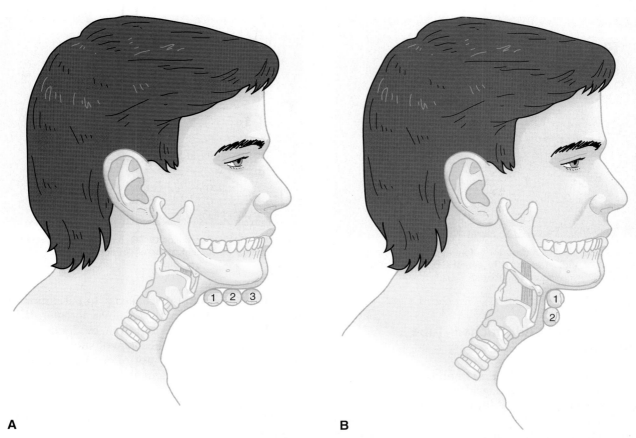

A

B

Figure 1-1. Final two steps of the 3-3-2 rule. **A,** Three fingers are placed along the floor of the mouth beginning at the mentum. **B,** Two fingers are placed in the laryngeal prominence (Adam's apple). (Adapted from Murphy MF, Walls RM: Identification of the difficult airway. In Walls RM, et al [eds]: *Manual of Emergency Airway Management*. Philadelphia, Lippincott Williams & Wilkins, 2004. The 3-3-2 Rule is copyrighted © 2004 by The Airway Course and Lippincott Williams & Wilkins, publishers of *The Manual of Emergency Airway Management*.)

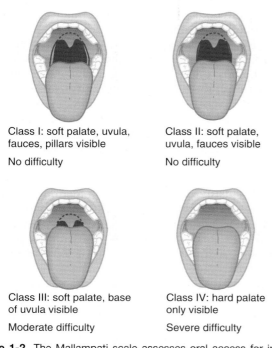

Class I: soft palate, uvula, fauces, pillars visible

No difficulty

Class II: soft palate, uvula, fauces visible

No difficulty

Class III: soft palate, base of uvula visible

Moderate difficulty

Class IV: hard palate only visible

Severe difficulty

Figure 1-2. The Mallampati scale assesses oral access for intubation. (From Whitten CE: *Anyone Can Intubate,* 4th ed. San Diego, KW Publication, 2004.)

Research has relied on laryngoscopic view to characterize the intubation difficulty, and the most widely used system is that of Cormack and Lehane, which grades laryngoscopy according to the extent to which laryngeal and glottic structures can be seen. In grade 1 laryngoscopy, the entire glottic aperture is seen. Grade 2 laryngoscopy visualizes only a portion of the glottis (arytenoid cartilages alone or arytenoid cartilages plus part of the vocal cords). Grade 3 laryngoscopy visualizes only the epiglottis. In grade 4 laryngoscopy, even the epiglottis is not visible.

Research conducted on elective anesthesia patients suggests that true grade 4 laryngoscopy, which is associated with impossible intubation, occurs in less than 1% of patients. Grade 3 laryngoscopy, which represents extreme intubation difficulty, is found in less than 5% of patients. Grade 2 laryngoscopy, which occurs in 10% to 30% of patients, can be subdivided further into grade 2a, in which arytenoids and a portion of the vocal cords are seen, and grade 2b, in which only the arytenoids are seen. Intubation failure occurs in 67% of grade 2b cases but only 4% of grade 2a cases.[29] Approximately 80% of all grade 2 laryngoscopies are grade 2a; the rest are grade 2b. A grade 1 view is associated with virtually 100% intubation success.

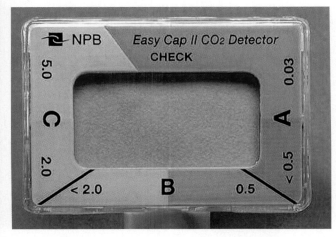

Figure 1-3. End-tidal CO_2 detector before application. The indicator is purple, which indicates failure to detect CO_2. This is the appearance when the esophagus is intubated.

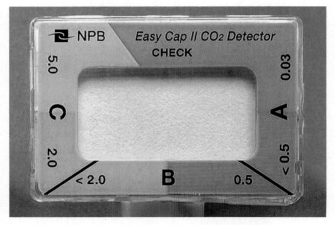

Figure 1-4. Positive detection of CO_2 turns the indicator yellow, indicating tracheal placement of the endotracheal tube.

Confirmation of Endotracheal Tube Placement

The most serious complication of endotracheal intubation is unrecognized esophageal intubation with resultant hypoxic brain injury. Although direct visualization of the ETT passing through the vocal cords is generally a reliable indicator of tracheal intubation, such clinical anatomic observations are fallible, and additional means are required to ensure correct placement of the tube within the trachea. Traditional methods, such as chest auscultation, gastric auscultation, bag resistance, exhaled volume, visualization of condensation within the ETT, and chest radiography, all are prone to failure as means of confirming tracheal intubation.[30] Other clinical techniques are readily available for detecting tracheal or esophageal intubation.

Immediately after intubation, the intubator should apply an end-tidal carbon dioxide (CO_2) detection device to the ETT and assess it through six manual ventilations. Disposable, colorimetric end-tidal CO_2 detectors are highly reliable, convenient, and easy to interpret, indicating adequate CO_2 detection by color change (Figures 1-3 and 1-4) (see Chapter 3). End-tidal CO_2 detection is highly reliable in identification of tracheal and esophageal intubation in patients with spontaneous circulation.[31] These devices indicate the CO_2 content in exhaled air either qualitatively or quantitatively. The persistence of detected CO_2 after six manual breaths indicates tracheal intubation. Rarely, BMV before intubation or ingestion of carbonated beverages may lead to release of CO_2 from the stomach after esophageal intubation, causing a false indication of tracheal intubation. Washout of this phenomenon occurs within six breaths, however, so persistence of CO_2 detection after six breaths indicates tracheal intubation.

Although end-tidal CO_2 detection is highly sensitive and specific for detecting esophageal intubation, caution is required for patients with cardiopulmonary arrest. Insufficient gas exchange may hamper CO_2 detection in the exhaled air, even when the tube is correctly placed within the trachea.[31] In patients with cardiopulmonary arrest, a CO_2 level greater than 2% should be considered definitive evidence of correct ETT placement, but the absence of such CO_2 cannot be used reliably as an indicator of esophageal intubation. This circumstance arises in approximately 25% to 40% of intubated cardiac arrest patients.[31,32] In all other patients, absence of CO_2 detection indicates failure to intubate the trachea, and immediate reintubation is indicated.

The other method of tube placement confirmation is the aspiration technique, which is based on the anatomic differences between the trachea and the esophagus. The esophagus is a muscular structure with no support within its walls. The trachea is held patent by cartilaginous rings. Vigorous aspiration of air through the ETT with the ETT cuff deflated results in occlusion of the ETT orifices by the soft walls of the esophagus, whereas aspiration after tracheal placement of the tube is easy and rapid.

Bulb or syringe aspiration devices may be used in cardiac arrest patients with no detectable CO_2, but although they are highly reliable at detecting esophageal intubation (high sensitivity), false-positives occur (poor specificity) and may indicate esophageal intubation when the tube is in the trachea. Aspiration devices may be useful in the out-of-hospital setting when poor lighting hampers colorimetric end-tidal CO_2 determination. They also are good backup devices when cardiac arrest confounds attempts to assess placement using end-tidal CO_2. Detection of expired CO_2 is more reliable and should be considered the standard for confirmation of tracheal placement of an ETT and for early detection of accidental esophageal intubation. Aspiration devices have a valuable, secondary role.

It is generally not sufficient to perform laryngoscopy to "confirm" that the tube is through the glottis because error and misinterpretation can occur, especially if the clinician confirming the intubation is the same person who intubated in the first place. The objective instrument (end-tidal CO_2) should be considered correct. In the absence of complete upper or lower (trachea, main stem bronchi) obstruction with inability to ventilate the patient with even small tidal volumes, failure of CO_2 detection should not be ascribed to other causes, such as severe asthma, in which the physician might postulate that adequate CO_2 exchange is not occurring for physiologic reasons. Absent equipment failure, this does not occur, and detection failure should be equated with intubation failure. A positive CO_2 reading also can occur when the tube has been misplaced above the glottis or in a main stem bronchus, where gas exchange can occur despite the lack of tracheal intubation.

End-tidal CO_2 detection with aspiration as backup should be considered the primary means of ETT placement confirmation. Secondary means include physical examination findings, oximetry, and radiography. The examiner should auscultate both lung fields and the epigastric area. Auscultation of typical hollow, gurgling, gastric sounds in the epigastrium is highly suggestive of esophageal intubation and should prompt consideration of immediate extubation for reintubation. Diminished or absent breath sounds on one side (usually the left side) indicate main stem bronchus intubation, in the absence of pneumothorax or an alternate cause of unilateral loss of breath sounds. Persistent, obvious leak despite positive end-tidal CO_2 detection indicates cuff malfunction or supraglottic placement of the ETT, such that the tube is in the airway, detecting CO_2, but above the vocal cords. In either case (main stem bronchus intubation or supraglottic intubation), tube repositioning is indicated.

Pulse oximetry is indicated as a monitoring technique in all critically ill patients, not just those patients who require intubation. Oximetry is useful in detecting esophageal intubation, but may not show a decreasing oxygen saturation for several minutes after a failed intubation because of the oxygen reservoir (preoxygenation) created in the patient before intubation.[33] Oximetry may be particularly misleading in a spontaneously breathing patient who has had an inadvertent nasal-esophageal intubation. In this case, oxygen saturation may be preserved because of spontaneous respirations, but catastrophe ensues if the patient is later paralyzed or heavily sedated in the mistaken belief that the tube is in the trachea.

Although chest radiography is universally recommended after ETT placement, its primary purpose is to ensure that the tube is well positioned below the cords and above the carina. A single anteroposterior chest radiograph is not sufficient to detect esophageal intubation, although esophageal intubation may be detected if the ETT is clearly outside the air shadow of the trachea. In doubtful cases, a fiberoptic scope can be passed through the ETT to identify tracheal rings, a "gold standard" for confirmation of tracheal placement.

MANAGEMENT

Approach to Intubation

After it is determined that the patient requires intubation, an approach must be planned. The algorithm in

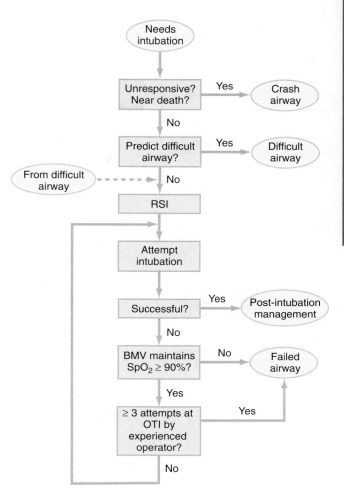

Figure 1-5. Main emergency airway management algorithm. RSI, rapid sequence intubation; BMV, bag/mask ventilation; SpO_2, pulse oximetry; OTI, orotracheal intubation. (Adapted from: Walls RM: The emergency airway algorithms. In Walls RM, et al [eds]: *Manual of Emergency Airway Management.* Philadelphia, Lippincott Williams & Wilkins, 2004. Copyright © 2004 The Airway Course and Lippincott Williams & Wilkins.)

Figure 1-5 assumes that a decision to intubate has been made and outlines such an approach. The approach is predicated on two key determinations that must be made before active airway management is begun (see Figure 1-5). The first determination is whether the patient is in cardiopulmonary arrest or a state near to arrest and is predicted to be unresponsive to direct laryngoscopy. Such a patient (agonal, near death) is called a "crash airway" patient for the purposes of airway management and is managed using the crash airway algorithm by immediate intubation without use of drugs, supplemented by a single dose of succinylcholine if the attempt to intubate fails and the patient is not sufficiently relaxed (Figure 1-6). The second determination is whether the patient represents a difficult intubation as determined by the "LEMON" evaluation. If so, the difficult airway algorithm is used (Figure 1-7).

For all other cases, that is, for all patients who require emergency department intubation but who have neither a "crash" airway nor a difficult airway, RSI is

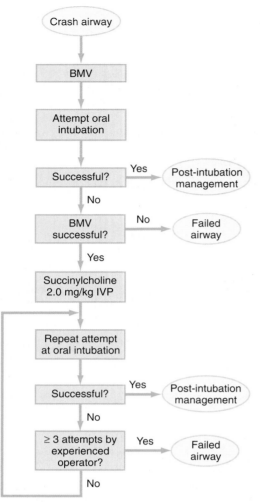

Figure 1-6. Crash airway algorithm. BMV, bag/mask ventilation; IVP, intravenous push. (Adapted from: Walls RM: The emergency airway algorithms. In Walls RM, et al [eds]: *Manual of Emergency Airway Management*. Philadelphia, Lippincott Williams & Wilkins, 2004. Copyright © 2004 The Airway Course and Lippincott Williams & Wilkins.)

recommended. RSI provides the safest and quickest method of achieving intubation in such patients.[1,19,34] After administration of the RSI drugs, intubation attempts are repeated until the patient is intubated or a failed intubation is identified. If more than one intubation attempt is required, oxygen saturation is monitored continuously, and if saturation falls to 90% or less, BMV is performed until saturation is recovered for another attempt. If the operator cannot maintain the oxygen saturation at 90% or greater, or at least stable if beginning at less than 90%, despite optimal use of a two-person, two-handed technique with an oral airway in place, a failed airway exists. This is referred to as a "can't intubate, can't oxygenate" situation. In addition, if three attempts at direct laryngoscopy have been unsuccessful, a failed airway exists because subsequent attempts at laryngoscopy by the same operator are unlikely to succeed. The three failed laryngoscopy attempts are defined as attempts by an experienced operator, using optimal patient positioning and best

possible technique. A further attempt at direct laryngoscopy by the same operator or one of equivalent experience is not advisable, unless the operator identifies a specific situation on the third laryngoscopy that is amenable to correction, justifying a fourth attempt. Also, if the operator ascertains after even a single attempt that intubation would be impossible (e.g., grade IV laryngoscopic view despite optimal patient positioning), a failed airway is present. The failed airway is managed according to the failed airway algorithm.

Difficult Airway

When preintubation evaluation has identified a potentially difficult airway, a different approach is used (see Figure 1-7).[6] The approach is based on the fact that NMBAs should not be administered to a patient for intubation unless the operator believes that (1) intubation is likely to be successful and (2) BMV is likely to be successful if a first intubation attempt does not succeed.

The perception of a difficult airway is relative, and many emergency department intubations could be considered "difficult." The judgment regarding whether to treat the airway as a typical emergency airway or whether to use the difficult airway algorithm is based on the degree of perceived difficulty and the individual circumstances of the case.[35] The LEMON assessment provides a systematic framework to assist in identifying the potentially difficult airway.

When a difficult airway approach is used, the first step is to ensure that oxygenation is sufficient to permit a planned, sequential approach (see Figure 1-7). If oxygenation is inadequate and cannot be made adequate by supplementation with bag and mask, the airway should be considered a failed airway. The failed airway algorithm should be used because the predicted high degree of intubation difficulty combined with failure to maintain oxygen saturation is analogous to the "can't intubate, can't oxygenate" situation. When oxygenation is adequate, the next consideration is whether RSI is appropriate, based on the operator's assessment of the likelihood of (1) successful intubation and (2) successful ventilation if intubation is unsuccessful. In some cases, a double setup can be used in which RSI is performed, but all preparations are undertaken for rescue cricothyrotomy before the drugs are administered. If RSI is not advisable, an "awake" technique can be used. In this context, *awake* means that the patient continues to breathe and is able to respond to caregivers. Usually the technique involves sedation and topical anesthesia. The awake technique is usually direct laryngoscopy, assisted by topical anesthesia and sedation, with the purpose of ascertaining whether intubation using direct laryngoscopy is possible. If the glottis is adequately visualized, the patient can be intubated at that time, or, in a stable difficult airway situation, the operator may proceed with planned RSI, now assured of intubation success. Alternatives to awake direct laryngoscopy include rigid and flexible fiberoptic intubation and video laryngoscopy. If the awake laryngoscopy determines that oral intubation using a standard laryngo-

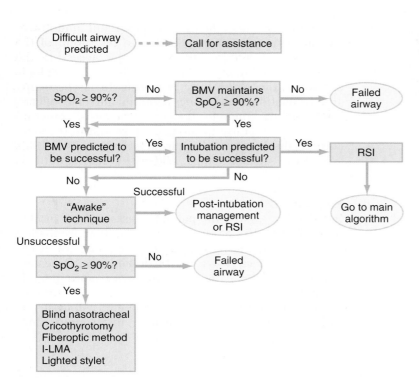

Figure 1-7. Difficult airway algorithm. SpO$_2$, pulse oxime-try; BMV, bag/mask ventilation; RSI, rapid sequence intu-bation; I-LMA, intubating laryngeal mask airway. (Adapted from: Walls RM: The emergency airway algorithms. In Walls RM, et al [eds]: *Manual of Emergency Airway Management.* Philadelphia, Lippincott Williams & Wilkins, 2004. Copyright © 2004 The Airway Course and Lippin-cott Williams & Wilkins.)

scope would not be successful, the patient is intubated using any of numerous techniques shown in the last box in Figure 1-7. For each of these methods, the patient is kept breathing but variably sedated with topical anes-thesia, and each of the methods results in placement of a cuffed ETT in the trachea. The choice among these methods depends on operator experience and prefer-ence and patient attributes.

Failed Airway

Management of the failed airway is dictated by whether or not the patient can be oxygenated.[6] If adequate oxy-genation cannot be maintained, the rescue technique of first resort is cricothyrotomy (Figure 1-8). Multiple attempts at other methods in the context of failed oxy-genation delay cricothyrotomy and place the patient at increased risk for hypoxic brain injury. If an alternative device (e.g., supra-glottic airway, laryngeal mask airway [LMA]) is readily at hand, however, it can be attempted simultaneously with preparations for imme-diate cricothyrotomy.

If adequate oxygenation is possible, several options are available for the failed airway. In almost all cases, cricothyrotomy is the definitive rescue technique for the failed airway if time does not allow for other approaches or if they fail. The fundamental difference in philosophy between the difficult airway and the failed airway is that the difficult airway is planned for, and the standard is to place a cuffed ETT in the trachea. The failed airway is *not* planned for, and the standard is to achieve an airway that provides adequate oxy-genation to avert the immediate problem of hypoxic brain injury. Some of the devices used in the failed airway (e.g., supraglottic airways) are temporary and do not provide airway protection.

THERAPEUTIC MODALITIES

Methods of Intubation

Although many techniques are available for intubation of the emergency patient, four methods represent most emergency department intubations, with RSI being the most frequently used in non-arrested patients.[1,19,36]

Rapid Sequence Intubation

RSI is the cornerstone of modern emergency airway management and is defined as the virtually simultane-ous administration of a potent sedative (induction) agent and an NMBA, usually succinylcholine, for the purpose of endotracheal intubation. This approach pro-vides optimal intubating conditions, while minimizing the risk of aspiration of gastric contents.

The central concept of RSI is to take the patient from the starting point (e.g., conscious, breathing sponta-neously) to a state of unconsciousness with complete neuromuscular paralysis, then to achieve intubation *without* interposed assisted ventilation. The risk of aspiration of gastric contents is significantly higher for patients who have not fasted before induction. Appli-cation of positive-pressure ventilation can cause air to pass into the stomach, resulting in gastric distention and increasing the risk of aspiration.[37] The purpose of RSI is to avoid positive-pressure ventilation until the ETT is placed correctly in the trachea with the cuff inflated. This requires a preoxygenation phase, during which the nitrogen reservoir in the functional residual capacity in the lungs is replaced with oxygen, permit-ting at least several minutes of apnea in the normal adult before oxygen desaturation to 90% ensues (Figure 1-9).[33]

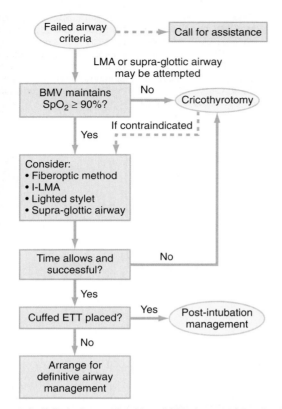

Figure 1-8. Failed airway algorithm. LMA, laryngeal mask airway; BMV, bag/mask ventilation; SpO₂, pulse oximetry; I-LMA, intubating laryngeal mask airway; ETT, endotracheal tube. (Adapted from: Walls RM: The emergency airway algorithms. In Walls RM, et al [eds]: *Manual of Emergency Airway Management*. Philadelphia, Lippincott Williams & Wilkins, 2004. Copyright © 2004 The Airway Course and Lippincott Williams & Wilkins.)

Use of RSI also facilitates successful endotracheal intubation by causing complete relaxation of the patient's musculature, allowing better access to the airway.[24,38,39] Finally, RSI permits pharmacologic control of the physiologic responses to laryngoscopy and intubation, mitigating potential adverse effects. These effects include further intracranial pressure increase in response to the procedure and to the sympathetic discharge resulting from laryngoscopy.[40] RSI is a series of discrete steps, and every step should be planned (Box 1-3).

Preparation

In the initial phase, the patient is assessed for intubation difficulty (if not already done), and the intubation is planned, including dosages and sequence of drugs, tube size, and laryngoscope blade and size. Drugs are drawn up and labeled. All necessary equipment is assembled. All these patients require continuous cardiac monitoring and pulse oximetry. At least one and preferably two good-quality intravenous lines

---

BOX 1-3. The Six "Ps" of RSI

1. Preparation
2. Preoxygenation
3. Pretreatment
4. Paralysis with induction
5. Placement of tube
6. Post-intubation management

Figure 1-9. Desaturation time for apneic, fully preoxygenated patients. Children, patients with comorbidity, and obese patients desaturate much more rapidly than healthy, normal adults. The box on the lower right-hand side of the graph depicts time to recovery from succinylcholine, which in almost all cases exceeds safe apnea time. Note also the precipitous decline of oxygen saturation from 90% to 0% for all groups. (Modified from Benumof J, et al: Critical hemoglobin desaturation will occur before return to unparalyzed state following 1 mg/kg intravenous succinylcholine. Anesthesiology 87:979, 1997.)

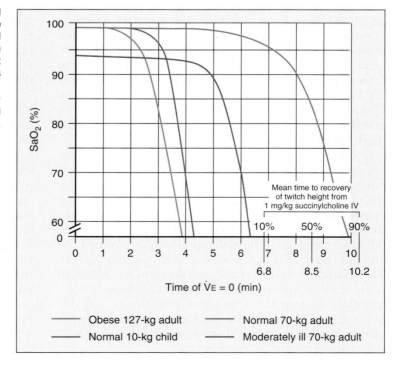

should be established. Redundancy is always desirable in case of equipment or intravenous access failure.

Preoxygenation

Administration of 100% oxygen for 3 minutes of normal, tidal volume breathing in a normal, healthy adult results in the establishment of an adequate oxygen reservoir to permit 8 minutes of apnea before oxygen desaturation to less than 90% occurs (see Figure 1-9).[33] The time to desaturation to less than 90% in children, obese adults, late-term pregnant women, and patients with significant comorbidity is considerably less. Desaturation time also is reduced if the patient does not inspire 100% oxygen.[41] Nevertheless, adequate preoxygenation usually can be obtained, even in emergency department patients, to permit several minutes of apnea before oxygen desaturation to less than 90% occurs. In children and adults, preoxygenation is essential to the "no bagging" approach of RSI. If time is insufficient for a full 3-minute preoxygenation phase, eight vital capacity breaths using high-flow oxygen can achieve oxygen saturations and apnea times that match or exceed those obtained with traditional preoxygenation.[42] Preoxygenation should be done in parallel with the preparation phase and can be started in the field for high-risk patients. Oxygen saturation monitors permit earlier detection of desaturation during laryngoscopy, but preoxygenation remains an essential step in RSI.

Pretreatment

During this phase, drugs are administered 3 minutes before administration of the succinylcholine and induction agent to mitigate the effects of laryngoscopy and intubation on the patient's presenting condition or underlying conditions. Intubation is intensely stimulating and results in sympathetic discharge (the reflex sympathetic response to laryngoscopy), elevation of intracranial pressure in patients with intracranial pressure disturbance, reactive bronchospasm, and bradycardia in children. In certain circumstances, mitigation of these adverse effects is desirable.

The pretreatment agents can be recalled by using the mnemonic *LOAD* (as in "load the patient before intubation") (Box 1-4). There is evidence supporting the physiologic benefits of these agents, but outcome data are lacking, so individualization is necessary, and critical time should not be lost administering pretreatment drugs if the patient requires immediate intubation. Despite the lack of outcome studies, there is considerable inferential evidence supporting this approach, and these agents probably provide protection for vulnerable patients against the adverse hemodynamic and intracranial effects of laryngoscopy and intubation.[43] Although many variations are possible for pretreatment regimens in various conditions, pretreatment can be simplified to these few basic indications.

When possible, 3 minutes should elapse between the administration of the pretreatment drug and the administration of the induction drug and NMBA. If time is insufficient to wait 3 minutes, even a reduced time may provide some benefit.

Paralysis with Induction

In this phase, a potent sedative agent is administered by rapid intravenous push in a dose capable of rapidly producing unconsciousness. This is immediately followed by rapid administration of an intubating dose of an NMBA, usually succinylcholine. The patient should be positioned for intubation as consciousness is lost, and Sellick's maneuver should be initiated.[44] Sellick's maneuver is the application of pressure to the anterior cricoid cartilage, causing posterior displacement of the cartilage to occlude the esophagus and prevent passive regurgitation of gastric contents. Although the patient is unconscious and apneic, BMV should not be initiated unless the patient is unable to maintain an oxygen saturation of 90%.

Placement of Tube

Approximately 45 seconds after the administration of succinylcholine, the patient is relaxed sufficiently to permit laryngoscopy; this is assessed most easily by moving the mandible to test for absence of muscle tone. The ETT is placed under direct visualization of the glottis. If intubation is unsuccessful or if the cords are not visualized, and the oxygen saturation is approaching 90%, the patient may be ventilated briefly with a bag and mask between attempts to reestablish the oxygen reservoir. In such cases, Sellick's maneuver must be continued; proper use of this maneuver during BMV of a paralyzed patient prevents passage of air into the stomach.[37] As soon as the ETT is placed, the cuff should be inflated and its position confirmed as described earlier. After confirmation of correct tracheal placement of the tube, Sellick's maneuver may be discontinued.

Post-intubation Management

A chest radiograph should be obtained to confirm that main stem intubation has not occurred and to assess

Table 1-1. Sample Rapid Sequence Intubation Using Etomidate and Succinylcholine

Time	Step
Zero minus 10 min	**Preparation**
Zero minus 5 min	**Preoxygenation**
	100% oxygen for 3 min *or* eight vital capacity breaths
Zero minus 3 min	**Pretreatment**
	as indicated "LOAD"
Zero	**Paralysis with induction**
	Etomidate, 0.3 mg/kg
	Succinylcholine, 1.5 mg/kg
Zero plus 45 sec	**Placement**
	Sellick's maneuver
	Laryngoscopy and intubation
	End-tidal carbon dioxide confirmation
Zero plus 2 min	**Post-intubation management**
	Midazolam 0.1 mg/kg, *plus*
	Pancuronium, 0.1 mg/kg, *or*
	Vecuronium, 0.1 mg/kg

the lungs. Long-acting NMBAs (e.g., pancuronium, vecuronium) usually are indicated and should be accompanied by adequate doses of a sedative agent (e.g., benzodiazepine). Mechanical ventilation should be initiated. Table 1-1 presents a sample RSI protocol using etomidate and succinylcholine. "Zero" refers to the time at which the induction agent and succinylcholine and pushed.

Blind Nasotracheal Intubation

Blind nasotracheal intubation (BNTI) historically was used extensively in the emergency department and prehospital setting, but has fallen out of favor largely because of the superiority of RSI. Success rates have been about 80% and high complication rates are reported, most often epistaxis or delayed or incorrect tube placement.[45] Long-term complications (e.g., sinusitis, turbinate destruction, laryngeal perforation) are uncommon and related to multiple attempts or prolonged intubation. Basilar skull fracture and facial trauma have been considered contraindications to nasotracheal intubation because of the risk of entering the cranial vault or increasing the incidence of intracranial infection. These contraindications are not based on scientific study, however, and two studies failed to detect a difference in complications between orally and nasally intubated facial trauma patients.[46,47] Two prehospital studies compared the success rates of RSI and BNTI performed by physicians or paramedics on helicopter services. Results differed, with one study showing essentially equivalent success rates and the other showing a significant advantage for neuromuscular blockade over BNTI.[48,49] Emergency department studies have shown superiority of RSI over BNTI.[36] Also, the incidence and severity of oxygen desaturation are increased in BNTI compared with RSI.[50]

BNTI is a valid and useful method of intubation in the prehospital setting and is still widely used there. In the emergency department, where NMBAs and RSI are available, BNTI should be considered a second-line approach and reserved for patients in whom presence of a difficult airway makes RSI undesirable or contraindicated. Use of BNTI in the emergency department has declined sufficiently that it is doubtful that emerging emergency medicine residents will be adequately trained in the technique.[45]

Awake Oral Intubation

Awake oral intubation is a deliberate technique in which sedative and topical anesthetic agents are administered to permit management of a difficult airway. Sedation and analgesia are achieved in a manner analogous to that for painful procedures in the emergency department. Topical anesthesia may be achieved by spray, nebulization, or local anesthetic nerve block. After the patient is sedated and topical anesthesia has been achieved, gentle direct or fiberoptic laryngoscopy is performed to determine whether the glottis will be visible and intubation will be possible. The patient may be intubated during the laryngoscopy, or the laryngoscopy may show that oral intubation will be possible, permitting safe use of RSI.

Awake oral intubation is distinct from the practice of oral intubation using a sedative or opioid agent to obtund the patient for intubation without neuromuscular blockade, which has been a typical emergency department practice. This latter technique can be referred to as "intubation with sedation alone." Proponents of intubation with sedation alone argue that administration of a benzodiazepine, opioid, or both to a patient provides improved access to the airway, decreases patient resistance, and avoids the risks inherent in neuromuscular blockade. This technique is actually more hazardous than RSI, however. Intubating conditions achieved even with deep anesthesia are significantly inferior to the conditions achieved when neuromuscular blockade is used.[34,51] The same superiority of neuromuscular blockade–assisted intubation over intubation with sedation alone has been observed in pediatric emergency medicine and in prehospital care.[52,53] In general, the technique of administering a potent sedative agent to obtund the patient's responses and permit intubation in the absence of neuromuscular blockade is ill advised and inappropriate for endotracheal intubation in the emergency department.

Oral Intubation without Pharmacologic Agents

The unconscious, unresponsive patient may not require pharmacologic agents for intubation. If the patient is comatose and fully relaxed, administration of any pharmacologic agent, including an NMBA, may needlessly delay intubation. Even an unconscious patient may retain sufficient muscle tone to render intubation difficult, however. If the glottis is not adequately visualized, administration of a single dose of succinylcholine alone may facilitate laryngoscopy.

Pharmacologic Agents

Neuromuscular Blocking Agents

Muscle contraction is the result of membrane depolarization, which causes massive intracellular release of calcium ions from the sarcoplasmic reticulum, leading to active contraction of myofibrils. The inciting incident is the depolarization of portions of the myocyte membrane, called the motor end plates, which are adjacent to the innervating axons. Action potentials conducted down the innervating axons cause release of the neurotransmitter acetylcholine (ACh) from the terminal axon. The ACh traverses the synaptic cleft, binds reversibly to receptors on the motor end plate, and opens channels in the membrane to initiate depolarization.

NMBAs are highly water-soluble, quaternary ammonium compounds that mimic the quaternary ammonium group on the ACh molecule. Their water solubility explains why these agents do not readily cross the blood-brain barrier or placenta. The NMBAs are divided into two main classes. The *depolarizing* agent, succinylcholine, exerts its effects by binding noncompetitively with ACh receptors on the motor end plate and causing sustained depolarization of the myocyte. The other major class of NMBA comprises the *competitive,* or *nondepolarizing,* agents, which bind competitively to ACh receptors, preventing access to ACh and preventing muscular activity. The competitive agents are of two pharmacologically distinct types, steroid-based agents (aminosteroid compounds) and benzylisoquinolines. Each of these basic chemical types has distinct properties.

Succinylcholine

Succinylcholine is a chemical combination of two molecules of ACh. Succinylcholine is rapidly hydrolyzed by plasma pseudocholinesterase to succinylmonocholine, which is a weak NMBA, then to succinic acid and choline, which have no NMBA activity. Pseudocholinesterase is not present at the motor end plate and exerts its effects systemically before the succinylcholine reaches the ACh receptor.[54] Only a small amount of the succinylcholine that is administered survives to reach the motor end plate. When attached to the ACh receptor, succinylcholine is active until it diffuses away. Decreased plasma pseudocholinesterase activity can increase the amount of succinylcholine reaching the motor end plate, prolonging succinylcholine block. This occurs in two ways. Pseudocholinesterase activity can be reduced, or the enzyme can be (rarely) genetically defective or deficient. The activity of pseudocholinesterase is reduced in several conditions (Box 1-5).[54,55] Reduced pseudocholinesterase activity is of little significance in the emergency setting because the prolongation of action is rarely significant, reaching only 23 minutes at the extreme.

Uses. Succinylcholine is rapidly active, typically producing intubating conditions within 60 seconds of administration by rapid intravenous bolus injection.[56] The clinical duration of action is 6 to 10 minutes, but adequate spontaneous respirations may occur within 7 minutes (see Figure 1-9).[33] Full recovery of normal neuromuscular function occurs within 15 minutes. The combination of rapid onset, complete reliability, short duration of action, and absence of serious side effects maintains succinylcholine as the drug of choice for most emergency department intubations.[1,19,52] The use of a competitive NMBA for RSI may be desirable when succinylcholine is contraindicated and in certain other settings.

Cardiovascular Effects. As an ACh analogue, succinylcholine binds to ACh receptors throughout the body, not just at the motor end plate. It is difficult to separate the effects of succinylcholine on the heart that are caused by direct cardiac muscarinic stimulation from the effects caused by stimulation of autonomic ganglia by succinylcholine and from the effects that are induced by the autonomic responses to laryngoscopy and intubation. Succinylcholine is a weak negative inotrope, which is not clinically significant. It is also a negative chronotrope, however, especially in children, and sinus bradycardia may ensue after succinylcholine administration. Sinus bradycardia is prevented by prior administration of atropine, which is recommended for all children younger than 10 years old and as a standby for adults receiving a second dose of succinylcholine.[57] Other cardiac dysrhythmias, including ventricular fibrillation and asystole, have been reported with succinylcholine, but it is impossible to distinguish the effects of the drug itself from the effects caused by the intense vagal stimulation and catecholamine release that accompany laryngoscopy and intubation. In addition, many of these catastrophic complications occur in critically ill patients, further confounding attempts to identify whether the illness or any particular drug or procedure is the cause.

Fasciculations. The depolarizing action of succinylcholine results in fine, chaotic contractions of the muscles throughout the body for several seconds at the onset of paralysis. Although fasciculations have been linked temporally to several adverse side effects of succinylcholine, such as increases in intracranial pressure (ICP), intragastric pressure, and intraocular pressure, evidence of a cause-and-effect relationship is lacking.[54] Muscle pain occurs in many patients who receive succinylcholine. Although it is widely believed that muscle pains are reduced or abolished by prior administration of a defasciculating dose of a competitive NMBA, the evidence is not conclusive.[58] Administra-

---

BOX 1-5. Conditions and Drugs that Reduce Pseudocholinesterase Activity

Pregnancy
Liver disease
Cancer
Cytotoxic drugs
Metoclorpramide
Phenelzine
Other drugs

Table 1-2. Conditions Associated with Hyperkalemia After Succinylcholine Administration

Condition	Period of Concern
Burns >10% BSA	>5 days until healed
Crush injury	>5 days until healed
Denervation (stroke, spinal cord injury)	>5 days until 6 mo
Neuromuscular disease (ALS, MS)	Indefinitely
Intra-abdominal sepsis	>5 days until resolution

BSA, body surface area; ALS, amyotrophic lateral sclerosis; MS, multiple sclerosis.

tion of a defasciculating dose of a competitive NMBA is desirable for certain patients, such as patients with elevated ICP, but there is little or no benefit in others. In patients other than those with elevated ICP, abolition of fasciculation is primarily a cosmetic issue, and the decision is appropriately left to the individual clinician.

Hyperkalemia. Succinylcholine has been associated with severe, fatal hyperkalemia when administered in specific clinical circumstances (Table 1-2).[59,60] Although the hyperkalemia occurs within minutes after administration of succinylcholine and may be severe or fatal, the patient's vulnerability to succinylcholine-induced hyperkalemia does not begin until at least 5 days after the inciting injury or burn. Succinylcholine remains the agent of choice for RSI in acute burn, trauma, stroke, spinal cord injury, and intra-abdominal sepsis patients if intubation occurs less than 5 days after onset of the condition. If doubt exists regarding the onset time, competitive RSI should be used. Denervation syndromes (e.g., multiple sclerosis, amyotrophic lateral sclerosis) can be particularly troubling, however, because the risk begins with the onset of the disease and continues indefinitely, regardless of the apparent stability of the symptoms. Stroke patients and patients with spinal cord injury are stabilized after 6 months, and thereafter can receive succinylcholine safely.[55] Potassium release does not occur to any significant extent in the general population. Succinylcholine is not contraindicated in renal failure but probably should not be used in patients known to have significant hyperkalemia. The only published series of patients with hyperkalemia, many of whom had renal failure, failed to show a single adverse event related to succinylcholine administration.[61]

Increased Intraocular Pressure. Succinylcholine may cause a modest increase in intraocular pressure and historically has been considered relatively to absolutely contraindicated in penetrating globe injury. There is no published evidence to support this view, however, and several large series show safety when succinylcholine is used in patients with open globes. The admonition to avoid succinylcholine in open globe injuries is unjustified and should be abandoned.[62]

Masseter Spasm. Succinylcholine has been reported rarely to cause masseter spasm, primarily in children.[54]

The clinical significance of this phenomenon is unclear, but administration of a competitive NMBA terminates the spasm. Severe, persistent spasm should raise suspicion of malignant hyperthermia.

Malignant Hyperthermia. Succinylcholine has been associated with malignant hyperthermia, a perplexing syndrome of rapid temperature rise and aggressive rhabdomyolysis. Malignant hyperthermia occurs in genetically predisposed individuals who receive certain volatile anesthetic agents or succinylcholine. The condition is extremely rare and has not been reported in the context of emergency department intubation. Treatment consists of cessation of any potential offending agents; administration of dantrolene, 2 mg/kg intravenously every 5 minutes to a maximum dose of 10 mg/kg; and attempts to reduce body temperature by external means.[63] A national malignant hyperthermia hot line is available for emergency consultation at 1-800-644-9737 (then dial zero).

Refrigeration. The standard recommendation to keep succinylcholine refrigerated creates problems related to its storage, timely retrieval, and ready availability on intubation carts or kits in the emergency department. Succinylcholine undergoes degradation beginning at the time of manufacture, and the rate of this degradation is much lower when the drug is refrigerated. Succinylcholine retains more than 90% of its original activity when stored at room temperature for 3 months; it retains even more if protected from light.[64] Succinylcholine may be kept at room temperature in the emergency department, provided that a proper inventory control system ensures that all supplies are replaced not more than 3 months after introduction.

Competitive Agents

Competitive NMBAs are classified according to their chemical structure. The aminosteroid agents include pancuronium, vecuronium, and rocuronium. Rapacuronium (Raplon) was withdrawn from use because of histamine release that induced fatal bronchospasm. The benzylisoquinolines include tubocurarine, atracurium, cisatracurium, mivacurium, doxacurium, and metocurine. Histamine release, which may be important in hemodynamically compromised patients and patients with reactive airways disease, is caused by the benzylisoquinolines, primarily tubocurarine.[54] Pancuronium is widely used because of its familiarity, absence of histamine release, and low cost. Although its muscarinic effects almost universally cause a modest tachycardia, this is rarely of consequence. Vecuronium neither releases histamine nor exhibits cardiac muscarinic blockade. Rocuronium seems to be the best agent for use in RSI when succinylcholine is contraindicated. Atracurium is advocated for use in patients with renal failure because its excretion is completely independent of renal function, but this is rarely an issue in the emergency department.

Rapid Sequence Intubation with a Competitive Agent. Competitive agents, especially vecuronium and rocuronium, have been studied extensively for RSI. Although

Table 1-3. Sample Rapid Sequence Intubation Using Etomidate and Competitive Neuromuscular Blocking Agent

Time	Step
Zero minus 10 min	**Preparation**
Zero minus 5 min	**Preoxygenation**
	100% oxygen for 3 min *or* eight vital capacity breaths
Zero minus 3 min	**Pretreatment**
	as indicated "LOAD"
Zero	**Paralysis with induction**
	Etomidate, 0.3 mg/kg
	Rocuronium, 1.0 mg/kg
Zero plus 60 sec	**Placement**
	Sellick's maneuver
	Laryngoscopy and intubation
	End-tidal carbon dioxide confirmation
Zero plus 2 min	**Post-intubation management**
	Midazolam 0.1 mg/kg *plus*
	Rocuronium (one third of intubating dose as needed at signs of recovery of muscle function)

vecuronium was the first competitive NMBA to establish a role in RSI, the dose required to achieve rapid intubating conditions, 0.3 mg/kg, results in almost 2 hours of paralysis, making it less desirable for emergency department RSI. Alternatively, vecuronium can be given in a split dose. First, 0.01 mg/kg is administered as a "priming" dose. Three minutes later, 0.15 mg/kg is given for paralysis, which is achieved in about 75 to 90 seconds. Rocuronium bromide, 1 mg/kg intravenously, achieves intubating conditions closely approaching those of succinylcholine, lasts approximately 50 minutes, and has been used in the emergency department with success (Table 1-3).[51,65]

Paralysis After Intubation. After intubation, longer paralysis usually is desired for patient control and to permit mechanical ventilation. In most cases, one agent is comparable to another, and cost or convenience may be a consideration. A good choice is vecuronium, 0.1 mg/kg intravenously. Longer term neuromuscular blockade must not be undertaken without attention to appropriate sedation of the patient. An adequate dose of a benzodiazepine, such as midazolam 0.1 mg/kg intravenously, is often the best initial choice for sedation accompanying use of longer acting NMBAs. Often an opioid analgesic, such as fentanyl, 3 µg/kg intravenously, or morphine, 0.1 mg/kg intravenously, is added to improve patient comfort and decrease sympathetic response to the ETT. Additional medication may be required if the patient's blood pressure and heart rate indicate excessive sympathetic tone.

Induction Agents

Virtually every patient who is receiving an NMBA for intubation requires a potent sedative to induce unconsciousness. Neuromuscular paralysis without sedation can lead to undesirable psychological and physiologic effects. A patient who presents with any degree of clin-ical responsiveness, including reactivity to noxious stimuli, requires a sedative or induction agent at the time of administration of any NMBA. Patients who already are deeply unconscious and unresponsive may not require an induction agent if drugs or alcohol are the cause of the unconscious state. Patients who are unconscious because of a central nervous system insult should receive an induction agent to optimize the attenuation of adverse responses to airway manipulation. Induction agents also enhance the effect of the NMBA and improve intubation conditions because the intubation is done at the earliest phase of neuromuscular blockade, and the relaxation effects of the induction agent are additive to those of the NMBA.[66]

Etomidate

Etomidate is an imidazole derivative that has been in use since 1972. It has a similar profile of activity to thiopental, with rapid onset, rapid peak activity, and brief duration, but is remarkably hemodynamically stable.[67] The induction dose is 0.3 mg/kg intravenously. Because etomidate is able to decrease ICP, cerebral blood flow, and cerebral metabolic rate without adversely affecting systemic mean arterial blood pressure and cerebral perfusion pressure, it is an excellent induction agent for patients with elevated ICP, even with hemodynamic instability.[68] Etomidate may cause brief myoclonus, but this is of no clinical significance. Etomidate has been reported to cause suppression of endogenous cortisol production, but not with single use or short periods of intravenous infusion. Diminished response to adrenocorticotropic hormone challenge has been documented 24 hours after a single use of etomidate, but the clinical significance of this is unknown.[69] Etomidate seems to have emerged as the agent of choice for emergency department RSI, and numerous reports attest to its effectiveness and safety.[1,19,66]

Barbiturates

Although both the thiobarbiturate, sodium thiopental, and the methylated oxybarbiturate, methohexital, have been used as induction agents for RSI, thiopental has been used more widely. The use of these agents has declined significantly, however, with the adoption of newer agents, particularly etomidate. These rapidly acting barbiturates are highly lipid soluble and readily cross the blood-brain barrier, acting on the γ-aminobutyric acid receptor neuroinhibitory complex to produce rapid depression of central nervous system activity. A single dose of 3 mg/kg of thiopental produces loss of consciousness in less than 30 seconds, has a peak effect at 1 minute, and has a clinical duration of 5 to 8 minutes. Methohexital may have a slightly shorter duration of action but is more prone to cause central nervous system excitatory side effects, such as myoclonus. Thiopental is a negative inotrope and a potent venodilator and should be used with caution in patients whose cardiovascular reserve is diminished. For the same reason, thiopental should be avoided in a hypotensive patient who would not tolerate further compromise of circulation. Thiopental can release histamine and probably should not be used in asthmatic patients.

Benzodiazepines

Of the benzodiazepines, only midazolam is well suited to use as an induction agent, with a normal induction dose of 0.2 to 0.3 mg/kg intravenously. In a dose of 0.2 mg/kg intravenously, midazolam produces loss of consciousness in about 30 seconds and has a clinical duration of 15 to 20 minutes.[70] Midazolam is a negative inotrope comparable to thiopental and should be used with caution in hemodynamically compromised patients and elderly patients, for whom the dose can be reduced to 0.1 mg/kg or 0.05 mg/kg. Onset is slower at these reduced doses. Much lower doses than indicated often are used in emergency department intubations, perhaps because practitioners are familiar with the sedation doses, but not the anesthetic induction doses, of midazolam.[71] These inadequate doses reduce the effectiveness of laryngoscopy, do not provide optimal blunting of adverse physiologic effects of laryngoscopy and intubation, and may compromise the patient's amnesia for the intubation. Midazolam is cerebroprotective, but less so than etomidate or thiopental.

Ketamine

Ketamine, a phencyclidine derivative, has been widely used as a general anesthetic agent since 1970. After an intravenous dose of 1 to 2 mg/kg, ketamine produces loss of consciousness within 30 seconds, peaks in approximately 1 minute, and has a clinical duration of 10 to 15 minutes. As a dissociative anesthetic agent, ketamine induces a cataleptic state rather than a true unconscious state. The patient has profound analgesia but may have open eyes. Many protective reflexes, including airway reflexes, are preserved.

The principal use of ketamine in emergency airway management is for the induction of patients with asthma and for hemodynamically unstable trauma patients without head injury. Ketamine is exceptionally hemodynamically stable, more so than etomidate, and this latter indication capitalizes on ketamine's superior cardiovascular stability.[70] Controversy exists regarding the use of ketamine in patients with elevated ICP because ketamine has been documented to increase cerebral metabolic rate, ICP, and cerebral blood flow.[72] There is conflicting evidence that ketamine can produce harm in this way, however, and its role as an induction agent in trauma is significant because of its superior hemodynamic stability.[16] Ketamine tends to produce unpleasant emergence phenomena, especially disturbing or frightening dreams in the first 3 hours after awakening. These reactions, which are more prominent in adults than in children, in women than in men, in patients receiving larger doses, and in certain personality types, are mitigated by benzodiazepine administration. Patients (e.g., with asthma) who undergo RSI with ketamine should receive a sufficient dose of a benzodiazepine, such as 0.05 mg/kg of lorazepam or 0.1 mg/kg of midazolam, as part of postintubation management.

Special Clinical Circumstances

Status Asthmaticus

Status asthmaticus with supervening respiratory failure is a preterminal event. Respiratory failure in the asthmatic patient is not caused primarily by progressive worsening of the bronchospasm, but rather by eventual exhaustion and fatigue secondary to the effort of breathing against severe airway resistance. All patients who are intubated for status asthmaticus are heavily sedated and paralyzed and receive mechanical ventilation. RSI permits the most rapid attainment of intubation, protects against aspiration, and induces the unconsciousness and motor paralysis necessary for mechanical ventilation; it is the superior technique for intubation of a patient in status asthmaticus. BNTI takes longer, results in greater oxygen desaturation, and has a higher complication and lower success rate than RSI[73]; it should be reserved for rare cases with compelling reasons to avoid neuromuscular blockade. Difficult airway considerations are complex in an asthmatic patient because of impending respiratory arrest and the patient's inability to tolerate attempts at awake intubation. Even when a difficult airway is identified in an asthmatic patient, RSI is usually the intubation method of choice, with a double setup for rescue cricothyrotomy when indicated.

The asthmatic patient has highly reactive airways, and steps should be taken to minimize any additional bronchospasm that may occur during intubation. Lidocaine has been shown to suppress the coughing that occurs in response to airway manipulation and may improve ETT tolerance and reduce reactive bronchospasm in asthmatic patients.[74] The balance of evidence indicates that lidocaine, 1.5 mg/kg, is indicated as a pretreatment drug before intubation in status asthmaticus and in asthmatic patients being intubated for reasons other than their asthma. High-dose, inhaled β-agonists may provide maximal protection against reactive bronchospasm during intubation in asthmatics without active bronchospasm, and lidocaine may provide little additional benefit in this setting.[75] This approach has not been tested in patients in status asthmaticus, however. Ketamine has been shown to produce bronchodilation in humans and animal models and may be the ideal induction agent in asthma. Although reports to date have been limited, there is a growing body of experience with ketamine as an induction agent for the emergency intubation of patients with status asthmaticus. Ketamine also has been reported to mitigate bronchospasm in patients who are not intubated and in patients who are already intubated and who are not improving with mechanical ventilation (Table 1-4).

Hemodynamic Consequences of Intubation

Laryngoscopy and intubation are potent stimuli for the reflex release of catecholamines.[73] This reflex sympathetic response to laryngoscopy (RSRL) produces only modest increases in blood pressure and heart rate and

Table 1-4. Rapid Sequence Intubation for Status Asthmaticus

Time	Step
Zero minus 10 min	**Preparation**
Zero minus 5 min	**Preoxygenation** (as possible)
	Continuous albuterol nebulizer
	100% oxygen for 3 min *or* 8 vital capacity breaths
Zero minus 3 min	**Pretreatment**
	Lidocaine, 1.5 mg/kg
Zero	**Paralysis with induction**
	Ketamine, 1.5 mg/kg
	Succinylcholine, 1.5 mg/kg
Zero plus 45 sec	**Placement**
	Sellick's maneuver
	Laryngoscopy with intubation
	End-tidal carbon dioxide confirmation
Zero plus 2 min	**Post-intubation management**
	Midazolam, 0.1 mg/kg *plus*
	Pancuronium, 0.1 mg/kg, *or*
	Vecuronium, 0.1 mg/kg
	In-line albuterol nebulization
	Additional ketamine as indicated

is of little consequence in otherwise healthy patients. The RSRL is of potential clinical significance in two settings: acute elevation of ICP and certain cardiovascular diseases (e.g., intracerebral hemorrhage, subarachnoid hemorrhage, aortic dissection or aneurysm, ischemic heart disease). In these settings, the reflex release of catecholamines, increased myocardial oxygen demand, and attendant rise in mean arterial blood pressure and heart rate may produce deleterious effects. The synthetic opioids (e.g., fentanyl) and β-adrenergic blocking agents (e.g., esmolol) are capable of blunting the RSRL and stabilizing heart rate and blood pressure during intubation.[76] Lidocaine also has been studied, but the results are contradictory and inconclusive.[77] In patients at risk from acute blood pressure elevation, administration of fentanyl, 3 µg/kg, during the pretreatment phase of RSI, attenuates the heart rate and blood pressure increase. The full sympatholytic dose of fentanyl is 5 to 9 µg/kg, but if this dose is administered as a single pretreatment bolus, hypoventilation or apnea can occur. The administration of 3 µg/kg is safer and can be supplemented with an additional 3 µg/kg immediately after intubation if full sympathetic blockade is desired or if hypertension and tachycardia ensue, providing evidence of excessive sympathetic activity. Fentanyl should be given as the last pretreatment drug over at least 60 seconds to prevent hypoventilation or apnea.

Elevated Intracranial Pressure

When ICP is elevated as a result of head injury or acute intracranial catastrophe, maintenance of cerebral perfusion pressure and avoidance of further increases in ICP are desirable.[40] Significant reductions in mean arterial blood pressure decrease cerebral perfusion pressure by reducing the driving gradient between arterial pressure and intracranial pressure, leading to increased cerebral ischemia.[78] Maintenance of the systemic mean

arterial blood pressure at 100 mm Hg or greater supports the cerebral perfusion pressure and reduces the likelihood of secondary injury. In addition, cerebral autoregulation may be lost, and increases in systemic blood pressure may lead to corresponding increases in cerebral blood flow and ICP. With elevated ICP, control of the reflex hemodynamic stimulation resulting from intubation is desirable to avoid further elevation of ICP. Fentanyl, 3 µg/kg, given as a pretreatment drug, is the best choice for this purpose.[40,79]

Evidence suggests a separate reflex that increases ICP in response to laryngoscopy and intubation, although the precise mechanism is not understood. Intravenous lidocaine reduces ICP and blunts the ICP response to laryngoscopy and intubation.[80] Lidocaine, 1.5 mg/kg intravenously during the pretreatment phase of RSI, is desirable to blunt the ICP response to laryngoscopy and intubation. Similarly, RSRL and ICP response to laryngoscopy and intubation relatively contraindicate BNTI, which should be undertaken only if RSI is not possible and fiberoptic intubation is not an option.

Succinylcholine may induce a modest increase in ICP.[81] Prior administration of a defasciculating dose of the competitive NMBA, metocurine, greatly reduces or abolishes this response, and this result has been interpreted to apply to any of the competitive NMBAs that blunt fasciculations.[79,82] Although pretreatment administration of a "mini" dose of succinylcholine has been shown to abolish fasciculation effectively, no evidence indicates that this technique protects against the potential ICP increase with succinylcholine.[83] An alternative approach would be to substitute rocuronium (1 mg/kg) for succinylcholine in RSI, avoiding the need for a defasciculating agent. The physician should choose an induction agent that balances a favorable effect on cerebral dynamics and ICP with a stable systemic hemodynamic profile. At present, etomidate (0.3 mg/kg) probably is the best choice for patients with elevated ICP, although thiopental also is an excellent choice when hypotension is not present (Table 1-5).

Potential Cervical Spine Injury

Historically, it was believed that oral endotracheal intubation carried an unacceptably high risk of injury to the cervical spinal cord in patients with blunt cervical spine injury and was relatively contraindicated, but this assertion was never subjected to scientific scrutiny. Numerous studies and reports have asserted the safety and effectiveness of controlled, oral intubation with in-line cervical spine immobilization, whether done as an awake procedure or with neuromuscular blockade.[84,85] The evidence favors RSI with in-line stabilization, which provides maximal control of the patient, the ability to mitigate adverse effects of the intubation, and the best conditions for laryngoscopy. In-line stabilization also seems to improve the laryngoscopic view of the larynx compared with conventional tape/collar/sandbag immobilization. The intubating laryngeal mask airway (ILMA) also has been compared to conventional laryngoscopy and may result in even less movement of the cervical spine during intubation than

Table 1-5. Rapid Sequence Intubation for Elevated Intracranial Pressure

Time	Step
Zero minus 10 min	**Preparation**
Zero minus 5 min	**Preoxygenation** (as possible) 100% oxygen for 3 min *or* 8 vital capacity breaths
Zero minus 3 min	**Pretreatment** Vecuronium, 0.01 mg/kg* Lidocaine, 1.5 mg/kg Fentanyl, 3 µg/kg (slowly)
Zero	**Paralysis with induction** Etomidate, 0.3 mg/kg Succinylcholine, 1.5 mg/kg*
Zero plus 45 sec	**Placement** Sellick's maneuver Laryngoscopy with intubation End-tidal carbon dioxide confirmation
Zero plus 2 min	**Post-intubation management** Fentanyl, 3 µg/kg (optional) Midazolam 0.1 mg/kg *plus* Vecuronium, 0.1 mg/kg *or* Pancuronium, 0.1 mg/kg

*May substitute rocuronium, 1 mg/kg for succinylcholine. If so, omit vecuronium dose during pretreatment phase.

that caused by direct laryngoscopy.[86] A comparison of methods on a cadaver model of unstable injury of the third cervical vertebra reinforced the potential role for fiberoptic intubation and raised questions about the safety of the Combitube because of significant cervical spine movement during its placement.[87] Cervical spine immobilization of patients with penetrating head and neck trauma is poorly addressed in the literature. It is uncertain whether patients with gunshot or shotgun injuries to the head or neck are at risk of exacerbation of cervical cord injury during intubation, but there is no report of such a patient, without spinal neurologic injury, who was injured by intubation. Unless the path of the missile has been established and there is no evidence of spinal cord injury, prudence would dictate immobilization of patients with gunshot wounds to the neck and patients with gunshot wounds to the head with secondary injury (e.g., fall from height) or with neurologic deficit suggesting spinal involvement.[88] Immobilization for intubation of patients with penetrating injury elsewhere in the body should be directed by the likelihood of secondary injury to the spine from a fall or other event distinct from the wounding.

Pediatric Intubation

Although many considerations in pediatric intubation are the same as for adults, a few differences exist in regard to airway management. The larynx is higher in the child's neck, causing a more acute angle between the oral pharynx and the larynx. Visualization is aided by gentle posterior pressure on the anterior aspect of the thyroid cartilage. The epiglottis is high and soft, making visualization of the cords more difficult. If the child is very small, the prominent occiput brings the mouth to a position far anterior to the larynx; an assistant can lift the chest gently by grasping both shoul-

ders, immobilizing the head at the same time. The airway in the small child is short, and care must be taken not to intubate either bronchus.

A straight laryngoscope blade is desirable, especially in young children, and positioning for intubation may be different. BNTI is relatively contraindicated in children younger than 12 years old. Although the product insert for succinylcholine now advises against its routine use in pediatric anesthesia, because of fatal hyperkalemia in children with undiagnosed congenital neuromuscular disorders (e.g., muscular dystrophy), it remains the drug of choice for emergency RSI of infants and children.[52] Rocuronium has been used in children, but experience is too limited to recommend that it replace succinylcholine for pediatric RSI in the emergency department. RSI may be used in children in a similar manner to adults, with two important differences. Excessive bradycardia may be seen with succinylcholine in children younger than 10 years old, and this is prevented by administration of atropine (0.02 mg/kg) during the pretreatment phase. The dose of succinylcholine in infants is 2 mg/kg. Induction agents may be selected using similar criteria as for adults. Successful RSI using vecuronium through an intraosseous needle has been reported.[78] The major difficulty in intubating children and infants is choosing the correct size of equipment and the correct drug doses for age or size. The best method for overcoming these obstacles is to use a length-based system (Broselow-Luten Color Coding for Kids; Vital Signs, Inc, Totowa, NJ), which provides dosing and equipment sizes based on the length of the child. Cricothyrotomy is impossible in small children, and alternative rescue airway devices (e.g., percutaneous transtracheal jet ventilation) are required.

Methods for the Difficult or Failed Airway

Regardless of the care taken by the intubator and the detailed assessment of the patient before intubation, some intubations are simply unsuccessful or impossible. In most circumstances when intubation is not possible, BMV provides adequate ventilation and oxygenation until a rescue airway can be established. This underscores the importance of evaluating the patient for ease of intubation and ventilation before deciding on the best approach and initiating the intubation sequence. Several airway options are available in the event of a difficult or failed intubation.

Special Airway Devices

Laryngeal Mask Airway

The LMA is an irregular, ovoid, silicone mask with an inflatable rim, connected to a tube that allows ventilation (Figure 1-10). The mask is inserted blindly into the pharynx, then inflated, providing a seal that permits ventilation of the trachea with minimal gastric insufflation. In elective anesthesia, the LMA has an extremely high insertion success rate and low complication rate, including a low incidence of tracheal aspiration.[89,90] In the emergency setting, studies to date

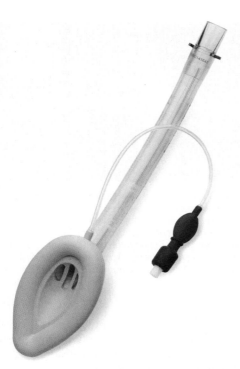

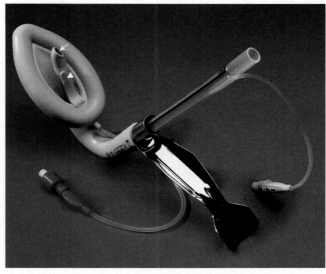

Figure 1-10. The standard laryngeal mask airway (LMA Classic) is available in sizes from infant to large adult. (Courtesy LMA North America, Inc, San Diego.)

Figure 1-11. The intubating laryngeal mask airway is modified to facilitate insertion of an endotracheal tube after placement and ventilation are achieved. The epiglottic elevater *(triangle)* lifts the epiglottis to allow passage of the special ETT *(arrow)*.

have focused on use during resuscitation from cardiopulmonary arrest. Evaluations of LMA insertion by experienced and inexperienced personnel consistently have shown ease of insertion, high insertion success rates, and successful ventilation.[91] The LMA may be a viable alternative to endotracheal intubation for in-hospital or pre-hospital cardiac arrest, particularly when responders are inexperienced airway managers. At a minimum, the device may serve a temporizing role equal or superior to BMV until definitive airway management can be achieved.

The ILMA is designed to facilitate intubation through the mask after correct placement (Figure 1-11). It differs from the LMA in two main ways: The mask is attached to a rigid, stainless steel ventilation tube that is bent almost to a right angle, and the mask incorporates an epiglottic elevator at its distal end. Placement of the ILMA results in successful ventilation in almost 100% of cases and successful subsequent intubation in 95%.[86,92,93,95] The ILMA has a special ETT and a stabilizer rod to remove the mask over the ETT after intubation is accomplished.

The ILMA is a better device than the standard LMA for use in the emergency department because it facilitates rescue ventilation and intubation. Intubation through the ILMA has compared favorably in terms of success with direct laryngoscopy.[92] When the ILMA is placed, intubation can be performed blindly or guided by a lighted stylet (Trachlight; Laerdal Medical AS, Stavanger, Norway) or a fiberoptic scope. The ILMA comes only in sizes 3, 4, and 5 and so is not suitable for use in patients weighing less than about 30 kg. For smaller patients, the standard LMA, which has sizes down to size 1 (infant), should be used. Intubation can be

achieved through the standard LMA, but the success rate is significantly less than when the ILMA is used.

In the emergency department, the primary use of the LMA or ILMA is as a rescue technique to provide a temporary airway when intubation has failed, bag ventilation is satisfactory, and the patient has been paralyzed or is otherwise in need of immediate airway management. In such cases, the LMA is one of numerous acceptable techniques, including lighted-stylet intubation and cricothyrotomy. In the "can't intubate, can't ventilate" situation, cricothyrotomy is indicated, but an ILMA may be placed rapidly in an attempt to achieve ventilation (converting the situation to "can't intubate, can ventilate") as long as this is done in parallel with preparations for cricothyrotomy and does not delay the initiation of a surgical airway.[94] Availability of the LMA and adequate prior training of the operator offer a legitimate option for the management of the failed airway, and the ILMA compares well with fiberoptic intubation in terms of successful intubation of difficult airways.[95] In the prehospital setting, where concerns about esophageal placement of ETTs has focused interest on methods used for airway management, the LMA and Combitube offer excellent placement and ventilation characteristics and may be preferable to endotracheal intubation in the prehospital setting, especially when intubation is relatively infrequently performed.[96] New LMA devices, from a number of manufacturers, are now available.

Lighted Stylet

The lighted stylet is a device that incorporates a handle, a fitting for mounting an ETT, and an intubating stylet with a fiberoptic light mounted on the end (Figure 1-12). The ETT is mounted as on a conventional intubating stylet, but transillumination of the soft tissues from within the neck permits identification of tracheal entry by the stylet and ETT. The lighted stylet has been

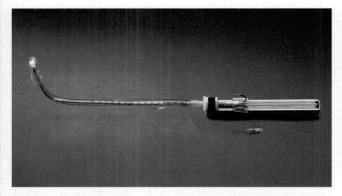

Figure 1-12. The Trachlight lighted stylet facilitates placement of the endotracheal tube when the glottis cannot be visualized by direct laryngoscopy. It also is used as a primary intubation device.

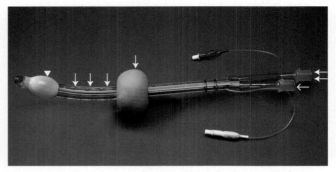

Figure 1-13. The Combitube is inserted through the mouth blindly, although a laryngoscope can be used, if desired. It seats itself in the esophagus more than 95% of the time, and ventilation is performed through the side ports *(white arrows)* after inflation of the two balloons. The lower balloon *(triangle)* occludes the esophagus. The upper (large) balloon *(thin arrow)* occludes the oropharynx. If the tube is in the trachea, the alternate lumen *(open arrows)* is used for ventilation.

used for oral and nasal intubation and has an excellent success rate.[97] The lighted stylet is less stimulating to the heart rate and blood pressure than conventional laryngoscopy and may be useful when sympathetic stimulation is not desirable.[98] Although overall success rates with the Trachlight have been high, it may be more difficult for novice intubators to learn than conventional laryngoscopy, if only minimal manikin training is used.[99] The Trachlight can be used as a primary intubating device or as a rescue device in the "can't intubate, can ventilate" failed airway. It is not appropriate for the "can't intubate, can't ventilate" failed airway, when cricothyrotomy is indicated. As a device for a difficult airway, the lighted stylet can be used as the intubating stylet for a standard oral intubation. The direct illumination by the stylet can aid in visualization during intubation. If direct laryngoscopy is unsuccessful, the first rescue procedure could be an immediate attempt at blind, oral intubation using the lighted stylet, as long as ventilation is possible.

Esophagotracheal Combitube

The Combitube is a plastic double-lumen tube with one lumen functioning as an airway after esophageal insertion and the other lumen functioning as a tracheal airway (Figure 1-13). The tube is placed blindly into the esophagus, and proximal and distal balloons are inflated to prevent escape of ventilatory gases through the pharynx to the mouth or nose or down the esophagus. The tube is placed into the esophagus, as designed, almost 100% of the time, but both lumens are patent, so ventilation is still possible if the tube has been placed inadvertently into the trachea.

The Combitube is primarily a substitute for endotracheal intubation by non–ETT-trained personnel, but has a role as a primary airway device in place of endotracheal intubation in the prehospital setting.[100] It also has been used as a rescue device or as a primary intubating device in difficult airways that have precluded endotracheal intubation, but most studies have focused on subjects in full cardiopulmonary arrest.[101] It seems that the tube may be difficult to insert blindly when the patient is in cervical spine precautions, raising concerns about prehospital use in trauma patients, but results have been conflicting.[102,103] Standard methods

for confirming tube placement, using end-tidal CO_2, seem to be reliable in identifying whether the tube has been passed into the esophagus or trachea and in confirming the correct ventilation port.

Although the Combitube has provided successful ventilation for several hours, it should be considered a temporizing measure only. Current use in the emergency department should be restricted to rescue placement after failed oral intubation with adequate BMV or a quick maneuver in the "can't intubate, can't oxygenate" patient simultaneous with preparation for a cricothyrotomy (analogous to the use of the ILMA in this situation). The Combitube has virtually no role in the emergency department as a primary airway management device except in cardiopulmonary arrest when expertise for endotracheal intubation is not available.

Retrograde Intubation

In retrograde intubation, a flexible wire is passed in retrograde fashion through a cricothyroid membrane puncture. The wire is retrieved through the mouth, then used to facilitate intubation by serving as a guide over which the ETT is passed. Purported advantages of retrograde intubation include ease of learning and application to the difficult airway. Although retrograde intubation theoretically may be useful when the upper airway is disrupted by trauma, rendering oral intubation difficult or impossible, it is unlikely to be used in the emergency department except in circumstances in which alternative devices, such as fiberoptic intubation, Trachlight, Combitube, and cricothyrotomy, are unavailable. Published reports of its use in emergency circumstances have been limited to case reports, very small series, and review articles. It is doubtful whether retrograde intubation would ever be the airway maneuver of first choice in the emergency department, but it may be a useful consideration in rare, unique difficult airway cases.

Fiberoptic Intubation

Fiberoptic intubation is widely used in the operating room for difficult airway cases, but its use is more vari-

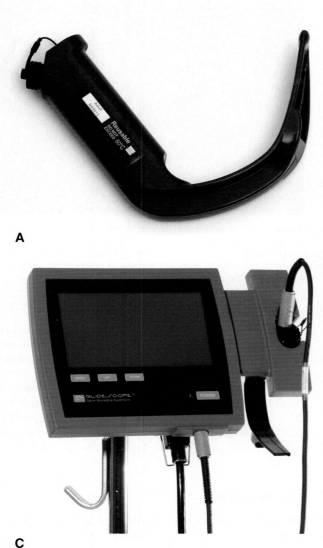

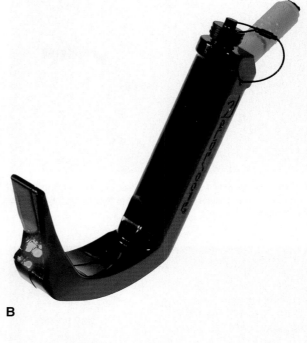

A

B

C

Figure 1-14. The GlideScope is a videolaryngoscope that uses a 60-degree deflection of the distal tip of the blade (which is otherwise similar to a MAC-3 blade) to direct the video camera and light source directly at the glottis without repositioning the head. The endotracheal tube insertion is done under direct vision via the video screen.

able in emergency departments. The intubating fiberoptic bronchoscope can be passed through the vocal cords under fiberoptic visualization, then can serve as an introducer over which the ETT is passed. The advantage of fiberoptic intubation is simultaneous airway assessment and intubation; for example, in a patient with smoke inhalation, examination with the fiberoptic scope might identify that intubation is not required. Fiberoptic intubation also can be used to complete the intubation if airway injury is identified. The fiberoptic scope also has been used successfully in concert with the ILMA to achieve intubation in difficult cases, including when the cervical spine is immobilized, where it significantly outperforms conventional laryngoscopy.[104]

Video and Rigid Fiberoptic Laryngoscopy

New devices incorporate video imaging into modified laryngoscopes to allow superior visualization of the glottis without the need to create a straight-line visual axis through the mouth (Figure 1-14). Although there is limited experience with these new devices, they offer

the ability to direct a video camera and light source at the glottis without extensive (or any) manipulation of the patient's head and neck. The potential advantages in difficult airway situations, including cervical spine immobilization, seem obvious, but additional study is needed before the role of these devices in the emergency department is fully elucidated.[105,106]

Two rigid fiberoptic intubating stylets have also been approved and adopted into clinical use. The Bonfils Intubating Fiberscope (Karl Storz Endoscopy of America, Culver City, Calif.) functions as an intubating stylet (Figure 1-15). The endotracheal tube is loaded directly onto the nonmalleable fiberoptic stylet, then guided through the glottic aperture by direct fiberoptic visualization, using a retro-molar approach.[107] The Shikani Optical Stylet (Clarus Medical, Minneapolis, Minn.) is similarly used. The endotracheal tube is placed over the malleable stylet, then advanced into the trachea using built-in fiberoptic visualization (Figure 1-16). Both devices show promise in difficult and failed airway applications, and they may also be used for routine "direct" laryngoscopy.[107]

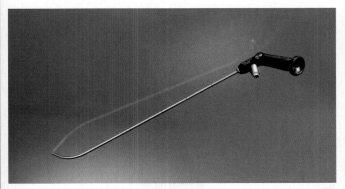

Figure 1-15. The Bonfils Intubating Fiberscope. The endotracheal tube is mounted on the stylet and intubation is facilitated through the eyepiece at right.

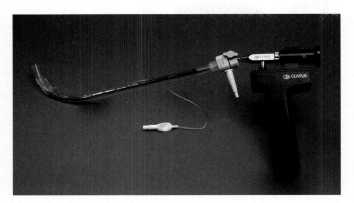

Figure 1-16. The Shikani Optical Stylet with endotracheal tube mounted. The eyepiece and battery pack are at the right.

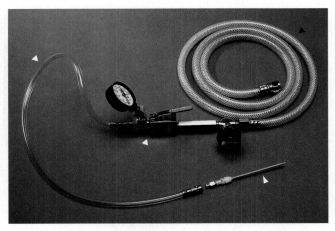

Figure 1-17. Transtracheal jet ventilation. High-pressure ventilation tubing *(black triangle)* attaches to standard wall oxygen outlet at 55 psi. Ventilation block *(middle arrow)* is used to control oxygen flow through tubing *(white triangle)* to catheter *(lower right arrow)*, which is inserted in the airway.

Needle Cricothyrotomy with Transtracheal Jet Ventilation

Needle cricothyrotomy involves the insertion of a large needle (ideally 10-gauge) through the cricothyroid membrane into the airway. When inserted, the needle is used to ventilate the patient with a standard wall oxygen source. Because of the high-velocity ventilation that ensues through the narrow catheter, this procedure is called *transtracheal jet ventilation.* Transtracheal jet ventilation has been used successfully in humans and has been subjected to various animal experiments to determine its uses and limitations. It rarely has been used in patients in emergency departments, however, where its role as a rescue device in the "can't intubate, can't ventilate" situation is vastly inferior to cricothyrotomy.

The jet ventilator should include a regulator and gauge so that pressures can be monitored and reduced, especially in children. Upper airway obstruction has been considered a contraindication to transtracheal jet ventilation, but ventilation still can be successful, although at the cost of higher intrapleural pressure and possibly pulmonary barotrauma. In general, when upper airway obstruction is present in adults, percutaneous or surgical cricothyrotomy is preferred.

The primary indication for transtracheal jet ventilation in the emergency department is the initiation of emergency ventilation for a pediatric patient who is apneic (either because of the presenting condition or because of administration of an NMBA) and in whom intubation and BMV are impossible. Cricothyrotomy is extremely difficult or impossible in children younger than 10 years old, and transtracheal jet ventilation should be considered the surgical rescue modality of choice in this age group. For children younger than 5 years old, bag ventilation is used with the percutaneous catheter, and pressurized devices are avoided (Figure 1-17).[57]

Cricothyrotomy

Cricothyrotomy is the creation of an opening in the cricothyroid membrane through which a cannula, usually a cuffed tracheostomy tube, is inserted to permit ventilation.[108] When surgical airway management is required, cricothyrotomy is the procedure of choice in the emergency setting, where it is faster, more straightforward, and more likely to be successful than tracheotomy.

Cricothyrotomy is indicated when oral or nasal intubation is impossible or fails and when BMV cannot maintain adequate oxygen saturation (the "can't intubate, can't ventilate" situation). Several large series have established that the incidence of cricothyrotomy is approximately 1% of all emergency department intubations.[1,36] Cricothyrotomy is relatively contraindicated by distorted neck anatomy, preexisting infection, and coagulopathy; these contraindications are relative, however, and the establishment of the airway takes precedence over all other considerations. Successful cricothyrotomy after systemic fibrinolytic therapy has been reported.[95,109] The procedure should be avoided in children younger than 10 years old, in whom anatomic considerations make it exceedingly difficult.[57]

Cricothyrotomes are devices used to perform percutaneous cricothyroidotomy. Percutaneous cricothyrotomy using the Seldinger technique may be comparable to formal surgical cricothyrotomy and may be easier to

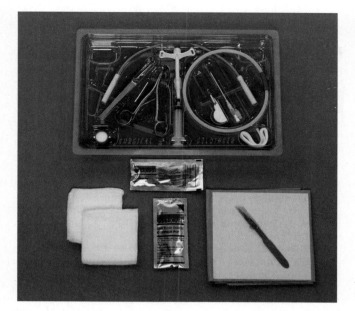

Figure 1-18. Melker universal cricothyrotomy kit. (Courtesy of Cook Critical Care.)

- Knowledge of the clinical course of the patient's condition and anticipation of possible deterioration are crucial to the decision to intubate, especially if the patient is to leave the emergency department for a time (e.g., interfacility transfer, diagnostic testing).
- Assessment of the patient for potential difficulty with intubation, bag/mask ventilation, or both is an essential step in planning airway management. The mnemonic *LEMON* is a useful aid.
- In the absence of a "crash" patient (agonal, unresponsive to laryngoscopy) or a difficult airway, RSI is the airway management method of choice for emergency department patients.
- Succinylcholine is the NMBA of choice for emergency department RSI, but it should be avoided in certain patient groups because of risk of significant hyperkalemia.
- Pretreatment drugs given during RSI can mitigate adverse responses to intubation and improve the patient's clinical condition.
- Tube placement confirmation using end-tidal CO_2 is essential after intubation, and failure to detect adequate quantities of exhaled CO_2 is evidence of esophageal intubation until proven otherwise.

perform.[110] The safety and effectiveness of other cricothyrotomes are not clearly established. Only two percutaneous cricothyrotomy sets on the market currently have the ability to place a cuffed tracheostomy tube. One is a dedicated Seldinger cricothyrotomy set; the other is a combination set that has all necessary equipment for either a Seldinger percutaneous cricothyrotomy or a standard surgical cricothyrotomy (Melker universal cricothyrotomy kit; Cook Critical Care Bloomington, Ind) (Figure 1-18).

OUTCOMES

Few studies of emergency airway management have characterized complications and outcomes. The largest single-institution series reported a success rate for emergency department RSI of 99% and a complication rate of 9.3%; most complications were minor.[1] Phase II of the large National Emergency Airway Registry Study (NEAR II) of more than 8500 patients reported success rates of approximately 99% for patients intubated in the emergency department for medical indications and greater than 97% for trauma patients.[111] The definition of a "complication" for emergency department intubation is also evolving, and the NEAR classification system characterizes potentially adverse occurrences during intubation as "events."[36,111,112] If a pneumothorax is identified after intubation of a patient with status asthmaticus, is the pneumothorax caused by the intubation or by the asthma?[96] Reclassification of complications as events will permit more appropriate comparisons of intubation outcomes in the future. In the NEAR study, the immediate complication rate was 2.3%; these are complications attributable to the intubation.[111] No studies have evaluated the long-term outcome of intubated emergency department patients.

REFERENCES

1. Sakles J, et al: Airway management in the emergency department: A one-year study of 610 tracheal intubations. *Ann Emerg Med* 31:325, 1998.
2. Ma O, et al: Airway management practices in emergency medicine residencies. *Am J Emerg Med* 13:501, 1995.
3. Levitan R, Kush S, Hollander J: Devices for difficult airway management in academic emergency departments: Results of a national survey. *Ann Emerg Med* 33:694, 1999.
4. American College of Emergency Physicians: Policy statement: Rapid sequence intubation. *Ann Emerg Med* 29:573, 1997.
5. Murphy MF, Walls RM: Identification of the difficult airway. In Walls RM, et al (eds): *Manual of Emergency Airway Management.* Philadelphia, Lippincott Williams & Wilkins, 2004, pp 70-81.
6. Walls RM: The emergency airway algorithms. In Walls RM, et al (eds): *Manual of Emergency Airway Management.* Philadelphia, Lippincott Williams & Wilkins, 2004, pp 8-21.
7. Walls R: The decision to intubate. In Walls RM, et al (eds): *Manual of Emergency Airway Management.* Philadelphia, Lippincott Williams & Wilkins, 2004, pp 1-7.
8. Davies A, et al: Pharyngeal sensation and gag reflex in healthy subjects. *Lancet* 345:487, 1995.
9. Moulton C, Pennycook A, Makower A: Relation between the Glasgow Coma Scale and the gag reflex. *BMJ* 303:1240, 1991.
10. Bleach N: The gag reflex and aspiration: A retrospective analysis of 120 patients assessed by videofluoroscopy. *Clin Otolaryngol* 18:303, 1993.
11. Kulig K, Rumack B, Rosen P: Gag reflex in assessing level of consciousness. *Lancet* 8271:565, 1982.
12. Lightowler J, et al: Non-invasive positive pressure ventilation to treat respiratory failure resulting from exacerbations of chronic obstructive pulmonary disease: Cochrane systematic review and meta-analysis. *BMJ* 326:185, 2003.

13. Cross A, et al: Non-invasive ventilation in acute respiratory failure: A randomised comparison of continuous positive airway pressure and bi-level positive airway pressure. *Emerg Med J* 20:531, 2003.

14. Omert L, et al: Role of the emergency medicine physician in airway management of the trauma patient. *J Trauma Injury Infection Crit Care* 51:1065, 2001.

15. Walls RM: Airway management. *Emerg Med Clin North Am* 11:53, 1993.

16. Walls R: Management of the difficult airway in the trauma patient. *Emerg Med Clin North Am* 16:45, 1998.

17. Walls RM, Wolfe R, Rosen P: Fools rush in? Airway management in penetrating neck trauma. *J Emerg Med* 11:479, 1993.

18. Mandavia DP, Qualls S, Rokos I: Emergency airway management in penetrating neck trauma. *Ann Emerg Med* 35:221, 2000.

19. Tayal V, et al: Rapid-sequence intubation at an emergency medicine residency: Success rate and adverse events during a two-year period. *Acad Emerg Med* 6:31, 1999.

20. Sagarin M, et al: Emergency medicine residents' skill development in airway management: Analysis of 8367 intubation attempts [abstract]. *Acad Emerg Med* 10:467, 2003.

21. Wheeler M, Ovassapian O: Prediction and evaluation of the difficult airway. In Hagberg CA (ed): *Manual of Difficult Airway Management.* Philadelphia, Churchill Livingstone, 2000, pp 15-30.

22. Benumof JL: Definition and incidence of the difficult airway. In Benumof JL (ed): *Airway Management Principles and Practice.* St Louis, Mosby-Year Book, 1996, pp 121-125.

23. Langeron O, et al: Prediction of difficult mask ventilation. *Anesthesiology* 92:1229, 2000.

24. Combes X, et al: Unanticipated difficult airway in anesthetized patients: Prospective validation of a management algorithm. *Anesthesiology* 100:1146, 2004.

25. American Society of Anesthesiologists Task Force on Management of the Difficult Airway: Practice guidelines for management of the difficult airway: An updated report by the American Society of Anesthesiologists Task Force on Management of the Difficult Airway. *Anesthesiology* 98:1269, 2003.

26. Naguib M, et al: Predictive models for difficult laryngoscopy and intubation: A clinical, radiologic and three-dimensional computer imaging study. *Can J Anaesth* 46:748, 1999.

27. Mallampati SR, et al: A clinical sign to predict difficult tracheal intubation: A prospective study. *Can Anaesth Soc J* 32:429, 1985.

28. Adnet F, et al: Randomized study comparing the 'sniffing position' with simple head extension for laryngoscopic view in elective surgery patients. *Anesthesiology* 95:836, 2001.

29. Yentis SM, Lee DJH: Evaluation of an improved scoring system for the grading of direct laryngoscopy. *Anaesthesia* 53:1041, 1998.

30. Knapp S, et al: The assessment of four different methods to verify tracheal tube placement in the critical care setting. *Anesth Analg* 88:766, 1999.

31. Takeda T, et al: The assessment of three methods to verify tracheal tube placement in the emergency setting. *Resuscitation* 56:153, 2003.

32. Tanigawa K, et al: The efficacy of esophageal detector devices in verifying tracheal tube placement: A randomized cross-over study of out-of-hospital cardiac arrest patients. *Anesth Analg* 92:375, 2001.

33. Benumof J, Dagg R, Benumof R: Critical hemoglobin desaturation will occur before return to unparalyzed state following 1 mg/kg intravenous succinylcholine. *Anesthesiology* 87:979, 1997.

34. Li J, et al: Complications of emergency intubation with and without paralysis. *Am J Emerg Med* 17:141, 1999.

35. Orebaugh SL: Difficult airway management in the emergency department. *J Emerg Med* 22:31, 2002.

36. Bair AE, et al: The failed intubation attempt in the emergency department: Analysis of prevalence, rescue techniques, and personnel. *J Emerg Med* 23:131, 2002.

37. Lawes EG, Campbell I, Mercer D: Inflation pressure, gastric insufflation and rapid sequence induction. *Br J Anaesth* 59:315, 1987.

38. Pace S, Fuller F: Out-of-hospital succinylcholine-assisted endotracheal intubation by paramedics. *Ann Emerg Med* 35:568, 2000.

39. Alexander R, et al: Comparison of remifentanil with alfentanil or suxamethonium following propofol anaesthesia for tracheal intubation. *Anaesthesia* 54:1032, 1999.

40. Walls RM: Rapid-sequence intubation in head trauma. *Ann Emerg Med* 22:1008, 1993.

41. Nimmagadda U, et al: Efficacy of preoxygenation with tidal volume breathing: Comparison of breathing systems. *Anesthesiology* 93:693, 2000.

42. Baraka A, et al: Preoxygenation: Comparison of maximal breathing and tidal volume breathing techniques. *Anesthesiology* 91:612, 1999.

43. Schneider RE, Caro D: Pretreatment agents. In Walls RM, et al (eds): *Manual of Emergency Airway Management.* Philadelphia, Lippincott Williams & Wilkins, 2004, pp 183-188.

44. Sellick B: Cricoid pressure to control regurgitation of stomach contents during induction of anesthesia. *Lancet* 2:404, 1961.

45. Roppolo L, et al: Nasotracheal intubation in the emergency department, revisited. *J Emerg Med* 17:791, 1999.

46. Rhee K, et al: Does nasotracheal intubation increase complications in patients with skull base fractures? *Ann Emerg Med* 22:1145, 1993.

47. Rosen C, et al: Blind nasotracheal intubation in the presence of facial trauma. *Ann Emerg Med* 23:617, 1994.

48. Vilke GM: Intubation techniques in the helicopter. *J Emerg Med* 12:217, 1994.

49. Rhee K, O'Malley R: Neuromuscular blockade-assisted oral intubation versus nasotracheal intubation in the prehospital care of injured patients. *Ann Emerg Med* 23:37, 1994.

50. Mateer J: Continuous pulse oximetry during emergency endotracheal intubation. *Ann Emerg Med* 22:675, 1993.

51. Kirkegaard-Nielsen H, et al: Rapid tracheal intubation with rocuronium. *Anesthesiology* 91:131, 1999.

52. Sagarin M, et al: Rapid sequence intubation for pediatric emergency airway management. *Pediatr Emerg Care* 18:417, 2002.

53. Rose WD, Anderson LD, Edmond SA: Analysis of intubations before and after establishment of a rapid sequence intubation protocol for air medical use. *Air Med J* 13:475, 1994.

54. Savarese J, et al: Pharmacology of muscle relaxants and their antagonists. In Miller RD, et al (eds): *Anesthesia.* London, Churchill Livingstone, 2000, pp 412-490.

55. Schneider RE, Caro D: Neuromuscular blocking agents. In Walls RM, et al (eds): *Manual of Emergency Airway Management.* Philadelphia, Lippincott Williams & Wilkins, 2004, pp 200-211.

56. Naguib M, et al: Optimal dose of succinylcholine revisited. *Anesthesiology* 99:1045, 2003.

57. Luten RC, Kissoon N: Approach to the pediatric airway. In Walls RM, et al (eds): *Manual of Emergency Airway Management.* Philadelphia, Lippincott Williams & Wilkins, 2004, pp 212-227.

58. McLoughlin C, et al: Muscle pains and biochemical changes following suxamethonium adminstration after six pretreatment regimens. *Anaesthesia* 47:202, 1992.

59. Gronert GA: Cardiac arrest after succinylcholine: Mortality much greater with rhabdomyolysis than receptor upregulation. *Anesthesiology* 94:523, 2001.

60. Gronert GA: Succinylcholine hyperkalemia after burns. *Anesthesiology* 91:320, 1999.

61. Schow A, et al: Can succinylcholine be used safely in hyperkalemic patients? *Anesth Analg* 95:119, 2002.

62. Vachon C, Warner D, Bacon D: Succinylcholine and the open globe: Tracing the teaching. *Anesthesiology* 99:220, 2003.

63. Gronert GA, Antognini J, Pessah I: Malignant hyperthermia. In Miller RD, et al (eds): *Anesthesia*. London, Churchill Livingstone, 2000, pp 1033-1052.

64. Schmutz D, Muhlebach S: Stability of succinylcholine chloride injection. *Am J Hosp Pract* 48:501, 1991.

65. Sakles JC, et al: Rocuronium for rapid sequence intubation of emergency department patients. *Ann Emerg Med* 32:S13, 1998.

66. Sivilotti M, et al: Does the sedative agent facilitate emergency rapid-sequence intubation? *Acad Emerg Med* 10:612, 2003.

67. Weiss-Bloom L, Reich D: Haemodynamic responses to tracheal intubation following etomidate and fentanyl for anaesthetic induction. *Can J Anaesth* 39:780, 1992.

68. Modica PA, Tempelhoff R: Intracranial pressure during induction of anaesthesia and tracheal intubation with etomidate-induced EEG burst suppression. *Can J Anaesth* 39:236, 1992.

69. Absalom A, Pledger D, Kong A: Adrenocortical function in critically ill patients 24 hours after a single dose of etomidate. *Anaesthesia* 54:861, 1999.

70. Reves J, Glass P, Lubarsky D: Nonbarbiturate intravenous anesthetics. In Miller RD, et al (eds): *Anesthesia*. London, Churchill Livingstone, 2000, pp 228-272.

71. Sagarin MJ, et al: Underdosing of midazolam in emergency endotracheal intubation. *Acad Emerg Med* 10:329, 2003.

72. Albanese J, et al: Ketamine decreases intracranial pressure and electroencephalographic activity in traumatic brain injury patients during propofol sedation. *Anesthesiology* 87:1328, 1997.

73. Dohi S, et al: End-tidal carbon dioxide monitoring during awake blind nasotracheal intubation. *J Clin Anesth* 2:415, 1990.

74. Groeben H, et al: Both intravenous and inhaled lidocaine attenuate reflex bronchoconstriction but at different plasma concentrations. *Am J Respir Crit Care Med* 159:530, 1999.

75. Maslow A, et al: Inhaled albuterol, but not intravenous lidocaine, protects against intubation induced bronchoconstriction in asthma. *Anesthesiology* 93:1198, 2000.

76. Adachi YU, et al: Fentanyl attenuates the hemodynamic response to intubation more than the response to laryngoscopy. *Anesth Analg* 95:233, 2002.

77. Helfman SM, et al: Which drug prevents tachycardia and hypertension associated with tracheal intubations: Lidocaine, fentanyl, or esmolol? *Anesth Analg* 72:482, 1991.

78. Woster PS, Leblanc K: Management of elevated intracranial pressure. *J Clin Pharm* 9:762, 1990.

79. Jagoda AS, Bruns JJ: Increased intracranial pressure. In Walls RM, et al (eds): *Manual of Emergency Airway Management*. Philadelphia, Lippincott Williams & Wilkins, 2004, pp 262-269.

80. Yano M, et al: Effect of lidocaine on ICP response to endotracheal suctioning. *Anesthesiology* 64:651, 1986.

81. Minton MD, et al: Increases in intracranial pressure from succinylcholine: Prevention by prior nondepolarizing blockade. *Anesthesiology* 65:165, 1986.

82. Stirt JA, et al: "Defasciculation" with metocurine prevents succinylcholine-induced increases in intracranial pressure. *Anesthesiology* 67:50, 1987.

83. Koenig KL: Rapid sequence intubation of head trauma patients: Prevention of fasciculations with pancuronium versus mini-dose succinylcholine. *Ann Emerg Med* 12:929, 1992.

84. Crosby E: Airway management after upper cervical spine injury: What have we learned? *Can J Anaesth* 49:733, 2002.

85. Criswell J, et al: Emergency airway management in patients with cervical spine injuries. *Anaesthesia* 49:900, 1994.

86. Walt B, et al: Tracheal intubation and cervical spine excursion: Direct laryngoscopy vs. intubating laryeal mask. *Anaesthesia* 56:221, 2001.

87. Brimacombe J, et al: Cervical spine motion during airway management: A cinefluoroscopic study of the posteriorly destabilized third cervical vertebrae in human cadavers. *Anesth Analg* 91:1274, 2000.

88. Chong CL, Ware DN, Harris JHJ: Is cervical spine imaging indicated in gunshot wounds to the cranium? *J Trauma Injury Infection Crit Care* 44:501, 1998.

89. Brimacombe JR, Berry A: The incidence of aspiration associated with the laryngeal mask airway: A meta-analysis of published literature. *J Clin Anesth* 7:297, 1995.

90. Choyce A, et al: A comparison of the intubating and standard laryngeal mask airways for airway management by inexperienced personnel. *Anaesthesia* 56:357, 2001.

91. Reinhart DJ, Simmons G: Comparison of placement of the laryngeal mask airway with endotracheal tube by paramedics and respiratory therapists. *Ann Emerg Med* 24:260, 1994.

92. Joo HS, Rose DK: The intubating laryngeal mask airway with and without fiberoptic guidance. *Anesth Analg* 88:662, 1999.

93. Baskett PJF: The intubating laryngeal mask: Results of a multicenter trial with experience of over 500 cases. *Anaesthesia* 53:1174, 1998.

94. Parmeet JL: The laryngeal mask airway reliably provides rescue ventilation in cases of unanticipated difficult tracheal intubation along with difficult mask ventilation. *Anesth Analg* 87:661, 1998.

95. Langeron O, et al: Comparison of the intubating laryngeal mask airway with fiberoptic intubation in anticipated difficult airway management. *Anesthesiology* 94:968, 2001.

96. Katz SH, Falk JL: Misplaced endotracheal tubes by paramedics in an urban emergency medical services system. *Ann Emerg Med* 37:32, 2001.

97. Hung OR, et al: Clinical trial of a new lightwand device (Trachlight) to intubate the trachea. *Anesthesiology* 83:509, 1995.

98. Nishikawa K, et al: A comparison of hemodynamic changes after endotracheal intubation by using the lightwand device and the laryngoscope in normotensive and hypertensive patients. *Anesth Analg* 90:1203, 2000.

99. Soh CR, et al: Trachlight intubation by novice staff: The direct vision laryngoscope or the lighted stylet (Trachlight)? *Emerg Med J* 19:292, 2002.

100. Lefrancois DP, Dufour DG: Use of the esophageal tracheal Combitube by basic emergency medical technicians. *Resuscitation* 52:77, 2002.

101. Vezina D: Complications associated with the use of the esophageal tracheal Combitube. *Can J Anaesth* 45:76, 1998.

102. Mercer MH, Gabbott DA: Insertion of the Combitube airway with the cervical spine immobilised in a rigid cervical collar. *Anaesthesia* 53:971, 1998.

103. Mercer MH, Gabbott DA: The influence of neck position on ventilation using the Combitube airway. *Anaesthesia* 53:146, 1998.

104. Asai T, et al: Ease of tracheal intubation through the intubating laryngeal mask during manual in-line head and neck stabilisation. *Anaesthesia* 55:79, 2000.
105. Cooper RM: Use of a new videolaryngoscope (GlideScope) in the management of a difficult airway. *Can J Anaesth* 50:611, 2003.
106. Sakles JC: Video laryngoscopy. In Walls RM, et al (eds): *Manual of Emergency Airway Management*. Philadelphia, Lippincott Williams & Wilkins, 2004, pp 151-157.
107. Gravenstein DA, Liem EB, Bjoraker DG: Alternative management techniques for the difficult airway: Optical stylets. *Curr Opin Anesth* 17:495, 2004.
108. Vissers RJ, Bair AE: Surgical airway techniques. In Walls RM, et al (eds): *Manual of Emergency Airway Management*. Philadelphia, Lippincott Williams & Wilkins, 2004, pp 158-182.
109. Pollack CV, Walls RM: Successful cricothyrotomy after thrombolytic therapy for acute myocardial infarction: A report of two cases. *Ann Emerg Med* 35:188, 2000.
110. Chan TC: Comparison of wire-guided cricothyrotomy versus standard surgical cricothyrotomy technique. *J Emerg Med* 17:957, 1999.
111. Walls RM, et al: Emergency department intubation of need patients: Report of the second phase of the National Emergency Airway Registry Project (NEAR II). *Ann Emerg Med* 2005 (in press).
112. Barton ED, et al: What is a complication? Classifying events during emergency intubations. *Acad Emerg Med* 6:365, 1999.

CHAPTER
2

Mechanical Ventilation and Noninvasive Ventilatory Support

Charles V. Pollack, Jr.

PERSPECTIVE

Invasive and noninvasive ventilation are essential tools for the management of critically ill patients. The indications for endotracheal intubation and for assisted ventilation in the emergency department are not always the same. Some patients are intubated simply for airway protection or as part of overall management of critical illness or injury; others are intubated specifically for failure of ventilation or oxygenation.

The objectives of assisted ventilation are to improve pulmonary gas exchange, relieve respiratory distress, alter adverse pressure-volume relationships in the lungs, permit lung healing, and avoid complications.[1] Acute respiratory failure can be defined by the presence of at least two of four criteria: (1) acute dyspnea, (2) arterial oxygen partial pressure (PaO_2) less than 50 mm Hg at room air, (3) arterial carbon dioxide partial pressure ($PaCO_2$) greater than 50 mm Hg, and (4) significant respiratory acidemia.[2] Abnormal pH and even relative hypoxemia should be tolerated sometimes in the short-term to avoid the complications of high inflation pressures with positive-pressure ventilation (PPV).[1] The consensus approach is to treat the specific patient and the underlying problem, not the arterial blood gas (ABG) disruption (see Chapter 1).

BASIC APPROACHES

Three basic concepts must be considered in the initial discussion of intensive ventilatory support: (1) negative-pressure ventilation versus PPV, (2) invasive versus noninvasive ventilatory management, and (3) volume-cycled versus pressure-cycled ventilators. Negative-pressure ventilation is no longer used in acute care and has no role in the emergency department management of respiratory emergencies. PPV occurs when a preset gas mixture is cyclically introduced at supra-atmospheric pressure into the upper airway. The pressure gradient created between the upper airway and the lungs entrains gases into the lungs. PPV can be delivered invasively through an endotracheal tube (ETT) or noninvasively via a face mask or nose mask. Forcing gases into the lungs with PPV involves assuming the risk of several potential adverse effects (Box 2-1).[3] Each of these potential complications must be anticipated and addressed when PPV, whether invasive or noninvasive, is used in the emergency department.

BOX 2-1. Potential Adverse Effects of Positive-Pressure Ventilation

Increased mean intrathoracic pressure
Decreased venous return to the heart and decreased cardiac output
Increased ventilation/perfusion ratio
Decreased renal blood flow and glomerular filtration rate with fluid retention
Air trapping and intrinsic positive end-expiratory pressure (iPEEP, auto-PEEP)
Barotrauma
Nosocomial infections of the lungs and sinuses
Respiratory alkalosis
Agitation and increased respiratory distress
Increased work of breathing

Ventilators that deliver PPV may be pressure or volume cycled. With *pressure-cycled ventilation,* a peak inspiratory pressure (PIP) is established for inspiration regardless of tidal volume (VT), inspiratory time, or inspiratory flow rate; when this preset pressure is reached, inspiration is terminated, and exhalation occurs passively. With *volume-cycled ventilation,* inhalation is terminated when a preset VT is delivered, even though peak airway pressures, inspiratory time, and inspiratory flow rates may vary. If the peak pressures in the patient's lungs increase, however, a greater proportion of the preset VT is left behind in the ventilator's circuit.[4]

No consensus in the literature exists regarding which approach to PPV is more efficacious. Pressure-cycled ventilators are less useful than volume-cycled respirators in critically ill patients with rapidly changing pulmonary mechanics because, if compliance decreases or airway resistance increases, hypoventilation might result. Pressure-cycled machines generally are much less expensive than their volume-cycled counterparts, however, and are in widespread clinical use.

VENTILATORY ASSISTANCE

Invasive Techniques

The most important of the clinically available modes of PPV are (1) controlled mechanical ventilation (CMV), (2) assist/control (A/C) ventilation, (3) intermittent mandatory ventilation (IMV), and (4) synchronized intermittent mandatory ventilation (SIMV), all of which can be supplied through either pressure-cycled or volume-cycled ventilators. Three main factors differentiate these modes from one another: (1) the initiation trigger for a breath (by timed cycle or by inspiratory effort sensed by the ventilator), (2) the target capacity (pressure or volume) for each breath, and (3) the cycling from inspiration to expiration. Pressure support ventilation (PSV), positive end-expiratory pressure (PEEP), and continuous positive airway pressure (CPAP) also can be supplied by a pressure-cycled ventilator through an ETT.

With CMV, the ventilator delivers breaths at a preset interval, regardless of any ventilatory effort made by the patient. The patient on CMV neither can trigger a positive-pressure breath nor can inspire gas spontaneously through the ventilator circuit, so this mode is appropriate only for apneic and pharmacologically paralyzed patients. In contrast, a ventilator set to A/C mode responds with a full VT breath to the patient's inspiratory effort, but in the absence of any such effort, it automatically cycles at a preset minimum background rate. If an A/C ventilator is set at 12 breaths/min, the machine cycles to inspiration every 5 seconds in the absence of spontaneous inspiratory effort. If the patient inspires and triggers an assisted breath, the ventilator's timer resets for another 5 seconds. The patient can breathe at a higher rate than the A/C rate, with an attendant increase in work of breathing over that anticipated. A/C ventilation is the preferred initial mode of mechanical ventilation in most emergency department patients, although potential disadvantages of this mode include poor toleration in awake patients and worsening of volume retention in patients with chronic obstructive pulmonary disease (COPD).[5]

IMV is a combination of spontaneous ventilation and CMV. A background CMV rate is set and triggers regardless of any inspiratory effort by the patient. When the patient breathes spontaneously, warmed, humidified, oxygen-enriched gas is supplied from the ventilator's circuit, but no preset volume or pressure is triggered. IMV is used because it allows the patient to adjust the $PaCO_2$, preserves ventilatory muscle tone, requires less sedation than CMV (and no paralysis), and facilitates *weaning,* the process by which patients are converted from mechanical ventilation to spontaneous ventilation.[2]

SIMV is a combination of spontaneous ventilation and A/C ventilation. The delivery of the mechanical breath is synchronized to support the patient's spontaneous breaths at a preset rate, preventing the patient from *stacking* (i.e., a mechanical breath being delivered at the same time as a spontaneous breath is taken, which is possible with IMV). Stacking may result in hyperinflation and barotrauma.[2] If spontaneous breathing occurs at a rate faster than the SIMV rate, the patient breathes gas from the ventilator circuit. If the patient's spontaneous efforts lapse, the ventilator breathes by default at the SIMV rate. SIMV is presumed to be more comfortable for the patient than IMV, but studies have failed to show any significant difference in ventilatory efficacy between the two modes.[6]

PSV is a partial ventilatory support mode in which breathing is controlled by the patient, and peak pressures are controlled by the ventilator. The primary goal of PSV is to support the patient's spontaneous breathing effort while providing satisfactory oxygenation. PSV provides for the prompt attainment of a preset PIP each time the patient initiates inspiratory effort. Inspiratory time, inspiratory flow rate, and VT are augmented, whereas inspiratory work of breathing is reduced. The machine likewise senses the end of inspiration or initiation of exhalation, at which time exhalation is allowed to proceed spontaneously. Increasing levels of PSV decrease work of breathing.[5] PEEP may be added to PSV, and a mandatory ventilation background rate can be set, in case spontaneous respirations deteriorate.

PSV initially was used as a weaning mode, but some authorities now recommend it as a primary means of ventilatory support. Careful monitoring is necessary during its use because VT is uncontrolled. Invasive ventilation with PSV is rarely used in the emergency department, but PSV may be applied noninvasively.

PEEP and CPAP refer to the maintenance of positive pressure after the completion of passive exhalation. Strictly defined, PEEP is pressure applied during mechanical ventilation, whereas CPAP is the application of positive pressure (invasively or noninvasively) during spontaneous breathing. Although many clinicians use the terms interchangeably, there is one significant difference: With CPAP, inspiratory and expiratory pressures are positive, although the inspiratory pressure is less than the expiratory pressure. With PEEP, airway pressure is subambient during inhalation but positive during exhalation. PEEP may be added to any of the ventilation modes discussed previously. The primary physiologic effect of PEEP is to increase functional residual capacity by maintaining patency of alveoli at the end of exhalation.

The best-supported indication for PEEP or CPAP is a need for augmentation of PaO_2 when the patient is severely hypoxemic or is at risk of oxygen toxicity, as in cardiogenic pulmonary edema or acute respiratory distress syndrome (ARDS). PEEP and CPAP increase PaO_2 at constant fraction of inspired oxygen (FIO_2) by decreasing intrapulmonary shunting and ventilation/perfusion (V/Q) mismatch.

Applied PEEP must be differentiated from *intrinsic PEEP* (iPEEP, or auto-PEEP), which may result from improper assisted ventilation when adequate time is not allowed between breaths for complete exhalation. The end-expiratory pressure in the alveoli becomes more positive than the positive pressure in the more proximal airways; this phenomenon further causes hemodynamic compromise, makes inspiratory efforts increasingly less effective, and may precipitate barotrauma.

Intrinsic PEEP also occurs in most patients with obstructive respiratory failure, at levels often exceeding 10 cm H_2O.[7] COPD-related iPEEP results from air trapping in the alveoli at the end of expiration. Intrinsic PEEP can add to the inspiratory work of breathing because the positive alveolar pressure must be overcome before a VT can be generated. When assisting the ventilation of patients with iPEEP, extrinsic PEEP should be set *below* iPEEP, and VT, rate, and expiratory time should be set to optimize adequate exhalation. Some newer ventilators can measure iPEEP directly; otherwise it also may be estimated by measuring pressure after end-expiratory occlusion of the expiratory line. Extrinsic PEEP is postulated to allow respiratory muscles previously used to maintain iPEEP to relax and be recruited to participate in inspiratory effort, decreasing work of breathing.[8] When iPEEP is not offset, breath stacking and barotrauma may result.

Noninvasive Techniques

Although the first is of historical interest only, the four modes of noninvasive intensive ventilatory support pertinent to emergency medicine are (1) intermittent positive-pressure breathing, (2) mask CPAP, (3) bilevel positive airway pressure (BL-PAP), and (4) mask mechanical ventilation (MMV). These sometimes are collectively termed *noninvasive positive-pressure ventilation* (NPPV). Intermittent positive-pressure breathing, previously a popular emergency department modality, withered under scientific scrutiny and is no longer used.[9]

Mask CPAP has extensive and well-documented use as a means of NPPV in the emergency department. Mask CPAP is efficacious as the sole ventilatory support in the treatment of pulmonary edema.[10]

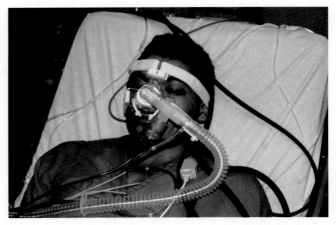

Figure 2-1. Patient wearing nose mask for noninvasive support with pressure support ventilation (bilevel positive airway pressure).

Battery-powered units have been used with success in the prehospital setting.[11] Some authors have suggested that CPAP provides benefits during acute asthma exacerbation by reducing inspiratory work of breathing, mean airway pressures, and air trapping, although there may be a higher risk of barotrauma when CPAP is used in these patients.[8]

BL-PAP conceptually combines inspiratory PSV and CPAP (Figure 2-1). The BL-PAP noninvasive ventilators provide differential preset support of spontaneous inspiration (inspiratory positive airway pressure [IPAP]) and expiration (expiratory positive airway pressure [EPAP]). The IPAP must be set higher than the EPAP, and the difference between the two settings is equivalent to the amount of pressure support provided. The BL-PAP is pressure limited and flow triggered; the machine senses the initiation of inspiration and immediately cycles to the preset IPAP, increasing VT with less work of breathing. IPAP levels are sustained for at least 200 msec and for as long as 3 seconds, or until the patient ceases inspiratory effort or begins to exhale. The machine cycles to the EPAP setting, below which it never drops, maintaining supra-atmospheric end-expiratory pressure. Analogous to PEEP/CPAP, EPAP reduces work of breathing.

Although the most extensive experience with BL-PAP is in the control of nocturnal hypoventilation, it has the widest potential emergency department applicability of all modes of NPPV. Its efficacy in acute respiratory failure has been documented in many series.[12-14] In selected patients in respiratory distress caused by COPD, pulmonary edema, pneumonia, and status asthmaticus, BL-PAP by face mask or nose mask may be an effective alternative to endotracheal intubation and mechanical ventilation. Similar to CPAP, it may be beneficial in acute asthma.[15,16] The BL-PAP ventilator is portable, and its settings are highly adjustable. These ventilators also can be programmed with a background cycling rate analogous to an invasive A/C mode, although this feature is not generally applicable to emergency department use; patients who may require untriggered ventilation should be intubated for definitive control while in the emergency department.

Table 2-1. General Guidelines for Initial Invasive Ventilator Settings in Various Clinical Settings

	Mode*	FIO$_2$ (%)	VT (mL/kg)	Rate (breaths/min)	I/E Ratio	PEEP (cm H$_2$O)
Overdose in otherwise healthy patient	CMV, A/C, IMV, SIMV	100	8-10	10-12	1:2	0-5
Status asthmaticus	CMV, A/C, IMV, SIMV	100	5-10	8-12	1:4	2.5-10[†]
	PHC[‡], CMV, IMV, SIMV	100	5-8	6-10	1:4	2.5-10[†]
COPD exacerbation, respiratory acidosis	CMV, A/C, IMV, SIMV	100	5-10	10-12	1:3-1:4	2.5-10[†]
	PHC[‡], CMV, IMV, SIMV	100	5-8	8-12	1:3-1:4	2.5-10[†]
Cardiogenic pulmonary edema	CMV, A/C, IMV, SIMV	100	8-10	10-12	1:2	2.5-15
ARDS	CMV, A/C, IMV, SIMV	100	6-8	20-25	1:2	2.5-10
	Inverse ratio	100	6-8	8-12	1:1-1:2.1	2.5-5
Hypovolemic shock	CMV, A/C, IMV, SIMV	100	8-10	§	1:2	0-5

*CMV is the appropriate mode when the patient is apneic or paralyzed. See text for abbreviations.
†PEEP in air-trapping diseases should not exceed measured intrinsic PEEP.
‡PHC is *permissive hypercapnia*, a ventilatory strategy that can be employed in multiple modes.
§Rate should be set based on desired PaCO$_2$.
FIO$_2$, fraction of inspired oxygen; VT, tidal volume; I/E, inspiratory/expiratory; PEEP, positive end-expiratory pressure.
When using a pressure-cycled ventilator, set pressures to deliver desired VT. After 20 minutes on initial settings, arterial blood gases should be checked so that settings and down-titrations of FIO$_2$ can be modified appropriately.

MMV simply involves changing the ventilator-patient interface for a pressure-cycled or volume-cycled ventilator to a face mask instead of an ETT. Most awake patients tolerate MMV better than endotracheal intubation–mechanical ventilation. Patients in hypercapnic respiratory failure have been managed successfully with MMV alone using PSV, volume-cycled CMV, and A/C modes.[15-17] MMV and BL-PAP also are used in the ongoing management of less acute ventilatory insufficiency (e.g., daily or three or four times weekly in patients with severe but stable COPD).[18]

Patient Selection

Patients with a patent airway and an intact respiratory drive, even if that drive is clearly insufficient, may be candidates for NPPV. Patients most likely to respond to NPPV in the emergency department are patients with more readily reversible etiologies of their distress, such as COPD exacerbation or cardiogenic pulmonary edema.[13,14,19,20] Patient selection, comprehensive management of the underlying condition, and ongoing monitoring are essential for successful NPPV. The patient should be reassessed frequently for progress of therapy, tolerance of the mode of support, and any signs of clinical deterioration that indicate a need for intubation. NPPV also may be considered for a patient whose advance directives proscribe intubation. An individualized approach is important, and discussion with the patient and family members may be helpful.[21]

MANAGEMENT

Patients in the emergency department require assisted ventilation in one of three scenarios: (1) as a consequence of intubation, (2) as a resuscitative measure taken in anticipation of admission, and (3) as a stabilizing measure for short-term (≤24 hours) management in an inpatient unit or emergency department observation unit. In the latter two cases, either endotracheal intubation–mechanical ventilation or NPPV may be used as appropriate. Observation units may be suitable for improving chronically hypoventilatory patients with BL-PAP before discharge home; such a practice requires standing protocols and dedicated respiratory care personnel.[22]

Initial Settings and Ongoing Monitoring

Initial ventilator settings depend on the goal of the ventilatory intervention (mechanical ventilation, assist ventilation, or PSV) and on the underlying cause of deterioration. The basic parameters to be set in volume-cycled ventilators in CMV, A/C, IMV, and SIMV modes are FIO$_2$, VT, rate, and inspiratory/expiratory (I/E) ratio. (The I/E ratio reflects the duration of machine ventilations and rest periods between them.) If atelectasis is a problem, PEEP should be added; the addition of PEEP may allow direct reduction of FIO$_2$ as well. For an apneic or paralyzed patient, CMV, A/C, or IMV mode may be used. For a patient with inadequate ventilatory effort, A/C is usually the best initial approach.

Typical initial ventilator settings are a VT of 10 mL/kg body weight and a rate of 10 to 12 breaths/min. Increasing concern about barotrauma from such large, nonphysiologic VT, termed *volutrauma,* has resulted in recommendations that VT be initiated at less than 10 mL/kg in essentially all clinical scenarios resulting from primary lung disease, in which patients have decreased lung compliance (Table 2-1).[22] Initial FIO$_2$ should be set at 1 L/min, but generally can be titrated down quickly to maintain an oxygen saturation of 90% or greater. The ventilation can be initiated using the "rule of tens," which dictates 10 breaths/min, VT of 10 mL/kg, and FIO$_2$ of 1.0. Ventilator settings are adjusted dynamically using pulse oximetry, end-tidal carbon dioxide determination, ventilation pressures, clinical status, and ABGs as a guide. PEEP, if indicated, should be initiated at 2.5 to 5 cm H$_2$O. The usual I/E ratio is 1:2. In pressure-cycled ventilators, an inspiratory pressure should be chosen that results in a comparable VT, usually 25 to 40 cm H$_2$O. There are additional specific considerations for essentially every lung disorder (see Table 2-1).

Mechanical ventilation is a dynamic process that requires constant monitoring and regular adjustment of these parameters. Tachycardia and hypertension can indicate ventilator intolerance and a need for increased sedation or adjustment of the ventilator settings. Bradycardia and ventricular irritability must be considered to represent hypoxemia until this is absolutely disproved. Unless capnometry and pulse oximetry are in use, an ABG should be measured within 20 minutes of beginning ventilation. These results indicate the extent of ventilation (using the pH and $PaCO_2$) and oxygenation (using pulse oximetry or PaO_2). Adjustments in minute volume (product of V_T and rate) and FiO_2 can be guided by baseline measurements supplemented by ongoing monitoring. To avoid oxygen toxicity, FiO_2 should be lowered as rapidly as possible to less than 0.5 (50%) as long as oximetry indicates an acceptable ($\geq$90%) oxygen saturation. PEEP can be used to support PaO_2 at lower FiO_2.

ABG results also should be used to verify the accuracy of noninvasive (transcutaneous) pulse oximetry when doubt exists. Pulse oximetry does not always reflect PaO_2 accurately (see Chapter 3). When correlation is verified, however, the frequency of ABG determinations usually can be reduced. Concomitant use of capnography can reduce reliance on arterial sampling further.

Important ventilator parameters include PIP and expiratory volume. PIP is the most frequently measured variable of ventilatory function during mechanical ventilation. It depends on lung compliance and airway resistance; changes in the magnitude of PIP may reflect any of several potentially detrimental problems related to ventilation.[4] In a practical sense, PIP should be considered an additional vital sign for patients on a ventilator.

Decreases in PIP reflect inadequate volume delivery to the patient, which may be caused by insufficient gas supply to the ventilator, inadvertent change in settings, a leak in the breathing circuit, unintended extubation, or failure or disconnection of the ventilator. Increases in PIP may indicate ETT occlusion by secretions in or kinking of the tube, acute bronchospasm, pneumothorax, or conditions causing decreased lung compliance such as the development or worsening of pulmonary edema. PIP can serve as a useful measure of effectiveness of therapy in patients with asthma or COPD; as airway resistance lessens, the PIP decreases. High PIP may cause barotrauma and other acute lung injury.[23,24]

Measurement of expiratory volume and expiratory flow allows estimation of the effectiveness of spontaneous respiratory efforts and, by comparing expiratory volume with V_T, assessment of the effectiveness of ventilation and the integrity of the breathing circuit. The expiratory volume measurement is particularly important in assessing mechanical ventilation in children who may have air leaks around an uncuffed ETT.

Recommended initial settings for BL-PAP ventilators in the noninvasive support of patients in respiratory distress or failure are an IPAP of 8 cm H_2O and an EPAP of 3 cm H_2O, for a pressure support (IPAP − EPAP) of 5 cm H_2O. Either a face mask or a nose mask can be used (see Figure 2-1). The flow of supplemental oxygen bled into the circuit should be governed by pulse oximetry, as corroborated by ABG results; it is appropriate to initiate therapy with 3 to 5 L/min, but this should be adjusted with each titration of IPAP or EPAP. The ventilator should be in spontaneous mode to support the patient's respiratory effort.

As the patient's response to NPPV and other therapy is monitored (using cardiac and blood pressure monitors, ABG and oximetry, and the patient's own voiced assessment of tolerance and progress), support pressures are titrated. Although titration must be individualized, a reasonable approach for BL-PAP support in hypoxemic patients is to increase EPAP in 2-cm H_2O increments, with IPAP maintained at a fixed interval higher. Hypercapnic patients can be managed by increasing IPAP in 2-cm H_2O increments, with EPAP being increased in approximately a 1:2.5 ratio to IPAP.[12,20] Because iPEEP cannot be measured by a noninvasive ventilator, EPAP generally should be maintained at less than 8 to 10 cm H_2O to ensure that it does not exceed iPEEP in patients with COPD. The IPAP must be set higher than the EPAP.

Patient Management

Even if a ventilated patient's stay in the emergency department is brief, ventilatory management and intervention must be optimal. Important factors in this regard are sedation, neuromuscular paralysis, analgesia, and suctioning. Sedation and analgesia should be titrated to provide the best possible patient comfort and ventilation performance. Proposed scoring systems are too elaborate for emergency department use or do not provide information on the quality of sedation.

Careful attention must be paid to serial examination and vital signs. Persistent grimace, cough, and focused or random motor activity indicate a need for sedation, paralysis, or both. Lacrimation, diaphoresis, and increasing heart rate and blood pressure must be interpreted in context but often are manifestations of undersedation.

Although many parenteral sedatives are available, benzodiazepines have anxiolytic, hypnotic, amnestic, and muscle-relaxant properties and are the drugs of choice for sedation in ventilated patients in the emergency department. Diazepam, lorazepam, and midazolam all are appropriate; no clinical studies have shown any agent's relative superiority. Diazepam is inexpensive, consistent, and safe and may be the preferred drug based on cost considerations; an initial dose of 0.2 to 0.3 mg/kg is reasonable. Midazolam is the shortest acting of the three and the most likely benzodiazepine to cause transient hypotension after administration. All benzodiazepines exert a dose-dependent depressive effect on respiratory drive and should be used with caution in A/C and PSV modes. Other options include propofol and ketamine. Although ketamine may be a good choice for intubation of asthmatic patients because of its bronchodilatory effects, it is not indicated in adults for sedation after intubation because of the incidence of emergence phenomena. If ongoing ketamine therapy is planned, a benzodiazepine also should be administered.

Undersedation must be differentiated from inadequate analgesia. An indwelling ETT is itself a painful stimulus. Suctioning adds to the discomfort, and some ventilated patients have underlying painful problems as well (e.g., pleuritic chest pain in pulmonary embolus or fracture pain after trauma). Sedatives do not treat pain and are inappropriate as sole agents in the management of ventilated patients experiencing distress.

Opioids are the drugs of choice for analgesia in ventilated patients. From among the many available agents, the choice should be based on duration of action and effect on blood pressure. Shorter acting opioids (e.g., fentanyl, alfentanil, sufentanil), when available in the emergency department, may have theoretical advantages in terms of shorter duration of action (which may or may not be desirable) and less propensity to hypotension than morphine, but morphine is generally well tolerated and is reliable and inexpensive.

Endotracheal suctioning should be performed regularly on ventilated patients. The appropriate frequency of suctioning is a balance between the need for clearing secretions (especially in pulmonary edema or asthma) and the hazard of interrupting ventilation. Orally intubated patients should have a bite-block placed to protect the ETT.

"Fighting-the-ventilator" behavior by a previously calm patient ("bucking" may occur immediately after intubation and with the initiation of mechanical ventilation) may indicate undersedation, but sedation should not be given until a detailed evaluation excludes a specific problem with the patient or the ventilator. The differential diagnosis, after initial acclimatization, includes ETT migration, ETT occlusion, pneumothorax, bronchospasm, pulmonary edema, acute pulmonary embolism, dynamic hyperinflation, abdominal distention, ventilator problems, and patient-ventilator asynchrony.[25] Most of these problems also manifest an elevated PIP. ETT placement can be checked by capnometry, physical examination, and chest radiography. ETT patency should be assessed by passing a suction catheter.

The diagnoses of pulmonary edema, pneumothorax, and bronchospasm can be made clinically, with chest radiography used as an adjunct. Pulmonary embolism in a ventilated patient may be an even more elusive diagnosis than in other emergency department patients. Abdominal distention should be apparent clinically and is relieved by passage of a nasogastric or orogastric tube. Dynamic hyperinflation and ventilator problems may be diagnosed by momentarily disconnecting the ventilator. In the former, allowing full exhalation results in improvement; in the latter, the patient can be ventilated satisfactorily with a bag and 100% oxygen.

Patient-ventilator asynchrony results from excessive or asynchronous breathing by the patient, which impairs machine-driven inspiration. This problem indicates an improper mode selection, improper flow trigger sensitivity for A/C or SIMV modes, intolerance of PSV, dynamic hyperinflation, or poor tolerance of mechanical ventilation despite sedation. In the last case, there is an indication for increased sedation and often neuromuscular blockade.

Paralysis also is indicated for any condition in which complete rest of the patient's respiratory muscles is desired. Nondepolarizing neuromuscular blocking agents should be used for ventilator maintenance. An appropriate dose of pancuronium or vecuronium for paralysis is 0.08 to 0.10 mg/kg intravenously, or approximately 5 to 10 mg for the average patient. Additional doses, at approximately 25% of the paralyzing dose, can be given when patient response indicates return of motor activity. A reasonable initiating sedative/neuromuscular blocking agent regimen for intubated, mechanically ventilated patients in the emergency department is diazepam, 0.2 mg/kg, with pancuronium or vecuronium, 0.1 mg/kg, supplemented as needed by repeat doses of diazepam (0.1 mg/kg) and pancuronium or vecuronium (0.025 mg/kg), perhaps every 30 to 60 minutes.

Patients treated in the emergency department with NPPV generally should not be given sedatives or major analgesics because preservation of respiratory drive is essential to the use of these modes. Small, incremental doses of benzodiazepines for patients who have difficulty tolerating the face mask or nose mask may be useful.[26]

Special Clinical Circumstances

In the following five common clinical indications for mechanical ventilation in the emergency department, special fine-tuning adjustments to the guidelines offered previously may be appropriate (see Table 2-1).

Acute Exacerbation of Chronic Obstructive Pulmonary Disease

In managing patients with COPD on the ventilator, respiratory acidosis should be corrected gradually over hours. Overcorrection or too-rapid correction of hypercapnia and acidosis may result in metabolic alkalosis, hypokalemia, and hypophosphatemia.[27] Hypoxemia usually is easily correctable by increasing FIO_2. Target values for PaO_2, $PaCO_2$, and pH should reflect the patient's predicted (or known) baseline function rather than usual "normal" values.

The other major goal in the mechanical ventilation of patients with COPD is normalization of lung volume. Air trapping and resultant iPEEP in a patient with COPD increase work of breathing and the likelihood of barotrauma with mechanical ventilation. Strategies used to address this problem center on reducing iPEEP. When inadequate expiratory time is allowed in the COPD patient, air trapping is exacerbated with each inspiration; this *dynamic hyperinflation* eventually results in a sufficiently high iPEEP that the inhaled volume cannot overcome the exhaled volume. The immediate remedy for this problem is to disconnect the patient from the ventilator momentarily, allowing complete exhalation. The ongoing solution is to build adequate expiratory time into the ventilator settings. The rate should be kept as low as possible for patients with COPD, and the expiratory time should be maximized by increasing the I/E ratio to 1:3 or 1:4. The V_T also should be minimized to reduce exhaled volumes. Often patients with COPD require higher flow rates ($\geq$100 L/min) during inspiration to minimize inspiratory time. This approach allows more of the ventilatory cycle to be spent in exhalation. Each of these modifications in the settings reduces iPEEP.

The iPEEP also may be reduced by the use of bronchodilators and corticosteroids. These agents increase inspiratory muscle strength and reduce the amount of secretions in the bronchial lumen, both of which decrease work of breathing. Finally, iPEEP can be replaced in part by extrinsic PEEP. PEEP at a level of no more than the measured iPEEP (some authors suggest no more than 85% of iPEEP) unloads the work required to maintain iPEEP and allows the recruitment of the muscles providing the inspiratory effort. A consensus statement has suggested that BL-PAP should be the initial ventilatory assistance modality of choice in COPD exacerbation.[27]

Status Asthmaticus

Interventions aimed at reducing hypercapnia in ventilated patients with status asthmaticus may result in dynamic hyperinflation and barotrauma. The best approach to use in these patients, similar to that used in COPD, is small V_T and high inspiratory flow rates to reduce inspiratory time and peak airway pressures. Pressures also can be lowered by *permissive hypercapnia,* which uses a low V_T (5 to 8 mL/kg) *and* relatively low rates to prevent excessive alveolar distention. $PaCO_2$ is allowed to remain at greater than 40 mm Hg without ventilatory correction. The primary goal of permissive hypercapnia is the reduction of lung volume (and iPEEP) and the risk of barotraumas, while maintaining adequate oxygenation. This approach has not been studied thoroughly under controlled conditions, but permissive hypercapnia has potential applicability in status asthmaticus, ARDS, and severe COPD exacerbations.[28] Occasional external chest compression also may be useful in assisting exhalation in asthma. This concept has shown promise in animal and uncontrolled human trials.[29]

Acute Respiratory Distress Syndrome

ARDS typically develops over several hours, but may become evident in the emergency department. Pressure-limited special modes may be the optimal means of ventilating patients with ARDS, but these techniques are often unavailable in the emergency department. On standard ventilators, settings should be adjusted to keep PEEP and FiO_2 as low as possible. Small V_T (6 to 8 mL/kg) and fast rates (20 to 25 breaths/min) are indicated.[30] Although PEEP is considered primary therapy for ARDS, these patients are highly susceptible to barotrauma. The risk of oxygen toxicity in ARDS also is high and can be minimized by titrating the inspired oxygen concentration to less than 50% as rapidly as possible.

Cardiogenic Shock and Pulmonary Edema

The ventilatory management of pulmonary edema with cardiogenic shock is complicated by the adverse effect of applied PEEP, which is ordinarily a primary mode of therapy for pulmonary edema, on cardiac output. A reasonable compromise is to use only sufficient PEEP to allow titration of the inspired oxygen concentration down to 60% or less. Patients in cardiogenic shock require invasive hemodynamic monitoring. Hemodynamic and ventilatory parameters must be followed in tandem to achieve optimal benefit.

Patients with less severe pulmonary edema secondary to congestive heart failure often may benefit from noninvasive ventilatory support while receiving appropriate pharmacologic therapy. CPAP and BL-PAP have been studied in this setting, and a study indicated that there may be little difference between the two modes in either safety or efficacy.[31]

Hypovolemic Shock

Appropriate volume resuscitation is the optimal means of managing respiratory compromise after trauma or with other causes of hypovolemic shock (e.g., massive gastrointestinal hemorrhage). PPV may exacerbate hypotension in hypovolemic patients. Patients in shock should be ventilated with 100% oxygen at a rate and V_T predicted to produce near-physiologic $PaCO_2$. PEEP generally should be avoided until circulating volume is restored.

OUTCOMES

When NPPV is successful (i.e., when endotracheal intubation–mechanical ventilation is avoided), several potential therapeutic, patient comfort, and fiscal benefits are derived. The advantages of NPPV over endotracheal intubation–mechanical ventilation include (1) preservation of speech, swallowing, and physiologic airway defense mechanisms; (2) reduced risk of airway injury; (3) reduced risk of nosocomial infection; and (4) decreased length of stay in, and reduced need for admission to, the intensive care unit (ICU) because less weaning and less intensive monitoring are necessary.[26,32-35]

Patients treated with NPPV have an increased risk of pulmonary barotrauma, aerophagia, and pressure stress to the face compared with intubated and ventilated patients. (BL-PAP is a leak-tolerant system so that pressure sores are a much less common complication of extended BL-PAP support than of CPAP or MMV.) In two series, patients successfully supported in the emergency department with NPPV usually could be admitted to a telemetry unit instead of an ICU, with significant cost savings.[12,34] Uncontrolled studies without definitive inclusion criteria found NPPV successful in avoiding endotracheal intubation–mechanical ventilation in 60% to 90% of patients.[13,14] One study[36] showed increased mortality from the use of NPPV, which was attributed to a delay in necessary intubation; the study suffered from selection bias, however, and its results have not been corroborated.[20]

Management of mechanically ventilated patients usually extends beyond the emergency department. Adequate resuscitation and stabilization are the primary emergency department goals so that more focused therapy of the underlying problems can be pursued in the ICU. Occasionally, patients are extubated in the emergency department, most often patients intubated solely for airway protection when the initial insult has been reversed or adequately tolerated. Adequate ventilatory drive and oxygen must be confirmed before emergency department extubation; before attempting to discontinue mechanical ventilation, patients should have a respiratory rate less than 30 breaths/min, PEEP 5 cm H_2O or less, and PaO_2 greater than 60 mm Hg with FIO_2 less than 60%. NPPV may serve as a bridge between mechanical and spontaneous ventilation.

EVOLVING THERAPIES

Newer modes of ventilatory therapy gaining acceptance in the ICU eventually may become part of emergency department therapy. *Inverse ratio ventilation* (IRV) is mechanical ventilation with an extended inspiratory time (i.e., I/E ratio <1:2). The first efficacious use of IRV was in infants with hyaline membrane disease, but subsequently, ARDS has been the focus of most trials of IRV. In ARDS, I/E ratios of 4:1 have shown promise.[37] The purpose of IRV in ARDS is to maintain oxygenation at lower levels of PEEP and airway pressures, minimizing barotrauma. IRV can be accomplished with a volume-cycled, low inspiratory flow rate or by pressure-controlled ventilation, both of which can be used to prolong inspiratory time. Patients must be heavily sedated and usually paralyzed to permit effective use of IRV.

Airway pressure release ventilation may be used invasively or noninvasively. It augments spontaneous breathing with CPAP. The patient's inspiration is aided by CPAP, which reduces work of breathing, then expiration is allowed by periodically releasing the CPAP to a lower level. Spontaneous breathing is unrestricted at both levels, and the intended result is cardiostable ventilation. This modality was designed specifically for patients with severe restrictive lung disease, who poorly tolerate PPV because of their susceptibility to barotrauma and cardiac depression.[38]

High-frequency ventilation is a generic term for any mode of mechanical ventilation that supplies small V_T at rates of more than 60 breaths/min. High-frequency ventilation is jet ventilation that augments V_T by entraining additional airway gases and delivering 2 to 5 mL/kg at 60 to 80 breaths/min.[30,39,40] Although high-frequency ventilation has minimal potential utility in the emergency department, it may have utility in acute respiratory failure with circulatory shock, in which it may cause less cardiac depression than conventional mechanical ventilation plus PEEP.[41]

Proportional assist ventilation is an approach to ventilatory support in which the ventilator responds to each spontaneous breath in an independent manner. This modality augments patient effort, but leaves the patient completely in control of all aspects of breathing. For a given breath, the pressures, volumes, times, and flows may differ from previous and subsequent breaths. The use of proportional assist ventilation may allow for assisted ventilation with relatively low peak airway pressures and less risk of barotrauma or cardiac depression.[42]

Use of NPPV in the emergency department also is likely to expand. Although these techniques are used commonly in the ICU, they have been gaining acceptance among emergency physicians only more recently. The most promise for benefit to emergency department patients from NPPV use is simply expanding its application (i.e., wider use of BL-PAP and CPAP to avoid endotracheal intubation–mechanical ventilation and its attendant complications). Fiscal pressure to avoid unnecessary endotracheal intubation–mechanical ventilation and correspondingly long ICU stays also may drive expansion of this therapy.

Another potential area of development of NPPV is in the treatment of acute asthma. Although inspiratory pressure support for asthma seems reasonable, the application of CPAP or EPAP is less intuitive. Nevertheless, preliminary studies have shown potential benefits when BL-PAP is used to deliver β-agonist therapy or as respiratory support.[43] Better evidence is needed before conclusions can be drawn, but the persistent, significant mortality from status asthmaticus is a stimulus for further study.

 KEY CONCEPTS

- Patients who require intensive ventilatory support in the emergency department do not require endotracheal intubation–mechanical ventilation. Careful patient selection for noninvasive ventilatory support may spare some patients invasive therapy and its attendant risk of complications.

- The "rule of tens" (V_T of 10 mL/kg, rate of 10 breaths/min, FIO_2 of 1.0) is a reasonable starting point for mechanical ventilator settings for patients whose primary pathology is not pulmonary. For patients with pulmonary pathology, settings specific for the etiology of the patient's respiratory failure should be used, then carefully adjusted based on clinical response.

- Sudden difficulty in the management of patients receiving NPPV usually is the result of intolerance, barotrauma, or EPAP/CPAP exceeding iPEEP. Intolerance should not be assumed until other causes are excluded.

- Sudden difficulty in the management of patients receiving mechanical ventilation should prompt a quick and systematic evaluation for tube, ventilator, and physiologic problems; such difficulties must not be automatically assumed to result from undersedation.

- The goal of therapy in patients with obstructive lung disease is *not* prompt normalization of blood gas parameters. Slow correction to a patient-specific baseline likely results in significantly better clinical outcomes.

REFERENCES

1. Tobin MJ: Current concepts: Mechanical ventilation. *N Engl J Med* 330:1056, 1994.
2. Bone RC, Eubanks DH: The basis and basics of mechanical ventilation. *Dis Mon* 37:321, 1991.
3. Kacmarek RM, Hess DR: *Essentials of Mechanical Ventilation.* New York, McGraw-Hill/Appleton & Lange, 2002.
4. Banner MJ, Lampotang S: Mechanical ventilators: Fundamentals. In Stock MC, Perel A (eds): *Handbook of Mechanical Ventilatory Support,* 2nd ed. Philadelphia, Lippincott Williams & Wilkins, 1997.
5. Slutsky AS: ACCP Consensus Conference: Mechanical ventilation. *Chest* 104:1833, 1993.
6. Irwin RS: Mechanical ventilation. In Rippe JM, et al (eds): *Intensive Care Medicine,* 5th ed. Philadelphia, Lippincott Williams & Wilkins, 2003.
7. Rossi A, Polese G, De Sandre G: Respiratory failure in chronic airflow obstruction: Recent advances and therapeutic implications in the critically ill patient. *Eur J Med* 1:349, 1992.
8. Shivaram U, et al: Cardiopulmonary responses to continuous positive airway pressure in acute asthma. *J Crit Care* 8:87, 1993.
9. IPPB Trial Group: Intermittent positive pressure breathing therapy of chronic obstructive pulmonary disease. *Ann Intern Med* 99:612, 1983.
10. Bersten AD, et al: Treatment of severe cardiogenic pulmonary edema with continuous positive airway pressure delivered by face mask. *N Engl J Med* 325:1825, 1991.
11. Sullivan MP, et al: Continuous positive airway pressure in the prehospital treatment of acute pulmonary edema. *Ann Emerg Med* 25:129, 1995.
12. Pollack CV, Torres M, Alexander L: A feasibility study of the use of bilevel positive airway pressure for respiratory support in the emergency department. *Ann Emerg Med* 27:189, 1996.
13. Keenan SP, et al: Effect of noninvasive positive pressure ventilation on mortality in patients admitted with acute respiratory failure: A meta-analysis. *Crit Care Med* 25:1685, 1997.
14. Poponick JM, Renston JP, Bennett RP, Emerman CL: Use of a ventilatory system (BiPAP) for acute respiratory failure in the emergency department. *Chest* 116:166, 1999.
15. Fernandez MM, et al: Noninvasive mechanical ventilation in status asthmaticus. *Intens Care Med* 27:486, 2001.
16. Soroksky A, Stav D, Shpirer I: A pilot prospective, randomized, placebo-controlled trial of bilevel positive airway pressure in acute asthmatic attack. *Chest* 123:1018, 2003.
17. Vitacca M, et al: Non-invasive modalities of positive pressure ventilation improve the outcome of acute exacerbations in COPD patients. *Intensive Care Med* 19:450, 1993.
18. Carrey Z, Gottfried SB, Levy RD: Ventilatory muscle support in respiratory failure with nasal positive pressure ventilation. *Chest* 97:150, 1990.
19. Bott J, Carroll MP, Conway JH: Randomised controlled trial of nasal ventilation in acute ventilatory failure due to chronic obstructive airways disease. *Lancet* 341:1555, 1993.
20. Liesching T, Kwok H, Hill NS: Acute applications of noninvasive positive pressure ventilation. *Chest* 124:699, 2003.
21. Freichels TA: Palliative ventilatory support: Use of noninvasive positive pressure ventilation in terminal respiratory insufficiency. *Am J Crit Care* 3:6, 1994.
22. Ambrosino N, et al: Physiologic evaluation of pressure support ventilation by nasal mask in patients with stable COPD. *Chest* 101:385, 1992.
23. Dreyfuss D, Saumon G: Barotrauma is volutrauma, but which volume is the one responsible? *Intensive Care Med* 18:139, 1992.
24. Manning HL: Peak airway pressure: Why the fuss? *Chest* 105:242, 1994.
25. Tobin MJ, Fahey PJ: Management of the patient who is "fighting the ventilator." In Tobin MJ (ed): *Principles and Practice of Mechanical Ventilation.* New York, McGraw-Hill, 1994.
26. Hill NS: Noninvasive ventilation: Does it work, for whom, and how? *Am Rev Respir Dis* 147:1050, 1993.
27. Honig EG: Chronic obstructive pulmonary disease and asthma. In Stock MC, Perel A (eds): *Handbook of Mechanical Ventilatory Support,* 2nd ed. Philadelphia, Lippincott Williams & Wilkins, 1997.
28. Tuxen DV: Permissive hypercapnic ventilation. *Am J Respir Crit Care Med* 150:870, 1994.
29. Van der Touw T, et al: Cardiorespiratory consequences of expiratory chest wall compression during mechanical ventilation and severe hyperinflation. *Crit Care Med* 21:1908, 1993.
30. Eichacker PQ, et al: Meta-analysis of acute lung injury and acute respiratory distress syndrome trials with low tidal volumes. *Am J Respir Crit Care Med* 166:1510, 2002.
31. Cross AM, et al: Non-invasive ventilation in acute respiratory failure: A randomised comparison of continuous positive airway pressure and bi-level positive airway pressure. *Emerg Med J* 20:531, 2003.
32. Antonelli M, et al: A comparison of noninvasive positive-pressure ventilation and conventional mechanical ventilation in patients with acute respiratory failure. *N Engl J Med* 339:429, 1998.
33. Meyer TJ, Hill NS: Noninvasive positive pressure ventilation to treat respiratory failure. *Ann Intern Med* 120:760, 1994.
34. Celikel T, et al: Comparison of noninvasive positive pressure ventilation with standard medical therapy in hypercapnic acute respiratory failure. *Chest* 114:1636, 1998.
35. Keenan SP, et al: Noninvasive positive pressure ventilation in the setting of severe, acute exacerbations of chronic obstructive pulmonary disease: more effective and less expensive. *Crit Care Med* 28:2094, 2000.
36. Wood KA, et al: The use of noninvasive positive pressure ventilation in the emergency department: Results of a randomized clinical trial. *Chest* 113:1339, 1998.
37. Wang SH, Wei TS: The outcome of early pressure-controlled inverse ratio ventilation on patients with severe acute respiratory distress syndrome in the surgical intensive care unit. *Am J Surg* 183:151, 2002.
38. Sydow M, et al: Long-term effects of two different ventilatory modes on oxygenation in acute lung injury: Comparison of airway pressure release ventilation and volume-controlled inverse ratio ventilation. *Am J Respir Crit Care Med* 149:1550, 1994.
39. Derdak S, et al: High-frequency oscillatory ventilation for acute respiratory distress syndrome in adults: A randomized, controlled trial, Multicenter Oscillatory ventilation for Acute respiratory distress syndrome Trial (MOAT). *Am J Respir Crit Care Med* 166:801, 2002.
40. Burchardi H: New strategies in mechanical ventilation for acute lung injury. *Eur Respir J* 9:1063, 1996.
41. Herridge MS, Slutsky AS, Colditz GA: Has high-frequency ventilation been inappropriately discarded in adult acute respiratory distress syndrome? *Crit Care Med* 26:2073, 1998.
42. Wrigge H: Proportional assist versus pressure support ventilation: Effects on breathing pattern and respiratory work of patients with chronic obstructive pulmonary disease. *Intensive Care Med* 25:790, 1999.
43. Pollack CV, Fleisch KB, Dowsey K: Treatment of acute bronchospasm with beta-adrenergic aerosols delivered via a Bi-PAP circuit. *Ann Emerg Med* 26:547, 1995.

CHAPTER 3

Monitoring the Emergency Patient

Michael F. Murphy and Timothy A. D. Graham

PERSPECTIVE

To *monitor* means to measure or observe a physiologic parameter either continuously or intermittently. The monitoring device may provide a "snapshot in time" or may detect deterioration, track improvement, or measure the effects of interventions. Monitoring parameters, such as clinical observation, routine vital sign measurement, and electrocardiogram monitoring, are basic requirements in emergency medicine. This chapter addresses newer technologies, such as pulse oximetry, end-tidal carbon dioxide (CO_2) measurement, sublingual capnography, and noninvasive blood pressure (BP) measurement. Fetal monitoring immediately after maternal trauma also is discussed briefly. The following questions are important with respect to monitoring:

1. Which physiologic parameters are important indicators of status or progression?
2. What technology monitors that parameter?
3. Can the monitoring device be relied on to do so with precision and accuracy in this particular clinical situation? In other words, what are the limitations of the technology? (For example, is a noninvasive monitor of BP adequate for the management of a hypertensive crisis with sodium nitroprusside?) In which clinical situations are the data provided potentially inaccurate?
4. What is the role of the emergency department in the management of this particular problem? The best example of this question relates to the appropriateness of inserting pulmonary artery catheters in the emergency department. Is the emergency department an extension of the intensive care unit (ICU)?
5. Does the expected standard of care demand a certain level of monitoring?

NONINVASIVE BLOOD PRESSURE MEASUREMENT

Automatic, noninvasive measurement has become a popular and, if applied to appropriate clinical situations, an accurate method of determining BP. Advantages include (1) more time for staff to attend to other tasks; (2) timed repetition of BP measurements; (3) continuous display of the systolic pressure; and (4) a display of other several parameters (e.g., systolic, diastolic, and mean BP; pulse rate), depending on the machinery.

Noninvasive machines use a detection system based on auscultatory, oscillometric, or Doppler principles.[1,2] Automatic oscillometric devices determine BP by electronically determining the pulse amplitude. This method and Doppler are the most accurate of the indirect methods. The cuff is automatically inflated at predetermined intervals to a preset level. As the machine gradually deflates the cuff, it senses the amplitude of the oscillations (pulsations) transmitted to the cuff by movement of the arterial wall under the cuff. An abrupt increase in the magnitude of the oscillation signals an opening of the artery and an increase in volume under the cuff; this is the *systolic pressure*. The magnitude of the oscillation increases to a peak, then falls rapidly. The point where there is no longer an alteration in the magnitude of the oscillation is the *diastolic pressure*. Some machines calculate the *mean arterial pressure,* identified as the cuff pressure at the point of largest oscillation.[1]

Limitations

The shortcomings of noninvasive BP techniques are the same shortcomings of any cuff measurement technique, including patients with obese arms, uncooperative moving patients, and patients with very high or very low BP. Even with these limitations, automatic machines are more accurate, precise, and reliable than auscultation in patients with very low or very high BP, primarily because the sensing devices are more sensitive than the human ear.[2] The cycle length of the inflation-deflation sequence of the older machines was exceedingly long and led to frequent failure. Newer machines have rectified this problem.

The most accurate method of measuring BP is with an intra-arterial catheter transduced to an electronic display. The ability to identify beat-to-beat variability, respiratory variation, and longer trends is unsurpassed by any other currently available technology. In addition, the placement of the arterial catheter enables frequent sampling of arterial blood without additional arterial punctures. Arterial line pressure monitoring is used increasingly in emergency departments, particularly because lack of ICU bed availability mandates longer stays in the emergency department for critically ill patients. The risk of arterial injury or thrombosis related to arterial line insertion is low but real and can result in vascular compromise. Arterial line insertion should not delay transfer of patients to an operating room or critical care setting. Traditional methods of noninvasive BP measurement are often inadequate in the following situations, and invasive monitoring should be considered:

1. Exceedingly high (>250 mm Hg systolic) or low (<80 mm Hg systolic) BPs. Although the invasive method also is less accurate at these extremes than in the physiologic range, the error is significantly less.
2. Many clinicians believe that any patient receiving sodium nitroprusside should have continuous invasive monitoring because of rapid fluctuations in blood pressure, although this is unsupported in the literature.
3. In a patient who is rapidly going into shock, the best chance to insert an arterial line may be in the emergency department while the arterial pulse is still palpable, although this should not be allowed to delay transfer to a more appropriate location for definitive care.
4. Anatomic indications for invasive monitoring include patients who are critically ill and either have no limb or no have suitable limb (e.g., too obese) to undertake conventional measurement.
5. Frequent arterial sampling is required. The requirement in such cases is for vascular access rather than the monitoring modality per se. Patients who are ill enough to require frequent arterial sampling usually benefit from continuous arterial BP monitoring.

BLOOD GAS MONITORING

Although the ability to monitor oxygen usage at the level of the individual cell or group of cells might be considered ideal, current technology allows less precise measures of performance. Transcutaneous oxygen and CO_2 monitoring, conjunctival oxygen pressure, pulse oximetry, and end-tidal CO_2 measurements (capnography, capnometry) all are used to indicate the adequacy of pulmonary gas exchange and arterial blood gas tensions and to assess ventilatory efficacy. Sublingual capnography is emerging as a valuable modality in detecting early shock and visceral hypoperfusion.[3]

Transcutaneous and Conjunctival Monitors

Transcutaneous ($PtCO_2$) and conjunctival ($PcjO_2$) systems of oxygen pressure monitoring use the Clark polarographic oxygen electrode, the same device used in blood gas machines. The skin must be heated to obtain reliable PO_2 readings with rapid response times when transcutaneous devices are used. The sensor actually measures epidermal tissue PO_2. Conjunctival devices do not require heating.[4] $PtCO_2$ and $PcjO_2$ are significantly influenced by cardiac output, local tissue metabolism, and capillary blood flow. The utility of these devices in emergency medicine has been mostly in relation to their ability to reflect tissue perfusion in situations of reduced or absent cardiac output as an early indicator of gas exchange difficulty and cardiopulmonary deterioration.[5] This modality has been used most extensively and appropriately in the neonatal ICU and in medical air transport.[4] Slow calibration

and response times relative to other modalities (e.g., oximetry) make $PtCO_2$ and $PcjO_2$ devices less useful for the noninvasive monitoring of arterial oxygen saturation in the emergency department.

$PtCO_2$ monitors generally use a miniature, heated electrode that is pH sensitive. The same technical limitations apply to these devices. Technologic developments should eliminate these shortcomings in the future to make these devices more useful in the emergency department and field environment.

Pulse Oximetry

The pulse oximeter provides a noninvasive and continuous means of rapidly determining arterial oxygen saturation and its changes. The devices are easy to use and interpret, pose no risk to the patient, and are relatively inexpensive.[6] A reliable interpretation of the information given by these devices requires an appreciation of their limitations in certain situations.

Transmission oximetry is based on differences in the optical transmission spectrum of oxygenated and deoxygenated hemoglobin. Specifically, the physics and physiology of oximetry are based on the Beer-Lambert law, which relates the concentration of a solute to the intensity of light transmitted through a solution.[7] Light absorption is related to the concentration of the solute and a constant called the *extinction coefficient*. This extinction coefficient is constant for a given solute at a specified wavelength. At the wavelength of red light (660 nm), reduced hemoglobin absorbs about 10 times as much light as oxyhemoglobin, whereas at the infrared (IR) wavelength (940 nm), the extinction coefficient of oxyhemoglobin is near that of reduced hemoglobin.[7] In addition to arterial hemoglobin, other absorbers in the light path include skin, soft tissue, and venous and capillary blood. Pulse oximeters measure red and IR light transmitted through a tissue bed and in particular the pulse variations in that transmission.[6] The light sources are light-emitting diodes, and the detectors are photodiodes.[7] The light absorption is divided into a pulsatile (AC) component related to the pulsatile arterial blood and a nonpulsatile (DC) component related to the tissue bed, including venous and capillary blood and nonpulsatile arterial blood. The digital microprocessor of the pulse oximeter first determines the AC component of absorbance at each wavelength and divides this value by the corresponding DC component to obtain a "pulse-added" absorbance. The device calculates the ratio of these pulse-added absorbances, a nonlinear but reproducible function of the oxygen saturation of arterial blood. The microprocessor converts this pulse-added absorbance to saturation.[7] Data averaged over several arterial pulse cycles are presented as saturation (SpO_2).[6] Studies have shown an excellent correlation between arterial hemoglobin oxygen saturation and SpO_2.[6,7]

Limitations to the value of pulse oximetry exist with severe vasoconstriction (e.g., shock, hypothermia), excessive movement, synthetic fingernails and nail polish, severe anemia, or the presence of abnormal hemoglobins. The extinction coefficients for carboxyhemoglobin (COHb) and methemoglobin (MetHb) are not zero in the red and IR range. Their presence contributes to light absorption and causes errors in pulse oximetry readings.[7] The pulse oximeter senses COHb as though it were mostly oxyhemoglobin and provides a falsely high reading. The MetHb produces a large pulsatile absorbance signal at the red and the IR wavelengths. This signal forces the absorbance ratio toward unity, which corresponds to an SpO_2 of 85%.[7] With high levels of MetHb, the SpO_2 is erroneously low when the arterial saturation is greater than 85% and erroneously high when the arterial saturation is less than 85%. Erroneously high readings (about 3% to 5%) and a higher incidence of failure to detect signals have been reported in dark-skinned races.[6]

In general, signals are weaker from ears than from fingers except in hypotension or peripheral vasoconstriction, but ear responses are faster. Nasal bridge probes have been reported to read falsely high. In children particularly, it is essential to be certain the signals are adequate; a valid pulse reading can be of some reassurance.

Pulse oximetry is particularly useful in the emergency department evaluation of patients with acute cardiopulmonary disorders, such as bronchiolitis, asthma, heart failure, and chronic obstructive pulmonary disease (COPD), but is valuable in any patient for whom continuous knowledge of oxygen levels is of value in their management.[8] It is a standard monitoring parameter for patients undergoing procedural analgesia and sedation and in patients with a decreased level of consciousness, such as intoxication, overdose, and head injury.[8,9] The ability of pulse oximetry to decrease the frequency with which arterial blood gas readings are obtained also has been shown.[8] Improvements in pulse oximeter technology have resulted in significantly better accuracy and reliability during patient motion. Continuous monitoring may indicate the insidious development of shock as vasoconstriction and deterioration of signal detection develops. Continuous oximetry is mandatory in patients requiring definitive airway management. This valuable device has become an established component of the monitoring armamentarium of the emergency physician.[10,11] Adequate oxygen saturation does not ensure adequate *ventilation,* however, particularly in patients with decreased levels of consciousness. Also, a normal oxygen saturation does not preclude the presence of a pulmonary embolus.

Capnography/Capnometry: End-Tidal Carbon Dioxide

CO_2 concentration in exhaled gases is intrinsically linked to tissue metabolism, systemic circulation, and ventilation.[12] Capnography is the graphic record of instantaneous CO_2 concentrations (capnogram) in the respired gases during a respiratory cycle.[13] This record may be qualitative or quantitative, although typically only the end-tidal CO_2 concentration is displayed quantitatively. Capnometry is the measurement and display of CO_2 concentrations on a visual display; the usual concentration displayed is the end-tidal CO_2. Although traditionally a parameter followed during general anesthesia in the operating room, end-tidal CO_2 monitoring is becoming increasingly common in the emergency department and prehospital setting. More than 80% of emergency medicine training programs in the United States use CO_2 monitoring, with colorimetric devices being the most frequently used.[14] The remaining programs did not use them, in direct conflict with what some authorities would say is the standard of care for the verification of tracheal placement of an endotracheal tube (ETT).[15]

Four spectrographic methods are used to measure end-tidal CO_2 concentration in expired gases: IR, mass, Raman, and photoacoustic spectrography.[12,13] Most stand-alone units use the IR technique. CO_2 selectively absorbs IR light with a wavelength of 4.26 μm. The concentration of the CO_2 in a gas can be determined by passing filtered IR light through the gas in question and comparing the amount of light that is absorbed with a reference light beam passing through a CO_2-free chamber.[12]

Capnometers are either sidestream or mainstream in design. *Sidestream capnometers* are more likely to be encountered in the emergency department and work by aspirating a sample of gas through a small catheter into a measuring chamber. They are lightweight, can be used in intubated and nonintubated patients, and have been incorporated into commercially available nasal prong oxygen delivery apparatus to facilitate CO_2 monitoring during procedural sedation. Disadvantages include plugging by secretions, 2- or 3-second delays in response time, and air leaks, which can dilute the sample.[12] *Mainstream capnometers* are useful only in intubated patients; they are bulky and heavy; and because they must be heated to prevent condensation, they may burn patients.

Colorimetric capnometers use color scales to estimate ranges of end-tidal CO_2 but are not accurate enough to give quantitative measurements. They use pH-sensitive filter paper impregnated with metacresol purple, which changes color from purple (<4 mm Hg CO_2) to tan (4 to 15 mm Hg CO_2) to yellow (>20 mm Hg CO_2) depending on the concentration of CO_2, although there is some variability in absolute numbers based on the brand of device (see Chapter 1, Figures 1-3 and 1-4).[12,16] The indicator, housed in a plastic casing, is inserted between the ETT and the ventilator bag and responds quickly enough to detect changes on a breath-by-breath basis.[13] Colorimetric capnometers are inexpensive and easy to use and should be available in every emergency department for confirmation of ETT placement if quantitative methods are not available.

Usually a close correlation exists between end-tidal CO_2 and arterial CO_2 partial pressure ($PaCO_2$). In patients who are otherwise healthy, the end-tidal CO_2 is usually 2 to 5 mm Hg less than the $PaCO_2$ because of the contribution of physiologic dead space to the end-tidal gases.[12,14] Many conditions that affect ventilation-perfusion ratios can widen the $PaCO_2$–end-tidal CO_2 gradient, including pulmonary embolism, cardiac arrest, hypovolemia, asthma, COPD, and the lateral

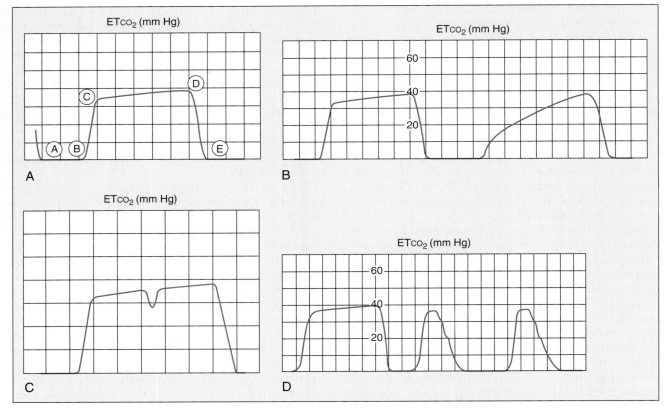

Figure 3-1. Four phases of a normal capnogram. **A-B,** The carbon dioxide–free portion of the respiratory cycle. **B-C,** The rapid upstroke of the curve, representing the transition from inspiration to expiration and the mixing of dead space and alveolar gas. **C-D,** The alveolar plateau, representing the alveolar gas rich in carbon dioxide and tending to slope gently upward with the uneven emptying of the alveoli. **D-E,** The respiratory downstroke, which is a nearly vertical drop to baseline.

decubitus position.[12,17] Although end-tidal CO_2 may not always reflect the absolute $PaCO_2$ in critically ill patients accurately, it is still valuable in detecting trends and sudden airway events.

Phases

A normal capnogram has four phases (Figure 3-1A). Phase A-B represents a *CO_2-free* portion of the respiratory cycle. Most often this is the inspiratory phase, although it may represent apnea or a disconnection of the device from the patient. Increase in this baseline implies rebreathing of CO_2, as in increased dead space in the circuit, hypoventilation, or contamination of the sensor.[12]

Phase B-C, the *rapid upstroke* of the curve, represents the transition from inspiration to expiration and the mixing of dead space and alveolar gas. Prolongation of phase B-C (Figure 3-1B) occurs with obstruction to expiratory gas flow (e.g., asthma, bronchospasm, COPD, kinked ETT[12]) or leaks in the breathing system.

Phase C-D, the *alveolar plateau,* represents alveolar gas rich in CO_2 and tends to slope gently upward with the uneven emptying of alveoli. The end-tidal CO_2 that is measured and read by capnometry represents *point D*. The slope of this phase can be increased by the same obstructive factors that increase the slope of phase B-C and is a normal physiologic variation in pregnancy.[13] A dip in the plateau indicates a spontaneous respiratory

effort during mechanical ventilation, as in hypoxia, hypercarbia, or oligoanesthesia (Figure 3-1C).[12,13]

Phase D-E, the *inspiratory downstroke,* is a nearly vertical drop to baseline. This slope can be prolonged and blend in with the expiratory phase with ETT cuff leaks (Figure 3-1D). Abnormal respiratory patterns that are fast or chaotic limit the usefulness of end-tidal CO_2 monitoring.

Uses

Capnography is used in the emergency department in several clinical scenarios. It can confirm ETT placement; estimate $PaCO_2$; monitor the effectiveness of cardiopulmonary resuscitation (CPR) and mechanical ventilation; and during procedural sedation. Capnography may be used in the future to diagnose asthma and pulmonary embolism and to measure cardiac output.

Along with visualizing an ETT going through the vocal cords, capnometry is the other "gold standard" used to confirm intubation of the trachea. Misleading end-tidal CO_2 readings can occur with esophageal intubation after bag/mask ventilation and ingestion of carbonated beverages or antacids. These tracings usually resolve after six breaths and look abnormal.[16,18] End-tidal CO_2 also is falsely elevated for about 5 minutes after the injection of bicarbonate.[18] In nonarrest settings, the end-tidal CO_2 approaches 100% sensitivity and specificity in confirming correct tube placement; conversely, it is also useful to monitor for accidental extubation.

End-tidal CO_2 can estimate $PaCO_2$ in hemodynamically stable patients who do not have rapidly progressive lung pathology.[18] The $PaCO_2$–end-tidal CO_2 gradient is usually 2 to 5 mm Hg, but this may increase to 15 mm Hg in patients with hemodynamic instability and pulmonary complications.[17,18] It may be helpful initially to compare a serum $PaCO_2$ determination with the end-tidal CO_2 to determine what magnitude of gradient is present in a particularly unstable patient. With correction for this gradient, trends in end-tidal CO_2 generally can be used as a substitute for $PaCO_2$ measurements.

Sidestream sampling of spontaneously breathing nonintubated patients is a reliable technique for monitoring hypoventilation and apnea.[12] It can be used to monitor patients undergoing procedural sedation in the emergency department.

Animal and human studies have shown that end-tidal CO_2 is a useful noninvasive measurement that is highly correlated with cardiac output and can help in predicting return of spontaneous circulation in CPR.[19] Return of spontaneous circulation is heralded by an almost immediate increase in end-tidal CO_2. Two studies showed that end-tidal CO_2 has prognostic value in terms of mortality during CPR.[19,20] No patient with an average end-tidal CO_2 level less than 10 mm Hg during CPR survived, giving end-tidal CO_2 measurement a high negative predictive value for failure of resuscitation. Capnography needs to be prospectively validated to confirm its utility as a monitor of adequacy of CPR and as a prognostic tool in prehospital arrest.

Asthma-induced bronchospasm can cause upward slanting of the expiratory plateau of the capnogram. Changes in end-tidal CO_2 over time have been shown to correlate well with 1-second forced expiratory volume measurements.[18] End-tidal CO_2 has the advantage of being independent of effort, gender, age, and height and might be a useful objective measure in asthmatic patients who are unwilling or unable to cooperate with 1-second forced expiratory volume testing (e.g., children, ventilated patients).

Pulmonary embolism results in the increase of the ratio of physiologic dead space in the lung to total tidal volume (V_D/V_T).[18] Hypovolemia, cardiac arrest, and the lateral decubitus position also increase V_D/V_T, but are uncommon ambulatory complaints. In the future, end-tidal CO_2 measurements correlated with V_D/V_T may allow the emergency physician to provide bedside testing to rule in or rule out pulmonary embolism in the appropriate clinical setting.[13,18]

The measurement of cardiac output requires invasive placement of pulmonary arterial catheters and is rarely done in the emergency department. Using modified forms of the direct Fick equation, animal and human studies have shown excellent correlation of end-tidal CO_2 measurements and cardiac output over a wide range of values. These measurements seem independent of changes in dead space (hypovolemia) or shunt (pulmonary edema) and might be adaptable to nonintubated patients.[18]

Sublingual Capnography

Studies in the mid-1990s identified that increases in esophageal and gastric PCO_2 ("gastric tonometry") were associated with tissue hypoxia, most commonly found in low-flow states, such as shock.[21] This finding occurred early in the clinical course of shock before more conventional global measures of tissue oxygenation, such as heart rate, blood pressure, serum lactate, and arterial blood gases, heralded tissue hypoxia. Sublingual capnography ($PslCO_2$) subsequently was found to correlate with gastric tonometry and to be a useful and noninvasive alternative to visceral PCO_2 monitoring.[3,21]

$PslCO_2$ is relatively simple to monitor. A noninvasive microelectrode CO_2 probe is placed under the tongue. A hand-held device similar in appearance to a digital thermometer (Tycohealthcare, Hazelwood, MO) provides a continuous $PslCO_2$ reading.[22] The device consists of three major components: a disposable CO_2 sensor, a fiberoptic cable that connects the disposable sensor to a blood gas analyzer, and a blood gas monitoring instrument.

Studies currently are under way to determine what absolute measures of $PslCO_2$ or trends in $PslCO_2$ would be useful in diagnosing early tissue dysoxia. One study of patients with penetrating torso trauma found that a $PslCO_2$ less than 45 mm Hg accurately predicted hemodynamic stability.[23] This technology is likely to prove useful in emergency medicine and prehospital care, where the early detection of tissue hypoxia is important and currently imprecise.

FETAL MONITORING

Trauma occurs in about 7% of pregnant women.[24] The maternal mortality in trauma is no different than that for nonpregnant women with comparable injury severity. The fetal mortality is increased, however, even with seemingly minor trauma. The American College of Obstetricians and Gynecologists recommends that a pregnant patient with a viable fetus undergo fetal monitoring for 2 to 6 hours after injury characterized as any degree of abdominal jarring.[25]

Emergency physicians usually use fetal monitoring in the emergency department to detect occult fetal distress and to inform therapy and referral. A study found that 92% of emergency medicine residents were taught the cardiotocographic findings indicative of fetal distress, although only 15% of the programs have this monitoring equipment available in the emergency department; however, 51% of programs have the sonographic equipment available to permit monitoring.[24] Figure 3-2A depicts a normal fetal heart trace with good baseline fetal heart rate. Persistent fetal tachycardia (Figure 3-2B), bradycardia, loss of baseline variability (Figure 3-2C), or decelerations after uterine contractions (Figure 3-2D) (e.g., Braxton Hicks contractions), and uterine hyperactivity are indications for referral to an obstetrician.

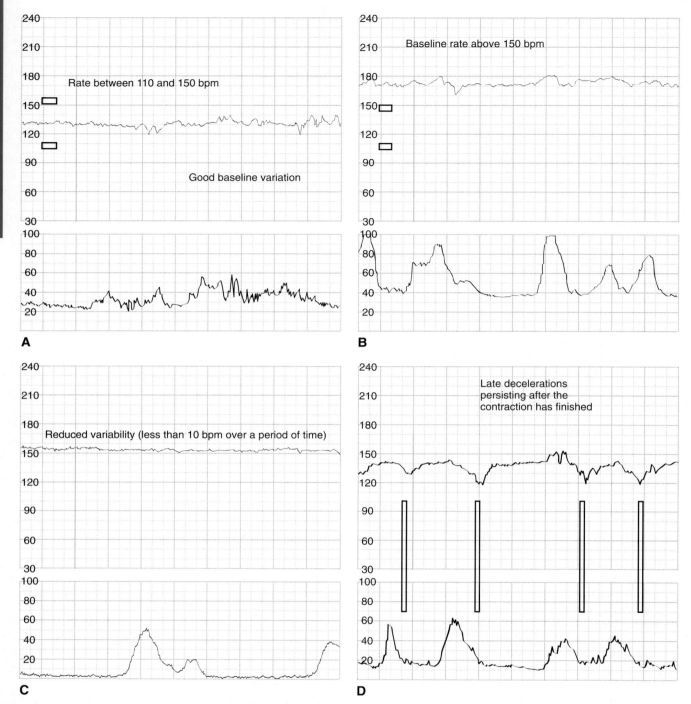

Figure 3-2. Examples of cardiotachographs. **A,** Normal trace. The fetal heart rate is the top trace; the bottom trace shows uterine activity. **B,** Fetal tachycardia. **C,** Reduced baseline heart rate variability. **D,** Late heart rate decelerations. (Courtesy Dr. C.J. Peters, Fetal Monitoring Tutorial, www.freeserve.co.uk)

KEY CONCEPTS

- Monitors do not replace the observations made by clinicians; these are decision support devices for aiding management, identifying the impacts of interventions, predicting deterioration, and following the patient's clinical course.

- Emergency personnel must know the limitations of the technology and the machinery in the clinical setting in which they work.

- Alarm limits should be adjusted to ensure reasonable warnings are delivered. Disabling alarms is dangerous.

REFERENCES

1. Ng KG: Automated noninvasive blood pressure measurement. *Intensive Care World* 12:89, 1995.
2. De Jong JR, Ros HH, De Lange JJ: Noninvasive continuous blood pressure measurement during anaesthesia: A clinical evaluation of a method commonly used in measuring devices. *Int J Clin Monit Comput* 12:1, 1995.
3. Jin X, et al: Decreases in organ blood flows associated with increases in sublingual Pco_2 during hemorrhagic shock. *J Appl Physiol* 85:2360, 1998.
4. Isenberg SJ, et al: Continuous oxygen monitoring of the conjunctiva in neonates. *J Perinatol* 22:46, 2002.
5. Abraham E, Ehrlich H: Conjunctival and transcutaneous oxygen monitoring during resuscitation. *Ann Emerg Med* 13:287, 1984.
6. Severinghaus JW: Oximetry: What does it tell you? *ASA Annual Refresher Course Lectures* 266:1, 1991.
7. Tremper KK, Barker SJ: Pulse oximetry. *Anaesthesiology* 70:98, 1989.
8. Sinex JE: Pulse oximetry: Principles and limitations. *Am J Emerg Med* 17:59, 1999.
9. Cote CJ, et al: Adverse sedation events in pediatrics: A critical incident analysis of contributing factors. *Pediatrics* 105:805, 2000.
10. Burillo-Putze G, et al: Transcranial oximetry as a new monitoring method for HEMS (Helicopter EMS). *Air Med J* 21:13, 2002.
11. Macnab AJ, et al: The cost-benefit of pulse-oximeter use in the prehospital environment. *Prehospital Disaster Med* 14:245, 1999.
12. Ward KR, Yealy DM: End-tidal carbon dioxide monitoring in emergency medicine: Part 1. Basic principles. *Acad Emerg Med* 5:628, 1998.
13. Buhre W, Rossaint R: Perioperative management and monitoring in anaesthesia. *Lancet* 29:1839, 2003.
14. Wang VJ, Krauss B: Carbon dioxide monitoring in emergency medicine training programs. *Pediatr Emerg Care* 18:251, 2002.
15. Schneider RE, Murphy MF: Bag mask ventilation and endotracheal intubation. In Walls RM, et al (eds): *Manual of Emergency Airway Management,* 2nd ed. Philadelphia, Lippincott Williams & Wilkins, 2004, pp 43-69.
16. Cardoso MM, et al: Portable devices used to detect endotracheal intubation during emergency situations: A review. *Crit Care Med* 26:957, 1998.
17. Wahba RWM, Tessler MJ: Misleading end-tidal CO_2 tensions. *Can J Anaesth* 43:862, 1996.
18. Ward KR, Yealy DM: End-tidal carbon dioxide monitoring in emergency medicine: Part 2. Clinical applications. *Acad Emerg Med* 5:637, 1998.
19. Ahrens T, et al: End-tidal carbon dioxide measurements as a prognostic indicator of outcome in cardiac arrest. *Am J Crit Care* 10:391, 2001.
20. Wayne MA, Levine RL, Miller CC: Use of end-tidal carbon dioxide to predict outcome in prehospital cardiac arrest. *Ann Emerg Med* 25:762, 1995.
21. Marik PE: Sublingual capnography: A clinical validation study. *Chest* 120:923, 2001.
22. Boswell SA, Scalea TM: Sublingual capnography: An alternative to gastric tonometry for the management of shock resuscitation. *AACN Clin Issues* 14:176, 2003.
23. Baron BJ, et al: Diagnostic utility of sublingual Pco_2 for detecting hemorrhage in patients with penetrating trauma. *Acad Emerg Med* 9:492, 2002.
24. Kolb JC, et al: Blunt trauma in the obstetric patient: monitoring practices in the ED. Am J Emerg Med 20:524, 2002.
25. An educational aid to obstetrician-gynecologists: Trauma during pregnancy. *ACOG Technical Bulletin* 161:1-5, 1991.

CHAPTER 4

Shock

Alan E. Jones and Jeffrey A. Kline

PERSPECTIVE

In philosophic terms, shock can be viewed as a transition between life and death. Whether shock results from hemorrhage, sepsis, or cardiac failure, mortality rates exceed 20%.[1,2] In scientific lexicon, shock results from the widespread failure of the circulatory system to oxygenate and nourish the body adequately. In the laboratory, the scientist defines the metabolic effect of shock quantitatively, by examining the mechanisms by which shock alters mitochondrial energy transfer, evokes the production of toxic chemicals, and reduces their removal. At the bedside, the clinician identifies shock by linking the clinical impression, synthesized from the patient's history of present illness, age, underlying health status, and general appearance, to quantitative data, including vital signs, blood chemistry, urine output, and direct measurements of oxygenation. When the clinical impression and the quantitative data suggest widespread inadequate organ perfusion, emergent resuscitation must restore normal tissue oxygenation and substrate delivery to prevent deterioration into systemic inflammation, organ dysfunction, and death.

Classification

For years, shock has been classified into four broad categories based on Blalock's 1934 description: hematological, neurologic, vasogenic, and cardiogenic.[3] Although it seems archaic to classify a gunshot wound as "hematologic" shock, this basic organization scheme remains useful today. Box 4-1 outlines five categories

BOX 4-1. Categories of Shock According to Primary Treatment

Causes That Require Primarily the Infusion of Volume
Hemorrhagic shock
 Traumatic
 Gastrointestinal
 Body cavity
Hypovolemia
 Gastrointestinal losses
 Dehydration from insensible losses
 Third-space sequestration from inflammation

Causes That Require Improvement in Pump Function by Either Infusion of Inotropic Support or Reversal of the Cause of Pump Dysfunction
Myocardial ischemia
 Coronary artery thrombosis
 Arterial hypotension with hypoxemia
Cardiomyopathy
 Acute myocarditits
 Chronic diseases of heart muscle (ischemic, diabetic, infiltrative, endocrinologic, congenital)
Cardiac rhythm disturbances
 Atrial fibrillation with rapid ventricular response
 Ventricular techycardia
 Supraventricular tachycardia
Hypodynamic septic shock (late sepsis)
Overdose of negative inotropic drug
 β-blocker
 Calcium channel antagonist overdose (e.g., verapamil)

Structural cardiac damage
 Traumatic (e.g., flail mitral valve)
 Ventriculoseptal rupture
 Papillary muscle rupture

Causes That Require Volume Support and Vasopressor Support
Hyperdynamic sepsis syndrome (early sepsis)
Anaphylactic shock
Central neurogenic shock
Drug overdose (dihydropyridines, α_1-antagonists)

Problems That Require Immediate Relief from Obstruction to Cardiac Output
Pulmonary embolism
Cardiac tamponade
Pneumothorax
Valvular dysfunction
 Acute thrombosis of prosthetic valve
 Critical aortic stenosis
Congenital heart defects in newborn (e.g., closure of patent ductus arteriosus with critical aortic coarctation)
Critical idiopathic subaortic stenosis

Cellular Poisons That Require Specific Antidotes
Carbon monoxide
Methemoglobinemia
Hydrogen sulfide
Cyanide

of shock that generally have specific mechanisms and treatments.

Epidemiology

The epidemiology of shock in the emergency department remains speculative because shock rarely is listed as a primary coding diagnosis and usually is hidden within another diagnosis. Patients presenting with traumatic, cardiogenic, or septic shock constitute about 1% of all emergency department visits. This chapter reviews the metabolic, systemic, and inflammatory responses that occur in all types of circulatory shock and discusses specific pathophysiology of the major causes of shock.

PATHOPHYSIOLOGY

At the subcellular level, shock first affects the mitochondria. Mitochondria function at the lowest oxygen tension in the body, but paradoxically, they consume almost all the oxygen used by the body. More than 95% of aerobic chemical energy comes from mitochondrial combustion of fuel substrates (fats, carbohydrates, ketones) plus oxygen into carbon dioxide and water. Mitochondria have been referred to as the "canaries in the coal mine" because they are affected first in conditions of inadequate tissue perfusion.[4,5] When mitochondria have inadequate oxygen, the cell converts fuels to lactate (Figure 4-1), which accumulates and diffuses into the blood.

Most cellular energy transfer derives from combustion of acetyl coenzyme A (CoA) in the tricarboxylic acid (TCA) cycle to form reduced pyridine and flavin nucleotides, which pass electrons along a series of proteins in the inner mitochondrial membrane, culminating in the reduction of molecular oxygen to form water. The mitochondrion harnesses energy from this process in an electromotive (proton) gradient to form adenosine triphosphate (ATP) from adenosine diphosphate plus inorganic phosphate. Acetyl CoA is primarily formed by one of two pathways: β-oxidation or decarboxylation of pyruvate. Either fatty acids or ketones are processed by β-oxidation. Pyruvate derives from either glycolysis or lactate dehydrogenation. In addition, almost every cell in the body possesses its own internal reserve of chemical energy in the form of triacylglycerol (fat) and glucose (glycogen), which it can expend in times of stress and inadequate tissue perfusion to allow continuous supply of acetyl CoA into the mitochondria.

In the early stage of shock, the skeletal muscle and splanchnic organs are affected more by oxygen deprivation than by a lack of delivery of fuel substrate. As a result, shock rapidly stalls transfer of electrons in the mitochondria and "jams" the pathways of acetyl CoA input into the TCA. The main byproduct of this jam in oxidative metabolism is lactic acid, which can exit the cell across the cell membrane by way of a specific protein transporter. In the resuscitated sepsis syndrome[6] and in resuscitated hemorrhagic shock,[7] skeletal muscle may produce lactate not entirely because of

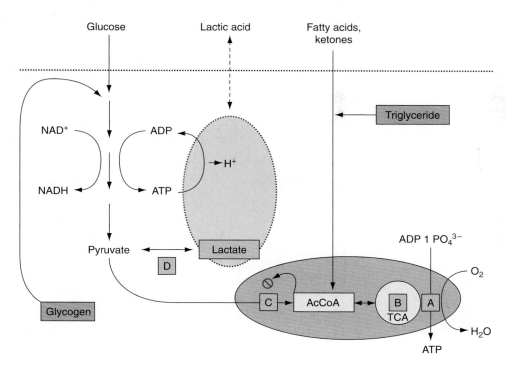

Glucose   Lactic acid   Fatty acids, ketones

Figure 4-1. Energy metabolism with special reference to the development of lactic acidosis in shock. At *site A*, oxygen availability to the mitochondrial electron transport system decreases. In the tricarboxylic acid (TCA) cycle *(site B)*, intermediary metabolites accumulate, including acetyl coenzyme A (AcCoA), which causes the pyruvate dehydrogenase enzyme complex *(site C)* to shut down, leading to accumulation in pyruvate. At *site D*, pyruvate is reduced to lactate, which generates oxidized nicotinamide adenine dinucleotide (NAD⁺) to permit anaerobic glycolysis to generate a marginal supply of adenosine triphosphate (ATP). Lactate can diffuse across the cell membrane through a specific monocarboxylase transporter in the cytosolic membrane *(dotted horizontal line)*. ADP, adenosine diphosphate; NADH, reduced nicotinamide adenine dinucleotide.

low mitochondrial oxygenation, but because the delivery of pyruvate from glycolysis overwhelms the ability of dehydrogenase enzymes in the TCA to dispose of pyruvate, which is converted to lactate. This scenario has been termed *aerobic glycolysis*.[8] Regardless of etiology, elevated concentrations of lactate in the blood serve as a sentinel marker of widespread inadequate tissue perfusion and disappear when adequate resuscitation has been achieved.

At the whole-body level, shock from any etiology initiates a sequence of stress responses that are intended to preserve flow to vital organs and to signal cells to expend internal energy stores (Figure 4-2). Shock initially reduces wall tension in the large intrathoracic arteries, which activates their baroreceptors, which activate adrenergic reflexes that have neural and circulating hormonal components. The two major arms of the neural component include sympathetic fibers from the stellate ganglion, which stimulates the heart, and sympathetic fibers from regional ganglia, which cause peripheral arterial vasoconstriction. Exceptions include certain toxic causes of shock (e.g., septic shock) and many drug overdoses, which can block these reflex sympathetic actions on the heart and vascular smooth muscle. The circulating "stress hormones" derive mainly from the hypothalamic-pituitary-adrenomedullary axis, which leads to secretion of epinephrine and norepinephrine from the adrenal medulla and corticosteroids from the adrenal cortex, renin from the kidney, and glucagon from the pancreas. These hormones signal the liver to break down glycogen to release glucose into the plasma and alert adipose tissue to release fatty acids via lipolysis. As a result, stress hormones increase the input of carbon substrates into the TCA throughout the body, often overwhelming the mitochondrial ability to oxidize them and leading to an

increase in lactic acid production and release into the bloodstream.

Although lactic acidosis is a unifying feature of shock, its exact source may depend on the cause of shock. Lactic acidosis from hemorrhagic shock probably arises largely from skeletal muscle during hypotension and after resuscitation,[9] whereas with sepsis the skeletal muscle probably extracts lactate until the late stage. Some evidence suggests that the viscera and the lung are the primary sources of lactic acidosis in septic shock.[10]

Initiation of inflammatory events constitutes a third unifying feature of shock. Shock causes neutrophil activation and liberation of adhesion molecules, which promote binding of neutrophils to vascular endothelium. Activated, sticky neutrophils can damage organs directly by liberating toxic reactive oxygen species, *N*-chloramines, and proteolytic enzymes. Neutrophils also can plug capillaries and cause microischemia.[11] Although much of the knowledge about the inflammatory responses in shock has evolved from the study of septic shock, the consensus is that any low-perfusion state that produces widespread cellular hypoxia can trigger systemic inflammation. Early in sepsis, multiple tissues (e.g., macrophages, endothelial and epithelial cells, muscle cells) are signaled to upregulate transcription of messenger RNA (mRNA) coding for cytokines, including tumor necrosis factors (TNF-α, TNF-β) and interleukins (IL-1, IL-6).

Figure 4-3 is a brief overview of some of the inflammatory changes that can occur in shock, using the action of TNF-α on a heart muscle cell as the prototype. Cytokines bind to surface receptors and cause changes that lead to the activation of nuclear factor κ B (NFκB), a protein that travels to the cell nucleus. NFκB upregulates the transcription of mRNA needed to synthesize

Figure 4-2. Overview of whole-body hormonal stress response to shock. *Upper left,* Stress hormones (catecholamines, glucagons) stimulate the liver to increase glucose output, derived from glycogen breakdown and by synthesis from lactate and alanine, which are released from skeletal muscle catabolism *(right side). Lower left,* Adrenal medulla secretes glucocorticosteroids and catecholamines, which induce glycogenolysis, insulin resistance, hypokalemia, and lipolysis. Juxtaglomerular cells of the kidney release renin, which activates the renin-angiotensin-aldosterone (RAA) system. *Upper right,* Skeletal muscle becomes more resistant to substrate uptake and continues to release lactate, which becomes the main fuel source for the heart in shock. FFA, free fatty acids.

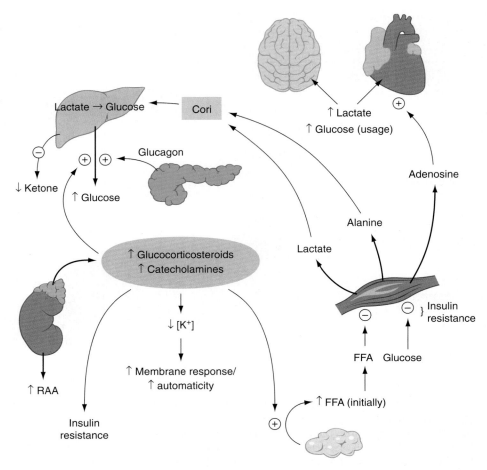

Figure 4-3. Overview of selected inflammatory mechanisms of shock, using the muscle cell as a prototype. Tumor necrosis factor α (TNF-α) causes upregulation of inducible nitric oxide synthase (iNOS), which overproduces nitric oxide (NO). In conditions of low oxygen tension, NO reacts with superoxide (O_2^-) generated from the mitochondria to form peroxynitrite ($ONOO^-$), which can damage mitochondria and decrease adenosine triphosphate (ATP) production. TNF-α also binds to a surface receptor and causes a shift of nuclear factor κ B (NFκB) protein into the nucleus, which further increases production of TNF-α and other inflammatory cytokines. TNF-α also causes production of sphingosine, which can directly block release of calcium from the sarcoplasmic reticulum (SR) and depress cardiac contraction. cGMP, cyclic guanosine monophosphate; IL, interleukin.

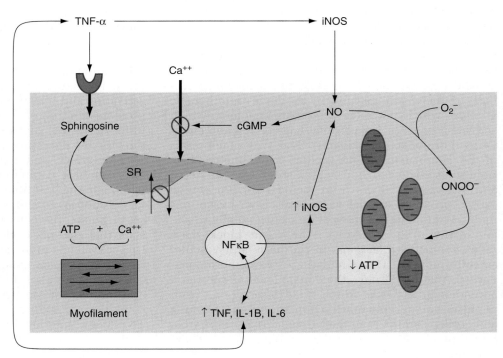

inflammatory cytokines and leads to production of inducible nitric oxide (NO) synthase, which liberates high concentrations of NO. NO causes vascular smooth muscle relaxation. Under healthy conditions, NO is produced in small amounts by a native enzyme, constitutive NO synthase. Constitutive NO synthase provides enough NO to help balance against naturally produced vasoconstrictors to maintain blood flow to autoregulated organs. When inducible NO synthase becomes upregulated, however, too much NO is produced, leading to pathologic vasodilation and eventually conversion of NO to a highly reactive free radical, peroxynitrite, which can damage cell membranes, DNA, and organelles and contribute to organ failure during shock.[12]

Heart Function

During resuscitation from shock, the heart must transition rapidly from a low-work, low-flow state to a higher workload and maintain adequate cardiac output in the presence of inflammatory injury to the cardiac myocyte. The degree to which the heart is affected by shock depends on the cause of shock, but the pathophysiologic effect of cytokine exposure, arterial hypotension, and acidosis on cardiac function can be generalized.

The heart generates its pumping power during systole by interaction of actin and myosin in the myofilament. For this interaction to occur, the contractile apparatus has two basic needs, calcium and chemical energy (ATP or creatine phosphate). Calcium reaches troponin C in the contractile apparatus by the mechanism of excitation-contraction. In this model, intracellular calcium release starts with an external electrical signal on the myocyte surface, which opens voltage-dependent calcium channels on the membrane. These slow, or L-type, channels conduct the current of calcium that causes the plateau phase (II) of the ventricular myocyte action potential. This relatively small influx of calcium triggers a larger release of calcium from the sarcoplasmic reticulum by way of a connection between involutions of the plasma membrane, called the *T tubules*. This connection is the ryanodine-sensitive pathway; the alkaloid agent ryanodine is used experimentally to evoke calcium release from the sarcoplasmic reticulum. The force of cardiac contraction varies in proportion to the amount of calcium bound to troponin C during systole. To increase strength of cardiac contraction, or cardiac contractility, the clinician either must increase calcium entry through the L channel or must increase calcium release from the sarcoplasmic reticulum. In almost all cases, clinically available inotropic drugs work by the former mechanism, by binding to cardiac membrane β_1-receptors (catecholamines), or by inhibition of cyclic adenosine monophosphate (cAMP) breakdown (phosphodiesterase inhibitors), which leads to phosphorylation of the L channel via the stimulatory G protein. Phosphorylation of the L channel increases its probability of opening, increasing calcium entry and myocardial contractility.

The other component of cardiac contraction, chemical energy, comes almost entirely from mitochondrial oxidative phosphorylation. Myocardial mitochondria must remain highly active to meet the mechanical energetic needs of the heart. The heart lives on a thin margin of high-energy phosphate supply; it has been estimated that the heart completely turns over its reserve of ATP and creatine phosphate every 5 to 10 beats.[13]

Cardiac function may be indirectly depressed in shock conditions by coronary hypotension. In an isolated working heart, the strength of cardiac contraction varies in proportion to the coronary perfusion pressure (the Gregg phenomenon). The cellular basis for the link between contractile strength and coronary perfusion pressure seems to be independent of the L-type calcium current.[14] Although decreased coronary perfusion aggravates cardiac performance in shock,[15] it is more difficult to determine if coronary hypotension causes myocardial ischemia in shock. While myocardial oxygen delivery decreases as coronary flow diminishes in shock, the oxygen requirement for the heart decreases in proportion to coronary flow because the external workload on the heart diminishes. With respect to oxygen, the heart seems to obtain what it needs during hypotensive shock. Whether shock is caused by hemorrhage,[16] sepsis,[17] or drug-induced cardiogenic shock,[18] the heart *extracts* lactate, indicating the absence of global myocardial hypoxia. A substantial body of evidence now suggests that specific actions of cytokines may decrease cardiac function, especially in hyperinflammatory causes of shock, such as sepsis (see Figure 4-3).[12,19,20] In addition, intracellular and extracellular acidosis can depress cardiac contraction, but in the whole picture of shock, the contribution of acidosis to depressed heart function is probably minimal.

Specific Causes

Hemorrhagic Shock

Hemorrhagic shock results from a rapid reduction in blood volume, which causes baroreceptor activation and leads to vasoconstriction, increased strength of cardiac contraction, and increased heart rate (HR). Cardiovascular response to hemorrhage can vary with underlying cardiopulmonary status, age, and presence of ingested drugs. Responses of HR and blood pressure (BP) are notoriously variable in hemorrhage, so no firm conclusion can be made at the bedside about the presence or absence of hemorrhagic shock simply by evaluating HR and BP.[21] In general, hemorrhage first increases pulse and cardiac contraction, then increases vasoconstriction. The first clinical manifestations of hemorrhage are tachycardia, then a slight increase in the diastolic BP, causing the pulse pressure (difference between systolic and diastolic BP) to narrow. With worsened bleeding, ventricular filling is compromised, and cardiac output decreases, followed by a reduction in systolic BP. Before the total cardiac output begins to decrease, blood flow to noncritical organs and tissues (e.g., skin, skeletal muscle, viscera) begins to decrease, and these tissues produce lactic acid.

Consequently a change in arterial acid-base status often precedes any significant decrease in cardiac output with hemorrhage.[22] The *base deficit* is defined as the amount of strong base that would have to be added to 1 L of blood to normalize the pH. In the clinical setting, the base deficit is indirectly calculated from the pH and arterial carbon dioxide partial pressure ($PaCO_2$) and is normally more positive than −2 mEq/L. Accordingly the arterial and venous blood base deficit worsens (the numeric measurement becomes more negative) early in hemorrhage even while pH and BP remain in the normal range. It can be scientifically rationalized that the threshold to distinguish simple hemorrhage from hemorrhagic shock occurs when the base deficit worsens (the total body base deficit increases, but the laboratory numeric measurement becomes more negative), indicating widespread tissue hypoperfusion. To maintain a normal arterial pH, the brainstem chemoreceptor responds to acidemia by increasing minute ventilation, leading to reduced $PaCO_2$. After approximately one third of the total blood volume is acutely lost, cardiovascular reflexes no longer can cause adequate filling of the arterial circuit, and frank hypotension supervenes. Arterial hypotension is generally and arbitrarily defined as a systolic arterial BP less than 90 mm Hg, but this threshold should be increased to 100 mm Hg in patients with known systemic hypertension and in patients older than age 60 years. Usually coincident with the development of hypotension, the patient no longer can hyperventilate sufficiently to maintain a normal arterial pH, and acidemia occurs. Hemorrhagic shock causes a large activation of the hypothalamic-pituitary-adrenomedullary axis, with release of stress hormones that cause glycogenolysis, lipolysis, and mild hypokalemia (see Figure 4-2). In the emergency department, patients sustaining traumatic hemorrhage generally have an arterial lactate concentration greater than 4 mmol/L, a $PaCO_2$ less than 35 mm Hg, and mild hyperglycemia (150 to 170 mg/dL) and hypokalemia (3.5 to 3.7 mEq/L). Although hemorrhagic hypotension does significantly alter ventilation-perfusion relationships in the lung, hemorrhagic hypotension seldom produces arterial hypoxemia if the airway is clear, the lungs are not injured, and respiratory effort is adequate.

The second phase of organ injury from hemorrhagic shock occurs during resuscitation. Many experts assert that the period of hemorrhage "cocks the gun," and resuscitation "pulls the trigger" to cause organ injury from hemorrhagic shock. During resuscitation, neutrophils become most aggressive, binding to the lung endothelium and initiating capillary leak, which can produce acute respiratory distress syndrome (ARDS). Inflammatory cytokines are liberated during resuscitation, and membrane injury occurs in many cells. In the liver, damage from inflammation and reactive oxygen species from neutrophils is compounded by persistent microischemia. During resuscitation from hemorrhagic shock, the normal balance of vasodilation by NO versus vasoconstriction by endothelins becomes distorted, producing patchy centrilobular ischemic damage in the liver, which may produce an immediate increase in blood transaminase levels. A growing body of evidence suggests that retransfusion from hemorrhage exerts greater injury to the heart than the actual hypotensive insult.[23,24] Depending on the degree of hypotensive insult, the kidney may manifest acute spasm of the preglomerular arterioles, causing acute tubular necrosis. Systemic metabolic changes can impair fuel delivery to the heart and brain, secondary to depressed hepatic glucose output, impaired hepatic ketone production, and inhibited peripheral lipolysis.[25]

Septic Shock

Septic shock can be produced by infection with any microbe. Previously, gram-negative aerobic bacteria were the primary organisms that caused septic shock; however, more recently the incidence of gram-positive infections has increased to a frequency equal to that of gram-negative infections.[1] In one third of cases of septic shock, no organism is identified. One of the chief mediators of sepsis is lipopolysaccharide, which is contained in the cell wall of gram-negative bacteria. Infusion of lipopolysaccharide into humans or animals produces cardiovascular, immunologic, and inflammatory changes identical to the changes observed with microbial infection. In recent years, multicenter trials have suggested the emergence of gram-positive organisms as the chief cause of sepsis in hospitalized patients. Further growth in primarily gram-positive sepsis occurs for two main reasons:

1. More patients are being treated at home for chronic immunocompromising diseases with indwelling catheters, which serve as excellent portals of entry into the vascular space for *Staphylococcus aureus* and coagulase-negative staphylococci.
2. The frequency of community-acquired infections caused by antibiotic-resistant, gram-positive organisms has increased greatly, including infections caused by *S. aureus, Streptococcus pneumoniae,* and *Streptococcus pyogenes.*

Septic shock causes three major effects that must be addressed during resuscitation: hypovolemia, cardiovascular depression, and induction of systemic inflammation. Septic shock always produces relative hypovolemia from increased venous capacitance, which reduces right ventricular filling. Septic shock often causes absolute hypovolemia from gastrointestinal volume losses, tachypnea, sweating, and decreased ability to drink during development of the illness. Sepsis also induces capillary leak, which leads to relative loss of intravascular volume into third spaces. Evidence has shown that septic shock causes myocardial depression simultaneously with vasodepression and capillary leak. For years it was thought that septic shock depressed the heart only in the later, hypodynamic stages because sepsis induces hyperdynamic heart function, characterized by an increase in cardiac output.[26] More sophisticated and direct measurements of cardiac contractility have shown, however, that cardiac mechanical function becomes impaired early in the course of septic shock, even in the hyperdynamic stages.[27] Evidence for multiple mechanisms may explain depressed heart function in sepsis, including actions of specific cytokines (most notably TNF-α and IL-1β),[20] overproduction of NO by inducible NO synthase,[12] and possibly impairment in mitochondrial oxidative phosphorylation[28] coincident with reduced mechanical efficiency.[29] Evidence indicates that circulating mediators, myocellular injury from inflammation, and deranged metabolism interact synergistically to injure the heart during septic shock. Systemic inflammation causes capillary leak in the lung, which may cause alveolar infiltration characteristic of ARDS early in the treatment of septic shock in 40% of patients.[1] With the potential for early development of ARDS, more profound ventilation-perfusion mismatching, and pneumonia or pulmonary aspiration, hypoxemia is more severe with septic shock than hemorrhagic shock.

Cardiogenic Shock

Cardiogenic shock results when more than 40% of the myocardium becomes necrosed from ischemia, inflammation, toxins, or immune destruction. The primary cause of cardiogenic shock is pump failure. Otherwise, cardiogenic shock essentially produces the same circulatory and metabolic alterations that are observed with hemorrhagic shock. Impaired baseline cardiac function can contribute to the development of circulatory shock state secondary to infection, hemorrhage, or vasodilatory drug overdose. When shock results from a pure cardiac cause, however, severe left ventricular dysfunction is evident on echocardiography early in the course. Patients with severe left ventricular dysfunction are far more likely to have a cardiogenic cause of shock than patients with normal or moderate left ventricular dysfunction.[30]

Acute massive pulmonary embolism produces circulatory shock by obstruction of the pulmonary vasculature, which leads to right ventricular overload and impairs left ventricular filling. Echocardiogram and electrocardiogram (ECG) observations suggest that selective right ventricular ischemia occurs with massive pulmonary embolism.[31] A pulmonary embolism large enough to cause shock always results in pulmonary ventilation-perfusion mismatching, so arterial hypoxemia becomes a significant problem. Hypoxemia, together with coronary hypoperfusion from arterial hypotension, and systemic acidosis may produce synergistic effects on cardiac function, resulting in a "stunning" effect on right and left ventricles.[32]

Anaphylactic Shock

Anaphylactic shock results from an IgE-mediated systemic response to an allergen. The mast cell plays a central role in the etiology of anaphylactic shock. IgE causes mast cells to release histamine, which results in vascular smooth muscle relaxation, bronchial smooth muscle constriction, and capillary leak of plasma into interstitial spaces. Platelets also participate in anaphylaxis by secreting platelet-activating factor (PAF),

which is derived from membrane phospholipid. PAF causes peripheral vasodilation, bronchial constriction, and pulmonary arterial and coronary vasoconstriction. Antagonists to PAF can reverse the negative inotropy and vasodilation observed with experimental anaphylaxis.[33] As such, PAF may be an important mediator of anaphylaxis that is refractory to antihistamine treatments.

CLINICAL FEATURES

Patients frequently present to the emergency department in shock with no obvious etiology. Rapid recognition of shock requires the integration of information from immediate history and physical examination. Shock can be strongly supported by the presence of a worsening base deficit or lactic acidosis. In general, patients in shock exhibit a stress response: They are ill appearing, pale, often sweating, usually tachypneic or grunting, and often with a weak and rapid pulse (Box 4-2). HR can be normal or low in shock, especially in cases complicated by prescribed drugs or profound hypoxemia that can depress HR. BP can be normal because of adrenergic reflexes or because of measurement errors from cuff sphygmomanometry.[21] As a result, arterial BP as a sole measurement remains an unreliable marker of circulatory status. The HR-to-systolic BP ratio may provide a better marker of shock than either measurement alone; a normal ratio is less than 0.8.[34] Urine output provides an excellent indicator of organ perfusion and is readily available with insertion of a Foley catheter into the bladder. Measuring urine output requires at least 30 minutes, however, to determine accurately if output is normal (>1 mL/kg/hr), reduced (0.5 to 1 mL/kg/hr), or severely reduced (<0.5 mL/kg/hr). Measurements of the arterial lactate concentration and the base deficit can be performed rapidly and provide accurate assessment of global perfusion status. An arterial lactate concentration greater than 4 mM/L or an arterial base deficit more negative than −4 mEq/L predicts the presence of circulatory insufficiency severe enough to cause subsequent multiple organ failure.[35]

When the empiric criteria for circulatory shock are discovered, the next step is to classify the cause of shock (Figure 4-4). Although the questions in Figure 4-4 are connected in sequence to allow logical organi-

---

BOX 4-2. Empiric Criteria for Diagnosis of Circulatory Shock*

- Ill appearance or altered mental status
- Heart rate >100 beats/min
- Respiratory rate >22 breaths/min or $PaCO_2$ <32 mm Hg
- Arterial base deficit <−5 mEq/L or lactate >4 mM/L
- Urine output <0.5 mL/kg/hr
- Arterial hypotension >20 minutes duration

---

*Regardless of cause. Four criteria should be met.

Figure 4-4. Flow diagram to classify undifferentiated shock.

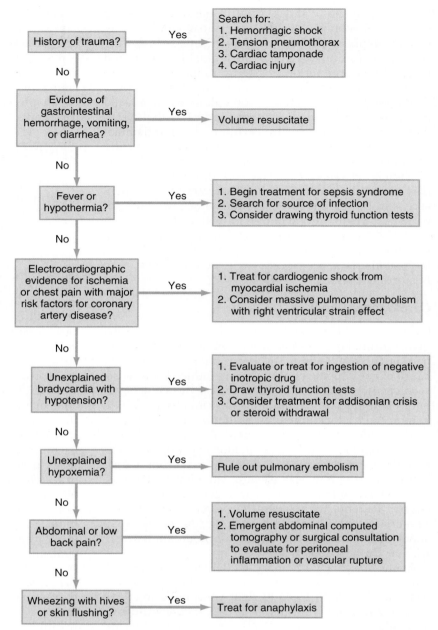

zation, parallel processing of all these questions is required to determine a cause rapidly in practice. The history, vital signs, and physical examination documented by prehospital providers represent a valuable insight into a patient's physiologic status before any medical intervention and can be useful in emergency department management. A study found that nontrauma patients with symptoms consistent with circulatory insufficiency and prehospital hypotension (systolic BP <100 mm Hg) have a threefold increase in in-hospital mortality than patients without hypotension.[36]

The primary survey must ensure presence of a patent airway and sufficient respiratory effort to ensure adequate oxygenation and ventilation. The physical examination should be performed on an undressed patient and should begin with general inspection of the body for visual or tactile evidence of trauma; odor of ethanol or other toxins; presence of any indwelling devices; and evidence of soft tissue or bone infection, rashes, or extremity edema. Dry mucous membranes suggest dehydration, whereas distended jugular veins suggest cardiac failure or obstruction from pulmonary embolism or cardiac tamponade. Muffled heart sounds suggest cardiac tamponade, whereas a loud machine-like systolic murmur indicates acute rupture of a papillary muscle or rupture of the interventricular septum. Bilateral pulmonary rales in a patient with a normal rectal temperature help to define the presence of left ventricular failure. Wheezing suggests bronchospasm from anaphylaxis or, less likely, cardiac failure or pulmonary embolism. Abdominal tenderness may indicate peritoneal inflammation or occult trauma. Rectal and pelvic examinations may disclose occult gastrointestinal hemorrhage or an unexpected adnexal mass or tenderness indicating an ectopic pregnancy. Rectal temperature should be performed on every patient with suspected shock.

The initial neurologic examination may be extremely helpful, especially to providers later during hospitalization, and should include notation of speech fluency and content, ability to follow one-step commands, pupillary function and cardinal eye movements, symmetry of extremity movements, and strength. In children, documentation should include level of alertness, response to parents, appropriateness of crying, pupillary function, symmetry of grimace, and symmetry of extremity movements (and motor tone in infants).

Laboratory, radiographic, and other ancillary data should be ordered (1) to assess tissue and vital organ perfusion and (2) to diagnose injury from trauma, find the source of infection with sepsis, or identify the cause of cardiac failure. A chest radiograph can identify significant thoracic trauma, pulmonary infection, pulmonary edema, or tension pneumothorax. In adults, an ECG helps to identify myocardial ischemia, cardiac failure from dysrhythmia, or pulmonary embolus. A finger-stick glucose measurement can identify unsuspected hyperglycemia or hypoglycemia, which might prompt further evaluation for myocardial ischemia or a source of infection. A hemoglobin level less than 8 g/dL strongly suggests the need for blood transfusion if other criteria for shock are present (see Box 4-2). Serum electrolytes can help identify a metabolic acidosis indicating lactic acidosis, an elevated blood urea nitrogen-to-creatinine ratio suggests dehydration or chronic gastrointestinal bleeding, and combined electrolyte abnormalities of hyponatremia and hyperkalemia suggest adrenal insufficiency. The complete blood count helps to diagnose anemia or identify neutropenia. Arterial blood gases are ordered for a base deficit calculation; a normal arterial oxygen partial pressure (PaO_2) from a patient breathing room air can rule out hypoxemia. Serum lactate measurement should be performed as early as possible in patients with suspected shock. Urinalysis can reveal dehydration (specific gravity >1.025 with ketones present) and can identify urinary infection as a cause of sepsis. Some emergency departments have bedside ultrasound capability, and cardiac and abdominal scanning can be performed rapidly at the bedside to screen for inadequate central venous volume, occult hemoperitoneum, abdominal aortic aneurysm, left ventricular failure, and cardiac tamponade. A systematic ultrasound protocol can improve significantly the physician's ability to diagnose accurately the etiology of undifferentiated shock in emergency department patients.[37]

Consensus definitions of shock show the spectra of hypoperfusion for the following three common causes of shock (Box 4-3):

1. *Septic shock*. The American College of Chest Physicians and Society for Critical Care Medicine[38] developed a consensus to distinguish septic shock from its precursor conditions, systemic inflamma-

---

BOX 4-3. Definitions and Criteria for Septic, Hemorrhagic and Cardiogenic Shock

Septic Shock
- Systemic inflammatory response syndrome (SIRS)
  Two or more of the following:
  1. Temperature >38° C or <36° C
  2. Heart rate >90 beats/min
  3. Respiratory rate >20 breaths/min or $PaCO_2$ <32 mm Hg
  4. While blood cell count >12,000/mm³, <4000/mm³, or >10% band neutrophilia
- Sepsis syndrome
  SIRS associated with organ dysfunction or hypotension; organ dysfunction may include presence of lactic acidosis, oliguria, or altered mental status
- Septic shock
  SIRS with hypotension despite adequate fluid resuscitation; septic shock should still be diagnosed if vasopressor therapy has normalized blood pressure

Hemorrhagic Shock
- Simple hemorrhage
  Suspected bleeding with pulse <100 beats/min, normal respiratory rate, normal blood pressure, and normal base deficit
- Hemorrhage with hypoperfusion
  Suspected bleeding with base deficit <−5 mEq/L *or* persistent pulse >100 beats/min
- Hemorrhagic shock
  Suspected bleeding with at least four criteria listed in Box 4-2

Cardiogenic Shock
- Cardiac failure
  Clinical evidence of impaired forward flow of the heart, including presence of dyspnea, tachycardia, pulmonary rales, peripheral edema, or cyanosis
- Cardiogenic shock
  Cardiac failure plus four criteria listed in Box 4-2

---

tory response syndrome and sepsis syndrome. Although this particular consensus requires persistent hypotension to define septic shock, initiation of treatment for empirically diagnosed septic shock should not await the onset of hypotension.

2. *Hemorrhagic shock*. The American College of Surgeons has divided hemorrhagic shock into four stages, depending on the severity of blood loss and the physiologic response to this loss, but such arbitrary divisions are of little value. A more useful approach defines hemorrhagic shock as being present when systemic hypoperfusion manifests as lactic acidosis with organ dysfunction.

3. *Cardiogenic shock*. Many experts reserve the definition of cardiogenic shock for cardiac failure with arterial hypotension that is refractory to inotropic/vasopressor therapy.[39] Cardiogenic shock should be thought to be present, however, whenever cardiac failure (ischemic, toxic, or obstructive) causes systemic hypoperfusion that manifests as lactic acidosis with organ dysfunction.

MANAGEMENT

Monitoring Perfusion Status

In the effort to resuscitate a patient with circulatory shock, the clinician must follow specific indices of systemic perfusion and organ function to know if the resuscitation effort is working. In all patients with shock, circulation must be monitored by continuous ECG and pulse oximetry to follow HR and to maintain arterial oxygenation. BP should be measured by cuff sphygmomanometer every 2 to 5 minutes during resuscitation. Because cuff sphygmomanometer measurement may be inaccurate in severe hypotensive states, the use of an arterial pressure monitoring line should be considered. Clinicians should remember that BP and HR correlate poorly with cardiac index in shock and often underestimate the severity of systemic hypoperfusion.[21] Children with hypovolemic shock frequently have a normal BP until they rapidly deteriorate to a near-arrest hemodynamic state.[40] Urine output should be measured as an index of vital organ perfusion in patients (about 1 mL/kg/hr in persons without renal disease). Normalization of the serum lactate concentration or the base deficit, when observed with improving vital signs and urine output, can gauge reliably the adequacy of resuscitation and prognosis in shock from any etiology.[35,41] An increasing lactate concentration (or refractory hypotension with worsening base deficit) with ongoing volume resuscitation portends high mortality and mandates more aggressive resuscitation or specific procedural intervention.

The method of achieving intravenous access in a patient with suspected shock has been controversial. Most patients with shock can be fully resuscitated and adequately monitored with peripheral venous access established either with two catheters of size 18-gauge or smaller or with one catheter 16-gauge or larger. Patients with cardiac failure or renal failure may require closer measurement of the central venous pressure (CVP) and insertion of a central venous catheter. An 8.5F central venous catheter allows for accurate measurement of the CVP and insertion of a pulmonary artery catheter or other monitoring device if needed. In children, a 3F or 5F bi-lumen catheter can be placed in the femoral vein with few complications.[42] To reduce the potential for limb damage from extravasation from a peripheral intravenous catheter, vasoactive medications optimally are administered through a central venous catheter. If vasoactive medications are administered, additional peripheral intravenous catheters are required for infusion of crystalloid and other treatments. Many patients with renal disease or cancer have indwelling catheters in place. In patients with empiric criteria for shock, this catheter should be used for intravenous access, unless satisfactory access already has been established. In emergency departments, where the standard practice is not to use these ports at the request of other physicians, a specific hospital policy and training session should be developed to make an exception in the case of circulatory shock. If such a policy does not exist, the threat to the patient from failure to administer fluids rapidly and in sufficient quantity outweighs considerations about preservation of the line for future therapy.

Goal-Directed Therapy

Goal-directed therapy refers to the practice of resuscitating patients to a defined physiologic endpoint indicating that systemic perfusion and vital organ function have been restored.[35] For many years in the intensive care unit (ICU), physicians have relied on the use of the pulmonary artery catheter to help optimize left ventricular filling indices. At present, the use of the pulmonary artery catheter is controversial, based on evidence suggesting that its insertion was associated with increased morbidity in ICU populations. One multicenter randomized, controlled trial evaluated using pulmonary artery catheters in ICU patients with shock or ARDS (or both), and there were no differences in the use of vasoactive agents, number of days of organ failure, or mortality.[43] When data from 16 randomized, controlled trials were aggregated in a meta-analysis, however, pulmonary artery catheterization was associated with significantly reduced morbidity in ICU populations.[44] Insufficient data have been published to support the use or avoidance of pulmonary artery catheters in emergency department patients.

Several alternative methods to the pulmonary artery catheter have been proposed as endpoints to resuscitation in the emergency department. The *lactate clearance index* refers to serial measurements of arterial lactate.[41] Lactate clearance involves measuring the blood lactate concentration at two or more times. If the lactate concentration has not decreased by 50% 1 hour after resuscitation has begun, additional steps must be taken to improve systemic perfusion. Resuscitation should continue until the lactate concentration decreases to less than 2 mM/L. Enthusiasm for lactate measurement as an endpoint must be tempered by the relative lack of data from emergency department studies and the lack of availability of the test.

Mixed venous oxygen saturation (SvO_2) measurements reflect the balance between oxygen delivery and oxygen consumption. Previous studies suggested that the SvO_2 can be used as a surrogate to cardiac index when targeting normalization of endpoints (SvO_2 70% or cardiac index 2.5 to 3.5 L/min/m^2) for therapeutic intervention in critically ill patients.[45] Although SvO_2 requires the use of a pulmonary artery catheter, the central venous oxygen saturation ($ScvO_2$) drawn from the central circulation has been shown to parallel the SvO_2 closely, especially when tracking changes or trends in the values.[46]

Gastric or rectal *tonography* also has been studied extensively in ICU populations. A buffer-filled balloon consisting of a permeable membrane is inserted into the stomach or rectum. The balloon has an electrode in the buffer solution and can estimate the intramucosal pH. Mucosal pH is used to estimate the perfusion status of the gut. Use of gastric tonography as an endpoint failed

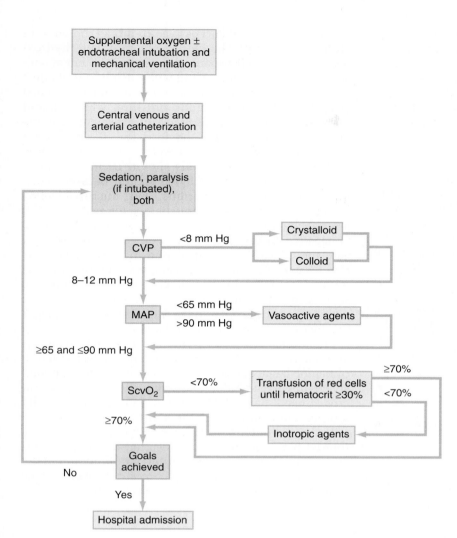

Figure 4-5. Flow diagram outlining the protocol for early goal-directed therapy when treating patients with severe sepsis or septic shock. This protocol outlines specific hemodynamic and physiologic parameters the clinician should seek to achieve within the first 6 hours of care. This protocol is focused on resuscitation and should be used in conjunction with standard clinical care for patients with suspected infection, such as appropriate diagnostic studies to determine the focus of infection and appropriate antimicrobial agents to treat the infection. CVP, central venous pressure; MAP, mean arterial pressure; ScvO₂, central venous oxygen saturation. (Redrawn from Rivers E, et al: Early goal-directed therapy in the treatment of severe sepsis and septic shock. N Engl J Med 345:1368, 2001.)

to predict organ dysfunction and mortality in one randomized, controlled study of heterogeneous ICU patients admitted from an emergency department.[47]

Goal-directed therapy incorporates multiple indices of circulatory status and oxygenation status. One study found that goal-directed therapy significantly reduced mortality and morbidity in emergency department patients with systemic inflammatory response syndrome and several criteria for severe sepsis or septic shock.[48] Patients were resuscitated within the first 6 hours of care to achieve several hemodynamic parameters and to maintain central venous oxygen saturation greater than or equal to 70% (Figure 4-5). This new treatment strategy has not been tested in other causes of shock, but it shows the value of using defined physiologic endpoints to measure systemic perfusion during resuscitation from shock in the emergency department. This approach also further substantiates the view that the real "make-or-break" time to treat shock occurs during the first 6 hours of resuscitation.

Ventilation

Rapid sequence intubation is the preferred method in most patients with shock (see Chapter 1). Anesthetic agents with a high degree of cardiovascular stability, such as ketamine or etomidate, should be used in reduced dosages (half of normal induction dose) with a full dose of succinylcholine to achieve intubation while minimizing cardiovascular depression. Intubation prevents aspiration, increases oxygenation, treats acute respiratory failure, provides initial treatment for metabolic or hypercarbic acidemia, and protects the patient who will be sent to an uncontrolled environment (e.g., for tests). Intubation also reduces the work of breathing, which, in the hypoperfused patient, further exacerbates lactic acidemia. Strenuous use of accessory respiratory muscles can increase oxygen consumption by 50% to 100% and decrease cerebral blood flow by 50%.[49,50] More importantly, if the patient has increased airway resistance (e.g., bronchospasm with anaphylaxis) or a decrease in lung compliance (e.g., pulmonary edema, ARDS), a more negative intrathoracic pressure must be generated to fill the lungs with each inspiration. The greater suction effect also is exerted on the left ventricle, impeding its ability to eject and increasing functional afterload. Positive-pressure ventilation removes this impedance and can improve ventricular function and cardiac output 30%.[49]

All intubated shock patients require at least 5 cm H_2O of positive end-expiratory pressure to prevent alveolar consolidation. In acute respiratory failure, ventilation at zero positive end-expiratory pressure can cause widespread alveolar collapse and lead to severe ventilation-perfusion mismatch and hypoxemia (see Chapter 2).

Volume Replacement

The next imperative in shock is to decide when "the tank is full." The goal in volume replacement is slightly elevated left ventricular end-diastolic *volume,* which is a difficult measurement to make in the emergency department. The CVP is used most often to estimate right ventricular filling pressure and is used in some goal-directed algorithms. Because both ventricles tend to stiffen during shock, a high CVP (10 to 15 cm H_2O) is often needed to produce adequate filling volume. It is a long way, however, from the CVP measurement to actual knowledge of left ventricular end-diastolic volume; a presumed adequate CVP must be substantiated by increases in urine output and BP and decreasing lactate concentrations.[51]

Treating Specific Causes

Box 4-4 summarizes the general treatment approach for the four common causes of shock.

Hemorrhagic Shock

Standard treatment for hemorrhagic shock consists of rapidly infusing several liters of isotonic crystalloid in adults or three successive 20-mL/kg boluses in children. Colloids, including albumin and hydroxyethyl hetastarch (Hespan), also can be used but at considerable increase in cost and without substantial effect on morbidity or mortality. Colloids offer the theoretical advantage of a high osmotic pressure, which should help to maintain a normal intravascular volume after retransfusion from hemorrhage. If criteria for shock persist despite crystalloid infusion (see Box 4-2), packed red blood cells should be infused (5 to 10 mL/kg). Type-specific blood should be used when the clinical scenario permits, but uncrossmatched blood should be used immediately for patients with arterial hypotension and uncontrolled hemorrhage. O-negative blood is used in women of childbearing age, and O-positive blood is used in all other patients (see Chapter 5). Substantial evidence supports the use of leukodepleted blood, which has been filtered to remove donor neutrophils.[52] Leukodepleted blood is used in countries outside the United States because it produces less retransfusion-related organ damage.[53]

The infusion of hemoglobin-based oxygen carriers as alternatives to packed red blood cells for resuscitation of hemorrhagic shock patients has been studied extensively. In a large randomized, controlled trial, diaspirin cross-linked hemoglobin, a purified and chemically modified human hemoglobin substrate, was compared with crystalloid for initial resuscitation in critically injured patients, and its use resulted in a higher mortality at interim analysis resulting in termination of the trial.[54] Other artificial hemoglobin substitutes may be available in the future but at present show no benefit over packed red blood cells.

BOX 4-4. Clinical Management Guidelines for Four Common Causes of Shock

Hemorrhagic Shock
- Ensure adequate ventilation/oxygenation
- Provide immediate control of hemorrhage, when possible (e.g., traction for long bone fractures, direct pressure)
- Initiate judicious infusion of lactated Ringer's solution (10-20 mL/kg) or 5% hydroxyethyl starch (5 mL/kg)
- With evidence of poor organ perfusion and 30-minute anticipated delay to hemorrhage control, begin packed red blood cell (PRBC) infusion (5-10 mL/kg)
- With suspected central nervous system trauma or Glasgow Coma Scale score <9, immediate PRBC transfusion may be preferable as initial resuscitation fluid
- Treat severe acidosis (pH <6.8) with THAM
- Treat coincident dysrhythmias (e.g., atrial fibrillation with synchronized cardioversion)

Cardiogenic Shock
- Ameliorate increased work of breathing; provide oxygen and positive end-expiratory pressure (PEEP) for pulmonary edema
- Begin inotropic support; dobutamine (5 μg/kg/min) is common empiric agent
- Seek to reverse the insult (e.g., initiate thrombolysis, arrange percutaneous transluminal angioplasty, or administer charcoal for drug overdose)
- Consider intra-aortic balloon pump counterpulsation for refractory shock

Septic Shock
- Ensure adequate oxygenation; remove work of breathing.
- Administer 20 mL/kg of crystalloid or 5 mL/kg of colloid, and titrate infusion to adequate urine output
- Begin antimicrobial therapy; attempt surgical drainage or debridement
- If volume restoration fails to improve organ perfusion, begin vasopressor support; initial choice includes dopamine, infused at 5-15 μg/kg/min, or norepinephrine, infused at 0.1-1 μg/kg/min

Anaphylactic Shock
- Control airway and ventilation
- Administer 10-20 mL/kg of crystalloid
- Test an intravenous bolus of epinephrine (50-100 μg), then mix 5 mg of epinephrine in 500 mL of normal saline. Begin infusion at 10 cc/hr, and titrate to arterial blood pressure response
- Administer 5-10 mg/kg of hydrocortisone or 1-2 mg/kg of methylprednisolone

More recent studies have endorsed the concept of either delayed resuscitation or hypotensive resuscitation for hemorrhagic shock. Bickell and associates[55] showed improved mortality among patients with penetrating torso trauma in whom all resuscitation was withheld until they reached the operating room compared with patients who received standard resuscitation in the prehospital and hospital setting. Other studies have found no mortality difference in patients with hemorrhagic shock who were resuscitated to either standard clinical parameters (systolic BP >100 mm Hg) or hypotensive parameters (systolic BP 70 mm Hg).[56] Although interesting concepts, further prospective controlled studies are needed before the concept of withholding or limiting volume resuscitation in patients with severe bleeding can be endorsed. Controlling hemorrhage remains the cornerstone of treating hemorrhagic shock, and evidence continues to support immediate surgery when direct vascular control cannot otherwise be obtained (see Chapter 34).

In rare instances, hypodynamic hemorrhagic shock may be treated with a positive inotropic drug. Amrinone and dopamine decrease mortality in crystalloid-resuscitated animals with hemorrhage.[57]

Septic Shock

Septic shock begins as an infectious nidus, which triggers a domino effect of cellular, microvascular, hematologic, and cardiovascular dysfunction. Treatment begins by establishing adequate ventilation to correct hypoxia and pH and to reduce systemic oxygen consumption and left ventricular work. Endotracheal intubation and sedation with or without chemical paralysis are often required.

The second goal is to achieve adequate ventricular filling. The choice of fluids in treating septic shock is probably less important than scrupulous monitoring for adequate tissue perfusion. Colloid solutions may decrease the incidence of postresuscitative pulmonary edema and degree of ARDS.[58] Choices for fluid resuscitation involve consideration of availability and the cost-to-benefit ratio. The initial volume replacement should include rapid infusion of 20 to 25 mL/kg of crystalloid, followed by 5- to 10-mL/kg boluses of the least expensive colloid available (usually 6% hydroxyethyl hetastarch) for persistent hypoperfusion. Blood should be transfused in the emergency department to restore hematocrit to at least 30% to 35%.

The third directive is to eradicate the infection with antimicrobial therapy and, when necessary, surgical or percutaneous drainage. If an infectious focus is found, the choice of antimicrobial agent can be directed by clinician experience and institutional minimal infective concentration data. When no focus can be found in septic shock, a semisynthetic penicillin with a β-lactamase inhibitor, in combination with an aminoglycoside plus vancomycin, or monotherapy with imipenem-cilastatin is a rational empiric choice. When neutropenia is suspected in a patient with sepsis syndrome, the progression to refractory, fatal septic shock

can be cataclysmic. Neutropenia should be suspected in patients who have recently undergone chemotherapy. Chemotherapy patients with sepsis represent a special challenge because the pathophysiology may be complicated by anemia, thrombocytopenia, dehydration from vomiting, and the effect of adjunctive steroid therapy. Chemotherapy patients often have indwelling catheters, which predispose them to more unusual causes of sepsis, including gram-positive bacteria and fungi.[59]

Septic shock refractory to volume restoration (urine output or BP remains low; lactate increases) requires vasopressor support. The primary goal of vasopressor support is to increase cardiac output and oxygen delivery to vital organs. Dopamine is a rational first-line therapy in septic shock at 5 to 15 µg/kg/min and titrated to urine output greater than 1 mL/kg/hr and mean arterial BP (two thirds diastolic plus one third systolic) greater than 70 mm Hg. Dopamine primarily stimulates HR and cardiac contractility in doses ranging from 3 to 8 µg/kg/min, then produces peripheral arterial vasoconstriction at doses greater than 10 µg kg/min. Dopamine also may improve splanchnic, renal, and systemic perfusion. If urine output remains low with high doses of dopamine (>10 µg/kg/min), dobutamine should be started at 5 µg/kg/min to increase cardiac output and increased to 20 µg/kg/min to maintain urine output.

Multiple agents have been directed against the biologic actions of lipopolysaccharide. Cytokines and autocoids have been investigated in animal studies and human trials of septic shock, but no antichemokine has been adopted for routine clinical use in the emergency department.[1] It seems that no single cytokine or mediator is the sole cause of septic shock, and no single agent treats it. Evidence has emerged to suggest that derangements in the coagulation cascade in addition to a robust inflammatory response contribute substantially to the development of organ dysfunction in the setting of sepsis. Drotrecogin alfa activated (or activated protein C), a recombinant human activated protein with anti-inflammatory, antithrombotic, and profibrinolytic properties, has shown promising preliminary results in the treatment of patients with systemic inflammation and organ failure from acute infection.[60] Patients who receive activated protein C have a lower 28-day mortality, but the use of activated protein C is associated with a greater risk of serious bleeding. Certain subgroups may derive additional benefit from the use of activated protein C, including patients older than 50 years, patients with more than one dysfunctional organ system, patients with an Acute Physiologic and Chronic Health Evaluation (APACHE) II score greater than 24, and patients with shock at the time of drug infusion.[61] In general, the institution of activated protein C therapy is not part of the routine emergency department management of sepsis because there is a large window of time for treatment initiation (within 24 hours of meeting criteria). If this therapy is considered, consultation with an ICU physician who would assume care of the patient is recommended because the therapy is continued for 96 hours.

The use of corticosteroids in the treatment of sepsis and septic shock has been investigated with mixed results. The results of two large randomized, controlled trials confirm that there is no role for high-dose, short-course corticosteroid therapy in septic shock.[62,63] Evidence has suggested, however, that some patients with septic shock have relative adrenal insufficiency when the hypothalamic-pituitary axis is tested with a corticotropin stimulation test. One multicenter randomized, controlled trial of patients with septic shock showed a reduction in the mortality rate and number of days on vasoactive medications in nonresponders to a corticotropin stimulation test (defined as an increase of serum cortisol ≤9 µg/dL after stimulation) who received low-dose hydrocortisone (50 mg every 6 hours for 7 days) versus placebo.[64] More trials are needed to investigate the potential benefit of low-dose hydrocortisone in subgroups of patients with septic shock, and specifically to identify any potential hazards from use of this agent, before any firm recommendations can be made.

Cardiogenic Shock

The immediate treatment of cardiogenic shock focuses on improving myocardial contractility and pump function. Cardiogenic shock traditionally is defined as the combination of systemic signs of hypoperfusion with arterial systolic BP less than 90 mm Hg (or 30% below a known baseline). If work of breathing is tiring the patient, if severe pulmonary edema is causing significant hypoxemia, or if respiratory failure is imminent, intubation and mechanical ventilation should be initiated, followed by emergent treatment of bradydysrhythymia or tachydysrhythmia and inotropic support. For sedation or anxiety, barbiturates, morphine, and benzodiazepines should be avoided in cardiogenic shock; when perfused into a failing heart, their negative inotropism is exaggerated.[65] Cautious doses of fentanyl may be used to manage pain, but the best approach to calm anxiety and restlessness is to improve perfusion. Etomidate has excellent hemodynamic stability and should be used (but in reduced doses) for intubation, accompanied by a full dose of succinylcholine. To improve myocardial contractility, dobutamine and dopamine are the agents of choice begun in order at the same doses used for septic shock. For refractory hypotension and shock, amrinone or milrinone may improve cardiac output. Amrinone and milrinone are biperiden derivatives that increase cAMP by inhibiting phosphodiesterase (complex F-III). These drugs exhibit little tachyphylaxis with no measurable increase in myocardial oxygen consumption.[66] A loading dose of 0.75 mg/kg for amrinone or 50 µg/kg for milrinone is necessary, followed by a titrated constant infusion for either drug (5 to 10 µg/kg/min for amrinone and 0.5 µg/kg/min for milrinone).

When pharmacologic support fails to improve indices of perfusion, the next step is to initiate intraaortic balloon pump counterpulsation (IABPC). IABPC requires the facilities and personnel of a high-level ICU or critical care unit. IABPC can augment diastolic coronary perfusion by 30% and may interrupt the vicious cycle of hypotension-induced myocardial hypoperfusion.[67] Controlled trials have shown IABPC to improve short-term survival, improve post-thrombolytic patency rates, and reduce stroke morbidity. IABPC increases cardiac output by a mean of 30% in refractory cardiogenic shock and can prolong survival until interventional procedures can be performed. IABPC may be contraindicated in patients with aortic insufficiency or severe peripheral vascular disease.

The dismal outcome of cardiogenic shock complicating acute myocardial infarction has been improved in recent years. Evidence from a randomized trial suggests that emergent revascularization is not superior to medical management in reducing short-term mortality; however, significant improvements in mortality are seen at 6 months and 1 year (see Chapter 77).[68,69] At present, the management of acute myocardial infarction with cardiogenic shock proceeds as follows and constitutes optimal therapy: (1) ensure adequate ventilation and oxygenation, (2) treat emergent dysrhythmias, (3) initiate inotropic support, (4) administer aspirin if the patient is not allergic, and (5) begin heparin anticoagulation (in absence of contraindications) and arrange for emergent percutaneous transluminal coronary angioplasty.

Anaphylactic Shock

Therapy for anaphylactic shock is aimed at reversing the effect of its mediators. Aggressive volume resuscitation with isotonic fluid should be initiated rapidly in any patient with suspected anaphylactic shock. Epinephrine effectively counteracts the vasodepression, bronchoconstriction, fluid transudation, and reduced cardiac function in anaphylaxis. Epinephrine should be administered intravenously in patients with hypotension, even in the presence of coronary artery disease. Initially, 1 mL of 1:10,000 epinephrine (100 µg) can be injected slowly and the response monitored. Afterward, 5 mg of epinephrine can be diluted in 500 mL of saline, with a starting infusion rate of 10 mL/hr (about 0.02 µg/kg/min) and titrated to maintain perfusion. Corticosteroids are integral to arresting synthesis and release of anaphylaxis mediators. Corticosteroids inhibit phospholipase A_2 and decrease prostanoid, leukotriene, and PAF synthesis. Corticosteroids also quench T-cell and mast cell triggering and reduce late-phase bronchial inflammation. Hydrocortisone (5 to 10 mg/kg intravenously) or methylprednisolone (1.5 to 2 mg/kg intravenously) are good choices in anaphylaxis. Histamine receptor antagonists (H_1 and H_2) prevent urticaria, aid in reducing bronchoconstriction, reduce fluid transudation, and may improve myocardial function. Diphenhydramine (0.5 mg/kg intravenously) and cimetidine (2 to 5 mg/kg intravenously) may be used. Nebulized β_2-agonists can be used to help reduce bronchospasm. For patients with profound bronchospasm, obvious increased work of breathing, and hypotension, mechanical ventilation is indicated. Ketamine is a logical agent to use for sedation during rapid sequence intubation with succinylcholine (see Chapter 1).

KEY CONCEPTS

- Circulatory shock often occurs with normal arterial BP, and not all patients with arterial hypotension have circulatory shock.
- A base deficit more negative than −4 mEq/L or a serum lactate greater than 4 mmol/L indicates the presence of widespread circulatory insufficiency in suspected shock.
- Urine output is a reliable index of vital organ perfusion in patients with suspected shock.
- Ill patients with tachycardia, a worsening base deficit, and low urine output should be diagnosed with circulatory shock.
- Use of defined physiologic endpoints to measure systemic perfusion during resuscitation (goal-directed therapy) is a valuable approach to optimal resuscitation in emergency department patients with shock.

REFERENCES

1. Astiz ME, Rackow EC: Septic shock. *Lancet* 351:1501, 1998.
2. Shoemaker WC, et al: Resuscitation from severe hemorrhage. *Crit Care Med* 24:S12, 1996.
3. Blalock A: *Principles of Surgical Care: Shock and Other Problems.* St Louis, Mosby, 1940.
4. Williams RS: Canaries in the coal mine: Mitochondrial DNA and vascular injury from reactive oxygen species. *Circ Res* 86:915, 2000.
5. Watts J, Kline J: Bench to bedside: The role of mitochondrial medicine in the pathogenesis and treatment of cellular injury. *Acad Emerg Med* 10:985, 2003.
6. Gore DC, et al: Lactic acidosis during sepsis is related to increased pyruvate production, not deficits in tissue oxygen availability. *Ann Surg* 224:97, 1996.
7. Luchette FA, et al: Increased skeletal muscle Na⁺, K⁺-ATPase activity as a cause of increased lactate production after hemorrhagic shock. *J Trauma* 44:796, 1998.
8. Hotchkiss RS, Karl IE: Reevaluation of the role of cellular hypoxia and bioenergetic failure in sepsis. *JAMA* 267:1503, 1992.
9. Daniel AM, Shizgal HM, MacLean LD: The anatomic and metabolic source of lactate in shock. *Surg Gynecol Obstet* 147:697, 1978.
10. Bellomo R, Kellum JA, Pinsky MR: Transvisceral lactate fluxes during early endotoxemia. *Chest* 110:198, 1996.
11. Kapoor R, Prasad K: Role of polymorphonuclear leukocytes in cardiovascular depression and cellular injury in hemorrhagic shock and reinfusion. *Free Rad Biol Med* 21:609, 1996.
12. Liaudet L, Soriano FG, Szabo C: Biology of nitric oxide signaling. *Crit Care Med* 28:N37, 2000.
13. Taegtmeyer H: Six blind men explore an elephant: Aspects of fuel metabolism and the control of tricarboxylic acid cycle activity in heart muscle. *Basic Res Cardiol* 79:322, 1984.
14. Kojima S, et al: Effects of perfusion pressure on intracellular calcium, energetics, and function in perfused rat hearts. *Am J Physiol* 264:H183, 1993.
15. Siegel HW, Downing SE: Contributions of coronary perfusion pressure, metabolic acidosis and adrenergic factors to the reduction of myocardial contractility during hemorrhagic shock in the cat. *Circ Res* 27:875, 1970.
16. Barbee RW, Kline JA, Watts JA: Depletion of lactate by dichloroacetate reduces cardiac efficiency after hemorrhagic sepsis. *Shock* 14:208, 2000.

17. Dhainaut JF, et al: Coronary hemodynamics and myocardial metabolism of lactate, free fatty acids, glucose, and ketones in patients with septic shock. *Circulation* 75:533, 1987.
18. Kline JA, et al: Insulin improves heart function and metabolism during non-ischemic cardiogenic shock in awake canines. *Cardiovasc Res* 34:289, 1997.
19. Kumar A, et al: Tumor necrosis factor alpha and interleukin 1beta are responsible for in vitro myocardial cell depression induced by human septic shock serum. *J Exp Med* 183:949, 1996.
20. Cain BS, et al: Tumor necrosis factor-alpha and interleukin-1beta synergistically depress human myocardial function. *Crit Care Med* 27:1309, 1999.
21. Wo CC, et al: Unreliability of blood pressure and heart rate to evaluate cardiac output in emergency resuscitation and critical illness. *Crit Care Med* 21:218, 1993.
22. Davis JW, Kaups KL, Parks SN: Base deficit is superior to pH in evaluating clearance of acidosis after traumatic shock. *J Trauma* 44:114, 1998.
23. McDonough KH, et al: Effects of blood resuscitation versus dextran resuscitation after hemorrhage on intrinsic myocardial function. *J Trauma* 48:1122, 2000.
24. Barbee RW, Kline JA, Watts JA: A comparison of resuscitation with packed red blood cells and whole blood following hemorrhagic shock in canines. *Shock* 12:449, 1999.
25. Maitra SR, Gestring M, el Maghrabi MR: Alterations in hepatic 6-phosphofructo-2-kinase/fructose-2,6-bisphosphatase and glucose-6-phosphatase gene expression after hemorrhagic hypotension and resuscitation. *Shock* 8:385, 1997.
26. Heineman FW, Balaban RS: *The Heart and Cardiovascular System.* New York, Raven, 1992.
27. Parker MM, et al: Profound but reversible myocardial depression in patients with septic shock. *Ann Intern Med* 100:483, 1984.
28. Tatsumi T, et al: Cytokine-induced nitric oxide production inhibits mitochondrial energy production and impairs contractile function in rat cardiac myocytes. *J Am Coll Cardiol* 35:1338, 2000.
29. Watts JA, et al: Metabolic dysfunction and depletion of mitochondria in hearts of septic rats. *J Mol Cell Cardiol* 36:141, 2004.
30. Moore CL, et al: Determination of left ventricular function by emergency physician echocardiography of hypotensive patients. *Acad Emerg Med* 9:186, 2002.
31. Goldhaber SZ, Visani L, De Rosa M: Acute pulmonary embolism: Clinical outcomes in the International Cooperative Pulmonary Embolism Registry (ICOPER). *Lancet* 353:1386, 1999.
32. Sullivan DM, Watts JA, Kline JA: Biventricular cardiac dysfunction after acute massive pulmonary embolism in the rat. *J Appl Physiol* 90:1648, 2001.
33. Terashita Z, et al: Beneficial effects of TCV-309, a novel potent and selective platelet activating factor antagonist in endotoxin and anaphylactic shock in rodents. *J Pharmacol Exp Ther* 260:748, 1992.
34. Rady MY, et al: A comparison of the shock index and conventional vital signs to identify acute, critical illness in the emergency department. *Ann Emerg Med* 24:685, 1994.
35. Porter JM, Ivatury RR: In search of the optimal end points of resuscitation in trauma patients: A review. *J Trauma* 44:908, 1998.
36. Jones AE, et al: Nontraumatic out-of-hospital hypotension predicts inhospital mortality. *Ann Emerg Med* 43:106, 2004.
37. Jones AE, et al: Randomized controlled trial of immediate versus delayed goal-directed ultrasound to identify the cause of nontraumatic hypotension in emergency department patients. *Crit Care Med* 32:1703, 2004.
38. Bone RC, et al: Definitions for sepsis and organ failure and guidelines for the use of innovative therapies in sepsis. The

ACCP/SCCM Consensus Conference Committee. American College of Chest Physicians/Society of Critical Care Medicine. *Chest* 101:1644, 1992.

39. Califf RM, Bengtson JR: Cardiogenic shock. *N Engl J Med* 330:1724, 1994.

40. Thomas NJ, Carcillo JA: Hypovolemic shock in pediatric patients. *New Horiz* 6:120, 1998.

41. Abramson D, et al: Lactate clearance and survival following injury. *J Trauma* 35:584, 1993.

42. Stenzel JP, et al: Percutaneous femoral venous catheterizations: A prospective study of complications. *J Pediatr* 114:411, 1989.

43. Richard C, et al: Early use of the pulmonary artery catheter and outcomes in patients with shock and acute respiratory distress syndrome. *JAMA* 290:2713, 2003.

44. Ivanov R, Allen J, Calvin JE: The incidence of major morbidity in critically ill patients managed with pulmonary artery catheters: A meta-analysis. *Crit Care Med* 28:615, 2000.

45. Gattinoni L, et al: A trial of goal-oriented hemodynamic therapy in critically ill patients. *N Engl J Med* 333:1025, 1995.

46. Reinhart K, et al: Comparison of central-venous to mixed-venous oxygen saturation during changes in oxygen supply/demand. *Chest* 95:1216, 1989.

47. Gomersall CD, et al: Resuscitation of critically ill patients based on the results of gastric tonometry: A prospective, randomized, controlled trial. *Crit Care Med* 28:607, 2000.

48. Rivers E, Nishikawa K, Havstad SRJ: Early goal-directed therapy in the treatment of severe sepsis and septic shock. *N Engl J Med* 345:1368, 2001.

49. Aubier M, Trippenbach T, Roussos C: Respiratory muscle fatigue during cardiogenic shock. *J Appl Physiol* 51:499, 1981.

50. Pinsky MR: Cardiopulmonary interactions: The effects of negative and positive changes in pleural pressure on cardiac output. *Cardiopulm Crit Care* 50:87, 1998.

51. Diebel L, et al: End-diastolic volume versus pulmonary artery wedge pressure in evaluating cardiac preload in trauma patients. *J Trauma* 37:950, 1994.

52. Cook LS: An overview of leukocyte depletion in blood transfusion. *J Intravenous Nurs* 18:11, 1995.

53. Schleuning M, et al: Complement activation during storage of blood under normal blood bank conditions: Effects of proteinase inhibitors and leukocyte depletion. *Blood* 79:3071, 1992.

54. Sloan EP, et al: Diaspirin cross-linked hemoglobin in the treatment of severe traumatic hemorrhagic shock. *JAMA* 282:1857, 1999.

55. Bickell WH, et al: Immediate versus delayed fluid resuscitation for hypotensive patients with penetrating torso injuries. *N Engl J Med* 331:1105, 1994.

56. Dutton RP, Mackenzie CF, Scalea TM: Hypotensive resuscitation during active hemorrhage: Impact on in-hospital mortality. *J Trauma* 52:1141, 2002.

57. Nordin A, Makisalo H, Hockerstedt K: Dopamine infusion during resuscitation of experimental hemorrhagic shock. *Crit Care Med* 22:151, 1994.

58. Rackow EC, et al: Fluid resuscitation in circulatory shock: A comparison of the cardiorespiratory effects of albumin, hetastarch, and saline solutions in patients with hypovolemic and septic shock. *Crit Care Med* 11:839, 1983.

59. Sarkodee-Adoo CB, Merz WG, Karp JE: Management of infections in patients with acute leukemia. *Oncology* 14:659, 2000.

60. Bernard GR, et al: Efficacy and safety of recombinant human activated protein C for severe sepsis. *N Engl J Med* 344:699, 2001.

61. Warren HS, et al: Risks and benefits of activated protein C treatment for severe sepsis. *N Engl J Med* 347:1027, 2002.

62. Veterans Administration Systemic Sepsis Cooperative Study Group: Effect of high dose glucocorticoid therapy on mortality in patients with clinical signs of systemic sepsis. *N Engl J Med* 317:659, 1987.

63. Bone RC, et al: A controlled clinical trial of high dose methylprednisolone in the treatment of severe sepsis and septic shock. *N Engl J Med* 317:653, 1987.

64. Annane D, et al: Effect of treatment with low doses of hydrocortisone and fludrocortisone on mortality in patients with septic shock. *JAMA* 288:862, 2002.

65. Riggs TR, Yano Y, Vargish T: Morphine depression of myocardial function. *Circ Shock* 19:31, 1986.

66. Benotti JR, et al: Effects of amrinone on myocardial energy metabolism and hemodynamics in patients with severe congestive heart failure due to coronary artery disease. *Circulation* 62:28, 1980.

67. Scheidt S, et al: Intra-aortic balloon counterpulsation in cardiogenic shock: Report of a co-operative clinical trial. *N Engl J Med* 288:979, 1973.

68. Hochman JS, et al: Early revascularization in acute myocardial infarction complicated by cardiogenic shock. SHOCK Investigators. Should We Emergently Revascularize Occluded Coronaries for Cardiogenic Shock. *N Engl J Med* 341:625, 1999.

69. Hochman JS, et al: One year survival following early revascularization for cardiogenic shock. *JAMA* 285:190, 2001.

CHAPTER

5 Blood and Blood Components

Gwendolyn L. Hoffman

PERSPECTIVE

The era of modern blood transfusion began in the early 1900s with the discovery of A, B, O, and AB blood types. The first blood bank in the United States was established in 1937.[1] Whole blood and plasma were widely used during World War II as resuscitative fluids. In the 1950s the introduction of plastic storage containers and apheresis instruments made component therapy possible. By the 1970s the use of blood components became more popular than whole blood.[2] The number of red blood cell (RBC) units transfused in the United States was 12.4 million in 2000, which was a 4% to 5% increase from 1999.[3]

Increased demand for the blood supply is expected in the future because of the predicted increase in population older than 65.[4] Currently, much research is being conducted on the development of blood substitutes. The two major classes are cell-free hemoglobin solutions that approximate the oxygen-carrying capacity and oxygen delivery of cellular hemoglobin and perfluorocarbon emulsions that act as synthetic oxygen carriers. Potential advantages of these products include a prolonged shelf life, ability to be stored at room temperature, universal biocompatibility, and reduced risk of disease transmission. They will help reduce the demand for banked blood.[5]

PATHOPHYSIOLOGIC PRINCIPLES

Blood Banking

Blood and blood products are provided to most institutions by specific blood bank services such as the American Red Cross. These services offer centralized testing laboratories and record keeping, area-wide inventories of blood components, and simplified medical control.

At the time of collection an anticoagulant-preservative of citrate, phosphate, dextrose, and adenine (CPDA-1) is added, ensuring a shelf life (viability of at least 70% of the RBCs 24 hours after infusion) of 35 days and hematocrit of 70% to 80% for packed red blood cells (PRBCs). An alternative additive solution containing higher concentrations of saline and glucose (e.g., Adsol) extends the shelf life to 42 days and decreases the hematocrit to 52% to 60%, which makes it easier to administer.[2]

Even though blood must be stored and refrigerated at 1° C to 6° C (usually at 4° C), cell metabolism continues and changes occur (*storage lesions*). A decrease in pH causes a degree of acidosis that is effectively buffered by the metabolism of the citrate preservative. Levels of 2,3-diphosphoglycerate (2,3-DPG) also decrease, resulting in a shift of the oxyhemoglobin dissociation curve to the left. The level soon rises again and within 24 hours of infusion is usually normal and of little clinical significance. Also, deformability of RBCs causes them to become more spherical and rigid, resulting in increased resistance to flow through capillary beds. This is also corrected with transfusion.[2]

The sodium-potassium adenosine triphosphatase–dependent pump also becomes less efficient, resulting in some cell leakage of potassium. In neonates and patients with renal impairment, this could result in hyperkalemia. Normally, the impact is not significant because the increased potassium load is excreted by the kidneys, absorbed by the remaining RBCs, or shifted intracellularly.[1]

After 24 hours of storage, granulocytes have no functional capacity and platelets have only 50% capacity, which becomes zero by 72 hours. Levels of factor V and factor VIII also decrease.[6]

Blood Typing

More than 400 RBC antigens have been identified. ABO identification and compatibility constitute the most important step of the type-and-crossmatch procedure because any incompatibility produces the most serious transfusion reaction, *acute hemolysis.* Patients who lack A or B red cell antigens have antibodies for the absent A (blood type B) or B (blood type A) antigen. Patients who lack both A and B antigens have antibodies against both A and B antigens (blood type O). Rh typing, antibody screening, and the testing of donor cells with recipient serum are also done. Antibody screening is performed with recipient serum to discover agglutinating or nonagglutinating antibodies. The antiglobulin (Coombs') test is also included.[2] The risk of disease transmission is extremely low because of the development of improved screening and testing techniques (Table 5-1).

Universal Donor Blood

In crisis situations in which there is no time for type and crossmatch, group O universal donor blood is indicated. RBCs of type O do not have A or B antigens on their surface and therefore are not agglutinated or hemolyzed by anti-A or anti-B antibodies. Because of the relative scarcity of group O–negative blood, its use is restricted to women of childbearing age who are at risk for Rh immunization against subsequent pregnancies. Universal donor group O–positive blood is recommended in all other patients.[6]

Massive Transfusion

In a patient's initial resuscitation in the emergency department, abnormalities from massive transfusion are rarely seen, but the physician should be aware of potential problems. Massive transfusion is defined as replacement of the patient's blood volume with stored RBCs in 24 hours or as a transfusion of greater than 10 units of blood over a few hours. A blood volume is estimated at 75 mL/kg or about 5000 mL in a 70-kg man.[7]

In addition to storage lesion problems, hypothermia may result when patients receive more than 100 mL/min of cold blood for 30 minutes, placing them at increased risk for ventricular dysrhythmias. This can be prevented by warming the blood to 37° C with a blood warmer.[8] Transiently decreased levels of ionized calcium may result from the citrate preservative. Clinical signs of hypocalcemia include circumoral tingling, skeletal muscle tremors, and a prolongation of the QT

Table 5-1. Risk of Transfusion-Transmitted Viruses

Virus	Risk per Unit Transferred
Hepatitis B	1:58,000 to 1:149,000
Hepatitis C	1:872,000 to 1:1.7 million
Human immunodeficiency virus	1:1.4 million to 1:2.4 million

Data from Goodnough LT, Shander A, Brecker ME: Transfusion medicine: Looking to the future. *Lancet* 361:162, 2003.

segment of the electrocardiogram (ECG). Most normothermic adults can tolerate 1 unit of RBCs every 5 minutes without calcium supplementation. Calcium administration should be used only when the patient's ionized calcium levels drop to abnormal values or when ECG changes occur.[1,6]

Dilutional thrombocytopenia may result, but platelet concentrate is not indicated unless there is evidence of microvascular bleeding in a normothermic patient. If disseminated intravascular coagulation (DIC) develops, large doses of platelet concentrate, fresh frozen plasma (FFP), and cryoprecipitate may be required.[1]

CLINICAL FEATURES

The need to administer blood component therapy in the emergency department is specific to the situation and the patient. The patient's stability and the time available before intervention is needed determine the specific product that is utilized.

Universal Donor Group O

Universal donor group O is immediately available and is used when blood must be given at once to hemorrhaging, unstable patients. Women of childbearing age need group O–negative blood, and all others can receive group O–positive blood, which is more readily available.

Type and Crossmatch

If the patient's condition can be initially stabilized with crystalloid infusion, type-specific blood should be available in 5 to 10 minutes. ABO grouping and Rh typing are sufficient.[7]

Incomplete type and crossmatch take approximately 30 minutes. They involve ABO and Rh compatibility as well as screening of the recipient's serum for unexpected antibodies. An immediate "spin" crossmatch is also performed at room temperature.[6]

When blood is not immediately needed, fully crossmatched blood, which takes approximately 45 minutes to process, should be used.[7]

Administration

Legal Aspects

Before a blood product can be infused, it must be checked at the bedside by two qualified personnel. This check includes recipient and unit identification, compatibility, and expiration.[8] The identification of the patient and the intended product prevents a potentially fatal clerical error.

At times a patient may arrive from a transferring facility with type and crossmatched blood. If the blood is administered immediately in the emergency department, the hospital blood bank is not involved and accepts no responsibility for the blood. If the blood is not used immediately and the blood bank is requested to hold the blood for the patient, the blood must be processed and crossmatched as for other issued blood

and quarantined for 24 hours. It can be sent back to the blood bank to have this done only if (1) it has been maintained at a temperature below 6° C, (2) all container seals are intact and have not been entered, and (3) segments have remained attached to the blood container.[8]

Infusion Adjuncts

Urgent transfusion situations require flow rates faster than gravity can provide. An administration set with an in-line pump that is squeezed by hand is the simplest method to speed infusion. Pressure bags are also available that completely encase the blood bag and apply pressure evenly to the blood bag surface. If external pressure is anticipated, large-bore needles are recommended for venous access to prevent hemolysis by manually forcing RBCs through a small-gauge line.[8]

If only a small-gauge needle is available, the transfusion may be diluted with normal saline (NS), but this may cause unwanted volume expansion. In elective transfusions, no significant hemolysis occurs when small-gauge needles are used and when the maximum rate of infusion is less than 100 mL/hr.[8]

MANAGEMENT

Decision Making

The decision to use blood component therapy must encompass the entire clinical picture. The patient's age, severity of symptoms, cause of the deficit, underlying medical condition, ability to compensate for decreased oxygen-carrying capacity, and tissue oxygen requirements must all be considered. Clinical evaluation, including appearance (pale color, pale conjunctiva, diaphoresis), mentation (alert, confused), heart rate, blood pressure, and the nature of the bleeding (active, controlled, uncontrolled), can be supplemented by laboratory evaluation of hemoglobin, hematocrit, platelets, and clotting functions.[9]

Transfusions are needed if a rapid loss is greater than 30% to 40% of blood volume and if tachycardia and hypotension are not corrected by crystalloid replacement alone. Transfusion is rarely needed with a hemoglobin concentration greater than 10 g/dL and almost always needed when the hemoglobin is less than 6 g/dL.[10,11]

Whole Blood

Whole blood is not as useful and economical as component therapy. In the United States it is essentially unavailable in the emergency department.[1]

Packed Red Blood Cells

PRBCs are administered for acute blood loss in an otherwise healthy patient with signs and symptoms of decreased oxygen delivery and at least two of the following: estimated or expected blood loss of 15% or more of total blood volume (750 mL in 70-kg man), hypotension, tachycardia, oliguria, and mental status changes.[1] PRBCs are also used for patients with symptomatic anemia and evidence of myocardial ischemia, including angina, shortness of breath or dizziness with mild exertion, tachycardia, and mental status changes.[12] RBCs are not indicated with a hemoglobin concentration greater than 10 g/dL (men) or 7 g/dL (women) in an otherwise stable asymptomatic patient.[1]

Fresh Frozen Plasma

FFP is indicated for emergent reversal of warfarin therapy and correction of known coagulation deficiencies when specific concentrates are unavailable. It is also useful in DIC when prothrombin and partial thromboplastin times are greater than 1.5 times normal. Empirical use during massive transfusion when the patient does not exhibit coagulopathy is questionable. FFP is not recommended for augmentation of plasma volume or albumin concentration.[1,11]

Platelets

On occasion, a patient may receive platelets in the emergency department. They are indicated prophylactically when the count is less than 20,000/mL or less than 50,000/mL if there is oozing or a planned invasive procedure. When platelet counts are below 10,000/mm³, spontaneous bleeding is common and may be severe. Patients taking abciximab (ReoPro) who develop bleeding may require platelet transfusion.[13] Prophylactic platelet transfusion is ineffective when the thrombocytopenia is caused by increased platelet destruction.[1,11] Also, no evidence indicates that prophylactic transfusion of platelets is beneficial in massive transfusion.[13]

Autotransfusion

Autotransfusion may be used in the event of severe chest trauma. There is immediate availability; blood compatibility; normothermic blood; elimination of risk of patient-to-patient disease transmission; higher levels of 2,3-DPG than in stored blood; less risk of circulatory overload; fewer direct complications, such as hyperkalemia, hypocalcemia, and metabolic acidosis; and greater acceptability to some patients whose religious convictions prohibit transfusions.[14,15] Widespread use has not occurred, however, because of the limited number of appropriate trauma patients, the training required to operate the autologous collection and reinfusion equipment, the time required for equipment setup, and the need for improving safety and availability of homologous blood.[2,16]

Therapeutic Modalities

Packed Red Blood Cells

In acute hemorrhage, PRBCs are used to supplement initial crystalloid replacement. In an average adult, 1 unit of PRBCs increases the hemoglobin by about 1 g/dL or the hematocrit by about 3%. A similar increase in pediatric patients is obtained by administering 3 mL/kg.[1,2,11] PRBCs must be run through a filter with a large-bore intravenous line with NS. Lactated Ringer's solution could lead to clotting secondary to the added calcium, and hemolysis may result with a hypotonic solution. From 50 to 100 mL of NS may be added for a dilutional effect to permit faster administration. Medications should never be added to the unit or pushed through the transfusion line unless it has been thoroughly flushed. Most transfusions are given over 60 to 90 minutes and no longer than 4 hours. Any excess units should be returned promptly to the blood bank because any units unrefrigerated for more than 30 minutes are discarded.[2,13]

Fresh Frozen Plasma

A unit of FFP typically has a volume of 200 to 250 mL, must be ABO compatible, and is given through blood tubing within 2 to 6 hours of thawing. It contains all clotting factors, including factors V and VIII, which are labile. One unit of activity for any coagulation factor is equal to 1 mL of FFP. It should be given in doses calculated to achieve a minimum of 30% of plasma factor concentration, which is usually 10 to 15 mL/kg of FFP. When used for the urgent reversal of warfarin anticoagulation, 5 to 8 mL/kg of FFP is usually sufficient.[2,11]

Platelets

Crossmatching is unnecessary, but Rh-negative patients should receive Rh-negative platelets because there may be enough cells in the platelet concentrate to cause Rh sensitization. Each bag contains at least 5.5×10^{10} platelets in 50 to 70 mL of plasma. On average, a single unit raises the platelet count by 5000/mm³. In adults the usual dose is 6 to 10 units, and in children it is 1 U/10 kg body weight. In situations in which human leukocyte antigen (HLA) matching of platelets is required, leukocyte-reduced apheresis platelets can be used to prevent HLA antibodies.[1,2]

OUTCOMES

Adverse effects of RBC transfusion can be divided into immune-mediated and non–immune-mediated categories, as well as acute, delayed, and chronic effects.

Immune-Mediated Adverse Effects

Acute

Intravascular Hemolytic Transfusion Reaction

Intravascular hemolytic transfusion reaction is the most serious transfusion reaction and is usually the result of ABO incompatibility. It is often the result of a clerical error. An antigen-antibody reaction results in the intravascular destruction of transfused cells. Lysis of the transfused RBCs causes hemoglobin to be released, producing hemoglobinemia and hemoglobinuria. The onset of symptoms is immediate, and the patient may have fever, chills, headache, nausea, vomiting, and a burning sensation at the site of the infusion. A sensation of chest restriction, shock, and severe joint or low back pain may also be present.[2,9,17] Treatment includes stopping the transfusion immediately, hanging all new tubing, and initiating vigorous crystalloid fluid therapy. Diuretic therapy should be used to maintain urine output at 1 to 2 mL/kg/hr. Dopamine in renal-sparing doses may be needed to sustain the blood pressure and protect the kidneys. The use of steroids is not currently recommended. Renal and coagulation status should be monitored.[2,17] Because acute tubular necrosis and DIC may develop, a urine and a blood specimen should be obtained and sent to the laboratory, as well as the remainder of the transfusion and the blood tubing.

Febrile Transfusion Reaction

This most common and least serious transfusion reaction is characterized by fever, chills, and malaise. Reactions are frequently related to antileukocyte and antiplatelet antibodies and seen in multiply transfused patients. Treatment is symptomatic with an analgesic-antipyretic and an antihistamine. If recurrent febrile reactions occur in a patient, leukocyte-poor RBCs (washed, frozen-thawed-deglycerolized, filtered) should be considered. If a febrile reaction occurs in a first-time transfusion, it should be treated in the same way as an extravascular hemolytic reaction until proved otherwise.[2,17]

Allergic Reactions (Urticaria to Anaphylaxis)

Urticaria or hives may occur during a transfusion without other signs or symptoms and no serious sequelae. It is generally attributed to an allergic, antibody-mediated response to a donor's plasma proteins. The transfusion does not need to be stopped, and treatment with an antihistamine is usually sufficient. If the patient has a known history of this, the antihistamine should be administered before the transfusion. Occasionally, full anaphylaxis may be caused by an anti–immunoglobulin A (IgA) reaction to IgA in the donor's blood components. The patient is likely to have a genetic IgA deficiency and display hypotension, respiratory and gastrointestinal symptoms, but no fever. Treatment is with epinephrine and corticosteroids. Future transfusions should be with washed RBCs, and plasma products should be from other IgA-deficient individuals.[17]

Transfusion-Related Acute Lung Injury

Transfusion-related acute lung injury (TRALI) results from transfusion of white blood cell antibodies (leukoagglutinins) that react with the recipient's leukocytes. Clinically, TRALI is indistinguishable from acute respiratory distress syndrome. The patient has acute respiratory distress, diffuse bilateral alveolar and interstitial infiltrates on the chest radiograph, and varying degrees of hypoxemia. Hypotension and fever are also present. Appearance is usually within 6 hours of transfusion and may occur after the infusion of relatively small quantities of blood or plasma. Treatment consists of stopping the transfusion and providing respiratory support, which may include intubation and mechanical ventilation.[17-19]

Delayed

Extravascular Hemolytic Transfusion Reaction

The onset of an extravascular hemolytic transfusion reaction is likely to be delayed by several days to weeks. High titers of antibodies to erythrocyte antigens other than anti-A and anti-B are not present in the plasma of most individuals. For a non–ABO-mediated transfusion reaction to occur, an anamnestic immune response must first develop. In other words, a prior exposure to a foreign RBC antigen must occur, followed by rechallenge with the same antigen. The patient may have fever, anemia, and jaundice. Symptoms are not usually severe, and no specific treatment is needed. Because the hemolysis is extravascular, hemoglobinemia and hemoglobinuria are rarely present.[17]

Transfusion-Associated Graft-versus-Host Disease

During a transfusion the recipient is exposed to a variety of cells and proteins from the donor, including viable lymphocytes, which in an immunocompromised patient can result in graft-versus-host disease. These multiplying, immunocompetent, histoincompatible lymphocytes attack the recipient, causing further bone marrow suppression. High fever, erythematous maculopapular skin rash (frequently postauricular), anorexia, nausea and vomiting, profuse diarrhea, hepatomegaly, elevated liver enzymes, and pancytopenia may be seen. No effective treatment exists and death ensues, usually the result of overwhelming sepsis. Efforts are therefore directed at prevention by using gamma irradiation of all cellular components, which renders the donor lymphocytes incapable of proliferating. The use of leukocyte-poor components is also advocated. This condition is rarely encountered in the emergency department but should be kept in mind when considering transfusion in anemic leukemia or lymphoma patients, especially those who have recently received chemotherapy.[1,2,17]

Non–Immune-Mediated Adverse Effects

Acute

Circulatory Overload

Chronically anemic, normovolemic elderly patients are at greatest risk for developing congestive heart failure with the rapid infusion of blood. Taking 4 hours to infuse a unit and using diuretics (if needed) should prevent this complication.[2,17]

Bacterial Contamination

Bacterial contamination of stored blood is rare but can be a severe risk to the transfusion recipient. Both gram-negative and gram-positive organisms may grow in units of RBCs and more commonly in pooled platelet concentrates.[20] This contamination may result from faulty preparation of collection equipment, contamination of the anticoagulant solution, or poor technique while collecting or administering the blood. *Yersinia enterocolitica* is the organism most often implicated in RBC contamination, and *Staphylococcus aureus* is the most common organism in platelet contamination.[19] During or after the transfusion the patient may develop rigors, severe fever, hypotension, and shock.

Hemoglobinuria and hemoglobinemia are rarely present. When a septic transfusion reaction is considered, aggressive resuscitative therapy and broad-spectrum antibiotics should be started and the transfusion stopped.[13]

Other Effects

Although infrequent, the following complications may occur secondary to multiple unit transfusions: hypocalcemia, hyperkalemia and acidosis, hypothermia, microembolization, and coagulopathies. Treatment is specific to the symptom and problem.[2,13]

Chronic

Risk of Transmission-Transmitted Viruses

Improved techniques for selecting and testing blood donors have dramatically reduced the risk of viral transmission of disease by transfusion. The blood supply in the United States has never been safer.[19,21-23] The current rates of transmission of viral infections are too low to measure, so mathematical models have been used to estimate the risks of transmission of human immunodeficiency virus, hepatitis C virus, hepatitis B virus, and human T cell lymphotropic virus types I and II.[19-22] Cytomegalovirus can be transmitted by blood transfusion as well and is largely a problem associated with neonatal or intrauterine transfusions and with immunocompromised patients.[9]

Transfusional Hemosiderosis

Transfusional hemosiderosis is a condition of iron overload that may develop in chronically transfused patients. Each milliliter of PRBCs contains 1 mg of iron, and with continued transfusions, iron can accumulate, causing liver and heart damage. Patients may require chelation therapy.[13]

 KEY CONCEPTS

- Type and screen should be ordered rather than type and crossmatch unless transfusion is inevitable. Crossmatched blood is reserved for specific patients for 48 hours.
- Normal saline (0.9% NS) is the only approved solution for use with blood. Lactated Ringer's solution is not used with PRBCs.
- O-positive blood can be used if type specific or type and crossmatch blood is not yet available. O-negative blood should only be used in women of childbearing age.
- If the transfusion is not begun within 30 minutes of issue, the blood should be returned to the blood bank.
- Most PRBC transfusions are given over 60 to 90 minutes and no longer than 4 hours.
- Patients may need to be pretreated with an antihistamine, antipyretic, or steroid 30 minutes before the transfusion to reduce risk of reaction.
- Intravascular hemolytic transfusion reaction is life threatening and most often secondary to a clerical error.

REFERENCES

1. Fakhry SM, Sheldon GF: Blood administration, risks, and substitutes. *Adv Surg* 28:71, 1995.
2. Labadie LL: Transfusion therapy in the emergency department. *Emerg Med Clin North Am* 11:379, 1993.
3. Goodnough LT, Shander A, Brecker ME: Transfusion medicine: Looking to the future. *Lancet* 361:161, 2003.
4. Vamvakan EC: Epidemiology of red blood cell utilization. *Transfus Med Rev* 10:44, 1996.
5. Stowell CP, Levin J, Spress BD, Winslow RM: Progress in the development of RBC substitutes. *Transfusion* 41:287, 2001.
6. Storer DL: Blood and blood component therapy. In Rosen P et al (eds): *Emergency Medicine: Concepts and Clinical Practice*, 4th ed. St Louis, Mosby, 1998.
7. American Association of Blood Banks: *Standards for Blood Banks and Transfusion Services*, 16th ed. Bethesda, Md, The Association, 1994.
8. American Association of Blood Banks: *Technical Manual*, 13th ed. Bethesda, Md, The Association, 1999.
9. Simon TL, et al: Practice parameter for the use of red blood cell transfusions. *Arch Pathol Lab Med* 122:130, 1998.
10. Stehling L, Simon TL: The red blood cell transfusion trigger. *Arch Pathol Lab Med* 118:429, 1994.
11. American Society of Anesthesiologists Task Force: Practice guidelines for blood component therapy. *Anesthesiology* 84:732, 1996.
12. Spence RK, Swisher SN: Red cell transfusion—The transfusion trigger. In Petz LD et al (eds): *Clinical Practice of Transfusion Medicine*, 3rd ed. New York, Churchill Livingstone, 1996.
13. Lan TA (ed): *Blood Transfusion Therapy, a Physician's Handbook*, 5th ed. Bethesda, Md, American Association of Blood Banks, 1996.
14. Goodnough LT, et al: Transfusion medicine. Part II. *N Engl J Med* 340:525, 1999.
15. Wilcox P: Jehovah's Witnesses and blood transfusions. *Lancet* 353:757, 1999.
16. National Heart, Lung, and Blood Institute Autologous Transfusion Symposium Working Group: Autologous transfusion: Current trends and research issues. *Transfusion* 35:525, 1995.
17. Jenner PW, Holland PV: Diagnosis and management of transfusion reactions. In Petz LD et al (eds): *Clinical Practice of Transfusion Medicine*, 3rd ed. New York, Churchill Livingstone, 1996.
18. Florell SR, Velasco SE, Fine PG: Perioperative recognition, management, and pathologic diagnosis of transfusion-related acute lung injury. *Anesthesiology* 81:508, 1994.
19. Goodnough LT, et al: Transfusion medicine. Part I. *N Engl J Med* 340:438, 1999.
20. Jacobs MR, Palavecino E, Yomtovian R: Don't bug me: The problem of bacterial contamination of blood components—Challenge and solution. *Transfusion* 41:1331, 2001.
21. Au Buchon JP, Birkmeyer JD, Bursch MP: Safety of the blood supply in the United States: Opportunities and controversies. *Ann Intern Med* 127:904, 1997.
22. Kleinman S, Bursch MP: General overview of transfusion-transmitted infections. In Petz LD et al (eds): *Clinical Practice of Transfusion Medicine*, 3rd ed. New York, Churchill Livingstone, 1996.
23. Perkins H: Transfusion reactions: The changing priorities. *Immunol Invest* 24:289, 1995.

Brain Resuscitation

Robert Silbergleit and Norman S. Abramson

From the brain and from the brain only, arise our pleasures, joys, laughter, and jests, as well as our sorrow, pain, grief, and tears.

Hippocrates, *The Sacred Disease*

PERSPECTIVE

Recognition of the dominant role of the brain in determining the quality of human life dates back to the dawn of recorded medical history. Until more recently, however, medical efforts after cardiac arrest have focused exclusively on cardiac resuscitation. Advances in the understanding of the pathophysiologic mechanisms of brain ischemia have directed attention to cerebral resuscitation. This chapter reviews the pathophysiology of postischemic encephalopathy and discusses accepted, newly proven, and promising future therapies for improving neurologic recovery after cardiac arrest.

PATHOPHYSIOLOGY

The human brain consists of 10 billion neurons, each with multiple connections to other cells, totaling an estimated 500 trillion synapses. Although the brain composes only 2% of body weight, it receives 15% of the body's cardiac output and accounts for 20% of the body's overall oxygen use because of its high metabolic activity. Although no mechanical or secretory work is performed, energy expenditures include the synthesis of cellular constituents (e.g., an estimated 2000 mitochondria are reproduced each day by each cell) and neurotransmitter substances, the axoplasmic transport of these substances, and the transmembrane pumping of ions.

When the brain is deprived of adequate blood flow, the resulting ischemia is characterized by a bewildering array of interrelated physiologic and cellular responses that ultimately result in neuronal cell death (Figure 6-1).[1] Although this complex cascade of events can be triggered by periods of ischemia lasting only a few minutes, the resulting neuronal death usually is delayed by hours or days. The biology of cerebral cell death after global cerebral ischemia follows (with slight variations) the pattern of delayed cerebral cell death that follows stroke, traumatic brain injury, and other forms of hypoxic or toxic brain injury. Increased understanding of the brain's response to injury during the period between insult and neuronal cell death

eventually will allow more specific brain resuscitation therapies.

Physiologic Responses to Cerebral Ischemia

The primary pathologic event in global cerebral ischemia is loss of adequate blood flow to the brain. Autoregulation allows the brain to compensate initially for decreases in systemic perfusion and oxygenation during cardiogenic shock, but as cerebral perfusion pressure decreases to less than about 30 to 60 mm Hg, cerebral blood flow (CBF) also decreases. As cerebral oxygen delivery is compromised, cerebral oxygen extraction from the blood increases until reaching a maximum extraction of about 70% to 80%. Cerebral oxygen delivery and brain function generally are maintained until CBF decreases to about 35% of baseline.[2] At this level, the electroencephalogram becomes flat, and sensory-evoked responses cannot be elicited, but membrane ionic potentials and cellular viability can be maintained for some time. When CBF decreases to 20% or less of baseline during cardiac arrest, loss of cerebral oxygen delivery causes the brain to use much less efficient anaerobic metabolic pathways, which are unable to meet the brain's metabolic demands. Neurons are unable to maintain ionic gradients, and widespread depolarization occurs, interstitial pH decreases, and brain edema forms. Prolonged or severe hypoperfusion triggers neuronal cell death through a cascade of cellular responses.

In all areas of the brain, neurons are typically more susceptible to ischemic injury than are surrounding glial and endothelial cells. Some areas of the brain, such as certain levels of the hippocampus, basal ganglia, and cortex, are more susceptible to neuronal cell death than others.[3] The reasons for the anatomic pattern of injury seen after global cerebral ischemia are unclear but may be related to afferent pathways of excitatory neurons or areas at risk for vascular insufficiency (boundary zones) or hemorrhage.

Reperfusion

Restoration of blood flow after cardiac arrest allows reperfusion of the ischemic brain. Reperfusion itself has characteristic pathophysiologic responses. Immediately after the onset of reperfusion, CBF is greater than normal for several minutes, followed by the gradual onset of delayed hypoperfusion for several hours.[4] The exact cause of this delayed hypoperfusion, which can be heterogeneous and is also called *no*

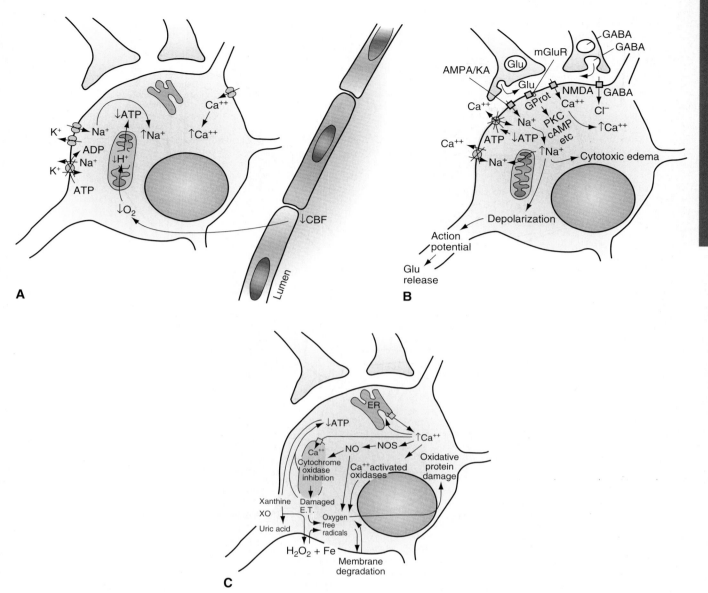

Figure 6-1. Synopsis of events contributing to neuron cell death cascade after ischemia. **A,** Decreased cerebral flow (DCF) and arterial oxygen content during ischemia cause decreased adenosine triphosphate (ATP) production, failure of ATP-driven ion pump efflux of potassium ions (K^+), and influx of sodium ions (Na^+) and calcium ions (Ca^{++}) through voltage-gated channels. ADP, adenosine diphosphate. **B,** Na^+ influx causes depolarization and glutamate (Glu) release, opening Glu receptor α-amino-3-hydroxy-5-methyl-4-isoxazolepropionate (AMPA) and kainate (KA) channels and exacerbating intracellular Na^+ overload. Increased sodium ion concentration ($[Na^+]i$) leads to cytotoxic edema. Glu-mediated *N*-methyl-D-aspartate (NMDA) channels allow intracellular Ca^{++} overload. Insufficient ATP causes failure of energy-dependent Ca^{++} pumps, and high $[Na^+]i$ prevents removal of Ca^{++} by Na^+/Ca^{++} exchange pumps. γ-Aminobutyric acid (GABA) release can attenuate excitatory changes by opening a receptor-gated Cl^-. $[Ca^{++}]i$, calcium ion concentration; cAMP, cyclic adenosine monophosphate; PKC, protein kinase C. **C,** Increased $[Ca^{++}]i$ is amplified by calcium-induced release of Ca^{++} from the endoplasmic reticulum (ER). Mitochondria may be injured attempting to buffer increasing $[Ca^{++}]i$, resulting in further metabolic failure and diminished ATP. Ca^{++} activates nitric oxide synthase (NOS) to make it nitric oxide (NO), which is amplified by NO activation of NOS. NO contributes to the formation of damaging oxygen free radicals and inhibits mitochondrial cytochrome oxidase function. ATP degradation to xanthine and then uric acid by xanthine oxidase (XO) yields hydrogen peroxide (H_2O_2), which reacts with iron to form dangerous oxygen radicals. Oxygen free radicals react with lipids in the cell membrane, which produces membrane degradation and more free radicals. Oxygen free radicals also can damage proteins.

reflow, is poorly understood, but may be related to vasospasm from endothelial-derived vasoconstrictors such as endothelin, from clumping of activated leukocytes, or from coagulation of blood in the microcirculation. Cerebral oxygen consumption is low during the hyperemic period immediately after reperfusion, but then gradually increases. During the period of delayed hypoperfusion, oxygen extraction may increase signif-

icantly, and no reflow may represent a secondary period of ischemia.[4]

The return of oxygen consumption in the brain during reperfusion allows global restoration of adenosine triphosphate (ATP) and improved pH, as determined by magnetic resonance spectroscopy. Tissue metabolic rate generally is depressed by about 50% for several hours after reperfusion, then gradually returns

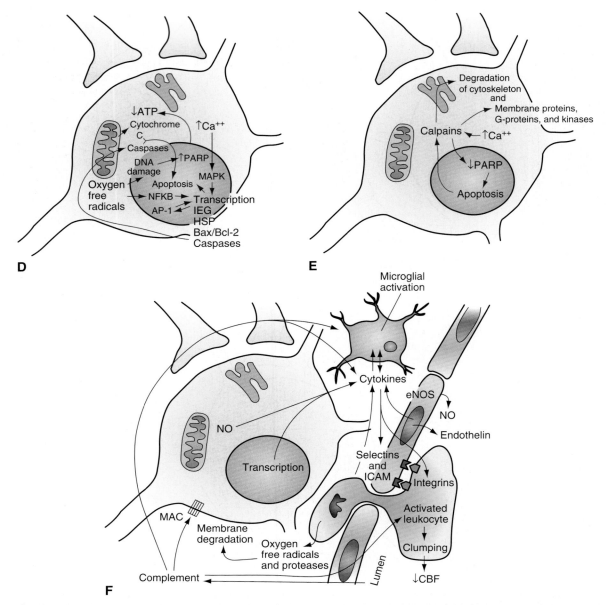

Figure 6-1, cont'd. D, Ca^{++} also activates kinase transcription factors, such as mitogen-activated protein kinase (MAPK). Oxygen radicals trigger nuclear factor κ B (NFκB), another transcription factor. Many genes, including immediate early genes (IEG), heat-shock protein (HSP) genes, genes for caspases, and the *Bax/Bcl-2* systems, are activated. IEG products include AP-1, another transcription factor. Mitochondrial release of cytochrome *c,* existing and newly formed caspases, and other factors trigger apoptosis. DNA is damaged by oxygen free radicals and by endonucleases formed in apoptosis. DNA damage activates poly(ADP-ribose) polymerase (PARP), which further depletes ATP stores. **E,** Ca^{++} and apoptosis activate calpains, proteases that degrade a variety of structural elements (e.g., cytoskeletal and membrane proteins), signaling elements (e.g., G proteins, kinases), and PARP. **F,** Transcription and NO contribute to neuronal expression of cytokines, chemokines, and growth factors. These intercellular signals activate complement, epithelial cells, leukocytes, and microglia. Complement can amplify chemotactic signals, activate microglia directly, or cause cellular damage by creation of the membrane attack complex (MAC). Leukocyte integrins, epithelial cell selectins, and intercellular adhesion molecules (ICAM) allow demargination. Activated leukocytes cause neuronal injury by releasing potent oxidants and protease. Cerebrovascular resistance may be affected by epithelial release of NO and endothelin and by leukocyte clumping. eNOS, endothelial nitric oxide synthase.

toward baseline. Failure to resume significant oxygen consumption after reperfusion, with subsequently low rates of cerebral oxygen extraction, is an ominous sign of globally irreversible cerebral metabolic failure.[5,6] Such failure, presumably because of destruction of the mitochondria or other cellular respiratory components, is an early predictor of a brain that cannot be resuscitated despite reperfusion.

Brain Edema

Brain edema begins during ischemia and continues during reperfusion. Swelling from cytotoxic edema generally predominates and reduces the intracellular space with little effect on intracranial pressure (ICP), whereas vasogenic edema is associated with increased ICP and secondary hemorrhage.[7] Cytotoxic brain edema occurs during ischemia and may continue during reperfusion because of increased cellular membrane ion permeability. Vasogenic brain edema occurs almost exclusively during reperfusion as a result of damage to the blood-brain barrier (BBB). Cellular responses to ischemia and reperfusion (inflammation), nitric oxide (NO), and other reactive oxygen species (ROS) attack the BBB from the luminal side, whereas protease degradation of the extracellular matrix and damage to astrocytes forming the BBB occur from the parenchymal (or abluminal) side.[8] Vasogenic edema may be bimodal, with an initial opening of the BBB several hours after reperfusion, followed by a second episode days later. Edema may cause increases in ICP that peak 24 to 72 hours after acute brain ischemia, but ICP monitoring and surgical decompression typically are not indicated in survivors of global cerebral ischemia.[7] Edema may be greater after focal cerebral ischemia, and decompressive hemicraniectomy has been used experimentally in selected patients with massive stroke.

Cellular Responses to Cerebral Ischemia

Cellular responses to ischemia are complex. They occur simultaneously at the cell surface, within the cytosol, and within the nucleus. Interactions between different pathways, or cascades, occur at multiple levels. These responses generally are categorized in this chapter as (1) *trigger events,* which initiate the ischemic cascades but are easily reversed with reperfusion; (2) *second messengers,* which mediate the ischemic responses during reperfusion; and (3) *perpetrators of functional or structural damage,* which are the final common pathways of cellular destruction.[1] The categories are illustrative but are not definitive. Many processes may fit into more than one category, and signaling may be bidirectional between different parts of this paradigm.

Trigger Events

Trigger events are the initial, often reversible, biochemical changes that result from ischemia and activate other intracellular and extracellular signals, which persist after reperfusion. Within seconds of the onset of ischemia, the decline in blood flow and the accompanying loss of oxygen supply result in a reduction of high-energy metabolites, such as ATP and phosphocreatine. ATP breakdown and compensatory activation of anaerobic glycolysis increase the levels of inorganic phosphate and lactate and cause cellular acidification.[1,9]

Without adequate ATP, the energy-dependent ionic gradients across neuronal membranes begin to collapse. Potassium efflux through ATP-sensitive channels begins shortly after the onset of ischemia. As ATP levels decrease by greater than 50%, there is a pronounced influx of sodium ions (Na^+) and calcium ions (Ca^{++}) through voltage-gated channels, causing cellular depolarization.[9] Depolarization subsequently causes axonal release of neurotransmitters, including the excitatory amino acid glutamate. *Glutamate* is a funda-

mental trigger of ischemic neuronal injury because it activates a ligand-gated Ca^{++} channel called the *N*-methyl-D-aspartate (NMDA) receptor. The NMDA receptor allows additional rapid Ca^{++} influx into postsynaptic neurons. This increase in intracellular Ca^{++} serves as the most prominent second messenger in ischemic cells. Glutamate also activates other receptors, including α-amino-3-hydroxy-5-methyl-4-isoxazolepropionate, a ligand-gated Na^+ channel, and metabotropic receptors that activate G protein–mediated second messengers, such as phospholipases and cyclic adenosine monophosphate.

After reperfusion, ATP levels and glutamate reuptake usually are restored quickly.[1] Other potential trigger events may be caused directly by depletion of ATP, but are even more strongly activated by Ca^{++} or other second messengers of ischemia. These events include inhibition of overall neuronal protein synthesis and production of ROS, including oxygen free radicals.[1] Because these events are more pronounced during reperfusion than during ischemia, they are unlikely to be important as trigger events.

Second Messengers

Second messengers are intracellular or intercellular signals initiated during ischemia by trigger events, which then activate other second messengers and perpetrators of functional or structural damage to cells.

Calcium
Intracellular Ca^{++} overload is a predominant second messenger of neuronal ischemia. Ca^{++} influx, initially through voltage-gated channels and by glutamate–NMDA receptor channels during ischemia, is maintained through several mechanisms, including inhibition of efflux by calcium-adenosine triphosphatase transporters owing to low levels of ATP and additional Ca^{++} influx from Na^+/Ca^{++} exchange. Calcium-induced Ca^{++} release from the endoplasmic reticulum also occurs, amplifying cytosolic Ca^{++} levels. Mitochondria initially may buffer increases in cytosolic Ca^{++}, but also may be a source of continued release of Ca^{++} after reperfusion. Intracellular calcium remains elevated for hours after reperfusion. Elevations of intracellular Ca^{++} trigger several other second messenger and perpetrator pathways.[10]

Nitric Oxide
Intracellular Ca^{++} elevations in ischemia activate nitric oxide synthase (NOS) to form NO. NO may block mitochondrial uptake of Ca^{++}, creating another positive feedback amplification loop. NO also may be amplified by NO activation of NOS. NO itself is implicated in a variety of protective and destructive processes after ischemia,[11] including interaction with superoxide (O_2^-) to form peroxynitrite ($ONOO^-$), an extremely damaging ROS. NO also specifically may inhibit the recovery of mitochondrial respiration by binding to the oxygen-binding site of cytochrome oxidase. NO has been implicated in the activation of cytokines and chemokines that are intercellular proinflammatory

signals. NO also can cause single-stranded DNA nicks and DNA nitration and may activate transcription factors of immediate early genes or genes responsible for programmed cell death. Endothelial release of NO may have beneficial vascular effects, including vasodilation and inhibition of platelet aggregation. There are at least three forms of NOS with different anatomic distributions within the brain, and the relative balance between destructive and protective effects of NO may be determined partially by the form of NOS activated.[12]

Protein Kinases and Gene Activation

Rapid transcription of many genes occurs within minutes of brain ischemia and reperfusion. These genes may be mediated by Ca^{++}-triggered phosphorylation of protein kinase systems, such as mitogen-activated protein kinase, protein kinase C, or other transcription factors, such as the free radical–activated nuclear factor κ B (NFκB) or AP-1. Several classes of genes are expressed, including immediate early genes (e.g., *c-fos, c-jun, junB*), heat-shock proteins, *Bcl-2/Bax* genes, growth factors, NOS, cyclooxygenase 2, and cytokines, such as interleukin-1β and tumor necrosis factor-α.[1,12] Some of these genes are thought to contribute to cellular destruction, whereas others may mediate protective processes. The relative contributions of each after global cerebral ischemia are still unclear.

Perpetrators

Perpetrators of functional and structural damage represent the final common pathways by which neurons die after an ischemic insult. Although the categories overlap, perpetrators may be considered generally as necrotic, inflammatory, or apoptotic mechanisms.

Necrotic Mechanisms

Cell swelling, membrane disruption, and random DNA breaks characterize necrotic neuronal death. Necrotic neuronal loss generally occurs relatively quickly (usually within the first day) after ischemic insult and is caused primarily by damage to the extranuclear cellular infrastructure, including the mitochondria, cytoskeleton, and cell membrane.

Free radicals and other ROS are formed in neurons and surrounding cells after ischemia by several mechanisms.[13] Even during ischemia, the breakdown of adenine nucleotides leads to accumulation of hypoxanthine, which is converted (with the scant available tissue oxygen) by xanthine oxidase to superoxide ion, hydrogen peroxide, and urate. This reaction is accelerated by Ca^{++}-activated proteolytic cleavage of xanthine dehydrogenase to make more xanthine oxidase, then accelerated further by the return of oxygen during reperfusion. Superoxide and hydroxyl radicals also are formed from the metabolism (by the lipoxygenase or cyclooxygenase systems) of arachidonic acid and other free fatty acids that accumulate from phospholipid breakdown during ischemia.[1,12] This process then propagates itself because the ROS formed can attack membranes and cause further phospholipid breakdown. The formation of NO and $ONOO^-$ was described earlier. After reperfusion, monoamine oxidase converts accumulated catecholamines into hydrogen peroxide, which can produce hydroxyl radicals through the iron-mediated Fenton reaction. Finally, leakage of ROS can occur from mitochondrial electron transport.

All these processes form highly reactive oxygen radicals that react with proteins and lipids to increase membrane rigidity and failure, disable necessary metabolic enzymes, or otherwise directly damage important cellular structures, causing necrotic cell death. By inactivation of some proteins, however, ROS also can act as second messengers that activate nonoxidative perpetrators, and they can enter the nucleus and damage DNA, activating apoptotic processes.[1]

Autodigestion by activated proteases is another important perpetrator of necrotic neuronal cell death. *Calpains,* a class of Ca^{++}-activated cysteine protease, may play a particularly important role. Calpain substrates include cytoskeletal proteins, plasma membrane–associated proteins (mostly receptors), and signal transduction proteins and transcription factors.[12] The timing of proteolytic damage is unclear but may be bimodal, with a peak shortly after reperfusion and a second peak 24 or more hours later. Calpain may represent a relatively late-acting or persistent necrotic perpetrator that may be more amenable to treatment than other processes occurring immediately after reperfusion. In addition to their role in necrotic cell death, calpains may be important in apoptosis.[12]

Metabolic failure is a functional injury causing necrotic cell death. Damage to mitochondria during ischemia or reperfusion (caused by oxidative or proteolytic processes) increases mitochondrial membrane permeability and decoupling of oxidative phosphorylation. Rates of metabolism and ATP levels in reperfused ischemic tissue may remain low even when the cytochromes at the end of the electron transport chain (aa_3) remain oxidized. Impaired electron transport is another source of oxygen free radicals. Damage also may occur to specific tricarboxylic acid cycle enzymes, such as pyruvate dehydrogenase, inhibiting metabolism. Mitochondria also may be damaged or may lyse as a result of Ca^{++} uptake while attempting to buffer cytosolic Ca^{++} overload.[14] In addition to causing necrotic cell death from metabolic failure, damaged mitochondria release cytochrome *c,* a factor that is a crucial element in apoptosis.[15]

Inflammatory Mechanisms

Inflammatory responses after ischemia are complex and can cause cellular death by several mediators. Complement activation is the most rapidly initiated inflammatory response, but its role after global cerebral ischemia is unclear. Complement activation turns dormant microglia into brain macrophages, attracts activated leukocytes, and can itself lead to cellular lysis and death through the membrane attack complex.[16] Cytokines upregulated by ischemia (e.g., interleukin-1β, tumor necrosis factor-α) cause expression of membrane selectins and integrins, which are adhesion molecules that cause activation, rolling, adhesion, emigration, and chemotaxis of circulating leukocytes.[17] Activated leukocytes can induce damage by causing capillary vascular occlusion or by direct toxic attack on injured neurons. Micro-occlusions by clumps of leukocytes and platelets are seen often after focal cerebral ischemia but may be less prominent after global ischemia.[18] Direct toxic attacks by neutrophils cause extensive oxidative injury through powerful oxidases and the resulting free radicals and through release of proteases that act against cellular proteins and extracellular matrix proteins.[12,19]

Apoptotic Mechanisms

Apoptosis, also called *programmed cell death,* is an orderly, genetically controlled, energy-consuming process of cellular suicide that has a normal physiologic role in brain development and possibly in other processes, such as cancer surveillance. After cerebral ischemia, neuronal apoptosis can occur for many days and can contribute significantly to total neuronal loss. Apoptotic cell death involves chromatin condensation, DNA fragmentation, membrane blebbing, cell shrinkage, and disassembly into membrane-enclosed vesicles (apoptotic bodies).[9] The mechanism of apoptosis in cerebral ischemia includes transcription of several cell death genes and inhibition of several protective genes, activation of caspases, a precise and orderly pattern of DNA destruction, and activation and degradation of poly(ADP-ribose) polymerase. Apoptosis can be caused by intercellular inflammatory signaling and can cause inflammation through caspase-activated cytokines.

Summary

Ultimately, apoptosis and necrotic cellular destruction occur in the injured brain and may represent opposite ends of a spectrum of mechanisms in which neurons can die after global cerebral ischemia.[20] Despite the complex array of biochemical processes and signals surrounding neuronal cell death, understanding of these mechanisms is increasing rapidly. Much of this complex pathophysiology occurs in patients while they are being treated in the emergency department, inspiring hope of more effective and more specific brain resuscitation in the future.

MANAGEMENT

Standard management of a patient with cardiac arrest and subsequent ischemic brain damage involves restoring CBF and preventing secondary insult. These treatments generally have not been studied in prospective, randomized controlled trials, but are supported by clinical experience and limited experimental data. Although proposed and experimental therapies generally are aimed at specific molecular interventions in the pathophysiology of ischemic brain injuries, none of these have proved effective as yet.

Standard Strategies

Return of Spontaneous Circulation

Cardiac resuscitation is the first priority in cerebral resuscitation. The degree of brain injury after cardiac arrest depends on the duration of complete cerebral ischemia (the "down time," or time before the initiation of cardiopulmonary resuscitation [CPR]) and the duration of relative ischemia that occurs during CPR and that may occur from cardiogenic shock preceding or subsequent to the period of cardiac arrest.[21] Extensive clinical evidence on hospital discharge rates and neurologic recovery rates supports the concept first proposed nearly 100 years ago that success in resuscitation is inversely proportional to the duration of cardiac arrest. Although duration of arrest generally predicts outcome in the population of patients with sudden cardiac death, it cannot be used reliably to predict the outcome of individual patients. The epidemiology of neurologic outcome of survivors is influenced by patient comorbidity and other individual characteristics. Depending on their timing and severity, low-flow states, hypotension, or hypoxia preceding cardiac arrest may provide protective preconditioning or may increase the risk of poor neurologic outcome.

As originally envisioned in the 1950s, the purpose of closed-chest CPR is to provide adequate artificial circulation to the myocardium during ventricular fibrillation until electric countershock can be administered. Since then, prehospital clinical experience has shown that the key to successful resuscitation is the early initiation of CPR and early defibrillation.

The efficacy of closed-chest CPR in generating adequate cerebral perfusion is controversial. Cardiac output during optimal standard closed-chest CPR has been estimated previously to be only 20% to 30% of normal, but more recent data suggest that higher cardiac outputs are possible in clinical practice.[22] Experimental measurement of CBF during CPR has led to estimates ranging from 1% to 60% of prearrest CBF, depending on the experimental model and technique and the duration of arrest.[23] The CBF achieved with standard closed-chest CPR is inversely proportional to the duration of cardiac arrest preceding the initiation of CPR.[24] Researchers have obtained 50% of normal (prearrest) CBF in animals when CPR was started within 2 minutes of the onset of ventricular fibrillation, but they obtained only 28% of normal CBF if the circulatory arrest persisted for 5 minutes before CPR was started. After 10 minutes of arrest, CBF was 0 with standard CPR. Although some experimental work suggests that about 20% of normal CBF is necessary to maintain neuronal viability, the real issue is not the degree of biochemical, electric, or physiologic abnormality measured in animal experiments of brain ischemia, but whether functional recovery will occur (i.e., whether "the cat will ever catch mice again"). Approached from this perspective, clinical evidence overwhelmingly confirms the beneficial effects of CPR in terms of improvement in survival and neurologic recovery.[25,26]

Considerable effort has been directed toward the investigation of improved CPR techniques that would be even more effective for longer periods (see Chapter 7).

Treatment of Hypotension, Hypoperfusion, and Hypoxia

Maintaining cerebral oxygen delivery after cardiac resuscitation is a mainstay of therapy. Oxygen delivery requires a sufficiently high cerebral perfusion pressure, a sufficiently low cerebrovascular resistance, and adequate blood oxygen saturation.

Hypotension in the postarrest period can reduce cerebral perfusion pressure to dangerously low levels. Although CBF is normally independent of perfusion pressure over a wide range of arterial blood pressures, such autoregulation is often lost in the injured brain. As a result, perfusion of ischemic tissue becomes passively dependent on arterial pressure, and hypotension can compromise CBF and result in significant additional brain damage.[21] After restoration of spontaneous circulation, low arterial pressures should be normalized rapidly, using intravascular volume administration and vasopressors as needed. Because elevated arterial pressures may be needed to provide sufficient CBF, hypertension usually should not be treated in the postresuscitation period. Very high blood pressures may require treatment, but specific cutoffs are controversial. Generally, diastolic pressures may be 120 mm Hg without requiring treatment. Hypertension sometimes is induced clinically or experimentally with vasopressors in an attempt to increase cerebral perfusion pressure and improve neurologic recovery.[27] Because it is unproved, and because risks of this therapy include BBB disruption and worsening of vasogenic edema, induced hypertension is not currently a standard therapy.

Cerebrovascular resistance after resuscitation from cardiac arrest is another determinant of CBF and may be affected by hyperventilation and microvascular patency. Although the cerebral circulation may lose its ability to adjust to blood pressure changes after ischemia, attenuated responsiveness to carbon dioxide and oxygen levels in arterial blood still can be present.[28,29] Carbon dioxide is a potent vasoactive agent, and lowering of the arterial carbon dioxide partial pressure ($PaCO_2$) by hyperventilation results in rapid reduction of CBF. Because reductions in CBF decrease total cerebral blood volume, hyperventilation can transiently abort brainstem herniation in the presence of critically elevated ICP until osmotherapy or ventriculostomy can be initiated. When ICP is not elevated, however, the vasoconstriction and increased cerebrovascular resistance caused by hyperventilation can cause potentially dangerous decreases in CBF. Although controversy surrounds whether increases in ICP are clinically significant after global ischemia, the measurement of ICP generally is not recommended in the management of adult cardiac arrest survivors.[7] Generally, ventilation to maintain a $PaCO_2$ between 35 and 40 mm Hg is safe and appropriate. Cerebrovascular resistance also may be elevated after cardiac arrest by

endothelin-induced vasospasm or microvascular occlusion by leukocyte clumping or coagulation. Hemodilution, anticoagulation, and antiplatelet agents have been studied in animals for effectiveness in mitigating microvascular occlusion with mostly negative results.[30] Acute use of these agents to improve microcirculatory flow has not been studied in human cerebral ischemia.

Normal arterial oxygen saturation should be maintained after resuscitation from cardiac arrest. Because the injured brain may not be able to compensate for hypoxia by augmenting CBF, cerebral oxygen delivery may diminish rapidly as the oxygen content of blood decreases. Hyperoxia secondary to the use of 100% oxygen in the immediate postarrest period also has been shown to increase oxidative brain injury in animal models of cardiac arrest and resuscitation.[31] Normoxia or mild hyperoxia (PaO_2 80 to 120 mm Hg) should be maintained using the lowest fraction of inspired oxygen possible. The use of 100% oxygen is appropriate during cardiac arrest, but fraction of inspired oxygen should be titrated downward shortly after the return of spontaneous circulation. Because hypoxia and hypercapnia must be avoided, controlled ventilation is appropriate in the period after resuscitation, with muscle relaxation and sedation if needed.

Maintenance of Body Temperature

Hyperthermia (or fever) exacerbates brain injury and worsens neurologic outcome.[32,33] Elevated body temperature increases cerebral metabolic demand by 8% to 13% per degree Celsius, escalates glutamate release, increases oxygen free radical production, and increases cytoskeletal and BBB breakdown with increased vasogenic edema.[34,35] Core body temperature (usually rectal, bladder, or esophageal) should be accurately measured in patients resuscitated from cerebral ischemia.[36] Hyperthermia may be treated with antipyretics, circulating air or water cooling systems, or evaporative cooling using water mist and fans.[36] Aggressive treatment, at a minimum, should be used to prevent temperature increases in the postischemic period in all patients, and the practice of inducing therapeutic hypothermia is now emerging as a therapy for comatose survivors of cardiac arrest.

Resuscitative Mild Hypothermia

Hypothermia was first reported more than 50 years ago to have a protective effect in global and focal brain ischemia[37] and ranges from mild (32°C to 34°C) to profound (5°C). The mechanism by which hypothermia conveys protection is uncertain, but several possibilities have been suggested. Hypothermia reduces glutamate release, metabolic demand, free radical formation, and production of inflammatory cytokines.[34] Cell-signaling and genetic responses to cellular injury also are affected by hypothermia and may protect the brain from programmed neuronal cell death.[38,39]

Mild hypothermia is easier to achieve and has fewer adverse effects than lower temperatures and has been found consistently to be neuroprotective in experimental cerebral ischemia.[38,40] Two multicenter prospective, randomized, controlled trials of mild hypothermia have shown marked improvements in neurologic outcome in comatose survivors of out-of-hospital cardiac arrest (Table 6-1).[41,42] In these trials, the number needed to treat to have one additional patient with a good neurologic outcome was only about seven. The American Heart Association and other members of the International Liaison Committee on Resuscitation now recommend cooling unconscious adult patients after cardiac arrest to 33°C for 12 to 24 hours.[43]

Mild hypothermia can be induced through a variety of techniques. In both clinical trials of hypothermia after cardiac arrest, hypothermia was achieved by cooling the body surface with ice packs and cooling blankets. Surface cooling is noninvasive, and a variety of specialized devices have been developed to make it less labor intensive and more rapid.[44,45] Some difficulties inherent with surface cooling are well described,[46] however, including slower than desired rates of cooling (0.3°C/hr to 0.6°C/hr ± SD 0.3°C/hr),[41,42] overshooting and undershooting the temperature target (SD usually >1°C),[47] and uncontrolled rewarming with frequent rebound hyperthermia.[46] Alternative core cooling methods have been investigated. A promising technique using infusions of ice cold intravenous fluids has been shown and is more effective than would be expected based on the transfer of heat content alone.[48] Endovascular cooling with a heat exchange catheter, although more invasive, provides the most rapid cooling (1.4°C/hr to 6.3°C/hr ± SD 0.3°C/hr) and offers the tightest control of body temperature (SD usually <0.3°C) at the target temperature and during controlled rewarming.[47,49-51] Designed to induce hypothermia or maintain normothermia in surgical patients, this new type of commercially available device is placed in the inferior vena cava through a femoral introducer and cools or heats passing blood. Endovascular systems promise to be far less nursing-labor intensive than surface cooling because they monitor core temperature and are automatically controlled through a feedback loop. Although temperature control also can be achieved by extracorporeal bypass devices, this is not pragmatic in most circumstances and does not offer the same promise as simpler core cooling techniques. The optimal method of cooling patients resuscitated from cardiac arrest has not been established.

The rate of cooling needed for effective neuroprotection, the optimal duration of cooling, and the best process for rewarming after hypothermia are all unknown.[52] Animal experiments and the consensus recommendations suggest that cooling should be initiated as early and as rapidly as possible.[43] Cooling may begin during the prehospital phase of resuscitation and may be initiated before the return of spontaneous circulation. In the positive clinical trials, hypothermia at 33°C ± 1°C was achieved by 2 hours[42] or 8 hours[41] after return of spontaneous circulation and was maintained for either 12 hours[42] or 24 hours.[41] Patients were then allowed to rewarm passively[41] or with a combination of passive and active rewarming.[42] Rebound hyperthermia is common with passive rewarming and must be avoided.[46] Although the clinical trials enrolled only patients resuscitated from cardiac arrest caused by ventricular fibrillation, there is clinical experience with resuscitative hypothermia in patients with cardiac arrest from other etiologies,[53] and consensus recommendations support its use in such cases.[43]

Cooling of comatose survivors of out-of-hospital cardiac arrest requires a multidisciplinary hospital policy and should be initiated as early as possible. In hospitals capable of hypothermic resuscitation, it is likely to be started in the emergency department and maintained in the intensive care unit. Regardless of cooling technique, patients cooled after cardiac arrests require pharmacologic therapy to prevent shivering because shivering effectively warms the patient. In the two clinical trials, shivering was prevented with a nondepolarizing paralytic, and sedation was maintained with midazolam with or without fentanyl.[41,42] When paralysis is not clinically desired, it may be possible to lower the shivering threshold sufficiently in awake patients with meperidine, buspirone, dexmedetomidine, or a combination of these.[54,55] Shivering sometimes also can be reduced in a patient cooled by an endovascular catheter even when the core temperature is 33°C by applying a warming blanket because surface temperature receptors control thermoregulation to a much greater extent than core temperature receptors. Other pharmacologic treatments that may be used during induced hypothermia include antipyretics, which lower the core body temperature set point, even in normothermic patients, although to such a small degree

Table 6-1. Clinical Outcomes in Randomized Controlled Trials of Hypothermia in Comatose Survivors of Cardiac Arrest

Clinical Trial	Hypothermia, *N* (%)	Normothermia, *N* (%)	*P* Value
HACA[41]	*N* = 137	*N* = 138	
Good neurologic outcome*	75 (55)	54 (39)	<0.01
Death	56 (41)	76 (55)	0.02
Bernard[42]	*N* = 43	*N* = 34	
Good neurologic outcome†	21 (49)	9 (26)	0.05
Death	22 (51)	23 (68)	0.14

*Defined as recovery with no neurologic deficits or with moderate disability but living independently and working at least part time at 6 months.
†Defined as recovery with moderate, minimal, or no neurologic deficits at hospital discharge, and discharge to home or acute rehabilitation facility.

that the effect is unlikely to be clinically relevant.[56] More effective pharmacologic lowering of core body temperature is being investigated. Neurotensin is an endogenous neuropeptide involved in thermoregulation that can induce hypothermia and neuroprotection in experimental models of cerebral ischemia.[57]

Clinical trials of mild hypothermia in the resuscitation of patients with acute ischemic stroke and a new clinical trial of mild hypothermia in patients with traumatic brain injury are being performed and may expand the indications of this therapy in the near future. Ongoing efforts to develop feasible methods of selective cooling of the brain after cardiac arrest[58,59] and studies of profound systemic hypothermia are still experimental.

Treatment of Hyperglycemia

Postischemic hyperglycemia has detrimental effects on CBF, metabolism, edema formation, and neurologic outcome. In experimental focal cerebral ischemia, profound hyperglycemia (>500 mg/dL) causes a more pronounced decrease in intracellular pH, increases brain lactate, and increases neuronal loss. Increased neuronal damage from hyperglycemia in global cerebral ischemia also may be glutamate mediated. Observational studies in patients with stroke and survivors of cardiac arrest have shown that hyperglycemia after brain ischemia is strongly associated with worse outcomes in diabetics and nondiabetics.[60,61] In experimental studies, normoglycemia and mild insulin-induced hypoglycemia have been shown to improve neurologic function after focal and global ischemia. Insulin itself may have a neuron growth factor–like effect that theoretically also may be neuroprotective. The best available evidence supports active treatment of hyperglycemia after global brain ischemia, and the administration of glucose should be avoided except in verified hypoglycemia.

Seizure Management

Seizures may result from global cerebral ischemia and may exacerbate the underlying brain injury. Seizure activity can increase brain metabolism by 300% to 400%, worsening the mismatch between oxygen delivery and demand in the postarrest period, with greater metabolic failure and neuronal loss and worsened neurologic outcome. Although prevention of seizures has not proved to improve neurologic recovery, seizures are not desirable in the postischemic period. The prophylactic use of anticonvulsant drugs in patients resuscitated from cardiac arrest is controversial and is not standard care, but it is generally agreed that seizures should be treated quickly and effectively. Common therapeutic agents include benzodiazepines, phenytoin, and barbiturates. Each of these anticonvulsant drugs also has been considered as a specific therapy for cerebral ischemia because of the antagonism of excitatory amino acids, sodium channel blockade, or effects on cerebral metabolism. Although these drugs are of proven value as anticonvulsants, other uses in cerebral ischemia are experimental and unproved.

Immobilization, Sedation, and Head Position

The comatose brain responds to external stimuli (e.g., physical examination, airway suctioning) with increases in cerebral metabolism. This elevation of regional brain metabolism requires increased regional CBF at a time when the oxygen demand-to-perfusion ratios may be precariously balanced. Protection from afferent sensory stimuli with administration of titrated doses of sedative-anesthetic drugs and muscle relaxants may prevent oxygen supply/demand imbalance and improve the chances for neuronal recovery.

All activity that increases ICP (e.g., straining, coughing) should be restricted, and tracheal suction should be performed only when necessary and with care. There is no evidence to support the commonly recommended practice of elevating the head of the bed to reduce intracranial venous pressure, and this practice may even be harmful.[62] Torsion or compression of neck veins should be avoided by eliminating compressive dressings and not rotating or flexing the head.[63]

Experimental and Potential Specific Therapies

Profound and Selective Hypothermia

Although mild systemic hypothermia now is clinically recommended to improve outcome in victims of cardiac arrest, the use of profound systemic hypothermia and localized cooling of the brain still are being studied. Profound to moderate hypothermia (5°C to 28°C) during and after experimental cerebral ischemia consistently preserves neurologic function in a variety of laboratory models.[64] Adverse systemic effects of this level of hypothermia can be significant, however, and include increased blood viscosity, decreased cardiac output, and dysrhythmias. Over several decades, the induction of profound to moderate hypothermia for neuroprotection has produced mixed results in clinical settings.[34]

Efforts are continuing to develop feasible methods of selective cooling of the brain after cardiac arrest to obviate the need for systemic hypothermia.[58,59] In neonates with birth asphyxia, randomized clinical trials of localized cooling of the brain through the scalp (the Olympic trial) and of systemic hypothermia (NICHD Neonatal Research Network trial) have been completed, but the results of these have not been published. The applicability of these results to other clinical situations would be limited in any case because selective cooling of neonatal brains is technically easier than cooling of brains of older children or adults.

Research on profound and selective hypothermia continues to be promising, but further laboratory and clinical investigations are needed. At present, only mild systematic hypothermia is ready for routine clinical use after cardiac arrest.

Free Radical Scavengers and Other Antioxidants

Oxygen free radicals act as second messengers and perpetrators of cellular damage after global cerebral ischemia. Endogenous antioxidant systems (e.g., superoxide dismutase, catalase, glutathione) detoxify free radicals formed as side products of oxygen metabolism in normal physiology but are quickly exhausted after ischemic injury. Pharmacologic supplementation of these systems with exogenous antioxidant enzymes and free radical scavengers can reduce brain injury in animal models of cerebral ischemia but have not yet been proved effective in clinical trials.[65]

Tirilazad, a 21-amino steroid, reduces cerebral damage in various models of brain injury, but has been found ineffective in clinical trials of patients with stroke.[66] Superoxide dismutase attached to polyethylene glycol (PEG-SOD) also has been beneficial in models of traumatic and ischemic brain injury, but has not been effective in clinical trials. N-acetyl cysteine increased availability of the endogenous free radical scavenger glutathione but did not improve neurologic outcome in a clinically realistic animal model of cardiac arrest and resuscitation.[67] Although they have not been tested clinically, other experimental antioxidants effective in some animal models of cerebral ischemia include nitron spin traps (e.g., α-phenyl-N-tert-butyl nitrone [PBN]), other nonglucocorticoid steroids (21-amino steroids, also called *lazaroids*), and phenolic free radical scavengers.[65,68] Other free radical scavengers with therapeutic potential include ascorbic acid, vitamin E, dimethyl sulfoxide, mannitol, and thiopental. The more recently synthesized, extremely aromatic class of molecules called *fullerenes* (50 or 60 carbon molecules arranged as geodesic spheres) theoretically may create ideal free radical scavengers.[69] Chelation of iron (Fe^{++}) to prevent Fenton-type conversion of hydrogen peroxide to the much more damaging hydroxyl radical is another antioxidant strategy, but few of the many potential agents have been used for neuroprotection.[68] Deferoxamine has been found to reduce neuronal injury after experimental cardiac arrest, but is associated with significant cardiovascular side effects.[70]

Glutamate Antagonists

Release of glutamate and subsequent receptor activation are important early processes in the cascade of ischemic neuronal injury. For this reason, attempted pharmacologic intervention at the level of glutamate release and at the glutamate receptor has been popular. Glutamate release may be inhibited by hypothermia or other "upstream" drugs, such as ion channel blockers, or by a more specific endogenous inhibitor of presynaptic excitatory amino acid release, such as adenosine.[71] Exogenous adenosine is unlikely to be clinically useful as a neuroprotective agent because of cardiovascular side effects, but more selective adenosine receptor subtype agonists and antagonists are being studied.

NMDA receptor activity can be reduced endogenously by glycine, magnesium, and polyamines or exogenously by many other drugs. Although there have not been clinical trials of all of these putative NMDA blockers, magnesium given by paramedics immediately after return of spontaneous circulation failed to show any improvement in neurologic outcome in 300 patients resuscitated from cardiac arrest in Seattle.[72] A large trial of magnesium given by paramedics for acute ischemic stroke is ongoing. Synthesized receptor antagonists show mixed but promising results in animal models, but clinical trials of NMDA receptor antagonists (aptiganel [Cerestat/CNS 1102], selfotel/CGS 19755, eliprodil) generally have failed primarily because of neurobehavioral and cardiovascular side effects.[66] Newer, more specific agents with fewer side effects are being developed and tested.[65] Glutamate blockade remains a conceptually appealing goal with prolific pharmacologic opportunities, but the early peak and the transience of glutamate elevation after resuscitation from cardiac arrest may limit its success, at least as monotherapy.

Calcium Channel Antagonists

In the wake of expanding knowledge of the role of voltage-dependent calcium channels in the development of intracellular calcium overload during cerebral ischemia, investigators have been examining the potential usefulness of drugs that block calcium entry after circulatory arrest. After promising results in animal models, human clinical trials of calcium channel blockers were organized, but neither lidoflazine nor nimodipine provided any benefit in large, well-designed human outcome studies.[73-75] Post-hoc subgroup analyses from these trials suggest that calcium channel blockers may work in carefully selected patients, but these hypotheses have not been tested clinically. Work continues on more neuron-specific agents and combination therapies.

Sodium and Potassium Channel Antagonists

Lubeluzole is a benzothiazole sodium channel blocker that improves neurologic outcome in animal models of focal cerebral ischemia. Other possible mechanisms of action for lubeluzole include inhibition of glutamate release, decreased potassium-related calcium influx, and decreased NO synthesis. The drug has been tested in two large clinical trials of patients with acute focal cerebral ischemia with encouraging but mixed results.[66] Further studies in global and focal cerebral ischemia are warranted. Other sodium channel blockers, including lidocaine, lamotrigine, and fosphenytoin, have proved beneficial in animal models of global and focal cerebral ischemia, and clinical trials are under way.[75,76]

Barbiturates and Other γ-Aminobutyric Acid Agonists

γ-Aminobutyric acid (GABA) is the major inhibitory neurotransmitter in the brain. Activation of the GABA receptor, a ligand-mediated chloride channel, reduces brain metabolism and may antagonize the damaging effects of glutamate excitotoxicity. Barbiturates are prototypical GABA agonists.

Barbiturate therapy was among the first experimental brain resuscitation measures specifically aimed at reversing the secondary, postreperfusion pathophysiology that occurs after prolonged cardiac arrest. After some promising early evidence that barbiturates might be capable of reducing cerebral metabolism, edema formation, ICP, seizure activity, and damage induced by focal and incomplete ischemia, a large human trial was undertaken, which failed to show any benefit of barbiturate loading in patients after resuscitation from cardiac arrest.[77] Other GABA antagonists, including diazepam and clomethiazole, have undergone human trials without evidence of benefit.

Calpain and Caspase Inhibitors

Inhibitors of these two classes of cysteine proteases have been developed and are being studied in models of global and focal cerebral ischemia.[12] Because calpain and caspase inhibitors seem to inhibit pivotal steps in necrotic and apoptotic cell death, their therapeutic potential is significant. Calpain inhibition is a relatively end-stage process in the ischemic cascade and seems to be effective 6 hours after transient focal ischemia and in global ischemia.[78] Specific caspase inhibition is even more recent and has been shown to reduce neuronal damage after global and focal brain ischemia. Evidence also suggests that the combination of calpain and caspase inhibition may be synergistic.[12] Clinical experimentation with these drugs in patients with brain injury is needed.

Anti-inflammatory Therapies

The importance of inflammatory changes after global cerebral ischemia is less clear than after focal cerebral ischemia, but antileukocyte therapies have improved CBF in the postischemic period and have reduced neurologic deficit in animal models of global and focal cerebral ischemia.[79] Inflammatory changes after brain injury may be modulated at several levels, but more recent clinical trials have studied antibodies to cell surface molecules. Enlimomab is a murine monoclonal antibody to intercellular adhesion molecule 1 that was found to exacerbate rather than reduce injury when tested in a large randomized trial of patients with focal cerebral ischemia.[1,53,80] Worsened outcomes may have been the result of fevers generated in response to the murine antibody, a problem that may not occur in "humanized" antibodies. A humanized antibody to the CD11/CD18 β-integrin also has been tested in stroke patients with apparently negative results. Other pharmacologic agents, including the glycoprotein portions of heparin[81] and inhibitors of proinflammatory cytokines and chemokines,[82] also have been shown to have neuroprotective antileukocyte properties in animal models of cerebral ischemia. One of these, neutrophil inhibitory factor, was ineffective, however, in a clinical trial in patients with focal cerebral ischemia.[83]

Anti-inflammatory treatments for ischemia require further study.

Other Experimental Treatments

Several other classes of agents have been studied for treatment of ischemic brain injury. Metabolic promoters, such as acetyl-L-carnitine, may prevent metabolic failure by improving the efficiency of oxidative phosphorylation and are neuroprotective in animal models of global and focal cerebral ischemia.[84] Metabolic agents, such as dichloroacetate, or buffering compounds, such as sodium carbonate/sodium bicarbonate, can reduce cerebral acidosis and improve neuronal survival after global cerebral ischemia.[85,86] Endogenous opioid peptides have been implicated in the pathophysiology of neurotrauma, and opioid receptor antagonists (e.g., naloxone) may have beneficial effects in some animal models of central nervous system injury and have been studied in focal cerebral ischemia in humans.[87] Estrogens have been shown to reduce ischemic brain injury by a variety of transcriptional and nongenomic mechanisms.[88] Other possible treatments for cerebral ischemia include growth factors, gangliosides, and serotonin receptor agonists.[66,76]

CLINICAL OUTCOMES

Global cerebral ischemia resulting from a period of cardiac arrest is a frequently fatal and highly morbid condition, but the prognosis for its victims is not universally poor. An increasing body of data is providing more complete and precise estimates of the functional outcomes and quality of life of survivors of cardiac arrest, and the results are better than many physicians assume.

The published experience in Olmsted County, Minnesota, between 1990 and 2000 may represent the best possible outcomes with currently available therapy.[89] First responders (including police and firefighters) with automated external defibrillators in that county responded to 330 patients with cardiac arrest, 200 (61%) of whom had ventricular fibrillation at presentation. Most patients with ventricular fibrillation (145 patients, 44% of all arrests) survived to hospital admission, and 84 patients (25%) were discharged alive. Among these 84 survivors, 79 (24% of all arrests) left the hospital neurologically intact.[89]

More typical outcomes were identified by a large cohort study of outcomes in 8091 patients with cardiac arrest in Ontario.[90] Survival was 5.2% at hospital discharge and was 4% at 1 year. Most 1-year survivors (3% of all patients with cardiac arrest) had no or minimal neurologic deficits, however, and the average quality-of-life indices of all survivors was as good as patients without a history of cardiac arrest.[90] The Ontario experience echoes that of a Portuguese study,[91] but other more recent data on 6240 patients from studies in the Netherlands,[92] Norway,[93] and Switzerland[94] all confirm a rate of survival to discharge home with minimal or no deficit of 8% of all out-of-hospital cardiac arrests.

Quality of life among long-term survivors of cardiac arrest is consistently high in all of these studies with low rates of patients in persistent vegetative states or requiring skilled nursing care. Overall, among patients surviving to hospital admission, 14% to 55% have good long-term neurologic outcomes.[89,91]

Despite these data, nihilism is common among physicians treating patients with cardiac arrest and ischemic brain injury. This attitude may be due in part to the fact that most survivors of cardiac arrest are comatose at the time of admission and are without early prognostic findings suggestive of a favorable outcome. Although predicting the outcome of coma is difficult, a meta-analysis suggests that the absence of pupillary and corneal reflexes at 24 hours and the absence of motor responses at 72 hours on physical examination are the best predictors of a poor neurologic outcome.[95] Nihilism is of particular concern, however, and should be avoided because of the potential for poor prognoses to be self-fulfilling.[95] In the near future, serum biomarkers of brain injury may identify the potential for neurologic recovery early in a patient's course and help guide therapy. Until early predictions of outcome can be made accurately, the emergency physician should consider every survivor of cardiac arrest as having a significant chance of full recovery (14% to 55%) and should know that bad neurologic outcomes are usually fatal rather than chronically debilitating.

SUMMARY

Rapidly expanding knowledge about the pathophysiology of postischemic brain injury has stimulated the search for effective cerebral resuscitation therapies. Newly proven therapies, such as resuscitative hypothermia, will continue to be developed and will improve the outcomes of patients with ischemic brain injury in future years. Although experimental work suggests many potentially promising brain resuscitation therapies, attention also should be paid to determining the benefits of existing "standard" therapies. Because of the complexity and interconnectedness of the pathophysiologic cascades that occur after global cerebral ischemia, it is likely that a multifaceted therapeutic approach, or "cocktail" rather than a single pharmacologic agent, will be needed to reduce neurologic damage after cardiac arrest.

It is crucial that the emergency physician recognize that the patient resuscitated from cardiac arrest is, contrary to outward appearance, in a dynamic stage of brain injury. At present, patients must be protected from further brain injury caused by hypotension, hypoperfusion, hypoxia, hyperthermia, hyperglycemia, or seizures. Comatose survivors of out-of-hospital cardiac arrest now also should undergo resuscitative hypothermia. In the future, cerebral resuscitation also may involve other specific pharmacologic interventions to derail the process by which brain cells slowly die after ischemic brain injury.

KEY CONCEPTS

- Neuronal injury is a dynamic process that continues for hours or days after an ischemic insult to the brain.
- Hypotension, hypoperfusion, and hypoxia must be avoided during brain resuscitation.
- Hyperthermia, hyperglycemia, and seizures should be treated promptly during brain resuscitation.
- Comatose survivors of out-of-hospital cardiac arrest should be rapidly cooled in the emergency department and maintained at 33°C in the intensive care unit for 12 to 24 hours after resuscitation.

REFERENCES

1. Lipton P: Ischemic cell death in brain neurons. *Physiol Rev* 79:1431, 1999.
2. Ginsberg M: The new language of cerebral ischemia. *AJNR Am J Neuroradiol* 18(8):1435, 1997.
3. Fujioka M, et al: Specific changes in human brain following reperfusion after cardiac arrest. *Stroke* 25:2091, 1994.
4. Oku K-I, et al: Cerebral and systemic arteriovenous oxygen monitoring after cardiac arrest: Inadequate cerebral oxygen delivery. *Resuscitation* 7:141, 1994.
5. Rivers E, et al: Venous hyperoxia after cardiac arrest: Characterization of a defect in systemic oxygen utilization. *Chest* 102:1787, 1992.
6. Takasu A, Yagi K, Ishihara S, Okada Y: Combined continuous monitoring of systemic and cerebral oxygen metabolism after cardiac arrest. *Resuscitation* 29:189, 1995.
7. Rosenberg G: Ischemic brain edema. *Prog Cardiovasc Dis* 42:209, 1999.
8. del Zoppo G, Hallenbeck J: Advances in the vascular pathophysiology of ischemic stroke. *Thromb Res* 98:V73, 2000.
9. Small D, Morley P, Buchan A: Biology of ischemic cerebral cell death. *Prog Cardiovasc Dis* 42(3):185, 1999.
10. Kristian T, Siesjo B: Calcium in ischemia cell death. *Stroke* 29:705, 1998.
11. Dalkara T, Moskowitz M: The complex role of nitric oxide in the pathophysiology of focal cerebral ischemia. *Brain Pathol* 4:49, 1994.
12. Schaller B, Graf R: Cerebral ischemia and reperfusion: The pathophysiologic concept as a basis for clinical therapy. *J Cereb Blood Flow Metab* 24:351, 2004.
13. Cohen G: Enzymatic/nonenzymatic sources of oxyradicals and regulation of antioxidant defenses. *Ann N Y Acad Sci* 738:8, 1994.
14. Fiskum G, Murphy A, Beal M: Mitochondria in neurodegeneration: Acute ischemia and chronic neurodegenerative diseases. *J Cereb Blood Flow Metab* 19:351, 1999.
15. Green D, Kroemer G: The pathophysiology of mitochondrial cell death. *Science* 305:626, 2004.
16. del Zoppo GJ: In stroke, complement will get you nowhere. *Nat Med* 5:995, 1999.
17. Stanimirovic D, Satoh K: Inflammatory mediators of cerebral endothelium: A role in ischemic brain inflammation. *Brain Pathol* 10:113, 2000.
18. Uhl E, et al: Leukocyte-endothelium interactions in pial venules during the early and late reperfusion period after global cerebral ischemia in gerbils. *J Cereb Blood Flow Metab* 20:979, 2000.
19. del Zoppo G, et al: Inflammation and stroke: Putative role for cytokines, adhesion molecules and iNOS in brain response to ischemia. *Brain Pathol* 10:95, 2000.

20. Zeng Y, Xu Z: Co-existence of necrosis and apoptosis in rat hippocampus following transient forebrain ischemia. *Neurosci Res* 37:113, 2000.

21. Jorgensen E, Holm S: The course of circulatory and cerebral recovery after circulatory arrest: Influence of pre-arrest, arrest and post-arrest factors. *Resuscitation* 42:173, 1999.

22. Fodden DI, Crosby AC, Channer KS: Doppler measurement of cardiac output during cardiopulmonary resuscitation. *J Acad Emerg Med* 13:379, 1996.

23. Shaffner DH, et al: Effect of arrest time and cerebral perfusion pressure during cardiopulmonary resuscitation on cerebral blood flow, metabolism, adenosine triphosphate recovery, and pH in dogs. *Crit Care Med* 27:1335, 1999.

24. Szmolensky T, et al: Organ blood flow during external heart massage. *Acta Chir Acad Sci Hung* 15:283, 1974.

25. Eisenberg MS, et al: Cardiac arrest and resuscitation: A tale of 29 cities. *Ann Emerg Med* 19:179, 1990.

26. Bur A, et al: Effects of bystander first aid, defibrillation and advanced life support on neurologic outcome and hospital costs in patients after ventricular fibrillation cardiac arrest. *Intensive Care Med* 27:1474, 2001.

27. Marzan AS, et al: Feasibility and safety of norepinephrine-induced arterial hypertension in acute ischemic stroke. *Neurology* 62:1193, 2004.

28. Brian J: Carbon dioxide and the cerebral circulation. *Anesthesiology* 88:1365, 1998.

29. Olsen TS, et al: Blood flow and vascular reactivity in collaterally perfused brain tissue: Evidence of an ischemic penumbra in patients with acute stroke. *Stroke* 14:332, 1983.

30. Chaves C, Caplan L: Heparin and oral anticoagulants in the treatment of brain ischemia. *J Neurol Sci* 173:3, 2000.

31. Liu Y, et al: Normoxic ventilation after cardiac arrest reduces oxidation of brain lipids and improves neurologic outcome. *Stroke* 29:1679, 1998.

32. Hajat C, Hajat S, Sharma P: Effects of poststroke pyrexia on stroke outcome: A meta-analysis of studies in patients. *Stroke* 31:410, 2000.

33. Hickey RW, et al: Induced hyperthermia exacerbates neurologic neuronal histologic damage after asphyxial cardiac arrest in rats. *Crit Care Med* 31:531, 2003.

34. Corbett D, Thornhill J: Temperature modulation (hypothermic and hyperthermic conditions) and its influence on histologic and behavioral outcomes following cerebral ischemia. *Brain Pathol* 10:145, 2000.

35. Globus M, et al: Detection of free radical activity during transient global ischemia and recirculation: Effects of intraischemic brain temperature modulation. *J Neurochem* 65:1250, 1995.

36. Marion DW: Controlled normothermia in neurologic intensive care. *Crit Care Med* 32(2 Suppl):S43, 2004.

37. Marshall SB, Owens JC, Swan H: Temporary circulatory occlusion to the brain of the hypothermic dog. *Arch Surg* 72:98, 1956.

38. Hicks S, DeFranco D, Callaway C: Hypothermia during reperfusion after asphyxial cardiac arrest improves functional recovery and selectively alters stress protein expression. *J Cereb Blood Flow Metab* 20:520, 2000.

39. Yenari MA, et al: Gene therapy and hypothermia for stroke treatment. *Ann N Y Acad Sci* 993:54, 2003.

40. Sterz F, et al: Mild hypothermic cardiopulmonary resuscitation improves outcome after prolonged cardiac arrest in dogs. *Crit Care Med* 19:379, 1991.

41. The Hypothermia after Cardiac Arrest Study Group: Mild therapeutic hypothermia to improve the neurologic outcome after cardiac arrest. *N Engl J Med* 346:549, 2002.

42. Bernard SA, et al: Treatment of comatose survivors of out-of-hospital cardiac arrest with induced hypothermia. *N Engl J Med* 346:557, 2002.

43. Nolan JP, et al: Therapeutic hypothermia after cardiac arrest: An advisory statement by the Advanced Life Support Task Force of the International Liaison Committee on Resuscitation. *Circulation* 108:118, 2003.

44. Bernard SA, Buist M: Induced hypothermia in critical care medicine: A review. *Crit Care Med* 31:2041, 2003.

45. Zweifler RM, Voorhees ME, Mahmood MA, Parnell M: Rectal temperature reflects tympanic temperature during mild induced hypothermia in nonintubated subjects. *J Neurosurg Anesthesiol* 16:232, 2004.

46. Felberg RA, et al: Hypothermia after cardiac arrest: Feasibility and safety of an external cooling protocol. *Circulation* 104:1799, 2001.

47. Keller E, et al: Endovascular cooling with heat exchange catheters: A new method to induce and maintain hypothermia. *Intensive Care Med* 29:939, 2003.

48. Bernard S, Buist M, Monteiro O, Smith K: Induced hypothermia using large volume, ice-cold intravenous fluid in comatose survivors of out-of-hospital cardiac arrest: A preliminary report. *Resuscitation* 56:9, 2003.

49. Georgiadis D, Schwarz S, Kollmar R, Schwab S: Endovascular cooling for moderate hypothermia in patients with acute stroke: First results of a novel approach. *Stroke* 32:2550, 2001.

50. Doufas AG, et al: Initial experience with a novel heat-exchanging catheter in neurosurgical patients. *Anesth Analg* 95:1752, 2002.

51. Dae MW, et al: Safety and efficacy of endovascular cooling and rewarming for induction and reversal of hypothermia in human-sized pigs. *Stroke* 34:734, 2003.

52. Bernard S: Hypothermia after cardiac arrest: How to cool and for how long? *Crit Care Med* 32:897, 2004.

53. Silfvast T, Tiainen M, Poutiainen E, Roine RO: Therapeutic hypothermia after prolonged cardiac arrest due to non-coronary causes. *Resuscitation* 57:109, 2003.

54. Mokhtarani M, et al: Buspirone and meperidine synergistically reduce the shivering threshold. *Anesth Analg* 93:1233, 2001.

55. Doufas AG, et al: Dexmedetomidine and meperidine additively reduce the shivering threshold in humans. *Stroke* 34:1218, 2003.

56. Kasner SE, et al: Acetaminophen for altering body temperature in acute stroke: A randomized clinical trial. *Stroke* 33:130, 2002.

57. Katz LM, et al: Neurotensin-induced hypothermia improves neurologic outcome after hypoxic-ischemia. *Crit Care Med* 32:806, 2004.

58. Kuhnen G, Bauer R, Walter B: Controlled brain hypothermia by extracorporeal carotid blood cooling at normothermic trunk temperatures in pigs. *J Neurosci Methods* 89:167, 1999.

59. Wang H, et al: Rapid and selective cerebral hypothermia achieved using a cooling helmet. *J Neurosurg* 100:272, 2004.

60. Capes SE, et al: Stress hyperglycemia and prognosis of stroke in nondiabetic and diabetic patients: A systematic overview. *Stroke* 32:2426, 2001.

61. Skrifvars MB, Pettila V, Rosenberg PH, Castren M: A multiple logistic regression analysis of in-hospital factors related to survival at six months in patients resuscitated from out-of-hospital ventricular fibrillation. *Resuscitation* 59:319, 2003.

62. Feldman Z, et al: Effect of head elevation on intracranial pressure, cerebral perfusion pressure and cerebral blood flow in head injured patients. *J Neurosurg* 76:207, 1992.

63. Shapiro H: Brain protection: Fact or fancy. In Shoemaker W (ed): *Critical Care: State of the Art,* vol 6. Fullerton, Calif, Society of Critical Care Medicine, 1985.

64. Marion D, et al: Resuscitative hypothermia. *Crit Care Med* 24(Suppl):S81, 1996.

65. Danton G, Dietrich WD: The search for neuroprotective strategies in stroke. *AJNR Am J Neuroradiol* 25:181, 2004.

66. Kermer P, Klocker N, Bahr M: Neuronal death after brain injury: Models, mechanisms, and therapeutic strategies in vivo. *Cell Tissue Res* 298:383, 1999.
67. Silbergleit R, Haywood Y, Fiskum G, Rosenthal R: Lack of a neuroprotective effect from N-acetyl cysteine after cardiac arrest and resuscitation in a canine model. *Resuscitation* 40:181, 1999.
68. Gassen M, Youdim M: Free radical scavengers: Chemical concepts and clinical relevance. *J Neural Transm* 56:193, 1999.
69. Lai HS, Chen WJ, Chiang LY: Free radical scavenging activity of fullerenol on the ischemia-reperfusion intestine in dogs. *World J Surg* 24:450, 2000.
70. Rosenthal R, Chanderbhan R, Marshall G, Fiskum G: Prevention of post-ischemic brain lipid conjugated diene production and neurological injury by hydroxyethyl starch-conjugated deferoxamine. *Free Radic Biol Med (US)* 12:29, 1992.
71. Sweeney M: Neuroprotective effects of adenosine in cerebral ischemia: Window of opportunity. *Neurosci Biobehav Rev* 21:207, 1997.
72. Longstreth WT Jr, et al: Randomized clinical trial of magnesium, diazepam, or both after out-of-hospital cardiac arrest. *Neurology* 59:506, 2002.
73. Schwartz AC: Neurological recovery after cardiac arrest: Clinical feasibility trial of calcium blockers. *Am J Emerg Med* 3:1, 1985.
74. Brain Resuscitation Clinical Trial II Study Group: A randomized clinical study of a calcium-entry blocker (lidoflazine) in the treatment of comatose survivors of cardiac arrest. *N Engl J Med* 324:1225, 1991.
75. Koroshetz W, Moskowitz M: Emerging treatments for stroke in humans. *Trends Pharm Sci* 17:227, 1996.
76. Hickenbottom S, Grotta J: Neuroprotective therapy. *Semin Neurol* 18:485, 1998.
77. Abramson N, et al: Randomized clinical study of thiopental loading in comatose cardiac arrest survivors. *N Engl J Med* 314:397, 1986.
78. Rami A, Agarwal R, Botez G, Winckler J: Mu-calpain activation, DNA fragmentation, and synergistic effects of caspase and calpain inhibitors in protecting hippocampal neurons from ischemic damage. *Brain Res* 866:299, 2000.
79. Hartl R, Schurer L, Schmid-Schonbein G, del Zoppo G: Experimental antileukocyte interventions in cerebral ischemia. *J Cereb Blood Flow Metab* 16:1108, 1996.
80. DeGraba TJ: The role of inflammation after acute stroke: Utility of pursuing anti-adhesion molecule therapy. *Neurology* 51(3 Suppl 3):S62, 1998.
81. Yanaka K, et al: Reduction of brain injury using heparin to inhibit leukocyte accumulation in a rat model of transient focal cerebral ischemia: II. Dose-response effect and the therapeutic window. *J Neurosurg* 85:1108, 1996.
82. Pantoni L, Sarti C, Inzitari D: Cytokines and cell adhesion molecules in cerebral ischemia: Experimental bases and therapeutic perspectives. *Arterioscler Thromb Vasc Biol* 18:503, 1998.
83. Krams M, et al: Acute Stroke Therapy by Inhibition of Neutrophils (ASTIN): An adaptive dose-response study of UK-279,276 in acute ischemic stroke. *Stroke* 34:2543, 2003.
84. Rosenthal R, et al: Prevention of postischemic canine neurological injury through potentiation of brain energy metabolism by acetyl-L-carnitine. *Stroke* 23:1312, 1992.
85. Katz L, Wang Y, Rockoff S, Bouldin T: Low-dose carbicarb improves cerebral outcome after asphyxial cardiac arrest in rats. *Ann Emerg Med* 39:359, 2002.
86. Peeling J, Sutherland G, Brown RA, Curry S: Protective effect of dichloroacetate in a rat model of forebrain ischemia. *Neurosci Lett* 208:21, 1996.
87. Olinger CP, et al: High-dose intravenous naloxone for the treatment of acute ischemic stroke. *Stroke* 21:721, 1990.
88. Merchenthaler I, Dellovade T, Shughrue P: Neuroprotection by estrogen in animal models of global and focal ischemia. *Ann N Y Acad Sci* 1007:89, 2003.
89. Bunch TJ, et al: Long-term outcomes of out-of-hospital cardiac arrest after successful early defibrillation. *N Engl J Med* 348:2626, 2003.
90. Stiell I, et al: Health-related quality of life is better for cardiac arrest survivors who received citizen cardiopulmonary resuscitation. *Circulation* 108:1939, 2003.
91. Granja C, Cabral G, Pinto AT, Costa-Pereira A: Quality of life 6-months after cardiac arrest. *Resuscitation* 55:37, 2002.
92. van Alem AP, Waalewijn RA, Koster RW, de Vos R: Assessment of quality of life and cognitive function after out-of-hospital cardiac arrest with successful resuscitation. *Am J Cardiol* 93:131, 2004.
93. Naess A-C, Steen PA: Long term survival and costs per life year gained after out-of-hospital cardiac arrest. *Resuscitation* 60:57, 2004.
94. Saner H, et al: Quality of life in long-term survivors of out-of-hospital cardiac arrest. *Resuscitation* 53:7, 2002.
95. Booth CM, Boone RH, Tomlinson G, Detsky AS: Is this patient dead, vegetative, or severely neurologically impaired? Assessing outcome for comatose survivors of cardiac arrest. *JAMA* 291:870, 2004.

CHAPTER

7 Adult Resuscitation

Robert W. Neumar and Kevin R. Ward

PERSPECTIVE

Background

Most effective techniques used in resuscitation today were described more than 100 years ago. The modern era of cardiopulmonary resuscitation (CPR) began in the late 1950s with the rediscovery of closed-chest cardiac massage and mouth-to-mouth ventilation coupled with technical advances in external defibrillation. The first successful electrical reversal of ventricular fibrillation (VF) by externally applied paddles was reported by Zoll in 1956.[1] Safar and Elam[2,3] described effective techniques of airway management and mouth-to-mouth ventilation in 1958. Closed-chest cardiac massage was rediscovered by Kouwenhoven and colleagues[4] in 1960. The synthesis of these three non-invasive techniques greatly increased the number of people who could be trained to administer CPR and the locations where it could be performed. The realization that most sudden deaths occur outside the hospital led to the extension of CPR and emergency cardiac care to the out-of-hospital setting. Despite intensive research efforts since the 1970s, the only clinically feasible interventions consistently shown to improve survival from cardiac arrest are early CPR, early defibrillation, CPR before defibrillation after prolonged arrest, and prolonged hypothermia induced after return of spontaneous circulation.

Epidemiology

Sudden unexpected death, defined as death within 24 hours of symptom onset in a previously functional individual, accounts for one third of all nontraumatic deaths, with most occurring outside the hospital.[5] Of these, 75% are attributed to cardiovascular disease, with the remaining 25% attributed to noncardiac causes. Based on these numbers, an estimated 670,000 of the 2 million nontraumatic deaths each year in the United States occur suddenly, making incidence of sudden death 0.26%. Of these, 500,000 could be attributed to cardiovascular disease and the remaining 170,000 to noncardiac causes.

PRINCIPLES OF DISEASE

Although cardiac arrest results in global cessation of blood flow, vulnerability to ischemic injury varies among different organs and by region within the same organ. The brain is the most susceptible organ to ischemic injury, with neurons in the cerebral cortex, hippocampus, and cerebellum being selectively vulnerable. The heart is the second most susceptible organ to ischemic injury, with the endocardium being more sensitive than the epicardium. The renal, gastrointestinal, musculoskeletal, and integumentary systems are much more resistant to ischemia than the heart and brain and rarely sustain irreversible primary damage after durations of cardiac arrest compatible with successful resuscitation.

Traditionally, irreversible ischemic brain damage is thought to begin after 5 minutes of normothermic cardiac arrest. Most experimental data suggest, however, that the potential exists for neuronal survival after 20 minutes of ischemia. In the clinical setting, restoration of prearrest neurologic function rarely occurs after durations of untreated cardiac arrest longer than 10 minutes. The pathophysiologic mechanisms causing cellular injury during global ischemia and reperfusion from cardiac arrest can be broken down into four phases: prearrest, arrest, resuscitation, and postresuscitation.

Prearrest

Underlying disease and precipitating factors can significantly affect the metabolic state of cells before the onset of complete ischemia and may alter cells' ability to recover from a prolonged ischemic insult. A period of hypoxia or hypotension immediately preceding cardiac arrest, as occurs in respiratory arrest, depletes cell energy stores and causes tissue acidosis, both of which worsen the insult severity. In contrast, cells may be "preconditioned" by chronic or intermittent ischemia, rendering them more resistant to subsequent prolonged ischemic insults.

Arrest

Total circulatory arrest results in tissue hypoxia and cessation of aerobic metabolism within seconds. In an attempt to maintain viability, cells revert to anaerobic metabolism, which is less efficient and produces inadequate adenosine triphosphate (ATP) to maintain cellular ionic gradients. The rate of energy depletion varies among tissues and depends on their energy stores and metabolic requirements. Myocardial energy depletion during cardiac arrest also is likely to depend on the cardiac rhythm. The fibrillating heart depletes its energy stores more rapidly than a heart in asystole or electromechanical dissociation (EMD). When energy depletion occurs, cell membranes depolarize, and a cascade of metabolic events is initiated, including intracellular calcium overload, generation of free radicals, mitochondrial dysfunction, altered gene expression, activation of catabolic enzymes (phospholipases, endonucleases, proteases), and inflammation. Most injury pathways triggered during ischemia progress during the resuscitation and postresuscitation periods.

Resuscitation

CPR represents a period of ongoing global ischemia. Cardiac output generated by standard chest compressions is at best less than 30% of baseline and decreases precipitously with time to initiation and duration of chest compressions.[6] Most animal studies have shown that myocardial and cerebral blood flows generated during standard CPR are inadequate to meet baseline energy demands. The distribution of blood flow during CPR depends on arterial vascular tone. Endogenous mechanisms to direct blood flow preferentially to the heart and brain during the early minutes of resuscitation include release of catecholamines (epinephrine, norepinephrine) and vasoactive peptides (angiotensin, vasopressin), which increase arterial vascular tone in nonessential tissue beds. This response becomes ineffective within minutes of circulatory arrest, however, and administration of exogenous vasoconstrictors becomes essential to optimize myocardial and cerebral perfusion. This preferential distribution of blood flow is ideal during CPR because the goal is to generate myocardial perfusion adequate to restore organized electrical activity and effective mechanical function of the heart, while minimizing ischemic brain injury. When vasoconstriction persists after return of spontaneous circulation (ROSC), however, the hemodynamic impact is potentially detrimental. Increased afterload puts additional strain on an already weakened heart, and prolonged vasoconstriction may contribute to ongoing ischemia in nonessential tissue beds, such as the gastrointestinal tract.

Since the 1960 description of the standard method of chest compressions,[4] the mechanism of blood flow has been debated continuously. Predominant theories include the thoracic pump mechanism versus direct cardiac compression.[7] By either mechanism, the valve system in the heart allows forward rather than retrograde blood flow when a pressure gradient is created between the ventricles and the arterial system.

In the *cardiac compression model,* the heart is squeezed between the sternum and the thoracic spine, creating a pressure gradient between the ventricles and the great arteries. This pressure causes blood to flow into the systemic and pulmonary arterial circulation. The heart valves prevent retrograde flow. Transesophageal echocardiography has shown mitral valve closure during chest compressions and anterograde flow across the mitral valve during the relaxation phase of chest compressions in humans. Valve function deteriorates, however, during the course of cardiac arrest, with the exception of the aortic valve.

In the *thoracic pump model,* chest compression causes an increase in intrathoracic pressure that creates a pressure gradient between the intrathoracic vascular bed and the extrathoracic arterial bed. Blood flows down the pressure gradient into the peripheral arterial system. Retrograde flow into the cerebral venous circulation is limited by Niemann's valve at the junction of the superior vena cava and internal jugular vein.[8] Theoretically, because no pressure gradient is created between the right ventricle and the pulmonary artery, the right-sided circulation acts as a passive conduit.

Current evidence suggests that the cardiac compression and the thoracic pump mechanisms are working during standard chest compressions, but the impact of the thoracic pump is dominant. The contribution of each mechanism may be determined by body habitus and duration of CPR.

Postresuscitation

The postresuscitation period is a physiologically complex shock state characterized by persistent ischemia-induced metabolic derangements and initiation of reperfusion-induced metabolic cascades, both of which mediate secondary cellular injury. Cells that survive the initial ischemic insult may succumb to secondary injury after reperfusion. The *postresuscitation syndrome* is defined as multiorgan injury and failure occurring after severe global ischemia, exemplified but not limited to various degrees of neurologic injury.[9]

Myocardial function is depressed after resuscitation from cardiac arrest.[10] The degree and reversibility of postarrest myocardial dysfunction are related to the events preceding the arrest, arrest rhythm, arrest dura-

tion, and amount of adrenergic agonists used during resuscitation. The reversible component of postischemic myocardial dysfunction is termed *myocardial stunning.*[10,11] Global myocardial dysfunction also may be exacerbated by myocardial depressant factors released from the visceral organs after cardiac arrest.[12] In many patients, antecedent or ongoing regional myocardial ischemia (angina or myocardial infarction [MI]) causes additional regional myocardial dysfunction.

Despite being subjected to the same duration of ischemia during cardiac arrest and almost no blood flow during CPR, the visceral organs rarely sustain irreversible primary ischemic injury during durations of arrest compatible with successful resuscitation. Cardiac arrest sets the stage for metabolic events leading to multiorgan dysfunction, however, and unrecognized ongoing ischemia after ROSC contributes to the development of multiorgan dysfunction.

Etiology

Understanding the causes of cardiac arrest directs therapy and diagnostic testing during resuscitation and in the immediate postresuscitation period (Table 7-1). Cardiac arrest from a primary cardiac etiology typically presents as VF or less often as pulseless ventricular tachycardia (VT). Coronary artery disease is the most common pathologic condition found in patients who die suddenly from VF; autopsy studies show a 75% incidence of previous MI and a 20% to 30% incidence of acute MI.[13] Other anatomic abnormalities associated with sudden cardiac death caused by VF or VT include myocardial hypertrophy, cardiomyopathy, and specific structural abnormalities. Pulseless electrical activity (PEA) and asystole are less common initial presenting rhythms in patients with a cardiac etiology of arrest. These rhythms most often occur as a deterioration of VF or VT or develop in response to resuscitation treatments, such as defibrillation.

Primary respiratory failure generally causes initial hypertension and tachycardia, followed by hypotension and bradycardia and progressing to PEA, VF, or asystole. Circulatory obstruction (e.g., tension pneumothorax, pericardial tamponade) and hypovolemia generally present with initial tachycardia and hypotension, progressing through bradycardia to PEA, but also may deteriorate to VF or asystole.

The most common metabolic cause of cardiac arrest is *hyperkalemia,* which is seen most frequently in patients with renal failure. Hyperkalemia results in progressive widening of the QRS complex, which can deteriorate to VT, VF, asystole, or PEA. Other electrolyte abnormalities (e.g., hypomagnesemia, hypermagnesemia, hypokalemia) may lead to significant dysrhythmias, but the frequency with which they cause cardiac arrest is not documented.

Cardiac arrest from drug toxicity has specific characteristics depending on the drug involved. Specific therapy directed at drug toxicity is essential but may not be immediately effective. Prolonged resuscitation efforts may be needed using a method that provides adequate perfusion.

Table 7-1. Common Causes of Nontraumatic Cardiac Arrest

General	Specific	Disease/Agent
Cardiac		Coronary artery disease
		Cardiomyopathies
		Structural abnormalities
		Valve dysfunction
Respiratory	Hypoventilation	CNS dysfunction
		Neuromuscular disease
		Toxic and metabolic encephalopathies
	Upper airway obstruction	CNS dysfunction
		Foreign body
		Infection
		Trauma
		Neoplasm
	Pulmonary dysfunction	Asthma, COPD
		Pulmonary edema
		Pulmonary embolus
		Pneumonia
Circulatory	Mechanical obstruction	Tension pneumothorax
		Pericardial tamponade
		Pulmonary embolus
	Hypovolemia	Hemorrhage
	Vascular tone	Sepsis
		Neurogenic
Metabolic	Electrolyte abnormalities	Hypokalemia or hyperkalemia
		Hypermagnesemia
		Hypomagnesemia
		Hypocalcemia
Toxic	Prescription medications	Antidysrhythmics
		Digitalis β-Blockers
		Calcium channel blockers
		Tricyclic antidepressants
	Drugs of abuse	Cocaine
		Heroin
	Toxins	Carbon monoxide
		Cyanide
Environmental		Lightning
		Electrocution
		Hypothermia or hyperthermia
		Drowning/near-drowning

CNS, central nervous system; COPD, chronic obstructive pulmonary disease.

Electrocution causes cardiac arrest through primary dysrhythmias or apnea. Alternating current in the range of 100 mA to 1 A generally causes VF, whereas currents greater than 10 A can cause ventricular asystole. Lightning produces a massive direct current electrocution that can result in asystole and prolonged apnea.

Hypothermia-induced cardiac arrest can present with any electrocardiogram (ECG) rhythm, and successful resuscitation depends on rapid rewarming, which often requires aggressive and invasive measures (e.g., peritoneal lavage, cardiopulmonary bypass [CPB], open-chest cardiac massage [OCCM]). Drowning is a form of asphyxia usually resulting in bradyasystolic arrest. Because drowning often is accompanied by hypothermia, the victim may benefit from prolonged resuscitation efforts similar to resuscitation efforts for hypothermia.

CLINICAL FEATURES AND MANAGEMENT

Most cardiac arrest cases managed in the emergency department initially occur outside the hospital. An increasing number of first responders, nontraditional providers, and public venues are being equipped with automated defibrillators. Dramatic resuscitation rates have been achieved when these programs enable providers to deliver countershock within less than 4 to 5 minutes of arrest onset.[14-17] Programs that fail to enable a significant number of patients to be defibrillated within this critical time window have limited or no impact on survival.[18,19]

Advanced life support (ALS) units staffed by paramedics often have standing orders to follow advanced protocols. In general, there is no advantage to interrupting properly performed advanced measures to transport a patient who is still in cardiac arrest. In cases of cardiac arrest refractory to properly performed advanced measures, the patient may be pronounced dead at the scene if appropriate protocols have been outlined within the system.[20]

Simultaneous assessment and management of a patient in cardiac arrest must occur in an orchestrated effort by a health care team led by an emergency physician who can synthesize the ongoing assessment and monitor the efficacy and response to therapeutic interventions. It is often difficult or impossible to determine the cause of cardiac arrest at presentation. Although a differential diagnosis can be formulated based on history, physical examination, and ECG rhythm on arrival, key information often is not available or is unreliable.[21] The differential diagnosis potentially can be narrowed by the patient's age, underlying diseases, and medications.

History and Physical Examination

Historical information from the family, bystanders, and emergency medical services (EMS) personnel provides key information regarding etiology and prognosis. Information surrounding the event includes whether the arrest was witnessed, the time of arrest, what the patient was doing (e.g., eating, exercising, trauma), the possibility of drug ingestion, time of initial CPR, initial ECG rhythm, and interventions by EMS providers. Important past medical history includes baseline health and mental status; previous heart, lung, renal, or malignant disease; hemorrhage; infection; and risk factors for coronary artery disease and pulmonary embolism. The patient's current medications and allergies also should be obtained.

Physical examination of a cardiac arrest patient is essential to (1) ensure adequacy of airway maintenance and ventilation, (2) confirm the diagnosis of cardiac arrest, (3) find evidence of etiology, and (4) monitor for complications of therapeutic interventions. This examination must occur in descending order of importance, simultaneous with therapeutic interventions, and must be repeated frequently to assess for response to therapy and occurrence of complications (Table 7-2).

Table 7-2. Physical Examination Findings Indicating Potential Cause of Cardiac Arrest and Complications of Therapy

Physical Examination	Abnormalities	Potential Causes
General	Pallor	Hemorrhage
	Cold	Hypothermia
Airway	Secretions, vomitus, or blood	Aspiration
		Airway obstruction
	Resistance to positive-pressure ventilation	Tension pneumothorax
		Airway obstruction
		Bronchospasm
Neck	Jugular venous distention	Tension pneumothorax
		Cardiac tamponade
		Pulmonary embolus
	Tracheal deviation	Tension pneumothorax
Chest	Median sternotomy scar	Underlying cardiac disease
Lungs	Unilateral breath sounds	Tension pneumothorax
		Right main stem intubation
		Aspiration
	Distant or no breath sounds or no chest expansion	Esophageal intubation
		Airway obstruction
		Severe bronchospasm
	Wheezing	Aspiration
		Bronchospasm
		Pulmonary edema
	Rales	Aspiration
		Pulmonary edema
		Pneumonia
Heart	Audible heart tones	Hypovolemia
		Cardiac tamponade
		Tension pneumothorax
		Pulmonary embolus
Abdomen	Distended and dull	Ruptured abdominal aortic aneurysm or ruptured ectopic pregnancy
	Distended, tympanitic	Esophageal intubation
		Gastric insufflation
Rectal	Blood, melena	Gastrointestinal hemorrhage
Extremities	Asymmetric pulses	Aortic dissection
	Arteriovenous shunt or fistula	Hyperkalemia
Skin	Needle tracts or abscesses	Intravenous drug abuse
	Burns	Smoke inhalation
		Electrocution

Cardiopulmonary arrest is defined by the triad of unconsciousness, apnea, and pulselessness. The pulse must be palpated in a large artery (carotid or femoral). If any question exists as to the diagnosis of pulselessness, CPR should be initiated and pulselessness confirmed with measures such as a hand-held vascular Doppler or end-tidal carbon dioxide monitoring. Rapid bedside ultrasound may confirm loss of cardiac activity. With sudden onset of circulatory arrest, as in VF, loss of consciousness occurs within 15 seconds, although agonal gasping respirations may persist for 60 seconds. A brief seizure may result from cessation of cerebral blood flow. Primary respiratory arrest results in transient tachycardia and hypertension that progress to loss of consciousness, bradycardia, and pulselessness, usually within 5 minutes.

After the initial minutes of cardiac arrest, physical examination may provide little evidence of the duration of arrest. Pupils dilate within 1 minute but constrict if CPR is initiated immediately and performed effectively. Dependent lividity and rigor mortis develop after hours of cardiac arrest. Temperature is an unreliable predictor of duration of cardiac arrest because it does not decrease significantly during the first hours of arrest. Moderate to severe hypothermia may cause

cardiac arrest or may be caused by prolonged arrest, with opposite prognostic implications.

Monitoring

Traditional monitoring during CPR has relied on evaluation of the ECG in one or more leads and palpation of carotid or femoral artery pulses. Although the lack of a palpable pulse during CPR may indicate inadequate forward flow, the degree of forward flow cannot be estimated accurately in the presence of a palpable pulse because pressures generated during CPR may be transmitted equally to the venous and the arterial vasculatures. In addition, myocardial blood flow does not depend on the palpated arterial systolic pressure, but does depend on the difference between aortic diastolic pressure and right atrial diastolic pressure. ECG monitoring during cardiac arrest indicates the presence or absence of electrical but not mechanical activity. Although these two monitoring modalities may be the best attainable in certain circumstances, they do not provide reliable information regarding the effectiveness of CPR and interventions or prognosis.

Although no ideal monitoring technique provides all the information that might be desired during resuscitation, the modalities discussed next can provide valuable treatment and diagnostic information during CPR. In particular, coronary perfusion pressure (CPP), partial pressure end-tidal carbon dioxide (PetCO₂), and central venous oxygen saturation (ScvO₂) monitoring can be used to detect inadequate CPR with high specificity (Table 7-3). In addition, several of these techniques are useful in the immediate postresuscitation period.

Arterial Blood Pressure and Coronary Perfusion Pressure

Successful resuscitation of the arrested heart depends on generating adequate CPP during CPR, which has been directly correlated with myocardial blood flow.[20] Animal and human studies indicate that a minimum CPP of 15 mm Hg is necessary to achieve ROSC if initial defibrillation attempts have failed.[22,23] Although CPP monitoring is the most reliable predictor of CPR adequacy, its main disadvantages are that (1) no method currently exists to monitor CPP noninvasively, and (2) proper instrumentation requires adequate resources and time. CPP measurement requires placement of an intra-arterial catheter to monitor arterial diastolic pressure and a central venous catheter (preferably at or near the right atrium) to monitor right atrial diastolic pressure. CPP tracings show positive and negative

CPP during human CPR that are indistinguishable by palpation of pulse alone (Figure 7-1). Although CPP measurement has limited feasibility, it is the gold standard by which all other monitoring modalities are compared and the effectiveness of vasopressor therapy is evaluated.

Although not ideal, arterial blood pressure monitoring alone also may be helpful. Studies have indicated that achievement of an arterial diastolic pressure of 40 mm Hg is highly predictive of ROSC.[24] Additional benefits of arterial cannulation during CPR include ability to distinguish EMD from pseudo-EMD, immediate confirmation of ROSC, and facilitation of serial arterial blood gas monitoring. Arterial and central

Table 7-3. Indicators of Inadequate Blood Flow During Cardiopulmonary Resuscitation

Monitoring Technique	Indicator
Carotid or femoral pulse	Not palpable
CPP	<15 mm Hg
PetCO₂	<10 mm Hg (before vasopressor)
ScvO₂	<40%

CPP, coronary perfusion pressure; PetCO₂, end-tidal carbon dioxide partial pressure; ScvO₂, central venous oxygen saturation.

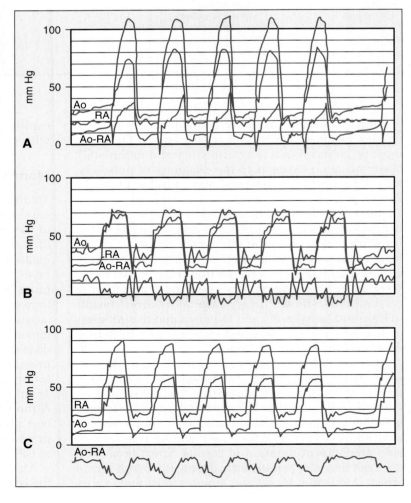

Figure 7-1. Aortic (Ao), right atrial (RA), and coronary perfusion (Ao-RA) pressure tracings during human cardiopulmonary resuscitation. **A,** Positive coronary perfusion pressure (CPP) generated during compression and relaxation phases of chest compressions. **B,** Positive CPP generated only during the relaxation phase of chest compressions. **C,** Negative CPP throughout the compression cycle. (From Martin GB, et al: Aortic and right atrial pressures during standard and simultaneous compression and ventilation CPR in human beings. *Ann Emerg Med* 15:125, 1986.)

venous monitoring are needed to optimize postresuscitation care.

End-Tidal Carbon Dioxide

Experimental and clinical studies have shown that $PetCO_2$ is a reliable indicator of cardiac output during CPR. Several conditions must be met or assumed to use $PetCO_2$ as a correlate of cardiac output during CPR. $PetCO_2$ depends on CO_2 production, alveolar ventilation, and pulmonary blood flow (i.e., cardiac output). If ventilation and CO_2 production are held constant, any increase or decrease in $PetCO_2$ should reflect an increase or decrease in cardiac output. Although CO_2 production during cardiac arrest and CPR probably is not constant, small changes in CO_2 production are not likely to cause appreciable changes in $PetCO_2$ because of the extremely high mixed-venous CO_2 levels and large dead space created by cardiac arrest and CPR. Administration of sodium bicarbonate ($NaHCO_3$) during CPR may cause a sudden large increase in mixed-venous CO_2, however, which may produce a variable but transient increase in $PetCO_2$. Otherwise, with minute ventilation held constant, only increased cardiac output during CPR and ROSC significantly increases $PetCO_2$.

In addition to correlations with cardiac output, animal and human studies show that $PetCO_2$ correlates with CPP and cerebral perfusion pressure during CPR.[25,26] This correlation would be predicted based on the known relationship between mean arterial pressure and cardiac output when peripheral vascular resistance (PVR) is constant. With dramatic increases in PVR, however, as may occur with high-dose vasopressor therapy, cardiac output and $PetCO_2$ may decrease despite increased CPP.[27]

$PetCO_2$ can be used to adjust compression force and rate, maximizing forward flow, and to detect CPR provider fatigue (Figure 7-2).[28] Resuscitation of cardiac arrest is likely to fail if $PetCO_2$ values are less than 10 mm Hg.[29,30] In the absence of high-dose vasopressor therapy, $PetCO_2$ values less than 10 mm Hg should prompt the clinician to modify the ongoing resuscitation. After large doses of vasopressors, a more reliable measure (e.g., CPP, $ScvO_2$) should be used to titrate therapy.

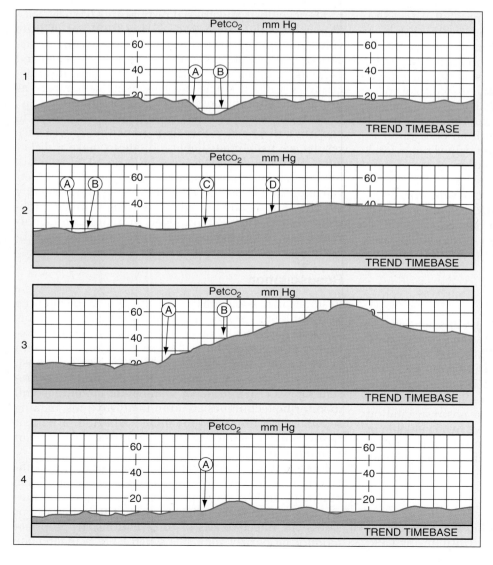

Figure 7-2. Capnogram tracings of end-tidal carbon dioxide pressure ($PetCO_2$) during human cardiopulmonary resuscitation (CPR). **1,** Effect of rescuer fatigue is shown at point *A.* Point *B* shows the effect of changing to a fresh rescuer. **2,** Patient with pseudo–electromechanical dissociation. At point *A,* the patient is pulseless but has a persistent $PetCO_2$ value of 20 mm Hg without CPR; at point *B,* CPR is restarted; at point *C,* dopamine infusion is started; and at point *D,* CPR is stopped, and a pulse is palpated. **3,** Sudden increase in $PetCO_2$ (point *A*) heralds the return of spontaneous circulation; pulses are palpated at point *P.* **4,** Point *A* shows a transient increase in $PetCO_2$ such as occurs during bolus administration of sodium bicarbonate.

PetCO$_2$ monitoring also can aid in the diagnosis and treatment of PEA. Patients in a state of pseudo-EMD (cardiac contraction that does not generate a pulse) are likely to have higher PetCO$_2$ values than patients in EMD (absence of cardiac contraction). PetCO$_2$ monitoring also is useful in rapidly detecting success of tension pneumothorax decompression, pericardiocentesis for pericardial tamponade, and fluid resuscitation for hypovolemia. ROSC causes immediate and significant increases in PetCO$_2$ before detection of a pulse by palpation. Finally, PetCO$_2$ monitoring is valuable in patients after cardiac arrest to detect sudden hemodynamic deterioration. Undetectable PetCO$_2$ during CPR indicates failure to intubate the trachea, massive pulmonary embolism, or inadequate chest compressions. Undetectable PetCO$_2$, even after prolonged cardiac arrest, cannot be attributed to cessation of CO$_2$ production.

Central Venous Oxygen Saturation

ScvO$_2$ provides an additional method to monitor adequacy or resuscitative measures.[31] The mixed-venous blood oxygen saturation in the pulmonary artery (SvO$_2$) represents the oxygen remaining in the blood after systemic extraction. Studies have shown a close correlation between ScvO$_2$ and SvO$_2$ during CPR.[32] Because oxygen consumption remains relatively constant during CPR, as does arterial oxygen saturation (SaO$_2$) and hemoglobin, changes in ScvO$_2$ reflect changes in oxygen delivery by means of changes in cardiac output.

Multilumen oximetric ScvO$_2$ catheters are placed in the same manner as regular central venous catheters and can be used to monitor ScvO$_2$ continuously in real time. ScvO$_2$ values normally range from 60% to 80%. During cardiac arrest and CPR, these values range from 25% to 35%, indicating the inadequacy of blood flow produced during CPR. Failure to achieve a ScvO$_2$ of 40% or greater has a negative predictive value for ROSC of almost 100%.[31] ScvO$_2$ also helps to confirm ROSC rapidly (Figure 7-3). ScvO$_2$ monitoring also is useful in the postresuscitation period to help titrate therapy and recognize any sudden deterioration in the patient's clinical condition.

Echocardiography

The main usefulness of echocardiography is diagnostic, especially in patients with PEA. Echocardiography distinguishes EMD from pseudo-EMD. It also may be helpful in diagnosing mechanical causes of PEA, such as tension pneumothorax, pericardial tamponade, and pulmonary embolism. Echocardiography also is useful in guiding pericardiocentesis. In the postresuscitation period, echocardiography could prove to be valuable in determining the need for postresuscitation cardiac intervention or mechanical assistance of the failing heart.

Laboratory Testing

Intermittent arterial and venous blood sampling for gas or chemistry analysis is of limited utility during CPR.

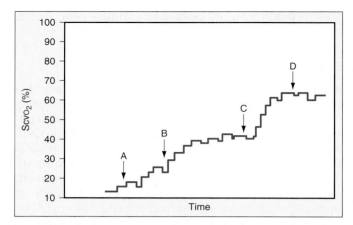

Figure 7-3. Central venous oxygen saturation (ScvO$_2$) monitoring during human cardiopulmonary resuscitation in a pulseless asystolic patient. Standard advanced cardiac life support is being performed at point *A*. High-dose epinephrine is administered at points *B* and *C*. Point *D* represents the return of spontaneous circulation. (From Ander DS, et al: Continvous central venous oxygen saturation monitoring as an adjunct in the treatment of cardiac arrest and shock: Principles and practice. *Crit Intensive Care* 5:236, 1994.)

Typical blood gas findings during CPR are venous respiratory acidosis and arterial respiratory alkalosis. SaO$_2$ is usually greater than 94% during CPR and of little value in titrating resuscitation therapy except in the case of massive pulmonary embolism or unrecognized esophageal intubation. Although ScvO$_2$ indicates adequacy of CPR, a single measurement may not be as useful as continuous oximetric ScvO$_2$ monitoring.

Other laboratory studies during CPR serve more to confirm a diagnosis rather than guide therapy because results are usually available too late to make a difference. Serum electrolytes may be ordered to rule out hyperkalemia, hypokalemia, hypomagnesemia, hypercalcemia, and hypocalcemia; however, empiric therapy should be initiated immediately if a high clinical probability exists. Hemoglobin levels may indicate hemorrhage, but initial hemoglobin may be normal even in acute exsanguinating hemorrhage.

Resuscitation

Restoration of adequate cardiac function is the defining factor of ROSC. Restoration of normal brain function is the defining factor of successful resuscitation. The likelihood of achieving both of these goals decreases with every minute the patient remains in cardiac arrest. Although many interventions are specific to the presenting ECG rhythm, most therapeutic modalities and monitoring techniques are used in all rhythms, making separate algorithms redundant. In addition, a patient rarely remains in one ECG rhythm during the course of prolonged resuscitation.

Interventions must be performed rapidly and efficiently to maximize the chances of a good neurologic outcome. Unless appropriate monitoring techniques are used, there is no reliable way to titrate therapy or assess the effectiveness of interventions. Appropriate monitoring clearly indicates when CPR is inadequate

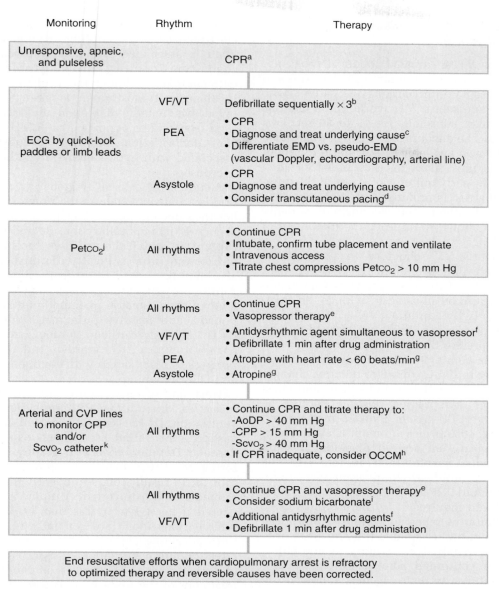

Monitoring	Rhythm	Therapy

Unresponsive, apneic, and pulseless — CPRᵃ

ECG by quick-look paddles or limb leads

VF/VT
Defibrillate sequentially × 3ᵇ

PEA
- CPR
- Diagnose and treat underlying causeᶜ
- Differentiate EMD vs. pseudo-EMD (vascular Doppler, echocardiography, arterial line)

Asystole
- CPR
- Diagnose and treat underlying cause
- Consider transcutaneous pacingᵈ

Petco₂ʲ — **All rhythms**
- Continue CPR
- Intubate, confirm tube placement and ventilate
- Intravenous access
- Titrate chest compressions Petco₂ > 10 mm Hg

All rhythms
- Continue CPR
- Vasopressor therapyᵉ

VF/VT
- Antidysrhythmic agent simultaneous to vasopressorᶠ
- Defibrillate 1 min after drug administration

PEA
- Atropine with heart rate < 60 beats/minᵍ

Asystole
- Atropineᵍ

Arterial and CVP lines to monitor CPP and/or Scvo₂ catheterᵏ — **All rhythms**
- Continue CPR and titrate therapy to:
  - AoDP > 40 mm Hg
  - CPP > 15 mm Hg
  - Scvo₂ > 40 mm Hg
- If CPR inadequate, consider OCCMʰ

All rhythms
- Continue CPR and vasopressor therapyᵉ
- Consider sodium bicarbonateⁱ

VF/VT
- Additional antidysrhythmic agentsᶠ
- Defibrillate 1 min after drug administation

End resuscitative efforts when cardiopulmonary arrest is refractory to optimized therapy and reversible causes have been corrected.

Figure 7-4. Emergency treatment algorithm for treatment of cardiac arrest. ᵃIf arrest is witnessed and known to be of short duration, immediate rhythm assessment and defibrillation of ventricular fibrillation/ventricular tachycardia (VF/VT) precede cardiopulmonary resuscitation (CPR). In cases of prolonged untreated VF/VT, 1 to 2 minutes of CPR before defibrillation may enhance the ability to achieve return of spontaneous circulation. PEA, pulseless electrical activity; EMD, electromechanical dissociation. ᵇConsider using biphasic impedance-corrected defibrillation (150 J three times) versus monophasic defibrillation (200 J, 200-300 J, or 360 J). ᶜSee Table 7-4. ᵈGenerally ineffective unless initiated immediately after onset of asystole. ᵉEpinephrine, initial dose of 1 mg intravenous (IV) push or 2.5 mg by endotracheal tube (ETT). Repeat every 3 to 5 minutes. Subsequent doses may be increased up to 0.1 mg/kg. An alternative to epinephrine is vasopressin, 40 U IV push. Vasopressin is potentially more effective if the presenting rhythm is asystole. The dose (40 U) can be repeated once in 3 minutes, followed by administration of epinephrine every 3-5 minutes. ᶠAmiodarone, 300 mg IV push followed by 150 mg every 30 minutes. Alternative antidysrhythmics include lidocaine and bretylium (see text for dosing). Magnesium sulfate, 1 to 2 mg IV push in torsades de pointes or known hypomagnesemia. ᵍAtropine, 1 mg IV push or 2.5 mg by ETT. Repeat dose every 3 to 5 minutes to a total dose of 0.04 mg/kg. ʰOpen chest cardiac massage (OCCM) should be considered if (1) there are clear indications of inadequate blood flow during standard CPR, (2) duration of arrest is less than 20 minutes, and (3) the clinician judges that a potential exists for good neurologic outcome. AoDP, aortic diastolic pressure; CPP, coronary perfusion pressure; CVP, central venous pressure; Scvo₂, central venous oxygen saturation. ⁱSodium bicarbonate, 1 mEq/kg after prolonged rest or high dose of epinephrine. ʲChanges in end-tidal carbon dioxide partial pressure (Petco₂) may not be predictive of myocardial blood flow after high-dose vasopressor therapy. ᵏInvasive monitoring should be performed only if adequate personnel are available and if it would not delay therapeutic interventions.

(see Table 7-3). If the inadequacy of CPR is recognized early in the resuscitation despite optimized therapy, the treating physician in charge should consider OCCM, if a good neurologic outcome is possible. After prolonged arrest, however, clear indications that CPR is inadequate (based on appropriate monitoring techniques) should prompt cessation of resuscitation efforts. Figure 7-4 presents an algorithm for management of cardiac arrest. Interventions specific to each rhythm are discussed in the following sections.

Ventricular Fibrillation and Pulseless Ventricular Tachycardia

VF and pulseless VT are treated identically because they are generally caused by the same mechanisms and respond to the same interventions. A patient who develops VF or pulseless VT while on a cardiac monitor may remain conscious for 15 to 30 seconds. The patient should be encouraged to cough vigorously until a defibrillator is available. Defibrillation without antecedent CPR is most likely to result in ROSC when administered in the early minutes of arrest. If the duration of untreated arrest is prolonged (>4 to 5 minutes), a brief period of CPR (90 to 180 seconds) before defibrillation has been shown to improve the likelihood of ROSC and survival.[33,34]

VF and pulseless VT refractory to three initial attempts at defibrillation should be treated with assisted ventilation and chest compression. Chest compression force should be adjusted to achieve the greatest level of $PetCO_2$ (with a minimal value >10 mm Hg). Intravenous (IV) access and intubation should be performed, and vasopressor therapy (epinephrine or vasopressin) should be administered and repeated every 3 to 5 minutes. After initial vasopressor therapy, changes in $PetCO_2$ may be unpredictable, and subsequent chest compressions and vasopressor dosages should be adjusted to achieve CPP greater than 15 mm Hg and $ScvO_2$ greater than 40% if measurement is available. If CPP cannot be measured, arterial diastolic pressure should be titrated to greater than 40 mm Hg. The administration of an antidysrhythmic agent (e.g., amiodarone) with the initial dose of vasoconstrictor is not contraindicated and may result in more rapid ROSC. Defibrillation should be repeated 2 minutes after drug administration to allow reasonable time for peak drug effect. Subsequent therapy for refractory VF and pulseless VT includes continued administration of vasopressors and antidysrhythmic agents, followed by repeated countershocks. Antidysrhythmics should be administered up to their maximum loading dose. The use of magnesium sulfate during VF and pulseless VT is of no proven efficacy except in torsades de pointes and suspected hypomagnesemia. Specific indications for $NaHCO_3$ therapy include hyperkalemia, tricyclic antidepressant overdose, and preexisting severe metabolic acidosis. If a patient is defibrillated into a different pulseless rhythm, such as PEA or asystole, subsequent treatment should be modified to address those specific rhythms.

Pulseless Electrical Activity

PEA is defined as coordinated electrical activity of the heart (other than VT/VF) without a palpable pulse. This group of dysrhythmias includes EMD, in which no myocardial contractions occur, and pseudo-EMD, in which myocardial contractions occur but no pulse can be palpated. Although distinguishing EMD from pseudo-EMD may be useful in determining etiology and guiding treatment, in most cases of primary PEA there is a natural progression from hypotension to pseudo-EMD to EMD.

True EMD is the result of a primary disorder of electromechanical coupling in myocardial cells. It often is associated with abnormal automaticity and conduction resulting in bradycardia and a wide QRS complex. Although the mechanism of uncoupling is unclear, it most often is associated with global myocardial energy depletion and acidosis resulting from ischemia or hypoxia. True EMD typically occurs after defibrillation following prolonged VF and is associated with hyperkalemia, hypothermia, and drug overdose.

Pseudo-EMD caused by global myocardial dysfunction is a transient state in the progression to EMD and has the same etiologies. An additional cardiac cause of pseudo-EMD is papillary muscle and myocardial wall rupture, in which the ventricle continues to contract, but forward flow is greatly diminished. Pseudo-EMD also may be caused by primary supraventricular VT. Additional extracardiac causes of pseudo-EMD include hypovolemia, tension pneumothorax, pericardial tamponade, and massive pulmonary embolism. Pseudo-EMD of extracardiac etiology most often has narrow-complex tachycardia initially, which can progress to bradycardia with conduction abnormalities and QRS widening.

Treatment of PEA requires all general resuscitation measures, including CPR, intubation with assisted ventilation, IV access, and repeated administration of vasopressors. Initial assessment also should include vascular Doppler, echocardiography, or $PetCO_2$ monitoring to distinguish EMD and pseudo-EMD. PEA thought to result from supraventricular VT should be immediately cardioverted. Atropine should be administered if heart rate is less than 60 beats/min. These interventions alone are generally inadequate, unless the underlying cause of PEA is primary respiratory arrest or supraventricular VT. Successful resuscitation of patients with PEA hinges on rapid diagnosis and treatment of the underlying cause. Physical examination may provide valuable clues to the underlying etiology (Table 7-4). In several cases, such as hypoxia and hypovolemia, the diagnosis is based on response to empiric therapy, whereas other etiologies, such as pericardial tamponade, tension pneumothorax, and hypothermia, can be definitively diagnosed during resuscitation. After chest decompression for pneumothorax, CPR efficacy may be reduced in patients dependent on the thoracic pump mechanism of forward flow. All monitoring techniques previously described should be considered to guide ongoing resuscitation efforts.

Asystole

Asystole represents complete cessation of myocardial electrical activity. Although asystole may occur early in cardiac arrest as a consequence of progressive bradycardia, asystole generally represents the end-stage rhythm after prolonged cardiac arrest caused by VF or PEA. Because the potential exists for an organized rhythm or VF to appear as asystole in a single lead (if the rhythm vector is completely perpendicular to the

Table 7-4. Diagnosis and Treatment of Common Causes of Pulseless Electrical Activity

Cause	Diagnosis	Palliative Therapy	Definitive Therapy
Hypovolemia	Response to volume infusion	Volume infusion, consider OCCM	Hemostasis if hemorrhage
Hypoxia	Response to oxygenation	Oxygenation, assisted ventilation	Treat underlying cause
Cardiac tamponade	Echocardiogram, pericardiocentesis	Pericardiocentesis	Thoracotomy and pericardiotomy
Tension pneumothorax	Asymmetric breath sounds, tracheal deviation	Needle thoracostomy	Tube thoracostomy
Hypothermia	Rectal temperature		Warm peritoneal or thoracic lavage, OCCM or CPB
Pulmonary embolus	Risk factors or evidence of deep venous thrombosis	OCCM or CPB	Lytic therapy, pulmonary embolectomy
Drug overdose	History of drug ingestion	Drug specific	Drug specific
Hyperkalemia	History of renal failure or elevated serum potassium	Calcium chloride, insulin and glucose, sodium bicarbonate	Hemodialysis
Acidosis	Arterial blood gas	Hyperventilation, sodium bicarbonate	Treat underlying cause

CPB, cardiopulmonary bypass; OCCM, open-chest cardiac massage.

lead vector), asystole always should be confirmed in at least two limb leads. It may be difficult to distinguish between extremely fine VF and asystole. Routine countershock of asystole to treat possible fine VT has not been shown to improve outcome, however.

Treatment of asystole requires all general resuscitation measures, including CPR, intubation with assisted ventilation, IV access, and repeated administration of vasopressors. In one randomized prospective prehospital trial, improved survival to hospital admission and discharge was observed in patients presenting in asystole when two doses of vasopressin (40 IU) were given initially during resuscitation compared with standard-dose epinephrine (1 mg) followed by additional epinephrine if needed.[35] Atropine should be administered with the first dose of vasopressor and repeated to a total dose of 0.04 mg/kg. When asystole occurs early in cardiac arrest, proper diagnosis and treatment of the underlying cause are essential for successful resuscitation. Extensive research has shown that asystole in the out-of-hospital setting seldom responds to pacing. To be effective, pacing must be initiated within several minutes of arrest. CPR and vasopressor administration should be titrated to appropriate monitoring. All monitoring techniques previously described should be considered to guide ongoing resuscitation efforts.

Postresuscitation

Resuscitation of a cardiac arrest victim does not end with ROSC. Rapid diagnosis and proper management of the pathologic conditions that precipitated and resulted from the arrest are essential for optimal outcome. Because of the historically poor neurologic prognosis of patients resuscitated from out-of-hospital cardiac arrest, clinicians may be inclined to withhold aggressive postresuscitation management because the patient is judged to have no hope of a good neurologic outcome. Although the epidemiologic data cannot be ignored, no reliable way exists to determine the neurologic prognosis of an individual patient immediately after resuscitation. Every patient initially resuscitated deserves aggressive postresuscitation management to optimize the outcome. This management includes rapid diagnosis and treatment of the disorders that caused the arrest and the complications of prolonged global ischemia. Simultaneous management of these two entities makes caring for a postresuscitation patient particularly challenging.

Induction of prolonged therapeutic hypothermia in comatose survivors of cardiac arrest has been shown to improve survival and functional outcome in two prospective randomized clinical trials.[36,37] Both studies enrolled only prehospital patients with witnessed arrest and an initial rhythm of VF. The time to achieve target temperature (32° C to 34° C) ranged from less than 2 hours[36] to a median of 8 hours (interquartile range 4-16 hours),[37] suggesting a broad therapeutic window. Hypothermia was maintained 12 to 24 hours followed by gradual rewarming over 12 to 24 hours. Although these parameters provide guidelines within which postresuscitation hypothermia is effective, additional preclinical and clinical data are needed to determine the optimal temperature, time to achieve target temperature, and duration of therapy. In both studies, the rates of complications were not statistically different between groups, but the frequency of coagulopathy, pneumonia, and sepsis were slightly increased in patients treated with hypothermia.[37] Although there are no absolute contraindications, relative contraindications include severe cardiogenic shock, life-threatening dysrhythmias, uncontrolled bleeding, preexisting coagulopathy, pregnancy, another obvious reason for coma (i.e., drug overdose or status epilepticus), known end-stage terminal illness, and a preexisting do-not-resuscitate status. Thrombolytic therapy does not preclude the use of hypothermia.[37] Finally, although the current data are limited to patients with witnessed VF prehospital cardiac arrest, induced postresuscitation hypothermia potentially could be effective in patients resuscitated from other cardiac arrest presentations.

When the decision is made to treat the patient with therapeutic hypothermia, cooling efforts should be initiated as soon as possible. Practical methods of rapidly inducing hypothermia include ice packs (applied to the neck, femoral groins, and axilla), fan cooling of dampened exposed skin, cooling blankets underneath and on top of the patient, and rapid IV infusion of limited volumes (1 to 2 L) of 4° C saline, and reducing ambient temperature in the room.[38,39] Newer invasive methods, including endovascular venous catheters, are now available and allow for rapid and precise control of temperature, but they require time and additional resources to institute. Shivering must be prevented, and the most effective technique is sedation and paralysis. Target core body temperature should be 32° C to 34° C and is best monitored by an indwelling temperature-sensitive Foley catheter or pulmonary artery catheter. When the patient is stabilized and cooling efforts are initiated, transfer to a critical care unit should occur as soon as possible. Although the optimal duration of postresuscitation hypothermia is unknown, target temperature should be actively maintained for a minimum of 12 to 24 hours followed by gradual passive rewarming, which generally takes 12 to 24 hours. Effective application of therapeutic hypothermia in comatose cardiac arrest survivors requires a coordinated interdisciplinary effort and is best carried out using a predetermined goal-directed algorithm developed with input from emergency medicine, cardiology, and critical care physicians and nurses.

A simultaneous immediate concern in a comatose cardiac arrest survivor is whether the patient has an acute coronary syndrome. Diagnosing acute coronary syndrome in an unconscious patient after cardiac arrest presents a unique challenge. A standard 12-lead ECG should be obtained as soon as feasible after ROSC, with a right-sided 12-lead ECG also considered. Forty percent of postresuscitation patients without complaint of chest pain before arrest or ST segment elevations on the initial ECG may have an acute coronary occlusion responsible for their arrest.[21] In addition, patients with critical coronary lesions may have arrested from other causes but exhibit ECG evidence of acute myocardial ischemia precipitated from the arrest and resuscitation itself. Transient ST segment elevations also may be caused by electrical countershock.

Relative exclusion criteria for fibrinolytic therapy unique to the resuscitated patient include CPR duration greater than 10 minutes and evidence of significant CPR trauma (e.g., pneumothorax, flail chest, pulmonary contusion with hemorrhage). Immediate angioplasty should be considered in patients with evidence of acute myocardial ischemia who have exclusion criteria for thrombolytic therapy, drug-resistant hypertension, or cardiogenic shock. Given the potentially high incidence of occult critical coronary stenosis and myocardial ischemia, patients without evidence of acute myocardial ischemia represent a greater dilemma. Angioplasty of acute coronary lesions regardless of history or initial postresuscitation ECG has been shown to be an independent predictor of survival after cardiac arrest.[21]

Antiplatelet and anticoagulant therapy should be administered to all patients after ROSC if no evidence of hemorrhage exists and profound hypertension is absent. The choice of antiplatelet and anticoagulant therapy depends in part on the presence of active ischemia, renal function, and plans for acute angioplasty.[40] Antidysrhythmic therapy should be administered in all patients resuscitated from VF or VT and considered in patients experiencing significant ectopy. Concomitant therapies (e.g., nitrates, β-blockers) are best performed in conjunction with careful hemodynamic monitoring. If indicated, IV preparations of nitrates and short-acting β-blockers (e.g., esmolol) should be used because they have a brief duration of action and are easily titrated. Patients with new left bundle branch blocks, right bundle branch blocks with left anterior or posterior hemiblocks, second-degree type II blocks, or third-degree blocks should have transthoracic pacing pads immediately applied to use if needed. Placement of transvenous pacing catheters also should be considered.[41]

Effective postresuscitation care requires a basic understanding of the oxygen delivery (Do$_2$)/consumption (Vo$_2$) curve (Figure 7-5). Vo$_2$ is normally fixed over a wide range of Do$_2$ because tissues can regulate the

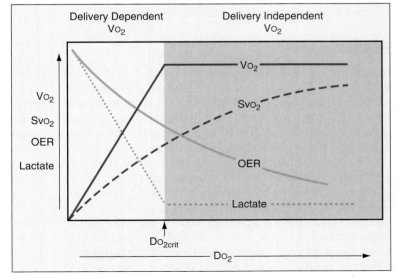

Figure 7-5. Oxygen delivery (Do$_2$)/oxygen consumption (Vo$_2$) curve. Oxygen extraction ratio (OER) increases, and mixed-venous oxygen saturation (Svo$_2$) decreases in response to decreased Do$_2$. Below the critical Do$_2$ (Do$_{2crit}$), Vo$_2$ becomes dependent. Do$_2$ below Do$_{2crit}$ results in anaerobic metabolism and lactate production. Do$_2$ = CO × O$_2$ (normal range 460-650 mL/min/m^2); Vo$_2$ = CO × (Cao$_2$ − Cvo$_2$) (normal range 96-170 mL/min/m^2); Cao$_2$ (arterial oxygen content) = (Hb × 1.39 × Sao$_2$) + (0.003 × Pao$_2$); Cvo$_2$ = (Hb × 1.39 × Svo$_2$) + (0.003 × Pvo$_2$). Svo$_2$ normal range 65% to 70%. CO, cardiac output; Pao$_2$, arterial oxygen tension; Hb, hemoglobin.

amount of oxygen extracted from arterial blood. A global increase in oxygen extraction results in decreased mixed-venous oxygen saturation (SvO_2). A critical DO_2 (DO_{2crit}) exists, however, below which VO_2 demand cannot be met despite maximized oxygen extraction. At this point, VO_2 becomes delivery dependent. DO_2 below DO_{2crit} causes cells to convert to anaerobic metabolism, resulting in increases in lactate production (dysoxia). Continued resuscitation efforts to optimize DO_2 and oxygen use stabilize the patient and potentially prevent subsequent multiorgan dysfunction and recurrent arrest.

During cardiac arrest and CPR, DO_2 is well below DO_{2crit}. On ROSC, resuscitation efforts should continue until DO_2 exceeds DO_{2crit}. Serum lactate levels provide an indirect measure of whether DO_2 is adequate to prevent anaerobic metabolism. A single lactate level almost universally is elevated after resuscitation from cardiac arrest. Detection of ongoing lactate production requires following serial lactate levels. Insufficient DO_2 also causes increased oxygen extraction, resulting in decreased SvO_2. Low SvO_2 coupled with persistently elevated lactate levels indicates inadequate DO_2. Patients subjected to prolonged CPR times or high-dose vasopressor therapy during CPR also may develop impaired tissue oxygen extraction.[42] In such patients, SvO_2 is abnormally high (venous hyperoxia) in the face of inadequate DO_2 and likely represents a state of severe systemic shunting resulting in an increase in non-nutritive blood flow. Lactate levels in these circumstances continue to be elevated.

The use of combined hemodynamic and metabolic endpoints to guide resuscitation in the emergency department has been shown to improve the outcome of patients with other shock states.[43] This strategy is straightforward and requires only the insertion of a supradiaphragmatic central venous catheter. $ScvO_2$ can be used as a reliable surrogate for SvO_2, which eliminates the need for a pulmonary artery catheter.[32] If $ScvO_2$ is abnormally low (<65%), but hemoglobin and SaO_2 values are normal, cardiac output is insufficient. Central venous pressure (CVP) should be used to deduce whether inadequate cardiac output is secondary to hypovolemia or impaired myocardial function. Augmenting CVP to levels between 10 and 15 mm Hg ensures adequate preload in most patients. If CVP is adequate and a mean arterial pressure of at least 70 mm Hg exists, therapy with an inotropic agent, such as dobutamine, should be initiated while considering reperfusion strategies. CVP measurements may decrease rapidly on initiation of dobutamine therapy. Additional volume expansion while maintaining a hemoglobin value of at least 10 g/dL should be provided as needed to maintain an adequate CVP.

The response to DO_2-optimizing interventions can be monitored by continuous or serial $ScvO_2$ measurements and serial lactate levels. An increase in $ScvO_2$ coupled with a decrease in lactate levels indicates improved DO_2. An unchanging $ScvO_2$ level indicates the need to continue to increase delivery. Repeat measurements of $ScvO_2$ and lactate should be performed to optimize DO_2.

Persistently elevated lactate levels and low $ScvO_2$ despite maximum pharmacologic support and volume management signal the need for additional interventions to optimize DO_2 to prevent accumulation of oxygen debt, which leads to either death or the development of sepsis and multisystem organ failure. Options to consider include revascularization or mechanical assistance in the form of intra-aortic balloon pumping or extracorporeal support. The induction of mild hypothermia may assist in lowering the metabolic demands of tissues in the postresuscitation state. Figure 7-6 provides a goal-directed guide to the postresuscitation care of a cardiac arrest patient. Similar options should be considered in a patient with venous hyperoxia and elevated levels of lactate because the combination of these findings indicate severe microvascular dysfunction, which also leads to the accumulation of oxygen debts incompatible with survival. The incidence of these patients may increase as the use of potent vasopressors, such as vasopressin, increases. Although not well studied, vasopressin potentially may result in a prolonged reduction in visceral organ blood flow in the postresuscitation period. Use of special monitoring modalities, such as gastric tonometry as an indicator of gastric mucosal perfusion, may be indicated.

Systems should ensure prompt transfer of postresuscitation patients from the emergency department to the cardiac catheterization laboratory or an intensive care unit, where intensive monitoring can guide subsequent therapy to achieve the optimal patient outcome. Family members should be fully informed of the circumstances and the patient's transfer. Deferring postresuscitation care until the patient arrives at the intensive care unit is ill conceived, however, and does not recognize the impact of early interventions, as initiated for other critical illnesses (e.g., acute MI, stroke).

Therapeutic Modalities

Airway and Breathing

The amount of ventilation required during CPR is not well established. Although minute ventilation requirements may be decreased because of the low cardiac output during CPR, an excess load of CO_2 returning from ischemic tissue beds must be cleared by ventilation. Chest compressions alone do not generate adequate or consistent ventilation in humans, even after intubation.[44] In the emergency department, bag/valve/mask ventilation with 100% oxygen should be instituted immediately and followed rapidly by endotracheal tube (ETT) intubation. ETT intubation is the most effective method of ensuring adequate ventilation, oxygenation, and airway protection during cardiac arrest. It also provides a route of drug administration. If ETT intubation cannot be performed successfully, an alternative technique must be used (see Chapter 1). When an airway has been secured, 10 to 12 ventilations should be provided per minute; these can be superimposed on chest compressions so that chest compressions need not be interrupted.[45]

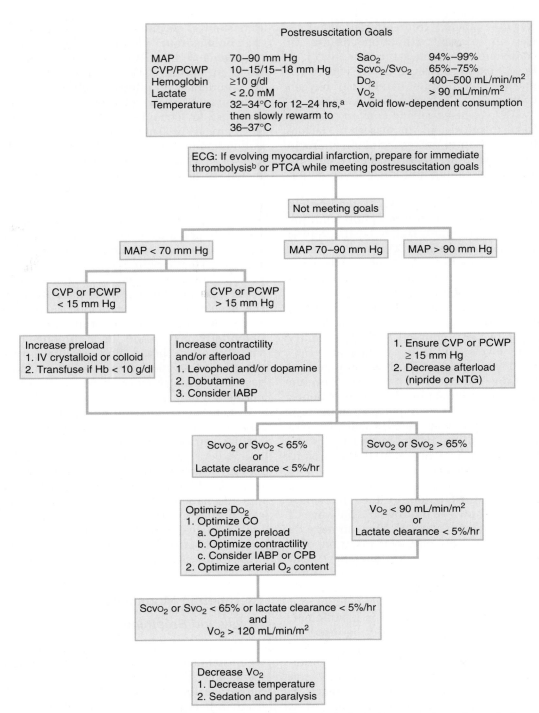

Figure 7-6. Goal-directed postresuscitation algorithm. [a]Therapeutic hypothermia is indicated in comatose survivors of witnessed cardiac arrest that had a presenting rhythm of ventricular fibrillation. It may also be effective in patients resuscitated from other cardiac arrest presentations. Relative contraindications include an unwitnessed cardiac arrest, severe cardiogenic shock, life-threatening dysrhythmias, uncontrolled bleeding, pre-existing coagulopathy, pregnancy, another obvious reason for coma (i.e., drug overdose or status epilepticus), known end-stage terminal illness, and a pre-existing do-not-resuscitate status. [b]Initiation of therapeutic hypothermia is not a contraindication to thrombolytic therapy. MAP, mean arterial pressure; CVP, central venous pressure; PCWP, pulmonary capillary wedge pressure; SaO_2, mixed-venous oxygen saturation; DO_2, oxygen delivery; VO_2, oxygen consumption; ECG, electrocardiogram; PTCA, percutaneous transluminal angioplasty; IABP, intra-aortic balloon pulsation; CPB, cardiopulmonary bypass; Hb, hemoglobin.

Circulation

After unsuccessful initial defibrillation of VT or VF, reperfusion of the heart is the main controllable factor determining successful resuscitation. Standard chest compression remains the mainstay of artificial circulation during cardiac arrest because of its simplicity, noninvasiveness, and lack of sufficient evidence for improved outcome with other methods. Modifications of standard chest compressions, including interposed abdominal compressions, active compression-decompression, and circumferential or vest CPR, have shown improved hemodynamics, but there is no compelling evidence for improved survival or neurologic outcome.

Invasive methods of artificial circulation, including OCCM and CPB, generate superior blood flow during cardiac arrest but have logistic and technical limitations, and no clinical trials have shown improved survival or neurologic outcome.

Standard Chest Compressions

Standard chest compressions are performed with the patient in supine position and consist of serial rhythmic compressions over the lower half of the sternum. The optimal rate, depth, and duration of compression are controversial and likely to vary from patient to patient. The sternum should be depressed at least 2 inches, after which pressure on the chest should be released completely to allow complete re-expansion of the chest. Experimental studies have shown a threshold compression force that is required for maximum forward flow during CPR.[46] Compression force should be adjusted to optimize forward flow based on hemodynamic monitoring techniques discussed in this chapter. The optimal duration of compression is 50% of the compression/release cycle.[47] Although the currently recommended rate of compressions is 80 to 100, human data indicate that if the duration of compression is maintained at 50% of the compression/release cycle, changes in compression rate in the range of 60 to 140 compressions/min have little effect on aortic pressures or cardiac output.[46,47] Standard mechanical CPR devices generate equal hemodynamics without increased complications, but no difference in resuscitation rate or long-term survival has been shown.[48] The main advantage of mechanical CPR is that chest compression force does not deteriorate because of provider fatigue, and compression/release cycle is accurately maintained at 50/50.

Common complications of standard CPR include (1) aspiration, resulting in hypoxia, pneumonia, and acute respiratory distress syndrome; (2) hepatic trauma, which can lead to rapid exsanguination; (3) gastroesophageal damage, which carries the risk of fatal mediastinitis or hemorrhage; (4) cardiac trauma, including cardiac contusion, hemopericardium, and pericardial effusions; and (5) bone trauma, including rib and sternal fractures, resulting in hemothorax and bone marrow emboli.

Interposed Abdominal Compression– Cardiopulmonary Resuscitation

Interposed abdominal compression (IAC)–CPR was first described by Ohomoto and associates in 1976.[49] Theoretical benefits of IAC during CPR include increased intrathoracic pressure and aortic compression producing retrograde aortic flow, which potentially augments coronary flow.[50] However, Increased right atrial pressure caused by abdominal compression may decrease CPP or cause negative CPP.[51] Two human studies reported improved short-term survival of in-hospital cardiac arrest patients with IAC-CPR.[52,53] These results should be interpreted with caution because chest compression force was not controlled between groups, and the etiology of in-hospital cardiac arrest may differ significantly from out-of-hospital cardiac arrest, particu-

larly with respect to the frequency of PEA. The only out-of-hospital study evaluating IAC-CPR failed to show an improvement in rates of ROSC, survival, or neurologic outcome.[54]

Active Compression-Decompression– Cardiopulmonary Resuscitation

First reported as a case report in 1990 by Lurie and colleagues,[55] active compression-decompression (ACD)–CPR is a modification of standard CPR in which the chest is actively expanded during relaxation by using a suction cup device to pull up on the chest between compressions. Proposed mechanisms of improved tissue perfusion with ACD-CPR include increased venous return as a result of negative intrathoracic diastolic pressure, decreased right atrial diastolic pressure resulting in increased CPP, and increased air trapping caused by improved lung filling during relaxation resulting in greater systolic intrathoracic pressure. Although this method has been shown to improve hemodynamic variables during CPR in animals and humans, many out-of-hospital clinical trials of ACD-CPR have failed to show improved initial resuscitation rates, long-term survival, or neurologic outcome.[56-59] More recently, ACD-CPR combined with an inspiratory impedance threshold device, which enhances negative pressures during the decompression phase, was shown to result in improved ROSC and 24-hour survival compared with standard CPR but no difference in survival to hospital discharge or neurologic outcome.[60]

Vest or Circumferential Cardiopulmonary Resuscitation

Methods of circumferential chest compression have been studied in an attempt to generate more effective intrathoracic pressure fluctuations during CPR.[61] More effective intrathoracic pressure fluctuations have been accomplished in humans with a pneumatically driven vest[62] or circumferential band.[63] Improved hemodynamics with circumferential CPR are attributed to greater intrathoracic pressure through increased chest compression force and air trapping in the lungs.[64] Human studies have shown improved aortic pressure and CPP and short-term survival when circumferential CPR devices are used late in resuscitation.[62,63] The U.S. Food and Drug Administration approved a device that uses a band across the anterior chest anchored to a rigid backboard, which has been shown to generate improved hemodynamics during CPR in humans.[65] Clinical trials designed to evaluate the impact of circumferential or vest CPR devices on survival and neurologic outcome have yet to be performed.

Open-Chest Cardiac Massage

OCCM was first described in animals in the late 1800s and until the 1960s was the standard method of in-hospital resuscitation. In humans, initial resuscitation rates of 19% to 46% and hospital discharge rates of 3% to 19% were reported with OCCM.[66,67] Since the acceptance of closed-chest CPR, little clinical research has been performed to determine the relative efficacy of the two techniques. Animal studies clearly indicate that compared with standard CPR, OCCM generates higher cardiac output, CPP, and tissue blood flows[68,69]; this has translated into improved resuscitation rates, survival, and neurologic outcome in animals.[70,71] Human studies have shown improved hemodynamics with open-chest CPR compared with closed-chest CPR.[6,72,73]

To date, controlled human data are lacking on the hemodynamics, long-term survival, neurologic outcome, and cardiac disability associated with OCCM. Based on the existing data, OCCM should not be a first-line therapy or a last resort after all other noninvasive resuscitation measures have failed. The potential does exist for improved outcome, however, if myocardial perfusion is inadequate despite optimized closed-chest CPR and if OCCM is initiated early during the resuscitation. Specific nontraumatic causes of cardiac arrest in which standard CPR is likely to be inadequate include hypothermia, pulmonary embolism, pericardial tamponade, abdominal hemorrhage, third-trimester pregnancy, toxic etiologies, and chest deformity preventing effective chest compressions. Regardless of the cause of cardiac arrest, OCCM is a potentially effective intervention when (1) the clinician has a clear indication, preferably through the use of reliable hemodynamic monitoring techniques, that noninvasive measures are generating inadequate myocardial perfusion despite optimized therapy; (2) the duration of cardiac arrest is less than 20 minutes; and (3) in the clinician's judgment a realistic potential for a good neurologic outcome exists.

Cardiopulmonary Bypass

Emergency CPB is feasible as a method of artificial circulation during cardiac arrest. CPB can be applied by either an open-chest method, requiring thoracotomy, or a closed-chest method, in which the bypass pump is applied by femoral artery and vein cutdowns. CPB is capable of providing adequate tissue perfusion during cardiac arrest and has the added advantages of rapidly controlling body temperature and providing prolonged circulatory support during postresuscitation cardiogenic shock. Animal studies have shown improved hemodynamics and survival with the use of CPB after prolonged cardiac arrest, and its feasibility has been shown in humans.[74,75] The current limitations of this technique are the availability of equipment and personnel and the time required to place the patient on bypass. No clinical trial has been performed to show improved survival or neurologic outcome using emergency CPB. Numerous case reports have shown benefit from emergency CPB in cardiac arrest caused by hypothermia.[76] As with OCCM, clinical trials in which CPB is initiated early in cardiac arrest are required to determine its potential impact on outcome. Considering the inevitable delay in initiating CPB, OCCM may be an essential bridge to the institution of this therapy.

Cough Cardiopulmonary Resuscitation

Cough CPR, in which patients witnessed experiencing cardiac arrest are immediately induced to cough intermittently and vigorously, has been shown to maintain arterial pressures and consciousness for several minutes until definitive therapy can be administered.[8,77] Because unconsciousness usually occurs within 15 seconds of cardiac arrest, the clinical use of cough CPR in the emergency department is limited to the rare case in which a monitored patient is witnessed having a nonperfusing rhythm but remains conscious. Although the optimal rate of cough CPR is unknown, clinical studies showing the effectiveness of cough CPR use rates of at least one cough every 2 seconds.[77] Cough CPR can be used only as a temporizing method until definitive restoration of circulation is accomplished.

Defibrillation

Timing

The goal of defibrillation in cardiac arrest is to terminate VF or pulseless VT electrically, in the hope that an organized perfusing rhythm will follow. The success rate of electrical conversion of VF to an effective rhythm decreases with increasing duration of ischemia. The rationale for defibrillation as the initial intervention in patients with VF is based on clinical data showing that the time to initial defibrillation is the major determinant of survival in out-of-hospital cardiac arrest caused by VF. Postdefibrillation asystole or PEA occurs in 60% of patients, however, with out-of-hospital VF.

Re-energizing the heart before defibrillation enhances the possibility of achieving a perfusing rhythm after prolonged cardiac arrest. Cobb and coworkers[33] reported that modifying the resuscitation protocol of first-responding emergency medical technicians to perform 90 seconds of CPR before the initial countershock resulted in improved survival to hospital discharge after out-of-hospital cardiac arrest compared with historical controls. This effect was most pronounced in patients with arrest durations longer than 4 minutes before intervention. Wik and colleagues[34] showed that performing 3 minutes of CPR before defibrillation in patients with response times greater than 5 minutes resulted in improved rate of ROSC and 1-year survival. Overall, these data strongly support performing a brief period of CPR (90 to 180 seconds) before defibrillation when the estimated duration of VF exceeds 4 to 5 minutes.

The major limitation of general application of reperfusion before defibrillation is that currently no means exist for determining when defibrillation would be successful. This obstacle soon may be overcome by the use of VF ECG signal analysis.[78-80] This emerging technology may allow therapy during CPR to be titrated to maximize potential for successful countershock and may decrease the incidence of postcountershock asystole and PEA.

Technique

Successful defibrillation depends on transmyocardial current, which is proportional to the energy output of the defibrillator and inversely proportional to transthoracic impedance. Human transthoracic impedance is variable and depends on chest size, phase of respiration, paddle/pad placement, and conductance between the paddles/pads and skin. Transthoracic impedance also declines with rapid sequential countershocks (8% with second shock) resulting in increased current delivery at any given energy setting.[81] Inadequate current does not stop myocardial fibrillation, and excessive current can result in myocardial injury. Defibrillation has been shown to cause morphologic and functional damage to the myocardium, which is directly related to the total cumulative energy delivered.[82] The minimal effective energy should be used for defibrillation.

Traditional monophasic defibrillators using either a monophasic truncated exponential (MTE) waveform or a monophasic dampened sinusoidal (MDS) waveform rapidly are being replaced by defibrillators that use a biphasic truncated exponential waveform. With biphasic defibrillation, the energy required for successful defibrillation, or the "defibrillation threshold," is less than with monophasic defibrillation. This translates into an increased likelihood of initial defibrillation success and a decreased likelihood of postcountershock myocardial dysfunction.

A prospective prehospital clinical trial comparing efficacy of three consecutive 150-J biphasic truncated exponential (BTE) countershocks with escalating energy (200 W-sec, 300 W-sec, 360 W-sec) monophasic countershocks showed improved rates of defibrillation and ROSC with biphasic countershock but no overall improvement in survival to admission or hospital discharge.[83] This study used two forms of monophasic defibrillation, however, 79% MTE and 21% MDS. A subsequent prehospital study by Carpenter and associates[84] provided evidence that MDS is superior to MTE defibrillation and is nearly equivalent to BTE defibrillation. The improved ROSC rate with BTE defibrillation observed by Schneider and colleagues[83] may be due to predominant use of MTE rather than MDS in that study. A subsequent randomized, double-blind, prospective prehospital trial comparing MDS and BTE defibrillation detected a higher rate of defibrillation into an organized rhythm with BTE, but no difference in ROSC or survival.[85] Despite documented advantages of lower defibrillation threshold and reduced myocardial injury, data currently are inadequate to conclude that BTE defibrillation is superior to MDS defibrillation in prehospital cardiac arrest based on clinically meaningful outcome measures.

The recommended energy settings for monophasic defibrillation are based on prehospital clinical trials showing efficacy of an initial countershock with 200 W-sec[86] and equivalence of 175 W-sec compared with 320 W-sec.[87] Escalation from 200 W-sec for initial defibrillation to 300 W-sec and 360 W-sec without intercedent CPR optimizes delivered current by taking advantage of the decrease in thoracic impedance that occurs with rapidly repeated countershocks.[81]

If the initial three attempts of electrical defibrillation are unsuccessful, interventions to reperfuse the heart, including CPR and vasopressors, should be instituted before repeated defibrillation. Antidysrhythmic therapy can be administered either before or after subsequent countershocks. If a patient reverts to VF or pulseless VF after successful defibrillation, subsequent defibrillations should begin at the energy used for previous successful defibrillation.

The *precordial thump* has been reported to have a 10% to 25% efficacy in converting pulseless VT to a perfusing rhythm. VF is rarely converted by this method, however. Administration of a precordial thump is an optional technique if an arrest is witnessed and no defibrillator is available. A precordial thump should not be administered to patients with VT and a pulse in the absence of a defibrillator because it can result in deterioration to a more malignant rhythm, such as VF, asystole, or EMD.

Pacing

Although the development of transcutaneous pacing devices has expanded greatly the rapidity with which emergency cardiac pacing can be performed, extensive research has shown that asystole in the out-of-hospital setting seldom responds to pacing. To be effective in asystole, pacing must be initiated within several minutes at maximal current.

Pharmacologic Therapy

Drug Administration Routes

Potential sites of access to the circulation during CPR include peripheral and central venous, endotracheal, intra-arterial, intracardiac, and intraosseous. During CPR, drugs should be administered through the most rapidly available access to the circulation. In the out-of-hospital setting and emergency department, this generally is the peripheral venous or endotracheal route.

Drugs that can be given by ETT include epinephrine, atropine, and lidocaine. Because of decreased bioavailability, 2 to 2.5 times the recommended intravenous dosage should be administered, and the dose should be diluted in 10 mL of normal saline or distilled water. Optimal drug bioavailability is achieved by passing a catheter beyond the tip of the ETT, temporarily holding chest compressions, and injecting the drug through the cannula while delivering several deep breaths with the Ambu-bag.[88]

A peripheral vein (antecubital or external jugular) should be the first choice for venous access during ongoing CPR. Although lower peak drug levels and increased circulation times occur with peripheral venous drug administration compared with central venous administration during CPR, these differences can be minimized by administering drugs by rapid bolus followed by a 20-mL bolus of IV fluid and elevation of the extremity.[89]

Central venous access provides the advantages of more rapid drug delivery and the ability to perform invasive monitoring. The risk of complication is greater, however, and failed central access is a relative contraindication for subsequent fibrinolytic therapy. If central access is to be obtained, internal jugular or supraclavicular routes are preferred over the subclavian route because CPR does not have to be interrupted. Because subdiaphragmatic blood flow is minimal during CPR, femoral vein cannulation should be avoided, unless a cannula long enough to pass above the diaphragm is used.

Intraosseous drug infusion during CPR is effective, but access may be difficult in adults, is associated with delayed circulation, and may be complicated by marrow emboli. Intracardiac injection is recommended only when other routes are not readily available or during open-chest CPR, when the heart can be directly visualized.[45]

Vasopressors

Epinephrine is the most useful drug currently available for the treatment of cardiac arrest. The most important mechanism of action of epinephrine during CPR is to increase PVR through direct α-adrenergic activity on arteriolar smooth muscle. Although increased PVR during CPR decreases overall cardiac output, it increases aortic systolic and aortic diastolic pressures, resulting in higher CPP and cerebral perfusion pressure and improved coronary and cerebral blood flows. A higher rate of ROSC in asphyxial and VF cardiac arrest models also results. The β$_1$-adrenergic activity of epinephrine also may be important in enhancing myocardial contractile force in the immediate postresuscitation period; however, the increase in myocardial oxygen consumption with β$_1$-adrenergic stimulation may compromise the myocardial oxygen supply-to-demand ratio during CPR and after resuscitation, resulting in post-ROSC myocardial dysfunction. Epinephrine dosages in excess of what is necessary to optimize CPP may be detrimental to myocardial resuscitation. Mean epinephrine levels (baseline 160 pmol/L) during cardiac arrest reach 56,217 pmol/L before exogenous epinephrine administration; 829,616 pmol/L after administration of 1 mg of epinephrine; and 12,400,000 pmol/L after administration of 10 mg.[90,91]

The currently recommended initial IV dose of epinephrine for clinical use is 1 mg (0.014 mg/kg) in a 70-kg person.[45] The endotracheal dosage is 2 to 3 mg. Epinephrine also may be administered as a continuous infusion via a central line.[45] Clinical trials have shown that higher epinephrine doses during CPR do not improve survival to hospital discharge, and there is no indication for high-dose epinephrine in cardiac arrest in adults or children.[92-94]

Experimental evaluation of other catecholamines (e.g., norepinephrine, methoxamine, phenylephrine) during CPR has not shown improved efficacy or decreased side effects compared with epinephrine. *Vasopressin* has been shown to be an effective alternative to epinephrine in animal and human studies.[35,95,96] Vasopressin is a peptide hormone normally released from the posterior pituitary gland in response to hypovolemia and hypotension or increased plasma osmolarity. Vasopressin is a potent vasoconstrictor whose action is mediated through the G protein–linked V$_{1a}$ receptor on vascular smooth muscle. Vasoconstriction results from second messenger–mediated increases in cytosolic calcium causing smooth muscle contraction.

In one prehospital clinical trial, IV vasopressin (40 U) was compared with IV epinephrine (1 mg) and resulted in improved ROSC and 24-hour survival.[95] A subsequent in-hospital study using single-dose vasopressin and a prehospital study using repeated-dose vasopressin showed no overall improvement in survival compared with standard-dose epinephrine.[35,96] Subset analysis revealed, however, that prehospital patients presenting in asystole did have improved survival to admission and hospital discharge when treated with vasopressin compared with epinephrine.[35] In this prehospital trial, patients received two 40-U doses of vasopressin 3 minutes apart followed by additional epinephrine as needed. The preponderance of evidence suggests that vasopressin is at least as effective as standard-dose epinephrine during cardiac arrest and is potentially more effective in patients presenting in asystole.

Antidysrhythmics

To be effective in terminating VF, drugs should alter the electrophysiologic mechanisms that sustain the dysrhythmia. The mechanisms initiating VF are different from the mechanisms sustaining VF.[97] Initiation of VF is multifactorial and includes inhomogeneity in ventricular activation and recovery and shortening of refractoriness. VF is believed to be sustained by multiple wave fronts, creating a pattern of rapid and irregular excitation through constantly changing reentrant pathways. Early in VF, the number of activation pathways is small, but their size is large. Late in VF, the number of activation pathways is large, but their size is small. Sustained VF requires a critical mass of myocardium and an appropriate relationship between conduction velocity and refractoriness of the ventricle.

Amiodarone is a class III antidysrhythmic agent but has characteristics of all four Vaughan-Williams classes. Amiodarone administered to prehospital patients with persistent VF after three countershocks, orotracheal intubation, and 1 mg of epinephrine has been shown to improve survival to hospital admission compared with placebo[98] or lidocaine.[99] Neither study showed improved survival to hospital discharge, however.

Significant side effects of amiodarone therapy include bradycardia and hypotension. The 300-mg bolus given during cardiac arrest is expected to provide sufficient levels for 30 minutes. If VF or VT persists for longer than 30 minutes, an additional bolus of 150 mg is indicated. Recommended postresuscitation dosing is 360 mg over 6 hours (1 mg/min) followed by 540 mg (0.5 mg/min) over the next 18 hours. If breakthrough VT or VF occurs, the patient should receive another bolus of 150 mg over 15 to 30 minutes. Based on the available data, amiodarone should be considered the first-line antidysrhythmic in the treatment of refractory VF and pulseless VT.

Lidocaine is an amide local anesthetic and class IB antidysrhythmic agent. Electrophysiologic effects of lidocaine on ischemic myocardial cells include extinguishing very slow conduction, prolonging recovery time, and reducing excitability in severely depressed cells. Lidocaine also has been shown to shorten action potential duration in nonischemic zones and to slow conduction and prolong refractoriness in ischemic zones.

Lidocaine increases the VF threshold, which decreases the likelihood of fibrillation. It also increases the defibrillation threshold, or minimum electrical dose, required for defibrillation. Its beneficial effect is likely mediated by preventing recurrence of VF after successful defibrillation, rather than improving the likelihood of successful defibrillation. A plasma level of 6 μg/kg is necessary to achieve antifibrillatory effects and can be achieved in animals after IV doses of 2 mg/kg.[100] The dosage of lidocaine during VF or pulseless VT refractory to defibrillation is a 1.5-mg/kg initial bolus followed by 0.5- to 1.5-mg/kg boluses every 5 to 10 minutes if necessary, up to a total dose of 3 mg/kg. It is recommended as an alternative to amiodarone.[45]

Magnesium deficiency is associated with sudden cardiac death, and hypomagnesemia can precipitate refractory VF. Although magnesium may have antidysrhythmic properties, it is known to cause smooth muscle relaxation, and administration during CPR in humans has been shown to decrease CPP. To date, no prospective clinical trial of magnesium sulfate therapy in cardiac arrest has been published. In the event of torsades de pointes and severe magnesium deficiency, 1 to 2 g of magnesium sulfate diluted in 100 mL of 5% dextrose in water may be administered over 1 to 2 minutes.

Atropine

Atropine acts as a competitive antagonist of acetylcholine at the muscarinic receptor. Cholinergic input to the heart is mediated through the vagus nerve, which releases acetylcholine at the sinus and atrioventricular nodes, causing decreased conduction and automaticity. The use of atropine in bradyasystolic arrest is based on the belief that parasympathetic tone is increased as a result of vagal stimulation, possibly resulting from hypoxia and acidosis of the carotid body. Atropine blocks the depressant effects of vagally released acetylcholine at the sinus and atrioventricular nodes. Limited human studies suggest a possible benefit of atropine in bradyasystolic arrest. The maximum vagolytic dosage in healthy human volunteers is 0.04 mg/kg (3 mg in a 70-kg person). The benefit of higher dosages in cardiac arrest has not been studied clinically. Based on the available data, a total dose of 0.04 mg/kg should be used in asystole.[45]

Buffers

Historically, controversy surrounded the use of buffer therapy in CPR. Cardiac arrest causes progressive respiratory and metabolic tissue acidosis as a result of accumulation of CO_2 and lactate. Neither respiratory nor metabolic tissue acidosis can be corrected without adequate ventilation, oxygenation, and tissue perfusion. Adequate tissue perfusion is generally not accomplished when CPR is initiated late or is continued for prolonged periods, as shown by persistent venous hypercarbia and metabolic acidemia despite arterial hypocarbic alkalemia.

The historical rationale for buffer therapy was to provide additional buffering capacity to correct persistent metabolic acidosis. Theoretical advantages to correcting metabolic acidosis during CPR include improving vascular response to pressors and lowering the ventricular defibrillation threshold. In the immediate postresuscitation period, correction of metabolic acidosis may improve myocardial contractility and increase the VF threshold. One theoretical disadvantage of buffer therapy is that it shifts the oxyhemoglobin saturation curve to the right, inhibiting the release of oxygen at the tissue level. The only prospective clinical trial to date of buffer therapy in out-of-hospital cardiac arrest showed no effect on resuscitation rate or survival.[101]

At present, no clinical data support the empiric routine use of buffer therapy during CPR except in cases of known or strongly suspected hyperkalemia, tricyclic antidepressant overdose, or preexisting metabolic acidemia. Similarly, no clinical evidence supports the use of alternative buffers (e.g., tromethamine [Tham], Carbicarb, Tibonate). When indicated (i.e., hyperkalemia, cyclic antidepressant overdose), the recommended dosage of $NaHCO_3$ is 0.5 to 1 mEq/kg initially and every 10 minutes during CPR or as guided by arterial blood gases.[45]

Calcium Chloride

The use of calcium during CPR should be limited to specific cases of known efficacy. No evidence exists that empiric calcium use during cardiac arrest improves resuscitation or survival. Increases in intracellular calcium are thought to be an important mechanism of ischemic cellular injury; calcium administration may have detrimental effects. Calcium administration is likely to be beneficial in cases of hyperkalemia, hypocalcemia, and calcium channel blocker toxicity and in cases in which arrest occurs after massive, rapid blood replacement therapy for exsanguinating hemorrhage. If required, 4 mg/kg of calcium chloride (0.04 mL/kg of 10% solution) may be administered every 10 minutes.[45]

Oxygen

Although SaO_2 is maintained for 30 minutes in untreated VF, this rapidly decreases to hypoxic range within 2 minutes of chest compressions without ventilation.[102] Oxygenation is required, but the optimal fraction of inspired oxygen for resuscitation remains to be determined. Because it is often unclear whether cardiac arrest was precipitated by hypoxia resulting from pulmonary dysfunction, and because a high incidence of pulmonary edema has been reported during and after CPR, the most prudent course of action at this time is to use 100% oxygen during initial resuscitation until oxygenation state can be assessed. When assessed, either by arterial blood gas or by pulse oximetry, fraction of inspired oxygen should be adjusted immediately to maintain adequate hemoglobin saturation, while avoiding excessively high arterial oxygen tension.

OUTCOMES

Epidemiologic data from studies of out-of-hospital cardiac arrest show a wide range of outcomes. ROSC long enough to result in hospital admission ranges from 9% to 65%, whereas only 1% to 31% of patients survive to hospital discharge.[103-105] This wide range of outcomes has been attributed to differences in emergency medical systems and inclusion criteria used in these studies. Adoption of the Utstein method of uniform reporting should improve the interpretation of future epidemiologic studies of out-of-hospital cardiac arrest.[106]

The type of prehospital care system seem to have a significant effect on outcome; systems using emergency medical technician and paramedic units have the highest resuscitation and survival rates.[103] Several retrospective studies have shown that patients who fail prehospital ALS measures have less than 2% chance of survival to hospital discharge.[107-109] Individual factors that increase the likelihood of ROSC and survival include witnessed arrest, early bystander CPR, early ALS, an initial rhythm of VF or VT, early defibrillation, and CPR before defibrillation if estimated duration of cardiac arrest exceeds 4 to 5 minutes.[17,34,110,111]

Of patients admitted to the hospital after prehospital cardiac arrest, less than 50% survive to discharge.[112,113] Early in-hospital deaths are caused by cardiogenic shock and dysrhythmias, whereas later in-hospital deaths most often are attributed to complications of anoxic encephalopathy, respiratory failure, and sepsis. Only 1% to 2% of admitted patients meet criteria for brain death, however. Of patients surviving to hospital discharge, one third have persistent neurologic deficits, and less than one half return to prearrest function. In patients meeting the inclusion criteria of the more recent clinical hypothermia trials, favorable outcome was reported in approximately 50% of cardiac arrest survivors who were admitted comatose and treated with hypothermia.[36,37]

KEY CONCEPTS

- CPR for 90 to 180 seconds should precede defibrillation when the arrest "downtime" is greater than 4 to 5 minutes.
- Biphasic defibrillators require less energy to terminate VF and are less likely to cause myocardial damage.
- There is currently no compelling clinical evidence to prove that any alternative or mechanical forms of CPR improve outcome over traditional chest compressions.
- Restoration of adequate cardiac function is the defining factor of ROSC. Restoration of normal brain function is the defining factor of successful resuscitation.
- Resuscitation of a cardiac arrest victim does not end with ROSC. Rapid diagnosis and proper management of the pathologic conditions that precipitated and resulted from the arrest are essential for optimal outcome.
- Induced prolonged hypothermia (32° C to 34° C for 12 to 24 hours) is the first and only post-ROSC intervention shown to improve survival and functional outcome of comatose cardiac arrest survivors.

REFERENCES

1. Zoll PM, et al: Termination of ventricular fibrillation in man by externally applied electric countershock. *N Engl J Med* 254:727, 1956.
2. Safar P, Escarraga LA, Elam JO: A comparison of the mouth-to-mouth and mouth-to-airway methods of artificial respiration with the chest-pressure arm-lift methods. *N Engl J Med* 258:671, 1958.
3. Elam JO, et al: Oxygen and carbon dioxide exchange and energy cost of expired air resuscitation. *JAMA* 167:328, 1958.
4. Kouwenhoven WB, Jude JR, Knickerbocker GG: Closed-chest cardiac massage. *JAMA* 173:1064, 1960.
5. Kuller L, Lilienfeld A, Fischer R: An epidemiological study of sudden and unexpected deaths in adults. *Medicine* 46:341, 1967.
6. Del Guercio LRM, et al: Comparison of blood flow during external and internal cardiac massage in man. *Circulation* 31/32(Suppl I):171, 1965.
7. Halperin HR: Mechanisms of forward flow during CPR. In Paradis N, Nowak R, Halperin H (eds): *Cardiac Arrest: The Science and Practice of Resuscitation Medicine.* Baltimore, Williams & Wilkins, 1996.
8. Niemann JT, et al: Cough-CPR: Documentation of systemic perfusion in man and in an experimental model: A "window" to the mechanism of blood flow in external CPR. *Crit Care Med* 8:141, 1980.
9. Safar P: Effects of the postresuscitation syndrome on cerebral recovery from cardiac arrest. *Crit Care Med* 13:932, 1985.
10. Tang W, et al: Progressive myocardial dysfunction after cardiac resuscitation. *Crit Care Med* 21:1046, 1993.
11. Deantonio HJ, Kaul S, Lerman BB: Reversible myocardial depression in survivors of cardiac arrest. *Pacing Clin Electrophysiol* 13:982, 1990.
12. Haglund UH: Myocardial depressant factors. In Marston A, et al (eds): *Splanchnic Ischemia and Multiple Organ Failure.* St Louis, Mosby, 1989.
13. Myerburg RJ, Kessler KM, Castellanos A: Sudden cardiac death: Structure, function, and time-dependence of risk. *Circulation* 85(Suppl I):2, 1992.
14. Valenzuela TD, et al: Outcomes of rapid defibrillation by security officers after cardiac arrest in casinos. *N Engl J Med* 343:1206, 2000.
15. Page RL, et al: Use of automated external defibrillators by a U.S. airline. *N Engl J Med* 343:1210, 2000.
16. Caffrey SL, et al: Public use of automated external defibrillators. *N Engl J Med* 347:1242, 2002.
17. Hallstrom AP, et al: Public-access defibrillation and survival after out-of-hospital cardiac arrest. *N Engl J Med* 351:637, 2004.
18. Myerburg RJ, et al: Impact of community-wide police car deployment of automated external defibrillators on survival from out-of-hospital cardiac arrest. *Circulation* 106:1058, 2002.
19. van Alem AP, et al: Use of automated external defibrillator by first responders in out of hospital cardiac arrest: Prospective controlled trial. *BMJ* 327:1312, 2003.
20. Bonnin M, et al: Distinct criteria for termination of resuscitation in the out-of-hospital setting. *JAMA* 270:1457, 1993.
21. Spaulding CM, et al: Immediate coronary angiography in survivors of out-of-hospital cardiac arrest *N Engl J Med* 336:1629, 1997.
22. Niemann JT, et al: Predictive indices of successful cardiac resuscitation after prolonged arrest and experimental cardiopulmonary resuscitation. *Ann Emerg Med* 14:521, 1985.

23. Paradis NA, et al: Coronary perfusion pressure and the return of spontaneous circulation in human cardiopulmonary resuscitation. *JAMA* 263:1106, 1990.

24. Sanders AB, Ewy GA, Taft TV: Prognostic and therapeutic importance of the aortic diastolic pressure in resuscitation from cardiac arrest. *Crit Care Med* 12:877, 1984.

25. Sanders AB, et al: Expired P_{CO_2} as an index of coronary perfusion pressure. *Am J Med* 3:147, 1985.

26. Lewis LM, et al: Correlation of end-tidal CO_2 to cerebral perfusion during CPR. *Ann Emerg Med* 21:1131, 1992.

27. Callaham M, Barton C, Matthay M: Effect of epinephrine on the ability of end-tidal carbon dioxide readings to predict initial resuscitation from cardiac arrest. *Crit Care Med* 20:337, 1992.

28. Ward KR, et al: A comparison of chest compressions between mechanical and manual CPR by monitoring end-tidal P_{CO_2} during human cardiac arrest. *Ann Emerg Med* 22:669, 1993.

29. Sanders AB, et al: End-tidal carbon dioxide monitoring during cardiopulmonary resuscitation: A prognostic indicator of survival. *JAMA* 262:134, 1989.

30. Callaham M, Barton C: Prediction of outcome of cardiopulmonary resuscitation from end-tidal carbon dioxide concentration. *Crit Care Med* 18:358, 1990.

31. Rivers EP, et al: The clinical implications of continuous central venous oxygen saturation during human CPR. *Ann Emerg Med* 21:1094, 1992.

32. Emerman CL, et al: A comparison of venous blood gases during cardiac arrest. *Am J Emerg Med* 6:580, 1988.

33. Cobb LA, et al: Influence of cardiopulmonary resuscitation prior to defibrillation in patients with out-of-hospital ventricular fibrillation. *JAMA* 281:1182, 1999.

34. Wik L, et al: Delaying defibrillation to give basic cardiopulmonary resuscitation to patients with out-of-hospital ventricular fibrillation: A randomized trial. *JAMA* 289:1389, 2003.

35 Wenzel V, et al: A comparison of vasopressin and epinephrine for out-of-hospital cardiopulmonary resuscitation. *N Engl J Med* 350:105, 2004.

36. Bernard SA, et al: Treatment of comatose survivors of out-of-hospital cardiac arrest with induced hypothermia. *N Engl J Med* 346:557, 2002.

37. Hypothermia after Cardiac Arrest Study Group: Mild therapeutic hypothermia to improve the neurologic outcome after cardiac arrest. *N Engl J Med* 346:549, 2002.

38. Bernard S, et al: Induced hypothermia using large volume, ice-cold intravenous fluid in comatose survivors of out-of-hospital cardiac arrest: A preliminary report. *Resuscitation* 56:9, 2003.

39. Nolan JP, et al: Therapeutic hypothermia after cardiac arrest: an advisory statement by the advanced life support task force of the international liaison committee on resuscitation. *Circulation* 108:118. 2003.

40. Braunwald E, et al: ACC/AHA 2002 guideline update for the management of patients with unstable angina and non-ST-segment elevation myocardial infarction—summary article: A report of the American College of Cardiology/American Heart Association Task Force on Practice Guidelines (Committee on the Management of Patients with Unstable Angina). *J Am Coll Cardiol* 40:1366, 2003.

41. Ryan TJ, et al: 1999 update: ACC/AHA guidelines for the management of patients with acute myocardial infarction—executive summary and recommendations: A report of the American College of Cardiology/American Heart Association Task Force on Practice Guidelines (Committee on Management of Acute Myocardial Infarction). *Circulation* 100:1016, 1999.

42. Rivers EP, et al: Venous hyperoxia after cardiac arrest: characterization of a defect in systemic oxygen utilization. *Chest* 102:1787, 1992.

43. Rivers E, et al: Early goal-directed therapy in the treatment of severe sepsis and septic shock. *N Engl J Med* 345:1368, 2001.

44. Safar P, et al: Ventilation and circulation with closed-chest cardiac massage in man. *JAMA* 176:92, 1961.

45. American Heart Association: Guidelines for cardiopulmonary resuscitation emergency cardiovascular care. *Circulation* 102(Suppl I):I-1, 2000.

46. Taylor GJ, et al: Importance of prolonged compression during cardiopulmonary resuscitation in man. *N Engl J Med* 296:1515, 1977.

47. Ornato JP, et al: Effect of cardiopulmonary resuscitation compression rate on end-tidal carbon dioxide concentration and arterial pressure. *Crit Care Med* 16:241, 1988.

48. Ward KR, et al: A comparison of chest compressions between mechanical and manual CPR by monitoring end-tidal PCO_2 during human cardiac arrest. *Ann Emerg Med* 22:669, 1993.

49. Ohomoto T, Miura I, Konno S: A new method of external cardiac massage to improve diastolic augmentation and prolong survival time. *Ann Thorac Surg* 21:284, 1976.

50. Halperin HR, et al: Determinants of blood flow to vital organs during cardiopulmonary resuscitation in dogs. *Circulation* 73:539, 1986.

51. Adams CP, et al: Hemodynamics of interposed abdominal compression during human cardiopulmonary resuscitation. *Acad Emerg Med* 1:498, 1994.

52. Sack JB, Kesselbrenner MB, Bregman D: Survival from in-hospital cardiac arrest with interposed abdominal counterpulsation during cardiopulmonary resuscitation. *JAMA* 267:379, 1992.

53. Sack JB, Kesselbrenner MB, Jarrad A: Interposed abdominal compression cardiopulmonary resuscitation and resuscitation outcome during asystole and electromechanical dissociation. *Circulation* 86:1692, 1992.

54. Mateer JR, et al: Pre-hospital IAC-CPR versus standard CPR: Paramedic resuscitation of cardiac arrest. *Am J Emerg Med* 3:143, 1985.

55. Lurie KG, Lindo C, Chin J: CPR: The P stands for plumber's helper [letter]. *JAMA* 264:1661, 1990.

56. Cohen TJ, et al: Active compression-decompression: A new method of cardiopulmonary resuscitation. Cardiopulmonary Resuscitation Working Group. *JAMA* 267:2916, 1992.

57. Cohen TJ, et al: A comparison of active compression-decompression cardiopulmonary resuscitation with standard cardiopulmonary resuscitation of cardiac arrests occurring in the hospital. *N Engl J Med* 329:1918, 1993.

58. Lurie KG, et al: Evaluation of active compression-decompression CPR in victims of out-of-hospital cardiac arrest. *JAMA* 271:1405, 1994.

59. Schwab TM, et al: A randomized clinical trial of active compression-decompression CPR vs standard CPR in out-of-hospital cardiac arrest in two cities. *JAMA* 273:1261, 1995.

60. Halperin HR, et al: Vest inflation without simultaneous ventilation during cardiac arrest in dogs: Improved survival from prolonged cardiopulmonary resuscitation. *Circulation* 74:1407, 1986.

61. Wolcke BB, et al: Comparison of standard cardiopulmonary resuscitation versus the combination of active compression-decompression cardiopulmonary resuscitation and an inspiratory impedance threshold device for out-of-hospital cardiac arrest. *Circulation* 108:2201, 2003.

62. Halperin HR, et al: A preliminary study of cardiopulmonary resuscitation by circumferential compression of the chest with use of a pneumatic vest. *N Engl J Med* 329:1918, 1993.

63. Halperin H, et al: Cardiopulmonary resuscitation with a hydraulic-pneumatic band. *Crit Care Med* 28(11 Suppl):N203, 2000.

64. Halperin HR, et al: Air trapping in the lungs during cardiopulmonary resuscitation in dogs: A mechanism for generating changes in intrathoracic pressure. *Circ Res* 65:946, 1989.

65. Timmerman S, et al: Improved hemodynamic performance with a novel chest compression device during treatment of in-hospital cardiac arrest. *Resuscitation* 61:273, 2004.

66. Stephenson HE Jr, Reid LC, Hinton JW: Some common denominators in 1200 cases of cardiac arrest. *Ann Surg* 137:731, 1953.

67. Osborn H: Introduction to proceedings of a conference on resuscitative thoracotomy. *Resuscitation* 15:1, 1987.

68. Ditchey RV, Winkler JV, Rhodes CA: Relative lack of coronary blood flow during closed-chest resuscitation in dogs. *Circulation* 66:297, 1982.

69. Bartlett RL, et al: Comparative study of three methods of resuscitation: closed-chest, open-chest manual, and direct mechanical ventricular assistance. *Ann Emerg Med* 13:773, 1984.

70. Bircher N, Safar P: Cerebral preservation during cardiopulmonary resuscitation. *Crit Care Med* 13:185, 1985.

71. Kern KB, et al: Long-term survival with open chest massage after ineffective closed-chest compressions in a canine model. *Circulation* 75:498, 1987.

72. Geehr EC, Lewis FR, Auerbach PS: Failure of open-heart massage to improve survival after prehospital non-traumatic cardiac arrest [letter]. *N Engl J Med* 314:1189, 1986.

73. Boczar ME, et al: A technique revisited: Hemodynamic comparison of closed- and open-chest cardiac massage during human cardiopulmonary resuscitation. *Crit Care Med* 23:498, 1995.

74. Martin GB, et al: Cardiopulmonary bypass in the treatment of cardiac arrest in humans. *Crit Care Med* 18:S247, 1990.

75. Tisherman AS, et al: Feasibility of emergency cardiopulmonary bypass for resuscitation from CPR-resistant cardiac arrest: A preliminary report. *Ann Emerg Med* 20:491, 1991.

76. Vretenar DF, et al: Cardiopulmonary bypass resuscitation for accidental hypothermia. *Ann Thorac Surg* 58:895, 1994.

77. Criley JM, Blaufuss AH, Kissel GL: Cough-induced cardiac compression: Self-administered form of cardiopulmonary resuscitation. *JAMA* 236:1246, 1976.

78. Brown CG, Dzwonczyk R: Signal analysis of the human electrocardiogram during ventricular fibrillation: Frequency and amplitude parameters as predictors of successful countershock. *Ann Emerg Med* 27:184, 1996.

79. Callaway CW, et al: Scaling exponent predicts defibrillation success for out-of-hospital ventricular fibrillation cardiac arrest. *Circulation* 103:1656, 2001.

80. Menegazzi JJ, et al: Ventricular fibrillation scaling exponent can guide timing of defibrillation and other therapies. *Circulation* 109:926, 2004.

81. Kerber RE, et al: Transthoracic resistance of human defibrillation: Influence of body weight, chest size, serial shocks, paddle size and paddle contact pressure. *Circulation* 63:676, 1981.

82. Doherty PW, et al: Cardiac damage produced by direct current countershock applied to the heart. *Am J Cardiol* 43:225, 1979.

83. Schneider T, et al: Multicenter, randomized, controlled trial of 150-J biphasic shocks compared with 200- to 360-J monophasic shocks in the resuscitation of out-of-hospital cardiac arrest victims. *Circulation* 102:1780, 2000.

84. Carpenter J, et al: Defibrillation waveform and post-shock rhythm in out-of-hospital ventricular fibrillation cardiac arrest. *Resuscitation* 59:189, 2003.

85. van Alem AP, et al: A prospective, randomised and blinded comparison of first shock success of monophasic and biphasic waveforms in out-of-hospital cardiac arrest. *Resuscitation* 58:17, 2003.

86. Tacker WA, Ewy GA: Emergency defibrillation dose: Recommendations and rationale. *Circulation* 60:223, 1979.

87. Weaver WD, et al: Ventricular defibrillation: A comparative trial using 174-J and 320-J shocks. *N Engl J Med* 307:1101, 1982.

88. Aitkenhead AR: Drug administration during CPR: What route? *Resuscitation* 22:191, 1991.

89. Emerman CL, et al: The effect of bolus injection on circulation times during cardiac arrest. *Am J Emerg Med* 8:190, 1990.

90. Prengel A, et al: Plasma catecholamine concentrations after successful resuscitation in patients. *Crit Care Med* 20:609, 1992.

91. Wortsman J, et al: Functional responses to extremely high plasma epinephrine concentrations in cardiac arrest. *Crit Care Med* 21:692, 1993.

92. Brown CG, et al: A comparison of standard-dose and high-dose epinephrine in cardiac arrest outside the hospital. *N Engl J Med* 327:1051, 1992.

93. Stiell IG, et al: High-dose epinephrine in adult cardiac arrest. *N Engl J Med* 327:1045, 1992.

94. Callaham M, et al: A randomized clinical trial of high-dose epinephrine and norepinephrine vs standard-dose epinephrine in prehospital cardiac arrest. *JAMA* 268:2667, 1992.

95. Lindner KH, et al: Randomised comparison of epinephrine and vasopressin in patients with out-of-hospital ventricular fibrillation. *Lancet* 349:535, 1997.

96. Stiell IG, et al: Vasopressin versus epinephrine for inhospital cardiac arrest: A randomised controlled trial. *Lancet* 358:105, 2001.

97. Tomaselli G: Etiology, electrophysiology, and myocardial mechanisms of ventricular fibrillation. In Paradis N, Nowak R, Halperin H (eds): *Cardiac Arrest: The Science and Practice of Resuscitation Medicine.* Baltimore, Williams & Wilkins, 1996.

98. Kudenchuk PJ, et al: Amiodarone for resuscitation after out-of-hospital cardiac arrest due to ventricular fibrillation. *N Engl J Med* 341:871, 1999.

99. Dorian P, et al: Amiodarone as compared with lidocaine for shock-resistant ventricular fibrillation. *N Engl J Med* 346:884, 2002.

100. White RD: Antifibrillatory drugs: The case for lidocaine and procainamide. *Ann Emerg Med* 13:802, 1984.

101. Vukmir RB, et al: Sodium bicarbonate may improve outcome in dogs with brief or prolonged cardiac arrest. *Crit Care Med* 23:515, 1995.

102. Lesser R, et al: Sternal compression before ventilation in cardiopulmonary resuscitation (CPR). *Disaster Med* 1:239, 1983.

103. Eisenberg MS, et al: Cardiac arrest and resuscitation: A tale of 29 cities. *Ann Emerg Med* 19:179, 1990.

104. Becker LB, et al: Outcome of CPR in a large metropolitan area: Where are the survivors? *Ann Emerg Med* 20:355, 1991.

105. Lombardi G, Gallagher J, Gennis P: Outcome of out-of-hospital cardiac arrest in New York City: The Pre-Hospital Arrest Survival Evaluation (PHASE) study. *JAMA* 272:1573, 1994.

106. Cummins RO, Task Force of the American Heart Association, European Resuscitation Council, Heart and Stroke Foundation of Canada, and Australian Resuscitation Council: Recommended guidelines for uniform reporting

of data from out-of-hospital cardiac arrest: The Utstein style. *Ann Emerg Med* 20:861, 1991.

107. Kellerman AL, Staves DR, Hackman B: In-hospital resuscitation following unsuccessful prehospital advanced cardiac life support: "Heroic efforts" or an exercise in futility? *Ann Emerg Med* 17:589, 1988.

108. Bonnin MJ, Swor RA: Outcomes in unsuccessful field resuscitation attempts. *Ann Emerg Med* 18:507, 1989.

109. Gray WA, Capone RJ, Most AS: Unsuccessful emergency medical resuscitation: Are continued efforts in the emergency department justified? *N Engl J Med* 325:1393, 1991.

110. Eisenberg M, Bergner L, Hallstrom A: Paramedic programs and out-of-hospital cardiac arrest: I. Factors associated with successful resuscitation. *Am J Public Health* 69:30, 1979.

111. Cummins RO, et al: Survival of out-of-hospital cardiac arrest with early initiation of cardiopulmonary resuscitation. *Am J Emerg Med* 3:114, 1985.

112. Longstreth WT Jr, et al: Neurologic recovery after out-of-hospital cardiac arrest. *Ann Intern Med* 98:588, 1983.

113. Roine RO: *Neurologic Outcome of Out-of-Hospital Cardiac Arrest.* Helsinki, Yliopistopaino, 1993.

CHAPTER

8 Pediatric Resuscitation

Brian P. Gilligan and Robert C. Luten

PERSPECTIVE

Resuscitation of the pediatric patient is challenging because of the technical demands of vascular access and airway control as well as the cognitive demands of managing the many age- and size-related issues particular to children.[1] In addition, the causes of pediatric cardiac arrest are different from those seen in adults. This chapter reviews pediatric cardiac arrest, resuscitation terms, basic and advanced life support techniques, drug therapy, pediatric applications and measurements, and discontinuation of resuscitative efforts.

The outcome after cardiac arrest in children is poor. Despite earlier studies suggesting a better outcome, more recent studies, clearly differentiating between cardiac and respiratory arrest, report a poor prognosis.[2-10] *Cardiac arrest* is the cessation of cardiac mechanical activity, determined by the absence of a *detectable* pulse, unresponsiveness, and apnea. *Respiratory arrest* is the absence of respiratory effort with ongoing cardiac activity (i.e., apnea). *Agonal respiration* requiring immediate assisted ventilation is a form of respiratory compromise but is not respiratory arrest.[11] Cardiac arrest usually results from profound hypoxemia, hypercarbia, or ischemia; it rarely results from an acute dysrhythmia unless the patient has underlying cardiac disease or the dysrhythmia stems from drug or metabolic toxicity.

The overall survival after pediatric cardiac arrest is only 13%.[12] Patients with an out-of-hospital cardiac arrest have a significantly lower survival rate (8.4%) than patients with in-hospital cardiac arrest (24%).[12,13] Clearly, prevention of a cardiac arrest is of much greater benefit than the use of advanced resuscitation skills in a cardiac arrest victim.

BASIC LIFE SUPPORT TECHNIQUES

Airway

Opening the airway is the first basic life support step. In the pediatric patient, the relatively large tongue may cause airway obstruction. Forward movement of the tongue is achieved by a head tilt–chin lift or jaw-thrust maneuver. The *jaw-thrust maneuver* is recommended with possible cervical spine injury because the airway may be effectively opened without extending the neck. With bag/mask ventilation, the jaw-thrust procedure requires a two-person technique: one rescuer secures the mask, using a bilateral jaw lift, while the other rescuer compresses the resuscitation bag.

The *head tilt–chin lift maneuver* is designed to move the mandible forward, which then displaces the tongue forward. Although this procedure is reportedly as effective as the jaw-thrust maneuver, lack of care in performing the technique may result in an obstructed airway. The fingers must be carefully placed on the underside of the mandible. If the soft tissues of the submental triangle (area under chin) are compressed instead, the tongue may be displaced into the floor of the mouth, resulting in airway obstruction.

Despite concern over infectious disease transmission during cardiopulmonary resuscitation (CPR), no cases of human immunodeficiency virus, hepatitis B virus, hepatitis C virus, or cytomegalovirus infections have been documented during mouth-to-mouth ventilation.[14] However, alternative airway techniques are becoming routine basic life support procedures. The most popular technique is use of a *pocket mask.* The single-sized pocket mask can be used in infants, older children, and adults. In the small child, turning the mask upside down, so that the side intended for the nose is placed over the chin, usually permits an adequate mask fit. In the small child and infant the top of the mask extends above the eyes; care is needed to avoid compressing the mask over the eyes.

Breathing

Rescue breathing is essential for successful resuscitation. Adequate ventilation depends on using an adequate volume to move the patient's chest. Two slow (1- to 1.5-second) rescue breaths are recommended to provide effective air delivery.[15] More rapid delivery of the breath results in high airway pressure that overcomes esophageal resistance, directing gas into the stomach rather than the lungs. The rate of rescue breathing in pediatric patients has not been carefully studied; current recommendations are based on a compromise between a practical rate of chest compression and the desire to ventilate the pediatric victim more rapidly because of a higher rate of carbon dioxide (CO_2) production and oxygen consumption.

Rescue breaths are given at a rate of 30 breaths/min in neonates, 20 breaths/min in infants and children, and 12 breaths/min in older children and adolescents. Breaths should be given in a breath/compression ratio of 1:3 in a neonate and 1:5 in infants and children. Only in single-rescuer CPR of an adolescent should the adult technique be used (compression/breath ratio of 15:2).[16] Rescue breaths are given with a pause during the compressions rather than attempting to deliver the breath on the upstroke of the fifth compression.

Chest Compressions

The purpose of chest compressions is to circulate an adequate volume of blood that has been oxygenated by rescue breathing and to return blood to the lungs from the peripheral tissues. From adult studies, effective chest compressions must achieve a diastolic pressure of at least 20 mm Hg or a coronary perfusion pressure of at least 15 mm Hg to provide minimally adequate coronary blood flow.[17] The mechanism of chest compression–induced cardiac output has been much debated (see Chapter 7). The earliest theory stated that the heart was simply compressed between the sternum and vertebral bodies. This proposed mechanism was replaced by the *thoracic pump mechanism,* wherein blood flow results from a global increase in intrathoracic pressure. During compression, blood contained within intrathoracic structures is at a higher pressure than that contained in extrathoracic vessels, and blood flow occurs. Retrograde blood flow into the venous system is prevented by collapse of the relatively thin-walled veins with the increase in intrathoracic pressure; the thicker arteries maintain their lumen, permitting flow.

Although numerous studies supported the thoracic pump mechanism, more recent human studies suggest that direct cardiac compression is important.[18] In children, *direct cardiac compression* is more likely to be important because of the infant's and child's compliant chest. For example, in piglets, whose anatomy and physiology closely mimic those of humans, closed-chest compression produces cardiac outputs that are equal to normal values early after cardiac arrest. Pediatric studies also show that changes in hand position have an important effect on the blood pressure produced during chest compression; direct compression over the heart produces the highest pressures. If direct cardiac compression is important in the pediatric patient, compression should be directly over the heart. Heart position was thought to be higher in infants and young children, as evidenced by morgue studies of children. More recent data show that the position of the heart relative to external landmarks is the same as for adults; the heart is located behind the lower third of the sternum. Thus, the chest should be compressed one fingerbreadth below the intermammary line in infants and over the lower third of the sternum in older children.[15]

The optimal rate of cardiac compression remains uncertain. High compression pressure and rate improve cardiac output in some experimental studies, whereas other studies have not shown a benefit from this technique.[19] A disadvantage of using rates in excess of 100 compressions/min is the increased potential for rescuer fatigue unless an automated chest compression device is available. Furthermore, the optimal *duty cycle* (duration of compression as a percentage of the time between compressions) may be only 30% at the faster compression rates used in children.[20] The recommended compression rates are 100 to 120 compressions/min in newborns and 100 compressions/min in infants and children.[15]

The alternative compression techniques, *interposed abdominal compression* CPR (IAC-CPR) and *active compression-decompression* CPR (ACD-CPR), have been suggested in adults to improve the rate of return of spontaneous circulation (ROSC) and in some cases the outcome.[21-24] Currently, the use of these techniques in children is not recommended because of lack of data; however, research in this area may be indicated, especially ACD-CPR.[22,23]

Extracorporeal membrane oxygenation (ECMO) has been used successfully in both adult and pediatric patients in cardiac arrest. A large study showed 88% survival (to hospital discharge) for neonatal respiratory patients ($n = 586$), 70% survival for pediatric respiratory patients ($n = 132$), and 48% survival for pediatric cardiac or shock patients ($n = 105$). Survival to hospital discharge for adults was 56% (respiratory, $n = 146$) and 33% (cardiac or shock, $n = 31$).[25] One center also reported survival with good neurologic outcome in a 3.5-year-old with out-of-hospital cardiac arrest who received ECMO in the emergency department.[26] Overall, however, the use of this technology in the emergency department for witnessed arrest has not been as successful and cannot be recommended at present.[27]

ADVANCED LIFE SUPPORT TECHNIQUES

Vascular Access

Rapid vascular access is often difficult to achieve in the pulseless victim but is essential to deliver resuscitation medication. Rapid delivery of a drug to the central circulation, combined with effective chest compression–induced blood flow, is necessary to deliver epinephrine to its site of action in the arterial vascular bed. Central venous drug administration is ideal but difficult to achieve in the arrest setting. Peripheral venous administration may not be equivalent, but any available venous route should be used in arrest situations. When using peripheral venous routes, it is essential to flush the catheter with at least 5 mL of saline to help deliver the drug to the central circulation.

The intraosseous (IO) route is also effective for rapid drug delivery.[28] IO injections are usually given in the proximal tibia, but the distal femur, distal tibia, and anterior superior iliac spine may also be used. Any drug or fluid that can be given intravenously (IV) can be given by the IO route. Some studies suggest that the IO route is superior to the IV route; higher central venous and arterial drug concentrations are obtained. Although complications such as anterior compartment syndromes, bilateral tibial fractures, and fat and marrow emboli to the lungs have been reported, more recent data suggest that the risk of pulmonary fat emboli is not increased by the use of IO access for emergent fluid and drug administration.[29] To minimize complications, IO needles should not be placed in fractured long bones or into the same extremity where a needle was previously placed and then displaced. In both cases, the drugs or fluid may egress from the defect in the bony cortex.

Endotracheal Drug Administration

The IV and IO routes are the preferred sites for drug administration during cardiopulmonary arrest. In infants and children in whom IO access is delayed, certain drugs may be given by the endotracheal (ET) route.[30] These include lidocaine, epinephrine, atropine, and naloxone (LEAN). Although the ET route has the theoretical advantage of more rapid drug delivery to the arterial circulation by absorption from the pulmonary capillaries, the kinetics of drug absorption do not favor this route.

The ET route needs about 10 times the amount of drug (epinephrine) given IV to achieve equal plasma concentrations and peak drug action. Unfortunately, the lung acts as a depot for these large doses of drugs. Thus, if ROSC occurs, the patient may have prolonged and profound hypertension. Profound hypertension

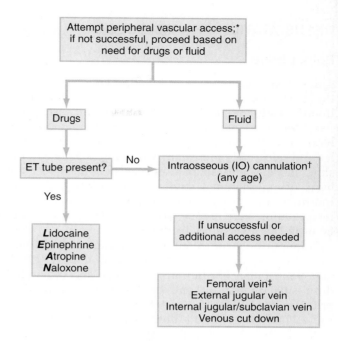

* Attempt site you are most successful with.
† Pursue IO cannulation immediately if CPR/severe shock.
‡ Femoral vein is safest central venous site during CPR.

Figure 8-1. Vascular access and drug delivery algorithm in pediatric advanced life support. CPR, cardiopulmonary resuscitation; ET, endotracheal.

after restoration of circulation may be harmful to cerebral recovery, and excessive afterload may further compromise cardiac function when it is already diminished by arrest-induced myocardial ischemia.

The optimal dose and method of drug delivery by the ET route have not been determined. Current recommendations are based on anecdotal reports and limited experimental data. On the basis of poor absorption, ET epinephrine doses of 0.1 mg/kg are recommended, given as 0.1 mL/kg of the 1:1000 concentration.[15]

Although administration of ET drugs through a catheter has been recommended, data show that direct instillation followed by 2 to 5 mL of saline flush is just as effective and is simpler.[31] Alternatively, the drug may be diluted to a final volume of 2 to 5 mL with normal saline. With any technique, it is important to follow drug administration with several deep positive-pressure breaths to help distribute the drug into the lower airways.

Drug injection into an intravascular location (IV or IO) is always preferred over the ET route (Figure 8-1). Central venous injection is always preferred over peripheral venous injection. When the IO and IV routes are not immediately available, the first dose of epinephrine should be given by the ET route, but an IV dose should be given as soon as a line is secured because the ET route is unreliable.[32,33]

RESUSCITATION PHARMACOLOGY

Epinephrine

Epinephrine has both α- and β-adrenergic actions, but the large doses used in cardiac arrest produce predominantly α-adrenergic effects. This action increases coronary perfusion pressure and myocardial and cerebral blood flow by preventing collapse of intrathoracic arteries and selectively increasing vascular resistance in the skin, muscle, and splanchnic vascular beds. On the basis of experimental studies, epinephrine's positive inotropic and chronotropic actions are not important in resuscitation from cardiac arrest, but these actions can be useful to reverse bradycardia.[34]

Epinephrine is indicated in all cardiac arrest settings, including asystole, pulseless electrical activity (PEA), and ventricular fibrillation (VF). The recommended dose is 0.01 mg/kg (0.1 mL/kg of 1:10,000 solution) IV or 0.1 mg/kg (0.1 mL/kg of 1:1000 solution) by the ET route (Table 8-1). If this dose is not effective after 3 to 5 minutes, 10 times the initial dose, or 0.1 mg/kg (0.1 mL/kg of the 1:1000 solution), may be tried, but it is unlikely that high doses of epinephrine improve outcome.[35-37] Clinical data show that patients who do not have restoration of organized spontaneous cardiac activity with two rounds of epinephrine do not survive to leave the hospital.[9] Immediate use of high-dose epinephrine is not recommended.[38,39]

Epinephrine is also the drug of choice in the treatment of bradycardia caused by a hypoxic or ischemic insult to the heart; a dose of 0.01 mg/kg is recommended.[15]

Vasopressin

Vasopressin, an endogenous hormone, produces vasoconstriction by action on specific V_1 receptors and reabsorption of water in the renal tubule (V_2 receptor). In the early 1990s vasopressin levels were found to be elevated in survivors of cardiac arrest compared with patients who died.[40] This led investigators to evaluate vasopressin in experimental cardiac arrest models. Vasopressin has been found to increase blood flow preferentially to the heart and brain with improved long-term survival compared with epinephrine.[41,42] It was also shown to improve survival after hypothermic CPR and to restore spontaneous circulation after hypothermia or near-drowning cardiac arrest.[43,44] Vasopressin is equally absorbed and effective whether administered IV, IO, or by endobronchial routes.[45,46]

Vasopressin has been shown to be an effective vasopressor in children in noncardiac arrest settings and may prove beneficial in pediatric cardiac arrest.[47,48] In one small study of prolonged, in-hospital, pediatric cardiac arrest, two of four patients receiving vasopressin survived longer than 24 hours with one surviving to hospital discharge with baseline neurologic function.[49] A large, prospective, multicenter study randomly assigned 1186 adult patients to receive vasopressin or epinephrine for out-of-hospital cardiac arrest.[50] The effects were similar for VF and PEA, but vasopressin was superior in patients with asystole. In addition, 732 of these patients had refractory cardiac arrest (not responding to two doses of the study drug) and were subsequently given epinephrine. In this subgroup, vasopressin followed by epinephrine was superior to epinephrine alone in survival to admission (25.7% versus 16.4%, $P = .002$) and hospital discharge (6.2% versus 1.7%, $P = .002$) with similar neurologic outcomes. Although currently not a first-line agent in pediatric cardiac arrest, vasopressin shows some promise for use in the future. A dose of 0.4 to 1 U/kg may have a role in shock-refractory VF and 0.005 to 0.01 U/kg/hr as a vasopressor for circulatory shock.[47-49]

Sodium Bicarbonate

Sodium bicarbonate ($NaHCO_3$) buffers metabolic acidosis through a mechanism represented by the following reaction:

$$NaHCO_3 + H^+ \rightarrow Na^+ + H_2CO_3 \rightarrow H_2O + CO_2$$

Unless ventilation is adequate, the reaction cannot proceed to the right by the elimination of formed CO_2. Unfortunately, ventilation is not usually the limiting factor; instead, inadequate blood flow results in poor CO_2 elimination. Administration of $NaHCO_3$ increases CO_2 production, which may worsen intracellular acidosis, even when the measured arterial pH improves. An unfavorable change in intracellular pH results from the increased permeability of the cell membrane to CO_2 compared with bicarbonate.[51] A negative inotropic effect, acute vasodilation, and acute exacerbation of myocardial intracellular acidosis may result from the administration of $NaHCO_3$.[52,53]

No evidence shows an improvement in outcome when $NaHCO_3$ is administered during resuscitation from cardiac arrest.[15] Because of this and the potential for harm, $NaHCO_3$ is not thought to be useful for patients in cardiac arrest. However, guidelines still allow bicarbonate administration in a dose of 1 mEq/kg IV or IO only *after* the airway has been secured, the victim is ventilated, effective chest compressions are being delivered, and epinephrine administration and defibrillation are ineffective (see Table 8-1). Subsequent doses (0.5 mEq/kg; 0.5 mL/kg) may be given every 10 minutes of continued arrest. Administration of $NaHCO_3$ in the postarrest setting to correct acidosis may be injurious if the patient has poor myocardial function but may be helpful if effective perfusion and ventilation are maintained. Sodium bicarbonate may be used to antagonize the adverse electrophysiologic effects of hyperkalemia, hypermagnesemia, sodium channel blocker poisonings, and cyclic antidepressants.

Because catecholamines are inactivated and calcium salts precipitate in $NaHCO_3$ solutions, careful flushing of the IV line is necessary after administration. Acute alkalosis may depress ionized calcium concentrations.

Glucose

Glucose is the major energy substrate of the brain and the myocardium; vigorous myocardial contractility

Table 8-1. Primary and Secondary Measures in Pediatric Resuscitation

Drug Availability	Dose/Route	Indications	Adverse Reactions	Comments
Adenosine (Adenocard) (3 mg/mL)	0.1 mg/kg rapid IV push (maximum: 12 mg/dose)	Supraventricular tachycardia	Hypotension, chest pain, dyspnea, dysrhythmia, heart block	Monitor carefully; do not use in second- or third-degree heart block or sick sinus syndrome
Albuterol (Proventil, Ventolin) (0.5%-5 mg/mL)	Inhalation 0.03 mL/kg/dose (maximum: 0.5-1.0 mL/dose) diluted in 2 mL NS	Bronchoconstriction, hyperkalemia	Tachycardia, nausea	β_2-Agonist
Amiodarone	5 mg/kg IV	Ventricular tachycardia/fibrillation	Hypotension, bradycardia Prolongs the QT interval	Do not combine with procainamide Give rapid push in pulseless VT
Atropine (0.1, 0.4, 1.0 mg/mL)	0.01-0.02 mg/kg/dose (minimum: 0.1 mg/dose; maximum: 2.0 mg) q5 min prn IV, ET, IO	Bradycardia, asystole, ↑ vagal tone Heart block (temporary)	Tachycardia, dysrhythmias, anticholinergic	Parasympatholytic; use 2-3 times dose ET
Bicarbonate, sodium (NaHCO$_3$) (8.4%-50 mEq/50 mL) (7.5%-44.5 mEq/50 mL)	1 mEq/kg/dose q10 min prn IV, IO	Metabolic acidosis Hyperkalemia	Metabolic alkalosis, hyperosmolality, hypernatremia	Incompatible with calcium, catecholamine infusion; monitor ABGs
Calcium chloride (CaCl$_2$) (10%-100 mg/mL) (1.36 mEq Ca^{++}/mL)	20-30 mg (0.2-0.3 mL/kg/dose (maximum: 500 mg/dose) q10 min prn IV slowly	Hyperkalemia Calcium channel blocker overdose	Rapid infusion causes bradycardia, hypotension Extravasation—necrosis	Inotropic; monitor; use caution with digitalized patient; probably no benefit in asystole or electromechanical dissociation
Crystalloid 0.9% NS, LR, D5W 0.9% D5NS, D5LR	20 mL/kg over 20-30 min IV	Hypovolemia	Fluid overload and pulmonary edema	Monitor volume status
Defibrillation	2-4 J/kg (maximum: 200 J)	Ventricular fibrillation		Use correct paddle size and paste; cardioversion (0.5-1.0 watt-sec/kg)
Dexamethasone (Decadron) (4, 24 mg/mL)	0.15-0.60 mg/kg/dose IV, IM, PO	Croup, asthma, meningitis	Hyperglycemia	Delayed onset
Dextrose (D50W-0.5 g/mL)	0.5-1.0 g (2-4 mL D25W or 1-2 mL D50W)/kg/dose IV	Hypoglycemia, with coma or seizure	Hyperglycemia	Check glucose; if possible use D25W
Diazepam (Valium) (5 mg/mL)	0.2-0.3 mg/kg/dose (maximum: 10 mg/dose) IV	Status epilepticus	Respiratory depression	Also begin maintenance medication; may give higher dose rectally (0.5 mg/kg)
Diazoxide (Hyperstat) (15 mg/mL)	1-3 mg/kg q4-24 hr IV	Hypertension	Hypotension, hyperglycemia	Monitor (very prompt onset)
Digoxin (0.1, 0.25 mg/mL)	Premie: 0.01-0.02 mg/kg TDD IV 2 wk-2 yr: 0.03-0.05 mg/kg TDD IV Newborn and >2 yr: 0.04 mg/kg TDD IV. $^1/_2$ TDD initially, then $^1/_4$ TDD q4-8 hr IV ×2	Congestive heart failure (CHF) Supraventricular tachycardia	Dysrhythmia, heart block, vomiting	Monitor electrocardiogram; may also load PO in stable, nonurgent situation; if mild CHF, may give PO without loading
Dobutamine (Dobutrex) (vial: 250 mg)	2-20 µg/kg/min IV	Cardiogenic shock	Tachycardia, dysrhythmia, hypotension, hypertension	β-Adrenergic; positive inotropic; may be synergistic with dopamine or isoproterenol
Dopamine (200 mg/5 mL)	Low: 2-5 µg/kg/min IV Mod: 5-20 µg/kg/min IV High: >20 µg/kg/min IV	Cardiogenic shock (moderate dose) Maintain renal perfusion Septic shock	Tachycardia, bradycardia, vasoconstriction (increase with higher doses)	β-Adrenergic; avoid in hypovolemic shock; may use in combination with epinephrine or levarterenol (norepinephrine)
Epinephrine (1 : 10,000) (0.1 mg/mL)	Initial: 0.01 mg (0.1 mL; 1 : 10,000)/kg/dose (maximum: 10 mL/dose) IV ET: 0.1 mg (0.1 mL; 1 : 1,000)/kg/dose q3-5 min prn	Asystole Ventricular fibrillation (fine) Anaphylaxis Hemodynamically significant bradycardia	Tachycardia, dysrhythmia, hypertension, decreased renal and splanchnic blood flow	α- and β-adrenergic; inotropic

Continued

Table 8-1. Primary and Secondary Measures in Pediatric Resuscitation—cont'd

Drug Availability	Dose/Route	Indications	Adverse Reactions	Comments
Epinephrine (1:1,000) (1 mg/mL)	0.01 mL/kg/dose SC (maximum: 0.35 mL/dose) q10-20 min SC ×3 prn	High-dose epinephrine or ET epinephrine for cardiac arrest (above) Reactive airway disease	Tachycardia, headache, nausea	Rarely used because of side effects; may use for ET or second IV dose (above and text)
Epinephrine racemic (Vaponefrin) (2.25% solution)	0.25-0.75 mL/dose by inhalation	Croup, airway edema	Tachycardia, palpitations, dysrhythmia, nausea, vomiting	Monitor; observe over time
Fentanyl (Sublimaze) (50 μg/mL)	1-5 μg/kg/dose IV, IM	Analgesia	Respiratory depression, apnea, muscle rigidity, bradycardia, nausea, vomiting, cardiac arrest	Monitor; be prepared to manage the airway
Flumazenil (Romazicon) (0.1 mg/mL) (5, 10 mL)	0.01-0.03 mg/kg IV (maximum: 1 mg)	Benzodiazepine overdose	May precipitate benzodiazepine withdrawal, seizures	Onset: 1-3 min; duration of action: 1 hr
Fosphenytoin (Cerebyx) (50 mg/mL) (2, 10 mL)	15-20 phenytoin equivalents (PE)/kg IV/IM Give slowly IV (2 PE/kg/min)	Seizures	Hypotension, bradycardia (less common than with phenytoin)	1 PE ≈ 1 mg phenytoin; less side effects; can administer more rapidly than phenytoin
Furosemide (Lasix) (10 mg/mL)	1 mg/kg/dose q6-12 hr IV up to 6 mg/kg; may repeat q2hr prn	Fluid overload, pulmonary edema, cerebral edema	Hypokalemia, hyponatremia, prerenal azotemia	Reduce interval in newborn to q12 hr; if no response in urine output in 30 min, repeat; do not use if hypovolemic
Glucagon (1 mg [1 unit]/mL)	0.1 mg/kg/dose q20 min prn IV, SC, IM	β-Blocker overdose Hypoglycemia	Hypotension, nausea, vomiting	Not adequate as only glucose support in neonate; inotropic
Hydrocortisone (Solu-Cortef) (100, 250, 500 mg)	1-5 mg/kg/24 hr (max: 100 mg IV	Adrenal failure		Check electrolytes/glucose, replace fluid loss, treat hyperkalemia
Labetalol	0.2 mg/kg IV Double dose q15 min prn (Max 2-3 mg/kg/dose)	Hypertension	Bronchospasm	α- and β-blocker Does not increase ICP
Lidocaine (1%-10 mg/mL) (2%-20 mg/mL)	1 mg/kg/dose q5-10 min IV, ET up to 5 mg/kg, then 20-50 μg/kg/min	Ventricular dysrhythmias Cardiac arrest caused by ventricular fibrillation	Hypotension, bradycardia with block, seizures	Decreased automaticity; for ET, give 1:1 dilution, with 2-3 times IV dose
Lorazepam (Ativan) (2, 4 mg/mL)	0.05-0.10 mg/kg/dose IV (maximum: 4 mg/dose); may repeat	Status epilepticus	Respiratory depression	Longer acting than diazepam
Methylprednisolone (Solu-Medrol) (40, 125, 500, 1000 mg)	Asthma: 1-2 mg/kg/dose q6 hr IV; usual maximum: 125 mg	Adrenal failure Asthma	Hyperglycemia	
Midazolam (Versed) (1, 5 mg/mL)	0.05-0.1 mg/kg/dose (maximum: 6 mg) IV	Sedation	Respiratory depression, hypotension, bradycardia	Antidote: flumazenil (Romazicon) Monitor: be prepared to manage the airway
Milrinone	Load: 50-75 μg/kg Infuse: 0.5-1.0 μg/kg/min	Inotrope	Hypotension during load	Inodilator (inotrope/vasodilator)
Morphine (8, 10, 15 mg/mL)	0.1-0.2 mg/kg/dose (maximum: 15 mg/dose) q2-4 hr IV	Analgesia Pulmonary edema Tetralogy spell Reduce preload and afterload	Hypotension, respiratory depression	Antidote: naloxone (Narcan)
Naloxone (Narcan) (0.4 mg/mL) (1 mg/mL)	For a drug overdose 0.1 mg/kg/dose (maximum: 0.8 mg) IV, ET; if no response in 10 min give 2 mg IV To reverse adverse effects of therapeutic narcotics, 0.05-0.01 mg/kg/dose	Narcotic overdose		Give empirically in suspected opiate overdose; may be given ET

Drug Availability	Dose/Route	Indications	Adverse Reactions	Comments
Nicardipine	0.03 mg/kg Then 1-5 µg/kg/min	Hypertension	Increases ICP, HR	Ca channel blocker
Nitroprusside (50 mg/vial)	0.5-10 µg (average: 3 µg)/kg/min IV	Hypertensive emergency Afterload reduction	Hypotension, nausea, vomiting, thiocyanate toxicity, cyanide poisoning	Monitor closely; light sensitive Thiocyanate toxicity common in patient with impaired renal function
Oxygen	100% mask, ET	Hypoxia Major injury	Toxicity not a problem with acute short-term use	Use high flow (3-6 L/min); monitor ABGs
Pancuronium (Pavulon) (1, 2 mg/mL)	0.04-0.1 mg/kg/dose IV; may repeat 0.01-0.02 mg/kg/ dose q20-40 min IV prn	Muscle relaxation	Tachycardia	Rapid onset; support respirations; lower dose in newborn
Phenobarbital (65 mg/mL)	15-20 mg/kg load IV/IM (adult: 100 mg/ dose q20 min prn ×3), then 5 mg/ kg/24 hr PO, IV, IM	Seizures	Sedation	If not controlled after load, repeat 10 mg/kg/dose IV; administer <1 mg/ kg/min IV; IM erratically absorbed
Phenytoin (Dilantin 50 mg/mL)	15-20 mg/kg load IV slowly, then 5- 10 mg/kg/24 hr PO, IV q12-24 hr	Seizures	Hypotension, bradycardia when given too rapidly; cerebral disturbance	Not to exceed 1.0 mg/ kg/min; dilute in normal saline
Procainamide	15 mg/kg IV over 30-60 min	Recurrent or refractory VT/SVT	Hypotension, bradycardia Prolongs the QT interval	Do not combine with amiodarone
Succinylcholine (20 mg/mL)	1 to 2 mg/kg/dose IV (larger dose in children <20 kg)	Neuromuscular blockade	Hyperkalemia Malignant hyperthermia Dysrhythmia	Must be able to control ventilation; requires advanced airway skills
Vasopressin	0.4-1.0 units/kg 0.005-0.001 units/kg/hr	Shock-refractory VT/VF Vasopressor		Still investigational in VT/VF
Vecuronium (Norcuron) (10 mg/mL)	0.08-0.1 mg/kg/dose IV	Nondepolarizing neuromuscular blockade		Monitor; requires advanced airway skills

ABG, arterial blood gas; *HR*, heart rate; *ICP*, intracranial pressure; *NS*, normal saline; *SVT*, supraventricular tachycardia; *VF*, ventricular fibrillation; *VT*, ventricular tachycardia.

may not be possible when hypoglycemia occurs. Infants and small children, especially if they have been chronically ill, are predisposed to hypoglycemia because they have limited glycogen stores.[54] If hypoglycemia is present, the dose of glucose is 0.5 to 1.0 g/kg IV (see Table 8-1). This is most conveniently administered by using 50% dextrose in water (D50W), but this solution should be diluted because it is hyperosmolar. A 1:1 dilution with sterile water results in D25W; the recommended dose is then 2 to 4 mL/kg of D25W IV. Repeated administration is usually not required and may result in a hyperosmolar state.

The major side effect of glucose administration is related to local irritation from infusion of this hypertonic solution. Moreover, both experimental and clinical data suggest that hyperglycemia predisposes the brain to a more severe ischemic insult by providing increased substrate for lactate formation during anaerobic glycolysis.[55] The increased production of lactate produces a severe intracellular acidosis that injures the cell. Therefore, the goal of treatment is to normalize glucose concentration and avoid hyperglycemia.

Atropine

Atropine is a competitive antagonist at muscarinic receptors and therefore inhibits vagal activity. This action increases sinoatrial node firing rate and atrioventricular (AV) conduction, producing tachycardia. At low doses, atropine has central and peripheral parasympathomimetic actions that may produce paradoxical vagotonic effects.

Atropine is recommended in the treatment of symptomatic bradycardia caused by AV block or increased vagal tone (ET intubation). It may also be helpful in the treatment of bradycardia accompanied by poor perfusion and hypotension, but epinephrine is generally more effective. The initial treatment of bradycardia in any patient is ensuring adequate oxygenation, ventilation, and temperature (treat hypothermia).[15]

If bradycardia persists despite adequate oxygenation and ventilation and administration of epinephrine, administration of atropine may be appropriate. Atropine may be given by the IV, IO, or ET route (see Table 8-1). A minimum dose of 0.1 mg is used to avoid paradoxical bradycardia. A maximum single dose of 0.5 mg in a child and 1.0 mg in an adolescent may be used and repeated to a total maximum dose of 1.0 mg and 2.0 mg, respectively. These maximum doses produce complete vagal inhibition, and additional doses are not helpful, except in special circumstances (organophosphate poisoning).

Tachycardia may follow atropine administration but is usually well tolerated in pediatric patients. Although atropine causes mydriasis, fixed and dilated pupils after an arrest and resuscitation should not be attributed to atropine.[56]

Calcium

Calcium is essential in excitation-contraction coupling. Normally, calcium entry into the cardiac myocyte stimulates calcium release from the endoplasmic reticulum; the increase in intracellular calcium concentration stimulates actin-myosin coupling. In infants, intracellular calcium release is deficient, and cardiac contractility depends more on extracellular calcium influx, as demonstrated by the greater inhibition of cardiac contractility in infants by calcium channel blockers. Thus, hypocalcemia may arise with poor contractility and a clinical picture of cardiogenic shock.

No evidence from adult studies supports the use of calcium in asystole, and its use in PEA is questionable. The incidence of hypocalcemia is increased in out-of-hospital arrest victims, but the benefit of calcium administration in this setting remains controversial. Only limited data are available for pediatric patients. Ionized hypocalcemia occurs in pediatric cardiac arrest patients but is associated with septic shock in most of these patients.[9] Hypocalcemia is also relatively common in the pediatric intensive care unit, occurring in 35% of patients in one study.[57] Because calcium can antagonize the action of epinephrine and other adrenergic agents and because accumulation of intracellular calcium appears to mediate the final common pathway of cell death, calcium is indicated only (1) to correct documented hypocalcemia, (2) to antagonize the adverse cardiovascular actions of hyperkalemia and hypermagnesemia, and (3) to reverse the hypotension produced by calcium channel blocker toxicity.

For indicated conditions, calcium is given IV or IO in a dose of 20 mg/kg of calcium chloride ($CaCl_2$, 0.2 mL/kg of 10% solution) (see Table 8-1). Repeated doses increase the risk of morbidity, and the initial dose should be repeated only once in 10 minutes if needed; subsequent doses should be based on measured deficiencies of ionized calcium concentration. Total calcium concentrations are unreliable indicators of ionized calcium concentration in critically ill patients.

Rapid calcium administration should be avoided because bradycardia or sinus arrest may occur, especially in patients receiving digoxin. $CaCl_2$ solution is hyperosmolar and sclerosing; severe chemical burns may occur if the solution extravasates from peripheral injection sites.

Magnesium

Magnesium is an important intracellular cation and acts as a cofactor in many enzymatic reactions. It causes smooth muscle relaxation by inhibition of calcium channels. Through this mechanism and other membrane-stabilizing effects, magnesium has proved useful in the treatment of torsades de pointes. Torsades de pointes is a unique form of ventricular tachycardia (VT) with characteristic changes of QRS amplitude on electrocardiogram tracings. It is seen in conditions that prolong the QT interval (congenital prolonged QT), drug toxicity (quinidine, sotalol, amiodarone, digitalis), and drug interactions (cisapride and erythromycin).[15]

In children, the indications for magnesium therapy include torsades de pointes and symptomatic hypomagnesemia. Although the optimal dose is uncertain, a slow infusion over 15 minutes of 25 to 50 mg/kg (up to 2 g) IV or IO has been recommended.[58] Rapid administration may result in hypotension, bradycardia, and decreased cardiac contractility.[59]

Adenosine

Adenosine acts at specific myocardial receptors to (1) decrease sinoatrial node and AV node automaticity, (2) decrease atrial contractility, (3) decrease atrial action potential duration, and (4) suppress norepinephrine release.[60] It effectively blocks conduction through the AV node and interrupts reentry circuits that involve the AV node, thus interrupting the majority of supraventricular tachycardia (SVT) episodes in infants and children.[15] Adenosine is the drug of choice in the treatment of SVT in children and is approximately 70% effective.[61] With a half-life of only 10 seconds, adenosine must be administered as a rapid IV bolus. The site of administration should be as close to the heart as possible and followed immediately by a saline flush. This enhances delivery to the site of action. An initial dose of 0.1 mg/kg is given (up to 6 mg) and, if not effective, may be doubled and repeated once (up to 12 mg) during continuous electrocardiogram monitoring.

Amiodarone

Amiodarone is an antiarrhythmic agent with shared characteristics of class Ia, II, III, and IV antiarrhythmic drugs. Amiodarone inhibits sodium channels (class Ia), which slows conduction in the ventricles, prolonging the QRS duration. It inhibits α- and β-adrenergic receptors (class II), producing vasodilation and AV node suppression. Amiodarone also blocks K^+ channels (class III), prolonging the QT interval, and has some Ca^{++} channel blocking effects as well (class IV).[36]

The clinical use of amiodarone is based on adult data with shock-resistant VT/VF[62] and experience with nonarresting children in the intensive care unit.[63,64] It has been effective for treatment of infants and children with VT, SVT, and postoperative junctional tachycardia.[65-69] One study also demonstrated that amiodarone is safe and effective treatment for drug-refractory fetal tachycardia.[70] In the setting of pulseless arrest, 5 mg/kg is given as a rapid bolus. This may be repeated up to a maximum of 15 mg/kg/day. Hypotension is a significant side effect of rapid IV administration. For VT with adequate or poor perfusion and SVT with poor perfusion, one should consider amiodarone 5 mg/kg over 20 to 60 minutes and repeated as before. Amiodarone should not be given concurrently with other medications that prolong the QT interval (procainamide) to prevent VT.

Procainamide

Procainamide is a class I antiarrhythmic agent that works by blocking sodium channels. Procainamide prolongs the refractory period of both atria and ventricles and slows conduction velocity, thereby prolonging PR, QRS, and QT intervals. It also has vasodilatory and negative inotropic properties.

Procainamide is recommended as an alternative therapy for refractory or recurrent VT/VF. It is not used in pulseless VT/VF. Procainamide should be administered slowly, 15 mg/kg over 30 to 60 minutes, to avoid heart block, myocardial depression, hypotension, and prolongation of the QT interval.[36] Procainamide should not be administered concurrently with other medications that prolong the QT interval (amiodarone).

Lidocaine

Lidocaine is a class Ib antiarrhythmic agent with membrane-stabilizing effects mediated through inhibition of sodium channels. Sodium channel inhibition reduces automaticity and the difference in effective refractory period between normal and ischemic tissue; these effects inhibit the propagation of re-entrant dysrhythmias.[71]

Lidocaine is now considered an alternative to amiodarone for stable VT and pulseless VT/VF. VF is seen in fewer than 10% of pediatric cardiac arrest victims.[9] When VF is seen in a young patient, a search for a metabolic etiology is indicated unless the patient is known to have an underlying cardiac disorder (e.g., structural heart disease, myocarditis, digoxin toxicity). Metabolic causes of ventricular dysrhythmias include hyperkalemia, hypermagnesemia, and hypothermia, as well as toxin-induced causes (e.g., cyclic antidepressant overdose).

Lidocaine is administered as an initial bolus of 1.0 mg/kg; a repeated dose of 1.0 mg/kg may be given in 10 to 15 minutes (see Table 8-1). If a second dose is required, a lidocaine infusion is started at 20 to 50 µg/kg/min; lower infusion rates are used in patients with liver disease or persistent low cardiac output states because lidocaine clearance is depressed in these conditions. Lidocaine is rapidly redistributed from the plasma compartment after bolus injection, and the plasma concentration may transiently fall to subtherapeutic levels on initiation of infusion. If not already given, a second bolus may be required.

High lidocaine plasma concentrations can depress myocardial contractility and produce hypotension through peripheral vasodilation. Additional toxicities result from central nervous system effects. Toxic symptoms range from drowsiness and disorientation to muscle twitching and generalized seizures. Discontinuation of the infusion is usually effective treatment for toxicity. If necessary, lorazepam or phenobarbital may be given to control seizure activity.

MANAGEMENT

The most obvious difference between pediatric and adult resuscitation is related to etiology. Adult cardiopulmonary arrest is primarily cardiac in etiology. Conversely, pediatric cardiopulmonary arrest is usually a *secondary* phenomenon, most often occurring after either respiratory failure or shock. Therefore, recognition of shock and respiratory failure and their appropriate treatment are both key to prevention of cardiac arrest in children.

Airway

The most notable difference between the adult and pediatric airways is related to the small size and variability of the airway with age. Major differences are most prominent in the infant or young child; the airway becomes more similar to the adult's as the child grows. The opening of the larynx assumes a superior and anterior position in the neck in infancy and descends with age, assuming an adult position at approximately 8 to 10 years of age. The narrowest portion of the trachea in the infant is at the cricoid ring; in the adult, the smallest cross-sectional area of the larynx is at the level of the vocal cords.

Features related to the size of the head, the large tongue, and the submandibular tissue are important in pediatric airway management. The head is approximately equal to the width of the shoulders in an infant. As the child grows, the head gradually assumes normal adult proportions. Because of a prominent occiput, a child placed in a supine position has a tendency to flex the neck, which can occlude the airway. The correct position for maximal airway patency is the sniffing position (Figure 8-2). A towel or other support often needs to be placed under the neck or upper shoulders to maintain this position. Overflexion of the neck or extension of the head can occlude the airway. Occlusion occurs at the level of the posterior pharynx because of the large floppy tongue falling back against the pharynx.

The chin-lift and the jaw-thrust maneuvers elevate the mandible anteriorly, separating the tongue from the pharynx and opening the airway. If these maneuvers fail to open a patient's airway, an oral or nasal pharyngeal airway may be placed. Care must be taken in using oral airways in pediatric patients. If the wrong size is selected, it can exacerbate airway obstruction by pushing the tongue and submandibular tissues posteriorly against the posterior pharynx. In addition, a child who is not unconscious may gag or vomit during the placement of an oral airway. Nasal pharyngeal airways are appropriate in semiconscious patients and can be used in patients with a gag reflex as long as the airway is sized appropriately.

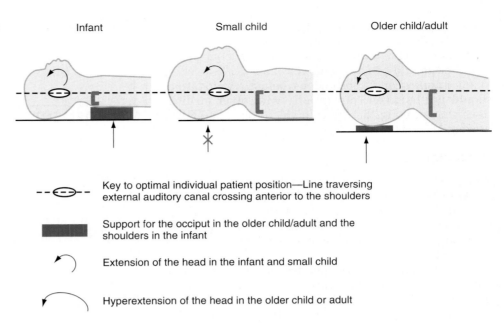

Figure 8-2. Correct (sniffing) position for maximal airway patency.

Infant   Small child   Older child/adult

Key to optimal individual patient position—Line traversing external auditory canal crossing anterior to the shoulders

Support for the occiput in the older child/adult and the shoulders in the infant

Extension of the head in the infant and small child

Hyperextension of the head in the older child or adult

Intubation

ET intubation in children requires choosing the proper laryngoscope blade type and size and the correct ET tube size. Body length can be used to predict the correct tube size.[72] The length intervals associated with a specific tube size are included on the Broselow emergency tape (see Figure 8-8). As noted earlier, the sniffing position is preferred for intubation. Because of the superior and anterior position of the tracheal opening as well as the large tongue and relatively large floppy epiglottis, visualization of the glottic opening can be obstructed in children younger than 4 years if a curved blade is used. The straight blade lifts these tissues superiorly so that the glottic opening can be visualized.

Uncuffed ET tubes are generally used in children younger than 6 to 8 years. Because the subglottic area of the trachea is narrow in this age group, an uncuffed tube usually forms an adequate subglottic seal. If a cuffed tube is used, a high-volume, low-pressure cuff is preferred, and the cuff should be inflated to permit an audible air leak at 20 to 30 cm H_2O pressure. Ideally, cuff pressure should be measured to minimize the risk of subglottic injury. In children older than 8 years, the narrowest portion of the trachea is at the level of the vocal cords; a cuff is typically used to produce a satisfactory seal and prevent air leakage and aspiration of foreign material. After successful ET intubation, the next step is to maintain tube position until the tube is securely fastened to the patient.

Besides using body length, several formulas may be used to establish the proper tube size: (age/4) + 4 yields the internal diameter of the ET tube in millimeters for children older than 1 year. Also, the tube may be selected by choosing a size similar to that of the patient's little finger or nares. These formulas are only approximations, and auscultation reveals whether the tube is too small; a large glottic air leak occurs with small tubes. If the tube is too large, excessive force is

required to insert the tube; the intubation should be aborted and a smaller tube inserted.

Another common problem is determining the proper insertion length for the ET tube. A useful rule is that the position of the tube at the lips in centimeters should be equal to three times the internal diameter of the tube in millimeters. For example, if the patient is intubated with a 4.0-mm ET tube, it should be inserted to a distance of 12 cm at the lips. This formula assumes that the proper size of ET tube is selected. End-tidal CO_2 detection by disposable device or capnography must be used in children to confirm proper tube placement with a high degree of specificity. In children with cardiac arrest, absence of color change indicates either an esophageal intubation or a child who will not survive (see Chapter 2).[73] The latter results from the correlation between end-tidal CO_2 and cardiac output.[74]

Common errors after intubation include the following:

1. Failure to secure the ET tube. The procedure requires both taping or securing the tube at the lips and immobilization of the neck to prevent head movement, which may also cause tube dislodgement.
2. Failure to confirm tube position by end-tidal CO_2 detection for tracheal placement and careful auscultation for main stem intubation.
3. Failure of the patient to improve because of a distended abdomen from gastric air insufflation during bag/mask ventilation; corrected by placement of a nasogastric tube.
4. Selection of a tube that is too small, resulting in a large glottic air leak; reintubation with a larger tube is required.

The differential diagnosis of clinical deterioration in a previously stable intubated patient receiving positive-pressure ventilation can be remembered by the mnemonic DOPE: (1) a *d*islodged tube, either in the esophagus or in the right main stem bronchus; (2) a

Table 8-2. Drugs for Pediatric Rapid-Sequence Intubation

Drug	Dosage	Comments
Pretreatment*		
Atropine	0.02 mg/kg IV (min/max dose)	Prevents bradycardia caused by airway maneuvers or succinylcholine
Lidocaine	1.5 mg/kg IV	Head injury
Defasciculating agent (pancuronium/vecuronium)	0.01 mg/kg IV	Never <5 yr/20 kg
		Over 5 yr/20 kg: use for head injury
Fentanyl	0.1-0.3 mg/kg kg IV	
Induction agents		
Midazolam	0.3 mg/kg IV	Use 0.1 mg/kg if hypotensive
Thiopental	3-5 mg/kg IV	Lower dose to 1 mg/kg or delete if perfusion poor
Etomidate	0.3 mg/kg IV	
Ketamine	1-2 mg/kg IV *or* 4 mg/kg IM	
Propofol	1-2 mg/kg IV	
Neuromuscular Blocking Agents		
Succinylcholine	2 mg/kg IV	Always precede with atropine
Pancuronium/vecuronium		
Defasciculation	0.01 mg/kg IV	
Paralysis	0.2 mg/kg IV	
Maintenance	0.1 mg/kg IV	
Rocuronium	1.0 mg/kg IV	

*In general the same indications (LOAD) apply equally to adults and children (see Chapter 1), with the following exceptions:
Lidocaine: not used for prevention of bronchospasm in children.
Opioid (fentanyl): use only with extreme caution; infants and young children may be very sensitive to the respiratory depressant and sympathetic blunting effects of opioids.
Atropine is used for all children less than 10 years old.
Defasciculating agents may be given to children over 20 kg (5 years).

BOX 8-1. Alternatives for Failed or Difficult Pediatric Airway Intubation

Surgical cricothyroidotomy: may be difficult to perform in children <6-8 years old
Blind nasotracheal intubation (BNTI): contraindicated until age 10 years
Combitube (esophagotracheal tube): only if over 4 feet (1.2 m) tall
Laryngeal mask airway (LMA) for age: acceptable
Needle cricothyrotomy: acceptable

Table 8-3. Sequence for Pediatric RSI

Time	Step
Zero minus 10 minutes	Preparation
Zero minus 5 minutes	Preoxygenation: 100% oxygen
Zero minus 3 minutes	Pretreatment: atropine
Zero	Paralysis with induction: etomidate + succinylcholine
Zero plus 15 seconds	Protection: Sellick's maneuver, positioning
Zero plus 45 seconds	Placement with proof: perform intubation, confirm placement clinically and with end-tidal CO_2
Zero plus 1 minute	Postintubation management: long-acting paralytics, sedation

tube that has been blocked or *o*bstructed by a mucus plug or by kinking; (3) a tension *p*neumothorax; or (4) *e*quipment failure.

Rapid Sequence Intubation

As in adults, rapid sequence intubation (RSI) is emerging as the primary technique for intubation (see Chapters 1 and 2). Because the indications for and doses of some drugs in Table 8-1 may vary in RSI, they are also listed separately in Table 8-2, along with pretreatment considerations particular to children.

As in adults, the decision to use RSI in a pediatric patient is based on an assessment of the patient's clinical condition, the indication for intubation, and predicted airway difficulty. Most children have normal anatomy and do not have the various alterations (e.g., cervical arthritis) that may make adult intubation difficult. For patients with an airway that is perceived as difficult, certain alternatives are available, not all of which can be used in pediatric patients (Box 8-1). Table

8-3 outlines the standard RSI sequence used in pediatric patients. Modifications to the sequence, depending on the clinical situation, are the same for adults and children, with few exceptions, as already described. The most clinically important difference between the adult and pediatric sequences is probably the potential for desaturation even with adequate preoxygenation. This is the result of the doubled rate of oxygen consumption in children and a proportionally decreased functional residual capacity (see Figure 1-5). Bag/mask ventilation with cricoid pressure is usually sufficient to restore oxygenation after desaturation. Failure to ventilate or oxygenate requires institution of a failed airway protocol; although rarely required, this may consist of the use of an alternative device, such as a laryngeal mask airway or a needle cricothyroidotomy.

The protocol in Table 8-3 represents the RSI sequence, including drug selection, used in the

National Emergency Airway Management course. This protocol uses succinylcholine as the neuromuscular blocking agent of choice for adults and children. Although years of experience demonstrate the safety of this medication for emergency intubation, some authors recommend the use of a nondepolarizing (competitive) neuromuscular blocking agent for RSI. The agent of choice for competitive RSI is rocuronium bromide, 1 to 1.2 mg/kg IV.

In summary, RSI is the technique of choice for emergency airway management of the pediatric patient, with little variation from adult airway management.

Breathing

Because of infectious disease considerations, mouth-to-mouth resuscitation by health care workers is not recommended unless no other means of ventilation is available. Whether to use mouth-to-mouth or mouth-to-nose-and-mouth ventilation is determined by the size of the patient and rescuer. The method that most easily produces chest rise should be used. Ventilation rates are as follows:

1. 20 breaths/min (one breath every 3 seconds) for infants and children younger than 8 years
2. 12 breaths/min (one breath every 5 seconds) for adolescents and adults

Bag-Mask Ventilation

Correct use of the bag/mask apparatus or manual resuscitator is essential for airway management of the pediatric patient, and proper technique must be learned and practiced. One common problem is inadequate maneuvers to open the airway. Often, rescuers tend to seal the mask tightly to the face without performing an adequate jaw thrust to open the airway. To minimize barotrauma, excessive tidal volumes must be avoided to prevent excessive pressures. Rescuers may say "squeeze-release-release" while ventilating the patient. The manual resuscitator (bag device) is squeezed just until chest rise is initiated and then released to allow exhalation. Infants should not be ventilated more than 30 times per minute and children no more than 20 times per minute. Certain patients occasionally require higher than normal inspiratory pressures for adequate ventilation; if a BVM apparatus has a pop-off valve, the valve needs to be occluded to allow higher pressures for adequate chest rise.

When ventilating a pediatric patient, an adequate tidal volume is determined by the presence of normal chest rise, auscultation of good air movement, and improvement of color. An adequate minute volume is delivered when the struggling patient relaxes and becomes apneic or breathes with the delivered breaths. Although epiglottitis is rarely encountered in the post–*Haemophilus influenzae* type b (Hib) vaccine era, airway management in the apneic patient with suspected epiglottitis involves the following progressive steps:

1. Position the airway to see whether the patient ventilates with repositioning only.

2. Most children respond to bag/mask ventilation provided a two-person technique is used; ensure that one person concentrates on the mask seal while the other compresses the ventilation bag.
3. For intubation, use a tube (with stylet) one size smaller than usually selected for a child of that size. Applying gentle pressure over the chest wall can produce an air bubble at the tracheal opening to help guide tube placement.
4. Needle cricothyrotomy is used for supraglottic obstruction only if the previous measures fail. A commercially available device or a 14-gauge Angio-cath can be used. When the cricoid membrane is entered, a 3-mm ET tube adapter can be attached followed by attachment of a bag device or manual resuscitator. The clinician must realize that airway resistance is great through the catheter when attempting ventilation with the manual resuscitator. The use of a jet ventilation device has been suggested by some sources but may be associated with a high degree of complications in the small child. This technique provides adequate ventilation in small animals but has not been evaluated in children.[75]

Endotracheal Tube

After the patient is intubated, a number of factors are important to achieve adequate ventilation and avoid complications. Besides confirming proper tube position, the application of appropriate tidal volumes and the use of appropriate ventilation rates are important. Careful auscultation over the peripheral lung fields and axilla ensures proper tube placement and adequate tidal volumes. In children, breath sounds may be heard over the stomach, which is caused by transmission of sounds throughout the thorax. One should not remove the ET tube but should continue the clinical assessment of tube placement. If gurgling sounds are heard over the stomach, they indicate esophageal placement of the ET tube and the tube should be removed.

If the patient has bronchiolitis, asthma, or another airway disease characterized by air trapping, it is important to ventilate at a relatively slow rate to permit adequate time for exhalation. Even if the patient has hypercapnia, rapid rates are not indicated. It is more important to ensure adequate oxygenation; hypercapnia is well tolerated even at very high carbon dioxide pressure levels.[76] Effective ventilation in this setting requires heavy sedation or paralysis of the patient. Typical ventilatory rates for patients with air-trapping diseases are 8 to 12 breaths/min for older children, 15 breaths/min for children, and about 20 breaths/min for young children and infants. Regardless of the rate and tidal volume used, it is essential that adequacy of ventilation be objectively determined by arterial blood gases, pulse oximetry, and continuous capnography. Use of pulse oximetry alone does not ensure adequate CO_2 elimination.

If the patient is placed on a volume ventilator, the peak inspiratory pressure should equal 20 to 25 cm

H_2O. This assumes that lung compliance is normal, appropriate tidal volumes are used, and the inspiratory time is at least 0.6 second. Shorter inspiratory times produce higher peak inspiratory pressures, which incorrectly suggests that an adequate tidal volume is being delivered. Lower peak pressures suggest that the tidal volume is inadequate. In patients with poor lung compliance, peak inspiratory pressures of 30 cm H_2O or higher may be needed. Typical initial tidal volumes are 8 to 12 mL/kg, recognizing that the inspiratory volume may need to be larger if an adult ventilator circuit is used in a child because more of the tidal volume is lost as compressible volume in the high-volume, higher compliance ventilator circuit.

If a pressure-limited ventilator is used, the peak inspiratory pressure should be similar to the parameters just noted. Improper tube position or tube obstruction is *not* detected on a pressure-limited ventilator because high pressure does not occur. Therefore, continuous monitoring with a pulse oximeter is essential, along with confirmation of adequate ventilation by checking arterial blood gases or using an end-tidal CO_2 monitor.

Circulation

External Cardiac Compression

From a practical viewpoint, use of two fingers, three fingers, or the heel of the hand for compression depends on the size of the child. It is important to compress 33% to 50% of the anteroposterior diameter of the chest to achieve effective circulation. The rate of compression is at least 100 times/min for infants and 100 times/min in older children. The ventilation/compression ratio for both one- and two-person CPR is 1:5. A pause of at least 1 to 1.5 seconds should be allowed for ventilation. If the patient is intubated, it is probably not important to sequence ventilation and compression as carefully.

Pharmacologic Therapy

Fluids

If the pediatric patient is in full arrest, IV access and fluids are used only to provide a vehicle for drug delivery. In general, IV lines should be maintained at a minimal keep-open rate.

If the patient has an organized rhythm and detectable pulse but is hypotensive, a fluid bolus of 20 mL/kg should be given. If hypotension persists after two or three boluses of fluids (maximum of 50 mL/kg) or if the patient develops pulmonary edema, vasoactive drugs are started. Complicated fluid calculations based on maintenance and deficit therapy are reserved for the postresuscitation phase.

Isotonic non–glucose-containing fluid should be used for fluid boluses in resuscitation; a glucose-containing solution running at a maintenance rate is appropriate for maintenance fluids. A microdrip or infusion pump should be standard equipment for pediatric resuscitation preparedness.

Cardiac Rhythm and Etiology of Arrest

The greatest difference between pediatric and adult resuscitation may be in the area of dysrhythmia management. Dysrhythmias are often a secondary phenomenon in the pediatric patient. Most rhythm disturbances encountered in the resuscitation of infants and children are secondary to hypoxia, acidosis, or metabolic derangements. Correction of ventilation and oxygenation through appropriate airway management is usually adequate therapy. VF in adult patients, especially in a monitored arrest, is usually amenable to therapy. Unfortunately, most pediatric patients present to the emergency department in full arrest with either asystole or severe bradycardia. The outcome, even with appropriate treatment, is uniformly poor. Figure 8-3 classifies rhythm treatment on the basis of the presence or absence of a pulse and whether the pulse rate is slow or fast.

Rapid Heart Rate

If the patient has a fast heart rate, it is critical to decide whether the rapid rate is caused by a primary rhythm disturbance or is a secondary phenomenon. Table 8-4 provides parameters for making this distinction between the two most common types of fast heart rates, sinus tachycardia and SVT. Indications for the use of

Table 8-4. Sinus Tachycardia versus Supraventricular Tachycardia

	Sinus Tachycardia	Supraventricular Tachycardia
History	Consistent with volume loss (vomiting, diarrhea, bleeding)	Nonspecific, lightheaded, "heart rate too fast to count"
Physical examination	Clinical dehydration or pallor	Signs of congestive heart failure (rales, cardiomegaly), low cardiac output, shock
Chest radiograph	Small heart, clear lungs	Normal to large heart, pulmonary edema
Electrocardiogram	<220 in infants, <180 in children	>220 in infants, >180 in children
	Beat-to-beat variability (rate changes with stimulation/fluids)	No beat-to-beat variability (no rate change with stimulation/fluids)
	P wave may be hard to identify in both SVT and VT	
Treatment	IV fluids 20 mL/kg bolus IV/IO	Vagal maneuvers, adenosine
	Repeat as needed	Cardioversion if unstable (0.5-1.0 J/kg)

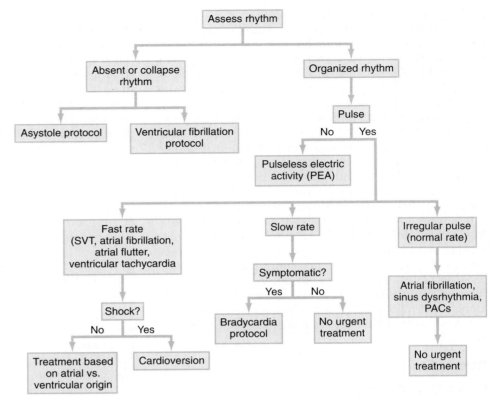

Figure 8-3. Management algorithm for the assessment and treatment of pediatric rhythm disorders. PACs, premature atrial contractions; SVT, supraventricular tachycardia.

Table 8-5. Summary of Therapy of Unstable Rhythms in Pediatric Patients

Heart Rate	Specific Rhythms	Treatment
Slow	Sinus bradycardia	Assess airway and ventilation, then administer epinephrine followed by atropine* (infant or child) or epinephrine alone in the neonate.
	Nodal or idioventricular rhythm	Epinephrine if no response to ventilation and oxygenation.

	Blocks
	    Type I or II second-degree
	    Third-degree
		Atropine first, then isoproterenol or epinephrine infusion and transcutaneous or transvenous pacemaker.

Fast	Narrow QRS complex
	    Supraventricular tachycardia
	    Atrial fibrillation or flutter
		Cardioversion.

	Wide QRS complex
	    Ventricular tachycardia
	    Any supraventricular rhythm with aberrant conduction†
		Cardioversion. If not successful, search for metabolic/toxic cause. Lidocaine, bretylium, then magnesium should be considered.

Collapse (no pulse present)	Ventricular fibrillation Asystole	Defibrillation. If not successful, use epinephrine or lidocaine. Bretylium and magnesium are second-line drugs. Bicarbonate may be considered.
	Pulseless electrical activity (PEA)	Epinephrine. Atropine and bicarbonate may be used if epinephrine is not effective. Bicarbonate, calcium, and fluid bolus are considered if no response to epinephrine.

*Epinephrine is recommended in newborns for bradycardia unresponsive to airway management.
†Differentiation between supraventricular and ventricular rhythm disturbances is difficult in the unstable patient with a wide-complex rhythm. When in doubt, treat the child for ventricular tachycardia.

cardiac drugs are the same for children as for adults: only unstable patients with cardiac rhythm disturbances require immediate drug or electrical treatment. The clinical definition of "instability" is usually based on evidence of poor perfusion (cyanosis, altered mental status, hypotension, prolonged capillary refill). To make an objective determination of a symptomatic dysrhythmia (i.e., measuring blood pressure and pulse), the lower limit of normal hemodynamic parameters from adolescents to newborns must be known. A blood pressure of 70 mm Hg or less in infants or 70 + (2 × the age in years) mm Hg or less in children, combined with evidence of poor tissue perfusion, indicates a patient with an unstable rhythm disturbance (Table 8-5). In newborns the blood pressure is often difficult to obtain; a heart rate less than 80 beats/min rather than a specific blood pressure is usually used as the objective measurement of instability.

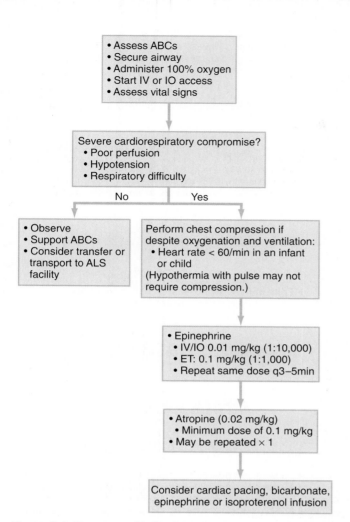

• Assess ABCs
• Secure airway
• Administer 100% oxygen
• Start IV or IO access
• Assess vital signs

↓

Severe cardiorespiratory compromise?
• Poor perfusion
• Hypotension
• Respiratory difficulty

No ← → Yes

No:
• Observe
• Support ABCs
• Consider transfer or transport to ALS facility

Yes:
Perform chest compression if despite oxygenation and ventilation:
• Heart rate < 60/min in an infant or child
(Hypothermia with pulse may not require compression.)

↓

• Epinephrine
  • IV/IO 0.01 mg/kg (1:10,000)
  • ET: 0.1 mg/kg (1:1,000)
  • Repeat same dose q3–5min

↓

• Atropine (0.02 mg/kg)
  • Minimum dose of 0.1 mg/kg
  • May be repeated × 1

↓

Consider cardiac pacing, bicarbonate, epinephrine or isoproterenol infusion

Figure 8-4. Treatment algorithm for bradycardia. ABCs, airway, breathing, and circulation; ALS, advanced life support; ET, endotracheal route; IO, intraosseous; IV, intravenous. (Modified from Guidelines for cardiopulmonary resuscitation and emergency cardiac care. Emergency Cardiac Care Committee and Subcommittees, American Heart Association. Part VI. Pediatric advanced life support. *JAMA* 268:2262, 1992.)

Bradycardia

Bradycardic rhythms are the second most common type of arrest rhythm seen in children. Their management is based on the underlying cause of the bradycardia. When precipitated by an arrest from a severe hypoxic-ischemic (HI) insult, the resulting rhythm is often wide complex and not preceded by identifiable p waves. Children with structural cardiac disease may develop bradycardia because of heart block or sinus node dysfunction, or bradycardia may be caused by drug intoxication, such as β-blocker or calcium channel blocker toxicity. Bradycardia resulting from these conditions accounts for only a small fraction of cases. The therapeutic approach to children with primary cardiac causes of bradycardia differs from that used with HI-induced bradycardia. Figure 8-4 outlines the therapeutic approach to symptomatic bradycardia; support of oxygenation and ventilation always precedes drug therapy.

Immediate correction of airway compromise and delivery of high concentrations of oxygen are the primary treatments for HI-induced bradycardia. After the airway is established, usually by intubation, and oxygen delivery is optimal, epinephrine may be used. Epinephrine is the drug of choice in HI-induced, refractory bradycardia; atropine is unlikely to be helpful in this setting. If bolus administration of epinephrine is only transiently effective in postarrest bradycardia, a continuous infusion is needed. A bolus of 0.01 mg/kg of 1:10,000 epinephrine solution IV may be repeated every 3 to 5 minutes with the same dose. If required, an infusion of epinephrine should start at 0.1 μg/kg/min and should be titrated to achieve the desired heart rate and blood pressure. Epinephrine infusion is preferable to isoproterenol for this indication because isoproterenol often compromises coronary perfusion pressure, whereas epinephrine maintains coronary blood flow.

Although uncommon, primary cardiac disease and drug intoxication must be considered as a cause of symptomatic bradycardia after hypoxemia has been excluded. Calcium channel blocker, β-blocker, and digitalis overdose as well as intrinsic nodal disease may produce bradycardia. In this setting, atropine may be useful to accelerate the pacemaker rate in primary cardiac conditions such as heart block; epinephrine infusion may also be effective. Epinephrine infusions are given in a wide dosage range of 0.05 to 1.0 μg/kg/min; the infusion rate is adjusted to the patient's need. β-Blocker toxicity may also be managed by glucagon administration. Calcium channel blocker toxicity may respond to calcium administration, although severe intoxication often requires vasopressor infusions as well.

Cardiac pacing may be helpful in primary cardiac bradycardia. It can be rapidly accomplished by external (transcutaneous) pacing and by transvenous or esophageal pacing. Pacing the postarrest patient with HI-induced bradycardia is rarely successful.[77] Even if electrical capture of the heart is achieved, pacing does not improve contractility and myocardial blood flow.

Sodium bicarbonate administration may be considered in the patient who fails to respond to the therapy just outlined or in the patient whose response is suboptimal because of severe acidosis. The limitations of $NaHCO_3$ therapy are detailed earlier.

Asystole

Asystole is the most common pediatric arrest rhythm (Figure 8-5). Epinephrine is the drug of choice; no clinical data show that any other drug is more effective in the treatment of asystole. Optimal ventilation, oxygenation, and circulation (chest compressions) are essential and always precede drug administration. Epinephrine is given in a dose of 0.01 mg/kg (0.1 mL/kg of 1:10,000 solution) IV or 0.1 mg/kg (0.1 mL/kg of 1:1000 solution) by the ET route. If this dose is not effective after 3 to 5 minutes, 10 times the initial dose may be given.

Sodium bicarbonate has long been used in asystolic arrest, but no data support this. If it is used, the IV line

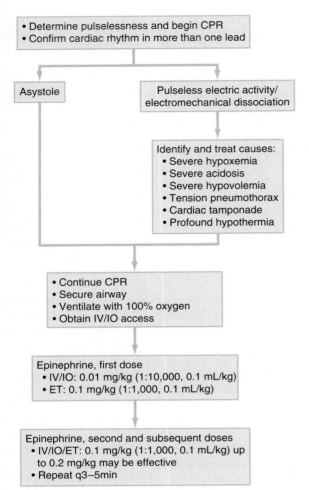

Figure 8-5. Treatment algorithm for asystole or pulseless electric activity/electromechanical dissociation. CPR, cardiopulmonary resuscitation. (Modified from Guidelines for cardiopulmonary resuscitation and emergency cardiac care. Emergency Cardiac Care Committee and Subcommittees, American Heart Association. Part VI. Pediatric advanced life support. *JAMA* 268:2262, 1992.)

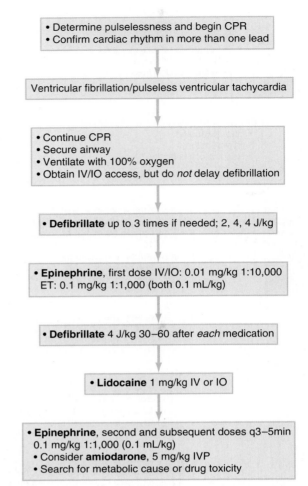

Figure 8-6. Treatment algorithm for ventricular fibrillation and pulseless ventricular tachycardia. CPR, cardiopulmonary resuscitation. (Modified from Guidelines for cardiopulmonary resuscitation and emergency cardiac care. Emergency Cardiac Care Committee and Subcommittees, American Heart Association. Part VI. Pediatric advanced life support. *JAMA* 268:2262, 1992.)

must be flushed with normal saline after $NaHCO_3$ administration to prevent precipitation with subsequent drugs. The dose of $NaHCO_3$ is 1 mEq/kg.

No evidence indicates that atropine or calcium is useful in asystolic arrest. Calcium is given only to treat documented or suspected hypocalcemia and to reverse the effects of hyperkalemia, hypermagnesemia, and calcium blocker toxicity.

Electromechanical Dissociation and Pulseless Electrical Activity

Electromechanical dissociation (EMD) is classified as a subset of PEA. PEA is a clinical state characterized by organized cardiac activity but absent pulses; EMD is characterized by narrow QRS complexes. PEA is most often seen as a wide-complex bradycardia in the postarrest setting. Drug therapy is the same as for asystole (i.e., epinephrine is the drug of choice), with an important caveat. The emergency physician must consider three correctable causes of PEA: hypovolemia, tension pneumothorax, and pericardial tamponade. When severe hypovolemia causes EMD, a narrow-complex

tachycardia or normal heart rate may be seen. Similarly, tension pneumothorax and pericardial tamponade may produce narrow-complex rhythms, particularly in the early phase of these conditions.

Ventricular Fibrillation and Pulseless Ventricular Tachycardia

VF and pulseless VT are uncommon pediatric rhythms. Electrical defibrillation (2 J/kg) is the initial treatment of choice for both rhythms (Figure 8-6). If defibrillation is unsuccessful after three attempts, epinephrine is used to manage VF for the same reason it is used in asystole: it increases coronary perfusion pressure and therefore myocardial blood flow. Augmenting myocardial blood flow helps restore myocardial cellular function and makes the heart more susceptible to subsequent defibrillation. Epinephrine should be repeated every 3 to 5 minutes as required, with subsequent doses being larger (as described for asystole).

Amiodarone is helpful in a wide range of atrial and ventricular arrhythmias. For pulseless VT/VF, a loading dose of 5 mg/kg IV may be given if defibrillation and epinephrine have not converted the rhythm. This should be followed by repeated defibrillation (4 J/kg) and ongoing CPR. Lidocaine is an alternative to amiodarone and may be given as a 1 mg/kg bolus and repeated in 10 to 15 minutes if required. If there is evidence of torsades de pointes VT, magnesium sulfate 25 to 50 mg/kg IV (maximum 2 g) should be given over 10 to 20 minutes. Again, defibrillation should occur 30 to 60 seconds after each medication, and CPR should be continued.

In pediatric patients, it is important to consider correctable causes of VT and VF. These include hypoxemia, metabolic abnormalities (e.g., hyperkalemia, hypomagnesemia, hypocalcemia), drug intoxication (e.g., cyclic antidepressant, digoxin overdose), and profound hypothermia (core temperature less than 33°C).

Defibrillation and Cardioversion

Electrical conversion of dysrhythmias on an emergent basis is rarely employed in the pediatric population. Tachydysrhythmias usually affect relatively stable patients, allowing elective drug therapy or cardioversion.

Because children vary in size, paddle sizes vary for a given patient. To improve energy delivery, the adult-size paddle should be used as soon as the child's chest permits adequate contact without the paddles touching; this typically corresponds to a weight of greater than 10 kg.[78] The interface substance from one paddle must not come in contact with the substance from the other paddle. This is most likely to occur in small children and infants, creating a short circuit and precluding energy delivery to the heart.

In infants and small children, it is sometimes difficult to have the heart interposed between the paddles when one paddle is to the right of the sternum at the second intercostal space and the other is at the left midclavicular line at the level of xiphoid process. If the infant's size precludes positioning of the heart between the paddles by this method, an anteroposterior paddle position may be used. The defibrillation dose is 2 J/kg. If this is unsuccessful, the energy dose should be doubled and attempted twice at the higher energy level. If the second attempt at the higher level is unsuccessful, epinephrine and amiodarone should be given, with attention to oxygenation and the acid-base status; increasing the energy dose further is usually not helpful.

For cardioversion of tachydysrhythmias such as atrial fibrillation or SVT, small energy doses of 0.5 to 1.0 J/kg can be used. The higher energy dose is used in the treatment of VT.

Automated external defibrillators (AEDs) are commonly used in the prehospital setting in adults and have been available to use in children older than 8 years. Recent recommendations suggest that AEDs may be used in children from 1 to 8 years who have no signs of circulation. There are insufficient data to support or recommend against AED use in infants younger than 1 year.[79]

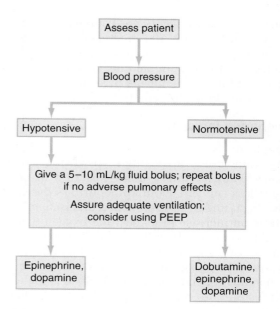

Figure 8-7. Treatment algorithm for cardiogenic (postarrest) shock. PEEP, positive end-expiratory pressure.

Postresuscitation Stabilization

After successful resuscitation, patients often require additional support to maintain a stable rhythm and improve perfusion. This section provides a practical approach to drug selection in the postresuscitation phase. The information provided is also applicable to the general management of critically ill infants and children with cardiogenic shock.

The goals of postresuscitation drug therapy are rapid restoration of adequate blood pressure and effective perfusion and correction of hypoxia and acidosis. These goals are vital to neurologic resuscitation after an HI insult. Therefore, we recommend using potent drugs initially to stabilize the patient. If the patient does well, less potent agents can be substituted. Figure 8-7 summarizes this treatment approach to postarrest stabilization by outlining the treatment plan for cardiogenic shock.

Postresuscitation patients are often poorly perfused, hypotensive, and very acidotic. After a cardiac arrest, a common reason for persistent poor perfusion is cardiogenic shock.[78] The latter results from arrest-associated myocardial ischemia. Some postarrest patients may also have poor lung compliance because of aspiration, pulmonary edema, or underlying lung pathology. Poor respiratory function complicates the ability to achieve adequate oxygenation and ventilation. In all patients, the primary focus is to ensure a stable airway and provide adequate oxygenation and ventilation.

Pharmacologic treatment of poor tissue perfusion is based on the patient's hemodynamic state as reflected by physical examination. In all patients, administration of a 20 mL/kg fluid bolus over several minutes with careful observation is reasonable; acidosis and severe shock can cause vasodilation and thus relative hypovolemia.

Three vasoactive agents are commonly used in the postarrest setting for the treatment of hypotension and poor perfusion: epinephrine, dobutamine, and dopamine. Although dopamine is often the drug of choice in adults, epinephrine by infusion is the initial treatment of choice in pediatric patients.

Epinephrine Infusion

Epinephrine is a potent vasoactive agent that effectively increases myocardial perfusion pressure. Because coronary artery disease is rare in children, there is less concern about epinephrine's dysrhythmogenic effects and the risk of myocardial ischemia resulting from an increase in myocardial oxygen demand in excess of coronary blood flow. The infusion rate of epinephrine varies from 0.05 to 1.0 μg/kg/min. An initial infusion of 0.1 μg/kg/min is a good starting dose, which can then be titrated to the desired effect. A higher starting infusion dose may be required in the hypotensive patient.

Dobutamine Infusion

Dobutamine may be an effective agent in the *normotensive* postarrest patient who remains poorly perfused. Dobutamine tends to decrease systemic vascular resistance (SVR), which is not helpful in the hypotensive patient. In children with cardiogenic shock, dobutamine increases cardiac output and decreases pulmonary wedge pressure, central venous pressure, SVR, and pulmonary vascular resistance (PVR).[80] An initial infusion of 5 μg/kg/min may be titrated to the desired effect. The normal range is 5 to 20 μg/kg/min. Dobutamine may produce hypotension and tachycardia. Hypotension may require epinephrine or epinephrine with dopamine to increase SVR.

Dopamine Infusion

Dopamine may be a limited inotropic agent in patients with poor myocardial function.[58] It has positive inotropic and chronotropic effects and tends to increase SVR and PVR, especially at the high infusion rates often required in the postarrest patient. An initial infusion of 5 to 10 μg/kg/min may be increased to 20 μg/kg/min if required for adequate blood pressure support. The advantage of dopamine when used at low infusion rates (2 to 5 μg/kg/min) is its selective effect to enhance renal and splanchnic perfusion.[81]

Caveats of Drug Infusion Therapy

Any of the vasoactive agents given at the recommended infusion rates may take 20 or more minutes to reach the patient, depending on where the infusion is connected to the IV line. Therefore, the drip should be run at 5 to 10 times the initial starting rate while the heart rate and blood pressure are carefully monitored. When the heart rate begins to increase, the drip rate is quickly decreased to the desired infusion dose. The rapid clearance of these drugs minimizes drug toxicity from the higher infusion rates as long as the rate is readjusted when a drug effect is first seen.

An alternative approach is to administer the vasoactive infusion through a Y connector, with an IV infusion flowing at a faster rate to carry the vasoactive infusion to the patient more rapidly. Although effective, this may be dangerous because an increase in the carrier infusion rate may result in a sudden bolus of a potent drug if the drug source is not controlled by an infusion pump.

Tape Measurement

To facilitate rapid weight estimation, drug dose calculation, and airway equipment selection, a length-based emergency tape system has been validated.[72,82] The *Broselow emergency tape* is based on the relationship between body length (readily measured in an emergency) and body weight (Figure 8-8A). Other length-based systems to estimate body weight for selection of pediatric resuscitation drugs and equipment have also been described.[83] The tape permits direct measurement of the patient and accurate estimation of the patient's weight when accurate weight cannot be obtained and estimations are inexact. The most recent edition of the tape, called the Rainbow tape, divides patients by color-coded zones for equipment selection and drug dosing (Broselow-Luten system) (Figure 8-8B). The cognitive burden or cognitive load associated with managing a pediatric resuscitation can be reduced by implementing such a resuscitation aid.[1,84]

FAMILY PRESENCE DURING RESUSCITATION

The presence of family members during pediatric resuscitation is an area of ongoing discussion. Surveys suggest that family members want to be present[85] and that it may help the grieving process in the event of a loved one's death.[86] Emergency department personnel have not uniformly supported this idea, however, citing medicolegal concerns, bedside teaching issues, and

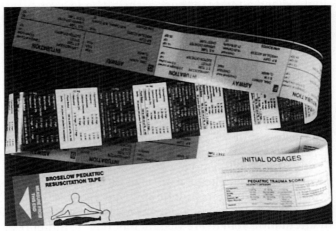

A

Figure 8-8. A, Broselow emergency tape.

GREEN

Resuscitation		Rapid sequence intubation	
		Premedications	
Epinephrine 1st dose (1:10,000)	0.33 mg/3.3 mL		
Epinephrine high dose/TT (1:1,000)	3.3 mg/3.3mL	Atropine	0.5 mg
Atropine	0.5 mg	Pan/vecuronium	
Sodium bicarbonate	33 mEq	(Defasiculating agent)	0.33 mg
Lidocaine	33 mg	Lidocaine	50 mg
Defibrillation		Fentanyl	100 mcg
First dose	66 Joules	**Induction agents**	
Second dose (may repeat)	132 Joules	Etomidate	10 mg
Cardioversion	33 Joules	Ketamine	66 mg
Adenosine		Midazolam	10 mg
1st dose	3.3 mg	Propofol	100 mg
2nd dose if needed	6.6 mg	**Paralytic agents**	
Amiodarone	165 mg	Succinylcholine	66 mg
Calcium chloride	660 mg	Pancuronium	6.6 mg
Magnesium sulfate	1650 mg	Vecuronium	6.6 mg
		Rocuronium	33 mg
		Maintenance	
		Pancuronium/vecuronium	3.3 mg
		Lorazepam	1.7 mg

30 KG	32 KG	34 KG	36 KG

GREEN

Seizure		Fluids	
Lorazepam	3.3 mg	Volume Expansion	
Diazepam IV	6.6 mg	Crystalloid (NS or LR)	660 mL
Diazepam - rectal	16.5 mg	Colloid/blood	330 mL
Phenobarbital load	660 mg	Maintenance	
Phenytoin load	500 mg	D5W + 1/4 NS + 20 meq KC/L	75 mL/HR
Fosphenytoin load	500 mg-PE	**Infusions**	
Overdose		20 mg Epi or Norepi fill to 100 mL	
Dextrose	16.5 gm	EPI . . . . at 1–10 mL/hr	
Naloxone	2 mg	NOREPI . . . . at 1–20 mL/hr	
Flumazenil	0.2 mg	200 mg Dopa or Dobut fill to 100 mL	
Glucagon	1 mg	DOPA . . . . .at 2–20 mL/hr	
Charcoal	33 gm	DOBUT . . . . .at 2–20 mL/hr	
ICP		1980 mg Lido fill to 100 mL	
Mannitol	33 gm	LIDO . . . . at 2–5 mL/hr	
Furosemide	33 mg		

Equipment

E.T. tube	6.5 Cuffed	0₂ mask	Pediatric/adult NRB
E.T. insertion length	18.5–19.5 cm	*ETCO₂	Adult
Stylet	14 French	*Urinary catheter	12 French
Suction catheter	10–12 French	*Chest tube	32–38 French
Laryngoscope	3 straight or curved	NG tube	18 French
*BVM	Adult	Vascular access	16–20 Ga
Oral airway	80 mm	Intraosseous	15 Ga
*Nasopharyngeal airway	30 French	BP cuff	Small adult
*LMA	3	*May not be included in organizer system(s).	

B

Figure 8-8.—cont'd B, Green section of the tape (front and back). The figures represent corresponding drug doses and equipment selection for patients weighing 30 to 36 kg using the Broselow-Luten system.

increased anxiety or distraction of the CPR team among the reasons for not wanting families present.[87,88] However, these concerns have not been validated in studies of family presence. The American College of Emergency Physicians supports the idea of family presence in resuscitation and encourages emergency physicians to educate staff on the option for family presence during procedures and resuscitations in the emergency department.[89] If family members are allowed to be present during a resuscitation, they should be:
1. Situated in an area that does not interfere with the resuscitation effort

2. With a member of the health care team for support and to answer questions
3. Be given the opportunity to ask questions and discuss the resuscitation efforts with the emergency physician upon completion of CPR

TERMINATION OF RESUSCITATION EFFORTS

The decision to terminate resuscitation efforts in the pediatric patient is often much more difficult than in the adult because of the emotional responses associated with the death of a child. Unfortunately, the outcome of cardiac arrest in pediatric patients is poor. Prolonged aggressive resuscitative efforts may restart the heart, but they do not restore brain function. This is particularly true if the patient has an out-of-hospital cardiac arrest.

There are limited data to guide the clinician. Studies have shown that requirements for more than two doses of epinephrine during resuscitation portend a dismal prognosis.[3,9] The application of prehospital advanced life support leading to ROSC in the field is the best predictor of survival.[10] Children who are asystolic on emergency department arrival or who experience cardiac arrest in the context of multiple trauma have a very poor prognosis.[5,10] In children with blunt trauma presenting with pulseless arrest to the emergency department, no survivors were seen in a large series.[5]

KEY CONCEPTS

- Pediatric cardiopulmonary arrest is usually a *secondary* phenomenon, most often occurring after either respiratory failure or shock. Recognition and aggressive treatment of shock and respiratory failure are key to prevention of cardiac arrest in children.
- Any drug or fluid that can be given IV can be given by the IO route.
- The *LEAN* drugs (lidocaine, epinephrine, atropine, naloxone) can be given by the ET route. ET administration of epinephrine requires about 10 times the IV dose, diluted to 5 mL or flushed with 5 mL of normal saline, and followed by three to five positive-pressure breaths.
- Administration of $NaHCO_3$ increases CO_2 production, which may worsen intracellular acidosis, even when the measured arterial pH improves. No evidence shows an improvement in outcome when $NaHCO_3$ is administered during resuscitation from cardiac arrest.
- RSI is the technique of choice for emergency airway management of the pediatric patient, with little variation from adult airway management.
- Length-based dosing and equipment selection systems facilitate pediatric resuscitation, reduce the need for error-prone dosage recall or calculation, and reduce the overall cognitive burden of the pediatric resuscitative process.

REFERENCES

1. Luten R, et al: Managing the unique size related issues of pediatric resuscitation: Reducing cognitive load with resuscitation aids. *Acad Emerg Med* 9:840, 2002.
2. Gausche M, et al: Effect of out-of hospital pediatric endotracheal intubation on survival and neurological outcome: A controlled clinical trial. *JAMA* 283:783, 2000.
3. Kyriacou DN, et al: Effect of immediate resuscitation on children with submersion injury. *Pediatrics* 94:137, 1994.
4. Mogayzel C, et al: Out-of-hospital ventricular fibrillation in children and adolescents: Causes and outcomes. *Ann Emerg Med* 25:484, 1995.
5. Hazinski MF, et al: Outcome of cardiovascular collapse in pediatric blunt trauma. *Ann Emerg Med* 23:1229, 1994.
6. Hickey RW, et al: Pediatric patients requiring CPR in the prehospital setting. *Ann Emerg Med* 25:495, 1995.
7. Teach SJ, et al: Death and resuscitation in the pediatric emergency department. *Ann Emerg Med* 25:799, 1995.
8. Schindler MB, et al: Outcome of out-of-hospital cardiac or respiratory arrest in children. *N Engl J Med* 335:1473, 1996.
9. Zaritsky A, et al: CPR in children. *Ann Emerg Med* 16:1107, 1987.
10. Ronco R, et al: Outcome and cost at a children's hospital following resuscitation for out-of-hospital cardiopulmonary arrest. *Arch Pediatr Adolesc Med* 149:210, 1995.
11. Zaritsky A, et al: Recommended guidelines for uniform reporting of pediatric advanced life support: The pediatric Utstein style. *Pediatrics* 96:765, 1995.
12. Young KD, Seidel JS: Pediatric cardiopulmonary resuscitation: A collective review. *Ann Emerg Med* 33:195, 1999.
13. Zaritsky A: Outcome of pediatric cardiopulmonary resuscitation. *Crit Care Med* 21(Suppl):S325, 1993.
14. Mejicano GC, et al: Infections acquired during cardiopulmonary resuscitation: Estimating risk and defining strategies for prevention. *Ann Intern Med* 129:813, 1998.
15. American Heart Association Subcommittee on Pediatric Resuscitation: Guidelines for pediatric advanced life support. *Circulation* 102:I-291, 2000.
16. Nadkarni V, et al: Pediatric resuscitation: An advisory statement from the Pediatric Working Group of the International Liaison Committee on Resuscitation. *Circulation* 95:2185, 1997.
17. Paradis NA, et al: Coronary perfusion pressure and the return of spontaneous circulation in human cardiopulmonary resuscitation. *JAMA* 263:1106, 1990.
18. Redberg RF, et al: Physiology of blood flow during cardiopulmonary resuscitation: A transesophageal echocardiographic study. *Circulation* 88:534, 1993.
19. Kern KB, et al: A study of chest compression rates during cardiopulmonary resuscitation in humans. *Arch Intern Med* 152:145, 1992.
20. Dean JM, et al: Improved blood flow during prolonged cardiopulmonary resuscitation with 30% duty cycle in infant pigs. *Circulation* 84:896, 1991.
21. Sack JB, et al: Survival from in-hospital cardiac arrest with interposed abdominal counterpulsation during cardiopulmonary resuscitation. *JAMA* 267:379, 1992.
22. Cohen TJ, et al: A comparison of active compression-decompression cardiopulmonary resuscitation with standard cardiopulmonary resuscitation for cardiac arrests occurring in the hospital. *N Engl J Med* 329:1918, 1993.
23. Plaisance P, et al: Benefit of active compression-decompression cardiopulmonary resuscitation as a prehospital advanced cardiac life support. *Circulation* 95:955, 1997.
24. Stiell IG, et al: The Ontario trial of active compression-decompression cardiopulmonary resuscitation for in-hospital and prehospital cardiac arrest. *JAMA* 275:1417, 1996.

25. Bartlett RH, et al: Extracorporeal life support: The University of Michigan experience. *JAMA* 283:904, 2000.

26. Posner JC, et al: Extracorporeal membrane oxygenation as a resuscitation measure in the pediatric emergency department. *Pediatr Emerg Care* 16:413, 2000.

27. Younger JG, et al: Extracorporeal resuscitation of cardiac arrest. *Acad Emerg Med* 6:700, 1999.

28. Fiser D: Intraosseous infusion. *N Engl J Med* 322:1579, 1990.

29. Fiallos M, et al: Fat embolism with the use of intraosseous infusion during cardiopulmonary resuscitation. *Am J Med Sci* 314:73, 1997.

30. Johnston C: Endotracheal drug delivery. *Pediatr Emerg Care* 8:94, 1992.

31. Jasani MS, et al: Endotracheal epinephrine administration technique effects in pediatric porcine hypoxic-hypercarbic arrest. *Crit Care Med* 22:1174, 1994.

32. Orlowski JP, Gallagher JM, Porembka DT: Endotracheal epinephrine is unreliable. *Resuscitation* 19:103, 1990.

33. Kleinman ME, et al: Comparison of intravenous and endotracheal epinephrine during cardiopulmonary resuscitation. *Crit Care Med* 12:2839, 1999.

34. Brown CG, Werman HA: Adrenergic agonists during cardiopulmonary resuscitation. *Resuscitation* 19:1, 1990.

35. Perondi M, et al: A comparison of high-dose and standard-dose epinephrine in children with cardiac arrest. *N Engl J Med* 350:1722, 2004.

36. Hazinski M (ed): *Pediatric Advanced Life Support Provider Manual.* Chicago, American Heart Association/American Academy of Pediatrics, 2002.

37. Brown CG, et al: A comparison of standard-dose and high-dose epinephrine in cardiac arrest outside the hospital. *N Engl J Med* 327:1051, 1992.

38. Hörnchen U, Christoph L, Schüttler J: Potential risks of high-dose epinephrine for resuscitation from ventricular fibrillation in a porcine model. *J Cardiothorac Vasc Anesth* 7:184, 1993.

39. Berg RA, et al: High-dose epinephrine results in greater early mortality after resuscitation from prolonged cardiac arrest in pigs: A prospective, randomized study. *Crit Care Med* 22:282, 1994.

40. Lindner KH, et al: Stress hormone response during and after cardiopulmonary resuscitation. *Anesthesiology* 77:662, 1992.

41. Lindner KH, et al: Vasopressin improves vital organ flow during closed-chest cardiopulmonary resuscitation in pigs. *Circulation* 91:215, 1995.

42. Wenzel V, et al: Survival with full neurologic recovery and no cerebral pathology after prolonged cardiopulmonary resuscitation with vasopressin in pigs. *J Am Coll Cardiol* 35:527, 2000.

43. Schwarz B, et al: Vasopressin improves survival in a pig model of hypothermic cardiopulmonary resuscitation. *Crit Care Med* 30:1311, 2002.

44. Sumann G, et al: Cardiopulmonary resuscitation after near drowning and hypothermia: Restoration of spontaneous circulation after vasopressin. *Acta Anaesthesiol Scand* 47:363, 2003.

45. Wenzel V, et al: Endobronchial vasopressin improves survival during cardiopulmonary resuscitation in pigs. *Anesthesiology* 86:1375, 1997.

46. Wenzel V, et al: Intraosseous vasopressin improves coronary perfusion rapidly during cardiopulmonary resuscitation in pigs. *Crit Care Med* 27:1565, 1999.

47. Rosenzweig EB, et al: Intravenous arginine-vasopressin in children with vasodilatory shock after cardiac surgery. *Circulation* 100(19 Suppl):182, 1999.

48. Katz K, et al: Vasopressin pressor effects in critically ill children during evaluation for brain death and organ recovery. *Resuscitation* 47:33, 2000.

49. Mann K, Berg RA, Nadkami V: Beneficial effects of vasopressin in prolonged pediatric cardiac arrest: A case series. *Resuscitation* 52:149, 2002.

50. Wenzel V, et al: A comparison of vasopressin and epinephrine for out-of-hospital cardiopulmonary resuscitation. *N Engl J Med* 350:105, 2004.

51. Nakanishi T, et al: Effect of acidosis on intracellular pH and calcium concentration in the newborn and adult rabbit myocardium. *Circ Res* 67:111, 1990.

52. Kette F, Weil MH, Gazmuri RJ: Buffer solutions may compromise cardiac resuscitation by reducing coronary perfusion pressure. *JAMA* 266:2121, 1991.

53. Gazmuri RJ, et al: Cardiac effects of carbon dioxide–consuming and carbon dioxide–generating buffers during cardiopulmonary resuscitation. *J Am Coll Cardiol* 15:482, 1990.

54. Losek J: Hypoglycemia and the ABC'S (sugar) of pediatric resuscitation. *Ann Emerg Med* 35:43, 2000.

55. Sieber FE, Traystman RJ: Special issues: Glucose and the brain. *Crit Care Med* 20:104, 1992.

56. Goetting MG, Contereas E: Systemic atropine administration during cardiac arrest does not cause fixed and dilated pupils. *Ann Emerg Med* 20:55, 1991.

57. Singhi SC, Singh J, Prasad R: Hypocalcaemia in a paediatric intensive care unit. *J Trop Pediatr* 49:298, 2003.

58. Zaritsky AL: Resuscitation pharmacology. In Chernow B (ed): *The Pharmacologic Approach to the Critically Ill Patient.* Baltimore, Williams & Wilkins, 1994.

59. Brown CG, et al: The effect of intravenous magnesium administration on aortic, right atrial and coronary perfusion pressures during CPR in swine. *Resuscitation* 26:3, 1993.

60. Bertolet BD, Hill JA: Adenosine: Diagnostic and therapeutic uses in cardiovascular medicine. *Chest* 104:1860, 1993.

61. Losek JD, et al. Adenosine and pediatric supraventricular tachycardia in the emergency department: Multicenter study and review. *Ann Emerg Med* 33:185, 1999.

62. Kudenchuk PJ, et al: Amiodarone for resuscitation after out-of-hospital cardiac arrest due to ventricular fibrillation. *N Engl J Med* 341:871,1999.

63. Perry JC, et al: Pediatric use of intravenous amiodarone: Efficacy and safety in critically ill patients from a multicenter protocol. *J Am Coll Cardiol* 27:1246,1996.

64. Perry JC, et al: Intravenous amiodarone for life-threatening tachyarrhythmias in children and young adults. *J Am Coll Cardiol* 22:95, 1993.

65. Figa FH, et al: Clinical efficacy and safety of intravenous amiodarone in infants and children. *Am J Cardiol* 74:573, 1994.

66. Mazic U, Berden P, Podnar T: Repetitive paroxysms of supraventricular tachyarrhythmias triggered during pediatric cardiac interventions: Suppression after short infusion of amiodarone. *Pediatr Cardiol* Jan 28, 2004. [Epub ahead of print]

67. Burri S, et al: Efficacy and safety of intravenous amiodarone for incessant tachycardias in infants. *Eur J Pediatr* 162:880, 2003.

68. Etheridge S, et al: Amiodarone is safe and highly effective therapy for supraventricular tachycardia in infants. *Am Heart J* 141:105, 2001.

69. Laird W, et al: Use of intravenous amiodarone for postoperative junctional ectopic tachycardia in children. *Pediatr Cardiol* 24:133, 2003.

70. Strasburger J, et al: Amiodarone therapy for drug-refractory fetal tachycardia. *Circulation* 109:375, 2004.

71. Roden DM: Antiarrhythmic drugs. In Hardman JG et al (eds): *Goodman and Gilman's the Pharmacological Basis of Therapeutics*, 10th ed. New York, McGraw-Hill, 2001, pp 933-970.

72. Luten RC, et al: Length-based endotracheal tube and emergency equipment in pediatrics. *Ann Emerg Med* 21:900, 1992.

73. Bhende MS, Thompson AE: Evaluation of an end-tidal CO_2 detector during pediatric cardiopulmonary resuscitation. *Pediatrics* 95:395, 1995.

74. Ornato JP, Garrett AR, Glauser FL: Relationship between cardiac output and the end-tidal carbon dioxide tension. *Ann Emerg Med* 19:1104, 1992.

75. Coté CJ, et al: Cricothyroid membrane puncture: Oxygenation and ventilation in a dog model using an intravenous catheter. *Crit Care Med* 16:615, 1988.

76. Bellomo R, et al: Asthma requiring mechanical ventilation: A low morbidity approach. *Chest* 105:891, 1994.

77. Quan L, et al: Transcutaneous cardiac pacing in the treatment of out-of-hospital pediatric cardiac arrests. *Ann Emerg Med* 21:905, 1992.

78. Atkins DL, Kerber RE: Pediatric defibrillation: Current flow is improved by using "adult" electrode paddles. *Pediatrics* 94:90, 1994.

79. Samson R, et al: Use of automated external defibrillators for children: An update—An Advisory Statement from the Pediatric Advanced Life Support Task Force, International Liaison Committee on Resuscitation. *Pediatrics* 112:163, 2003.

80. Martinez AM, Padbury JF, Thio S: Dobutamine pharmacokinetics and cardiovascular responses in critically ill neonates. *Pediatrics* 89:47, 1992.

81. Zaritsky AL: Catecholamines, inotropic medications, and vasopressor agents. In Chernow B (ed): *The Pharmacologic Approach to the Critically Ill Patient.* Baltimore, Williams & Wilkins, 1994.

82. Lubitz DS, et al: A rapid method for estimating weight and resuscitation drug dosages from length in the pediatric age group. *Ann Emerg Med* 17:576, 1988.

83. Garland A, et al: A rapid and accurate method of estimating body weight. *Am J Emerg Med* 4:390, 1986.

84. Shah AN, et al: Reduction in error severity associated with use of a pediatric medication dosing system: A crossover trial involving simulated resuscitation events. *Arch Pediatr Adolesc Med* 157:229, 2003.

85. Boie E, et al: Do parents want to be present during invasive procedures performed on their children in the emergency department? A survey of 400 parents. *Ann Emerg Med* 34:70,1999.

86. Robinson S, et al: Psychological effect of witnessed resuscitation on bereaved relatives. *Lancet* 352:614, 1998.

87. Sacchetti A, et al: Acceptance of family members presence during pediatric resuscitations in the emergency department: Effects of personal experience. *Pediatr Emerg Care* 16:85, 2000.

88. McClenathan B, et al: Family member presence during cardiopulmonary resuscitation. A survey of US and international critical care professionals. *Chest* 122:2204, 2002.

89. American College of Emergency Physicians Policy Statement: The role of emergency physicians in the care of children, June 2001 (www.acep.org).

CHAPTER

9 Neonatal Resuscitation

Eileen Klein and Linda Quan

PERSPECTIVE

Approximately 6% of all newborns require some resuscitative assistance at delivery.[1] Appropriate equipment and preparation, knowledge of neonatal physiology and response to stress, and skill in performing necessary procedures in managing these infants are essential to successful resuscitation. Preparation for neonatal resuscitation requires an understanding of how it differs from pediatric and adult resuscitation, as follows:

1. Newborns have rapidly changing cardiopulmonary physiology, their own range of normal vital signs (Table 9-1), and unique responses to stress.[1,2]

2. The approach to newborn resuscitation focuses almost *entirely* on respiratory, not cardiac, management.

3. Equipment needs are specific owing to the infant's size.

PATHOPHYSIOLOGY

Transition from Fetal to Extrauterine Life

The successful transition from the fetal to the extrauterine environment requires two major cardiorespiratory changes: (1) removal of fluid from unexpanded alveoli to allow ventilation and (2) redistribution of cardiac output to provide lung perfusion. Failure of the development of either adequate ventilation or adequate perfusion leads to shunting, hypoxia, and ultimately reversion to fetal physiology.[1]

In utero, the pulmonary alveoli are filled with pulmonary fluid. Removal of this fluid is partially accomplished by vaginal delivery, which compresses the fluid into the bronchi, trachea, and pulmonary capillary bed. Most pulmonary fluid is removed by the first few breaths; the amount of fluid removed depends on the

Table 9-1. Normal Vital Signs in the Newborn

Weight	Heart rate (beats/min)	Respiratory rate (breaths/min)	Systolic blood pressure (mm Hg, mean)
≥3 kg (full term)	>100 (100-180)	40-80	60-70 (45-55)
<3 kg (premature)	>100 (100-180)	40-80	40-60 (35-45)

forcefulness of these breaths. Expansion of alveoli requires the generation of high intrathoracic pressures and the presence of surfactant to maintain alveolar patency. The quality of the first few breaths is crucial to the establishment of adequate ventilation.

The fetal lung is poorly perfused. Because the pulmonary arterial bed is intensely vasoconstricted, the fetal lung receives only 40% of the right ventricular cardiac output; most of the right ventricular output is shunted from the pulmonary artery through the ductus arteriosus to the descending aorta. After the first few breaths, with exposure to diffused alveolar oxygen, pulmonary vascular resistance decreases. The fetal shunt through the ductus arteriosus reverses as systemic vascular resistance increases, then the shunt ceases by 15 hours of age as the ductus also constricts. This reversal of flow allows all right ventricular output to perfuse the lungs. If hypoxia or severe acidosis occurs, however, the muscular pulmonary vascular bed constricts again, and the ductus may reopen. The reinstitution of fetal circulation, with its attendant shunting, leads to ongoing hypoxia and is termed *persistent fetal circulation*. The role of the resuscitator is to facilitate the first few breaths, prevent and reverse ongoing hypoxia and acidosis, and assist the newborn in the transition to extrauterine life.

Neonatal Responses

Hypoxia

The newborn's clinical response to severe hypoxia is unique.[3] In utero or intrapartum asphyxia (pathologic lack of oxygen to the fetus before or during delivery) precipitates a sequence of events termed *primary apnea* and *secondary apnea*. After initial hypoxia, the infant has rapid gasping, followed by cessation of respirations (primary apnea) and a decreasing heart rate. At this point, only simple stimulation and oxygen are needed to reverse bradycardia and assist the development of ventilation. With ongoing asphyxia, however, the infant takes several final deep, gasping respirations, followed by secondary apnea, worsening bradycardia, and decreasing blood pressure. More vigorous and prolonged resuscitation is needed to restore ventilation and an adequate circulation. Apnea in the newborn should be assumed to be secondary apnea and treated rapidly with ventilatory assistance.

The presence of respirations *may not* ensure adequate ventilation. In addition, signs of hypoxia (e.g., cyanosis, lethargy, unresponsiveness) may have other causes. Bradycardia in the newborn (heart rate <100 beats/min) almost always reflects inadequate ventilation and oxygenation. *Bradycardia is a major indicator of hypoxia.*[4-6]

Hypothermia

The newborn's inability to maintain body temperature (36.5° C to 37° C) has severe physiologic consequences. The newborn cannot generate heat by shivering, cannot retain heat because of low fat stores, and has a relatively large surface-to-volume area. In addition, the newborn is at risk for heat loss because of a high metabolic rate, wet amniotic fluid covering, and exposure to a relatively cool environment, especially in contrast to intrauterine temperature. The body temperature easily decreases, and low body temperatures can lead to metabolic acidosis, increased oxygen consumption, hypoglycemia, and apnea.[1,7] Hypothermia may have a protective effect in an asphyxiated infant. Some studies have suggested that selective cerebral hypothermia in asphyxiated infants may protect against brain injury, but there is not enough evidence to implement such a therapy until further study is performed.[8] Current recommendations are to avoid hypothermia in the newborn infant.[9-11]

Hypoglycemia

The newborn is at risk for developing hypoglycemia (defined as glucose level <40 mg/dL if >2.5 kg or <30 mg/dL if <2.5 kg) when stressed because of poor glycogen stores and immature liver enzymes. Hypoglycemia is common in premature or small-for-gestational-age infants and infants born to diabetic mothers. It also develops in response to respiratory illness, hypothermia, asphyxia, and sepsis. Hypoglycemia may be asymptomatic or may cause an array of symptoms, including apnea, color changes, respiratory distress, lethargy, jitteriness, seizures, acidosis, and poor myocardial contractility.[12]

INDICATIONS FOR RESUSCITATION

Any infant born outside of the controlled environment of the delivery room should be considered to need resuscitation.[13] Minimal intervention may be required, but a standardized approach as described in this chapter should be used. Specific conditions increase the likelihood that resuscitation will be required. Premature infants pose a special problem because of immature lungs and susceptibility to hypothermia. Adequate ventilation and warming are essential to a successful resuscitation.

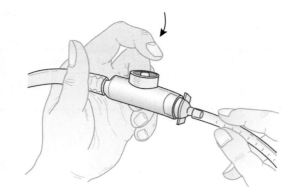

Figure 9-1. One form of adapter (meconium aspirator) placed between endotracheal tube and suction tubing. (From Chameides L, Hazinski MF (eds): *Textbook of Pediatric Advanced Life Support*. Dallas, American Heart Association, 1994.)

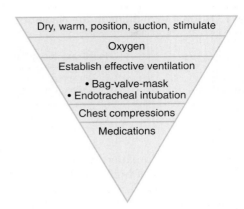

Figure 9-2. Inverted pyramid reflecting relative frequencies of neonatal resuscitation efforts for a newborn who does not have meconium-stained amniotic fluid. Most newborns respond to simple measures. (From Chameides L, Hazinski MF (eds): *Textbook of Pediatric Advanced Life Support*. Dallas, American Heart Association, 1994.)

The presence of meconium in the amniotic fluid at delivery indicates that the infant has been stressed before delivery and poses a special problem in resuscitation. All infants with meconium should have their nose and mouth suctioned at the perineum before full delivery. When delivered, a nonvigorous infant with meconium in the amniotic fluid must have the trachea suctioned before other steps in resuscitation to prevent aspiration of meconium.

Medications given to the mother or illicit drugs taken before delivery can lead to respiratory depression in the newborn. Maternal opioid administration or opioid use should be considered in any newborn with isolated respiratory depression. Naloxone reverses respiratory depression caused by opioids, although its use may precipitate acute withdrawal in infants who have prolonged intrauterine exposure.[14] Support of ventilation may be preferable to reversal using naloxone.

Hemorrhage caused by abruptio placentae, placenta previa, trauma, or other complications can lead to respiratory depression and shock. Hemorrhage is one of the few situations in which fluid resuscitation is required.

No reliable set of parameters identifies newborns who would *not* benefit from resuscitative efforts.[15] Current recommendations for infants in whom not initiating resuscitation may be appropriate include neonates with confirmed gestational age less than 23 weeks; neonates with weight of less than 400 g; and neonates with confirmed anencephaly, trisomy 13, or trisomy 18.[9,10] In the out-of-hospital setting or in the emergency department, every attempt should be made to stabilize the neonate until it is clear that attempted or continued resuscitation would not improve the patient's chance of survival. Discontinuation of resuscitative efforts may be appropriate after 15 minutes because a newborn with cardiac arrest and failure of return of spontaneous circulation after 15 minutes of resuscitation is unlikely to survive.[9,10]

Few situations require deviations from the approach described here. The presence of meconium is common and requires intervention to prevent aspiration. Other anatomic anomalies require special care and include diaphragmatic hernia, meningomyelocele, abdominal anomalies (e.g., gastroschisis, omphalocele), and upper airway obstructive lesions (e.g., bilateral choanal atresia, Pierre Robin syndrome).

SPECIFIC DISORDERS

Meconium Aspiration

Meconium in the amniotic fluid is a sign of in utero distress, and the presence of thick or particulate meconium before or at delivery immediately should raise concern about the potential for aspiration. Aspiration of meconium and its consequences can be avoided by aggressive intervention to avoid aspiration. Intervention should begin when the neonate is still at the perineum. As soon as the infant's head is delivered, the mouth and the nose should be suctioned. Immediately after delivery of the body, the infant should be positioned on the radiant warmer and assessed. Recommendations for the need for endotracheal intubation with tracheal suctioning after delivery of the infant should be made based on the vigor of the infant, rather than on the consistency of the meconium (e.g., thick or particulate versus thin). Infants with meconium-stained fluid and with any of the following are candidates for tracheal suctioning: (1) absent or depressed respirations, (2) poor muscle tone, or (3) heart rate less than 100 beats/min.[9-11] In such newborns, a meconium aspirator should be attached to the endotracheal tube (ETT) and connected to wall suction at 100 mm Hg or less (Figure 9-1). The ETT is withdrawn as suction is being applied. The ETT with meconium aspirator serves as the ideal suction catheter. Because of its narrower width, a suction catheter placed in the ETT does *not* suction meconium effectively. Reintubation and suction should be repeated until the meconium clears. Two passes are usually sufficient. When these steps are completed, the resuscitation should continue, beginning with the steps at the top of the inverted pyramid (Figure 9-2).

Anatomic Anomalies

The neonate should be intubated immediately if there has been a prenatal diagnosis of diaphragmatic hernia or if a diaphragmatic hernia is diagnosed on chest radiograph. Bag/mask ventilation distends the stomach and worsens respiratory distress because of the presence of the stomach in the chest cavity.

Infants with meningomyelocele should not be placed on their backs to avoid pressure on the defect, but on their stomachs or sides. The resuscitation should be conducted in this position if possible. The spinal defect should be covered with warm sterile gauze pads soaked in warm sterile saline and covered with a plastic covering. Infants with gastroschisis or omphalocele should be resuscitated as needed; as in patients with meningomyelocele, the defect should be covered with an occlusive plastic covering to decrease water and heat loss.

Because newborns are obligate nose breathers, bilateral choanal atresia causes upper airway obstruction and respiratory distress. It is diagnosed by the inability to pass a catheter through either naris into the oropharynx. An oral airway bypasses the obstruction. Patients with Pierre Robin syndrome have small jaws and large tongues leading to upper airway obstruction. A nasal or oral airway should be able to bypass the obstruction; if not, intubation may be necessary. It is technically difficult to intubate a patient with Pierre Robin anomaly, and an anesthesiologist may be needed.

PREPARATION

To maximize effectiveness of the resuscitation, the emergency department should have a prestocked drug pack, standardized equipment (Box 9-1), and staff familiar with newborn resuscitation.[3,10,15,16] The pediatric Broselow Emergency Tape has a section for infants weighing greater than or equal to 3 kg that can be used to determine equipment size and drug dosages for newborn resuscitation.

It is crucial to use universal precautions and to wear gown, gloves, and eye protection during neonatal resuscitation. For adequate preparation, the heat source must be turned on early, and the resuscitation table must be warm when the newborn is placed on it. Equipment of proper size is essential, especially respiratory equipment because it is most likely to be used, and ventilation is the key to most resuscitative efforts. Appropriate-size bag/masks decrease complications from overventilation and prevent injury or inability to ventilate because of improper mask fit.

If available, additional information may be helpful in preparing for resuscitation (Box 9-2). The estimated gestational age provides information about possible prematurity and associated complications. Multiple births require more equipment and personnel, and the newborns are at greater risk for prematurity and its complications. Meconium present in the amniotic fluid may require suctioning of the neonate's trachea to prevent aspiration of meconium. A history of vaginal

> ### BOX 9-1. Equipment Needed for Neonatal Resuscitation
>
> 1. Gown, gloves, and eye protection (universal precautions)
> 2. Blankets (to warm and dry infant)
> 3. Radiant warmer
> 4. Bulb syringe
> 5. Suction and suction catheters (5 F, 8 F, and 10 F)
> 6. Self-inflating bags (450 and 750 mL)
> 7. Masks (premature, newborn, and infant sizes)
> 8. Laryngoscope with straight blades (numbers 0 and 1)
> 9. Endotracheal tubes with stylets (2.5, 3, and 3.5 mm)
> 10. Scissors and tape to stabilize endotracheal tube
> 11. Meconium aspirator
> 12. Umbilical catheters (3.5 F and 5 F)
> 13. Hemostats, sterile drapes and gloves, povidone-iodine solution, scalpel, umbilical tape, suture, and three-way stopcock for umbilical vessel catheterization

> ### BOX 9-2. Maternal History Questions
>
> 1. What is the estimated gestational age?
> 2. Is this a multiple gestation?
> 3. Is meconium present?
> 4. Is there a history of vaginal bleeding?
> 5. Were medications given or drugs taken?

bleeding increases the likelihood of hypovolemic shock and respiratory distress in the newborn. A history of medication administration or drug use may provide clues to the cause of respiratory depression in the neonate.

MANAGEMENT

An organized approach is key to successful resuscitation outside and inside the delivery room. The American Heart Association describes the inverted pyramid in the *Textbook of Pediatric Advanced Life Support* (see Figure 9-2), showing the steps of resuscitation and the relative frequency with which each step is required.[17] These steps are discussed in this section and follow the guidelines of the American Heart Association and American Academy of Pediatrics.[3,17,18]

Dry, Warm, Position, Suction, Stimulate, Assess Need for Further Intervention

To prevent complications caused by hypothermia, all newborns except infants with meconium present immediately should be dried off and placed under a radiant heat source. Wet blankets should be replaced after drying with dry, preferably warm blankets. Currently there is inadequate evidence that selective cerebral hypothermia protects against brain injury in

Table 9-2. Apgar Score

Sign	0	1	2
Heart rate (beats/min)	Absent	Slow (<100)	>100
Respirations	Absent	Slow, irregular	Good, crying
Muscle tone	Limp	Some flexion	Active, good flexion
Reflex irritability	No response	Grimace	Cough, sneeze
Color	Blue, pale	Pink body, blue hands/feet	Pink

asphyxiated infants, although studies are ongoing.[9-11] Current recommendations include the avoidance of hypothermia. Next, the neonate should be positioned to attain maximal air entry and avoid obstruction of airflow. Because of the infant's relatively large occiput and anterior airway, an open airway is best achieved with the neck in slight extension. The slightly extended position is best accomplished by placing a rolled diaper or small towel *under the infant's shoulders.* Placement under the neck is not useful, and a towel that is too large and under the shoulders leads to hyperextension at the neck and possible airway occlusion.

Ideally the infant's airway should be suctioned initially while on the perineum during delivery. This suctioning is especially important when meconium is present. With meconium and the presence of poor respirations, poor tone, or bradycardia (heart rate <100 beats/min), the trachea should be suctioned with an ETT before any other intervention. If no meconium is present, the newborn may be suctioned with bulb or mechanical suction (<100 mm Hg wall suction). The mouth should be suctioned first, followed by the nose. The mouth is suctioned first to avoid aspiration of material if the infant takes in a breath after suctioning of the nose. Vigorous or deep suctioning can lead to a vagal response, with subsequent bradycardia, or to apnea and should be avoided.[19]

Usually these measures adequately stimulate the infant to breathe effectively and may be the only measures needed to resuscitate a newborn. If adequate respirations are not present at this point, stimulation of the infant is needed; this is best done by flicking the soles of the feet and rubbing the back. It is important to avoid stimulation that is too vigorous because it does not aid in initiation of respirations and may stress the newborn. If stimulation is not effective in initiating respirations, bag/mask ventilation is required followed by intubation if necessary.

The Apgar score, comprising heart rate, respiratory effort, muscle tone, reflex irritability, and color, has been used as a prognostic indicator in newborns (Table 9-2). The Apgar score is not useful in resuscitation management.[20] Muscle tone and reflex irritability do not aid in the assessment of the newborn during resuscitation.[20] Heart rate, respiratory effort, and color are the important indicators of hypoxia and should be monitored continuously. Further resuscitative efforts are required if respiratory effort is insufficient, heart rate is less than 100 beats/min, or central cyanosis is present.

Oxygen, Ventilation, Intubation

Any infant who is cyanotic or appears to be in respiratory distress (grunting, nasal flaring, tachypnea) should be given 100% oxygen. If the infant is apneic, appears to be in severe respiratory distress, has a heart rate of less than 100 beats/min, or has central cyanosis despite oxygen administration, bag/valve/mask ventilation (with a manometer, if available) should be initiated. Although resuscitation with 100% oxygen is recommended, more recent studies support the effectiveness of room air if 100% oxygen is not available for bag/valve/mask ventilation.[9,10,21] The initial breaths require higher pressure (30 to 40 mm Hg) to remove lung fluid. Subsequent breaths generally require 20 mm Hg. In addition to heart rate and color, one of the best indicators of adequate ventilation is chest wall movement, which should be observed during efforts at ventilation.[3] An appropriate-size mask with a good seal (covering the mouth and nose, but not the eyes), proper positioning of the infant, and use of appropriate pressure to attain chest wall movement are essential for effective ventilation. The newborn should be bagged at 40 breaths/min, unless blood gases dictate otherwise. If bag/valve/mask ventilation is required for more than 2 minutes, an orogastric tube should be placed to prevent respiratory compromise from stomach distention.[3]

Endotracheal intubation is indicated for prolonged positive-pressure ventilation or the inability to bag effectively because of facial or other anatomic anomalies (e.g., diaphragmatic hernia). The presence of thick or particulate meconium is an indication for immediate endotracheal intubation and tracheal suctioning. Box 9-1 lists the equipment needed for endotracheal intubation. Confirmation of proper ETT placement should include detection of expired carbon dioxide. Currently data are insufficient to recommend the use of the esophageal detector device as a tool to confirm tracheal intubation in the neonate.[22]

Acute deterioration (bradycardia, decreased oxygen saturation) after intubation should suggest one of the following problems (*DOPE*)[17]:

1. *D*islodgment: The ETT is no longer in the trachea (right main stem bronchus or esophagus).
2. *O*bstruction: Secretions are obstructing airflow through the ETT.
3. *P*neumothorax
4. *E*quipment: Oxygen is not being delivered to the patient (check equipment).

If the patient acutely deteriorates after intubation, the equipment should be checked quickly; if no explanation is obvious, the patient should be extubated and ventilated with bag/valve/mask. Time should not be wasted adjusting or suctioning the ETT if the patient is bradycardic. If unequal breath sounds are present after extubation, or if the patient is not improving with effective ventilation, needle aspiration of the chest should be considered for treatment of a possible pneumothorax.

Table 9-3. Resuscitation Medications

Medication	Concentration	Dose	Route	Considerations
Oxygen	100%		Blowby, ET	
Epinephrine	1:10,000	0.01-0.03 mg/kg (0.1-0.3 mL/kg)	IV, ET	
Naloxone	0.4 mg/mL	0.1 mg/kg (0.25 mL/kg)	IV, ET, IM, SC	
Glucose	D10W	2-4 mL/kg	IV	Avoid higher concentrations
Volume expanders	Whole blood Normal saline Ringer's lactate 5% albumin/saline	10 mL/kg	IV	Give over 5-10 min; repeat as needed 5% albumin/saline no longer recommended for use during initial resuscitation efforts
Dopamine	60 × wt (kg) = amount in mg per 100 mL Then 0.1 mL/hr = 1 µg/kg/min If 6 × wt, 1 mL/hr = 1 µg/kg/min		Continuous IV infusion at 5 µg/kg/min Increase to 20 µg/kg/min as needed	

ET, endotracheal; IV, intravenous; IM, intramuscular; SC, subcutaneous; D10W, 10% dextrose in water.

The laryngeal mask airway has been touted as a possible adjunct for neonatal resuscitation.[23] Use of the laryngeal mask airway is controversial, however, and experience is insufficient to recommend it for neonatal resuscitation at this time, although it may be an appropriate alternative to the ETT in a full-term newborn.[10,23]

Chest Compressions

Bradycardia (heart rate <100 beats/min) is the major indicator of hypoxia. Most infants respond promptly to effective ventilation with 100% oxygen. If a neonate has a heart rate of less than 60 beats/min despite oxygen and adequate ventilation (good air movement and chest rise) for at least 30 seconds, chest compressions also should be provided.[10] Chest compressions should be performed at a rate of 90/min, with 30 breaths/min for a total of 120 events/min. The two methods of performing chest compressions are as follows:

1. The fingers of both hands encircle the chest and support the back. The thumbs of both hands are placed side by side or one over the other on the sternum just below the nipple line.
2. The ring and middle fingers of one hand are placed on the sternum just below the nipple line with the other hand supporting the infant's back. The depth of compression is one third the anteroposterior diameter of the chest.

The pulse rate with compressions (to assess adequacy of compressions) and the spontaneous pulse rate should be checked frequently. Chest compressions may be discontinued when the spontaneous pulse rate is greater than 60 beats/min.[10]

Medications

Few neonates require the use of medications during resuscitation. Medications are indicated for bradycardia or asystole that does not respond to effective ventilation and chest compressions and hemorrhage (maternal, fetal, or placental) that requires fluid resuscitation.[24] Naloxone may be needed for respiratory depression caused by maternal ingestion of opioids before delivery.

The only medications that should be used during the early phase of neonatal resuscitation are oxygen, epinephrine, and volume expanders (Table 9-3). Albumin has been removed as an initial resuscitation drug but may be used afterward. Dopamine should be reserved for prolonged resuscitation. Naloxone should be used only after the neonate is adequately ventilated. Sodium bicarbonate should not be used in most resuscitations; it may be beneficial in the rare instance of a prolonged resuscitation when metabolic acidosis has been documented and ventilation is adequate.[25] No current evidence supports the use of atropine or calcium in neonatal resuscitation.

Vascular access is a challenge in neonatal resuscitation. The preferred route of immediate vascular access is the umbilical vein because it is easily identified and cannulated. Because of potentially serious complications (infection, portal vein thrombosis), the umbilical vein cannula should be removed immediately after stabilization after other access (e.g., umbilical artery catheterization) has been attained. Other routes include peripheral veins and the femoral vein. Intraosseous access can be problematic in neonates (especially premature infants) because of bone fragility and the small size of the intraosseous space.[10] If access cannot be achieved, many resuscitation drugs (e.g., lidocaine, epinephrine, naloxone) can be given through the ETT, with dosages the same as for intravenous administration. The medication should be diluted to a total volume of 2 mL and injected directly into the ETT, followed by several positive-pressure ventilations.[3,17]

Oxygen

The first resuscitation medication that should be used is 100% oxygen. Indications for oxygen use include central cyanosis and respiratory distress (nasal flaring, grunting, tachypnea, apnea).

Epinephrine

Epinephrine is indicated for asystole and for heart rate less than 60 beats/min despite effective ventilation with 100% oxygen and chest compressions. Epinephrine may be given intravenously or by ETT. The dose is 0.01 to 0.03 mg/kg or 0.1 to 0.3 mL/kg of 1:10,000 solution. Repeat doses may be given every 3 to 5 minutes.[10,26,27] Given the lack of data for its use and possible complications (e.g., intracranial hemorrhage), high-dose epinephrine cannot be recommended at this time, even through the ETT.[10]

Naloxone

Respiratory depression induced by opioids given or taken within 3 to 4 hours of delivery can be reversed with naloxone. If respiratory depression is present, and if it is unclear whether the mother took opioids before delivery, reversal with naloxone may be attempted. The dose is 0.1 mg/kg by ETT, intravenously, intramuscularly, or subcutaneously. The duration of action of naloxone is 1 to 4 hours depending on route of administration. Repeat dosing may be necessary, and the patient should be monitored carefully. Naloxone is not always needed in a newborn with respiratory depression. It may precipitate withdrawal seizures in an infant born to a drug-addicted mother.[26] The priority of care is support with bag/valve/mask and intubation if necessary. Naloxone should be considered only after ventilatory support is achieved.

Glucose

Hypoglycemia should *always* be considered in a neonate undergoing resuscitation. Hypoglycemia is diagnosed with a rapid bedside glucose or serum glucose measurement. Treatment is indicated only for documented hypoglycemia: glucose less than 40 mg/dL in a full-term infant (>2.5 kg) and less than 30 mg/dL in a premature infant (<2.5 kg). Hypoglycemia is treated with 2 to 4 mL/kg of 10% dextrose in water. Higher concentrations of glucose (e.g., 25% dextrose in water) are hyperosmolar and should be avoided. Repeat glucose measurement should be obtained 10 to 20 minutes after glucose administration.

Volume Expanders

Volume expanders are indicated when acute bleeding is evident with signs of hypovolemia (pallor despite oxygenation, weak pulses with a good heart rate, poor response to resuscitation), or the newborn appears to be in shock.[9,10] Volume expanders include whole blood (O-negative blood crossmatched with the mother's blood), normal saline, or Ringer's lactate solution. Whole blood is preferred in the setting of significant blood loss but may be difficult to obtain quickly. Normal saline and Ringer's lactate (e.g., isotonic crystalloid solutions) should be readily available and may be considered the fluid of choice overall for volume expansion. Expanders are given in small intravenous boluses of 10 mL/kg over 5 to 10 minutes. Higher volume bolus volumes are recommended for older infants (e.g., 20 mL/kg). Boluses may be repeated several times, guided by patient assessment. The use of albumin 5% with saline is currently not recommended for the initial resuscitation.

Dopamine

Dopamine is indicated only when signs of shock (e.g., poor peripheral perfusion, thready pulses) still are present despite adequate volume replacement. Given as a continuous infusion beginning at 5 µg/kg/min, dopamine may be increased to 20 µg/kg/min as necessary (see Table 9-3 for method of preparation).

DISPOSITION

Early consultation with a neonatologist can assist in the resuscitation and postresuscitation phases of care. When the neonate has been stabilized, monitoring of oxygenation, ventilation, perfusion, temperature, and glucose must continue. Preparations should be made for transport of the newborn to a neonatal intensive care unit. A transport team with personnel skilled in neonatal resuscitation should be employed. Ideally, before transport, parents should see and touch (and hold if medically appropriate) their newborn.

 KEY CONCEPTS

- The necessary equipment must be readily available for neonatal resuscitation in the emergency department.
- Preparation is most effective with an adequate maternal and prenatal history.
- The inverted pyramid for neonatal resuscitation provides a guide for management.
- Drying, warming, positioning, and stimulating the infant are usually sufficient resuscitative measures in most deliveries.
- Endotracheal suctioning for neonates at risk for meconium aspiration is reserved for nonvigorous infants after suctioning of the mouth and nose at the perineum.
- Transport of the neonate to an neonatal intensive care unit allows continued management.

REFERENCES

1. Avery ME, Treusch HW (eds): *Schaffer's Diseases of the Newborn.* Philadelphia, WB Saunders, 1984.
2. Hodson WA, Truog WE: *Critical Care of the Newborn.* Philadelphia, WB Saunders, 1989.
3. Bloom RS, Cropley C, AHA/AAP Neonatal Resuscitation Program Steering Committee: *Textbook of Neonatal Resuscitation.* Elk Grove Village, Ill, American Academy of Pediatrics, 1994.
4. Anderson RH, et al: *Paediatric Cardiology.* London, Churchill Livingstone, 1987.
5. Long WA: *Fetal and Neonatal Cardiology.* Philadelphia, WB Saunders, 1990.
6. Emmanouilides GC, Baylen BG: *Neonatal Cardiopulmonary Distress.* Chicago, Year Book Medical Publishers, 1988.
7. Jain L, Vidyasagar D: Cardiopulmonary resuscitation of newborns: Its application to transport medicine. *Pediatr Clin North Am* 40:287, 1993.
8. Gunn AJ: Cerebral hypothermia for prevention of brain injury following perinatal asphyxia. *Curr Opin Pediatr* 12:111, 2000.

9. Niermeyer S, et al: Resuscitation in newborns. *Ann Emerg Med* 37:S110, 2001.
10. Kattwinkel J, et al: ILCOR advisory statement: Resuscitation of the newly born infant. *Pediatrics* 103:1, 1999 (URL: http://www.pediatrics.org/cgi/content/full/103/4/e56).
11. Anonymous: Guidelines 2000 for cardiopulmonary resuscitation and emergency cardiovascular care. Part 11: Neonatal resuscitation. The American Heart Association in collaboration with the International Liaison Committee on Resuscitation. *Circulation* 102(8 Suppl):I343, 2000.
12. Yeh TF: *Neonatal Therapeutics*. St Louis, Mosby, 1991.
13. Boychuk RB: The critically ill neonate in the emergency department. *Emerg Med Clin North Am* 9:507, 1991.
14. Landwirth J: Ethical issues in pediatric and neonatal resuscitation. *Ann Emerg Med* 22:502, 1993.
15. American Heart Association Emergency Cardiac Care Committee and subcommittees: Neonatal resuscitation. *JAMA* 268:2276, 1992.
16. Khan NS, Luten RC: Neonatal resuscitation. *Emerg Med Clin North Am* 12:239, 1994.
17. Chameides L, Hazinski MF (eds): *Textbook of Pediatric Advanced Life Support*. Dallas, American Heart Association, 2002.
18. Kattwinkel J, et al (eds): *Textbook of Neonatal Resuscitation*, 4th ed. Elk Grove Village, Ill, American Academy of Pediatrics and American Heart Association, 2000.
19. Cordero L, Hon EH: Neonatal bradycardia following nasopharyngeal stimulation. *J Pediatr* 78:441, 1971.
20. Marlow N: Do we need an Apgar score? *Arch Dis Child* 67:765, 1992.
21. Saugstad OD, Rootwelt T, Aalen O: Resuscitation of asphyxiated newborn infants with room air of oxygen—an international controlled trial: The Resair 2 study. *Pediatrics* 102:1, 1998 (URL: http://www.pediatrics.org/cgi/content/full/102/1/e1).
22. Zideman D, et al: Airways in pediatric and newborn resuscitation. *Ann Emerg Med* 37:S126, 2001.
23. Berry AM, Brimacombe JR, Verghese C: The laryngeal mask airway in emergency medicine, neonatal resuscitation, and intensive care medicine. *Int Anesthesiol Clin* 36:91, 1998.
24. Burchfield DJ, et al: Medications in neonatal resuscitation. *Ann Emerg Med* 22:435, 1993.
25. Hein HA: The use of sodium bicarbonate in neonatal resuscitation: Help or harm? *Pediatrics* 91:496, 1993.
26. Quinton DN, O'Byrne G, Aitkenhead AR: Comparison of endotracheal and peripheral intravenous adrenaline in cardiac arrest: Is the endotracheal route reliable? *Lancet* 1:828, 1987.
27. American Academy of Pediatrics: Emergency drug doses for infants and children and naloxone use in newborns: Clarification. *Pediatrics* 83:803, 1989.

Section II CARDINAL PRESENTATIONS

CHAPTER

10 Clinical Decision Making

Dane M. Chapman, Douglas M. Char, and Chandra D. Aubin

PERSPECTIVE

Physicians must continually integrate vast amounts of medical information with their skills in clinical decision making. They must be thorough yet efficient in gathering data and use strategies that promote maximal diagnostic proficiency while limiting costs. These unique skills are neither adequately taught nor measured in medical schools and residencies. Emergency physicians have become some of the most facile and rapid decision makers in medicine. This is probably due to the nature of the specialty. Emergency physicians are bombarded by diagnostic and management decisions throughout a clinical shift. Many pertain directly to diagnosing and managing a patient's problem. Others are related to managing the staff, clinical environment, and educational responsibilities (Box 10-1). By better understanding the decision-making process, improved decision-making strategies can be developed and taught.

Both an adequate knowledge base of medical information and a repertoire of decision-making skills are necessary to diagnose and manage medical problems. Expert emergency physicians have learned to recognize disease and injury patterns and have developed sets of heuristics (rules of thumb) to make rapid decisions.[1,2] When patients' presentations do not fit an existing pattern or heuristic, emergency physicians move between several levels of clinical decision making depending on their clinical experience, the clinical situation, and time constraints.[3] Most errors in mental functioning affecting patients' care can be traced to defects in pattern recognition or in one or more of these levels of clinical decision making.[4-6]

Mental effort saved through improved decision making provides a "cognitive reserve" for emergency physicians to control their hectic environment with decreased occupational stress and potential burnout. With greater mental energy reserve, physicians are better able to expand their knowledge base and to consider patients' values and concerns.

DIAGNOSTIC APPROACH

When diagnosing or managing a patient's problem, there are decisions relating to both *medical inquiry* and *clinical decision making*. Medical inquiry refers to the

BOX 10-1. Typical Emergency Physician Decisions during a Clinical Shift

Diagnostic and Patient Management Decisions

Triage decisions: What patients need to be seen first?

Stabilization decisions: What management interventions are needed to stabilize the patient?

Diagnostic decisions: What clinical findings are needed to make the diagnosis?

Therapeutic decisions: What ongoing therapy is needed?

Disposition decisions: Will the patient need to be admitted? Where?

Other Decisions

Administrative decisions: What needs to change to maintain a safe working environment for patients and staff (e.g., diversion, call in backup, transfer, or discharge by ambulance)?

Educational decisions: How much do I inform the patient of his or her illness? When and how should medical students, residents, or staff be assigned to see a patient with an important clinical finding? Should the attending take time to teach if the emergency department is busy?

Interpersonal decisions: What do I do when conflicts arise with nursing, consultants, patients, or family members?

Well-being decisions: When and where will I go to the bathroom, take a lunch break, wash hands, or share uplifting humor?

Feedback decisions: Were my decisions today correct? Will I do things differently next time? If so, how? Did the diagnostic test help in my decision making?

cognitive and psychomotor skills or techniques used to gather medical data (i.e., data gathering) and includes history taking, physical examination, and diagnostic testing. *Clinical decision making* refers to the cognitive processes required to utilize the medical data obtained to evaluate, diagnose, or manage medical problems. *Clinical reasoning* involves both *medical inquiry* and *clinical decision making* and has been described as the scientific method of clinical medicine.[1,7]

Diagnostic and Management Processes of Clinical Decision Making

Emergency physicians operate in situations in which even small mistakes may cause high morbidity or mortality. The difficulty in teaching decision making in these situations is that experienced clinicians may have little insight into their own thought processes because much of their decision making occurs at preconscious levels using pattern recognition.[4,8,9]

Human factor specialists and cognitive scientists have intensely studied the diagnostic and management decision making of expert physicians to understand the underlying processes and to better teach them to novices. Four consistent diagnostic and management decision-making processes or strategies have emerged: (1) pattern recognition, (2) "rule-using" algorithm, (3) hypothetico-deductive, and (4) naturalistic or event driven.[1-3] The expert emergency physician utilizes all four diagnostic and management decision-making processes depending on the clinical situation.

Clinical Decision Making by the Pattern Recognition Process

Pattern recognition requires the memorization of a critical number of facts. A *fact* or *concept* is a group of objects, symbols, or events that are grouped together with common characteristics referred to by a collective name (e.g., acidosis, myocardial infarction). Facts relating to a certain disease may be memorized without knowing how to use them. Over time, experienced physicians can group together related facts such as disease-specific history and physical examination findings that allow pattern recognition or the "doorway diagnosis." To develop this expertise, most practitioners must experience hundreds or even thousands of encounters with patients.

For each new patient, the physician's task is to build a representation that links the patient's case to an existing knowledge structure (i.e., the disease pattern) and facilitates recall of important disease entities and patient-related information. Disease-oriented patterns contain little knowledge about pathology or physiology but a wealth of clinically relevant information about the disease, its consequences, and associated signs and symptoms.

This pattern recognition (or "skill-based") process corresponds to the lowest level of the clinical decision-making hierarchy.[2] Without conscious effort, pattern recognition decision making is automatic, operates briefly, and processes information rapidly and in parallel after being activated by sensory input or conscious thought.[1,2] Clinical acumen related to the skill of pattern recognition is cognitive rather than psychomotor and is developed over time and after exposure to many patients and disease presentations.

Clinical Decision Making by the Rule-Using Process

Higher on the clinical decision-making hierarchy is the ability to "use rules," which requires greater understanding than memorization or pattern recognition alone. The recognition of the pattern, however, is a prerequisite to applying the correct rule. At this level of decision making, solutions to familiar problems are governed by previously memorized rules of the "if X then Y" variety.[3,9] These rules include heuristics, algorithms, and clinical pathways. When clinicians are faced with atypical presentations or unusual symptom complexes not previously memorized, they may resort to using rules, heuristics, or algorithms to discriminate or classify symptoms, signs, or diagnostic study results into previously defined diagnostic or therapeutic groups. Similarly, related heuristics can be grouped into algorithms, such as those developed for the advanced cardiac life support course, allowing the physician to use agreed-upon rules of action in critical or high-stress situations in which higher levels of decision making are difficult. This is not unlike the situation in the airline industry, where pilots are required to follow the same algorithm or checklist before takeoff, thus minimizing the chance for human error.

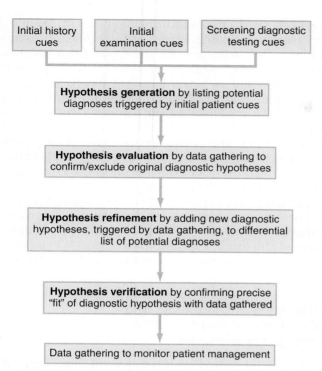

Figure 10-1. Relationship between medical inquiry (data gathering) and clinical decision making by the hypothetico-deductive process. Data gathering can include history taking, physical examination, or diagnostic testing.

Clinical Decision Making by the Hypothetico-Deductive Process

Highest in the clinical decision-making hierarchy is the intellectual ability to make clinical decisions by problem solving using previous knowledge to create new solutions ("knowledge based"). The physician must originate a novel solution to a problem that requires conscious, analytic processing of stored knowledge, for example, finding a solution to a difficult disposition of a patient. Any departure from the routine clinical presentation where the disease pattern is recognized requires either a rule-based or hypothetico-deductive solution (Figure 10-1).[1,8,9]

Initial cues are perceived from the patient and the environment, and multiple diagnostic hypotheses are rapidly generated (*hypothesis generation*). Next, data-gathering inquiry strategies are used to collect relevant history, physical examination, and diagnostic study information. The cues and data are interpreted to confirm or reject the provisional hypotheses (*hypothesis evaluation*), a process that may lead to additional diagnostic hypotheses being generated (*hypothesis refinement*). Finally, the physician chooses and verifies the most likely diagnosis (confirmed by data) from among the provisional diagnostic hypotheses (*hypothesis verification*). Strategies useful in clinical decision making of the hypothetico-deductive variety include: generating *new and unusual ideas* (hypotheses) that relate to the problem; *avoiding premature judgment or closure*, such as labeling with a diagnosis that does not exactly "fit"; *breaking mental sets*, such as dismissing initial disease patterns to look at the problem differently (i.e., outside the box); and *classifying the essentials* by attending to relevant facts and conditions of the problem, such as pertinent positive and negative historical, physical examination, and diagnostic study findings.

Clinical Decision Making by the Naturalistic, or Event-Driven, Process

Clinical decision making by the naturalistic (event-driven) process characterizes emergency physicians who treat patients' signs or symptoms before definitive diagnoses have been determined.[2] This dynamic process is more likely to be utilized in emergency medicine than any other specialty. When presented with an unstable patient, certain therapeutic actions are necessary to stabilize the patient long before the cause of the instability is known. The atypical presentation is compared with an existing schema, and if no match is found on the basis of presenting cues, the expert clinician switches decision making from an evaluation of diagnostic possibilities to an evaluation of possible courses of action or therapeutic trials. In general, the number of available therapeutic or management options is smaller than the number of possible diagnoses. The emergency physician often uses a strategy of ruling out the worst-case scenario.[10] This strategy, coupled with a focus on stabilizing actions and not diagnoses, can rapidly prune the decision tree. When a satisfactory response to intervention is obtained, the search for the definitive diagnosis can often be truncated. The physician must be willing to accept a good or likely presumptive diagnosis instead of the definitive diagnosis.

Which Clinical Decision-Making Process Is Best?

Determining which clinical decision-making process is best depends on the experience of the clinician and difficulty or uniqueness of the medical problem. Inexperienced physicians who lack a broad mental set of disease patterns or schema may be exhaustive in their history taking and physical examination to discern sufficient cues to develop a differential diagnosis. They are often unfocused in ordering diagnostic tests because they cannot eliminate diagnostic possibilities on the basis of their undeveloped association of presenting signs, symptoms, and diagnostic study findings with clinical diagnoses. Experienced physicians, when faced with a complex patient who does not "fit" into their memorized set of disease frames, use details of history, physical examination, diagnostic tests, or therapeutic trials to assess the possibility of significant or life-threatening disease.

Many presentations of patients that require physicians to use the highest level of diagnostic decision making (hypothetico-deductive) early in their career are gradually "pushed down" to classification or discrimination tasks (pattern recognition) requiring little conscious thought or mental processing.

BOX 10-2. Heuristics for Optimal Decision Making in Emergency Medicine

Sit at patient's bedside to collect a thorough history.

Perform an uninterrupted physical examination.

Generate life-threatening and most likely diagnostic hypotheses.

Use information databases and expert systems to broaden diagnostic hypotheses.

Collect data to confirm or exclude life threats first, then most likely diagnoses.

Avoid diagnostic testing whenever possible by using readily available decision making algorithms (e.g., Ottawa ankle rules).

Order only those tests that will affect disposition or that will confirm or exclude diagnostic hypotheses.

Include decision rules on diagnostic testing order forms.

Use guidelines and protocols for specific therapeutic decisions to conserve mental energies while on duty.

Allow 2 to 3 minutes of uninterrupted time to mentally process each patient.

Mentally process one patient at a time to disposition.

Avoid decision making when overly stressed or angry. Take 1 to 2 minutes out, regroup, then make the decision.

Carry a maximum of 4 or 5 "undecided" category patients. Stop—make some dispositions.

Use evidence-based medicine techniques to substantiate decisions with evidence, understand the limitations of the evidence, and to answer specific questions, such as usefulness of diagnostic testing, management plans, and disease prognosis.

By eventually emphasizing the lower cognitive processes of recognizing disease patterns and using decision-making algorithms and clinical pathways, clinicians can efficiently and proficiently diagnose and manage undifferentiated patients with less mental effort. When lower cognitive processes are consistently utilized, discrete facts previously memorized about a particular disease are often forgotten by the expert who easily retains the ability to diagnose and manage patients efficiently but must struggle to maintain "the edge" in factual recall. Following heuristic rules of thumb in clinical decision making can create a framework for gaining the information and insight necessary to make the best decision (Box 10-2).

Multitasking–Simultaneous Processing

Multitasking is a key characteristic of the emergency physician who can process simultaneous workups on from five to seven patients. Time and motion observations of emergency physicians at an academic medical center suggest that only 10% to 20% of their time is spent multitasking.[11] By increasing the degree of multitasking, physicians can significantly improve their clinical decision-making efficiency without necessarily having to decrease their decision-making thoroughness and proficiency.[12] Optimally, emergency physicians would see patients upon arrival to the emergency department because the time between the arrival and first seeing a physician is a major determinant in patients' satisfaction and throughput times. An initial evaluation, including a brief history, physical examination, and selection of the appropriate clinical decision-making pathway, maximally affects patients' throughput and decreases length of stay (LOS).

Data-gathering techniques that permit multitasking, such as the complaint-based templates with specific prompts and other forms of bedside charting, decision-making algorithms included as part of physician ordering forms, on-line order entry, and the problem-oriented medical record can all contribute to increased decision-making efficiency and to decreased LOS for the patient. With Center for Medicare-Medicaid Studies documentation requirements for attending physician supervision, and increased emphasis on patient-focused and timely care, multitasking needs to increase to degrees not yet achieved at most academic medical centers.

Heuristics of Diagnostic and Management Decision Making in Emergency Medicine

A number of important heuristics guiding diagnostic and management decision making have been identified by emergency medicine decision-making experts.[8-10] We have combined several of these rules into an emergency medicine decision-making algorithm (Figure 10-2).

1. *Rule out life or limb threats first (i.e., think the worst)*. Upon identifying life or limb threats, the emergency physician must also decide whether direct intervention is necessary to mediate or prevent the patient's deterioration. These decisions are typically based on incomplete data. If no life threat is identified, the physician must consider other serious diseases consistent with the patient's complaint and work to exclude them before accepting less serious, plausible diagnostic hypotheses.

2. *Determine whether more than one active pathologic process is present*. A single diagnosis, although appealing, is not always appropriate. The physician must remain open minded with a continually probing data-gathering approach: "Is this all there is?"

3. *Try a diagnostic-therapeutic trial*. Administering a stabilizing therapy that also provides diagnostic information is an important decision-making strategy in the emergency department. The results of the trial may provide precise information or may just help differentiate the seriously ill patient from others, for example, glucose in the unconscious patient.

4. *Determine the bottom line*. Practicing emergency medicine is filled with uncertainty. Is a diagnosis possible or even necessary when life threats have been ruled out? Is hospitalization appropriate for the patient, even without making a final diagnosis? When the emergency department workup is complete, the physician is often left with unanswered questions that may not really affect the bottom line. If the bottom line is affected, that is, patients' safety,

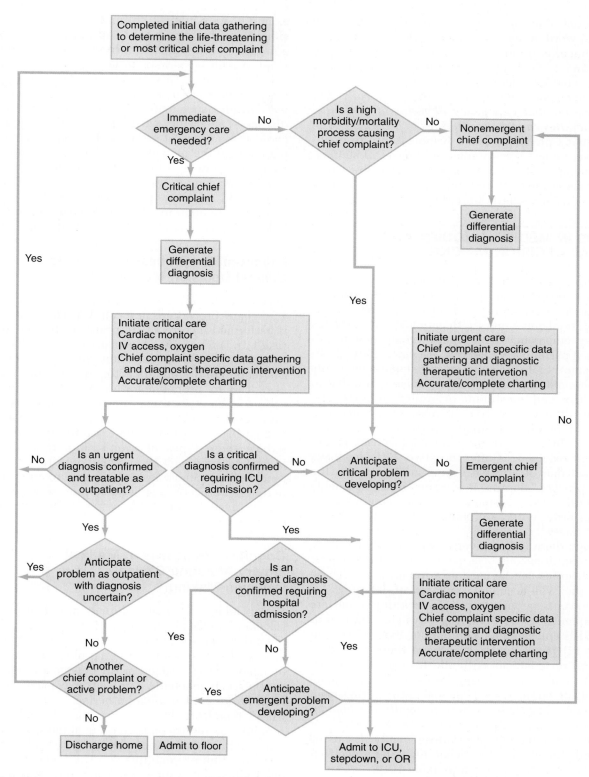

Figure 10-2. Emergency medicine clinical decision-making algorithm. ICU, intensive care unit; OR, operating room.

the answers must be addressed before making the disposition.

5. *Close the disposition and follow-up loop.* Emergency physicians have a unique relationship with other physicians. This relationship is based on the concept of "our" patient. We share responsibility for

the health and welfare of the patients in our care with other providers.

6. *Understand fully why the patient is in the emergency department, and then meet the patient's expectation.* The stated chief complaint may not be the real reason for the visit. The emergency physi-

cian must often look beyond the written chart and spoken word to uncover which of the patient's fears and concerns prompted the visit to the emergency department. Such clues are easily missed in our hectic work environment.

7. *Use emergency department resources fully but understand that emergency department personnel and facilities cannot be all things to all people.* The emergency physician has a responsibility to maintain the highest level of quality in terms of staffing, equipment, and care. Recognizing what the emergency department is not and knowing the facility limitations are equally important.

ERRORS IN MEDICAL INQUIRY AND CLINICAL DECISION MAKING

According to a landmark Institute of Medicine report on medical error, 44,000 people die in U.S. hospitals each year as a result of medical error.[13] With overcrowding, brief encounters with patients, and the chaos of a busy emergency department, emergency physicians are at particularly high risk. An emergency physician frequently reflects upon recently completed shifts hoping that nothing significant was missed and that in all the chaos and constraints of limited resources, no injury might have occurred because of an incorrect decision or missed (or misinterpreted) information.[2] Because of the nature of the practice, feedback is rare and, when received, is often negative. Still, feedback and knowledge of adverse events are crucial to the learning process.[8] Because it is assumed that avoidable events will occur, systems, such as computerized physician order entry, are being designed to enhance patients' safety.[14]

Although there is no universally accepted classification of practitioner adverse events in medicine, three broad categories can be used as a framework.[2-5] These parallel the well-accepted domains of learning: (1) *affective events* pertain to physician attitude and are most frequently those involving physician communication skills and patients' complaints about physician conduct; (2) *psychomotor events* are those related to procedural or technical skill; and (3) *cognitive events* are those that occur during medical inquiry (data gathering) or clinical decision making resulting from a faulty knowledge base (pattern recognition or memorization of facts); faulty use of rules, heuristics, or protocols (rule-using); or faulty synthesis using the hypothetico-deductive decision-making process. A more detailed listing is given in Table 10-1.

Affective Processes Affecting Clinical Decision Making

Affective events occur not because of deficient medical knowledge or faulty decision making directly but rather because of physician perception or attitude.[9] Anger, overconfidence, prejudice, or fear may bias a physician's mental set during decision making. What is perceived during history taking and the physical examination may be influenced by *attitudinal bias*. For

example, stereotypical cultural differences in expression of severity of pain may lead a physician to develop a negative bias, which in turn may lead to undertreatment of pain or perhaps to failure to consider a more severe diagnosis. This can also occur when we have a negative personal reaction, such as anger, or because we consider such patients responsible for their own disease—called the *attribution error*. Techniques to avoid these types of errors include approaching each patient as if the patient were a blank slate (no impression) and viewing the patient as if he or she were a family member. If we can recognize these personal biases and separate ourselves from them, we can remain more open to alternative diagnoses and potentially reduce errors in medical decision making.

Psychomotor Processes Affecting Clinical Decision Making

Psychomotor adverse events usually occur during emergency procedures and can directly harm a patient if performed incorrectly. Improper technique may also result in emergency physician morbidity, such as a needlestick-induced infectious disease inoculation. Distraction omission and acting out of "force of habit" also lead to psychomotor events in that undesired actions occur that cause injury or subject patients to unnecessary risk. Reviewing procedures beforehand and letting staff know when to avoid interruptions can reduce these types of events. Important diagnostic information may not be obtained or critical treatments rendered in a timely fashion because of an improperly performed procedure or because a necessary procedure was delayed or withheld owing to lack of technical competence.

Cognitive Processes in Medical Inquiry Affecting Clinical Decision Making

History taking, physical examination, and diagnostic test selection are data-gathering skills that form the basis of potential cognitively based adverse events. A thorough review of systems and screening physical examination of major organ systems of all emergency department patients can markedly limit adverse events resulting from *faulty clinical data gathering*. Use of complaint-based templates for charting that include specific prompts can reduce omissions but at the same time may impair clinical decision making by providing a structured but limited cognitive domain. Emergency department efficiency is directly related to diagnostic testing strategy. A common, significant error in data gathering is to order tests without completing an adequate history or performing a physical examination. This *unfocused diagnostic testing error* wastes time and resources and may confound optimal decision making. Often a rapid but thorough history and physical examination eliminate the need for expensive and time-consuming diagnostic tests. Another source of inefficiency is the practice of using the *"trial and error" diagnostic testing* approach in which diagnostic tests are ordered sequentially.

Table 10-1. Errors Influencing Clinical Decision Making

Domain of Learning	Cognitive Control Mode	Cognitive Deficiency	Faulty Process Leading to Error
Affective domain: attitude, communication			Fear or anger can lead to negative, impulsive, or irrational behavior Cultural stereotyping Attribution error; blaming patients for their illness
Psychomotor domain: technical motor skill			Distraction omissions; taking one action, intending another Force of habit; invoking an action unconsciously Improper technique can lead to morbidity or mortality
Cognitive domain: I. Medical inquiry (data gathering)			Faulty history and physical examination data gathering Confirmation bias; only seeing what you want to see, "ignoring cues" Unfocused diagnostic testing; tests ordered do not help rule in or rule out hypothesis "Trial-and-error" test ordering "Shotgun" test ordering
II. Diagnostic decision making: 1. Pattern recognition	Schematic control mode, automatic, parallel processing, rapid, preconscious	Memory-based, error of actions, "slips," "lapses"	"Slips"; well practiced preconscious mental routine improperly applied "Lapses"; failures in memory that result in omissions and inefficiencies Coning of attention; overfocus on single source of information despite other sources Revision under stress; recently learned behavior replaced by older familiar one Missed cues; tendency to recognize only what has been memorized Biased memory; relying only on what you "know" from prior experience, discounting other possibilities
2. Using rules/ heuristics	Attentional control mode, conscious, sequential processing	Rule based, misapplied expertise, using wrong rule, "mistake"	Using wrong heuristic—incorrect rule or clinical pathway Using correct heuristic incorrectly Representativeness error; patient atypical for given diagnosis—discounted Availability heuristic; using the first information that comes to mind
3. Hypothetico-deductive A. Hypothesis generation	Attentional control mode, effortful, slow, conscious, difficult to sustain, sequential processing	Problem-solving, knowledge-based, error of conscious thought, "mistakes"	*Faulty hypothesis generation—failure to consider a diagnostic hypothesis, maintaining a narrow view of possible diagnoses or hypotheses* Context or situational bias; "patients in urgent care, thus not really sick" "Sutton's slip"; consider only the "obvious" (i.e., bank is where the money is) "Psych out"; failure to consider medical diagnosis due to psychiatric diagnosis "Playing the odds"; faulty estimate of disease prevalence "Anchoring"; accepting previously applied labels without questioning diagnosis "Ying-yang out"; presuming you have nothing to add to a prior workup
B. Hypothesis evaluation			*Faulty hypothesis evaluation—failure to interpret cues and data properly (wrong hypotheses are confirmed or rejected)* "Posterior probability"; misinterpret history, physical, or laboratory results due to prior label
C. Hypothesis refinement			*Faulty hypothesis refinement—failure to revise list of diagnostic hypotheses to explain results of data gathered* Overconfidence; unquestionable belief in the validity of chosen course
D. Hypothesis verification			*Faulty hypothesis verification—failure to verify "fit" of diagnosis to data* "Zebra retreat"; rare diagnosis considered but not pursued despite cues "Premature closure"; latching onto a presumptive diagnosis and not considering other possibilities
III. Management decision making	Naturalistic, event-driven process	Rigid, unwilling to act without complete data	Unwilling to accept a good or likely presumptive diagnosis before making critical time-dependent therapeutic decisions

Preparing a differential diagnosis and determining the data necessary to refine the list will determine what tests or interventions need to be ordered.

Finally, emergency physicians are also subject to *confirmation bias*, that is, diagnosing what is preconceived and interpreting test results in that light. Therefore, in the patient with an atypical presentation of chest pain, T wave changes on the electrocardiogram might be labeled "nonspecific" rather than "possibly ischemic."

Cognitive Defects in Pattern Recognition Decision Making

If physicians do not have an adequate knowledge base or if their knowledge is not organized for appropriate retrieval when presented with a novel, undiagnosed patient, cues that may be obvious to the expert are missed (i.e., *error of "missed cues"*). Later, when interviewing and examining patients, cues characteristic of the disease are missed because the clinician does not know what to look for. To be most useful, typical and atypical symptoms and signs of disease processes need to be organized in such a way that they can be recalled when the clinician uncovers the distinguishing cues of a disease. Pattern recognition errors may be due more to lack of having memorized a sufficient number of disease frames than to inability to recall details within a particular disease frame. The clinician need only develop broader lists of diagnostic hypotheses that are associated with presenting symptoms and signs to avoid this error. The clinician should not be afraid to stop and ask the question, "What am I missing?" Physicians are also more likely to make errors under stressful situations. Recently learned behaviors are often replaced by older familiar outdated ones. The physician may also gain additional prompts of potential diagnostic hypotheses using heuristics or the hypothetico-deductive process of decision making or by making an appropriate referral to someone who can.

Cognitive Defects in Using Rules (Protocols, Practice Guidelines, and Clinical Pathways)

Common errors in decision making at the level of using rules, protocols, and clinical pathways typically result from either not having the correct rule or applying the correct rule improperly. The challenge is to determine which clinical rule can be most appropriately applied to generate a diagnosis and management plan for the constellation of symptoms and signs of each patient's presentation. Faulty application of the wrong rule or heuristic leads to errors in diagnosis and management similar to those of the premature closure variety. Common sense suggests that if the rule does not fit the situation, it is probably the wrong rule.

Cognitive Problems in Hypothetico-Deductive Clinical Decision Making

When presenting symptoms, signs, and diagnostic test results do not fit any validated clinical rule or proto-col, decision-making strategies must be used to create new facts or rules not previously originated or created. Making a correct diagnosis in an as yet unrecognized disease process or in an unrecognized association among multiple disease processes requires problem-solving skills similar to those used in scientific research. Using "peripheral brains" such as readily available reference texts, handheld electronic databases, and real-time, on-line literature searches frees up mental capacity to allow physicians to focus on creative decision making.

Errors at this level of the clinical decision-making process are typically related to misjudging either the need for novel diagnostic hypotheses (hypothesis generation, hypothesis evaluation, and hypothesis refinement) or diagnostic accuracy (hypothesis verification). Termed *mistakes*, such errors can occur whenever the clinician's analytic processing activities are disturbed, interrupted, or missing key data.[2,4] Mistakes are triggered by personal stress, fatigue, task overload, environmental distractions, and lack of clinical knowledge. Perfect execution of a faulty management plan for a patient is an example of a mistake. In contrast, poor execution of an appropriate management plan could be due to errors in pattern recognition (a "slip" or "lapse" in memory) or to errors in rule using.

Problems in Management Processes of Clinical Decision Making

Errors can lead to inappropriate management and often result in bad outcomes for patients. Making the right management decision is often more important than making the right diagnostic decision. This is often the case with critically ill or injured patients. Intervention based on very limited data supercedes an exhaustive evaluation. Being rigid or unwilling to act without complete data leads to errors of omission. Use of guidelines and protocols to "drive" actions and interventions (advanced trauma life support, advanced cardiac life support, pediatric advanced life support) can reduce this type of error.[3] The complex management decision to admit or discharge a patient can be "pushed down" from the synthetic, knowledge-based decision-making process to the rule-using process by implementing a heuristic designed to prevent inappropriate discharges when diagnoses are uncertain (see Figure 10-2).

Decision analysis, the methodology of weighing mathematically the pros and cons of various options in complex decision making, may be most useful for choosing from various therapeutic options when a diagnosis has been made. Decision analysis utilizes a branching decision tree in which probabilities are calculated for each step of the decision tree.[1] This technique has not yet significantly affected emergency medicine because of the lack of real-time computing, the limited number of predetermined clinical pathways, and the difficulty of fitting psychological or social factors into the mathematical models. However, these limitations are rapidly dissolving, and this technique may greatly facilitate emergency physician management decision making in the future.

BOX 10-3. Heuristics for Minimizing Errors in Clinical Decision Making

Avoid the biggest obstacle to the correct diagnosis—a previous diagnosis.

Avoid inheriting someone else's thinking whether it is related to diagnostic or personal bias.

Check for critical past medical history and risk factors for serious disease or poor outcome.

Pay attention to vital signs and nurses' and Emergency Medical Service (EMS) notes.

Avoid premature closure if the diagnosis is not certain—enlist the patient as a partner in that uncertainty, arrange for appropriate follow-up, and give specific precautions in written form.

Beware of high-risk times—patient sign out (see and touch all), high-volume or high-acuity times, and times of personal fatigue.

Beware of high-risk patients—hostile, violent, or abusive patients, patients with alcohol or drug abuse, psychiatric patients, and patients who elicit a negative visceral response.

Beware of the return visit—this is an opportunity to correct what was missed during the previous visit.

Beware of high-risk diagnoses—myocardial infarction (MI), pulmonary embolism (PE), subarachnoid hemorrhage (SAH), tendon and nerve injuries, retained foreign bodies, intracranial hemorrhage (ICH) in intoxicated patients, vascular catastrophes in elderly patients, appendicitis, meningitis, ectopic pregnancy, and testicular torsion. Rule out the worst-case scenario or high-risk diagnoses first.

Beware of the *nonfit*—when the presumptive diagnosis does *not* match the symptoms, signs, or diagnostic tests—recognize the nonfit and reevaluate and refine diagnostic hypotheses.

Using Heuristics to Reduce Adverse Events

Emergency physicians can limit their adverse events related to clinical decision making by recognizing potential bias and sources of error and developing "error-reducing heuristics" (Box 10-3). By identifying subsets of patients in whom clinicians are more likely to make errors, associated bias and negative emotional reactions that could cloud clinical judgment can be avoided. Such subsets would include patients with a different cultural or language background; patients who elicit a negative emotional reaction, such as the abusive or potentially drug-seeking patient; and chemically altered or psychiatric patients. Physicians can choose to avoid inheriting someone else's diagnostic or personal bias by "seeing and touching all" patients who are signed out to them. When faced with a case in which "something is not quite right" or the fit is not precise, clinicians need to rethink their diagnostic hypothesis generation and verification strategy. To limit the adverse effect of personal fatigue and workload on their clinical judgment, emergency physicians can choose to adjust their own clinical schedules. Physicians can also use *metacognition*, the process by which one reflects upon and regulates what one is thinking, and, in so doing, incorporate error avoidance techniques presented in Table 10-1.[3,6,9] Perhaps most important, when mistakes occur, clinicians must be willing to admit their mistakes and discuss them with others so that all can learn to minimize human error in the emergency department setting.

ACKNOWLEDGMENTS

The authors would like to thank the Emergency Medicine faculty and residents at Washington University in St. Louis, York Hospital, Pennsylvania State University, the University of California-Davis, and Denver Health Medical Center Residencies in Emergency Medicine, who have taught us much of what we know about the clinical decision-making process in emergency medicine.

REFERENCES

1. Elstein AS, Schwarz A: Clinical problem solving and diagnostic decision making: Selective review of the cognitive literature. *BMJ* 324:729, 2002.
2. Wears RL: Comments on clinical decision making: An emergency medicine perspective. *Acad Emerg Med* 7:411, 2000.
3. Kovacs G, Croskerry P: Clinical decision making: An emergency medicine perspective. *Acad Emerg Med* 6:947, 1999.
4. Wears RL, Leape LL: Human error in emergency medicine. *Ann Emerg Med* 34:370, 1999.
5. Leape LL: Error in medicine. *JAMA* 272:1851, 1994.
6. Graber M, Gordon R, Franklin N: Reducing diagnostic errors in medicine: What's the goal? *Acad Med* 77:981, 2002.
7. Chapman DM, Calhoun JG, Davis WK, VanMondfrans AP: Acquiring clinical reasoning competency: Group versus individual practice using patient management computer simulations. *Acad Emerg Med* 4:511, 1997.
8. Cosby KS, Croskerry P: Patient safety: A curriculum for teaching patient safety in emergency medicine. *Acad Emerg Med* 10:69, 2003.
9. Croskerry P: Achieving quality in clinical decision making: Cognitive strategies and detection of bias. *Acad Emerg Med* 9:1184, 2002.
10. Hamilton G: *Emergency Medicine: An Approach to Clinical Problem Solving*, 2nd ed. Philadelphia, WB Saunders, 2003.
11. Moche JA, Gauer KA, Chapman DM: Emergency medicine faculty time utilization: Implications for faculty funding and medical student and resident education. *Acad Emerg Med* 6:413, 1999.
12. Chisholm CD, Collison EK, Nelson DR, Cordell WH: Emergency department workplace interruptions: Are emergency physicians "interrupt-driven" and "multitasking"? *Acad Emerg Med* 7:1239, 2000.
13. Kohn LT, Corrigan JM, Donaldson MS (eds): To Err Is Human: Building a Safer Health System. Institute of Medicine report. Washington, DC, National Academy Press, November 21, 1999.
14. Kyriacou DN, Coben JH: Errors in emergency medicine: Research strategies. *Acad Emerg Med* 7:1201, 2000.

PERSPECTIVE

Epidemiology

Fever is part of the presenting complaint in 6% of all adult (age 18 to 65) visits to the emergency department, 10% to 15% of all elderly (older than 65 years) visits, and 20% to 40% of all pediatric visits.[1,2] Morbidity and mortality vary dramatically with age. Younger adults with fever usually have benign self-limited disease with less than 1% mortality. The challenge in this group is to identify the rare meningitis or septic conditions when confronted with a predominance of self-limited viral and focal bacterial diseases. Patients older than 65, or those with chronic disease who present with fever, represent a group at high risk for serious disease. Morbidity and mortality in this group are significant. Between 70% and 90% are hospitalized, and 7% to 9% die within 1 month of admission. Infection is the most common cause of fever in these patients, and most of these infections are bacterial in nature. Three body systems; the respiratory tract, the urinary tract, and the skin and soft tissue, are the target for more than 80% of these infections.[3] The relative mortality and morbidity for any given infection are much higher in the geriatric population. For example, they are 5 to 10 times higher for urinary tract infections and 15 to 20 times higher for appendicitis.[4,5] Even viral illnesses that are generally not fatal, such as influenza, can be highly lethal in elderly persons.

Pathophysiology

Body temperature is normally controlled within a narrow range by the preoptic area of the hypothalamus. This range is usually between 36.0° C and 37.8° C (96.8° F and 100.4° F). There is a circadian rhythm within this range, with lower temperatures in the morning and higher temperatures in the late afternoon. Fever occurs when this normal range is reset to a higher value. Fever is typically defined as a core temperature greater than 38.0° C. Fever should not be confused with hyperthermia. Hyperthermia is an elevation of the temperature related to the inability of the body to dissipate heat. Almost all cases of temperatures higher than 41.0° C (105° F) are due to hyperthermia rather than to fever.

In the anterior hypothalamus, neurons directly sense the blood temperature. Temperature is subsequently controlled by a combination of vasomotor changes, shivering, changes in metabolic heat production, and behavioral changes.

Fever may be produced by a number of endogenous and exogenous substances referred to as *pyrogens*. Endogenous pyrogens include a variety of cytokines released by leukocytes in response to infectious, inflammatory, and neoplastic processes. Exogenous pyrogens include a large number of bacterial and viral products and toxins. Toxins induce fever by stimulating cells of the immune system to release endogenous pyrogens. These cytokines, such as interleukin 1, interleukin 6, tumor necrosis factor, and interferon, travel to the hypothalamus and induce the production of prostaglandin E_2 (PGE_2).

PGE_2 raises the set point of the temperature range by a combination of effects including peripheral vasoconstriction, increased metabolic heat production, shivering, and behavioral changes that conserve heat. Fever is maintained as long as the levels of endogenous pyrogens and PGE_2 are high. Cyclooxygenase inhibitors, such as aspirin, decrease fever by blocking the production of PGE_2. Age, malnutrition, and chronic disease may also blunt the febrile response.

Moderate elevations of the body temperature may serve to aid the host defense by increasing chemotaxis, decreasing microbial replication, and improving lymphocyte function. Elevated temperatures directly inhibit the growth of certain bacteria and viruses.

Fever also results in certain costs to the host including increased oxygen consumption, increased metabolic demands, increased protein breakdown, and increased gluconeogenesis. These costs are particularly problematic in elderly persons, who typically have a smaller margin of reserve for any given body system. It has not been proved that treatment of fever with antipyretics has a beneficial effect on outcome or prevents complications.

The initial step in the process of fever is the resetting of the thermostatic set point in the hypothalamus to a higher temperature while actual body temperature remains normal. This mismatch of the thermostat with the "sensed" body temperature causes the patient to feel chilled or chills. If the chills are reported to a caregiver and the skin is touched or the temperature is taken, it is usually noted to be normal or minimally elevated. The patient remains chilled until the body temperature rises, through the preceding mechanisms, to match the elevated set point. At this point, the patient feels euthermic (but may feel fatigued or ill), but to the caregiver the skin temperature or thermometer reading

Table 11-1. Differential Diagnoses—Infectious Causes

Organ System	Critical Diagnoses	Emergent Diagnoses	Nonemergent Diagnoses
Respiratory	Bacterial pneumonia with respiratory failure	Bacterial pneumonia, peritonsillar abscess, retropharyngeal abscess, epiglottitis	Otitis media, sinusitis, pharyngitis, bronchitis, influenza, tuberculosis
Cardiovascular		Endocarditis, pericarditis	
Gastrointestinal	Peritonitis	Appendicitis, cholecystitis, diverticulitis, intraabdominal abscess	Colitis/enteritis
Genitourinary		Pyelonephritis, tubo-ovarian abscess, pelvic inflammatory disease	Cystitis, epididymitis, prostatitis
Neurologic	Meningitis, cavernous sinus, thrombosis	Encephalitis, brain abscess	
Skin and soft tissue		Cellulitis, infected decubitus ulcer, soft tissue abscess	
Systemic	Sepsis/septic shock, meningococcemia		

BOX 11-1. Differential Diagnosis—Noninfectious Causes of Fever

Critical Diagnoses
Acute myocardial infarction
Pulmonary embolism/infarction
Intracranial hemorrhage
Cerebrovascular accident
Neuroleptic-malignant syndrome
Thyroid storm
Acute adrenal insufficiency
Transfusion reaction
Pulmonary edema

Emergent Diagnoses
Congestive heart failure
Dehydration
Recent seizure
Sickle cell disease
Transplant rejection
Pancreatitis
Deep venous thrombosis

Nonemergent Diagnoses
Drug fever
Malignancy
Gout
Sarcoidosis
Crohn's disease
Postmyocardiotomy syndrome

is now elevated. When the thermostatic set point is reduced to normal, the patient suddenly feels hot and sweats until the body temperature falls to match the (now normal) set point.

DIAGNOSTIC APPROACH

Differential Considerations

The complete differential diagnosis of the patient presenting to the emergency department with fever is extensive. The major infectious and noninfectious etiologies are summarized in Table 11-1 and Box 11-1, respectively. The vast majority of serious causes are infectious in origin. Immediate threats to life result from decompensated shock (usually septic), respiratory failure (related to shock or pneumonitis), or central nervous system infection (meningitis). There are some critical noninfectious causes of fever (see Box 11-1), but these are relatively rare and frequently do not occur with fever as the primary symptom.

Rapid Assessment and Stabilization

Patients with life-threatening signs and symptoms, including significant alterations in mental status, respiratory distress, and cardiovascular instability, require rapid, aggressive treatment. Prompt establishment of airway management, monitoring, intravenous access, fluid resuscitation, supplemental oxygen, and respiratory support are often necessary despite incomplete information concerning etiology. Sustained temperatures above 41.0° C are rare but can be damaging to neural tissue and require rapid, aggressive cooling (e.g., misting, fans, cooling blankets).

In the younger, otherwise healthy patient with fever, immediate threats to life such as toxic or septic shock, meningitis, meningococcemia, and peritonitis should be considered and treated empirically.

In the older, chronically ill population with fever, most of the serious illnesses originate from infections in the respiratory tract, the genitourinary tract, and the skin and soft tissues. Meningitis, although less common, can also be a significant cause of morbidity and mortality in this group.

Pivotal Findings

Although the differential diagnosis of fever is broad, most of the treatable causes are of infectious origin. Up to 85% of these may be diagnosed by careful history and physical examination alone. Age and the presence of underlying medical conditions can substantially influence the evaluation and subsequent decision making regarding management.

Younger and otherwise healthy adults have self-limited, localized bacterial infections or benign systemic viral infections as the cause of their fever.

The challenge with this group is to identify the rare life-threatening illness, such as meningococcemia or meningitis. In this population, one should beware of a sense of complacency supported by the fact that most patients have benign illness.

In the older or chronically ill population, fever is frequently a sign of severe illness. Usually, the etiology is infectious. Eighty percent have respiratory infections, urinary tract infections, or soft tissue infections as the cause. Infections such as meningitis, cholecystitis, appendicitis, and diverticulitis may arise with atypical signs and symptoms in the elderly or immunosuppressed patient. In this population, subtle changes in behavior may be the only sign of severe infection. Abnormal vital signs, especially tachypnea and hypotension, may portend a complicated and severe course. Seventy-five percent of the cases of functional decline in nursing home patients are due to infection.[6,7]

History

The *onset* of the fever and its *duration* and *magnitude* and any *associated symptoms* help identify possible causes and severity of illness. Localizing symptoms such as dysuria and productive cough are especially helpful. The *timing* of the fever and its *patterns* may implicate certain diseases (such as malaria). *Recent or remote travel*, *chronic illnesses*, past surgeries, hospitalizations, and treatment modalities may raise the suspicion of exotic or nosocomial infections. The presence of cardiac valves or any prosthetic or indwelling device may be critical to the diagnosis.

Also important is a list of all the patient's medications, including any antipyretic medication. Family members are frequently an important source of information. They are often the first to notice a functional decline in the patient, such as difficulty ambulating, anorexia, decreased activity, or new urinary incontinence.

Atypical symptoms are the rule in elderly patients. The most common symptoms of pneumonia or urinary tract infection in the older patient are a change in mental status, difficulty ambulating, or some other functional decline. Dysuria, frequency, and flank pain are often absent in elderly patients with urinary tract infection. Patients with pneumonia may inconsistently present with productive cough or shortness of breath. Other frequent but nonspecific symptoms include anorexia, weight loss, weakness, lethargy, nausea, and recurrent falls.[8,9] A history of cancer with recent chemotherapy or radiation therapy may be a clue to leukopenia or other immunodepressed states.[4]

Physical Examination

The presence of fever is an obvious critical element of the examination, but the elderly or chronically ill patient may not mount a febrile response to significant infection. Temperatures may fluctuate, and regular rechecks are necessary.

Rectal temperatures are the most accurate. Axillary and tympanic temperatures are often unreliable. Oral temperatures may be distorted by recent ingestion of hot or cold liquids, smoking, or hyperventilation. Rectal temperatures are typically 0.7° C to 1.0° C degree higher than oral temperatures.

Fever is inconsistently associated with tachycardia and tachypnea. The heart rate may increase by 10 beats/min for each 0.55° C degree rise in temperature. Relative bradycardia may be caused by medication but can suggest factitious or drug-related fevers, typhoid fever, brucellosis, or leptospirosis. Frank bradycardia may occur with rheumatic fever, Lyme disease, viral myocarditis, and endocarditis. The respiratory rate may increase 2 to 4 breaths per minute per degree centigrade. More significant tachypnea may be due to respiratory infection or the acidosis related to shock.

Recognizing a decline in mental status is critical in the older patient and may be the only clue to the presence of significant infection. The emergency physician frequently does not know the patient's baseline mental function.

The head and neck examination focuses on treatable foci of infection such as otitis media, sinusitis, pharyngitis, peritonsillar abscess, retropharyngeal abscess, and dental infections. A muffled, "hot potato" voice may be a clue to adult epiglottitis or upper airway abscess. Funduscopy may reveal evidence of disseminated candidiasis, miliary tuberculosis, endocarditis, toxoplasmosis, or leukemia.

The neck should be examined for lymphadenopathy, masses, or thyroid pathology. Nuchal rigidity should be assessed but may not be prominent in the debilitated or elderly patient even if meningitis is present. Conversely, cervical arthritis or Parkinson's disease may involve preexisting nuchal rigidity.

The lungs are examined for rales, egophony, pleural rubs, or dullness to percussion. Localized wheezing or rhonchi may be more subtle clues to the presence of pneumonia. The presence of concomitant chronic obstructive pulmonary disease or congestive heart failure, as well as poor respiratory effort, may hamper the diagnosis of pneumonia in the elderly patient. The heart should be examined for pericardial rubs or new murmurs.

The abdominal examination may be deceptively benign in older patients, patients with diabetes, or patients taking immunosuppressives or steroids.[10] All patients should receive a rectal examination to check for evidence of enteritis, perirectal abscess, or prostatitis. The external genitalia examination may reveal evidence of Bartholin's abscess, urethral or vaginal discharge, or evidence of epididymitis or orchitis.

Females with appropriate symptoms should have a pelvic examination to evaluate for pelvic inflammatory disease or tubo-ovarian abscess. The skin and extremities should be evaluated for rash, petechiae, joint inflammation, or evidence of soft tissue infection. In the absence of trauma, tenderness over the long bones or the spine may be evidence of osteomyelitis or neoplastic processes.

Elderly and bedfast patients should be checked for the presence of pressure sores or decubitus ulcers.[3]

The two most important ancillary tests, especially in elderly patients, are urinalysis and chest radiography. Chest radiographs are often helpful in the diagnosis of pulmonary infection but may be deceptive in the patient with concurrent chronic obstructive pulmonary disease, congestive heart failure, dehydration, or other chronic lung disease. The urinalysis, although not foolproof, is highly sensitive and reasonably specific for urinary tract infection. Although the white blood cell count is almost universally used in the evaluation of febrile patients, it lacks the sensitivity and specificity to be of discriminatory value. The white blood cell count may incorrectly indicate serious infection when none is present or may be normal in the presence of life-threatening infection.[11] Other indirect tests of infection and inflammation, such as the erythrocyte sedimentation rate, are also plagued with irregular sensitivity and poor specificity and should be used sparingly. Culture and Gram's stain of appropriate specimens may be helpful. In the elderly or chronically ill patient with fever of unknown source, blood and urine cultures are frequently appropriate. Outpatient blood cultures should rarely, if ever, be done. A patient ill enough to require blood cultures generally requires hospitalization and empirical antibiotic coverage. Cerebrospinal fluid evaluation should be considered with the presence of mental status changes, headache, meningismus, or other unexplained neurologic symptoms.

Plain films of the abdomen are rarely indicated or helpful. Abdominal computed tomography (CT) is helpful if appendicitis, diverticulitis, cholecystitis, or intraabdominal abscess is suspected. Ultrasonography may be helpful in the patient with potential cholecystitis.

Cranial CT scanning may be indicated prior to lumbar puncture in patients with focal neurologic findings or an embolic source, such as suspected endocarditis, to exclude mass lesions such as tumor or brain abscess. This test should not delay antibiotics in patients with suspected meningitis.

Other ancillary testing is directed by the findings of the history and physical examination.

DIFFERENTIAL DIAGNOSIS

The differential diagnoses of infectious causes of fever are summarized in Table 11-1. The differential diagnoses of noninfectious causes of fever are listed in Box 11-1.

EMPIRICAL MANAGEMENT

Patients with temperatures greater than 41.0° C require prompt and aggressive treatment with antipyretics. Temperatures above this range can result in damage to neuronal tissue. Patients with signs and symptoms of shock require aggressive treatment with isotonic fluids. Only after adequate hydration is provided should pressors be considered. Frequently, hemodynamic monitoring is required to guide therapy. Patients with evidence of respiratory failure from shock or pneumonia require ventilatory support. Soft tissue infections of the head and neck may compromise the airway because of mechanical obstruction. These may require acute intervention to provide a secure airway.

In many cases, early empirical antibiotic therapy is appropriate. The choice of antibiotics is based on the likely cause of the fever as well as concomitant conditions such as absolute neutropenia and end-stage renal disease. If a specific infection is identified, antibiotic therapy should be specific to that infection. In the absence of a clear source of infection, broad-spectrum coverage of gram-positive and gram-negative aerobic and anaerobic bacteria is indicated.

DISPOSITION

Localized bacterial infections can most frequently be treated with outpatient oral antibiotics. Relatively young, healthy patients with systemic viral illness can be treated as outpatients. These illnesses are often accompanied by vomiting and poor oral intake, and treatment in the emergency department with antipyretics, antinausea medications, and intravenous hydration may help prepare the patient for a successful outpatient course.

When no clear infection is identified in older patients or those with chronic illness such as diabetes or chronic renal failure, admission to the hospital is almost always indicated. In this subset of patients, a diligent search for evidence of bacterial infection is required. Blood and urine cultures and broad-spectrum antibiotics with cerebrospinal fluid coverage are necessary to ensure that life-threatening infection is rapidly identified and treated. Patients with indwelling devices frequently require those to be cultured and removed. Neutropenic patients with fever require prompt treatment with broad-spectrum parenteral antibiotics pending cultures. Patients with unstable vital signs or life-threatening infections require admission to a special care unit.

REFERENCES

1. Strange GR, Chen EH: Use of the emergency department by elder patients: Five-year follow-up study. *Acad Emerg Med* 5:1157, 1998.
2. Shah SM, Searls L, Weihl AC: The febrile adult—Parts 1 and 2. *Emerg Med Rep* 19:17, 1998.
3. Norman DC, Yoshikawa TT: Fever in the elderly. *Infect Dis Clin North Am* 10:93, 1996.
4. Marco CA, et al: Fever in geriatric emergency patients: Clinical features associated with serious illness. *Ann Emerg Med* 26:18, 1995.
5. Leinicke T, Navitsky R, Cameron S, Brillman J: Fever in the elderly. *Emerg Med Pract* 1:5, 1999.
6. Gallagher EJ, Brooks F, Gennis P: Identification of serious illness in febrile adults. *Am J Emerg Med* 12:129, 1994.

7. Keating HJ, et al: Effect of aging on the clinical significance of fever in the ambulatory adult patient. *J Am Geriatr Soc* 32:282, 1984.
8. Fein AM, Niederman MS: Severe pneumonia in the elderly. *Clin Geriatr Med* 10:121, 1994.
9. Stamm WE: Protocol for diagnosis of urinary tract infection. *Urology* 32:6, 1988.
10. Elangovan S: Clinical and laboratory findings in acute appendicitis in the elderly. *J Am Board Fam Pract* 9:75, 1996.
11. Badgett RG, Hanson CJ, Rodgers CS: Clinical usage of the leukocyte count in emergency room decision making. *J Gen Intern Med* 5:198, 1990.

CHAPTER

12 Weakness

Robert C. Reiser

PERSPECTIVE

Weakness is defined as "lacking physical strength, energy, or vigor; feeble." This definition, in including the sensation of lost energy or vigor, highlights the largely subjective component of the symptom. Most cases of generalized weakness do not represent true neuromuscular transmission failure; cases that do may prove fatal. Weakness as a symptom may be manifested by a wide spectrum of disease states (Table 12-1), including psychiatric disorders. This chapter focuses on the initial approach to a patient with generalized symmetric weakness and excludes trauma, strokes, and space-occupying lesions.[1]

Epidemiology

The World Health Organization reported 1831 new cases of acute flaccid paralysis in the United States in 2003 that were not due to trauma, stroke, or tumor. The epidemiology of acute symmetric weakness ranges from the near extinction of poliomyelitis in the world (no new cases in the Western Hemisphere since 1991, 682 new cases worldwide in 2003) to myasthenia gravis, the most commonly occurring disease of neuromuscular transmission, with a prevalence of 5 to 14.2 cases per 100,000 people. The most common cause of acute symmetric paralysis is Guillain-Barré syndrome, with an incidence of 0.75 to 2 cases per 100,000 people.[2]

Pathophysiology

The stimulus for muscle contraction is generated in the brain. It is transmitted to the anterior horn cells in the spinal cord and travels as a wave of depolarization via myelinated peripheral nerves to the motor end plate. When the impulse reaches the motor end plate, the peripheral nerve releases packets of acetylcholine (quanta), which cross the synaptic cleft and bind to receptors on the muscle fiber. This release of acetylcholine is calcium dependent. Binding of the acetylcholine opens Ca^{++} channels in the muscle fiber, leading to an influx of Ca^{++} and depolarization of the muscle fiber. This spreading wave of depolarization causes contraction of the muscle fiber. Acetylcholine rapidly diffuses away or is degraded by plasma acetylcholinesterase in 1 msec. Lesions at any level of this motor unit can cause weakness; this chapter presents examples of diseases at each level and shows how to distinguish them.

DIAGNOSTIC APPROACH

Differential Considerations

When the neurologic symptom is generalized weakness, the first question should be, "Is there a neuromuscular cause?" (see Table 12-1). Is the patient describing a systemic, nonspecific fatigue, or is the patient describing a specific, well-defined muscular weakness? Common non-neurologic entities that may present as weakness include infections (e.g., urinary tract infection, influenza, pneumonia); myocardial infarction; and endocrine, metabolic, and psychiatric disease states. If a lesion of the central nervous system or peripheral nervous system is suggested, including the neuromuscular junction, the focus is on differentiating upper motor neuron from lower motor neuron, or neuromuscular, disorders.[3]

Rapid Assessment and Stabilization

All patients presenting to the emergency department complaining of weakness should be evaluated for protective airway reflexes (swallowing, managing secretions, and phonation) and for adequacy of ventilation (Figure 12-1). Profound weakness, manifested by inadequate forced expiratory volume or negative inspiratory pressure, mandates early intubation before progressive ventilatory insufficiency supervenes.

Two groups of muscles are crucial for maintaining normal respiration. The upper airway muscles (palatal, pharyngeal, and lingual) receive their innervation from the cranial nerves and are responsible for maintaining airway patency and handling secretions and swallowing. Patients with primarily weakness of the upper airway muscles typically present with a hoarse or nasal

Table 12-1. Differential Diagnosis of Weakness: Non-neuromuscular versus Neuromuscular Causes

Non-neuromuscular	Neuromuscular
Critical	
Myocardial infarction	Rabies
Impending respiratory failure	Botulism
Sepsis	Tetanus
Emergent	
Dehydration	Guillain-Barré syndrome
	Electrolyte imbalance
	Myasthenia gravis crisis
	Periodic paralysis
	Transverse myelitis
Other	
Simple fatigue	Lambert-Eaton syndrome
Anxiety	Poliomyelitis
Fibromyalgia	ALS
Chronic fatigue syndrome	Multiple sclerosis
Malignancy	Diphtheria
	Porphyria
	Seafood toxins
	Tick paralysis

ALS, amyotrophic lateral sclerosis.

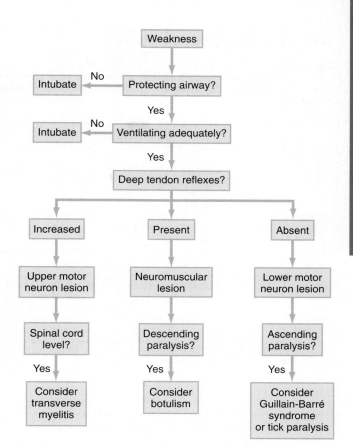

Figure 12-1. Diagnostic-management algorithm: an approach to weakness.

voice, difficulty swallowing fluids or saliva, other cranial nerve palsies, and a history of a descending weakness. Botulism, myasthenia, and multiple sclerosis are important differential diagnoses.

The inspiratory muscles (sternocleidomastoids, diaphragm, scalenes, and external intercostals) receive innervation from cranial nerve XI in the case of the sternocleidomastoid, the phrenic nerve for the diaphragm, and C4-T8 for the scalenes and intercostals. Patients with primarily weakness of the inspiratory muscles present with tachypnea, paradoxical abdominal movement (inward movement of the abdomen during inspiration), and a history of an ascending paralysis. Guillain-Barré syndrome is the most important differential diagnosis in these patients.[4,5] The tachypnea is a physiologic attempt to maintain minute ventilation in the face of decreased tidal volume, and the paradoxical abdominal movement is a sign of diaphragmatic weakness.

Subtle weakness occasionally can progress quickly to ventilatory failure requiring mechanical support. A careful history of the onset and speed of progression of the weakness suggests which patients are at risk of rapid progression. In general, descending weakness tends to be more worrisome for rapid progression to ventilatory failure than ascending weakness.

Pivotal Findings (Table 12-2)

History

The history should focus on the manifestations of weakness in the patient. What does the patient mean when he or she reports weakness? Are there specific activities or muscle groups that seem to be involved, or is the feeling one of systemic fatigue? The temporal course of the symptoms and the progression, if any, of

the weakness are important clues to separate neuromuscular disease from systemic fatigue resulting from other causes. The presence or absence of fever and any preceding infectious syndromes should be elicited. Chest pain, shortness of breath, cough, urinary symptoms, or other localizing symptoms should be explored. A history of malignancy should be sought.[1]

Physical Examination

If neuromuscular disease is suspected, the physical examination helps answer the most important question of where the lesion may be (Box 12-1; see Table 12-2).

Ancillary Testing

Rapid bedside tests are available, usually through respiratory therapy, to measure forced vital capacity, negative inspiratory force, and peak expiratory force. Forced vital capacity less than 10 to 12 mL/kg or negative inspiratory force less than 20 cm H_2O is an indication for intubation.[5] In addition, electrolytes, calcium, magnesium, blood urea nitrogen, and creatinine tests should be ordered if true weakness is found. Electrocardiography may assist in gauging the cardiac impact of an abnormal potassium or calcium value. Arterial blood gases, computed tomography, magnetic resonance imaging, electromyography, and lumbar puncture may aid in the evaluation.

Table 12-2. Pivotal Findings in Weakness

Appearance	History	Physical	Laboratory Findings	Diagnoses
Respiratory distress, fatigued	SOB, weak	Tachypnea, paradoxical breathing, abnormal phonation	Increasing PaCO₂, decreased PFTs	Impending respiratory failure
Prostrated	Fever, cough, weak	Febrile, lung findings	CXR abnormal or CBC elevated	Pneumonia, influenza
Delirious or demented	Fever, altered mental status, weak	No local findings	UA or CBC abnormal	Sepsis, UTI
Normal	Globally weak, sometimes worsened by meal, exercise	Strength 4/5, reflexes normal	Electrolytes abnormal (especially K⁺)	Hypokalemia (including familial periodic paralysis), other metabolic disarray
Normal	Preceding viral infection, ascending paralysis	Absent DTRs, flaccid paralysis	CSF albuminocytologic dissociation	Guillain-Barré syndrome
Normal	Globally weak	Strength 4/5, reflexes normal	Electrolytes normal	Botulism, Lambert-Eaton syndrome, myasthenia gravis
Normal	Rapidly progressive paralysis	Demarcated spinal cord level DTRs hyperreflexic	Normal	Transverse myelitis
Normal	Ascending paralysis	Absent DTRs, flaccid paralysis, ataxia	Tick found imbedded	Tick paralysis

CBC, complete blood count; CSF, cerebrospinal fluid; CXR, chest x-ray; DTR, deep tendon reflex; PFT, pulmonary function test; SOB, shortness of breath; UA, urinalysis; UTI, urinary tract infection.

BOX 12-1. Physical Signs to Localize Neuromuscular Lesions

Upper Motor Neuron Lesions
Plantar reflex upgoing
Deep tendon reflexes increased
Normal to increased muscle tone or spasticity (late finding)

Lower Motor Neuron Lesions
Plantar reflex normal or absent
Deep tendon reflexes decreased, usually absent
Decreased to flaccid muscle tone

Neuromuscular Junction or Muscle Lesions
Plantar reflex normal or absent
Deep tendon reflexes usually preserved, may be decreased
Decreased to flaccid muscle tone

BOX 12-2. Neurologic Levels of Common Causes of Neuromuscular Weakness

Upper Motor Neuron Lesions
Transverse myelitis
Poliomyelitis
Amyotrophic lateral sclerosis (mixed upper and lower)
Multiple sclerosis

Lower Motor Neuron Lesions
Guillain-Barré syndrome
Toxic neuropathies
Impingement syndromes
Diphtheria
Porphyria
Ciguatera, shellfish, or puffer fish toxin

Myoneural Junction/Muscle Fiber Lesions
Myasthenia gravis
Lambert-Eaton syndrome
Botulism
Periodic paralyses
Electrolyte imbalances
Tick paralysis

DIFFERENTIAL DIAGNOSIS

The history and physical examination with attention to certain patterns of neurologic findings often lead to a presumptive diagnosis of neuromuscular disease (Box 12-2; see Box 12-1). If the weakness is due to other causes, the diagnosis may be found in the electrocardiogram or the laboratory studies.[6]

If the level of a neurologic lesion has been determined, the differential diagnosis can be narrowed considerably. Frequently the specific diagnosis can be reasonably inferred from the history and associated physical findings. Ancillary studies may aid in the evaluation. A pattern of ascending paralysis after a viral syndrome with absent deep tendon reflexes and an albumin-cytologic dissociation in the cerebrospinal fluid (protein > 400 mg/dL, white blood cell count < 10 mL) is virtually diagnostic of Guillain-Barré syndrome.[2,7] Early in the course of an acute presentation of generalized weakness, the history and physical examination may suggest several processes, and definitive diagnosis is often not possible in the emergency department.[2]

EMPIRIC MANAGEMENT

The immediate life threats associated with acute presentations of weakness are an inability to maintain

---

BOX 12-3. Indications for Intubation in Patients with Weakness and Ventilatory Insufficiency

Severe fatigue
Inability to protect airway or handle secretions
Rapidly rising $PaCO_2$
Hypoxemia despite supplemental O_2
FVC < 12 mL/kg
NIF < 20 cm H_2O

Note: If paralytics are used to facilitate intubation, depolarizing agents should be avoided because of the potential for hyperkalemia.
FVC, forced vital capacity; NIF, negative inspiratory force.

---

or protect the upper airway, inadequate strength to breathe, and circulatory collapse resulting from autonomic instability. Initial empiric management consists of repeated assessment beyond initial stabilization of the patient for airway protective reflexes and for adequacy of ventilatory effort (see Figure 12-1). Most decisions about intubation can be made based on clinical assessment (Box 12-3). Patients with neuromuscular weakness have an intact respiratory drive, and the decrease in tidal volume is offset by an increase in respiratory rate. Because of a subjective sense of dyspnea at low tidal volumes, patients often maintain arterial partial pressure of carbon dioxide ($PaCO_2$) in the range of 35 mm Hg, and a critically low vital capacity develops. When the $PaCO_2$ begins to increase in these circumstances, abrupt respiratory failure is imminent. Rapid sequence intubation is the preferred approach to the airway in the absence of identified difficult airway markers, but if a progressive denervation syndrome is suspected, succinylcholine should be avoided because of the potential for hyperkalemia. Intravenous access should be established to support circulation as needed.[3] A thorough search for a tick should be performed, especially in the hair. Tick removal is rapidly curative in cases of tick paralysis.[8]

DEFINITIVE MANAGEMENT

When the diagnosis is known, specific therapies can be applied. Specific antitoxins exist for botulism and diphtheria and can shorten the course of the disease and avoid the need for intubation in the case of botulism.[9] Potassium supplements can be given orally or intravenously if hypokalemia is a contributing cause.

Good results have been obtained with plasma exchange and intravenous immunoglobulin G in Guillain-Barré syndrome. Consultation with a neurologist or intensivist helps direct the application of these therapies. Steroids have no role in the management of Guillain-Barré syndrome.[10,11]

Most cases of myasthenia present to the emergency department with the diagnosis already established, but exacerbations of the weakness may be seen and present a diagnostic challenge to determine if the weakness is due to a myasthenic crisis or a cholinergic crisis caused by cholinesterase inhibitor therapy. About 20% of patients with myasthenia gravis experience a myasthenic crisis that requires intubation and mechanical ventilation. Although a Tensilon (edrophonium chloride) test may help distinguish between myasthenic and cholinergic crises, the interpretation of this test is complex and best left to an experienced neurologist. Most cholinergic crises occur superimposed on an underlying myasthenic crisis, and in questionable cases it is best to protect the airway, support ventilation, and withdraw all anticholinergic medications.[12-14]

DISPOSITION

Most patients with complaints of weakness in the emergency department have nonspecific, non-neuromuscular problems and are simply reporting subjective weakness that is neither focal nor progressive. A thorough assessment, including directed ancillary testing, allows most of these patients to be discharged with follow-up care planning through a primary physician.

Patients with known neuromuscular problems who are in the emergency department for exacerbations or complications should be treated in consultation with their primary physician or a neurologist. Most of these patients can be discharged with prearranged follow-up.

Patients with new-onset neuromuscular problems usually are admitted for definitive studies. Selected patients with limited manifestations of disease may be discharged after consultation and planned follow-up with a neurologist. In cases in which toxin-mediated paralyses, such as botulism, are suspected, patients should be hospitalized in an intensive care setting for close ventilatory monitoring and support. Consultation with a clinical toxicologist or regional poison center is advisable.

REFERENCES

1. LoVecchio F, Jacobson S: Approach to generalized weakness and peripheral neuromuscular disease. *Emerg Med Clin North Am* 15:605, 1997.
2. Bolton CF: The changing concepts of Guillain-Barré syndrome. *N Engl J Med* 333:1415, 1995.
3. Abrunzo TJ, Bowman MJ: Acute presentation of muscle weakness. *Pediatr Emerg Med Rep* 4:29, 1999.
4. Cheng BC, et al: Predictive factors and long-term outcome of respiratory failure after Guillain-Barré syndrome. *Am J Med Sci* 327:336, 2004.
5. Lawn ND, et al: Anticipating mechanical ventilation in Guillain-Barré syndrome. *Arch Neurol* 58:893, 2001.
6. Miller JD, Quillian W, Cleveland WW: Nonfamilial hypokalemic periodic paralysis and thyrotoxicosis in a 16-year-old male. *Pediatrics* 100:412, 1997.
7. Sladky JT: Guillain-Barré syndrome in children. *J Child Neurol* 19:191, 2004.
8. Felz MW, Smith CD, Swift TR: A six-year-old girl with tick paralysis. *N Engl J Med* 342:90, 2000.
9. Robinson RF, et al: Management of botulism. *Ann Pharmacother* 37:127, 2003.
10. van Koningsveld R, et al: Effect of methylprednisolone when added to standard treatment with intravenous immunoglobulin for Guillain-Barré syndrome: Randomized trial. *Lancet* 363:192, 2004.

11. Hughes RA, et al: Practice parameter: Immunotherapy for Guillain-Barré syndrome: Report of the Quality Standards Subcommittee of the American Academy of Neurology. *Neurology* 61:736, 2003.
12. Keesey JC: Clinical evaluation and management of myasthenia gravis. *Muscle Nerve* 29:484, 2004.
13. Younger DS, et al: Medical therapies in myasthenia gravis. *Chest Surg Clin N Am* 11:329, 2001.
14. Bedlack RS, et al: How to handle myasthenic crisis: Essential steps in patient care. *Postgrad Med* 107:211, 2000.

CHAPTER

13 Dizziness and Vertigo

Jonathan S. Olshaker

PERSPECTIVE

Dizziness is an imprecise term with multiple meanings. It is a common complaint in the emergency department, especially in the elderly. Dizziness in older persons is associated with a variety of cardiovascular, neurosensory, and psychiatric conditions and with the use of multiple medications.[1] Among patients older than 60 years, 20% have experienced dizziness severe enough to affect their daily activity.[2] In a study of 1000 outpatients, dizziness was the third most common complaint. *Vertigo* is defined more clearly as a sensation of disorientation in space combined with a sensation of motion. In 1921, Bárány published the first detailed description of benign paroxysmal positional vertigo, the most common disorder of the peripheral vestibular system.

Most of these patients have an organic basis for these symptoms. The diagnostic process is consistently based on two basic concepts: deciding whether the patient has true vertigo and, if vertigo exists, deciding whether the cause is central or peripheral.[3]

Pathophysiology

The maintenance of equilibrium and awareness of the body in relationship to its surroundings depend on the interaction of three systems: visual, proprioceptive, and vestibular. The eyes, muscles, joints, and otic labyrinths continuously supply information about the position of the body. Visual impulses, mediated through the higher brain centers, provide information about body position in space. Impulses from proprioceptors of the joints and muscles supply data about the relative positions of the parts of the body. Impulses from the neck are of special importance in relating the position of the head to the rest of the body. The sense organs of the visual, vestibular, and proprioceptive systems are connected with the cerebellum by way of the vestibular nuclei in the brainstem. Any disease that interrupts the integration of these three systems may give rise to symptoms of vertigo and disequilibrium.

The vestibular apparatus helps maintain head position and stabilize head movement. It is housed in the inner ear, or labyrinth, which lies embedded in the petrous portion of the temporal bone, where it is vulnerable to trauma; blood-borne toxins; and infections in nearby structures, including the middle ear and meninges. The vestibular apparatus consists of three semicircular canals with their cristae and two otolithic structures—the utricle and saccule. The semicircular canals provide information about movement and angular momentum; the otoliths provide information about the orientation of the body with respect to gravity.

The semicircular canals are paired structures that normally respond to motion in a symmetric manner. With inner ear disease, the resting discharge or the discharge stimulated by motion can be altered in one ear. This alteration produces asymmetric responses and results in the perception of vertigo. Freely moving debris within the semicircular canals can produce positional vertigo as the debris moves under the influence of gravity.

Impulses leave the vestibular apparatus by the vestibular part of the acoustic nerve (cranial nerve VIII), enter the brainstem just below the pons and anterior to the cerebellum, and proceed to the four vestibular nuclei of the brainstem and to the cerebellum. From there, impulses travel along two pathways that contribute to the clinical manifestations of vertigo—the medial longitudinal fasciculus and the vestibulospinal tract. In individuals with healthy vestibular systems, these connections allow the eyes to compensate for body movement in different directions and to maintain a visual axis that is stable with respect to the environment.

Nystagmus occurs when the synchronized vestibular information becomes unbalanced. Typically, it results from unilateral vestibular disease, which causes asymmetric stimulation of the medial and lateral rectus muscles. This unopposed activity causes a slow movement of the eyes toward the side of the stimulus, regardless of the direction of deviation of the eyes. The cerebral cortex then corrects for these eye movements and rapidly brings the eyes back to the midline, only to have the process repeated.

By convention, the direction of nystagmus is denoted by the direction of the fast "cortical" component. Nystagmus caused by vestibular disease tends to be unidirectional and horizontorotary. If the nystagmus is vertical, a central lesion (either brainstem or cerebral) is usually the cause.

The vestibular nuclei send information to the lateral vestibulospinal tract, where they connect with motor neurons that supply the muscles of the extremities. This phenomenon explains the false steps or other body movements made by people with a defective vestibular apparatus who are making attempts to correct for an imagined change in position. Connections between the vestibular nuclei and the autonomic system account for the perspiration, nausea, and vomiting that commonly accompany an attack of vertigo. Connections between the vestibular nuclei and the cerebellum account for the modulating influence of this organ on motor activity.

DIAGNOSTIC APPROACH

Differential Considerations

Patients use the term *dizzy* to describe a variety of experiences, including sensations of motion, weakness, fainting, lightheadedness, unsteadiness, and depression. To clarify the picture, it is often helpful to have patients describe the sensation without using the word *dizzy*. True vertigo may be defined as a sensation of disorientation in space combined with a sensation of motion. There is a hallucination of movement either of the self (subjective vertigo) or the external environment (objective vertigo). Descriptions of lightheadedness or feeling faint are more consistent with presyncope. The differential diagnosis for these patients should include dysrhythmias, myocardial infarction, sepsis, hypovolemia, drug side effects, and pulmonary embolism. For some patients, dizziness is simply a metaphor for malaise, representing a variety of other causes, such as anemia, viral illness, or depression. The primary focus of this chapter is to review the evaluation of the vertiginous patient.

If the patient has true vertigo, the clinician must determine whether the cause is a peripheral lesion (e.g., of the inner ear) or a central process, such as cerebrovascular disease or a neoplasm. In most cases, peripheral disorders are benign, and central processes have more serious consequences. Occasionally, as in the case of a cerebellar hemorrhage, immediate therapeutic intervention is indicated. Acute suppurative labyrinthitis is the only cause of peripheral vertigo that requires urgent intervention. Box 13-1 lists causes of vertigo and identifies the peripheral, central, and systemic diagnoses. Table 13-1 summarizes the different characteristics of peripheral and central vertigo.

BOX 13-1. Causes of Vertigo

Peripheral Causes
Foreign body in ear canal
Cerumen or hair against tympanic membrane
Acute otitis media
Labyrinthitis (suppurative, serous, toxic, chronic)
Benign positional vertigo
Ménière's disease
Vestibular neuronitis
Perilymphatic fistula
Trauma (labyrinth concussion)
Motion sickness
Acoustic neuroma*

Central Causes
Infection (encephalitis, meningitis, brain abscess)
Vertebral basilar artery insufficiency
Subclavian steal syndrome
Cerebellar hemorrhage or infarction
Vertebral basilar migraine
Posttraumatic injury (temporal bone fracture)
Postconcussive syndrome
Temporal lobe epilepsy
Tumor
Multiple sclerosis
Cervical spine muscle and ligamentous injury

Systemic Causes
Diabetes mellitus
Hypothyroidism

---

*Cause of peripheral vertigo that proceeds centrally.

Table 13-1. Characteristics of Peripheral and Central Vertigo

Characteristic	Peripheral	Central
Onset	Sudden	Gradual
Intensity	Severe	Mild
Duration	Usually seconds or minutes; occasionally hours, days (intermittent)	Usually weeks, months (continuous)
Direction of nystagmus	One direction (usually horizontorotary), never vertical	Horizontal, rotary, or vertical (different directions in different positions)
Effect of head position	Worsened by position, often single critical position	Little change, associated with more than one position
Associated neurologic findings	None	Usually present
Associated auditory findings	May be present, including tinnitus	None

Pivotal Findings

History

The medical history is the most important source of information in the evaluation of the dizzy patient. Does true vertigo exist? Does the patient have a sensation of disorientation in space or a sensation of motion? The sensation of spinning usually indicates a vestibular disorder. Some nausea, vomiting, pallor, and perspiration accompany almost all but the mildest forms of vertigo. The presence of these symptoms without vertigo should suggest a different cause. The labyrinth has no effect on the level of consciousness. The patient should not have an associated change in mentation or syncope.

Because nystagmus accompanies acute vertigo, it is often helpful to ask members of the patient's family if they have noted any unusual eye movements during the dizzy spells. This question is especially important in children unable to offer a concise history.[4] Occasionally, the patient may be able to describe a flickering or oscillating visual field immediately after a change in position, such as rolling over in bed.

The *time of onset* and the *duration of vertigo* are important clues to the cause. Episodic vertigo that is severe, lasts several hours, and has symptom-free intervals between episodes suggests a peripheral labyrinth disorder. Vertigo produced primarily by a change in position also suggests a peripheral disorder. Vestibular neuronitis and benign positional vertigo fit this pattern.

The presence of *auditory symptoms* suggests a peripheral cause of the vertigo, as in middle and inner ear problems, or a peripheral cause that progresses centrally, such as an acoustic neuroma. The abnormally hearing ear is usually the side of end-organ disturbance. Progressive unilateral hearing loss of several months' duration may be the earliest symptom of an acoustic neuroma. Tinnitus occurs in most patients with acoustic neuroma and, along with vertigo, is what often prompts patients to seek medical attention. Hearing loss, vertigo, and tinnitus form the characteristic triad of Ménière's disease.

Are there associated neurological symptoms? The patient or family members should be questioned about the time of onset of ataxia or gait disturbances. Ataxia of recent and relatively sudden onset suggests cerebellar hemorrhage or infarction in the distribution of the posterior inferior cerebellar artery or the superior cerebellar artery. The salient feature of chronic cerebellar disorders is a slowly progressive ataxia. True ataxia may be difficult to discern from the unsteadiness that occurs when a patient with significant vertigo attempts to walk.

Vertiginous symptoms are common after head injury. The presence of recent head or neck trauma should be explored because vertiginous symptoms are common after both.[5] Head injury can cause vertigo occasionally from intercerebral injury and more commonly from labyrinth concussion. Neck injury can cause vertigo from strain of muscle proprioceptors. In addition, vertebral artery injury has been seen resulting from activities such as chiropractic manipulation and even hair shampooing with marked hyperextension in a salon.[6]

Past Medical History

Many *medications* have direct vestibulotoxicity. The most commonly encountered are the aminoglycosides, anticonvulsants, alcohols, quinine, quinidine, and minocycline. In addition, caffeine and nicotine can have wide-ranging autonomic effects that may exacerbate vestibular symptoms. The history of *past and present illnesses* should be explored, with specific questioning about the existence of diabetes and drug or alcohol use.

Physical Examination

Vital Signs

In some cases, pulses and blood pressure should be checked in both arms. Most patients with subclavian steal syndrome, which also can cause vertebrobasilar artery insufficiency, have pulse or systolic blood pressure differences between the two arms.

Head and Neck

Carotid or vertebral artery bruits suggest atherosclerosis. The neck is auscultated along the course of the carotid artery from the supraclavicular area to the base of the skull.

Vertigo can be caused by impacted cerumen or a foreign object in the ear canal. Accumulation of fluid behind the eardrum as a result of a middle ear infection may cause mild vertigo, as can occlusion of the eustachian tubes associated with an upper respiratory tract infection. A perforated or scarred eardrum may indicate a perilymphatic fistula, especially if the history includes previous trauma.

Examination of the eyes is key in assessing a patient with vertigo or disequilibrium. The focus is on any pupillary abnormalities indicating third cranial nerve or descending sympathetic tract involvement or optic disk signs of early increased intracranial pressure. Extraocular movements should be assessed carefully. Relatively subtle ocular movement abnormalities can be the only clue to a cerebellar hemorrhage. A sixth cranial nerve palsy ipsilateral to the hemorrhage may result from early brainstem compression by the expanding hematoma. Internuclear ophthalmoplegia is recognized when the eyes are in a normal position on straight-ahead gaze, but on eye movement the adducting eye (cranial nerve III) is weak or shows no movement while the abducting eye (cranial nerve VI) moves normally, although often displaying a coarse nystagmus. This finding indicates an interruption of the medial longitudinal fasciculus on the side of the third cranial nerve weakness. It indicates brainstem pathology and is virtually pathognomonic of multiple sclerosis.

Abnormal nystagmus is the cardinal sign of inner ear disease and the principal objective evidence of abnormal vestibular function. In nystagmus, the patient has difficulty maintaining the conjugate deviation of the eyes or has a postural-control imbalance of eye movements.[7]

The abnormal jerk nystagmus of inner ear disease consists of slow and quick components. The eyes slowly "drift" in the direction of the diseased, hypoactive ear, then quickly jerk back to the intended direc-

Table 13-2. Distinguishing Characteristics of Nystagmus with Central and Peripheral Vertigo

Characteristic	Central	Peripheral
Direction	Any direction	Horizontal or horizontotory
Laterality	Unilateral or bilateral	Bilateral
Position testing effects:		
Latency	Short	Long
Duration	Sustained	Transient
Intensity	Mild	Mild to severe
Fatigability	Nonfatigable	Fatigable
Effect of visual fixation	Not suppressed, may be enhanced	Suppressed

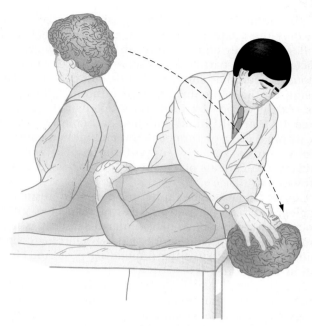

Figure 13-1. Testing for positional vertigo and nystagmus

tion of gaze. Positional nystagmus, induced by rapidly changing the position of the head, strongly suggests an organic vestibular disorder. The characteristics of nystagmus are one of the most valuable tools to distinguish peripheral from central causes of vertigo (Table 13-2).

Positional Testing

If nystagmus is not present at rest, positional testing can be helpful to determine its existence and characteristics. In the Hallpike maneuver, the patient is moved quickly from an upright seated position to a supine position, and the head is turned to one side and extended (to a head-down posture) approximately 30 degrees from the horizontal plane off the end of the stretcher. The eyes should be observed for nystagmus and the patient queried for the occurrence of symptoms. This test should be repeated with the head turned to the other side. Positive elicitation of symptoms and signs to one side or the other generally indicates vestibular pathology on that same side. This test should be performed with caution if vertebrobasilar insufficiency (VBI) is suspected because sudden twisting movements theoretically might dislodge atheromatous plaques (Figure 13-1).

Neurologic Examination

The presence of cranial nerve deficits suggests a space-occupying lesion in the brainstem or cerebellopontine angle. The corneal reflex is a sensory cranial nerve V and motor cranial nerve VII circuit. Its diminution or absence can be one of the early signs of an acoustic neuroma. Vertigo caused by eighth cranial nerve involvement is likely to be accompanied by a unilateral hearing loss. Patients cannot hear a tuning fork when it is held alongside the affected ear, but they can hear it when it is held against the mastoid process. Involvement of the eighth cranial nerve should suggest an acoustic tumor. Seventh cranial nerve involvement causes facial palsy that affects the entire side of the face. In supranuclear facial paralysis, the forehead is spared because these muscles receive bilateral cortical innervation.

The patient should be evaluated specifically for evidence of cerebellar dysfunction. This examination must be performed in bed and standing because truncal ataxia may be occult on testing of limbs in bed and may become obvious only when the patient has to sit, stand, or walk unaided. *Dysmetria* is the inability to arrest a muscular movement at the desired point. Dysmetria should be assessed using finger-to-finger/finger-to-nose pointing, and dysdiadochokinesia (an inability to perform coordinated muscular movement smoothly) is checked with rapid alternating movements. The gait must be evaluated when the patient gives a history suggesting ataxia, although examination may be impossible during an attack of vertigo. Any marked abnormality (e.g., consistent falling or a grossly abnormal gait) should arouse suspicion of a central lesion, especially in a patient whose vertiginous symptoms have subsided. The main features of a cerebellar gait are a wide base (separation of legs), unsteadiness, irregularity of steps, tremor of the trunk, and lurching from side to side. The unsteadiness is most prominent on arising quickly from a sitting position, turning quickly, or stopping suddenly while walking. Patients with gait ataxia cannot perform heel-to-toe walking.

Ancillary Testing

Most routine laboratory testing is not helpful in the evaluation of a vertiginous patient. A finger stick blood glucose test should be performed in most cases because hypoglycemia can present as vertigo.[8] Blood counts and blood chemistries are sometimes helpful in cases in which it is difficult to distinguish whether "dizziness" is vertigo or near-syncope. An electrocardiogram should be obtained if there is any suspicion of myocardial ischemia.

Radiologic Imaging

If cerebellar hemorrhage, cerebellar infarction, or other central lesions are suspected, emergent computed tomography (CT) or magnetic resonance imaging (MRI) of the brain is indicated. MRI, when available, has become the diagnostic modality of choice when cerebellar processes other than acute hemorrhage are suspected. MRI is particularly useful for the diagnosis of acoustic neuromas and for sclerotic and demyelinating lesions of the white matter, as seen in multiple sclerosis. Acute vertigo by itself does not usually warrant urgent CT or MRI in all patients, particularly patients in whom a clear picture of peripheral vertigo emerges. Many studies strongly support the use of imaging, however, in patients of advanced age or at risk for cerebrovascular disease.[9,10]

Conventional angiography or magnetic resonance angiography can be used in cases of suspected VBI to document the presence of vascular disease. It is used most often in patients with changing neurologic signs and symptoms, suggesting impending posterior circulation occlusion.

Audiology and electronystagmography are helpful in the follow-up evaluation of a vertiginous patient. Audiology can locate the anatomic site of a lesion causing vertigo. Electronystagmography is a collection of examinations that, when abnormal, suggest vestibular dysfunction but do not yield the specific diagnosis.

DIFFERENTIAL DIAGNOSIS

The differential diagnosis for other peripheral, central, and systemic causes of vertigo is large (see Box 13-1). More detailed information is given on selected causes in Table 13-3, including the most common peripheral causes of true vertigo: benign positional vertigo, labyrinthitis, Ménière's disease, and vestibular neuronitis.

Diagnostic Algorithm (Figure 13-2)

Most cases of vertigo are of peripheral origin and do not usually represent a life threat. The diagnostic approach must focus on identifying entities that either immediately or in the near future can lead to death or significant morbidity.

MANAGEMENT

Management is based on an accurate diagnosis that distinguishes the serious central causes of vertigo from the less serious, albeit more debilitating, peripheral causes (Figure 13-3). Any suspicion of cerebellar hemorrhage should warrant immediate imaging with CT or MRI and neurosurgery consultations. VBI should be considered in any patient of advanced age or at high risk of cerebrovascular disease with isolated, new-onset vertigo without an obvious cause.[11,12] Because of the possibility of progression of new-onset VBI in the first 24 to 72 hours, hospital or observation unit admission and consideration of early magnetic resonance angiography probably are warranted, even in a stable patient. Changing or rapidly progressive symptoms should raise suspicions of impending posterior circulation occlusion. If CT or MRI excludes hemorrhage as the source of the patient's symptoms, an immediate neurologic consultation, emergency angiography, and possibly anticoagulation are indicated.

Acute bacterial labyrinthitis requires admission, intravenous antibiotics and, occasionally, surgical drainage and debridement. In cases of toxic labyrinthitis, the offending medication should be discontinued immediately.

Some cases of Ménière's disease have been treated successfully by vasodilation and diuretic therapy. Diets low in sodium and caffeine and cessation of smoking also have been helpful. Chemical ablation of vestibular function with gentamicin and streptomycin is an option in severe Ménière's disease. In one small controlled study, corticosteroids were more effective than placebo in treating the acute symptoms of vestibular neuritis.

The treatment of acute attacks of vertigo caused by peripheral disorders is symptomatic. Intravenous diazepam in 2- to 10-mg doses is extremely effective in stopping vertigo. It has a sedative effect that acts on the limbic system, the thalamus, and the hypothalamus. Outpatient treatment with benzodiazepines can be continued at doses of 5 to 10 mg three times daily.

The neurons involved in vestibular reactions are mediated by acetylcholine. Anticholinergic drugs or antihistamines with anticholinergic activity are extremely useful in treating vertigo. Meclizine hydrochloride (Antivert) is usually prescribed as 25 mg every 8 hours, but has a wide therapeutic margin and can be taken much more frequently to control symptoms. Diphenhydramine hydrochloride (Benadryl), 25 to 50 mg every 6 to 8 hours, and dimenhydrinate (Dramamine, Gravol) are also effective, but are more sedating than meclizine. Either drug also can be given intravenously. Transdermal scopolamine has shown disappointing results for treatment of peripheral vertigo but may be considered a third-line or fourth-line option. Promethazine hydrochloride (Phenergan), 25 mg orally or rectally every 6 to 8 hours, is effective because of its strong antiemetic and mild anticholinergic properties; it also can be used intravenously in doses of 12.5 to 25 mg. Buccal prochlorperazine (Compazine, Stemetil) also has been shown to be a safe and effective treatment for vertigo. Avoidance of stimulants (e.g., caffeine, pseudoephedrine, nicotine) may ease symptoms in some cases. In addition, canalith repositioning procedures, such as the Epley and Semont maneuvers, have been shown to be extremely effective in treating benign paroxysmal positional vertigo.[13-15]

One of the most useful tools the physician has is patient reassurance. Most patients with vertigo have self-limited disease processes that have a specific organic cause. By combining patient education and reassurance with judicious use of medications, the treatment of a dizzy patient can be rewarding for the patient and the physician.

DISPOSITION

Documented or suspected cerebellar hemorrhage or infarction, VBI, and acute bacterial labyrinthitis require

Table 13-3. Differential Diagnosis of Patients with True Vertigo

Cause	History	Associated Symptoms	Physical
Peripheral			
1. Benign paroxysmal positional vertigo	Short-lived, positional, fatigable episodes	Nausea, vomiting	Single position can precipitate vertigo. Horizontorotary nystagmus often can be induced at bedside
2. Labyrinthitis			
A. Serous	Mild to severe positional symptoms. Usually coexisting or antecedent infection of ear, nose, throat, or meninges	Mild to severe hearing loss can occur	Usually nontoxic patient with minimal fever elevation
B. Acute suppurative	Coexisting acute exudative infection of the inner ear. Severe symptoms	Usually severe hearing loss, nausea, vomiting	Febrile toxic patient. Acute otitis media
C. Toxic	Gradually progressive symptoms: Patients on medication causing toxicity	Hearing loss that may become rapid and severe, nausea and vomiting	Hearing loss. Ataxia common feature in chronic phase
3. Ménière's disease	Recurrent episodes of severe rotational vertigo usually lasting hours. Onset usually abrupt. Attacks may occur in clusters. Long symptom-free remissions	Nausea, vomiting, tinnitus, hearing loss	Positional nystagmus not present
4. Vestibular neuronitis	Sudden onset of severe vertigo, increasing in intensity for hours, then gradually subsiding over several days. Mild positional vertigo often lasts weeks to months. Sometimes history of infection or toxic exposure that precedes initial attack. Highest incidence is found in third and fifth decades	Nausea, vomiting. Auditory symptoms do not occur	Spontaneous nystagmus toward the involved ear may be present
5. Acoustic neuroma	Gradual onset and increase in symptoms. Neurologic signs in later stages. Most occur in women between 30 and 60	Hearing loss, tinnitus. True ataxia and neurologic signs as tumor enlarges	Unilateral decreased hearing. True truncal ataxia and other neurologic signs when tumor enlarges. May have diminution or absence of corneal reflex. Eighth cranial nerve deficit may be present
Central			
1. Vascular disorders			
A. Vertebrobasilar insufficiency	Should be considered in any patient of advanced age with isolated new-onset vertigo without an obvious cause. More likely with history of atherosclerosis. Initial episode usually seconds to minutes	Often headache. Usually neurologic symptoms including dysarthria, ataxia, weakness, numbness, double vision. Tinnitus and deafness uncommon	Neurologic deficits usually present, but initially neurologic examination can be normal
B. Cerebellar hemorrhage	Sudden onset of severe symptoms	Headache, vomiting, ataxia	Toxic patient. Dysmetria, true ataxia. Ipsilateral sixth cranial nerve palsy may be present
C. Occlusion of posterior inferior cerebellar artery (Wallenberg's syndrome)	Vertigo associated with significant neurologic complaints	Nausea, vomiting, loss of pain and temperature sensation, ataxia, hoarseness	Loss of pain and temperature sensation on the side of the face ipsilateral to the lesion and on the opposite side of the body, paralysis of the palate, pharynx, and larynx. Horner's syndrome (ipsilateral ptosis, miosis, and decreased facial sweating)
D. Subclavian steal syndrome	Classic picture is syncopal attacks during exercise, but most cases present with more subtle symptoms	Arm fatigue, cramps, mild lightheadedness may be only other symptoms than vertigo	Diminished or absent radial pulses in affected side or systolic blood pressure differentials between the two areas occur in most patients
2. Head trauma	Symptoms begin with or shortly after head trauma. Positional symptoms most common type after trauma. Self-limited symptoms that can persist weeks to months	Usually mild nausea	Occasionally, basilar skull fracture
3. Neck trauma	Usual onset 7 to 10 days after whiplash injury. Symptoms may last weeks to months. Episodes seconds to minutes when turning head	Neck pain	Neck tenderness, pain on movement, and positional nystagmus and vertigo when head is turned to side of the whiplash

Continued

Table 13-3. Differential Diagnosis of Patients with True Vertigo—cont'd

Cause	History	Associated Symptoms	Physical
4. Vertebrobasilar migraine	Vertigo almost always followed by headache. Patient has usually had similar episodes in past. Most patients have a family history of migraine. Syndrome usually begins in adolescence	Dysarthria, ataxia, visual disturbances, or paresthesias usually precede headache	No residual neurologic or otologic signs are present after attack
5. Multiple sclerosis	Vertigo presenting symptoms in 7% to 10% and appears in the course of the disease in a third. Onset may be severe and suggest labyrinth disease. Disease onset usually between ages 20 and 40. Often history of other attacks with varying neurologic signs or symptoms	Nausea and vomiting, which may be severe	May have horizontal, rotary, or vertical nystagmus. Nystagmus may persist after the vertiginous symptoms have subsided. Bilateral internuclear ophthalmoplegia and ataxic eye movements suggest multiple sclerosis
6. Temporal lobe epilepsy	Can be initial or prominent symptom in some patients with the disorder	Memory impairment, hallucinations, trancelike states, seizures	May have aphasia or convulsions
7. Hypoglycemia	Should be suspected in diabetics and any other patient with unexplained symptoms	Sweating, anxiety	Tachycardia, mental status change may be present

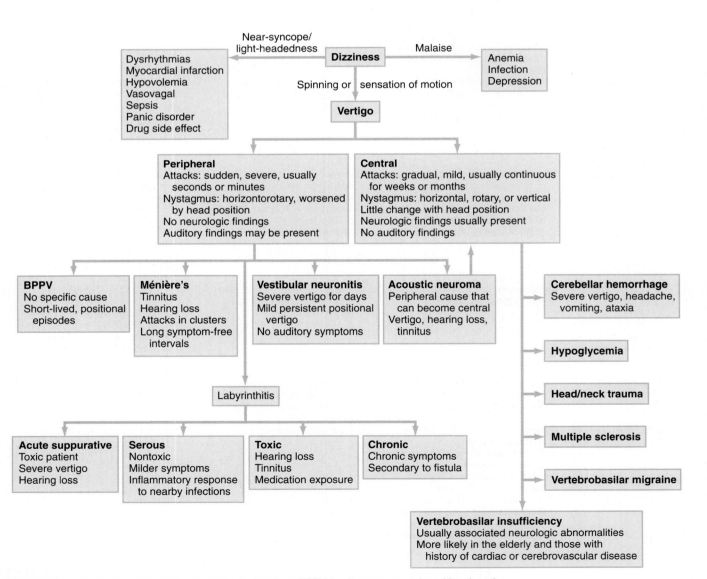

Figure 13-2. Diagnostic algorithm for dizziness and vertigo. BPPV, benign paroxysmal positional vertigo.

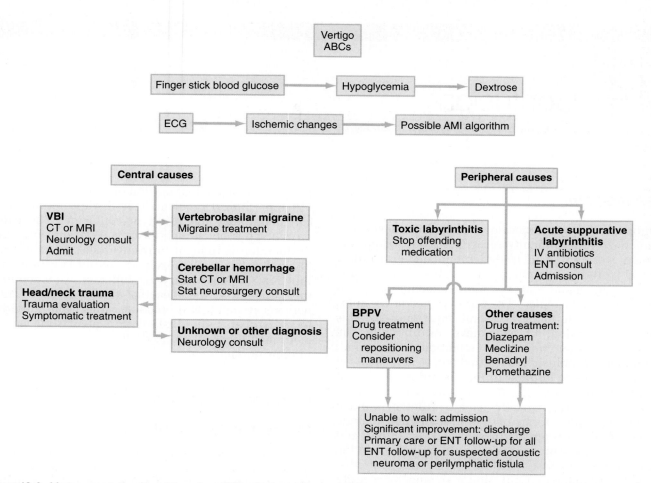

Figure 13-3. Management algorithm for vertigo. ECG, electrocardiogram; ENT, ear, nose, and throat; AMI, acute myocardial infarction; VBI, vertebrobasilar insufficiency; CT, computed tomography; MRI, magnetic resonance imaging; BPPV, benign paroxysmal positional vertigo.

workup and hospitalization. In patients older than age 55 years, particularly patients with vascular disease, admission for observation and imaging of cerebral vasculature is often warranted. Most younger patients with peripheral causes of vertigo can be discharged from the emergency department after symptoms are controlled. Some patients may have such severe symptoms (e.g., vomiting, inability to walk) despite a trial of medication that they require admission for intravenous hydration and observation. All discharged patients should receive primary care, neurology, or ear, nose, and throat specialist follow-up. This follow-up is especially important for suspected cases of acoustic neuroma and toxic labyrinthitis.

REFERENCES

1. Sloan P, Coeytaux R, Beck R, Dallar J: Dizziness: State of the science. *Ann Intern Med* 134(part 2):823, 2001.
2. Lawson J, et al: Diagnosis of geriatric patients with severe dizziness. *J Am Geriatr Soc* 47:113, 1999.
3. Baloh RW: Dizziness: Neurological emergencies. *Neurol Clin North Am* 16:305, 1998.
4. Eviatar L: Dizziness in children. *Otolaryngol Clin North Am* 27:557, 1994.
5. Mallinson AI, Longridge NS: Dizziness from whiplash and head injuries: Differences between whiplash and head injury. *Am J Otol* 19:814, 1998.
6. Young Y, Chen C: Acute vertigo following cervical manipulation. *Laryngoscope* 113:659, 2003.
7. Derebery MD: The diagnosis and treatment of dizziness. *Med Clin North Am* 83:10, 1999.
8. Herr RD, Zun L, Mathews JJ: A directed approach to the dizzy patient. *Ann Emerg Med* 18:664, 1989.
9. Fife TD, Baloh RW, Duckwiler GR: Isolated dizziness in vertebrobasilar insufficiency: Clinical features, angiography, and follow-ups. *J Stroke Cerebrovasc Dis* 4:4, 1994.
10. Gizzi M, Riley E, Molinari S: The diagnostic value of imaging the patient with dizziness: A Bayesian approach. *Arch Neurol* 53:1299, 1996.
11. Norving B, Magnusson M, Holta S: Isolated vertigo in the elderly: Vestibular or vascular disease? *Acute Neurol Scand* 91:43, 1995.
12. Rathore S, et al: Characterization of incident stroke signs and symptoms: Findings from the Atherosclerosis Risk in Communities Study. *Stroke* 33:2718, 2002.
13. Koelliker P, Summers R, Hawkins B: Benign paroxysmal positional vertigo: Diagnosis and treatment in the emergency department—A review of the literature and discussion of canalith-repositioning maneuvers. *Ann Emerg Med* 37:392, 2001.
14. Yimantae K, Srirompotong S, Srirompotong S, Saeseau P: A randomized trial of the canalith repositioning procedure. *Laryngoscope* 113:828, 2003.
15. Wolf JS, et al: Success of the modified Epley maneuver in treating benign paroxysmal vertigo. *Laryngoscope* 109:900, 1999.

J. Stephen Huff and William J. Brady

PERSPECTIVE

Confusion is a symptom, not a diagnosis. Most clinicians have little difficulty recognizing the "confused" patient, yet confusion is difficult to define. Clinical jargon includes "altered mental status," "delta MS" (change in mental status), "altered mentation," and "change from baseline." The term *confusion* connotes an alteration in higher cerebral functions, such as memory, attention, or awareness. Additionally, the ability to sustain and focus attention is impaired. Symptoms of confusion may fluctuate, as may the level of consciousness. Implicit in the definition is a recent change in behavior. Chronic mental status changes such as dementia typically have a different clinical chronology. Other forms of altered mentation include states of diminished alertness, such as stupor and coma; these presentations may result from some of the same disease processes causing confusion and are discussed in Chapter 15. Confusion may range in severity from a mild disturbance of short-term memory to a global inability to relate to the environment and process sensory input. This extreme state is termed *delirium*. It is characterized as an acute confusional state associated with increased alertness, increased psychomotor activity, and disorientation and is often accompanied by hallucinations. There are many causes of confusion, and an orderly approach is necessary to discover the causative diagnosis.

Epidemiology

Clinicians underestimate the incidence of confusion in patients. Often, confusion is accepted as an incidental or secondary component of another condition. A patient with injuries from a motor vehicle accident or with dyspnea may be confused, but the primary condition overshadows the underlying abnormal mental status. When confusion exists as an isolated or unexplained finding, it is more likely to receive full and immediate consideration by the clinician. Confusion is estimated to occur in 2% of emergency department patients, 10% of all hospitalized patients, and 50% of elderly hospitalized patients.[1,2]

Pathophysiology

Conceptually, consciousness may be divided into elements of alertness or arousal and elements constituting content of consciousness. Confusion is largely a problem of the content portion of consciousness. Many different clinical problems may disrupt optimal cortical functioning and result in confusion. The pathophysiology is not straightforward. Widespread cortical dysfunction is thought to result from substrate deficit (hypoglycemia or hypoxemia), neurotransmitter dysfunction, or circulatory dysfunction. Compounding this problem is the idea that the reserve of central nervous system (CNS) function varies from individual to individual; individuals with a preexisting impairment may become confused after even minor changes in their normal state.

DIAGNOSTIC APPROACH

Differential Considerations

The observation of acute confusion prompts a search for an underlying cause. Four groups of disorders encompass most causes of diffuse cortical dysfunction: (1) systemic diseases secondarily affecting the CNS, (2) primary intracranial disease, (3) exogenous toxins, and (4) drug withdrawal states (Box 14-1).[3] Focal cortical dysfunction, such as from tumor or stroke, typically does not cause confusion, although exceptions are encountered. Likewise, subcortical or brainstem dysfunction often results not in confusion, but in a diminished level of alertness and consciousness.

Rapid Assessment and Stabilization

Most patients with acute confusion do not require immediate interventions. Two crucial exceptions are patients with hypoglycemia and patients with hypoxemia. All confused patients should have early bedside blood glucose testing and pulse oximetry. Oral or intravenous glucose therapy is indicated if low blood glucose is found. Supplemental oxygen is administered as necessary. Other early assessments include vital signs, a rapid overview examination for focal neurologic signs, and a demonstrated ability of the patient to protect the airway by assessing speech and swallowing.

Patients must be protected from harming themselves or others. Close observation may need to be supplemented by physical or chemical restraint. Competent family members may offer valuable assistance in observing the patient and providing reassurance.

In a patient with abnormal or unstable vital signs, initial diagnostic and management efforts are directed toward treatment of the systemic condition. A confused

BOX 14-1. Major Categories: Differential Considerations

Primary intracranial disease
Systemic diseases secondarily affecting the central nervous system
Exogenous toxins
Drug withdrawal

BOX 14-2. Findings that Can Help Differentiate between Organic and Functional Causes of Confusion

Organic	Functional
History:	*History:*
Acute onset	Onset over weeks to months
Any age	Onset ages 12 to 40 years
Mental status examination:	*Mental status examination:*
Fluctuating level of consciousness	Alert
	Oriented
Disoriented	Agitated, anxious
Attention disturbances	Poor immediate memory
Poor recent memory	Hallucinations: most commonly auditory
Hallucinations: visual, tactile, auditory	Delusions, illusions
Cognitive changes	*Physical examination:*
Physical examination:	Normal vital signs
Abnormal vital signs	No nystagmus
Nystagmus	Purposeful movement
Focal neurologic signs	No signs of trauma
Signs of trauma	

patient with acute pulmonary edema, hypoxia, and confusion requires evaluation and treatment of the pulmonary edema, not a screening test for cognitive functions. In a patient with extreme hypertension, efforts must be directed at discovering the cause of the hypertensive emergencies, intracerebral hemorrhage.

Generally, in patients with schizophrenia and other psychiatric disorders, tests of cognition, orientation, and attention are normal unless the condition is severe. The term *psychosis* implies a disorder of reality testing and thought organization severe enough to interfere with normal daily functioning. Psychosis is a nonspecific syndrome, and careful evaluation is required to differentiate between psychiatric and organic origins (e.g., drug intoxication or other systemic process) (Box 14-2).

Pivotal Findings

A patient with an altered state of consciousness including confusion is evaluated by performing a focused history and pertinent examination, performing rapid bedside screening investigations, and observing the response to certain therapies (e.g., dextrose or naloxone). Additional evaluation may include laboratory testing and diagnostic imaging with various modalities. Useful information that provides the diagnosis or strongly suggests a cause is found roughly in descending order from the patient's history, the examination including results of rapid bedside testing, and the response to emergency department therapies; the results of laboratory testing and diagnostic imaging are less often useful.[4]

History

Confusion most often is reported by family members or caregivers; often the patient is not aware of the confusion and seemingly glosses over problems. Families may articulate the complaint as confusion but also may describe rambling, disorientation, speaking to persons not there, the patient's inability to find his or her way around familiar surroundings, or simply "not being right." An essential goal of the history is to determine when the patient last exhibited "normal" thinking and behavior.

Attention deficit is the common denominator in confusional states. The initial task in evaluating the patient is to define the symptoms and severity of confusion. The specific behaviors that are concerning to the patient or caregivers should be defined. Often, the family is the most valuable source for information; a physician or other caregiver with an established relationship with the patient also may be helpful. The duration of the confusion, any recent changes in medications, and recent illnesses are important points in the clinical history. Most importantly, what is meant by the term *confusion* should be clarified. Hallucinations are not unique to psychiatric illness and can commonly occur in confusion states, especially delirium. Hallucinations in delirium tend to be visual (with or without auditory components), fleeting, and poorly organized. A history of medication or substance abuse and any recent changes, especially cessation of benzodiazepines or ethanol, should be sought in all cases.

Physical Examination

The patient's confusion may be obvious at the bedside. In other cases, confusion may be subtle, and informal assessment of mental status and cognitive abilities may fail to detect it. The mini-mental state examination (MMSE) (Figure 14-1) commonly is recommended as a screening instrument but is used infrequently in the emergency department because of the time required to administer it.[5,6] A more rapidly performed screening tool, the Quick Confusion Scale (Figure 14-2), has been developed and tested in emergency department patients.[7-9] This tool objectively measures elements of the patient's mental status in 2 to 3 minutes and correlates well with the MMSE. The tasks measured by either the MMSE or the QCS require adequate attention.

If attention span is greatly impaired, more detailed testing may be impossible. Digit repetition forward (five or six digits) and backward (four digits) is a brief screen for attention function. Alternatively, spelling a commonly used word backward ("world" is frequently used) measures a patient's ability to concentrate. Screening tests may detect confusion not obvious in casual conversation, identifying the need for further investigations.[10,11]

The physical examination may suggest a cause such as congestive heart failure or pneumonia. A fever suggests an infection as the cause of confusion and should prompt a search for the source. Any focal neurologic findings suggest a possible mass lesion or stroke and should trigger investigations along those lines. Aphasia, fluent or nonfluent, is a focal sign suggesting a lesion in the dominant cerebral hemisphere. In confusional states, speech may be abnormal and is often incoherent, and the rate of speech may be either rapid or slowed. Involuntary movements, such as asterixis or tremor, may be present. The various toxidromes must be sought on the examination, perhaps assisting in the identification of an intoxication or drug effect as the cause of confusion.

Laboratory Tests

The results of the history and physical examination frequently guide the clinician in the choice of laboratory tests most likely to yield valuable diagnostic information. Pulse oximetry may reveal hypoxia, or bedside glucose testing may reveal hypoglycemia or hyperglycemia. In the presence of a fever, chest radiography and urinalysis often reveal the source of the infection that may be causing the altered mentation. In elderly patients, urinalysis should be performed whether or not fever is present. Other tests commonly available in the emergency department and useful in the evaluation of a confused patient are serum electrolyte testing (especially sodium) and electrocardiography. Electrocardiography is indicated in elderly patients because myocardial infarction may present as confusion. The complete blood count, although commonly performed, is unlikely to provide useful diagnostic clues. Arterial blood gas testing is rarely indicated or useful.

If common and simple tests do not suggest a solution, more complex testing should be done in the emergency department, observation unit, or inpatient service. The clinical situation and overall condition of the patient determine the speed and direction of evaluation. Additional laboratory work is often of decreasing yield but may reveal the cause of confusion. Serum ammonia, calcium, thyroid, various drug, and selected toxicologic testing may be ordered in this second tier of evaluation. Blood and urine cultures should be obtained in the febrile patient when hospital admission is anticipated and a clear infectious source is not evident. Paracentesis or thoracentesis may be appropriate if ascites or pleural effusion is present. Cranial computed tomography (CT) scanning is often done to screen for CNS lesions. Focal findings on CT increase the yield of this test, but unanticipated abnormalities are often found on neuroimaging. No clear guidelines for CT use exist in this patient group, but if the cause of the altered mental status is not discovered, liberal use of CT is common practice. Lumbar puncture may discover or exclude CNS infection if no other source has been identified. Cerebrospinal fluid examination is important not only to discover bacterial meningitis, but also for alternative diagnoses, such as encephalitis, aseptic men-

ITEM	SCORE (highest number in category indicates correct response; decreased scoring indicates increased number of errors)	WEIGHT	SCORE
What year is it now?	0 or 1 (score 1 if correct; 0 if incorrect)	×2	
What month is it?	0 or 1 (score 1 if correct; 0 if incorrect)	×2	
Repeat phrase and remember it: "John Brown, 42 Market Street, New York"			
About what time is it? (answer correct if within the hour)	0 or 1 (score 1 if correct; 0 if incorrect)	×2	
Count backwards from 20 to 1	0, 1, or 2 (score 2 if correct; 1 if 1 error; score 0 if more than 2 errors)	×1	
Say the months in reverse	0, 1, or 2 (score 2 if correct; 1 if 1 error; score 0 if more than 2 errors)	×1	
Repeat the memory phrase (each underlined portion is worth 1 point)	0, 1, 2, 3, 4, 5 (score 5 if correctly performed; each error drops score by one)	×1	
		TOTAL	——

Final score is sum of the totals; score less than 15 suggests the presence of altered cognition and need for further assessment.

Figure 14-2. Quick Confusion Scale.

ingitis, or subarachnoid hemorrhage. If the cause of confusion remains unclear, admission may be necessary for additional ongoing assessment, including diagnostic testing not usually available in the emergency department, such as magnetic resonance imaging or electroencephalography.[4]

DIFFERENTIAL DIAGNOSIS

Certain critical and emergent diagnoses require prompt recognition to prevent morbidity or mortality (Box 14-3). The diagnosis of confusion implies the exclusion of other states of altered mental status, such as coma and decompensated psychiatric syndromes. A new focal neurologic deficit points to a focal defect of the CNS, which is less likely to cause the global cortical dysfunction necessary for confusion. Stroke rarely causes confusion, but resulting disturbances in speech or understanding may mimic a confusional state. The

diagnosis of stroke is relatively straightforward if a new motor deficit is present. Occasionally, other focal neurologic abnormalities may mimic the global dysfunction typical of a confusional state. A person with a new visual field deficit and visual neglect with lack of awareness of the deficit may have difficulty ambulating in familiar surroundings and be labeled as confused, but this reflects focal neurologic injury and not a confusional state from global CNS dysfunction. Careful assessment of mental status assists in resolving the diagnostic dilemma. Frontal lobe dysfunction from stroke, subdural hematoma, or tumor may result in personality changes and the report of "confusion" by family or friends.

Altered mental status may be divided into three different categories depending on the findings of diminished level of consciousness, acute focal neurologic deficit, or abnormal attention span. Placement into one of these categories may guide the differential assessment and therapy (Figure 14-3).

BOX 14-3. Critical and Emergent Diagnoses

Critical
Hypoxia/diffuse cerebral ischemia
  Respiratory failure
  Congestive heart failure
  Myocardial infarction
Systemic processes
  Hypoglycemia
CNS infections
Hypertensive encephalopathy
Elevated intracranial pressure—medical and surgical origin

Emergent
Hypoxia/diffuse cerebral ischemia
  Severe anemia
Systemic diseases
  Electrolyte and fluid disturbance
  Endocrine disease
    Thyroid
    Adrenal

Hepatic failure
Nutrition/Wernicke's encephalopathy
Sepsis, infection
Intoxications and withdrawal
  CNS sedatives
  Ethanol
  Other medication side effects, particularly anticholinergics
CNS disease
  Trauma
  Infections
  Stroke
  Subarachnoid hemorrhage
  Epilepsy/seizures
    Postictal state
    Nonconvulsive status epilepticus
    Complex partial status epilepticus
Neoplasm

Note: These represent a partial diagnosis; causes are myriad. "Critical" in this case means conditions that need immediate assessment and correction within moments, such as oxygenation and ventilation problems or hypoglycemia. Because confusion represents CNS failure, other problems may be considered critical as well and may require intensive care unit admission, depending on severity.
CNS, central nervous system.

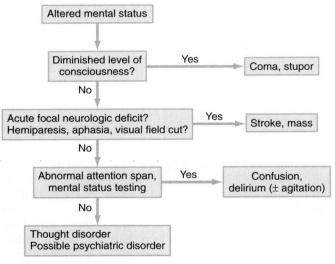

Figure 14-3. Diagnostic algorithm for confusion.

EMPIRIC MANAGEMENT

Ideally, treatment is directed at the underlying cause of the confusion. Investigations continue until a likely diagnosis is discovered or consultation and admission are deemed necessary (Figure 14-4). Many febrile patients are found to have a systemic infectious cause of the confusion. Urinary tract infections and pneumonia are the more common sources, but soft tissue infections also warrant consideration. CNS infections are encountered less frequently but have potentially devastating consequences if not recognized promptly. Antibiotic treatment for coverage of common causes of meningitis may be considered in ill febrile patients while definitive evaluation is in progress.

Postictal confusion is common in patients with seizures but should improve within 20 to 30 minutes. If the patient remains unconscious or confused after a seizure, the possibility of ongoing or intermittent seizure activity—nonconvulsive seizures—should be considered. Nonconvulsive status epilepticus, an epileptic twilight state, is unusual but does occur (see Chapter 16).

Sometimes it may be necessary to treat confusion or agitation for patient safety. Environmental manipulations, such as dim lighting or psychosocial support, may be helpful. Confinement or physical restraint may be necessary at times for patient safety; institutional guidelines should be followed. Benzodiazepines or butyrophenones may be used if necessary to decrease agitation. These medications may alter mental status further, making evaluation more difficult.

DISPOSITION

Most patients presenting with confusion are admitted for additional diagnostic procedures, extended observation, and treatment. Exceptions include patients

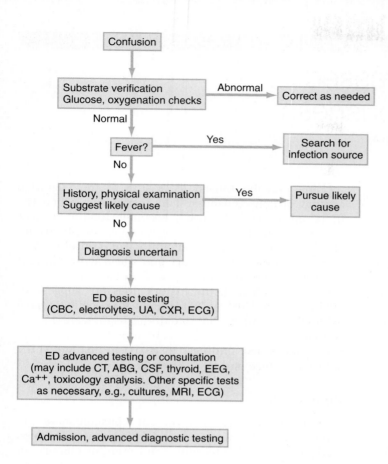

Figure 14-4. Management algorithm for confusion. ABG, arterial blood gas; CBC, complete blood count; CT, computed tomography; CSF, cerebrospinal fluid; CXR, chest x-ray; ECG, electrocardiogram; MRI, magnetic resonance imaging; UA, urinalysis.

with rapidly resolved confusional states after treatment for insulin-induced hypoglycemia, after generalized seizures of known origin, or after recovering from self-limiting intoxicants, such as ethanol or recreational drugs. These patients may be observed and then discharged after successful identification and resolution of acute confusional state. Unresolved confusion or unexplained findings on repeat mental status screen should prompt admission or a careful re-evaluation before considering discharge.

REFERENCES

1. Hustey FM, Meldon SW: The prevalence and documentation of impaired mental status in elderly emergency department patient. *Ann Emerg Med* 39:248, 2002.
2. Wofford L, Loehr LR, Schwartz E: Acute cognitive impairment in elderly ED patients: Etiologies and outcomes. *Am J Emerg Med* 14:649, 1996.
3. Lipowski ZJ: Delirium (acute confusional states). *JAMA* 258:1789, 1987.
4. American College of Emergency Physicians: Clinical policy for the initial approach to patients presenting with altered mental status. *Ann Emerg Med* 33:251, 1999.
5. Folstein MF, Folstein SE: "Mini-mental state": A practical method for grading the cognitive state of patients for the clinician. *J Psychiatr Res* 12:189, 1975.
6. Zun L, Gold I: A survey of the form of the mental status examination administered by emergency physicians. *Ann Emerg Med* 15:916, 1986.
7. Huff JS, et al: The quick confusion scale in the ED: Comparison with the mini-mental state examination. *Am J Emerg Med* 19:461, 2001.
8. Irons MJ, Farace E, Brady WJ, Huff JS: Mental status screening of emergency department patients: Normative study of the quick confusion scale. *Acad Emerg Med* 9:989, 2002.
9. Kaufman DM, Zun L: A quantifiable, brief mental status examination for emergency patients. *J Emerg Med* 13:449, 1995.
10. Dziedzic L, Brady WJ, Lindsay R, Huff JS: The use of the mini-mental status examination in the ED evaluation of the elderly. *Am J Emerg Med* 16:686, 1998.
11. Hustey FM, Meldon SW, Smith MD, Lex CK: The effect of mental status screening on the care of elderly emergency department patients. *Ann Emerg Med* 41:678, 2003.

Coma and Depressed Level of Consciousness

Richard E. Wolfe and David F. M. Brown

PERSPECTIVE

Epidemiology

Coma is a relatively rare presenting symptom in the emergency department; depressed level of consciousness occurs much more often. Both conditions are caused by a wide variety of disorders, ranging from structural central nervous system (CNS) problems to diffuse systemic diseases. Most patients presenting with either coma or depressed level of consciousness have an underlying metabolic or systemic disorder rather than a structural lesion.

Pathophysiology

Knowledge of the anatomic structures of consciousness and the pathophysiology of mentation helps interpret physical findings and distinguish between structural and systemic causes. Consciousness integrates two functions: arousal and cognition. These two functions are based in two different neuroanatomic locations—arousal in the brainstem and cognition in the cerebral cortex.

Arousal occurs by a nonspecific physiologic mechanism that can be selectively impaired by toxins, anesthetics, or compression or injury of the brainstem. An intact brainstem is essential for arousal. Small focal lesions within the pons can alter mental status and induce coma, whereas extensive unilateral lesions of the cerebral hemispheres do not blunt consciousness even as they destroy selective psychological functions. Both cerebral hemispheres must be structurally damaged or metabolically depressed to induce coma.

The ascending reticular activating system (ARAS) is the neuroanatomic structure responsible for arousal. The ARAS is located in the paramedian tegmental gray matter immediately ventral to the ventricular system in the pons and extends continuously from the posterior hypothalamic reticular formation to approximately the lower third of the pontine tegmentum. This architecture creates an ideal environment for stimulation by collaterals from many different afferent pathways and from adjacent brainstem nuclear masses. This structure is stimulated by every somatic and special sensory pathway.

The ARAS acts as a gateway for sensory and somatic stimuli to the cerebral cortex and as a trigger for arousal from sleep. The cerebral cortex in return provides feedback that modulates the activity of the reticular formation. When the ARAS is dysfunctional, coma occurs because the cerebral cortex cannot be aroused.[1]

Coma may be caused by a loss of the cognitive content of consciousness. This loss occurs when the functioning cerebral cortex becomes totally or near totally impaired. When both cerebral hemispheres are affected, the degree of alteration of consciousness depends on the size of injury and speed with which it progresses. Disorders may be diffuse or focal.

In cases in which the history does not suggest an obvious cause, 50% to 70% of comatose patients have metabolic disorders. Supratentorial lesions are a more common cause of coma than subtentorial lesions. Associated neurologic findings can assist in distinguishing between diffuse and focal disorders.

Definitions

Specific definitions of levels of consciousness are needed to communicate accurately between providers, establish a patient's baseline, and monitor changes in the patient's mental status. Different presentations of altered mental status suggest differences in management and outcome.

Coma, in the broad sense, refers to any depression of the level of consciousness. In the narrow sense, it is defined as a complete failure of the arousal system with no spontaneous eye opening. Patients in light coma respond to noxious stimuli with a variety of protective reflexes, whereas patients in deep coma do not respond at all. Coma is distinct from a *vegetative state,* characterized by a complete absence of behavioral evidence for self or environmental awareness. Patients with inconsistent but discernible evidence of consciousness do not meet diagnostic criteria for either coma or a vegetative state. This condition defines a *minimally conscious state* in which patients have an altered mental status but are able to follow simple commands, verbalize yes/no responses (regardless of accuracy), or show purposeful behavior.[2] *Clouding of consciousness* is a disturbance characterized by impaired capacity to think clearly and to perceive, respond to, and remember stimuli. *Confusion* connotes an alteration in higher cerebral functions, such as memory, awareness, and attention. *Delirium* is a state of disturbed consciousness with motor restlessness, transient hallucinations, disorientation, or delusions. *Obtundation* is the state wherein patients are awake but not alert and exhibit psychomotor retardation. *Stupor* is the state in which the patient, although conscious, exhibits little or no spontaneous activity. Stuporous patients awaken with stimuli but have little motor or verbal activity when aroused.

Table 15-1. Glasgow Coma Scale

Eye Opening	Talking	Motor	Score
Does not open eyes	Makes no noise	No motor response to pain	1
Opens eyes with pain	Moans, makes unintelligible sounds	Exterior response (decerebrate)	2
Opens eyes with loud verbal command	Talks, but nonsensical	Flexor response (decorticate)	3
Opens eyes on own	Seems confused, disoriented	Moves part of body, but does not remove noxious stimulus	4
	Alert and oriented	Pushes away noxious stimulus	5
		Follows simple motor commands	6

Table 15-2. Mnemonic for Treatable Causes of Altered Mental Status (AEIOU-TIPS)

Alcohol	**T**rauma
Epilepsy, electrolytes, encephalopathy	**I**nfection
Insulin, intussusception	**P**sychiatric
Opioids/overdose	**S**hock, subarachnoid hemorrhage, snake bite
Urea (metabolic)	

Graded scoring methods based on neurologic findings have been developed to define altered mentation. The Glasgow Coma Scale (GCS) is the most widespread method (Table 15-1), and a GCS of 8 or less has been used as an alternative definition of coma. This definition is valid, however, only when associated with the absence of eye opening to verbal command. Significant limitations of the GCS include variable reproducibility, inaccurate measure of level of consciousness, excessive focus on left-sided brain function, and limited clinical relevance. Other scales have been developed to address these problems (e.g., Liege coma scale, APACHE II scale, Swedish reaction level scale). Because of its ease, familiarity, and widespread acceptance, however, the GCS continues to be the standard scoring system in the United States.

Common misuse of terms by physicians and other health care professionals further adds to the confusion in describing a depressed level of consciousness. To avoid miscommunication, the most effective strategy is to state whether the patient is alert, awake, or unresponsive and to describe the ocular and motor response to verbal commands and painful stimuli.

DIAGNOSTIC APPROACH

Differential Considerations

The differential diagnosis of coma and depressed mental status is vast, and causes can be found across a wide range of categories (Box 15-1). The early goals in the emergency department are to provide supportive care, identify rapidly and treat reversible and life-threatening causes, and establish a methodical approach to definitive diagnosis (Table 15-2). Although there are many systematic ways to approach the diagnosis of coma or profoundly depressed mental status, the most life-threatening causes should be considered first.

If there is fever or other significant evidence of CNS infection (e.g., rash, hypotension, compatible history, immunocompromise), antimicrobial (and antiviral, if indicated) agents should be administered in advance of definitive diagnosis, usually imaging or spinal fluid analysis. CNS mass lesions, suggested by focal neurologic findings or evidence or history of trauma or cancer, warrant early computed tomography scanning. Similarly, intracranial hemorrhage is suggested by sudden onset of coma or complaint of headache before coma ensued. Toxic causes of CNS depression often require only supportive care, but carbon monoxide, cyclic antidepressants, methanol, and ethylene glycol require specific management, and historical or physical examination evidence suggestive of these poisonings is specifically sought.

Excepting glucose disorders metabolic/endocrine causes of coma are generally uncommon. Hyponatremia should be suspected if a delirium-like state or bizarre behavior preceded the coma or in patients taking psychotropic medications. Electrolyte determination is important early in the course of all patients because this provides information about plasma sodium level, acidemia, and anion gap.

Many psychiatric disorders may result in psychiatric unresponsiveness and mimic a comatose state. Psychogenic unresponsiveness is an extremely rare disorder, however, and should be considered only after an extensive evaluation fails to identify an organic cause of coma and a compatible history supports the diagnosis. Conversion disorder is the most common cause of these rare causes of psychogenic unresponsiveness and occurs most often in patients with significant psychiatric and behavioral history.

Rapid Assessment and Stabilization

All comatose patients should be placed on high-flow oxygen and fully undressed. Assessing responsiveness, pupillary reactivity to light, and movement of extremities completes a rapid neurologic screening examination to differentiate diffuse disease from structural causes.

Early use of point-of-care blood glucose testing or empiric administration of dextrose (25 to 50 g) intravenously is mandatory, even in the presence of focal neurologic findings, to prevent the sequelae from pro-

BOX 15-1. Etiology of Coma

Diffuse Brain Dysfunction
Neuronal damage caused by deprivation of oxygen, glucose, or metabolic cofactor
  Hypoxia with an intact CBF, severe pulmonary disease, anemia
  Decreased CBF (e.g., postcardiac arrest, cardiogenic and hypovolemic shock)
  Cellular toxins: carbon monoxide, cyanide, hydrogen sulfide
  Hypoglycemia
  Thiamine deficiency (Wernicke-Korsakoff syndrome)
Endogenous CNS toxins
  Hyperammonemia (hepatic coma, postureterosigmoidostomy, prune belly syndrome)
  Uremia
  CO_2 narcosis
  Hyperglycemia
Exogenous CNS toxins
  Alcohols: ethanol, isopropyl alcohol
  Acid poisons (methanol, ethylene glycol, salicylates)
  Sedatives and narcotics
  Anticonvulsants
  Psychotropics
  Isoniazid
  Heavy metals
Endocrine disorders
  Myxedema coma, thyrotoxicosis
  Addison's disease, Cushing's disease, pheochromocytoma
Abnormalities of ionic environment of CNS
  Hyponatremia, hypernatremia
  Hypocalcemia, hypercalcemia
  Hypomagnesemia, hypermagnesemia
  Hypophosphatemia
  Acidosis, alkalosis
Environmental disorders and disordered temperature regulation
  Hypothermia
  Heat stroke
  Neuroleptic malignant syndrome
  Malignant hyperthermia
Intracranial hypertension
  Hypertensive encephalopathy
  Pseudotumor cerebri

CNS inflammation or infiltration
  Meningitis
  Encephalitis
  Encephalopathy
  Cerebral vasculitis
  Subarachnoid hemorrhage
  Carcinoid meningitis
  Traumatic axonal shear injury
Primary neuronal or glial disorders
  Creutzfeldt-Jakob disease
  Marchiafava-Bignami disease
  Adrenoleukodystrophy
  Gliomatosis cerebri
  Progressive multifocal leukoencephalopathy
Seizures and postictal state

Focal Lesions of the CNS
Supratentorial Lesions
Hemorrhage (traumatic and nontraumatic)
  Intracerebral
  Epidural
  Subdural
  Pituitary apoplexy
Infarction
  Thrombotic arterial occlusion
  Embolic arterial occlusion
  Venous occlusion
Tumors
Abscess

Subtentorial Lesions
Compressive
  Cerebellar hemorrhage
  Posterior fossa subdural or extradural hemorrhage
  Cerebellar infarct
  Cerebellar tumor
  Cerebellar abscess
  Basilar aneurysm
Destructive
  Pontine hemorrhage
  Brainstem infarct
  Basilar migraine
  Brainstem demyelination

CBF, cerebral blood flow; CNS, central nervous system.

longed neuroglycopenia. Administration of dextrose should not be delayed for thiamine administration in nutritionally compromised patients because the theoretical concern of inducing a Wernicke-Korsakoff syndrome has not been validated. There is little risk of treating all comatose patients with naloxone other than inducing opioid withdrawal and possibly a violent reaction by the patient, but generally clinical evidence of opioid ingestion (e.g., miosis, depressed respirations, "track" marks) can guide decision making. A rapid response to naloxone may obviate the need for endotracheal intubation.[3]

If coma is not rapidly reversible, immediate airway management is indicated to prevent aspiration and ensure adequate ventilation and oxygenation. In the absence of concerning difficult airway attributes (see Chapter 1), rapid sequence intubation is the recommended method, with appropriate modification for elevated intracranial pressure if this is suspected. Evidence of trauma prompts cervical spine immobilization throughout management, including intubation, until cervical spine injury can be excluded.

Pivotal Findings

History

Although comatose patients cannot respond to questioning, the circumstances that lead to a comatose state are crucial to determine the underlying disorder. Information must be sought from a variety of sources (e.g., family, friends, coworkers, prehospital personnel). People are asked to describe the environment in which

Table 15-3. Pertinent Physical Examination in the Comatose Patient

Area	Findings	Comment/Interpretation
Vital signs	Blood pressure—hypotension	Decreased cerebral perfusion pressure alone can result in severe depression of mental status. Highly suggestive of systemic disease
	Blood pressure—hypertension	Systolic pressures > 200 mm Hg, diastolic > 130 mm Hg may suggest intracranial structural lesions. True hypertensive encephalopathy rarely presents as coma. Intracranial hemorrhage is the first consideration
	Respiratory rate—tachypnea	A sign of hypoxemia, brainstem herniation, or metabolic acidosis
	Respiratory rate—bradypnea	Most commonly associated with opiate or sedative-hypnotic poisoning
	Respiratory pattern	Of limited benefit diagnostically
Airway	Intact patency and protection; breath odor may suggest cause	Essential examination to anticipate need for airway management. Unique breath odors take some training and prior exposure to interpret
Skin	Cyanosis, pallor, jaundice, petechiae/purpura, surgical scars, needle tracks	Full exposure necessary to look for wide variety of visual clues
Head	Palpation for trauma, previous craniotomy, or ventricular shunt	External injury may reflect internal damage; previous surgery may be for hematoma, tumor, or hydrocephalus
ENT	Signs of infection, hemotympanum, tongue lacerations	May reveal source of meningitis or basilar skull fracture or indicate seizure activity
Eyes	Pupillary changes	May be significant in identifying specific toxic or structural causes. Reactivity usually presumed in metabolic causes
	Eye movement	Roving eye movement connotes intact brainstem. Oculocephalic testing may assist in locating level of structure damage
	Funduscopy	Papilledema, hemorrhage, findings of hypertension or DM
Neck	Rigidity	Usually assess after cervical spine clearance (historical or imaging) Meningismus must be considered meningitis or SAH until proved otheriwise
Lung	Varied	Findings consistent with acute or chronic hypoxia source or acute infection
Cardiovascular	Varied	Possible murmurs (embolic), dysrhythmias (cerebral perfusion pressure), or aneurysms (dissection or rupture)
Neurologic	Level and content of consciousness Posture	As per text, posture (decorticate, decerebrate) may indicate neurologic level of injury
	Movement	Movement—specifically looking for purpose (e.g., protective) and asymmetry and spontaneous patterns (e.g., subtle seizure activity)
	Deep tendon reflexes	Reflect spinal cord function; asymmetry may be useful

DM, diabetes mellitus; ENT, ear, nose, and throat; SAH, subarachnoid hemorrhage.

the patient was found (e.g., exposure to extremes of temperature or products of combustion) and the last time the patient was "normal." An attempt should be made to establish the onset and progression of the altered mental state. Abrupt onset, with or without antecedent headache, nausea, or vomiting, suggests CNS hemorrhage. Declining mental status over hours to days suggests other disorders (e.g., hyperosmolar non-ketotic coma, hyponatremia, infection). The patient's state before the onset of coma may provide clues to the underlying cause. Coma preceded by delirium suggests toxin ingestion, alcohol or sedative withdrawal, hyponatremia, or encephalitis. Other crucial elements in the history include drug use (prescription, nonprescription, illicit), antecedent trauma, fever, headache, and any known prior similar episodes.

Medical history (especially regarding diabetes, seizures, hypertensive vascular disease, thyroid disease, stroke, malignancy, liver disease, or renal failure) should be determined. The patient's wallet may contain clues to medications or appointment cards for medical specialists (e.g., oncologist, endocrinologist), and the patient should be checked for identifiers (e.g., a Medic-Alert bracelet).[1,4]

Physical Examination

The initial goal of the physical examination is to discriminate between focal structural CNS pathology and global metabolic processes. Concomitant with stabilization, vital signs, including a core temperature, are checked (Table 15-3). A special probe is necessary to record accurate temperatures less than 35°C. Signs of trauma are sought immediately after obtaining the patient's vital signs. Cervical immobilization is maintained until trauma has been excluded or the cervical spine has been cleared radiographically and clinically. The patient should be completely exposed, visually inspected, and manually palpated. Special attention should be given to the face and scalp. Hemotympanum, suggestive of a basilar skull fracture, is assessed on ear examination.

A focused neurologic examination should follow the general examination and any necessary initial resuscitation. The neurologic examination of a comatose patient of necessity differs from the examination of an awake, communicative patient. Detailed sensory and motor testing is foregone, and extra attention is given to eye findings, posture, and movement. The approach must be systematic to document a baseline, define the lesion, and determine the diagnosis. The presence or absence of focal or lateralizing neurologic signs guides the differential diagnosis. If all signs can be explained by a single anatomic lesion, the differential diagnosis narrows toward structural CNS causes. If there is neuroanatomic inconsistency, toxic and metabolic causes become more likely.

The patient's response to voice, touch, and noxious stimuli immediately focuses the examiner's attention on the patient's level of consciousness. Verbal stimuli should be graded, beginning with a whisper and progressing to a shout. A variety of noxious stimuli have been used, but perhaps the best stimulus is to tickle the nasal passage with a cotton swab. This is not harmful or painful, does not leave a mark, and can be reproduced accurately by subsequent examiners. The patient's response to any stimulus is carefully recorded. In particular, mumbling even a few words must be distinguished from nonsensical grunting because the ability to speak words indicates high cortical functioning and carries a good prognosis. In a nonverbal patient, motor responses are equally important to note; avoidance or protective movements by an extremity is a purposeful cortically mediated response, whereas adduction, flexion, or extension of a limb may occur

as a reflex response and does not imply an intact corticospinal system. Triple-flexion withdrawal of the lower extremity (i.e., flexion of the hip, knee, and ankle) is a spinal cord–mediated reflex and implies nothing about the status of brainstem and cortical function.

Spontaneous and elicited eye movements should be evaluated carefully; this is the cornerstone of the neurologic examination, providing information on a large portion of the brainstem near the reticular activating system. In addition, extraocular movement testing permits evaluation of the interaction between the cortex and the brainstem. Eye movements are controlled by the cortex and the medial longitudinal fasciculus in the brainstem and mediated by cranial nerves III, IV, and VI (Figure 15-1). This evaluation begins with observation of the resting position of the eyes and notation of any spontaneous movements. Dysconjugate gaze in the horizontal plane is normally observed in drowsiness and in various sedated states, including alcohol intoxication, with parallel ocular axes re-emerging when the patient awakens or slips deeper into coma. Dysconjugate gaze in the vertical plane, called *skew deviation,* generally results from pontine or cerebellar lesions. Sustained conjugate downward eye deviation may occur with a variety of neurologic disorders and

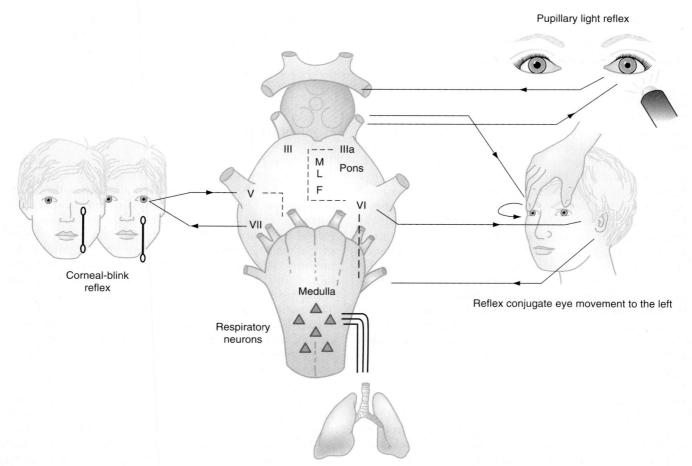

Figure 15-1. Schematic representation of major brainstem reflexes used in coma examination. MLF, medial longitudinal fasciculus.

is nonlocalizing. Sustained conjugate upward gaze is usually the result of hypoxic encephalopathy and is thought to indicate an intact brainstem. A persistently adducted eye indicates cranial nerve VI paresis, whereas a persistently abducted eye indicates cranial nerve III paresis. These findings in isolation are nonlocalizing because either may be a result of a pontine lesion or of elevated intracranial pressure causing extrinsic compression. Spontaneous eye movements, when present, often consist of conjugate horizontal roving. Such full, slow, left-right conjugate roving movements exclude the midbrain and pontine causes of coma. Numerous other uncommon spontaneous eye movements are described. *Ocular bobbing* is the term for cyclic, brisk, conjugate caudal jerks of the globes followed by a slow return to midposition. Although classic for bilateral pontine damage, it also is reported in cases of metabolic derangement and brainstem compression caused by cerebellar hemorrhage. *Ocular dipping* describes a slow, cyclic, conjugate downward movement of the eyes followed by a rapid return to midposition and is usually the result of diffuse cortical anoxic damage.

Oculocephalic movements, commonly called *doll's eyes,* are movements of the eyes that occur in response to movements of the head. Doll's eyes are tested by moving the head from side to side or vertically, first slowly, then briskly. This maneuver is strictly contraindicated when there is a possibility of cervical instability. Normal reflex eye movements are evoked in the direction opposite to the head turning, tending to maintain or return gaze to the forward position. This response is mediated by brainstem pathways originating in the labyrinths and vestibular nuclei and involving the high cervical spinal cord and medulla. It also requires integrity of the area of the midbrain and pons surrounding cranial nerves III and VI and an intact medial longitudinal fasciculus.

In a normal, awake subject, reflex eye movements are suppressed by visual fixation mechanisms in the cerebral cortex, maintaining forward gaze with respect to head turning. In a comatose patient, the response to head movement depends on the site of CNS dysfunction. In patients with primary or secondary cortical disease, the reflex mechanism remains intact, and the eyes move freely in the direction opposite the head turning, appearing to remain fixed on an object. The so-called intact doll's eyes show the functional integrity of a large portion of the brainstem, excluding it as the cause of coma. In patients with brainstem dysfunction, the eyes remain fixed in the orbits, moving with the head. Occasionally, oculocephalic testing yields specific information regarding brainstem function. Absent abduction of an eye implies a sixth cranial nerve lesion caused by either ipsilateral pontine damage or compression from elevated intracranial pressure. Incomplete adduction is much harder to assess with oculocephalic maneuvers; when present, it suggests damage to the midbrain in the area of cranial nerve III or to the pathways coursing through the pons in the medial longitudinal fasciculus. The presence of a dilated pupil distinguishes the former from the latter. A variety of drug intoxications can cause sluggish responses to oculocephalic maneuvers and should not be taken as an indicator of structural brainstem dysfunction.

Bedside Testing

Cold water testing of the vestibular apparatus, called the *oculovestibular response,* is an adjunct to the oculocephalic test and, although less easily performed, is more accurate in determining oculomotor reflexes. It presents a strong stimulus to the brainstem for reflex eye movements and can be performed safely in comatose patients regardless of the status of the cervical spine. Tympanic membrane perforation and cerumen impaction should be excluded before performing the test. The external auditory canal is irrigated with 10-30 mL of ice-cold water after elevating the head to 30 degrees above supine. If the spine is immobilized, this can be accomplished safely by placing the patient in the reverse Trendelenburg position; this isolates endolymph movement to the horizontal semicircular canal of the labyrinth. The normal response is transient conjugate slow deviation of gaze toward the side of the stimulus (brainstem mediated) followed by a quick beating motion with corrective efforts back to midline alignment (cortically mediated). The mnemonic "COWS" stands for "Cold—Opposite, Warm—Same" and describes the direction of the fast component of the nystagmus in response to caloric testing. Bilateral tonic deviation of the eyes toward the stimulus lasting 30 to 120 seconds indicates an intact brainstem without cortical correction (Figure 15-2). No response to the stimulus implies brainstem dysfunction. The oculovestibular response cannot be voluntarily resisted; a normal response in an otherwise comatose patient casts doubt on the presumptive diagnosis of coma.

Ancillary Testing

An accurate interpretation of the clinical presentation leads to a preliminary classification of coma as metabolic or structural and directs a more appropriate approach in ordering ancillary studies. Avoid performing radiologic studies before treating hypoglycemia or instituting elaborate metabolic investigations in patients with intracranial hemorrhage.

Whenever possible, a *serum* or *blood glucose* level should be obtained on all comatose patients before empirically administering dextrose. A prompt reversal of coma with intravenous dextrose followed by laboratory confirmation of hypoglycemia often obviates the need for further diagnostic studies. A glucose level should be obtained in all cases of coma, but is of particular value in patients with diabetes or ethanol intoxication (chronic ethanol abuse may deplete glycogen storage and precipitate coma).

Serum electrolytes should be obtained to assess patients for acid-base and electrolyte disturbances. The differential diagnosis of a metabolic acidosis in a comatose patient is extensive. Evaluation of electrolytes in patients who present with possible metabolic coma is needed to diagnose hyponatremia, hypernatremia,

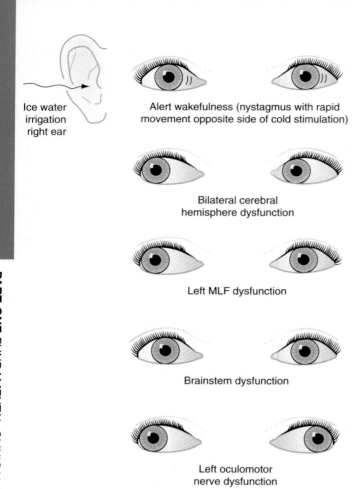

Ice water
irrigation
right ear

Alert wakefulness (nystagmus with rapid
movement opposite side of cold stimulation)

Bilateral cerebral
hemisphere dysfunction

Left MLF dysfunction

Brainstem dysfunction

Left oculomotor
nerve dysfunction

Figure 15-2. Oculocephalogyric (caloric) responses to various central nervous system pathologic conditions. MLF, medial longitudinal fasciculus.

and uremia. The serum calcium level also should be measured in patients with possible metastases or when another cause cannot be determined by the initial screening tests. In insulin-dependent diabetic patients with hypoglycemia, measurement of *creatinine* and *blood urea nitrogen* levels is useful because an insulin reaction may occur secondary to delayed insulin excretion as a result of worsening renal failure.

Pulse oximetry should be performed on all patients with altered mentation because this is more rapid and inexpensive in detecting hypoxemia than arterial blood gas measurements. *Supplemental arterial blood gas* measurements may be necessary to classify acid-base disturbances. Occasionally, arterial blood gas results reveal a discrepancy between the calculated and measured oxygen saturation, suggesting an occult carbon monoxide poisoning. If the history suggests carbon monoxide poisoning, the arterial or venous blood carboxyhemoglobin level should be obtained.

A *complete blood count* is rarely useful in comatose patients. The white blood cell (WBC) count is an insensitive and nonspecific marker of infection. A low WBC count may suggest a fulminant infection coupled with immunosuppression that mandates immediate broad-spectrum antibiotic coverage. Rarely, an extremely

elevated WBC count may identify leukemic crisis. Thrombocytopenia raises concern for an intracranial hemorrhage or sepsis. Until the thrombocytopenia can be corrected, lumbar puncture may be contraindicated because of the risk of iatrogenic spinal subarachnoid hemorrhage.

Urinalysis may be helpful in many settings. The presence of urine glucose with or without ketones implies hyperglycemia and suggests diabetic ketoacidosis or hyperosmolar coma. The presence of WBCs, nitrite, or bacteria suggests urosepsis, a common cause of altered mental status in the elderly. Microscopy may reveal calcium oxalate crystals, suggesting ethylene glycol poisoning. Fluorescent compounds detected by use of an ultraviolet light can lead to an early diagnosis of ethylene glycol poisoning.

Blood and *urine toxicology screens* should be obtained when an obvious cause for coma (e.g., hypoglycemia or alcohol intoxication) is absent. The toxicology screen rarely facilitates the management and disposition of patients with findings highly suggestive of a focal cause; screening should be performed only if radiologic studies are unrevealing.

A *head CT scan* should be ordered when an intracranial cause of coma is suspected. Head CT scanning is not necessary if a metabolic cause of coma is identified on initial evaluation, but should not await laboratory results unless there is strong suspicion of a metabolic cause and the neurologic examination does not indicate a focal lesion. Non–contrast-enhanced CT is the modality of choice because it is rapidly obtainable and identifies blood and masses sufficient to induce coma. Contrast-enhanced CT may be performed later, if indicated. A CT scan is less reliable than magnetic resonance imaging when attempting to visualize structural brainstem lesions. When neurologic examination indicates a possible brainstem problem, the patient should undergo magnetic resonance imaging.

Electroencephalography (EEG) has rarely been of use in the emergency department evaluation of a comatose patient. EEG can facilitate the diagnosis of nonconvulsive status epilepticus, however, reported as a cause of coma in 8% of intensive care unit patients.[5] Barbiturate coma and hypothermia suppress EEG responses significantly. An initial "silent" electroencephalogram may not represent clinical death in this circumstance. An algorithmic approach to the differential diagnosis of the patient with coma is given in Figure 15-3.

EMPIRIC MANAGEMENT

After initial treatment with glucose and naloxone, additional therapies may have value in selected cases. Although Wernicke's encephalopathy is rare, chronic alcoholism and malnourishment are common, and the empiric administration of 100 mg of intravenous thiamine is indicated. Thiamine deficiency has a role in causing Wernicke's encephalopathy in patients with depleted nutritional stores.

Flumazenil is a central antagonist of benzodiazepines. It binds benzodiazepine receptors and

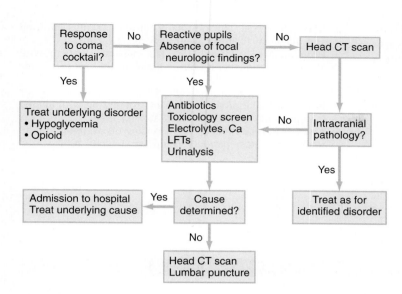

Figure 15-3. Diagnostic algorithm for approach to the patient in coma. Ca, calcium; CT, computed tomography; LFTs, liver function tests.

competitively blocks benzodiazepine activation of the inhibitory γ-aminobutyric acid synapses. The empiric use of flumazenil in all patients with coma of unknown cause is contraindicated because of the high cost of the drug and the risk of seizures in chronic benzodiazepine users. Some overdose patients who have co-ingested cyclic antidepressants are particularly at risk. In an isolated, acute benzodiazepine overdose, most commonly iatrogenic in origin, or rarely in a patient known not to be on long-term benzodiazepine (>1 week) therapy, flumazenil can be used and reverses coma within 1 to 2 minutes. Despite a return of normal mentation and protective airway reflexes, the therapeutic benefit of flumazenil is limited with a single dose, and respirations may remain depressed. The short half-life when compared with some benzodiazepine agents often leads to re-sedation within 45 to 60 minutes after administration. Repeat doses can be given safely to reverse the recurrent effects of the longer acting benzodiazepines. It is administered as a 0.2-mg dose in the first minute followed by 0.2-mg doses every minute until a response is obtained or a total dose of 1 mg is given. The need for tracheal intubation may be eliminated with a continuous intravenous flumazenil drip.

The empiric use of *physostigmine* is not indicated. Physostigmine specifically reverses anticholinergic effects and has nonspecific analeptic activities. A response to physostigmine does not confirm the diagnosis of anticholinergic poisoning because the induced cholinergic action may provoke arousal nonspecifically in other conditions.

Thyroxine may be given in comatose patients with characteristic findings consistent with myxedematous skin changes, mild hypothermia, bradycardia, and pseudomyotonic stretch reflexes (delayed relaxation phase). Treatment must be initiated based on clinical diagnosis because delaying for laboratory confirmation places the patient at significant risk. Steroids usually are given in advance because the potential for a combined adrenal and thyroid insufficiency exists.

Antibiotics should be considered in all patients with coma of unknown cause, particularly if fever or hypothermia is present. The key is early administration. Antibiotics administered before a lumbar puncture have little effect on cerebrospinal fluid cell count, differential, glucose, and protein for 68 hours. Blood cultures reveal the pathogen in 80% of patients with meningitis. Broad-spectrum antibiotics that cross the blood-brain barrier (e.g., third-generation cephalosporins) should be administered when the blood cultures are obtained. The actual risk of tonsillar herniation caused by a lumbar puncture in patients with a mass lesion or subarachnoid hemorrhage is unresolved. If meningitis is clinically probable, antibiotics should be started before the lumbar puncture and before the patient is sent for head CT scanning.

If an overdose is suspected, the empiric treatment of a potential toxic ingestion is indicated. The administration of 1 g/kg of activated charcoal through a nasogastric tube after airway protection is a benign and potentially beneficial intervention that should be performed in all cases in which poisoning is strongly suspected. Gastric lavage is not beneficial beyond 1 hour postingestion, but the retrieval of pill fragments confirms the diagnosis of poisoning and helps direct the evaluation and management.

The definitive diagnosis of depressed mental status is often uncertain in the emergency department. The patient's neurologic examination should be serially reassessed and aggressive assessment pursued until the final diagnosis is established, and definitive treatment and disposition are secured.

DISPOSITION

Patients with reversible causes of coma, such as hypoglycemia or heroin overdose, may be discharged after a period of observation and sustained consciousness. Even after normal mentation can be restored with antidotes, however, if the duration of action of the offending action exceeds that of the antidote, as with methadone or certain oral hypoglycemics, admission to the hospital is warranted. Patients with alcohol or other CNS depressants may be safely observed in the emergency department and discharged when they are sober. Patients with all other causes of coma are admitted to the hospital for observation and definitive treatment.

REFERENCES

1. Plum F, Posner JB: The pathologic physiology of signs and symptoms of coma. In: *The Diagnosis of Stupor and Coma.* Philadelphia, FA Davis, 1980, pp 1-73.

2. Giacino GT, et al: The minimally conscious state: Definition and diagnostic criteria. *Neurology* 58:349, 2002.
3. Hoffman RS, Goldfrank LR: The poisoned patient with altered consciousness: Controversies in the use of a coma cocktail. *JAMA* 274:562, 1995.
4. American College of Emergency Physicians: Clinical policy for the initial approach to patients presenting with altered mental status. *Ann Emerg Med* 33:251, 1999.
5. Towne AR, et al: Prevalence of nonconvulsive status epilepticus in comatose patients. *Neurology* 54:340, 2000.

CHAPTER

16 Seizures

Charles V. Pollack, Jr.

PERSPECTIVE

Seizure is defined as abnormal neurologic functioning caused by abnormally excessive activation of neurons, either in the cerebral cortex or in the deep limbic system. *Epilepsy* is defined as recurrent seizures; it is not an appropriate term for seizures that occur intermittently and predictably after a known insult, such as alcohol intoxication and withdrawal.

Presentation to the emergency department with generalized convulsive seizure prompts immediate concern for airway protection and neurologic stabilization, followed by a focused search for etiology. Nonconvulsive seizures, on the other hand, may be relatively obscure in their presentation, more diverse in their etiology, and are sometimes more difficult to control acutely.

Epidemiology and Classification

It is estimated that 6% of the U.S. population experience at least one afebrile seizure during their lifetime; the annual incidence among adults is 84 per 100,000 population, and more than half of these individuals develop epilepsy.[1] In one study, approximately 1% of emergency department visits were for seizure-related complaints.[2] Nearly half of these patients had alcohol or low antiepileptic drug levels implicated as contributing factors.

"Seizure" is not a diagnosis but rather a series of signs and symptoms. Similar seizures can result from a variety of cerebral processes. They may be the only manifestations of those processes or one of several signs and symptoms.

Seizures can be classified as primary or secondary (also termed *reactive*), as generalized or focal (partial), or as convulsive or nonconvulsive. Table 16-1 shows the distribution of primary generalized seizures in a typical population of patients. A generalized seizure is defined as abnormal neuronal activity in both cerebral hemispheres. They may be divided into tonic-clonic, absence, and myoclonic. Partial seizures or focal seizures usually involve one hemisphere. They are divided into simple partial (in which consciousness is maintained), complex partial (in which consciousness is lost), and those that become secondarily generalized. Some seizures are impossible to classify because of inadequate or inaccurate description of the ictal activity.[1,2]

Secondary seizures may occur as a result of a vast array of injuries and of illnesses such as intoxication or poisoning, encephalitis, encephalopathy, organ failure, other metabolic disturbances, infections of the central nervous system, cerebral tumors, pregnancy, and, paradoxically, supratherapeutic levels of anticonvulsants.

Seizures in children follow a different distribution, primarily because of the relatively high incidence of febrile seizures and the frequently uncertain observational history of possible ictal activity. Febrile seizure is the most common pediatric seizure, occurring in 2% to 5% of children between 6 months and 5 years of age; 20% to 30% of those children have at least one recurrence. It is important to differentiate between febrile seizure and seizure with fever.[3] First time seizures in infants younger than 6 months may indicate significant underlying pathology and warrant a full assessment.[4]

Pathophysiology

The pathophysiology of seizures at the neuronal level is not well understood. Neuronal recruitment is demonstrated in some studies. It occurs when the abnormal increased electrical activity of the initiating neurons activates adjacent neurons and propagates until the thalamus and other subcortical structures are similarly stimulated. Recruitment may follow contiguous paths or extend along diverse integrated circuits both deep and across the midline. The clinical seizure activity typically, but not always, reflects the initiating focus.

When the ictal discharge extends below the cortex to deeper structures, the reticular activating system in the brainstem may be affected, altering consciousness. In generalized seizures, the focus is often deep and midline, which explains the prompt loss of consciousness and bilateral involvement. Seizures are typically self-limited; at some point the hyperpolarization subsides and the bursts of electrical discharges from the focus terminate. This cessation may be related to reflex inhibition, neuronal exhaustion, or alteration of the local balance of neurotransmitters.

Partial seizures may represent a similar pathophysiologic process in which less recruitment occurs and the ictal activity does not cross the midline. Because of the more limited focus of abnormal activity, convulsive motor activity may not be the predominant clinical manifestation.[2]

DIAGNOSTIC APPROACH

Differential Considerations

Whether the patient is having a "true" seizure is the first differential consideration. Ictal activity can be irrefutably verified only by electroencephalography (EEG). Other abnormal movements and states of consciousness can be confused with ictal activity. Synchronized EEG and videotaping may be required to differentiate pseudoseizures (also called psychogenic seizures) from seizures, and both may coexist in the same patient. Other disorders mimicking seizures are listed in Table 16-2.[4]

Syncope, whether vasodepressive (vagal syncope), orthostatic, or arrhythmogenic, is often confused with ictal events by observers. A sudden loss of consciousness followed by abnormal movements can be ictal or syncopal in origin, hence the consideration "fit versus faint." One video analysis of 56 brief syncopes showed myoclonic activity in 90% of patients, together with frequent head turns, upward gaze, oral automatisms, and righting movements. Generally, ictal tonic-clonic movements are more forceful and prolonged than the "twitches" sometimes associated with fainting. In addition, most generalized seizures are characterized by a

Table 16-1. Classification of Seizures in a General Adult Population

Seizure Type	Percentage
Generalized	
Tonic-clonic	35
Absence	1
Myoclonic	<1
Others	2-3
Partial	
Simple partial	3
Complex partial	11
Secondarily generalized	27
Mixed partial	12
Unclassified	9

Table 16-2. Differential Considerations for the Diagnosis of Seizure*

Disorder	Classification	Ictal-like Manifestations
Syncope	Vasodepressive vs dysrhythmogenic (including long QT syndrome) vs orthostatic	"Fit versus faint"
Hyperventilation syndrome		Preictal or postictal twitching
		Mood disturbances
		Posturing of extremities
Prolonged breath-holding	Typically in children	Tonic-clonic movements
		Loss of urinary continence
Toxic and metabolic disorders	Alcohol abuse/withdrawal	Delirium tremens, blackout
	Hypoglycemia	Abnormal behavior
	Phencyclidine	Buccolingual spasms
	Tetanus	Myotonic spasms
	Strychnine and camphor	Myotonic spasms
	Extrapyramidal reactions	Posturing, deviation of eyes
Nonictal CNS events	Transient ischemic attacks	Drop attacks, "fit versus faint"
	Transient global amnesia	Similar to postictal state, absence status
	Hemiparetic migraine	Todd's paralysis
	Carotid sinus hypersensitivity	Drop attacks, "fit versus faint"
	Narcolepsy	Drop attacks, "fit versus faint"
Movement disorders	Hemiballismus, tics	Convulsions
Psychiatric disorders	Fugue state	Similar to postictal state, absence status
	Panic attacks	Twitching, altered mental state
Functional disorders	Pseudoseizure	May closely resemble ictal activity; patients may have both true seizures and pseudoseizures

*Electroencephalography provides the definitive diagnosis in unclear cases.
CNS, central nervous system.

postictal state (an important exception being atonic drop attack ictus), which syncope patients do not manifest.[5]

The cause of an unwitnessed, unprovoked loss of consciousness with a fall, after which the patient presents to the emergency department, may be difficult to classify. Suggestions of an ictal diagnosis include retrograde amnesia, loss of continence, and evidence of tongue biting.[6]

Rapid Assessment and Stabilization

The patient who arrives with a history of possible seizure activity should be placed in a monitored area of the emergency department and prepared for prompt physician examination.[7] An intravenous (IV) line or saline lock catheter should be placed in case anticonvulsants must subsequently be emergently administered. Blood glucose is checked at the bedside, and a thorough list of all medications (prescription and over the counter, including nutritional supplements and homeopathic agents) currently being used by the patient is obtained.

If the patient is seizing in the emergency department, the first step is to confirm that a pulse is present and that the "seizure" activity is not the result of cerebral hypoxia from lack of blood flow. After this, attention is paid to protection and maintenance of the airway. The use of a bite block is no longer recommended. A nasopharyngeal airway is appropriate because an oropharyngeal airway may stimulate vomiting. Availability of suction should be assured in anticipation of the need for clearing vomitus from the oral cavity. If possible, dentures should be removed. The patient should be protected from self-injury during this time.[7]

A pulse oximeter should be applied and oxygen administered as necessary. Optimally, the patient is turned on his or her side to protect the airway from aspiration. If the patient is immobilized on a spine board after trauma, the entire board is tipped up to one side. Preparation should be made for endotracheal intubation in case anticonvulsant drugs fail to terminate the seizure. While these procedures are accomplished, an assistant should be establishing IV access.[7]

Hypoglycemia is the most common metabolic cause of seizure activity. The only treatment required for the patient may be IV glucose. *Prolonged* seizure activity may also *cause* hypoglycemia, so that the cause-and-effect relationship may sometimes be reversed and further therapy is required. The optimal first-line agents for stopping seizure activity in patients of all ages are the benzodiazepines. Available agents include diazepam (Valium), lorazepam (Ativan), and midazolam (Versed). All three are efficacious in terminating seizure activity (see Table 16-3 for dosing), but if IV access cannot be achieved, diazepam may be given rectally, endotracheally, or intraosseously; and midazolam can be given intramuscularly.[8] Lorazepam, because of its relatively longer duration of action, is specifically recommended for alcohol withdrawal seizures.[9]

If benzodiazepines do not abort seizure activity, the airway should be reevaluated. If the patient's ability to protect the airway or oxygen saturation remains persistently below 90%, emergent intubation should be performed. Second-line therapy for adults with persistent seizure activity is phenytoin; its prodrug fosphenytoin can be administered more quickly and has less tendency to cause hypotension but is significantly more expensive and has not come into widespread use because of this.[10] Either may be given intramuscularly (see Table 16-3).[11,12] Second-line therapy for children

Table 16-3. Drugs and Dosages for Abortive Treatment of Seizures in the Emergency Department*

Drug	Adult Dose	Pediatric Dose	Comments
Diazepam	0.2 mg/kg IV at 2 mg/min up to 20 mg	0.2-0.5 mg/kg IV/IO/ET or 0.5-1.0 mg/kg PR up to 20 mg	Monitor airway protection and respiratory drive
Lorazepam	0.1 mg/kg IV at 1-2 mg/min up to 10 mg	0.05-0.1 mg/kg IV	Monitor airway protection and respiratory drive
Midazolam	0.1 mg/kg given at 1 mg/min up to 10 mg IV 0.2 mg/kg IM	0.15 mg/kg IV, then 2-10 µg/kg/min	Monitor airway protection and respiratory drive
Phenytoin	20 mg/kg IV at ≤40 mg/min	20 mg/kg IV at 1 mg/kg/min	During infusion patient should have continuous cardiac and blood pressure monitoring
Fosphenytoin	15-20 mg/kg IV at 100-150 mg/min or 20 mg/kg IM	Under investigation	Level of monitoring directed by patient's status, not drug use
Phenobarbital	20-30 mg/kg IV at 60-100 mg/min or as single IM dose		Intubation may be required
Valproate	20 mg/kg PR or 10-15 mg/kg IV (initial dose)		Maximum dosage 60 mg/kg/day Dilute 1 : 1 with water; onset is slow
Pentobarbital	5 mg/kg IV at 25 mg/min, then titrate to EEG		Intubation, ventilation, and pressor support are required.
Isoflurane	Via general endotracheal anesthesia		Monitor with EEG

*Although alternative routes of administration (e.g., IO, PR) have not all been studied in adults, appropriate weight or length based dosing by pediatric guidelines can be used when the clinical situation dictates.
EEG, electroencephalogram; ET, endotracheal; IM, intramuscular; IO, intraosseous; IV, intravenous; PR, rectal administration.

is phenobarbital. Third-line therapy is phenytoin for children and phenobarbital for adults.[13-16] Patients with seizures refractory to benzodiazepines should be screened for isoniazid overdose because the only effective pharmacologic treatment is pyridoxine. Likewise, females of childbearing age are considered at risk for eclampsia, although eclamptic seizures typically respond to benzodiazepines with or without phenytoin. Children and psychiatric patients at risk for water intoxication should be considered potential candidates for hypertonic saline therapy, preferably after laboratory confirmation of hyponatremia.

Status epilepticus is defined as prolonged or repetitive seizures without intervening neurologic recovery. Patients who remain unresponsive to the third-level choice of pharmacologic intervention are by definition in status epilepticus. Further choices for therapy at that juncture are barbiturate coma and isoflurane anesthesia; both of these interventions mandate endotracheal intubation.[15-17]

Pivotal Findings

When the patient is stabilized with a secure airway and ictal activity is controlled, attention is turned to more complete data gathering.

History

History taking in the patient with seizure is determined by two related factors: Does the patient have a previous history of diagnosed seizures? If not, was the reported ictal activity witnessed by a reliable observer? The latter question is of particular importance because of the broad differential diagnosis for seizures (see Table 16-2) and the notoriously inaccurate descriptions of seizure-like activity from laypersons.[6]

In the patient with a documented previous history of seizures, emergency department evaluation may be limited to a thorough history and consideration of measurement of anticonvulsant drug levels. History should focus on intercurrent illness or trauma, drug or alcohol use, potential adverse drug-drug interactions with anticonvulsants, medication compliance, a recent change in anticonvulsant dosing regimens, or a change in ictal pattern or characteristics.[1,7]

Supratherapeutic and toxic levels of some anticonvulsants such as phenytoin and carbamazepine, whether attained chronically or after acute overdose, may *cause* seizures. If empirical anticonvulsant therapy is indicated before the serum level is available, only 50% of a full loading dose should be given unless the patient is known reliably not to be taking anticonvulsant medication.

In evaluating the patient with a first-time seizure, the first step is to confirm, to the degree possible, that the occurrence in question was an ictal event by obtaining a careful description. Even when the event is witnessed in the emergency department, the true nature of the "spell" may not be entirely clear. In general, ictal events have six properties:

1. *Abrupt onset*: Generalized seizures typically occur without an aura.

2. *Brief duration*: Seizures rarely last longer than 90 to 120 seconds, although bystanders typically overestimate the duration.

3. *Altered mental status*: Present by definition, except for simple partial seizures.

4. *Purposeless activity*: For example, automatisms and undirected tonic-clonic movements.

5. *Unprovoked*: Especially with regard to emotional stimuli; fever in children and substance withdrawal in adults are notable exceptions.

6. *Postictal state*: An acute confusional state that typically occurs with all seizures except simple partial and absence; atypical postictal states include neurogenic pulmonary edema and Todd's paralysis.

Particularly useful, however, are any indications of focality of onset and the extent of any potential trauma before or during the episode. A history of febrile seizures in children should be sought.

When an actual ictal event is suspected, the history should focus on potential underlying medical, toxicologic, or neurologic causes. It must not be assumed that a first-time seizure is idiopathic in origin.

The history should also focus on potential exposure to any of the causes. Evidence for a toxicologic cause may be difficult to elicit because of fear of legal repercussions for both the patient and close observer. Any recent illness, particularly if fever was a feature, may be significant. Travel history may be significant because of possible exposure to unusual diseases such as cysticercosis or malaria. The familial transmission of seizures is inconsistent. Finally, a personal history from the patient, close friend, relative, or medical record may reveal potential ictogenic factors such as recent or remote head trauma, developmental abnormalities, metabolic diseases, drug or alcohol abuse, sleep deprivation, or pregnancy. When no witness or family member is available, extensive questioning must await clearance of the postictal confusional state.

Physical Examination

The physical manifestations of convulsive ictal activity include hypertension, tachycardia, and tachypnea from sympathetic stimulation. These signs typically resolve quickly after the seizure activity ceases. With more prolonged convulsions, skeletal muscle damage, lactic acidosis, and, rarely, frank rhabdomyolysis may ensue. Autonomic discharges and bulbar muscle involvement may result in urinary or fecal incontinence, vomiting (with significant aspiration risk), tongue biting, and airway impairment. All of these signs are helpful discriminators in the evaluation of seizure-like spells.

After the seizure activity has ceased, resting vital signs should be evaluated. Fever and underlying infection can cause seizures, although there may be a low-grade temperature elevation immediately after a convulsive generalized seizure. Tachypnea, tachycardia, or an abnormal blood pressure that persists beyond the immediate postictal period may indicate toxic exposure, hypoxia, or a central nervous system lesion. Pertinent physical findings may include nuchal rigidity, stigmata of substance abuse, lymphadenopathy suggestive of human immunodeficiency virus (HIV) disease or malignancy, dysmorphic features, or skin lesions such as café-au-lait spots and neurofibromata. The examination should also focus on potential adverse sequelae of convulsive seizures, such as tongue injury, posterior shoulder dislocation, or back pain.

Finally, a complete neurologic examination must be performed. A persistent focal deficit after a seizure (e.g., Todd's paralysis) often indicates the focal origin of the event but also can be the only evidence of an underlying stroke. The patient should be carefully examined for papilledema; elevated intracranial pressure can both cause and result from ictal activity. Failure to note steady improvement of postictal depression of consciousness suggests the possibility of an underlying encephalopathy.

Ancillary Testing

Laboratory

Routine screening studies such as a complete blood count and chemistry profile have little use in the neurologically normal, otherwise healthy, postictal patient with a known seizure disorder for whom a reliable history can be obtained. Bedside blood glucose is measured early. Anticonvulsant levels are appropriate in the patients known or suspected to take anticonvulsant medication. Febrile patients are evaluated for the source of the fever. For medically ill adults (e.g., diabetic patients, cancer patients, patients with liver disease, patients taking medications that can affect serum electrolyte levels) and in those presenting with a first-time seizure, appropriate chemistry studies are ordered.[1,7] Toxicologic screens should be obtained if there is a suspicion of substance abuse. Serum sodium should be evaluated, particularly if mental status remains altered after apparent recovery from the postictal state. Pregnancy testing is useful if toxemia is suspected. If there is *any* suspicion of meningitis or subarachnoid hemorrhage, lumbar puncture should be performed, with or without a preceding cranial computed tomography (CT) scan.

Imaging

In the fully recovered patient without headache and with fully normal mental status and neurologic examination who has had a single, brief seizure, a cranial CT scan can be obtained in the emergency department or at a follow-up visit, at the discretion of the treating physician.[7,17]

The literature on this issue for first-time nonfebrile seizures in children is also inconclusive.[18] A cranial CT scan is indicated in any age group when there is suspicion of head trauma, elevated intracranial pressure, intracranial mass, persistently abnormal mental status or focal neurologic abnormality, or HIV disease.

Electroencephalography

EEG is not consistently available in the emergency department. It may be particularly useful in specific cases, such as the diagnosis of nonconvulsive status epilepticus, to monitor seizure activity after intubation and neuromuscular blockade, and to help differentiate seizures from other similar presentations. In general, EEGs are most appropriate for the follow-up evaluation of first-time seizures without clear cause after a complete emergency department evaluation.[12]

MANAGEMENT

Abortive therapy for seizures in the emergency department begins with active, anticipatory airway protection. Rapidly reversible ictal insults (e.g., hypoglycemia, hypoxemia, isoniazid ingestion) should be considered and, if found, treated. Primary abortive therapy in the emergency department is accomplished with benzodiazepines; second-line therapy includes phenytoin (and fosphenytoin) and phenobarbital. Resistant status epilepticus may require barbiturate coma or deep inhalational anesthesia with EEG monitoring. Although a number of newer antiepileptic medications have become available, their therapeutic purpose is directed toward chronic rather than acute seizures.[19]

Identifying a new-onset seizure in the emergency department generates consideration for further management. The choice to initiate anticonvulsant therapy is dependent on the risk of seizure recurrence, any underlying predisposing disease, and the risk of anticonvulsant therapy and is typically not made by the emergency physician. The initiation of anticonvulsant therapy after a single seizure is an issue of considerable controversy. Prompt treatment of any apparent ictal source discovered in the emergency department, however, is always appropriate.

DISPOSITION

Disposition plans must be individualized according to the findings of the emergency department evaluation and the presence or absence of underlying disease. One quarter of adult patients presenting with seizure-related complaints has new-onset seizures.[2] Almost half of them require admission, most because of abnormal CT scans or persistent focal abnormalities; 95% of those who retrospectively required admission were correctly identified by using an emergency department evaluation consistent with that recommended. Patients discharged home from the emergency department should receive appropriate state-specific guidance regarding driver's license privileges. Outpatient therapy for seizure disorders should be initiated in consultation with a neurologist, if possible.

REFERENCES

1. Engel J, Starkman S: Overview of seizures. *Emerg Med Clin North Am* 12:895, 1994.
2. Huff JS, et al: Emergency department management of patients with seizures: A multicenter study. *Acad Emerg Med* 8:62, 2001.

3. Hirtz D, et al: Practice parameter: Treatment of the child with the first unprovoked seizure: Report of the Quality Standards Subcommittee of the American Academy of Neurology and the Practice Committee of the Child Neurology Society. *Neurology* 60:166, 2003.

4. Bui TT, et al: Infant seizures not so infantile: First-time seizures in children under six months of age presenting to the ED. *Am J Emerg Med* 20:518, 2002.

5. Schmidt D: Syncopes and seizures. *Curr Opin Neurol* 9:78, 1996.

6. Morrell MJ: Differential diagnosis of seizures. *Neurol Clin* 11:737, 1993.

7. American College of Emergency Physicians: Clinical policy for the initial approach to patients presenting with a chief complaint of seizure who are not in status epilepticus. *Ann Emerg Med* 29:706, 1997.

8. Cereghino JJ, et al: Treating repetitive seizures with a rectal diazepam formulation: A randomized study. *Neurology* 51:1274, 1998.

9. D'Onofrio G, et al: Lorazepam for the prevention of recurrent seizures related to alcohol. *N Engl J Med* 340:915, 1999.

10. Ramsey RE, DeToledo J: Intravenous administration of fosphenytoin: Options for the management of seizures. *Neurology* 46(Suppl 1):S17, 1996.

11. Uthman BM, Wilder BJ, Ramsey RE: Intramuscular use of fosphenytoin: An overview. *Neurology* 46(Suppl 1):S24, 1996.

12. Quigg M, Shneker B, Domer P: Current practice in administration and clinical criteria of emergent EEG. *J Clin Neurophysiol* 18:162, 2001.

13. Haafiz A, Kissoon N: Status epilepticus: Current concepts. *Pediatr Emerg Care* 15:119, 1999.

14. Hanhan UA, Fiallos MR, Orlowski JP: Status epilepticus. *Pediatr Clin North Am* 48:683, 2001.

15. Lowenstein DH, Alldredge BK: Status epilepticus. *N Engl J Med* 338:970, 1998.

16. Smith BJ: Treatment of status epilepticus. *Epilepsy* 345:631, 2001.

17. Alldredge BK, et al: The comparison of lorazepam, diazepam, and placebo for the treatment of out of hospital status epilepticus. *N Engl J Med* 345:631, 2001.

18. Sharma S, et al: The role of emergent neuroimaging in children with new-onset afebrile seizures. *Pediatrics* 111:1, 2003.

19. French JA, et al: Efficacy and tolerability of the new antiepileptic drugs I. Treatment of new onset epilepsy. *Neurology* 62:1252, 2004.

CHAPTER 17

Headache

Gregory L. Henry and Christopher S. Russi

PERSPECTIVE

Epidemiology

As many as 85% of the U.S. adult population complains of significant headaches at least occasionally and 15% on a regular basis. Headache as a primary complaint represents between 3% and 5% of all emergency department visits. The vast majority of patients who have the primary complaint of headache do not have a serious medical cause for the problem. Tension headache accounts for approximately 50% of patients presenting to the emergency department, another 30% have headache of nonidentified origin, 10% have migraine-type pain, and 8% have headache from other potentially serious causes (e.g., tumor, glaucoma). It is estimated that less than 1% of patients who present to the emergency department with headache have a life-threatening organic disease.[1] The percentages can create a false sense of security, and headache is disproportionately represented in emergency medicine malpractice claims. Although still rare, the most commonly encountered cause of severe sudden head pain is subarachnoid hemorrhage (SAH); approximately 20,000 potentially salvageable cases of SAH present to emergency departments each year. It is estimated that between 25% and 50% of these are missed on the first presentation to a physician.[2] The other significant, potentially life-threatening causes of headache occur even less frequently. Meningitis, carbon monoxide poisoning, temporal arteritis, acute angle closure glaucoma, and increased intracranial pressure often have specific historical elements and physical findings that facilitate their diagnosis.

Pathophysiology

The brain parenchyma is insensitive to pain. The pain-sensitive areas of the head include the coverings of the brain—the meninges—and the blood vessels, both arteries and veins supplying the brain, and the various tissues lining the cavities within the skull. The ability of the patient to localize head pain specifically is often poor. Much of the pain associated with headache, particularly with vascular headache and migraines, is mediated through the fifth cranial nerve. Such pain may proceed back to the nucleus and then be radiated through various branches of the fifth cranial nerve to areas not directly involved. A specific inflammation in a specific structure (e.g., periapical abscess, sinusitis, or tic douloureux) is much easier to localize than the relatively diffuse pain that may be generated by tension or traction headaches. Pains in the head and neck may easily overlap. They should be thought of as a unit when considering complaints of headache.

DIAGNOSTIC APPROACH

Differential Considerations

The differential diagnosis of headache is complex because of the large number of potential disease entities and the diffuse nature of many types of pain in the head and neck region (Table 17-1). However, in evaluating the patient with a headache complaint, the first focus is on excluding intracranial hemorrhage, meningitis, encephalitis, and mass lesions. Carbon monoxide is an exogenous toxin that may be reversible by removing the patient from the source and administering oxygen. It is a rare example of a headache in which a simple intervention may quickly improve a critical situation. On the contrary, returning the patient to the poisoned environment without diagnosis could be lethal.

Rapid Assessment and Stabilization

If the patient presents in a critical state, a fundamental approach to airway, breathing, and circulatory management must supercede any other initial intervention.

Included in the primary survey is a focused and rapid assessment of the patient's mental status. For purposes of the initial assessment, headache can be divided into two categories: accompanied by altered mental status and without altered mental status. Whenever a patient's mental status is decreased, it must be initially assumed that brain tissue is being compromised. The principles of care centered on cerebral resuscitation address the seven major causes of evolving brain injury: lack of substrate (glucose, oxygen), cerebral edema, mass lesion intracranially, endogenous or exogenous toxins, metabolic alterations (fever, seizure), ischemia, or elevated intracranial pressure.

Pivotal Findings

History

The history is the pivotal part of the workup for the patient with headache (Table 17-2).
1. A patient should be asked to describe the *pattern and onset of the pain*. Patients often relate frequent and recurrent headaches similar to the one they have on this emergency department visit. A marked

Table 17-1. Differential Diagnosis

Organ System	Critical Diagnoses	Emergent Diagnoses	Nonemergent Diagnoses
Neurologic, CNS, vessels	Subarachnoid hemorrhage	Shunt failure Traction headaches Tumor/other masses Subdural hematomas	Migraine, various types Vascular, various types Trigeminal neuralgia Posttraumatic Post–lumbar puncture Headaches
Toxic/metabolic Environmental	Carbon monoxide poisoning	Mountain sickness	
Collagen vascular disease Eye/ENT	Temporal arteritis	Glaucoma/sinusitis	Dental problems/temporomandibular joint disease
Musculoskeletal			Tension headaches Cervical strain
Allergy			Cluster/histamine headaches
Infectious disease	Bacterial meningitis/encephalitis	Brain abscess	Febrile headaches/nonneurologic source of infection
Pulmonary/O₂		Anoxic headache Anemia	
Cardiovascular		Hypertensive crisis	Hypertension (rare)
Unspecified			Effort-dependent/coital headaches

CNS, central nervous system; ENT, ear, nose, and throat.

Table 17-2. Significant Symptoms

Symptom	Finding	Possible Diagnoses
Sudden onset pain	Lightning strike or thunder clap with any decreased mentation, any positive focal finding and/or intractable pain	Subarachnoid hemorrhage
"Worst headache of their life"	Associated with sudden onset	Subarachnoid hemorrhage
Near syncope or syncope	Associated with sudden onset	Subarachnoid hemorrhage
Increase with jaw movement	Clicking or snapping. Pain with jaw movement	Temporomandibular joint disease
Facial pain	Fulminant pain of the forehead and area of maxillary sinus. Nasal congestion.	Sinus pressure or dental infection
Forehead and/or temporal area pain	Tender temporal arteries	Temporal arteritis
Periorbital or retroorbital pain	Sudden onset with tearing	Temporal arteritis or acute angle closure glaucoma

variance in a headache pattern can signal a new or serious problem. The rate of onset of pain may have significant value. Pain with rapid onset of a few seconds to minutes is more likely to be vascular in origin than pain that developed over several hours or days.

Almost all studies dealing with subarachnoid bleeding report that patients have moved from the pain-free state to severe pain within seconds to minutes. The "thunder clap" or "lightning strike" headache is a real phenomenon, and this response to questioning may lead to the correct diagnosis of subarachnoid bleeding, even if the pain is improving at the time of evaluation.[3]

2. The patient's *activity at the onset of the pain* may be helpful. Certainly, headaches that come on during severe exertion have a relationship to vascular bleeding, but again, there is enough variation to make assignment to any specific cause highly variable. The syndrome of coital or postcoital headache is well known, but coitus is also a common time of onset for SAH. These headaches require the same evaluation on initial presentation as any other exertion-related head pain. If the patient can recall the precise activity in which he or she was engaging at the time of the onset of the headache (e.g., "I was just getting up out of the chair to answer the doorbell"), sudden onset is extremely likely and evaluation for SAH is warranted.

3. If the patient or prehospital personnel can relate a *history of head trauma*, the differential diagnosis and emergent causes have narrowed significantly. The considerations now focus on epidural and subdural hematoma, skull fracture, and closed head injury (i.e., concussion and diffuse axonal injury).

4. Toxoplasmosis, cryptococcal meningitis, and abscess are considered higher in the differential in patients with a *history of human immunodeficiency virus (HIV) or immunocompromised state*. Although such entities are rare, it is important to remember this subset of patients may have serious disease without typical signs or symptoms of systemic illness, that is, fever and meningismus.

5. The *intensity of head pain* is difficult to quantify objectively. Almost all patients who present to the emergency department consider their headache to be "severe." Use of a pain scale of 1 to 10 may help differentiate patients initially but has more value in monitoring their response to therapy.

6. The *character of the pain*, that is, throbbing, steady, and so forth, although statistically helpful, may not be adequate to differentiate one type of headache from another.

7. The *location of head pain* is helpful when the patient can identify a specific area. It is useful to have the patient point or try to indicate the area of pain and the emergency physician then properly examine that area. Unilateral pain is more suggestive of migraine or a localized inflammatory process in the skull (e.g., sinus) or soft tissue.[4] Occipital headaches are classically associated with hypertension. Certainly, temporal arteritis, tem-

poromandibular joint disease, dental infections, and sinus infections frequently have a highly localized area of discomfort. Meningitis, encephalitis, SAH, and even severe migraine, although intense in nature, are usually more diffuse in their localization.

8. *Exacerbating* or *alleviating factors* may be important. Patients whose headaches rapidly improve when they are removed from their environment may have carbon monoxide poisoning. Most other severe causes of head pain are not rapidly relieved or improved when they get to the emergency department. Intracranial infections, dental infections, and other regional causes of head pain tend not to be improved or alleviated before therapy is given.

9. *Associated symptoms and risk factors* may relate to the severity of headache but rarely point to the specific causes (Box 17-1). Because head pain is medi-

---

BOX 17-1. Risk Factors Associated with Potentially Catastrophic Illness

1. Carbon Monoxide Poisoning
   a. Breathing in enclosed or confined spaces with engine exhaust or ventilation of heating equipment
   b. Multiple family members with the same symptoms
   c. Wintertime and working around machinery or equipment producing carbon monoxide, furnaces, etc.
2. Subarachnoid Hemorrhage
   a. History of polycystic kidney disease
   b. Family history of subarachnoid hemorrhage
   c. Hypertension—severe
   d. Previous vascular lesions in other areas of the body
   e. Middle aged
3. Meningitis/Encephalitis/Abscess
   a. History of sinus or ear infection or recent surgical procedure
   b. General debilitation with decreased immunologic system function
   c. Acute febrile illness—any type
   d. Extremes of age
   e. Impacted living conditions (e.g., military barracks, college dormitories)
   f. Lack of primary immunizations
4. Temporal Arteritis
   a. Age > 50
   b. Females > males 4:1
   c. History of other collagen vascular diseases (e.g., systemic lupus)
   d. Previous chronic meningitis
   e. Previous chronic illness such as tuberculosis, parasitic infection, fungi
5. Glaucoma—sudden angle closure
   a. Not associated with any usual or customary headache pattern
   b. History of previous glaucoma
   c. Age > 30
   d. History of pain increasing in a dark environment
   e. Hypertension—mild statistical association
6. Increased intracranial pressure
   a. History of previous benign intracranial hypertension
   b. Presence of a cerebrospinal fluid shunt
   c. History of congenital brain or skull abnormalities

ated largely through the cranial nerves, outflow through other cranial nerves is common. Nausea and vomiting are completely nonspecific. Migraine headaches, increased intracranial pressure, temporal arteritis, and glaucoma can all be manifested through severe nausea and vomiting, as can some systemic viral infections with headache. Such factors may point toward the intensity of the discomfort but are not specific in establishing the diagnosis.

10. A *prior history of headache,* although helpful, does not rule out current serious problems. It is extremely helpful, however, to know that the patient has had a workup for severe disease. Previous emergency department visits, computed tomography (CT) scanning, magnetic resonance imaging, and other forms of testing should be sought. Patients with both migraine and tension headaches tend to have a stereotypical recurrent pattern. Adherence to these patterns is also helpful in deciding the degree to which a patient's symptoms are pursued.

Physical Examination

Physical findings associated with various forms of headache are listed in Table 17-3.

Ancillary Testing

The vast majority of headache patients do not require additional testing (Table 17-4). The single largest consistent mistake made by emergency physicians in the workup of the headache patient is believing a single CT scan clears the patient of the possibility of SAH. The CT scan is at least 6% to 8% insensitive in SAH, especially in patients with minor (grade I) SAH, who are most salvageable.[5] The sensitivity of CT scanning for SAH is reduced by nearly 10% if over 12 hours and by almost 20% at 3 to 5 days. The basic approach to integrating CT scanning and lumbar puncture in assessing the headache patient is outlined in Figure 17-1.[6] When the decision has been made to obtain a CT scan and do a lumbar puncture, short-term sedation of the patient is appropriate as necessary.

Obtaining cerebrospinal fluid should not delay antimicrobial treatment if intracranial infection is suspected. Intravenous antibiotics should precede lumbar puncture. Any abnormal mental status, signs of increased intracranial pressure, focality, focal findings on the neurologic examination, or any other suspicion of focal intracranial lesion would require CT scanning before lumbar puncture.

Table 17-3. Pivotal Findings on Physical Examination

Sign	Finding	Diagnoses
General appearance	Alteration of mental status—nonfocal	Meningitis/encephalitis
		Subarachnoid hemorrhage
		Anoxia
		Increased CSF pressure
	Alterations of mental status with focal findings	Intraparenchymal bleed
		Tentorial herniation
		Stroke
	Severe nausea/vomiting	Increased CSF pressure
		Acute angle closure glaucoma
		Subarachnoid hemorrhage
Vital signs	Hypertension with normal or bradycardia	Increased CSF pressure
		Subarachnoid hemorrhage
		Tentorial herniation
		Intraparenchymal bleed
	Tachycardia	Anoxia/anemia
		Febrile headache
		Exertional/coital headaches
	Fever	Febrile headaches
		Meningitis/encephalitis
HEENT	Tender temporal arteries	Temporal arteritis
	Fundi—loss of spontaneous venous pulsations and/or presence of papilledema	Increased CSF pressure
		Mass lesions
	Subhyaloid hemorrhage	Subarachnoid hemorrhage
	Acute red eye (severe ciliary flushing) and poorly reactive pupils	Acute angle closure glaucoma
	Enlarged pupil with third nerve palsy	Tentorial pressure cone
		Mass effect (i.e., subdural, epidural, tumor, intraparenchymal hemorrhage)
Neurologic	Lateralized motor or sensory deficit	Stroke (rare)
		Subdural hematoma, epidural hematoma, hemiplegic or anesthetic migraine (rare)
	Acute cerebellar ataxia	Acute cerebellar hemorrhage
		Acute cerebellitis (mostly children)
		Chemical intoxication—various types

CSF, cerebrospinal fluid; HEENT, head, eyes, ears, nose, and throat.

Table 17-4. Diagnostic Adjuncts in Headache Assessment

Test	Finding	Diagnosis
Erythrocyte sedimentation rate (ESR)	Significant elevation	Temporal arteritis
ECG	Nonspecific ST-T wave changes	Subarachnoid hemorrhage
		Increased CSF pressure
CBC	Severe anemia	Anoxia
CT—head	Increased ventricular size	Increased CSF pressure
	Blood in subarachnoid space	Subarachnoid hemorrhage
	Blood in epidural or subdural space	Epidural/subdural hematoma
	Bleeding into parenchyma of brain	Intraparenchymal hemorrhage
	Areas of poor vascular flow	Pale infarct
	Structural/mass lesion	Traction headache secondary to mass effect
Lumbar puncture/ CSF analysis	Increased pressure	Pseudotumor cerebri
		Mass lesions
		Shunt failure
	Increased protein	Tumor/other structural lesions
	Increased RBCs	Subarachnoid hemorrhage
	Increased WBCs	Infection
	Positive Gram's stain	Infection
	Decreased glucose	Infection

CBC, complete blood count; CSF, cerebrospinal fluid; CT, computed tomography; ECG, electrocardiogram; RBC, red blood cell; WBC, white blood cell.

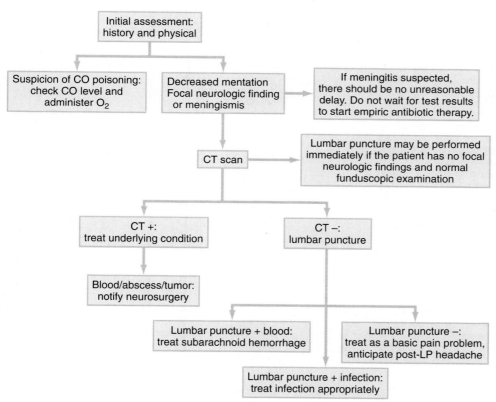

Figure 17-1. Initial assessment and treatment of headache. CT, computed tomography.

DIFFERENTIAL CONSIDERATIONS

Certain historical and physical findings can help decide whether the patient falls into an "all clear" or a "warning signal" group. In the warning group, further investigation and testing should be performed on all patients who present with any of the following: (1) sudden onset of headache, (2) "the worst headache ever," (3) decreased or altered mental status, (4) true meningismus, (5) unexplained abnormal vital signs, (6) focal neurologic deficits on examination, (7) worsening under observation, (8) new onset of headache with exertion, or (9) history of HIV. This group of patients represents those who are at high risk for significant disease.

In addition, a group of responsible "all clear signals" indicates patients who do not require further investigation when all are present: (1) previous identical headaches, (2) normal alertness and cognition by both examination and history of the event, (3) normal examination of the neck showing no meningismus, (4)

Table 17-5. Causes and Differentiation of Potentially Catastrophic Illness Presenting with Nontraumatic Headache

Disease Entities	Pain History	Associated Symptoms	Support History	Prevalence	Physical Examination	Useful Tests	Atypical or Important Aspects
Carbon monoxide poisoning	Usually gradual, subtle, dull, nonfocal throbbing pain	May wax and wane as they leave and enter the involved area of carbon monoxide Throbbing may vary considerably	Exposure to engine exhaust, old or defective heating systems, most common in winter months	Rare	No focal neurologic findings. May need cognitive testing	Carbon monoxide level, cognitive testing	May improve on the way to the hospital. Occurs in groups, may involve entire families or groups of people exposed to the carbon monoxide
Subarachnoid hemorrhage	Sudden onset, "thunder clap" or "lightning strike," severe throbbing	Whenever altered mental status is present the outcome is decidedly worse	History of polycystic kidney disease History of chronic hypertension	Uncommon	Frequently decreased mentation—meningismus, increased blood pressure, decreased pulse, decreased spontaneous venous pulsations, rarely subhyaloid hemorrhage	CT Lumbar puncture	If CT positive, immediate involvement of neurosurgery If CT negative, lumbar puncture
Meningitis/ encephalitis/ abscess	Gradual—as general symptoms increase headache increases—nonfocal	Decreased mentation prominent, irritability prominent With abscess focal neurologic findings may be present	Recent infection Recent facial or dental surgery or other ENT surgery	Uncommon	Fever—late in course decreased spontaneous venous pulsations	CT Lumbar puncture	When such infection suspected, treat Do not delay antibiotics and steroids awaiting laboratory results
Temporal arteritis	Often pain developing over a few hours from mild to severe Virtually always focal in nature	Decreased vision, nausea, vomiting intense—may confuse diagnosis	Age over 50 Other collagen vascular diseases or inflammatory diseases	Uncommon	Tender temporal arteries	Sedimentation rate	Usually unrelated rapidly progressive
Acute angle closure glaucoma	Sudden in onset	Nausea, vomiting, decreased vision	History of glaucoma History of pain going into dark area	Rare	"Steamy" cornea Midposition pupil poorly reactive Acute red eye	Measurement of intraocular pressure	Rapid intervention with medications required—if no relief, immediate surgery may be required
Increased intracranial pressure syndromes	Gradual, dull, nonfocal	Vomiting, decreased mentation	History of CSF shunt or other congenital brain or skull abnormality	Uncommon	Papilledema Loss of spontaneous venous pulsations	CT Shunt function study If OK, lumbar puncture	Shunt failure or other cause of significant increased CSF pressure requires involvement of neurosurgery

CSF, cerebrospinal fluid; CT, computed tomography; ENT, ear, nose, and throat.

normal vital signs, (5) normal or nonfocal neurologic examination, and (6) improvement under observation or with treatment.

Several risk factors for aneurysmal SAH were demonstrated in a case-control study. In a population of 26 cases of known aneurismal SAH, smoking, hypertension, and excessive caffeine intake (>5 cups of coffee daily) showed statistical significance as risk factors in a logistic regression analysis.[7]

After initial history taking, physical examination, and stabilization, findings should match the classical atypical patterns of the various potentially critical diseases causing headache. This sequential evaluation and assessment of data are ongoing processes and should be reevaluated when a patient is under observation in the department. Inconsistency in findings may require a rapid review of the situation and rethinking of the diagnosis (Table 17-5).[8]

MANAGEMENT

Empirical

Patients with headache represent a spectrum of disease. Patients with headache need to be placed for evaluation according to their symptoms. Clearly, patients with abnormal vital signs or altered mental status require evaluation before patients with less severe symptoms. If history and physical examination point toward potentially lethal causes, however, effort should be made to establish the diagnosis rapidly with ancillary testing. Pain treatment should be started early. The pain medication of choice depends on the particular patient, underlying vital signs, allergies, and general condition; but relief of pain is still an essential part of the physician's job and should have little effect on the workup of the patient.

Specific

Specific management for the patient with headache is described in Chapter 101. The challenge in emergency medicine, however, is to eliminate life-threatening causes of headache and to treat the patient's pain.

DISPOSITION

Most patients presenting with headache are discharged from the emergency department with appropriate analgesia and follow-up. These represent patients in the all clear category or those found to have no serious disease after a careful evaluation and testing. Any patients in whom warning findings are noted require more extensive assessment.

REFERENCES

1. Barton CW: Evaluation and treatment of headache patients in the emergency department: A survey. *Headache* 34:91, 1994.
2. Mayer PL, et al: Misdiagnosis of symptomatic cerebral aneurysm: Prevalence and correlation with outcome at four institutions. *Stroke* 27:1558, 1996.
3. Day JW, et al: Thunderclap headache: Symptom of unruptured cerebral aneurysm. *Lancet* 2:1247, 1986.
4. Olesen J, et al: Migraine classification and diagnosis: International Headache Society criteria. *Neurology* 44(Suppl 4):S6, 1994.
5. Edlow J, Caplan L: Avoiding pitfalls in the diagnosis of subarachnoid hemorrhage. *N Engl J Med* 342:29, 2000.
6. Edmeads J: Emergency management of headache. *Headache* 28:675, 1988.
7. Isaksen J, et al: Risk factors for aneurysmal subarachnoid haemorrhage: The Tromso study. *J Neurol Neurosurg Psychiatry* 73:185, 2002.
8. Silberstein SD: Evaluation and emergency treatment of headache, review article. *Headache* 32:396, 1992.

CHAPTER

18 Dyspnea

Sabina Braithwaite and Debra Perina

PERSPECTIVE

Dyspnea is a sign and a symptom and is manifested by physical signs of labored breathing. *Dyspnea* is the term applied to the sensation of breathlessness and the patient's reaction to that sensation. It is an uncomfortable awareness of breathing difficulties that in the extreme manifests as "air hunger." Dyspnea is often ill defined by patients, who may describe the feeling as shortness of breath, chest tightness, or difficulty breathing. Dyspnea results from a variety of conditions ranging from nonurgent to life-threatening. The clinical severity does not correlate well with the seriousness of underlying pathology and may be affected by emotions, behavioral and cultural influences, and external stimuli.

The following terms may be used in the assessment of the dyspneic patient:

Tachypnea: A respiratory rate greater than normal. Normal rates range from 44 cycles/min in a newborn to 14 to 18 cycles/min in adults.

Hyperpnea: Greater than normal minute ventilation to meet metabolic requirements.

Hyperventilation: A minute ventilation (determined by respiratory rate and tidal volume) that exceeds metabolic demand. Arterial blood gases characteristically show a normal PO_2 with an uncompensated respiratory alkalosis (low PCO_2 and elevated pH).

Dyspnea on exertion: Dyspnea provoked by physical effort or exertion. It often is quantified in simple terms, such as the number of stairs or number of blocks a patient can manage before the onset of dyspnea.

Orthopnea: Dyspnea in a recumbent position. It usually is measured in number of pillows the patient must use to lie in bed (e.g., two-pillow orthopnea).

Paroxysmal nocturnal dyspnea: Sudden onset of dyspnea occurring while reclining at night, usually related to the presence of congestive heart failure.

Epidemiology

Dyspnea is a common presenting complaint among emergency department patients of all ages. Causes vary widely and may be due to a benign, self-limited condition or significant pathology that can produce long-term morbidity and mortality.

Pathophysiology

The actual mechanisms responsible for dyspnea are unknown. Normal breathing is controlled by the respiratory control center in the medulla oblongata, peripheral chemoreceptors located near the carotid bodies, and mechanoreceptors in the diaphragm and skeletal muscles. Any imbalance between these sites is perceived as dyspnea. This imbalance generally results from ventilatory demand being greater than capacity.

The sensation of dyspnea is believed to occur by one or more of the following mechanisms: increased work of breathing, such as the increased lung resistance or decreased compliance that occurs with asthma or chronic obstructive pulmonary disease (COPD), or increased respiratory drive, such as results from severe hypoxemia, acidosis, or centrally acting stimuli (toxins, central nervous system events). Pulmonary stretch receptors also are thought to play a role.

DIAGNOSTIC APPROACH

Differential Considerations

Dyspnea is subjective, and there are many different potential causes.[1] The differential diagnosis list can be divided into acute and chronic causes, of which many are pulmonary. Other etiologies include cardiac, metabolic, infectious, neuromuscular, traumatic, and hematologic (Table 18-1).

Pivotal Findings

History

Duration of Dyspnea

Chronic or progressive dyspnea usually denotes cardiac disease,[2] asthma, COPD, or neuromuscular dis-

Table 18-1. Differential Diagnoses for Acute Dyspnea

Organ System	Critical Diagnoses	Emergent Diagnoses	Nonemergent Diagnoses
Pulmonary	Airway obstruction Pulmonary embolus Noncardiogenic edema Anaphylaxis	Spontaneous pneumothorax Asthma Cor pulmonale Aspiration Pneumonia	Pleural effusion Neoplasm Pneumonia COPD
Cardiac	Pulmonary edema Myocardial infarction Cardiac tamponade	Pericarditis	Congenital heart disease Valvular heart disease Cardiomyopathy
Primarily Associated with Normal or Increased Respiratory Effort			
Abdominal		Mechanical interference Hypotension, sepsis from ruptured viscus, bowel obstruction, inflammatory/infectious process	Pregnancy Ascites Obesity
Psychogenic			Hyperventilation syndrome Somatization disorder Panic attack
Metabolic/endocrine	Toxic ingestion DKA	Renal failure Electrolyte abnormalities Metabolic acidosis	Fever Thyroid disease
Infectious	Epiglottitis	Pneumonia	Pneumonia (less severe)
Traumatic	Tension pneumothorax Cardiac tamponade Flail chest	Simple pneumothorax, hemothorax Diaphragmatic rupture	Rib fractures
Hematologic	Carbon monoxide poisoning	Anemia	
Primarily Associated with Decreased Respiratory Effort			
Neuromuscular	CVA, intracranial insult Organophosphate poisoning	Multiple sclerosis Guillain-Barré syndrome Tick paralysis	ALS Polymyositis Porphyria

ALS, amyotrophic lateral sclerosis; COPD, chronic obstructive pulmonary disease; CVA, cerebrovascular accident; DKA, diabetic ketoacidosis.

eases such as multiple sclerosis. Acute dyspneic spells may result from asthma exacerbation; infection; pulmonary emboli; intermittent cardiac dysfunction; psychogenic causes; or inhalation of irritants, allergens, or foreign bodies.

Onset of Dyspnea

Sudden onset of dyspnea should lead to consideration of pulmonary embolism or spontaneous pneumothorax. Dyspnea that builds slowly over hours or days may represent pneumonia; recurrent, small pulmonary emboli; congestive heart failure; or malignancy.

Positional Changes

Orthopnea can result from left heart failure, COPD, or neuromuscular disorders. One of the earliest symptoms seen in patients with diaphragmatic weakness from neuromuscular disease is orthopnea.[3] Paroxysmal nocturnal dyspnea is most common in patients with left heart failure,[2] but also can be found in COPD. Exertional dyspnea commonly is associated with COPD, but also can be seen with poor cardiac reserve and abdominal loading. Abdominal loading, caused by ascites, obesity, or pregnancy, leads to elevation of the diaphragm, resulting in less effective ventilation and dyspnea.

Trauma

Trauma can cause fractured ribs, flail chest, hemothorax, pneumothorax, pericardial effusion, or cardiac tamponade resulting in dyspnea.

Associated Symptoms

Fever suggests an infectious cause. Anxiety may point to panic attack or psychogenic dyspnea, if no organic cause can be isolated. Associated chest pain may indicate pulmonary embolism or myocardial infarction, particularly if it is constant, dull, or visceral. If the pain is sharp and worsened by movements or deep breathing, musculoskeletal origins or pleural effusion/pleurisy should be suspected. Spontaneous pneumothorax also may produce sharp pain with deep breathing that is not worsened by movement.

Physical Examination

Physical examination findings in dyspneic patients may be consistent with specific illnesses (Table 18-2). Physical findings found in specific diseases also can be grouped as presenting patterns (Table 18-3).

Ancillary Studies

Specific findings obtained from the history and physical examination should be used to determine which ancillary studies are needed (Table 18-4). Bedside oxygen saturation determinations, supported by selective use of arterial blood gases, are useful in determining the degree of hypoxia and the need for supplemental oxygen or assisted ventilation. An electrocardiogram may be useful if the etiology is cardiac or suggests acute pulmonary hypertension.

Serum electrolytes may suggest less common etiologies, such as hypokalemia, hypophosphatemia, diabetic ketoacidosis, or hypocalcemia. A complete blood count may identify severe anemia or thrombocytopenia associated with sepsis. Cardiac markers and d-dimer may be useful in pursuing etiologies such as cardiac ischemia or pulmonary embolism. Specialized tests, such as ventilation-perfusion scans, spiral chest computed tomography scan, or pulmonary angiography, may confirm the diagnosis of pulmonary embolus.[4] If dyspnea is believed to be upper airway in origin, direct laryngoscopy, bronchoscopy, or a soft tissue lateral radiograph of the neck may be useful.

DIFFERENTIAL DIAGNOSIS

The range and diversity of pathophysiologic states that produce dyspnea make a simple algorithmic approach difficult.[5] After initial stabilization and assessment, findings from the history, physical examination, and ancillary testing are collated to match patterns of disease that produce dyspnea. This process is updated periodically as new information becomes available. Table 18-3 presents recognizable patterns of disease for common dyspnea-producing conditions, along with specific associated symptoms.

Critical Diagnoses

Several critical diagnoses must be considered immediately to determine the best treatment options to stabilize the patient. Tension pneumothorax is a critical diagnosis that requires immediate treatment. If a dyspneic patient has diminished breath sounds on one side, ipsilateral hyperresonance, severe respiratory distress, hypotension, and oxygen desaturation, immediate decompression of presumptive tension pneumothorax is necessary. If obstruction of the upper airway is suspected, as evidenced by dyspnea and stridor, early aggressive assessment must occur in the emergency department or operating room. Complete obstruction by a foreign body warrants the Heimlich maneuver and efforts to secure and protect the airway, including surgical approaches. Congestive heart failure and pulmonary edema can produce dyspnea and respiratory failure and should be treated immediately if severe.[6] Significant dyspnea and wheezing can be seen in anaphylaxis and must be treated immediately to prevent further deterioration. Severe bronchospastic exacerbations of asthma at any age may lead rapidly to respiratory failure and arrest and should be managed aggressively, including continuous or frequent β-agonist aerosolization.[7]

Emergent Diagnoses

Asthma and COPD exacerbations can result in marked dyspnea with bronchospasm and decreased ventilatory volumes.[8] Sudden onset of dyspnea with a decreased oxygen saturation on room air accompanied by sharp chest pain may represent a pulmonary embolus.[4] Dyspnea accompanied by decreased breath sounds

Table 18-2. Pivotal Findings in Physical Examination

Sign	Physical Finding	Diagnoses to Consider
Vital signs	Tachypnea	Pneumonia, pneumothorax
	Hypopnea	Intracranial insult, drug/toxin ingestion
	Tachycardia	Pulmonary embolism, traumatic chest injury
	Hypotension	Tension pneumothorax
	Fever	Pneumonia, pulmonary embolism
General appearance	Cachexia, weight loss	Malignancy, acquired immune disorder, mycobacterial infection
	Obesity	Hypoventilation, sleep apnea, pulmonary embolism
	Pregnancy	Pulmonary embolism
	Barrel chest	COPD
	"Sniffing" position	Epiglottitis
	"Tripoding" position	COPD/asthma with severe distress
	Traumatic injury	Pneumothorax (simple, tension), rib fractures, flail chest, hemothorax, pulmonary contusion
Skin/nails	Tobacco stains/odor	COPD, malignancy, infection
	Clubbing	Chronic hypoxia, intracardiac shunts or pulmonary vascular anomalies
	Pallid skin/conjunctivae	Anemia
	Muscle wasting	Neuromuscular disease
	Bruising	Chest wall: rib fractures, pneumothorax
		Diffuse: thrombocytopenia, chronic steroid use, anticoagulation
	Subcutaneous emphysema	Rib fractures, pneumothorax, tracheobronchial disruption
	Hives, rash	Allergic reaction, infection, tick-borne illness
Neck	Stridor	Upper airway edema/infection, foreign body, traumatic injury, anaphylaxis
	JVD	Tension pneumothorax, COPD or asthma exacerbation, fluid overload/CHF, pulmonary embolism
Lung examination	Wheezes	CHF, anaphylaxis
		Bronchospasm
	Rales	CHF, pneumonia, pulmonary embolism
	Unilateral decrease	Pneumothorax, pleural effusion, consolidation, rib fractures/contusion, pulmonary contusion
	Hemoptysis	Malignancy, infection, bleeding disorder, CHF
	Sputum production	Infection (viral, bacterial)
	Friction rub	Pleurisy
	Abnormal respiratory pattern (e.g., Cheyne-Stokes)	Intracranial insult
Chest examination	Crepitance or pain to palpation	Rib or sternal fractures
	Subcutaneous emphysema	Pneumothorax, tracheobronchial rupture
	Thoracoabdominal desynchrony	Diaphragmatic injury with herniation; cervical spinal cord trauma
	Flail segment	Flail chest, pulmonary contusion
Cardiac examination	Murmur	Pulmonary embolism
	S₃ or S₄ gallop	Pulmonary embolism
	S₂ accentuation	Pulmonary embolism
	Muffled heart sounds	Cardiac tamponade
Extremities	Calf tenderness, Homans' sign	Pulmonary embolism
	Edema	CHF
Neurologic examination	Focal deficits (motor, sensory, cognitive)	Stroke, intracranial hemorrhage causing central abnormal respiratory drive; if long-standing, risk of aspiration pneumonia
	Symmetric deficits	Neuromuscular disease
	Diffuse weakness	Metabolic or electrolyte abnormality (hypocalcemia, hypomagnesemia, hypophosphatemia), anemia
	Hyporeflexia	Hypermagnesemia
	Ascending weakness	Guillain-Barré syndrome

CHF, congestive heart failure; COPD, chronic obstructive pulmonary disease; JVD, jugular venous distention.

Table 18-3. Diagnostic Table: Patterns of Diseases Often Resulting in Dyspnea

Disease	History: (Dyspnea +)	Associated Symptoms	Signs and Physical Findings	Tests
Pulmonary embolism	HPI: abrupt onset, pleuritic pain, immobility (travel, recent surgery) PMH: malignancy, DVT, PE, hypercoagulability, oral contraception, obesity	Diaphoresis, exertional dyspnea	Tachycardia, tachypnea, low-grade fever	ABG (A-a gradient), d-dimer, ECG (dysrhythmia, right heart strain) CXR (Westermark sign, Hampton's hump) V/Q, spiral CT Pulmonary angiogram
Pneumonia Bacterial	Fever, productive cough, chest pain SH: tobacco use	Anorexia, chills, nausea, vomiting, exertional dyspnea, cough	Fever, tachycardia, tachypnea, rales or decreased breath sounds	CXR, CBC, sputum and blood cultures ABG if hypoxia suspected or if altered mental status
Viral	Exposure (e.g., influenza, varicella)			
Opportunistic	Immune disorder, chemotherapy			
Fungal/parasitic	Exposure (e.g., birds), indolent onset	Episodic fever, nonproductive cough		
Pneumothorax Simple	Abrupt onset ± trauma, chest pain, thin males more likely to have spontaneous pneumothorax	Localized chest pain	Decreased breath sounds, subcutaneous emphysema, chest wall wounds or instability	CXR: pneumothorax, rib fractures, hemothorax
Tension	Decompensation of simple pneumothorax	Diaphoresis	Above + JVD, tracheal deviation, muffled heart sounds, cardiovascular collapse	Clinical diagnosis: requires immediate decompression
COPD/asthma	Tobacco use, medication noncompliance, URI symptoms, sudden weather change PMH: environmental allergies FH: asthma	Air hunger, diaphoresis	Retractions, accessory muscle use, tripoding, cyanosis	CXR: rule out infiltrate, pneumothorax, atelectasis (mucus plug)
Malignancy	Weight loss, tobacco or other occupational exposure	Dysphagia	Hemoptysis	CXR, chest CT: mass, hilar adenopathy, focal atelectasis BNP elevation
Fluid overload	Gradual onset, dietary indiscretion or medication noncompliance, chest pain PMH: recent MI, diabetes, CHF	Worsening orthopnea, PND	JVD, peripheral edema, S_3 or S_4 gallop, new cardiac dysrhythmia, hepatojugular reflux	CXR: pleural effusion, interstitial edema, Kerley B lines, cardiomegaly ECG: ischemia, dysrhythmia
Anaphylaxis	Abrupt onset, exposure to allergen	Dysphagia	Oral swelling, stridor, wheezing, hives	

ABG, arterial blood gas; BNP, brain natriuretic peptide; CBC, complete blood count; CHF, congestive heart failure; CT, computed tomography; CXR, chest x-ray; DVT, deep vein thrombosis; ECG, electrocardiogram; FH, family history; HPI, history of present illness; JVD, jugular venous distention; MI, myocardial infarction; PE, pulmonary embolism; PMH, past medical history; PND, paroxysmal nocturnal dyspnea; SH, social history; URI, upper respiratory infection.

Table 18-4. Ancillary Testing in the Dyspneic Patient

Category	Test	Findings/Potential Diagnoses
Laboratory	Pulse oximetry, selective ABG use	Hypoxia, hyperventilation (muscular weakness, intracranial event) CO_2 retention (COPD, sleep apnea) Metabolic versus respiratory acidosis (DKA, ingestions) A-a gradient (pulmonary embolism) Elevated carboxyhemoglobin (inhalation injury or CO poisoning)

	Complete blood count	WBC
		    Increase: infection, stress demargination, hematologic malignancy
		    Decrease: neutropenia, sepsis
		Hgb/Hct: anemia, polycythemia
		Smear: abnormal Hgb (i.e., sickling), inclusions
		Platelets: thrombocytopenia (marrow toxicity)

	Chemistry	BUN/Cr: acute/chronic renal failure K/Mg/Phos: low levels resulting in muscular weakness Glucose: DKA D-dimer: abnormal clotting activity BNP: possible CHF
Cardiac	ECG	Ischemia, dysrhythmia, S1Q3T3 (pulmonary embolism), right heart strain
	Echocardiogram	Pulmonary hypertension, valvular disorders Wall motion abnormalities related to ischemia, intracardiac shunts
Radiologic	Chest radiograph	Bony structures: fractures, lytic lesions, pectus, kyphoscoliosis Mass: malignancy, cavitary lesion, infiltrate, foreign body Diaphragm: eventration, elevation of hemidiaphragm, bowel herniation Mediastinum: adenopathy (infection, sarcoid), air Cardiac silhouette: enlarged (cardiomyopathy, fluid overload) Soft tissue: subcutaneous air Lung parenchyma: blebs, pneumothorax, effusions (blood, infectious), interstitial edema, local consolidation, air bronchograms, Hampton's hump, Westermark's sign
	V/Q scan	Pulmonary embolism
	Pulmonary angiogram	Pulmonary embolism, intervention (thrombolysis)
	CT	Mass lesion, adenopathy, trauma, pulmonary embolism
	Soft tissue neck	Epiglottitis, foreign body
Fiberoptic	Bronchoscopy	Mass lesion, foreign body Intervention (stenting, biopsy)
	Laryngoscopy	Mass lesion, edema, epiglottitis, foreign body

ABG, arterial blood gas; BNP, brain natriuretic peptide; BUN, blood urea nitrogen; CHF, congestive heart failure; CO, carbon monoxide; COPD, chronic obstructive pulmonary disease; Cr, creatinine; CT, computed tomography; DKA, diabetic ketoacidosis; ECG, electrocardiogram; WBC, white blood cell.

and tympany to percussion on one side is seen with spontaneous pnemothorax. Dyspnea associated with decreased respiratory effort may represent a neuromuscular process, such as multiple sclerosis, Guillain-Barré syndrome, or myasthenia gravis.[3] Unilateral rales, cough, fever, and dyspnea most often represent pneumonia.

Figure 18-1 provides an algorithm for assessment and stabilization of a dyspneic patient. The initial division is based on the degree of breathing effort associated with the symptoms. The most critical diagnoses must be considered first and appropriate intervention taken as necessary. The clinician must perform rapid assessment and stabilization of all dyspneic patients.

All patients experiencing dyspnea, regardless of suspected cause, should be transported immediately to the treatment area. Bedside pulse oximetry should be obtained, and the patient should be placed on a cardiac monitor. If the pulse oximetry is less than 98% saturated on room air, the patient should be placed on supplemental oxygen either by nasal cannula or mask depending on the degree of desaturation detected. An adequate airway and ventilation are paramount. If necessary, the patient should be intubated, and breathing should be assisted with manual or mechanical ventilation.

When the airway has been secured, rapid assessment of the patient's appearance and vital signs can help determine the need for further stabilization. Decreased mental alertness, inability to speak in more than one-word syllables, or certain body positioning signals the presence of significant respiratory distress and the need for rapid intervention. After stabilization has occurred, one can determine further the etiology of the dyspnea.

EMPIRIC MANAGEMENT AND DISPOSITION

The primary treatment for patients with dyspnea is to identify and treat the underlying pathology. Critical problems must be identified and treated before proceeding to complete diagnostic workup and definitive treatment.

The management algorithm for dyspnea (Figure 18-2) outlines the approach to treatment for most identifiable diseases. Unstable patients or patients with critical diagnoses must be stabilized and admitted to an intensive care unit. Emergent patients who have improved in the emergency department may be admitted to an intermediate care unit. Patients diagnosed

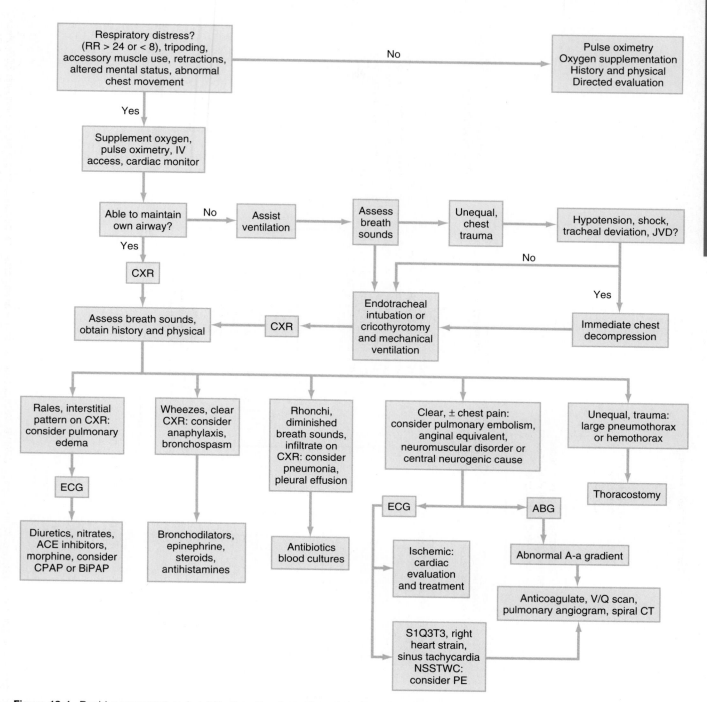

Figure 18-1. Rapid assessment and stabilization of a dyspneic patient. RR, respiratory rate; IV, intravenous; CXR, chest x-ray; ECG, electrocardiogram; ACE, angiotensin-converting enzyme; CPAP, continuous positive airway pressure; BiPAP, biphasic positive airway pressure; JVD, jugular venous distention; ABG, arterial blood gas; CT, computed tomography; NSSTWC, nonspecific ST wave changes (on ECG); PE, pulmonary embolus.

with urgent conditions in danger of deterioration without proper treatment or patients with stable conditions and comorbidities, such as diabetes, immunosuppression, or cancer, should be admitted for observation and treatment.

Most patients in the nonurgent category can be managed as outpatients if good medical follow-up can be arranged. If dyspnea persists despite therapy and no definitive cause has been delineated, the best course of action is hospitalization for observation and ongoing evaluation. If no definitive diagnosis can be obtained and the symptoms have abated, the patient may be discharged with good medical follow-up and instructions to return if symptoms recur.

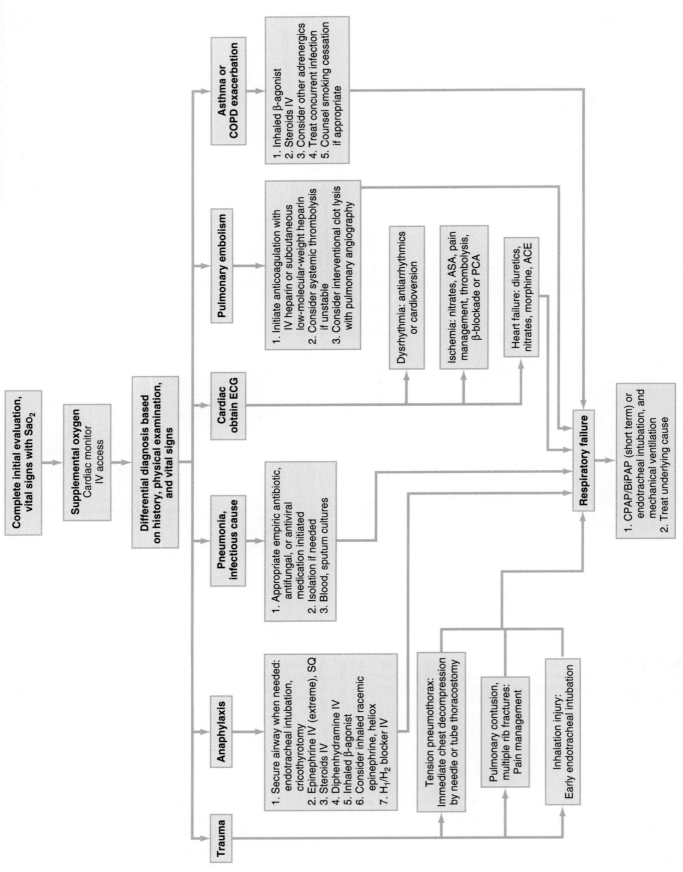

Figure 18-2. Clinical guidelines for emergency department management of dyspnea. IV, intravenous; CPAP/BiPAP, continuous positive airway pressure/ biphasic positive airway pressure; ECG, electrocardiogram; ASA, acetylsalicylic acid; PCA, patient-controlled analgesia; ACE, angiotensin-converting enzyme; COPD, chronic obstructive pulmonary disease. SQ, subcutaneously.

REFERENCES

1. Fletcher K, Forch W: Acute symptom assessment: Determining the seriousness of the presentation. *Prim Care Pract* 3:216, 1999.
2. Ailani RK, et al: Dyspnea differential index: A new method for rapid separation of cardiac versus pulmonary dyspnea. *Chest* 119:1100, 1999.
3. Sivak ED, Shefner JM, Sexton J: Neuromuscular disease and hypoventilation. *Curr Opin Pulm Med* 5:335, 1999.
4. Kline JA, Wells PS: Methodology for a rapid protocol to rule out pulmonary embolism in the emergency department. *Ann Emerg Med* 42:266, 2003.
5. Michelson E, Hollrah S: Evaluation of the patient with shortness of breath: Evidence based approach. *Emerg Clin North Am* 17:221, 1999.
6. Murray S: Bi-level positive airway pressure (BiPAP) and acute cardiogenic pulmonary oedema (ACPO) in the emergency department. *Aust Crit Care* 15:51, 2002.
7. Rodrigo GJ: Inhaled therapy for acute adult asthma. *Curr Opin Allergy Clin Immunol* 3:169, 2003.
8. Peigang Y, Marini JJ: Ventilation of patients with asthma and chronic obstructive pulmonary disease. *Curr Opin Crit Care* 8:70, 2002.

CHAPTER

19 Chest Pain

James E. Brown and Glenn C. Hamilton

PERSPECTIVE

More than 5 million patients present to the emergency department each year with complaints of chest pain; this represents nearly 5% of all patients seen in emergency departments in the United States.[1] Chest pain is a symptom caused by several life-threatening diseases and has a broad differential diagnosis. It is complicated by a frequent disassociation between intensity of signs and symptoms and seriousness of underlying pathology. Accurately discerning the correct diagnosis and treatment of a patient with chest pain is one of the most difficult tasks for the emergency physician.

Epidemiology

The epidemiology of the critical diagnoses causing chest pain varies widely. Acute coronary syndromes (ACS), aortic dissection, pulmonary embolus, pneumothorax, pericarditis with tamponade, and esophageal rupture are potentially catastrophic causes of chest pain. Because of its high incidence and high potential lethality, ACS is the most significant potential diagnosis in the emergency department. Of all deaths in the United States, 35% are attributed to atherosclerosis; this accounts for nearly 1 million deaths per year.[2] Historically, emergency physicians reportedly have missed approximately 3% to 5% of myocardial infarctions (MIs), accounting for 25% of malpractice losses in emergency medicine.[3,4] Thoracic aortic dissection has an incidence of 0.5 to 1 per 100,000 population with a mortality rate exceeding 90% if misdiagnosed. Because of difficulties in making the diagnosis, the true incidence of pulmonary embolus is unclear. Estimates of 70 per 100,000 are published; this would equate to approximately 100,000 pulmonary embolism cases per year in the United States.[5] Although the incidence of tension pneumothorax is unclear, the incidence of spontaneous pneumothorax ranges from 2.5 to 18 per 100,000 total patients, depending on the study. The total incidence of esophageal rupture is 12.5 cases per 100,000 persons. The true incidence of pericarditis is unknown, but the diagnosis is made in 1 in every 1000 hospital admissions.[6] Most patients with chest pain presenting to the emergency department have a benign origin of their pain; the challenge is in separating out and appropriately treating patients with serious causes.

Pathophysiology

Afferent fibers from the heart, lungs, great vessels, and esophagus enter the same thoracic dorsal ganglia. Through these visceral fibers, each organ produces the same indistinct quality and location of pain. The quality of visceral chest pain varies widely and has been described as "burning," "aching," "stabbing," or "pressure." Because dorsal segments overlap three segments above and below a level, disease of a thoracic origin can produce pain anywhere from the jaw to the epigastrium. Radiation of pain is explained by somatic afferent fibers synapsing in the same dorsal root ganglia as the thoracic viscera. This stimulation can "confuse" the patient's central nervous system into thinking the pain originates in the arms or shoulders.

DIAGNOSTIC APPROACH

Differential Considerations

Owing to the indistinct nature of visceral pain, the differential diagnosis of chest pain covers many organ systems and disease entities within those systems. The

Table 19-1. Differential Diagnosis of Chest Pain

Organ System	Critical Diagnoses	Emergent Diagnoses	Nonemergent Diagnoses
Cardiovascular	Acute myocardial infarction Acute coronary ischemia Aortic dissection Cardiac tamponade	Unstable angina Coronary spasm Prinzmetal's angina Cocaine induced Pericarditis Myocarditis	Valvular heart disease Aortic stenosis Mitral valve prolapse Hypertrophic cardiomyopathy
Pulmonary	Pulmonary embolus Tension pneumothorax	Pneumothorax Mediastinitis	Pneumonia Pleuritis Tumor Pneumomediastinum
Gastrointestinal	Esophageal rupture (Boerhaave)	Esophageal tear (Mallory-Weiss) Cholecystitis Pancreatitis	Esophageal spasm Esophageal reflux Peptic ulcer Biliary colic
Musculoskeletal			Muscle strain Rib fracture Arthritis Tumor Costochondritis Nonspecific chest wall pain
Neurologic			Spinal root compression Thoracic outlet Herpes zoster Postherpetic neuralgia
Other			Psychologic Hyperventilation

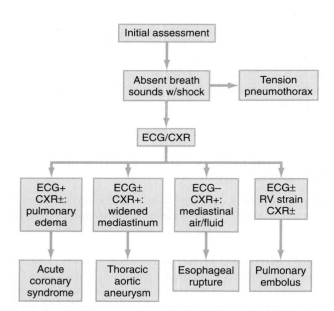

Figure 19-1. Initial assessment of critical diagnoses. ECG, electrocardiogram; CXR, chest x-ray; RV, right ventricular.

differential diagnosis of chest pain includes many of the most critical diagnoses in medicine and many nonemergent conditions (Table 19-1).

Rapid Assessment and Stabilization

The first questions the physician must ask are, "What are the life-threatening possibilities in this patient, and must I intervene immediately?" These questions usually can be answered within the first few minutes of the patient encounter. By assessing the patient's appearance and vital signs, the physician knows whether immediate intervention is needed. The one critical diagnosis that needs to be treated at this stage is tension pneumothorax. If a patient presents with chest pain, respiratory distress, shock, and unilateral reduction or absence of breath sounds, immediate intervention with needle/tube thoracostomy is required. Additionally, patients with severe derangements in vital signs require stabilizing treatment while a search for the precipitating cause is begun. Patients who present with respiratory distress require immediate intervention and lead the physician to suspect a more serious cause of the pain (Figure 19-1).

All patients except those with obvious benign causes of chest pain are transported as promptly as possible to the treatment area. The patient is placed on the cardiac monitor, oxygen therapy is initiated, and an intravenous line is placed. If the patient shows signs and symptoms of tension pneumothorax, immediate needle/tube thoracostomy is performed. If there are symptomatic derangements in vital signs, these are treated as appropriate. If vital signs are stable, a brief history and physical examination are performed. If the patient is older than age 30 years, an electrocardiogram (ECG) should be ordered and interpreted by the responsible physician promptly. Most patients also require a chest radiograph to evaluate the chest pain. If a cardiac cause is suspected, and vital signs are stable, pain relief with nitroglycerin (0.4 mg sublingual every 3 to 5 minutes) may be appropriate. Aspirin (81 to 325 mg) is given to patients without bleeding disorders or known allergies. Clopidrogrel (loading dose 300 mg) is given to patients with a contraindication to aspirin. Patients with low voltage on the ECG, diffuse ST segment elevation, elevated jugular venous pressure on examination,[7] and signs of shock should undergo prompt cardiac ultrasound or pericardiocentesis or both. The evaluation then proceeds. When a diagnosis is established, appropriate treatment is rendered.

Pivotal Findings

The broad and complex nature of chest pain defies application of a simple algorithmic approach. An organized approach to a patient with chest pain is essential, however, to ensure that all causes are evaluated appropriately. The history and physical examination are key to diagnosis. In all, 80% to 90% of information pertinent to the differential diagnosis is obtained by the history, physical examination, and ECG.

History

1. The patient is asked to describe the character of the pain or discomfort. Descriptions such as "squeezing," "crushing," or "pressure" lead the physician to suspect a cardiac ischemic syndrome, although cardiac ischemia can be characterized by nonspecific discomfort, such as "bloating" or "indigestion." "Tearing" pain that may migrate from the front to back or back to front classically is described in aortic dissection. "Sharp" or "stabbing" pain is seen more in pulmonary and musculoskeletal diagnoses. Patients complaining of a "burning" or "indigestion" type of pain lead the physician to think of gastrointestinal etiologies. Because of the visceral nature of chest pain, however, any cause of pain may present with any of the preceding descriptions.

2. Additional history about the patient's activity at the onset of pain may be helpful. Pain occurring during exertion would cause the physician to suspect an ischemic coronary syndrome, whereas progressive onset of pain at rest suggests acute MI. Pain of sudden onset would make the physician more suspicious of aortic dissection, pulmonary embolus, or pneumothorax. Pain after meals is more indicative of a gastrointestinal cause.

3. The severity of pain is quantified. A 1-to-10 pain scale is commonly used. Alterations in pain severity are documented at times of onset, peak, present, and after intervention.

4. The location of the discomfort is described. Pain that is localized to a small area is more likely to be somatic versus visceral in origin. Pain localized at the periphery of the chest makes a cardiac cause less likely and a pulmonary cause more likely. Lower chest/upper abdominal pain may be of cardiac or gastrointestinal origin.

5. Any description of radiation of pain is noted. Pain that goes through to the back makes the diagnoses of aortic dissection and gastrointestinal causes, especially pancreatitis or posterior ulcer, more likely. Inferior/posterior myocardial ischemia also may present primarily as thoracic back pain. Radiation to the arms, neck, or jaw increases the physician's suspicion of cardiac ischemia as a cause.[8,9]

Pain located primarily in the back, especially interscapular back pain that migrates to the base of the neck, suggests aortic dissection.[10]

6. Duration of pain is an important historical factor. Pain that lasts a few seconds is rarely of cardiac origin.[11] Pain that is exertional but lasts for only a few minutes after rest may be a manifestation of cardiac ischemia.[8] Pain that is maximal at onset may be due to aortic dissection.[10] Pain that is not severe and constantly persists over the course of days is less likely to be of serious origin. Pain that is severe or has a stuttering or fluctuating course is more likely to be serious, and this includes a cardiac origin.

7. Aggravating or alleviating factors need be considered. Pain that worsens with exertion and is better with rest is more likely related to coronary ischemia.[8] Pain related to meals makes the physician more suspicious of a gastrointestinal cause. Pain that worsens with respiration is seen more often with pulmonary, pericardial, and musculoskeletal causes.

8. Other associated symptoms may give a key to the visceral nature of the pain (Table 19-2). The symptoms may appear as the initial chief complaint. Diaphoresis should lead to an increased clinical suspicion for a serious or visceral cause. Hemoptysis, a classic, although rarely seen symptom, would lead the physician to consider pulmonary embolus.[12] Syncope and near-syncope lead to higher suspicion for a cardiovascular cause or pulmonary embolus. Dyspnea is seen in cardiovascular and pulmonary disease. Nausea and vomiting may be seen in cardiovascular and gastrointestinal complaints.

9. A history of prior pain and the diagnosis of that episode can facilitate the diagnostic process, but the physician must be wary of prior presumptive diagnoses that may be misleading. A prior history of cardiac testing, such as stress testing, echocardiography, or angiography, may be useful in determining if the current episode is suspicious for cardiac disease. Similarly, patients with previous spontaneous pneumothorax or pulmonary embolus[13] are at increased risk of recurrence.

10. The presence of risk factors for a particular disease is primarily of value as an epidemiologic marker for large population studies (Box 19-1). Still, positive risk factors in a patient without established disease may increase or decrease the clinical likelihood (pretest probability) of a specific disease process.

Physical Examination

Specific findings may be found in a variety of causes (Table 19-3).

Ancillary Studies

The two most commonly performed studies in patients with chest pain are chest radiograph and 12-lead ECG (Table 19-4). ECG should be performed as soon as pos-

Table 19-2. Significant Symptoms of Chest Pain

Symptom	Finding	Diagnosis
Pain	Severe, crushing, pressure, substernal, exertional, radiation to jaw, neck, shoulder, arm	Acute MI Coronary ischemia Unstable angina Coronary spasm
	Tearing, severe, radiating to or located in back, maximum at onset, may migrate to upper back or neck	Aortic dissection
	Pleuritic	Esophageal rupture Pneumothorax Cholecystitis Pericarditis Myocarditis
	Indigestion or burning	Acute MI Coronary ischemia Esophageal rupture Unstable angina Coronary spasm Esophageal tear Cholecystitis
Associated syncope/near-syncope		Aortic dissection Pulmonary embolus Acute MI Pericarditis Myocarditis
Associated dyspnea (SOB, DOE, PND, orthopnea)		Acute MI Coronary ischemia Pulmonary embolus Tension pneumothorax Pneumothorax Unstable angina Pericarditis
Associated hemoptysis		Pulmonary embolus
Associated nausea/vomiting		Esophageal rupture Acute MI Coronary ischemia Unstable angina Coronary spasm Esophageal tear Cholecystitis

DOE, dyspnea on exertion; MI, myocardial infarction; PND, paroxysmal nocturnal dyspnea; SOB, shortness of breath.

BOX 19-1. Risk Factors Associated with Potentially Catastrophic Causes of Chest Pain

Acute coronary syndromes
  Past history of coronary artery disease
  Family history of coronary artery disease
  Age
    Men >33 years
    Women >40 years
  Diabetes mellitus
  Hypertension
  Cigarette use/possible passive exposure
  Elevated cholesterol (LDL)/triglycerides
  Sedentary lifestyle
  Obesity
  Postmenopausal
  Left ventricular hypertrophy
  Cocaine abuse
Pulmonary embolism
  Prolonged immobilization
  Surgery > 30 days 3 mo
  Prior deep vein thrombosis or pulmonary embolus
  Pregnancy or recent pregnancy
  Pelvic or lower extremity trauma
  Oral contraceptives with cigarette smoking
  Congestive heart failure
  Chronic obstructive pulmonary disease
  Obesity
  Past medical or family history of hypercoagulability
Aortic dissection
  Hypertension
  Congenital disease of the aorta or aortic valve
  Inflammatory aortic disease
  Connective tissue disease
  Pregnancy
  Arteriosclerosis
  Cigarette use
Pericarditis/myocarditis
  Infection
  Autoimmune disease (e.g., systemic lupus erythematosus)
  Acute rheumatic fever
  Recent myocardial infarction or cardiac surgery
  Malignancy
  Radiation therapy to mediastinum
  Uremia
  Drugs
  Prior pericarditis
Pneumothorax
  Prior pneumothorax
  Valsalva's maneuver
  Chronic lung disease
  Cigarette use

sible in all patients with chest pain in whom myocardial ischemia is suspected; this generally includes all patients 30 years old and older who complain of chest pain unless the cause is obviously noncardiac. Rapid acquisition of the ECG facilitates the diagnosis of acute MI and expedites the National Heart, Lung, and Blood Institute's recommended "door to drug" time of less than 30 minutes from arrival to administration of thrombolytic therapy or percutaneous coronary intervention in acute MI. Patients with a new injury pattern on ECG (Table 19-5), with the appropriate history, should have therapy instituted for acute MI. New ischemic ECG changes indicate acute coronary ischemia or spasm, and appropriate therapy is instituted at this point (Figure 19-2). An ECG showing right ventricular strain pattern, in the appropriate setting, should raise the clinical suspicion for pulmonary embolus. Diffuse ST segment elevation helps make the diagnosis of pericarditis.

A portable chest radiograph is performed for patients with suspected serious cause of chest pain. Pneumothorax is definitively diagnosed at this point. A wide mediastinum or ill-defined aortic knob increases the clinical suspicion for acute aortic dissection. Pleural effusion, subcutaneous air, or mediastinal air-fluid level may be seen in esophageal rupture. Increased

Table 19-3. Pivotal Findings in Physical Examination

Sign	Finding	Diagnoses	Sign	Finding	Diagnoses
Appearance	Acute respiratory distress	Pulmonary embolus, Tension pneumothorax, Acute MI, Pneumothorax	Cardiovascular examination	Significant difference in upper extremity blood pressures	Aortic dissection
	Diaphoresis	Acute MI, Aortic dissection, Coronary ischemia, Pulmonary embolus, Esophageal rupture, Unstable angina, Cholecystitis, Perforated peptic ulcer		Narrow pulse pressure	Pericarditis (with effusion)
				New murmur	Acute MI, Aortic dissection, Coronary ischemia
Vital signs	Hypotension	Tension pneumothorax, Pulmonary embolus, Acute MI, Aortic dissection (late), Coronary ischemia, Esophageal rupture, Pericarditis, Myocarditis		S_3/S_4 gallop	Acute MI, Coronary ischemia
				Pericardial rub	Pericarditis
				Audible systolic "crunch" on cardiac auscultation (Hamman's sign)	Esophageal rupture, Mediastinitis
	Tachycardia	Acute MI, Pulmonary embolus, Aortic dissection, Coronary ischemia, Tension pneumothorax, Esophageal rupture, Coronary spasm, Pericarditis, Myocarditis, Mediastinitis, Cholecystitis, Esophageal tear (Mallory-Weiss)		JVD	Acute MI, Coronary ischemia, Tension pneumothorax, Pulmonary embolus, Pericarditis
			Pulmonary examination	Unilateral diminished/absent breath sounds	Tension pneumothorax, Pneumothorax
				Pleural rub	Pulmonary embolus
				Subcutaneous emphysema	Tension pneumothorax, Esophageal rupture, Pneumothorax, Mediastinitis
	Bradycardia	Acute MI, Coronary ischemia, Unstable angina		Rales	Acute MI, Coronary ischemia, Unstable angina
	Hypertension	Acute MI, Coronary ischemia, Aortic dissection (early)	Abdominal examination	Epigastric tenderness	Esophageal rupture, Esophageal tear, Cholecystitis, Pancreatitis
				Left upper quadrant tenderness	Pancreatitis
	Fever	Pulmonary embolus, Esophageal rupture, Pericarditis, Myocarditis, Mediastinitis, Cholecystitis		Right upper quadrant tenderness	Cholecystitis
			Extremity examination	Unilateral leg swelling, warmth, pain, tenderness, or erythema	Pulmonary embolus
	Hypoxemia	Pulmonary embolus, Tension pneumothorax, Pneumothorax	Neurologic examination	Focal findings	Aortic dissection
				Stroke	Acute MI, Coronary ischemia, Aortic dissection, Coronary spasm

JVD, jugular venous distention; MI, myocardial infarction.

Table 19-4. Ancillary Testing of Patients with Chest Pain

Test	Finding	Diagnosis
ECG	New injury	Acute MI
		Aortic dissection
	New ischemia	Coronary ischemia
		Coronary spasm
	RV strain	Pulmonary embolus
	Diffuse ST segment elevation	Pericarditis
CXR	Pneumothorax with mediastinal shift	Tension pneumothorax
	Wide mediastinum	Aortic dissection
	Pneumothorax	Esophageal rupture Pneumothorax
	Effusion	Esophageal rupture
	Increased cardiac silhouette	Pericarditis
	Pneumomediastinum	Esophageal rupture Mediastinitis
ABG	Hypoxemia, A-a gradient	Pulmonary embolus
V/Q scan or spiral CT	High probability or any positive in patient with high clinical suspicion	Pulmonary embolus

ABG, arterial blood gas; CT, computed tomography; ECG, electrocardiogram; MI, myocardial infarction; RV, right ventricular.

Table 19-5. Electrocardiogram Findings in Ischemic Chest Pain

Classic myocardial infarction	ST segment elevation (>1 mm) in contiguous leads; new LBBB; Q waves ≥0.04 sec duration
Subendocardial infarction	T wave inversion or ST segment depression in concordant leads
Unstable angina	Most often normal or nonspecific changes; may see T wave inversion
Pericarditis	Diffuse ST segment elevation; PR segment depression

LBBB, left bundle-branch block.

cardiac silhouette may indicate pericarditis or cardiomyopathy.

Pneumomediastinum is seen with esophageal rupture and mediastinitis. Serum D-dimer assay may help discriminate patients with pulmonary embolus. A low serum D-dimer in a patient believed to be at low pretest probability of pulmonary embolus effectively excludes the diagnosis.[12,14]

Patients at moderate or high pretest probability should undergo diagnostic imaging (multidetector computed tomography scan, pulmonary angiography, or ventilation-perfusion lung scan). High pretest probability warrants initiation of anticoagulation (heparin or low-molecular-weight heparin) therapy in the emergency department before the imaging study, in the absence of a contraindication.

Laboratory testing may be useful in the evaluation of ACS. Creatine kinase (CK) has been used for many years. Although it is 95% sensitive for all MIs, it is less than 40% sensitive at 4 hours. CK also is associated with multiple false-positive results and has no use in the evaluation of unstable angina. CK-MB, an isoform of CK, is more specific for cardiac ischemia. There are fewer false-positive results, and peak sensitivity approaches 98%. Sensitivity at 4 hours is only about 60%, however. CK-MB isoforms improve sensitivity at 4 hours to 80%, approaching 93% at 6 hours. Myoglobin is an enzyme released in all muscle damage. Although its measurement is sensitive (90% at 4 hours), its false-positive rate is estimated at 50%. These markers and their corresponding sensitivities and specificities are used only for the diagnosis of MI, and none are useful in diagnosing other acute ischemic coronary syndromes, including unstable angina.

Troponins (I and T), when elevated, identify patients with ACS who have the highest risk for adverse outcome. Sensitivity for ACS is 35%, but most of these patients are at high risk for complications.[15] Sensitivity for acute MI at 4 hours is 60% (similar to CK-MB). Studies have shown an advantage to serial enzyme testing over the course of 2 to 4 hours. A significant increase (two to three times the baseline value) has been shown to be more sensitive than isolated measurements of any enzyme. Single values of any enzyme cannot be used to exclude coronary ischemia as a cause of pain.[16,17]

DIAGNOSTIC TABLE

After the patient is stabilized and assessment has been completed, the findings are matched to the classic and atypical patterns of the seven potentially critical diseases causing chest pain. This matching process is continual while evaluating the patient and monitoring the response to therapy. Any inconsistency in findings with the primary working diagnoses requires a rapid review of the pivotal findings and the potential diagnoses (Table 19-6).

MANAGEMENT AND DISPOSITION

The management of ACS is discussed in Chapter 77. Figure 19-3 outlines the approach to treatment of critical noncardiac diagnoses. Patients with critical diagnoses generally are admitted to the intensive care unit. Patients with emergent diagnoses typically are admitted to the hospital, most often on telemetry units. Patients with nonemergent diagnoses most frequently are managed as outpatients. Hospitalization is required in certain circumstances, particularly when patients have other comorbid conditions.

Frequently, no definitive diagnosis is found at the end of the workup. Any patient with almost any type of chest pain may be having coronary ischemia, pulmonary embolus, or aortic dissection. When a clear pattern does not emerge to allow the emergency physician to make an alternative diagnosis confidently, continued evaluation, hospitalization, or observation admission may be the best course.

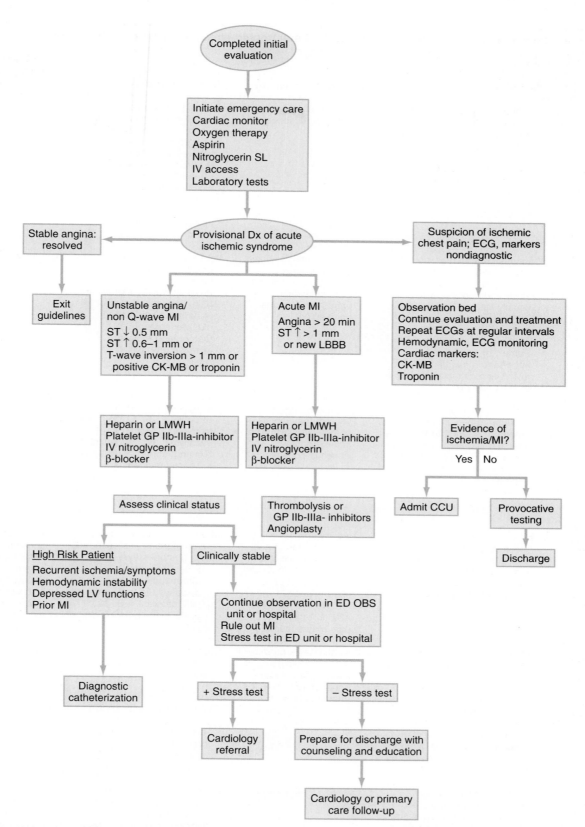

Figure 19-2. Clinical guidelines for emergency department management of myocardial ischemic origin chest pain. SL, sublingual; IV, intravenous; ECG, electrocardiogram; MI, myocardial infarction; LBBB, left bundle-branch block; LMWH, low-molecular-weight heparin; CCU, critical care unit; OBS, observation; LV, left ventricular.

Table 19-6. Causes and Differentiation of Potentially Catastrophic Illness Presenting with Central Chest Pain or

	Pain History	Associated Symptoms	Supporting History	Prevalence in Emergency Department
Myocardial Infarction	Discomfort is usually moderately severe to severe and rapid in onset. May be more "pressure" than pain. Usually retrosternal, may radiate to neck, jaw, both arms, upper back, epigastrium, and sides of chest (left more than right). Lasts more than 15-30 min and is unrelieved by NTG	Diaphoresis, nausea, vomiting, dyspnea	May be precipitated by emotional stress or exertion. Often comes on at rest. May come on in early awakening period. Prodromal pain pattern often elicited. Previous history of MI or angina. >40 years old, positive risk factors, and male sex increase possibility	Common
Unstable Angina	Changes in pattern of preexisting angina with more severe, prolonged, or frequent pain (crescendo angina). Pain usually lasts >10 min. Angina at rest lasting 15-20 min or new-onset angina (duration <2 mo) with minimal exertion. Pattern of pain change important in gauging risk for AMI. Unpredictable responses to NTG and rest	Often minimal. May have mild diaphoresis, nausea, dyspnea with pain. Increasing pattern of dyspnea on exertion	Not clearly related to precipitating factors. May be a decrease in amount of physical activity that initiates pain. Previous history of MI or angina. Over 40 years old, presence of risk factors, and male sex increase probability	Common
Aortic Dissection	90% of patients have rapid-onset severe chest pain that is maximal at beginning. Radiates anteriorly in chest to the back interscapular area or into abdomen. Pain often has a "tearing" sensation, and may migrate	Neurologic complications of stroke, peripheral neuropathy, paresis or paraplegia, abdominal and extremity ischemia possible	Median age 59 years. History of hypertension in 70-90% of patients. 3 : 1 ratio males to females. Marfan's syndrome and congenital bicuspid aortic valves have increased incidence	Rare
Pulmonary Embolism	Pain is more often lateral-pleuritic. Central pain is more consistent with massive embolus. Abrupt in onset and maximal at beginning. May be episodic or intermittent	Dyspnea and apprehension play a prominent role, often more than pain. Cough accompanies about half the cases Hemoptysis occurs in <20%. Angina-like pain may occur in 5%	Often some period of immobilization has occurred, e.g., postoperative. Pregnancy, oral contraceptives, heart disease, and cancer are all risk factors. Previous DVT or PE is the greatest risk factor	Uncommon in ambulatory patients, but common in departments with high volumes of elderly or medically complex patients
Pneumothorax	Pain is usually acute and maximal at onset. Most often lateral-pleuritic, but central pain can occur in large pneumothorax	Dyspnea has a prominent role. Hypotension and altered mental states occur in tension pneumothorax	Chest trauma, previous episode, or asthenic body type	Infrequent
Esophageal Rupture	Pain usually is preceded by vomiting and is abrupt in onset. Pain is persistent and unrelieved, localized along the esophagus, and increased by swallowing and neck flexion	Diaphoresis, dyspnea (late), shock	Older individual with known gastrointestinal problems. History of violent emesis, foreign body, caustic ingestion, blunt trauma, alcoholism, esophageal disease	Rare
Pericarditis	Dull, aching recurrent pain unrelated to exercises or meals. Or it may be a sharp, stabbing, pleuritic-type pain that does not change with chest wall motion. May be severe. Not relieved by NTG	Dyspnea, diaphoresis	Pain is often worse when supine, but improves sitting up. Often preceded by viral illness or underlying disease (SLE or uremia)	Rare Tamponade even more rare complication

NTG, nitroglycerin; CK-MB, an isoform of creatine kinase; AMI, acute myocardial infarction; ECG, electrocardiogram; CT, computed tomography; MRI, magnetic resonance imaging; DVT, deep vein thrombosis; PE, pulmonary embolus; COPD, chronic obstructive pulmonary disease; SLE, systemic lupus erythematosus; NSAID, nonsteroidal anti-inflammatory drug.

Physical Examination	Useful Tests	Atypical or Additional Aspects
Patients are anxious and uncomfortable. Blood pressure usually is elevated, but normotension and hypotension are seen. The heart rate is usually mildly increased, but bradycardia can be seen. Patients may be diaphoretic and show peripheral poor perfusion. There are no diagnostic examination findings for MI, although S_3 and S_4 heart sounds and new murmur are supportive	ECG changes (new Q waves or ST segment–T wave changes) occur in 80% of patients. CK-MB and troponins are helpful if elevated, but may be normal	Pain may present as "indigestion" or "unable to describe." Other atypical presentations include altered mental status, stroke, angina pattern without extended pain, severe fatigue, syncope. Elderly may present with weakness, congestive heart failure, or chest tightness. 25% of nonfatal MIs are unrecognized by patient. The pain may have resolved by the time of evaluation
Nonspecific findings of a transient nature, may have similar cardiac findings as in MI, especially intermittent diaphoresis	Often no ECG or enzyme changes. Variant angina (Prinzmetal's) has episodic pain, at rest, often severe, with prominent ST segment elevation	May be pain-free at presentation. Full history is essential. Fewer than 15% of patients hospitalized for unstable angina go on to acute MI. May respond to nitroglycerin. May manifest similarly to non–Q wave infarction
Often poorly perfused peripherally but with elevated BP. In 50–60% of cases, there is asymmetric decrease or absence of peripheral pulses. 50% of proximal dissections cause aortic insufficiency. Other vascular occlusions: coronary (1-2%), mesentery, renal, spinal cord. New-onset pericardial friction rub or aortic insufficiency murmur supportive of diagnosis	ECG usually shows left ventricular hypertrophy, nonspecific changes. Chest film shows abnormal aortic silhouette (90%). Aortic angiography has diagnostic accuracy of 95-99%. Transesophageal echocardiogram, CT, MRI most useful in screening	Rare for patient to present pain-free. May present with neurologic complications. Physical examination findings may be minimal. Dissection into coronary arteries can mimic MI Ascending aortic aneurysms are approached more surgically. Descending are generally managed medically
Patients are anxious and often have a respiratory rate >16/min. Tachycardia, inspiratory rales, and an increased pulmonic second sound are common. Fever, phlebitis, and diaphoresis are seen in 30-40% of patients. Wheezes and peripheral cyanosis are less common	Arterial blood gases show P_{O_2} <80 mm Hg in 90%. Widened A-a gradient is helpful. Chest film is usually normal, although 40% show some volume loss, oligemia, or signs of consolidation due to pulmonary infarction. Lung perfusion scan rules out, if truly negative	Patients may present with dyspnea with or without bronchospasm. Acute mortality rate is 10%. Emboli usually from lower extremities above knee, prostate/pelvis venous plexus, right heart. May be subtle cause of COPD exacerbation
Decreased breath sounds, increased resonance on percussion. Elevated pressure in neck veins occur in tension pneumothorax	Chest film definitive. Inspiratory and expiratory films may enhance contrast between air and lung parenchyma. Tension pneumothorax should be diagnosed on physical examination	May be subtle in COPD, asthma, cystic fibrosis. Can be complicated by pneumomediastinum
Signs of lung consolidation, subcutaneous emphysema may be present	Chest film usually has mediastinal air, a left-sided pleural effusion, pneumothorax, or a widened mediastinum. pH of pleural effusion is < 6.0. Diagnosis supported by water-soluble contrast esophagram or esophagoscopy	Patient may present in shock state. This entity often considered late in differential diagnostic process
Friction rub may be heard, often fleeting, position dependent (50% of patients).	ECG pattern typical for ST segment elevation across the precordial leads. Erythrocyte sedimentation rate may be elevated	More common in 20- to 50-year-olds. May have associated tachycardias, ventricular dysrhythmias. Idiopathic most common (80%). Treated with aspirin, NSAID

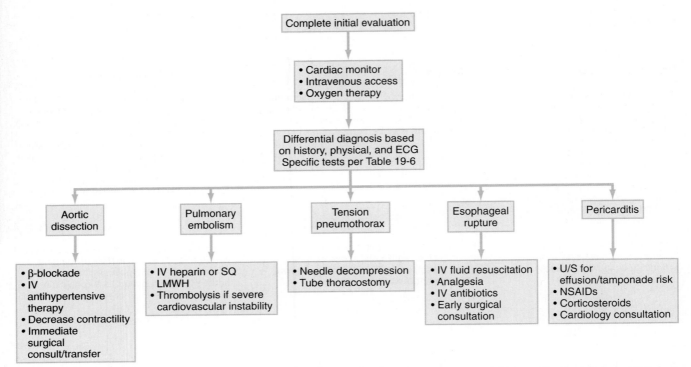

Figure 19-3. Clinical guidelines for emergency department management of chest pain from potentially catastrophic nonmyocardial origins. ECG, electrocardiogram; U/S, ultrasound; IV, intravenous; NSAIDs, nonsteroidal anti-inflammatory drugs; SQ, subcutaneous; LMWH, low-molecular-weight heparin.

REFERENCES

1. McCaig LF, Burt CW: National Hospital Ambulatory Medical Care Survey: 2001 emergency department summary. *Adv Data* 335:1, 2003.

2. Kochanek KD, Smith BL: Deaths: Preliminary data for 2002. *Natl Vital Stat Rep* 52:1, 2004.

3. Karcz A, et al: Malpractice claims against emergency physicians in Massachusetts: 1975-1993. *Am J Emerg Med* 14:341, 1996.

4. Pope JH, et al: Missed diagnoses of acute cardiac ischemia in the emergency department. *N Engl J Med* 342:1163, 2000.

5. Silverstein MD, et al: Trends in the incidence of deep vein thrombosis and pulmonary embolism: A 25-year population-based study. *Arch Intern Med* 158:585, 1998.

6. Lorell BH: Pericardial disease. In Brunwald E (ed): *Heart Disease: A Textbook of Cardiovascular Medicine,* 5th ed. Philadelphia, WB Saunders, 1997, pp 1478-1534.

7. McGhee S: *Evidence-Based Physical Diagnosis.* Philadelphia, WB Saunders, 2001.

8. Goodacre S, Locker T, Morris F, Campbell S: How useful are clinical features in the diagnosis of acute, undifferentiated chest pain? *Acad Emerg Med* 9:203, 2002.

9. Panju AA, Hemmelgarn BR, Guyatt GH, Simel DL: Is this patient having a myocardial infarction? *JAMA* 280:1256, 1998.

10. Klompas M: Does this patient have an acute thoracic aortic dissection? *JAMA* 287:2262, 2002.

11. Lee TH, et al: Acute chest pain in the emergency room: Identification and examination of low-risk patients. *Arch Intern Med* 145:65, 1985.

12. Kline J, Wells P: Methodology for a rapid protocol to rule out pulmonary embolism in the emergency department. *Ann Emerg Med* 42:266, 2003.

13. Eichinger S, et al: Symptomatic pulmonary embolism and the risk of recurrent venous thromboembolism. *Arch Intern Med* 164:92, 2004.

14. Clinical policy: Critical issues in the evaluation and management of adult patients presenting with suspected pulmonary embolism. *Ann Emerg Med* 41:257, 2003.

15. Ohman EM, et al: Cardiac troponin T levels for risk stratification in acute myocardial ischemia. *N Engl J Med* 335:1333, 1996.

16. Clinical policy: Critical issues in the evaluation and management of adult patients presenting with suspected acute myocardial infarction or unstable angina. American College of Emergency Physicians. *Ann Emerg Med* 35:521, 2000.

17. Karras DJ, Kane DL: Serum markers in the emergency department diagnosis of acute myocardial infarction. *Emerg Med Clin North Am* 19:321, 2001.

CHAPTER

20 Syncope

Robert A. De Lorenzo

PERSPECTIVE

Syncope is the sudden transient loss of consciousness with a loss of postural tone. Syncope is a common presenting complaint among patients in the emergency department, yet consensus on diagnostic approach and disposition remains elusive. This lack of consensus is due in part to its varied etiology and a lack of definitive diagnostic studies. Diagnostic accuracy relies largely on the synthesis of patient risk factors and reported symptoms, with limited reliance on the physical examination and ancillary testing.

Epidemiology

At some time in their lives, 12% to 48% of people may experience syncope.[1] Up to five percent of patients presenting to the emergency department complain of syncope, and 1% to 6% of hospitalized patients have syncope as a reason for admission.[2,3] Institutionalized patients older than age 75 have a 6% annual incidence of syncope.[3] Of children, 15% to 50% experience at least one episode of syncope.

Most causes of syncope are benign and are associated with favorable outcomes. Patients with preexisting cardiovascular disease and syncope from any cause are at the greatest risk of short-term and long-term mortality.[2,4] Syncope from cardiovascular causes also has a high risk of death, with a 1-year mortality rate of 18% to 33%.[1,3,5] Increasing age and other serious comorbidities are important cofactors in raising this rate.[2] In contrast, reported 1-year mortality for syncope of unknown etiology is 6%, and 1-year mortality from other, noncardiovascular causes is 12%.[3,4] Recurrence of syncope, particularly among the elderly, is common, reported to be 30%.[6] Benign causes of syncope predominate in adolescents and young adults. Approximately 30% of athletes dying during exercise had syncope as a sentinel event, however.[7] Prospective outcome studies in children are lacking, but most reports suggest that mortality is low overall.[8] Significant trauma may result from syncope and can contribute to mortality and morbidity, particularly in the elderly.[9,10]

Pathophysiology

The final common pathway resulting in syncope is dysfunction of both cerebral hemispheres or the brainstem (reticular activating system), usually from acute hypoperfusion. Reduced blood flow may be regional (cerebral vasoconstriction) or systemic (hypotension). Loss of consciousness results in loss of postural tone, with the resulting syncopal episode. By definition, syncope is transient; the cause of central nervous system dysfunction likewise must be transient.[4,11] Persistent causes of significant central nervous system dysfunction result in coma or altered mental status. These causes may overlap with causes of syncope.

Hypoperfusion resulting in approximately 35% or more reduction in cerebral blood flow usually produces unconsciousness, and any mechanism that adversely affects the components of perfusion (cardiac output, systemic vascular resistance, blood volume, regional vascular resistance) can cause or contribute to syncope. Other mechanisms of central nervous system dysfunction resulting in syncope include hypoglycemia, toxins, metabolic abnormalities, failure of autoregulation, and primary neurologic derangements.

DIAGNOSTIC APPROACH

Differential Considerations

There are numerous potential causes of syncope (Box 20-1). The chief differential consideration in syncope is to distinguish life-threatening causes, primarily cardiovascular in origin, from more benign forms. Chief among the serious causes of syncope are dysrhythmias and myocardial ischemia.[3] Less frequently encountered but equally serious is cerebrovascular disease, toxic-metabolic abnormalities, and structural cardiac lesions, such as critical aortic stenosis.[11] Rarely encountered as a primary presentation of syncope, but potentially catastrophic if not diagnosed promptly, are thoracic dissection of the aorta, massive pulmonary embolus, and subarachnoid hemorrhage.[3]

Pivotal Findings

Because most cases of syncope arise from benign causes, the evaluation is focused largely on excluding serious pathology. Young, healthy patients with clearly benign causes of syncope may require no formal diagnostic evaluation other than a thorough history and physical examination.[12] The clinical examination alone can suggest the diagnosis in 45% of cases. Nevertheless, 50% of patients may not have a clear diagnosis for syncope after an initial evaluation in the emergency department.[13]

Symptoms

The patient is asked to describe the *character* of the syncopal event.[11] Witnesses may be able to supplement

BOX 20-1. Causes of Syncope

Focal Hypoperfusion of CNS Structures
Cerebrovascular disease
Hyperventilation
Subclavian steal
Subarachnoid hemorrhage
Basilar artery migraine
Cerebral syncope

Systemic Hypoperfusion Resulting in CNS Dysfunction
Outflow obstruction
  Mitral, aortic, or pulmonic stenosis
  Hypertrophic cardiomyopathy
  Atrial myxoma
  Pulmonary embolism
  Pulmonary hypertension
  Cardiac tamponade
  Congenital heart disease
Reduced cardiac output
  Tachycardias
  Supraventricular tachycardia
  Ventricular tachycardia
  Ventricular fibrillation
  Wolff-Parkinson-White syndrome
  Torsades de pointes
Bradycardias
  Sinus node disease
  Second-degree and third-degree blocks
  Long Q-T syndrome
  Pacemaker malfunction
  Implanted cardioverter-defibrillator malfunction
  Other cardiovascular disease
  Aortic dissection
  Myocardial infarction
  Cardiomyopathy

Vasomotor—neurally mediated (reflex vasodepressor)
  Neurocardiogenic (vasovagal)
    Emotion
    Pain
    Situational
  Carotid sinus sensitivity
    Necktie syncope
    Shaving syncope
  Miscellaneous reflex
    Cough, sneeze
    Exercise/postexercise
    Gastrointestinal—swallowing, vomiting, defecation
    Postmicturition
    Raised intrathoracic pressure (weightlifting)
  Other causes of hypoperfusion
    Orthostatic hypotension—volume depletion
    Anemia
    Drug-induced

CNS Dysfunction Not as a Result of Hypoperfusion
Hypoglycemia
Hypoxemia—asphyxiation
Seizure
Narcolepsy
Psychogenic
  Anxiety disorder
  Conversion disorder
  Somatization disorder
  Panic disorder
  Breath-holding spells
Toxic
  Drugs
  Carbon monoxide
  Other agents
Undetermined causes

CNS, Central nervous system.

and corroborate the patient's incomplete recall, and their history should be solicited. Key characteristics include the setting (e.g., postprandial), any possible prodrome, rate of onset (gradual or abrupt), position on symptom onset (e.g., standing, sitting, or supine), duration, and rate of recovery. Abrupt onset, occurrence while sitting or supine, and duration of more than a few seconds are usually ascribed to serious, often cardiac causes of syncope.[3] Similarly, incomplete syncope, or near-syncope, may be less serious, but definitive studies linking symptom characteristics and outcome have not been performed. The diagnostic approach to presyncope is the same as for syncope.

Additional history on the events *preceding* the syncope is helpful.[11] Occurrence during significant exertion suggests outflow obstruction, whereas occurrence after exercise or a prolonged exposure to heat stress suggests orthostasis. The myriad mechanisms that may mediate a neurocardiogenic response (e.g., vagal stimulation) must be addressed, including significant emotional events, micturition, bowel movements, emesis, and movement or manipulation of the neck causing stimulation of the carotid sinus. Seizures may be preceded by an aura.

Events *during* the syncopal episode may suggest a cause.[11] Tonic-clonic movements suggest seizure, although a few brief hypoxic-mediated myoclonic jerks are common in uncomplicated syncope. Trauma from a fall or other mechanism may mask the underlying syncope that caused the incident.[10]

The patient should be queried about postsyncopal events. Symptoms consistent with a postictal state are characteristic of seizures. Initial vital signs and electrocardiogram (ECG) monitoring by prehospital providers may provide clues to primary cardiac dysrhythmias.

Associated symptoms can offer potentially important clues.[3] Chest pain or shortness of breath can suggest myocardial ischemia or pulmonary embolus. Diaphoresis and light-headedness are nonspecific, but if prominent and accompanied by a graying of vision may suggest orthostasis or vasovagal causes. Tongue biting and incontinence of urine or stool suggest seizures.

The *past medical history* is important in stratifying risk.[14] Among hospitalized patients, syncope was associated with orthostatic hypotension, complete heart block, chronic cerebral disease, migraine headache, aortic stenosis, and gastrointestinal bleeding. Prior coronary artery or cerebrovascular disease, diabetes, hypertension, or other significant disease increases the risk of mortality after syncope.[15]

Certain *medications* are well established to be associated with syncope (Box 20-2). Q-T interval–prolonging agents, β-blockers, insulin, and oral hypoglycemics, in particular, deserve attention because of the likelihood of repeated syncope without careful medication monitoring.[15]

Signs

The physical examination focuses primarily on the elements affecting the cardiovascular and neurologic systems (Table 20-1).[14] Signs of orthostasis should be sought in all cases in which this mechanism is suspected.[16] Rectal examination and testing stool for occult blood are recommended in all patients with syncope.

Ancillary Studies

The chief diagnostic adjunct in evaluating syncope is the 12-lead ECG (Table 20-2). ECG is warranted in all cases of syncope except cases with a clear cause occurring in otherwise healthy, young adults or adolescents.[12] New ischemic ECG changes indicate acute coronary ischemia and warrant appropriate therapy at this point. Dysrhythmias, shortened P-R intervals, or prolonged Q-T intervals may be identified on the 12-lead ECG. Continuous limb-lead ECG monitoring in the emergency department also may identify transient dysrhythmias. An ECG showing a right ventricular strain pattern may suggest pulmonary embolus, whereas diffuse ST segment elevation or electrical

alternans helps diagnose pericarditis associated with pericardial tamponade.

Routine blood, serum, and urine studies have limited utility in the evaluation of syncope and are generally unrewarding.[17] When suggested by the history and physical examination, however, selective use of

---

BOX 20-2. Drugs That May Induce Syncope

Cardiovascular
β-Blockers
Vasodilators (α-blockers, calcium channel blockers, nitrates, hydralazine, angiotensin-converting enzyme inhibitors, phenothiazines, phosphodiesterase inhibitors)
Diuretics
Central antihypertensives (clonidine, methyldopa)
Other antihypertensives (guanethidine)
Q-T prolonging (amiodarone, disopyramide, flecainide, procainamide, quinidine, sotalol, encainide)
Other antidysrhythmics

Psychoactive
Anticonvulsants (carbamazepine, phenytoin)
Antiparkinsonians
Central nervous system depressants (barbiturates, benzodiazepines)
Monoamine oxidase inhibitors
Tricyclic antidepressants
Narcotic analgesics
Sedating and nonsedating antihistamines
Cholinesterase inhibitors (donepezil, tacrine)

Drugs with Other Mechanisms
Drugs of abuse (cannabis, cocaine, alcohol, heroin)
Digitalis
Insulin and oral hypoglycemics
Neuropathic drugs (vincristine)
Nonsteroidal anti-inflammatory drugs
Bromocriptine

Table 20-1. Directed Physical Examination in Syncope

System	Pivotal Finding	Significance
Vital signs	Pulse rate and rhythm	Tachycardia, bradycardia, other dysrhythmias
	Respiratory rate and depth	Tachypnea suggests hypoxia, hyperventilation, or pulmonary embolus
	Blood pressure	Shock may cause decreased cerebral perfusion, hypovolemia may lead to orthostasis. May contribute to cause of syncope in up to 15–30% of patients
	Temperature	Fever from sepsis, may cause orthostasis
Skin	Color, diaphoresis	Signs of decreased organ perfusion
HEENT	Tenderness and deformity	Signs of trauma
	Papilledema	Increased intracranial pressure, head injury
	Breath	Ketones from ketoacidosis
Neck	Bruits	Source of cerebral emboli
	Jugular venous distention	Right heart failure from myocardial ischemia, tamponade or pulmonary embolus
Lungs	Breath sounds, crackles, wheezes	Infection, left heart failure from myocardial ischemia; pulmonary embolus
Heart	Systolic murmur	Aortic stenosis, hypertrophic cardiomyopathy
	Rub	Pericarditis, tamponade
Abdomen	Pulsatile mass	Abdominal aortic aneurysm
Rectum	Hematest stool	Anemia, hypovolemia
Pelvis	Uterine bleeding, adnexal tenderness	Anemia, ectopic pregnancy, hypovolemia
Extremities	Pulse equality in upper extremities	Subclavian steal, thoracic dissection of the aorta
Neurologic	Mental status, focal neurologic findings	Seizure, stroke, or other primary neurologic disease

HEENT, head, eyes, ears, nose, and throat.

Table 20-2. Ancillary Studies in Syncope

Study	Indication
12-lead ECG	Cardiac dysrhythmia, ischemia
Limb-lead ECG monitoring	Dysrhythmia
Tilt-table test, orthostatic vital signs	Orthostatic hypotension
Hemogram	Anemia
Electrolytes, serum	Metabolic abnormality
Glucose, serum or blood	Hypoglycemia
β-hCG	Pregnancy
Drug screen, urine	Drug syncope
Ethanol, serum	Drug syncope
Arterial blood gas	Hypoxemia, hyperventilation
CXR	Thoracic dissection
Computed tomography, head	New-onset or focal seizure, head trauma
Echocardiogram	Cardiac outflow obstruction, tamponade, thoracic dissection
Ventilation-perfusion scan	Pulmonary embolus
Abdominal ultrasound	Abdominal aortic aneurysm
Pelvic ultrasound	Ectopic pregnancy
Tests Usually Performed as Part of an Outpatient Evaluation	
Holter or loop ECG	Dysrhythmia
Exercise/thallium ECG	Myocardial ischemia
Electrophysiologic study	Dysrhythmia
Carotid ultrasound	Stroke, TIA
Magnetic resonance imaging, head	Seizures, stroke
Tilt-table test	Orthostatic hypotension
Electroencephalogram	Seizures

CXR, chest radiograph; ECG, electrocardiogram; hCG, human chorionic gonadotropin; TIA, transient ischemic attack.

Table 20-3. Critical Diagnoses to Consider in Syncope

Myocardial infarction
Life-threatening dysrhythmias
Aortic dissection
Critical aortic stenosis
Hypertrophic cardiomyopathy
Cardiac tamponade
Abdominal aortic aneurysm
Pulmonary embolism
Subarachnoid hemorrhage
Stroke
Toxic-metabolic derangements
Severe hypovolemia or hemorrhage

hemogram, serum electrolytes and glucose, urine drug screen, and pregnancy test may exclude some uncommon causes of syncope. As a general rule, radiographic studies offer limited yield in most cases of syncope and unless specific pathology is suspected are not routinely indicated.

In cases of syncope in which outpatient evaluation is warranted, several modalities are useful. Transient dysrhythmias can be detected with either Holter or loop ECG long-term monitoring. In selected patients, stress testing, electrophysiologic studies, or magnetic resonance imaging may be indicated. Electroencephalography has a low yield unless seizure is suspected. Tilt-table testing, although infrequently used, may have diagnostic value in elderly patients and children in whom chronic orthostatic hypotension is suspected.

Although not technically an ancillary study, formal psychiatric evaluation deserves mention as an important diagnostic tool in syncope.[18] In patients with compatible signs and symptoms or negative medical evaluation and continued syncope, psychiatric evaluation may be revealing.

DIFFERENTIAL DIAGNOSIS

Critical Diagnoses

The critical diagnoses to consider are listed in Table 20-3.

Emergent Diagnoses

The emergent causes of syncope are protean (see Box 20-1). Many other causes, such as neurocardiogenic and reflex-mediated syncope, have benign mechanisms. Any cause of syncope may recur, however, and result in falls or accidents. A thorough evaluation for treatable causes is warranted.

Diagnostic Algorithm

After stabilization and assessment, the findings are matched to the likely causes of syncope (Table 20-4). In many cases of syncope, it is possible to use a stepwise approach to diagnose the cause and risk-stratify the patient (Figure 20-1).

EMPIRIC MANAGEMENT

Rapid Assessment and Stabilization

The patient's acute symptoms and status of vital signs dictate the need for immediate stabilization. Because syncope is by definition a transient event, most patients are asymptomatic on presentation. Most asymptomatic patients do not need immediate attention, but consideration should be given to bringing elderly patients and patients with preexisting cardiovascular disease directly into the treatment area of the emergency department. If these patients have normal or near-normal vital signs, they require no immediate stabilization, and a brief history and physical examination are performed. The subset of patients with repeated episodes of syncope or associated symptoms of a concerning nature (e.g., chest pain) should undergo a rapid search for the cause. Significantly abnormal vital signs (in particular, severe bradycardia or tachycardia and hypotension) demand immediate attention.

Patients with repeated episodes of syncope, significant associated symptoms, or abnormal vital signs should be placed on pulse oximetry and ECG monitoring. Intravenous access, preferably with a large-bore catheter, should be accomplished. Most patients presenting with syncope require confirmatory bedside diagnostic evaluation or testing to exclude life-threatening causes. The 12-lead ECG is the principal

Table 20-4. Clinical Features of Common and Serious Causes of Syncope

Cause	Onset and Recovery	Features
Dysrhythmia	Abrupt onset, rapid recovery	Past cardiac history, risk factors for CAD more common in elderly; implanted pacemaker or cardioverter-defibrillator
Cardiac outflow obstruction	Exertion causes rapid symptoms; rapid recovery	Murmurs not always audible; mechanical valves warrant close monitoring
Myocardial infarction	Exertion or at rest; recovery often incomplete with chest pain persisting	Past cardiac history, risk factors for CAD; chest pain and shortness of breath common but occasionally absent in diabetics and the elderly
Pulmonary embolus	Abrupt onset; recovery often incomplete with dyspnea persisting	Chest pain, dyspnea, hypercoagulable state, DVT, pregnancy
Aortic dissection	Spontaneous; recovery often incomplete with abdominal pain persisting	Tearing chest pain; associated with hypertension, Marfan's syndrome, cystic medial necrosis
Abdominal aortic aneurysm	Spontaneous; recovery often incomplete with abdominal pain persisting	Abdominal or back pain; associated with peripheral vascular disease
Pericardial tamponade	Penetrating chest trauma or thoracic cancer	Beck's triad of hypotension, JVD, muffled heart sounds
Anomalous left coronary artery	Exercise	Left coronary artery arises from right of Valsalva; usually detected in childhood
Stroke	Unpredictable; TIAs may resolve over hours	Focal neurologic findings; vertebrobasilar ischemia may present with ataxia, vertigo, "drop attacks"; history of atherosclerosis
Subarachnoid hemorrhage	Rapid onset; sentinel event may resolve	Focal neurologic findings; "thunderclap" worst headache; nuchal rigidity
Vertebrobasilar insufficiency	Posture change or neck movement	Vertigo, nausea, dysphagia, dysarthria, blurry vision common associated symptoms
Hypovolemia	Bleeding, emesis, heat stress, dehydration; gradual onset	Orthostatic hypotension
Anemia	Bleeding, often occult or gradual from menses or gastrointestinal sources; iron deficiency or decreased red blood cell production	Orthostatic hypotension commonly associated
Hypoglycemia	Gradual onset; incomplete spontaneous recovery common	Diabetes, ingestion/injection of hypoglycemics/insulin; diaphoresis, anxiety, jitteriness
Hypoxemia	Usually gradual; spontaneous recovery if asphyxiating circumstance is reversed	Carbon monoxide, natural gas, sewer gas, bleach/ammonia mix
Subdural hematoma	Onset with or after trauma (which may be trivial)	Elderly, alcoholics at greater risk
Air embolus	Diving	Hyperbaric oxygen key treatment
Pulmonary hypertension	Associated with myocardial infarction or pulmonary embolus	Risk factors for myocardial infarction or pulmonary embolus
Drug syncope	Medication associated with syncope	Consider illicit and alternative drug use; elderly at risk for polypharmacy and drug interactions
Ruptured ectopic pregnancy	Patient often unaware of pregnancy	Abdominal pain, abnormal tenderness; positive β-hCG test
Seizure	Abrupt or with aura postictal state common	Past history common
Carotid sinus sensitivity	Carotid sinus sensitivity; rapid onset and recovery	Shaving, necktie, sudden neck movement; carotid massage may provoke symptoms
Reflex syncope	Gastrointestinal, genitourinary, or thoracic stimulation	Urination, defecation, cough, eating, swallowing, weight lifting
Neurocardiogenic (vasovagal)	Emotion, pain are common triggers; upright posture; gradual onset; rapid recovery once supine	Prodrome of light-headedness, graying or blurring of vision, nausea, sweats common
Hyperventilation	Emotion, pain; gradual onset; patient often unaware of rapid respirations	Perioral tingling, carpopedal spasms, extremity numbness
Narcolepsy	Often spontaneous	Known history
Basilar artery migraine	Specific triggers often known to patient	Visual prodrome often absent. More common in young women; vertigo and nausea common
Trigeminal or glossopharyngeal neuralgia	Sudden onset; specific triggers often known to patient	Lancinating pain in characteristic location
Subclavian steal	Moving affected arm	Thoracic outlet syndrome
Psychogenic	Variable	Anxiety or psychiatric history; diagnosis by examining symptom pattern and excluding organic cause
Breath holding	Deliberate breath holding	Usually toddlers or young children
Drop attack	Unpredictable	Not true syncope—no loss of consciousness; usually elderly; loss of tone, ataxia, vertigo

CAD, Coronary artery disease; DVT, deep vein thrombosis; hCG, human chorionic gonadotropin; JVD, jugular venous distention; TIA, transient ischemic attack.

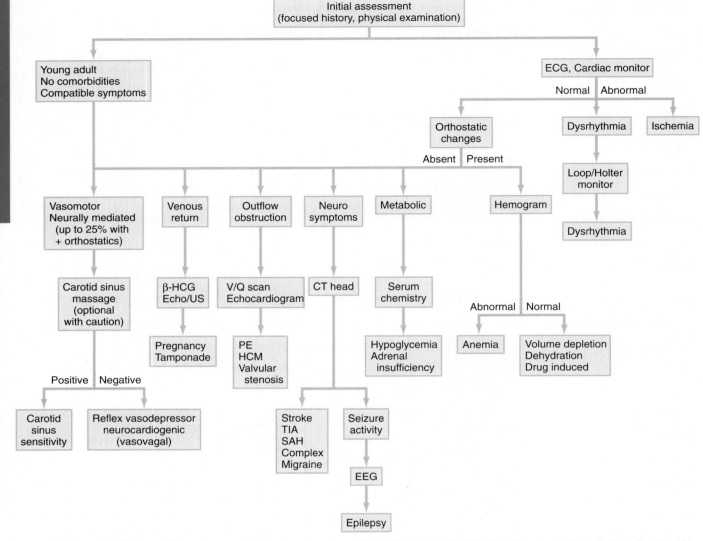

Figure 20-1. Management approach for patients with syncope. ECG, electrocardiogram; β-hCG, β-human chorionic gonadotropin; US, ultrasound; V/Q, ventilation-perfusion; CT, computed tomography; EEG, electroencephalogram; TIA, transient ischemic attack; SAH, subarachnoid hemorrhage; PE, pulmonary embolus; HCM, hypertrophic cardiomyopathy.

tool to evaluate cardiac causes of syncope, and the orthostatic vital signs may support a diagnosis of volume depletion.[17] Figure 20-2 shows an approach to the diagnosis and general management of syncope.

The treatment of syncope is directed toward the underlying cause, if known. Patients with critical diagnoses generally are admitted to the intensive care unit with appropriate consultation. Patients with emergent or unknown diagnoses typically are admitted to the hospital, most often on telemetry units. Patients with nonemergent diagnoses most frequently are managed as outpatients.

Hospitalization is required in patients with associated chest pain, significant signs of congestive heart failure, or valvular disease.[11,12,19] Patients with ECG evidence of ventricular dysrhythmias, ischemia, pro-

longed Q-T interval, or new bundle-branch block also are admitted.[11,12] Admission to a monitored setting also should be considered in patients with any of the following characteristics: age older than 60 years, preexisting cardiovascular or congenital heart disease, family history of sudden death, or exertional syncope.[12,17,19]

Frequently, emergency department evaluation of patients complaining of syncope is inconclusive. After a history, physical examination, and 12-lead ECG, 50% of patients do not have a firm diagnosis.[13,19] Patients younger than age 45 and without worrisome signs, symptoms, or ECG findings are generally at lower risk for an adverse outcome and often may be managed as an outpatient. Discharged patients should be warned of the hazards of recurrent syncope occurring during activities such as driving or working at heights.

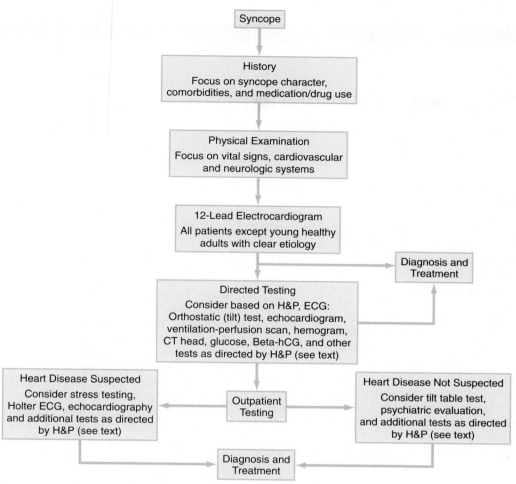

Figure 20-2. General approach to the management of syncope. H&P, history and physical examination; β-hCG, β-human chorionic gonadotropin; ECG, electrocardiogram.

REFERENCES

1. Kapoor WN: Evaluation and management of the patient with syncope. *JAMA* 268:2553, 1992.
2. Colivicchi F, et al: Development and prospective validation of a risk stratification system for patients with syncope in the emergency department: The OESIL risk score. *Eur Heart J* 24:811, 2003.
3. Hayes OW: Evaluation of syncope in the emergency department. *Emerg Med Clin North Am* 16:601, 1998.
4. Soteriades ES, et al: Incidence and prognosis of syncope. *N Engl J Med* 347:878, 2002.
5. Junaid A, Dubinsky IL: Establishing an approach to syncope in the emergency department. *J Emerg Med* 15:593, 1997.
6. Silverstein MD, et al: Patients with syncope admitted to medical intensive care units. *JAMA* 248:1185, 1982.
7. Maron BJ, Epstein SE, Roberts WC: Causes of sudden death in competitive athletes. *J Am Coll Cardiol* 7:204, 1986.
8. Prodinger RJ, Reisdorff EJ: Syncope in children. *Emerg Med Clin North Am* 16:617, 1998.
9. Rubenstein LZ, Josephson KR: The epidemiology of falls and syncope. *Clin Geriatr Med* 18:141, 2002.
10. Rehm CG, Ross SE: Syncope as etiology of road crashes involving elderly drivers. *Am Surg* 61:1006, 1995.
11. Kapoor WN: Syncope. *N Engl J Med* 343:1856, 2000.
12. American College of Emergency Physicians: Clinical policy: Critical issues in the evaluation and management of patients presenting with syncope. *Ann Emerg Med* 37:771, 2001.
13. Linzer M, et al: Clinical guideline: Diagnosing syncope: Part 1. Value of history, physical examination, and electrocardiography. *Ann Intern Med* 126:989, 1997.
14. Alboni P, et al: Diagnostic value of history in patients with syncope with or without heart disease. *J Am Coll Cardiol* 37:1921, 2001.
15. Chen L, et al: Risk factors for syncope in a community-based sample (the Framingham study). *Am J Cardiol* 85:1189, 2000.
16. Sarasin FP, et al: Prevalence of orthostatic hypotension among patients presenting with syncope in the ED. *Am J Emerg Med* 20:497, 2002.
17. Meyer MD, Handler J: Evaluation of the patient with syncope: An evidence based approach. *Emerg Med Clin North Am* 17:189, 1999.
18. Kouakam C, et al: Prevalence and prognostic significance of psychiatric disorders in patients evaluated for recurrent unexplained syncope. *Am J Cardiol* 89:530, 2002.
19. Sarasin FP, et al: A risk score to predict arrhythmias in patients with unexplained syncope. *Acad Emerg Med* 10:1312, 2003.

21 Nausea and Vomiting

Leslie S. Zun and Amardeep Singh

PERSPECTIVE

Nausea and vomiting may represent the primary presentation of many gastrointestinal (GI) disorders (e.g., bowel obstruction, gastroenteritis) or the secondary presentation of numerous systemic conditions (1) caused by severe pain, especially visceral pain; (2) caused by or related to severe systemic illness, such as myocardial infarction, sepsis, or shock; or (3) related to specific conditions by specific mechanisms, such as pregnancy (hormones), increased intracranial pressure (central mechanism), and chemotherapy (chemoreceptor trigger zone [CTZ]). Additionally, vomiting may cause serious sequelae, such as aspiration pneumonia, Mallory-Weiss syndrome, esophageal rupture, volume depletion, and metabolic derangement. Classification by vomiting duration and acute, recurrent, chronic, or cyclic vomiting may assist in determination of the etiology.[1]

Epidemiology

The most common causes of nausea and vomiting are acute gastroenteritis, febrile systemic illnesses, and drug effects. Acute viral gastroenteritis is the most common GI disease in the United States. In adult medicine, nausea and vomiting are caused most often by medications. Emesis associated with pregnancy is common, but hyperemesis gravidarum is not.

Pathophysiology

The act of vomiting can be divided into three distinct phases: nausea, retching, and actual vomiting. Nausea may occur without retching or vomiting, and retching may occur without vomiting. *Nausea* is defined as a vague and extremely unpleasant feeling that often precedes vomiting. The exact neural pathways mediating nausea are not clear, but they are likely the same pathways that mediate vomiting. Mild activation of the pathways may result in nausea, whereas more intense stimulation results in vomiting. During nausea, there is an increase in tone in the duodenum and jejunum, with a concomitant decrease in gastric tone; this leads to reflux of intestinal contents into the stomach. There is often associated hypersalivation, repetitive swallowing, and tachycardia.

Retching is characterized as rhythmic, synchronous contractions of the diaphragm, abdominal muscles, and intercostals, which occur against a closed glottis. There is a resultant increase in abdominal pressure with a concurrent decrease in intrathoracic pressure. This pressure gradient causes gastric contents to move up into the esophagus.

Vomiting is the forceful expulsion of gastric contents through the mouth. There is contraction of the external oblique and abdominal rectus muscles, and the hiatal portion of the diaphragm relaxes; this increases the pressure in the abdominal and the thoracic compartments. There is contraction of the pyloric portion of the stomach. Simultaneously, there is relaxation of the gastric fundus, cardia, and upper esophageal sphincter as the vomitus is brought up and out the mouth. The glottis closes to prevent aspiration.

The complex act of vomiting is coordinated by a vomiting center located in the lateral reticular formation of the medulla (Figure 21-1). The efferent pathways from the vomiting center are mainly through the vagus, phrenic, and spinal nerves. These pathways are responsible for the integrated response of the diaphragm, intercostals, abdominal muscles, stomach, and esophagus. The vomiting center is activated by afferent stimuli from a variety of sources. These include vagal and sympathetic impulses directly from the GI tract. Direct irritation of the stomach causes vomiting in this way. Other GI sources of afferent impulses include the pharynx, small bowel, colon, biliary system, and peritoneum. Receptors also are found outside the GI tract in the vestibular system, heart, and genitalia.

The other major source of impulses to the vomiting center is from the CTZ. The CTZ is located in the area postrema, the floor of the fourth ventricle. It is activated by medications or toxins in the circulation, including opiates, digitalis, chemotherapy agents, salicylate, syrup of ipecac, and dopamine neurotransmitters.

The discovery of various neurotransmitters and their receptor sites within the medulla has improved the understanding and development of therapeutic agents. The CTZ area is rich in dopamine D_2 receptors, which are antagonized by drugs such as prochlorperazine, metoclopramide, and droperidol. The serotonin receptor has been found widely in the area postrema and the GI tract. It may act directly and through the release of dopamine. Serotonin receptor antagonists, ondansetron and granisetron, have been shown to be effective in preventing chemotherapy-induced nausea and vomiting. Concentrations of cholinergic and histamine receptors are found in the lateral vestibular nucleus and are important in motion sickness. Meclizine, diphenhydramine, and scopolamine act by antagonizing these receptors.

Rumination is regurgitation of ingested food that subsequently is reswallowed or ejected. Rumination syndrome is found in infants, children, and mentally challenged adults, but rarely in adults with normal intelligence.

DIAGNOSTIC APPROACH

Differential Considerations

The differential diagnosis for nausea and vomiting is particularly broad; almost any organ system can be involved (Table 21-1). Vomiting also can result in complications; the causes and complications must be considered. The sequelae of vomiting may include the following:

Hypovolemia is caused by loss of water and sodium chloride in the vomitus. The contraction of the extracellular fluid space leads to activation of the renin-angiotensin-aldosterone system.

Metabolic alkalosis is produced by loss of hydrogen ions in the vomitus. Many factors serve to maintain the alkalosis, including volume contractions, hypokalemia, chloride depletion, and increased aldosterone.

Hypokalemia is produced primarily by loss of potassium in the urine. The metabolic alkalosis leads to large amounts of sodium bicarbonate being delivered to the distal tubule. Secondary hyperaldosteronism from volume depletion causes reabsorption of sodium and excretion of large amounts of potassium in the urine.

Mallory-Weiss tears typically follow a forceful bout of retching and vomiting. The lesion itself is a 1- to 4-cm tear through the mucosa and submucosa; 75% of cases occur in the stomach with the remainder near the gastroesophageal junction. Bleeding usually is mild and self-limited; however, 3% of deaths from upper GI bleeds are due to Mallory-Weiss tears.

Boerhaave's syndrome refers to a perforation of all layers of the esophagus as a result of forceful retching or vomiting. The overlying pleura is torn so that there is free passage of esophageal contents into the mediastinum and thorax; 80% of cases involve the

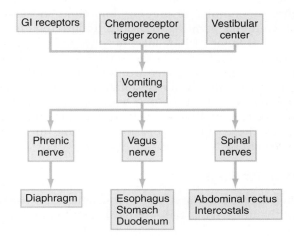

Figure 21-1. Pathophysiology of nausea and vomiting. GI, gastrointestinal.

Table 21-1. Differential Diagnosis of Nausea and Vomiting

Organ System	Critical Diagnoses	Emergent Diagnoses	Nonemergent Diagnoses
Gastrointestinal	Boerhaave's syndrome Ischemic bowel	Gastric outlet obstructed Pancreatitis Cholecystitis Bowel obstruction/ileus Ruptured viscus Appendicitis Peritonitis	Gastritis Gastroparesis Peptic ulcer disease Gastroenteritis Biliary colic Hepatitis
Neurologic	Intracerebral bleed Meningitis	Migraine CNS tumor Raised ICP	
Endocrine	DKA	Adrenal insufficiency	Thyroid
Pregnancy		Hyperemesis gravidarum	Nausea and vomiting of pregnancy
Drug toxicity		Tylenol Digoxin Aspirin Theophylline	
Therapeutic drug use			Aspirin Erythromycin Ibuprofen Chemotherapy
Drugs of abuse			Narcotics Narcotic withdrawal Alcohol
Genitourinary		Gonadal torsion	Urinary tract infection Kidney stone
Miscellaneous	Myocardial infarction Sepsis	Carbon monoxide Electrolyte disorders	Motion sickness Labyrinthitis

CNS, central nervous system; DKA, diabetic ketoacidosis; ICP, intracranial pressure.

posterolateral aspect of the distal esophagus. Boerhaave's syndrome is a surgical emergency. Mortality is 50% if surgery is not performed within 24 hours. *Aspiration* of gastric contents is a concern in patients who have altered mental status or pulmonary findings after an episode of vomiting. Patients with pulmonary findings after vomiting need further evaluation for aspiration.

Rapid Assessment and Stabilization

The initial assessment is directed toward the patient's hemodynamic status and identifying the critical causes or sequelae of vomiting (see Table 21-1). Data gathered include duration of vomiting, whether blood is in the vomitus, symptoms of volume depletion, and associated symptoms pointing to serious underlying disease. Physical findings include level of consciousness, status of abdomen, rapid neurologic screen for focality, and serial vital signs. Initial stabilization may include intravenous access and fluid resuscitation if there are signs of volume depletion, cardiac monitoring, and therapeutic measures directed toward specific underlying diseases (e.g., blood pressure control in severe hypertension).

Pivotal Findings

A thorough history and physical examination usually yield the underlying cause of nausea and vomiting.

History

Content of the vomitus may provide clues. The presence of bile indicates a patent connection between the duodenum and the stomach and essentially rules out a gastric outlet obstruction. Regurgitation of undigested food can suggest achalasia, esophageal stricture, or Zenker's diverticulum. Feculent material usually suggests a distal bowel obstruction, but also may be seen with gastrocolic fistula or bacterial overgrowth of stomach contents in long-standing outlet obstruction.

Timing of the vomiting may be important. An acute onset of nausea and vomiting suggests gastroenteritis, pancreatitis, cholecystitis, or a drug-related side effect. Symptoms occurring primarily in the morning suggest pregnancy, although this pattern also may be seen in uremia, alcohol ingestion, or increased intracranial pressure. Delayed vomiting more than 1 hour after eating suggests gastric outlet obstruction or gastroparesis. Vomiting of material eaten more than 12 hours previously is pathognomonic for outlet obstruction. Nausea and vomiting for more than 1 month are considered chronic.

Associated symptoms may be helpful. Hypersalivation, defecation, tachycardia, bradycardia, atrial fibrillation, and termination of ventricular tachyarrhythmias are associated phenomena with nausea and vomiting. Chronic headaches with nausea and vomiting should raise the suspicion for an intracranial lesion. Also, vomiting without preceding nausea is typical of central nervous system pathology. The *social history* should include inquiries about alcohol or other substance abuse. The *past medical history* should include any GI disease or surgeries. Nutritional history is valuable in the consideration of failure to thrive in infancy. Finally, a thorough *medication list,* including over-the-counter drugs, should be included.

Physical Examination

The important physical examination findings are outlined in Table 21-2. During evaluation, findings of jaundice, lymphadenopathy, abdominal masses, and occult blood in stool can help determine the etiology of the disease. Orthostatic vital signs should be obtained in patients with signs of dehydration, lightheadedness, generalized weakness, or toxic appearance. It also is important to evaluate neurologic status to rule out a central cause of a patient's symptoms, which includes cranial nerves, funduscopic examination, and gait observation.

Ancillary Studies

Because of the broad differential diagnosis of nausea and vomiting, there is no standard panel of laboratory tests. Appropriate testing is determined by the specifics of the history and physical examination. The following are general guidelines:

Table 21-2. Physical Examination of Patient with Nausea and Vomiting

Organ System	Finding	Suggested Diagnosis
General	Poor skin turgor Dry mucous membranes	Dehydration
Vital signs	Fever	Gastroenteritis, cholecystitis, appendicitis, hepatitis Bowel perforation
	Tachycardia/ orthostatic changes	Dehydration
HEENT	Nystagmus	Labyrinthitis Vertebro-basilar insufficiency Cerebellar infarct or bleed CPA tumor
	Papilledema	Increased ICP from CNS tumor or bleeding
Abdomen	Abdominal distention Peristaltic waves	Bowel obstruction, gastroparesis
	High-pitched bowel sounds	Gastric outlet obstruction
	Decreased bowel sounds	Bowel obstruction Ileus
	Hernias or surgical scars	Possible bowel obstruction
	Peritoneal signs	Appendicitis, cholecystitis Perforated viscus
Neurologic	Abnormal mental status	CNS pathology
	Cerebellar findings Cranial nerve findings	

CNS, central nervous system; CPA, cerebellar pontine angle; HEENT, head, eyes, ears, nose, throat; ICP, intracranial pressure.

Complete blood count: Most patients do not require a complete blood count. Elevated hemoglobin may suggest dehydration, but other tests are better for this purpose. An elevated white blood count is entirely nonspecific and of no discriminatory value.

Serum electrolytes: Measurement of serum electrolytes is not indicated in most cases of vomiting. Severe, protracted vomiting can cause a hypochloremic, hypokalemic, metabolic alkalosis. Patients with this history or clinical findings of dehydration should have electrolyte testing ordered. In general, serum electrolyte testing is indicated only in patients with symptoms lasting longer than 3 days or who require intravenous fluid to replenish vascular volume.

Blood urea nitrogen and creatinine: Classically a blood urea nitrogen-to-creatinine ratio greater than 20:1 implies significant dehydration.

Serum lipase: Lipase is indicated in cases of suspected pancreatitis.

Urine tests: A urine pregnancy test should be performed on all women of childbearing age. Nitrites, leukocyte esterase, white blood cells, and bacteria indicate a urinary tract infection. Ketones may support a diagnosis of diabetic ketoacidosis. Hematuria indicates a possible renal calculus.

Liver function tests: Liver function tests are indicated in cases of suspected hepatitis or biliary disease.

Serum drug levels: Serum drug levels may be important in patients on theophylline, digoxin, or salicylates, especially in elderly patients who are taking medication without supervision.

Abdominal imaging: Flat and upright films are indicated only in cases of suspected bowel obstruction or ileus. Computed tomography scan of the abdomen has supplanted plain films in the evaluation of many patients with suspected obstruction because of the improved ability to discern the cause of the problem in addition to the presence of obstruction. An abdominal ultrasound study is indicated in cases of suspected choledocholithiasis or cholecystitis in adults, suspected pyloric stenosis, and intussusception in children.

Electrocardiogram: Electrocardiogram is indicated in cases of suspected coronary ischemia.

DIFFERENTIAL DIAGNOSIS

Clinical and diagnostic findings are helpful in differentiating the common and catastrophic causes of nausea and vomiting (Table 21-3). An algorithmic approach to the assessment of nausea and vomiting is given in Figure 21-2.

PEDIATRIC CONSIDERATIONS

The evaluation and management of pediatric patients with nausea and vomiting depends on age and probable etiologies (Table 21-4). Mild degrees of reflux and associated regurgitation are common in the first few months of life, but vomiting in infancy can be associated with life-threatening illness. In the first week of life, obstructive lesions of the alimentary tract, inborn errors of metabolism, and serious infectious processes are associated with vomiting. After the first week of life, pyloric stenosis needs to be considered. The diagnosis of "feeding problems" should be considered a diagnosis of exclusion. After the first month of life, infections, metabolic diseases, cow's milk intolerance, and subdural hematoma from abuse should be prime considerations. Thereafter, recurrent cyclic vomiting of varying etiologies, acute surgical emergencies, food poisoning, toxic ingestion, Henoch-Schönlein purpura, pneumonia, and diabetic ketoacidosis are likely causes of nausea and vomiting. Anorexia nervosa should be considered in teenagers with recurrent vomiting.[2,3]

MANAGEMENT

Management of patients with nausea and vomiting is outlined in Figure 21-2. Decreased oral intake is a major cause of dehydration and malnutrition. Hypokalemia is rarely of clinical significance, but may be found with profound vomiting secondary to contraction alkalosis. Placement of a nasogastric tube is important in cases such as persistent vomiting or gastroparesis. The pharmacologic therapies available may be classified to allow the physician to make an appropriate choice for each patient (Box 21-1 and Table 21-5).[4]

The phenothiazines are widely used as general-purpose antiemetics. These agents have multiple complex mechanisms of action. The antiemetic effect is apparently through blockage of the dopamine D_2 receptor in the CTZ. Prochlorperazine (Compazine) and promethazine (Phenergan) are the most commonly used medications in this class. Mild to moderate side effects are fairly common and include dystonic reactions and feelings of restlessness. These side effects may be treated with diphenhydramine (Benadryl). Although prochlorperazine was found to be more effective in reducing vomiting than promethazine, prochlorperazine has been reported in association with a 16% incidence of akathisia and a 4% incidence of dystonia, and patients should be advised of this potential and its mitigation with diphenhydramine or benztropine (Cogentin). Neuroleptic malignant syndrome, blood dyscrasias, and cholestatic jaundice have been documented rarely with phenothiazines. The serotonin receptor antagonists, such as ondansetron, are a new class of agents that generated much interest because of their effect on chemotherapy-induced emesis. Their principal site of action is the area postrema, although they also affect receptors in the GI tract. Several small series have looked at their effect in overdoses of theophylline and acetaminophen. Both of these overdoses cause vomiting, and both require oral intake as part of therapy (multiple-dose charcoal and *N*-acetyl cysteine). It is well documented that the vomiting often prevents effective oral therapy in these patients. These small studies showed that ondansetron stopped the vomiting and allowed oral therapy to proceed. The dose was 8 mg given intravenously over 20 minutes. The side effects of the serotonin receptor antagonists are mild and include headache and constipation.[5,6]

Table 21-3. Differential Diagnoses in Patient with Vomiting

	History	Prevalence	Physical Examination	Useful Tests	Comments
Nausea and vomiting of pregnancy (NVP)	Vomiting occurs predominantly in the morning. Associated breast tenderness and late menses. NVP typically starts in week 4-7, peaks in week 10-16, and disappears by week 20. Vomiting that begins after week 12 or continues past week 20 should prompt a search for another cause	Very common Affects 75% of all pregnancies	Benign abdomen	Urine pregnancy test Serum electrolytes, urine ketones to exclude hyperemesis gravidarum	Consider NVP in all females of childbearing age. Prognosis for mother and infant is excellent. NVP is associated with a decreased risk of miscarriage, fetal growth retardation, and fetal mortality
Hyperemesis gravidarum	Severe, protracted form of NVP. No universally accepted definition of the disease. Generally accepted hallmarks include 5% weight loss, ketonuria, and electrolyte disturbance. Hyperemesis is associated with multiple gestation, molar pregnancy, and nulliparity	Uncommon Affects < 1% of pregnancies	Signs of dehydration Benign abdomen	β-HCG Urinalysis for ketones Serum electrolytes Ultrasound to exclude molar pregnancy or multiple gestation	Most studies have found no adverse outcomes for the fetus. A few studies, however, have shown a correlation with fetal growth retardation
Gastroenteritis	Fever, diarrhea, and crampy abdominal pain. Vomiting and pain occur early, followed by diarrhea within 24 hr	Very common	Benign abdomen	Usually not necessary	Early gastroenteritis, when only vomiting and periumbilical pain are present, may be confused with early appendicitis. Diarrhea must be present to make the diagnosis of gastroenteritis
Gastritis	Epigastric pain, belching, bloating, fullness, heartburn, and food intolerance. Use of NSAIDs or ETOH common	Very common	Mild epigastric tenderness may be present	Lipase and pregnancy test may be necessary to exclude other diagnoses	Removal of inciting agent along with antacid therapy will resolve symptoms in most patients
Peptic ulcer disease	Epigastric pain present in 90% of cases. Classically, duodenal ulcer pain is relieved by food while gastric ulcer pain is made worse. Presence of severe pain should raise suspicion of perforation	Very common	Mild epigastric tenderness Heme positive stool	Hemoglobin if bleeding is suspected Upright abdominal film if perforation is suspected	Three major causes of PUD are NSAIDs, *H. pylori* infection, and hypersecretory states.
Biliary disease	Abdominal pain may be midepigastric or right upper quadrant (RUQ). Onset frequently after a fatty meal. May have history of similar episodes in the past	Very common	RUQ tenderness present in most cases. If instructed to breathe deeply during palpation in the RUQ, the patient experiences heightened tenderness and inspiratory arrest (Murphy's sign)	WBC Lipase Serum bilirubin Alkaline phosphatase RUQ ultrasound	Normal temperature, WBC, and spontaneous resolution of symptoms suggest biliary colic. Fever, Murphy's sign, elevated WBC, and suggestive ultrasound indicate cholecystitis

Table 21-3. **Differential Diagnoses in Patient with Vomiting—cont'd**

	History	Prevalence	Physical Examination	Useful Tests	Comments
Myocardial infarction	Patients typically have substernal chest pain that may radiate to left arm or jaw. Often associated with dyspnea, diaphoresis, or dizziness	Common	Patients are often anxious and in distress from pain. No diagnostic examination findings	ECG (new Q waves, ST segment changes or T wave inversions) CPK/troponin	Not all patients present with chest pain. A subset of patients, particularly diabetics and the elderly, may present with only nausea, vomiting, and epigastric discomfort
Diabetic ketoacidosis	Polydipsia and polyuria occur early. If not treated, altered mental status and coma may develop. In long-standing diabetics, DKA may be triggered by infection, trauma, MI, or surgery	Common	"Fruity" breath odor results from serum acetone. Tachypnea occurs as the patient attempts to blow off carbon dioxide to compensate for metabolic acidosis. Signs of dehydration may be present. Severe cases often present with altered mental status or coma	Serum glucose, urine ketones, ABG	DKA may be the first manifestation of diabetes in some patients. These patients often do not recognize the importance of polydipsia and polyuria. They often present complaining only of nausea, vomiting, and epigastric pain
Pancreatitis	Patients present with epigastric pain, which often radiates to the back. Most cases are caused by gallstones or alcoholism. Other causes include hypercalcemia, hyperlipidemia, drugs (sulfas and thiazides), ERCP	Common	Epigastric tenderness is present. Associated paralytic ileus may cause abdominal distention and decreased bowel sounds. Frank shock may be present in severe cases	Lipase WBC, serum glucose, LDH, AST Hematocrit, BUN, calcium, ABG	Criteria correlating with higher mortality include: At admission—Age >55, WBC >16,000, glucose >200, base deficit >4, LDH >350, AST >250 Within 48 hours—Hct drop of 10%, BUN increase of 5, P_{O_2} < 60, calcium <8, fluid sequestration >6 L
Appendicitis	Abdominal pain classically begins in periumbilical region and later moves to right lower quadrant Anorexia is common	Common	Localized tenderness over right lower quadrant. Low-grade fever may be present	WBC Abdominal CT	Early appendicitis can be a difficult diagnosis to make. It is still frequently missed on the first physician encounter
Bowel obstruction	Classically, abdominal pain consists of intermittent cramps occurring at regular intervals. The frequency of the cramps varies with the level of the obstruction; the higher the level, the more frequent the cramps. The location of the pain also varies with the level of the obstruction; high obstruction causes epigastric pain, mid-level obstruction causes periumbilical pain, colonic obstruction causes hypogastric pain	Common	Abdominal distention, mild diffuse tenderness, and high-pitched "tinkling" bowel sounds may be present. Thorough search for hernias should be performed	Supine and upright plain abdominal films Abdominal CT	Adhesions, hernias, and tumors account for 90% of bowel obstructions. Other causes include intussusception, volvulus, foreign bodies, gallstone ileus, inflammatory bowel disease, stricture, cystic fibrosis, and hematoma

Continued

Table 21-3. Differential Diagnoses in Patient with Vomiting—cont'd

	History	Prevalence	Physical Examination	Useful Tests	Comments
Carbon monoxide (CO) poisoning	Headache is usually present. CO poisoning often occurs during winter months when furnaces are turned on. Family members may have similar symptoms if they also have been exposed	Uncommon	No reliable signs of early CO poisoning	CO level	Because CO is a tasteless, odorless gas, patients may not realize they have been exposed. It is important to keep a high index of suspicion during the winter months
Boerhaave's syndrome	Patients may have neck, chest, or epigastric pain. Forceful, protracted vomiting usually causes the tear. Most cases follow a bout of heavy eating and drinking. Other reported causes include childbirth, defecation, seizures, and heavy lifting	Uncommon	Tachypnea, tachycardia, and hypotension may be present. Escaped air from the esophagus may produce subcutaneous emphysema. Air in the mediastinum produces a "crunching" sound as the heart beats (Hamman's sign)	CXR may show pleural effusion, widened mediastinum, pneumothorax, or pneumomediastinum. Esophagogram using water-soluble contrast is definitive	The classic presentation includes forceful vomiting, severe chest pain, subcutaneous emphysema, and multiple CXR findings. There is a growing body of evidence that most cases do not have this "classic" picture. In more subtle presentations, the diagnosis can be difficult to make

ABG, arterial blood gas; AST, aspartate aminotransferase; β-hCG, β-human chorionic gonadotropin; BUN, blood urea nitrogen; CPK, creatine phosphokinase; CT, computed tomography; CXR, chest radiography; DKA, diabetic ketoacidosis; ECG, electrocardiogram; ERCP, endoscopic retrograde cholangiopancreatography; ETOH, ethyl alcohol; LDH, lactate dehydrogenase; MI, myocardial infarction; NSAID, nonsteroidal anti-inflammatory drug; PUD, peptic ulcer disease; WBC, white blood cell.

The prokinetic agents are useful in patients with gastroparesis, gastroesophageal reflux disease, and other putative dysmotility syndromes. Metoclopramide (Reglan) has the most applicability in the emergency department. It has dopamine antagonist activity at the CTZ and anticholinergic and antiserotonin effects. The primary effect is increased gastric emptying; the exact mechanism for this is not understood. Metoclopramide has multiple antiemetic actions and may be used as a general-purpose agent. Newer prokinetic agents, such as cisapride (Propulsid), do not cross the blood-brain barrier. They are not useful as general-purpose antiemetics. Prokinetic agents are used in patients with isolated gastric motility disorders. The most common side effects of metoclopramide are restlessness, drowsiness, and diarrhea. These effects are usually mild and transient. Prophylactic administration of metoclopramide, prochlorperazine, or any other agent to prevent vomiting in the administration of opioid analgesics has been shown to be of no benefit and has fallen out of favor.[7]

Antihistamines are useful in nausea and vomiting associated with motion sickness and vertigo. Agents such as dimenhydrinate (Gravol, Dramamine) and meclizine (Antivert) directly inhibit vestibular stimulation and vestibular-cerebellar pathways. Their anticholinergic effect also may contribute to their effectiveness in vertigo and motion sickness. Antihistamines have some use as general antiemetics, but are better in the prevention of motion sickness; for nausea and vomiting, they are less effective than the phenothiazines. The most common side effects of antihistamines are drowsiness, blurred vision, dry mouth, and hypotension.

The anticholinergic agent scopolamine in a transdermal patch (Transderm Scōp) is used for prophylaxis and treatment of motion sickness. It also has mild efficacy in preventing cytotoxic chemotherapy-related nausea and vomiting, but it is not a useful antiemetic agent in the emergency department.

Many agents have been advocated for the treatment of nausea and vomiting in pregnancy. For severe symptoms, hospitalization, fluids, electrolyte replacement, thiamine supplementation, and administration of antiemetics including antihistamines (e.g., meclizine, and phenothiazines) may be used. Hyperemesis gravidarum begins early in pregnancy, and other causes for severe vomiting after the first trimester must be considered.

Metoclopramide, cisapride, serotonin receptor antagonists, domperidone, and bethanecol are commonly used in pediatric patients for nausea and vomiting. Domperidone blocks dopamine in the area postrema and in the gut. Bethanecol, a selective muscarinic ester, is used frequently in children with gastroesophageal reflux because of the reduction in vomiting episodes with its use.

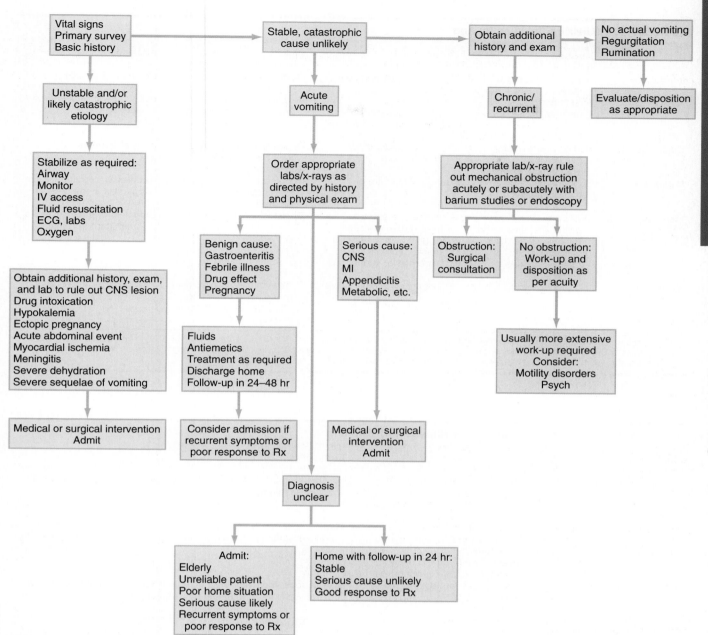

Figure 21-2. Algorithmic approach to nausea and vomiting. IV, intravenous; ECG, electrocardiogram; CNS, central nervous system; MI, myocardial infarction; Psych, psychiatric origin.

DISPOSITION

Admitting the patient to the hospital is appropriate when the patient has a significant underlying disease, the patient has an unclear diagnosis and responds poorly to fluid and antiemetic therapy, the patient has uncontrolled emesis refractory to medication, or the patient is at the extremes of age with poor response to treatment. A category subject to broad interpretation is when the diagnosis is unclear and there are poor prospects for timely follow-up (e.g., the patient has no family, no transportation, is indigent, is a drug abuser or an alcoholic, or has a language barrier). Patients are considered for discharge if no serious underlying illness is present, there is a good response to fluid and antiemetic therapy, the patient is able to take clear liquids before discharge, and there are good prospects for follow-up and observation at home.

Close follow-up is arranged for all discharged patients, preferably with their primary physician, in 24 to 48 hours. At discharge, the gradual return to a normal diet is explained, as are doses of any prescribed medications. Clear instructions are given to return to the emergency department if recurrence, change or deterioration in symptoms occurs.

Causes for nausea and vomiting frequently remain undiagnosed. Some cases declare themselves or resolve over time; re-evaluation and close follow-up are imperative. In patients with persistent symptoms, psy-

Table 21-4. Pediatric Etiologies by Age

	Newborn	Infant	Child	Adolescent
Infectious	Sepsis, meningitis, UTI, thrush	Pneumonia, otitis media, thrush	Gastroenteritis	Gastroenteritis, URI
Anatomic	Atresia and webs, malrotation, stenosis, meconium ileus, Hirschsprung's disease	Pyloric stenosis, intussusception, Hirschsprung's disease	Bezoars, chronic granulomatous disease	PUD, superior mesenteric syndrome
Gastrointestinal	Reflux, overfeeding, gastric outlet obstruction, volvulus	Reflux, gastritis, milk intolerance	Appendicitis, pancreatic, hepatitis, other food intolerance	Achalasia, hepatitis
Neurologic	Subdural hematoma, hydrocephalus	Subdural hematoma	Neoplasia, migraine, Reye syndrome, motion sickness, hypertension	Neoplasia, migraine, motion sickness, hypertension
Metabolic	Organic or amino acidemias, urea cycle defects, galactosemia, hypercalcemia, phenylketonuria, kernicterus	Hereditary fructose intolerance, disorders of fatty acid metabolism, uremia, adrenal hyperplasia, kernicterus	Diabetes, vitamin A excess	Diabetes, pregnancy, acute intermittent porphyria
Other	Idiopathic, cardiac failure	Rumination, cardiac failure	Cyclic vomiting syndrome, toxins, food poisoning, Munchausen syndrome by proxy	Psychogenic, anorexia

PUD, peptic ulcer disease; URI, upper respiratory infection; UTI, urinary tract infection.
Adapted from Li BUK: Common symptoms and signs of gastrointestinal disease; and Dodge, JA: Vomiting and regurgitation. In Walker WA, Durie PR, Hamilton JR, et al (eds): *Pediatric Gastroenterology.* Philadelphia, BC Decker, 1991.

Table 21-5. Symptomatic Treatment of Nausea and Vomiting

Medication	Dose	Comments
Promethazine (Phenergan)	*Adult:* 12.5-25 mg IV, IM, PO, or by rectum *Pediatric:* 0.5 mg/pound IV, IM, PO, or by rectum	May be repeated every 6 hr, until cessation of vomiting. Dry mouth, dizziness, blurred vision
Prochlorperazine (Compazine)	*Adult:* 5-10 mg IM, or PO; 2.5-10 mg IV; 25 mg by rectum *Pediatric:* 2.5 mg PO or by recturm; 0.06 mg/pound IM	May be repeated every 4 hr by IV or IM or every 12 hr by rectum, until cessation of vomiting. Lethargy, hypotension, extrapyramidal effects
Haloperidol (Haldol)	*Adult:* 0.5-5 mg PO; 2-5 mg IM *Pediatric:* 0.075-0.15 mg/kg/day bid or tid	May be repeated every 8-12 hr, until cessation of vomiting. Known extrapyramidal effects, lethargy, confusion

IM, intramuscular; IV, intravenous.

BOX 21-1. Antiemetic Therapy of Specific Diseases

Phenothiazines or 5-HT Antagonists	Antihistamines	Phenothiazines or 5-HT Antagonists	Prokinetics
CTZ	Vestibular	GI irritation	Gastroparesis
DKA	Motion sickness	Gastritis	
Opiates	Labyrinthitis	Appendicitis	
Chemotherapy		Biliary disease	
Theophylline		Gastroenteritis	
Digoxin			

CTZ, chemoreceptor trigger zone; DKA, diabetic ketoacidosis; GI, gastrointestinal.

chogenic causes or cyclic vomiting syndrome should be ruled out.

REFERENCES

1. Quigley E, Hasler W, Parkman H: American Gastroenterological Association technical review on nausea and vomiting. *Gastroenterology* 120:263, 2001.
2. Koletzko S: Dysmotilities. In Walker WA, et al (eds): *Pediatric Gastroenterology*. Philadelphia, BC Decker, 2004, pp 1016-1030.
3. Sondheimer JM: Vomiting. In Walker WA, et al (eds): *Pediatric Gastroenterology*. Philadelphia, BC Decker, 2004, pp 203-209.
4. Allan S: Antiemetics. *Gastroenterol Clin North Am* 21:597, 1992.
5. Sage TA, Jones WN, Clark RF: Ondansetron in the treatment of intractable nausea associated with theophylline toxicity. *Ann Pharmacother* 27:584, 1993.
6. Reed M, Marx C: Ondansetron for treating nausea and vomiting in the poisoned patient. *Ann Pharmacother* 28:331, 1994.
7. Reynolds J, Putnam P: Prokinetic agents. *Gastroenterol Clin North Am* 21:567, 1992.

CHAPTER

 Abdominal Pain

Kelly E. King and John M. Wightman

PERSPECTIVE

The nature and quality of abdominal pain are often difficult for the patient to convey and may be subject to a wide range of patients' and physicians' perceptions. The physical examination is often not helpful. Pain perception may be remote from the site of pathology, and the examination can change over time as the disease process evolves. Seemingly routine symptoms and signs may stem from life-threatening problems, and benign processes can present with severe symptoms. All of these factors make the evaluation of patients with acute abdominal pain a continuing challenge in emergency care.

Epidemiology

Abdominal pain is a common presenting complaint, accounting for up to 10% of all emergency department visits. Some of the most common causes of acute abdominal pain are listed in Table 22-1. Many patients present with pain and other symptoms that are not typical of any specific disease process. A specific diagnosis may not be possible in about one in every four individuals presenting with this chief complaint.[1] In addition, two groups deserve special consideration: elderly people (age older than 65 years) and women of reproductive age.

Elderly patients with acute abdominal pain are more likely to have a life-threatening process as the cause of their pain, which can also be more rapidly progressive. Atypical symptoms and clinical findings in elderly patients make specific diagnoses difficult to determine. Decreased diagnostic accuracy, coupled with increased probability of severe disease, results in increased mortality in elderly patients with abdominal pain.[2]

Pain in pelvic organs is commonly perceived as abdominal in origin. The possibility of ectopic pregnancy in women of reproductive age greatly increases the risk of serious disease with a high potential for misdiagnosis. During pregnancy the uterus becomes an abdominal rather than pelvic organ. It may displace the normal intraperitoneal contents, adding complexity to the evaluation of these patients.[3]

Pathophysiology

Pathology in the gastrointestinal and genitourinary tracts remains the most common source of pain perceived in the abdomen. Also, pain can arise from a multitude of other intraabdominal and extraabdominal locations (Box 22-1). Abdominal pain is derived from one or more of three distinct pain pathways: visceral, somatic, and referred.

Visceral pain results from stimulating autonomic nerves invested in the visceral peritoneum surrounding internal organs. It is often the earliest manifestation of a particular disease process. Hollow-organ distention by fluid or gas and capsular stretching of solid organs from edema, blood, cysts, or abscesses are the most common stimuli. This discomfort is poorly characterized and difficult to localize. If the involved organ is affected by peristalsis, the pain is often described as intermittent, crampy, or colicky. In general, visceral pain is perceived from the abdominal region that correlates with the embryonic somatic segment:

- Foregut structures (stomach, duodenum, liver, and pancreas) cause upper abdominal pain.
- Midgut derivatives (small bowel, proximal colon, and appendix) cause periumbilical pain.

Table 22-1. Common Causes of Abdominal Pain

	Epidemiology	Etiology	Presentation	Physical Examination	Useful Tests
Peptic ulcer	Occur in all age groups. Peak at age 50. Men affected twice as much as women. Severe bleeding or perforation in less than 1% of patients.	May be associated with *Helicobacter pylori* infection. Risk factors include COPD, NSAID use, tobacco and alcohol use.	Nonradiating epigastric pain that starts 1–3 hours after eating and is relieved by food or antacids. Pain frequently awakens patient at night.	Epigastric tenderness without rebound or guarding. Perforation or bleeding leads to more severe clinical findings.	Uncomplicated cases are treated with antacids or H_2 blockers before invasive studies are contemplated. Gastroduodenoscopy is valuable in diagnosis and biopsy. Valuable in diagnosing *H. pylori*. Also blood test for *H. pylori*. US, barium enema, or CT with contrast may have diagnostic benefit.
Acute appendicitis	Peak age: adolescence and young adulthood. Less common in children and elderly. Higher perforation rate in women, children, and elderly. Mortality rate is 0.1% but increased to 2%–6% with perforation.	Appendiceal lumen obstruction leads to swelling, ischemia, infection, and perforation.	Epigastric or periumbilical pain migrates to RLQ over 8–12 hours (50%–60%). Later presentations associated with higher perforation rates. Pain, low-grade fever (15%), and anorexia (80%) common; vomiting less common (50%–70%).	Mean temperature 38° C (100.5° F). Higher temperature associated with perforation. RLQ tenderness (90%–95%) with rebound (40%–70%) in majority of cases. Rectal tenderness in up to 30%.	Leukocyte count usually elevated or may show left shift. Urine may show sterile pyuria. C-reactive proteins sensitive, but accuracy varies. CT is sensitive and specific. US may have use in women with RLQ pain.
Biliary tract disease	Peak age 35–60. Rare in patients younger than 20. Female-to-male ratio of 3 : 1. Risk factors include multiparity, obesity, alcohol intake, and birth control pills.	Passage of gallstones causes biliary colic. Impaction of a stone in cystic duct or common duct causes cholecystitis or cholangitis.	Crampy RUQ pain radiates to right subscapular area. Prior history of pain is common. Longer duration of pain favors diagnosis of cholecystitis or cholangitis.	Temperature normal in biliary colic, elevated in cholecystitis, cystitis, and cholangitis. RUQ tenderness, rebound, and jaundice (less common) may be present.	WBC count elevated in cholecystitis and cholangitis. Amylase and liver function tests may help differentiate this from gastritis or ulcer disease. Ultrasound shows anatomy, stones, or duct dilatation. Hepatobiliary scintigraphy diagnoses gallbladder function.
Ureteral colic	Average age 30–40, primarily in men. Prior history or family history of stones is common.	Family history, gout, *Proteus* sp infections. Renal tubular acidosis and cystinuria lead to stone formation.	Acute onset of flank pain radiating to groin. Nausea, vomiting, and pallor are common. Patient usually writhing in pain.	Vital signs usually normal. Tenderness on CVA percussion with benign abdominal examination.	Urinalysis usually shows hematuria. Intravenous pyelography is the mainstay of diagnosis. Helical or spiral CT may be more appropriate in older patients or patients with elevated renal functions. US ± KUB with fluid bolus useful diagnostically.
Diverticulitis	Incidence increases with advancing age; occurs in males more than females. Recurrences are common. Often called "left-sided" appendicitis.	Colonic diverticula become infected or perforated or cause local colitis Obstruction, peritonitis, abscesses, fistulas result from infection or swelling.	Common to have change in stool frequency or consistency. Left lower quadrant pain is common. Associated fever, nausea/vomiting, rectal bleed may be seen.	Fever usually low grade. Left lower quadrant pain without rebound is common. Stools may be heme positive.	Most testing usually normal. Plain films may show obstruction or mass effect. Barium enema is often diagnostic.

Table 22-1. Common Causes of Abdominal Pain—cont'd

	Epidemiology	Etiology	Presentation	Physical Examination	Useful Tests
Acute gastroenteritis	Common diagnosis. Seasonal. Most common misdiagnosis of appendicitis. May be seen in multiple family members.	Usually viral.	Pain usually poorly localized. Intermittent, crampy diffuse pain. Diarrhea is key element in diagnosis, usually large volume, watery. Nausea and vomiting usually begin before pain. Sense of increased peristalsis may be noted.	Abdominal examination usually nonspecific without peritoneal signs. Watery diarrhea or no stool noted on rectal examination. Fever is usually present.	Usually symptomatic care with antiemetics and volume repletion. Key is not using this as a "default" diagnosis and missing more serious disease.
Nonspecific abdominal pain	More common in persons of young and middle age, women of childbearing years, or low social class and those with psychiatric disorders. Up to 10% of patients over 50 years of age prove to have intraabdominal cancer.	Unknown.	Variable but tends to be chronic or recurrent.	Variable but no peritoneal signs.	Variable and can often be done on an outpatient basis.

COPD, chronic obstructive pulmonary disease; CT, computed tomography; CVA, costovertebral angle; KUB, kidney, ureters, and bladder; NSAID, nonsteroidal anti-inflammatory drug; RLQ, right lower quadrant; RUQ, right upper quadrant; US, ultrasonography; WBC, white blood cell.

BOX 22-1. Important Extraabdominopelvic Causes of Abdominal Pain

Thoracic
Myocardial infarction/unstable angina
Pneumonia
Pulmonary embolism
Herniated thoracic disc (neuralgia)

Genitourinary
Testicular torsion

Abdominal Wall
Muscle spasm
Muscle hematoma
Herpes zoster

Infectious
Strep pharyngitis (more often in children)
Rocky Mountain spotted fever
Mononucleosis

Systemic
Diabetic ketoacidosis
Alcoholic ketoacidosis
Uremia
Sickle cell disease
Porphyria
Systemic lupus erythematosus
Vasculitis
Glaucoma
Hyperthyroidism

Toxic
Methanol poisoning
Heavy metal toxicity
Scorpion bite
Black widow spider bite

Adapted from: Purcell TB: Nonsurgical and extraperitoneal causes of abdominal pain. *Emerg Med Clin North Am* 7:721, 1989.

■ Hindgut structures (distal colon and genitourinary tract) cause lower abdominal pain.

Visceral pain can be perceived in a location remote from the actual disease process. Localization occurs with the extension of the disease process beyond the viscera. A classical example is the early periumbilical pain of appendicitis (midgut). When the parietal peritoneum becomes involved, the pain localizes to the right lower quadrant of the abdomen, the usual location of the appendix.

Somatic pain occurs with irritation of the parietal peritoneum. This is usually caused by infection, chemical irritation, or other inflammatory processes. Sensations are conducted by the peripheral nerves and are

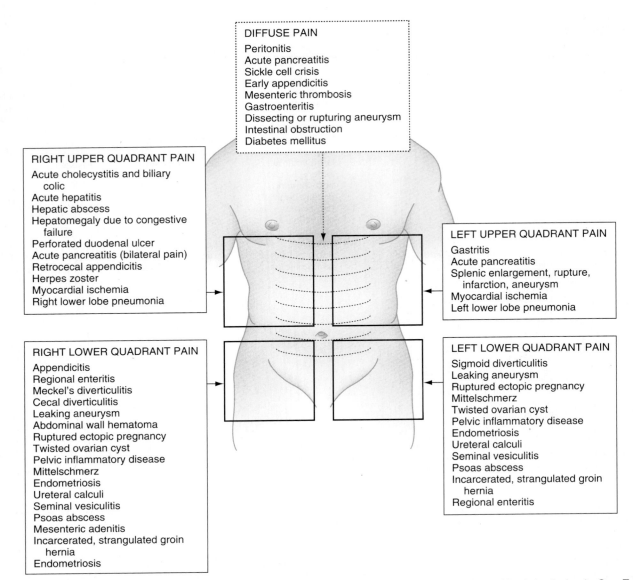

DIFFUSE PAIN

Peritonitis
Acute pancreatitis
Sickle cell crisis
Early appendicitis
Mesenteric thrombosis
Gastroenteritis
Dissecting or rupturing aneurysm
Intestinal obstruction
Diabetes mellitus

RIGHT UPPER QUADRANT PAIN

Acute cholecystitis and biliary
  colic
Acute hepatitis
Hepatic abscess
Hepatomegaly due to congestive
  failure
Perforated duodenal ulcer
Acute pancreatitis (bilateral pain)
Retrocecal appendicitis
Herpes zoster
Myocardial ischemia
Right lower lobe pneumonia

LEFT UPPER QUADRANT PAIN

Gastritis
Acute pancreatitis
Splenic enlargement, rupture,
  infarction, aneurysm
Myocardial ischemia
Left lower lobe pneumonia

RIGHT LOWER QUADRANT PAIN

Appendicitis
Regional enteritis
Meckel's diverticulitis
Cecal diverticulitis
Leaking aneurysm
Abdominal wall hematoma
Ruptured ectopic pregnancy
Twisted ovarian cyst
Pelvic inflammatory disease
Mittelschmerz
Endometriosis
Ureteral calculi
Seminal vesiculitis
Psoas abscess
Mesenteric adenitis
Incarcerated, strangulated groin
  hernia
Endometriosis

LEFT LOWER QUADRANT PAIN

Sigmoid diverticulitis
Leaking aneurysm
Ruptured ectopic pregnancy
Mittelschmerz
Twisted ovarian cyst
Pelvic inflammatory disease
Endometriosis
Ureteral calculi
Seminal vesiculitis
Psoas abscess
Incarcerated, strangulated groin
  hernia
Regional enteritis

Figure 22-1. Differential diagnosis of acute abdominal pain. (From Wagner DK: Approach to the patient with abdominal pain *Curr Top* 1:3, 1978, with permission)

better localized than the visceral pain component. Figure 22-1 illustrates some more typical pain locations corresponding to specific disease entities. Somatic pain is often described as intense and constant. As disease processes evolve to peritoneal irritation with inflammation, better localization of the pain to the area of pathology generally occurs.

Referred pain is defined as pain felt at a distance from its source because peripheral afferent nerve fibers from many internal organs enter the spinal cord through nerve roots that also carry nociceptive fibers from other locations. This makes interpretation of the location of noxious stimuli difficult for the brain. Both visceral pain and somatic pain can manifest as referred pain. Two examples of referred pain are the epigastric pain associated with an inferior myocardial infarction and the shoulder pain associated with blood in the peritoneal cavity irritating the diaphragm.

Gynecologic and obstetric presentations are discussed in other chapters. Notably, any abdominal pain in a female could be referred pain from pelvic structures or an extension of a pelvic process, as in the case of perihepatic inflammation with pelvic inflammatory disease.

DIAGNOSTIC APPROACH

The clinical approach should focus on early stabilization, history, physical examination, and any ancillary tests collectively facilitating appropriate management and disposition plans.

Differential Considerations

Classically, potential diagnoses are divided into intraabdominopelvic (intraperitoneal, retroperitoneal, and pelvic) causes (e.g., appendicitis, cholecystitis, pancreatitis) and extraabdominopelvic processes (e.g., pneumonia, myocardial infarction, ketoacidosis).

Although significant morbidity and mortality can result from many causes of abdominal pain, a few processes warrant careful consideration in the emergency department. Table 22-2 lists the six most important potentially life-threatening nontraumatic causes of abdominal pain. This group represents the major etiologies likely to arise with hemodynamic compromise and for which early therapeutic intervention is critical.

Rapid Assessment and Stabilization

As with any complaint, triage is the first critical step in management. Most patients presenting with abdominal pain do not have hemodynamic instability, but up to 7% of these patients may have a life-threatening process. This percentage is higher in elderly and immunocompromised patients.[1]

Physiologically compromised patients should be brought to a treatment area immediately and resuscitation initiated. Profound shock or protracted emesis can lead to airway compromise and require intubation. Volume repletion, if necessary for the patient's stabilization, is usually accomplished with an isotonic crystalloid solution and titrated to a physiologic endpoint.

Extreme conditions such as ruptured abdominal aortic aneurysm, massive gastrointestinal hemorrhage, ruptured spleen, and hemorrhagic pancreatitis may require blood or blood product replacement. Bedside ultrasonography can be used to establish the presence of free intraperitoneal fluid quite rapidly and can aid in directing the initial stabilization phase. Because all of the immediately life-threatening entities could require surgical intervention or management, early surgical consultation is necessary.

Pivotal Findings

History

A careful and focused history is central to unlocking the puzzle of abdominal pain. Box 22-2 lists some historical questions with high yields for serious pathology. Language and cultural differences may influence accurate communication and mutual understanding.

Abrupt onset is often indicative of a more serious cause; however, delayed presentations may also represent a surgical condition. Surgical causes of abdominal pain are more likely to arise with pain first followed by nausea and vomiting, rather than nausea and vomiting followed by pain. Localization and pain migration are also helpful. Diffuse pain is generally nonsurgical, but it may represent the early visceral component of a surgical process.

The severity and descriptive nature of the pain are the most subjective aspects of the pain history, but there are a few classical descriptions, such as the following:

- The diffuse, severe, colicky pain of bowel obstruction
- The "pain out of proportion to examination" observed in patients with mesenteric ischemia
- The radiation of pain from the epigastrium straight through to the midback associated with pancreatitis,

either related to primary organ inflammation or secondary to a penetrating ulcer

Physical Examination

The objective evaluation begins with measurement of the vital signs. Significant tachycardia and hypotension are indicators that shock may be present. Tachypnea may be an indication of metabolic acidosis from gangrenous viscera or sepsis, hypoxemia from pneumonia, or simply a catecholamine-induced reaction to pain. Elevated temperature is often associated with intraabdominal infections. However, fever does not accurately predict significant abdominal pathology. For example, the temperature is often normal in elderly patients with laparotomy-proven intraperitoneal infections.[4]

The abdomen and pelvis are examined to identify the area of maximal tenderness, anticipating some correspondence with the location of the diseased organ. This can be true, but it is often not the case. Although 80% of suspected appendicitis cases manifest right lower quadrant abdominal tenderness, 20% of patients with proven appendicitis do not.[5]

Rectal examination may have limited use in abdominal pain, except when associated with intraluminal gastrointestinal hemorrhage, prostatitis, and perirectal disease. Its main utility is in the detection of heme-

---

BOX 22-2. High-Yield Historical Questions

1. *How old are you?* Advanced age means increased risk.
2. *Which came first—pain or vomiting?* Pain first is worse (i.e., more likely to be caused by surgical disease).
3. *How long have you had the pain?* Pain for less than 48 hours is worse.
4. *Have you ever had abdominal surgery?* Consider obstruction in patients who report previous abdominal surgery.
5. *Is the pain constant or intermittent?* Constant pain is worse.
6. *Have you ever had this before?* A report of no prior episodes is worse.
7. *Do you have a history of cancer, diverticulosis, pancreatitis, kidney failure, gallstones, or inflammatory bowel disease?* All are suggestive of more serious disease.
8. *Do you have human immunodeficiency virus (HIV)?* Consider occult infection or drug-related pancreatitis.
9. *How much alcohol do you drink per day?* Consider pancreatitis, hepatitis, or cirrhosis.
10. *Are you pregnant?* Test for pregnancy—consider ectopic pregnancy.
11. *Are you taking antibiotics or steroids?* These may mask infection.
12. *Did the pain start centrally and migrate to the right lower quadrant?* High specificity for appendicitis.
13. *Do you have a history of vascular or heart disease, hypertension, or atrial fibrillation?* Consider mesenteric ischemia and abdominal aneurysm.

From Colucciello SA, Lukens TW, Morgan DL: Abdominal pain: An evidence-based approach. *Emerg Med Pract* 1:2, 1999.

Table 22-2. Potentially Life-Threatening Causes of Abdominal Pain

Cause	Epidemiology	Etiology	Presentation	Physical Examination	Useful Tests
Ruptured ectopic pregnancy (critical)	Occurs only in females of childbearing age without bilateral oophorectomy. No method of contraception prevents ectopic pregnancy. Approximately 1 in every 100 pregnancies.	Risk factors include nonwhite race, older age, history of STD or PID, infertility treatment, intrauterine contraceptive device within the last year, tubal sterilization, and previous ectopic pregnancy.	Severe, sharp constant pain localized to the affected side. More diffuse abdominal pain with intraperitoneal hemorrhage. Signs of shock may be present. Midline pain tends not to be ectopic pregnancy.	Shock or evidence of peritonitis may be present. Lateralized abdominal tenderness. Localized adnexal tenderness or cervical motion tenderness increase the likelihood of ectopic pregnancy. Vaginal bleeding does not have to be present.	βHCG testing necessary for all women of childbearing ages (10-55). This combined with ultrasonography, preferably transvaginal, is usually diagnostic. Culdocentesis reserved for circumstances where other more sophisticated testing is not available.
Ruptured or leaking abdominal aneurysm (critical)	Incidence increases with advancing age. More frequent in men. Risk factors include HTN, DM, smoking, COPD, and CAD.	Atherosclerosis in over 95%. Intimal dissection causes aortic dilatation and creation of a false lumen. Leakage or rupture causes shock.	Patient often asymptomatic until rupture. Acute epigastric and back pain often associated with or followed by syncope or signs of shock. Pain may radiate to back, groin, or testes.	Vital signs may be normal (in 70% of patients) to severely hypotensive. Palpation of a pulsatile mass is usually possible in aneurysms 5 cm or greater. If suspected, the physical examination should not be relied on only. CT or US usually indicated. Bruits or inequality of femoral pulses may be evident.	Abdominal plain films abnormal in 80% of cases. Lateral abdominal film may be helpful. Ultrasound can define diameter and length but limited by obesity and gas. Spiral CT test of choice if patient is stable.
Mesenteric ischemia (emergent)	Occurs most commonly in elderly people with CV disease, CHF, cardiac dysrhythmias, DM, sepsis, and dehydration. Responsible for 1 of 1000 hospital admissions. Mortality 70%. Mesenteric venous thrombosis associated with hypercoagulable states, hematologic inflammation, and trauma.	20%–30% of lesions are nonocclusive. The causes of ischemia are multifactorial, including transient hypotension tension in the presence of preexisting atherosclerotic lesion. The arterial occlusive causes (65%) are secondary to emboli (75%) or acute arterial thrombosis (25%).	Severe pain, colicky, that starts in periumbilical region and then becomes diffuse. Often associated with vomiting and diarrhea.	Early examination results can be remarkably benign in the presence of severe ischemia. Bowel sounds often still present. Rectal examination important because mild bleeding with positive guaiac stools can be present.	Often a pronounced leukocytosis is present. Elevations of amylase and creatine phosphokinase levels are seen. Metabolic acidosis due to lactic acidemia is often seen with infarction. Plain films of limited benefit. CT, MRI, and angiography are accurate to varying degrees.
Intestinal obstruction (urgent)	Peaks in infancy and elderly. More common with history of previous abdominal surgery.	Adhesions, carcinoma, hernias, abscesses, volvulus, and infarction. Obstruction leads to vomiting, third spacing of fluid, strangulation, and necrosis of bowel.	Crampy diffuse abdominal pain associated with vomiting.	Vital signs usually normal unless dehydration or bowel strangulation has occurred. Abdominal distention, hyperactive bowel sounds, and diffuse tenderness. Local peritoneal signs indicate strangulation.	WBC count may indicate strangulation if elevated. Electrolytes may be abnormal if associated with vomiting or prolonged symptoms. Abdominal films are useful for identifying level of obstruction. US or CT rarely needed to make diagnosis.

Table 22-2. Potentially Life-Threatening Causes of Abdominal Pain—cont'd

Cause	Epidemiology	Etiology	Presentation	Physical Examination	Useful Tests
Perforated viscus (urgent)	Incidence increases with advancing age. History of peptic ulcer disease or diverticular disease common.	More often a duodenal ulcer that erodes through the serosa. Colonic diverticula, large bowel, small bowel, and gallbladder perforations are rare. Spillage of bowel contents causes peritonitis.	Acute onset of epigastric pain is common. Vomiting in 50%. Fever may be present later. Pain may localize with omental walling off of peritonitis. Shock may be present with bleeding or sepsis.	Fever, usually low grade, is common, higher fever occurs with time. Tachycardia is common. Abdominal examination reveals diffuse guarding and rebound. A "boardlike" abdomen in later stages. Bowel sounds are decreased.	WBC count usually elevated due to peritonitis. Amylase may be elevated as well. LFT results are variable. Upright view of radiographs reveals free air in 70%–80% of cases with perforated ulcers.
Acute pancreatitis (urgent)	Peak age in adulthood. Rare in childhood and elderly. Male preponderance. Alcohol abuse and biliary tract disease are risk factors.	Alcohol, gallstones, hyperlipidemia, hypercalcemia, or endoscopic retrograde pancreatography causes pancreatic damage, saponification, and necrosis. ARDS, sepsis, hemorrhage, and renal failure are secondary.	Acute onset of epigastric pain radiating to the back. Nausea and vomiting common. Pain disproportionate to physical findings. Adequate volume repletion is important in the initial therapy.	Low-grade fever common. Patient may be hypotensive or tachypneic. Some epigastric tenderness usually present. Since retroperitoneal organ, guarding or rebound not present unless severe. Flank ecchymoses may be seen if hemorrhagic.	Lipase is test of choice. Amylase 3× normal more specific for diagnosis. Ultrasound may show edema or pseudocyst. CT scan may show abscesses, necrosis, hemorrhage, or pseudocysts. CT is ordered if severe acute pancreatitis is suspected.

CAD, coronary artery disease; CHF, congestive heart failure; COPD, chronic obstructive pulmonary disease; CV, cardiovascular; DM, diabetes mellitus; HTN, hypertension; PID, pelvic inflammatory disease; STD, sexually transmitted disease.

positive stool. Rectal examination has not been shown to increase diagnostic accuracy for appendicitis when added to external physical examination of the abdomen.[6]

The abdominal evaluation should include a pelvic examination in female patients with lower abdominal pain or an otherwise uncertain diagnosis. Male patients should receive a genital examination as well as evaluation for the presence of inguinal or femoral hernias.

Given the evolving nature of abdominal pain, repetitive examinations may be used. This is common practice with respect to suspected appendicitis and has improved the diagnostic accuracy in patients whose presentations were atypical.[2]

Ancillary Testing

Urinalysis and testing for pregnancy are perhaps the most time- and cost-effective adjunctive laboratory tests available (Table 22-3). Results can often be obtained quickly, so the former can lead to an early diagnosis and the latter may significantly affect further evaluation and management approaches. It is necessary to interpret urinalysis results within the entire spectrum of the patient's clinical picture. Pyuria, with or without bacteriuria, is often present in a variety of conditions besides a simple urinary tract infection. Hematuria can also be misleading. Up to 30% of patients with appendicitis have an abnormal urinalysis.[7]

Complete blood counts are frequently ordered for patients with abdominal pain. Despite elevated white blood cell (WBC) counts being associated with many infectious and inflammatory processes, the WBC count is neither sufficiently sensitive nor specific to be considered a discriminatory test to help establish the cause of the abdominal pain. Even serial WBC counts have failed to differentiate surgical versus nonsurgical conditions. The WBC count is, therefore, not helpful for diagnosis. Serum electrolytes, even in the presence of protracted emesis or diarrhea, are abnormal in less than 1% of patients. These studies are not indicated for most patients in the absence of another indication. Blood urea nitrogen concentrations can be elevated in gastrointestinal hemorrhage and dehydration, but such conditions are better detected and quantified by history and physical examination. Increased serum creatinine is usually indicative of renal dysfunction. Blood glucose, anion gap, and serum ketone determinations are useful in diabetic ketoacidosis, one cause of acute abdominal pain and tachypnea.

Liver enzymes and coagulation studies are helpful only in a small subset of patients with suspected liver disease.[8] If pancreatitis is suspected, the most useful diagnostic result is serum lipase elevated to at least double the normal value because it is more specific and more sensitive than serum amylase for this process. There is no value to obtaining a serum amylase if a serum lipase level is available.[9] Serum phosphate

Table 22-3. Diagnostic Studies for Common Abdominal Presentations

Common Testing	CBC	Lytes	UA	Plain Films	U/S	CT Scan	Other
Abdominal aortic aneurysm	A		A		Y	Y	Angiography, MR imaging*
Appendicitis	Y		A		Y	Y	C-reactive protein
Biliary tract disease	A		A		Y*	Y	HIDA scan
Bowel obstruction, perforation	A		A	Y*	Y	Y	
Cholecystitis	A		A		Y*	Y	
Diverticulitis	A		A		Y	Y	Barium enema
Ectopic pregnancy	A		A		Y*		HCG, progesterone
Gastroenteritis	Y	Y	A				Fecal leukocytes
Hernia			A				Physical examination
Intestinal infarction/ischemia	A		A	A		Y	Angiography, ECG, MR imaging
Ovarian torsion	Y		A		Y		Doppler ultrasound
Pancreatitis	A		A		Y	Y	Lipase*, amylase
Pelvic inflammatory disease	Y		A		A		ESR, CRP
Pyelonephritis	Y		Y				
Renal colic	A	Y	Y		A	Y	Helical CT, IVP
Testicular torsion			Y		Y		Doppler, nuclear scan
Urinary tract infection	Y		Y*			A	

*Diagnostic test of choice to detect the particular disease entity.
A, helpful adjunct to testing for disease but not necessarily indicated; Y, indicated for establishing diagnosis.
CT, computed tomography; CRP, C-reactive protein; ECG, electrocardiogram; ESR, erythrocyte sedimentation rate; hCG, human chorionic gonadotropin; HIDA, hepatoiminodiacetic acid; IVP, intravenous pyelography; MR, magnetic resonance.
From Gaff LG, Robinson D: Abdominal pain and the emergency department evaluation. Emerg Med Clin North Am 19(1), 2001.

and serum lactate levels are elevated late in bowel ischemia and may be useful if this entity is suspected but cannot be considered either sufficiently sensitive or specific to establish or exclude the diagnosis on their own.

Plain radiography of the abdomen has limited utility in the evaluation of acute abdominal pain. Suspected bowel obstruction, foreign body, and perforated viscus are the main indications. Helical computed tomography of the abdomen has become the imaging modality of choice with respect to nonobstetric abdominal pain. It allows visualization of both intraperitoneal and extraperitoneal structures and has a high degree of accuracy, establishing a diagnosis in more than 95% of cases in one study[10] and increasing the confidence of diagnosis in another.[11] In the elderly subpopulation, computed tomography results changed management or disposition decisions in a significant proportion of patients.[12]

Transabdominal and transvaginal ultrasonography have emerged as extremely useful adjuncts. Bedside emergency department ultrasonography applications with utility in life-threatening abdominopelvic processes include the following:

- Identification of an intrauterine pregnancy, effectively lowering the chances of an ectopic pregnancy to less than 1 in 20,000
- Measurement of the cross-sectional diameter of the infrarenal aorta to determine whether an abdominal aortic aneurysm exists
- Detection of free intraperitoneal fluid indicating hemorrhage, pus, or extrusion of gut contents

Uses as a diagnostic aid in non–life-threatening conditions include the following:

- Detection of gallstones or a dilated common bile duct, which may aid in diagnosis of cholecystitis
- Detection of free intraperitoneal fluid indicating ascites

The results of sonographic examinations are operator dependent and misdiagnosis can occur because of failure to detect or identify pathology, incorrect identification of normal anatomy as pathologic, and over-interpretation of correctly identified findings (e.g., the mere presence of gallstones does not indicate that cholelithiasis is the etiology of the pain).

DIFFERENTIAL DIAGNOSIS

A simple algorithmic approach to acute abdominal pain is difficult, given the broad range of potential etiologies. The differential considerations include a significant number of potentially life- or organ-threatening entities, particularly in the setting of a hemodynamically unstable or toxic-appearing patient. This is particularly important when dealing with elderly or potentially pregnant patients (see Tables 22-1 and 22-2).

Traditionally, despite the limitations already described, the approach to the differential diagnosis of abdominal pain is based on the location of maximal tenderness. Figure 22-1 shows locations of subjective pain and maximal tenderness on palpation related to various underlying causes.

Women of reproductive age should undergo pregnancy testing early, and a known pregnancy or a positive urine or serum pregnancy test in the emergency department should be considered to represent an ectopic pregnancy until proved otherwise. If evidence of blood loss is present, early obstetric consultation and diagnostic ultrasonography should be promptly sought. Bedside, transabdominal sonography may identify free intraperitoneal fluid during the evaluation of shock, which may be sufficient evidence to justify operative intervention in the context of a positive pregnancy test and appropriate history and physical findings.

In patients who are hemodynamically normal and stable, including women with a negative pregnancy test, the diagnostic algorithm then proceeds to identify the general region of the abdomen that contains the point of maximal tenderness. In the hemodynamically stable patient, a positive pregnancy test may indicate ectopic pregnancy, but the entire spectrum of intraabdominal conditions remains in the differential diagnosis, as for the nonpregnant patient. When the very broad differential list is compartmentalized by both history and physical examination, ancillary testing should proceed to either confirm or support the clinical suspicion. Table 22-3 lists the ancillary tests used in the evaluation of specific causes of abdominal pain.

Despite the significant variety of tests available, close to one half of the patients presenting to the emergency department with acute abdominal pain have no conclusive diagnosis. It is incumbent upon the clinician to reconsider the extraabdominal causes of abdominal pain (see Box 22-1), with special consideration for the elderly and the immunocompromised patient subsets, before arriving at the diagnosis of "nonspecific abdominal pain."

EMPIRICAL MANAGEMENT

The main therapeutic goals in managing acute abdominal pain are physiologic stabilization, mitigation of symptoms (e.g., emesis control, pain relief), and expeditious diagnosis, with consultation, if required (Figure 22-2).

Gastric emptying by nasogastric tube with suction is appropriate for suspected small bowel obstruction. Antiemetics, such as promethazine or trimethobenzamide, can be useful for intractable vomiting, but they can also cause mental status changes in some patients. Granisetron and ondansetron are alternative antiemetics with less potential for mental status changes, but these agents are more expensive.

If intraabdominal infection is suspected, broad-spectrum antibiotic therapy should be initiated promptly. Abdominal infections are often polymicrobial and coverage for enteric gram-negative, gram-positive, and anaerobic bacteria must be included. In the choice of antibiotic or combination, the following should be considered:

- Unless local antibiotic resistance surveillance indicates otherwise, second-generation cephalosporins (e.g., cefamandole, cefotetan, cefoxitin) may be combined with metronidazole for the initial dose of antibiotics in the emergency department. Other noncephalosporin, β-lactam agents with β-lactamase antagonists (e.g., ampicillin-sulbactam, piperacillin-tazobactam, ticarcillin-clavulanate) are alternatives.

- Many enteric gram-negative bacilli mutate rapidly to produce β-lactamases that are poorly antagonized by specific drug combinations containing clavulanate, sulbactam, or tazobactam. A carbapenem (e.g., imipenem, meropenem) or cefepime is an alternative for patients who may have recently received other antibiotics.[5,13]

The need to cover *Enterococcus* species is still a subject of debate, and the decision to treat these bacteria specifically can be made after consultation. Immunocompromised patients may require antifungal agents.

There is no evidence to support withholding analgesics for patients with acute abdominal pain to prevent potentially limiting the effectiveness of subsequent physical examinations by consultants not present in the emergency department. Pain relief may facilitate the diagnosis in patients ultimately requiring surgery.[14-16] In the acute setting, analgesia is usually accomplished with intravenously titrated opioids. Meperidine (Demerol) has an unfavorable side-effect profile and should be avoided. Intravenous ketorolac, the only parenteral nonsteroidal anti-inflammatory drug available in North America, is useful for both ureteral and biliary colic,[17,18] as well as some gynecologic conditions, but is not indicated for general treatment of undifferentiated abdominal pain. Relative to patients with gastrointestinal hemorrhage and potential surgical candidates, ketorolac has been shown to increase bleeding times in healthy volunteers.[19]

Aside from analgesics, a variety of other medications may be helpful to patients with abdominal pain. The burning pain caused by gastric acid may be relieved by antacids.[20] Intestinal cramping may be diminished with oral anticholinergic agents such as atropine-scopolamine-hyoscyamine-phenobarbital (Donnatal).

DISPOSITION

Because up to 40% of patients presenting with acute abdominal pain receive the diagnosis of nonspecific abdominal pain, the dispositions of patients with abdominal pain can be as difficult as their diagnoses. Categories for disposition may include surgical versus nonsurgical consultation and management, admission for observation, and discharge to home with follow-up evaluation.[21] The decision to admit a patient to an observation unit or a hospital bed must factor in the following:

- Information gained from the history, physical examination, and test results
- The likelihood of any suspected disease
- Any potential ramifications, if a known disease progresses or the patient is incorrectly diagnosed or managed
- Whether follow-up evaluation can occur in a timely manner if the patient is discharged home

Clinically stable patients may be discharged from the emergency department with appropriate follow-up

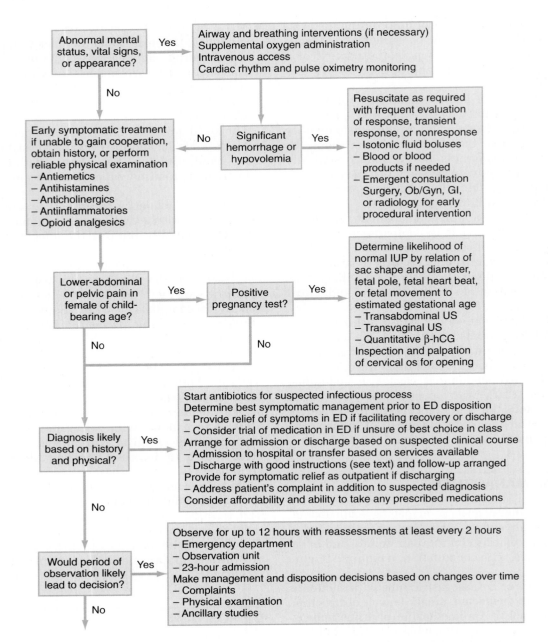

Figure 22-2. Management algorithm for acute abdominal pain. β-hCG, β subunit of human chorionic gonadotropin; ED, emergency department; EMTALA, Emergency Medical Treatment and Active Labor Act; GI, gastroenterology; IUP, intrauterine pregnancy; Ob/Gyn, obstetrics and gynecology; US, ultrasonography.

care, possibly to include repeated or additional diagnostic imaging.

In the case of nonspecific abdominal pain that is considered potentially worrisome, it is prudent to have the patient reevaluated after 8 to 12 hours. This can be done through a return visit to the emergency department, an appointment with a primary care physician, or an observation unit protocol.

If a patient is to be discharged home without a specific diagnosis, clear instructions to the patient must include the following information:

- What the patient has to do to improve his or her symptoms or chances of resolving the condition

(e.g., avoiding exacerbating food or activities, taking medications as prescribed)

- Under what circumstances, with whom, and in what time frame to seek follow-up evaluation, if all goes as desired on the basis of what is known when the patient is in the emergency department

- Under what conditions the patient should seek more urgent care, if there are unexpected changes in his or her condition (e.g., natural progression of the process before improvement, incorrect diagnosis made in the emergency department, untoward reactions to medications)

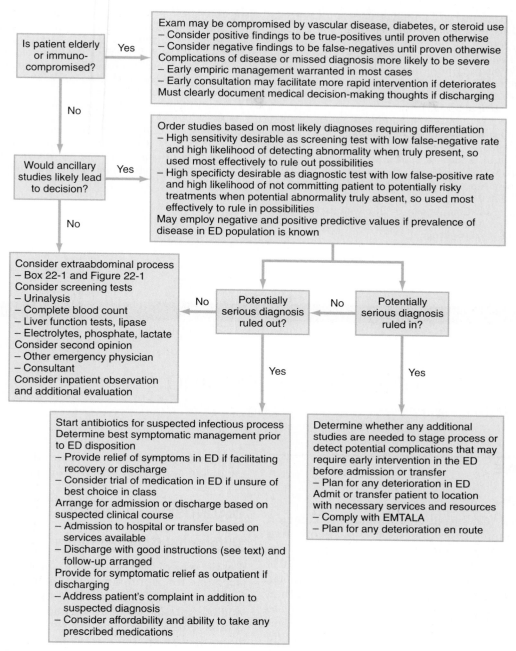

Figure 22-2, cont'd.

REFERENCES

1. Powers RD, Guertler AT: Abdominal pain in the ED: Stability and change over 20 years. *Am J Emerg Med* 13: 301, 1995.
2. Sanson TG, O'Keefe KP: Evaluation of abdominal pain in the elderly. *Emerg Med Clin North Am* 14:615, 1996.
3. Dart RG, Kaplan B, Varaklis K: Predictive value of history and physical examination in patients with suspected ectopic pregnancy. *Ann Emerg Med* 33:283, 1999.
4. Cooper GS, Shales DM, Salata RA: Intraabdominal infection: Differences in presentation and outcome between younger patients and the elderly. *Clin Infect Dis* 19:146, 1994.
5. Wagner JM, McKinney WP, Carpenter JL: Does this patient have appendicitis? *JAMA* 276:1589, 1996.
6. Dixon JM, et al: Rectal examination in patients with pain in the right lower quadrant of the abdomen. *BMJ* 302:386, 1991.
7. Scott JH, et al: Abnormal urinalysis in appendicitis. *J Urol* 129:1015, 1983.
8. Chase CW, et al: Serum amylase and lipase in the evaluation of acute abdominal pain. *Am Surg* 62:1028, 1996.
9. Pratt DS, Kaplan MM: Evaluation of abnormal liver-enzyme results in asymptomatic patients. *N Engl J Med* 342:1266, 2000.
10. Gore RM, et al: Helical CT in the evaluation of the acute abdomen. *AJR Am J Roentgenol* 174:901, 2000.
11. Rosen MP, et al: Impact of abdominal CT on the management of patients presenting to the emergency department with acute abdominal pain. *AJR Am J Roentgenol* 174:1391, 2000.

12. Esses D, et al: Ability of CT to alter decision making in elderly patients with acute abdominal pain. *Am J Emerg Med* 22:270, 2004.
13. Johnson CC, Baldessare J, Levison ME: Peritonitis: Update on pathophysiology, clinical manifestations, and management. *Clin Infect Dis* 24:1035, 1997.
14. Attard AR, et al: Safety of early pain relief for acute abdominal pain. *BMJ* 305:554, 1992.
15. Pace S, Burke TF: Intravenous morphine for early pain relief in patients with acute abdominal pain. *Acad Emerg Med* 3:1086, 1996.
16. Thomas SH, et al: Effects of morphine analgesia on diagnostic accuracy in emergency department patients with abdominal pain: A prospective, randomized trial. *J Am Coll Surg* 196:18, 2003.
17. Cordell WH, et al: Comparison of intravenous ketorolac, meperidine, and both (balanced analgesia) for renal colic. *Ann Emerg Med* 28:151, 1996.
18. Henderson SO, et al: Comparison of intravenous ketorolac and meperidine in the treatment of biliary colic. *J Emerg Med* 23:237, 2002.
19. Singer AJ, et al: The effect of IM ketorolac tromethamine on bleeding time: A prospective, interventional, controlled study. *Am J Emerg Med* 21:441, 2003.
20. Berman DA, et al: The GI cocktail is no more effective than plain liquid antacid: A randomized, double blind clinical trial. *J Emerg Med* 25:239, 2003.
21. American College of Emergency Physicians: Clinical policy: Critical issues for the initial evaluation and management of patients presenting with a chief complaint of nontraumatic abdominal pain. *Ann Emerg Med* 36:406, 2000.

CHAPTER

23 Gastrointestinal Bleeding

Philip L. Henneman

PERSPECTIVE

Epidemiology

Gastrointestinal (GI) bleeding is a relatively common problem encountered in emergency medicine that requires early consultation and often admission. The overall mortality of GI bleeding is approximately 10% and has not changed significantly since the 1960s. Diagnostic modalities have improved much more than therapeutic techniques. GI bleeding is often easy to identify when there is clear evidence of vomiting blood or passing blood in the stool, but it may present subtly with signs and symptoms of hypovolemia, such as dizziness, weakness, or syncope.

The approach to GI bleeding depends on whether the hemorrhage is located in the proximal or distal segments of the GI tract (i.e., upper or lower GI bleeding). These segments are defined by the ligament of Treitz in the fourth section of the duodenum. In the United States, upper GI bleeding (UGIB) affects 50 to 150 people per 100,000 population each year and results in 250,000 admissions at an estimated annual cost of almost $1 billion. Lower GI bleeding (LGIB) affects a smaller portion of patients and results in proportionally fewer hospital admissions than UGIB.

GI bleeding can occur in individuals of any age, but most commonly affects people in their 40s through 70s (mean age 59 years). Most deaths caused by GI bleeding occur in patients older than age 60 years. UGIB is more common in men than women (2:1), whereas LGIB is more common in women. Significant UGIB requiring admission is more common in adults, whereas LGIB requiring admission is more common in children.[1]

DIAGNOSTIC APPROACH

Differential Considerations

Peptic ulcer disease, gastric erosions, and varices account for approximately three fourths of adult patients with UGIB (Box 23-1). Diverticulosis and angiodysplasia account for approximately 80% of adults with LGIB. Esophagitis, gastritis, and peptic ulcer disease are the most common causes of UGIB in children, and infectious colitis and inflammatory bowel disease are the most common causes of LGIB in children (Box 23-2). In children younger than age 2 years, massive LGIB is most often a result of Meckel's diverticulum or intussusception. At all ages, anorectal abnormalities are the most common cause of minor LGIB. Despite improved diagnostic techniques, no source of bleeding is identified in approximately 10% of patients with GI bleeding. Patients who have abdominal aortic grafts who present to the emergency department with GI bleeding should receive prompt surgical consultation in the emergency department for the possibility of aortoenteric fistula.

Rapid Assessment and Stabilization

Most patients with GI bleeding are easy to diagnose because they present to the emergency department complaining of vomiting blood or passing black or

BOX 23-1. Etiology of Significant Gastrointestinal (GI) Bleeding in Adults*

Upper	Lower
Peptic ulcer disease	Upper GI bleeding
Gastric erosions	Diverticulosis
Varices	Angiodysplasia
Mallory-Weiss tear	Cancer/polyps
Esophagitis	Rectal disease
Duodenitis	Inflammatory bowel disease

*Listed in decreasing frequency.

BOX 23-2. Etiology of Gastrointestinal Bleeding in Children*

Upper	Lower
Esophagitis	Anal fissure
Gastritis	Infectious colitis
Ulcer	Inflammatory bowel
Esophageal varices	Polyps
Mallory-Weiss	Intussusception

*Listed in decreasing frequency.

bloody stool. The diagnosis is confirmed quickly by examination of the stool for the presence of blood.

Patients with suspected GI bleeding who are hemodynamically unstable should undergo rapid evaluation and resuscitation. They should be undressed quickly, placed on cardiac and oxygen saturation monitors, and given supplemental oxygen as needed. At least two large-bore peripheral intravenous lines should be placed (minimum 18-gauge); blood should be drawn for hemoglobin or hematocrit, platelet count, prothrombin time (PT), and type and screen or type and crossmatch; and crystalloid resuscitation should be initiated. Intravenous crystalloid fluid should be given as a 2-L bolus in adults or 20 mL/kg in children until the patient's vital signs have stabilized or the patient has received 40 mL/kg of crystalloid. Patients who remain unstable after 40 mL/kg of crystalloid should be given type O, type-specific, or crossmatched blood depending on availability. Persistently unstable patients should receive immediate consultation—patients with UGIB with a gastroenterologist and surgeon and patients with LGIB with a surgeon.[2]

Pivotal Findings

History, physical examination, testing stool for blood, and measuring hemoglobin or hematocrit are the keys to diagnosing GI bleeding in most patients.

History

Patients usually complain of vomiting red blood or coffee ground–like material or passing black or bloody stool. *Hematemesis* (vomiting blood) occurs with bleeding of the esophagus, stomach, or proximal small bowel. Approximately 50% of patients with UGIB present with this complaint. Hematemesis may be bright red or darker (i.e., coffee ground–like) as a result of conversion of hemoglobin to hematin or other pigments by hydrochloric acid in the stomach. The color of vomited or aspirated blood from the stomach cannot be used to determine if the bleeding is arterial or venous in nature.

Melena, or black tarry stool, occurs from approximately 150 to 200 mL of blood in the GI tract for a prolonged period. Melena is present in approximately 70% of patients with UGIB and a third of patients with LGIB.

Black stool that is not tarlike may result from 60 mL of blood from the upper GI tract. Blood from the duodenum or jejunum must remain in the GI tract for approximately 8 hours before turning black. Occasionally, black stool may follow bleeding into the lower portion of the small bowel and ascending colon. Stool may remain black and tarry for several days, even though bleeding has stopped. Black stool also may be seen after ingestion of bismuth (e.g., Pepto-Bismol), which can confuse the situation because it is often taken for UGI distress. In contrast to melena, stool rendered black by bismuth is not positive on Hemoccult testing.

Hematochezia, or bloody stool (bright red or maroon), most often signifies LGIB, but may be due to brisk UGIB with rapid transit time through the bowel. Because UGIB is much more common than LGIB, a more proximal source of significant bleeding must be excluded before assuming the bleeding is from the lower GI tract. Approximately two thirds of patients with LGIB present with red blood per rectum. Small amounts of red blood (e.g., 5 mL) from rectal bleeding, such as bleeding due to hemorrhoids, may cause the water in the toilet bowl to appear bright red. Bright red stools also can be seen after ingestion of a large quantity of beets, but Hemoccult testing would be negative.

When taking the history, specific questions should address the duration and quantity of bleeding, associated symptoms, previous history of bleeding, current medications, alcohol, nonsteroidal anti-inflammatory drug and long-term aspirin ingestion, allergies, associated medical illnesses, previous surgery, treatment by prehospital personnel, and the response to that treatment.[3,4] Patients with GI bleeding may complain of symptoms of hypovolemia, such as dizziness, weakness, or loss of consciousness, most often after standing up. Other nonspecific complaints include dyspnea, confusion, and abdominal pain. Rarely an elderly patient may present with ischemic chest pain from significant anemia. One in five patients with GI bleeding may have only nonspecific complaints.

History is of limited help in predicting the site or quantity of bleeding. Patients with a previously documented GI lesion bleed from the same site in only 60% of cases. Gross estimates of blood loss based on the volume and color of the vomitus or stool (e.g., brown or black, pink or red) or the number of episodes of hemorrhage are notoriously inaccurate.

Physical Examination

Vital Signs

Vital signs and postural changes in heart rate have been used to assess the amount of blood loss in patients with GI bleeding but are notoriously insensitive and nonspecific, with the exception of significant, sustained heart rate increase. All patients with a history suggesting GI bleeding who are hypotensive, are tachycardic, or have sustained postural changes of greater than 20 beats/min in heart rate should be assumed to have significant hemorrhage. Normal vital signs do not exclude significant hemorrhage, however, and postural changes in heart rate and blood pressure may occur in individuals who are not bleeding (e.g., elderly people, many normal individuals, individuals with hypovolemia from other causes).

General Examination

The physical examination is valuable in making the diagnosis and assessing the severity of blood loss and a patient's response to that loss. Careful attention is given to the patient's general appearance, vital signs, mental status (including restlessness), skin signs (e.g., color, warmth, and moisture to assess for shock and lesions such as telangiectasia, bruises, or petechiae to assess for vascular diseases or hypocoagulable states), pulmonary and cardiac findings, abdominal examination, and rectal and stool examination. Frequent reassessment is important because a patient's status may change quickly.

Rectal Examination

Rectal and stool examination are often key to making or confirming the diagnosis of GI bleeding. The finding of red, black, or melenic stool early in the assessment is helpful in prompting early recognition and management of patients with GI bleeding. The absence of black or bloody stool does not exclude the diagnosis of GI bleeding. Regardless of the apparent character and color of the stool, occult blood testing is indicated.

Ancillary Testing

Tests for Occult Blood

The presence of hemoglobin in occult amounts in stool is confirmed by tests such as guaiac (e.g., Hemoccult) Stool tests for occult blood may have positive results 14 days after a single, major episode of UGIB. False-positive results have been associated with ingestion of red fruits and meats, methylene blue, chlorophyll, iodide, cupric sulfate, and bromide preparations. False-negative results are uncommon but can be caused by bile or ingestion of magnesium-containing antacids or ascorbic acid. Tests to evaluate gastric contents for occult blood (e.g., Gastroccult) can be unreliable and should not be used for this purpose. In newborns, maternal blood that is swallowed may cause bloody stools; the Apt test may show that it is maternal in origin.

Clinical Laboratory Tests

Blood should be drawn for evaluation of baseline hematocrit or hemoglobin, coagulation studies (PT and platelet count), and type and crossmatch (or type and screen if the patient is stable). Hematocrit and hemoglobin are clinically useful tests that may be obtained at the patient's bedside, but they have significant limitations. The initial hematocrit may be misleading in patients with preexisting anemia or polycythemia. Changes in the hematocrit may lag significantly behind actual blood loss. Infusion of normal saline speeds equilibration of the hematocrit; however, rapid infusion of crystalloid in nonbleeding patients also may cause a decrease in hematocrit by hemodilution. The optimal hematocrit with respect to oxygen-carrying capacity and viscosity in critically ill patients has been reported to be 33%. In general, patients with hemoglobin of 8 g/dL or less (hematocrit <25%) from acute blood loss usually require blood therapy. After transfusion and in the absence of ongoing blood loss, the hematocrit can be expected to increase approximately 3% for each unit of blood administered (hemoglobin increases by 1 mg/dL).

PT should be used to determine whether a patient has a preexisting coagulopathy. An elevated PT may indicate vitamin K deficiency, liver dysfunction, warfarin therapy, or consumptive coagulopathy. Patients receiving therapeutic anticoagulants or patients with an elevated PT and evidence of active bleeding should receive sufficient fresh frozen plasma to correct the PT. Serial platelet counts are used to determine the need for platelet transfusions (i.e., if <50,000/mm^3).

Blood Bank

Blood should be sent for type and hold or type and crossmatch early in the patient's care. Immediate transfusion needs in unstable patients can be met with O-positive packed red blood cells (O-negative packed red blood cells in women of childbearing age whose Rh status is unknown). Within 10 to 15 minutes, type-specific blood is usually available. Group O and type-specific blood are safe for patients and result in few transfusion reactions. Fully crossmatched blood may take 60 minutes to prepare. Stable patients can be managed more cost-effectively by ordering "type and hold" for several units of blood.

Other Laboratory Tests

Determination of electrolytes, blood urea nitrogen, and creatinine may be useful in a small percentage of patients with GI bleeding when indicated. Electrolytes usually are normal in patients with GI bleeding. Patients with repeated vomiting may develop hypokalemia, hyponatremia, and metabolic alkalosis, which usually correct with adequate hydration and resolution of vomiting. Patients with shock often have metabolic acidosis from lactate accumulation. The blood urea nitrogen is elevated in many patients with UGIB as a result of the absorption of blood from the GI tract and hypovolemia causing prerenal azotemia. After 24 hours, hypovolemia is probably the sole determinant of azotemia unless there has been recurrent bleeding.

Electrocardiogram

An electrocardiogram should be obtained on all patients older than age 50; patients with preexisting ischemic cardiac disease; patients with significant anemia; and all patients with chest pain, shortness of breath, or severe hypotension. Asymptomatic myocardial ischemia (ST segment depression >1 mm) or injury (ST segment elevation >1 mm) may develop in the setting of GI bleeding. Patients with GI bleeding and clinical or electrocardiogram evidence of myocardial ischemia should receive packed red blood cells as soon as they are available and appropriate treatment for ischemia.

Imaging

GI hemorrhage is not an indication for plain abdominal radiography. An upright chest radiograph should be performed in patients with UGIB suspected of aspiration or with signs and symptoms of bowel perforation (shock with significant abdominal/peritoneal tenderness). Subdiaphragmatic air consistent with bowel perforation is a rare finding with UGIB, but it is an indication for immediate surgical consultation and operative repair.

DIFFERENTIAL DIAGNOSIS

Not all patients complaining of vomiting blood or passing blood in the stool have GI bleeding. Swallowing blood from the nose or oral cavity may cause hematemesis or melena. Red vomitus may be due to food products (e.g., Jell-O, tomato sauce, wine), and black stool may be due to iron therapy or bismuth (e.g., Pepto-Bismol). Hypovolemia (and its symptoms) may be due to vomiting and diarrhea without bleeding. Poor oral intake with or without fever also may result in hypovolemia. Usually the patient's hemoglobin or hematocrit is normal or elevated until hemodilution can occur. There are many causes of anemia other than GI bleeding, and the absence of suggestive symptoms or blood in the stool makes GI bleeding less likely the cause.[2]

MANAGEMENT

Quick identification, aggressive resuscitation, risk stratification, and prompt consultation are the keys to appropriate emergency management. When the diagnosis of GI bleeding is made, emergency management of patients can proceed (Figure 23-1).

Reassurance

Patients who present to the emergency department with symptoms and signs of GI bleeding are often frightened. They may be concerned about the possibility of painful procedures and of the real or perceived risk of death. These patients and their families should

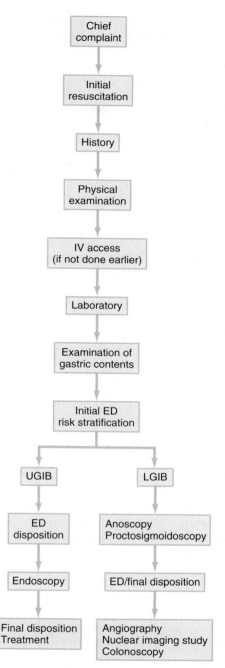

Figure 23-1. Emergency management of patients with gastrointestinal bleeding. IV, intravenous; UGIB, upper gastrointestinal bleeding; LGIB, lower gastrointestinal bleeding; ED, emergency department.

be treated in a supportive and reassuring manner. They should be provided with accurate information about their problem, and all aspects of the care they are receiving should be explained in a way that they understand.

Nasogastric Tube and Gastric Lavage

After initial resuscitation of the patient, it is important to identify whether the hemorrhage is proximal or distal to the ligament of Treitz (i.e., UGIB or LGIB). If the patient's vomitus can be inspected for blood or has been reported by the patient as bloody or "coffee grounds" or if melenic stool is present, an upper GI bleed should be the first consideration. Placement of a nasogastric tube is generally not necessary and rarely yields information that is independently useful for either diagnosis or risk stratifications. Aspiration of bloody contents diagnoses UGIB (or bleeding from nasal or oral passageways), but it does not differentiate if the bleeding is ongoing or has already stopped. There is a 10% incidence of failure to aspirate blood in established UGIB. False-negative results may occur if the bleeding is intermittent or has already stopped and the stomach cleared or if the bleeding is in the duodenum, and edema or spasm of the pylorus has prevented reflux of blood into the stomach. The presence of bile in an otherwise clear aspirate excludes the possibility of active bleeding above the ligament of Treitz, but is rarely seen and should not be used to exclude UGIB in a patient with documented melena. False-positive results may occur from nasal bleeding. Gastric contents should not be tested for occult blood because visual inspection of the vomitus or aspirate is insufficient to diagnose subtle bleeding, and testing is unreliable. In patients who have hematochezia, an upper GI origin for the bleeding is often associated with signs and symptoms of shock because rapid transit time of large quantities of blood is producing the hematochezia. Because up to 11% of patients with hematochezia have UGIB, a nasogastric tube is indicated in most cases of LGIB.[1,5] If the gastric aspirate does not appear bloody, the nasogastric tube should be removed, LGIB should be considered, and anoscopy/proctosigmoidoscopy performed.

Gastric tubes are safe in most patients, but pharyngeal and esophageal perforation, cardiac arrest, ethmoid sinus fracture with brain trauma, and bronchial intubation have been reported. Care must be exercised in placing gastric tubes only in patients in whom they are clearly indicated and ensuring optimal location. The old approach of placing a nasogastric tube in all patients with suspected UGIB predated endoscopy and has no place in modern emergency medicine. No evidence exists that gastric tube placement aggravates hemorrhage from varices or Mallory-Weiss tears.

Gastric lavage may be necessary to prepare a patient for endoscopy. Before gastric lavage, patients with evidence of a possible perforated viscus (e.g., severe pain, peritoneal signs) should undergo radiologic assessment looking for free air. Lavage should not be performed in the presence of pneumoperitoneum. Gastric lavage does not reduce blood loss in patients with UGIB, and iced lavage is not recommended. Gastric lavage, in preparation for endoscopy, is best performed with a large-bore Ewald tube, passed orally while the patient is in the left lateral decubitus position with the bed in Trendelenburg position. Additional holes may be cut in the distal portion of the Ewald tube to improve aspiration of blood and clots. Clots that cannot be aspirated continue to cause pink return and give the false impression of continued bleeding. The irrigant need not be sterile; regular tap water may be used. The irrigant should be delivered and removed by gravity in volumes of 200 to 300 mL until the return is clear. Little irrigant is absorbed by the patient. Gastric rupture has been reported as a rare complication of gastric lavage.[6,7]

Anoscopy/Proctosigmoidoscopy

Patients with mild rectal bleeding who do not have obviously bleeding hemorrhoids should have anoscopy/proctosigmoidoscopy performed. If bleeding internal hemorrhoids are discovered, and the patient does not have portal hypertension, the patient may be discharged with appropriate treatment and follow-up evaluation for hemorrhoids. If hemorrhoids are not detected, it is important to determine if the stool above the rectum contains blood. The absence of blood above the rectum in a patient who is actively bleeding indicates that the source of bleeding is in the rectum. The presence of blood above the anoscope or sigmoidoscope does not invariably indicate a proximal source of bleeding because retrograde passage of blood into the more proximal colon commonly occurs. Such patients need further evaluation.

Endoscopy

Endoscopy is the most accurate diagnostic tool available for the evaluation of UGIB. It identifies a lesion in 78% to 95% of patients with UGIB if it is performed within 12 to 24 hours of the hemorrhage. Accurate identification of the bleeding site allows for risk stratification with respect to predicting rebleeding and mortality. Endoscopy-based triage significantly reduces hospitalization rates and costs of treating upper GI bleeding.[8] Significant advances in endoscopic hemostasis also make it of therapeutic value in select patients (e.g., banding or sclerosing of varices). Colonoscopy is an effective tool for diagnosis and selected treatment of LGIB.[9]

Angiography

Angiography can detect the location of UGIB in two thirds of patients studied. Since the advent of endoscopy, however, the use of angiography has decreased significantly, and today angiography is used in only 1% of patients with UGIB. Angiography is used more commonly in patients with LGIB and usually in consultation with a general surgeon. Although angiography rarely diagnoses the cause of bleeding, it does identify the site of bleeding in approximately 40% of patients who have LGIB and 65% of patients who eventually require surgical intervention. Angiography ideally is performed during active bleeding; this may be apparent by persistently unstable vital signs or continued transfusion requirements to establish or maintain an optimal hemoglobin or hematocrit level. Arterial embolization can be used in selected cases of LGIB.[10]

Gastric Acid Secretion Inhibition

All patients with documented peptic ulcer disease should be treated with a proton-pump inhibitor (e.g., omeprazole).[11] There is no benefit to initiating this therapy or administering H_2 antihistamines in the emergency department for patients with UGIB. When the diagnosis of peptic ulcer has been confirmed by endoscopy, it is appropriate to start a proton-pump inhibitor. Medical therapy is an adjunct, not a substitute for endoscopic evaluation, as appropriate.

Octreotide (Somatostatin Analogues)

Patients with documented esophageal varices should be treated with an intravenous infusion of octreotide at 50 µg/hr for a minimum of 24 hours while being observed in the intensive care unit (ICU). It is a useful addition to endoscopic sclerotherapy and decreases rebleeding occurrences.[12,13]

Vasopressin

Intravenous vasopressin has been used in the treatment of patients with UGIB, most commonly in patients with variceal hemorrhage. Controlled studies have not shown a positive effect of vasopressin on overall mortality, however. These results, combined with a relatively high rate of serious complications (9% major and 3% fatal), suggest that use of vasopressin should be limited. A trial of vasopressin may be warranted in an exsanguinating patient with suspected variceal bleeding, especially if endoscopy is unavailable. The recommended dose of vasopressin is 20 U IV over 20 minutes, then 0.2-0.4 unit/min. Consultation with a gastroenterologist is advisable.

Sengstaken-Blakemore Tube

The Sengstaken-Blakemore tube stops hemorrhage in approximately 80% of patients bleeding from esophageal varices. The Linton tube is superior to the Sengstaken-Blakemore tube in patients with bleeding gastric varices. Both of these tubes are rarely used. In general, these tubes should not be used without endoscopic documentation of the source of bleeding because complications are common and significant (14% major, 3% fatal). A trial of balloon tamponade should be considered, however, in an exsanguinating patient with probable variceal bleeding in whom endoscopy is not immediately available and vasopressin has not slowed the hemorrhage. Consultation with a surgeon or gastroenterologist is advisable.

Surgery

Surgery is indicated for all hemodynamically unstable patients with active bleeding who do not respond to appropriate intravascular volume replacement, correction of any coagulopathy, and endoscopic intervention (if available). The mortality for patients undergoing emergency operations for GI bleeding is approximately 23%. Generally, surgery is indicated whenever the risk of ineffective medical therapy and continued hemorrhage outweighs that of surgical morbidity and mortality.[14] Emergency surgery should be considered when blood replacement exceeds 5 U within the first 4 to 6 hours or when 2 U of blood is needed every 4 hours

---

BOX 23-3. Very-Low-Risk Criteria for Patients Complaining of Gastrointestinal Bleeding Who Can Be Discharged Home

No comorbid diseases
Normal vital signs
Normal or trace positive stool guaiac
Negative gastric aspirate, if done
Normal or near-normal hemoglobin/hematocrit
No problem home support
Proper understanding of signs and symptoms of significant bleeding
Immediate access to emergent care if needed
Follow-up arranged within 24 hr

---

after replacing initial losses to maintain normal cardiac output.

DISPOSITION

Risk Stratification

Risk stratification involves combining historical, clinical, and laboratory data to determine the risk of death and rebleeding in patients presenting to an emergency department with GI bleeding. Patients can be sorted into four categories: very low, low, moderate, and high risk. Some patients present to the emergency department with a chief complaint of vomiting blood or passing blood from their rectum but with little or no objective evidence of significant GI bleeding. These patients can be categorized as very low risk and can be sent home without further diagnostic tests (Box 23-3).[1,6,15]

Before discharge, patients should be educated about the signs and symptoms of significant GI bleeding and when to return to the emergency department or call their primary care physician. They should be given specific education about the possible or actual cause of the bleeding and specific treatment for the cause of the bleeding. They should be educated about the side effects of any medications. Patents should be given specific follow-up evaluation within 24 to 36 hours. They should be instructed to avoid aspirin, nonsteroidal anti-inflammatory drugs, and alcohol.[1]

Patients with low-risk, moderate-risk, and high-risk criteria are more complicated. Historically, nearly all patients with significant GI bleeding were admitted to the hospital. As health care has changed, a greater emphasis has been placed on outpatient management of select low-risk patients with GI bleeding. Studies have shown that combining clinical and endoscopic criteria provides an accurate estimation of the risk of rebleeding and mortality in patients with UGIB. These combined criteria have been used to identify patients with UGIB who are at low risk and can be discharged home and patients at moderate or high risk who need to be admitted to an appropriate care site in the hospital. Risk stratification for patients with LGIB is not as well studied, and so nearly all patients with significant

Table 23-1. Initial Emergency Department Risk Stratification for Patients with Gastrointestinal Bleeding

Low Risk	Moderate Risk	High Risk
Age <60	Age >60	
Initial SBP ≥100 mm Hg	Initial SBP <100 mm Hg	Persistent SBP <100 mm Hg
Normal vitals for 1 hr	Mild ongoing tachycardia for 1 hr	Persistent moderate/severe tachycardia
No transfusion requirement	Transfusions required ≤4 U	Transfusion required >4 U
No active major comorbid diseases	Stable major comorbid diseases	Unstable major comorbid diseases
No liver disease	Mild liver disease—PT normal or near-normal	Decompensated liver disease—i.e.,
No moderate-risk or high-risk clinical features	No high-risk clinical features	coagulopathy, ascites, encephalopathy

PT, prothrombin time; SBP, systolic blood pressure.
Data from Lindenauer GF, Terdiman JP: Acute gastrointestinal bleeding. In Wachter RM, Goldman L, Hollander H (eds): *Hospital Medicine*, Philadelphia, Lippincott Williams & Wilkins, 2000.

Table 23-2. Final Risk Stratification for Patients with Upper Gastrointestinal Bleeding After Endoscopy

	Clinical Risk Stratification		
Endoscopy	*Low Risk*	*Moderate Risk*	*High Risk*
Low risk hospitalization	Immediate discharge*	24-hr inpatient stay (floor)†	Close monitoring for 24 hr‡; ≥48-hr
Moderate risk	24-hr patient stay†	24-48 hr inpatient stay (floor)†	Close monitoring for 24 hr; ≥48-hr hospitalization
High risk	Close monitoring for 24 hr; 48-72 hr hospitalization	Close monitoring for 24 hr; 48-72 hr hospitalization	Close monitoring ≥72-hr hospitalization

*Patients with low-risk clinical and endoscopic findings can be discharged home with appropriate treatment based on diagnosis, scheduled follow-up evaluation within 24 hours, and proper patient education to ensure immediate return if signs of rebleeding.
†Patients may be discharged after 24 to 48 hours of in-hospital observation if there is no evidence of rebleeding, vital signs are normal, there is no need for further transfusion, and the hemoglobin or hematocrit has remained stable. They should be provided with appropriate treatment based on diagnosis, scheduled follow-up evaluation within 24 hours, and proper patient education to ensure immediate return if signs of rebleeding.
‡Patients with high-risk clinical or endoscopic findings should be admitted and monitored closely for evidence of rebleeding.
Data from Lindenauer GF, Terdiman JP: Acute gastrointestinal bleeding. In Wachter RM, Goldman L, Hollander H (eds), *Hospital Medicine,* Philadelphia, Lippincott Williams & Wilkins, 2000.

LGIB are admitted. Risk stratification can be used for patients with LGIB, however, to decide an appropriate inpatient care site.

Table 23-1 presents an initial risk stratification tool for patients with upper and lower GI bleeding. Combining clinical and endoscopic findings allows for a final risk stratification (Table 23-2) to decide patient disposition, inpatient care site, and treatment.[1,5,15-18]

Patients with clinical evidence of GI bleeding should undergo endoscopy as soon as it is available for final risk stratification, inpatient triage, and determination of appropriate treatment (see Table 23-2). If endoscopy is not immediately available, patients with low clinical risk may be admitted to an emergency department observation unit or short-stay hospital bed until endoscopy can be performed. Patients with moderate clinical risk criteria may be admitted to an inpatient floor, intermediate care unit, or ICU depending on the individual patient and the capabilities of the institution. Patients with high clinical risk should be admitted to a closely monitored step-down unit or an ICU. The timing of endoscopy depends on availability, the acuity of the patient, the need for emergent therapy, the need to determine final care site, and the need to minimize length of stay.[2]

Patients with LGIB that is not clearly due to hemorrhoids, fissure, or proctitis should be admitted to an inpatient bed. Patients with low risk may be admitted to the floor and set up for a nuclear medicine imaging study (e.g., red blood cell–labeled study) or colonoscopy. Patients with high-risk criteria should be admitted to a step-down unit or ICU and be considered for angiography to identify the site of LGIB. Patients with moderate-risk criteria need to be individualized for the most appropriate inpatient care site (floor, intermediate care bed, or ICU), and the best diagnostic studies (nuclear imaging or angiography).

Consultation with a surgeon should be obtained if it appears that more than 2 U of blood will be required after the initial emergency department resuscitation or if there is reasonable suspicion that operative intervention may be needed. This is especially true of patients older than 65 years of age. In general, the older the patient, the more aggressive the surgical management ought to be. Patients with a history of varices, persistent postural changes in heart rate, or significant bright red blood per rectum are more likely to require surgery than patients without these findings. Patients who have abdominal aortic grafts who enter the emergency department with GI bleeding should receive prompt vascular surgical consultation in the emergency department for the possibility of aortoenteric fistula.

REFERENCES

1. Lindenauer PK, Terdiman JP: Acute gastrointestinal bleeding. In Wachter RM, Goldman L, Hollander H (eds): *Hospital Medicine*. Philadelphia, Lippincott Williams & Wilkins, 2000, pp 599-610.
2. Westhoff JL, Holt KR: Gastrointestinal bleeding: An evidence-based ED approach to risk stratification. *Emerg Med Pract* 6:1, 2004.
3. Derry S, Loke YK: Risk of gastrointestinal haemorrhage with long term use of aspirin: Meta-analysis. *BMJ* 321:1183, 2000.
4. Ofman JJ, et al: A metaanalysis of severe upper gastrointestinal complications of nonsteroidal antiinflammatory drugs. *J Rheumatol* 29:804, 2002.
5. Eisen GM, et al: American Society for Gastrointestinal Endoscopy: Standard of Practice Committee: An annotated algorithmic approach to acute lower gastrointestinal bleeding. *Gastrointest Endosc* 53:859, 2001.
6. Podila PV, et al: Managing patients with acute, nonvariceal gastrointestinal hemorrhage: Development and effectiveness of a clinical care pathway. *Am J Gastroenterol* 96:208, 2001.
7. Kollef MH, et al: BLEED: A classification tool to predict outcomes in patients with acute upper and lower gastrointestinal hemorrhage. *Crit Care Med* 25:11125, 1997.
8. Bleau BL, et al: Recurrent bleeding from peptic ulcer associated with adherent clot: A randomized study comparing endoscopic treatment with medical therapy. *Gastrointest Endosc* 56:1, 2002.
9. Jensen D, Machiado GA: Colonoscopy for diagnosis and treatment of severe lower gastrointestinal bleeding: Routine outcomes and cost analysis. *Gastrointest Endosc Clin N Am* 7:477, 1997.
10. Gordon RL, et al: Selective arterial embolization for the control of lower gastrointestinal hemorrhage: A population based study. *Am J Gastroenterol* 92:419, 1997.
11. Lau JY, et al: Effect of intravenous omeprazole on recurrent bleeding after endoscopic treatment of bleeding peptic ulcers. *N Engl J Med* 343:310, 2000.
12. Zuberi BF, Baloch Q: Comparison of endoscopic variceal sclerotherapy alone and in combination with octreotide in controlling acute variceal hemorrhage and early rebleeding in patients with low-risk cirrhosis. *Am J Gastroenterol* 95:768, 2000.
13. Schoenfeld PS, Butler JA: An evidence-based approach to the treatment of esophageal variceal bleeding. *Crit Care Clin* 14:441, 1998.
14. Stabile BE, Stamos MJ: Surgical management of gastrointestinal bleeding. *Gastroenterol Clin North Am* 29:189, 2000.
15. Hay JA, et al: Prospective evaluation of a clinical guideline recommending hospital length of stay in upper gastrointestinal tract hemorrhage. *JAMA* 278:2151, 1997.
16. Eisen GM, et al: American Society for Gastrointestinal Endoscopy: Standard of Practice Committee: An annotated algorithmic approach to acute lower gastrointestinal bleeding. *Gastrointest Endosc* 53:859, 2001.
17. Lee JG, et al: Endoscopy-based triage significantly reduces hospitalization rates and costs of treating upper GI bleeding: A randomized controlled trial. *Gastroenterol Endosc* 50:755, 1999.
18. Longstreth GF, Feitelberg SP: Outpatient care of selected patients with acute non-variceal upper gastrointestinal haemorrhage. *Lancet* 345:108, 1995.

CHAPTER 24 Diarrhea

John E. Gough and Phillip A. Clement

PERSPECTIVE

Diarrhea is a common presenting symptom in the emergency department and can account for 5% of visits, especially during the fall and winter. Although the differential diagnosis is broad, most cases (85% by some estimates) have infectious causes.[1] Most cases of diarrhea are self-limiting and require only supportive care and symptomatic treatment. Infectious diarrhea has the potential for serious illness, however, and when combined with susceptible patient populations may lead to significant morbidity and mortality.[2] There are numerous noninfectious causes of diarrhea, which may pose an even greater threat to patient well-being and survival. Diarrhea may be a presenting symptom of abdominal and endocrine pathology, toxic exposures or ingestions, and other systemic illnesses. The diagnosis of gastroenteritis, of presumed viral origin, should be applied only after the more serious causes have been considered and eliminated.

Epidemiology

Worldwide, diarrhea remains a major health problem, accounting for more than 4 million deaths each year. In developing countries, diarrhea is estimated to claim the lives of 10,000 children younger than 5 years old every day.[3] In the United States, children younger than age 5 experience 20 million episodes of diarrhea annually, resulting in 200,000 hospitalizations and 300 deaths per year.[4] Among adults, the incidence is one episode of diarrhea per person per year. Diarrhea accounts for 1.5% of total hospitalizations and is second only to the common cold in days lost from work. Patients at risk for significant morbidity and mortality are at the extremes of age, have hospital-associated or antibiotic-associated diarrhea, have significant underlying illness, have certain invasive etiologies, or have immunodeficiencies. An estimated 60% of patients infected with human immunodeficiency virus (HIV) experience significant diarrhea during the course of their illness.[5]

Pathophysiology

The term *diarrhea* is derived from the Greek words *dia* ("through") and *rhein* ("to flow"). A clinically useful definition is an increase in the volume, frequency, or fluidity of the stool, relative to the patient's normal pattern. It is important to determine each patient's understanding and use of the term *diarrhea* because lay definitions vary widely. *Dysentery* is an inflammatory diarrhea caused by pathogens, which invade the intestinal mucosa, resulting in the presence of blood, mucus, and protein in the stool. It often is associated with other indications of systemic illness, such as fever, abdominal pain, anorexia, dehydration, and weight loss.

Diarrhea can be characterized as acute or chronic. Acute diarrhea is defined as being present for less than 4 weeks.[1] Diarrhea can be divided further into four major types: osmotic, secretory, inflammatory, and abnormal motility.

Osmotic diarrhea occurs with the ingestion of nonabsorbable, osmotically active solutes. These solutes cause the osmotic movement of water into the intestinal lumen. This movement may be caused by exogenous agents, such as laxatives; magnesium-containing antacids; dietetic foods containing sorbitol, mannitol, or xylitol; and certain drugs (e.g., colchicine, cholestyramine, neomycin). If exogenous agents are the cause, fasting results in the eventual resolution of the diarrhea. Congenital and acquired causes of malabsorption or maldigestion may result in an excess of osmotically active solutes, causing diarrhea.

In secretory diarrhea, cytotoxins produce an increased cellular permeability resulting in the secretion of water and electrolytes (mainly chloride) into the intestinal lumen. In contrast to osmotic diarrhea, secretory diarrhea usually persists with fasting. Stool studies examining electrolyte concentrations and osmolality can help to differentiate between osmotic and secretory diarrhea but are of little value in the acute setting. Secretory diarrhea may be induced by bacterial cytotoxins (*Vibrio cholerae*), enteropathogenic viruses (viral gastroenteritis), hormonal hypersecretion, and certain drugs. Fecal erythrocytes and leukocytes are uncommon, as are significant systemic symptoms. Most cases of diarrhea encountered in the emergency department are secretory.

Inflammatory diarrhea results from cellular damage to the intestinal mucosa, leading to the secretion of water, electrolytes, blood, mucus, and plasma proteins. This diarrhea is caused most commonly by invasive bacterial and parasitic pathogens that produce dysenteric illnesses (Table 24-1). Epithelial damage can occur with chemotherapy, radiation therapy, hypersensitivity reactions, autoimmune disorders, and inflammatory bowel disease. Fecal leukocytes and erythrocytes are typically present, as are systemic symptoms, and the diarrhea continues despite fasting.

Abnormal motility is generally seen in patients with chronic diarrhea. This is a diagnosis of exclusion. Hypermotility decreases contact time between luminal contents and the absorbing mucosa, limiting water and electrolyte absorption. Hypomotility may be associated with bacterial overgrowth and results in steatorrhea.

DIAGNOSTIC APPROACH

Differential Considerations

Diarrhea can be classified as infectious (85%) or noninfectious (15%). Infectious diarrhea can be divided into viral, bacterial, and parasitic causes (Box 24-1), with estimates of the relative contributions of the infectious causes being viral, 70%; bacterial, 24%; and parasitic, 6%.[6]

Bacterial agents can be characterized further as agents that cause a dysenteric, inflammatory diarrhea by invading the colonic mucosa and agents that cause a secretory diarrhea by the production of cytotoxins. Viral and parasitic agents may cause either inflammatory or secretory diarrhea. Most viral and many bacterial agents cause a self-limiting, secretory diarrhea, with only mild dehydration and minimal systemic symptoms. Although the greatest pathology generally is seen with bacterial and parasitic pathogens that cause invasive, inflammatory disease, any infectious agent may be associated with significant morbidity and mortality.[1] This is especially true with susceptible patient populations or patients not provided with adequate supportive care. Several invasive bacterial pathogens, most notably *Salmonella* and *Shigella,* may result in bacteremia, sepsis, and death. Acute amebic dysentery, caused by *Entamoeba histolytica,* may be difficult to distinguish clinically from bacterial dysentery. The specific causative agent of infectious diarrhea is rarely identified in the emergency department.

Noninfectious causes of diarrhea (Box 24-2) are responsible for about 15% of total cases and can be a significant threat to patient well-being and survival. Although the distinction between infectious and noninfectious causes may not always be clinically apparent, it is imperative to consider entities such as surgical pathology of the abdomen, including gastrointestinal bleeding, ischemic bowel, acute appendicitis, intussusception, ectopic pregnancy, and bowel obstruction.[7] Thought should be given to possible toxic exposures or ingestions, such as heavy metal poisoning and ingestion of plant-borne or fish-borne toxins. Endocrine pathology, such as adrenal insufficiency, and other systemic illnesses should be in the differential diagnosis. Special attention should be given to underlying medical conditions, medication use, and past surgical history.

Rapid Assessment and Stabilization

The evaluation and treatment of patients with diarrhea should begin with a rapid assessment of the overall

Table 24-1. Infectious Causes of Dysenteric Colitis

Agents	Historical Features	Clinical Features	Comments	Treatment
Campylobacter sp.	Contaminated food/water, summer months Backpacker's diarrhea, 2-5 days incubation, 1 wk duration, 10% relapse, 1-5 yr-olds and college students	3-4 day prodrome of fever, HA, myalgia and abdominal cramps, minimal vomiting Fecal RBC/WBC	Most common diagnosed bacterial cause of diarrhea May mimic appendicitis or IBD	Rx debilitated or septic patients: Ciprofloxacin (Cipro) 500 mg po BID × 5 days Azithromycin (Zithromax) 500 mg po qd × 3 days Erythromycin 500 mg po qid × 5 days
Salmonella sp.	Contaminated food/water, eggs/poultry/milk, summer months Cafeteria outbreaks, family gatherings Esp. children <5, elderly, compromised 8-24 hr incubation, 2-5 day duration	Several-hour prodrome of fever, HA, abdominal pain, myalgia, minimal vomiting, 5-10% bacteremia Fecal WBC, rarely RBC	Increased risk of sepsis, osteomyelitis, meningitis, infected aneurysms in the elderly, neonates, SS disease, HIV, IVDU, asplenic, prosthesis, malignancies, immunocompromised	Rx septic, elderly or compromised: IV ceftriaxone Ciprofloxacin (Cipro) 500 mg po bid 3-7 days TMP/SMX DS po bid 3-7 days
Shigella sp.	Very contagious, person to person, day care, families, institutions, poor sanitation Children 1-5 yrs old, institutionalized patients, 24-48 hr incubation, 4-7 day duration	Sudden-onset fever, HA, myalgia, irritability, abdominal pain, diarrhea, minimal vomiting, bacteremia rare Fecal RBC and WBC sheets	Severe dysentery/ dehydration in elderly, very young, febrile seizures common, diarrhea may start during LP	Rx if severe dysentery or institutional outbreak: Ciprofloxacin (Cipro) 500 mg po bid × 3 days TMP/SMX DS po bid × 3 days
Yersinia enterocolitica	Contaminated food/water, milk, pork, person to person, children and young adults, 12-48 hr incubation, 3-12 day duration	RLQ abdominal pain, anorexia, low-grade fever, vomiting with little initial diarrhea, mimics appendicitis Fecal RBC/WBC	Bacteremia rare except elderly/infants, also mimics IBD, adults may develop postinfectious complications, Reiter's syndrome	Usually self-limiting, Rx if septic: Ciprofloxacin (Cipro) 500 mg po bid × 3 days
Vibro parahaemolyticus	Raw or undercooked seafood, shrimp and oysters, summer months Any age, more common in adults 10-24 hr incubation, 1-2 day duration	Sudden onset of diarrhea, mild abdominal cramps, low-grade fever, HA, nausea with little vomiting Fecal RBC/WBC	Self-limiting, bacteremia rare, common in Japan, no fatalities in U.S., septicemia from *V. vulnificus* in compromised patients	Supportive care, usually self-limiting, Rx if severe disease or immunocompromised: Tetracycline or doxycycline × 7 days
Enterohemorrhagic *E. coli* 0157 : H7	Contaminated food/water, raw beef, milk, meats, outbreaks in institutions, day care, nursing homes; children and elderly. 3-8 day incubation, 5-10 day duration	Severe abdominal cramps, vomiting, low-grade fever, grossly bloody stool, shigella-like toxins, not invasive Fecal RBC/WBC	Hemorrhagic gastroenteritis, grossly bloody, may mimic GI bleed/ischemic colitis, complicated by HUS or TTP 5-20% of cases, 5-20 day postinfection	Supportive care Rx with antibiotics associated with increased risk of HUS in children and elderly
Plesiomonas shigelloides	Uncooked shellfish, raw oysters, travel in Mexico or Asia, 1-2 day incubation, 5-20 day duration	Severe abdominal cramps, diarrhea, vomiting and dehydration Fecal RBC/WBC	Common in immunocompromised, sporadic in normal host	Usually not required normal host, Ciprofloxacin (Cipro) 500 mg po bid 3-7 days TMP/SMX DS po bid 3-7 days
Aeromonas hydrophila	Contaminated water, more acute onset and severe disease in children than adults 1-5 day incubation, 2-10 wk duration	Diarrhea, abdominal cramps, vomiting occasional fever, chronic in adults 2-10 wk, may mimic IBD Fecal RBC/WBC	10-15% cases of diarrhea in children, common in elderly or immunocompromised, HIV	Ciprofloxacin (Cipro) 500 mg po bid × 3-7 days TMP/SMX DS po bid × 3-7 days Tetracycline 500 mg po qid × 7 days
Entamoeba histolytica	Fecal contaminated food/ water, history of travel in developing countries, institutions, poor hygiene, 1-12 wk incubation	Acute amebic dysentery, abrupt onset fever, severe abdominal cramps, bloody diarrhea, minimal vomiting, fecal RBC/WBC	Rare pathogen in HIV, no eosinophilia Chronic amebic colitis mimics IBD Steroids potentially fatal causing perforation/ toxic megacolon	For dysentery Metronidazole Flagyl 750 mg po tid × 10 days followed by Iodoquinol 650 mg po tid × 20 days

Continued

Table 24-1. Infectious Causes of Dysenteric Colitis—cont'd

Agents	Historical Features	Clinical Features	Comments	Treatment
Strongyloides stercoralis	Fecal contaminated soil, southern US, tropics, institutions, poor sanitation Incubation weeks to months	Sepsis in immunocompromised, fever, vomiting, diarrhea, abdominal pain	Cutaneous and pulmonary symptoms, eosinophilia, pneumonia, meningitis	Thiabendazole 25 mg/kg po bid × 3-5 days
Clostridium difficile	Rx with antibiotic especially clindamycin Hospitalized patients, constipating agents More common adults, more severe children Onset during or up to 10 wk after Rx	May produce systemic toxicity, fever, abdominal pain, dysenteric stools Significant morbidity/ mortality, especially children Fecal RBC/WBC	Cytopathic toxin, destroys colonic mucosa, dx by *C. difficile* toxin in stool Avoid antimotility agents, 10-20% relapse	Discontinue causative antibiotic Flagyl 500 mg po tid × 7-14 days Vancomycin 125 mg po qid × 10-14 days

HA, headache; HIV, human immunodeficiency virus; HUS, hemolytic uremic syndrome; IBD, inflammatory bowel disease; IVDU, intravenous drug use; LP, lumbar puncture; RBC/WBC, red blood cells/white blood cells; RLQ, right lower quadrant; TMP/SMX, trimethoprim/sulfamethoxazole; TTP, thrombotic thrombocytopenic purpura.

BOX 24-1. Etiologic Agents of Infectious Diarrhea

Viral (60%)
Astrovirus
Calicivirus
Coronavirus
Cytomegalovirus*
Enteric adenovirus
Hepatitis A-G
Herpes simplex virus
HIV enteropathy
Norwalk-like agents
Norwalk virus
Pararotavirus
Picornavirus
Rotavirus
Small round viruses

Bacterial (20%)
Invasive:
  Aeromonas sp.
  Campylobacter sp.
  Clostridium difficile
  Enteroinvasive *E. coli*
  Mycobacterium sp.
  Plesiomonas shigelloides
  Salmonella sp.
  Shigella sp.
  Vibrio fluvialis
  Vibrio parahaemolyticus
  Vibrio vulnificus
  Yersinia enterocolitica
  Yersinia pseudotuberculosis
Toxigenic:
  Food poisoning with preformed toxins
    Bacillus cereus
    Clostridium botulinum
    Staphylococcus aureus
  Toxin formation after colonization
    Aeromonas hydrophila

Clostridium perfringens
Enterohemorrhagic *E. coli** 0157:H7
Enterotoxigenic *E. coli*
Klebsiella pneumoniae
Shigella sp.
Vibrio cholerae
Other bacteria
  Listeria monocytogenes
  Neisseria gonorrhoeae
  Treponema pallidum

Parasitic (5%)
Protozoa:
  *Balantidium coli**
  Blastocystis hominis
  Cryptosporidium
  Cyclospora
  Dientamoeba fragilis
  *Entamoeba histolytica**
  Entamoeba polecki
  Enteromonas hominis
  Giardia lamblia
  Isospora belli
  Microsporidia
  Sarcocystis hominis
Helminths:
  Angiostrongylus costaricense
  Anisakiasis
  Ascaris lumbricoides
  Diphyllobothrium latum
  Enterobius vermicularis
  Hookworms
  Schistosoma sp.
  Strongyloides stercoralis
  Taenia sp.
  Trichinella spiralis
  Trichuris trichiura

---

*Associated with fever, abdominal pain, and fecal red blood cell/white blood cell. % indicates the estimated contribution to total cases.

BOX 24-2. Differential Diagnosis of Noninfectious Diarrhea

Toxins

Drugs
ACE inhibitors
Alprazolam (Xanax)
Antacids (Mg)
Antibiotics
Antidepressants
Antiepileptic drugs
Antihypertensives
Antiparkinson drugs
β-blockers
Caffeine
Cardiac antiarrhythmics
Chemotherapy agents
Cholesterol-lowering drugs
Cholinergic agents
Cholinesterase inhibitors
Colchicine
Digitalis
Diuretics
Fluorouracil
Fluoxetine (Prozac)
H_2-receptor antagonist
Hydralazine
Lactulose
Laxatives/cathartics
Levodopa
Lithium
NSAIDs
Neomycin
Podophyllin
Procainamide
Prostaglandins
Quinidine
Ricinoleic acid
Theophylline
Thyroid hormone
Valproic acid

Dietetic foods
Mannitol
Sorbitol
Xylitol

Fish-associated toxins
Amnestic shellfish poisoning
Ciguatera
Echinoderms
Neurotoxic shellfish poisoning
Paralytic shellfish poisoning
Scombroid
Tetroton

Plant-associated toxins
Herbal preparations
Horse chestnut
Mushrooms—*Amanita* sp.
Nicotine
Other plant toxins
Pesticides—organophosphates
Pokeweed
Rhubarb

Miscellaneous
Allergic reactions
Carbon monoxide poisoning
Ethanol
Heavy metals
Monosodium glutamate (MSG)
Opiate withdrawal

Gastrointestinal Pathology
Appendicitis
Autonomic dysfunction

Bile acid malabsorption
Blind loop
Bowel obstruction
Celiac disease
Cirrhosis
Defects in amino acid transport
Diverticular disease
Familial dysautonomia
Fecal impaction
Fecal incontinence
GI bleed
GI cancer
Hirschsprung's disease
Inflammatory bowel disease (ulcerative colitis, Crohn's disease)
Intussusception
Irritable bowel syndrome
Ischemic bowel
Lactose/fructose intolerance
Malabsorption syndromes
Malrotation
Postsurgical
Postvagotomy
Radiation therapy
Short-gut syndrome
Small bowel resection
Strictures
Toxic megacolon
Tropical sprue
Volvulus
Whipple's disease

Endocrine Pathology and Systemic Illness

Hormonal hypersecretion
Carcinoid syndrome (serotonin)
Hyperthyroidism (thyroid hormone)
Medullary carcinoma of the thyroid (calcitonin)
Pancreatic cholera (VIP)
Somatostatinoma (somatostatin)
Systemic mastocytosis (histamine)
Zollinger-Ellison syndrome (gastrin)

Endocrine pathology
Adrenal insufficiency
Diabetes enteropathy
Hypoparathyroidism
Pancreatic insufficiency

Systemic Illness/Other
Alcoholism
Amyloidosis
Connective tissue disease
Cystic fibrosis
Ectopic pregnancy
Hemolytic-uremic syndrome
Henoch-Schönlein purpura
Lymphoma
Otitis media—infants
Pelvic inflammatory disease
Pneumonia/sepsis
Pyelonephritis
Scleroderma/SLE
Severe malnutrition
Stevens-Johnson syndrome
Toxic shock syndrome
Wilson's disease
Miscellaneous
Factitious diarrhea
Runner's diarrhea

ACE, angiotensin-converting enzyme; GI, gastrointestinal; NSAIDs, nonsteroidal anti-inflammatory drugs; SLE, systemic lupus erythematosus.

health of the patient, the severity of volume depletion, and the initiation of appropriate resuscitative measures. Complete vital signs should be obtained, including blood pressure, pulse rate, respiratory rate, pulse oximetry, and rectal temperature. If severe dehydration is present, and intravenous fluid replenishment is anticipated, serum electrolytes may be helpful. In short-duration diarrhea, especially when volume depletion is not an issue, electrolytes rarely provide useful information.

The physician should search for evidence of hemodynamic instability, such as hypotension, tachycardia, cool pale skin, oliguria, tachypnea, or altered mental status. Signs of systemic illness, such as fever, abdominal pain, dehydration, bloody stools, myalgia, cephalgia, and anorexia, should be sought. The physician should evaluate for evidence of sepsis, gastrointestinal bleeding, surgical abdomen, toxic exposures, endocrine pathology, or anaphylaxis. Unstable patients should receive supplemental oxygen, intravenous access, continuous cardiac monitoring, and pulse oximetry, together with normal saline volume resuscitation. Rarely, transfusion of blood and blood products may be necessary. If the diarrhea is believed to be of an infectious nature, and there are associated signs of systemic infection, early antibiotic use is indicated. Antibiotic choice should be based on the suspected cause of the diarrhea (see Table 24-1), although empiric treatment often is necessary. If heavy metal ingestion is suspected, specific antidotes may be warranted. An unstable or critically ill patient should be hospitalized for supportive treatment, continuous monitoring, and further investigation if the cause is uncertain. When the cause is determined, specific treatment is initiated.

Pivotal Findings

After the initial assessment and stabilization, history, physical examination, and laboratory investigations are conducted to identify further the cause of diarrhea.

History

1. Characterize the volume, frequency, and character of the stools.
2. Identify the onset and duration of the diarrhea: Is this episode acute or chronic?
3. Conduct a review of symptoms. Inquire about vomiting; fever; abdominal pain; anorexia; constipation; myalgia; cephalgia; tenesmus; and neurologic symptoms such as paresthesias, weakness, or cranial nerve palsies.
4. Inquire about the onset of diarrhea in relation to other symptoms. Abdominal cramps after copious, watery diarrhea is consistent with gastroenteritis, whereas the onset of pain followed by a single loose stool may suggest surgical pathology.
5. Determine the severity or significance of the diarrhea in relation to other symptoms. Is diarrhea a major or minor aspect of this presentation?
6. Identify any pattern to defecation. Does eating or drinking exacerbate the diarrhea?
7. Identify the presence of blood or mucus in the stool.
8. Ask about prior treatments for diarrhea, either self-medicated or prescribed by a physician. Note the response to such treatment.
9. Inquire about the patient's past medical and surgical history. Give special attention to immunocompetency. Ask about a history of HIV, diabetes mellitus, gastrointestinal bleeds, malignancies, abdominal surgeries, and endocrine disease. Ask about recent chemotherapy or radiation therapy.
10. Identify medications used by the patient, including medications prescribed by a physician, over-the-counter medications, herbal remedies, and drugs of abuse. Pay particular attention to recent antibiotic therapy or laxative use.
11. Ask about sexual contacts. Heterosexual and homosexual contact may be associated with the transmission of amebic dysentery and *Salmonella, Shigella, Giardia,* and *Campylobacter* infections. Lower gastrointestinal symptoms may be caused by sexually transmitted diseases, such as *Chlamydia trachomatis,* herpes simplex, and *Neisseria gonorrheae.* In HIV-positive patients, *Cryptosporidium, Mycobacterium avium-intracellulare,* and cytomegalovirus may be the cause of diarrhea.
12. Inquire about a personal or family history of diarrheal diseases.
13. Ask about contact with persons associated with daycare centers, and inquire about community outbreaks.
14. Inquire about hospitalizations or institutional exposures.
15. Give special attention to dietary history. Ask about unusual foods; dairy products; eggs; seafood; and unpasteurized, undercooked, or poorly prepared foods. Ask about the ingestion of mushrooms or other plant products.
16. Inquire about recent travel, especially to developing countries. Ask about recent outdoor activities, including backpacking and exposure to new water sources.
17. Determine any known exposure to toxins, including heavy metals, carbon monoxide, salicylates, and digoxin. Consider occupational exposures. In farm workers, consider pesticides (organophosphate poisoning) and nicotine (green tobacco syndrome). Inquire about a history of allergic reactions.

Physical Examination

The physical examination should assess the patient's overall health, look for signs of volume depletion and a toxic appearance, rule out the surgical abdomen, and determine the presence of blood in the stool. Fever is consistent with dysentery, but also could indicate an acute surgical process. Fever is less commonly associated with viral or noninvasive bacterial gastroenteritis. Hypotension and tachycardia may indicate volume depletion. Young healthy adults may maintain a normal blood pressure and heart rate even with significant dehydration. In elderly patients and patients who are taking antidysrhythmic or β-blocker medications, the heart rate may not be a reliable indicator of volume status. The physician should assess the moistness of the mucosa, skin turgor, and the presence of any mental status changes. Additionally, in children, the physician should look for sunken eyes, depression of the fontanel, and decrease in urine output (number of wet diapers) and attempt to determine percent weight loss from pre-morbid condition.[7]

Particular attention should be given to the abdominal examination. In patients with significant abdominal pain, causes other than infectious gastroenteritis are actively sought. Signs and symptoms consistent with surgical pathology include focal tenderness, evidence of peritoneal inflammation (rebound), and pain that precedes the diarrhea. Subjective, diffuse, and crampy abdominal pain may occur after extensive vomiting or diarrhea and is consistent with gastroenteritis. *Yersinia enterocolitica* and *Campylobacter* sp. may cause right lower quadrant pain, low-grade fever, anorexia, and vomiting, preceding the onset of diarrhea, and mimic acute appendicitis. Early acute abdominal emergencies with diarrhea may be differentiated from gastroenteritis with serial abdominal examination in the emergency department or, when indicated, by abdominal computed tomography.

A rectal examination should be performed to detect fecal impaction, melena, or hematochezia. Gross blood is consistent with gastrointestinal bleed, ischemic bowel, intussusception, radiation therapy, and infection with enterohemorrhagic *Escherichia coli* 0157:H7. Stool smear may be sent for fecal cell count. A search for specific toxidromes, such as cholinergic or sympathomimetic, should be conducted.

Ancillary Testing

Because most cases of diarrhea are self-limiting, laboratory and diagnostic tests are of limited value and should be kept to a minimum. Testing should be carried out, as indicated, in patients who are hemodynamically unstable, patients with a toxic appearance, patients at the extremes of age, immunocompromised patients, and patients suspected to have a noninfectious cause of diarrhea. In addition, testing may be necessary in patients with a prolonged course or in patients not responding to conservative management.[1] A complete blood count is rarely helpful and is not sensitive or specific enough to aid in diagnostic decision making. Renal and liver function studies, serum lipase, and a pregnancy test may be helpful in selected cases.

Hemoccult and fecal cell count: The presence of fecal leukocytes, by stool smear, often has been used inappropriately to decide which patients with presumed gastroenteritis should be treated empirically with antibiotics. The finding of fecal leukocytes is suggestive, but not specific for bacterial colitis. Many causes of inflammatory diarrhea produce red and white fecal blood cells. Included are bacterial, parasitic, and noninfectious causes, such as chemotherapy, radia-

tion therapy, hypersensitivity reactions, autoimmune disorders, and inflammatory bowel disease. The presence of fecal leukocytes has not been shown to delineate which patients would benefit from empiric antimicrobial therapy. The presence of blood does not always correlate with the presence of fecal leukocytes so that reliance on guaiac alone is not recommended. The presence of blood without fecal leukocytes may indicate amebiasis, malignancies, heavy metal poisoning, fissures, hemorrhoids, bowel ischemia, or gastrointestinal bleeding.

Clostridium difficile toxin: This test is considered if the patient reports recent antibiotic use. *C. difficile*-associated diarrhea most commonly occurs during the antibiotic course. In 25% to 40% of cases, however, the diarrhea may be delayed 12 weeks after antibiotic therapy. The most commonly implicated antibiotics are cephalosporins, penicillins, and clindamycin. Although *C. difficile* accounts for only 10% to 20% of antibiotic-associated diarrhea, an assay for *C. difficile* toxin is positive in nearly all cases of antibiotic-associated pseudomembranous colitis.[8] Approximately 3% of adult patients and 65% of newborns may be colonized with *C. difficile*.

E. coli 0157:H7 toxin: This test is considered in endemic areas and in patients with suspected hemolytic-uremic syndrome.

Stool for bacterial culture: Stool cultures may be warranted in patients who are febrile, toxic appearing, immunocompromised, at the extremes of age, experiencing a prolonged course, or not responding to conventional treatment. Studies have shown a 2% positive rate, making routine cultures of virtually no value.

Stool for ova and parasites: The assessment of stool for ova and parasites is not routinely recommended. This study is used in patients with chronic diarrhea (*E. histolytica, Cryptosporidium*); patients with a history of travel to developing countries, particularly to Nepal or areas of Russia (*Cryptosporidium, Giardia, Cyclospora*)[9]; patients with exposure to infants in daycare centers (*Cryptosporidium, Giardia*); and patients with HIV infection (*E. histolytica, Giardia*).[5]

Giardia antigen: This test is considered in patients exposed to poor sanitation, HIV-infected patients, patients with a history of travel to developing countries, patients with a history of backpacking, and patients with daycare exposures.

Urinalysis: A urinalysis and a urine pregnancy test should be obtained only when urinary tract infection is suspected, a gastrointestinal origin for the symptoms is not clear, or pregnancy is suspected.

Radiographic studies: Radiographic studies may be indicated for patients thought to have a surgical abdomen and to identify anatomic abnormalities, such as tumor, obstructions, fistulae, blind loops, and Crohn's disease.

Gastrointestinal referral: Referral may be indicated in the evaluation of chronic diarrhea and for workup beyond the scope of the emergency department (e.g., endoscopy, further stool studies).

DIFFERENTIAL DIAGNOSIS

The causes of diarrhea are numerous, and a specific cause may be difficult to determine in the acute setting (see Boxes 24-1 and 24-2). The most common diagnosis is gastroenteritis, although it is often applied incorrectly. Gastroenteritis is a clinical syndrome that manifests as nausea, vomiting, and diarrhea. The upper gastrointestinal symptoms are often most prominent, and the diarrhea is of variable severity. The term *gastroenteritis* generally implies an uncertain cause and is often used to indicate a self-limiting, presumably viral process.

The diagnosis of gastroenteritis has been applied inappropriately to entities such as acute appendicitis, ectopic pregnancy, carbon monoxide poisoning, and subarachnoid hemorrhage. This misdiagnosis can be avoided by a careful and systematic approach, beginning with a thorough history and physical examination. Special attention should be given to details such as the onset and severity of diarrhea and the relationship to other symptoms.

Although abdominal cramps after copious, watery diarrhea are consistent with gastroenteritis, abdominal pain followed by nausea and a loose stool could represent acute appendicitis. Profuse diarrhea, nausea, fever, myalgias, and cephalgia are consistent with dysentery, whereas a sudden severe headache, nausea, vomiting, and a loose stool could represent a process such as subarachnoid hemorrhage.

EMPIRIC MANAGEMENT

Patients with evidence of systemic illness, patients who appear toxic, and patients who are hemodynamically unstable require aggressive management (Figure 24-1). Patients who are elderly, are very young, have significant underlying medical conditions, are severely ill, or are immunocompromised should be admitted to the hospital.[5] Young healthy adults rarely require admission.

Initial therapy for patients with diarrhea from any cause consists of supportive care with special attention given to the patient's hydration status. This may be the only treatment necessary for many patients. Oral rehydration is the treatment of choice for mild to moderate fluid losses. In pediatric patients, oral rehydration can

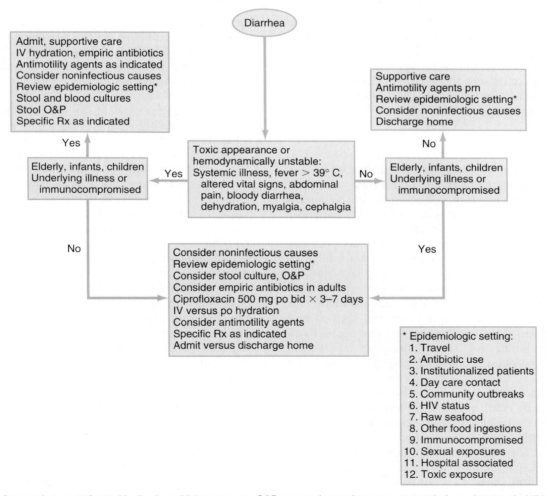

Figure 24-1. Approach to a patient with diarrhea. IV, intravenous; O&P, ova and parasites; prn, as needed; po, by mouth; HIV, human immunodeficiency virus.

be accomplished by giving 50 to 100 mL/kg of a glucose-electrolyte solution over 4 hours.[10] Replacement of micronutrients, particularly copper and zinc, has been recommended, especially in developing countries.[11] The concept of bowel rest should be abandoned because it may worsen diarrhea and lead to more severe dehydration. The choice of oral rehydration fluids depends on the extent of dehydration and the underlying health of the patient. In otherwise healthy patients, with mild to moderate dehydration, fluids such as sports drinks, diluted fruit juices, and soft drinks supplemented with soups, broths, or crackers may be sufficient to replace the fluid and sodium losses associated with acute diarrhea. Such frequently used "clear liquids" may contain excess sugars and insufficient sodium content, however, leading to an osmotic diarrhea. Beverages containing caffeine should be avoided because caffeine increases cyclic adenosine monophosphate levels and may cause a secretory diarrhea. Milk and other products containing lactose also should be avoided because viral and bacterial pathogens, responsible for many cases of diarrhea, may cause a transient lactase deficiency, leading to malabsorption. Food intake is encouraged, but foods high in simple sugars should be avoided, owing to the tendency to promote an osmotic diarrhea. Foods with a high fat content may delay gastric emptying and should be avoided. The BRAT (bananas, rice, apples, and toast) diet has long been recommended, particularly with pediatric patients. Although no controlled studies have examined the efficacy of the BRAT diet, it remains a commonly recommended strategy. The pectin in the apples is constipating (pectin, found in fruit peel, is the "pectate" in Kaopectate), and bananas provide potassium. If this diet is used for extended periods, there is concern it would not adequately provide for the protein and energy needs of the patient.

In patients with evidence of more severe dehydration, intravenous fluid resuscitation with normal saline or lactated Ringer's solution is the preferred treatment. Pediatric patients should receive a bolus of 20 mL/kg of normal saline, which may be repeated as needed. Specific treatment for diarrhea must be directed toward the suspected cause. For patients with suspected surgical pathology, further diagnostic testing and surgical consultation may be required. For toxic exposures, treatment consists of early decontamination, supportive care, and, if appropriate, administration of specific antidotes. Other noninfectious causes of diarrhea are treated as indicated.

Specific treatment of infectious diarrhea in the emergency department also begins with supportive care and fluid resuscitation. Because the specific pathogen causing infectious diarrhea is rarely identified in the emergency department, and the results of cultures are usually unavailable, any antimicrobial treatment must be empiric and guided by knowledge of the common causes of infectious diarrhea (see Box 24-1). Viral and noninvasive bacterial gastroenteritis tend to be self-limiting and to require only supportive therapy. Empiric antibiotic treatment is directed against invasive bacterial and parasitic organisms that cause the greatest harm (see Table 24-1). Antibiotic treatment is initiated in patients with a suspected invasive process and severe diarrhea, systemic symptoms, fever, or abdominal pain and in patients who appear toxic. Fecal cell count is of limited utility in deciding whom to treat. Current recommendations for empiric treatment of a systemically ill–appearing adult include ciprofloxacin, 500 mg orally twice a day for 3 to 7 days. Ciprofloxacin is efficacious against most organisms that cause dysenteric illnesses (see Table 24-1) and has been shown to be more effective than trimethoprim-sulfamethoxazole.[2,9] Ciprofloxacin should not be administered to pregnant patients or children, however. The treatment of enteritis in children with ciprofloxacin and trimethoprim-sulfamethoxazole has been associated with the development of hemolytic-uremic syndrome and thrombotic thrombocytopenic purpura. These complications are most commonly associated with the treatment of enterohemorrhagic *E. coli* 0157:H7, although *Salmonella, Shigella,* and *Campylobacter* also have been implicated. If possible, the treatment of pediatric patients should be based on culture results.

If amebic dysentery is of concern (chronic diarrhea, a travel history, institutionalized or immunocompromised patients), treatment with metronidazole, after stool analysis for ova and parasites, is recommended. A second agent (see Table 24-1) is needed after initial treatment. In patients with a history of recent antibiotic use suspected of having *C. difficile* colitis, a *C. difficile* toxin assay followed by vancomycin or metronidazole is appropriate.[9]

The use of antimotility agents in the treatment of acute enteritis has been controversial with the literature divided over this issue. In patients with ulcerative colitis or antibiotic-associated colitis, the use of opioids, loperamide, or diphenoxylate with atropine has been associated with the precipitation of toxic megacolon, but these patients usually are easily identified or already carry the diagnosis. Because most beneficial effects are modest, these agents are used, if at all, with caution in patients with inflammatory bowel disease, antibiotic-associated colitis, or dysentery and in pediatric patients. In other patients, antimotility agents may be used, as needed, especially in conjunction with antibiotics, and often provide significant relief of symptoms (Table 24-2).

DISPOSITION

Most patients with diarrhea can be discharged home after assessment and symptomatic relief. Hospitalization rarely is required for diarrhea secondary to viral and many forms of bacterial gastroenteritis, which tend to be self-limiting. Often the exact etiologic agent of diarrhea is not identified in the emergency department. An understanding of common causes and their treatment and recognizing patients at risk for a more severe course of the disease are essential to make the appropriate disposition. In patients with severe dehydration, hemodynamic instability, or a toxic appearance and in

Table 24-2. Symptomatic Treatment of Acute Diarrhea

Medication	Dosage	Action	Comments

Bismuth subsalicylate (Pepto-Bismol)	30 mL or 2 tablets q 30 min for 8 doses × 2 days	Not known
		May bind enterotoxins
			Commonly used for traveler's diarrhea
			Potential for:
			  Salicylate toxicity
			  Bismuth
			  Encephalopathy (especially in HIV)

Koalin/pectin (Kaopectate)	60-120 mL after each loose stool	Decrease gastric motility
		Bulk forming
		May bind enterotoxins
			Adverse effects:
			  Bloating
			  Flatus
			  Constipation
			  Intestinal obstruction (if preexisting stricture)

Loperamide (Imodium)	4 mg initially, then 2 mg after each stool
	Maximum dose:
	  8 mg/day OTC
	  16 mg/day Rx
		Impairs peristalsis	Use for <2 days
			Adverse effects:
			  Drowsiness
			  Abdominal pain
			  Fatigue
			Contraindications:
			  Ulcerative colitis
			  PM colitis
			  E. coli diarrhea

Diphenoxylate with atropine (Lomotil)	4 mg qid for <2 days	Increase GI transit time	CNS depression May enhance invasion/delay clearance of microorganisms May precipitate toxic megacolon in severe inflammatory bowel disease

Tincture of opium	0.5-1.0 mL po q4-6h for <2 days	Impairs peristalsis	CNS depressant
			Contraindications:
			  PM colitis
			  Ulcerative colitis

Octreotide (Sandostatin)	100-500 µg SC tid	Similar to hormone somatostatin	AIDS-associated diarrhea not responding to other therapy

AIDS, acquired immunodeficiency syndrome; CNS, central nervous system; HIV, human immunodeficiency virus; OTC, over the counter; PM, pseudomembranous.

high-risk groups, admission is warranted for continuous monitoring, further treatment, and definitive management when the initial evaluation and stabilization is complete.

REFERENCES

1. Aranda-Michel J, Giannella RA: Acute diarrhea: A practical review. *Am J of Med* 106:670, 1999.
2. Oldfield EC, et al: The role of antibiotics in the treatment of infectious diarrhea. *Gastroent Clin North Am* 30:817, 2001.
3. Black RE, Morris SS, Bryce J: When and why are 10 million children dying every year? *Lancet* 361:2226, 2003.
4. King CK, Glass R, Bresee JS, Duggan C: Managing acute gastroenteritis among children: Oral rehydration, maintenance, and nutritional therapy. *MMWR Recommend Rep* 52(RR-16):1, 2003.
5. Oldfield EC: Evaluation of chronic diarrhea in patients with human immunodeficiency virus infection. *Gastroenterol Disord* 2:176, 2002.
6. Clement PA, Gardiner JA: Diarrhea and vomiting. In Stone CK, Humphries RL (eds): *Current Emergency Diagnosis and Treatment*, 5th ed. New York, Lange/McGraw-Hill, 2004, pp 296-310.
7. Armon K, et al: An evidence and consensus based guideline for acute diarrheoa management. *Arch Dis Child* 85:132, 2001.
8. Hogenauer C, et al: Mechanisms and management of antibiotic-associated diarrhea. *Clin Infect Dis* 27:702, 1998.
9. Gomi H, et al: In vitro antimicrobial susceptibility testing of bacterial enteropathogens causing traveler's diarrhea in four geographic regions. *Antimicrob Agents Chemother* 45:212, 2001.
10. Duggan C, et al: Oral rehydration solution for acute diarrhea prevents subsequent unscheduled follow-up visits. *Pediatrics* 104:e29, 1999.
11. Patel AB, Dhande LA, Rawat MS: Economic evaluation of zinc and copper use in treating acute diarrhea in children: A randomized controlled trial. *Cost Eff Resour Alloc* 1:7, 2003.

CHAPTER

25 Constipation

Natalie Cullen

PERSPECTIVE

The American Academy of Gastroenterologists defines *constipation* as any two of the following: (1) straining to pass stool 25% of the time, (2) lumpy or hard stools 25% of the time, (3) incomplete sensation of evacuation 25% of the time, and (4) two or fewer stools per week. The Rome II criteria constitute a well-accepted definition of constipation used in research (Table 25-1).[1] Constipation is a symptom, not a diagnosis. It is usually necessary to identify the cause of this symptom to effect proper treatment and disposition. A definitive diagnosis often is not possible in the emergency department, and appropriate follow-up evaluation should be arranged.

Constipation is a common complaint that is often injudiciously and incorrectly self-diagnosed and treated by patients. The more than 700 over-the-counter laxative preparations available attest to the misguided premium people place on "regularity." The complaint of "constipation" should be of concern when there has been a significant change from a patient's own normal pattern that is creating unease or discomfort for the patient. This change may manifest as a decrease in frequency of defecation, sudden and persistent change in the character or amount of stools (especially decrease in stool caliber), blood in the stool, or problems expelling the stool.[1]

Epidemiology

Approximately 20% of the population at one time complains of constipation; 98% are elderly individuals. Constipation is more common in women than in men, nonwhites than whites, and children than adults. Twenty-six percent of elderly men and 34% of elderly women are affected by constipation. This symptom accounts for almost 2.5 million visits a year to health care providers. It is estimated that 30% of the general population, 60% of all elderly individuals, and 75% of all elderly individuals hospitalized or in nursing homes use laxatives on a regular basis. Laxative use is greater in women than in men.

The high prevalence in the elderly population is multifactorial and related to a diet low in fiber, sedentary habits, multiple medications, and various disease processes that impair neurologic and motor control. The elderly have a decreased thirst mechanism even in the presence of dehydration; inadequate fluid intake may play a role. Constipation also is common with patients who are institutionalized, debilitated, or neurologically impaired for any reason.[2,3]

Pathophysiology

Normally the gastrointestinal tract is presented with 9 to 10 L/day of secretions and ingested fluids. The small intestine usually absorbs all of this except 500 to 600 mL, and further absorption by the colon results in only 100 mL/day of fluid lost in the stool. Water is passively absorbed, following the osmotic gradient produced by the absorption of sodium. Sodium is actively absorbed even against large concentration gradients.

Normal defecation consists of a complex coordinated series of events: (1) distention of the rectum, (2) relaxation of the internal sphincter, (3) contraction of the external sphincter, (4) relaxation of the puborectalis muscle with Valsalva, (5) mild ascent of the pelvic floor causing straightening of the anorectal angle and opening of the anal canal, and (6) increased intraluminal pressure by straining. The pathophysiology of constipation is often multifactorial. Some authors classify constipation into three broad groups: normal-transit (e.g., functional constipation), slow-transit (e.g., colonic inertia, Hirschsprung's disease), and disorders of defecatory or rectal evacuation (e.g., dysfunction of pelvic floor or anal sphincter).

Constipation is primarily a consequence of a motility imbalance between the churning nonpropulsive forces that regulate stool consistency and fluid absorption and the propulsive forces that propel the feces toward the rectum. Studies of normal patients show intestinal transit time and bowel frequency are independent of age. Elderly patients with idiopathic chronic constipation do have prolonged total gut transit times, however, referred to as *colonic inertia*. This colonic inertia often is accompanied by a decrease in rectal sensitivity. The prolonged transit time allows increased time for colonic absorption of fluids from the fecal material, producing hard stools that may be difficult to pass. An abnormality in the sensory defecation reflexes has been documented in elderly patients and patients with spinal cord lesions. Ignoring the urge to defecate also may occur because of inconvenience; incapacity; or painful lesions in the anorectal area, such as hemorrhoids, fissures, or perirectal abscesses. Repeatedly resisting the urge to defecate suppresses the normal sensory stimuli evoked by rectal distention from feces, which leads to chronic rectal distention and eventually decreased motor tone.[4,5] By far the most important external factor governing colonic function is diet. An adequate intake of fluid and fiber is essential in preventing constipation.

Table 25-1. Rome II Criteria for Constipation

Adult
≥2 of the following for at least 12 wk (not consecutive) in the preceding 12 mo:
  Straining during >25% of bowel movements
  Lumpy or hard stools for >25% of bowel movements
  Sensation of incomplete evacuation for >25% of bowel movements
  Manual maneuvers of facilitate >25% of bowel movements (e.g., digital evacuation or support of the pelvic floor)
  <3 bowel movements per week
  Loose stools not present, and insufficient criteria for irritable bowel syndrome met[10]
Infants and Children
Pebble-like, hard stools for most bowel movements for at least 2 wk
Firm stools ≤2 times/wk for at least 2 wk
No evidence of structural, endocrine, or metabolic disease

DIAGNOSTIC APPROACH

Differential Consideration

The causes of constipation are numerous (Box 25-1). In the emergency department, patients most often present with acute constipation due to drugs or painful perianal lesions.[6]

Pivotal Findings

History

A thorough, detailed history usually identifies the most likely cause of a patient's constipation. Patients may present with abdominal cramping or distention, which leads to a diagnosis of constipation. Defining what the patient means by the term *constipation* is the essential beginning. Historical information can be separated into five categories:

1. The *character of the stools* can provide a clue to diagnosis and suggest the seriousness of the disorder. Diarrhea alternating with constipation suggests an obstructing colonic mass lesion, often cancer, but also is highly suggestive of an irritable bowel syndrome.
2. *Timing and frequency of stools* are important in diagnosis.
3. *Exogenous factors* may induce acute constipation. Innumerable medications can produce constipation. Changes in diet and exercise are important historical clues. Any newly prescribed medication is suspect if its administration precedes the onset of constipation.
4. *Associated symptoms* may give important clues regarding the cause of constipation and the patient's clinical status. Questions should be asked about the patient's job, sleep habits, appetite, daily activities, and associated symptoms of depression. Studies have indicated that depression is relatively common in the elderly population and may compound the problem of constipation. Flatulence and bloating are common with constipation and may represent a malabsorption syndrome. Significant temperature

BOX 25-1. Causes of Constipation

Acute Constipation (Four Ds)
Diet
  Deficient fluid intake
  Deficient fiber intake
Drugs
  Anticholinergics, e.g., antihistamines, tricyclic antidepressants, phenothiazines, antiparkinsonian agents, antispasmodics
  Antacids, e.g., aluminum hydroxide, calcium carbonate
  Antihypertensives, e.g., diuretics, calcium-channel blockers, clonidine
  Narcotics
  Sympathomimetics, e.g., ephedrine, phenylephedrine, phenylpropanolamine, terbutaline
  Laxative abuse
  Nonsteroidal anti-inflammatory drugs
  Others such as iron, phenytoin, barium, bismuth, sucralfate
Daily routine
  Immobility, lack of exercise
  Travel
  Psychosocial stress, depression, psychosis
  Failure to respond to the urge to defecate
Disease
  Anatomic
    Painful perianal lesion, e.g., hemorrhoids, abscesses, fissures, herpes
    Intrinsic bowel lesions, e.g., diverticulitis, carcinoma, obstruction
  Metabolic
    Hypothyroidism, hypoadrenalism
    Hypokalemia, hypercalcemia, chronic renal failure

Chronic Constipation (Three Hs)
Hypertonic
  Irritable bowel syndrome
  Diverticulosis
Hypotonic
  Neurogenic
    Dementia, stroke
    Diabetic autonomic neuropathy
    Multiple sclerosis, amyotrophic lateral sclerosis
    Spinal cord lesions
    Parkinson's disease
  Psychogenic, e.g., chronic schizophrenia or chronic psychosis
  Debilitated, bedridden, or institutionalized
Habit—toilet training

elevation suggests invasive infection, inflammatory disease, or prolonged fecal impaction. Nausea and vomiting are generally nonspecific symptoms. When they occur, acute obstruction should be considered. Weakness suggests dehydration or electrolyte imbalance. Weight loss and decreased appetite suggest the possibility of a debilitating disease (e.g., cancer, inflammatory bowel disease). Abdominal pain may accompany constipation. The location and character of the pain may localize a specific disease process, but are not diagnostic of constipation. The pain associated with constipation may be dull, crampy, and visceral in nature. Other symptoms associated with constipation include excessive gas, anorexia, fatigue, headache, low back pain, weakness, depression, and restlessness. If fecal impaction is present, the patient may present with low-grade fever, fecal incontinence, or alternating diarrhea and constipation. The most concerning symptoms associated with constipation are rectal bleeding and change in the caliber of the stool. These are warning signals suggesting possible colorectal cancer.

5. A history of concurrent or related disease states can help in establishing a diagnosis. The current constipated state may represent an acute exacerbation of a chronic intestinal disease (see Box 25-1).[6-8]

Physical Examination

The physical examination should include evaluation for systemic diseases and a search for organic causes of the constipation. The abdominal examination is usually normal but may reveal tenderness, a mass, or distention and evidence of obstruction. The perineum should be examined for fissures, inflamed hemorrhoids, or perirectal abscesses. Anal fissures are a common cause of constipation in young children.

The rectal examination for anorectal conditions and an evaluation of the stool are the most important parts of the physical assessment. Patients with acute constipation generally have large amounts of hard stool in the rectum. Obstructive disease or hypertonic constipation generally is associated with an empty ampulla. A rectum full of soft, putty-like stools in a patient lacking the sensation to defecate is characteristic of hypotonic or habit constipation. Results of rectal examinations have not been shown, however, to correlate with complaints of constipation or with evidence of colonic loading on abdominal radiographs. The rectal examination alone should not be used to confirm or exclude the presence of constipation. The stool should be checked for occult blood, which may indicate a colon carcinoma or simply the trauma of repeated attempts to defecate.[8,9]

Ancillary Testing

Plain abdominal radiographs are accurate in documenting colonic loading. These films provide information about extent of retention, bowel obstruction, megacolon, volvulus, or mass lesions. Masses of stool typically have a bubbly or speckled appearance and are usually readily visible on plain film.

Clinical laboratory studies are indicated only as dictated by the history and physical examination. Patients on diuretics or patients with known carcinoma who have constipation may have hypokalemia or hypercalcemia. When blood is found in the stool, a hemoglobin level may reveal an accompanying anemia, suggesting an occult carcinoma. The white blood cell count is nonspecific and not helpful.[3]

Patients with acute constipation for which the cause is not readily apparent should be treated symptomatically and referred for outpatient diagnostic evaluation. This evaluation usually includes a sigmoidoscopy and a barium enema, preferably air contrast in nature, to evaluate for an underlying intrinsic bowel lesion. Possible endocrinologic or metabolic causes are usually investigated on an outpatient basis.

Chronic laxative abuse can present as acute constipation, and patients often do not volunteer their laxative use. If laxative abuse is suspected, a sodium hydroxide test of the stool may be revealing. If 3% sodium hydroxide turns stool red, and if the reaction is abolished by the addition of hydrochloric acid, it indicates the presence of phenolphthalein, the most commonly abused laxative.

DIFFERENTIAL DIAGNOSIS

The cause of acute constipation is usually readily apparent from a complete history and physical examination. Any patient with recent-onset constipation, the cause of which is not obvious, should undergo a complete evaluation. In these cases, the problem is often due to an intrinsic bowel lesion, such as diverticulitis or an obstructing carcinoma. Figure 25-1 outlines a diagnostic approach.[10,11]

For patients who have chronic constipation, the specific reason for their being in the emergency department should be assessed before symptomatic relief is provided. These patients should be referred to their private physician for continued evaluation and therapy.

Critical and Emergent Diagnoses

Constipation rarely is associated with morbidity or mortality. Most bad outcomes are due to missed diagnosis of bowel obstruction or perforation. These conditions are diagnosed easily with flat and upright abdominal radiographs, when indicated.

Complications of constipation can be classified as nonobstructive or obstructive. Nonobstructive complications occur secondary to straining at stools and the resulting changes in intrathoracic pressure and include hernias; exacerbation or gastroesophageal reflux; and decreases in coronary, cerebral, or peripheral arterial circulation. Obstructive complications include fecal impaction, idiopathic megacolon, volvulus, and intestinal obstruction.

EMPIRIC MANAGEMENT

Treatment of acute constipation is directed toward eradicating the underlying cause and providing adjunctive symptomatic therapy (Box 25-2; see Figure 25-1). Symptomatic therapy includes adequate intake of fluids and fiber and, if necessary, additional sources of bulk in the form of synthetic bulk agents (Table 25-2). Specific therapy may include withholding of a causative medication, correction of hypokalemia, management of an anal fissure, or draining of a perirectal abscess.

Acutely, manual disimpaction may be necessary, especially if fecal impaction is noted. Enemas should not be used routinely but may be necessary in some

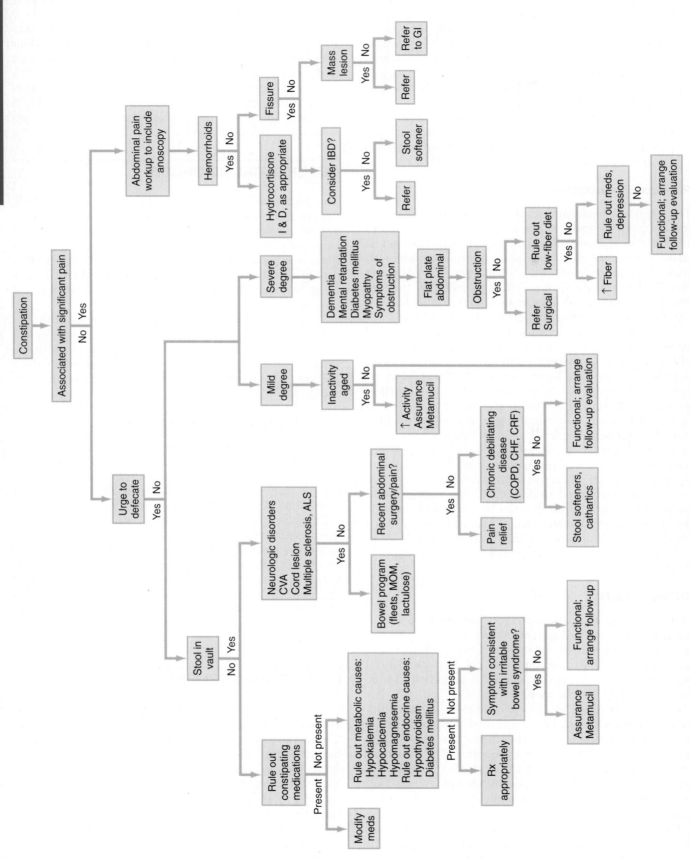

Figure 25-1. Algorithmic approach to constipation. I&D, incision and drainage; CVA, cerebrovascular accident; ALS, amyotrophic lateral sclerosis; IBD, inflammatory bowel disease; MOM, milk of magnesia; COPD, chronic obstructive pulmonary disease; CHF, congestive heart failure; CRF, chronic renal failure.

Table 25-2. Preparations Used in the Symptomatic Treatment of Constipation or Fecal Impaction

Type	Action	Generic Agent	Brand	Daily Dose	Precautions
Bulk agents	Increase in stool water, bulk, and rate of bowel transit	Bran/fiber		10 g/day × 7 days, then 20 g/day PO	Bulk agents require adequate fluid intake, 1.5-2 L/day, to prevent worsening of the constipation or development of obstruction or impaction
		Psyllium	Metamucil Hydrocil Fiberall	Up to 30 g/day in divided doses PO	
		Methylcellulose	Citrucel Cologel Hydrolase	Up to 6 g/day in divided doses PO	
Lubricants	Inhibit colonic water absorption and coat stool for easier passage	Mineral oil	Zymenol Kondremul	15-30 mL once or twice per day PO	Contraindicated in debilitated patients or patients with swallowing problems; aspiration causes lipoid pneumonia; may impair absorption of fat-soluble vitamins
Stool softener	Soften stool and some gut secretory and stimulant effect	Docusate sodium Docusate calcium Docusate potassium	Colace Surfak Dialose	50-360 mg PO	Little evidence in literature supporting effectiveness; may be directly hepatotoxic or potentiate hepatotoxicity of other drugs
Irritants	Stimulate motility and increase gut mucosal secretion of sodium and water	Senna extract Phenolphthalein	Senekot Ex-Lax Feen-a-Mint Correctol	1-2 tabs or tsp PO 130-275 mg PO	Chronic use may cause myenteric plexus neuronal damage and major motility dysfunction, "cathartic colon"
		Bisacodyl	Dulcolax Carter's Pills	5-15 mg PO	
		Danthron	Dorbane	75-150 mg PO	
		Castor oil	Neoloid	50-60 mL PO	
Osmotic agents	Osmotically draw fluid into the bowel lumen, increasing intraluminal pressure and stimulating peristalsis	Magnesium salts Citrate Hydroxide Sulfate	Citrate of Magnesia Milk of Magnesia Epsom salts	200 mL PO 15-30 mL PO 240-300 mL PO	Magnesium toxicity in patients with renal insufficiency All osmotic agents require good fluid intake for maximal effect Monitor glucose level
		Nonabsorbable sugars Lactose	Cephulac Chronulac	15-30 mL PO bid	
		Sorbitol (70% sol) Polyethylene glycol–saline solution	GoLYTELY CoLyte	15-30 mL PO bid 2-6 L PO	
Suppositories	Local irritant or osmotic effect	Glycerine Bisacodyl	Dulcolax	3 g PR 10 mg PR	May cause rectal irritation
Enemas	Local irritant, osmotic, or lubricating effect	Tap water or saline enemas Sodium salts Phosphate Sulfate Mineral oil	Fleet Enema Phospho-Soda	100-200 mL PR 120 mL PR 60-120 mL PR	Hot water, soap, or hydrogen peroxide enemas should never be used beause they irritate the rectal mucosa and may cause bleeding; sodium salts may cause fluid overload in patients with congestive heart failure; phosphates may affect the serum phosphorus and calcium levels; phosphate enemas should not be used in patients with renal insufficiency

PO, by mouth; PR, per rectum.

BOX 25-2. Approach to Treatment of Constipation

For specific agents, dosages, and precautions, see Table (25-2).

I. Core program for all patients
   A. Adequate intake of fluid and fiber is the key to preventing constipation. Fiber is available primarily from grains and bran cereals. Fiber is not the same as roughage; fiber increases fecal bulk but roughage does not. Most fruits and vegetables have high roughage content but relatively low amounts of dietary fiber. Flatulence, bloating, or cramps are common side effects encountered when bran fiber is introduced; bacterial metabolism of bran forms methane gas in some patients.
   B. Another source of bulk is from synthetic bulk agents. Bulk agents require an adequate amount of fluid intake or they may worsen constipation.
   C. Avoid irritant laxatives because long-term use may decrease bowel motility. Encourage the patient to exercise and respond promptly to the urge to defecate.

II. Individualized program—specific indications for the use of other agents
   A. *Lubricants:* Oral mineral oil lubricants are particularly helpful in patients who have acute painful perianal lesions. The softening and coating of the stool can make passage much easier and less painful, preventing constipation. It is also helpful in elderly patients who have chronically hard stools and is usually well tolerated. Mineral oil is contraindicated in patients with swallowing problems or patients particularly debilitated to prevent aspiration leading to lipid pneumonia.
   B. *Stool softeners:* Stool softeners are wetting agents believed to enhance the moisture content of fecal material. Evidence exists that stool softeners are no more effective than placebo and certainly not any better than other agents available. Evidence also exists that stool softeners themselves can be hepatotoxic or may enhance the absorption of other liver toxins; it is recommended that stool softeners not be used chronically in the treatment of constipation.
   C. *Irritants:* Short-term use of irritant laxatives can be beneficial in acute constipation caused by diminished gut motility, such as with constipating drugs, hypokalemia, or immobility caused by illness or injury. In chronic constipation, the use of these stimulant laxatives should be limited to patients with weakened abdominal perineal muscles, diminished bowel motility from constipating medications that cannot be eliminated, loss of rectal refluxes, or severely delayed gut transit or megacolon.
   D. *Osmotic agents:* These agents are most often used for colonic preparation for bowel procedures or in combination with activated charcoal in overdose cases. Magnesium salts are contraindicated in patients with renal failure and are not recommended for chronic use. The nonabsorbable sugars, particularly lactulose or sorbitol, are often the mainstay treatment for chronically constipated patients. Polyethylene glycol is a colonic lavage solution most often used in preparation for bowel procedures. It has been found to be effective in the treatment of fecal impaction.
   E. *Suppositories and enemas:* These agents are especially helpful in patients who tend to have trouble expelling soft stool from the rectum. Glycerine suppositories may have a soothing effect and be helpful in patients with constipation caused by local, painful perianal lesions. Tap-water enemas or oil-retention enemas are helpful when disimpaction is necessary.

cases, especially if the patient already has failed a trial of outpatient laxatives. Warm tap water enemas are probably the safest (see Table 25-2). Repeated enemas have the potential to cause myenteric plexus damage, resulting in motility dysfunction. Specialists may perform balloon expulsion, or surgery may be necessary in recalcitrant cases.[1,7,8]

DISPOSITION

Constipation is appropriately treated at home, and only the most obstinate cases require disimpaction or enema treatment in the emergency department. If complications or serious causes of constipation exist, such as fecal impaction, megacolon, volvulus, or bowel obstruction, the patient usually is admitted to the hospital for further intervention.[9]

REFERENCES

1. Gattuso JM, Kamm A: Review article: The management of constipation in adults. *Aliment Pharmacol Ther* 7:487, 1999.
2. Wilson J: Constipation in the elderly. *Gastroenterology* 15:499, 1999.
3. Soffer E: Constipation: An approach to diagnosis, treatment, referral. *Cleve Clin J Med* 66:41, 1999.
4. Shafik A: Constipation: Pathogenesis and management. *Drugs* 45:528, 1993.
5. Lembo A, et al: Chronic constipation. *N Engl J Med* 349:1360, 2003.
6. Arce DA, et al: Evaluation of constipation. *Am Fam Physician* 65:2283, 2002.
7. Dosh SA: Evaluation and treatment of constipation. *J Fam Pract* 51:555, 2002.
8. Holten KB, et al: Diagnosing the patient with abdominal pain and altered bowel habits: Is it irritable bowel syndrome? *Am Fam Physician* 67:2157, 2003.
9. Prather C, Ortiz-Camacho C: Evaluation and treatment of constipation and fecal impaction in adults. *Mayo Clin Proc* 73:881, 1998.
10. Browning SM: Constipation, diarrhea, and irritable bowel syndrome. *Prim Care North Am Clin* 26:113, 1999.
11. Bulloch B, et al: Constipation: Diagnosis and management in the pediatric emergency department. *Pediatr Emerg Care* 18:254, 2002.

CHAPTER 26 Jaundice

Katherine L. Heilpern and Tammie E. Quest

PERSPECTIVE

Epidemiology and Pathophysiology

Jaundice affects patients of all ages, from neonates to elderly persons. An understanding of the metabolism of bilirubin is crucial for the diagnosis and evaluation of jaundice, which is usually a manifestation of hepatic or hematopoietic disease.

Bilirubin Metabolism

Bilirubin is generated from heme products, primarily senescent red blood cells. A small portion is derived from myoglobin and maturing erythroid cells. Within the reticuloendothelial system, heme is oxidized to biliverdin, which is then converted to bilirubin. Unconjugated bilirubin forms a tight but reversible bond with albumin. It is observed clinically in tissues with high albumin concentrations, for example, the skin and eyes. It is absent in albumin-poor fluids, such as tears or saliva. Successful excretion of bilirubin from the body requires hepatic conjugation.

Pathophysiology

Clinical jaundice is usually not evident until the serum bilirubin concentration rises above 2.5 mg/dL. The physiology of bile metabolism may be altered on four principal levels: overproduction of heme products, failure of the hepatocyte to take up the bilirubin for processing, failure of the hepatocyte to conjugate or excrete bilirubin, or an obstruction of biliary excretion into the intestine. Unconjugated bilirubin that is not bound to albumin can cross the blood-brain barrier, causing adverse neurologic effects ranging from subtle developmental abnormalities to encephalopathy and death. The risk of neurotoxicity is increased by conditions that favor the unbound fraction of unconjugated bilirubin, including hemolysis, hypoalbuminemia, acidemia, and drugs that bind competitively to albumin. Conjugated bilirubins are not neurotoxic, although they may indicate serious disease.

DIAGNOSTIC APPROACH

Differential Considerations

The three major diagnostic categories to consider are liver injury or dysfunction (cholestasis), biliary obstructive disorders, and disorders of hemolysis. Figure 26-1 outlines a laboratory-based approach to differentiating among these three categories.

Pivotal Findings

The pivotal findings related to history, physical examination, and ancillary testing are listed in Figure 26-2.

History

Patients may present with jaundice and abdominal pain. This presentation suggests biliary obstruction or significant hepatic inflammation. New-onset painless jaundice is the classical presentation for a neoplasm involving the head of the pancreas. Patients may complain of pruritus, a consequence of bile pigment deposition in the skin. Constitutional symptoms are common and include fatigue, fever, and anorexia. Patients may complain of ill-fitting clothing because of weight loss or increasing abdominal girth related to ascites. The patient or caregiver may note personality changes or confusion, suggestive of hepatic encephalopathy.

Physical Examination

Fever with right upper quadrant tenderness suggests cholangitis or cholecystitis.[1] In this instance, the liver should not be engorged. A large tender liver could represent an exacerbation of acute or chronic hepatitis or malignant infiltration. A palpable gallbladder, a rare finding, suggests chronic cholestasis or malignancy. The presence of splenomegaly suggests hemolysis, malignancy, or portal hypertension. Ascites may be associated with acute or chronic liver disease. Ascites associated with abdominal tenderness raises suspicion for spontaneous bacterial peritonitis. Rapid onset of hepatomegaly and ascites may indicate portal vein thrombosis (Budd-Chiari syndrome).[2] Jaundice associated with a large pulsatile abdominal mass may indicate a rapidly enlarging or ruptured abdominal aortic aneurysm. The patient's mental status should be assessed for evidence of hepatic encephalopathy.

Physical examination findings associated with chronic liver disease and cirrhosis include spider angiomas, gynecomastia, testicular atrophy, and caput medusa. Excoriations from pruritus suggest chronic liver disease. Asterixis, a sign of hepatic encephalopathy, is usually found only in patients with chronic liver disease. Table 26-1 addresses the clinical stages of hepatic encephalopathy.

Ancillary Testing

Figure 26-1 lists the laboratory tests that should be considered in the evaluation of a patient with jaundice.[3,4]

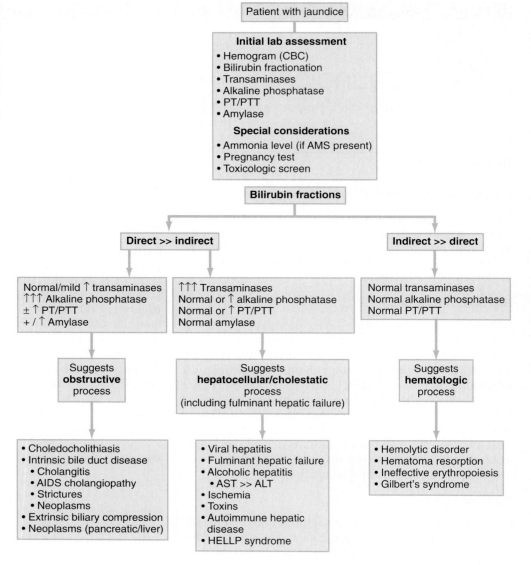

Figure 26-1. Laboratory approach to differential diagnosis of jaundice. AIDS, acquired immunodeficiency syndrome; ALT, alanine aminotransferase; AMS, altered mental status; AST, aspartate aminotransferase; CBC, complete blood count; HELLP, hemolysis, elevated liver enzymes, and low platelets; PT, prothrombin time; PTT, partial thromboplastin time.

The figure content:

Patient with jaundice

Initial lab assessment
- Hemogram (CBC)
- Bilirubin fractionation
- Transaminases
- Alkaline phosphatase
- PT/PTT
- Amylase

Special considerations
- Ammonia level (if AMS present)
- Pregnancy test
- Toxicologic screen

Bilirubin fractions

Direct >> indirect

Normal/mild ↑ transaminases
↑↑↑ Alkaline phosphatase
± ↑ PT/PTT
+ / ↑ Amylase

Suggests **obstructive** process

- Choledocholithiasis
- Intrinsic bile duct disease
  - Cholangitis
  - AIDS cholangiopathy
  - Strictures
  - Neoplasms
- Extrinsic biliary compression
- Neoplasms (pancreatic/liver)

↑↑↑ Transaminases
Normal or ↑ alkaline phosphatase
Normal or ↑ PT/PTT
Normal amylase

Suggests **hepatocellular/cholestatic** process (including fulminant hepatic failure)

- Viral hepatitis
- Fulminant hepatic failure
- Alcoholic hepatitis
  - AST >> ALT
- Ischemia
- Toxins
- Autoimmune hepatic disease
- HELLP syndrome

Indirect >> direct

Normal transaminases
Normal alkaline phosphatase
Normal PT/PTT

Suggests **hematologic** process

- Hemolytic disorder
- Hematoma resorption
- Ineffective erythropoiesis
- Gilbert's syndrome

A reticulocyte count and evaluation of the peripheral blood smear may identify hemolysis. If a toxic ingestion is suggested, a quantitative acetaminophen level may be indicated. Rapid stool guaiac testing should be performed to assess the presence of gastrointestinal bleeding. Patients with altered mental status should have a rapid bedside glucose assessment in addition to a quantitative ammonia level. Although a quantitative ammonia level may help with the diagnosis, the level has not been shown to correlate with the degree of encephalopathy.[5] In the presence of abdominal tenderness and ascites, ascitic fluid should be tested for cell count, Gram's stain, culture, and protein.[6] Two sets of blood cultures should be obtained for patients with fever and jaundice. If the patient appears ill or there is evidence of gastrointestinal bleeding, a type and crossmatch should be performed by the laboratory.

Imaging

The first choice radiologic study for obstructive biliary disease remains somewhat controversial. Both ultrasonography and computed tomography are helpful, depending on the information sought. Ultrasonography is preferred if cholecystitis or biliary obstruction related to choledocholithiasis is thought most likely and is superior to computed tomography for these diagnoses. Ultrasonography with Doppler flow can detect obstruction in the hepatic, portal, and splenic veins. Sonographic features that suggest acute cholecystitis include pericholecystic fluid and gallbladder wall thickening.[7] If gallstones are present on ultrasonography, a sonographic Murphy sign has a positive predictive value of 90% for acute cholecystitis.

Computed tomography imaging can detect extrabiliary (including retroperitoneal) conditions with greater accuracy, such as obstructing mass lesions, erosive complications of gallbladder disease, and other intraabdominal pathology. Endoscopic retrograde cholangiopancreatography (ERCP) is the "gold standard"; it provides direct visualization of the biliary system and may be indicated for both diagnostic and therapeutic reasons.

DIFFERENTIAL DIAGNOSIS

Utilizing a systems approach, one can categorize jaundice into critical, emergent, and nonemergent categories (Table 26-2). Patients are considered critical if they present with jaundice and any of the following: altered level of consciousness, hypotension, fever with abdominal pain, or active bleeding. Any patient with a *new* triad of jaundice, encephalopathy, and coagulopathy is considered to have fulminant hepatic failure.[8] In general, these patients have no prior history of liver disease and develop a sudden illness or toxic exposure that leads to hepatic necrosis. The time course from exposure to fulminant hepatic failure ranges from 1 to 8 weeks.

One specific presentation warrants discussion. Women in the third trimester of pregnancy can present with jaundice, complicating two critical diseases, both of which require emergent delivery. The preeclampsia-eclampsia syndrome may progress to the syndrome of hemolysis, elevated liver enzymes, and low platelets (HELLP). This is heralded by nausea, vomiting, and right upper quadrant pain. Mental status is usually normal. Rarely, these patients may suffer spontaneous rupture of the liver, a grave complication. Acute fatty liver of pregnancy arises with jaundice, encephalopathy, and coagulopathy, and the pathology resembles that of Reye's syndrome. Patients with the HELLP syndrome and acute fatty liver of pregnancy require intensive care unit monitoring pending fetal delivery.[2]

EMPIRICAL MANAGEMENT AND DISPOSITION

Intravenous access should be obtained immediately (Figure 26-3). The patient with depressed mental status should have pulse oximetry performed and undergo bedside testing of blood glucose levels. Empirical naloxone and thiamine should be considered. If the mental status remains significantly depressed, endotracheal intubation for maintaining airway patency or protection is usually indicated.

Crystalloid infusion may be indicated in the hypotensive patient with jaundice. A quick assessment of volume status is required because hepatic congestion with jaundice can occur in the setting of congestive heart failure. Central venous pressure monitoring may be helpful. Significant bleeding from any source requires aggressive management. Crystalloid infusion is initiated until blood products become available. Coagulopathy should be corrected with fresh frozen plasma and blood volume repleted with packed red blood cells.

If ascites is present, diagnostic paracentesis is recommended to rule out spontaneous bacterial peritoni-

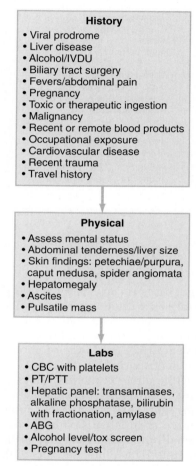

Figure 26-2. Pivotal points in the assessment of the jaundiced patient. ABG, arterial blood gas; CBC, complete blood count; IVDU, intravenous drug use; PT, prothrombin time; PTT, partial thromboplastin time.

Table 26-1. Clinical Stages of Hepatic Encephalopathy

Clinical Stage	Intellectual Function	Neuromuscular Function
Subclinical	Normal examination but work or driving may be impaired	Subtle changes in psychometric testing
Stage 1	Impaired attention, irritability, depression, or personality changes	Tremor, incoordination, apraxia
Stage 2	Drowsiness, behavioral changes, poor memory, disturbed sleep	Asterixis, slowed or slurred speech, ataxia
Stage 3	Confusion, disorientation, somnolence, amnesia	Hypoactive reflexes, nystagmus, clonus, muscular rigidity
Stage 4	Stupor and coma	Dilated pupils and decerebrate posturing; oculocephalic reflex

From Fitz G: Systemic complications of liver disease. In Feldman M, Sleisenger M (eds): *Gastrointestinal and Liver Disease.* Philadelphia, WB Saunders, 1998.

Table 26-2. Jaundice: Differential Diagnosis of Critical and Emergent Diagnoses

System	Critical	Emergent	Nonemergent

Hepatic	Fulminant hepatic failure
	  Toxin
	  Virus
	  Alcohol
	  Ischemic insult
	  Reye's syndrome
		Hepatitis of any etiology with confusion,
		  bleeding, or coagulopathy
		Wilson's disease
		Primary biliary cirrhosis
		Autoimmune hepatitis
		Liver transplant rejection
		Infiltrative liver disease
		Drug-induced (isoniazid, phenytoin,
		  acetaminophen, ritonavir, halothane,
		  sulfonamides)
		Toxin ingestion or exposure
			Hepatitis with normal mental status,
			  normal vital signs, and no active
			  bleeding

Biliary	Cholangitis	Bile duct obstruction (stone, inflammation, stricture, neoplasm)	
Systemic	Sepsis Heatstroke	Sarcoidosis Amyloidosis Graft-versus-host disease	Posttraumatic hematoma resorption Total parenteral nutrition
Cardiovascular	Obstructing AAA Budd-Chiari syndrome Severe congestive heart failure	Right-sided congestive heart failure Veno-occlusive disease	
Hematologic-Oncologic	Transfusion reaction	Hemolytic anemia Massive malignant infiltration Inborn error of metabolism Pancreatic head tumor Metastatic disease	Gilbert's syndrome Physiologic neonatal jaundice
Reproductive	Preclampsia//HELLP syndrome Acute fatty liver of pregnancy	Hyperemesis gravidarum	Cholestasis of pregnancy

AAA, abdominal aortic aneurysm; HELLP, hemolysis, elevated liver enzymes, and low platelets.

tis (SBP). This disease can have a subtle presentation and may be missed without a screening diagnostic tap. The presence of more than 250 polymorphonuclear cells per cubic millimeter of ascitic fluid is diagnostic for SBP. The empirical antibiotic of choice is a third-generation cephalosporin.[6]

Patients with altered mental status, fulminant hepatic failure, or unstable vital signs should be admitted to the hospital. Patients with encephalopathy are usually managed as inpatients. Oral or rectal lactulose may be initiated in the emergency department. On the basis of laboratory data alone, patients with new-onset jaundice should be hospitalized if transaminases are greater than 1000 IU/L, the bilirubin exceeds 10 mg/dL, or there is evidence of coagulopathy. Any of these laboratory abnormalities suggests significant hepatic dysfunction.

In general, patients with uncomplicated cholecystitis should receive intravenous fluids in the emergency department, parenteral analgesics, and antiemetics as needed and should be hospitalized. For uncomplicated cholecystitis, antibiotic therapy is usually not indicated. Patients with temperature greater than 38.8° C (102° F), a toxic appearance, or frank sepsis should receive broad-spectrum antibiotic therapy to cover enteric pathogens, streptococcal species, and anaerobes. These patients should undergo emergent imaging and consultation with a surgeon or gastroenterologist.[7]

Choledocholithiasis, stones in the common bile duct, is not as easily visualized by sonography but is suggested by significant obstructive signs and symptoms and a common bile duct dilated beyond 6 mm. These patients require hospitalization for possible ERCP and cholecystectomy. If cholangitis is suspected, blood cultures should be obtained immediately, followed by prompt administration of broad-spectrum antibiotics covering gram-negative aerobes and anaerobes. These patients usually require emergent ERCP with decompression, which dramatically improves survival.[9]

Patients with hepatitis or cholestatic jaundice may be managed as outpatients if they have a normal mental status, stable vital signs, ability to take oral fluids, no evidence of acute bleeding, and no complicating infectious process. Intravenous fluids and antiemetics may be required in the emergency department. Medications with potential hepatotoxicity, particularly acetaminophen, should be avoided.

In immune-mediated hemolytic anemia, the appropriate crossmatch may be difficult and fatal if not done properly. The decision to transfuse should be based on the patient's ability to oxygenate and the ability to institute alternative treatments. An urgent hematology consultation is recommended. In the case of drug-induced hemolytic anemia, the mainstay of treatment involves removal of the offending agent. For patients with glucose-6-phosphate deficiency, blood transfusions are rarely indicated and the focus of management should be on maintaining urine output to prevent renal failure. Patients with hemoglobinopathies rarely require transfusion therapy unless they present with severe anemia without evidence of reticulocytosis. Fluids, oxygen, and analgesics often abort an acute crisis.[10]

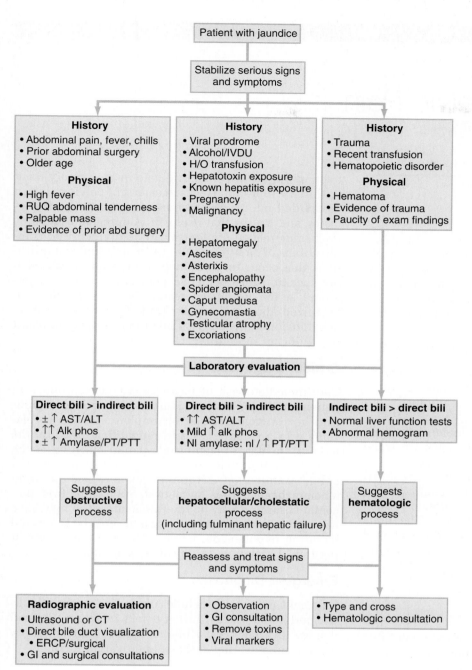

Figure 26-3. Management of the patient with jaundice. ALT, alanine aminotransferase; AST, aspartate aminotransferase; CT, computed tomography; ERCP, endoscopic retrograde cholangiopancreatography; GI, gastrointestinal; H/O, history of; IVDU, intravenous drug use; nl, normal; PT, prothrombin time; PTT, partial thromboplastin time; RUQ, right upper quadrant.

REFERENCES

1. Trowbridge RL, Rutkowski NK, Shojania KG: Does this patient have acute cholecystitis? *JAMA* 289:80, 2003.
2. Lee WM: Acute liver failure. *N Engl J Med* 329:1862, 1993.
3. Pratt DA, Kaplan MM: Primary care: Review of abnormal liver enzyme results in asymptomatic patients. *N Engl J Med* 342:1266, 2000.
4. Case 2-2000: A 74-year-old man with painless jaundice 10 years after renal transplantation. *N Engl J Med* 342:192, 2000.
5. Menon KV, Kamath PS: Managing the complications of cirrhosis. *Mayo Clin Proc* 75:501, 2000.
6. Gines P, et al: Management of cirrhosis and ascites. *N Engl J Med* 350:1646, 2004.
7. Indar AA, Beckingham IJ: Acute cholecystitis. *BMJ* 325:639, 2002.
8. Starzl TE: Fulminant hepatic failure. *Surg Clin North Am* 79:77, 1999.
9. Yusoff IF, Barkun JS, Barkun AN: Diagnosis and management of cholecystitis and cholangitis. *Gastroenterol Clin North Am* 32:1145, 2003.
10. Tabbara IA: Hemolytic anemias: Diagnosis and management. *Med Clin North Am* 76:649, 1992.

PERSPECTIVE

Epidemiology

Acute pelvic pain is common in women of childbearing age and is the second most common gynecologic complaint after vaginal bleeding.[1] Pelvic pain can be secondary to a variety of different causes, many of which do not require definitive diagnosis or treatment on an emergent basis. Disease is suspected more often than it is found on laparoscopy.

Causes of acute pelvic pain vary widely depending on the age and socioeconomic status of the patient. Most cases are due to salpingitis, ectopic pregnancy, ruptured corpus luteum cyst, adnexal torsion, tubo-ovarian abscess, and appendicitis. No pathologic condition is found in 20% of women.[2]

Many causes of pelvic pain have potentially serious sequelae. Salpingitis carries the risk of acute tubo-ovarian abscess, subsequent infertility, and an increased frequency of ectopic pregnancy. In one study, approximately 40% of women not using contraception were unable to conceive 2 to 9 years after an index episode of pelvic inflammatory disease.[3] The odds of ectopic pregnancy were increased by a factor of 3.4 in women with a confirmed prior episode of salpingitis.[4] Ruptured ectopic pregnancy may lead to life-threatening hemorrhage.

Pathophysiology

The pelvis contains the vagina, uterus, fallopian tubes and ovaries, ureter and urinary bladder, and sigmoid colon and rectum. Although pelvic pain often originates from the reproductive organs, it also may arise from structures that lie adjacent to or course through the pelvis. Visceral pain afferents supplying the pelvic organs share a common innervation of the appendix, ureters, and colon. Their significant overlap makes accurate localization difficult for the patient and clinician. Pain may be initiated by inflammation, distention, or stretching of an organ. Parietal pain develops when the afferent nerves in the parietal peritoneum adjacent to an affected organ become stimulated.

DIAGNOSTIC APPROACH

The differential diagnosis of pelvic pain is broad (Box 27-1). Most causes of pelvic pain fit into three categories, however: (1) causes that originate in the reproductive tract, (2) causes that originate in the intestinal tract, and (3) causes that originate in the urinary tract. Within the reproductive tract, causes of pelvic pain can be divided into causes that are complications of pregnancy and causes that occur in nonpregnant patients. Pregnancy-related etiologies can be divided into complications of first-trimester pregnancy and complications that occur further along in pregnancy. Although the specific cause of pelvic pain is not always determined at the initial emergency department visit, an organized approach usually leads to the confirmation or exclusion of the causes that are most likely to result in significant morbidity.

Critical Diagnoses

The immediate risk of death or serious morbidity in patients with pelvic pain is from hemorrhage. Significant hemorrhage from an incomplete abortion or placenta previa usually is readily identified based on the patient's history of significant vaginal bleeding or the identification of evidence of significant hemorrhage at pelvic examination. Ectopic pregnancy, bleeding from a hemorrhagic corpus luteal cyst, or bleeding from placental abruption may be life-threatening, but may have minimal or no vaginal bleeding and must be suspected based on hypotension, pelvic pain, and tenderness or peritoneal irritation on physical examination.

Emergent Diagnoses

Emergent diagnoses include appendicitis, diverticulitis, perforated viscus, urinary tract infection, ureteral stones, ovarian cysts/tumors, pelvic inflammatory disease/tubo-ovarian abscess, and ovarian torsion.

Pivotal Findings

History

Numerous historical findings are useful in evaluating a patient with pelvic pain. The *location* of pain and the *radiation pattern* are often helpful in determining a specific cause. Lateral pelvic pain often is related to a process in the tube or ovary. Appendicitis needs to be considered if the pain is right sided. Diverticulitis is considered in older (>40 years old) patients with left lower quadrant pain. Central pelvic pain often is related to conditions involving the uterus or bladder. Pain radiating to the rectum is often secondary to fluid or blood pooling in the cul-de-sac. Diffuse pain may occur with a bilateral process, such as pelvic inflammatory disease, or when diffuse peritonitis occurs secondary to infection or intra-abdominal hemorrhage.

BOX 27-1. Differential Diagnosis of Acute Pelvic Pain

Reproductive Tract
Nonpregnant
Salpingitis/tubo-ovarian abscess
Ovarian cyst
Ovarian torsion
Endometriosis
Uterine fibroids
Uterine perforation
Round ligament pain

Pregnant
First trimester
    Ectopic pregnancy
    Threatened abortion
    Nonviable pregnancy
    Endometritis
    Corpus luteal cyst
    Ovarian hyperstimulation syndrome
    Ovarian torsion
Second and third trimester
    Placenta previa
    Placental abruption

Intestinal Tract
Appendicitis
Diverticulitis
Inflammatory bowel disease
Gastroenteritis
Ischemic bowel
Bowel obstruction
Perforated viscus
Incarcerated/strangulated hernia

Urinary Tract
Pyelonephritis
Cystitis
Ureteral stone

The *onset and duration of pain* also can be useful in the patient evaluation. Patients with uncomplicated appendicitis (without perforation or abscess) typically present within 48 hours of symptom onset.[5] Sudden-onset pain suggests acute intrapelvic hemorrhage, cystic rupture, or ovarian torsion. Gradual-onset pain is more consistent with inflammation or obstruction. Chronic or recurrent pain is consistent with endometriosis, recurrent ovarian cysts, or a persistent ovarian mass. The *quality of pain* may differentiate the crampy, intermittent pattern of hollow versus muscular contractions from the steady, progressive pain associated with inflammatory or neoplastic causes. Pain associated with pelvic inflammatory disease often presents at the end of menses; ovarian cyst pain may fluctuate through several menstrual cycles, finally presenting as rupture, which often occurs in the middle phase of the menstrual cycle.

During a review of *associated symptoms,* a complaint of fever and chills is found more commonly with an infectious process. Nausea and vomiting occur more frequently when the process originates from the gastrointestinal tract, but commonly may accompany ovarian torsion, ureteral colic, and early pregnancy. Dysuria, frequency, or urgency suggests *urinary tract infection*; however, these also are often found in young women with pelvic inflammatory disease or herpes infection.

All women of childbearing age presenting with lower abdominal or pelvic pain must have a pregnancy test. The patient's last menstrual period, pattern of menses, and sexual activity pattern are potentially useful, but do not obviate the need for a pregnancy test. In a pregnant patient, the obstetric history may provide some helpful diagnostic clues. Patients with a history of recurrent spontaneous abortions are at increased risk for having another spontaneous abortion. Patients with a prior history of ectopic pregnancy are at increased risk for having a recurrent ectopic pregnancy. Patients with a history of infertility are at increased risk for ectopic pregnancy. In addition, patients who are actively undergoing infertility treatment are at increased risk for ectopic pregnancy, heterotopic pregnancy, ovarian torsion, and ovarian hyperstimulation syndrome.[6,7]

The *presence, quantity, and duration* of associated *vaginal bleeding* should be ascertained. In a nonpregnant patient, bleeding can be associated with pelvic inflammatory disease, dysfunctional uterine bleeding, or cervical or uterine cancer. In a pregnant patient, bleeding may be associated with a subchorionic hemorrhage in an otherwise viable pregnancy, with an ectopic pregnancy, with a nonviable intrauterine pregnancy, or later in pregnancy with placenta previa or abruption. In some cases, the amount of bleeding may be substantial enough to require uterine evacuation and blood transfusion.

As part of the *past medical history,* the performance of any recent procedures should be ascertained. The onset of abdominal pain recently after uterine instrumentation increases the possibility of uterine perforation. *Sexual history* is essential, with an emphasis on recent sexual contact and previous history of potential infections.

Physical Examination

The physical examination is directed toward the pelvis and abdomen (Table 27-1). Based on laparoscopic findings, two thirds of patients with pain but a "normal" pelvic examination have some pelvic pathology.[2] Patients with abnormal pelvic examinations or ultrasound findings are much more likely to have an abnormal laparoscopic examination.[2,8] All stable patients less than 20 weeks' gestational age should have a pelvic examination performed. An urgent obstetric consultation should be obtained for patients greater than 20 weeks' gestational age. If the patient complains of vaginal bleeding, a transabdominal pelvic ultrasound study should be done for placental localization before the performance of a pelvic examination to exclude the diagnosis of placenta previa. Manipulation of the cervix in these patients may precipitate significant hemorrhage.

Table 27-1. Pivotal Findings at Physical Examination in Acute Pelvic Pain

Sign	Finding	Diagnoses
Vital signs	Hypotension	Ruptured ectopic pregnancy
		Ruptured cyst
		Secondary to heavy vaginal bleeding from a variety of causes
		Pelvic peritonitis with sepsis
	Fever	PID
		Appendicitis
		UTI
		Ovarian torsion
		Uterine perforation
Peritonitis	Localized	Appendicitis
		Ovarian torsion
	Diffuse	PID
		Ruptured appendix
		Generalized intra-abdominal hemorrhage
Cervical motion tenderness	Present	PID
		Ovarian cyst
		Ovarian torsion
		Endometriosis
Pus from cervical os	Present	PID
Open os (pregnant patient)		Incomplete or inevitable abortion
Adnexal mass		Ovarian cyst
		Ovarian torsion
		Tubo-ovarian abscess
		Ovarian tumor

PID, pelvic inflammatory disease; UTI, urinary tract infection.

Ancillary Studies

In addition to the pregnancy test, bedside urine dipstick testing can be used to identify pyuria or hematuria to suggest the presence or absence of a urinary tract infection or of a ureteral stone. History and physical examination do not reliably exclude the diagnosis of ectopic pregnancy, and ultrasonography should be considered in all pregnant patients in the first trimester with abdominal pain or vaginal bleeding.[9] Identification of an intrauterine pregnancy by ultrasound excludes ectopic pregnancy with a high degree of certainty. Concomitant intrauterine and ectopic (heterotopic) pregnancy is rare, except in the context of infertility treatment. Abnormal cul-de-sac fluid or an adnexal mass is often present with ectopic pregnancy, but the absence of specific findings does not exclude this diagnosis in patients without a confirmed intrauterine pregnancy at ultrasound.[10]

In a nonpregnant patient, ultrasound can support the diagnosis of acute salpingitis or a tubo-ovarian abscess, identify the size and character of any adnexal mass, quantify grossly the amount of pelvic fluid, and assess the status of ovarian blood flow in suspected ovarian torsion. Although ultrasound can be a useful test in the evaluation of appendicitis or ureteral colic, abdominal computed tomography is a more sensitive and specific test for either of these diagnoses.[11,12] Computed tomography is generally inferior to ultrasound, particularly

transvaginal ultrasound, in the diagnosis of pelvic pathology. Laparoscopy remains the gold standard for the diagnosis and, in many cases, the treatment of acute pelvic pathology.

DIFFERENTIAL DIAGNOSIS

The potential life threats related to various causes of pelvic pain (Table 27-2) can be divided into two main areas—hemorrhage and sepsis. The primary life threat from hemorrhage occurs from intra-abdominal bleeding caused by a ruptured ectopic or a hemorrhagic ovarian cyst or from vaginal bleeding related primarily to a uterine process. Life-threatening causes of sepsis include a perforated viscus such as a ruptured appendix, salpingitis or tubo-ovarian abscess, and urinary tract infection. In a patient who presents with stable vital signs, the evaluation may proceed in a less hurried fashion.

EMPIRIC MANAGEMENT

The two common pathways that place a patient at risk for death secondary to pelvic pathology are (1) shock secondary to hemorrhage and (2) sepsis with associated shock from a condition causing pelvic peritonitis. Stable versus unstable hemodynamic status (Figure 27-1) is the first critical decision in all patients with acute pelvic pain.

In an unstable patient, resuscitative efforts should focus on supplemental oxygen, cardiac monitoring, aggressive volume resuscitation with isotonic crystalloid, and blood products as needed. Patients should have a complete blood count, urinalysis, type and crossmatch, and a rapid pregnancy test ordered. Consultation with obstetrics/gynecology should be done on an emergent basis. If the patient is thought to be in hemorrhagic shock and cannot be stabilized rapidly, she should be transported directly to the operating room. A laparoscopy or laparotomy may be done in the operating room for diagnostic and therapeutic reasons. In patients who respond to volume resuscitation, an immediate bedside pelvic ultrasound scan often clarifies the diagnosis. Patients with a ruptured ectopic pregnancy still need operative intervention. Patients with a hemorrhagic corpus luteum might avoid operative intervention if their vital signs stabilize and serial hematocrits do not show evidence of severe anemia or continued blood loss.

The specific management of a hemodynamically stable patient usually is directed at the underlying cause of pelvic pain (Figure 27-2). Patients with clinical evidence of diffuse peritoneal irritation require admission in most cases. Broad-spectrum antibiotics should be initiated as early as possible if peritoneal irritation is from a presumed infectious cause. More specific treatment is directed at the underlying cause of the peritonitis.

Patients less than 16 weeks' pregnant typically have an ultrasound performed. Patients with a viable intrauterine pregnancy and no significant adnexal

Table 27-2. Differentiation of Common or Potentially Catastrophic Causes of Pelvic Pain

	Pain History	Associated Symptoms	Supporting History	Prevalence in Emergency Department	Physical Examination	Useful Tests	Atypical or Additional Aspects
Ovarian torsion	Acute onset of moderately severe lateral pain	Nausea and vomiting	History of ovarian mass	Uncommon	Adnexal tenderness possible peritonitis (+) CMT adnexal mass	Ultrasound with Doppler flow studies, laparoscopy	Torsion can be intermittent
Appendicitis	Duration often <48 hr. Generalized followed by localized RLQ	Low-grade fever, nausea, anorexia	Abdominal pain before vomiting, anorexia, migration of pain to RLQ	Common	RLQ tenderness with or without peritoneal signs	WBC often elevated, ultrasound or CT in equivocal cases	Early in course tenderness may be minimal or poorly localized
Ectopic pregnancy	Classically severe sharp lateral pelvic pain, but severity, location, and quality often variable	Vaginal bleeding common	Missed period; history of previous ectopic, infertility, tubal ligation, or IUD use	Common	Variable, classically lateral adnexal tenderness (+) CMT, adnexal mass	Pelvic ultrasound, quantitative β-hCG, progesterone, laparoscopy	Cannot reliably exclude diagnosis based on history and physical; severe pain, hypotension, or peritonitis suggest rupture
PID/TOA	Without TOA pain usually bilateral. May present acutely within 48 hr or have more subacute presentation 1-2 wk of pain	Fever, vaginal discharge	Vaginal discharge, prior history of PID, lack of nausea vomiting or anorexia	Common	Pus from cervical os, (+) CMT. If peritonitis present usually bilateral adnexal mass with TOA	CBC, ESR, pelvic ultrasound, laparoscopy, cervical cultures, cervical smear looking for WBC	History and physical alone inaccurate, particularly in patients presenting subacutely
Ruptured corpus luteal cyst	Abrupt moderately severe lateral pain	Lightheadedness if bleeding is severe; rectal pain from fluid in cul-de-sac		Uncommon	Hypotension and tachycardia if blood loss is significant possible peritonitis	Pelvic ultrasound, CBC	Physical examination findings often do not correlate with volume of blood in pelvis at ultrasound
Nonruptured ovarian cyst/tumor	Lateral ache, gradual onset	Often minimal	Prior history similar pain	Common	Lateral pelvic tenderness, with or without a mass, (+) CMT	Pelvic ultrasound, CBC	
UTI	Pain with urination usually not severe unless has flank pain from associated pyelonephritis	Urinary urgency and frequency; fever and vomiting if has associated pyelonephritis	Recent urologic procedure, prior history UTI	Common	Suprapubic tenderness, flank tenderness and fever with pyelonephritis	Urinalysis, urine culture	WBC can be present in urine with PID and appendicitis
Endometriosis	Unilateral or bilateral pelvic pain, often recurrent	Dysmenorrhea, dyspareunia	Prior history of same type of pain in association with the menstrual cycle	Common	Unilateral or bilateral adnexal tenderness, occasionally pelvic mass present, peritoneal findings uncommon	Pelvic ultrasound, laparoscopy	Symptoms can mimic other types of pelvic pathology, laparoscopy often needed for confirmation

Continued

Table 27-2. Differentiation of Common or Potentially Catastrophic Causes of Pelvic Pain—cont'd

	Pain History	Associated Symptoms	Supporting History	Prevalence in Emergency Department	Physical Examination	Useful Tests	Atypical or Additional Aspects
Ureteral colic	Acute onset presents within hours. Pain is lateral usually moderate to severe. Often radiates into the groin	Nausea and vomiting	Prior history of stones	Common	Patient often appears uncomfortable but physical examination can be otherwise unremarkable	Urinalysis—hematuria present in about 90% of cases, abdominal CT	If stone is at junction of ureter and bladder, can have localized tenderness that can mimic appendicitis or other acute pelvic pathology

β-hCG, β-human chorionic gonadotropin; CBC, complete blood count; CMT, cervical motion tenderness; CT, computed tomography; ESR, erythrocyte sedimentation rate; IUD, intrauterine device; PID, pelvis inflammatory disease; RLQ, right lower quadrant; TOA, tubo-ovarian abscess; UTI, urinary tract infection; WBC, white blood cell count;

Figure 27-1. Management algorithm for patients who are hemodynamically unstable. IV, intravenous; OB/GYN, obstetrics/gynecology; β-hCG, β-human chorionic gonadotropin; CT, computed tomography.

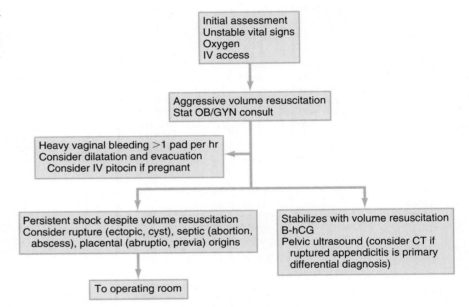

pathology by ultrasound, a normal urinalysis, and no symptoms consistent with appendicitis typically are discharged with obstetric/gynecologic follow-up. Patients more than 16 weeks' pregnant should be evaluated by the obstetric service before discharge. Important considerations in these patients include the possibility of an incompetent cervix, placental abruption, and premature labor.

Nonpregnant patients without shock or peritonitis should have a focused assessment to exclude many specific causes. A normal urinalysis excludes a urologic cause in most cases. The combination of cervical motion tenderness and either pus coming from the cervical os or a fever suggests the diagnosis of acute salpingitis. The presence of an adnexal mass on pelvic examination in these patients suggests the presence of a tubo-ovarian abscess, which can be delineated better at ultrasound. Ovarian torsion should be considered in

patients with moderate to severe unilateral adnexal pain and tenderness. In addition, an adnexal mass is often palpated. These patients are best evaluated with ultrasound. Appendicitis is a difficult diagnosis to confirm or exclude in women of childbearing age because there is a considerable amount of overlap between symptoms present with appendicitis and symptoms related to a variety of other conditions affecting the female reproductive organs. Clinicians should have a low threshold for consulting a surgeon or obtaining a computed tomography scan to exclude this diagnosis in patients presenting with acute onset of right lower quadrant pain.

After emergent and critical diagnoses have been excluded, most patients do not require specific treatment other than a prescription for an appropriate analgesic. These patients require gynecologic follow-up, however. Laparoscopic studies of patients with acute

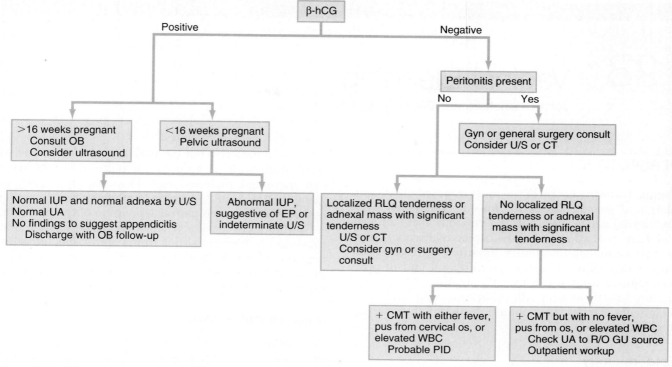

Figure 27-2. Management algorithm for patients who are hemodynamically stable. β-hCG, β-human chorionic gonadotropin; OB, obstetrics; IUP, intrauterine pregnancy; US, ultrasound; UA, urinalysis; EP, ectopic pregnancy; CT, computed tomography; RLQ, right lower quadrant; CMT, cervical motion tenderness; WBC, white blood cell count; PID, pelvic inflammatory disease; GU, genitourinary.

pelvic pain have revealed that a specific cause can be identified in about 75% of cases.[2]

REFERENCES

1. Jamieson D, Steege J: The prevalence of dysmenorrhea, dyspareunia, pelvic pain and irritable bowel syndrome in primary care practices. *Obstet Gynecol* 87:55, 1996.
2. Cunanan R, Courey N, Lippes J: Laparoscopic findings in patients with pelvic pain. *Am J Obstet Gynecol* 46:589, 1983.
3. Pavletic AJ, et al: Infertility following pelvic inflammatory disease. *Infect Dis Obstet Gynecol* 7:145, 1999.
4. Bouyer J, et al: Risk factors for ectopic pregnancy: A comprehensive analysis based on a large case-control, population-based study in France. *Am J Epidemiol* 157:185, 2003.
5. Bergeron E, Richer B, Charib R, Giard A: Appendicitis is a place for clinical judgement. *Am J Surg* 177:460, 1999.
6. Beerendonk CC, et al: Ovarian hyperstimulation syndrome. *Obstet Gynecol Surv* 53:439, 1998.
7. Soriano D, et al: Diagnosis and treatment of heterotopic pregnancy compared with ectopic pregnancy. *J Am Assoc Gynecol Laparosc* 9:352, 2002.
8. Cacciatore B, et al: Transvaginal sonographic findings in ambulatory patients with suspected pelvic inflammatory disease. *Obstet Gynecol* 80:912, 1992.
9. Dart R, Kaplan B, Varaklis K: Predictive value of history and physical examination in patients with suspected ectopic pregnancy. *Ann Emerg Med* 33:283, 1999.
10. Dart R: Role of pelvic ultrasonography in the evaluation of the symptomatic first trimester pregnancy. *Ann Emerg Med* 33:310, 1999.
11. Styrud J, Josephson T, Eriksson S: Reducing negative appendectomy: Evaluation of ultrasonography and computed tomography in acute appendicitis. *Int J Qual Health Care* 12:65-68, 2000.
12. Sheafor DH, et al: Nonenhanced helical CT and US in the emergency evaluation of patients with renal colic: Prospective comparison. *Radiology* 217:792, 2000.

28 Vaginal Bleeding

John C. Bradford and Christ G. Kyriakedes

PERSPECTIVE

Vaginal bleeding is one of the most frequent chief complaints of women presenting for emergency care. The underlying causes are multiple and can occur in girls and women of all ages. Causes can be relatively benign or carry significant morbidity and mortality risks. Typically, vaginal bleeding during childhood and in postmenopausal women is clinically significant but rarely acutely life-threatening. Bleeding as a complication of pregnancy carries the potential for life-threatening hypovolemic shock.

Epidemiology

Approximately 20% of all pregnant patients have vaginal bleeding in the first 20 weeks of gestation; more than 50% of these women miscarry. Ectopic pregnancy is less common but more serious, occurring in nearly 2% of all pregnancies in the United States. Refractory hemorrhagic shock from an ectopic pregnancy is the most common cause of maternal death in the first trimester of pregnancy. Gestational trophoblastic disease is rare (1 in 1700 pregnancies in North America).[1]

Vaginal bleeding after 20 weeks' gestation occurs in about 4% of pregnancies; about 30% of cases are due to abruptio placentae, and 20% are due to placenta previa. Postpartum hemorrhage results in nearly 30% of pregnancy-related deaths. The most common early cause in the first 24 hours is uterine atony. After 24 hours postpartum, retained products of conception is frequently the cause. The most common cause of postmenopausal uterine bleeding is atrophic endometrium. The incidence of malignancy as a source of postmenopausal bleeding ranges from 3% to 14% of cases.

Pathophysiology

Pregnant Patients

Anatomic or functional abnormalities of the fallopian tube are considered the most important cause of ectopic pregnancies. Disruption of the placental blood supply causes hemorrhage into the tube, with subsequent rupture of the aborting fetus through the tubal wall.

In first-trimester vaginal bleeding, spontaneous abortion occurs when embryo death causes a decline in placental hormone production and separation of the products of conception from the uterus.

Abruptio placentae occurs spontaneously or may be caused by abdominal trauma with transmission of

forces to the uterus. An increased incidence is seen in association with cocaine use, hypertension, smoking, and increased maternal age. Placenta previa occurs when the implanted placenta overlaps the os. Bleeding is thought to be from partial separation of the placenta.

Uterine atony occurs when myometrial dysfunction prevents the uterine corpus from contracting, allowing continued bleeding at the placental site. Atony is more likely to occur with multiple gestations, hydramnios, multiparity, and prolonged or precipitous labor.[2]

Nonpregnant Patients

The pathophysiology of vaginal bleeding unrelated to pregnancy varies with cause and age group. Children may present with foreign bodies, genital trauma, or severe vulvovaginitis causing mucosal breakdown and hemorrhage. Sexual abuse always must be considered. In adolescent girls and women, anovulatory uterine bleeding occurs when estrogen stimulates endometrium proliferation without the stabilizing effect of progesterone, causing spontaneous sloughing of the endometrium.

Submucosal leiomyomas cause hemorrhage by disrupting the endometrial vascular supply. Cervical and endometrial polyps have vascular pedicles that are prone to bleed. Malignant tumors of the cervix, endometrium, and vagina bleed with invasion and proliferation. Coagulopathies associated with leukemia, thrombotic thrombocytopenic purpura (TTP), von Willebrand's disease, or aplastic anemia are rare causes of severe hemorrhage.[3,4]

DIAGNOSTIC APPROACH

Differential Considerations

The differential diagnosis can be categorized as critical, emergent, or nonemergent. An organ system approach can identify the origin of these hemorrhage categories (Table 28-1).

Rapid Assessment and Stabilization

Patients presenting with hemodynamic instability require intravenous access, fluid resuscitation, and stabilization with blood components. Concurrently, steps must be taken to prevent further vaginal bleeding. In causes considered "critical," surgical intervention is often necessary to control bleeding effectively.[5]

Blood should be obtained for routine preoperative testing and should include complete blood count,

Table 28-1. Differential Diagnosis of Vaginal Bleeding

Organ System	Critical Diagnosis	Emergency Diagnosis	Nonemergent Diagnosis
Uterus	Abruptio placentae Placenta previa Vasa previa	Threatened abortion Uterine atony Uterine prolapse	DUB Uterine fibroids Atrophic endometrium, endometrial carcinoma Polyps, IUD Endometrial hyperplasia Infections
Fallopian tube/ovaries	Ectopic pregnancy	Ruptured ovarian cyst	Infections Polycystic ovarian disease
Vagina/cervix		Vagina lacerations	Vaginal cancer Cervical cancer Infections Foreign bodies
Perineum/bladder		Genital trauma	Genital tumors Lichen sclerosis Urethral prolapse Secondary anovulation Infection
Systemic	TTP DIC		Coagulopathy Estrogen ingestion, estrogen-producing ovarian cysts Drugs—tamoxifen Endocrinopathies

DIC, disseminated intravascular coagulopathy; DUB, dysfunctional uterine bleeding; IUD, intrauterine device; TTP, thrombotic thrombocytopenic purpura.

platelet count, prothrombin time, partial thromboplastin time, ABO and Rh typing, and crossmatching of at least 4 U of blood. Vital signs are obtained concurrently while fluid resuscitation continues. In prepubertal patients with significant bleeding, a coagulopathy workup should be initiated.

Pivotal Findings

Although a critical diagnosis may be readily apparent, a careful history and physical examination are often key to establishing emergent and noncritical causes of vaginal bleeding. The most important question to answer is, "Is the patient pregnant?"[1]

History

1. The *volume and duration of bleeding* should be ascertained. Generally the estimated amount of blood does not indicate the diagnosis and may not correlate with actual loss. Menstrual blood does not normally clot; the presence of clots may indicate significant bleeding.
2. The *menstrual history* should include regularity of the cycle, date of the last menstrual period, timing, and duration. Amenorrhea may not indicate pregnancy, and bleeding around the time of the expected period does not exclude pregnancy. Bleeding during or after intercourse may indicate a cervical lesion.
3. *Contraception methods* used can raise suspicion of certain clinical diagnoses. Use of an intrauterine contraceptive device or progesterone-only pill increases the likelihood of ectopic pregnancy and increases the incidence of erratic bleeding. Recent changes in oral contraception may affect the bleeding cycle.
4. *Clinical risk factors for ectopic pregnancies* should be noted (see Table 28-4), but are neither diagnostic nor exclusive of the diagnosis. Risk factor analysis applies only to populations and not to individual patients. Its role is to increase the clinical index of suspicion regarding further evaluation or consultation. About 25% to 50% of ectopic pregnancies occur in women with a previous history of pelvic inflammatory disease, tubal surgery, or previous ectopic pregnancy or after assisted conception; however, the remaining 50% to 75% of women presenting with ectopic pregnancy have none of these "risk factors." An abnormal Pap smear history may indicate possible malignancy.
5. A history of *recent delivery or therapeutic abortion* may indicate retained products of conception or infection.
6. A history of *previous cesarean sections* in a patient in active labor, a patient abusing cocaine, or a patient who has received high doses of oxytocin or prostaglandins raises suspicion of uterine rupture.
7. *Past medical history* may alert the clinician to medical causes of vaginal bleeding. Heavy bleeding can arise secondary to a bleeding diathesis resulting from liver disease or can be induced by anticoagulant medication. Idiopathic or thrombotic thrombocytopenic purpura and von Willebrand's disease may present in women as menorrhagia.
8. A history of *trauma* should be considered in an adolescent with bleeding, and *sexual assault* should be considered in an adult in whom abuse is present. If the pregnancy is unwanted and vaginal bleeding is associated with amniotic fluid leakage in the second trimester, illegal abortion should be considered.
9. *Associated symptoms* of nausea, breast tenderness, urinary frequency, and fatigue may indicate that

Table 28-2. Selected Physical Examination Findings in Patients with Vaginal Bleeding

Sign	Finding	Diagnosis
Appearance	Anxiety/diaphoresis	Ruptured ectopic, vasa previa
	Hypovolemic shock	Placenta previa, abruptio placentae, placenta accreta, uterine rupture
Vital signs	Hypotension	Same as above
	Tachycardia	Ruptured ectopic, vasa previa
		Placenta previa, abruptio placentae, placenta accreta, uterine rupture, plus threatened abortion, uterine atony, retained products of conception, ruptured ovarian cysts, lacerations, and trauma
Dermatologic	Ecchymosis, petechiae	Coagulation defects, von Willebrand's disease, DIC, TTP, ITP
Abdominal examination	Fetal heart tones	Pregnancy viable
	Tenderness severe with peritoneal irrtation	Ruptured uterus, placenta accreta
Pelvic examination	Heavy/significant bleeding	Placenta previa, vasa previa, ectopic pregnancy, abruptio placentae, uterine rupture
	Heavy/significant bleeding with delivery of placenta	Placenta accreta
	Adnexal/uterine mass or enlargement	STD/abscess, uterine cancer, fibroid, cervical/vaginal cancer, benign tumors, ovarian tumors, ectopic pregnancy
	Cervical motion or uterine tenderness	STD, uterine masses, cervical lesions, ectopic pregnancy
	Bleeding vulvar/vaginal lesions	Trauma, atrophic vaginitis secondary to anovulation, infection
	Open internal cervical os, with or without products of conception	Inevitable miscarriage

DIC, disseminated intravascular coagulation; ITP, idiopathic thrombocytopenic purpura; STD, sexually transmitted disease; TTP, thrombotic thrombocytopenic purpura.

Table 28-3. Vaginal Bleeding: Ancillary Testing

Test	Finding	Diagnosis
β-hCG	Positive	Ectopic pregnancy
		Placenta previa
		Vasa previa
		Abruptio placentae
		Threatened abortion
		Uterine rupture
		Placenta accreta
Pelvic ultrasound	Adnexal mass	Ectopic pregnancy
	Low-lying placenta	Placenta previa
	Placental separation	Abruptio placentae
	Umbilical cord at os	Vasa previa
	Peritoneal fluid or peritoneal fetal part	Uterine rupture
	Uterine "snowstorm" appearance	Molar pregnancy
	Uterine mass	Fibroids, leiomyomas, molar pregnancy, polyps, adenomyosis, endometrial carcinoma, endometrial hyperplasia
	Ovarian mass	Ectopic, ovarian cyst/ovarian pregnancy, cancer
	No ovarian mass Blood flow	Ovarian torsion
Culdocentesis	Nonclotting blood	Ruptured ectopic Ruptured ovarian cyst

β-hCG, β-human chorionic gonadotropin.

the patient is pregnant. A pregnancy test is indicated in all cases. Abdominal pain may indicate critical, noncritical, or emergent causes, depending on the severity of pain, bleeding, and hemodynamic state. Vaginal discharge, pelvic pain, and fever may suggest pelvic inflammatory disease.

10. In a *prepubertal patient,* history should include symptom onset, infections, possibility of abuse, foreign bodies, trauma, associated abdominal pain, urinary or bowel symptoms, precocious puberty, or potential ingestion of estrogen-containing compounds.[6]

Physical Examination

Specific findings may be found in a variety of causes of vaginal bleeding (Table 28-2).[7]

Ancillary Testing

β-human chorionic gonadropin (β-hCG) levels should be obtained in women of childbearing age regardless of their sexual, contraception, or menstrual history (Table 28-3). A positive β-hCG test necessitates a pelvic ultrasound study in the following situations: (1) vaginal bleeding with or without pelvic pain in a patient who has not had a pelvic ultrasound confirming intrauterine pregnancy, (2) vaginal bleeding in a near-term pregnancy with or without pelvic pain, and (3) significant vaginal bleeding in a patient in active labor. Transvaginal ultrasonography can identify intrauterine pregnancies (gestational sac) at approximately 35 days' gestation or during the first week after a missed period and in most or all cases when the serum β-hCG is greater than 2000 U.[8] Serial quantitative β-hCG levels every 48 hours are beneficial only in distinguishing ectopic pregnancy from threatened abortion in pregnancies less than 5 to 7 weeks' gestation.

β-hCG is useful in identifying intrauterine pregnancy, ectopic pregnancy, molar pregnancy, or tubo-ovarian abscess in the emergency department. Transabdominal ultrasound is less accurate in assessing vaginal bleeding causes.[9] Culdocentesis is rarely indicated. It may be considered when there is no possibility of obtaining transvaginal or transabdominal ultrasound in a hemodynamically stable patient with a positive pregnancy test and suspicion of hemorrhage from ruptured ectopic pregnancy. Hemodynamically unstable patients in this setting should be taken directly to the operating room for laparoscopy or laparotomy. Molar pregnancy may be suspected when the uterus is significantly larger than would be expected for gestational age and is confirmed easily by the characteristic appearance on ultrasound.

DIFFERENTIAL DIAGNOSIS

Table 28-4 summarizes the causes and differentiation of seven potentially life-threatening conditions presenting as vaginal bleeding.

EMPIRIC MANAGEMENT

All patients who present in shock with a surgical abdomen should be resuscitated and expeditiously moved from the emergency department to the operating suite (Figures 28-1 and 28-2).

Pregnant Patients

If ectopic pregnancy is suspected, a positive serum or urine β-hCG confirms the pregnancy, and immediate laparotomy may be required to control the bleeding. If third-trimester bleeding is present with shock, stabilization is performed while obtaining an ultrasound to evaluate the placenta (location in placenta previa, separation and hemorrhage in placentae abruptio). Bimanual or speculum vaginal examination should not be undertaken until placenta previa is excluded. High-grade third-trimester bleeding should prompt immediate obstetric consultation, even before diagnostic studies elucidate the possible cause. Vaginal delivery is preferred, but cesarean section is indicated in the following cases: (1) if fetal distress is present and vaginal delivery is not imminent, (2) if there is severe abruption with a viable fetus, (3) if life-threatening hemorrhage exists, or (4) if the patient has failed a trial of labor.[10]

Uterine rupture may present with excessive vaginal bleeding, uterine pain, and a boggy uterine fundus that seems to be expanding. Urgent surgical delivery is indicated.

Urgent cesarean section is performed if excessive vaginal bleeding accompanies the rupture of membranes. The bleeding suggests vasa previa. If after delivery of the fetus there is an indistinct placental cleavage plane and excessive hemorrhage, placenta accreta is present and requires urgent hysterectomy. Firm bimanual compression of the uterus may limit

Table 28-4. Causes and Differential Diagnoses of Potentially Catastrophic Illness Presenting with Vaginal Bleeding

	Pain History	Associated Symptoms	Supporting History	Emergency Department Prevalence	Physical Examination	Useful Tests	Atypical or Additional Aspects
Ectopic pregnancy	Lower abdominal pain almost always present (97%). Variable equality and character. Often sudden onset and unilateral. Occasional radiation into back or flank	Vaginal bleeding (55–86%). Tenesmus. Weakness, syncope, or near-syncope. Abdominal hemorrhage may be significant, with minimal associated vaginal bleeding	First-trimester pregnancy, amenorrhea, irregular menses, prior ectopic pregnancy, PID, STD, tubal ligation or other tubal procedures increase risk In vitro fertilization or ovulation indication Recent elective abortion	Common	Tenderness on pelvic and lower abdominal examination. Vaginal bleeding. Peritoneal irritation if intra-abdominal hemorrhage has occurred	Using β-hCG as screen for possible ectopic gestation Serum qualitative β-hCG if stable Vaginal ultrasound for detection of intrauterine gestational sac or possible detection of extrauterine gestational sac. Culdocentesis	Methotrexate sometimes used in the nonsurgical treatment of unruptured ectopic pregnancies 2% of ectopic pregnancies are intra-abdominal Incidence of concomitant intrauterine and extrauterine pregnancies 1:30,000

Table 28-4. Causes and Differential Diagnoses of Potentially Catastrophic Illness Presenting with Vaginal Bleeding—cont'd

	Pain History	Associated Symptoms	Supporting History	Emergency Department Prevalence	Physical Examination	Useful Tests	Atypical or Additional Aspects
Abruptio placentae	Uterine tenderness and irritability. Intermittent or steady abdominal cramping. Back pain	Dark, variable bleeding, Hemorrhage may be more intrauterine and occult. 20% have no vaginal bleeding Fetal distress often present Hypotension, DIC	>20 weeks gestation. Increased maternal age, hypertension, smoking, cocaine use, abdominal trauma	Rare	Abdominal and uterine tenderness. Variable (or absent) dark red uterine bleeding	CBC, type and crossmatch, coagulation profile Vaginal ultrasound often normal. May help rule out placenta previa	Frequently misdiagnosed as preterm labor. Nontraumatic causes are more common than trauma
Placenta previa	Usually very little pain	Bright red vaginal bleeding, rarely severe	>20 weeks gestation. Incidence increased with multiparity and prior cesarean-section	Rare	Gravid uterus. abdominal examination usually benign. Withhold vaginal examination until gynecologic backup and ultrasound examination	CBC, type and crossmatch, coagulation profile Utrasound often diagnostic	Vaginal probe ultrasound believed to be safe due to wide angle between cervical canal and vaginal axis Speculum or manual pelvic examination should not be done until placenta previa is ruled out
Postpartum hemorrhage (first 24 hr postdelivery	Often minimal. Can be severe with uterine inversion	Vaginal bleeding, often brisk, but much blood loss can be hidden in uterus	Difficult, traumatic delivery (vaginal lacerations). Previous cesarean-section, curettage, multiple fetuses (uterine rupture). Multiple gestations, hydramnios, multiparity, precipitous or prolonged labor (uterine atony). Premature assisted delivery of placenta (retained placental fragments)	Rare	Tender abdomen with guarding (uterine rupture). Enlarged, doughy uterus (uterine atony). Inability to palpate uterus (uterine inversion). Vaginal bleeding without uterine bleeding (vaginal lacerations)	DIC profile if suspect coagulopathy	Pregnancy-induced hypertensive disease, amniotic fluid embolus, or abruption can induce consumptive coagulopathies
Uterine rupture	Uterine pain without contraction	Vaginal bleeding	Previous cesarean section Cocaine use Prostaglandins	Rare	Tender. Boggy uterine fundus. Expanding uterus	Ultrasound, nonmeasuring fetal tracing	Urgent surgery
Placenta accreta	Very little	Bright red vaginal bleeding, brisk	During delivery of placenta—difficult placental delivery	Rare	Placental cleavage plane indistinct	Clinical only	Fist in uterus with anterior compression for stasis/surgery
Vasa previa	Very little	Bright red vaginal bleeding, brisk, more than bloody show	Abrupt-onset vaginal bleeding with rupture of membranes	Rare	Decrease fetal movement	Nonmeasuring fetal tracing	Can be caused iatrogenically with fetal monitoring

PID, pelvic inflammatory disease; STD, sexually transmitted disease; β-hCG, β-human chorionic gonadotropin; DIC, disseminated intravascular coagulation; CBC, complete blood count.

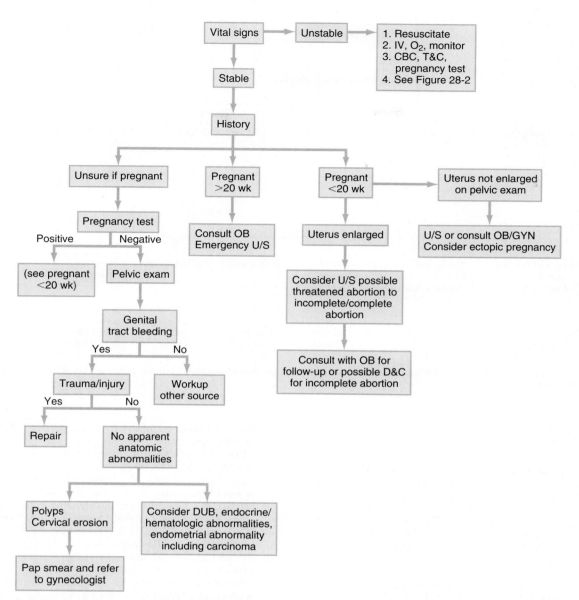

Figure 28-1. Management algorithm for patients with vaginal bleeding. IV, intravenous; CBC, complete blood count; T&C, type and cross-match; U/S, ultrasound; D&C, dilation and curettage; DUB, dysfunctional uterine bleeding.

hemorrhage until surgery is arranged. Uterine atony often responds to vigorous uterine massage and intravenous oxytocin.[8]

Nonpregnant Patients

In nonpregnant patients, most vaginal bleeding is related to dysfunctional (anovulatory) uterine bleeding and nonsteroidal anti-inflammatory drugs. This bleeding usually is managed with estrogen supplementation in consultation with a gynecologist. Patients with other causes, such as neoplasm, suspected endometriosis, or ovarian cysts, are referred to a gynecologist. Before discharge, it is important to assess the patient's tolerance of the hemorrhage by measuring vital signs, including orthostatics. A baseline hemoglobin/hematocrit is recommended. Finally, other medical causes, such as hypothyroidism, hemostasis disorders, or anticoagu-

lant therapy, must be considered and appropriate consultation obtained.

DISPOSITION

In a patient with postpartum uterine atony or coagulopathy, medical management often is sufficient. Obstetrics consultation is indicated. In a preadolescent patient, abuse must be ruled out before the patient is discharged to her current environment. In a nonpregnant stable patient, malignancy always should be suspected, and additional inpatient or timely outpatient gynecologic workup is indicated. Laboratory studies, such as thyroid function and prolactin levels, may be helpful to the consultant, but are rarely indicated in the initial workup.[11]

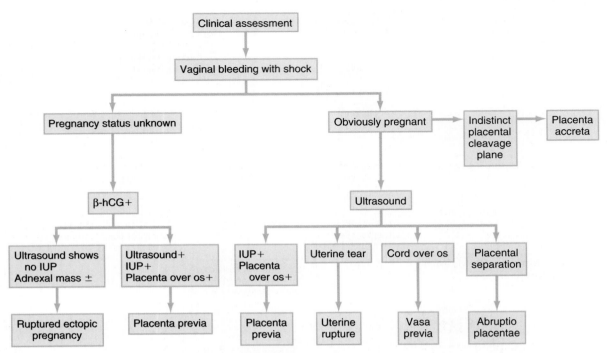

Figure 28-2. Rapid assessment and stabilization of critical diagnoses of vaginal bleeding. β-hCG, β-human chorionic gonadotropin; IUP, intrauterine pregnancy.

REFERENCES

1. ACEP Committee: Clinical policy for the initial approach to patients presenting with a chief complaint of vaginal bleeding. *Ann Emerg Med* 29:435, 1997.
2. Khong TY, Khong TK: Delayed postpartum hemorrhage: A morphologic study of causes and their relation to other pregnancy disorders. *Obstet Gynecol* 82:17, 1993.
3. Daniels R, McCuskey C: Abnormal vaginal bleeding in the nonpregnant patient. *Emerg Med Clin North Am* 21:45, 2003.
4. Jutras ML, Cowan BD: Abnormal bleeding in the climacteric. *Obstet Gynecol Clin North Am* 17:409, 1990.
5. Papp Z: Massive obstetric hemorrhage. *J Perinat Med* 31:408, 2003.
6. Kilbourn C, Richards C: Abnormal uterine bleeding. *Postgrad Med* 109:1371, 2001.
7. Coppola P, Coppola M: Vaginal bleeding in the first 20 weeks of pregnancy. *Emerg Med Clin North Am* 21:41, 2003.
8. Munro MG: Abnormal uterine bleeding in the reproductive years. *J Am Assoc Gynecol Laparosc* 6:393, 1999.
9. Williams P, Laifer-Narin S, Ragavendra N: US of abnormal uterine bleeding. *Radiographics* 23:703, 2003.
10. Turner LM: Vaginal bleeding during pregnancy. *Emerg Med Clin North Am* 12:45, 1994.
11. Minjarez D, Bradshaw K: Abnormal uterine bleeding in adolescents. *Obstet Gynecol Clin North Am* 27:63, 2000.

CHAPTER

29 Back Pain

Kevin G. Rodgers and James B. Jones

PERSPECTIVE

Back pain is a common symptom causing patients to seek care in the emergency department. It accounts for 1% of emergency department visits. Although mechanical low back is the most common cause, the differential diagnosis is broad and contains several life-threatening conditions. Developing a systematic approach that examines all the potential causes of back pain is the key to accurate clinical decision making.

Epidemiology

"Acute low back strain" is the most common condition that initiates an emergency department visit for "back pain." Of all individuals, 70% to 90% experience debilitating back pain at some point in their lifetime, and 5% of these have chronic pain. About 1% of all patients with back pain have true sciatica.[1] Back pain is the second most common cause of lost time in the workplace, and in 1998, total health care expenditures for patients with back pain in the United States were estimated at $90.7 billion.[2,3]

Before considering mechanical causes, several emergent causes must be excluded, including aortic dissection or aneurysm, cauda equina syndrome, epidural abscess, osteomyelitis, and spinal cancer.[4] Aortic dissection is the most common catastrophic event involving the aorta, with an incidence of 10 per 1 million population per year, and mortality exceeds 90% if it is not diagnosed. Although cauda equina syndrome (bilateral leg pain and weakness, urinary retention with overflow incontinence, fecal incontinence/decreased rectal tone, and "saddle anesthesia") is seen in less than 1% of all herniated disks, it also may occur as a result of infectious or metastatic diseases.[5] Epidural abscess (0.02% of hospitalized patients) and vertebral osteomyelitis (0.1% of hospitalized patients) are rare infectious conditions that present primarily with back pain. Spinal carcinoma is uncommon (<1%) in the general population presenting with back pain. Of cancer patients, 80% who present with back pain have spinal metastases. Metastasis to bone is seen commonly in breast, lung, prostate, kidney, and thyroid carcinomas.

Pathophysiology

The pathophysiology of back pain is as diverse as its etiology. Pain may emanate from various structures within the back, including muscles, joints, tendons, periosteum, fascia, vascular structures, and nerves. Any innervated structure may produce pain based on mechanical irritation, inflammation, compression of adjacent pressure-sensitive structures, or increased vascular pressure. Often a specific origin for the pain cannot be identified, although about 80% of pain occurs in the L4-5 area.[6] Radicular pain is described as resulting from direct compression, microvascular ischemia, and inflammation of the involved nerve root. Although the mechanism is poorly understood, facet joint discomfort typically is localized to the level involved, whereas sacroiliac joint pain can be local and referred to the lower abdominal quadrants and inguinal area.

Pain associated with vascular catastrophes may be migratory (dissection) or diffuse (expanding/ruptured aneurysm). The presentation may vary based on secondary insults involving the spinal cord, kidney, heart, or bowel. Patients with oncologic and infectious causes of back pain present with persistent and localized pain. This pain results from inflammation, compression, and erosion of adjacent structures. Finally, visceral disorders involving the pancreas, kidney, duodenum, colon, and gallbladder may produce poorly localized back pain based on a shared segmental innervation.

> ### BOX 29-1. Common Historical and Physical Examination "Red Flags"
>
> **Historical Information**
> Recent significant trauma
> Recent mild trauma in patients >50 years old
> History of prolonged steroid use
> History of osteoporosis
> Patients >70 years old
> Syncope
> Prior history of cancer
> History of recent infection
> Fever >38° C (>100° F)
> Intravenous drug use or immunocompromised patients
> Low back pain worse at rest
> Unexplained weight loss
> Acute onset of back, flank, or testicular pain
> Diaphoresis or nausea associated with pain
>
> **Physical Examination**
> Abnormal vital signs—hypotension, tachycardia
> Unequal blood pressure readings in the upper extremities
> Pulsatile abdominal mass
> Pulse deficit or circulatory compromise of the lower extremities
> Loss of rectal sphincter tone, urinary retention, or focal lower extremity weakness
> Focal back pain with fever

DIAGNOSTIC APPROACH

Differential Considerations

The goal of the initial assessment of patients who present to the emergency department with a complaint of back pain is similar to that for headache—to determine whether the back pain is "benign" in its cause or whether a potentially serious or lethal disorder is underlying the presentation. Most of these conditions can be screened for with an accurate history and complete physical examination to identify findings that should raise concern about a more serious underlying pathologic process (Boxes 29-1 and 29-2).[7,8]

Rapid Assessment and Stabilization

If the initial history and physical examination identify any concerns about serious disease, immediate stabilization measures should ensue consistent with the cause of concern (Figure 29-1). A vascular cause (abdominal aortic aneurysm or aortic dissection) requires early surgical consultation, intravenous access, supplemental oxygen, cardiac monitoring, blood samples for type and crossmatching, and careful monitoring and control of blood pressure. Dissection is managed with β-blockers and nitroprusside or with labetalol alone. If an infectious cause is suspected (epidural abscess), emergent magnetic resonance imaging (MRI) and neurosurgical consultation should be obtained. Blood cultures typically are obtained but have limited sensitivity. Intravenous antibiotics should be initiated immediately. For all patients with signifi-

BOX 29-2. Differential Considerations in Acute Low Back Pain

Emergent
Aortic dissection
Cauda equina syndrome
Epidural abscess/hematoma
Ruptured/expanding aortic aneurysm
Spinal fracture with cord/nerve impingement

Urgent
Back pain with neurologic deficits
Intervertebral disk herniation
Malignancy
Meningitis
Sciatica with potential of nerve root compression
Spinal fractures without cord impingement
Spinal stenosis
Transverse myelitis
Vertebral osteomyelitis

Common/Stable
Acute ligamentous injury
Acute muscle strain
Ankylosing spondylitis
Degenerative joint disease
Intervertebral disk disease without impingement
Pathologic fracture without impingement
Seropositive arthritis
Spondylolisthesis

Referred/Visceral
Cholecystitis
Esophageal disease
Nephrolithiasis
Ovarian torsion/mass/tumor
Pancreatitis
Peptic ulcer disease
Pleural effusion
Pneumonia
Pulmonary embolism
Pyelonephritis
Retroperitoneal hemorrhage/mass

cant pain, including patients with "benign" causes for back pain, effective analgesia should be provided early in the evaluation.

Pivotal Findings

History

History of Present Illness

Questions are asked to attempt to localize pain to the most likely structure and mechanism.[9] The answers are useful to separate mechanical from nonmechanical causes.

Where is the pain? The patient is asked to point with one finger to the one spot where it hurts the most. Does the pain radiate to the legs and, if so, where in the legs? Does the pain conform to a specific dermatomal area? Radicular pain in a dermatomal distribution implies nerve root involvement. Pain mainly in the paralumbar musculature without dermatomal radiculopathy implies muscular or liga-

mentous strain. Any associated abdominal pain is reviewed because this added history may indicate a possible visceral cause.

When did the pain start? The patient should describe in detail what he or she was doing when the pain started. Is there any past history of back pain, and what therapeutic modalities were used to treat it? If there is a history of back pain, is there any difference between present and past pain? Acute onset associated with a specific task suggests a mechanical cause. Sudden-onset, severe back pain suggests aortic dissection. Slow onset or onset unrelated to activity suggests a nonmechanical cause (e.g., tumor). Nonmechanical pain may improve then recur, but the trend is progressive worsening.

Are there any aggravating or alleviating factors? Cough or Valsalva's maneuver that aggravates the pain in general favors a mechanical cause and may point specifically to a herniated disc. Patients with muscular strain tend to become stiff with rest and vary position while at rest. Patients with back pain associated with tumors and infectious etiologies often present with nighttime pain and persistent pain unrelieved by rest and analgesics. Spinal stenosis presents with diffuse back discomfort and pain, numbness, and tingling in one or both legs (pseudo-claudication). Symptoms are aggravated by ambulation (especially "uphill") and relieved with spinal flexion (sitting or pushing a grocery cart).

Is there other pertinent history? Other pertinent history should include work history, past and present (a history of repeated loading would suggest mechanical cause); pain associated with neurologic symptoms (suggesting nerve root impingement); presence of urinary retention or bowel incontinence (requires emergent decompression if related to disk prolapse); fever (suggesting infectious cause); medications (anticoagulants associated with epidural hematomas, steroids associated with infection and compression fractures); and pending litigation or worker's compensation status (possible secondary gains).

Past Medical History

In addition to any history of back disorders, a thorough inquiry about any systemic disease is important. The following are queried: history of cancer (metastatic disease), collagen vascular disease, intravenous drug abuse (diskitis), arthropathies, endocrinopathies (hyperparathyroidism), bleeding disorders, and sickle cell disease. Knowledge of medications used to treat present and past symptoms helps direct treatment decisions. Knowledge of current medications used by the patient gives clues about the presence of other systemic disease. The family history also is assessed. Diseases such as spondyloarthropathies (e.g., ankylosing spondylitis) have a familial component.

Physical Examination

Vital Signs

Vital signs are important because alterations may suggest a life-threatening process (e.g., hypotension

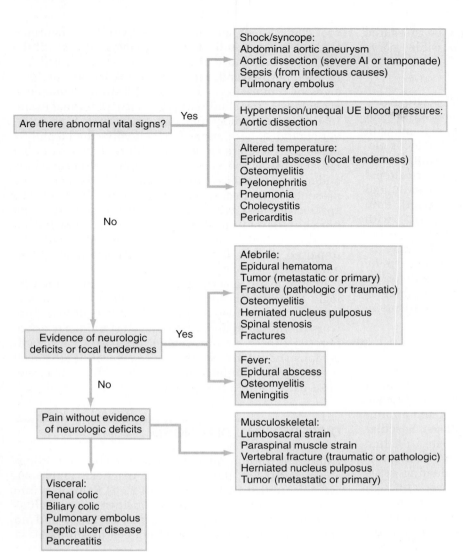

Figure 29-1. Rapid assessment of acute low back pain. AI, aortic insufficiency; UE, upper extremity.

Are there abnormal vital signs? — Yes →

Shock/syncope:
Abdominal aortic aneurysm
Aortic dissection (severe AI or tamponade)
Sepsis (from infectious causes)
Pulmonary embolus

Hypertension/unequal UE blood pressures:
Aortic dissection

Altered temperature:
Epidural abscess (local tenderness)
Osteomyelitis
Pyelonephritis
Pneumonia
Cholecystitis
Pericarditis

No ↓

Evidence of neurologic deficits or focal tenderness — Yes →

Afebrile:
Epidural hematoma
Tumor (metastatic or primary)
Fracture (pathologic or traumatic)
Osteomyelitis
Herniated nucleus pulposus
Spinal stenosis
Fractures

Fever:
Epidural abscess
Osteomyelitis
Meningitis

No ↓

Pain without evidence of neurologic deficits →

Musculoskeletal:
Lumbosacral strain
Paraspinal muscle strain
Vertebral fracture (traumatic or pathologic)
Herniated nucleus pulposus
Tumor (metastatic or primary)

↓

Visceral:
Renal colic
Biliary colic
Pulmonary embolus
Peptic ulcer disease
Pancreatitis

and tachycardia with ruptured abdominal aortic aneurysm, hypertension with aortic dissection, fever with osteomyelitis/diskitis).

Lower Back Inspection

1. The gait of the patient entering the department and preparing for examination is observed. Does the patient move cautiously, protecting himself or herself, or freely and appear to be in little pain?
2. The patient is examined first while standing. A careful search is made for scoliosis (may be structural or secondary to muscle spasm), increase or decrease of lumbar lordosis or thoracic kyphosis (may predispose to mechanical pain), or pelvic obliquity (may indicate muscle spasm, leg-length discrepancy, or uncompensated scoliosis).
3. The range of motion for the low back is assessed. Patients with significant mechanical pain usually flex without reversing the normal lumbar lordosis, and extension may aggravate facet causes or nerve root impingement.
4. Palpation is done in an orderly fashion with the fingertips to localize the area of greatest tenderness (e.g., specific spinous process, paravertebral musculature).

Other Examinations, Including Neurologic Examination

1. The neurologic assessment evaluates the asymmetry of reflexes (clinically reflexes diminish with age, and uncovering asymmetry is key), dermatomal sensory loss, and focal muscle weakness (suggests nerve root impingement). A patient with a long history of back pain is asked about previous motor, sensory, or reflex abnormality. The presence of clonus, hyper-reflexia, or upgoing toes (Babinski's sign) indicates an upper motor neuron lesion.
2. A rectal examination can assess sphincter tone and anal wink. Testing for perianal sensation is necessary if there is any history of bowel or bladder dysfunction.
3. A head-to-toe screening examination looking for signs of systemic disease should include an abdominal examination for aneurysm or masses.
4. The hips and sacroiliac joints are examined for a musculoskeletal focus other than the back.

5. The thigh or calf circumference may be measured for muscle atrophy, suggesting possible nerve impingement.

Straight Leg Raise

The straight leg raise is the classic test for sciatic nerve root irritation, but is neither sensitive nor specific for disk disease. This test is often negative in patients with spinal stenosis. With the knee extended, the leg is elevated until pain is elicited. A positive result is pain radiating down the leg below the knee in a dermatomal distribution when the leg is elevated between 30 and 70 degrees (not back, buttocks, or thigh pain). Pain referred to an affected leg ("crossover pain") with straight leg raise of the unaffected leg is highly specific for nerve root irritation.[5] In a patient who may be malingering, the straight leg raise can be done with the patient sitting with the knees flexed on the side of the bed and passively straightening the legs. If there is true nerve root irritation, results should be positive in the sitting and the supine positions.

Ancillary Testing

Laboratory Tests

For mechanical causes of back pain, laboratory studies are of little use. For nonmechanical causes, erythrocyte sedimentation rate, complete blood count, and antinuclear antibody titers may be useful if collagen vascular disease is suspected. Calcium, phosphate, alkaline phosphatase, protein electrophoresis, and acid phosphatase determinations may aid in evaluating cases with metabolic and tumor-related causes, although these are not best done in the emergency department. Urinalysis may be helpful in patients suspected of having renal disease with referred back pain (nephrolithiasis, pyelonephritis, urinary tract infection).

Imaging

Plain radiographs, including lateral and oblique views and spot films of the L5-S1 region, are not useful in uncomplicated mechanical low back pain with no history of trauma, lack of neurologic deficits, pain of less than 6 weeks' duration, or no history of cancer or in recurrent back pain that has been previously evaluated.[10] MRI, computed tomography, or myelogram (in order of preference) may be indicated if an acute, significant neurologic deficit is present.[11] Emergency imaging is indicated if cauda equina syndrome is suspected to be present (i.e., progressive lower extremity weakness and bowel or bladder involvement). Without cauda equina presentation, imaging may be done on an urgent or outpatient basis and can be arranged in conjunction with a consultant.

For patients in whom infection or tumor is suspected, MRI (or bone scan followed by MRI) has become the diagnostic test of choice.[12] The degree of neurologic impairment and patient stability dictates whether these tests are obtained on an emergent or urgent basis.

Other

Electromyography may be useful to document neurologic deficit and to delineate between specific nerve root compression and generalized peripheral neuropathy, but it is not indicated on an emergent basis. If the patient has a history of trauma, cancer, advanced age, or osteoporosis and shows bony tenderness or focal signs of trauma (e.g., soft tissue swelling, hematoma, ecchymosis, abrasion) with an otherwise normal examination, plain radiographs may be helpful. Most intervertebral disk herniations (95%) involve the L5 and S1 nerve roots and are associated with radicular pain that radiates below the knee, paresthesias or sensory loss, and muscle weakness. Involvement of the L5 nerve root presents with decreased sensation in the first web space, weakness with extension of the great toe, and normal reflexes. An S1 radiculopathy is characterized by diminished sensation of the lateral small toe, impaired plantar flexion, and a decreased or absent ankle jerk.[5]

In atraumatic, afebrile patients with a normal neurologic examination, indications for plain films include age older than 70 years; unexplained weight loss; pain worse at rest; or history of prolonged steroid use, osteoporosis, cancer, or intravenous drug use. Plain radiographs should not be obtained, however, if advanced imaging (e.g., computed tomography, MRI) is planned. Most patients do not require radiographic evaluation.[13]

DIFFERENTIAL DIAGNOSIS

After stabilization and assessment, the clinical findings aid in narrowing the differential diagnosis (Table 29-1).[5,14-20] An algorithm (see Figure 29-1) that takes into account important differential considerations, such as abnormal vital signs, the presence of fever, and an abnormal neurologic examination, is a useful tool.

EMPIRIC MANAGEMENT

The initial empiric management of acute back pain depends on the presenting vital signs and overall appearance of the patient. There are specific management considerations for unstable patients (Figure 29-2).[14-20] For a stable patient, early pain management can be of significant value. While waiting for radiographic evaluation, pain medications should be initiated. The choice of analgesic is dictated by the patient's and physician's perception of the degree of pain. Physicians notoriously underestimate and undertreat pain, especially acute low back pain. If the pain is severe, opioids are the preferred analgesic and should be given intravenously in a titrated fashion. Frequent reassessment of the patient for an adequate response is required. Morphine and the newer synthetic opioids, such as fentanyl, offer more potent analgesia while minimizing side effects, such as hallucinations, sedation, and respiratory depression. Meperidine (Demerol) is not recommended because of its significantly higher adverse event rate. After adequate response to the initial intravenous opioid, an oral agent can be administered in preparation for discharge. For patients with less acute symptoms, an oral opioid, such as hydromorphone/*N*-

Table 29-1. Classic Findings in Selected Serious Causes of Acute Back Pain

	Diagnoses	History	Important Physical Examination Findings	Ancillary Testing	Comments
Critical Vascular	Aortic dissection	Often sudden-onset, "tearing" severe pain. Associated nausea, vomiting, acute anxiety are common. Syncope can occur	Associated diaphoresis, unstable vital signs. Hypertension is common. Unequal upper extremity blood pressure. New-onset aortic insufficiency murmur. Central and peripheral neurologic deficits secondary to ischemia	Choice of CT, MRI, aortogram depends on patient stability and availability	More common as a chest pain cause, but low back pain may be only complaint
	Abdominal aortic aneurysm (ruptured/expanding)	Pain may radiate to back, flank, or testicle. May present with syncope	Pulsatile abdominal mass (especially if right of midline), abdominal bruits. Diminished lower extremity pulses or hypoperfusion or both	Bedside ultrasonography. If "stable," abdominal CT with contrast. Plain films may show a calcified enlarged aortic contour	Can also mimic renal colic, GI bleeding, diverticulitis, and myocardial infarction. 30% of signs are misdiagnosed
Infectious	Spinal epidural abscess	At-risk population with diabetes, chronic renal failure, intravenous drug use, alcoholism, cancer, or recent spinal surgery or trauma. Sepsis-linked history is common	Fever, reproducible radicular pain, other signs of sepsis. Localized body tenderness along spine. Focal neurologic deficits are late findings (<50% patients). Rare cauda equina–like syndrome	CBC, blood cultures useful but nonspecific. MRI modality of choice. CT or myelography can be used. Search for source of infection. *Staphylococcus aureus* most common cause (70%)	Presents as mass-occupying lesion compressing spinal cord, may be hematoma, malignancy, disk. Often begins as focal pyogenic infection in disk. Biopsy may be necessary
Mechanical	Cauda equina syndrome	Usually a history of back pain. Symptoms may develop over hours	Urinary retention and fecal incontinence. Saddle anesthesia, bilateral leg pain. Lower extremity weakness with hyperreflexia	CT with or without contrast, MRI useful	Can result in severe dysfunction. An emergent condition caused by compression of lumbosacral nerve roots
	Spinal fracture with cord impingement	Acute onset, localized pain. Usually trauma history. Older population with osteoporosis also at risk	Bone tenderness, radicular, or cord compression findings	Plain films initially, then CT or MRI.	Symptoms/signs depend on level
	Epidural hematoma	Usually patient with coagulation disorder, hereditary or acquired, e.g., anticoagulants. May occur after epidural anesthesia	Radicular findings (neurologic defects). Similar neurologic pattern as abscess	Similar imaging as abscess	Can also occur in AV malformations
Emergent Infectious	Vertebral osteomyelitis	Similar group at risk as epidural abscess. Onset may be insidious. Back pain, tenderness, and stiffness may precede neurologic findings by significant time period	Fever and other constitutional symptoms. Localized body tenderness of two adjacent vertebrae	CBC, blood cultures generally low yield. Plain films diagnostic 80-95%, but MRI more accurate and detailed	Biopsy may be necessary for diagnosis. *S. aureus* is common
Immune	Transverse myelitis	Back pain and neurologic deficits. Almost 50% of patients worsen maximally in 24 hr	Partial/total loss sensory, motor, autonomic and sphincter function below the level of the lesion. Leg weakness more common, arm involvement is rare. Bladder (bowel control) involved in most patients	Goal is to rule out mass lesion compressing the cord. Thought to be autoimmune origin. MRI is imaging modality of choice. Contrast CT and CT myelogram may be obtained	May be associated with multiple sclerosis, SLE, sarcoidosis. Also associated with Lyme disease. Epstein-Barr virus, and after other viral (herpes, enterovirus) or bacterial (tuberculosis syphilis) infections.

Continued

Table 29-1. Classic Findings in Selected Serious Causes of Acute Back Pain—cont'd

	Diagnoses	History	Important Physical Examination Findings	Ancillary Testing	Comments
Mechanical	Back pain with neurologic deficits Intervertebral disk herniation Spinal stenosis Spinal fractures without cord impingement Malignancy Sciatica with potential of nerve root compression	Most patients recall atraumatic mechanisms (lifting, twisting). Common complaints are stiffness, tenderness, decreased range of motion	Positive straight leg raise test. Muscular weakness. Potential for sensory deficits. Absent or diminished deep tendon reflexes	Selective use of pain films. CT or MRI performed for complete assessment	Search for "red flags" (see Box 29-1) to rule out serious underlying disease

AV, arteriovenous; CBC, complete blood count; CT, computed tomography; GI, gastrointestinal; MRI, magnetic resonance imaging; SLE, systemic lupus erythematosus.

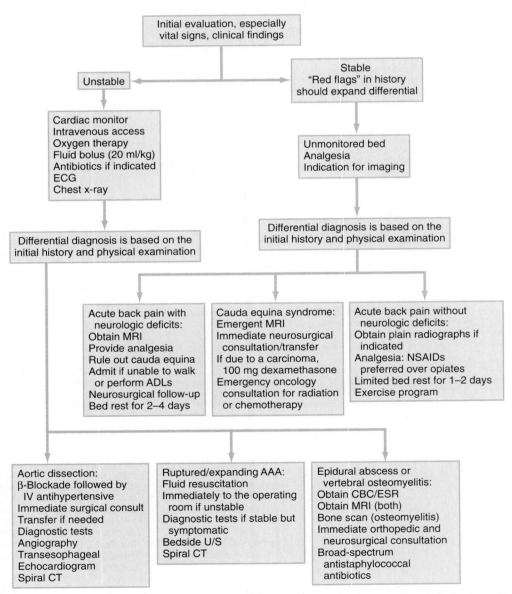

Figure 29-2. Management of acute low back pain. ECG, electrocardiogram; MRI, magnetic resonance imaging; ADL, activities of daily living; NSAIDs, nonsteroidal anti-inflammatory drugs; IV, intravenous; AAA, abdominal aortic aneurysm; U/S, ultrasound; CT, computed tomography; CBC, complete blood count; ESR, erythrocyte sedimentation rate.

acetyl-*p*-aminophenol (APAP) or hydrocodone/APAP is appropriate.

Patients presenting with chronic pain, without evidence of disk herniation, usually are treated with nonsteroidal anti-inflammatory drugs (NSAIDs). NSAIDs also are the most common prescribed drug for the acute phase after a back injury; however, their effectiveness seems to be limited after 48 hours.[21,22] Benzodiazepines may be of some adjunctive help in managing back pain, functioning as nonspecific sedative agents with perhaps some muscle relaxation properties. Evidence supporting the use of cyclobenzaprine (Flexeril) is scanty at best, and the high side-effect profile of this agent suggests that it be used with caution, if at all.[23]

DISPOSITION

The disposition of patients with back pain depends on the underlying cause. Patients who present with abnormal vital signs and evidence of shock probably require admission to the operating room or intensive care unit. In addition, patients with acute cord compression from a fracture, disk protrusion, abscess, or hematoma may require urgent neurosurgical evaluation and early surgical intervention.

Patients who are unable to ambulate or who require additional intravenous analgesics for adequate pain control should be considered for admission. If pain control can be obtained using oral analgesics, patients can be discharged with appropriate follow-up. For patients with chronic or continued acute low back pain, massage therapy seems to be cost-effective and clinically effective compared with acupuncture or spinal manipulation.[24]

REFERENCES

1. Borenstein DG: Epidemiology, etiology, diagnostic evaluation, and treatment of low back pain. *Curr Opin Rheumatol* 11:151, 1999.
2. Stewart WF, et al: Lost productive time and cost due to common pain conditions in the US workforce. *JAMA* 290:2443, 2003.
3. Luo X, et al: Estimates and patterns of direct health care expenditures among individuals with back pain in the United States. *Spine* 29:79, 2004.
4. Braddom RL: Perils and pointers in the evaluation and management of back pain. *Semin Neurol* 18:197, 1998.
5. Deyo RA, Rainville J, Kent DL: What can the history and physical examination tell us about low back pain? *JAMA* 268:760, 1992.
6. Deyo RA: Diagnostic evaluation of back pain: Reaching a specific diagnosis is often impossible. *Arch Intern Med* 162:1444, 2002.
7. Bigos S, et al: *Acute Low Back Pain in Adults: Clinical Practice Guideline #14* (AHCPR Publication No. 95-0642). Rockville, Md, Agency for Health Care Policy and Research, 1994.
8. Deyo RA, Weinstein JN: Primary care: Low back pain. *N Engl J Med* 344:363, 2001.
9. Linton SJ, Hallden K: Can we screen for problematic back pain? A screening questionnaire for predicting outcome in acute and subacute back pain. *Clin J Pain* 14:209, 1998.
10. Kendrick D, et al: Radiography of the lumbar spine in primary care patients with low back pain: Randomized controlled trial. *BMJ* 322:400, 2001.
11. Saal JS: General principles of diagnostic testing as related to painful lumbar spine disorders: A critical appraisal of current diagnostic techniques. *Spine* 27:2538, 2002.
12. Joines JD, et al: Finding cancer in primary care outpatients with low back pain. *J Gen Intern Med* 16:14, 2001.
13. Atlas SJ, Deyo RA: Evaluating and managing acute low back pain in the primary care setting. *J Gen Intern Med* 16:120, 2001.
14. Klompas M: Does this patient have an acute thoracic aortic dissection? *JAMA* 287:2262, 2002.
15. Lederle FA, Simel DL: Does this patient have abdominal aortic aneurysm? *JAMA* 281:77, 1999.
16. Nienaber CA, Eagle KA: Aortic dissection: New frontiers in diagnosis and management: Part I. From etiology to diagnostic strategies. *Circulation* 108:628, 2003.
17. Kuhn M, et al: Emergency ultrasound scanning for abdominal aortic aneurysm: Accessible, accurate and advantageous. *Ann Emerg Med* 36:219, 2000.
18. Lyu RK, et al: Spinal epidural abscess successfully treated with percutaneous, computed tomography-guided, needle aspiration and parenteral antibiotic therapy: Case report and review of the literature. *Neurosurgery* 51:509, 2002.
19. Orendacova J, et al: Cauda equina syndrome. *Prog Neurobiol* 64:613, 2001.
20. Kerr D, and the Transverse Myelitis Consortium Working Group: Proposed diagnostic criteria and nosology of acute transverse myelitis. *Neurology* 59:499, 2002.
21. Cherkin DC, et al: Medication use for low back pain in primary care. *Spine* 23:607, 1998.
22. van Tulder MV, et al: Non-steroidal anti-inflammatory drugs for low back pain. *Cochrane Database Syst Rev* 2:CD000396, 2000.
23. van Tulder MW, et al: Muscle relaxants for nonspecific back pain: A systematic review within the framework of the Cochrane Collaboration. *Spine* 28:1978, 2003.
24. Cherkin DC, et al: A review of the evidence for the effectiveness, safety and cost of acupuncture, massage therapy, and spinal manipulation for back pain. *Ann Intern Med* 138:898, 2003.

30 Cyanosis

Jennifer Bocock and Joan Kolodzik

PERSPECTIVE

Cyanosis is a blue or purple appearance of the skin or mucous membranes. This clinical finding is secondary to inadequately oxygenated blood perfusing peripheral tissues or the presence of abnormal hemoglobin forms unable to bind oxygen or to supply adequate oxygen to end organs and tissues. Cyanosis is a relatively rare presenting chief complaint in the emergency department and most commonly noted in patients with a hypoperfused state or known cardiopulmonary disease, including congenital heart disease.[1]

Pathophysiology

Cyanosis is visible when there is an elevated absolute amount of desaturated (nonoxygenated) hemoglobin in the circulating capillary blood (>4 to 5 g/dL in whole blood). It is not a percent of desaturated total hemoglobin mass or a decreased amount of oxyhemoglobin. Cyanosis is not a sensitive indicator of tissue oxygenation, and although its presence suggests hypoxia, its absence does not exclude it.

Abnormal hemoglobin forms are significant contributors to cyanotic disease. Cyanosis results when greater than 10% to 15% of the total hemoglobin is methemoglobin (≥ 1.5 g/dL). Methemoglobin has a dark purple to brown color, even on exposure to room air. This form of hemoglobin has a high affinity for oxygen molecules and does not readily release oxygen to the peripheral tissues. The normal oxygen dissociation curve is shifted to the left, resulting in hypoxia and lactic acid production (Figure 30-1).

Under normal conditions, red blood cells (RBCs) contain hemoglobin with iron molecules in the reduced state (ferrous [Fe^{2+}]). The iron molecule may be oxidized (ferric state [Fe^{3+}]) to produce methemoglobin, which is normally less than 1% of total hemoglobin. Elevated methemoglobin levels occur when excess amounts of hemoglobin are oxidized to the ferric state, causing cyanosis.[2] Methemoglobin is degraded primarily by reduced nicotinamide adenine dinucleotide (NADH) cytochrome-b_5 reductase, an enzyme present within RBCs, reducing ferric state methemoglobin to the ferrous hemoglobin.

Primary methemoglobinemia is a congenital error of enzyme metabolism, with diminished levels of NADH reductase or an abnormally functioning enzyme.[3] Patients may present with cyanosis in a stable compensated state. Acquired methemoglobinemia occurs when methemoglobin production (hemoglobin oxidation) is accelerated beyond the normal level of NADH reductase activity. Direct oxidant stressors or indirect oxidants may be causative agents. Newborns are at risk for the development of methemoglobinemia because their levels of NADH reductase are low, making them susceptible to oxidant stress and the development of cyanosis (Box 30-1).

DIAGNOSTIC APPROACH

Differential diagnoses to be considered are listed in Box 30-2.

Pivotal Findings

History

The onset of symptoms, including duration, time of day, abruptness of onset, association with exercise, and any previous episodes, should be noted. Precipitating factors, including exposure to cold air, water, exercise (patients with history of cardiopulmonary disease), or high altitude and association with chemicals, drugs, or fumes in the home or workplace, should be reviewed. The potential of pseudocyanosis resulting from exposure to dyes, heavy metals, or topically absorbed pigments should be explored.

Additional history should include known congenital heart disease or cardiopulmonary disease (i.e., myocardial infarction, atrial fibrillation, congestive heart failure, aortic disease, pulmonary embolus, chronic obstructive pulmonary disease, pneumonia, oxygen dependency), hypercoagulable states, and any family history of cyanotic disease or hematologic illness.[1,2] A history of home or occupational exposures to chemicals should be obtained, including aniline, azo dyes (pyridium), phenacetin, and nitrates. Drug history is reviewed, including use of prescription drugs, over-the-counter substances, health food supplements, and herbal or alternative preparations. Associated symptoms, such as headache, nausea, vomiting, and weakness, suggest carbon monoxide toxicity, especially occurring in multiple patients from a single scene location (from a home or single job site). Other symptoms may include chronic fatigue, weakness, or dyspnea.

In infants, fatigue is suggested by difficulty feeding, excessive somnolence, poor weight gain, or respiratory distress. Episodic cyanotic events, or "Tet spells," may be seen in the emergency department, often in children. Cyanosis, tachypnea, and anxiety present secondary to decreased pulmonary blood flow with shunting of nonoxygenated blood into the peripheral circulation.

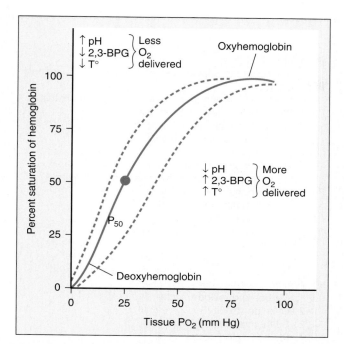

Figure 30-1. Hemoglobin-oxygen dissociation curve. Deoxyhemoglobin does not bind oxygen efficiently. Methemoglobin has a high affinity for oxygen molecules and does not readily release oxygen to the peripheral tissues. This shifts the normal oxygen dissociation curve to the left, resulting in hypoxia and lactic acid production. Typically, when acid is produced in the tissues, the dissociation curve shifts back to the right, facilitating oxygen release; however, the high affinity of methemoglobin prevents this normal process. (Redrawn from Benz EJ Jr: Hemoglobinopathies. In *Harrison's online*.)

These spells are characteristic in patients with tetralogy of Fallot, which includes ventricular septal defect, pulmonary stenosis, an overriding aorta, and a right ventricular outlet obstruction and right ventricular hypertrophy with or without pulmonary atresia.

Physical Examination

There is significant interobserver variability in detecting cyanosis on physical examination. Subjective factors affecting detection include the skill of the physician examiner and the awareness of other potential medical problems. Room lighting and ambient temperature may affect examination of the skin and mucous membranes. A patient's normal/natural skin tone, skin thickness, and pigmentation also may alter findings.

Physical findings of cyanosis vary, and presentation patterns provide clues to the cause of the symptom complex. Central cyanosis is often secondary to the shunting of venous unsaturated hemoglobin or abnormal hemoglobin into the arterial circulation. The amount of oxygen available peripherally is decreased, and a bluish discoloration appears on the skin and mucous membranes, best seen on perioral skin, oral mucosa, or conjunctivae.

Peripheral cyanosis is secondary to vasoconstriction and slow flow of normally oxygenated hemoglobin in arterial blood, allowing for greater oxygen extraction. Peripheral cyanosis affects capillary beds and typically is seen on the extremities and nail beds. Differential

BOX 30-1. Common Etiologies of Methemoglobinemia

Hereditary
Hemoglobin M
NADH methemoglobin reductase deficiency (homozygote and heterozygote)

Acquired
Medications
Amyl nitrite
Benzocaine
Dapsone
Lidocaine
Nitroglycerin
Nitroprusside
Phenacetin
Phenazopyridine
Prilocaine (local anesthetic)
Quinones (chloroquine, primaquine)
Sulfonamides (sulfanilamide, sulfathiazide, sulfapyridine, sulfamethoxazole)

Chemical Agents
Aniline dye derivatives (shoe dyes, marking inks)
Butyl nitrite
Chlorobenzene
Fires (heat-induced denaturation)
Food adulterated with nitrites
Food high in nitrates
Isobutyl nitrite
Naphthalene
Nitrophenol
Nitrous gases (seen in arc welders)
Silver nitrate
Trinitrotoluene
Well water (nitrates)

Pediatric
Reduced NADH methemoglobin reductase activity in infants (4 mo).
Seen in association with low birth weight, prematurity, dehydration, acidosis, diarrhea, and hyperchloremia

NADH, reduced nicotinamide adenine dinucleotide.
From Goldfrank LR: Toxicologic Emergencies, 6th ed. Stamford, Conn, Appleton and Lange, 1998.

cyanosis may occur in either the upper or the lower (or the right or the left) half of the body, with the remainder appearing well oxygenated. This form of cyanosis usually is seen in cases of cyanotic heart disease with multiple anomalies.

Vital signs are obtained on all patients. Temperature is typically normal. Blood pressure may be normal or low if hypovolemia is present. Heart sounds are assessed for tachycardia or abnormal rhythm. Upper airway obstruction and other signs of respiratory insufficiency should be sought. Intermittent apnea in infants suggests central nervous system immaturity or a central lesion. Infants with cyanosis, increased respiratory depth, periodic apnea episodes, or diaphoresis with feeds may have congenital heart disease.[4] Tachypnea (>100 breaths/min) in a newborn may be a marker for a pulmonary disorder versus congenital heart disease.[5]

BOX 30-2. Differential Diagnosis of Cyanosis

I. Peripheral cyanosis
  A. Low cardiac output states
    1. Shock
    2. Left ventricular failure
    3. Hypovolemia
  B. Environmental exposure (cold)
    1. Air or water
  C. Arterial occlusion
    1. Thrombosis
    2. Embolism
    3. Vasospasm (Raynaud's)
    4. Peripheral vascular disease
  D. Venous obstruction
  E. Redistribution of blood flow from extremities
II. Central cyanosis
  A. Decreased arterial oxygen saturation
    1. High altitude >8000 ft
    2. Impaired pulmonary function
      a. Hypoventilation
      b. Impaired oxygen diffusion
      c. Ventilation-perfusion mismatching
      d. Respiratory distress
        (1) Upper airway obstruction
        (2) Pneumonia
        (3) Diaphragmatic hernia
        (4) Tension pneumothorax
        (5) Polycythemia

  B. Anatomic shunts
    1. Pulmonary arteriovenous fistulae and intrapulmonary shunts
    2. Cerebral, hepatic, peripheral arteriovenous-fistulae
    3. Cyanotic congenital heart disease
      a. Endocardial cushion defects
      b. Ventricular septal defects
      c. Coarctation of aorta
      d. Tetralogy of Fallot
      e. Total anomalous pulmonary venous drainage
      f. Hypoplastic left ventricle
      g. Pulmonary vein stenosis
      h. Tricuspid atresia and anomalies
      i. Premature closure of foramen ovale
      j. Dextrocardia
      k. Pulmonary stenosis of atrial septal defect
      l. Patent ductus arteriosis with reversed shunt
  C. Abnormal hemoglobin
    1. Carbon monoxide toxicity
    2. Cyanide toxicity
    3. Sulfhemoglobinemia
    4. Methemoglobinemia
      a. Hereditary
      b. Acquired
    5. Mutant hemoglobin with low oxygen affinity (e.g., hemoglobin Kansas)

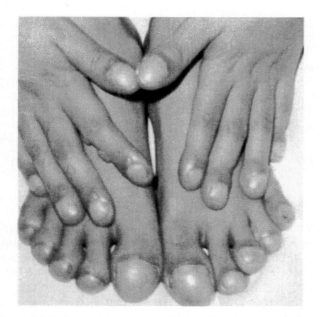

Figure 30-2. Symmetric cyanosis. Equal cyanosis and clubbing of hands and feet resulting from transposition of great vessels and a ventricular septal defect without patent ductus arteriosus.

Interpretation of pulse oximetry values is difficult in the context of cyanosis. Assessment of distal perfusion usually determines if poor circulation is a cause of low pulse oximetry. Pulse oximetry reads light absorbance of tissue at 660 nm (red; reduced hemoglobin) and at 940 nm (infrared; oxyhemoglobin). The ratio of these two readings is the basis of pulse oximetry calculation. Methemoglobin absorbs well at both wavelengths, closing the ratio difference to 1, with a saturation approximation of 85%, regardless of actual PaO_2 and SaO_2.[6,7] Carboxyhemoglobin absorbs light at approximately the same wavelength as oxyhemoglobin, and pulse oximetry overestimates the oxygen content of blood when compared with co-oximetry testing.[8]

General appearance and mental status evaluation, including the tolerance of the problem causing the cyanosis, are evaluated. The head, eyes, ears, nose, and throat examination may reveal central cyanosis. Funduscopic examination may detect retinopathy, especially dilated tortuous veins. Jugular venous distention may be seen on the neck examination in patients with pulmonary edema.

The chest examination may reveal sounds of consolidation, wheezing, or inadequate ventilation. Abnormal heart sounds (gallop or dysrhythmia), the presence and quality of murmurs (especially in newborns), and central pulse strength are noted. The abdomen may have findings of hepatosplenomegaly. Palpation of the abdominal aorta may reveal the presence of a pulsatile mass or abdominal bruit.

Extremity examination includes evaluation of nail beds for peripheral cyanosis and strength of distal pulses. Clubbing of the nails may be present secondary to increased soft tissue and expansion of the capillary beds (Figure 30-2). Clubbing occasionally may be idiopathic or hereditary, but is commonly the result of chronic hypoxemic states, such as cyanotic heart disease, infective endocarditis, pulmonary disease (chronic obstructive pulmonary disease, cystic fibrosis), and some gastrointestinal disorders (cirrhosis, Crohn's disease, and regional enteritis). Thrombotic events should be considered, with findings of skin and nail bed hemorrhages or end-organ damage (eye, kidney). Chronic vascular disease stigmata are sought, and skin temperature, distal pulses, and capillary refill are assessed (pulsation strength and symmetry).

A complete neurologic examination is completed. The neurologic examination is done with a focus on mental status, symmetry of motor and sensory function, or gross deficit.[9,10]

Ancillary Testing

Laboratory

Arterial blood gas testing assesses arterial oxygen saturation, often sampled when the patient is breathing room air (see Figure 30-1). Co-oximetry measurements should be specifically ordered for blood gas testing. If carbon monoxide exposure or methemoglobinemia is suspected, specific levels are ordered. If sulfhemoglobinemia is suspected, measured oxygen saturation should be specifically requested. The complete blood count is analyzed to assess for polycythemia or anemia. Smear evaluation assesses RBC morphology, RBC fragments, and white blood cell differential count. Cyanide levels should be ordered if there is suspicion of exposure, but elevations may not be measured until 4 to 6 hours after exposure. Patients should be treated empirically based on the clinical situation.[11]

Imaging

A chest radiograph may be ordered to evaluate lung fields for consolidation, infiltrates, and increased vasculature or pulmonary edema. The cardiac silhouette and mediastinum may assist in the diagnosis of congenital heart disease.

Electrocardiogram and Echocardiogram

An electrocardiogram should be completed on all patients with cyanosis. Rhythm abnormalities may be detected (e.g., atrial fibrillation), and acute ischemic changes should be sought. Right-axis deviation or right ventricular hypertrophy may be seen with significant cardiac disease (e.g., cor pulmonale, acute pulmonary hypertension). An echocardiogram may be helpful to assist detection of septal defects in infants or valvular disease in adults.

DIFFERENTIAL DIAGNOSIS

When the initial assessment of the patient is completed, the distribution of cyanosis is noted. The clinician begins 100% oxygen therapy and follows steps to determine the etiology of the cyanosis (Figure 30-3). Clinical improvement with oxygen may be a useful differential observation. Patients with improvement have an increase of arterial PO_2 by the supplemental oxygen, suggesting diffusion impairments. Patients who do not respond are more likely to have ventilation-perfusion ratio abnormalities. An extreme example is shunting from a consolidated pulmonary lobule or congenital heart disease with right-to-left shunting. A chest radiograph is reviewed, particularly if improvement with oxygen is noted. Cardiac size and silhouette may be a clue to the presence of congenital cardiac disease. If heart size is normal, impaired pulmonary function, pulmonary embolus, or other noncardiac etiology is considered. If an abnormal cardiac silhouette is seen, congenital or acquired cardiac disease becomes more prominent in the differential diagnosis.

If no improvement occurs with 100% oxygen administration, the patient's respiratory status should be reevaluated. Acute respiratory distress is managed for the etiology, including tension pneumothorax (decompression and tube thoracostomy) or upper airway obstruction (airway opening and clearance of obstruction or emergency surgical airway). Pulmonary embolus may present in this scenario, and ventilation-perfusion scan or spiral computed tomography of the chest (pulmonary embolus protocol) is recommended. If a patient is without respiratory distress and remains resistant to oxygen therapy, cardiac shunting or abnormal hemoglobin should be considered.

Critical Diagnoses

Acute cardiovascular and respiratory compromise must be considered in a patient presenting with cyanosis and signs and symptoms of shock. The differential diagnoses for these critical presentations include acute congestive heart failure, acute coronary syndromes or ischemia, hypovolemic or cardiogenic shock, acute respiratory insufficiency or failure, pulmonary embolism, an exacerbation or decompensation of a patient with known congenital heart disease, or the first presentation of pediatric congenital heart disease. These patients require emergent management, critical therapeutic intervention, and admission to the intensive care unit.

Emergent Diagnoses

Cyanide poisoning occurs after exposures to cyanide-containing products (i.e., sodium nitroprusside), combusted plastics (fire and inhalation victims), or direct cyanide compounds. Cyanide has a high affinity for the iron and protein components of the mitochondrial cytochrome aa_3. This affinity renders the cytochrome oxidase system unable to function normally, with resultant anaerobic metabolism. A patient with history of suspected exposure accompanied by profound refractory hypoxia and metabolic acidosis (lactic acid >8 mmol/L) should have cyanide poisoning high in the differential diagnosis.

Carboxyhemoglobin is formed after carbon monoxide exposures—typically cigarette smoke, automobile exhaust, combustion byproducts, or industrial fumes—and is the most common cause of death by poisoning in the United States. Carbon monoxide has a 240 times greater affinity for hemoglobin than does oxygen.[12] Car-

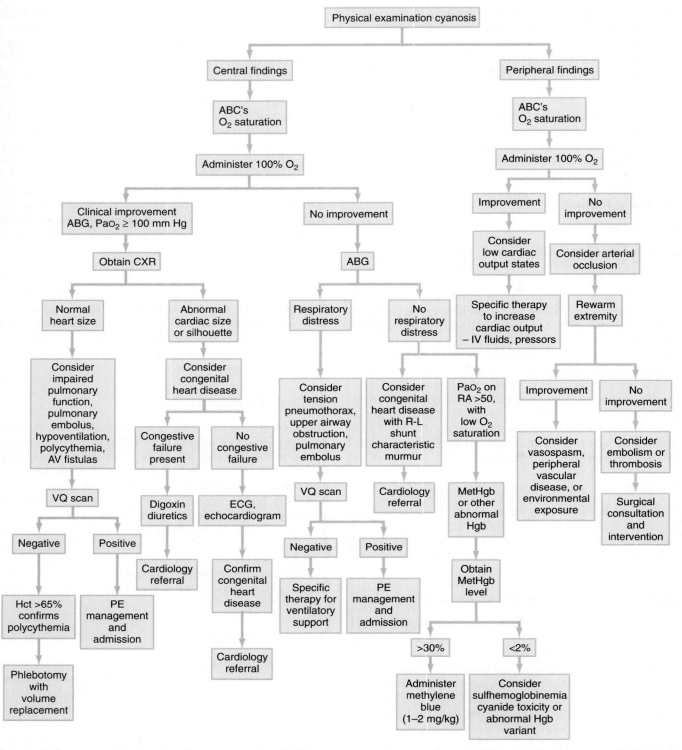

Figure 30-3. An algorithmic approach to cyanosis. ABCs, airway, breathing, circulation; ABG, arterial blood gas; CXR, chest radiograph; AV, arteriovenous; VQ, ventilation-perfusion scan; Hct, hematocrit; PE, pulmonary embolus; ECG, electrocardiogram; R-L, right-to-left; RA, room air; MetHgb, methemoglobin; Hgb, hemoglobin; IV, intravenous.

boxyhemoglobin does not transport oxygen and shifts the oxygen dissociation curve to the left (see Figure 30-1). The remaining oxyhemoglobin increases its affinity for oxygen, decreasing delivery to peripheral tissues. Blood with high carboxyhemoglobin levels has a bright red color, and cyanosis may not be noted.

Sulfhemoglobin is an infrequent cause of cyanosis, most commonly occurring after exposure to hydrogen sulfide from organic sources, medications that are sulfonamide derivatives, or gastrointestinal sources (bacterial overgrowth). Patients suspected to have hydrogen sulfide toxicity have pulse oximetry that does not correlate to PaO_2 measurements. In patients with cyanotic findings and abdominal disorders, strong consideration should be given to sulfhemoglobin toxicity.

Polycythemia is defined as an elevated RBC mass. It usually has one of three etiologies. Polycythemia vera is a hematologic disorder of bone marrow stem cells, with increased RBC mass, cyanosis, and splenomegaly. Patients may present with hyperviscosity syndrome. Secondary polycythemia occurs with either an appropriate or inappropriate increase of erythropoietin,[10] a physiologic response to chronic hypoxemia (≤92% oxygen saturation), cyanotic congenital heart disease, cigarette smoking, or high altitude exposures. Relative polycythemia is an increased RBC mass, often a result of dehydration or reduced plasma volumes. Because cyanosis is a direct reflection of the absolute amount of unsaturated hemoglobin, patients with polycythemia manifest cyanosis earlier in the course of compromised oxygen binding capacity than patients with a normal or low RBC count. The latter patients may have severe hypoxemia without cyanosis occurring.

Finally, vascular disease states, such as Raynaud's phenomenon, may present with a cyanotic appearance. Raynaud's phenomenon occurs in 15% of the population and has a female predominance. Patients have an abnormal response to excessive cold or emotional stressors and report vasoconstriction, profound cold sensitivity, and recurrent events of sharply demarcated pallor or cyanosis of the digits. Most commonly, the cutaneous arterial capillary beds of the fingers and toes are affected, but tongue, ear, and other distal areas have been reported.[13]

EMPIRIC MANAGEMENT

Administration of oxygen is a diagnostic and therapeutic procedure and may be lifesaving for some patients with cyanosis. Any clinical improvement, or lack thereof, with 100% oxygen administration should be noted. At this point, consideration of abnormal hemoglobin and toxin-induced cyanosis is crucial because the administration of appropriate antidotes and systemic therapies may decrease morbidity and improve patient outcomes.

Intravenous fluid resuscitation should be started in patients with hypovolemic presentations. As diagnostic testing is completed, the differential is narrowed, and specific therapies may be instituted as the patient's condition indicates. Treatment of congestive heart failure, arrhythmia, or poor cardiac output occurs as indicated by clinical condition. Cardiology consultation is needed when patients are admitted to the hospital. Although several specific treatments are discussed here, the etiology of the cyanosis may be elusive, and these patients require hospitalization.

Specific Strategies

Methemoglobinemia

If cutaneous exposure with an inciting agent occurred (i.e., aniline dyes), complete decontamination with

soap and water is needed. The staff should use appropriate protective equipment. Urgent treatment with methylene blue is indicated for patients with symptomatic hypoxia (dysrhythmias, angina, respiratory distress, seizures, or coma) and methemoglobin levels greater than 30%.

Other Causes of Cyanosis

Carbon monoxide and cyanide poisoning are covered elsewhere. Acute therapy for patients with symptomatic hyperviscosity syndrome and secondary polycythemia includes phlebotomy and volume expansion.[10] Isotonic crystalloid replacement volumes should be two to three times the volume of blood removed. The goal of therapy is a hematocrit less than 60% and symptom improvement.

Raynaud's phenomena may be treated with warming the affected distal digits and extremities and maintaining that temperature. Management therapies focus on increasing cardiac output and improving vascular perfusion with oxygen, intravenous fluid resuscitation, and pressor agents if necessary. If there is no improvement of peripheral cyanosis with administration of 100% oxygen, arterial insufficiency or occlusion may be present. Systemic vasodilating agents (e.g., calcium channel blockers [nifedipine] or nitrates) may be useful in the acute setting. In cases of critical ischemia, intravenous prostaglandins that vasodilate distal vasculature may be beneficial while the patient is managed in the hospital.[9] If there is no improvement with emergent management in the emergency department, urgent surgical intervention should be initiated.

PATIENT DISPOSITION

Admission

All patients with a first episode of cyanosis, whose diagnosis is obscure, and all patients who are unstable require admission. Urgent cardiology consultation and referral is necessary for children with a first episode of congestive heart failure and newly diagnosed or suspected congenital heart disease. Surgical consultation and intervention is indicated for acute arterial occlusion from embolic or thrombotic sources.

Discharge

Patients with peripheral cyanosis resulting from vasospasm, patients with methemoglobinemia less than 15% who remain asymptomatic, and stable patients with primary pulmonary disease may be managed as outpatients, after several hours of monitoring in the emergency department. Unless the patient is known to have chronic cyanosis from a previous diagnosis, follow-up must be arranged within the next 24 hours. Instructions need to state clearly that if the cyanosis worsens, or if dyspnea, altered mentation, or chest pain occur after discharge, the patient must return immediately to the emergency department.

REFERENCES

1. Da Silva SS, Sajan IS, Underwood JP 3rd: Congenital methemoglobinemia: A rare cause of cyanosis in the newborn—a case report. *Pediatrics* 112:e158, 2003.
2. Priest JR, et al: Mutant fetal hemoglobin causing cyanosis in a newborn. *Pediatrics* 83:734, 1989.
3. Kedar PS, et al: Congenital methemoglobinemia due to NADH-methemoglobin reductase deficiency in three Indian families. *Haematologia* (Budap) 32:543, 2002.
4. McCollough M, Sharieff GQ: Common complaints in the first 30 days of life. *Emerg Med Clin North Am* 20:27, 2002.
5. Fuloria M, Kreiter S: The newborn examination: Part I. Emergencies and common abnormalities involving the skin, head, neck, chest, and respiratory and cardiovascular systems. *Am Fam Physician* 65:61, 2002.
6. Li AM, et al: Normal pulse oximeter reading in a cyanotic infant. *J Paediatr Child Health* 37:94, 2001.
7. Gold NA, Bithoney WG: Methemoglobinemia due to ingestion of at most three pills of pyridium in a 2-year-old: Case report and review. *J Emerg Med* 25:143, 2003.
8. Mokhlesi B, Corbridge T: Toxicology in the critically ill patient. *Clin Chest Med* 24:689, 2003.
9. Hamilton GC: *Presenting Signs and Symptoms in the Emergency Department: Evaluation and Treatment.* Baltimore, Williams & Wilkins, 1993.
10. Berlin NI: Polycythemia vera. *Hematol Oncol Clin North Am* 17:1191, 2003.
11. Mutlu GM, et al: An unresponsive biochemistry professor in the bathtub. *Chest* 122:1073, 2002.
12. Mokhlesi B, et al: Adult toxicology in critical care: Part II. Specific poisonings. *Chest* 123:897, 2003.
13. Flavahan NA, et al: The vasculopathy of Raynaud's phenomenon and scleroderma. *Rheum Dis Clin North Am* 29:275, 2003.

CHAPTER

31 Sore Throat

Jonathan I. Singer and Mark E. Gebhart

PERSPECTIVE

Epidemiology

Sore throat is among the most frequent complaints that cause patients to visit the emergency department. Annually, physicians see approximately 27 million cases of pharyngitis.[1] The chief complaint is seen throughout all age groups evaluated in the emergency setting.[2] Despite the frequent occurrence of sore throat in the population of patients, estimates suggest that less than 20% present for assessment by a physician.[1]

Pathophysiology

Sore throat results from irritation or inflammation on any anatomic surface within the oropharynx. The oropharynx is defined posteriorly by the prevertebral fascia, laterally by the buccinator muscle groups, superiorly by the base of the skull, and inferiorly by the vocal cords. Within these boundaries, pain may emanate from the buccal mucosa, tongue, palatine tonsils, lingual tonsils, adenoids, soft palate, and posterior pharyngeal wall. Pain results from inflammatory or infiltrative invasion of potential spaces such as peritonsillar, retropharyngeal, sublingual, submental, lateral pharyngeal, parotid, buccal, and pretracheal. Sore throat also occurs with inflammatory changes of the epiglottis, aryepiglottic folds, vocal cords, and subglottic region. It can result from irritation or inflammation from structures outside the confines of the oropharynx (referred pain). Examples include infectious diseases of dental structures, cervical nodes, and middle ear fluid. In all cases of sore throat, pain is perceived through the 9th and 10th cranial nerves, which provide sensory input from the oropharynx, larynx, middle ear, and external auditory canal.[3] Systemic diseases, such as hepatitis, infectious mononucleosis, and neutropenia, may also have sore throat as part of their symptom complex.

Sore throat most often results from infectious disease within the oropharynx (Table 31-1; see also Chapter 74). The majority of infections are self-limited, unassociated with morbidity and mortality. Occasionally, these pathogens may give rise to airway obstructions, systemic invasion with distant manifestations or sepsis, and postinflammatory immune manifestations. In the course of acute sore throat from an infectious disease, a single microorganism typically causes the complaint. A virus accounts for sore throat in an estimated 50% to 60% of cases. Enterovirus infection accounts for the majority of sore throats in all age groups from late spring through autumn. Adenovirus, rhinovirus, parainfluenza virus, influenza virus, and respiratory syncytial virus predominate during winter months. Epstein-Barr virus (EBV), herpes simplex, and varicella-zoster virus have less seasonal predilection.

Bacterial infection of the oropharynx occurs less often than viral infection.[4] Aerobes typically cause superficial infection. Aerobes and anaerobes or only anaerobes cause infection within the deeper planes. Of all the bacterial pathogens, group A beta-hemolytic

Table 31-1. Differential Diagnosis for Sore Throat

Infectious Causes				
	Aerobes			
Viral	**Common**	**Uncommon**	**Anaerobes**	**Others**
Rhinovirus	Streptococcus pyogenes (GABHS)	Haemophilus influenzae	Bacteroides sp	Candida sp
Adenovirus	GABHS	Haemophilus parainfluenzae	Peptostreptococcus sp	Coccidioides sp
Coronavirus	Non–group A streptococcus	Corynebacterium diphtheriae	Peptococcus sp	
Herpes simplex 1, 2	Neisseria gonorrhoeae	Streptococcus pneumoniae	Clostridium sp	
Influenza A, B	Neisseria meningitidis	Yersinia enterocolitica	Fusobacterium sp	
Parainfluenza	Mycoplasma pneumoniae	Treponema pallidum	Prevotella sp	
Cytomegalovirus	Arcanobacterium hemolyticum	Francisella tularensis		
Epstein-Barr	Chlamydia trachomatis	Legionella pneumophila		
Varicella-zoster	Staphylococcus aureus	Mycobacterium sp		
Hepatitis virus				

Noninfectious Causes			
Systemic	**Trauma**	**Tumor**	**Miscellaneous**
Kawasaki's disease	Penetrating injury	Tongue	Angioneurotic edema
Stevens-Johnson	Retained foreign body	Larynx	Anomalous aortic arch
Cyclic neutropenia	Laryngeal fracture	Thyroid	Calcific retropharyngeal tendinitis
Thyroiditis	Retropharyngeal hematoma	Leukemia	
Connective tissue disease	Caustic exposure		

GABHS, group A beta-hemolytic streptococcus.

streptococcus (GABHS) is the most common.[5] This microorganism is isolated as the offending pathogen in 10% to 15% of all patients with sore throat. The incidence of GABHS in school-age children with sore throat may reach 15% to 30%, and some indicate that the incidence may be as high as 50%.[1] GABHS is most often isolated from sore throat patients between late winter and spring. GABHS infection may cause coinfection with other viral agents. As an example, GABHS is isolated from the pharynx in up to 10% of patients who have EBV infection of the pharyngeal structures.

Fungal colonization and systemic infection with *Candida albicans* may occur throughout the oral cavity. Repeated or severe infections are typically seen in immunocompromised hosts. Recent antibiotic therapy, chemotherapy, and radiation therapy place individuals at risk for fungal colonization with *Candida* species.

Sore throat may rarely be seen as a manifestation of noninfectious systemic disease, trauma, tumor, or congenital anomaly. In these circumstances, additional manifestations may accompany sore throat.[6]

DIAGNOSTIC APPROACH

Differential Considerations

In the rare circumstance in which the sore throat patient presents with tenuous vital signs or evidence of airway compromise, the emergency physician must act before an acquisition of all data.

Pivotal Findings

In the absence of a life-threatening circumstance, the history and physical examination should focus on manifestations of systemic illness and concentrate on potential head and neck pathology. A child may handle secretions poorly or demonstrate apparent pain with swallowing, leading to the interpretation of a sore throat.

History

Characteristic of Pain

A brief duration associated with inordinate pain or hyperpyrexia suggests the possibility of invasive disease.[7] A duration of several days accompanied by fever suggests deeper plane infection or systemic, noninfectious causes. The location of the pain may be of utility. Infectious disease within Waldeyer's ring is accompanied by pain localized to the oropharynx. Pain that radiates to the back of the neck or between the shoulder blades suggests prevertebral or retropharyngeal pathology (abscess or calcific tendinitis). Sore throat with radiation to the jaw or ear may be seen with dental abscess or deeper tissue plane infection.[8]

Associated Complaints

Within the head and neck region, serious illness is considered if there is dysphagia, odynophagia, dysphonia, drooling, or difficulty breathing. In the afebrile patient, these findings suggest neurologic dysfunction or mass lesion.[6] In the febrile patient, they suggest glossal abscess, severe infection of the lingual tonsils or palatine tonsils (peritonsillar cellulitis or abscess), or Ludwig's angina (submental or sublingual space infection).[3, 8] The history of breathing difficulty when agitated or at rest suggests epiglottitis, retropharyngeal abscess, or suppurative obstruction of the tonsillar or adenoidal tissue.

Systemic Symptoms

The presence of prolonged fever for more than 5 to 7 days is seen in Kawasaki's disease. Cough, myalgia, and arthralgia are seen with influenza A and B, parainfluenza, *Neisseria meningitidis*, and *Mycoplasma pneumoniae* infection. Hepatitis and infectious mononucleosis are associated with fatigue, malaise, and loss of appetite.

Epidemiology

In children, exposure to contagion in the daycare or school setting may provide clue to infectious causes of sore throat. Secondary spread of disease is common for contacts exposed to *M. pneumoniae*, GABHS, *Haemophilus influenzae*, and *N. meningitidis*. Among adults, intrafamilial spread is common with all of the viral agents, *Mycoplasma* sp, and GABHS. Recent orogenital contact raises the question of gonococcal or herpetic infection.[2]

Trauma

Pursuit of a trauma history may uncover antecedent blunt or penetrating injury of the oropharynx, exposure to caustics, and the possibility of a retained foreign body.

Immunizations/Specific GABHS History

The patient's immunization status is assessed, and the currency of diphtheria, pertussis, and tetanus vaccines is discussed. Is there a past medical history of recurrent GABHS infection? Is the patient a chronic carrier of GABHS?

Immune Status

Is the patient immunocompromised by the presence of diabetes, any known immune disorders, or recent chemotherapeutic or radiation therapy? Does the patient have underlying alcoholism, malnutrition, or recent antibiotic use?

Physical Examination

The observation of the patient's color, hydration, alertness, preferred posture, and quality of vocalization can be rapidly and noninvasively accomplished. The presence of toxicity, air hunger, or stridor should lead the physician to consider life-threatening upper airway obstruction.[2,3] In these circumstances, head and neck examination must proceed deliberately and with great caution. In the absence of a compromised airway, a completed ear, nose, and throat (ENT) and general examination narrows the differential diagnosis (Table 31-2).

Airway compromise, either overt or impending, is the critical concern in the physician's initial examination and clinical decision making (Figure 31-1).

Table 31-2. Pivotal Findings in Physical Examination

Sign	Finding	Diagnoses
Appearance	Toxic	Epiglottitis
		Retropharyngeal abscess (RPA)
		Bacterial tracheitis
		Kawasaki's disease
Posturing	Fixed, upright, leaning forward	Epiglottitis
		RPA
		Tracheitis
		Laryngotracheobronchitis
	Torticollis	Parapharyngeal abscess
Phonation	Absent	Epiglottitis
	Muffled	RPA
		Peritonsillar cellulitis
		Peritonsillar abscess
Stridor, drool	Either present	Epiglottitis
		RPA
		Tracheitis
		Peritonsillar abscess
Noninvasive ENT	Conjunctivitis	Kawasaki's disease
		Stevens-Johnson
		Adenovirus
	Mucous membrane sore	Stevens-Johnson
		Behçet's disease
		Enterovirus
		Herpes simplex
	Submental, sublingual mass	Ludwig's angina
	Adenopathy	Adenovirus
		EBV
		Mycobacterium sp
		HIV
	Tender hyoid	Epiglottitis
	Tender thyroid	Thyroiditis
		Thyroglossal duct cyst infection
Augmented ENT findings	Trismus	Parapharyngeal abscess
		Peritonsillar abscess
	Tongue coating	Kawasaki's disease
		GABHS
	Palatal petechiae	GABHS
	Pharyngeal hyperemia	Infectious tonsillopharyngitis
		Caustic
		Trauma
	Exudative tonsillitis	GABHS
		Corynebacterium diphtheriae
		Fusobacterium sp
		EBV
		Adenovirus
	Bulged retropharynx	RPA
	Uvular erythema	Uvulitis
	Displaced uvula	Peritonsillar abscess
		Parapharyngeal abscess
	Inflamed epiglottis	Epiglottitis
Abdomen	Hepatosplenomegaly	EBV, hepatitis
Joint examination	Arthritis	Lemierre's syndrome
Rash	Scarlatiniform	GABHS
		Arcanobacterium sp
		EBV
		Kawasaki's disease

EBV, Epstein-Barr virus; ENT, ear, nose, throat; GABHS, group A beta-hemolytic streptococcus; HIV, human immunodeficiency virus.

A reduced functional caliber of the airway may occur acutely, subacutely, or insidiously, depending upon the cause of the disease process.[2,5] Ultimately, airway loss leads to air-preserving posturing. Infants unable to sit without support choose the lateral decubitus position

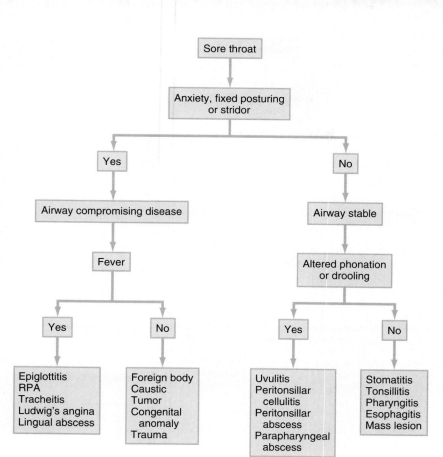

Figure 31-1. Diagnostic algorithm for the patient with a sore throat. RPA, retropharyngeal abscess.

Table 31-3. Centers for Disease Control and Prevention: Practice Guidelines for Acute Pharyngitis in Adults

Population: Adults (patients older than 15 years)
Patients with viral symptoms: Do not test or treat
Patients with symptoms of GABHS: Use Centor criteria*
  Centor score = 4: perform RADT or treat presumptively
  Centor score = 3: perform RADT or treat presumptively
  Centor score = 2: perform RADT or do not test or treat
  Centor score = 1 or 0: do not test or treat
In all cases in which an RADT is performed, only those with
  positive results are treated.
Culture after negative RADT? No
Recommended antibiotic: Penicillin (erythromycin if penicillin
  allergic)

*Centor criteria: history of fever; absence of cough; swollen, tender anterior cervical lymph nodes; and tonsillar exudate.
GABHS, group A beta-hemolytic streptococcus. RADT, rapid antigen detection test.

Ancillary Testing

In the patient with sore throat, the history and physical examination frequently provide sufficient information to support a presumptive diagnosis.[1,2] Laboratory procedures may not be necessary to support a working diagnosis of viral pharyngitis or GABHS pharyngitis (Table 31-3). Laboratory data may not be perceived to be cost effective.[5] Laboratory testing and its interpretation in the context of acute pharyngitis are discussed in detail in Chapter 74.

A complete blood count or serologic test for EBV may be useful for the patient with a compatible presentation. Hematologic findings of modest peripheral leukocytosis, lymphocytic predominance, and the presence of atypical lymphocytes constituting more than 10% of the total leukocyte count suggest EBV, cytomegalovirus, or toxoplasmosis as a cause of mononucleosis syndrome. A serologic test such as the Monospot may provide evidence of primary EBV infection.[9] Hepatitis testing is also appropriate to consider in these patients.

A lateral portable upright neck radiograph may be employed in the pediatric patient to narrow the differential diagnosis of infectious conditions associated with potential airway obstruction. Plain radiographic imaging is rarely warranted in the adult patient with acute, severe sore throat and has largely been supplanted by fiberoptic nasopharyngoscopy. Ultrasonography may be a useful tool to identify the size and internal characteristics of deep tissue abscesses, and localization may aid needle aspiration. Computed

with the neck hyperextended when obstruction occurs. Children capable of sitting maintain an upright posture. They may support their heads with their hands. Airway obstruction in an older child is typically associated with fixed upright posturing. The patient has forced flexion at the waist and maintains the neck flexed and the head extended with an open mouth. Alternatively, patients may assume tripod posturing, in which additional support is gained by hands held on a surface behind the patient's trunk.

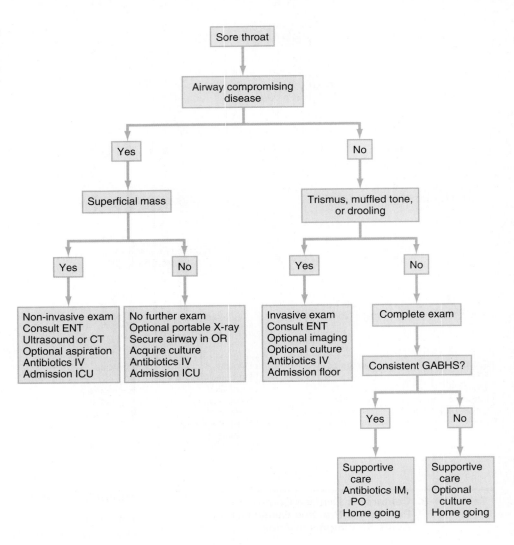

Figure 31-2. Management algorithm for the patient with a sore throat. CT, computed tomography; ENT, ear, nose, and throat; GABHS, group A beta-hemolytic streptococcus; ICU, intensive care unit.

tomography scanning also defines the extent of infection and is superior to ultrasonography for this purpose. It has the advantage of differentiating abscess from cellulitis. Magnetic resonance imaging provides superior resolution of deep tissue planes when ultrasound or CT scans have not been successful.

DIFFERENTIAL DIAGNOSIS

Inadequately recognized and treated GABHS pharyngitis can lead to localized epidemic spread (e.g., within a daycare population) and, rarely, to increased morbidity in the form of peritonsillar cellulitis or abscess.[8] GABHS pharyngitis, if untreated within the first week of onset of symptoms in children, may rarely lead to the delayed development of poststreptococcal complications, such as acute rheumatic fever.

EMPIRICAL MANAGEMENT
(Figure 31-2)

The management of the patient presenting with a sore throat revolves about the assessment for potential

airway compromise. If the patient is in extremis, immediate airway control is necessary. If the patient is preserving the airway and has adequate air exchange, the next decision is reached on the basis of the presence of an obvious mass. Infections within the parotid, buccal, parapharyngeal, submental, and sublingual spaces create masses that are readily apparent.[3,10] The purulent material rapidly expands the tissues but rarely occludes the airway. A thorough head and neck examination accompanied by fiberoptic nasopharyngoscopy is necessary to identify the severity and extent of the process. An ENT consultation may be advisable, particularly if the patient's condition is such that there appears to be sufficient time. Assessment with ultrasonography or CT imaging is often necessary. Needle aspiration of a peritonsillar abscess is both diagnostic and therapeutic. Intravenous antibiotics are begun that cover mixed infection with aerobic and anaerobic organisms.

If the febrile patient with sore throat appears toxic, evidences airway-preserving posturing, has an abnormal voice or prefers not to speak, and is drooling through a persistently open mouth, airway compromise may be imminent and immediate steps must be taken to secure the airway. The emergency physician remains at the bedside, and immediate transfer to the operating room is contemplated. This requires that the operating room be ready to receive the patient immediately and be close at hand (preferably not requiring elevator transport) and that the patient can be accompanied by a physician or surgeon capable of surgical cricothyrotomy and the equipment necessary to perform this procedure rapidly. Coordination with ENT and anesthesiology consultants is important. A preexisting protocol that gets the patient expeditiously to the operating room is optimal. If the patient is not considered appropriate for transport to the operating room, immediate fiberoptic intubation (nasal or oral) is the preferred route, with light sedation and topical anesthesia (see Chapter 1). A double setup with preparations in place for immediate surgical airway (cricothyrotomy) is essential. After the airway is secured, the infected surface and secretions can be swabbed for culture; tissue aspiration and blood culture specimens can be submitted for culturing.[6] Parenteral antibiotics are begun for mixed infection and the patient is transferred to the intensive care unit.

If the febrile patient evidences no compromise of the airway but has vocal changes (muffling or "hot potato" quality), it is likely that peritonsillar cellulitis or abscess is present, either condition easily identified during routine examination of the oropharynx. ENT need not be consulted for peritonsillar cellulitis or uvulitis. ENT may be consulted for peritonsillar abscess, even after needle aspiration, as tonsillectomy may be advisable after the acute infection subsides. Intravenous antibiotics are provided that cover *Streptococcus pyogenes*, non–group A streptococci, and *Staphylococcus aureus*. The patient can be admitted to a nonmonitored setting in the hospital.[11]

In the patient with a sore throat who has no evidence of airway compromise, the physician must determine whether the cause of the complaint is referred or rests within the oropharynx. Further diagnostic studies may be necessary to define the noninfectious causes of a sore throat. When infectious disease is likely, the patient is treated as outlined in Chapter 74.

REFERENCES

1. King BR, Charles RA: Pharyngitis in the ED: Diagnostic challenges and management dilemmas. *Emerg Med Pract* 6:5, 2004.
2. Lindberg EA: Acute sore throat. In Hamilton G, et. al (eds): *Emergency Medicine: An Approach to Clinical Problem Solving*, 2nd ed. Philadelphia, WB Saunders, 2003, pp 389-403.
3. Perkin RM, Swift JD: Infectious causes of upper airway obstruction in children. *Pediatr Emerg Med Rep* 7:117, 2002.
4. Pichichero ME: Group A streptococcal tonsillopharyngitis: Cost-effective diagnoses and treatment. *Ann Emerg Med* 25:390, 1995.
5. Attia M, et al: Multivariate predictive models for group A beta-hemolytic streptococcal pharyngitis in children. *Acad Emerg Med* 6:8, 1999.
6. Chen K, Varon J, Wenker OC: Malignant airway obstruction: Recognition and management. *J Emerg Med* 16:83, 1998.
7. Carey MJ: Epiglottis in adults. *Am J Emerg Med* 14:421, 1996.
8. Schraff S, McGinn JD, Derkay CS: Peritonsillar abscess in children: A ten-year review of diagnosis and management. *Int J Pediatr Otorhinolaryngol* 57:213, 2001.
9. Roberge RJ, et al: Lingual tonsillitis: An unusual presentation of mononucleosis. *Am J Emerg Med* 19:173, 2001.
10. Lee SS, Schwartz RH, Badori RS: Retropharyngeal abscess: Epiglottitis of the new millennium. *J Pediatr* 138:435, 2001.
11. Bisno AL, et al: Practice guidelines for the treatment of group A streptococcal pharyngitis. *Clin Infect Dis* 35:113, 2002.

CHAPTER

32 Hemoptysis

Brian Springer and Timothy G. Janz

PERSPECTIVE

Epidemiology

Hemoptysis is the expectoration of blood originating from the lower respiratory tract. Although most cases of hemoptysis are not immediately life-threatening, massive hemoptysis can occur, presenting extreme challenges to the physician trying to stabilize a patient's airway and identify and control the site of bleeding. Most cases of hemoptysis are relatively minor, such as a patient complaining of blood-streaked sputum. Massive hemoptysis lacks a universally accepted definition, but may be defined as blood loss ranging from 100 to greater than 600 mL of blood in a 24-hour period. It is estimated that 1.5% to 5% of patients with hemoptysis meet criteria for massive hemoptysis; mortality for these patients has been reported to be up to 80%.[1,2] Reasons for the high mortality may include difficulty in controlling the airway, the inability to access easily and tamponade the bleeding source, and the ability of even small amounts of blood in the alveolar space to inhibit oxygen exchange.

Pathophysiology

Bleeding may originate from the lungs or from the tracheobronchial tree. The lungs are supplied by the low-pressure pulmonary arteries and the high-pressure bronchial arteries. Most massive bleeding originates from the high-pressure bronchial arteries, although pathologic enlargement of the bronchial circulation (e.g., as in bronchiectasis) may create a lower pressure source of massive bleeding.

Mechanisms by which massive bleeding can occur include vascular alteration, chronic parenchymal inflammation, broncholithiasis, vascular invasion, and trauma.[3] Vascular mechanisms include erosion and rupture of enlarged vessels secondary to cavitary or bullous disease, immune-mediated vasculitis, and parenchymal infarction secondary to pulmonary embolism. Bronchiectasis previously was a common complication of patients with tuberculosis, inherited disorders such as cystic fibrosis, and other long-standing pulmonary disease. Chronic inflammation leads to hypertrophy of the bronchial arteries and loss of cartilaginous support of the bronchial wall.[4] Bleeding can occur because of rupture of a hypertrophied bronchial artery. Lung abscess resulting from anaerobic infection can lead to destruction of normal vessels. Broncholithiasis occurs in association with tuberculosis and histoplasmosis. Calcified lymph nodes may erode into a submucosal vessel, resulting in bleeding and expectoration of broncholiths. Centrally located tumors may invade the pulmonary vasculature, and blunt and penetrating trauma may cause disruption of the tracheobronchial tree. Other etiologies to consider include airway foreign bodies and the development of fistulae secondary to previous trauma or surgical manipulation of the airway or gastrointestinal tract.[5]

DIAGNOSTIC APPROACH

Differential Considerations

The location of bleeding is important in determining the approach to diagnosis and treatment. Hemoptysis refers to blood originating from below the vocal cords. Blood coming from the upper respiratory tract or from the gastrointestinal tract may spill into the lower airways and mimic hemoptysis. The physician should attempt to make an early determination if the bleeding source is tracheopulmonary. When possible, a thorough history and physical examination are the first step, although patient self-assessment is often unreliable, and physical examination is equivocal in up to 60% of patients.[4] Bronchoscopy and endoscopy may be required to localize the source of bleeding.

Examination of expectorated blood may be useful; expectorated blood in true hemoptysis is often bright red and mixed with sputum. Blood from the stomach is often dark red and may be mixed with food particles. Hematemesis is often acidic (barring medical conditions or medications that block gastric acid secretion), whereas hemoptysis has an alkaline pH.[1]

Rapid Assessment and Stabilization

The first step in the management of a patient presenting with hemoptysis is assessment of the patient's vital signs and cardiorespiratory status. Patients who die from hemoptysis die from asphyxiation rather than exsanguination. Even a relatively small amount of blood in the alveoli can impair oxygen exchange; patients may present hypoxemic and extremely agitated. In all but the most minor bleeding complaints, the patient is placed on a cardiac monitor, intravenous access is obtained, and pulse oximetry is instituted. Supplemental oxygen is delivered by nasal cannula or by mask, as necessary.

If the bleeding source is known and is unilateral, protection of the unaffected lung may be lifesaving. Placing the patient in a head-down angled position may help promote drainage of blood away from the lower airway. Positioning the patient with the affected side down may prevent spillover into the unaffected lung.[3,6]

The airway should be managed aggressively, and consideration should be given to early endotracheal intubation in all patients with massive hemoptysis. A large-bore (≥8.0 size), single-lumen tube should be placed to facilitate bronchoscopy. Airway landmarks may be difficult to visualize because of the presence of blood; the physician should have suction ready and have a backup plan to failed endotracheal intubation. These plans include consideration of nasotracheal or awake oral intubation, surgical airway, and fiberoptic laryngoscopy. The use of double-lumen tubes that allow each lung to be ventilated separately has become less common. These tubes are difficult to insert, and few physicians outside of anesthesiology are comfortable with their use.[7] Selective main stem intubation with a single-lumen endotracheal tube also is a consideration. However, airway anatomy generally limits this to intubation of the right main stem bronchus. Confirmation of endotracheal tube placement may be difficult. The presence of blood may impair the physician's ability to use auscultation, pulse oximetry, or capnography to ensure proper positioning within the airway. A postintubation radiograph should be obtained, although the presence of diffuse blood may make interpretation challenging. Following intubation, placement of a nasogastric or orogastric tube can help identify an upper gastrointestinal bleed. The emergency physician should be aware that despite intubation, the patient may continue to asphyxiate until bleeding is controlled. Ventilatory management should include maximal attempts to oxygenate the patient, and early consultation with a pulmonologist or intensivist is paramount. Blood should be obtained for laboratory analysis, including coagulation studies and type and crossmatch. Patients presenting with a coagulopathy should receive early treatment for reversal.

Pivotal Findings

History

History should be directed toward ascertaining the *etiology of bleeding*. An extensive past medical history should be obtained, including history of chronic obstructive pulmonary disease, cystic fibrosis, carcinoma, or other pulmonary diseases and if the patient has had any previous episodes of hemoptysis. *Risk factors* for pulmonary embolism should be obtained, including history of deep venous thrombosis or other hypercoagulable states. *History of infectious disorders,* such as pulmonary tuberculosis, fungal infections, or lung abscess, should be obtained. Foreign travelers or immigrants should be questioned carefully regarding *exposure to and symptoms of infectious disease.*

Patients with no underlying pulmonary disease may develop hemoptysis secondary to coagulopathy or anticoagulation therapy. *Medication lists* should be scrutinized, and the physician should inquire about over-the-counter medications, such as aspirin or non-steroidal anti-inflammatory drugs, and use of nutritional supplements. History of recent or past trauma and invasive airway procedures should be obtained. An attempt should be made to ascertain the *duration and volume of bleeding,* although patient reporting is unreliable and the amount of blood expectorated may not correlate with the volume of blood in the lungs. *Associated symptoms* may include chest pain, wheezing, abdominal pain, and lower extremity pain or swelling or both. *Review of systems* should focus on respiratory symptoms and symptoms of infectious disease, malignancy, or gastrointestinal disorders.

Physical Examination

The physical examination, although often equivocal, may contribute clues in isolating the source and cause of bleeding. The clinician should listen for wheezing or stridor secondary to a foreign body or mass. Sequelae of long-standing pulmonary disease, such as clubbing of the digits or hyperexpansion of the chest wall, should be sought. Examination of patients with autoimmune vasculitis may reveal the presence of oral or genital ulcerations, cutaneous nodules, or septal perforation. Examination of the abdomen may assist in detecting gastrointestinal pathology, and rectal examination may reveal evidence of gastrointestinal bleeding.[8]

Ancillary Testing

Chest radiography is obtained in all cases of hemoptysis. Radiographic findings may help pinpoint the bleeding source in 50% to 80% of patients[6]; however, distribution of the blood throughout the lung parenchyma via coughing may result in diffuse abnormalities. Other useful radiographic findings include presence of neoplasm, focal infection, or evidence of pulmonary infarction. Laboratory studies include hemoglobin and hematocrit (useful as a baseline measure and determinant of bleeding chronicity), platelet count, type and screen or type and crossmatch (depending on the patient's hemodynamic state), coagulation studies, and urinalysis and renal function (to look for evidence of vascular diseases, such as Wegener's granulomatosis or Goodpasture's syndrome).

The use of high-resolution computed tomography (CT) of the chest is preferred before bronchoscopy by many pulmonary and critical care physicians. Newer generation scanners are more sensitive and specific than chest radiographs in delineating major causes of life-threatening hemoptysis and may help guide later bronchoscopic evaluation.[4,7] Despite the availability of faster, open machines, CT use should be limited to stable patients. Decisions regarding CT scan before bronchoscopy should be made in consultation with the physician who will be assuming care of the patient.

DIFFERENTIAL DIAGNOSIS

Many disease states may lead to the development of massive hemoptysis. Box 32-1 lists some of the most common causes. A good history and physical examination help narrow the differential and direct diagnostic testing and treatment.

BOX 32-1. Differential Diagnosis: Hemoptysis

Airway Disease
Bronchitis (acute or chronic)
Bronchiectasis
Neoplasm (primary or metastatic)
Airway trauma
Foreign body

Parenchymal Disease
Infectious
  Tuberculosis
  Pneumonia
  Fungal disease
  Lung abscess
Autoimmune Disorders
  Goodpasture's syndrome
  Systemic lupus erythematosus
  Wegener's granulomatosis

Pulmonary Vascular
Pulmonary embolism
Arteriovenous malformation
Pulmonary hypertension
Aortic aneurysm

Hematologic Disease
Coagulopathy
Disseminated intravascular coagulation
Platelet dysfunction
Thrombocytopenia

Cardiac Disease
Mitral stenosis
Tricuspid endocarditis

Miscellaneous
Crack cocaine
Iatrogenic injury
Tracheal-arterial fistula

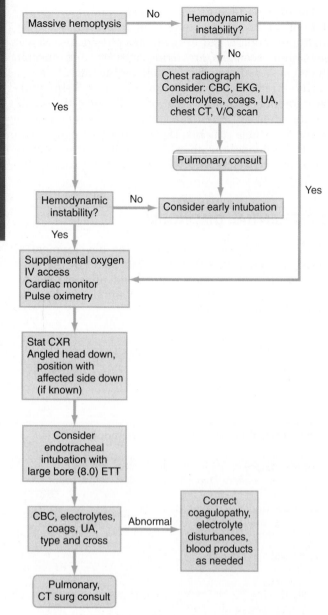

Figure 32-1. Emergency department management of hemoptysis. CBC, complete blood count; ECG, electrocardiogram; coags, coagulation studies; UA, urinalysis; CT, computed tomography; V/Q, ventilation-perfusion; IV, intravenous; CXR, chest radiograph; ETT, endotracheal tube.

MANAGEMENT

Little has changed since the 1990s in the management of massive hemoptysis; no consensus exists regarding optimal treatment.[2] As emphasized previously, the role of the emergency physician is early control of the airway, preferably with insertion of a large-bore, single-lumen endotracheal tube. When the airway has been secured and the patient relatively stabilized, consultation with pulmonary, critical care, and surgical colleagues determines further management strategy (Figure 32-1).

Bronchoscopy

Most pulmonologists favor early (within 24 hours) bronchoscopic evaluation.[7] Early bronchoscopy allows for localization of the bleeding site and protection of the unaffected lung and in some cases may facilitate specific therapy. Rigid bronchoscopy is recommended in cases of massive bleeding because of its ability to maintain airway patency and facilitate suctioning, although many intensivists prefer flexible scopes, primarily owing to familiarity. Numerous therapies exist for bleeding control through the bronchoscope, including balloon tamponade, thermocoagulation and photocoagulation, and use of hemostatic agents. Some specialists prefer the use of a CT "virtual bronchoscopy" before actual bronchoscopy. The use of CT depends on the wishes of the consultant and the stability of the patient.

Surgery

In general, surgery should be reserved for patients with rapid, uncontrollable, unilateral bleeding that is unresponsive to other measures. Morbidity and mortality are high. Consideration needs to be given to the patient's ability to tolerate lung resection. In general, patients with severe, diffuse underlying lung disease or with diffuse alveolar bleeding are not ideal surgical candidates.[2]

Percutaneous Embolotherapy

Embolization of the bronchial arteries may be used to control bleeding, especially in patients too unstable to tolerate surgery. Some studies have shown immediate control of the bleeding in 94% of patients. Embolization may serve as definitive treatment or serve as an interim treatment until surgery. Rarely is the bleeding heavy enough to be visualized during angiography. Most patients who undergo embolization first need bronchoscopy to locate the bleeding source.[8] Complications of embolization include arterial perforation or dissection secondary to guidewire injury, inadvertent spinal artery occlusion, and a relatively high rate of rebleeding.[9,10]

DISPOSITION

All patients who present with massive hemoptysis require admission to an intensive care unit. Patients who present with massive, uncontrollable bleeding may need to go directly to the operating room for bronchoscopy or for surgery. The emergency physician should not delay in contacting the intensivist, anesthesiologist, and cardiothoracic surgeon when dealing with an unstable patient.

Healthy, stable patients with only minor bleeding (presence of blood-streaked sputum) may be discharged after evaluation. If history, physical examination, and ancillary studies such as chest radiograph are normal or lead to a suspicion of a relatively minor entity, such as bronchitis, discharge with close follow-up may be reasonable. Patients should be advised to return immediately for worsening bleeding or for any difficulties breathing. If the workup leads to suspicion of a more serious diagnosis, such as carcinoma, vasculitis, or tuberculosis, admission is warranted and should be done in consultation with an appropriate physician.

REFERENCES

1. Cahill BC, Ingbar DH: Managing massive hemoptysis: A rational approach. *J Crit Illness* 11:604, 1996.
2. Ingbar DH: Causes and management of massive hemoptysis. *Up To Date* (11.2). Available at: www.uptodateonline.com. Accessed September 30, 2003.
3. Sternbach G, Varon J: Massive hemoptysis. *Intensive Care World* 12:74, 1995.
4. Cahill BC, Ingbar DH: A systematic approach to evaluating massive hemoptysis. *J Crit Illness* 11:446, 1996.
5. Weinberger SE: Etiology and evaluation of hemoptysis. *Up To Date* (11.2). Available at: www.uptodateonline.com. Accessed September 30, 2003.
6. Jean-Baptiste E: Clinical assessment and management of massive hemoptysis. *Crit Care Med* 28:1642, 2000.
7. Haponik EF, Fein A, Chin R: Managing life-threatening hemoptysis: Has anything really changed? *Chest* 118:1431, 2000.
8. Ingbar DH: Diagnostic approach to massive hemoptysis. *Up To Date* (11.2). Available at: www.uptodateonline.com. Accessed September 30, 2003.
9. Swanson K, et al: Bronchial artery embolization: Experience with 54 patients. *Chest* 121:789, 2002.
10. Wong ML, Szkup P, Hopely MJ: Percutaneous embolotherapy for life-threatening hemoptysis. *Chest* 121:95, 2002.

CHAPTER

33 Red and Painful Eye

John M. Wightman and Glenn C. Hamilton

PERSPECTIVE

Epidemiology and Pathophysiology

Most eye complaints are not immediately sight threatening and can be managed by an emergency physician. Nontraumatic diseases, such as glaucoma and peripheral vascular disease leading to retinal ischemia, are more common with advancing age. Ocular injuries are the leading cause of visual impairment and blindness in the United States.[1] More patients with postoperative complications can be expected to present to the emergency department as more vision correction surgeries are performed.

The external and internal anatomy of the eye is depicted in Figure 33-1A and B. The globe has a complex layering of blood vessels in the conjunctiva, sclera, and retina. Redness reflects vascular dilation and may occur with processes that produce inflammation of the eye or surrounding tissues. Eye pain may originate from the cornea, conjunctiva, iris, and vasculature. Each is sensitive to processes causing irritation or inflammation.

DIAGNOSTIC APPROACH

Rapid and accurate triage is the most critical consideration in the approach to the red and painful eye. The first question should be, "Did anything get in your eye?" If so, the second question should be, "What do you think it is?" This helps separate trauma from nontrauma but, more important, seeks to identify quickly eyes that may have been exposed to a caustic substance. These patients require immediate decontamination to prevent permanent loss of visual acuity.

Differential Considerations

Diagnoses are classically divided into traumatic and nontraumatic. Traumatic pain and redness can be caused by caustic fluids and solid materials, low-velocity contact with a host of materials that can fall or be rubbed into the eye, higher velocity blunt force impacts to the orbit or globe, or potential penetrating injuries. Causes of nontraumatic pain and redness require a more detailed history, including systemic illnesses.

Pivotal Findings

Measurement of the patient's best corrected visual acuity (i.e., with glasses on, if available) with each eye individually and with both eyes provides a vital sign when evaluating eye complaints. Only a few situations preclude early and accurate visual acuity testing. Eyes exposed to caustic materials must be decontaminated immediately. Patients with sudden and complete visual loss in one eye require an immediate funduscopic examination for the possibility of acute central retinal artery occlusion. This condition is readily apparent as a diffusely pale retina with indistinct or unseen retinal arteries (Figure 33-2).

Other pivotal findings, which are more likely to be associated with a serious diagnosis, in patients with a red or painful eye are listed in Box 33-1.

Figure 33-1. External (A) and internal (B) anatomy. (From Ragge NK, Easty DL: *Immediate Eye Care*. St. Louis, Mosby–Year Book, 1990.)

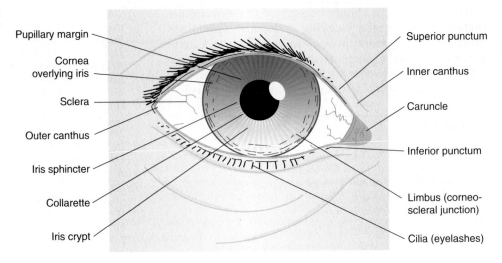

Pupillary margin
Cornea overlying iris
Sclera
Outer canthus
Iris sphincter
Collarette
Iris crypt

Superior punctum
Inner canthus
Caruncle
Inferior punctum
Limbus (corneo-scleral junction)
Cilia (eyelashes)

A   External appearance of the eye

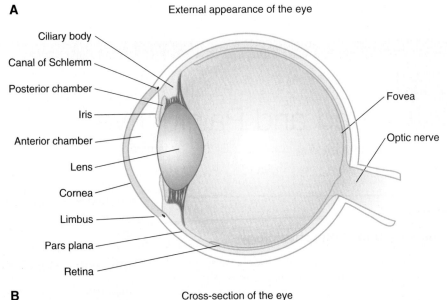

Ciliary body
Canal of Schlemm
Posterior chamber
Iris
Anterior chamber
Lens
Cornea
Limbus
Pars plana
Retina

Fovea
Optic nerve

B   Cross-section of the eye

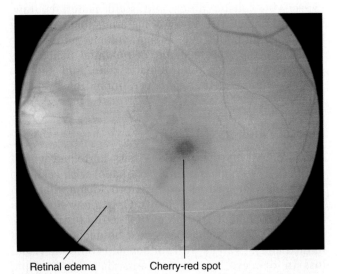

Retinal edema   Cherry-red spot

Figure 33-2. Key funduscopic findings in acute central retinal artery occlusion include general pallor of the retina (except for a characteristic cherry-red spot where the perfused choroid shows through the thinner fovea) and attenuation of retinal arteries (possibly with retinal veins preserved as in the photograph). (From Kaiser PK, Friedman NJ, Pineda R II: *The Massachusetts Eye and Ear Infirmary Illustrated Manual of Ophthalmology*, 2nd ed. Philadelphia, WB Saunders, 2004, p 297.)

BOX 33-1. Pivotal Findings More Likely Associated with a Serious Diagnosis in Patients with a Red or Painful Eye

Severe ocular pain
Photophobia
Persistently blurred vision
Proptosis
Reduced ocular light reflection
Corneal epithelial defect or opacity
Limbal injection (i.e., ciliary flush)
Pupil unreactive to a direct light stimulus
Wearer of soft contact lenses
Neonate
Immunocompromised host
Worsening signs after 3 days of pharmacologic treatment

Adapted and reprinted, with permission, from Trobe JD: *The Physician's Guide to Eye Care*. San Francisco, Foundation of the American Academy of Ophthalmology, 2001.

History

Chief complaints of pain can be manifestations of a variety of sensations. When carefully questioned, some patients may differentiate between itching, burning, dull pain, sharp pain, and perception of a foreign body. Foreign body sensation, in particular, is a distinct sensation and one with which most patients are familiar. Itching tends to be more often due to blepharitis, conjunctivitis, or dry eye syndrome. Burning includes these and other mostly extraocular problems such as irritation of a pterygium or pinguecula, episcleritis, or limbic keratoconjunctivitis. Dull pain may be a manifestation of increased intraocular pressure (IOP) or referred from an extraorbital process such as sinusitis, migraine headache, or temporal arteritis. Sharp pain generally results from abnormalities of the anterior eye such as keratitis, uveitis, and acute angle-closure glaucoma. A foreign body sensation is more typical of corneal irritation or inflammation.

A chief complaint of redness commonly results from palpebral or limbal injection of the conjunctiva but can also represent visible blood behind the bulbar conjunctiva or in the anterior chamber. Subconjunctival hemorrhage and hyphema can be spontaneous or post-traumatic. Spontaneous subconjunctival hemorrhages may follow coughing or straining or may be due to systemic hypertension. Often, it occurs without any identifiable precipitating incident and is simply noticed by the patient upon looking in the mirror. Spontaneous subconjunctival hemorrhage is painless, and the presence of pain raises concern for a more serious cause of the hemorrhage, such as direct globe injury. Hyphema of sufficient size to be noted by the patient or bystander usually arises with pain and blurred vision.

Other subjective findings may be transient and detected only by history. The patient may relate lid swelling, tearing, discharge, crusting, or sensitivity to light. Lid swelling can be caused by inflammatory and noninflammatory processes. Concurrent erythema of the lid favors the former. In the absence of trauma or other external irritant (e.g., contact dermatitis), inflammatory processes include primary lid problems such as hordeolum (i.e., stye) or blepharitis as well as extension from concomitant conjunctivitis or cellulitis in orbital or periorbital structures. When pain is present, tearing is usually secondary. Discharge and crusting are most commonly associated with conjunctivitis, whether allergic, viral, or bacterial. Blepharitis, dacryocystitis, and canaliculitis are other inflammatory processes that may create a discharge and subsequent crusting.

Other eye status review questions include the following:

- Are contact lenses used? If so, what type, how are they cleaned, and how old are the lenses? Has there been a change in the pattern of use (especially increased use)? Were the lenses worn for a particularly long time period recently? Are there problems with the lenses drying out? Does insertion of the lenses worsen or relieve the symptoms?
- Are glasses worn? If so, when was last assessment?

- Has previous eye surgery or injury occurred?
- Usual state of health?
- Current medications? Allergies, including environmental allergies?

Physical Examination

A complete eye examination usually includes eight components.[2] The mnemonic VVEEPP (pronounced "veep") plus slit-lamp and funduscopic examinations represent these components (Box 33-2).[3] Slit-lamp examination is recommended for any complaint involving trauma and for any medical presentation involving foreign body sensation or alteration of vision. Funduscopic examination is usually pursued if there is visual loss, visual alteration, or suggestion of serious pathology in the history and initial physical examination. A thorough physical examination can be conducted in the order presented next.

Visual Acuity

A patient's initial visual acuity determination provides a baseline from which deterioration or improvement may be followed. It is also predictive of functional outcome after ocular trauma. Visual acuity is quantitatively assessed by use of a Snellen chart test at a distance of 20 feet (6 m) or a Rosenbaum chart at a distance of 14 inches. Young patients who cannot yet read letters and numbers should be tested with an Allen chart that depicts easily recognizable shapes. Each eye is tested separately with the opposite eye carefully covered. Patients who present without their prescribed corrective lenses may be evaluated by having them view the chart through a pinhole eye cover, which negates most refractive errors in vision.

If the patient cannot distinguish letters or shapes on a chart, visual acuity must be determined qualitatively. Any printed material suffices. The result may be recorded as, for example, "patient able to read

---

BOX 33-2. Complete Eye Examination

Visual acuity (best possible using correction)
Visual fields (tested by confrontation)
External examination
    Globe position in orbit
    Conjugate gaze
    Periorbital soft tissues, bones, and sensation
Extraocular muscle movement
Pupillary evaluation (absolute and relative)
Pressure determination (tonometry)
Slit-lamp examination
    Lids and lashes
    Conjunctiva and sclera
    Cornea (with fluorescein in some cases)
    Anterior chamber
    Iris
    Lens
Funduscopic examination

Adapted from Wightman JM, Hurley LD: Emergency department management of eye injuries. *Crit Decis Emerg Med* 1998;12:1-11.

newsprint at 3 feet." If this is not possible, visual acuity is recorded as:

- Unable/able to count fingers (CF)
- Unable/able to perceive hand motion (HM)
- Unable/able to perceive light (LP/NLP)

Visual Field Testing

Confrontation is the most common method of testing visual fields in the emergency department.[4] Detection of a scotoma usually represents a retinal problem. However, glaucoma may cause scotomata that can be crescent shaped, involve just the binasal visual fields, or affect all peripheral vision. Hemi- or quadrantanopsia is more commonly a problem of the neural pathways to the brain.

External Examination

Gross abnormalities are assessed by a visual inspection of both eyes simultaneously. Findings may be more apparent if compared to the opposite side.

Globe position is part of the external examination. Subtle exophthalmos and enophthalmos are rare and are best detected by looking inferiorly, tangentially across the forehead, from over the patient's scalp.[5] Exophthalmos may have traumatic or nontraumatic causes but is due to increased pressure or a space-occupying lesion within the orbit, which may arise as pain. Medical causes include cellulitis, intraorbital or lacrimal tumors. Hyperthyroidism may cause enlargement of extraocular muscles. The most important cause of exophthalmos in the emergency department is retrobulbar hematoma, a condition characterized by hemorrhage within the bony orbit, behind the globe. The hemorrhage pushes the globe forward, stretching the optic nerve and retinal artery and increasing IOP. It is sight threatening if sufficiently severe and persistent. Orbital emphysema and inflammation caused by a retained foreign body behind the eye are other causes of exophthalmos. The discovery of exophthalmos should prompt ocular tonometry measurements to determine the urgency of intervention. Trauma, particularly penetrating globe injury with extrusion of vitreous, can cause the globe to recede into the orbit, but the most common etiology of enophthalmos is actually pseudoenophthalmos when the contralateral globe is proptotic.

Inspection also involves examination of the upper and lower palpebral sulci for foreign bodies or other abnormalities. The lower sulcus is easily viewed after manual retraction of the lower lid toward the cheek and having the patient gaze upward. The upper sulcus is inspected by pulling its lashes directly forward and looking under the lid with white light. The lid can be everted by pressing a cotton-tipped applicator in the external lid crease and folding the lid margin over the applicator.

Extraocular Muscle Function

Limitation of ocular movement in one eye may be detected by having the patient follow the examiner's finger or a bright light through the cardinal movements of gaze. The eyes may move in a disconjugate fashion, or the patient may admit to diplopia if asked. Diplopia on extreme gaze in one direction may indicate entrapment of one of the extraocular muscles within a fracture site but more often is caused simply by edema or hemorrhage related to the injury and is functional rather than actual entrapment. In the absence of trauma, diplopia is rarely associated with redness or pain.

Pupillary Evaluation

The pupils are inspected for abnormalities of shape, size, and reactivity. These examinations are conducted with light specifically directed into the pupil and by means of the swinging flashlight test.

Previous surgery (e.g., iridotomy for cataract extraction) and synechiae from prior iritis or other inflammatory condition are the most common causes of irregularly shaped pupils. Asymmetrically sized pupils may represent normal or pathologic conditions. Physiologic anisocoria is a slight difference in pupil size that occurs in up to 10% of the population. Topical or systemic medications, drugs, and toxins may cause abnormal pupillary constriction or dilation.

Pathologic reasons for failure of one pupil to constrict with a direct light stimulus include globe injury, abnormalities of afferent or efferent nerves, and paralysis of the ciliaris or sphincter pupillae muscles in the iris. Potentially serious problems, which also cause pain and redness, include uveitis and acute angle-closure glaucoma.

The swinging flashlight test is used to determine whether a relative afferent pupillary defect (RAPD) exists.[4] The patient fixes the gaze on a distant object and the examination room is darkened. The size of the pupils in lowered light is noted, and unless there is physiologic anisocoria, the pupils should be equal in size. The direct and consensual light responses of the eyes are compared as a light source, angled into the pupil from in front of the cheeks, is swung back and forth between the two. When the light source shines into an eye with an RAPD, the pupil dilates because the consensual response from withdrawal of light from the opposite eye with normal afferent activity is stronger than the direct constrictive response to light in the affected eye with inhibited afferent activity. It is termed "relative" because the response is compared with that of the opposite side as the light source is alternated between eyes. An RAPD may be partial or complete and due to inhibition of light transmission to the retina because of vitreous hemorrhage, loss of some or all of the retinal surface for light contact because of ischemia or detachment, or presence of lesions affecting the prechiasmal optic nerve (e.g., optic neuritis).

Pressure Determination

Ocular tonometry is usually the last examination performed in the emergency department. Common methods of determining the IOP in the emergency department include use of electronic, manual (e.g.,

Schiøtz), or applanation tonometers. IOPs in the 10-20 mm Hg range are considered normal. Causes of intraocular hypertension include glaucoma in its many forms, suprachoroidal hemorrhage, and space-occupying retrobulbar pathology. Patients with presenting IOPs exceeding 20 mm Hg should have ophthalmologic consultation. Acute treatment is usually not necessary until the pressure exceeds 30 mm Hg.

Slit-Lamp Examination

The slit lamp permits a magnified, binocular view of the conjunctivae and anterior globe for diagnostic purposes and to facilitate delicate procedures. It allows depth perception in otherwise clear structures, such as the cornea, aqueous humor, and lens. The slit-lamp examination can include the following:

- Lids and lashes may be inspected for blepharitis and pointing of a lid abscess (i.e., hordeolum). The inner canthus and lacrimal punctum may be better viewed for evidence of dacryocystitis.
- Punctures, lacerations, and inflammatory patterns of the conjunctiva or sclera may be discovered with magnification.
- Corneal abrasions, ulcers, foreign bodies, and other abnormalities may be seen. The depth of these lesions may be accurately assessed with an angled beam. Edema, which appears as a white haze or cloudiness within clear structures, can be differentiated as within the epithelium or deeper stroma.
- The anterior chamber may be examined for cells (e.g., red and white blood cells) and "flare." Flare is a diffuse haziness, related to cells and proteins suspended in the aqueous humor, that is often visible only when illuminated directly (Figure 33-3). It usually represents deep inflammation of the eye and is often seen in iritis. Collections of layered blood or pus in the dependent portions of the anterior chamber are called hyphema or hypopyon, respectively, and are graded by the percentage of the verti-

cal diameter of the visible iris. Foreign bodies that have penetrated the cornea may be found floating in the anterior chamber.

- The trabeculated pattern of the iris can be seen in detail. Spiraling muscle fibers may be seen in acute angle-closure glaucoma. If the beam is shown almost coaxially with the examiner's line of sight such that the red reflex is elicited, tears in the iris may be seen by light returning through the iris itself instead of just through the pupil.
- The lens should be examined for general clarity and the presence of opacities or foreign bodies. The type and position of any lens implants can also be better assessed during a slit-lamp examination.

Direct Funduscopic Examination

Emergency physicians most commonly perform a non-dilated funduscopic examination because there are several eye conditions in which dilation may be harmful (e.g., glaucoma). Iridodialysis, lens dislocation, and conditions requiring early intervention are usually identifiable along the visual axis.

Inability to obtain a red reflex or visualize the fundus of the eye can be due to:

- Opacification of the cornea, most commonly by edema secondary to injury or infection
- Hyphema or hypopyon within the anterior chamber
- Extremely miotic pupil
- Cataract of the lens
- Blood in the vitreous or posterior eye wall
- Retinal detachment

In the absence of trauma, there are few posterior findings associated with chief complaints of external redness. Findings associated with visual loss include pallor of the retina indicating ischemia, "cupping" of the optic disk indicating glaucoma, indistinctness of disk margins indicating papilledema or optic neuritis or neuropathy, air or plaque emboli in retinal arteries, and a host of other signs indicating more chronic ocular or systemic pathology not normally amenable to management in the emergency department.

Bedside Testing

Fluorescein solution and the cobalt blue lamp are the best means for identifying damage to the corneal epithelium, including that which cannot be seen with conventional slit-lamp examination. Fluorescein binds to exposed lipid in damaged membranes and pools in defects, making them easy to identify. Use of fluorescein may reveal corneal abrasions and ulcers as well as keratitides related to chemicals, ultraviolet light, or infections (e.g., herpes).

Relief of discomfort after instillation of a topical anesthetic can be used as a diagnostic test for an external source of pain. In general, abolition of pain by local anesthetic drops indicates pain of corneal origin. Modest but incomplete relief suggests a conjunctival process. Intraocular pain is not diminished by local anesthetic solution.[6] When ocular penetration is suspected, Seidel's test can be used. This test involves placing a fluorescein strip directly over an area of sus-

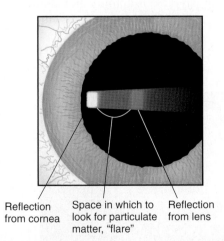

Reflection from cornea   Space in which to look for particulate matter, "flare"   Reflection from lens

Figure 33-3. Technique of slit-lamp examination with a short, narrow light beam projected from an extreme temporal angle across the contrasting black pupil to better find cells or "flare" indicative of acute anterior uveitis. (From Ragge NK, Easty DL: *Immediate Eye Care.* St. Louis, Mosby–Year Book, 1990.)

pected corneal penetration. The high localized concentration of fluorescein may facilitate identification of the corneal defect with a slit lamp by allowing visualization of leaking aqueous fluid diluting the fluorescein. This test does not work on the conjunctiva overlying the sclera, and a negative test result does not rule out a full-thickness corneal injury.

Ancillary Testing

An erythrocyte sedimentation rate may be used to evaluate for temporal arteritis, which may arise with eye pain and decreased visual acuity.

Infections are usually evident by examination, and laboratory tests such as a complete blood count are not necessary. Microbiologic cultures are rarely ordered in the emergency department.

Plain radiography is used to identify facial fractures associated with facial or ocular trauma or indirectly by detecting an air-fluid level in the orbit or fluid in the paranasal sinuses.

Computed tomography (CT), using 1.5-mm axial and coronal cuts, can reliably localize metal and many non-radiopaque foreign bodies in the globe and orbit. It can also detect small amounts of intraocular air following penetrating trauma. Magnetic resonance imaging (MRI) clearly delineates the orbital and retroorbital structures. It is less often used in emergency eye assessment, for which, in general, CT scanning is the imaging modality of choice.[7]

When the visual axis is obscured by blood during a nondilated funduscopic examination after trauma, ultrasonographic examination may assist in imaging vitreal and choroidal injuries. Ultrasonography is more sensitive for detecting intraocular foreign bodies, but CT is better at delineating the damage caused by them, so they are complementary tests.[8]

DIFFERENTIAL DIAGNOSIS

Clinical findings most indicative of serious eye disorder are listed in Box 33-1.

Critical Diagnoses

Caustic injury to the eye can rapidly lead to a destructive keratoconjunctivitis (Figure 33-4 A and B) if the agent is not removed immediately. The diagnosis is made on history alone, before any other examination is performed. Early and copious irrigation is indicated. Many patients have already undergone extensive irrigation at the job site, but when the exposure has occurred in the home, irrigation prior to arrival in the emergency department is uncommon. Alkaline caustic agents cause a liquefactive necrosis of the cornea by progressively reacting with the corneal layers, and destruction is severe and relentless. Continuous irrigation is the only effective method to terminate the reaction and should be continued for at least 30 minutes. Acid injury is much less severe and requires less irrigation than alkaline exposures, but irrigation should continue until the pH of the tears is neutral or the patient is essentially asymptomatic.

Acute angle-closure glaucoma is a relatively rare but important critical diagnosis to make in the emergency department. Patients present with pain, the onset of which is often sudden in low-light conditions requiring pupillary dilation through contraction and thickening of the iris peripherally. The iris becomes immobile and often irregular, and the pupil is commonly fixed at 5 to 6 mm in diameter. Inability of the pupil to constrict may result in photophobia, and accommodation may be affected. These and the increased IOP can lead to frontal headache, nausea, and vomiting. As inflammation progresses, limbal injection of the conjunctiva is almost universally seen. Figure 33-5 demonstrates many of these findings. Immediate medical intervention in the emergency department and urgent ophthalmological consultation are warranted.

Retrobulbar hematoma (blood) is usually caused by orbital trauma, but it can also occur spontaneously in patients with coagulopathy. Retrobulbar abscess (pus) or emphysema (air) can also occur.[9] Elevated IOP in any of these conditions constitutes a surgical emergency. Emergency intervention is to decompress the orbit by performing lateral canthotomy and cantholysis.

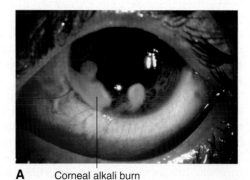

A   Corneal alkali burn

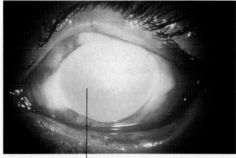

B   Corneal alkali burn

Figure 33-4. A, Alkali burn demonstrating corneal burns and conjunctival injection on the day of the accident. **B,** Complete corneal tissue destruction 7 days after alkali burn. (From Kaiser PK, Friedman NJ, Pineda R II: *The Massachusetts Eye and Ear Infirmary Illustrated Manual of Ophthalmology*, 2nd ed. Philadelphia, WB Saunders, 2004.)

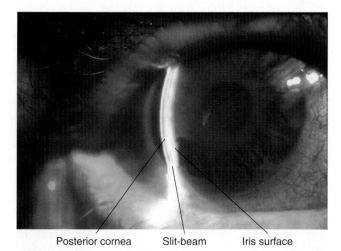

Posterior cornea   Slit-beam   Iris surface

Figure 33-5. Primary angle-closure glaucoma with very shallow anterior chamber and iridocorneal touch (no space between slit beam view of cornea and iris). (From Kaiser PK, Friedman NJ, Pineda R II: *The Massachusetts Eye and Ear Infirmary Illustrated Manual of Ophthalmology*, 2nd ed. Philadelphia, WB Saunders, 2004.)

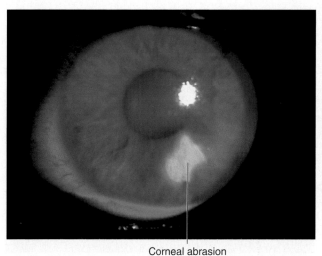

Corneal abrasion

Figure 33-6. Corneal abrasion demonstrating fluorescein pooling of a small inferior epithelial defect. (From Kaiser PK, Friedman NJ, Pineda R II: *The Massachusetts Eye and Ear Infirmary Illustrated Manual of Ophthalmology*, 2nd ed. Philadelphia, WB Saunders, 2004.)

Emergent Diagnoses

Most emergent diagnoses involve some kind of inflammation secondary to trauma, infection, or systemic disease. These include keratitis, anterior uveitis, scleritis, and endophthalmitis. Any of these may be complications of surgical procedures, and an appropriate ophthalmologic history must be obtained.

Keratitis, or inflammation of the cornea, is most commonly viral in origin but can also be caused by exposure to intense ultraviolet light (e.g., snow blindness, arc welder's blindness), various chemicals, or ischemia related to contact lens use. Patients present with an intense foreign body sensation, ciliary spasm causes photophobia that is often severe, and the affected eyes are often clenched shut. Topical anesthesia provides immediate (but temporary) relief of pain, thus reinforcing the corneal origin of the process and facilitating examination and definitive diagnosis.[6] Corneal abrasions are very common and may be identified by white light or fluorescein-facilitated blue light using a slit lamp or any other magnification (Figure 33-6). Following thorough irrigation, thermal and chemical burns must receive a careful slit-lamp examination for potential full-thickness injury. If this is not found, the corneal injury may be treated similarly to an abrasion.

In immunocompetent hosts, corneal ulcerations are most commonly due to overuse of contact lenses. They are seen as a denuding of epithelium with surrounding edema, the increased interstitial water of which is seen as whitish clouding of the normally clear tissue (Figure 33-7). Almost all ulcerations require same-day evaluation by an ophthalmologist. Infections of the cornea with herpes simplex virus can rapidly lead to opacification and significant visual loss. It is most commonly recognized by a characteristic dendritic pattern of fluorescein pooling under blue light (Figure 33-8). Anterior uveitis, which includes iritis and iridocyclitis, often occurs secondary to a traumatic injury or

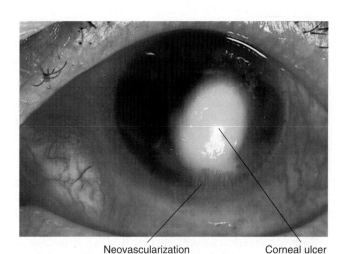

Neovascularization   Corneal ulcer

Figure 33-7. Bacterial keratitis demonstrating large, central *Streptococcus pneumoniae* corneal ulcer. Note the dense, white corneal infiltrate and the extreme conjunctival injection. (From Kaiser PK, Friedman NJ, Pineda R II: *The Massachusetts Eye and Ear Infirmary Illustrated Manual of Ophthalmology*, 2nd ed. Philadelphia, WB Saunders, 2004.)

infectious process or can be associated with serious systemic immune diseases such as adult and juvenile rheumatoid arthritis, sarcoidosis, and ankylosing spondylitis.

Scleritis is rare and may be difficult to differentiate from episcleritis, which is somewhat more common and a more benign inflammation. The former is commonly idiopathic but may be associated with a systemic inflammatory process such as a connective tissue disease, gout, or infection (e.g., Lyme disease, syphilis, tuberculosis). Eye redness in episcleritis results from dilation of the episcleral blood vessels just underneath the conjunctiva, usually in a small sector of the visible portion of the globe. If the location of the involved layer is in doubt, a topical anesthetic allows the examiner to

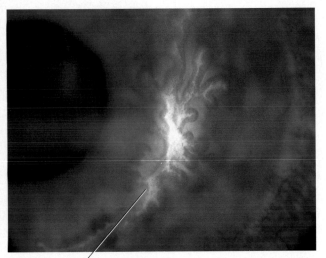

Herpes simplex virus dendrite

Figure 33-8. Patient demonstrating fluorescein pooling of herpes simplex virus dendrite. (From Kaiser PK, Friedman NJ, Pineda R II: *The Massachusetts Eye and Ear Infirmary Illustrated Manual of Ophthalmology*, 2nd ed. Philadelphia, WB Saunders, 2004.)

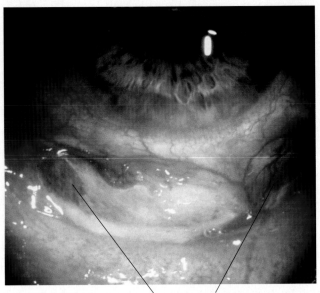

Necrotizing scleritis

Figure 33-9. Diffuse scleritis with slight bluish region in addition to injection of scleral, episcleral, and conjunctival vessels. (From Kaiser PK, Friedman NJ, Pineda R II: *The Massachusetts Eye and Ear Infirmary Illustrated Manual of Ophthalmology*, 2nd ed. Philadelphia, WB Saunders, 2004.)

move the conjunctiva and its contained vessels with a cotton-tipped applicator, thus differentiating between vessels of scleral or conjunctival origin. The pain of scleritis is typically slower in onset but is often described as a severe "boring" pain that radiates to the ipsilateral forehead, cheek, or jaw. Engorgement of scleral vessels is usually more prominent and more diffuse than that of the episcleral vessels in episcleritis. A bluish hue may be seen as the underlying pigmented epithelium shows through the edematous and more translucent sclera (Figure 33-9). Scleritis may be associated with anterior uveitis, cataract, and secondary glaucoma.

Endophthalmitis usually results from an infection of structures inside the globe. It is most common following penetrating trauma but may begin after hematogenous seeding from a remote or systemic infection, particularly in immunocompromised hosts. Unless it is detected early and is responsive to aggressive antimicrobial therapy, endophthalmitis is a devastating process that results in enucleation.

Urgent Diagnoses

Penetrating ocular trauma is evaluated by history (e.g., working with high-speed grinding equipment), examination (extrusion of aqueous humor or other globe content; direct visualization of a foreign body in the anterior chamber, vitreous, or retina), or identification of the offending object by biplanar plain radiography, thin-cut CT scan, or ultrasonography. MRI should not be used because magnetic particles can migrate and cause additional damage. Indirect indicators of globe penetration are hyphema, an irregularly shaped pupil from traction on the iris as an object passed its attachments, or lack of a red reflex. If penetrating ocular injury is confirmed or if suspicion persists after evaluation, ophthalmologic consultation is indicated.[4]

Spontaneous or traumatic hyphema is usually managed conservatively. Blood in the anterior chamber is usually the result of direct ocular trauma and may be associated with traumatic mydriasis or an obvious tear of the iris. If penetration and rupture can be reasonably excluded, the hyphema should be graded and IOP determined. Intraocular hypertension (or hypotension in the case of occult globe rupture) following trauma must also be evaluated by an ophthalmologist urgently. Inability to view posterior structures through the anterior blood may necessitate radiologic imaging.

Diagnostic Algorithm

A recommended algorithmic approach to the patient with an acute red eye is provided in Figure 33-10.

EMPIRICAL MANAGEMENT

Irrigation

Any clean water is appropriate for irrigation, and prompt initiation takes precedence over procurement of a particular irrigating solution. The most important principles are *immediate and copious* dilution and removal of the offending material. An eyewash station or faucet with tap water may be employed. Normal saline may be instilled through the end of macrodrip intravenous administration tubing. If there is no gross eye injury, a Morgan lens may be attached to this tubing, and emergency department staff do not have to help the patient hold the eye open. Quickly administering two drops of topical anesthetic greatly facilitates patients' tolerance of the prolonged irrigation required.

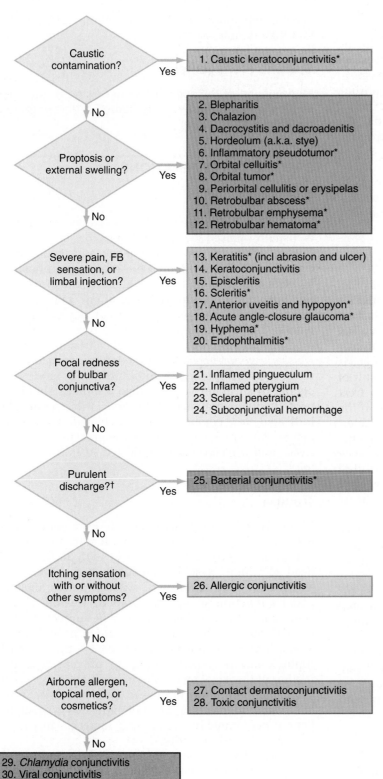

Figure 33-10. Diagnostic algorithm for red eyes *Indicates potentially serious diagnoses if not identified on initial emergency department evaluation).†Purulent implies true pus, as opposed to the mucoid discharge more commonly associated with nonbacterial etiologies of conjunctivitis. a.k.a., also known as; FB, foreign body; incl, including. (Modified from Trobe JB: *The Physician's Guide to Eye Care*. San Francisco, Foundation of the American Academy of Ophthalmology, 2001.)

It is recommended that the first 500 to 1000 mL of irrigation fluid be administered while examining the eye; then the Morgan lens may be placed.

Pain Relief

Pain often interferes with obtaining an adequate assessment. A topical anesthetic, such as proparacaine 0.5%, may facilitate cooperation in patients with suspected injury or inflammation of the anterior eye by reducing pain and blepharospasm long enough to obtain a targeted history and focused examination. Topical anesthetic agents should not be given to patients to use at home. Parenteral or oral analgesics can be used for severe deep pain not amenable to topical relief in the emergency department or for outpatient management of discomfort after the patient's discharge.

Mydriatic and Cycloplegic Agents

Dilation of the pupil is not usually necessary in the emergency department for funduscopic examination but may relieve pain associated with ciliary spasm in anterior uveitis. Mydriatic agents (e.g., phenylephrine, tropicamide) merely prevent constriction of the pupil by paralyzing the sphincter pupillae muscle of the iris. Cycloplegic agents (e.g., cyclopentolate, homatropine) paralyze the ciliaris muscle, with an accompanying mydriatic effect. The agent chosen should be guided by the desired length of time of mydriasis for the particular condition being treated (Table 33-2). Mydriatic agents are contraindicated in patients with narrow-angle glaucoma.[10]

Antimicrobial Prophylaxis

There is no evidence to support the widespread practice of administering antibiotic solution or ointment for surface infections. Antimicrobial prophylaxis is best reserved for penetrating wounds to prevent bacterial keratitis or endophthalmitis. Similarly, most conjunctivitis, regardless of the character of the discharge, is viral, and antibiotic administration is more a result of habit than science. Antibiotics are best used to treat identified or suspected bacterial infections, even if the exact bacterial agent has not been determined. Bacterial keratitis is rare; it is usually caused by streptococcus or staphylococcus and is treated with appropriate antibiotics (see Table 33-1, no. 25). Therapy of viral infections is discussed in Chapter 128.[11,12] The most common organisms cultured from deeper eye structures, particularly in cases with a retained foreign body, are *Bacillus cereus*, enterococcus, and various species of *Bacillus* and *Staphylococcus*.[13] While awaiting emergent ophthalmologic consultation for possible vitrectomy, empirical parenteral antibiotic combinations include cefazolin plus gentamicin or vancomycin plus cefotaxime, ceftazidime, or ceftriaxone. Suspected mycotic endophthalmitis must be treated with amphotericin B.

Open wounds also require tetanus prophylaxis if the patient's immunization status is not up to date. There is no current evidence supporting the practice of administering tetanus immunization to patients with superficial corneal abrasions.

Other Protective Interventions

Increased IOP must be reversed as rapidly as possible, often before the specific cause is known. After placing the patient in at least a 30-degree head-up position, two drops of timolol 0.5%, a topical β-adrenergic blocking medication, should be administered as a first-line agent to decrease the production of aqueous humor. This may be followed by two drops of dorzolamide 2%, a topical carbonic anhydrase inhibitor, to reduce aqueous humor production further. If not available, 500 mg of acetazolamide may be given orally or intravenously. If the patient has sickle cell disease or trait, oral methazolamide 50 mg must be used instead. Patients with suspected intraocular hypertension who also have nausea or vomiting should receive a parenteral antiemetic so that they do not gag or vomit.

Specific Management

Management of the specific entities listed in the diagnostic algorithm presented in Figure 33-10 is presented in Table 33-1.

SPECIAL CONSIDERATIONS

Pediatrics

A red eye in a neonate or infant is always abnormal. It is usually caused by corneal abrasion or infection. Corneal abrasions can also be a cause of inconsolable crying in an infant. Fluorescein examination helps to identify abrasions and herpes keratitis, acquired from the birth canal. *Chlamydia* infections may also be acquired during vaginal deliveries but may not arise for weeks. These infections should be treated with oral erythromycin as well as parenteral ceftriaxone to cover *Neisseria gonorrhoeae*. Conjunctivitis associated with respiratory symptoms or infiltrates on a chest radiograph in an infant younger than 3 months should be treated with an oral macrolide. Oral antibiotics are also indicated for conjunctivitis associated with otitis media. *Mycoplasma* is a common infection in these cases, and a macrolide is indicated in this syndrome too.[14]

Trauma

Blunt trauma is a common cause of a red and painful eye. Large hyphemas and those with clots are likely to require hospitalization for bed rest with 30 degrees of head elevation. Systemic analgesia and, if required, antiemetics are indicated. Medications affecting platelet function should be avoided. Treatment as in acute angle-closure glaucoma may be indicated when the IOP exceeds 30 mm Hg. If there is no iris injury, a long-acting cycloplegic agent (e.g., topical homatropine) may be recommended to prevent repetitive motion of the iris. Some reliable adult patients may be discharged with daily follow-up by a specialist. Strong analgesia and patching are not indicated so that the patient may immediately identify increases in pain or decreases in visual acuity.

Corneal abrasions are common problems in the emergency department. When the emergency physician is convinced that the cornea has not received a full-thickness laceration or penetration by a foreign body, management is relatively simple. Foreign bodies (on or in the epithelium only) should be removed when possible. These may frequently adhere to a saline-moistened cotton-tipped applicator. Ones that do not may sometimes be lifted off with a blunt-tipped tool ("spud") under the binocular magnification of a slit lamp. The common use of hypodermic needle removal may damage surrounding cornea and is not recommended. Whether or not the object can be successfully removed, management is the same as for corneal abra-

	Diagnosis from Figure 33-11	Management	Consultation	Disposition
1.	Caustic keratoconjunctivitis	Immediate and copious irrigation with tap water or sterile normal saline until tear-film pH = 7. *Solids*: lift particles out with dry swab before irrigation *Acids*: minimum of 2 L *and* 20 minutes *Alkalis*: minimum of 4 L *and* 40 minutes	Ophthalmologist must come to ED if there is any abnormal visual acuity or objective finding on examination after sufficient irrigation with exception of expected injection of conjunctiva secondary to treatment.	May discharge only if tear-film pH = 7 *and* no findings on examination except conjunctival injection *and* ophthalmologist can re-evaluate next day.
2.	Blepharitis Inflammation of eyelid margins often a/w crusts on awakening, foreign body sensation, and tearing	None except artificial tears for dry eye.	Outpatient referral only for treatment failure after 2 weeks.	Discharge with instructions to apply warm compresses to eyelids for 15 minutes four times/day and scrub lid margins and lashes with mild shampoo on wash-cloth two times/day.
3.	Chalazion Inflammation of meibomian gland causing subcutaneous nodule within the eyelid.	None.	Outpatient referral only for treatment failure after 2 weeks.	Discharge with instructions to apply warm compresses to eyelids for 15 minutes and gently massage nodule four times/day.
4.	Hordeolum (a.k.a. stye) Abscess in eyelash follicle or modified sebaceous gland at lid margin: *external* or *internal* based on side of lid margin that abscess is pointing.	*External*: Warm compresses often all that is needed, may Rx anti-*Staph* ointment two times/day. *Internal*: oral Rx for β-lactamase *Staph.*	Outpatient referral only for treatment failure after 2 weeks.	Discharge with instructions to apply warm compresses to eyelids for 15 minutes and gently massage abscess four times/day.
5.	Dacrocystitis and dacroadenitis Eye tearing and inflammation of lower eyelid inferior to lacrimal punctum finding redness and tenderness over nasal aspect of lower lid and adjacent periorbital skin.	First r/o periorbital cellulitis (#9) and orbital cellulitis (#7). Inspect for obstruction of punctum by SLE, may express pus by pressing on sac, oral Rx for nasal and skin flora if not admitting.	Ophthalmologist may admit if systemically ill, case is moderate or severe, or no social support for patient. Ask about culturing before Rx if admitting, then Rx same as periorbital cellulitis (#9).	May discharge mild cases with oral analgesics and antibiotics (such as amoxicillin/clavulanate), and instructions to apply warm compresses to eyelids for 15 minutes and gently massage inner canthal area four times/day.
6.	Inflammatory pseudotumor* Nonspecific, idiopathic, retrobulbar inflammation with eyelid swelling, palbebral injection of conjunctiva, chemosis, proptosis, blurred vision, painful or limited ocular mobility, binocular diplopia, edema of optic disk, or venous engorgement of retina.	Measure IOP. Evaluate for infection, diabetes mellitus, and vasculitis with CBC, BMP, UA, and ESR. Obtain axial CT of brain and axial and coronal CT of orbits and sinuses.	IOP > 20 mm Hg may be surgical emergency, Rx to decrease IOP in ED.	May discharge if no systemic problems, no findings of particular concern on CT, and IOP < 20 mm Hg. Start high-dose oral steroids after discussion with ophthalmologist and ensure re-evaluation in 2 to 3 days.
7.	Orbital cellulitis* Eyelid swelling, redness and warmth of skin overlying orbit, tenderness of skin overlying bone palbebral injection of conjunctiva, and chemosis. Differentiated from periorbital cellulitis by *presence* of any finding of fever, ill appearance, blurred vision, proptosis, painful or limited ocular mobility, binocular diplopia, edema of optic disk, or venous engorgement of retina.	Measure IOP. Start IV Rx with second-generation cephalosporin (such as cefuroxime, cefoxitin, or cefotetan) or with ampicillin/sulbactam to cover sinus and skin flora. Alternative Rx is ticarcillin/clavulanate, piperacillin/tazobactam, vancomycin, or clindamycin *plus* third-generation cephalosporin (such as cefotaxime or ceftriaxone).	IOP > 20 mm Hg may be surgical emergency, Rx to decrease IOP in ED. Obtain blood cultures and start antibiotics. Axial and coronal CT of orbits and sinuses to r/o FB, retrobulbar abscess, orbital gas, subperiosteal abscess, osteomyelitis, and changes in cavernous sinus. Consider LP.	Admit all cases of orbital cellulitis.

CHAPTER 33 Red and Painful Eye

	Diagnosis from Figure 33-11	Management	Consultation	Disposition
8.	Orbital tumor* Blurred vision, proptosis or other displacement of globe, painful or limited ocular mobility, or binocular diplopia (but can be asymptomatic).	Measure IOP. Evaluate for extraocular signs of malignancy. Obtain axial CT of brain and axial and coronal CT of orbits and sinuses.	IOP > 20 mm Hg may be surgical emergency, Rx to decrease IOP in ED. Ophthalmologist may want MRI, MRA, or orbital US.	Based on findings and discussion with consultant.
9.	Periorbital cellulitis or erysipelas Eyelid swelling, redness and warmth of skin overlying orbit, tenderness of skin overlying bone, palbebral injection of conjunctiva, and chemosis. Differentiated from orbital cellulitis by *absence* of any other finding listed in #7.	First r/o orbital cellulitis (#7). Oral Rx for sinus and skin flora if not admitting.	Ophthalmologist may admit if systemically ill, case is moderate or severe, or no social support for patient.	May discharge mild cases with oral antibiotics. Ophthalmologist must re-evaluate next day to ensure, no orbital extension.
10.	Retrobulbar abscess* Findings of orbital cellulitis (#7) but a/w increased IOP.	Measure IOP unless possibility of ruptured globe. IOP > 30 mm Hg, may require emergent needle aspiration or lateral canthotomy and cantholysis in ED. *Abscess*: Antibiotics as in orbital cellulitis (#7). *Emphysema*: Prophylax with antibiotics to cover sinus flora. *Hematoma*: Correct any coagulopathy or thrombocytopenia.	IOP > 20 mm Hg may be surgical emergency, Rx to decrease IOP in ED. Obtain axial CT of brain and axial and coronal CT of orbits and sinuses.	Admit all cases of retrobulbar pathology causing increased IOP. Others might be candidates for discharge depending on cause of problem.
11.	Retrobulbar emphysema* Findings of pseudotumor (#6) but a/w increased IOP.			
12.	Retrobulbar hematoma* Findings of pseudotumor (#6) but occurs due to trauma, coagulopathy, or thrombocytopenia and a/w diffuse subconjunctival hemorrhage anteriorly and extending posteriorly as well as increased IOP.			
13.	Keratitis (abrasion or UV injury) Pain, foreign body sensation, blepharospasm, tearing, photophobia, epithelial disruption on inspection under white light or fluorescein pooling under blue light. Superficial punctuate keratitis (SPK) appears as stippling of corneal surface [often lower 2/3 of cornea if due to light exposure].	First r/o corneal penetration either grossly or employing Seidel's test. Relieve pain and blepharospasm with topical anesthetic. Inspect all conjunctival recesses and superficial cornea for any foreign material that can be removed by irrigation or manually lifted from surface. Tetanus prophylaxis is standard of care even if cornea not penetrated.	Ophthalmologist must come to ED if there is any concern for globe penetration. Otherwise consult for follow-up examination in 1 or 2 days. One-time administration of cycloplegic agent may limit photophobia until follow-up examination.	May discharge cases not infected or ulcerated on topical antibiotic prophylaxis using polymyxin B combinations with bacitracin (ointment) or trimethoprim (solution). Gentamicin and sulfacetamide are less desirable single-agent alternatives. Oral NSAIDs or narcotics for analgesia. Patching not necessary.
	Keratitis (ulceration)* Symptoms and signs as above. Ulceration from complications of contact wear or neglected corneal abrasion has "scooped out" epithelium with surrounding edema appearing as white "cloudiness" in clear tissue.	Relieve pain and blepharospasm with topical anesthetic. *Staph.* and *Strep.* species still most common organisms, but *Pseudomonas* greater percentage in existing infections (especially contact lens wearer), so Rx with topical fluoroquinolone is preferred.	Discuss any potential need to debride or culture before starting antibiotic.	Based on findings and discussion with consultant. Typical ciprofloxacin dosing is 1 drop every 15 minutes for 1 hour, then 1 drop every hour for 8 hours, then 1 drop every 4 hours until seen by consultant next day. Oral NSAIDs or narcotics for analgesia. No patch.

Table 33-1. Management Algorithm for Red Eyes Extended from Diagnostic Algorithm in Figure 33-10—cont'd

	Diagnosis from Figure 33-11	Management	Consultation	Disposition
	Keratitis (herpetic infection)* Symptoms and signs as above. Look for other signs of herpes, varicella, zoster (or CMV infection in immunocompromised patient). Look for "dendritic" defects of cornea with fluorescein under blue light.	Relieve pain and blepharospasm with topical anesthetic. Rx with trifluridine 1% solution, vidarabine ointment, or acyclovir ointment. Varicella-zoster and CMV not normally given antivirals if immunocompetent.	Discuss any potential need to debride or culture before starting antiviral, with ophthalmologist.	Based on findings and discussion with consultant. Typical trifluridine dosing is 1 drop every 2 hours for 7 days, then taper over next 2 more weeks. Typical vidarabine or acyclovir dosing is five times a day for 7 days then taper over 2 more weeks. Oral NSAIDs or narcotics for analgesia. No patch.
14.	Keratoconjunctivitis Conjunctivitis with subepithelial infiltrates in cornea causing pain and decreased vision, possibly with halos reported.	Treat for conjunctivitis by likely etiologic category (#25–30).	Discuss findings and use of prednisolone acetate 1% (frequency determined by ophthalmologist).	May discharge patient with medications recommended by ophthalmologist and ensure re-evaluation in 2 to 3 days.
15.	Episcleritis Rapid onset of localized pain, injection of episcleral vessels, and localized tenderness.	Relieve irritation with artificial tears and decrease inflammation with ketorolac drops.	Outpatient referral only for treatment failure after 2 weeks.	May discharge patient with oral NSAIDs alone or in combination with topical ketarolac drops.
16.	Scleritis* Progressively increasing eye pain with radiation to ipsilateral face and decreasing vision, photophobia, tearing, and possible pain with eye motion.	Decrease inflammation with oral NSAIDs.	Discuss findings and use of topical or oral steroids.	May discharge patient with medications recommended by ophthalmologist and ensure re-evaluation in 2 to 3 days.
17.	Anterior uveitis and hypopyon* Eye pain, photophobia, tearing, limbal injection of conjunctiva, and cells or flare in anterior chamber. Hypopyon is layering of white cells (pus) in anterior chamber.	First r/o glaucoma with IOP measurement. Rx in ED if IOP > 20 mm Hg. Otherwise OK to dilate pupil with 2 drops of cyclopentolate 1%.	Discuss findings and use of prednisolone acetate 1% (frequency determined by ophthalmologist but range is every 1 to 6 hours).	May discharge patient with medications recommended by ophthalmologist and ensure re-evaluation in 2 to 3 days. Patients with hypopyon are generally admitted.
18.	Acute angle-closure glaucoma* Sudden-onset eye pain and blurred vision that may be a/w frontal headache, nausea, and vomiting. Anterior eye may manifest shallow or closed angle between iris and cornea, pupil fixed in mid-dilation, or limbal injection of conjunctiva. Rx in ED if IOP > 30 mm Hg.	Decrease production of aqueous humor Timolol 0.5% 1 drop then repeat in 30 min Apraclonidine 1% 1 drop once Dorzolamide 2% 2 drops *or if sickle cell disease or trait then methazolamide 50 mg orally* Decrease inflammation Prednisolone 1% 1 drop every 15 min four times Constrict pupil Pilocarpine 4% 1 drop then repeat in 15 min Consider establishing osmotic gradient Mannitol 2 g/kg IV.	Discuss any IOP > 20 mm Hg with ophthalmologist.	Based on findings and discussion with consultant, which primarily depends on speed of onset and response to treatment.

Continued

	Diagnosis from Figure 33-11	Management	Consultation	Disposition
19.	Hyphema* Pain, decreased visual acuity, gross or microscopic blood in anterior chamber, may be a/w dilated and fixed pupil following blunt trauma. Graded by amount of blood Percentage of vertical diameter of anterior chamber when blood layers with patient in upright position. Microhyphema shows no layering and only suspended red blood cells.	First r/o globe rupture. May require ultrasound if cannot visualize posterior structures. Measure IOP unless possibility of ruptured globe. IOP > 30 mm Hg, may require acute treatment as in glaucoma (#18). If IOP < 20 mm Hg and no iridodialysis, may use cycloplegic to prevent iris motion.	Discuss findings and use of ε-aminocaproic acid and steroids, other medical therapy, best disposition, and follow-up examination by ophthalmologist within 2 days. Some patients may be admitted for observation, bed rest, head elevation, and frequent medication administration.	Most patients can be discharged with careful instructions to return for any increased pain or change in vision. Patients should decrease physical activity and sleep with an eye shield in place. Eyes should be left open while awake, so any change in vision can be immediately recognized. Oral NSAIDs or narcotics for analgesia.
20.	Endophthalmitis* Progressively increasing eye pain and decreasing vision, diminished red reflex, cells and flare (and possibly hypopyon) in anterior chamber, chemosis, and eyelid edema.	Empirical parenteral antibiotic administration with cefazolin *plus* gentamicin *or* vancomycin *plus* cefotaxime, ceftazidime, *or* ceftriaxone to cover *Bacillus*, enterococcus, and *Staphylococcus* species.	Ophthalmologist must admit for parenteral and possibly intraocular antibiotics.	Admit all cases of endophthalmitis.
21.	Inflamed pingueculum Inflammation of soft yellow patches in temporal and nasal edges of limbal margin.	Decrease inflammation with naphazoline or ketorolac drops.	Outpatient referral only for treatment failure after 2 weeks.	Discharge to follow-up with ophthalmologist for possible steroid therapy or surgical removal.
22.	Inflamed pterygium Inflammation of firmer white nodules extending from limbal conjunctiva onto cornea.	Same as above	Same as above	Same as above
23.	Scleral penetration* Localized redness at site of entry, teardrop pupil, blood in anterior chamber or loss of red reflex.	Protect eye from further pressure, provide pain relief, and prevent vomiting. Tetanus prophylaxis.	Ophthalmologist must come to ED if there is any concern for globe penetration.	Admit for IV antibiotics and possible procedural intervention.
24.	Subconjunctival hemorrhage Red blood beneath clear conjunctival membrane.	Exclude coagulopathy or thrombocytopenia, if indicated by history.	None required if no complications.	Reassure patient that red should resolve over 2 to 3 weeks.
25.	Bacterial conjunctivitis* Hyperpurulent discharge not typical of common "pink eye" and more commonly unilateral in adults. Inflammation of eyelid margins a/w lid edema, chemosis, and possibly subconjunctival hemorrhage, but usually no follicular "cobblestoning."	Topical polymyxin B + trimethoprim in infants and children, because more *Staph.* species. Topical sulfacetamide or gentamicin clinically effective in 90% of uncomplicated adult cases. Use ciprofloxacin if *Pseudomonas* possible.	Culture drainage and consult ophthalmology in all neonates and those at risk for vision loss or systemic sepsis. *Neisseria gonorrhoeae* can be rapidly sight threatening.	Discharge uncomplicated cases with 10 days of topical antibiotics in both eyes, regardless of laterality of apparent infection. Use ointments in infants and drops in others.
26.	Allergic conjunctivitis Often bilateral palpebral injection of conjunctiva and follicular cobblestoning of inner surface of lids that may be seasonal and a/w other allergic symptoms such as rhinitis.	Decrease irritation with naphazoline drops.	Outpatient referral only for treatment failure after 2 weeks.	Identify antigen if possible. Consider treating other allergic symptoms with oral antihistamines.
27.	Contact dermatoconjunctivitis Localized lid and conjunctival redness and edema.	Irrigation with tap water or sterile normal saline. Decrease irritation with naphazoline drops.	Outpatient referral only for severe cases or treatment failure after 2 weeks.	Identify offending agent and avoid subsequent exposure. Discharge uncomplicated cases on continued naphazoline.

Table 33-1. Management Algorithm for Red Eyes Extended from Diagnostic Algorithm in Figure 33-10—cont'd

	Diagnosis from Figure 33-11	Management	Consultation	Disposition
28.	Toxic conjunctivitis Diffuse conjunctival injection, chemosis, and lid edema.	Same as above	Same as above	Same as above
29.	*Chlamydia* conjunctivitis Often bilateral palpebral injection of conjunctiva in neonate or other individual at risk for sexually transmitted disease.	Rx oral erythromycin for *Chlamydia*. Consider parenteral ceftriaxone for concurrent *Neisseria gonorrhoeae*.	Culture drainage and consult ophthalmology in all neonates and those at risk for vision loss or systemic sepsis.	Discharge uncomplicated cases on 14 days of oral erythromycin.
30.	Viral conjunctivitis Often bilateral palpebral injection of conjunctiva and follicular cobblestoning of inner surface of lids. Inflammation of eyelid margins often a/w crusts on awakening, foreign body sensation, and tearing.	Decrease irritation with artifical tears, naphazoline, or ketorolac drops.	Culture drainage and consult ophthalmology in all neonates and those at risk for vision loss or systemic sepsis.	Ask about pregnant mothers, infants, and immunocompromised individuals in close contact. Discharge uncomplicated cases with instructions on respiratory and direct-contact contagion for 2 weeks.

*Potentially serious diagnoses if not identified on initial emergency department evaluation. Antibiotic choices should be based on current practice.
a.k.a., also known as; a/w, associated with; BMP, basic metabolic profile (includes electrolytes, glucose, and renal function tests); CBC, complete blood count; CMV, cytomegalovirus; CT, computed tomography; IOP, intraocular pressure; LP, lumbar puncture; MRA, magnetic resonance angiography; MRI, magnetic resonance imaging; NSAIDs, nonsteroidal anti-inflammatory drugs; r/o, rule out; Rx, prescribe; SLE, slit-lamp examination; *Strep.*, *Streptococcus*; *Staph.*, *Staphylococcus*; US, ultrasonography; UV, ultraviolet.

Table 33-2. Duration of Action for Common Mydriatic and Cycloplegic Medications

Name	Concentation	Common Duration	Maximum Duration
Ephedrine*	5.0%	½-1 hour	3 hours
Phenylephrine*	2.5%	½-1 hour	3 hours
Tropicamide	0.5%	3-4 hours	6 hours
Cyclopentolate	0.5%	12-18 hours	24 hours
Homatropine	1.0%	1-2 days	3 days
Scopolamine	0.5%	2-5 days	7 days
Atropine	0.5%	5-10 days	14 days

*Mydriatic action only, no cycloplegic effect. Combination products are also available, such as Cyclomydril which is cyclopentolate 0.2% and phenylephrine 10%.

sions. Rust staining of the corneal epithelium does not require removal in the emergency department. The patient is referred to be seen by a specialist within 3 days. Prophylactic topical antibiotics are indicated for all epithelial defects of the cornea. Patching is not necessary and may be harmful. Systemic analgesia appropriate to the patient's level of pain should be provided. Larger lesions may require a prophylactic mydriatic or cycloplegic agent anticipating a secondary iritis. Topical anesthetics should not be given to the patient for home use.[4]

DISPOSITION

Most emergency department patients with eye complaints are candidates for discharge and, if indicated, follow-up in the emergency department or with an ophthalmologist in 1 to 2 days. Others may require referral only if there is lack of resolution or treatment failures. A few patients require admission for procedural intervention, parenteral antibiotic regimens, management of intractable pain, or further diagnostic evaluation. General consultation and disposition considerations for the most important entities are outlined in Table 33-1.

REFERENCES

1. Parver LM, et al: Characteristics and causes of penetrating eye injuries reported to the National Eye Trauma Registry, 1985-91. *Public Health Rep* 108:625, 1993.
2. Rhee DJ, Pyfer MF: Differential diagnosis of ocular symptoms. In *The Wills Eye Manual: Office and Emergency Room Diagnosis and Treatment of Eye Diseases*, 3rd ed. Philadelphia, Lippincott, Williams and Wilkins, 1999, pp 1-6.
3. Wightman JM, Hurley LD: Emergency department management of eye injuries. *Crit Decis Emerg Med* 12:1, 1998.
4. Trobe JD: The screening examination. In *The Physician's Guide to Eye Care*, 2nd ed. San Francisco, Foundation of the American Academy of Ophthalmology, 2001, pp 1-16.
5. Ragge NK, Easty DL: Methodology. In *Immediate Eye Care: An Illustrated Manual.* St. Louis, Mosby, 1990, pp 11-31.
6. Sklar DP, Lauth JE, Johnson DR: Topical anesthesia of the eye as a diagnostic test. *Ann Emerg Med* 18:1209, 1989.
7. Dobler AA, et al: A case of orbital emphysema as an ocular emergency. *Retina* 13:166, 1993.
8. McNicholas MM, et al: Ocular trauma: Evaluation with US. *Radiology* 195:423, 1995.
9. Birrer RB, Robinson T, Papachristos P: Orbital emphysema: How common, how significant? *Ann Emerg Med* 24:1115, 1994.
10. Howes DS, Hinkebein MK: The red painful eye. In Hamilton GC et al (eds): *Emergency Medicine: An Ap-*

proach to Clinical Problem Solving, 2nd ed. Philadelphia, WB Saunders, 2003, pp 417-435.

11. Barequet IS, O'Brien TP: Therapy of herpes simplex viral keratitis. *Ophthalmol Clin North Am* 12:63, 1999.

12. Miedziak AI, O'Brien TP: Therapy of varicella-zoster virus ocular infections. *Ophthalmol Clin North Am* 12:51, 1999.

13. Thompson JT, et al: Infectious endophthalmitis after penetrating injuries with retained foreign bodies. *Ophthalmology* 100:1468, 1993.

14. Diamant JI, Hwang DG: Therapy for bacterial conjunctivitis. *Ophthalmol Clin North Am* 12:15, 1999.

PART TWO
Trauma

CHAPTER

34 Multiple Trauma

Susan L. Gin-Shaw and Robert C. Jorden

PERSPECTIVE

The management of patients with multiple trauma is a complex undertaking that requires broad knowledge, sound judgment, technical skill, and leadership capabilities. Few patients offer a greater challenge to the emergency physician than do critical trauma patients. These patients benefit from skillful resuscitation; they are healthy, young individuals who, if salvaged, have a normal life expectancy.[1,2]

Emergency physicians play a vital role in the stabilization and diagnostic phases of trauma care. Often the emergency physician is the sole physician in attendance during the initial phase of resuscitation; what happens in this period often determines the outcome of care.

Epidemiology

Fatalities from motor vehicle crashes (MVCs) in 2002 numbered 42,815, and an additional 2,920,000 people suffered nonfatal injuries.[3] There were 4808 pedestrians killed in traffic collisions and 3244 motorcycle fatalities.[3] Data for firearm-related injuries in 2002 reveal 29,737 fatalities and more than 64,000 nonfatal firearm injuries annually.[4] Trauma, for the most part, is a disease of the young and is the leading cause of death in those 1 to 37 years old.[4]

Traumatic injuries have a large impact on society. For the victim and his or her immediate family there are physical, emotional, and medical costs as well as lost earnings during recovery. One study estimated that the medical costs of treating gunshot wounds (GSWs) were $2.3 billion, of which taxpayers ultimately pay 49%. This estimate does not include lost productivity—$1.6 billion acutely and $17.4 billion because of death.[5]

Many traumatic injuries are preventable. Educational campaigns on the consequences of drinking and driving and the importance of the use of seatbelts, helmets, and gun locks are efforts to increase public awareness of these problems. Alcohol is associated with 41% of fatal MVCs and 31% to 49% of firearm-related assaults. Although the number of alcohol-related fatalities has been rising steadily since 1999, the rate per 100 million vehicle miles traveled has been declining. Seatbelts, another preventive measure, were not used in 59% of fatal MVCs.[3] Although it can be argued that seatbelt users are more likely to be involved in nonfatal collisions, the overall use of seatbelts remains at less than 50%. Firearm-related injury rates have shown a steady decline since peaking in 1993.

The annual death rate has fallen from 15.4 to 11.4 per 100,000 population and the nonfatal rate from 40.5 to 23.9 per 100,000 population.[6] Further studies are needed to determine the impact of legislation, sentencing guidelines, violence prevention programs, and the general economy on this decline.

The Trauma System

An individual institution that operates in isolation cannot exercise its full impact on improving trauma outcomes. Therefore, it is essential to incorporate regional planning with designated trauma centers to manage trauma victims efficiently. Since the first studies from Orange County, research indicates that such systems reduce the preventable trauma death rate.[7,8]

The American College of Surgeons (ACS) has made great strides with trauma center designation and regionalized care plans. In 39 states, state and local agencies have legal authority to designate and categorize trauma centers.[9,10] In other regions, hospitals are self-designated and typically seek credential affiliation with the ACS. At the end of 1998, 43 states had statewide or regional trauma systems.[10] Integral to a well-managed trauma system is an ambulance destination policy (Figure 34-1). Clinically useful trauma scores should be easily calculated from data obtained under less than ideal conditions at the accident scene. Although triage scores have not been shown to be superior to the general impressions of the paramedics, they offer the advantage of allowing data comparison. Regardless of how it is accomplished, proper field triage ensures that injured patients are taken to the closest facility capable of delivering definitive care.

Ongoing quality assurance programs are another important aspect of a regionalized trauma system. Level I centers should maintain an accurate trauma log and review the outcome of patients' care. Trauma scoring scales allow a comparison of an institution's outcomes with a national standard. Commonly used scores include the revised trauma score (RTS) and the injury severity score (ISS).[11,12] The RTS assigns values from zero to four to defined intervals of the Glasgow Coma Scale, systolic blood pressure, and respiratory rate. The ISS is based on anatomic injury and is calculated by adding the sum of the squared scores on the abbreviated injury scale for the three most severely injured body regions. On the basis of a patient's age, RTS, and ISS scores, the probability of survival may be computed and the patient's outcome compared with that of similar patients (Box 34-1).

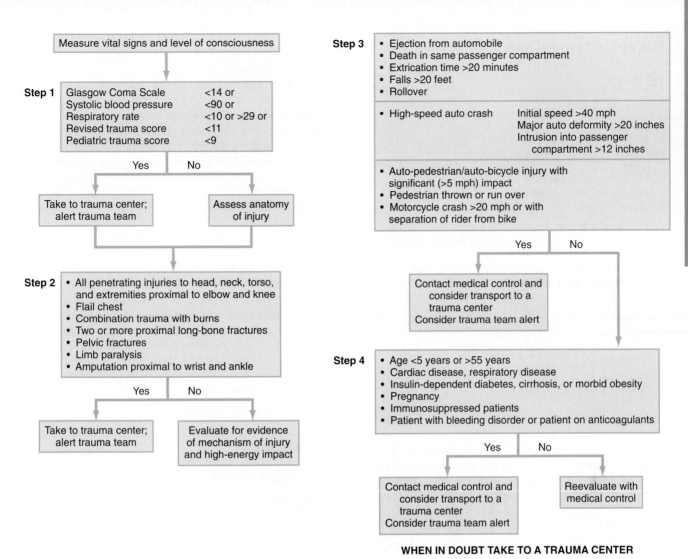

WHEN IN DOUBT TAKE TO A TRAUMA CENTER

Figure 34-1. Triage decision scheme. *Note*: It is the general intention of these triage guidelines to select severely injured patients for trauma center care. When there is doubt, the patient is best evaluated in a trauma center.

Step 1: Physiologic status thresholds are values of the Glasgow Coma Scale, blood pressure, and respiratory rate from which further deviations from normal are associated with less than a 90% probability of survival. Used in this manner, prehospital values can be included in the admission trauma score and the quality assessment process.

A variety of physiologic severity scores have been used for prehospital triage and have been found to be accurate. The scores contained in the triage guidelines are believed to be the simplest to perform and provide an accurate vasis for field triage based on physiologic abnormality.

Deterioration of vital signs would necessitate transport to a trauma center.

Step 2: A patient who has normal vital signs at the scene of the accident may still have a serious or lethal injury.

Step 3*: It is essential to look for indications that significant forces were applied to the body. Evidence of damage to the automobile can be a helpful guide to the change in velocity. Intrusion into the passenger compartment from any direction should prompt consideration of the potential for major injury.

Step 4*: Certain other factors that might lower the threshold at which patients should be treated in trauma centers must be considered in field triage. These include the following:

A. Age: Patients older than age 55 have an increased risk of death from even moderately severe injuries. Those younger than age 5 have certain characteristics that may merit treatment in a trauma center with special resources for children.

B. Comorbid factors: The presence of significant cardiac, respiratory, or metabolic diseases is an additional factor that may merit the triage of patients to trauma centers.

*Each trauma system and its hospitals should use quality improvement programs to determine use of mechanism of injury and comorbid factors as activators for bypass and trauma team action. (Redrawn and modified from American College of Surgeons: Resources for optimal care of the injured patient. In: *Field Triage*. Chicago, American College of Surgeons, 1993.)

The benefits of a coordinated trauma system are not as easily demonstrated in rural communities. Despite greater availability of air transport, long transport times often mandate that the initial trauma stabilization occurs in local hospitals. Medical providers in more remote areas vary widely in their level of experience in the management of trauma. The advanced trauma life support (ATLS) course is specifically designed to train such providers.

Even in large metropolitan areas, a regionalized trauma system can be limited by hospital overcrowding, which leads to ambulance diversion. Diversions force ambulance crews to transport critically injured patients longer distances to the nearest open trauma

BOX 34-1. Abbreviated Injury Scale

AIS Scores
1—minor, 2—moderate, 3—serious, 4—severe, 5—critical, 6—maximum (fatal)

Body Region
A. Head/neck
B. Face
C. Chest
D. Abdomen/pelvic contents
E. Extremities/pelvic girdle
F. External (skin)

Injury Severity Score
- Sum of the squared AIS scores of the three most severely injured body regions
- A score of 6 in any region is automatically assigned an injury severity score (ISS) of 75
- >20% blood loss generally raises the score by 1 in the most severely injured region
- Example: A patient with a grade 4 splenic laceration, closed femur fracture, and hand laceration:

$$D^2 + E^2 + F^2 = 4^2 + 3^2 + 1^2 = 26$$

center. Contributing to this dilemma is the triage of minimally injured patients to these centers.[13] This problem is ideally addressed at a local level with continuing education of prehospital personnel, cooperation of all regional hospitals, and the development of protocols for downgrading a given institution's trauma response to a minimally injured patient.[13,14]

Resources at existing Level I trauma centers are also overextended with the closure of similar facilities in a catchment area. Between 1980 and 1991, 58 trauma centers were discontinued; most were Level II centers in California and Florida.[9,15] Lack of adequate reimbursement and physician availability for trauma care are often the underlying reasons for such closures. In some regions, patients with multiple trauma are often uninsured and require extraordinary levels of personnel and specialty services. The 1995 near closure of Los Angeles County/USC Medical Center, one of the three largest trauma centers in the nation, threatened to overwhelm other area emergency departments. The Los Angeles county health system avoided this scenario by negotiating a $364 million federal bailout package.[16] Even for patients with insurance, only a fraction of actual costs is reimbursed for trauma patients under current diagnosis-related groups (DRGs) and Medicaid payment plans.[17,18]

PRINCIPLES OF DISEASE

Etiology: Mechanism of Injury

Knowledge of the mechanism of injury greatly enhances the management of trauma patients. It enables the emergency physician to anticipate specific injuries and therefore be more effective and timely in detection and treatment. Table 34-1 lists several mechanisms of injury and the accompanying potential

diagnoses. This list includes injuries commonly or classically associated with the particular mechanism and is by no means exhaustive.

A few guidelines are worth mentioning regarding GSWs. Nearly all handgun injuries are considered low velocity and are not likely to cause widespread injury. Conversely, hunting and military rifles are high-velocity weapons that produce immense kinetic energy and cause extensive internal damage to a victim that may not be apparent on general inspection. Similarly, close-range shotgun wounds produce massive injuries that are grossly contaminated by expelled components of the shot shell.

With injuries caused by a fall, there is a general correlation between the severity of injury and the height from which the fall took place. Using 12 feet as an average floor or story, the estimated heights lethal to 50% and 90% of the population (LD_{50} and LD_{90}) for falls are four and seven stories, respectively. Lower extremity, pelvis, and spine fractures are common after falls from heights, and shock is often present. Unlike other blunt trauma mechanisms, falls with feet-first or buttocks landings tend to produce retroperitoneal hemorrhage from pelvic fractures more commonly than intra-abdominal bleeding.[19]

MANAGEMENT

Prehospital Phase

Perspective

The clinical management of a trauma patient begins at the scene of the trauma. Currently, standards established by the Department of Transportation require all ambulance attendants to be trained at least to the basic emergency medical technician level. Paramedic ambulance systems have further advanced the quality and level of sophistication of treatment in the field. The role of the prehospital care team in cases of trauma includes prevention of additional injury, rapid transportation to the hospital, advance notification to the hospital, initiation of treatment, and triage.

Prevention of Additional Injury

The prevention of additional injury is accomplished through careful handling of the patient and splinting of both real and potential injuries. Patients must be extricated, moved to a stretcher, and placed in the ambulance with caution. Cervical immobilization, log-rolling techniques, and backboards ensure the protection of the spinal cord. Splinting extremity fractures can minimize neurovascular injury, prevent the conversion of a closed fracture into an open one, and minimize the amount of blood lost at the fracture site.

Rapid Transport

The philosophy of stabilization and transfer to the hospital may be reasonable for selected medical cases, but the rule of rapid transport remains unchanged for trauma care. Because critical patients often require sur-

Table 34-1. Trauma Mechanisms and Anticipated Injuries

Mechanism	Injury to Rule Out
Motor Vehicle Crashes	
Broken windshield	Closed head injury, facial fractures, skull fractures, cervical spine fractures
Broken steering wheel	Deceleration injuries of the chest, including myocardial contusion, aortic rupture, pulmonary contusion, fractured sternum, flail chest, and hemopneumothorax
	Upper abdominal injury, liver and spleen injury, diaphragmatic rupture, and pancreaticoduodenal injury
Knees to dashboard	Dislocated hip, fractured hip or femur, fractured acetabulum
Improper lap belt	Mid-lumbar spine fracture, hollow viscus injury
Three-point belt restraint	Fracture of ribs, clavicle, sternum; pulmonary contusion
Rollover with entrapment of lower body under vehicle	Crush injury, severe pelvic and other lower extremity fractures, compartment syndromes
Rear-end collision	Hyperextension injuries of the cervical spine, including fractures and central cord syndrome
Falls	
Supine impact	In general, great potential for axial and appendicular skeletal injury
	Renal artery thrombosis from intimal tear (potentially bilateral)
Prone impact	Deceleration chest and abdominal injuries
Head injury	Closed head and cervical spine injury
Upright impact	Calcaneal fractures; thoracolumbar spine fractures; spinous process fractures; pelvis fracture; severe, comminuted leg and femur fractures
Auto-Pedestrian Collisions	
Low-speed, adult	Tibial plateau fracture, ligamentous injury of knee
Low-speed, child	Chest and abdominal injury, closed head injury
High-speed	Life-threatening multisystem injury
Selected Penetrating Injuries	
Periorbital	Intracranial penetration, carotid-cavernous sinus fistula
Anterior neck	Retropharyngeal hematoma with potential for airway compromise, esophageal injury
Central chest	Heart and great vessel injury
Buttocks	Rectal injury, peritoneal penetration
High-velocity gunshot	Injury distant to the entrance wound
Miscellaneous	
Strangulation	Crushed larynx, fractured hyoid, intimal injury of the carotid artery
Localized epigastric or right upper quadrant trauma (e.g., bicycle handlebar)	Intramural duodenal hematoma, solid organ injury
Patient buried (e.g., cave-in of a trench)	Traumatic asphyxia

Data from Grande CM, Stene JK: Mechanisms of injury: etiologies of trauma. In Stene JK, Grande CM (eds): *Trauma Anesthesia,* Baltimore, Williams & Wilkins, 1990; Mono J, Holienberg RD, Harvey JT: *Ann Emerg Med* 15:589, 1988; and Panjabi M, White A: *Spine* 13:838, 1988.

gical intervention to achieve stability, no time should be lost in reaching definitive care.[20]

Advanced Notification

Regardless of the level of personnel training, a prehospital care system with the capacity for advanced hospital notification provides an important service. Such notification allows the trauma team to assemble, to anticipate patients' needs, to prepare for procedures, and to provide a more organized and expeditious resuscitation in general. Moreover, appropriate consultants can be alerted, the operating room notified, the blood bank prepared, and a critical care bed arranged if necessary.

Approach

The primary field interventions are spinal immobilization, airway management, and restoration of the circulating volume. The benefit of addressing these concerns needs to be balanced against time spent on the scene and the resulting delay of definitive care. Necessary airway management should be performed before transport of the patient. A protected airway and optimal oxy-genation and ventilation should be achieved as quickly as possible. Similarly, temporary field treatment of a tension pneumothorax by needle thoracostomy may be life-saving.[21]

The benefit of initiating intravenous (IV) fluid resuscitation before departure is less clear. In urban areas where transport times are brief, little justification exists for prolonging time on the scene for this procedure unless it can be accomplished while other essential procedures are being performed.[22-25] In rural areas with long transport times, IV line placement can be briefly attempted and fluid resuscitation continued en route to the hospital. The issue of fluid replacement in cases of uncontrolled hemorrhage is still being debated.[26-28]

Triage

In the context of routine trauma care, as opposed to disaster management, triage is the determination of the appropriate hospital destination based on the patient's assessment. Triage decision making must be sensitive in detecting patients truly in need of a trauma center. Several triage tools have been proposed, including the

BOX 34-2. Principles of Trauma Management

Organized team approach
Priorities in management and resuscitation
Assumption of the most serious injury
Treatment before diagnosis
Thorough examination
Frequent reassessment
Monitoring

BOX 34-3. Priorities in Trauma

High-Priority Areas	Low-Priority Areas
Airway/breathing	Neurologic
Shock/external hemorrhage	Abdominal
Impending cerebral herniation	Cardiac
Cervical spine	Musculoskeletal
	Soft tissue injury

RTS, Field Triage Criteria developed by the ACS, and the CRAMS (circulation, respiration, abdomen, motor, and speech) scale.[11,29] Although each triage tool is reasonably accurate in predicting mortality, none is more than 70% sensitive or specific in identifying victims with major injuries who survive. Factoring in mechanism of injury and certain anatomic injuries may help improve sensitivity, but the ideal triage tool has not been defined.

Emergency Department Phase

The resuscitation of multiple trauma patients usually involves many personnel and too often takes place amid anxiety and confusion. A well-planned, organized approach to such patients provides optimal management. Specific principles govern the management of trauma (Box 34-2).

Organized Team Approach

Because of the complexity of multiple trauma patients and the need to perform several procedures simultaneously, trauma victims are best managed by a team approach. The team composition varies among institutions but generally consists of several physicians, nurses, and ancillary personnel. The mere presence of such a team, however, does not guarantee a smooth resuscitation.

The emergency physician, as team leader, coordinates and controls the resuscitation and provides the leadership necessary for success. The trauma captain (TC) should be a senior member of the team with previous experience in trauma care. The TC's main responsibilities include assessing the patient, ordering needed procedures and diagnostic studies, managing fluid administration, and monitoring the patient's progress. In addition, as team leader, the emergency physician controls the area by ordering extraneous personnel out of the trauma room and keeping noise and confusion to a minimum. The TC must be constantly aware of the overall picture and must be informed of any changes in vital signs and the status of fluid resuscitation, including central venous pressure (CVP) trends and urine output. The TC is responsible for making decisions concerning changes in therapy and the transportation of patients to other locations such as the radiology department and requests subspecialty consultations and coordinates the activities of these consultants. In short, the emergency physician, as TC, has the overall responsibility for patients during their stay in the emergency department and therefore should not be so involved with procedures that the TC loses perspective on the overall care of the patient. Procedures should be delegated to other physician team members, which is their primary role in the resuscitation.

The number of physicians in attendance in a Level II or smaller institution is usually one or two, depending on the time of day. Therefore, the same resuscitation procedure is required but may be accomplished less efficiently because the physician must perform procedures sequentially. Thus, the prioritization of actions by the TC becomes increasingly important. Nurses may also play a more active role in performing procedures in this configuration.

Priorities in Management and Resuscitation

Immediate and potential threats to life must be identified and promptly treated. It makes no sense to treat an open extremity fracture while a tension pneumothorax goes undetected. It is the responsibility of the TC to assess the patient properly and manage injuries on the basis of their immediate threat to survival.

The priorities in the treatment of trauma patients are similar to those in any other life-threatening condition (Box 34-3). Securing the airway, maintaining ventilation, controlling hemorrhage, and treating shock are first priorities because of their crucial importance for survival. Similarly, a patient with impending cerebral herniation requires immediate treatment. The cervical spine must be stabilized until it is radiographically or functionally cleared. The evaluation of neurologic function, the cardiac examination, and the status of the abdomen and musculoskeletal systems are in the second echelon of priorities and should be addressed after the more critical ones.

Assumption of the Most Serious Injury

Given the circumstances, the emergency physician should give consideration to the worst possible injury and act accordingly until the diagnosis is confirmed or excluded. The consequences of an overzealous evaluation are more acceptable than those of a missed injury.

Treatment before Diagnosis

The urgency of the situation in trauma cases often demands treatment based on an initial brief assessment without substantiation by radiographic or laboratory data. For example, a patient with agonal respirations needs immediate active airway management.

Thorough Examination

The presence of one injury is no guarantee that a second or third injury does not exist. Only a thorough examination can ensure that significant injuries are not overlooked. The evaluation of a trauma patient should consist of a brief initial survey of vital organ systems, followed by resuscitative interventions, and a more thorough and detailed examination when time and the patient's stability permit. This approach avoids common errors, such as overlooking paraplegia in a patient with a GSW of the abdomen.

Most missed injuries occur in severely injured patients, especially those taken quickly to the operating room, and in unconscious patients with traumatic brain injuries. Delays in the diagnosis of injuries to the heart, great vessels, and diaphragm frequently arise if not considered initially. Commonly overlooked musculoskeletal injuries involve the thoracolumbar spine, pelvis, hip, and knee.[30-32] Many trauma centers advocate implementing a tertiary survey to detect overlooked injuries when the patient has been stabilized and admitted.[33]

Frequent Reassessment

A patient's status after injury is dynamic. Only through frequent reassessment can an emergency physician detect significant changes in vital signs and overall condition and make appropriate adjustments in management. For a number of reasons, a patient may not be aware of or demonstrate significant injuries on admission. A patient may be intoxicated, hysterical, or distracted by pain or the performance of procedures. Furthermore, some injuries, such as pulmonary contusions and duodenal injuries, may take time to become manifest. In these situations, frequent examinations can help detect early changes in the physical findings and thus lead to prompt corrective actions.

Monitoring

Certain vital functions must be monitored frequently in trauma victims; the exact interval between measurements depends on the patient's condition. Vital signs should be determined on admission and at least every 15 minutes for the first hour. Unstable patients require vital sign determinations every few minutes and continuous pulse oximetry and end-tidal carbon dioxide (CO_2) monitoring when applicable. The vital signs should be reported to the TC and recorded on a flow sheet so that trends can be monitored.

Fluid intake and output should be recorded and the information conveyed to the physician after the delivery of predetermined aliquots. Precise knowledge of the type and amount of fluid the patient has received is needed in determining subsequent fluid orders. A systolic blood pressure of 90 mm Hg after the infusion of 500 mL of crystalloid has a meaning entirely different from the same pressure after administration of 3 L of fluid. In the urgency of a complicated resuscitation, it is easy to lose track of intake and output, sometimes resulting in adverse consequences.

Certain laboratory tests should also be obtained serially. This is particularly true for hemoglobin. Changes in the hemoglobin level can alert the physician to occult as well as ongoing bleeding and the need for a more thorough evaluation or for transfusion. Although the emergency physician need not wait for arterial blood gas (ABG) results before performing intubation, ABG or continuous pulse oximetry can reveal significant deteriorations in pulmonary function that may not be apparent on physical examination. Patients with significant pulmonary contusion, for example, may have initially adequate oxygenation that later deteriorates rapidly.

Advanced monitoring techniques include the placement of CVP monitors, Swan-Ganz catheters, and arterial lines. Although more sophisticated measurements—such as cardiac output, oxygen consumption, oxygen delivery, and left atrial pressure—may individualize management, especially for those with preexisting pulmonary and cardiac disease, this degree of monitoring is rarely needed in the emergency department. Most trauma victims are young, healthy people. Because the CVP is an accurate reflection of left atrial pressure in this population, more elaborate monitoring techniques are usually not necessary. For elderly patients, there may be an advantage to early invasive monitoring. Some of these patients have inadequate tissue perfusion despite maintaining a normal blood pressure.[34] Even in patients who might benefit from Swan-Ganz catheter insertion, the procedure can be time consuming and should be performed after stabilization.

Arterial pressure monitoring is also not usually necessary in the emergency department. An arterial line can be helpful for an accurate blood pressure recording as well as for ABG determinations. However, the time delay in placing such a line is usually not warranted because noninvasive blood pressure monitors are reliable and widely available.

Stabilization

On receiving field notification, the TC should assemble the team in the designated resuscitation area. On the basis of the nature of the trauma and the patient's vital signs, appropriate diagnostic and therapeutic procedures are assigned to team members. Equipment and surgical trays are made ready. The captain presents the case briefly to the group and discusses identified and potential problems.

On arrival of the patient, the paramedics give their reports, which should consist of the circumstances of the injury, pertinent physical findings, treatment given, and current status of the patient. The patient is carefully transferred to the cart from the ambulance stretcher and all clothing is removed. Most often the clothing is cut away to avoid unnecessary movement of the patient. Oxygen administration is continued, an electrocardiograph monitor and pulse oximeter are placed, and IV lines are checked or initiated. Blood is sent for a panel of studies, which varies among centers and generally includes a complete blood count (CBC), electrolytes, blood urea nitrogen (BUN), creatinine, prothrombin time (PT), partial thromboplastin time (PTT), an alcohol level, and a pregnancy test (as appropriate). Blood for typing should be sent for all patients with potentially serious injuries and fully cross-matched blood ordered for those in whom serious hemorrhage is apparent. For the severely injured, baseline fibrinogen, lactic acid, and, in some centers, the base deficit are obtained to monitor the adequacy of the resuscitation.[35,36]

After the patient is transferred to the gurney and while head and neck immobilization is maintained, the TC conducts a prioritized examination while a nurse measures the vital signs. If it is apparent that therapeutic measures are needed immediately, the TC orders these to be performed before completing the initial survey.

The initial evaluation consists of a rapid survey of the high-priority systems. During this evaluation and after its completion, initial resuscitative measures are ordered by the TC and carried out by team members.

Airway and Breathing

The assessment and management of airway and ventilatory adequacy are considered simultaneously. Airway obstruction is a clear indication for immediate intervention. Obstruction can result from blood, emesis, and teeth; from posterior retraction of the tongue in an unconscious patient; and from direct neck or facial trauma. The first two conditions can be readily managed by digital removal of debris, suction, and insertion of an oral or nasopharyngeal airway. Obstruction caused by neck or facial trauma, however, can be a difficult problem; appropriate management requires considerable judgment and technical skill. Such an obstruction may result from displaced anatomic structures, mucosal edema, compression by a hematoma, or transection of the trachea, and it may progress rapidly. Although the patient may be conscious on arrival, airway control—utilizing rapid sequence intubation techniques or surgical intervention as necessary—is often the safest strategy. Other indications for active airway management are airway protection in the obtunded patient and those with significant head injuries.[37]

Airway management is also required to correct inadequate ventilation or oxygenation, and the need for interventions for these indications is sometimes more subtle. The assessment includes determining the adequacy of the ventilatory effort and the presence of chest injuries that may compromise oxygenation. The former can be readily accomplished by observing the rate and quality of respirations. The latter requires careful inspection, palpation, and auscultation of the chest. Signs of compromise discernible on inspection include labored or accelerated respirations, penetrating wounds, flail segments, distended neck veins, and tracheal deviation. Agitation and restlessness are subtle signs of inadequate oxygenation. The information obtained from this assessment is then placed in the context of the overall presentation of the patient, which includes skin perfusion, level of consciousness, and the nature of other apparent injuries. These data are considered when determining the need for emergent airway management.

When the decision is made to intubate the patient, the emergency physician chooses the route that meets the needs of the patient. The options for immediate intubation are oral, nasal, and surgical. Other methods including fiberoptic intubation can be considered only if the necessary equipment and personnel are present and time permits. Factors affecting this choice include the status of the cervical spine, the level of consciousness, the presence of facial injuries or anterior neck trauma, and the urgency of the need for airway management. The cervical spine is of little concern in penetrating trauma other than high-velocity GSWs of the neck. In blunt trauma, however, a cervical spine injury is assumed until proved absent. For patients who need immediate intubation, head-stabilized oral intubation with rapid sequence induction is recommended before obtaining cervical spine radiographs. Retrospective and limited prospective data document no neurologic deficits after head-stabilized oral intubation in the presence of unstable cervical fractures.[38,39] If this route is unsuccessful or contraindicated, the emergency physician must choose between nasotracheal intubation, a surgical airway, or alternative airway techniques such as placement of a laryngeal airway mask device.

Nasotracheal intubation was once deemed useful in the trauma patient because it does not require manipulation of the head or neck. However, nasotracheal intubation is now rarely undertaken as it is difficult to perform in the uncooperative patient, frequently requires multiple attempts, is associated with abrupt rises in intracranial pressure (ICP), and has a higher complication rate than rapid sequence induction with oral intubation.[40] Apnea and midface and severe basilar skull fractures are contraindications to its use. The latter can be associated with cribriform plate disruption, which may allow the passage of any nasally placed tube (including nasogastric tubes) into the cranial cavity.[41]

Surgical airways are rarely required but are indicated when oral and nasal intubation approaches have failed or are contraindicated. Surgical options include cricothyrotomy, percutaneous transtracheal ventilation (PTV), and tracheostomy. PTV has the advantages of speed and simplicity but has the disadvantage of requiring special equipment.[42,43]

Cricothyrotomy has proven efficacy and is easier to perform than tracheostomy.[44] Therefore, it is the emergent surgical option of choice. Tracheostomy may be necessary with complete trachea transection, in which case cricothyrotomy may be impossible or useless.[45]

Ventilatory problems related to a pneumothorax or hemopneumothorax may require a thoracostomy tube. A chest radiograph may be obtained before tube placement if the patient's condition permits. However, any signs of cardiopulmonary compromise or a tension pneumothorax (tracheal deviation, distended neck veins, hypotension, or deteriorating oxygenation) require immediate treatment before a chest radiograph is obtained.

Shock and External Hemorrhage

External hemorrhage should be controlled by direct manual pressure. Blind clamping within a wound in the hope of occluding a bleeding vessel should not be performed, but clamping bleeding vessels under direct visualization is acceptable and effective. The careful use of a tourniquet to stop hemorrhage is reserved for cases of amputation or when other measures have been ineffective.

Shock requires prompt diagnostic and therapeutic intervention. Treatment is directed at improving perfusion by volume resuscitation and the control of any ongoing hemorrhage. Of these, the first priority is volume resuscitation unless massive external hemorrhage is apparent. Insertion of short, large-bore (14-gauge), over-the-needle catheters is preferred. There is no formula that indicates the correct number of lines to insert in a given trauma situation. Individualization on the basis of vital signs, the mechanism of injury, and the likelihood of continued bleeding is indicated. As a rule, it is better to have too many rather than too few lines.

Central Venous Pressure. Placement of a CVP line should be considered under specific circumstances. If peripheral access is limited or unavailable, a CVP line using an 8-Fr introducer should be placed using the Seldinger technique. Although subject to pulmonary and vascular complications, this is a reasonable alternative that permits rapid fluid infusion and CVP monitoring. CVP line placement is also indicated in penetrating thoracoabdominal trauma when pericardial tamponade is a concern, although bedside emergency cardiac ultrasonography (US) may provide a more expedient diagnosis. CVP monitoring may also be helpful in elderly patients or those with heart disease in an attempt to titrate fluid administration more carefully. Unfortunately, initial CVP readings may not be helpful in these patients unless they are low or normal because preexisting cardiac disease may prevent accurate correlation with intravascular volume.

Vascular Access. Obtaining peripheral IV access may be impossible in certain situations. Patients in profound shock often require venous cutdowns or large-bore central line placement. The choice of procedure somewhat depends on the operator's familiarity with the techniques. Both routes can provide large volumes of fluid in short periods of time, especially when administered with a pressure bag. There are many acceptable sites for cutdowns, but the most commonly chosen are the brachial and the proximal and distal saphenous veins. The distal saphenous vein offers the advantages of large size, superficial depth, and constancy of location[46]; however, upper extremity lines are preferred in cases in which intra-abdominal hemorrhage may be present.

Choice of Resuscitation Fluid. Fluid options for resuscitation include crystalloid, colloid, and blood. Immediate transfusion is rarely needed, but when it is, type O un-crossmatched blood should be given.[47] To conserve supplies of O-negative blood, O-positive blood may be safely given to males as well as females beyond the childbearing years. In most instances, shock is managed initially with a crystalloid solution, either normal saline or lactated Ringer's solution. Shed blood should be replaced with two to three times its volume in crystalloid. Realistically, however, the amount of blood lost is never precisely known, so fluids are run at a wide-open rate and titrated to a response in vital signs and overall condition. Although some prefer colloid to crystalloid, the former offers no advantage.[48] The greatest advantage of crystalloid over colloid is its low cost.

Hypertonic saline/dextran (HSD) is under investigation as a resuscitative agent especially in the prehospital setting. It is commonly given as 7.5% NaCl in 6% dextran. In animal studies, HSD improves cardiac output, promotes redistribution of extravascular fluid into the vascular compartment, and decreases ICP. In controlled clinical trials involving trauma patients, however, there is no difference in survival among patients receiving HSD in the field and those receiving the same volume of normal saline. A small subset of patients receiving HSD and requiring surgery had improved survival rates and fewer complications.[49]

Transfusion. When resuscitation is under way, the clinician is often faced with the question of when and whether to initiate blood transfusion. As a guide, if the patient remains hemodynamically unstable after 2 to 3 L or 40 to 50 mL/kg of crystalloid, blood should be started. Fully crossmatched blood is preferable, but it may take 30 to 45 minutes to obtain. Type-specific blood is a safe alternative and is usually ready in 5 to 15 minutes.

Occasionally, a patient requires massive transfusion in the emergency department, which creates several potential problems. A coagulopathy may develop related to ongoing bleeding and consumption, dilution of platelets and clotting factors, and the adverse effects of hypothermia. No specific formula is recommended for the periodic administration of fresh frozen plasma (FFP), cryoprecipitate, or platelets in the course of massive transfusion. Some clinicians advocate administration of 2 units of FFP after every 5 to 6 units of blood, which represents approximately one half the circulating blood volume of a 70-kg adult. Two to 3 units of FFP should raise the fibrinogen level to a target of 80 to 100 mg/dL.[50] Others use the PT, PTT, platelet count, and fibrinogen levels as guidelines.[51] A platelet count of less than $100,000/mm^3$ in the presence of bleeding is usually considered an indication for platelet transfusion. Ten units of platelets should increase the platelet count by 50,000 to $100,000/mm^3$.[51]

The transfusion of banked blood stored at 4° C often worsens hypothermia in trauma patients. One unit of packed red blood cells can reduce the core temperature by 0.25° C. Hypothermia exacerbates acidosis, increases blood viscosity, decreases flow in the microcirculation, and reduces platelet aggregation.[52] These factors predispose the patient to development of a coagulopathy and disseminated intravascular coagulation. Every effort should be made to prevent hypothermia, including use of warm blankets, heat lamps, and blood warmers for all transfused blood or saline.

Autotransfusion, a technique used regularly in many trauma centers, can be helpful in overcoming some of the problems associated with transfusion. Although the technology of autotransfusion is still evolving, its application in trauma cases is limited primarily to chest trauma. The simpler, less expensive apparatuses are best suited to emergency department use.

Source of Hemorrhage. After initiating treatment for shock, a thorough search for the source of shock is conducted. Although significant hemorrhage can occur with long-bone fractures, this bleeding is usually limited. Ongoing blood loss that creates instability is usually located in one of three body cavities: the chest, the abdomen, or the retroperitoneum. In the infant, intracranial bleeding can also produce shock. These cavities should be evaluated radiographically or invasively to determine the site of bleeding.

Emergency Thoracotomy. In the past, all victims of trauma-induced cardiac arrest, except those with isolated head injuries, underwent emergency department thoracotomy. Several studies have now documented the need for a selective approach in applying this procedure. It is clear that blunt trauma victims with no signs of life before arrival at the hospital have no chance for survival and should not undergo thoracotomy. Blunt trauma victims who experience arrest in the emergency department and victims of penetrating trauma with no signs of life at the scene also have a dismal prognosis.[53-55] Patients with penetrating trauma who experience arrest during transport or in the emergency department have the best prognosis and are most likely to benefit from emergency thoracotomy. In a review of 4620 published emergency department thoracotomies, survival was 16.8% for stab wounds, 4.3% for GSWs, and 1.4% for blunt trauma.[55] Overall, patients with pericardial tamponade or isolated injury to the heart or lungs have the highest survival rates after thoracotomy.

When the chest is open, a number of therapeutic measures can be undertaken, depending on the injuries present. After identifying the phrenic nerve, tamponade should be relieved by pericardotomy. Cardiac injuries are sutured or hemorrhage controlled with digital pressure or placement of a Foley catheter balloon. Compressing or cross-clamping the pulmonary hilum can control major pulmonary bleeding. The descending aorta is compressed or cross-clamped to maximize coronary and cerebral perfusion. The aorta should remain clamped until hemorrhage has been controlled and volume replaced. Open cardiac massage can also be instituted at this point.

Impending Herniation

Impending herniation is a neurosurgical emergency that requires immediate intervention to ensure survival of the patient. Ideally, the patient should be intubated using a rapid sequence technique, taking care to minimize any elevation in ICP.[56] Controlled hyperventilation is the fastest way to manage a precipitously high ICP, but its prophylactic use in traumatic brain injuries is not currently recommended.[57-59] Mannitol 0.5 to 1.0 g/kg, furosemide 0.5 mg/kg, or both can be considered depending on the patient's hemodynamic status.[60] Hypertonic normal saline is under investigation as another potential means of intervening during herniation.

An immediate head computed tomography (CT) scan should be arranged. The neurosurgeon, if not already in attendance, should be consulted. Trephination in the emergency department is rarely done, particularly if a CT scan has not been obtained.

Cervical Spine

Patients with real or potential cervical spine injuries must be protected from the outset. In cases of penetrating trauma remote from the neck, there is little concern about the status of the cervical spine. Patients with penetrating neck trauma should be assessed by neurologic examination. If a neurologic deficit is not immediately obvious, it is unlikely to develop because the spine is not rendered unstable by such injuries.[61]

In cases of blunt trauma, however, a cervical spine injury is always presumed present until it can be excluded. If the patient is alert, the criteria validated in the National Emergency X-Radiography Utilization Study (NEXUS), absence of midline neck tenderness, lack of focal neurologic signs, and a lack of competitive pain from other injuries, clinically exclude a spinal injury.[62] If the patient's mental status is abnormal or if a distracting injury exists, spinal injury cannot be ruled out clinically. If the mechanism of injury is trivial, it is safe to use a semirigid collar and await the patient's cooperation rather than spend fruitless hours trying to clear the cervical spine in an uncooperative or intoxicated patient.

Prehospital personnel are aware of these principles and treat patients accordingly. Proper immobilization, when indicated, must be maintained from the moment when the patient enters the emergency department. Although no technique is perfect, an acceptable approach combines a semirigid collar with tape and towel-roll immobilization. This approach is effective in the unconscious or cooperative patient but is inadequate for the combative, unruly patient. These patients require a team member to stabilize the head and neck manually. The use of chemical restraint and sedation, and possibly rapid sequence intubation, may be necessary in the more difficult cases to prevent injury or deterioration during diagnostic procedures, such as a CT scan.

As soon as feasible, a portable cross-table lateral radiograph of the cervical spine should be obtained. To ensure that the film is adequate, two persons are needed to position the patient: one maintains head immobilization without traction while the other grasps the patient's hands and pulls them caudally. Care should be taken to prevent a distraction injury. This is best accomplished by placing the patient's feet against the chest of the person pulling the arms. With this technique, the shoulders are pulled clear of the lower cervical vertebrae. If the resulting film is still inadequate, a "swimmer's view" with one arm extended above the head can be attempted. Even when this procedure is followed, obtaining adequate films can be a frustrating, time-consuming experience requiring multiple attempts. As a result, some trauma centers obtain only a lateral C-spine radiograph followed by a helical CT scan of the entire C spine if the patient needs a head CT.[63] This approach has yet to be verified.

It is worth emphasizing that a cervical spine film is not adequate unless all seven cervical vertebrae and the top of the first thoracic vertebra are visualized. If the lateral film is normal, one can assume with a high degree of confidence that there is no serious abnormality in the spine. Nevertheless, fractures not seen on the lateral view are sometimes diagnosed on anteroposterior or odontoid views; therefore, neck immobilization should be maintained until the cervical spine series is completed.

When the cervical spine is radiographically cleared, it should be clinically evaluated. Patients with significant neck pain may have a ligamentous injury or a radiographically inapparent one. These patients may need additional evaluation with a cervical CT scan or magnetic resonance imaging.[64,65] Until these additional studies can be obtained, the head and neck should remain immobilized and all appropriate precautions taken. Patients with an altered mental status, including those who are persistently obtunded, cannot be cleared until their mental function normalizes or additional studies are performed.

CLINICAL FEATURES

Perspective

On completion of the initial portion of the examination, the patient's overall status is reevaluated. Current vital signs are interpreted, taking into account the treatment already instituted, and further orders are given accordingly. The five high-priority areas are reassessed first, and any additional therapeutic or diagnostic measures deemed necessary are undertaken. A thorough but brief head-to-toe examination is then conducted, including a neurologic evaluation and an examination of the heart, abdomen, musculoskeletal system, and any soft tissue injury.

Neurologic Evaluation

After reassessing level of consciousness and pupillary responses, the head and face are carefully inspected and palpated to detect any evidence of injury that may alert the emergency physician to the possibility of an intracranial injury. Cranial nerves are tested, and the tympanic membranes are inspected. Next, spinal cord and peripheral nerve function are evaluated. The assessment of spinal cord function in an alert patient is straightforward. The ability to move all extremities and sense pain indicates an intact cord. However, subtle injuries, such as a central cord syndrome (sensory and motor loss, arms greater than legs), can be missed if a rectal examination and a careful sensory and motor examination are not performed. Rectal tone must be evaluated even in alert patients because its absence may be the only indication of a spinal cord injury. The spine should be palpated for bone defor-

mities and tenderness by reaching under or log-rolling the patient to each side. If there is any suspicion of injury, radiographic evaluation should be obtained before the patient is moved.

Spinal cord injury is more difficult to diagnose in patients with altered mental status. Injuries can easily be missed if they are not specifically sought. Important findings include priapism, diaphragmatic breathing, loss of rectal tone, and absence of deep tendon and cremasteric reflexes. If a spinal cord injury is diagnosed, high-dose methylprednisolone is recommended. If initiated within the first 8 hours after injury, administration of a large bolus (30 mg/kg) followed by a continuous infusion (5.4 mg/kg/hr) for 24 to 48 hours may result in improved neurologic recovery.[66] A review of the existing data, however, did not support the original conclusion of the studies upon which the recommendations were made.[67] Currently, revised guidelines have not been issued.

Peripheral nerve injuries may cause significant long-term morbidity but are not threats to the patient's survival and do not require immediate attention in the emergency department. Commonly overlooked nerve injuries are those associated with lacerations and sacral and long-bone fractures.

Thoracic Examination

The entire thorax should be reexamined, including the adequacy and rate of respirations. Seatbelt or other contusions should be inspected and the ribs and sternum palpated for bone crepitus, flail segments, or subcutaneous emphysema. A repeated chest radiograph should be obtained to confirm placement of the endotracheal or thoracostomy tubes.

Abdominal Examination

Death does not occur as rapidly from an intra-abdominal injury as from an occluded airway or ineffective ventilation. However, the abdomen is an important site of possible life-threatening hemorrhage and significant injuries. Its examination is an important part of the secondary trauma survey.

The key to the proper emergency department management of an intra-abdominal injury is rapid diagnosis and stabilization of vital signs. In the alert patient, complaints of abdominal pain or findings of tenderness or ecchymosis raise the possibility of intra-abdominal injury. In a patient with an altered mental status from any cause or in those with severe distracting injuries, an objective means of injury detection is essential. This is especially important because many solid organ injuries are now managed conservatively.[68,69]

Management of penetrating abdominal trauma differs from that of blunt injury (Figure 34-2). All GSWs that penetrate the peritoneal cavity require laparotomy because of the high incidence of significant intra-abdominal injury. With stab wounds, laparotomy is more selective. In stable patients, local wound exploration with diagnostic peritoneal lavage (DPL), bedside emergency department US, or CT scan for patients with

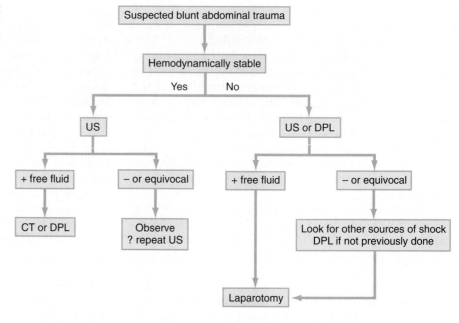

Figure 34-2. Algorithm for suspected blunt abdominal trauma. CT, computed tomography; DPL, diagnostic peritoneal lavage; US, ultrasonography.

fascial penetration has enabled more accurate performance of laparotomy and reduced the time needed for observation. Few physicians perform laparotomy on all penetrating wounds, most use imaging adjuncts and local wound exploration, and still others rely on serial examinations to determine the need for laparotomy. Laparoscopy has also been used in a limited number of stable patients with penetrating abdominal injuries.[70]

The insertion of a nasogastric tube and urinary bladder catheter should be routine in the management of patients with multiple trauma. The nasogastric tube permits the detection of gastric bleeding and decompression of the stomach. This latter function is important in preventing vomiting and aspiration and allows the safe performance of peritoneal lavage. Likewise, the Foley catheter should be placed after rectal and genital examinations have been performed. It is useful for detecting hematuria and for monitoring urine output. The Foley catheter must be placed before DPL to decompress the bladder.

The presence of hematuria may indicate renal injury. However, the indications for performing an intravenous pyelogram in the presence of hematuria are controversial. After blunt trauma, patients who have gross hematuria or microscopic hematuria with shock require study, as do those with penetrating trauma in proximity to the kidney.[71,72] In many instances, an abdominal CT scan or a helical CT scan with an IV contrast agent is useful for the evaluation of renal function and the presence of injuries not requiring surgical intervention.[71,72]

Cardiac Examination

The secondary cardiac effects of shock and hypoxia include myocardial depression and dysrhythmias. Penetrating injuries can result in tamponade or disruption of the cardiac septum or one of the valves. The detec-

tion of a murmur can indicate an incompetent valve or a septal defect, whereas hypotension, elevated jugular venous pressure, and muffled heart sounds are signs of tamponade. Blunt trauma can cause cardiac rupture and tamponade, but it is more likely to cause myocardial contusion or aortic transection. The former is difficult to discern by examination. The latter may be suspected by unequal pulses in the upper extremities, the presence of an aortic insufficiency murmur, or neurologic deficits.

An electrocardiogram should be obtained in all victims with serious torso injury. Other than electrical alternans and the low voltage that are occasionally seen in cases of pericardial effusion, no specific electrocardiographic findings are associated with traumatic cardiac tamponade. Cardiac contusion can produce virtually any dysrhythmia or bundle branch block and may cause T wave inversions or ST segment elevation in the area of injury.[73]

Musculoskeletal Examination

One goal of the musculoskeletal examination is to identify fractures by seeking any deformity, bone movement, crepitus, swelling, or area of tenderness. A second purpose is to check peripheral pulses and neurologic function. This examination assumes particular importance if lacerations, fractures, or dislocations are present. All patients need to be log-rolled to inspect the back, vertebrae, and buttocks.

Injuries to the musculoskeletal system are of low priority and do not generally require immediate, definitive management. Open fractures and knee and hip dislocations are exceptions that require immediate reduction because they can be associated with serious complications. Prophylactic antibiotics are recommended for open fractures.

Extremity and spinal injuries are among the most commonly overlooked injuries in multiple trauma patients. The emergency physician should ensure that these areas are appropriately evaluated even if this occurs after treatment of higher priority areas. Patients who have a significant mechanism of injury require radiographs of the thoracic and lumbosacral spine.[52]

Soft Tissue Examination

Soft tissue injuries hold the lowest priority in the multiple trauma patient. Except for the occasional injury with severe hemorrhage, such as a large scalp laceration, soft tissue injuries are not considered an immediate threat to survival. Treatment consists of inspecting wounds, clearing gross decontamination, and applying dressings. Tetanus immunization status should be verified.

DISPOSITION

The emergency department management of trauma victims, although critical, is just the beginning of their care. Regardless of the effectiveness of this management, the ultimate outcome for trauma victims is not optimal without the commitment of the hospital administration, nursing staff, surgical staff, and specialty consultants.

Surgeons can hardly be considered consultants in trauma care because they assume responsibility for the patient after he or she leaves the emergency department. Ideally, they should be present in the emergency department to interpret data and observe the evolution of the patient's course. Cooperation between emergency medicine and surgery services contributes to a smoothly run, effective resuscitation and an ideal working relationship. When surgical backup is not immediately available, the emergency physician must handle all aspects of the resuscitation, including invasive procedures. At times, this may require transfer of the patient to a higher level trauma center.

Consultants in surgical subspecialties—including neurosurgeons, otolaryngologists, urologists, ophthalmologists, plastic surgeons, and orthopedists—are obtained as needed. Consultants should not be called prematurely; too many physicians giving orders may detract from the efficient resuscitation of the patient. When the patient is stabilized, appropriate subspecialists can be consulted before final disposition. Regardless of the number of consultants, the emergency physician still has primary responsibility for the patient while in the department. Consultants must be carefully coordinated, and an ultimate plan for the patient's care should be developed with the surgeon and consultants.

Disposition is dictated by a number of factors, including the patient's condition, the nature of the injury, and the availability of surgeons, subspecialists, and anesthesiologists. Possible dispositions include transfer to the operating room, admission to the surgical service, limited observation in the emergency department, or transfer to another hospital. The level of care and monitoring established in the emergency department should be maintained throughout a transfer. All equipment and medications needed for resuscitation and maintenance of vital functions should be available during the transfer, as should qualified personnel to oversee the patient's care.

In cases of interhospital transfers, all arrangements should be carefully coordinated between the two institutions by the physicians. Stabilizing measures are begun before the patient's transfer, but decompensation in transit should be anticipated. Qualified personnel and necessary resuscitative equipment must accompany the patient. The only acceptable reason for transferring a patient with life-threatening trauma is lack of resources or personnel to care for the patient's particular injuries.

Many trauma victims who do not require immediate surgical intervention are admitted for intensive care or observation. Admission to the surgical service allows serial neurologic and abdominal examinations, cardiac monitoring, and further subspecialty consultations. In selected patients with limited injuries, shorter observation periods in the emergency department can be used. An isolated stab wound to the chest without apparent pneumothorax or hemothorax is an example of such a limited injury. Management may include observation for 3 to 8 hours followed by a repeated upright, expiratory chest radiograph before discharge.[74,75]

Third-party payers and utilization review panels at many hospitals are emphasizing outpatient management and reduced hospital length of stays. Partly in response to these pressures, an increasing number of trauma patients are being evaluated and discharged from the emergency department.[76] This approach should be viewed with caution. Many injuries, including duodenal hematomas, small bowel perforations, and intracerebral contusions, may have delayed presentations. By discharging a patient, one key diagnostic tool, the serial examination, is eliminated. This places a greater burden of proof on the interpretation of CT scans, US, and radiographs, none of which is 100% accurate. The decision to discharge a patient should be made after careful deliberation.

DIAGNOSTIC STRATEGIES

Radiology

Radiology plays an integral role in the evaluation of trauma victims. Unfortunately, obtaining appropriate studies can be time consuming, and the additional time required can be detrimental to the patient. In the ideal situation, permanent and versatile radiographic equipment is mounted in the trauma resuscitation room. Many centers, however, must rely on the portable radiograph machine for first-line studies. Fortunately, most films can be obtained with this device; only the more sophisticated studies must be performed in the radiology suite.

For the *critically injured* patient, chest and antero-posterior pelvis radiographs are obtained first to evaluate possible areas of life-threatening injury and to determine whether there is a possible source of hemorrhage either into the chest or from a pelvic fracture. The cervical spine radiograph can be delayed while maintaining immobilization.

In routine blunt trauma patients, radiographs of the cervical spine, chest, and pelvis are performed. Additional specific studies, such as extremity and thoracolumbar spine films, may be obtained as the individual case dictates. The first three areas, however, are essential for the moderately injured patient because they identify major pathologic conditions that dictate further resuscitative measures. The cervical spine film should be obtained early in the patient's course because the presence or absence of a fracture may affect subsequent procedures. According to the NEXUS rule, cervical spine radiographs may be omitted if the patient has no posterior midline tenderness or focal neurologic deficits, normal alertness, no intoxication, and no distracting, painful injury.[62] The Canadian C-spine rule stratifies patients into high and low risk for injury using slightly different criteria.[77] On the other end of the spectrum, concerns about ligamentous injuries and disk herniation have led some trauma centers to utilize the helical CT scan as the primary imaging modality. This approach is more expensive and exposes the thyroid to 14 times as much radiation as the standard three-view cervical spine series.[78] Further studies to clinically stratify patients at high risk for cervical injuries are ongoing.[79] The chest radiograph is ideally obtained in the radiology suite with the radiograph tube at a distance of 72 inches with the patient in an upright position. This technique minimizes the artifactual widening of the mediastinum commonly seen in portable supine films. Usually, however, the patient is not stable, the cervical spine has not been cleared for possible injury, or procedures are still being performed when it is desirable to obtain the chest radiograph. Therefore, the less than optimal supine film is often the only one available in the initial evaluation. A more definitive evaluation of the mediastinum can be performed subsequently if necessary.

The pelvis is the third area that should be routinely studied in moderately and severely injured blunt trauma cases. Pelvic fractures may not be clinically apparent, yet massive hemorrhage can result from such fractures. The pelvic film may be omitted if the patient denies pain and is awake, unintoxicated, without head injury, able to move the hips without pain, and free of other distracting injuries.[80,81] However, clinical indicators of patients at low risk for pelvic fractures have yet to be validated. In the stable patient who is undergoing a CT scan of the abdomen and pelvis, bone windows can be used to visualize the pelvis.

At present, three studies are used to evaluate blunt abdominal trauma: DPL, CT scanning, and US. DPL is a highly reliable means of detecting significant intra-abdominal injury. Its high sensitivity (98%) is offset by lack of specificity; that is, there is a 5% to 16% non-therapeutic laparotomy rate based on positive DPL

results.[82] Other drawbacks of DPL are that it is invasive, sometimes fraught with technical difficulties, and has occasional complications. A nasogastric tube and Foley catheter must be placed before it is safely performed. Nonetheless, it is widely available, can be performed quickly, and is relatively inexpensive. It is used predominantly for unstable patients with blunt trauma in whom bedside US cannot be obtained or is equivocal and for selected patients with penetrating trauma.

By comparison, CT scanning has the advantages of being noninvasive and capable of identifying the location and extent of solid visceral injury. Its drawbacks include expense, remoteness of the needed equipment from the resuscitation area, length of time to complete the study, and need for considerable expertise in interpreting the scans.[83]

Although proponents of both studies can argue superiority, both are reasonably reliable and both have shortcomings. However, bedside US or DPL is preferred when the patient is unstable because a move to a CT scanning suite would be ill advised under such circumstances. The exact definition of instability, however, still allows considerable disagreement and room for discussion concerning which study is indicated.

In the assessment of the abdomen, the utility of oral contrast material in abdominal CT scans is being reevaluated. Proponents argue that oral contrast material is safe and aids in the delineation of small bowel and pancreatic injuries.[84] Opponents contend that oral contrast material fails to reach the small bowel in a reasonable time, that its administration often delays the CT scan, that it induces vomiting or aspiration in 10% to 23% of patients, and that it does not increase the visualization of solid visceral injury.[85,86]

US has gained credibility and support as a diagnostic screening test for blunt abdominal trauma. Like DPL, it can be rapidly applied at the bedside. Like CT, US is less sensitive for bowel, mesentery, diaphragm, and pancreatic injuries. US is less expensive than CT and does not involve exposure to radiation or contrast agents. The chief role of US is in the detection of hemoperitoneum. Earlier studies reported sensitivities from 75% to 90% compared with CT for the presence of free intraperitoneal fluid.[87,88] The hepatorenal recess (Morison's pouch), splenorenal area, and rectovesicular recess (pouch of Douglas) are the areas most likely to demonstrate free intraperitoneal fluid (Figure 34-3).[88] Increasingly, the pericardium and pleural spaces are included in the initial scan. False-negative scans commonly involve bowel perforations or liver or spleen lacerations without free fluid.[87,89]

Can a patient with a negative US scan be safely discharged, or is a period of observation and repeated US study indicated? The accuracy and negative predictive value of US still warrant further investigation. Contemporary studies have emphasized the use of focused assessment with sonography for trauma (FAST) performed by surgeons or emergency physicians.[87,88] The amount of training and experience with US vary widely in these studies, and credentials in the use of US

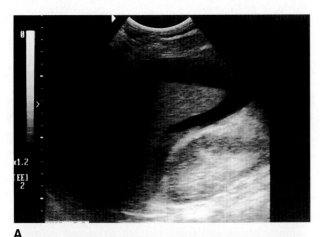

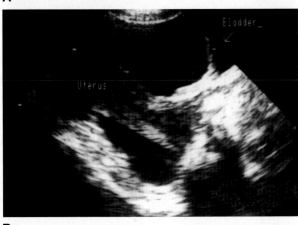

Figure 34-3. A, Intraperitoneal hemorrhage in the hepatorenal recess extends superiorly around the liver. **B,** Blunt abdominal trauma patient with blood in the retrovesicular and rectouterine recesses. (**B,** Courtesy of V. Tayal, MD.)

position of mediator of any conflicts arising between the neurosurgeons and trauma surgeons. Emergency physicians therefore need to remain current in the ongoing research on trauma resuscitations.

In the hemodynamically unstable patient with a depressed level of consciousness, when the need for urgent laparotomy is established, the operation should not be delayed in order to obtain a cranial CT scan unless there are focal neurologic findings.[94-96] A head CT scan may take 20 to 30 minutes, including mobilization and transportation of the patient, and an abdominal CT scan may take longer.[94] Less consensus exists about patients who respond to fluid resuscitation but nonetheless have indications from other diagnostic modalities for celiotomy. Some centers proceed with the cranial CT scan, whereas others maintain that abdominal injuries should still take precedence.[94-96] Alternatively, neurosurgeons at some trauma centers place a ventriculostomy catheter while the patient is undergoing a laparotomy. This approach allows the management of ICP until the patient is stabilized for transport to the CT scanner.[95]

The diagnostic evaluation of an abnormal mediastinum on a chest radiograph can also be problematic. For the hemodynamically unstable patient, DPL or US can be rapidly performed to exclude intra-abdominal injury. If the lavage is grossly bloody, celiotomy followed by arch aortography is performed. Conversely, in stable patients, a high-resolution helical CT scan or aortography followed by laparotomy is the recommended sequence.[97] A routine chest CT scan is not considered the definitive diagnostic procedure in suspected aortic injury.[97] However, the helical CT scan with an IV contrast agent appears to have sufficient specificity to exclude aortic injury in the stable patient with an equivocal chest radiograph.[98,99] Aortography or digital subtraction aortography remains the definitive test should abnormalities of the thoracic aorta or great vessels be found on helical CT.[98]

Transesophageal echocardiography (TEE) is being used more frequently in the evaluation of suspected aortic injury, cardiac contusion, or pericardial tamponade. TEE requires a cooperative patient with a protected airway and a normal or immobilized cervical spine but does not require transport of the patient from the resuscitation area.[100] TEE can be accomplished in less than half the time required for aortography, a distinct advantage in the unstable patient.[100,101] Although the sensitivity of TEE is improving, particularly with multiplanar scanners, it will not replace aortography as the diagnostic standard until more data are available.[100,101] Furthermore, at present, TEE is not widely available, nor are the personnel to perform the study.

Specialized radiographic studies such as CT scans, angiography, and intravenous pyelography are usually possible only in the radiology department. Patients sent to the radiology suite must be carefully monitored, just as they are in the emergency department. They should be accompanied by appropriate personnel, and full attention should be given to their vital signs as well as fluid intake and output.

remain a topic of debate.[90] How best to incorporate a FAST study into the management of abdominal trauma is a subject of ongoing clinical trials. Because US is less accurate than CT for the delineation of solid organ injuries, trials have focused on its use in the context of an algorithm.[91-93] Hemodynamically unstable patients can be rapidly assessed with US or DPL and taken directly for laparotomy. Stable patients with free intraperitoneal fluid on US are further evaluated by CT or DPL.[91-93] A CT scan under this circumstance can diagnose solid visceral injuries and allows for the option of nonoperative management.[93] For any given patient, the emergency physician must be aware of the strengths and limitations of the diagnostic modalities employed and proceed in a logical fashion.

Additional radiographic studies are usually obtained when the patient is stabilized. If the patient needs immediate surgery, most of these films may be obtained postoperatively. The sequence of diagnostic tests in multiply injured patients requires sound judgment by the emergency physician and surgeons. Common dilemmas arise in the hypotensive patient with a possible closed head injury or a widened mediastinum, and the emergency physician may be forced into the

KEY CONCEPTS

- The role of the prehospital care team in cases of trauma includes prevention of additional injury, rapid transportation to the hospital, advance notification to the hospital, initiation of treatment, and triage.
- Trauma victims are best managed by a team approach.
- Only a thorough examination can ensure that significant injuries are not overlooked.
- The priorities in the treatment of trauma patients include securing the airway, maintaining ventilation, controlling hemorrhage, and treating shock.
- For the *critically injured* patient, chest and anteroposterior pelvic radiographs are obtained first to evaluate possible areas of life-threatening injury and to determine whether there is a possible source of hemorrhage either into the chest or from a pelvic fracture.
- In the hemodynamically unstable patient with a depressed level of consciousness, once the need for urgent laparotomy is established, the operation should not be delayed in order to obtain a cranial CT scan unless there are focal neurologic findings.
- Patients sent to the radiology suite must be monitored just as in the emergency department.

REFERENCES

1. Kivioja AH, Myllynenn PJ, Rokkanen PU: Is the treatment of the most severe multiply injured patients worth the effort? *J Trauma* 30:480, 1990.
2. Van der Sluis CK, ten Duis HJ, Geertzen JH: Multiple injuries: An overview of the outcome. *J Trauma* 38:681, 1995.
3. *2002 Fatality Analysis Reporting System (FARS).* National Highway Transportation and Safety Administration, 2003.
4. Kochanek KD, Smith BL: Deaths: Preliminary data from 2002, National Center for Health Statistics. *Natl Vital Stat Rep* 52(13), 2004.
5. Cook PJ, et al: The medical costs of gunshot injuries in the United States. *JAMA* 282:447, 1999.
6. Gotsch KE, et al: Surveillance for fatal and nonfatal firearm-related injuries: United States 1993-1998. *MMWR Surveill Summ* 50(SS-2):1, 2001.
7. Nathens AB, et al: The effect of organized systems of trauma care on motor vehicle crash mortality. *JAMA* 283:1990, 2000.
8. Cayten CG, Quervalu I, Agarwal N: Fatality analysis reporting system demonstrates association between trauma system initiatives and decreasing death rates. *J Trauma* 46:751, 1999.
9. Bazzoli GJ, MacKenzie EJ: Trauma centers in the United States: Identification and examination of key characteristics. *J Trauma* 38:103, 1995.
10. Bass RR, Gainer PS, Carlini AR: Update on trauma system development in the United States. *J Trauma* 47:S15, 1999.
11. Champion HR, et al: A revision of the trauma score. *J Trauma* 29:623, 1989.
12. American Association for Automotive Medicine: *The Abbreviated Injury Scale (AIS), 1990 Revision.* Des Plaines, Ill, The Association, 1990.
13. Hoff WS, et al: Impact of minimal injuries on a level I trauma center. *J Trauma* 33:408, 1992.
14. Tinkoff GH, O'Connor RE, Falda GJ: Impact of a two-tiered trauma response in the emergency department: Promoting efficient resource utilization. *J Trauma* 41:735, 1996.
15. Dailey JT, Teter H, Cowley RA: Trauma center closures: A national assessment. *J Trauma* 33:539, 1992.
16. Cornwell EE, et al: Health care crisis from a trauma center perspective, the LA story. *JAMA* 276:940, 1996.
17. Flancbaum L, et al: DRGs and the "negative" trauma workup. *Ann Emerg Med* 19:741, 1990.
18. Henry MC, et al: Inadequate hospital reimbursement for victims of motor vehicle crashes due to health reform legislation. *Ann Emerg Med* 35:277, 2000.
19. Gruen GS, et al: The acute management of hemodynamically unstable multiple trauma patients with pelvic ring fractures. *J Trauma* 36:706, 1994.
20. Demetriades D, et al: Paramedic versus private transportation of trauma patients: Effect on outcome. *Arch Surg* 131:133, 1996.
21. Barton ED, et al: Prehospital needle aspiration and tube thoracostomy in trauma victims: A six-year experience with aeromedical crews. *J Emerg Med* 13:155, 1995.
22. Kaweski SM, Sise MJ, Virgilio RW: The effect of prehospital fluids on survival in trauma patients. *J Trauma* 30:1215, 1990.
23. Spaite DW, et al: The impact of injury severity and prehospital procedures on scene time in victims of major trauma. *Ann Emerg Med* 20:1299, 1991.
24. Pons PT, et al: Prehospital venous access in an urban paramedic system: A prospective on-scene analysis. *J Trauma* 28:1460, 1988.
25. Liberman M, et al: Advanced or basic life support for trauma: Meta analysis and critical review of the literature. *J Trauma* 49:584, 2000.
26. Stern SA, et al: Effect of blood pressure on hemorrhage volume and survival in a near fatal hemorrhage model incorporating a vascular injury. *Ann Emerg Med* 22:155, 1993.
27. Bickwell WH, et al: Immediate versus delayed fluid resuscitation for hypotensive patients with penetrating torso injuries. *N Engl J Med* 331:1105, 1994
28. Dutton RP, Mackenzie CF, Scalea TM: Hypotensive resuscitation during active hemorrhage: Impact on in-hospital mortality. *J Trauma* 52:1141, 2002.
29. Gormican SP: CRAMS Scale: Field triage of trauma victims. *Ann Emerg Med* 11:132, 1982.
30. Hirshberg A, et al: Causes and patterns of missed injuries in trauma. *Am J Surg* 168:299, 1994.
31. Laasonen EM, Kivioja A: Delayed diagnosis of extremity injuries in patients with multiple injuries. *J Trauma* 31:257, 1991.
32. Cooper C, Dunham CM, Rodriguez A: Falls and major injuries are risk factors for thoracolumbar fractures: Cognitive impairment and multiple injuries impede the detection of back pain and tenderness. *J Trauma* 38:692, 1995
33. Biffl WL, et al: Implementation of a tertiary trauma survey decreases missed injuries. *J Trauma* 54:38, 2003.
34. Scalea TM, et al: Geriatric blunt multiple trauma: Improved survival with early invasive monitoring. *J Trauma* 30:129, 1990.
35. Davis JW, et al: Admission base deficit predicts transfusion requirements and risk of complications. *J Trauma* 41:769, 1996.
36. Eberhard LW, et al: Initial severity of metabolic acidosis predicts the development of acute lung injury in severely traumatized patients. *Crit Care Med* 28:125, 2000.
37. Borel C, et al: Intensive management of severe head injury. *Chest* 98:180, 1990.
38. Holley JE, Jorden RC: Airway management in patients with unstable cervical spine fractures. *Ann Emerg Med* 18:151, 1989.
39. Rhee KJ, et al: Oral intubation in the multiply injured patient: The risk of exacerbating spinal cord damage. *Ann Emerg Med* 19:511, 1990.

40. Dronen SC, et al: A comparison of blind nasotracheal and succinylcholine-assisted intubation in the poisoned patient. *Ann Emerg Med* 16:650, 1987.

41. Horellou MF, Mathe D, Feiss P: A hazard of nasotracheal intubation. *Anaesthesia* 33:73, 1978.

42. Jorden RC, et al: A comparison of PTV and endotracheal ventilation in an acute trauma model. *J Trauma* 25:978, 1985.

43. Yealy DM, Stewart RD, Kaplan RM: Myths and pitfalls in emergency translaryngeal ventilation: Correcting misimpressions. *Ann Emerg Med* 17:690, 1988.

44. Hawkins ML, et al: Emergency cricothyrotomy: A reassessment. *Am Surg* 61:52, 1995.

45. Fuhrman GM, Stieg FH, Buerk CA: Blunt laryngeal trauma: Classification and management protocol. *J Trauma* 30:87, 1990.

46. Posner MC, Moore EE: Distal greater saphenous vein cutdown—Technique of choice for rapid volume resuscitation. *J Emerg Med* 3:395, 1985.

47. Schwab CW, et al: Saline-expanded group O uncrossmatched packed red blood cells as an initial resuscitation fluid in severe shock. *Ann Emerg Med* 15:1282, 1986.

48. Velanovich V: Crystalloid versus colloid fluid resuscitation: A meta-analysis of mortality. *Surgery* 105:65, 1989.

49. Mattox KL, et al: Prehospital hypertonic saline/dextran infusion for post-traumatic hypotension: The USA multicenter trial. *Ann Surg* 213:482, 1991.

50. Drummond JC, Petrovitch CT: The massively bleeding patient. *Anesthesiol Clin North America* 19:1, 2001.

51. Farringer PD, et al: Blood component supplementation during massive transfusion of AS-1 red cells in trauma patients. *J Trauma* 34:481, 1993.

52. Ferrara A, et al: Hypothermia and acidosis worsen coagulopathy in patients requiring massive transfusion. *Am J Surg* 160:515, 1990.

53. Durham LA, et al: Emergency center thoracotomy: Impact of prehospital resuscitation. *J Trauma* 32:775, 1992.

54. Branney SW, et al: Critical analysis of two decades of experience with postinjury emergency department thoracotomy in a regional trauma center. *J Trauma* 45:187, 1998.

55. Rhee PM, et al: Survival after emergency department thoracotomy: Review of published data from the past 25 years. *J Am Coll Surg* 190:288, 2000.

56. Walls RM: Rapid-sequence intubation in head trauma. *Ann Emerg Med* 22:1008, 1993.

57. Muizelaar JP, et al: Adverse effects of prolonged hyperventilation in patients with severe head injury: A randomized clinical trial. *J Neurosurg* 75:731, 1991.

58. Laffey JG, Kavanagh BP: Hypocapnia. *N Engl J Med* 347:42, 2002.

59. Coles JP, et al: Effect of hyperventilation on cerebral blood flow in traumatic head injury: Clinical relevance and monitoring correlates. *Crit Care Med* 30:1950, 2002

60. Schrot RJ, Muizelaar JP: Mannitol in acute traumatic brain injury. *Lancet* 359:1633, 2002.

61. Arishita GI, Vayer JS, Bellamy RF: Cervical spine immobilization of penetrating neck wounds in a hostile environment. *J Trauma* 29:332, 1989.

62. Hoffman JR, et al: Validity of a set of clinical criteria to rule out injury to the cervical spine in patients with blunt trauma. *N Engl J Med* 343:94, 2000.

63. Barba CA, et al: A new cervical spine clearance protocol using computed tomography. *J Trauma* 51: 652, 2001.

64. Ghanta MK, et al: An analysis of Eastern Association for the Surgery of Trauma practice guidelines for cervical spine evaluation in a series of patients with multiple imaging techniques. *Am Surg* 68:563, 2002.

65. Anglen J, et al: Flexion and extension views are not cost-effective in a cervical spine clearance protocol for obtunded trauma patients. *J Trauma* 52: 54, 2002.

66. Bracken MB, et al: Administration of methylprednisolone for 24 or 48 hours or tirilazad mesylate for 48 hours in the treatment of acute spinal cord injury. Results of the Third National Acute Spinal Cord Injury Randomized Controlled Trial. National Acute Spinal Cord Injury Study. *JAMA* 227:1597, 1997.

67. Nesathurai S: Steroids and spinal cord injury: Revisiting the NASCIS 2 and NASCIS 3 trials. *J Trauma* 45:1088, 1998.

68. Richardson JD, et al: Evolution in the management of hepatic trauma: A 25 year experience. *Ann Surg* 232:324, 2000.

69. Peitzmna AB, et al: Blunt splenic injury in adults: Multiinstitutional study of the Eastern Association for the Surgery of Trauma. *J Trauma* 49:177, 2000.

70. Sosa JL, et al: Laparoscopy in 121 consecutive patients with abdominal gunshot wounds. *J Trauma* 39:501, 1995.

71. Santucci RA, McAninch JW: Diagnosis and management of renal trauma: Past, present and future. *J Am Coll Surg* 191:443, 2000.

72. Lang EK: Intra-abdominal and retroperitoneal organ injuries diagnosed on dynamic computed tomograms obtained for assessment of renal trauma. *J Trauma* 30:1161, 1990.

73. Norton MJ, et al: Early detection of myocardial contusion and its complications in patients with blunt trauma. *Am J Surg* 160:577, 1990.

74. Kerr TM, et al: Prospective trial of the six hour rule in stab wounds of the chest. *Surg Gynecol Obstet* 169:223, 1989.

75. Ordog GJ, et al: Asymptomatic stab wounds of the chest. *J Trauma* 36:680, 1994.

76. Stephan PJ, et al: 23-hour observation solely for identification of missed injuries after trauma: Is it justified? *J Trauma* 53:895, 2002.

77. Stiell IG, et al: The Canadian C-spine rule for radiography in alert and stable trauma patients. *JAMA* 286:1841, 2001.

78. Rybicki F, et al: Skin and thyroid dosimetry in cervical spine screening: Two methods for evaluation and a comparison between a helical CT and radiographic trauma series. *AJR Am J Roentgenol* 179:933, 2002.

79. Hanson JA, et al: Cervical spine injury: A clinical decision rule to identify high-risk patients for helical CT screening. *AJR Am J Roentgenol* 174:713, 2000.

80. Gonzalez RP, et al: The utility of clinical examination in screening for pelvic fractures in blunt trauma. *J Am Coll Surg* 194:121, 2002.

81. Duane TM, et al: Blunt trauma and the role of routine pelvic radiographs: A prospective analysis. *J Trauma* 53:463, 2002.

82. Henneman PL, et al: Diagnostic peritoneal lavage: Accuracy in predicting necessary laparotomy following blunt and penetrating trauma. *J Trauma* 30:1345, 1990.

83. Marx JA, et al: Limitations of computed tomography in the evaluation of acute abdominal trauma: A prospective comparison with diagnostic peritoneal lavage. *J Trauma* 25:933, 1985.

84. Federle M, et al: Use of oral contrast material in abdominal trauma CT scans: Is it dangerous? *J Trauma* 38:51, 1995.

85. Tsang B, et al: Effect of oral contrast administration for abdominal computed tomography in the evaluation of acute blunt trauma. *Ann Emerg Med* 30:7, 1997.

86. Clancy T, et al: Oral contrast is not necessary in the evaluation of blunt abdominal trauma by computed tomography. *Am J Surg* 166:680, 1993.

87. McKenny MG, et al: 1000 consecutive ultrasounds for blunt abdominal trauma. *J Trauma* 40:607, 1996.

88. Ingeman JE, et al: Emergency physician use of ultrasonography in blunt abdominal trauma. *Acad Emerg Med* 3:931, 1996.

89. Chiu WC, et al: Abdominal injuries without hemoperitoneum: A potential limitation of FAST. *J Trauma* 42:617, 1997.

90. Mateer J, et al: Model curriculum for physician training in emergency ultrasonography. *Ann Emerg Med* 23:95, 1994.

91. Branney SW, et al: Ultrasound based key clinical pathway reduces the use of hospital resources for the evaluation of blunt abdominal trauma. *J Trauma* 42:1086, 1997.

92. Boulanger BR, et al: Prospective evidence of the superiority of a sonography-based algorithm in the assessment of blunt abdominal injury. *J Trauma* 47:632, 1999.

93. Hoff WS, et al: Practice management guidelines for the evaluation of blunt abdominal trauma: The EAST practice management guidelines work group. *J Trauma* 53:602, 2002.

94. Wisner DH, Victor NS, Holcroft JW: Priorities in the management of multiple trauma: Intracranial versus intraabdominal injury. *J Trauma* 35:271, 1993.

95. Thomason MH, et al: Head CT scanning versus urgent exploration in the hypotensive blunt trauma patient. *J Trauma* 34:40, 1993.

96. Winchell RJ, Hoyt DB, Simons RK: Use of computed tomography of the head in the hypotensive blunt-trauma patient. *Ann Emerg Med* 25:737, 1995.

97. Richardson JD, Wilson ME, Miller FB: The widened mediastinum: Diagnostic and therapeutic priorities. *Ann Surg* 211:731, 1990.

98. Mirvis SE, et al: Use of spiral computed tomography for the assessment of blunt trauma patients with potential aortic injury. *J Trauma* 45:922, 1998.

99. Dyer DS, et al: Thoracic aortic injuries: How predictive is mechanism and is chest computed tomography a reliable screening tool? A prospective study of 1561 patients. *J Trauma* 48:673, 2000.

100. Kearney PA, et al: Use of transesophageal echocardiography in the evaluation of traumatic aortic injury. *J Trauma* 34:696, 1993.

101. Smith MD, et al: Transesophageal echocardiography in the diagnosis of traumatic rupture of the aorta. *N Engl J Med* 332:356, 1995.

CHAPTER

35 Trauma in Pregnancy

John D. G. Neufeld

PERSPECTIVE

Emergency medical care of the pregnant woman is one of the special challenges in traumatology. Pregnancy produces changes that alter the usual course of trauma management. Obviously, the most dramatic difference is a second life that is both helpless and hidden from view.

Trauma occurs in 6% to 7% of all pregnancies. It is the leading cause of maternal death, accounting for 46.3% of fatalities in pregnant women.[1] Women stay active throughout pregnancy and are as likely to need trauma care during the third trimester as in the first or second trimester.[2,3] The most common causes of injury in pregnancy that result in emergency department visits involve motor vehicle crashes (MVCs), assaults, and falls.[4-8] Patients with penetrating injuries present more frequently to emergency departments in inner city medical centers.[9] Of note, 8% of women, aged 15 to 40, admitted to a trauma center do not yet know they are pregnant.[10]

PRINCIPLES OF DISEASE—CHANGES OF PREGNANCY

Physiology
Cardiovascular

The normal cardiovascular changes of pregnancy can alter the presentation of shock and vascular events (Table 35-1).

Some Alterations Mimic Shock. Blood pressure declines in the first trimester, levels out in the second trimester, and then returns to nonpregnant levels during the third trimester. The decline in systole is small, 2 to 4 mm Hg, whereas diastole falls 5 to 15 mm Hg. Heart rate increases in pregnancy but does not rise by more than 10 to 15 beats/min above baseline.[11]

More problematic is the supine hypotensive syndrome. After 20 weeks' gestation, the uterus has risen to the level of the inferior vena cava. Compression of this structure may occur when the pregnant patient is in the supine position. Such caval obstruction diminishes cardiac preload, which can decrease cardiac output 28% and reduce systolic blood pressure by 30 mm Hg.[11] In late pregnancy, it is common for the inferior vena cava to become completely occluded when the pregnant patient is supine. To determine whether observed hypotension is related to positioning, the pregnant woman's pelvis can be tilted to the left or the uterus can be manually pushed to the left. One study found that tilting limited to only about 15 degrees may only partially resolve vena caval obstruction.[12] Thus, putting the patient as far over on her left side as possible, once the spine is cleared, can be advantageous.

Similarly, central venous pressure (CVP) measurements can be lowered in the last two trimesters by inferior vena caval compression.

Some Alterations Hide Shock. Blood volume gradually increases during pregnancy to as much as 48% to 58% above normal, peaking at 32 to 34 weeks' gesta-

Table 35-1. Hemodynamic Changes of Pregnancy (Mean Values)

Parameter	Nonpregnant	Trimester 1	Trimester 2	Trimester 3
Heart rate (beats/min)	70	78	82	85
Systolic blood pressure (mm Hg)	115	112	112	114
Diastolic blood pressure (mm Hg)	70	60	63	70
Cardiac output (L/min)	4.5	4.5	6	6
Central venous pressure (mm Hg)	9.0	7.5	4.0	3.8
Blood volume (mL)	4000	4200	5000	5600
Hematocrit without iron (%)	40	36	33	34
Hematocrit with iron (%)	40	36	34	36
White blood cell (cell/mm³)	7200	9100	9700	9800

Data from deSwiet M: The cardiovascular system. In Hytten F, Chamberlain G (eds): *Clinical Physiology in Obstetrics.* Oxford, UK. Blackwell Scientific Publications, 1980: Colditz RB, Josey WE: Central venous pressure in supine position during normal pregnancy. Comparative determinations during first, second and third trimesters. *Obstet Gynecol* 36:769, 1970; Letsky E: The haematological system. In Hytten RF, Chamberlin G (eds): *Clinical Physiology in Obstetrics.* Oxford, UK. Blackwell Scientific Publications, 1980; and Cruikshank DP: Anatomic and physiologic alterations of pregnancy that modify the response to trauma. In Buchsbaum HJ (ed): *Trauma in Pregnancy.* Philadelphia, WB Saunders, 1979.

tion. Blood volumes become increasingly larger for multigravidas, twins, triplets, and quadruplets.[13] With this increased circulatory reserve, clinical signs of maternal hypotension from acute traumatic bleeding may be delayed.

Some Alterations Can Exacerbate Traumatic Bleeding. By the beginning of the second trimester and throughout the remaining pregnancy, cardiac output is increased 40%, to 6 L/min.[11] Blood flow to the uterus increases from 60 mL/min before pregnancy to 600 mL/min at term.[14] This hyperdynamic state is needed to maintain adequate oxygen delivery to the fetus. Because the mother's total circulating blood volume flows through the uterus every 8 to 11 minutes at term, this organ can be a major source of blood loss when injured. By the third trimester there is also marked venous congestion in the pelvis, increasing the potential for hemorrhage from both bony and soft tissue pelvic injuries.

Compression of the lower abdominal venous system by the gravid uterus increases peripheral venous pressure in the legs, creating the potential for brisk blood loss from leg wounds.

Pregnancy Is Associated with a Greater Risk of Thromboembolism. Stasis is potentiated by increased venous capacity, inferior vena cava compression from the gravid uterus, and posttrauma bed rest. By the third trimester, increases in coagulation factors V, VII, VIII, IX, X, and XII and fibrinogen exceed fibrinolytic activity.[15] One study found that pregnant women with an injury severity score exceeding 8 have a greater tendency for deep venous thrombosis and pulmonary embolism complications than their nonpregnant counterparts.[16]

Pulmonary

The pregnant woman has a significantly reduced oxygen reserve. This effect comes from a 20% reduction in functional residual capacity, at term, caused by diaphragm elevation and a 15% increase in oxygen consumption related to the growing fetus, uterus, and placenta.[17] Archer and Marx observed that mean arterial oxygen tension dropped by 29% in pregnant women during 60 seconds of apnea but just 11% in nonpregnant women. Labor accelerates this decline by a further 7%.[18]

Gastrointestinal

Gastroesophageal sphincter response is reduced in pregnancy and gastrointestinal motility is decreased, both of which increase the possibility of aspiration during reduced levels of consciousness and intubation.[19] The stomach's increased acid production in pregnancy makes aspiration more ominous than usual.[20]

Anatomic Changes in Pregnancy

The diaphragm progressively rises an extra 4 cm in pregnancy with compensatory flaring of the ribs.[21] Tension pneumothorax may develop more quickly in pregnancy because of this diaphragm elevation, combined with pulmonary hyperventilation. For thoracostomies done in the third trimester, the chest tube should be placed one or two interspaces higher than the usual fifth interspace site to allow for diaphragm elevation.

Abdominal viscera are pushed upward by the enlarging uterus, resulting in altered pain location patterns. The gravid uterus itself tends to protect abdominal organs from trauma but substantially increases the likelihood of bowel injury with penetrating trauma to the upper abdomen. The stretching of the abdominal wall modifies the normal response to peritoneal irritation. Therefore, expected muscle guarding and rebound can be blunted despite significant intraabdominal bleeding and organ injury.

The uterus grows from a 7-cm, 70-g organ to a 36-cm, 1000-g structure at term. Total weight for the gravid uterus and its contents typically reaches 4500 g.[14] In the first trimester the bony pelvis shields the uterus. After the third month, the uterus rises out of the pelvis and becomes vulnerable to direct injury. The bladder is also displaced into the abdominal cavity beyond 12 weeks' gestation, thereby becoming more vulnerable to injury. Like the uterus, the bladder becomes hyperemic, and injury may lead to a marked increase in blood loss compared with similar injury in a nonpregnant patient.

Imaging studies may show ureteral dilation that can be physiologic secondary to smooth muscle relaxation or caused by compression from the gravid uterus.

Changes in Laboratory Values with Pregnancy

The physiologic anemia of pregnancy, resulting from a 48% to 58% increase in plasma volume and only an 18% increase in red blood cells, causes hematocrits of 32% to 34% by the 32nd to 34th week. The leukocyte count averages 9000 to 10,000 in the last two trimesters and can sometimes reach 25,000 during labor or stress situations. The erythrocyte sedimentation rate (ESR) rises to a mean of 78 mm per hour at term. The high ESR is the result of increased levels of plasma globulins and fibrinogen in pregnancy.[13] Increased ESR and white blood cell counts make these usual hematologic markers of infection less reliable in pregnancy.

Increased coagulation factors shorten prothrombin times slightly from 13.5 seconds at 60 days' gestation to 11.2 seconds at term. Partial thromboplastin times are similarly shortened by a small amount.[22] Fibrinogen levels begin to rise in the third month of pregnancy. By term, fibrinogen levels are 400 to 450 mg per 100 mL (4 to 4.5 g/L), double those in the nonpregnant state.[23]

Placental progesterone directly stimulates the medullary respiratory center, producing a partial pressure of carbon dioxide in arterial blood ($PaCO_2$) of 30 mm Hg from the second trimester until term. The subsequent compensatory lowering of serum bicarbonate to 21 mEq/L slightly reduces blood-buffering capacity for stress situations.[17] A $PaCO_2$ of 40 mm Hg in the latter half of pregnancy reflects inadequate ventilation and potential respiratory acidosis that could precipitate fetal distress.

Electrocardiographic changes include a left-axis shift averaging 15 degrees, caused by diaphragm elevation. Consequently, Q waves in leads III and aVF may be seen.

CLINICAL FEATURES OF TRAUMA IN PREGNANCY

Blunt Trauma

Motor Vehicle Crashes

In numerous studies of trauma in pregnancy, MVCs typically account for more than half of all injuries. Unbelted pregnant women are twice as likely to experience vaginal bleeding and two times more likely to give birth within 48 hours of a crash than properly belted pregnant women; fetal death is three to four times more likely to occur when pregnant women are unbelted.[24,25] For low- to moderate-severity crashes (constituting 95% of all MVCs) proper restraint use, with or without air bag deployment, generally leads to acceptable fetal outcomes. However, a higher risk of adverse fetal outcome after MVCs occurs if the pregnant occupant is not properly restrained. For high-severity crashes even proper restraint does not improve fetal outcome.[26]

Pregnant crash test dummy trials show that improper placement of the lap belt over the pregnant abdomen causes a three- to fourfold increase in force transmission through the uterus. The lowest force transmission readings through the uterus occur when a three-point seat belt is used properly.[27] Correct positioning places the lap belt underneath the pregnant abdomen against the pelvis and the shoulder belt to the side of the pregnant abdomen, between the breasts, and over the midportion of the clavicle. Women who receive information on seat belt use during pregnancy from a health care worker are more likely to use seat belts (83% versus 65%) and use them properly (77% versus 57%).[28]

In a related report, placental separation has been documented with loose seat belt application during severe turbulence in an airplane.[29]

Physical Abuse

The prevalence of physical abuse during pregnancy ranges from 4% to 17%.[30-32] The abuser is usually someone the woman knows, typically her husband or boyfriend.[33] Multiple perpetrators tend to be cited by teenagers, who may identify both a boyfriend and a parent as abusive.[31] Of previously abused women, 64% report increased attacks during pregnancy but 78% of this group still remain with the abuser.[30] The most common area of the body struck in an assault during pregnancy is the abdomen. Two thirds of women receive medical treatment for abuse, but only 3% tell the physician what really happened.[30] Most often, the patient states that she has fallen and this is the cause of her injuries. Therefore, a history of abuse should be sought in all patients when the mechanism of injury is obscure or sounds suspicious. Because assaults are often recurrent, domestic violence during pregnancy has great potential for morbidity and may be a harbinger of future child abuse.

Falls

Falls become more prevalent after the 20th week of pregnancy.[4] Protuberance of the abdomen, loosening of pelvic ligaments, strain on the lower back, and fatigability contribute to this problem. In a given pregnancy, about 2% of pregnant women sustain repeated direct blows to the abdomen because of falling more than once. Although repeated falls often trigger premature contractions, they seldom result in immediate labor and delivery.[34]

Penetrating Trauma

Trauma centers in large urban settings see a disproportionate number of penetrating trauma cases. About 46% of maternal deaths in Cook County are caused by trauma. Gunshot wounds are responsible for 23% of these deaths and stab wounds for another 14%. Homicide is involved more than half of the time, and, typically, the biologic father or another male associate is responsible for the wounds.[1]

The gravid uterus alters injury patterns to the mother. There is an increased probability of harm (approaching 100%) to the bowel, liver, or spleen if the entrance of the penetrating object is in the upper abdomen. When the entry site is anterior and below the uterine fundus, visceral injuries are less likely (0% in some studies). Although the enlarging uterus can act as a shield against intraabdominal injuries in the mother, it places the fetus in a position more susceptible to injury. Awwad and colleagues observed a 67% fetal death rate from penetrating trauma to the uterus but a lesser 38% fetal death rate for injuries above the uterus.[35]

Fetal Injury

Pregnancy does not alter rates of maternal mortality caused by trauma. However, trauma is associated with a high risk for fetal loss. When the mother suffers a severe level of injury, poor fetal outcome is predicted by maternal hypotension and acidosis (hypoxia, lowered pH, lowered bicarbonate) plus a fetal heart rate of less than 110 beats/min.[3,8,9,36-40] When the mother suffers life-threatening injuries, 40.6% of fetuses die, compared with only 1.6% in non–life-threatening maternal cases.[41]

For women with less severe trauma, fetal outcome is not predicted by maternal vital signs, abdominal tenderness, blood tests, or ultrasonography (US) results. Only cardiotocographic monitoring for a minimum of 4 hours is useful to predict fetal outcome.[5]

Fatal in utero fetal injuries from blunt trauma usually involve intracranial hemorrhage and skull fractures. Such head injury is often secondary to fractured maternal pelvic bones striking the fetal skull.[42,43] Pelvic and acetabular fractures during pregnancy are associated with a high maternal (9%) and a higher fetal (38%) mortality rate.[44] With penetrating trauma, gunshot wounds to the uterus are associated with a high incidence of fetal injury (59% to 89%) and fetal mortality (41% to 71%).[45] Stab wounds to the uterus can produce 93% morbidity and 50% mortality to the fetus.[46]

Placental Injury

In blunt trauma, 50% to 70% of all fetal losses result from placental abruption.[47,48] Nonseverely injured pregnant women have a 3.7-fold increased risk of placental abruption and a 5-fold increased risk of fetal death compared with noninjured pregnant patients. Severely injured pregnant women have a 17-fold increased risk of placental abruption and a 30-fold increased risk of fetal death.[49]

Placental separation results when the inelastic placenta shears away from the elastic uterus during sudden deformation of the uterus. Because deceleration forces can be as damaging to the placenta as direct uterine trauma, abruption can occur with little or no external sign of injury to the abdominal wall.[50] Because all gas exchange between the mother and fetus occurs across the placenta, abruption inhibits the flow of oxygen to the fetus and causes in utero CO_2 accumulation. Such hypoxia and acidosis can lead to fetal distress.[14] Sustained uterine contractions induced by

intrauterine hemorrhage also inhibit uterine blood flow, further contributing to fetal hypoxia.[51]

Classical clinical findings of abruption may include vaginal bleeding, abdominal cramps, uterine tenderness, maternal hypovolemia (up to 2 L of blood can accumulate in the gravid uterus), or a change in the fetal heart rate. However, in some trauma studies, as many as 63% of cases showed no evidence of vaginal bleeding.[52]

The most sensitive indicator of placental abruption is fetal distress. Hence, prompt fetal monitoring is a very important assessment technique in trauma during pregnancy. There is also a close linkage of abruption to uterine activity. One study reported that if 12 or more contractions occurred in any hour of a 4-hour cardiotocographic monitoring period, the risk of abruption was 14%; abruption did not occur in this study if contractions occurred less than once every 10 minutes.[5] US is less than 50% accurate as a first-line test in detecting placental abruption.[5,53] If the abruption bleeds externally, not enough blood collects to be seen sonographically. Even with significant intrauterine blood accumulation, accurate US diagnosis may be difficult because of placental position (i.e., posterior) and confounding uterine or placental structural conditions.[54]

Placental abruption is associated with an 8.9-fold increased risk of stillbirth (>20 weeks) and a 3.9-fold increased risk of preterm delivery (<37 weeks). The extent of placental separation affects stillbirth rates. This is initially evident at 50% separation with a 4-fold increased risk of stillbirth and more profoundly at 75% separation with a 31.5-fold increased risk. The risk of preterm delivery is substantially increased with even mild abruptions; a 25% separation carries a 5.5-fold increased risk.[55]

Where mother and fetus are stable, expectant management can be tried for partial placental abruptions. This usually applies to fetuses of less than 32 weeks' gestation in whom the morbidity and mortality associated with prematurity make delivery management risky. Expectant care in stable patients may allow further maturation and improved outcome. Metzger and associates recommended intervention if the fetus is older than 32 weeks' gestation because the risk of further placental separation outweighs the benefit of further fetal maturation.[56] If expectant management is pursued, close maternal and fetal monitoring is needed to ensure the well-being of both patients. The ability to perform an immediate cesarean section is necessary because there may be little time between the appearance of fetal distress from further placental separation and the occurrence of fetal death.[57]

Women with placental abruption are 54 times more likely to have coagulopathies than those without abruption.[58] The injured placenta can release thromboplastin into the maternal circulation, resulting in disseminated intravascular coagulation, whereas the damaged uterus can disperse plasminogen activator and trigger fibrinolysis.[59] The precipitation of disseminated intravascular coagulation is directly related to the degree of placental separation. Severe clotting disorders rarely occur unless separation of the placenta is significant enough to result in fetal demise.[60]

Uterine Injury

The most common obstetric problem caused by maternal trauma is uterine contractions.[5,6,61] Myometrial and decidual cells, irritated by contusion or placental separation, release prostaglandins that stimulate uterine contractions. Progression to labor depends on the extent of uterine damage, the amount of prostaglandins released, and the gestational age of the pregnancy. The routine use of tocolytics for premature labor has come under question because 90% of contractions stop spontaneously.[5] Contractions that are not self-limited are often induced by some pathologic condition, such as underlying placental abruption, which is a contraindication to tocolytic therapy. Others consider this contraindication relative and have used tocolysis successfully with careful evaluation and intensive monitoring to continue the pregnancy and enhance fetal maturity.[62] The option to use tocolytics ends when cervical dilation reaches 4 cm.

Uterine rupture is a rare event. It is most often caused by severe vehicular crashes in which pelvic fractures strike directly against the uterus. There have been a few reports of uterine rupture from stab wounds and gunshot injuries.[63] Maternal shock, abdominal pain, easily palpable fetal anatomy caused by extrusion into the abdomen, and fetal demise are typical findings on examination. Diagnosing uterine rupture can be difficult. A fractured liver or spleen can produce similar signs and symptoms of peritoneal irritation, hemoperitoneum, and unstable vital signs. Optimal treatment, between suturing the tear or performing a hysterectomy, depends on the extent of uterus and uterine vessel tears and the importance of future childbearing.

DIAGNOSTIC STRATEGIES— RADIOGRAPHY

Plain Films

Sensitivity to radiation is greater during intrauterine development than at any other time of life. However, the risk to the fetus of a 1 rad (1000 mrad) exposure, approximately 0.003%, is thousands of times smaller than the spontaneous risks of malformations, abortions, or genetic disease.[64] Studies show that intrauterine exposure to 10 rad causes no significant increase in congenital malformations, intrauterine growth retardation, or miscarriage but is associated with a small increase in the number of childhood cancers.[65-67] Pathologic conditions more readily appear with intrauterine radiation doses of 15 rad. At 15 rad there is approximately a 6% chance that the fetus could experience severe mental retardation, a less than 3% chance of developing childhood cancer, and a 15% chance of having a small head, although this does not necessarily affect normal cerebral function.[68]

Table 35-2. Estimated Radiation Dose to the Ovaries/ Pelvic Uterus

Type of Radiographic Examination	Dose (mrad)*
Low-Dose Group	
Head	<1
Cervical spine	<1
Thoracic spine	<1
Chest	<1
Extremities	<1
High-Dose Group	
Lumbar spine	204-1260
Pelvis	190-357
Hip	124-450
Intravenous pyelogram	503-880
Urethrocystogram	1500
KUB	200-503

*mrad, millirad; dose increases as the fetus grows to occupy more of the abdomen.
KUB, kidney, ureter, and bladder.
Data from Bureau of Radiological Health: *Gonad Doses and Genetically Significant Dose from Diagnostic Radiology. US 1964 and 1970.* Rockville, Md, U.S. Department of Health, Education, and Welfare, 1976; Eliot G: Pregnancy and radiographic examination. In Haycock CE (ed): *Trauma and Pregnancy.* Littleton, Mass. PSG Publishing, 1985; and United Nations Scientific Committee on the effects of atomic radiation: *Sources and Effects of Ionizing Radiation.* New York, United Nations, 1977.

Providing information on radiation exposure from diagnostic radiographs is difficult. The individual amount of fetal dosage may vary by a factor of 50 or more, depending on the equipment used, technique, number of radiographs done in a complete study, maternal size, and fetal-uterine size. In general, coned x-ray beams aimed more than 10 cm away from the fetus are not harmful.[69]

Diagnostic radiographic studies should be performed with regard for fetal protection, but necessary diagnostic studies should not be withheld out of concern for fetal radiation exposure. When appropriate, fetal irradiation should be minimized by limiting the scope of the examination and using technical means such as shielding and collimation.[65] Table 35-2 provides estimated radiation doses from various types of examinations.[70-72] For comparison, the amount of naturally occurring radiation that the fetus receives during 9 months of gestation is approximately 50 to 100 mrad.[68]

Ultrasonography

US is the best modality for simultaneous assessment of both the mother and the fetus.[73] It has a sensitivity of 88%, a specificity of 99%, and an accuracy of 97% for detecting intraabdominal injuries in blunt trauma.[74] It is most useful in screening for free intraperitoneal fluid in the mother's abdomen (sensitivity 83%, specificity 98%) plus establishing fetal well-being or demise, gestational age, and placental location.[75] US is not sensitive for identifying bowel and biliary tree lesions.

US is considered a safe procedure. Individual scans do not cause embryonic loss, congenital malformations, neurobehavioral damage, or low birth weight.[76]

Table 35-3. Upper Limit Fetal Dose from Angiography and Computed Tomography Scan Studies

Type of Examination	Dose (mrad)
Angiography	
Cerebral	<100
Cardiac catheterization	<500
Aortography	<100
Computed Tomography	
Head (1-cm slices)	<50
Chest (1-cm slices)	<1000
Upper abdomen	<3000
(20 1-cm slices < 2.5 cm from the uterus)	
Lower abdomen	3000–9000
(10 1-cm slices over the uterus/fetus)	

Data from Wagner LK, Lester RG, Saldana LR: *Exposure of the Pregnant Patient to Diagnostic Radiations: A Guide to Medical Management.* Philadelphia, JB Lippincott, 1985; and Esposito TJ et al: Evaluation of blunt abdominal trauma occurring during pregnancy. *J Trauma* 29:1628, 1989.

Computed Tomography and Magnetic Resonance Imaging Scans

Computed tomography (CT) and magnetic resonance imaging (MRI) scan studies should be used as a complement to US and diagnostic peritoneal lavage (DPL) in evaluating abdominal trauma in pregnancy. If US and DPL are indeterminate and the patient's condition is stable, CT and MRI scans have the potential to identify specific organ damage.[77] They are particularly useful in assessing penetrating wounds of the flank and back. CT can miss diaphragm and bowel injuries.[78] Both of these studies lack portability, and trauma patients may have to be taken from the closely monitored environment of the emergency department to a distant room.

Radiation from CT scanning is a concern in the pregnant trauma patient. However, with shielding, fetal exposure from head and chest CT scans can be kept below an acceptable 1 rad limit. CT scanning of the abdomen above the uterus can be done with less than 3 rad of exposure to the fetus.[68] Pelvic CT scans, centered over the fetus, produce a more prohibitive 3 to 9 rad dose.[79] Fortunately, spiral CT scans can reduce radiation dosage by a further 14% to 30%.[80] Radiation exposure ultimately depends on the patient, scanner, and technique used in performing the study (Table 35-3).

MRI scanners use no radiation and cause no fetal disease or disability.[81]

SPECIAL PROCEDURES

Diagnostic Peritoneal Lavage

Although being replaced by US and serial examinations, DPL can be done quickly and safely in any trimester by an open technique above the uterus. Blunt trauma studies indicate that the gravid uterus does not compartmentalize intraperitoneal hemorrhage and does not reduce the accuracy of DPL for selecting patients who need operative intervention for intraabdominal bleeding.[82] DPL is limited in detecting bowel perforations and does not assess retroperitoneal and intrauterine pathology.

Kleihauer-Betke Test and Fetomaternal Hemorrhage

Fetomaternal hemorrhage (FMH), the transplacental bleeding of fetal blood into the normally separate maternal circulation, is a unique complication of pregnancy. The reported incidence of FMH after trauma is 8% to 30% (with a range of 2.5 to 115 mL of blood) compared with 2% to 8% (range of 0.1 to 8 mL) for control studies. MVCs, anterior placental location, and uterine tenderness are associated with an increased risk of FMH, but gestational age is not.[5,7,83] Complications of FMH include Rh sensitization of the mother, fetal anemia, fetal distress, and fetal death from exsanguination.

In theory, it is possible that trauma can result in FMH as early as the fourth week of gestation, when the fetal and placental circulations first form. In practice, FMH is usually of more concern after 12 weeks' gestation, when the uterus rises above the pelvis and becomes susceptible to direct trauma.[5]

The Kleihauer-Betke (KB) test identifies fetal cells in a maternal blood sample. Most laboratories screen for FMH of 5 mL or more. Unfortunately, the amount of FMH sufficient to sensitize most Rh-negative women is well below this 5-mL sensitivity level. Therefore, all Rh-negative mothers who have a history of abdominal trauma should receive one prophylactic dose of Rh immune globulin (RhIG). In the first trimester, one 50-μg dose is used because total fetal blood volume is only 4.2 mL by 12 weeks' gestation and a 50-μg dose covers 5 mL of bleeding. During the second and third trimesters, a 300-μg dose of RhIG is given, which protects against 30 mL of FMH.

In the emergency department, the KB test is useful in screening Rh-negative women who are at risk for massive FMH that exceeds the efficacy of one 300-μg dose of RhIG. This first becomes possible at 16 weeks' gestation, when total fetal blood volume reaches 30 mL.

Trauma patients at risk for massive FMH present with major injuries or abnormal obstetric findings, such as uterine tenderness, contractions, or vaginal bleeding. Less than 1% of all pregnant trauma patients and only 3.1% of major trauma cases exceed the coverage of one 300-μg RhIG dose.[7]

Because RhIG can effectively prevent Rh isoimmunization when administered within 72 hours of antigenic exposure, the results of the KB test are not immediately needed in the emergency department.

MANAGEMENT

Advance notification by out-of-hospital personnel regarding an injured pregnant patient allows the trauma team time to assemble. An obstetrician can be called, and if the patient is in her last trimester, a

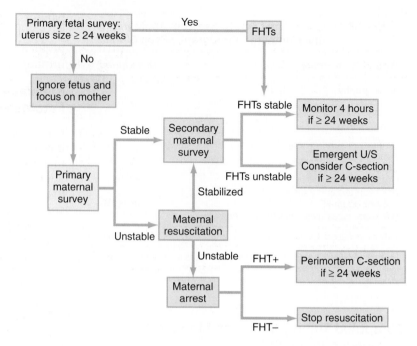

Figure 35-1. Decision-making algorithm in emergency obstetric care. C-section, cesarean section; FHTs, fetal heart tones; U/S, ultrasonography.

pediatrician's presence is desirable. A fetal monitor, portable US, and neonatal resuscitation equipment should be available in the emergency department.[73]

Maternal Resuscitation

Primary Survey

The primary survey focuses on the mother. However, because two patients are present, it is reasonable also to gather preliminary information about the fetus in the primary survey (Figure 35-1).

Airway and Breathing

Oxygen therapy should be instituted early. Because of reduced oxygen reserve and increased oxygen consumption, the traumatized pregnant woman can quickly become hypoxic. The fetus is very vulnerable to any reduction in oxygen delivery. Animal studies show that severe hypoxia causes a 30% reduction in uterine blood flow.[84] Therefore, supplemental oxygen should be continued throughout maternal resuscitation and evaluation. When maternal hypoxia, hypovolemia, and fetal distress have been ruled out, oxygen may be discontinued.[73]

A secure airway is critical to an optimum outcome. Not only does it enable proper oxygenation, but it negates the higher risk of aspiration in pregnancy. Rapid sequence intubation is recommended when intubation is performed. Mechanical respirators need to be adjusted for increased tidal volumes and respiratory alkalosis consistent with the physiologic $PaCO_2$ of 30 mm Hg in the last stage of pregnancy.

Circulation

Any time significant maternal injury is suspected from the mechanism of injury or clinical findings, early intravenous access for volume resuscitation is indi-

cated. Maternal blood pressure and heart rate are not consistently reliable predictors of fetal and maternal well-being.[73] Because of an expanded circulating volume, the mother can be bleeding but not show early signs of hypotension. The uterus is not a critical organ, and its blood flow is markedly reduced when the maternal circulation must be maintained. As a result, after an acute blood loss, uterine blood flow can be decreased 10% to 20% while maternal blood pressure remains normal.[85] Consequently, the mother who presents with borderline stability probably already has a jeopardized fetus. When traditional signs of shock appear, fetal compromise can be far advanced with fetal mortality rates as high as 85%.[2] Vasopressors should be avoided because they produce fetal distress by further decreasing uterine blood flow.

Lactated Ringer's solution is the preferred intravenous fluid for initial resuscitation. It is more physiologic than normal saline and has been shown to be more effective in restoring fetal oxygenation than other plasma expanders. Both the intravenous fluids and the mother may need to be warmed. Temperature losses are more significant in the emergency department than in the operating room,[86] and mortality in trauma patients is twice as high if core temperature is less than 32° C compared with a temperature of less than 34° C.[87]

Beyond 20 weeks' gestation, the patient should be tilted 15 to 30 degrees to the left when on a backboard or should have the right hip elevated. This reduces the compression on the inferior vena cava caused by the gravid uterus. Tilting to the right is less effective in removing the uterus from the inferior vena cava.

For severe injuries, a CVP line is helpful in assessing cardiac preload. CVP pressures decline as pregnancy progresses because of inferior vena caval compression by the gravid uterus. Therefore, correction to nonpregnant normal pressures may be unnecessary. Instead, it

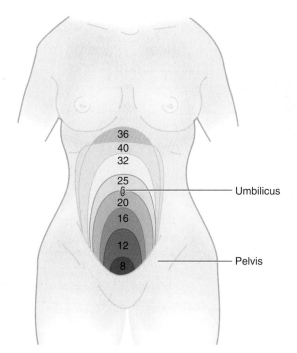

36
40
32
25
0 — Umbilicus
20
16
12
8 — Pelvis

Figure 35-2. Uterine size at different weeks of gestation. (From Kravis TC, Warner CG [eds]: *Emergency Medicine: A Comprehensive Review*. Rockville, Md, Aspen Publishers, 1979.)

Table 35-4. Fetal Viability

Weeks Gestation	6-Month Survival (%)	Survival with No Severe Abnormalities (%)
22	0	0
23	15	2
24	56	21
25	79	69

Data from Morris JA Jr et al: Infant survival after cesarean section for trauma. *Ann Surg* 223:481, 1996.

is more valuable to focus on trends of how the CVP responds to fluid challenges. A Foley catheter for measuring urine output provides further information on circulatory volume status.

With trauma in pregnancy, the primary survey can be modified to assess uterine size and the presence of fetal heart tones. Uterine size, measured from the symphysis pubis to the fundus, is the quickest means of estimating gestational age. This distance in centimeters equals the gestational age in weeks (e.g., 24 cm = 24 weeks), which allows some early indication of fetal viability if delivery is necessary (Figure 35-2). Usually, 24 to 25 weeks is used as the cutoff point for fetal viability[88] (Table 35-4). As a rough guide, the fetus is potentially viable when the dome of the uterus extends beyond the umbilicus. Fetal heart tones can be detected by auscultation at 20 weeks' gestation or by Doppler probe at 10 to 14 weeks. If either the uterus is less than 24 cm in size or fetal heart tones are absent, the pregnancy is probably too early to be viable, and treatment is directed solely at the mother.

Secondary Survey

The secondary survey involves a detailed examination of the patient but is also modified to gather additional information about the maternal abdomen and the fetus. Physical examination of the abdomen, frequently unreliable in the nonpregnant patient, is more inaccurate with changing organ position, abdominal wall stretching in advancing pregnancy, and uterine contraction pains. Still, information can be gathered about uterine tenderness, contraction frequency, and vaginal bleeding.

Pelvic examination begins with sterile speculum examination to allow direct visualization to detect trauma in the genital tract, the degree of cervical dilation, and the source of any observed vaginal fluid. Vaginal bleeding suggests placental abruption, and a watery discharge suggests rupture of the membranes. If a vaginal fluid sample placed on a slide dries and crystallizes in a ferning pattern, it is amniotic fluid and not urine. Cervical cultures for group B streptococci, *Neisseria gonorrhoeae*, and *Chlamydia* should be obtained if there is evidence of amniotic fluid leak. Bimanual examination should be limited to assessing for pelvic bone injury or progression of advanced labor.

Fetal Evaluation

Fetal evaluation in the secondary survey focuses on the fetal heart rate and detection of fetal movement. When the presence of fetal heart tones has been confirmed, intermittent monitoring of fetal heart rate is sufficient for the previable fetus. If the fetus is viable (i.e., 24 weeks or more), continuous external monitoring should be initiated quickly and maintained throughout all diagnostic and therapeutic procedures.[73] Such monitoring can also benefit the mother because fetal hemodynamics are more sensitive to decreases in maternal blood flow and oxygenation than are most maternal measures. Fetal distress can be a sign of occult maternal distress. Signs of fetal distress include an abnormal baseline rate, decreased variability of heart rate, and fetal decelerations after contractions.

The normal fetal heart rate ranges between 120 and 160 beats/min. Rates outside or trending toward these limits are ominous. Heart rate variability has two components. Beat-to-beat variability measures autonomic nervous function, whereas long-term variability indicates fetal activity. Heart rate variability increases with gestational age. The loss of beat-to-beat and long-term variability warns of fetal central nervous system depression and reduced fetal movement caused by fetal distress[73] (Figure 35-3).

Late decelerations are an indication of fetal hypoxia. These decelerations are relatively small in amplitude and occur after the peak or conclusion of a uterine contraction. By comparison, early decelerations are larger, occur with the contraction, and recover to baseline immediately after the contraction. Early decelerations may be vagally mediated when uterine contractions squeeze the fetal head, stretch the neck, or compress the umbilical cord. Variable decelerations are large,

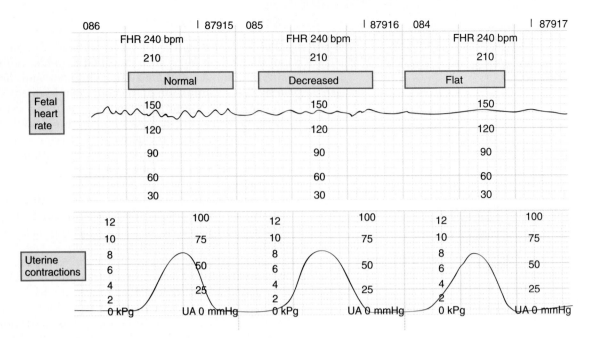

Figure 35-3. Types of fetal heart rate variability.

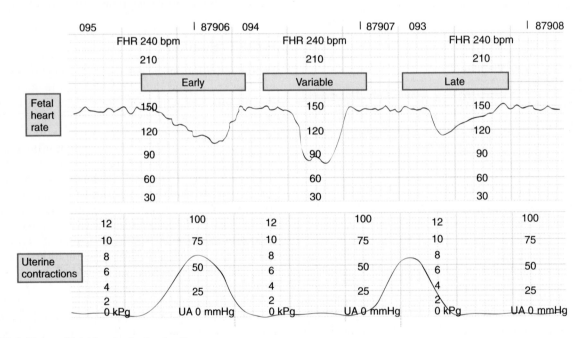

Figure 35-4. Types of fetal heart rate decelerations.

occur at any time, and are possibly caused by umbilical cord compression[73] (Figure 35-4).

Laboratory

Besides routine trauma blood work, emergency laboratory tests should include a blood type with Rh. In apparently stable pregnant patients, a low serum bicarbonate may indicate occult maternal shock.[89] Interpretation of bicarbonate results must consider that the normal bicarbonate level is 21 mEq/L in the later stages of pregnancy. Arterial blood gases can allow detection

of maternal hypoxia and acidosis, whereas pulse oximetry can be used to monitor oxygen saturation. Coagulation studies should be obtained for patients with multisystem trauma or when the diagnosis of placental abruption is considered.

Mother Stable, Fetus Stable

Minor trauma does not necessarily exempt the fetus from significant injury. It is estimated that 1% to 3% of all minor trauma results in fetal loss, typically from placental abruption.[28] Therefore, once the traumatized mother is stabilized, the focus of care is directed toward the fetus. For the viable fetus, monitoring is the next step. Because direct impact is not necessary for feto-placental pathology to occur, the mother with no obvious abdominal injury still needs monitoring.[5,7]

The recommended 4 hours of cardiotocographic observation of the viable fetus should be extended to 24 hours if, at any time during the first 4 hours, there are more than three uterine contractions per hour, persistent uterine tenderness, a worrisome fetal monitor strip, vaginal bleeding, or rupture of the membranes or if any serious maternal injury is present. In Pearlman's study, all cases of placental abruption after maternal trauma were detected within the first 4 hours of monitoring. These mothers typically had more than 12 uterine contractions per hour. Although 70% of patients required admission beyond the 4-hour observation period, all patients who are discharged at the end of the 4-hour or 24-hour monitoring periods have subsequent live births.[5]

On release from the hospital, the mother should be instructed to record fetal movements during the next week. If fewer than four movements per monitored hour are noted, the patient should see her obstetrician immediately and a nonstress test should be performed. The occurrence of preterm labor, membrane rupture, vaginal bleeding, or uterine pain also necessitates prompt re-evaluation. Serial US and fetal heart rate tests should be performed on viable fetuses a few days after all trauma episodes and periodically throughout the remaining portion of the pregnancy to monitor fetal well-being.

Mother Stable, Fetus Unstable

Fetal death rates following maternal trauma are three to nine times higher than maternal death rates.[8] If a viable fetus remains in distress despite optimization of maternal physiology, cesarean section should be performed.

Although fetal viability is first reached at 24 to 25 weeks, the ultimate determinant of the age of fetal viability is the level of neonatal care provided by the intensive care nursery unit in each hospital or accessible regional facility. Of note, determining gestational age for fetuses less than 29 weeks is difficult. Even with the best US criteria, unless the time of conception is known exactly, the assignment of gestational age is subject to 1 to 2 weeks of uncertainty.[90] Emergency decisions on fetal viability are, therefore, made on the basis of the best gestational age information available.

Morris and colleagues found that the presence of fetal heart tones is an important survival marker for fetuses about to undergo emergency cesarean section. No infant survives if there is no fetal heart tone before emergency cesarean section commences. If fetal heart tones are present and the gestational age is 26 weeks or more, then infant survival is 75%. Sixty percent of fetal deaths result from underuse of cardiotocographic monitoring and delayed recognition of fetal distress.[91]

Besides fetal distress, other reasons for a cesarean section include uterine rupture, fetal malpresentation during premature labor, and situations in which the uterus mechanically limits maternal repair. Fetal death is not an indication for cesarean section because spontaneous labor usually occurs within 1 week.

Mother Unstable, Fetus Unstable

If the mother's condition is critical, primary repair of her wounds is the best course. This may apply even when the fetus is in distress because a critically ill mother may not be able to withstand an additional operative procedure such as cesarean section, which prolongs laparotomy time and increases blood loss by at least 1000 mL. The best initial action on behalf of the fetus is early restoration of normal maternal physiology. If it is felt that the unstable mother can tolerate an emergency cesarean section, it can be attempted for the distressed, viable fetus.

As with nonpregnant patients, operative intervention for blunt trauma and above-the-uterus stab wounds is dictated by clinical findings and diagnostic testing results. Above-the-uterus intraperitoneal gunshot wounds should be explored.

It has been theorized that penetrating trauma to the gravid uterus can be managed expectantly. However, no prospective study has verified this. Damage to the uterus alone can be quite devastating because of its increased circulation. Meizner and Potashnik reported a shrapnel injury to only the uterus in a case in which an initially normal examination quickly changed to a hypotensive emergency. At celiotomy, 1000 mL of blood was found in the abdomen from a perforated corner injury to the uterus.[92] Without exploration it is impossible to know the occurrence, size, or depth of uterine penetration, and there are no guidelines indicating whether a uterine wound can be left unsutured without incurring an increased risk of infection or later uterine rupture. Laparotomy or laparoscopy seem to be the safest means of managing penetrating uterine wounds because missed maternal injuries can quickly compromise the fragile fetus.

Perimortem Cesarean Section

Restoration of maternal and thus fetal circulation is the optimal goal. However, extended and exclusive attention to the mother in cardiopulmonary arrest may prevent recovery of a potentially viable fetus. During maternal resuscitation, adequate oxygenation, fluid loading, and a 30-degree left tilting position should be tried to determine whether maternal circulation can be improved. If there is no response to advanced cardiac life support, a decision for perimortem cesarean section must be made. If there are no fetal heart tones, a cesarean section is not warranted.[91]

Perimortem cesarean section in the emergency department should be performed if uterine size exceeds the umbilicus (see Figure 35-2) and fetal heart tones are present. No time should be wasted obtaining consent for delivery. Time since maternal circulation ceased is the critical factor in fetal outcome. Katz and coworkers reported that 70% of children who survive perimortem cesarean sections are delivered in less than 5 minutes of emergency department arrival.[93]

The most experienced physician, preferably an obstetrician, should perform the procedure. However, this task ultimately may fall to the emergency physician or trauma surgeon, given the time constraints of the situation. A pediatric consultation should be obtained emergently.

While continuing CPR, a "classic midline vertical incision is made, using a large scalpel, extending from the epigastrium to the symphysis pubis and carried through all layers to the peritoneal cavity. A vertical incision is then made in the anterior uterus from the fundus to the bladder reflection. Assistants and other surgical instruments (e.g., clamps, retractors) are helpful but not required. If, when the uterus is entered, an anterior placenta is encountered, it should be incised in order to reach the fetus. The cord should be promptly clamped and cut following delivery of the child."[94]

Maternal revival after delivery of the fetus is reported in a few perimortem circumstances, presumably because vena caval compression is relieved.[95]

DISPOSITION

Any pregnant woman at 24 or more weeks of gestation who has suffered blunt body trauma should be admitted for fetal monitoring even if she looks well. Other admission and operative criteria are similar for pregnant and nonpregnant trauma patients. The emergency physician must always consider the stability of the mother and the viability of the growing fetus when making management and disposition decisions.

MISCELLANEOUS

Tetanus toxoid and immune globulin have no detrimental effect on the fetus. Proper immunization of pregnant women decreases the incidence of neonatal tetanus because the tetanus antibody crosses the placenta.

Electrical flow that bypasses the fetus has little effect on the pregnancy. Maternal elective and emergent cardioversion has been performed safely for cardiac dysrhythmias in all three stages of pregnancy. Energies up to 300 watt-seconds have been used without affecting the fetus or inducing premature labor. Cullhead reported no disruption of a monitored fetal heart rhythm during maternal cardioversion with 80 and 200 watt-seconds.[96] Although the amount of energy reaching the fetal heart is thought to be small, the fetal heart should be monitored during cardioversion.

KEY CONCEPTS

- Management of life- and limb-threatening injury in the mother comes first.
- Major trauma carries the highest risk for fetal demise.
- Minor trauma can cause fetal demise.
- The fetus is viable at 24 to 25 weeks' gestation. A fetus is estimated to be viable if the fundus is at or above the umbilicus.
- The fetus can be distressed even though the mother looks well. Therefore, continual fetal monitoring is vital to recognize early fetal distress.
- Stable pregnancies after trauma should be monitored for 4 hours.
- Keeping the mother tilted 30 degrees to the left or in the left lateral decubitus position may alleviate hypotension and improve perfusion for the mother and fetus.
- Perimortem cesarean section should be performed only for a viable fetus with positive life signs.
- Plain radiography is not contraindicated in pregnancy and should be performed as necessary in the pregnant trauma patient.
- US is the diagnostic abdominal test of choice in the stable pregnant patient, but a CT or MRI scan of the abdomen may be needed in selected cases.

REFERENCES

1. Fildes J, et al: Trauma: The leading cause of maternal death. *J Trauma* 32:643, 1992.
2. Esposito TJ, et al: Trauma during pregnancy: A review of 79 cases. *Arch Surg* 126:1073, 1991.
3. Hoff WS, et al: Maternal predictors of fetal demise in trauma during pregnancy. *Surg Gynecol Obstet* 172:175, 1991.
4. Connolly AM, et al: Trauma and pregnancy. *Am J Perinatol* 14:331, 1997.
5. Pearlman MD, Tintinalli JE, Lorenz RP: A prospective study of outcome after trauma during pregnancy. *Am J Obstet Gynecol* 162:1502, 1990.
6. Williams JK, McClain L, Rosemurgy AS: Evaluation of blunt abdominal trauma in the third trimester of pregnancy: Maternal and fetal considerations. *Obstet Gynecol* 75:33, 1990.
7. Goodwin TM, Breen MT: Pregnancy outcome and fetomaternal hemorrhage after noncatastrophic trauma. *Am J Obstet Gynecol* 162:665, 1990.
8. Kissinger DP, et al: Trauma in pregnancy: Predicting pregnancy outcome. *Arch Surg* 126:1079, 1991.
9. Rogers FB, et al: A multi-institutional study of factors associated with fetal death in injured pregnant patients. *Arch Surg* 134:1274, 1999.
10. Bochicchio GV, et al: Incidental pregnancy in trauma patients. *J Am Coll Surg* 192:566, 2001.
11. deSwiet M: The cardiovascular system. In Hytten F, Chamberlain G (eds): *Clinical Physiology in Obstetrics.* Oxford, Blackwell Scientific Publications, 1980.
12. Kerr MD, Scott DB, Samuel E: Studies of the inferior venae cavae in late pregnancy. *Br Med J* 1:532, 1964.
13. Letsky E: The haematological system. In Hytten F, Chamberlain G (eds): *Clinical Physiology in Obstetrics.* Oxford, Blackwell Scientific Publications, 1980.
14. Pearlman MD, Tintinalli JE, Lorenz RP: Blunt trauma during pregnancy. *N Engl J Med* 323:1609, 1990.
15. Sipes SL, Weiner CP: Venous thromboembolic disease in pregnancy. *Semin Perinatol* 14:103, 1990.

16. Shah KH, et al: Trauma in pregnancy: Maternal and fetal outcomes. *J Trauma* 45:83, 1998.

17. deSwiet M: The respiratory system. In Hytten F, Chamberlain G (eds): *Clinical Physiology in Obstetrics.* Oxford, Blackwell Scientific Publications, 1980.

18. Archer GW Jr, Marx GF: Arterial oxygen tension during apnoea in parturient women. *Br J Anaesth* 46:358, 1974.

19. Hytten FE: The alimentary system. In Hytten F, Chamberlain G (eds): *Clinical Physiology in Obstetrics.* Oxford, Blackwell Scientific Publications, 1980.

20. Chatterjee MS: Physiology of pregnancy. In Haycock CE (ed): *Trauma and Pregnancy*. Littleton, Mass, 1985, SG Publishing, 1985.

21. Cunningham FG, MacDonald PC, Gant NF (eds): Maternal adaptations to pregnancy. In *Williams Obstetrics*, 18th ed. Norwalk, Conn, Appleton & Lange, 1989.

22. Talbert LM, Langdell RD: Normal values of certain factors in the blood clotting mechanism in pregnancy. *Am J Obstet Gynecol* 90:44. 1964.

23. Biland L, Duckert F: Coagulation factors of the newborn and his mother. *Thromb Diath Haemorrh* 29:644, 1973.

24. Wolf ME, et al: A retrospective cohort study of seatbelt use and pregnancy outcome after a motor vehicle crash. *J Trauma* 34:116, 1993.

25. Hyde LK, et al: Effect of motor vehicle crashes on adverse fetal outcomes. *Obstet Gynecol* 102:279, 2003.

26. Desantis-Klinich K, et al: Investigations of crashes involving pregnant occupants. *Assoc Adv Auto Med* 44:37, 2000.

27. Pearlman MD, Viano D: Automobile crash simulation with the first pregnant crash test dummy. *Am J Obstet Gynecol* 175:977, 1996.

28. Pearlman MD, Phillips ME: Safety belt use during pregnancy. *Obstet Gynecol* 88:1026, 1996.

29. Fletcher HM, Wharfe GH, Mitchell SY: Placental separation from a seat belt injury due to severe turbulence during aeroplane travel. *J Obstet Gynecol* 23:73, 2003.

30. Stewart DE, Cecitto A: Physical abuse in pregnancy. *Can Med Assoc J* 149:1257, 1993.

31. McFarlane J, et al: Assessing for abuse during pregnancy. *JAMA* 267:3176, 1992.

32. Cokkinides VE, et al: Physical violence during pregnancy: Maternal complications and birth outcomes. *Obstet Gynecol* 93:661, 1999.

33. Poole GV, et al: Trauma in pregnancy: The role of interpersonal violence. *Am J Obstet Gynecol* 174:1873, 1996.

34. Runnebaum IB, Holcbery G, Katz M: Pregnancy outcome after repeated abdominal blunt abdominal trauma. *Eur J Obstet Gynecol Reprod Biol* 80:85, 1998.

35. Awwad JT, et al: High-velocity penetrating wounds of the gravid uterus: Review of 16 years of civil war. *Obstet Gynecol* 83:259, 1994.

36. Stafford PA, Biddinger PW, Zumwalt RE: Lethal intrauterine fetal trauma. *Am J Obstet Gynecol* 159:485, 1988.

37. Drost TF, et al: Major trauma in pregnant women: Maternal/fetal outcome. *J Trauma* 30:574, 1990.

38. Pak LL, Reece EA, Chan L: Is adverse pregnancy outcome predictable after blunt abdominal trauma? *Am J Obstet Gynecol* 179:1140, 1998.

39. Baerga-Varela Y, et al: Trauma in pregnancy. *Mayo Clin Proc* 75:1243, 2000.

40. Theodorou DA, et al: Fetal death after trauma in pregnancy. *Am Surg* 66:809, 2000.

41. Pearlman MD: Motor vehicle crashes, pregnancy loss and preterm labor. *Int J Gynecol Obstet* 57:127, 1997.

42. Landers DF, Newland M, Penney LL: Multiple uterine ruptures and crushing injury to the fetal skull after blunt maternal trauma. *J Reprod Med* 34:988, 1989.

43. Mudoch-Eaton DG, Ahmed Y, Dubowitz LM: Maternal trauma and cerebral lesions in preterm infants. Case reports. *Br J Obstet Gynaecol* 98:1292, 1991.

44. Leggon RE, Wood GC, Indeck MC: Pelvic fractures in pregnancy: Factors influencing maternal and fetal outcomes. *J Trauma* 53:796, 2002.

45. Buchsbaum HJ: Penetrating injury of the abdomen. In Buchsbaum HJ (ed): *Trauma in Pregnancy*. Philadelphia, WB Saunders, 1979.

46. Sakala EP, Kort DD: Management of stab wounds to the pregnant uterus: A case report and a review of the literature. *Obstet Gynecol Surv* 43:319, 1988.

47. Pearlman MD, Tintinalli JE: Evaluation and treatment of the gravida and fetus following trauma during pregnancy. *Obstet Gynecol Clin North Am* 18:371, 1991.

48. Corsi PR, et al: Trauma in pregnant women: Analysis of maternal and fetal mortality. *Injury* 30:239, 1999.

49. Schiff MA, et al: Maternal and infant outcomes after injury during pregnancy in Washington State from 1989 to 1997. *J Trauma* 53:939, 2002.

50. Lane PL: Traumatic fetal deaths. *J Emerg Med* 7:433, 1989.

51. Nyberg DA, et al: Placental abruption and placental hemorrhage: Correlation of sonographic findings with fetal outcome. *Radiology* 164:357, 1987.

52. Pepperel RJ, Rubinstein E, MacIssac IA: Motor-car accidents in pregnancy. *Med J Aust* 1:203, 1977.

53. Reis PM, Sander CM, Pearlman MD: Abruptio placentae after auto accidents. *J Reprod Med* 45:6, 2000.

54. Abu-Yousef MM, et al: Subchorionic hemorrhage: Sonographic diagnosis and clinical significance. *AJR Am J Roentgenol* 149:737, 1987.

55. Ananth CV, et al: Placental abruption and adverse perinatal outcomes. *JAMA* 282:1646, 1999.

56. Metzger DA, Bowie JD, Killam AP: Expectant management of partial placental abruption in previable pregnancies: A report of two cases. *J Reprod Med* 32:789, 1987.

57. Hurd WW, et al: Selective management of abruption placentae: A prospective study. *Obstet Gynecol* 61:467, 1983.

58. Saftlas AF, et al: National trends in the incidence of abruptio placentae, 1979-1987. *Obstet Gynecol* 78:1081, 1991.

59. Civil ID, Talucci RC, Scheab CW: Placental laceration and fetal death as a result of blunt abdominal trauma. *J Trauma* 28:708, 1988.

60. Twaalhoven FCM, et al: Conservative management of placental abruption complicated by severe clotting disorders. *Eur J Obstet Gynecol Reprod Biol* 46:25, 1992.

61. Towery R, English P, Wisner D: Evaluation pregnant women after blunt injury. *J Trauma* 35:731, 1993.

62. Henderson DE, Goldman B, Divon MY: Ritodrine therapy in the presence of chronic abruptio placentae. *Obstet Gynecol* 80:510, 1992.

63. Dash N, Lupetin AR: Uterine rupture secondary to trauma: CT findings. *J Comput Assist Tomogr* 15:329, 1991.

64. Brent RL: The effects of embryonic and fetal exposure to x-ray, microwaves, and ultrasound. *Clin Perinatol* 13:615, 1986.

65. National Council on Radiation Protection and Measurements: *Medical Radiation Exposure of Pregnant and Potentially Pregnant Women*, no 54. Washington, D.C., National Council on Radiation Protection and Measurements, 1979.

66. Harvey EB, et al: Prenatal x-ray exposure and childhood cancer in twins. *N Engl J Med* 312:541, 1985.

67. Ornoy A, Patlas N, Schwartz L: The effects of in utero diagnostic X-irradiation on the development of preschool-age children. *Isr J Med Sci* 32:112, 1996.

68. Wagner LK, Lester RG, Saldana LR: *Exposure of the Pregnant Patient to Diagnostic Radiations: A Guide to Medical Management.* Philadelphia, JB Lippincott, 1985.

69. Jacobson A, Conley JG: Estimation of fetal dose to patients undergoing diagnostic x-ray procedures. *Radiology* 120:683, 1976.

70. Bureau of Radiological Health: *Gonad Doses and Genetically Significant Dose from Diagnostic Radiology, US 1964*

and 1970. Rockville, Md, US Department of Health, Education, and Welfare, 1976.

71. Eliot G: Pregnancy and radiographic examination. In Haycock CE (ed): *Trauma and Pregnancy.* Littleton, Mass, PSG Publishing, 1985.

72. United Nations Scientific Committee on the Effects of Atomic Radiation: *Sources and Effects of Ionizing Radiation.* New York, United Nations, 1977.

73. Esposito TJ: Trauma during pregnancy. *Emerg Med Clin North Am* 12:167, 1994.

74. McKenney MG, et al: 1,000 consecutive ultrasounds for blunt abdominal trauma. *J Trauma* 40:607, 1996.

75. Goodwin H, Holmes JF, Wisner DH: Abdominal ultrasound examination in pregnant blunt trauma patients. *J Trauma* 50:689, 2001.

76. Salvesen KA: Epidemiology of diagnostic ultrasound exposure during pregnancy. *Eur J Ultrasound* 15:165, 2002.

77. Antuaco TL, et al: MR imaging in high-risk obstetric patients: A valuable complement to US. *Radiographics* 12:91, 1992.

78. Sherck JP, Oaks DD: Intestinal injuries missed by computed tomography. *J Trauma* 30:1, 1990.

79. Wagner LK, Archer BR, Zeck OF: Conceptus dose from two state-of-the-art CT scanners. *Radiology* 159:787, 1986.

80. Hidajat N: Radiation exposure in spiral computed tomography. Dose distribution and dose reduction. *Invest Radiol* 34:51, 1999.

81. Baker PN, et al: A three-year follow-up of children imaged in utero with echo-planar magnetic resonance. *Am J Obstet Gynecol* 170:32, 1994.

82. Esposito TJ, et al: Evaluation of blunt abdominal trauma occurring during pregnancy. *J Trauma* 29:1628, 1989.

83. Rose PG, Strohm PL, Zuspan FP: Fetomaternal hemorrhage following blunt trauma. *Am J Obstet Gynecol* 153:844, 1985.

84. Dilts PV, et al: Uterine and systemic hemodynamic interrelationships and their response to hypoxia. *Am J Obstet Gynecol* 103:138, 1969.

85. Greiss FC Jr: Uterine vascular response to hemorrhage during pregnancy. *Obstet Gynecol* 27:549, 1966.

86. Gregory JS: Incidence and timing of hypothermia in trauma patients undergoing operations. *J Trauma* 31:795, 1991.

87. Seekamp A: The role of hypothermia in trauma patients. *Eur J Emerg Med* 2:28, 1995.

88. Allen MC, Donohue PK, Dusman AE: The limit of viability—Neonatal outcome of infants born at 22 to 25 weeks' gestation. *N Engl J Med* 329:1597, 1993.

89. Scorpio RJ, et al: Blunt trauma during pregnancy: Factors affecting fetal outcome. *J Trauma* 32:213, 1992.

90. Hadlock FP, Harrist RB, Martinez-Poyer J: How accurate is second trimester fetal dating? *J Ultrasound Med* 10:557, 1991.

91. Morris JA Jr, et al: Infant survival after cesarean section for trauma. *Ann Surg* 223:481, 1996.

92. Meizner I, Potashnik G: Shrapnel penetration in pregnancy resulting in fetal death. *Isr J Med Sci* 24:431, 1988.

93. Katz VL, Dotter DJ, Droegemueller W: Perimortem cesarean delivery. *Obstet Gynecol* 68:571, 1986.

94. Jorden RC, Marx JA (eds): Urgent cesarean section following maternal death. *Case Studies in Emergency Medicine*, Vol 1. Rockville, Md, Aspen Publishers, 1985.

95. DePace NL, Betesh JS, Kotler MN: "Postmortem" cesarean section with recovery of both mother and offspring. *JAMA* 248:971, 1982.

96. Cullhead I: Cardioversion during pregnancy. *Acta Med Scand* 214:169, 1983.

CHAPTER

36 Pediatric Trauma

Richard M. Cantor

PERSPECTIVE

Half of all deaths in children 1 to 14 years old are the result of trauma. More than 15,000 traumatic deaths per year occur within this age group. More than half of these mortalities are directly related to motor vehicle crashes (MVCs). Injury accounts for approximately 30% of infant deaths as well.[1,2] U.S. estimates of mortality for children hospitalized after injury are uniformly low; however, most fatalities occur in the field before arrival at a health care facility, which contributes to an underestimation of the magnitude of overall mortality figures.

Patterns of injury help contribute to mortality factors. The most common single organ system injury associated with death in injured children is head trauma.[3]

Rates of 80% have been reported in patients with combined thoracoabdominal injuries.[1,4] Because multiple injuries are common in children, the emergency physician must evaluate all organ systems in any injured child, regardless of the actual mechanism of injury.

Within the subset of MVC, death rates increase steeply in adolescents (≥13 years old). MVC mortality statistics show that the youngest occupant in the vehicle is the most vulnerable to injury. Among school-age children (5 to 9 years old), pedestrian injuries and bicycle crashes predominate. Falls from heights account for 25% to 30% of injury; submersion injuries, 10% to 15%; and burns, 5% to 10%.[4,5] Across the United States, the number of children who are victims of violent acts has increased. Some children's hospitals report that 25% to 35% of all their trauma deaths are related to child abuse.[6]

BOX 36-1. Anatomic Differences in Adults and Children—Implications for Pediatric Trauma Management

The child's body size allows for a greater distribution of traumatic injuries, so multiple trauma is common.

The child's greater relative body surface area causes greater heat loss.

The child's internal organs are more susceptible to injury based on more anterior placement of liver and spleen and less protective musculature and subcutaneous tissue mass.

The child's kidney is less well protected and more mobile. making it susceptible to deceleration injury.

15% of pediatric patients presenting with hematuria after trauma have underlying congenital abnormalities.

Growth plates are not yet closed in pediatric patients, leading to Salter-type fractures with possible limb-length abnormalities with healing.

The child's head-to-body ratio is greater, the brain less myelinated, and cranial bones thinner, resulting in more serious head injury.

Table 36-1. Anatomic Differences in the Pediatric Airway—Implications in Pediatric Trauma Management

Differences	Implications
Relatively larger tongue, which can obstruct the airway	Most common cause of airway obstruction in children
	May necessitate better head positioning or use of airway adjunct (oropharyngeal or nasopharyngeal airway)
Larger mass of adenoidal tissues may make nasotracheal intubation more difficult	Nasopharyngeal airways may also be more difficult to pass in infants <1 year old
Epiglottis is floppy and more U-shaped	Necessitates use of a straight blade in young children
Larynx more cephalad and anterior	More difficult to visualize the cords; may need to get lower than the patient and look up at 45-degree angle or greater while intubating
Cricoid ring is the narrowest portion of the airway	Allows for use of uncuffed tubes in children up to size 6 mm or about 8 years old
Narrow tracheal diameter and distance between the rings, making tracheostomy more difficult	Needle cricothyrotomy for the difficult airway versus a surgical cricothyrotomy for the same reason
Shorter tracheal length (4–5 cm in newborn and 7–8 cm in 18-month-old)	Leads to intubation of right main stem or dislodgment of the endotracheal tube
Large airways more narrow	Leads to greater airway resistance (R α 1/radius^4)

PRINCIPLES OF DISEASE

There are major anatomic and physiologic differences between pediatric and adult patients that play a significant role in the evaluation and management of a pediatric trauma patient (Box 36-1 and Table 36-1). Compared with adults, any given force is more widely distributed through the body of a child, making multiple injuries significantly more likely to occur in children. The proportionately large surface area of infants and children relative to weight predisposes them to greater amounts of heat loss as a result of evaporation. Maintenance requirements for free water, trace metals, and minerals are magnified to a greater degree. All of these factors contribute to a significantly higher energy and caloric requirement for an injured child compared with an injured adult. Finally, a child's physiologic response to injury is different from an adult's response, depending on the age and maturation of the child and the severity of the injury. In contrast to adults, children have a great capacity to maintain blood pressure despite significant acute blood losses comprising 25% to 30% of total blood volume. Subtle changes in heart rate, blood pressure, and extremity perfusion may indicate impending cardiorespiratory failure and should not be overlooked.

CLINICAL FEATURES

Initial Assessment Priorities and Primary Survey

The highest priority in the approach to the injured child is ruling out the presence of life-threatening or limb-threatening injury. Treatment of these injuries must occur before proceeding with the rest of the physical examination. This initial assessment (the primary survey) and necessary initial resuscitation efforts must occur simultaneously. In general, the assessment and resuscitation should be addressed within the first 5 to 10 minutes of evaluation. Any infant or child with a potentially serious or unstable injury requires continual reassessment. Vital signs should be repeated every 5 minutes during the primary survey and every 15 minutes thereafter until the patient is considered stable. The primary survey for pediatric trauma patients can be remembered by *A, B, C, D, E, F.*

A—Airway and Cervical Spine Stabilization

The physician assesses for possible airway obstruction from injury, teeth, blood, or vomitus. Gurgling or stridor may indicate upper airway obstruction. While stabilizing the neck, the airway is opened with a jaw-thrust maneuver. Efforts should be directed toward clearing the oropharynx of debris. The clinician must consider the possibility of cervical cord injuries in all seriously traumatized children.

B—Breathing and Ventilation

The physician assesses for adequacy of chest rise; in a young child, this occurs in the lower chest and upper abdomen. The respiratory rate also is assessed. Rates that are too fast or slow can indicate respiratory failure. Treatment is assisted ventilation. If ventilation is necessary, a bag/valve/mask device is recommended initially. Only the volume necessary to cause the chest to rise should be provided because excessive volume or rate of ventilation can increase the likelihood of gastric distention and impair ventilation further. Cricoid pressure may be useful to decrease the amount of air entering the esophagus during positive-pressure ventilation.

Indications for endotracheal intubation of a pediatric trauma patient include (1) any inability to ventilate by bag/valve/mask methods or the need for prolonged control of the airway; (2) Glasgow Coma Scale (GCS) score of less than or equal to 9 to secure the airway and provide controlled hyperventilation as indicated; (3) respiratory failure from hypoxemia (e.g., flail chest, pulmonary contusions) or hypoventilation (injury to airway structures); and (4) the presence of decompensated shock resistant to initial fluid administration. Compared with adults, intubation of pediatric patients involves special considerations. Uncuffed tubes should be used in children younger than 8 years old because the narrowest portion of the pediatric airway in this age group is at the level of the cricoid cartilage (see Table 36-1). In general, the orotracheal approach is recommended. Problems associated with nasotracheal intubation include inherent difficulties in children, impairment of tube passage by the acute angle of the posterior pharynx, the potential for causing or worsening bleeding within the oral cavity, and increasing intracranial pressure (ICP) with insertion.

With regard to assessment of ventilation, early monitoring with pulse oximetry is useful; however, pulse oximetry measures adequacy of oxygenation only. There are many limiting factors that compromise ventilatory function in an injured child, including depressed sensorium, occlusion of the airway itself, painful restriction of lung expansion, and direct pulmonary injury. Determination of adequate ventilation is possible only in the face of airway patency and adequate air exchange. The diaphragm plays a special role in the maintenance of proper ventilatory status in children. It is easily fatigued in a young child and often is displaced by any process that promotes distention of the stomach. In this regard, it is advisable to consider early placement of a nasogastric tube to facilitate decompression of the stomach.

C—Circulation and Hemorrhage Control

Assessment of circulation in a child involves a combination of factors—pulse, skin color, and capillary refill time. In a child, maintenance of systolic blood pressure does not ensure that the patient is not in shock. The pediatric vasculature has the ability to constrict and increase systemic vascular resistance in an attempt to maintain perfusion. Signs of poor perfusion, such as cool distal extremities, decreases in peripheral versus central pulse quality, and delayed capillary refill time are signs of pediatric shock, even when blood pressure is maintained. Palpable pulses are detectable at a systolic blood pressure greater than 80 mm Hg. Normal capillary refill times are less than 2 seconds. Alteration

in a child's response to the environment or interaction with caregivers also may indicate respiratory failure or shock. External hemorrhage should be sought for and controlled with direct pressure.

D—Disability Assessment (Thorough Neurologic Examination)

To assess patient disability, a rapid neurologic evaluation is needed. Many methods are available to the clinician, specifically the AVPU (Box 36-2) and the GCS (Table 36-2).

E—Exposure and Thorough Examination

The final component of the primary survey involves fully undressing the patient to assess for hidden injury. Maintenance of normothermia is paramount in the undressed toddler and infant because metabolic needs are greatly increased by hypothermia.

F—Family

In the management of children, the family could be added to the primary survey. Rapidly informing the family of what has happened and the evaluation that is proceeding helps lessen the stress of the caregivers. Allowing family members to be present during resuscitations is acceptable and often preferred by families. Some caregivers choose not to be present, but that choice should be given to them. If a caregiver is present, it is advisable to assign a staff member to be with him or her during the trauma resuscitation to explain the process.

Secondary Survey

The secondary survey assesses the patient and treats additional injury not found on the primary survey and obtains a more complete and detailed history. Features of the detailed history that need to be obtained can be remembered by the mnemonic *AMPLE* (Box 36-3).

BOX 36-2. AVPU System

A *Alert*
V Responds to *verbal* stimuli
P Responds to *painful* stimuli
U *Unresponsive*

BOX 36-3. AMPLE History

A *Allergies*
M *Medications*
P *Past medical history*
L *Last meal*
E *Environments and events*

Table 36-2. Glasgow Coma Scale Modified for Pediatric Patients

Eye Opening Response

Score	>1 year	<1 year
4	Spontaneous	Spontaneous
3	To verbal command	To shout
2	To pain	To pain
1	None	None

Motor Response

Score	>1 year	<1 year
6	Obeys commands	Spontaneous
5	Localizes pain	Localizes pain
4	Withdraws to pain	Withdraws to pain
3	Abnormal flexion to pain (decerebrate)	Abnormal flexion to pain (decerebrate)
2	Abnormal extension to pain (decorticate)	Abnormal extension to pain (decorticate)
1	None	None

Verbal Response

Score	>5 years	2-5 years	0-2 years
5	Oriented and converses	Appropriate words and phrases	Babbles, coos appropriately
4	Confused conversation	Inappropriate words	Cries but is consolable
3	Inappropriate words	Persistent crying or screaming to pain	Persistent crying or screaming to pain
2	Incomprehensible sounds	Grunts or moans to pain	Grunts or moans to pain
1	None	None	None

Total score key: severe, <9; moderate, 9-13; mild, 14-15.

MANAGEMENT AND DIAGNOSTIC STRATEGIES

General Management Principles

All pediatric patients involved in major trauma should be placed on a cardiac monitor, receive supplemental oxygen, and have constant reassessment of vital signs and oximetry. Vascular access is best obtained by accessing the upper extremity for the establishment of two large-bore intravenous lines. In the absence of available upper extremity peripheral sites, lower extremity sites could be used. Many clinicians favor the femoral vein as a safe site for insertion of a central line, by use of a guidewire technique. If cutdowns are necessary, the antecubital or saphenous sites are preferred. If no other route for the delivery of fluids is easily obtained, intraosseous access may be obtained at the proximal tibia. The intraosseous route serves as an appropriate venous access site; however, delivery rate of large amounts of crystalloid solutions is limited based on maximal flow rates of approximately 25 mL/min.[7] Intraosseous placement in a fractured extremity is contraindicated.

Most hypovolemic pediatric trauma patients respond to infusions of 20-mL/kg boluses of isotonic crystalloid solutions. If 40 mL/kg has not reversed systemic signs of hypoperfusion, infusion of packed red blood cells at 10 mL/kg should be considered. In patients who present in decompensated shock or cardiopulmonary failure, and occult bleeding is a potential cause for the shock, crystalloid and blood products are administered simultaneously.

In contrast to an adult, cardiogenic shock is a rare event in the face of childhood injury.[3,8] Any degree of chest trauma associated with the presence of shock must alert the clinician, however, to the possibility of concomitant myocardial contusion or rupture. The classic presentation of neurogenic shock, involving hypotension without an increase in heart rate or compensatory vasoconstriction, should be considered in patients with head or neck injuries.

Specifics of the head examination include pupillary size and reactivity, funduscopic examination, and palpation of the skull. Assessment of the cervical spine must be done carefully, with the patient in full cervical spine immobilization.

Assessment of the chest and internal structures involves inspection for wounds and flail segments, palpation for tenderness and crepitance, and auscultation for asymmetry or poorly transmitted breath sounds or cardiac impulses.

Examination of the pediatric abdomen is most reliable when performed on a cooperative patient. It should be considered an insensitive screening process for the presence of an injury, however, with a low yield regarding which specific organ might be injured. The diagnostic test of choice to assess intra-abdominal injury in stable trauma patients is rapid abdominal computed tomography (CT).[9] The role of diagnostic peritoneal lavage (DPL) and bedside ultrasonography is more limited. As with all these tests, the finding of intraperitoneal hemorrhage alone is not an indication for surgery in a pediatric patient. Because of the desire for splenic salvage to maintain immunocompetency, an injured spleen often is left in place as long as the patient can be resuscitated adequately with crystalloid and blood products. Indications for surgery are listed in Box 36-4. Whatever the surgical preference within a health care facility, it is important to establish a

BOX 36-4. Indications for Surgery

Hemodynamic instability despite aggressive resuscitation
Transfusion of >50% of total blood volume
Radiographic evidence of pneumoperitoneum, intraperitoneal bladder rupture, grade V renovascular injury
Gunshot wound to the abdomen
Evisceration of intraperitoneal or stomach contents
Signs of peritonitis
Evidence of fecal or bowel contamination on diagnostic peritoneal lavage

Table 36-3. Airway: Assessment and Treatment

Assessment Priorities	Interventions
Airway patency	Jaw thrust, suction, airway adjuncts
Level of consciousness	Cervical spine immobilization
Maxillofacial injury	Apply 100% O_2 by mask
Stridor or cyanosis	Intubate for:
	Glasgow Coma Scale ≤8 or absent gag reflex or Po_2 <50 mm Hg or Pco_2 >50 mm Hg
	Needle cricothyrotomy if intubation impossible

protocol for approaching these challenging patients. Patients who remain hypotensive after adequate crystalloid infusion are candidates for early operative exploration.

A rectal examination provides information concerning sphincter tone, prostatic position, and the presence of blood in the stool. Although urethral injury is rare in children, all trauma patients should be assessed for a perineal or lower abdominal hematoma and blood from the urethral meatus. Examination of the extremities is directed toward the evaluation of any deformities, penetrations, and interruptions of perfusion. Most fracture sites may be stabilized with splinting until surgical intervention can be carried out. Early orthopedic consultation is advisable.

The pediatric patient is at great risk for the development of hypothermia. This risk is based on the large amount of surface area relative to body weight. Careful attention to core temperatures in these vulnerable patients is required, with early intervention as needed with supplemental external warming techniques. An overview of recommended interventions for a multiply traumatized child is contained in Tables 36-3 through 36-8.

Laboratory Studies

Blood sampling for a pediatric trauma patient is no different than that of an adult trauma patient; however, use of smaller blood collection tubes and microtechnique by laboratory staff may be necessary in infants and small children. All older children and adolescent trauma patients should be assessed for the possible use of drugs or alcohol as contributing factors to the traumatic event. In patients with hypovolemic shock, the

Table 36-4. Breathing: Assessment and Treatment

Assessment Priorities	Interventions
Respiratory rate	100% O_2 by nonrebreather mask or intubate if in respiratory failure; fast rates may indicate shock (fluid resuscitation) or pain (parenteral analgesics)
Chest wall movements	For pneumothorax or hemothorax: place chest tube
	Transfer to operating room if initial drainage >20 mL/kg or output >2 mL/kg/hr
Percussion	Open pneumothorax: seal with occlusive dressing (vaseline gauze) followed by tube thoracostomy
Paradoxical breathing	Contusion/flail chest: intubate if tachypneic or Po_2 <50 mm Hg or Pco_2 >50 mm Hg
Tracheal deviation	Tension pneumothorax: needle decompression at second intercostal space, midclavicular line, followed by placement of chest tube
Flail segments	O_2 by nonrebreather mask or intubate if in respiratory failure
Open wounds	Compress bleeding sites and cover as indicated

Table 36-5. Circulation: Assessment and Treatment

Assessment Priorities	Interventions
Capillary refill	Oximeter and cardiac monitor, O_2 and fluid resuscitation 20 mL/kg
Heart rate	Monitor vital signs every 5 min
Peripheral pulses	Two large-bore intravenous sites (above and below diaphragm)
Sensorium	Bolus with 20 mL/kg lactated Ringer's or normal saline solution (warm all intravenous fluids)
Pulse pressure	Repeat fluid bolus 2 times if necessary
Skin condition/perfusion	Packed red blood cells, 10–20 mL/kg for decompensated shock secondary to blood loss

Table 36-6. Disability: Assessment and Treatment

Assessment Priorities	Interventions
Level of consciousness	Maintain blood pressure and oxygenation and ventilation
AVPU scale or GCS	If head injury with GCS ≤9: RSI and intubate; head computed tomography, neurosurgical consult
	If normotensive, consider mannitol 0.25 g/kg
Pupil size and reactivity	Hyperventilate Pco_2 to 30-35 mm Hg with signs of hemiation
Extremity movement and tone	Stabilize spinal column
	If blunt cord trauma methylprednisolone sodium succinate (Solu-Medrol) 30 mm/kg IV bolus, then 5.4 mg/kg/hr for 23 hr IV
Posturing	Hyperventilate Pco_2 to 30-35 mm Hg
Reflexes	Assess for signs of respiratory failure

AVPU, alert, verbal, painful, unresponsive; GCS, Glasgow Coma Scale; RSI, rapid sequence intubation.

hemoglobin alone is unreliable because equilibration will not have occurred on presentation to the emergency department.[10]

Radiology

The most important "traditional" radiographs to obtain on moderately to severely injured children are of the chest and pelvis to assess for sites of blood loss or potential causes of shock. In stable, alert children without distracting injuries, the pelvic film may be eliminated. The radiographs of the cervical spine may be delayed until after further diagnostic studies are obtained, depending on the clinical presentation of the patient.

Other radiographs are obtained based on the physical examination. For patients sustaining minor trauma, no radiographs may be needed. Children younger than 2 years old with injuries consistent with child abuse need a skeletal survey, including skull, chest, abdomen, and long bone radiographs.

Secondary Survey

After performing the primary survey and correcting any detected abnormalities, the clinician proceeds with a careful complete assessment in an organized manner (Box 36-5). At this point, the past medical history may be obtained with regard to allergies, medications, past illnesses, and events preceding the injury.

Table 36-7. Exposure: Assessment and Treatment

Assessment Priorities	Interventions
Undress	Trauma examination including rectal examination
Look under collar and splints	
Log roll and examine back	
	Complete blood cell count, type and crossmatch, amylase, urinalysis, cervical spine, chest and pelvis radiographs, place urinary catheter and nasogastric or orogastric tube as indicated

SPECIFIC DISORDERS/INJURIES

Head Injury

Perspective

Head trauma is the leading cause of death among injured children and is responsible for 80% of all trauma deaths.[3] Each year, 29,000 children younger than 19 years old experience permanent disability from traumatic brain injury. Falls account for 37% of pediatric head injuries,[11] MVCs account for 18%,[12] pedestrian injuries account for 17%, and falls from bicycles account for 10%. On an age-related basis, infants and toddlers are more prone to falls from their own height, school-age children are involved in sports injuries and MVCs, and all ages are subject to the sequelae of abuse.

Principles of Disease

An important anatomic difference of a pediatric patient compared with an adult is that the cranial vault of a child is larger and heavier in proportion to the total body mass. This anatomic characteristic predisposes children, specifically toddlers and infants, to high degrees of torque that are generated by any forces along the cervical spine axis. Sutures within the pediatric skull are protective and detrimental to the outcome of head injury in these patients. Although the cranium may be more pliable relative to traumatic insult, forces are generated internally that predispose the pediatric patient to parenchymal injury in the absence of skull fractures. The pediatric brain is less myelinated, predisposing it to shearing forces and further injury.[3,13]

BOX 36-5. Tasks to be Completed after the Secondary Survey

- Complete head-to-toe examination
- Appropriate tetanus immunization
- Antibiotics as indicated
- Continued monitoring of vital signs
- Ensure urine output of 1 mL/kg/hr

Table 36-8. Emergent Management of Increased Intracranial Pressure

Therapy	Dose	Mechanism of Action
Head elevation (30 degrees)		Lowers intracranial venous pressure
Head in midline		Prevents jugular vein compression
Hyperventilation	Reduces $PaCO_2$ to 30-35 mm Hg	Promptly decreases cerebral blood volume and thus intracranial pressure
Mannitol	0.25-2 g/kg IV	Both agents effect rapid osmotic diuresis
or	0.5-2 g/kg IV	
Glycerol		
Pentobarbital	1-3 mg/kg (loading dose)	Thought to lower cerebral metabolism; also may have some effect on free radical formation
		Other barbiturates (phenobarbital) also have been used
Hypothermia (27° C-31° C)		Thought to decrease cerebral blood flow and metabolic rate; can cause cardiac dysrhythmias

Clinical Features

The clinician must obtain as many details surrounding the traumatic event as possible. The height of the fall or injury is particularly important with regard to the development of associated injury. Most children fall from their own height. Children involved in MVCs are best evaluated by the degree of restraint that was present during the time of the accident. An infant in a properly installed car seat is likely to have a good outcome in most cases. Unrestrained children involved in high-speed crashes are prone to serious injury. It is important to consider the quality of the surface at the point of impact, specifically the presence or absence of carpeting within the home or location of injury.

In most cases, it is important to establish whether there was loss of consciousness at the time of the injury event. With playground trauma, the history may be vague, and the interpretation of any change in consciousness of the child may be regarded as an actual loss of consciousness. The behavior of the child after the event should include questions related to the presence or absence of irritability, lethargy, abnormal gait, or alterations in behavior. Most importantly, establishment of a timeline from the point of insult is helpful in determining whether there have been changes in the mental status of the patient.

The prognostic significance of vomiting after pediatric head trauma is unclear. There is no adequate study defining an acceptable time frame in which vomiting after head injury is benign in nature. The development of seizures after head trauma, in contrast to vomiting, has been well studied.[13] A brief seizure that occurs immediately after the insult (with rapid return of normal level of consciousness) is commonly called an *impact seizure*. This seizure usually is not associated with intracranial parenchymal injury and does not mandate the institution of anticonvulsant therapy. Seizures that occur later (>20 minutes after the insult) portend the greater possibility of traumatic brain injury and the development of seizures at a later date. Patients who experience seizures later in the course of the post-traumatic event are best evaluated by the neurosurgical service. As in all instances of trauma, a careful history related to the possibility of substance abuse must be obtained.

The physical examination of a head-injured child must include strict attention to the ABCs of emergency care. Although internal injuries are important in the outcome of these patients, the maintenance of oxygenation and perfusion is paramount in eliminating further insult. Because the pediatric brain is sensitive to decreases in glucose, oxygen, and perfusion, their maintenance optimizes the chances of good recovery. Strict attention must be paid to the maintenance of euvolemia because cerebral perfusion pressure (CPP) is adequate only in the face of a normal mean arterial pressure (MAP). CPP is equal to the MAP minus the ICP (CPP = MAP − ICP). As the blood pressure is reduced, so is the CPP. Pediatric patients with any form of head injury should be evaluated and protected from cervical spine injury.

Several methods are available for evaluating head-injured patients, including AVPU and the GCS. The GCS has been modified for pediatric patients (see Table 36-2). Studies involving the reliability of the GCS in predicting the outcome in children with traumatic brain injury provide optimism compared with head-injured adults. In a study involving 80 children with traumatic brain injuries admitted to an intensive care unit (ICU), initial GCS scores were compared with eventual outcome.[14] ICU length of stay and time to cognition relative to GCS scores indicated that scores greater than or equal to 6 were associated with favorable outcomes and neurologic status. Although the number of patients in this study was small, the important message is that no matter how the patient presents neurologically, all efforts should be generated to ensure survival and maintain stable neurologic status in the emergency department.

Examining a brain-injured child involves cranial nerve testing, motor testing, and sensory testing. The evaluation of cranial nerve function is essentially no different from that of an adult. The most important aspect of motor and cranial nerve evaluation involves ruling out the presence of increased ICP. Common symptoms and signs of increased ICP in infants and children should be sought (Boxes 36-6 and 36-7).

Minor injury to the scalp of infants and children involves the development of three possible injury complexes. *Caput succedaneum* refers to injury to the connective tissue itself, *subgaleal hematoma* refers to injury to the tissue surrounding the skull, and *cephalhematoma* refers to a collection of blood under the periosteum.

Skull fractures in children occur in many different configurations.[11,13,15] Linear fractures, the most common

---

BOX 36-6. Common Symptoms and Signs of Increased Intracranial Pressure in Infants

- Full fontanel
- Split sutures
- Altered state of consciousness
- Paradoxical irritability
- Persistent emesis
- "Setting sun" sign (inability to open eyes fully)

BOX 36-7. Common Symptoms and Signs of Increased Intracranial Pressure in Children

- Headache
- Stiff neck
- Photophobia
- Altered state of consciousness
- Persistent emesis
- Cranial nerve involvement
- Papilledema
- Hypertension, bradycardia, and hypoventilation
- Decorticate or decerebrate posturing

type of skull fracture, rarely require therapy and often are associated with good outcomes. Factors favoring a poor outcome include the presence of the fracture overlying a vascular channel, a diastatic fracture, or a fracture that extends over the area of the middle meningeal artery. Diastatic fractures, or defects extending through suture lines, are different from linear fractures, in that leptomeningeal cysts (growing fractures) may develop at these sites. Fractures of the basilar portions of the occipital, temporal, sphenoid, or ethmoid bones commonly occur in children.[16] The presence of cerebrospinal fluid, rhinorrhea, and otorrhea has been associated with these injuries. Signs of basilar skull fractures in children are similar to signs in adults and include posterior auricular ecchymoses, or Battle's sign, and raccoon eyes, or the presence of periorbital subcutaneous bleeding.

Strictly speaking, *concussion* is defined as a brain insult with transient impairment of consciousness. Amnesia is often involved. Patients who sustain concussive insults have anorexia, vomiting, or pallor soon after the insult. This transitional period is followed by rapid recovery to baseline; if a CT scan of the head is obtained, it is most often normal. In contrast, contusions are often the result of coup and contrecoup forces at work. Contusions may not be associated with any loss of consciousness at the time of insult. Patients often present with associated symptoms, such as altered level of consciousness, severe headache, vomiting, or focal deficits on neurologic assessment. These injuries are clearly demonstrable on CT.

Traditional teaching regarding the development of epidural hematomas involves the typical triad of head injury followed by a lucid interval, followed by rapid deterioration as intracranial hemorrhage worsens. In contrast to epidural hematomas in adults, pediatric epidural hematomas may be the result of venous bleeding, which predisposes them to a subtle and more subacute presentation over days. In any event, epidural hematomas are associated with a high incidence of overlying skull fractures (60% to 80% of cases).

Special attention should be directed toward infants and toddlers to rule out the presence of subdural hematomas.[13] This clinical scenario is most often secondary to rupture of bridging veins and rarely is associated with the presence of overlying fractures (<30%). Subdural hematomas most commonly occur in patients younger than 2 years old, with 93% of cases involving children younger than 1 year old. Chronic subdural hematomas most often are encountered in patients who have been subjected to what has been termed the "shaken baby syndrome." This clinical complex involves forcible shaking of the child with acceleratory and deceleratory forces impacting the cranial vault. This syndrome is most often due to child abuse; 22% of abused children have central nervous system injuries. Patients present with nonspecific findings, such as vomiting, failure to thrive, change in level of consciousness, or seizures. Retinal hemorrhages are present in 75% of cases, and all patients should have careful funduscopic examinations to rule out the presence of these pathognomonic findings. Left to their own

development, the worst cases may manifest with signs of increased ICP. Retinal hemorrhages are not observed in children with mild to moderate trauma from other causes and are not associated with a prior history of cardiopulmonary resuscitation; the presence of retinal hemorrhages suggests child abuse.

Diagnostic Strategies and Management

As a basic rule, serial examinations are the most reliable indicators of clinical deterioration.[13,15] The presence of focality is a reliable indicator of a localized insult, whereas the absence of focality may be misleading. The signs of increased ICP usually develop late in the course of the process in infants. As in an adult, papilledema may require days to develop. The classic Cushing's response (bradycardia and hypertension) also is unreliable in children. If ICP elevation is suspected, emergency intervention must be immediately initiated (Box 36-8).

Most clinicians favor early and controlled intubation in pediatric patients with GCS scores that are deteriorating. Isolated head injury is uncommon; a careful search for other injury should be made using the principles of advanced trauma life support.

Herniation syndromes in children are similar to those in adults. Uncal herniation is suggested by the presence of a unilaterally dilated pupil, contralateral hemiplegia, and spontaneous hyperventilation. Small, sluggish pupils, decorticate posturing, and Cheyne-Stokes respirations characterize brainstem herniation. The final common pathway, brainstem herniation, presents with fixed and dilated pupils, flaccid muscle tone, and slow or apneic breathing. Management of suspected herniation is controlled hyperventilation. Clinical endpoints of hyperventilation are improved patient status or constriction of dilated pupils. Arterial blood gas determination is used to assess adequacy of hyperventilation with a target partial pressure of carbon dioxide (PCO_2) of 30 to 35 mm Hg. Excessive hyper-

---

BOX 36-8. Anatomic Differences in the Pediatric Cervical Spine

Relatively larger head size, resulting in greater flexion and extension injuries
Smaller neck muscle mass with ligamentous injuries more common than fractures
Increased flexibility of interspinous ligaments
Flatter facet joints with a more horizontal orientation
Incomplete ossification making interpretation of bony alignment difficult
Basilar odontoid synchondrosis fuses at 3-7 years of age
Apical odontoid epiphyses fuses at 5-7 years of age
Posterior arch of C1 fuses at 4 years of age
Anterior arch fuses at 7-10 years of age
Epiphyses of spinous process tips may mimic fractures
Increased preodontoid space 4-5 mm (3 mm in an adult)
Pseudosubluxation of C2 on C3 seen in 40% of children
Prevertebral space size may change because of variations with respiration

ventilation can result in excessive cerebral vasoconstriction and secondary brain injury; ventilation is started at an age-appropriate rate, then the rate is increased until pupillary constriction occurs.

Radiology

Skull Films

The role of skull films in the evaluation of pediatric patients was studied extensively before the advent of CT. The presence of a skull fracture on a plain radiograph does not predict the presence of underlying brain tissue damage. Previous studies have attempted to establish low and moderate risks for skull fractures on the basis of clinical presentations.[16,17] Low-risk groups include patients with a normal neurologic examination, with headache, dizziness, scalp lacerations, and the absence of baseline neurologic anomaly. Moderate-risk groups for skull fractures include patients with a history of a loss of consciousness or amnesia, a progressively worsening headache, age younger than 2 years, seizures, or protracted vomiting. Most clinicians agree that at present, firm indications for skull films alone include the skeletal survey involved with the evaluation of child abuse, establishment of a functioning ventricular peritoneal shunt, penetrating wounds of the scalp, or the suspicion of foreign bodies underlying scalp lacerations.

Computed Tomography of the Head

There has been a considerable amount of research on the indications and relative value of CT scanning in pediatric head-injured patients. A large study evaluated 185 children ages 2 to 17 years with loss of consciousness and GCS scores of 15 after mild head injury.[18] The children were grouped according to physical examination findings, neurologic status, and whether the head injury was isolated or nonisolated. Patients with obvious skull fractures were excluded. Two variables were highly associated with the presence of intracranial hemorrhage: the presenting neurologic status and presence of multiple injuries. None of the 49 neurologically normal children with isolated head injury had intracranial hemorrhages. All patients with intracranial hemorrhages were noted to have other traumatic insults on physical examination. The authors concluded that after isolated head injury with loss of consciousness, children older than 2 years of age who were neurologically normal may be discharged without a CT scan after careful physical examination alone.

Other studies contradict these findings, establishing a clear association with parenchymal injury and loss of consciousness.[19,20] At present, recommendations for CT scanning include the presence of neurologic deficits, GCS scores of less than 14, and injury patterns that are the result of major forcible insults. Children younger than 1 year of age are a special challenge to the clinician because their neurologic milestones are harder to evaluate. Within this age group, any loss of consciousness, protracted vomiting, irritability, poor feeding, or suspicion of abuse mandates CT scanning.

The evaluation of infants with minor closed head injury was studied in a series of 668 infants younger than 2 years who underwent CT scanning, in which a subset of 92 infants younger than 2 months old was scrutinized further. The presence of a significant scalp hematoma highly correlated with underlying parenchymal brain injury. The authors recommended CT scanning for these patients.[21]

Cervical Spine Injury

Perspective

In the United States, more than 1100 children sustain spinal injury annually, leading to an annual cost exceeding $4 billion.[22,23] Cervical injury patterns vary with the age of the patient. Fractures below the C3 level account for only 30% of spinal lesions in children younger than 8 years of age, which differs dramatically from the patterns seen in adults. Likewise, spinal cord injury (SCI) without radiographic abnormality has been found in 25% to 50% of spinal cord injuries in this same age group.[24-26]

Principles of Disease

Anatomic features of the cervical spine approach adult patterns between the ages of 8 and 10 years (see Box 36-8).[2] Injury patterns identical to those of adults are often not fully manifested, however, until age 15 years. The pediatric spine has greater elasticity of the supporting ligamentous structures than the adult spine. The joint capsules of the child have greater elastic properties, and the cartilaginous structures are less calcified than in adults. In the spine itself, there is a relatively more horizontal orientation of the facet joints and uncinate processes, and the anterior surfaces of the vertebral bodies have a more wedge-shaped appearance. Compared with adults, the child has relatively underdeveloped neck musculature and a head that is disproportionately large and heavy compared with the body. Both of these differences lead to an "anatomic fulcrum of the spine" in children that is at the level of the C2 and C3 vertebrae versus the lower cervical vertebrae as found in adults.[23]

Clinical Features

Any patient with severe multiple injuries should be considered to have a SCI until proved otherwise.[23] Likewise, significant head, neck, or back trauma and trauma associated with height, speed, MVCs, and falls from any height (especially falls with associated head injury) is suspicious for SCI and should be evaluated appropriately. The evaluation of a pediatric patient should begin with a primary survey to assess airway patency, ventilatory status, and perfusion. After initial evaluation and stabilization, the cervical region can be examined. Palpation of the neck for pain and bony deformity should be performed. Some factors, such as tenderness or pain with palpation, may be underappreciated, however, in a child who is not yet old enough to talk. Similarly, patients with head injury, decreased level of consciousness, intoxication, or distracting injury may not reliably localize pain in the cervical region, and spinal precautions should be maintained to avoid potential additional injury.

The neurologic examination in a pediatric patient can be difficult, but several factors should be evaluated in a patient with suspected cervical spine injury. Pain in the cervical region should raise suspicion of cervical spine injury. Likewise, paralysis, perceived paresthesias, ptosis, and priapism are neurologic signs highly correlated with spinal cord injuries. Finally, upper extremity positioning and function can help elucidate the presence and level of a SCI.

Several characteristic SCI syndromes can be diagnosed on initial emergency department evaluation.[22,24,25] Partial-cord syndrome is characterized by flaccid paralysis below the level of the spinal cord lesion, absent reflexes, decreased sympathetic tone, autonomic dysfunction with hypotension, and preservation of sensation. In complete-cord transection, all characteristics of partial-cord syndrome are present, and sensation is absent. Central-cord syndrome (seen commonly in extension injuries to the cervical spine) consists of decreased or absent upper extremity muscle tone with preservation of the lower extremity function at the level of the lesion. Anterior-cord syndrome (associated with flexion injuries to the cervical spine) is characterized by complete motor paralysis with loss of pain and temperature sensation; however, position and vibration sensation are preserved in this disorder. Finally, Brown-Séquard syndrome represents hemisection of the spinal cord with ipsilateral loss of motor function and proprioception. There is also contralateral loss of pain and temperature sensation. SCI syndromes are rare in children.

Radiology

Children with neck pain, involvement in an MVC, or any suspicion of cervical injury should receive radiographic evaluation; when present, these factors are 100% sensitive in identifying cervical spine injuries in this patient group.[25] Radiographic evaluation routinely should consist of three views: a cross-table lateral view, an anteroposterior view, and a Water's view to help visualize the odontoid process of C1. With these three plain film views of the cervical region, the sensitivity for detecting cervical fractures is 93%, and the specificity is 91%. The negative predictive value of these three views is 99%. Interpretation of plain cervical spine films in children may be challenging because of the anatomic changes that occur with growth (see Box 36-8). In addition, pseudosubluxation of C2 on C3 is common in children up to adolescence, occurring in approximately 40% of patients.[27] The emergency physician distinguishes between pseudosubluxation and true subluxation by the posterior cervical line or spinolaminar line, also called the *line of Swischuk*. A line is drawn from the anterior cortical margin of the spinous process of C1 down through the anterior cortical margin of C3. If this line at C2 crosses the anterior cortical margin of the spinous process at C2 or is off by less than 2 mm and no fractures are visualized, the

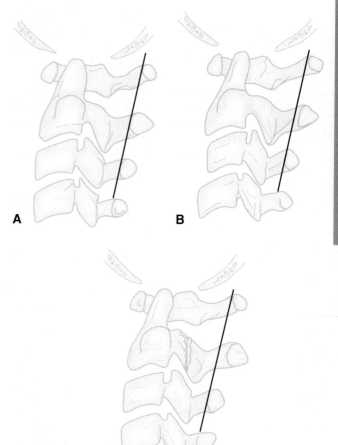

Figure 36-1. Posterior cervical line. Use only to access anterior displacement of C2 and C3. A line is drawn from the cortex of the spinous process of C1 to the cortex of the spinous process of C3, and the relationship of the spinous process of C2 is noted. **A,** Normal line passing through the cortex of C2. **B,** Normal line passing within 1.5 mm of the cortex of C2. **C,** Abnormal line passing greater than 2 mm anterior to the cortex of C2, suggesting underlying fracture of posterior elements of C2. (From American College of Emergency Physicians, American Academy of Pediatrics: APLS: The Pediatric Emergency Medicine Resource, 4th edition, Dallas, Elk Grove Village, IL, 2004, the College and the Academy.)

patient has pseudosubluxation versus true subluxation of the ligaments at that level (Figure 36-1).[28]

An important criterion for radiographic clearing of the cervical spine is complete visualization of all seven cervical vertebral bodies down to and including the C7-T1 interface. The predental space should not exceed 4 to 5 mm in children younger than 10 years old, and the prevertebral soft tissue space should not be greater than normal. The four cervical radiographic lines should be evaluated, and the atlanto-occipital alignment should be assessed for dislocation in this region. Other imaging modalities that can be used to delineate cervical fractures include thin-section CT and magnetic resonance imaging.

Management

There are two phases of SCI. Direct injury (initial phase) results in largely irreversible injury to the spinal cord. Indirect injury results from preventable or reversible injury to the spinal cord secondary to ischemia, hypoxemia, and tissue toxicity. Resuscitation of a patient with injury to the cervical spine should focus on prevention or minimization of the indirect causes of injury to the cervical spine. Management of the possible cervical injury should begin in the out-of-hospital phase of emergency treatment. Most injured children arrive at the emergency department with adequate immobilization. Some more recent evaluations of traditional cervical collars and rigid backboards have shown, however, less than adequate neutral positioning of pediatric patients related to their relatively large cranium in proportion to the rest of their body. Nevertheless, in the absence of modified backboards with cutouts for the occiput of the child, the child should be immobilized with stiff cervical collar, rigid backboard, and external fixation by means of head blocks, cloth tape, or straps to provide adequate precautions.

Breathing should be assessed to determine presence of hypoventilation. Patients with SCI may hypoventilate because of diminished diaphragmatic activity or intercostal muscle paralysis. Otherwise normal children held in a supine position have shown reduced ventilatory abilities as measured by the forced vital capacity. Head or chest injury or pulmonary compromise related to contusion, aspiration, or other causes likewise may contribute to relatively compromised ventilatory status. Supplemental oxygen should be given routinely, and ventilatory assistance by bag/valve/mask ventilation or definitive airway management should be considered in the presence of prolonged hypoventilation. Finally, circulatory status must be assessed because hypotension can be seen early in the traumatic patient and needs to be addressed promptly to prevent end-organ perfusion deficits. Hypotension can result from hypovolemia or be secondary to spinal shock. If the patient is hypotensive and is attempting to compensate for a lack of adequate volume, the normal response would be to increase the heart rate. Hypotension related to neurologic causes can occur in the presence of a relative bradycardia, however. In either case, fluid administration; chronotropic agents, such as atropine; and vasopressors, such as dopamine, may be required. Spinal shock remains a diagnosis of exclusion.

Any patient with definite SCI requires added precautions to ensure immobilization of the cervical spine. The use of intravenous steroids has been described in the neurosurgical literature, and steroids should be administered to decrease inflammatory infiltration and cord edema (see Table 36-8). Immediate evaluation by a spinal cord specialist should be sought. In the absence of such a specialist, the patient should be transported to a center with adequate facilities to care for spinal cord–injured patients.

Cardiothoracic Injury

Perspective

Most serious chest injuries in children (83%) are the result of blunt trauma.[6,29] Most result from MVCs with the remainder secondary to bicycle crashes. Isolated chest injury is a relatively infrequent occurrence when considering the typical mechanisms of blunt trauma in the pediatric patient. The presence of significant chest injury greatly enhances the potential for multisystem trauma mortality by a factor of 10. Sequelae of blunt injury include rib fractures and pulmonary contusion (50%), pneumothorax (20%), and hemothorax (10%).

Overall mortality is nearly equivalent for blunt versus penetrating trauma. Children subjected to penetrating trauma, in contrast to the injuries associated with blunt trauma, often die from the primary insult itself. Penetrating trauma accounts for only 15% of thoracic insults in children.[29-31] Nationwide use of firearms has resulted in an increasing incidence of penetrating trauma, often with children as victims. Specific clinical patterns should alert the clinician to the potential for concurrent abdominal and thoracic injury. Any patient with penetrating trauma at or below the level of the sixth rib falls into this category. Apparent isolated thoracic trauma does not exclude abdominal injury.

Principles of Disease

It is important to understand the physiology of pediatric respiration when considering the potential for early decompensation. Infants and young children are preferential diaphragm breathers, and any impairment of diaphragmatic mobility compromises ventilation. The presence of gastric distention elevates the diaphragm and severely lessens the vital capacity of a child. In addition, the particular types of muscle fibers involved in the diaphragm of infants and young children predispose to the sudden development of apnea when these muscles become fatigued. Most importantly, the presence of adequate oxygenation in a pediatric patient does not always ensure sufficiency of ventilation. It is important to rely on auscultatory and other physical findings rather than simple measurements of oximetry.

Infants and children are anatomically protected against blunt thoracic cage trauma because of the compliance of the rib cage.[32] Compressibility of the rib cage dissipates the force of impact, which lessens the likelihood of bony injury. These protective mechanisms also may mask fairly complex pediatric thoracic insults. The compliance of the rib cage allows significant injury to occur with little apparent external signs of trauma. Multiple rib fractures are a marker of serious injury in children, with child abuse being the most likely etiology and the mortality rate exceeding 40%. In addition, the pediatric mediastinum is mobile, which favors the development of rapid ventilatory and circulatory collapse in the presence of a tension pneumothorax.

Specific Disorders

Pneumothorax

The development of a traumatic pneumothorax commonly is associated with significant pulmonary injury.[29] In contrast to spontaneous pneumothoraces, these insults do not resolve spontaneously and often are associated with the presence of a hemothorax. Signs and symptoms include external evidence of chest trauma, such as abrasion, contusion, or ecchymoses; tachypnea; respiratory distress; hypoxemia; and chest pain. Decreased breath sounds may not be appreciated in children with pneumothoraces because of the wide transmission of breath sounds in the chest and upper abdomen.

Management of a simple pneumothorax noted on chest radiograph includes the placement of a large-caliber, laterally placed chest tube or close observation. Chest tube size can be estimated as four times the endotracheal tube size or can be found on a length-based resuscitation tape. Any patient with a pneumothorax who will be undergoing mechanical ventilation requires the placement of a chest tube. In the most conservative of scenarios—small (<20%), simple pneumothoraces that are not under tension in children who will not be mechanically ventilated—the children may be observed carefully for extended periods, with treatment of 100% oxygen supplementation and reassessment by repeat chest radiographs at selected intervals.

Open Pneumothorax. An open pneumothorax exists when the chest wall is injured sufficiently to allow bidirectional flow of air through the wound. The patient is unable to expand the lung because of equalization of pressures between the atmosphere and the chest cavity. Ventilation and oxygenation are severely impaired.

Management of an open pneumothorax is dictated by the size of the defect and the amount of respiratory compromise. Simple, small puncture wounds in a breathing patient may be treated by covering the chest wall defect with occlusive dressing, such as sterile petroleum gauze. An additional incision should be made for the placement of a thoracostomy tube. As in all cases, defects that are too large to seal adequately or patients who are severely impaired with regard to ventilation are candidates for intubation.

Tension Pneumothorax. Pulmonary air leaks that occur in a one-way valve arrangement favor the development of a tension pneumothorax. Increasing amounts of free air within the pleural cavity cause the mediastinal structures to shift toward the opposite side, compromising cardiac output. The final common pathway involves hypoxia, hypotension, and refractive shock. Most patients with tension pneumothoraces present with severe respiratory distress, decreased breath sounds, and a shift in the point of maximal cardiac impulse. In the worst scenario, the mediastinum shift forces contralateral tracheal deviation and distention of the neck veins. In pediatric patients, signs of tension pneumothorax are often subtle. A short neck and increased soft tissue may make detection of tracheal deviation difficult. The evaluation of pediatric patients for tension pneumothorax should consider skin signs and profound tachycardia suggesting shock. The emergency physician should consider the diagnosis of tension pneumothorax and, if detected or strongly suspected, should treat the patient immediately.

Without adequate decompression, circulatory collapse and hypotension occur.

Treatment for a tension pneumothorax involves rapid evacuation of the trapped air. In the out-of-hospital setting, treatment includes needle thoracostomy placed in the second intercostal space within the midclavicular line or possibly in the fourth intercostal space anterior to the axillary line (nipple line). The needle should be placed above the rib margin to avoid injuring the intercostal vessels. In the emergency department, definitive treatment involves the use of a large-caliber thoracostomy tube that favors drainage of the tension pneumothorax and any accompanying hemothorax.

Hemothorax

Significant bleeding may occur when injury is directed toward the intercostal, internal mammary vessels, or lung parenchyma. Without an upright chest film, it is difficult to quantify the degree of bleeding on plain radiographs. Development of a massive hemothorax is rare in children and is associated most often with severe impact, such as seen in high-velocity MVCs, falls from extreme heights, or use of high-powered firearms. These injuries must be evaluated and treated rapidly. Clinically, patients present with decreased breath sounds and dullness to percussion on the affected side. A pneumothorax may coexist with a hemothorax. The pediatric patient may present with early or late signs of hypovolemic shock.

Any alteration in cardiovascular sufficiency should be treated with rapid replacement of fluids with isotonic crystalloid solutions. The clinician also must prepare for transfusion with the institution of red blood cell replacement as necessary. Patients who present with profound shock may receive either type-specific or O-negative blood; crossmatched blood may be used for more stable patients. The amount of blood that is salvaged from the chest tube should be quantified to help determine the need for red blood cell replacement. Many centers have the capability to salvage blood from hemothoraces and reinfuse, using an autotransfuser. As in all cases of trauma, initial measurement of the hemoglobin is often unreliable for estimating the amount of blood loss because an adequate time interval for equilibration may not yet have passed.

The treatment of hemothorax includes a tube thoracostomy. The tube needs to be large enough to occupy most of the intercostal space and should be placed laterally and directed posteriorly. As in all interventions, repeat chest radiographs should be obtained to confirm positioning and document improvement in lung expansion. Indications for thoracotomy include evacuated blood volumes exceeding 10 to 15 mL/kg of blood, blood loss that exceeds 2 to 4 mL/kg/hr, or continued air leak. Emergency department thoracotomy is reserved for patients with penetrating trauma who deteriorate to cardiopulmonary failure despite maximal resuscitation in the out-of-hospital setting or emergency department. The emergency physician often is able to stabilize the patient with red blood cell replacement until surgical intervention is achieved.[33]

Pulmonary Contusion

Penetrating and blunt thoracic trauma may result in the development of a pulmonary contusion.[34] The compliance of the rib cage in children renders them susceptible to the development of pulmonary contusion even in the absence of external signs of chest trauma. Injury to capillary membranes allows the collection of blood within the interstitial spaces, resulting in hypoxia and respiratory distress. If bleeding is severe enough, oxygenation and ventilation are impaired. Initial chest radiographs may not show the classic findings of pulmonary consolidation. In addition, in the early stages of injury, blood gases may be normal.

Treatment of pulmonary contusions includes a careful evaluation for the presence of additional injuries because significant force is necessary to cause the contusion itself. Most patients may be treated with supplemental oxygen and close monitoring. Most pulmonary contusions resolve without sequelae. Rare cases are associated with the development of acute respiratory distress syndrome.

Traumatic Diaphragmatic Hernia

Children involved in MVCs who are wearing lap belts are predisposed to the development of diaphragmatic herniation.[31,35] Mechanisms of injury involve sudden increases in intra-abdominal pressure. Patients initially present in stable condition with the degree of respiratory distress directly proportional to the amount of abdominal contents that protrude into the pulmonary space. Presence of bruising, which is secondary to lap belt compression, should alert the clinician to the possibility of diaphragmatic hernia, other intra-abominal injuries (small bowel injury), and the possibility of associated thoracic spinal insults, such as Chance fractures.

Initial management for these patients involves placement of a nasogastric tube to decompress the stomach. In cases of severe respiratory distress, intubation is indicated. Surgery is required for repair of the injury.

Cardiac and Vascular Injuries

Injuries to the heart and large vessels are uncommon in children.[36-38] The most common traumatic cardiovascular injury sustained by children is myocardial contusion. Patients often present with chest wall tenderness or may have a complaint of generalized chest pain. Tachycardia is the most common finding. Elevation of myocardial enzymes may be diagnostic. Patients with myocardial contusions should be monitored closely for the development of dysrhythmias and impaired myocardial function; however, in most cases of myocardial contusion, there are no long-term sequelae. The most life-threatening scenario involving the cardiac structures is the development of cardiac tamponade. Extravasated blood fills the pericardial space and impairs cardiac filling during diastole. Tamponade is most often the result of a penetrating wound. Firearm insult often causes sudden death, and blunt trauma rarely results in the development of cardiac tamponade. Clinically, patients present with tachycardia, distant heart sounds, narrow pulse pressure, jugular venous distention, and pulsus paradoxus. In the scenario of profound hypovolemia, venous distention is absent. The final common pathway involves the development of pulseless electrical activity.

In cardiac and vascular injuries, the electrocardiogram may show anything from tachycardia with low voltage (pericardial tamponade) to findings consistent with acute myocardial infarction (ST segment elevation). In the subacute scenario, echocardiography often makes the diagnosis. Bedside transthoracic echocardiography defines the degree of pericardial effusion present and the significance of any diastolic dysfunction present. A simple single subxyphoid view provides the emergency physician with an excellent view of the pericardial sac and heart. Pericardiocentesis may be diagnostic and therapeutic. Definitive treatment involves drainage of the fluid from the pericardial sac. In certain situations, the amount of pericardial blood and clot necessitate the performance of a thoracotomy to evacuate the pericardium adequately.

Commotio Cordis. Commotio cordis is a disorder described in pediatric patients that results from sudden impact to the anterior chest wall (e.g., as seen in baseball injuries), which causes cessation of normal cardiac function.[39-41] The patient may have an immediate dysrhythmia or ventricular fibrillation that is refractory to resuscitation efforts. Significant morbidity and mortality are associated with this disorder, and although most recover completely, some patients require extended treatment with antiarrhythmic agents, cardiac pacemaker placement, inotropic agents, or intra-aortic balloon pumps. In patients with prolonged cardiac instability, cardiogenic shock and death are often frequent outcomes, despite maximal therapeutic interventions.[39,41]

Abdominal Injury

Perspective

Serious abdominal injury accounts for approximately 8% of admissions to pediatric trauma centers.[2] Abdominal trauma is the third leading cause of traumatic death in children after head and thoracic injuries. Abdominal trauma is the most common cause of unrecognized fatal injury in children. Pediatric abdominal trauma results from blunt causes in 85% of cases, and penetrating trauma accounts for the remaining 15%. Of patients presenting primarily for other associated injuries, 9% die from abdominal trauma associated with these injuries.

Blunt trauma related to MVCs causes more than 50% of abdominal injuries in children and is the most lethal. "Lap-belt" injury, including small bowel injury and Chance fractures, occurs in approximately 5% to 10% of restrained children involved in MVCs.[42-44] Another common cause of abdominal injury involves bicycle crashes. Handlebar injuries represent a serious cause of injury and subsequent hospitalization for the pediatric population, with patients requiring admission having a mean hospital stay greater than 3 weeks. Often the effects of bicycle injuries may not be seen on initial presentation, with the mean elapsed time to onset of symptoms being nearly 24 hours.

Sports-related injuries are another common cause of pediatric abdominal trauma. Sports-related injuries are associated most commonly with isolated organ injury as a result of a blow to the abdomen. At particular risk are the spleen, kidney, and intestinal tract in children.[43] Finally, significant abdominal injury occurs in only about 5% of child abuse cases, but it is the second most common cause of death in these cases, following deaths resulting from head injury.

Principles of Disease

The anatomy of the child lends special protection from some abdominal injury patterns and predisposes the child to other types of injuries in blunt and penetrating abdominal trauma.[45] Children have proportionally larger solid organs, less subcutaneous fat, and less protective abdominal musculature than adults and relatively more solid-organ injury from blunt and penetrating mechanisms. Children have relatively larger kidneys with fetal lobulations that predispose them to renal injury. Children also have a fairly flexible cartilaginous ribcage that allows for significant excursion of the lower chest wall, permitting compression of the internal organs. The combination of these factors provides the basis for the differences in abdominal injury patterns seen between children and adults.

Clinical Features

Pediatric patients with multiple injuries often present with blunt abdominal injury. In children, history is often limited, traditional signs of decompensation seen in adults are often not as evident, and physical examination can be difficult.[45] Subtle, early abdominal findings may be overlooked, leading to significant morbidity and mortality. The history and examination of young children who have sustained trauma is challenging because it may be difficult to know if the child hurts "all over" or has focal findings. The emergency physician may use distraction with toys, lights, or keys to get the child's mind off the examiner and onto the distraction; in this way, areas of tenderness may be located.

Signs and symptoms of abdominal injury in children include tachypnea from impaired diaphragmatic excursion, abdominal tenderness, ecchymoses, and signs of shock. Abdominal distention is a common nonspecific later finding, often the result of air swallowing subsequent to a painful event. Children with hepatic and splenic injuries may have trouble localizing their pain. Any abdominal tenderness on examination should prompt evaluation of the abdomen. Vomiting is usually a late sign or one associated with duodenal hematoma or traumatic pancreatitis. Signs of small bowel injury may be delayed and noted clinically only with serial examinations. Pelvic bone stability and a rectal examination looking for signs of urethral injury (rare) in boys or blood in the stool (girls and boys) need to be performed in all cases of serious trauma.

Even minor falls can result in significant splenic injury, but with only minimal findings on examination. Repeated examination, prolonged observation, and close attention to vital signs are warranted. Any child with a clinically suspicious abdominal examination should be evaluated further with additional radiologic and laboratory studies.

Diagnostic Strategies and Management

In patients with suspected abdominal injury or with mechanisms of possible injury, management and resuscitation must be rapid. Children, because of fear and pain, can compound the difficulties in the management of serious penetrating or blunt abdominal trauma. Children tend to distend the stomach greatly with ingested air, which can decrease the diaphragmatic excursion related to overdistention of the abdomen. This can compromise respiratory efforts, and early decompression via nasogastric or orogastric tube insertion should be considered. Children with a stable pelvis and who are not at risk of urethral trauma should have a urinary catheter inserted to decompress the bladder, evaluate for the presence of urinary retention, and examine for the presence of blood in the urine. Also, before any invasive evaluation of the abdomen, such as DPL, the bladder should be decompressed to prevent accidental laceration during the procedure.

Diaphragmatic Herniation

Acute diaphragmatic herniation secondary to trauma occurs from sudden compressive forces exerted over the abdomen causing an increase in the intra-abdominal pressure and resulting in tearing of the diaphragm. Most commonly, the herniation occurs over the left side and results from the lap-belt injury complex from restraint in a MVC. *Lap-belt injury complex* consists of bursting injury of solid or hollow viscera or disruption of the diaphragm or lumbar spine.[43] Lap-belt injury is characterized by ecchymosis across the abdomen and flanks.

Splenic Injury

Injuries to the spleen are the most common in pediatric abdominal trauma. Children involved in MVCs, sudden deceleration injuries, and contact sports–related injuries may sustain splenic trauma. Typical findings include left upper quadrant abdominal pain radiating to the left shoulder. The abdominal examination may show evidence for peritoneal irritation in the left upper quadrant of the abdomen. Patients may be hemodynamically stable or, after significant splenic rupture or laceration, may be persistently hypotensive or in fulminant cardiovascular collapse. All patients with suspected splenic injury should be evaluated by a surgeon. Stable patients may undergo CT for radiologic evaluation or a bedside ultrasound. Most often, with minor splenic trauma, bleeding is controlled spontaneously without operative intervention. In cases with a contained splenic subcapsular hematoma, bleeding may present days later. Patients with splenic injury should be admitted to the hospital for close observation and repeated examinations.

Liver Injury

The liver is the second most commonly injured solid organ in the pediatric patient with abdominal trauma. It is, however, the most common cause of lethal hemorrhage, carrying a mortality of 10% to 20% in severe liver injury. Mechanisms of injury causing splenic injury also may cause liver trauma. Tenderness on palpation of the right upper quadrant of the abdomen and the complaint of abdominal pain in this region or in the right shoulder are signs of possible liver injury. Patients managed conservatively often do well; however, patients who are initially treated as such but then go on to require delayed laparotomy often have significant morbidity and mortality. Close observation in the hospital, serial abdominal examinations, and serial hemoglobin are recommended.

Renal Injury

The kidney is less susceptible to trauma from forces applied to the anterior abdomen, but is often injured in a pediatric patient with multiple injuries.[46] Because this organ is retroperitoneal, signs and symptoms of kidney injury are often less obvious and more diffuse than signs and symptoms of other abdominal organ injuries. Often dull back pain, ecchymosis in the costovertebral region, and hematuria are the only clues to renal injury. Renal ultrasound and CT may be used in a stable patient to assess the degree of renal involvement.[47,48] Other organs, such as the pancreas and gastrointestinal tract, are less frequently injured in pediatric patients.

Penetrating Injury

Penetrating wounds to the abdomen usually require rapid evaluation by a surgeon and in some cases operative intervention. The role of DPL in the management of pediatric trauma is controversial. DPL provides the most rapid, objective evaluation of possible intraperitoneal injury. Patients who remain unstable despite fluid resuscitation may be candidates for DPL if they are too unstable for CT and there are multiple potential sites of blood loss. An important role for DPL is in the setting of an underlying small bowel injury. In some patients with small bowel injury, CT findings of free fluid may be ascribed improperly to underlying splenic bleeding. Finally, DPL may be considered in the operating room for patients undergoing emergent craniotomy, when adequate evaluation of the abdomen cannot take place because of the time urgency required for intervention for head injury.

Radiology

Because pediatric patients suffer more from injury to the spleen, liver, kidneys, and the gastrointestinal tract, CT of the abdomen can provide high sensitivity and specificity for identification of these injuries while being relatively noninvasive.[9] The necessity of using oral contrast media in CT has come under criticism because of delays in evaluation, difficulty with administration, and risk for aspiration.

Another useful procedure in an acutely traumatized pediatric patient is bedside abdominal ultrasound. When used by a properly trained emergency physician, ultrasonography can provide sensitive identification of intraperitoneal hemorrhage without invasive measures. Although radiologic evaluation can provide important diagnostic information in a pediatric patient with possible abdominal trauma, any patient with unstable vital signs should not be delayed in receiving operative intervention. Children with persistent or recurrent hypotension, continued abdominal pain, or persistent abdominal distention should have expedient evaluation by a surgeon.

DISPOSITION

The most important decision an emergency physician can make is whether to admit a pediatric trauma patient or transfer the patient to a tertiary care facility. The decision for admission should be based on consultation with the surgeon and the patient's primary care physician. Infants and children who are moderately to severely injured have improved outcomes in a pediatric ICU versus an adult ICU; the primary role of the emergency physician would be to evaluate and stabilize the patient before admission to a pediatric ICU or before transfer to a tertiary care facility. Before transport, it is vital that the child is appropriately stabilized and that the emergency physician communicates directly with the accepting physician at the transfer facility.

Indications for admission are many, but the main criterion is to admit patients requiring ongoing monitoring for deterioration or complications of their injuries. In addition, children with suspected physical injury from child abuse may be admitted for their protection and for medical treatment.

KEY CONCEPTS

- Trauma is the leading cause of death in children in the United States. It accounts for 64% of all deaths in children, totaling 1.5 million injuries per year and 250,000 hospitalizations annually.
- Proper management of a pediatric trauma patient involves most of the components of standard trauma protocols. By paying strict attention to the anatomic and physiologic differences in children, the clinician is assured of the best patient outcomes.
- The leading cause of traumatic shock in children is hypovolemia; management priorities include appropriate ventilation and oxygenation and fluid resuscitation to maintain perfusion.
- The diagnostic test of choice for the evaluation of intra-abdominal injury in a stable patient is CT of the abdomen.
- Controlled hyperventilation should be performed on children with signs of impending brain herniation, and Pco_2 levels should be maintained at 30 to 35 mm Hg to avoid secondary brain injury from excessive hyperventilation and subsequent cerebral vasoconstriction.

REFERENCES

1. Jaffe D: Emergency management of blunt trauma in children. *N Engl J Med* 324:1477, 1991.
2. Schafermeyer RW: Pediatric trauma. *Emerg Med Clin North Am* 11:187, 1993.
3. King DR: Trauma in infancy and childhood: Initial evaluation and management. *Pediatr Clin North Am* 32:1299, 1985.
4. Peclet MH, et al: Patterns of injury in children. *J Pediatr Surg* 25:85, 1990.
5. Sieben RL, Leavitt JD, French JH: Falls as childhood accidents: An increasing urban risk. *Pediatrics* 47:886, 1971.
6. Corey TS: Infant deaths due to unintentional injury: An 11-year autopsy review. *Am J Dis Child* 146:968, 1992.
7. Hodge D, Delgado-Paredes C, Fleisher G: Intraosseous infusion flow rates in hypovolemic "pediatric" dogs. *Ann Emerg Med* 16:305, 1987.
8. Furnival RA: Delayed diagnosis of injury in pediatric trauma. *Pediatrics* 98:56, 1996.
9. Meyer DM: Computed tomography in the evaluation of children with blunt abdominal trauma. *Ann Surg* 217:272, 1993.
10. Isaacman DJ: Utility of routine laboratory testing for detecting intra-abdominal injury (IAI) in the pediatric trauma patient. *Pediatrics* 92:691, 1993.
11. Lescholier I: Blunt trauma in children: Causes and outcomes of head vs extracranial injuries. *Pediatrics* 91:721, 1993.
12. Agran A, Dunkle DE: Motor vehicle occupant injuries to children in crash and noncrash events. *Pediatrics* 70:993, 1982.
13. Ghajar J: Management of pediatric head injury. *Pediatr Clin North Am* 39:1093, 1992.
14. Lieh-Lai MW: Limitations of the Glasgow Coma Scale in predicting outcome in children with traumatic brain injury. *J Pediatr* 120:195, 1992.
15. Hennes H: Clinical predictors of severe head trauma in children. *Am J Dis Child* 142:1045, 1988.
16. Kadish HA: Pediatric basilar skull fracture: Do children with normal neurologic findings and no intracranial injury require hospitalization? *Ann Emerg Med* 26:37, 1995.
17. Grove DL: Closed head injuries in children: Is hospital admission always necessary? *Pediatr Emerg Care* 11:86, 1995.
18. Davis RL: Cranial CT scans in children after minimal head injury with loss of consciousness. *Ann Emerg Med* 24:640, 1994.
19. Davis RL: The use of cranial CT scans in the triage of pediatric patients with mild head injuries. *Pediatrics* 95:345, 1995.
20. Livingston DH: The use of CT scanning to triage patients requiring admission following minimal head injury. *J Trauma* 31:483, 1991.
21. Greenes DS: Clinical indicators of intracranial injury in head-injured infants. *Pediatrics* 104:861, 2001.
22. Apple JS, et al: Cervical spine fractures and dislocations in children. *Pediatr Radiol* 17:45, 1987.
23. Chen LS, Blaw ME: Acute central cervical cord syndrome caused by minor trauma. *J Pediatr* 108:96, 1986.
24. Hadley MN, et al: Pediatric spinal trauma: Review of 122 cases of spinal cord and vertebral column injuries. *J Neurosurg* 68:18, 1988.
25. Hill SA, et al: Pediatric neck injuries: A clinical study. *J Neurosurg* 60:700, 1984.
26. Pang D, Wilberger JE: Spinal cord injury without radiographic abnormalities in children. *J Neurosurg* 57:114, 1982.
27. Cattell HS, Filtzer DL: Pseudosubluxation and other normal variations in the cervical spine in children. *J Bone Joint Surg Am* 47:1295, 1965.
28. Strange GR (ed): *APLS: The Pediatric Emergency Medicine Course.* Elk Grove Village, Ill, American Academy of Pediatrics and American College of Emergency Physicians, 1998.
29. Bender TM: Pediatric chest trauma. *J Thorac Imaging* 2:60, 1987.
30. Meller JL, Little AG, Shermeta DW: Thoracic trauma in children. *Pediatrics* 74:813, 1984.
31. Eichelberger MR: Trauma of the airway and thorax. *Pediatr Ann* 16:307, 1987.
32. Cooper A: Thoracic trauma. In Barkin RM (ed): *Pediatric Emergency Medicine: Concepts in Clinical Practice.* St Louis, Mosby, 1992.
33. Bonadio WA: Post-traumatic pulmonary contusion in children. *Ann Emerg Med* 18:1050, 1989.
34. Wiencek RG, Wilson RF, Steiger Z: Acute injuries of the diaphragm. *J Thorac Cardiovasc Surg* 92:989, 1986.
35. Eshel G: Cardiac injuries caused by blunt chest trauma in children. *Pediatr Emerg Care* 3:96, 1987.
36. Fishbone G, et al: Trauma to the thoracic aorta and great vessels. *Radiol Clin North Am* 11:543, 1973.
37. Tellez DW: Blunt cardiac injury in children. *J Pediatr Surg* 22:1123, 1987.
38. Abrunzo TJ: Commotio cordis: The single most common cause of traumatic death in youth baseball. *Am J Dis Child* 145:1279, 1991.
39. Maron BJ: Blunt impact to the chest leading to sudden death from cardiac arrest during sports activities. *N Engl J Med* 333:337, 1995.
40. Amerongen RV: Ventricular fibrillation following blunt chest trauma from a baseball. *Pediatr Emerg Care* 13:107, 1997.
41. Angran PF, Dunkle DE, Winn DG: Injuries to a sample of seat belted children evaluated and treated in a hospital emergency room. *J Trauma* 27:58, 1987.
42. Sivit CJ: Safety-belt injuries in children with lap-belt ecchymosis. *Am J Radiol* 157:111, 1991.
43. Sturm PF: Lumbar compression fractures secondary to lap-belt use in children. *J Pediatr Orthop* 15:521, 1995.
44. Saladino R: The spectrum of liver and spleen injuries in children: Failure of the PTS and clinical signs to predict isolated injuries. *Ann Emerg Med* 20:636, 1994.
45. Stalker HP: The significance of hematuria in children after blunt abdominal trauma. *Am J Radiol* 154:569, 1990.
46. Ablu-Jaude WA: Indicators of genitourinary tract injury or anomaly in cases of pediatric blunt trauma. *J Pediatr Surg* 31:86, 1996.
47. Bass DH: Investigation and management of blunt renal injuries in children. *J Pediatr Surg* 26:196, 1991.
48. Stein JP: Blunt renal trauma in the pediatric population: Indications for radiographic evaluation. *Urology* 44:406, 1994.

CHAPTER

37 Geriatric Trauma

Diane M. Birnbaumer

PERSPECTIVE

Background

At the beginning of the 21st century, nearly 13% of the population in the United States was older than 65 years, and by the year 2030 one in five people will be older than 65 years.[1] The financial impact of this aging has been tremendous; more than 35% of total health care dollars spent in the late 1990s was for medical care for patients older than 65 years.[1]

When it comes to trauma, elders (patients older than 65 years) account for only 10% to 14% of all victims, but they consume 25% to 33% of trauma-related health care dollars. Injury is the seventh leading cause of death in this age group because of a combination of physiologic changes that alter the older patient's response to trauma and injury mechanisms and patterns that are demographically different from those of younger trauma patients. Even among patients older than 65 years, risk stratification exists. Although the risk of death and significant injury is increased in patients 65 to 80 years of age, traumatized patients older than 80 years are four times more likely to die from their trauma than are younger patients.[2,3] Emergency practitioners must familiarize themselves with these differences among traumatized elder patients as well as understand the differences in resuscitation and stabilization of these patients.

Epidemiology

In younger patients, assault and motor vehicle crashes (MVCs) account for the vast majority of traumatic injuries. In elders, the most common cause of injury is falls, followed by MVCs, auto versus pedestrian incidents, and assaults.[4] In general, elder patients are more likely than younger patients to be injured as a result of activities of daily living.

Falls

Falls are the most common mechanism of injury in elders, accounting for 40% of trauma in patients older than 65 years. One third of elder patients suffer a significant fall each year, and serious injuries occur in up to one quarter. Risk factors for falls include sedative use, cognitive and visual impairment, history of stroke, and arthritis. Most falls occur at home and are same-level falls (i.e., falls from the standing position).

Because as many as a quarter of these falls occur as a result of an underlying medical problem,[5] it is critical that the cause of the fall be determined. An appropriate medical evaluation is indicated in addition to the trauma assessment and stabilization. Some of the medical causes of falls include strokes, syncope, near-syncope, medications, elder abuse, and hypovolemia (e.g., related to gastrointestinal bleeding, ruptured abdominal aortic aneurysm, or dehydration).

The most common injuries sustained in falls are fractures, occurring in 5% of fall victims.[6] Up to 10% of patients may sustain a major injury,[6] and head injury is the most concerning of these. Some studies have shown the incidence of trauma-related abnormalities on head computed tomography (CT) scans in this group of patients to be as high as 16%, with 1 in 50 requiring neurosurgery.[7] The most common abnormal head CT finding is a cerebral contusion, followed by subdural hematoma. The greater the height of the fall, the more likely the patient is to have an abnormal CT scan, but these injuries may also be seen in patients who suffer a same-level fall. Overall, the peri-injury mortality rate in elders from falls approaches 12%, and up to 50% die within a year of the fall,[6] often related to either recurrent falls or significant medical complications.

Motor Vehicle Crashes

MVCs are the second most common cause of trauma in elders, accounting for 20% to 59% of trauma in this age group.[8-11] Compared with younger patients, older drivers are more likely to be killed or hospitalized because of an MVC and are almost seven times more likely to be killed or hospitalized even when they are using seat belts.[10,11] Cognitive impairment, decreased hearing and vision, and slower reaction time are significant risk factors for MVCs

Most MVCs involving elders are daytime crashes occurring close to home. These crashes often occur at an intersection and usually involve two cars.[10] An elder is twice as likely as a younger person to be in an MVC when making a left-hand turn, and injuries sustained in these broadside crashes tend to be more severe. A single-vehicle crash should raise suspicion of a medical problem that may have caused the crash and requires a careful history, examination, and workup. MVCs in elders are less likely to involve alcohol, excessive speeds, or reckless driving than those involving younger patients. The overall fatality rate among elder MVC victims is as high as 21%.[10,11]

Auto Versus Pedestrian Incidents

The third most common cause of injury in elders is auto versus pedestrian incidents.[12] As with MVCs, poor eyesight and hearing as well as decreased mobility and longer reaction times make pedestrian elders more likely than younger patients to be hit by a motor vehicle. This mechanism accounts for 9% to 25% of trauma in elders and carries the highest fatality rate, reported to be from 30% to 55%.[13]

PRINCIPLES OF DISEASE

Physiology and Pathophysiology

Physiologic changes are inevitable with aging. These changes affect the mechanisms of trauma, types of injuries sustained, response to injury, approach to resuscitation, and prognosis for the injured elder patient.

Compared with younger patients, elders have a more severe injury response to any given trauma mechanism and have a decreased ability to respond to the trauma. In addition, preexisting medical problems may be exacerbated by the trauma, and morbidity and mortality may result from underlying diseases rather than the trauma itself.

Elders are more susceptible to trauma than their younger counterparts. Diminished hearing and sight increase the risk of falls, pedestrian injuries, and traffic collisions. Difficulty with gait and coordination because of impaired sensation and proprioception, muscle weakness, degenerative joint disease (DJD), neuromuscular disorders, and dementia lead to increased risk of falls and affect reaction times in pedestrians and MVCs. Finally, medications have a significant impact on the traumatized elder patient. Medications that may alter mental status (sedatives, antidepressants) make the elder patient more susceptible to traffic collisions and falls. Cardiac medications affect the response to hypovolemia and shock as well as resuscitation. Diuretics may lead to volume contraction and hypokalemia before the trauma occurs, and anticoagulants clearly affect the risk of bleeding. Many elder patients are taking these medications; one study of elder trauma patients showed that diuretics were taken by 50%, cardiac agents by 60%, psychotropic drugs by 38%, and anticoagulants by 17%.[14]

Cardiovascular System

Cardiovascular reserve decreases with age, and because the aging heart cannot easily increase cardiac output (the maximum achievable heart rate decreases with age), elders tend to respond to hypovolemia with increased systemic vascular resistance. In addition, they are less responsive to the increased circulating catecholamine response to shock, making them at risk for earlier decompensation from hypovolemia. Medications such as antihypertensives may affect their ability to increase systemic vascular resistance, and β-blockers, calcium channel blockers, and digoxin decrease their ability to develop a tachycardic response to shock. Underlying coronary artery disease increases the risk of myocardial ischemia from hypotension and blood loss. Overall, elders are less able to respond to fluctuations of blood pressure and blood volume that may accompany a traumatic injury than are younger patients.

Pulmonary System

Aging significantly affects the pulmonary system. Reductions in arterial partial pressure of oxygen (PaO_2), forced expiratory volume in 1 second (FEV_1), and vital capacity occur with aging; the lungs become less compliant; and the muscles of respiration weaken. As a result, elders are less tolerant of the volume resuscitation and spinal immobilization that are often needed in a trauma victim. In addition, the chest wall is more brittle because of osteoporosis and more rigid because of DJD, making injuries to the chest wall more likely in an elder patient. Combined with the decreased pulmonary reserve in elders, chest wall injuries may quickly lead to respiratory failure in this population of patients.

Central Nervous System

With aging, the dura mater adheres to the inside of the skull, making epidural hematomas more rare in elders. With age, the brain often atrophies, making it more mobile within the skull during trauma. This atrophy and the resultant stretching of the bridging veins seen in elders make them more susceptible to subdural hematomas than younger patients, even with seemingly minor injuries.

Skeletal System

Osteoporosis, a common condition in elders, is a significant risk factor for skeletal injuries such as compression fractures of the thoracic and lumbar spine and other injuries including hip and wrist fractures. These injuries may occur even with relatively minor trauma. Decreased mobility of the joints is also a problem, particularly in the spinal column. This limited mobility increases the risk of spinal injuries, and the locations of these injuries differ in the elder patient. Spinal stenosis, more common in elders than in younger patients, increases the risk of spinal cord damage even in the absence of spinal column injury.

SPECIFIC DISORDERS AND INJURIES

Perspective

Multiple trauma in the elder patient is more lethal than in younger patients; a multiply traumatized patient 70 years of age is three times more likely to die than a patient 20 years of age. The combination of comorbid illnesses, increased propensity to trauma, and decreased physiologic reserve often leads to exacerbation of underlying medical problems and a higher risk of multiple-system organ failure in the elder patient.[15,16]

Spinal Injuries

Physiologic changes with aging predispose the traumatized elder patient to both spinal column and spinal cord injury. DJD leads to decreased spinal mobility and a more brittle spinal column, and osteoporosis makes the bones more likely to fracture. Spinal stenosis increases the risk of cord injury even in the absence of a bone injury. Baseline cognitive impairment or acute brain injury may make evaluation of the spine in an elder trauma patient particularly difficult.

The most common mechanism of spinal injury in an older person is a fall.[17,18] Because of the relative immobility of the cervical spine related to DJD, the most common level of cervical spine injury in elders is C1 to C3,[19,20] a higher level than in younger patients. The most common fracture of the cervical spine in elders is a type 2 odontoid fracture,[19,20] which necessitates adequate visualization of this area of the cervical spine when imaging is performed. This may require CT scanning with reconstruction. Even if the patient does not suffer a fracture, spinal cord injuries may result from contusion of the cord. Contusion occurs most frequently in hyperextension injuries leading to central cord syndrome (upper extremity greater than lower extremity weakness and sensory loss). Overall mortality from cervical spinal injuries in elders is about 25%.[17] Compression fractures of the thoracic and lumbar spine commonly occur with falls, particularly in elder women with osteoporosis. Although spinal cord injuries are relatively rare with these fractures, disability from pain can be significant, and these patients may need admission for adequate pain control. It may also be necessary to differentiate compression fractures from burst fractures, and CT may be useful to make this distinction.

Head Injuries

Head injuries are the most common cause of mortality in elder trauma patients. The most common mechanism of significant head injury in elders is falls. Epidural hematomas are rare because of the adherence of the dura mater to the inside of the skull. Cerebral contusions, however, occur in up to one third of head-injured elder patients, and subdural hematomas become more common with age because of the stretching of the fragile bridging veins as the brain atrophies. This atrophied brain is more mobile within the skull, and head trauma may result in shearing of these veins. These patients may present with a broad range of symptoms, from frank coma to a relatively remote history of head trauma and slightly altered mental status.

Mortality from head injury is high in elders, and mortality from subdural hematoma in elders is four times higher than in younger patients. Only one in five elder patients with acute subdural hematomas survive to discharge.[21]

Head CT scanning is the diagnostic test of choice for brain injury, and a contrast study may be necessary if the injury is 7 to 20 days old and an isodense subdural hematoma is suspected.

Chest Injuries

Rigidity of the chest wall related to DJD and osteoporosis makes chest wall injuries more common in elders, even with relatively minor trauma. Because of the frailty of the chest in these patients, lap and shoulder belts in automobiles may actually cause injuries, including multiple rib fractures, flail chest, and sternal fractures. Rib fractures are the most common, and because elders have less pulmonary reserve than younger patients, they are more susceptible to respiratory insufficiency. They more frequently develop respiratory failure from their trauma and are more likely to require mechanical ventilation. In addition, elders may develop atelectasis, pneumonia, and acute respiratory distress syndrome. With proper care (including pain medication), meticulous attention to pulmonary hygiene, and careful hemodynamic management and monitoring, up to 90% of patients with chest injuries may return to normal life after their injuries.

Abdominal Injuries

Up to 30% of elder trauma patients may suffer a significant intra-abdominal injury, but the abdominal examination may be unreliable in these patients. Because mortality from abdominal injuries in elders is four to five times higher than in younger patients, a diligent search for potential intra-abdominal injuries is crucial. Often this requires CT scanning (in the stable patient) or ultrasonography. If the ultrasound study is inclusive or difficult, diagnostic peritoneal lavage can be used. The overall mortality is 27% in elder patients with intra-abdominal injuries.

Extremity Injuries

Because of the increased bone fragility and predisposition to falls with aging, the musculoskeletal system is the most commonly injured organ system in elder trauma patients. By the age of 75 years, 30% to 70% of patients with osteoporosis sustain a fracture. Although rarely life threatening, these injuries can severely limit the daily activities of elder patients to the degree that these patients may need admission for pain control as well as to arrange adequate home support.

Upper extremity fractures are common. Distal radial fractures are the most common upper extremity fractures in elders, accounting for up to 50% of fractures, followed by proximal humeral fractures (30%) and elbow injuries (radial head fractures and elbow dislocations) (15%).

Pelvic fractures are common in elder trauma patients, accounting for 25% of these injuries.[22] Pubic rami fractures, the most common pelvic fractures in this age group, may be seen with same-level falls. Although these injuries tend to be stable, pain control and gait training may necessitate hospitalization. High-velocity injury mechanisms (MVCs or auto versus pedestrian incidents) and falls from heights may result in unstable pelvic fractures, which are associated with a mortality of up to 80% if the fracture is open.[22]

Hip fractures are the most frequent lower extremity fractures and the most common cause of admission in elder trauma patients. These injuries are associated with an early mortality rate of 5% and a risk of death of 13% to 30% during the year after the injury (often related to other factors such as recurrent falls and underlying medical problems).[23] Plain films are often diagnostic, but CT or magnetic resonance imaging (MRI) scanning may be necessary to pick up subtle fractures in the elder patient with hip pain after a fall.

Tibial plateau fractures may occur with a fall or MVC and most commonly involve the lateral tibial plateau. Patellar fractures may result from a fall directly onto the kneecap, and sunrise views of the patella may be the only way to visualize these injuries. Ankle fractures account for 25% of all lower extremity fractures and most commonly involve the lateral malleolus; treatment often consists of a walking cast.

Soft Tissue Injuries

Elder patients are susceptible to skin injuries related to the thinning of the skin that occurs with aging. Treatment of these injuries often proves to be difficult, and débridement of devitalized tissue and careful local care are often necessary. Elder patients frequently are not up to date with their tetanus immunizations and are at risk for developing this infection. Treatment with both active and passive immunization is often indicated in this group.

Burns

Burns are particularly devastating in the elder patient. More than 90% of burns occur at home, and, as elder patients often live alone and have decreased reaction times, deeper and more extensive burns may occur in this age group. Flame burns account for 50% of all burns in this group and 20% of burn-related deaths. Some of these injuries are cooking related; scalds account for 19% and flammable liquid burns for 10%. Despite the fact that the incidence of burns is lower in elders than in younger patients, mortality from this injury is very high. Until the mid-1980s, Baux's formula (risk of mortality = age in years + percent body surface area burned)[24] provided a gross estimate of risk of death from burns, and although advances in burn care over the past two decades have decreased the mortality rate, elders are still at high risk for mortality from burns.[24] Thinning of the skin and decreased immunocompetence contribute to this higher risk of mortality as well as exacerbation of underlying medical conditions that the stress of an extensive burn injury and its treatment may precipitate.

CLINICAL FEATURES

Because elder patients may have significant injuries with subtle findings, a thorough examination supplemented by laboratory testing and radiographic studies is often the most prudent approach to even seemingly minor injuries, depending on the mechanism of injury.

History

A complete history of the events leading to the injury is needed and out-of-hospital personnel can be invaluable in providing this information. Falls and single-vehicle MVCs should trigger questioning about possible syncope, hypovolemia, cardiovascular or cerebrovascular events, or a complication of medications. The mechanism of injury itself should be considered and the different patterns of injury in elder patients evaluated (e.g., higher risk for subdural hematoma, high cervical spine injury, bone injuries).

Physical Examination

In patients with anything more than the most minor of mechanisms of injury, a thorough head-to-toe examination should be performed. Vital signs may be normal, even in the presence of significant blood loss. It is important to keep elder trauma patients warm, as they are more likely to develop hypothermia when disrobed for examination, and hypothermia increases the risk of mortality related to trauma.

DIAGNOSTIC STRATEGIES

Laboratory

Laboratory evaluation should include serial hemoglobin, hematocrit, or both; prothrombin time and partial prothromboplastin time; serum electrolytes; rapid and formal glucose measurements; and medication levels if indicated. An electrocardiogram is also useful to evaluate the patient for a precipitating event as well as to assess any cardiac ischemia that may be caused by the trauma and resultant injuries.

Radiology

Radiographic studies should be ordered as indicated by the history and physical examination. Plain films of the cervical spine are often difficult to interpret because of baseline DJD; therefore, CT scans of the neck, with particular attention to the more likely injured higher cervical spine, may be necessary to rule out spinal injury, notably if clinical findings warrant and plain films are inadequate or demonstrate suspicious areas. Plain films of the thoracic and lumbar spine should be obtained in patients with post-traumatic pain in these areas. A chest radiograph may be of particular importance both to evaluate the patient for traumatic injuries and to look for signs of congestive heart failure precipitated by the trauma or resuscitation efforts. Abdominal imaging may include CT scanning or abdominal ultrasonography to rule out significant intra-abdominal injury. Plain films of the pelvis are indicated in patients with suggestive mechanisms of injury or pain on examination of the pelvis. Extremity films should include all areas of concern, and CT or MRI scanning or bone scanning may be necessary to diagnose subtle hip fractures.

MANAGEMENT

Prehospital Considerations

Because elder patients may have significant injuries even with minor mechanisms of injury, prehospital management is particularly important. Scene assessment is important because prehospital personnel are often the "eyes and ears" for assessing the mechanism of injury and communicating this vital information. Rapid transport to the hospital is of prime importance. Because elder trauma patients are more likely to suffer significant injuries after even relatively minor events, the American College of Surgeons recommends that trauma patients older than 55 years be taken to trauma centers.

Emergency Department

Emergency department assessment of elder patients requires an organized and rapid evaluation for significant injuries and frequent reassessment to identify deterioration. Frequent monitoring of vital signs and maintaining a normal core temperature are important in the management of elder trauma patients.

Airway and Breathing

Supplemental oxygen should be administered to all elder trauma patients. Pulmonary insufficiency may develop quickly, and airway management equipment must be readily available. Airway management may be particularly difficult in elders, and potential problems should be anticipated. Cachectic or edentulous patients may be difficult to ventilate with bag, valve, and mask. Decreased mouth opening and limited neck mobility related to DJD may interfere with orotracheal intubation, and preexisting medical problems such as cerebrovascular accidents or renal failure may alter the choice of neuromuscular blocking agents used to facilitate intubation. Dosing of any agent that may affect cardiovascular stability must be carefully considered, and lower doses of these drugs may be prudent.

Circulation

Fluid and blood resuscitation is particularly challenging in the elder trauma patient. Underlying coronary artery disease or congestive heart failure may be exacerbated by aggressive circulatory resuscitation, but hypotension and hypovolemia are poorly tolerated and patients who go to the operating room before hemodynamic stabilization have an extremely high mortality rate. The most prudent approach is controlled boluses of warmed isotonic fluids with frequent assessment of physical examination, vital signs, pulse oximetry, and urine output. Hypotension is often an ominous finding and should be corrected, with attention to the potential effects of large fluid volumes on the respiratory system. Blood transfusion should be strongly considered when the hematocrit drops below 30, and there should be a diligent search for potential sites of blood loss.

Disability

Underlying hearing deficits and residual neurologic deficits from stroke, such as aphasia, motor deficit, or slurred speech, can make assessment of mental status and evaluation for neurologic injury problematic. Information on previous history of deafness or stroke or other neurologic disease should be obtained quickly from the patient or family, or both, and an assessment made of whether the patient's current condition represents new or old injury.

DISPOSITION

Typical criteria for admission related to traumatic injuries apply in elders, but other considerations often lower the threshold for hospitalization. If the patient does not have a support system or home situation amenable to careful observation and recovery from even relatively minor injuries, hospital admission may be required. Patients with significant underlying diseases may need admission until their injuries begin to heal. Often elder patients may need admission for pain control, particularly those with compression fractures of the spine who require high doses of narcotics for pain control. The use of narcotics can have additional adverse effects for elders that may put them at risk for additional injury, such as postural hypotension or confusion. Chest injuries may be particularly problematic and susceptible to complications, and elder patients with multiple rib fractures (three or more) or one or more displaced rib fractures should be admitted for aggressive pain management and supportive care. Elders with minor injuries, particularly extremity injuries, may be discharged with appropriate follow-up care and medications.

KEY CONCEPTS

- Elder patients are more susceptible to injuries than younger patients and have a higher mortality rate for any given injury.
- Mechanisms of injury are different in elders than in younger patients. Elder patients are more likely to sustain their injury from a fall, an MVC, or an auto versus pedestrian incident than from an assault.
- Physiologic changes that occur with aging alter the way in which these patients may manifest significant injuries as well as how they tolerate these injuries.
- Emergency physicians must remember that elder trauma patients may have suffered a medical event that precipitated their trauma and evaluate patients accordingly.
- Resuscitation of elder trauma patients requires oxygen supplementation, a lower threshold for advanced airway control (endotracheal intubation), and aggressive but judicious fluid and blood resuscitation with frequent reevaluation.

REFERENCES

1. U.S. Bureau of the Census: *The 65 Years and Over Population: 2000. Census 2000 Brief.* Washington, DC, Government Printing Office, 2000.
2. Knudson MM, et al: Mortality factors in geriatric blunt trauma patients. *Arch Surg* 129:448, 1994.
3. Tornetta P, et al: Morbidity and mortality in elderly trauma patients. *J Trauma* 46:702, 1999.
4. Santora TA, Schinco MA, Troskin SZ: Management of trauma in the elderly patient. *Surg Clin North Am* 74:163, 1994.
5. Kannus P, Parkkari J, Koskinen S: Fall-induced injuries and deaths among older adults. *JAMA* 281:1895, 1999.
6. Helling TS, et al: Low falls: An underappreciated mechanism of injury. *J Trauma* 46:453, 1999.
7. Rozzelle C, Wofforde JL, Branch CL: Predictors of hospital mortality in older patients with subdural hematoma. *J Am Geriatr Soc* 43:240, 1995.
8. Day RJ, Vinen J, Hewitt-Falls E: Major trauma outcomes in the elderly. *Med J Aust* 160:675, 1994.
9. Carrillo EH, et al: Long-term outcome of blunt trauma care in the elderly. *Surg Gynecol Obstet* 176:559, 1993.
10. Cook LJ, et al: Motor vehicle crash characteristics and medical outcomes among older drivers in Utah, 1992-1995. *Ann Emerg Med* 35:585, 2000.
11. Rehm CG, Ross SE: Elderly drivers involved in road crashes: A profile. *Am Surg* 61:435, 1995.
12. Kong LB, et al: Pedestrian-motor vehicle trauma: An analysis of injury profiles by age. *J Am Coll Surg* 182:17, 1996.
13. Schiller WR, Knox R, Chleborad W: A five-year experience with severe injuries in elderly patients. *Accid Anal Prev* 27:167, 1995.
14. Sartoretti C, et al: Comorbid conditions in old patients with femur fractures. *J Trauma* 43:570, 1997.
15. Hoyert DL, Kochanek KD, Murphy SL: Deaths: Final data for 1997, National Vital Statistics Reports from the Centers for Disease Control and Prevention. Available at: http://www.cdc.gov/nchs/pressroom/99facts/97mortal.htm
16. Zietlow SP, et al: Multisystem geriatric trauma. *J Trauma* 37:985, 1994.
17. Lieberman IH, Webb JK: Cervical spine injuries in the elderly. *J Bone Joint Surg Br* 76:877, 1994.
18. Spivak JM, et al: Cervical spine injuries in patients 65 and older. *Spine* 19:2302, 1994.
19. Mower WR, et al: Odontoid fractures following blunt trauma. *Emerg Radiol* 7:3, 2000.
20. Mann EA, et al: Improving the imaging diagnosis of cervical spine injury in the very elderly: Implications of the epidemiology of injury. *Emerg Radiol* 7:36, 2000.
21. Pennings JL, et al: Survival after severe brain injury in the aged. *Arch Surg* 128:787, 1993.
22. Alost T, Waldrop RD: Profile of geriatric pelvic fractures presenting to the emergency department. *Am J Emerg Med* 15:576, 1997.
23. Keil DP, et al: The outcomes of patients newly admitted to nursing homes after hip fractures. *Am J Public Health* 84:1281, 1994.
24. Ryan CM, et al: Objective estimates of the probability of death from burn injuries. *N Engl J Med* 338:362, 1998.

Section II SYSTEM INJURIES

CHAPTER

38   Head

William G. Heegaard and Michelle H. Biros

PERSPECTIVE

Epidemiology

Each year, more than 1.1 million patients in the United States undergo emergency evaluation for acute head injury.[1] The highest rates occur in children younger than 5 years old and persons older than 85 years. Eighty percent sustain minor head trauma (Glasgow Coma Scale [GCS] score of 14 to 15); 10% have moderate head injuries (GCS of 9 to 13); and 10% have severe head injuries (GCS of 8 or less). Almost 20% are hospitalized, and approximately 200,000 die or are permanently disabled because of their injury.[2,3]

Head injury is the leading cause of traumatic death in patients younger than 25 years and accounts for nearly one third of all trauma deaths.[4] Head injury from child abuse is common and estimated to represent up to two thirds of cases in the 0- to 4-year-old age group.[5] From 1989 to 1998, for all ages the leading causes of head injury deaths were firearm related (40%), motor vehicle related (34%), and fall related (10%). Head injury death rates declined by 11.4% during the period 1989 to 1998.[2]

Traumatic Brain Injury

The emergency physician sees patients with head injuries of different levels of clinical severity caused by a variety of mechanisms. External physical signs of head trauma only confirm that injury has occurred; they are not always present in the patient who has sustained serious underlying traumatic brain injury (TBI). The ultimate survival and neurologic outcome of the head trauma patient depend on the extent of TBI occurring at the time of injury, alone or in combination with secondary systemic insults that worsen the resulting neurochemical and neuroanatomic pathophysiology.

PRINCIPLES OF DISEASE

Anatomy and Physiology

Scalp and Cranium

The scalp consists of five tissue layers. The dermis is the outermost layer and is among the thickest layers of skin on the body. The underlying subcutaneous tissue contains the hair follicles and the rich blood supply of the scalp. The large blood vessels of the scalp do not fully constrict if they are lacerated and can be the source of significant blood loss. The middle scalp layer is the galea, which is made of tough fascial tissue. It contains the occipitofrontalis and temporoparietalis muscles, which move the scalp backward and forward, elevate the eyebrows, and wrinkle the forehead. Under the galea is a loose areolar tissue layer. Because the areolar attachments to the rest of the scalp are loose, scalp avulsions frequently occur through this layer. This is also the site for development of subgaleal hematomas, which can become quite large because blood easily dissects through the loose areolar tissue. The deepest layer of the scalp, the pericranium, is firmly adhered to the skull itself.

The skull comprises the frontal, ethmoid, sphenoid, and occipital bones and two parietal and two temporal bones. The unique layered architecture of the bones of the skull enhances its strength. Each bone consists of solid inner and outer layers, separated by a layer of cancellous bone tissue (the diploë). In adults the bones of the skull average between 2 and 6 mm in thickness; the bones in the temporal region are usually the thinnest of the skull.[6] The cranial bones form a smooth outer surface of the skull, but within the cranial vault are many bone protrusions and ridges. Contrecoup injuries and contusions far from the site of head impact often occur as the accelerating brain strikes against these uneven bone surfaces.

The inner aspect of the skull is lined with the periosteal dura, which is a thick connective tissue layer that adheres closely to the bone surface. The inner meningeal layer of the dura is the outermost covering of the brain. This dural membrane reflects back on itself to make folds within the cranial space. These folds serve to protect and compartmentalize different components of the brain. The midline falx cerebri separates the two cerebral hemispheres from each other. The tentorium cerebelli partitions the cerebellum and brainstem from the cerebral hemispheres. The U-shaped free margin of this dural fold is important in the pathology of the transtentorial herniation syndromes that can complicate severe head injury. Within the margins of the dural reflections, the two dural layers separate to form large dural venous sinuses. Injury to the dural sinuses is associated with significant morbidity and mortality because of the potential for uncontrolled hemorrhage and the difficulty in repairing these structures.

The cranial vault is rigid and nonexpandable, with an average volume in adults of about 1900 mL.[7] Cranial contents exit or enter the skull through many foramina. The largest, the foramen magnum, is the site of exit of the brainstem and spinal cord from the cranium.

Brain and Cerebrospinal Fluid

The brain is a semisolid structure, which weighs about 1400 g (3 lb) and occupies about 80% of the cranial vault.[7] It is covered by three distinct membranes: the meningeal dura, the arachnoid layer, and the pia. The location of traumatic hematomas relative to these membranes defines the pathologic condition and determines the consequences of the injury.

The major divisions of the brain are the cerebrum, cerebellum, and brainstem. Each lobe of the cerebrum is the source of highly specific neurobehavior, and specific injury to each lobe can disrupt normal behavior patterns. The brain is suspended in the cerebrospinal fluid (CSF), which provides some buffering for the brain during trauma. CSF is produced by the choroid plexus, located primarily in the lateral ventricles of the brain. CSF passes from the ventricular system into the subarachnoid space that surrounds the brain and spinal cord. CSF provides a fluid pathway for delivery of substances to brain cells, elimination of the products of brain metabolism, and transport of peptide hormones and hormone-stimulating proteins from their site of production within the central nervous system (CNS) to their peripheral sites of action.

The normal pressure exerted by the CSF is 65 to 195 mm H_2O or 5 to 15 mm Hg. Blood within the ventricles can obstruct the flow of CSF, causing a traumatic hydrocephalus. Brain injury and its complications can also alter the pH of CSF. Because the pH of the CSF influences pulmonary drive and cerebral blood flow (CBF), any alteration can produce detrimental neurophysiologic consequences.[7]

Cerebral Hemodynamics

Blood-Brain Barrier. The blood-brain barrier (BBB) maintains the microenvironment of the brain tissue. Extracellular ion and neurotransmitter concentrations are regulated by movement across this barrier. When the BBB is intact, the ability of neuroactive drugs to penetrate into the brain tissue usually depends on their lipid solubility. Posttraumatic cerebral edema and possibly the biomechanics of the injury itself can cause a prolonged disruption of the BBB for up to several hours after trauma.[8,9] Prolonged disruption of the BBB contributes to the development of posttraumatic vasogenic cerebral edema.

The brain has an extremely high metabolic rate, using approximately 20% of the entire oxygen volume consumed by the body. To provide for its high metabolic demands, the brain requires about 15% of the total cardiac output. Optimal regional CBF is maintained by the ability of cerebral vessels to alter their diameter in response to changing physiologic conditions.[9] Hypertension, alkalosis, and hypocarbia promote cerebral vasoconstriction; hypotension, acidosis, and hypercarbia cause cerebral vasodilation. In the normal brain, CBF is maintained at constant levels with a mean arterial pressure (MAP) of 60 to 150 mm Hg. This is referred to as *autoregulation*. Outside this range, the CBF varies linearly with MAP.

Cerebral vasoactivity is very sensitive to changes in systemic carbon dioxide and oxygen partial pressures (PCO_2, PO_2). The response to changes in PCO_2 is nearly linear between PCO_2 values of 20 and 60 mm Hg.[10] In this range, lowering PCO_2 by as little as 1 mm Hg decreases the diameter of cerebral vessels by 2% to 3%, which corresponds to an overall change in CBF of 1.1 mL per 100 g of tissue per minute. The physiologic response of blood vessels to PCO_2 is the rationale for the acute use of hyperventilation to control increased intracranial pressure (ICP) after head injury. As PCO_2 decreases with hyperventilation, cerebral vasoconstriction usually occurs. As a result, the volume of blood per unit area of brain tissue decreases. This decrease (even if small) may buffer the effects of increasing edema or an expanding hematoma within the rigid cranial vault. The vasoconstriction produced by

extreme changes in PCO_2 (20 mm Hg or less) can be so pronounced that some areas of brain experience ischemia; subsequently, tissue hypoxia can occur.[9,11,12] Therefore, hyperventilation must be controlled and monitored, with a goal of maintaining the PCO_2 between 30 and 35 mm Hg[11,12] and reserved for patients who are showing signs of acute herniation. Over time, injured vessels may lose their responsiveness to hyperventilation-induced hypocarbia and become vasodilated. Blood may then be shunted to the injured area, resulting in increased brain swelling and mass effect. Prolonged (i.e., beyond the acute resuscitation) or prophylactic hyperventilation is therefore not recommended as a treatment for increased ICP, and hyperventilation is not used for the routine management of head-injured patients with no signs of increased ICP.[11,12] The neurologic effects of hypocapnia are illustrated in Figure 38-1.

The cerebral vessels also respond to changes in PO_2. As PO_2 declines, cerebral vessels dilate to ensure adequate oxygen delivery to brain tissue.[10] When brain injury has occurred, increased CBF in the presence of

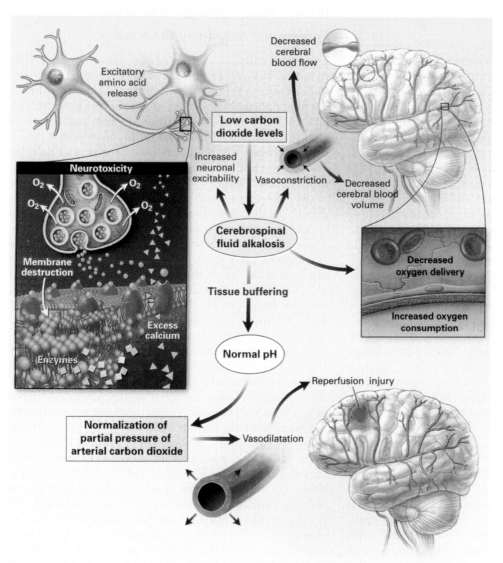

Figure 38-1. Neurologic effects of hypocapnia. Systemic hypocapnia results in cerebrospinal fluid alkalosis, which decreases cerebral blood flow, cerebral oxygen delivery, and to a lesser extent cerebral blood volume. The reduction in intracranial pressure may be lifesaving in patients in whom the pressure is severely elevated. However, hypocapnia-induced brain ischemia may occur because of vasoconstriction (impairing cerebral perfusion), reduced oxygen release from hemoglobin, and increased neuronal excitability, with the possible release of excitotoxins such as glutamate. Over time, cerebrospinal fluid pH and, hence, cerebral blood flow gradually return to normal. Subsequent normalization of the partial pressure of arterial carbon dioxide can then result in cerebral hyperemia, causing reperfusion injury to previously ischemic brain regions. (From Laffey JG, Kavanagh BP: Hypocapnia. *N Engl J Med* 347:43, 2002.)

a disrupted BBB can promote the formation of vaso-genic edema. Avoiding or reversing hypoxia is there-fore an essential goal in the acute management of the head-injured patient.[13] The responses of the cerebral vasculature to changing physiologic conditions protect the brain by increasing the delivery of oxygen to tissue, enhancing the removal of metabolic end products and allowing nearly instantaneous adjustments of regional blood flow to meet the changing metabolic demands.

Cerebral Perfusion Pressure. CBF also depends on cerebral perfusion pressure (CPP), which is the pres-sure gradient across the brain. The determinants of CPP are MAP and the resistance to CBF produced by mean systemic venous pressure and ICP. Because ICP is higher than mean systemic venous pressure, ICP effects predominate. Therefore, CPP is estimated as MAP minus ICP. CBF remains constant when CPP is 50 to 160 mm Hg. If CPP falls below 40 mm Hg, the autoreg-ulation of CBF is lost, CBF declines, and the resultant tissue ischemia critically affects cerebral metabolism.[7,9] It is essential to avoid or correct hypotension in the patient with multiple trauma who is also head injured so that the CPP can be maintained. Management must also be directed at reducing or preventing increased ICP to ensure adequate CPP to sustain cerebral metabolic needs.

Biomechanics of Head Trauma

Direct Injury. Direct impact head injury occurs when the head is struck by an object or its motion is arrested by another object. The resulting damage depends on the consistency, mass, surface area, and velocity of the object striking the head. Direct injury can also be caused by compression of the head. External signs of trauma are frequently noted at the site of application of the impact or compression force. The skull initially bends inward at the point of contact. If the force is suf-ficient, a skull fracture can occur. The cranium absorbs some of the applied energy, and some energy is trans-mitted to the brain by shock waves that travel distant to the site of impact or compression. These shock waves distort and disrupt intracranial contents and temporarily alter regional ICP as they propagate. In general, the more rapidly a force is applied, the greater the damage it causes. The extent of direct injury depends on the viscoelastic properties of the under-lying region of brain tissue, the duration of the force applied, the magnitude of the force reaching the brain tissue, and the surface area of the brain that is affected by the application of the force. In cases of penetrating trauma, the mass, shape, direction, and speed of the penetrating object also affect the extent of direct injury.

Direct injury from compression of the head requires significant force because the architecture of the skull provides substantial resistance to deformation. In the clinical setting, compression injury is less common than other types of direct impact. With sufficient and prolonged application of compression force, the ability of the skull to absorb the force is overcome, and mul-tiple linear skull fractures occur. Resulting fractures can be depressed if a high-energy rapid compression force is applied to a small area of the skull.

Isolated direct impact injury is rare; direct impact usually sets the head in motion, resulting in simulta-neous direct and indirect injury.

Indirect Injury. In indirect brain injury, the cranial contents are set into motion by forces other than the direct contact of the skull with another object. A common example is acceleration-deceleration injury, such as the shaken impact syndrome.[14] No direct mechanical impact is sustained, but the cranial con-tents are set into vigorous motion. The brain moves within the skull, and bridging subdural vessels are strained. Subdural hematomas may result. Differential acceleration of the cranial contents occurs, depending on the physical characteristics of the brain region. As one brain region slides past another, shear and strain injuries are produced. This movement results in diffuse injuries, such as diffuse axonal injury or concussion. Additional injury occurs as the movement of the intracranial contents is abruptly arrested and the brain strikes the skull or a dural structure. Contrecoup con-tusions are an example of the injury produced in this manner. In penetrating injury, the traversal of the object produces pressure waves that can strike structures distal to the path of the missile.

Brain Cellular Damage and Death

Primary and Secondary Brain Injury

The acute clinical picture of the patient with TBI is dynamic and represents the sum of primary and sec-ondary injury. Primary brain injury is mechanical irre-versible damage that occurs at the time of head trauma and includes brain lacerations, hemorrhages, contu-sions, and tissue avulsions. On the microscopic level, primary injury causes permanent mechanical cellular disruption and microvascular injury.[15] No specific intervention exists to repair or reverse primary brain injury; the only way to decrease brain injury is through public health interventions aimed at reducing the occurrence of head trauma.

The circumstances and extent of the primary injury are not the only contributors to the final neurologic outcome after head injury.[8,15,16] The traumatic event also produces injury at the functional and anatomic cellular level, which begins shortly after the impact and continues for several hours and even days after injury.[8,17] Secondary brain injury results from intracel-lular and extracellular derangements that are probably initiated at the time of trauma by a massive depolar-ization of brain cells and subsequent ionic shifts.[8,17] Animal studies have revealed a complicated series of neurochemical, neuroanatomic, and neurophysiologic reactions after head injury (Figure 38-2). The cell has some compensatory mechanisms to protect itself from widespread damage, such as endogenous free radical scavengers and antioxidants. With significant trauma, however, these systems are quickly overwhelmed, and the functional and structural integrity of the cell is threatened. Human studies document similar changes.[15,18] The relative importance and contribution of each adverse reaction to the final functional status of the damaged cell are uncertain, as are the rate and

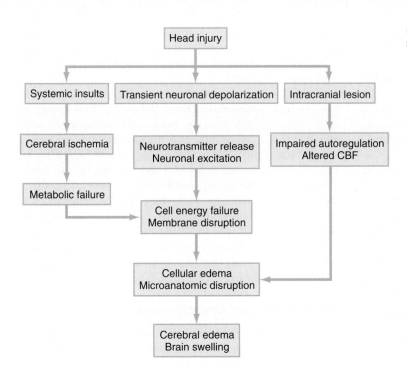

Figure 38-2. Contributing events in the pathophysiology of secondary brain injury. CBF, cerebral blood flow.

Head injury

Systemic insults | Transient neuronal depolarization | Intracranial lesion

Cerebral ischemia | Neurotransmitter release Neuronal excitation | Impaired autoregulation Altered CBF

Metabolic failure

Cell energy failure Membrane disruption

Cellular edema Microanatomic disruption

Cerebral edema Brain swelling

duration of each detrimental event. All currently used acute therapies for TBI are directed at reversing or preventing secondary injury. Experimental evidence for many investigational agents aimed at specific steps in the destructive processes suggests that some aspects of secondary brain injury may be reversed or modified. Multiple ongoing head injury trials are currently attempting to address numerous investigational therapeutic interventions.[19]

Secondary Systemic Insults

The final neurologic outcome after head trauma is influenced by the extent and degree of secondary brain injury. In turn, the amount of secondary brain injury depends on certain premorbid and comorbid conditions, such as the age of the patient and trauma-related systemic events.[20,21] A primary goal in the emergency care of the head-injured patient is prevention or reduction of systemic conditions that are known to worsen outcome after TBI.

Common secondary systemic insults in trauma patients include hypotension, hypoxia, and anemia. *Hypotension,* defined as a systolic blood pressure less than 90 mm Hg, is seen in up to 35% of all patients who have head injury.[21] Systemic hypotension reduces cerebral perfusion, thereby potentiating ischemia and infarction. The presence of hypotension nearly doubles the mortality from head injury and worsens the outcome of the patients who survive.[20,21]

Hypoxia, defined as a PO_2 less than 60 mm Hg, probably occurs often in the head-injured patient. Causes include (1) transient or prolonged apnea caused by brainstem compression or injury after the traumatic event; (2) partial airway obstruction caused by blood, vomitus, or other debris in the airway of the traumatized patient; (3) injury to the chest wall that interferes

with normal respiratory excursion; and (4) pulmonary injury that reduces effective oxygenation. The exact incidence of hypoxia in the head trauma patient is difficult to estimate because it is often unnoticed or undocumented in the out-of-hospital setting. When its occurrence is documented, the overall mortality from severe head injury doubles.[20,21] Increased recognition of the potentially devastating consequences of hypoxia has led to more vigilance in the out-of-hospital and emergency setting, and the occurrence of documented hypoxia in head-injured patients is declining.[20,21]

Anemia caused by blood loss can be detrimental to the head trauma patient by reducing the oxygen-carrying capacity of the blood, thus reducing the amount of necessary substrate delivered to the injured brain tissue. When anemia (hematocrit less than 30%) occurs in patients with severe head injury, the mortality rate increases.[21]

Other potential reversible causes of secondary injury in head injury include hypercarbia, hyperthermia, coagulopathy, and seizures.

Pathophysiology

Increased Intracranial Pressure

ICP represents a balance of the pressures exerted by the contents of the cranial cavity. Because the craniospinal intradural space is almost nonexpandable, the sum of the volume of brain, CSF, and blood within the cranium must remain constant. If the volume of any of these components increases, the volume of another must decrease to maintain a constant ICP. Increased ICP is defined as CSF pressure greater than 15 mm Hg (or 195 mm H_2O) and is a frequent consequence of severe head injury.[7] Initially, as ICP increases as a result of a mass lesion or edema formation, the CSF is displaced from the cranial vault to the spinal canal, offsetting the increased blood or brain volume. When this compensatory mechanism is overwhelmed, the elastic properties of the brain substance allow tissue compression to provide buffering for the increasing pressure. Depending on the location and the rate of expansion of the traumatic mass lesion and the rate of cerebral edema formation, the intracranial compensatory mechanisms can accommodate an increased volume of 50 to 100 mL. Beyond that, even small additional changes in intracranial volume relationships, such as those caused by vasodilation, CSF obstruction, or small areas of focal edema, cause a dramatic increase in ICP. If ICP increases to the point where CPP is compromised, vasoparalysis occurs and autoregulation is lost. The CBF then depends directly on the systemic MAP. With the loss of autoregulation, massive cerebral vasodilation occurs. Systemic pressure is transmitted to the capillaries, and the outpouring of fluids into the extravascular space can contribute to vasogenic edema and thus further increase ICP.[17] If ICP rises to the level of the systemic arterial pressure, CBF ceases and brain death occurs.

Methods to reduce elevated ICP include hyperventilation, use of osmotic and diuretic agents, and CSF drainage. Uncontrollable increased ICP is defined as an ICP of 20 mm Hg or higher refractory to treatment.[17] If ICP is not controlled, herniation syndromes can occur, resulting in brainstem compression and subsequent cardiorespiratory arrest.

Brain Swelling and Cerebral Edema

Two primary types of brain swelling occur after head injury. *Congestive brain swelling* results from an increased intracranial blood volume. Hyperemia occurs early after trauma and can persist for the first few days after injury.[22,23] It is especially common in children. The increased blood volume is most likely caused by vasodilation, which occurs as a compensatory mechanism to maintain optimal CBF in the presence of increased metabolic needs of the damaged brain tissue.

Cerebral edema is an increase in brain volume caused by an absolute increase in cerebral tissue water content. Diffuse cerebral edema may develop soon after head injury; however, its presence and extent do not always correlate with the severity of head injury.[17] On computed tomography (CT) scans, diffuse edema is manifest as bilateral compression of the ventricles, loss of definition of the cortical sulci, or effacement of the basal cisterns. Focal edema adjacent to traumatic mass lesions demonstrates decreased density on CT scans compared with normal tissue. CT can also detect a *mass effect,* caused by edema surrounding a traumatic lesion.

Both vasogenic and cytotoxic cerebral edema occur in the setting of trauma; the incidence and onset of each relative to the other depend on the nature of the injury. *Vasogenic edema* arises from transvascular leakage caused by mechanical failure of the tight endothelial junctions of the BBB.[22,23] Vasogenic edema accumulates preferentially in white matter and can become widespread. It is frequently associated with focal contusions or hematomas. Vasogenic edema eventually resolves as edema fluid is reabsorbed into the vascular space or the ventricular system.

Cytotoxic edema is an intracellular process that results from membrane pump failure.[22,23] It is common after head injury and is frequently associated with posttraumatic ischemia and tissue hypoxia. Normal membrane pump activity depends on adequate CBF to ensure adequate substrate and oxygen delivery to brain tissue. If the CBF is reduced to 40% or less of baseline, cytotoxic edema begins to develop. If CBF drops to 25% of baseline, membrane pumps fail and cells begin to die. Congestive brain swelling can contribute to cytotoxic edema if it becomes severe enough to increase ICP and reduce CPP so that cerebral circulation cannot be maintained.

Altered Levels of Consciousness

Consciousness is the state of awareness of the self and of the environment and requires intact functioning of the cerebral cortices and the reticular activating system (RAS) of the brainstem. An altered level of consciousness is the hallmark of brain insult from any cause and results from an interruption of the RAS or a global event that affects the cortices of both hemispheres.

A patient who has sustained TBI typically has an altered level of consciousness. Head trauma patients may be hypoxic from injury to respiratory centers or from concomitant pulmonary injury. Hypotension from other associated injuries can compromise CBF and affect consciousness. Global suppression may result from an intoxicant consumed before the injury. With increasing ICP from brain swelling or an expanding mass lesion, brainstem compression and subsequent RAS compression can occur.

Patients with altered levels of consciousness require careful monitoring and observation. Reversible conditions that can alter mental status, such as hypoxia, hypotension, or hypoglycemia, should be corrected as they are identified.

Cushing's Reflex

Progressive hypertension associated with bradycardia and diminished respiratory effort is a specific response to acute, potentially lethal rises in ICP. This response is called the Cushing reflex, or *Cushing's phenomenon,* and its occurrence indicates that the ICP has reached life-threatening levels. The Cushing reflex can occur whenever ICP is increased, regardless of the cause. The full triad of hypertension, bradycardia, and respiratory irregularity is seen in only one third of cases of life-threatening increased ICP.[22]

Cerebral Herniation

Cerebral herniation occurs when increasing cranial volume and ICP overwhelm the natural compensatory capacities of the CNS (Figure 38-3). Increased ICP may be the result of posttraumatic brain swelling, edema

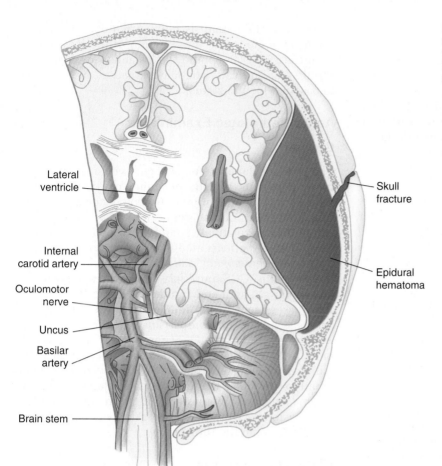

Figure 38-3. Anterior view of transtentorial herniation caused by large epidural hematoma. Skull fracture overlies hematoma. (From Rockswold GL: Head injury. In Tintinalli JE et al [eds]: *Emergency Medicine*. New York, McGraw-Hill, 1992, p 915.)

Lateral ventricle

Internal carotid artery

Oculomotor nerve

Uncus

Basilar artery

Brain stem

Skull fracture

Epidural hematoma

formation, traumatic mass lesion expansion, or any combination of the three. When increasing ICP cannot be controlled, the intracranial contents shift and herniate through the cranial foramen. Herniation can occur within minutes or up to days after TBI. When the signs of herniation syndrome are present, however, mortality approaches 100% without rapid implementation of temporizing emergency measures and definitive neurosurgical therapy.

Uncal

The most common clinically significant traumatic herniation syndrome is uncal herniation, a form of transtentorial herniation. Uncal herniation is often associated with traumatic extraaxial hematomas in the lateral middle fossa or the temporal lobe. The classical signs and symptoms are caused by compression of the ipsilateral uncus of the temporal lobe on the U-shaped edge of the tentorium cerebelli as the brain is forced through the tentorial hiatus. As compression of the uncus begins, the third cranial nerve is compressed; anisocoria, ptosis, impaired extraocular movements, and a sluggish pupillary light reflex develop on the side ipsilateral to the expanding mass lesion. This phase may last for minutes to hours, depending on how rapidly the expanding lesion is changing. As the herniation progresses, compression of the ipsilateral oculomotor nerve eventually causes ipsilateral pupillary dilation and nonreactivity.

Initially in the uncal herniation process, the motor examination can be normal, but contralateral Babinski's responses develop early.[22] Babinski's sign is dorsiflexion of the great toe and fanning of the other toes. Contralateral hemiparesis develops as the ipsilateral peduncle is compressed against the tentorium. With continued progression of the herniation, bilateral decerebrate posturing eventually occurs; decorticate posturing is not always seen with the uncal herniation syndrome.[24] In up to 25% of patients the contralateral cerebral peduncle is forced against the opposite edge of the tentorial hiatus. Hemiparesis is then detected ipsilateral to the dilated pupil and the mass lesion. This is termed *Kernohan's notch syndrome* and causes false-localizing motor findings.[24]

As uncal herniation progresses, direct brainstem compression causes additional alterations in the level of consciousness, respiratory pattern, and cardiovascular system. Mental status changes may initially be quite subtle, such as agitation, restlessness, or confusion, but soon lethargy occurs with progression to frank coma. The patient's respiratory pattern may initially be normal, followed by sustained hyperventilation. With continued brainstem compression, an ataxic respiratory pattern develops. The patient's hemodynamic status may change, with rapid fluctuations in blood pressure and cardiac conduction. Herniation that is uncontrolled progresses rapidly to brainstem failure, cardiovascular collapse, and death.

Central Transtentorial

The central transtentorial herniation syndrome is demonstrated by rostrocaudal neurologic deterioration caused by an expanding lesion at the vertex or the frontal or occipital pole of the brain. It is less common than uncal transtentorial herniation. Clinical deterioration occurs as bilateral central pressure is exerted on the brain from above. The initial clinical manifestation may be a subtle change in mental status or decreased level of consciousness, bilateral motor weakness, and pinpoint pupils (less than 2 mm). Light reflexes are still present but are often difficult to detect. Muscle tone is increased bilaterally, and bilateral Babinski's signs may be present. As central herniation progresses, both pupils become midpoint and lose light responsiveness. Respiratory patterns are affected and sustained hyperventilation may occur. Motor tone increases. Decorticate posturing is elicited by noxious stimuli. This progresses to bilateral decorticate and then spontaneous decerebrate posturing. Respiratory patterns initially include yawns and sighs and progress to sustained tachypnea, followed by shallow slow and irregular breaths immediately before respiratory arrest.

Cerebellotonsillar

Cerebellotonsillar herniation occurs when the cerebellar tonsils herniate downward through the foramen magnum. This is usually caused by a cerebellar mass or a large central vertex mass causing the rapid displacement of the entire brainstem.[22] Clinically, patients demonstrate sudden respiratory and cardiovascular collapse as the medulla is impinged. Pinpoint pupils are noted. Flaccid quadriplegia is the most common motor presentation because of bilateral compression of the corticospinal tracts. Mortality from cerebellar herniation approaches 70%.[24]

Upward Transtentorial

Upward transtentorial herniation occasionally occurs as a result of an expanding posterior fossa lesion. Level of consciousness declines rapidly. These patients may have pinpoint pupils from compression of the pons. Downward conjugate gaze is accompanied by absence of vertical eye movements.[24]

CLINICAL FEATURES AND DIAGNOSTIC STRATEGIES

History

Details regarding the mechanism of injury should be solicited from witnesses or the victim to determine whether the head-injured patient is at high risk for intracranial injury. The patient's condition before trauma may give clues to important, otherwise unsuspected, comorbid factors. Past medical history, medications, recent drug or alcohol use, and complaints immediately preceding the traumatic event should be determined.

The patient's current level of consciousness, as well as that immediately before and after the injury and at the arrival of first responders, should be determined. Witnessed posttraumatic seizures or apnea should be reported. If the patient is now awake but was unconscious at some point, the duration of the loss of consciousness (LOC) should be established. Witnesses should also indicate whether the patient has returned to baseline mental status.

Acute Neurologic Examination

General

The goals of the acute neurologic assessment of head-injured patients include detection of life-threatening injuries and identification of neurologic changes in the immediate posttrauma period. An awake, stable patient can undergo a relatively complete neurologic examination. In other patients an efficient neurologic examination in the emergency setting includes evaluation of mental status, GCS, pupillary size and responsiveness, and motor strength and symmetry. An accurate neurologic assessment in the immediate posttrauma period serves as a basis for comparison in subsequent examinations. If a formal GCS measure is not possible or is difficult because of comorbid confounders, the patient's mental status should be described in as much detail as possible. Declining mental status after head trauma suggests increasing ICP from an expanding mass lesion or worsening cerebral edema, which may rapidly become life threatening.

Glasgow Coma Scale

The GCS is an objective method of following the patient's neurologic status (Table 38-1). The GCS assesses a patient's best eye, verbal, and motor responsiveness. It was developed for the clinical evaluation of head trauma patients at 6 hours after trauma, and all initial validation studies investigated its application at this time. It was designed for assessment of patients with isolated head trauma who were hemodynamically stable and adequately oxygenated.[24] Because of its interrater reliability, reliance on objective clinical data, and ease of application, the GCS has become a standard acute measure of neurologic function in patients with altered mental status from any cause, including head trauma.

The acute application (less than 6 hours) of the GCS in head-injured patients has limitations. Hypoxia, hypotension, and intoxication can falsely lower the initial GCS.[25] Intubation lowers the patient's GCS by automatically assigning a score of 1 for verbal response, regardless of the actual contribution of head injury to the clinical examination. Periorbital edema from direct eye trauma may make assessment of spontaneous eye opening difficult. Extremity fractures or occult spinal cord injuries may interfere with the motor examination. Children and non–English-speaking patients are difficult to assess with the GCS. The GCS may miss subtle mental status changes and does not assess brainstem reflexes or pupillary reflexes. Decisions on continued resuscitation of severely head-injured patients should not be based on the initial GCS because of these limitations. Patients must be fully resuscitated, with evacuation of all surgical lesions, must remain hemo-

Table 38-1. Glasgow Coma Scale

Response	Score	Significance
Eye Opening		
Spontaneously	4	Reticular activating system is intact; patient may not be aware
To verbal command	3	Opens eyes when told to do so
To pain	2	Opens eyes in response to pain
None	1	Does not open eyes to any stimuli
Verbal Stimuli		
Oriented, converses	5	Relatively intact CNS, aware of self and environment
Disoriented, converses	4	Well articulated, organized, but disoriented
Inappropriate words	3	Random, exclamatory words
Incomprehensible	2	Moaning, no recognizable words
No response	1	No response or intubated
Motor Response		
Obeys verbal commands	6	Readily moves limbs when told to
Localizes to painful stimuli	5	Moves limb in an effort to remove painful stimuli
Flexion withdrawal	4	Pulls away from pain in flexion
Abnormal flexion	3	Decorticate rigidity
Extension	2	Decerebrate rigidity
No response	1	Hypotonia, flaccid: suggests loss of medullary function or concomitant spinal cord injury

CNS, central nervous system.

dynamically stable, and must not be intoxicated before the GCS can be used to predict their prognosis.[26]

Pupillary Examination

An evaluation of the patient's pupil size and responsiveness must be done early in the initial assessment of the head-injured patient. A large fixed pupil suggests herniation syndrome; it is usually on the side of the expanding lesion. Traumatic mydriasis, resulting from direct injury to the eye and periorbital structures, may confuse the assessment of the pupillary responsiveness.

Motor Examination: Posturing

The patient's acute motor examination assesses for strength and symmetry. Hemiparesis contralateral to a fixed and dilated pupil suggests herniation syndrome. A false-localizing motor examination can be caused by contralateral cerebral parenchymal injury occurring simultaneously with the expanding mass lesion or by Kernohan's notch syndrome (compression of the contralateral cerebral peduncle). False-localizing signs for the motor examination can also be caused by occult extremity trauma, spinal cord injury, or nerve root injury that makes the examination painful or difficult. If the patient is not cooperative or is comatose, motor movement should be elicited by application of noxious stimuli. Any movement should be recorded. Voluntary

purposeful movement must be distinguished from abnormal motor posturing. *Decorticate posturing* is abnormal flexion of the upper extremity and extension of the lower extremity. The arm, wrist, and elbow slowly flex, and the arm is adducted. The leg extends and internally rotates, with plantar flexion of the foot. Decorticate posturing implies injury above the midbrain. *Decerebrate posturing* is the result of a more caudal injury and therefore is associated with a worse prognosis.[22] The arms extend abnormally and become adducted. The wrist and fingers are flexed, and the entire arm is internally rotated at the shoulder. The neck undergoes abnormal extension, and the teeth may become clenched. The leg is internally rotated and extended, and the feet and toes are plantar flexed.

Brainstem Function

In the acute setting, brainstem activity is assessed by the patient's respiratory pattern, pupillary size, and eye movements. The *oculocephalic response* (doll's eyes maneuver) tests the integrity of the pontine gaze centers. This response cannot be tested until cervical spine fractures have been ruled out. The *oculovestibular response* (cold water calorics) also assesses the brainstem. Comatose patients no longer demonstrate nystagmus when cold water is placed in the ear canal; the only response is tonic deviation of the eyes toward the instilled cold water.[24] This response is dampened by cerumen or blood in the patient's ear canal, and the tympanic membrane must be intact to perform this test.

In the severely head-injured patient the cranial nerve (CN) examination is often limited to the pupillary responses (CN III), gag reflex (CNs IX and X), and corneal reflex (CNs V and VII). Facial symmetry (CN VII) can sometimes be assessed if the patient grimaces with noxious stimuli. In patients who are awake and can cooperate, a formal CN examination should be performed.

Deep Tendon Reflexes and Pathologic Reflexes

Tendon reflexes should be tested for symmetry. An extensor plantar reflex (Babinski's sign) is nonspecific and can be caused by injury anywhere along the corticospinal tract.[27] Rectal sphincter tone and anal reflexes should be determined to assess for spinal cord integrity.

Other Examination Findings

The head and neck should be carefully examined for external signs of trauma that may have also produced underlying TBI. A scalp laceration, contusion, abrasion, or avulsion may overlie a depressed skull fracture. Basilar skull fractures are usually diagnosed by the clinical examination (Box 38-1). Although not always related to severe brain injury, their presence implies that a significant impact force was sustained during head trauma. Carotid artery dissections caused by a hyperflexion-extension neck injury can occasionally be detected by auscultation of a carotid bruit.[22] In these

BOX 38-1. Clinical Characteristics of Basilar Skull Fractures

Blood in ear canal
Hemotympanum
Rhinorrhea
Otorrhea
Battle's sign (retroauricular hematoma)
Raccoon sign (periorbital ecchymosis)
Cranial nerve deficits
    Facial paralysis
    Decreased auditory acuity
    Dizziness
    Tinnitus
    Nystagmus

patients, a careful neurologic examination should assess for subtle asymmetry between the carotid arteries.

The incidence of concurrent cervical spine injury in patients with head trauma may be as high as 15%.[22] Often, other spinal regions are also injured.[27]

MANAGEMENT

Severe Head Trauma

The neurosurgical literature defines severe head injury as TBI manifested by a postresuscitation GCS of 8 or less within 48 hours. In the emergency setting, however, this definition is not practical because the outcome for the patient beyond the initial resuscitation is not known. Most emergency medicine research defines severe head injury by a GCS score of 8 or less at the acute presentation after injury. The presence of any intracranial contusion, hematoma, or laceration is also considered severe injury (Figure 38-4).

Approximately 10% of all head-injured patients who reach the emergency department alive have severe head trauma.[1,28] The clinical prognostic indicators in the acute setting are initial motor activity, pupillary responsiveness, the patient's age and premorbid condition, and the occurrence of secondary systemic insult during the acute period.[28-31] Up to 25% of these patients have lesions requiring neurosurgical evacuation.[29] The prognosis cannot be reliably predicted by the initial GCS or initial CT scan.

The overall mortality in severe head trauma approaches 60%.[1,28] Mortality for children is lower.[31] For nonsurvivors of head injury who reach the hospital alive, the average time to death is 2 days after trauma. Adult survivors of severe head trauma are usually severely disabled; currently, only 7% have moderate disability or a good outcome. Children older than 2 years who survive a severe closed-head injury have a better outcome than adults.[31-33]

Out-of-Hospital Care

The goals of the out-of-hospital management are necessary airway interventions to prevent hypoxia and establishing intravenous (IV) access to treat trauma-related hypotension. An accurate neurologic assessment provides a means to determine the subsequent effectiveness of treatment and should focus on the GCS, pupillary responsiveness and size, level of consciousness, and motor strength and symmetry.

Head trauma can produce profound effects on the cardiovascular system if compression of the brainstem and medulla occurs. Any cardiac dysrhythmia can occur and produce cardiac instability.[34] All head-injured patients should therefore have a cardiac monitor as they are transported from the accident scene.

The secondary survey of the head-injured patient should include a search for external signs of head trauma. Scalp lacerations may bleed a large volume into a bulky dressing. A less bulky dressing should be used with firm constant pressure applied to avoid excessive blood loss. Both hypoxia and hypotension in the prehospital setting have been found to have a negative impact on patients' outcome.[35]

Many severely head-injured patients are initially combative or agitated. Transporting an agitated patient who is fighting against physical restraints may exacerbate physical injury, cause a rise in ICP, and interfere with appropriate stabilization and management. It may be necessary to use out-of-hospital sedation or neuromuscular blockade for control. The use of sedatives or neuromuscular blockade may influence the initial emergency department evaluation of the neurotrauma patient. The risks and benefits of this acute intervention therefore must be carefully considered and decisions made on a case-by-case basis. Out-of-hospital protocols allowing the use of sedative agents for selected agitated head-injured patients should be established. Currently used agents include lorazepam (Ativan), diazepam (Valium), midazolam (Versed), etomidate, and other sedatives (i.e., haloperidol, droperidol).

Severe head injury is the most common reason for helicopter transfers in trauma care. Although the decision to transport by helicopter should be made on a case-by-case basis, considerations for helicopter use from an accident scene include a long extrication time, ground transport of longer than 30 minutes to an appropriate emergency department and trauma care facility, two or more severely injured patients at a scene, and assistance in performing expedient lifesaving procedures, especially airway management. Controversy exists regarding field intubation in patients with severe head injuries. It is unclear whether field intubations truly improve neurologic outcome or survival.[35-39] Unsuccessful attempts at field intubations may add to out-of-hospital time and increase the risk of aspiration or hypoxia. Ongoing education in airway intervention skills is especially important to avoid these potential problems in head-injured patients.

Emergency Department

Airway

Rapid sequence intubation (RSI) is an effective and the preferred method for securing the airway in combative

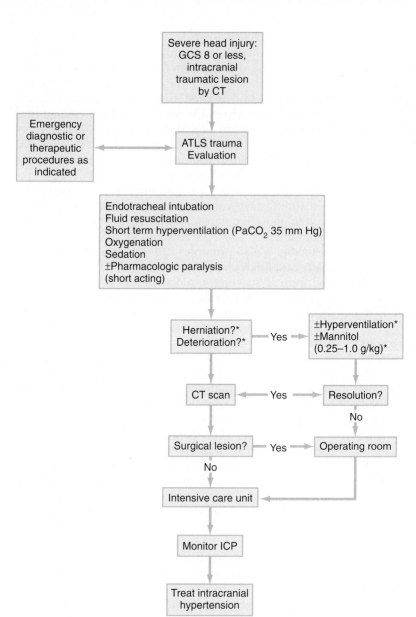

Figure 38-4. Initial resuscitation of patient with severe head injury: treatment options. ATLS, advanced trauma life support; CT, computed tomography; GCS, Glasgow Coma Scale; ICP, intracranial pressure; Paco₂, arterial carbon dioxide partial pressure. (From the Brain Trauma Foundation, American Association of Neurological Surgeons, Joint Section on Neurotrauma and Critical Care: *J Neurotrauma* 17:465, 2000.)

*Only in the presence of signs of herniation or progressive neurologic deterioration not attributable to extracranial factors.

or agitated patients. If possible, a brief neurologic examination should be performed before the patient is given any sedative or neuromuscular blocking agents. In general, the agents used for RSI in the head-injured patient are the same as those for other patients, although attention must be given to the increased ICP that can potentially occur with any physical stimulation of the respiratory tract. Lidocaine (1.5 to 2 mg/kg IV push) may attenuate the cough reflex, hypertensive response, and increased ICP associated with intubation. Thiopental may also be effective but should not be used in hypotensive patients. If succinylcholine is used, premedication with a subparalytic dose of a nondepolarizing agent should be considered if time permits because fasciculations produced by succinylcholine may increase ICP. The degree of ICP elevation and its clinical significance are unclear, however, and

must be balanced against the need for rapidly establishing an airway. Etomidate (0.3 mg/kg IV), a short-acting sedative-hypnotic agent, has beneficial effects on ICP by reducing CBF and metabolism.[40] In addition, etomidate has minimal adverse effects on blood pressure and cardiac output and fewer respiratory depressant effects than other agents.

Hypotension

If hypotension is detected at any time in the emergent management of a head-injured patient, a cause other than the head injury should be sought. Hypotension is rarely caused by head injury except as a terminal event and should prompt a search for occult blood loss in the acute setting. Some important exceptions occur. Profound blood loss from scalp lacerations can cause hypovolemic hypotension. In small children, hemorrhage into an epidural or subgaleal hematoma can produce profound hypovolemic shock. In the presence of concomitant spinal cord injury, neurogenic hypotension may occur. This is rare and can be differentiated from hypovolemic hypotension by its nonresponsiveness to fluid administration.

Systemic hypotension cannot be tolerated in the head-injured patient without profound worsening of neurologic outcome; fluids or blood transfusion should therefore be delivered to maintain a systolic blood pressure of at least 90 mm Hg. The delivery of large amounts of fluid to severely head-injured patients who are hypotensive from other injuries does not produce clinically significant increases in ICP; fluids should never be withheld in the head trauma patient with hypovolemic hypotension for fear of increasing cerebral edema and ICP. Hypotension may interfere with the accurate neurologic assessment of the brain-injured patient. Often, when blood pressure is restored, an improved neurologic status is observed.[41]

Traditionally, normal saline or lactated Ringer's solution has been used for resuscitation of trauma patients with hypovolemic hypotension. Although it is not yet included in practice guidelines on the management of head-injured patients, some researchers suggest that fluid resuscitation with hypertonic saline rather than normal saline may improve neurologic outcome after TBI.[42]

As many as 60% of patients with severe head injury are victims of multiple trauma.[30] The dramatic presentation of the head injury should not distract the clinician from a thorough search for other life threats.

The emergency department neurologic assessment should be compared with the initial out-of-hospital examination, focusing on evidence of neurologic deterioration or signs of increasing ICP. If the patient is deteriorating or has signs of increased ICP, active intervention must be initiated in the emergency department.

Hyperventilation

Hyperventilation to produce an arterial PCO_2 of 30 to 35 mm Hg temporarily reduces ICP by promoting cerebral vasoconstriction and subsequent reduction of CBF. The onset of action is within 30 seconds and probably peaks within 8 minutes after the PCO_2 drops to the desired range.[22] In most patients, hyperventilation lowers the ICP by 25%; if the patient does not rapidly respond, the prognosis for survival is generally poor. PCO_2 should not fall below 25 mm Hg because this may cause profound vasoconstriction and ischemia in normal as well as injured areas of the brain. As previously described, hyperventilation is recommended for brief periods during the acute resuscitation and only in patients demonstrating neurologic deterioration.[35,43]

Osmotic Agents: Mannitol

Additional therapy for increased ICP includes the use of osmotic diuretics, such as mannitol. With deepening coma, pupil inequality, or other deterioration of the neurologic examination, mannitol may be lifesaving.

Mannitol (0.25 to 1 g/kg) can effectively reduce cerebral edema by producing an osmotic gradient that prevents the movement of water from the vascular space into the cells during membrane pump failure and draws tissue water into the vascular space. This reduces brain volume and provides increased space for an expanding hematoma or brain swelling. The osmotic effects of mannitol occur within minutes and peak about 60 minutes after bolus administration. The ICP-lowering effects of a single bolus may last for 6 to 8 hours.[44]

Mannitol has many other neuroprotective properties. It is an effective volume expander in the presence of hypovolemic hypotension and therefore may maintain systemic blood pressure required for adequate cerebral perfusion. It also promotes CBF by reducing blood viscosity and microcirculatory resistance. It is an effective free radical scavenger, reducing the concentration of oxygen free radicals that may promote cell membrane lipid peroxidation. However, mannitol can produce renal failure or hypotension if given in large doses. It may also induce a paradoxical effect of increased bleeding into a traumatic lesion by decompressing the tamponade effect of a hematoma. Because of these and other potential problems, the use of mannitol should be reserved for head-injured patients with evidence of increasing ICP and neurologic deterioration.[45]

A potentially beneficial medical treatment for increased ICP is hypertonic saline even when the patient is not hypovolemic. Hypertonic saline at concentrations from 3.1% to as high as 23% has been studied as a potential brain diuretic agent in patients with intractable elevations of ICP.[46] The action of hypertonic saline also includes improved hemodynamics by plasma volume expansion, reduction of vasospasm by increasing vessel diameter, and reduction of the posttraumatic inflammatory response. It is possible that its benefits may prove different in pediatric compared with adult patients because of the increased prevalence and difference in the type of brain swelling and cerebral edema that occurs in head-injured children compared with adults.

Although this therapy looks promising in the few prospective studies that describe it, research to date has not evaluated its effectiveness compared head to head with mannitol or in the acute resuscitation of head-injured patients. Higher concentrations of saline must be administered through a central line, limiting its potential use in the out-of-hospital setting. Other concerns with its use are the potential for the precipitation of the osmotic demyelinization syndrome, acute renal failure, coagulopathies, hypernatremia, and red blood cell lysis.[46] Nevertheless, it is likely that the use of hypertonic saline will be increasingly investigated in the future for treatment of intractable increased ICP in the severely head-injured patient.

Barbiturates

Barbiturate therapy is occasionally used in severely head-injured patients to reduce cerebral metabolic demands of the injured brain tissue. Barbiturates also affect vascular tone and inhibit free radical–mediated cell membrane lipid peroxidation. The effects of barbiturates are delayed relative to other acute interventions for reducing ICP and therefore they are rarely initiated in the emergency department. If other methods of reducing ICP have been unsuccessful, barbiturates may be added in the hemodynamically stable patient. *Pentobarbital* is the barbiturate most often used.[47]

Steroids

Despite their popularity in the past, no evidence indicates that steroids are of benefit in head injury. They do not lower ICP or improve outcome and are therefore no longer recommended.[48]

Cranial Decompression

Under extreme circumstances when all other attempts at reducing ICP have failed, emergency cranial decompression must be considered in the deteriorating patient. Patients with signs of herniation who have not responded to other means of ICP reduction and who are rapidly deteriorating in the emergency department should be considered for placement of emergency burr holes. Emergency trephination is a blind invasive procedure, and the chances of localizing the expanding lesions are uncertain. In carefully considered patients, however, emergency cranial decompression may temporarily reverse or arrest the herniation syndrome, providing the time needed to prepare the patient for formal craniotomy.

Most patients who have been unconscious since the accident, with erratic or absent respiratory effort, bilateral fixed and dilated pupils, no spontaneous eye movements, and decerebrate posturing, have sustained diffuse massive brain injury with no focal lesion amenable to emergency decompression; these patients probably do not benefit from emergent burr holes. Instead, these patients should undergo rapid CT scanning or formal surgical decompression. The rapidity of obtaining CT scans in most institutions has reduced the frequency of the need for emergency cranial decompression in the emergency department. Some experts believe that early ventriculostomy and aggressive management of increased ICP improve outcome in the most severely head-injured patients. No prospective, randomized study has yet been performed on this important topic.

Seizure Prophylaxis

Up to 12% of all patients who sustain blunt head trauma and 50% of those with penetrating head injury develop early posttraumatic seizures.[48] Although the occurrence of seizures in the immediate posttrauma period has no predictive value for future epilepsy, early seizures can cause hypoxia, hypercarbia, release of excitatory neurotransmitters, and increased ICP, which can worsen secondary brain injury. Constantly firing neurons are soon depleted of their energy sources, and in the head trauma patient with compromised cerebral metabolism, uncontrolled seizures exacerbate the neurologic deficit.[22]

Box 38-2 lists accepted indications for early anticonvulsant therapy after head trauma. If the patient is actively seizing, benzodiazepines are administered as effective, rapid-acting first-line anticonvulsants. Lorazepam (0.05 to 0.15 mg/kg IV, over 2 to 5 minutes up to a total of 4 mg) has been found to be most effective at aborting status epilepticus.[49] Diazepam (0.1 mg/kg, up to 5 mg IV, every 10 minutes up to a total of 20 mg) is an alternative. For long-term anticonvulsant activity, phenytoin (13 to 18 mg/kg IV) or fosphenytoin (13 to 18 phenytoin equivalents/kg) can be given. In a review published in the Cochrane database, the use of antiepileptic drugs reduced the risk of early seizures by 66%.[50] Early seizure prophylaxis does not prevent late posttraumatic seizures; the goal is to prevent additional insult to the damaged brain.[50,51]

If the patient has been paralyzed to facilitate management, clinical manifestations of generalized seizures are obscured. Therefore, all paralyzed head-injured patients should have prophylactic anticonvulsant therapy in the acute phase. Continuous electroencephalographic monitoring is necessary for the ongoing assessment of seizure activity in paralyzed patients and, if available, should be initiated in the emergency department or the intensive care unit.

Antibiotic Prophylaxis

Infection may occur as a complication of penetrating head injury, open skull fractures, and complicated scalp lacerations. Prophylactic antibiotics may be used in these circumstances but are not recommended in patients with otorrhea or rhinorrhea from a basilar skull fracture.[48,52]

Ancillary Evaluation

Laboratory Tests. The acute management of the severely head-injured patient is directed by physical examination and diagnostic imaging. Ancillary laboratory tests that may provide useful information in the subsequent management of the patient include a urine toxicology screen, blood alcohol level, complete blood count, electrolytes, glucose, and coagulation studies.

Neuroimaging. The advantages and indications for neuroimaging techniques in the acute evaluation of head injury are listed in Table 38-2. In the acute phase the most useful imaging technique is a non–contrast-

Table 38-2. Comparison of Head Imaging Modalities

	Computed Tomography Scans	Magnetic Resonance Imaging	Angiography	Skull Radiography
Advantages	Fast Patient accessible for monitoring Defines acute hemorrhages, mass effects, bone injuries, hydrocephalus, intraventricular blood, edema	Defines contusions and pericontusion edema, posttraumatic ischemic infarction, brainstem injuries	Helps localize acute traumatic lesions Defines vascular injuries, injuries to venous sinuses Detects mass effects	Readily available May help screen some patients for further imaging studies
Disadvantages	Artifacts arise from patient's movement, foreign bodies Streak artifacts may obscure brainstem or posterior fossa	Slow Patients not easily accessible for monitoring Does not define most acute hemorrhagic lesions Not useful for bone injuries	Does not define nature of acute lesion Does not detect infratentorial masses	Does not indicate presence or absence of intracranial injury
Indications	Acute severe head trauma Acute moderate head trauma High-risk minor head trauma Deteriorating neurologic status	Persistent symptoms with postconcussive syndrome Suspected posttraumatic ischemic infarction Suspected contusions not seen on CT scan	Suspected vascular injury CT scan not available	CT scan may not be done Penetrating head trauma Suspected depressed skull fracture Suspected child abuse in minor head trauma

CT, computed tomography.

enhanced head CT scan.[53] This scan delineates acute intraaxial and extraaxial bleeding, subarachnoid blood, cerebral swelling, ischemic infarction caused by hypoxia after trauma, evidence of increased ICP, and pneumocephalus. Emergency management decisions are strongly influenced by these acute CT scan findings. The bone windows of the CT scan can detect skull fractures (including basilar fractures); plain skull radiographs are not necessary in patients who undergo CT scanning.

Magnetic resonance imaging (MRI) is better than CT in detecting posttraumatic ischemic infarctions, subacute nonhemorrhagic lesions and contusions, axonal shear injury , and lesions in the brainstem or posterior fossa.[53]

Angiography should be considered when CT scanning is unavailable. It demonstrates the vascular tree, and characteristic patterns can suggest the location but not always the nature of traumatic lesions. Mass effect, vascular disruptions or dissections, and venous sinus thromboses can also be detected, although angiography is not sensitive for the detection of infratentorial masses.

Disposition

Consultation. All patients with severe head trauma require an imaging modality to determine the extent and nature of the brain injury and the necessity of neurosurgical intervention. Neurosurgical consultation should be obtained as soon as possible to help direct the patient's subsequent management.

Transfer. Severely head-injured patients require admission to an institution capable of intensive neurosurgical care and acute neurosurgical intervention. If this is not available at the receiving hospital, the patient should be transferred to an appropriate institution by the most expedient transport method available.

Priority Management. The hemodynamically unstable patient with multiple trauma that includes head injury presents difficult emergency management decisions. The emergency physician must decide on the sequence that best addresses the most life-threatening pathologic conditions while still preventing morbidity and mortality from other serious injury. If the patient requires immediate surgical intervention for a life-threatening chest or abdominal injury, complete evaluation of the head injury may be curtailed; moreover, these patients are anesthetized for surgery, and any neurologic deterioration is not detected. Some patients may be too unstable to obtain even an abbreviated head CT scan before emergent surgical intervention for other life threats. In this circumstance, early neurosurgical and general surgical consultation should be coordinated by the emergency physician. Intraoperative ventriculostomies or bilateral trephinations may provide some temporary protection from increasing ICP while the patient undergoes surgical correction of the life-threatening injury. A CT scan can be performed later, after the primary life threats have been corrected.

Moderate Head Trauma

Approximately 10% of all patients with head injury have sustained moderate head trauma, defined as a postresuscitation GCS of 9 to 13.[28,54] Moderate head trauma is often caused by motor vehicle crashes. Most patients with moderate head trauma do not die at the scene from their initial head injury and present to the emergency department for stabilization and evaluation.

Moderate head trauma produces a number of physiologic abnormalities, including neuronal cell membrane dysfunction and a mild, brief acidosis with no concurrent depletion of adenosine triphosphate. These changes are probably reversible and therefore may be amenable to acute intervention to correct or prevent progression. The neuropathology of moderate brain injury probably represents the front end of the spectrum of pathophysiology seen with severe head trauma. Because of this, patients must be vigilantly monitored to avoid hypoxia and hypotension and other secondary systemic insults that could worsen neurologic outcome.

Clinical Features and Acute Management

A wide variety of clinical presentations occur with moderate head injury. Patients often have experienced a change in consciousness at the time of injury, a progressive headache, posttraumatic seizures, vomiting, and posttraumatic amnesia. On emergency department presentation, patients are often confused or somnolent, but most can still follow commands. Focal neurologic deficits may be present. Many patients with moderate head trauma have concurrent serious facial injuries that may interfere with attempts at securing their airway. Other systematic trauma must also be ruled out.

An important clinical scenario in the spectrum of moderate head injury is that of the "talk and deteriorate" patient. These patients speak after their head injury but deteriorate to a status of a severe head injury within 48 hours.[55] Approximately 75% of these patients have sustained subdural or epidural hematomas. Patients with an initial GCS of 9 or greater who later deteriorate to a GCS of 8 or less have a poorer outcome than those who originally present with a GCS less than 8.[55] Successful management of moderately head-injured patients involves close clinical observation for changing mental status or focal neurologic findings, early CT scanning, and aggressive neurosurgical intervention. When no neurosurgeon is available and the patient develops symptoms consistent with herniation syndrome not reversed by acute hyperventilation and mannitol, emergency department trephination and hematoma evacuation should be considered.[55]

Because of the varied presentation of the patient with moderate head trauma, the initial clinical examination alone cannot accurately predict who will have surgically correctable intracranial lesions. Approximately 40% of moderately head-injured patients have an abnormal CT scan, and 10% lapse into coma.[56] A CT scan is essential in patients with moderate head trauma to avoid delayed diagnosis of traumatic mass lesions or diffuse injury. Skull radiographs may be useful if the patient has sustained a depressed skull fracture or a penetrating injury but are otherwise rarely helpful.

Disposition

All patients with moderate head injury should be admitted for observation, even with an apparently normal CT scan. Ninety percent of patients improve over the first few days after injury.[22,56] Frequent neurologic checks should be initiated, and a repeated CT scan is indicated if the patient's condition deteriorates or fails to improve over the first 48 hours after trauma.

Complications

The overall mortality of patients with isolated moderate head trauma is about 20%, but the morbidity is substantial. Most moderate head trauma patients remain symptomatic for extended periods after head injury. At 3 months after trauma, up to 70% are unable to return to work, 90% have memory difficulties, and more than 90% complain of persistent headaches.[56,57] Almost 50% are left with a permanent disability that interferes with their previous daily activities. In patients with persistent symptoms of headache, confusion, or memory difficulties, delayed MRI may define lesions in the regions related to cognition that cannot be seen on CT. Although not useful in the acute setting, MRI has prognostic value during subsequent care and assists in directing the future rehabilitation of these patients.

Minor Head Trauma

Minor head trauma is defined as isolated head injury producing a GCS of 14 to 15.[58] It was previously believed that 75% to 80% of all head injuries seen for emergency medical evaluation are minor. More recent reports suggest that hospital managed care priorities may be changing this epidemiologic profile, such that now the number of emergency department patients with minor head injuries has decreased to about 60% of all head-injured patients seen.[59] An increasing proportion of these injuries are related to sports and other recreational activities.

Clinical and Historical Features

The most common complaint after minor head trauma is headache. Other common problems are nausea and emesis. Occasionally, patients may complain of disorientation, confusion, or amnesia after the injury, but these symptoms are usually transient. There has been little research to correlate these symptoms with the presence of intracranial lesions in patients with minor head injury, but most investigators believe these symptoms suggest potential TBI in adult patients. Most patients have no complaints by the time they reach the emergency department and present with a GCS of 14 or 15.

Careful and complete neurologic and mental status examinations are essential to detect subtle abnormalities after minor head trauma. Further diagnostic workup hinges on risk stratification in patients with minor head trauma (Box 38-3). The criteria are based on several large studies, but because of inconsistent methodology and reporting, they have limitations. For example, LOC in minor head trauma has historically been considered a risk factor for significant injury, and in minor head trauma patients with a GCS of 15 and a history of an LOC, the incidence of intracranial lesions may be increased by a factor of 5 compared with

BOX 38-3. Risk Stratification in Patients with Minor Head Trauma

High Risk

Focal neurologic findings
Asymmetric pupils
Skull fracture on clinical examination
Multiple trauma
Serious, painful, distracting injuries
External signs of trauma above the clavicles
Initial Glasgow Coma Scale score of 14 or 15
Loss of consciousness
Posttraumatic confusion/anemia
Progressively worsening headache
Vomiting
Posttraumatic seizure
History of bleeding disorder/anticoagulation
Recent ingestion of intoxicants
Unreliable/unknown history of injury
Previous neurologic diagnosis
Previous epilepsy
Suspected child abuse
Age >60 yr, <2 yr

Medium Risk

Initial Glasgow Coma Scale score of 15
Brief loss of consciousness
Posttraumatic amnesia
Vomiting
Headache
Intoxication

Low Risk

Currently asymptomatic
No other injuries
No focality on examination
Normal pupils
No change in consciousness
Intact orientation/memory
Initial Glasgow Coma Scale score of 15
Accurate history
Trivial mechanism
Injury >24 hr ago
No or mild headache
No vomiting
No preexisting high-risk factors

patients who have not sustained an LOC.[58] However, the negative predictive value for LOC has not been determined, and many patients who have TBI may have sustained only brief or no LOC. Anecdotal information suggests that the longer the duration of LOC, the more likely that an intracranial lesion exists, but the actual correlation between the duration of the LOC and the incidence of intracranial lesions has not been determined.[60] Other high-risk minor head trauma criteria have also been proposed. The key for the emergency physician, however, is to determine the low-risk patient, and these criteria are less controversial.

Imaging Studies

A major and controversial decision regarding the emergency department management of minor head trauma is whether imaging studies should be performed. Several approaches have been described in the literature, but the research behind these suggestions remains confusing primarily because of differences in study populations, definitions, and methods. Neurosurgical literature often advocates CT scanning of all patients with minor head trauma with a history of LOC (duration not clearly defined) or with amnesia for the traumatic event.[60,61] When interpreting this recommendation, however, emergency departments must recognize that their patients with minor head trauma requiring neurosurgical consultation probably represent a select, more injured population. Others advocate only hospital observation because the yield of initial abnormal scans requiring acute neurosurgical intervention is low, but patients who do deteriorate after minor head trauma have substantial morbidity and mortality. If resources allow, prolonged emergency department observation may be practical in some circumstances. For example, intoxicated patients with minor head injury who otherwise fulfill low-risk criteria should undergo meticulous serial evaluations in the emergency department until clinical sobriety is achieved. In these patients a CT scan may be unnecessary, and observation is beneficial. Some experts advocate both CT scanning and observation of all patients with minor head trauma to allow early detection of delayed complications or deterioration when the initial scan is normal.[60] Most experts, however, do not believe this is necessary. About 3% of all patients with minor head trauma deteriorate unexpectedly; fewer than 1% have surgically significant lesions.[62] The risk of intracranial lesions and delayed complications is minimal in low-risk patients with minor head trauma.

The most practical approach regarding CT scanning in the emergency department patient is probably selective scanning or observation based on risk stratification of the minor head trauma patient. If the low-risk patient is fully awake and not intoxicated, has no focal neurologic findings, no clinical evidence of skull fracture, and can be kept under competent observation for 12 to 24 hours, neuroimaging is usually not indicated.[58] Patients with moderate-risk minor head trauma (see Box 38-3) should probably undergo CT scanning or prolonged observation. Studies have prospectively identified and validated high-risk criteria for adult patients with minor head trauma that correlate with increased likelihood of intracranial lesions. These include the presence of a headache, vomiting, age older than 60, drug or alcohol intoxication, short-term memory deficits, external signs of trauma above the clavicles, and posttraumatic seizures.[63,64] A CT scan should therefore be considered for patients with these high-risk findings as well as the other criteria listed in Box 38-3.

Skull radiography after head trauma in adults has been largely replaced by more sophisticated imaging, when imaging is performed. Facial, scalp, or external signs of head trauma by themselves do not predict TBI in minor head trauma patients, but a skull fracture substantially increases the risk.[58] The skull fracture is therefore helpful to determine an increased risk for TBI, but its absence does not rule out TBI. Unless a specific skull lesion is suspected from physical examination, the yield of skull radiographs in minor head trauma patients is very low, and CT scanning is the preferred imaging study, when imaging is done. On rare occasions, minor head trauma patients who are deemed to be at indeterminate or moderate risk for intracranial injury and who cannot undergo a head CT scan (e.g., CT not immediately available) might be screened by plain skull radiographs to determine the need for a subsequent scan. Skull radiographs may reveal the presence of a skull fracture, pneumocephalus, fluid in the sinuses, depressed skull fracture, and penetrating foreign bodies.[65] Most fractures that are detected in minor head trauma patients are linear fractures with limited clinical significance in adults. Patients with clinical signs of a basilar skull fracture have a substantially increased incidence of intracranial lesions associated with their minor head trauma.[66] When the clinical examination shows evidence of skull fractures, CT scanning should be considered, forgoing plain radiographs.

Although CT scanning is extremely sensitive for acute blood, MRI is more sensitive than CT for detecting diffuse axonal injury, ischemia after TBI, and some hemorrhagic lesions, especially those located at the base of the skull or in the posterior fossa. Functional imaging, such as positron emission tomography (PET), can provide information on the metabolic and neurochemical state of the injured brain. Many studies suggest that significant long-term neuropsychiatric sequelae after minor head trauma can occur despite an initial negative head CT scan, and these may be related to lesions seen initially only by MRI or functional imaging.[67,68]

No routine laboratory tests are needed for patients with isolated minor head trauma. A urine toxicology screen and blood alcohol level may be useful in interpreting the patient's mental status. Alcohol can affect the GCS, but this effect is not observed until the blood alcohol concentration is greater than 200 mg/dL; until that level, changes in mental status cannot be explained solely by acute alcohol intoxication.[69]

Disposition

Most patients with low-risk minor head trauma can be discharged from the emergency department after a normal examination and observation of 4 to 6 hours.[59] If the emergency physician decides that the patient with moderate- or high-risk minor head trauma can be sent home, an appropriate early follow-up should be arranged. Patients should be discharged with instructions describing the signs and symptoms of delayed complications of head injury, should have access to a telephone, and should be monitored in the acute posttrauma period by a responsible, sober adult. If any doubt exists regarding the safety of the discharged patient with minor head injury, a brief inpatient observation period (i.e., 12 to 24 hours) is advisable.

If a patient with minor head trauma returns to the emergency department because of persistent symptoms, delayed complications of minor head injury should be sought.

Concussion

A concussion is a temporary and brief interruption of neurologic function after minor head trauma, which may involve LOC. Acute CT or MRI abnormalities are not usually found after concussions, but functional imaging (i.e., PET) shows abnormal glucose uptake and CBF when concussed patients perform spatial working memory tasks.[68] Many theories exist regarding the pathophysiology of concussion: shearing or stretching of white matter fibers at the time of impact, temporary neuronal dysfunction, transient alterations in levels of neurotransmitters, and temporary changes in CBF and oxygen use. A convulsive theory has been proposed to explain the physical and functional signs and symptoms following concussion.[70] Regardless of the underlying pathophysiology, levels of some neurotransmitters remain elevated and a hypermetabolic state may persist in the brain for several days to weeks after the initial injury.[67,68]

The most common complaints after concussion are headache, confusion, and amnesia, of variable duration and intensity. Approximately 300,000 yearly sports-related concussions are reported to the Centers for Disease Control and Prevention, usually a result of acceleration-deceleration forces to the head.[71] As many as 8% of U.S. high school and college football players sustain concussions each football season.[72] A study of concussed football players showed acute symptoms lasting at least 5 days, cognitive impairments lasting from 5 to 7 days, and balance deficits for 3 to 5 days after concussion; 91% were back to their preinjury baseline by 7 days, but some had deficits on verbal fluency tests as long as 90 days after injury.[72]

The demonstrated period of neurodysfunction and the delayed return to cognitive and physical baseline that follows concussive impact have lead to the development of several scoring systems to grade severity of concussions with the goal of determining when it is safe for an athlete to return to play. No single set of guidelines has emerged that has been universally accepted, but all are predicated on the concern about a period of vulnerability following impact. Football players sustaining concussion appear susceptible to an additional concussion,[73] with the majority of reinjury occurring within 10 days after the first injury, possibly because of balance defects, delayed reflexes, or delayed speed of information processing.[74]

The *second impact syndrome* occurs when an athlete sustains a second concussion before being completely asymptomatic from the first and then experiences a rapid, usually fatal, neurologic decline. It is postulated that persistent neurochemical disruptions and altered autoregulatory mechanisms after a first injury make the brain particularly vulnerable to marked brain swelling and subsequent herniation after a seemingly minor second impact.[74] Although the existence and frequency of the second impact syndrome are controversial and hotly debated in the sports medicine literature, its serious implications affect subsequent management decisions regarding head-injured athletes and others with concussion. All current recommendations for return to play after a sports-related concussion state that players with concussion should not return to play for at least 1 week after they have become asymptomatic. This is usually increased to at least a symptom-free month if an LOC or prolonged posttraumatic amnesia occurred at the time of concussion.[75]

Postconcussive symptoms may persistent for days to months after a concussion and are termed the *postconcussive syndrome* (PCS). The most common delayed or persistent postconcussive complaints are headache, sensory sensitivity, memory or concentration difficulties, irritability, sleep disturbances, and depression. It was long believed that persistent postconcussive symptoms were psychosomatic, litigious, or factitious. However, the presence of abnormalities on functional imaging and with sophisticated neuropsychometric testing suggests a pathophysiologic basis for the PCS. It was shown that emergency department patients who initially present with posttraumatic headache, nausea, or dizziness had an increased likelihood of having PCS. The duration of PCS was related to the number of initial complaints, with 50% of patients with three symptoms remaining symptomatic at 6 months after injury.[76]

Clinical Features

A wide spectrum of transient neurologic symptoms may occur with concussion; the most common complaints are headache, confusion, and amnesia for the traumatic event. The neurologic examination is nonfocal. The duration of the amnestic period suggests the severity of the sustained injury. Adults may complain of "seeing stars" or feeling nauseated, dizzy, or disoriented for a brief period. A brief LOC may last for seconds up to several minutes, but many patients report no LOC. In young children, acute symptoms of concussion differ from those in adults and may include restlessness, lethargy, confusion, or irritability. On presentation, they may be vomiting, be tachycardic, or appear pale. These signs and symptoms are usually completely resolved by 6 hours.

Disposition

The management decisions faced by the emergency physician are the same as those addressed when evaluating all patients with apparently minor head trauma: extent of workup to initiate in the emergency department and whether the patient can be safely discharged home. Emergency department patients who have a sports-related concussion should probably not be allowed to return to play from the emergency department; follow-up at 1 week determines the duration of symptoms and when the patient can safely return to sports. The possibility of the PCS should be considered in all concussed patients, regardless of their initially benign presentation, and it may be prudent to suggest scheduled primary care follow-up for reassessment if symptoms persist.

PEDIATRIC HEAD INJURIES

Epidemiology

Approximately 500,000 children are emergently evaluated yearly in the United States for head trauma, with approximately 100,000 hospital admissions and 7000 fatalities.[32] TBI accounts for the single largest source of childhood mortality, with an additional 29,000 children suffering permanent neurologic disability.[32] In children, transportation-related injuries or falls account for most head trauma. Child abuse is a common etiology of head injury in young children. Dunhaime and colleagues[77] found that nearly 25% of head-injured children younger than 2 had inflicted injuries. In head-injured children younger than 1 year, as many as 66% of all injuries and 95% of severe injuries may be nonaccidental.[78]

Pathophysiology

Until the cranial sutures close, children's skulls are more distensible than those of adults. As a result, young children may often sustain less TBI after head trauma than adults with comparable nonfatal mechanisms of injury.[32] Children, however, appear to have an age-dependent brain vulnerability. Very young children (younger than 1 year) have higher mortality after head trauma than older children with the same severity of injury.[32] Many factors contribute to this. Medical attention is often delayed in children with nonaccidental injuries. Because of limited language and comprehension, an accurate formal neurologic examination in young children is sometimes difficult. Medical personnel tend to underestimate the extent of the injuries in small children and are often reluctant to initiate invasive procedures, which may be necessary to aid in the diagnostic workup, such as IV access for sedation in CT scanning.

The types of TBI sustained after head trauma in children differ from those in adults. Children have fewer traumatic mass lesions, fewer hemorrhagic contusions, more diffuse brain swelling, and more diffuse axonal injury.[32] Of head-injured patients younger than 20 who talk and deteriorate, 39% have brain swelling only (i.e., no mass lesions), whereas 87% of patients older than 40 who talk and deteriorate have mass lesions.[79]

Clinical Features

As with adults, an accurate description of the mechanism of injury, the appearance of the child immediately before and after the injury, and subsequent events can provide useful information to assist in the evaluation and management of the acutely head-injured child.

In principle, the acute neurologic assessment of the head-injured child is the same as that of adults. Pupillary responsiveness and size, corneal reflexes, the presence of a gag or cough reflex, and spontaneous motor movements provide baseline neurologic information that can be followed over time. Additional neurologic assessment can be more challenging. Because of its reliance on developed language skills and the patient's attention and cooperation, the GCS is difficult to apply to children younger than 5 years. Modified scales have been developed, but none has been rigorously validated; as yet, no universally accepted coma scale exists for children.[32] Mental status changes, which may be the first symptom of head injury, are difficult to evaluate in children, and often the head-injured toddler has no deficit except irritability.

Children with severe and moderate head injury are clinically similar to adults with these degrees of injury, although children have an increased incidence of posttraumatic seizures after severe head injury. Infants appear at especially high risk for posttraumatic seizures.[80] Overall, up to 6% of all head-injured children and 35% of severely head-injured children have early (i.e., within the first week) posttraumatic seizures.[32] Most seizures occur within the first 24 hours and do not predict seizures later in the posttraumatic period.[32] However, early posttraumatic seizures can exacerbate secondary brain injury. Although long-term anticonvulsants are probably not indicated, acute prophylaxis with phenytoin is recommended in severely head-injured children to prevent early posttraumatic seizures.[80]

Children who sustain minor head trauma often have more pronounced physical signs and symptoms than adults. Despite apparently trivial trauma, children may appear pale, be lethargic, and have frequent emesis and complaints of headaches and dizziness. Concussive injuries in children produce two unique clinical circumstances. Many children experience a brief *impact seizure* at the time of relatively minor head injury. By the time the child is evaluated, he or she is at baseline neurologic function. Impact seizures do not appear to predict subsequent early posttraumatic seizures. However, a posttraumatic impact seizure may confuse the initial assessment of the severity of the head injury and prompt a more aggressive workup than needed. *Postconcussive blindness,* another serious complication of concussive injuries in children, is usually associated with impact to the back of the head.[81] Children experience a temporary loss of vision that can persist from minutes to hours before normal vision returns.

The clinical presentation of posttraumatic *intracranial lesions* in infants can be extremely subtle, especially in those younger than 6 months. Often these lesions are associated with scalp injuries and skull fractures but no other symptoms.[32,82] Toddlers are also difficult to assess; the only symptom of an intracranial injury may be irritability. Most authorities suggest that all head-injured infants and toddlers younger than 2 years should be considered at least at moderate risk for intracranial lesions, unless the injury was trivial.[82]

Inflicted head injury is the most common cause of head injury deaths in infants.[83] Child abuse must be considered in all children with unexplained head injuries or injuries not consistent with the history provided. The *shaken-baby syndrome* involves an acceleration-deceleration brain injury, with the moving brain striking against the interior of the skull.[32] Patients present with a broad range of symptoms, from nonspecific complaints to seizures and coma. Classically described findings include retinal hemorrhages, subdural hematomas, subarachnoid blood, and no signs of external trauma.[32]

Diagnosis and Management

As with adults, pediatric head-injured patients should be assessed for other major trauma and assumed to have cervical spine injury until proved otherwise. Goals of emergency department management are also generally the same: to prevent secondary injury and systemic insults, to prevent increasing ICP, and to detect traumatic mass lesions requiring emergency surgery. Airway management should be aggressive to prevent hypoxia and its complications and to allow brief hyperventilation if acute neurologic deterioration occurs.

In children, unlike adults, hypovolemic hypotension can occur because of head trauma. Hypotension from intracranial bleeding can occur in children younger than 1 year with a large linear skull fracture and an underlying large epidural hematoma.[32] The intracranial blood can seep through the fracture and produce a large galeal or subperiosteal hematoma. Hypotension from intracranial bleeding can also occur in a child with hydrocephalus and a functioning shunt. Blood may accumulate without much evidence of increased ICP. Scalp lacerations can also produce significant hemorrhage and subsequent hypotension.

Up to 80% of children with severe head trauma have elevated ICP.[32] In infants, a bulging fontanelle suggests elevated ICP. Other signs of elevated ICP include bradycardia, papilledema, declining level of consciousness, and seizures. When increased ICP is suggested by physical examination, methods to reduce ICP should be initiated. As with adults, acute hyperventilation has immediate effects but is never indicated for prophylaxis or for prolonged management of increased ICP.[32,80] Mannitol can also be used for reducing ICP but carries additional theoretical risks in children. Mannitol transiently increases CBF after administration. In children, increased CBF causes relatively more hyperemia than in adults.[32,80] When the hyperemic state develops, ICP increases. In brain-injured children who already have increased ICP, the additional increase can cause neurologic deterioration. This side effect may be lessened if mannitol is delivered at doses of 0.25 to 0.5 g/kg over 15 minutes rather than as an IV bolus.[80,81] Several studies have also renewed interest in 3% hypertonic saline, with some authorities advocating its use.[80] Severely head-injured children are less likely to have a surgically amenable lesion than adults. Because diffuse brain swelling is the most common finding in severely head-injured children, emergency burr holes are generally ineffective.

When considering minor head injury in children, it is important to differentiate children younger than 2 and older children. Children younger than 2 years with traumatic brain injuries are often difficult to assess and may have subtle clinical findings.[84,85] In general, the literature supports the conclusion that younger patients are at higher risk for intracranial injury.[32,82] One clinical sign of potential brain injury in children younger than 2 is the presence of a scalp hematoma, especially a large parietal scalp hematoma.[84-86] In an observational cohort study involving children with low risk for brain injuries,[87] scalp hematomas were present in 93% of children 2 years old or younger who had brain injuries.

The CT scan is the diagnostic imaging modality of choice in the evaluation of moderate or severe head trauma. It should also be strongly considered in pediatric patients with minor head trauma who have history of vomiting, abnormal mental status or lethargy, clinical signs of a skull fracture, obvious scalp hematomas in children 2 years old or younger, and increasing headache.[82,87] In these circumstances, the risks of sedating the child to obtain a high-quality image should be weighed against the likelihood of an intracranial lesion in the child with minor head trauma.

The use of skull radiographs in the diagnostic workup of head-injured children is controversial but may be appropriate under some circumstances. As with adults, when a CT scan is indicated, skull radiographs are not necessary. The presence of a skull fracture increases the likelihood of intracranial pathology up to 20-fold; conversely, a negative radiographic skull screen does not guarantee absence of TBI.[32,82] Parietal skull fractures are the most common.[82] Often, fractures occur in infants who sustain relatively minor head injury.[82] Skull films may be useful as a screening tool in determining the need for a CT scan, especially in children 2 years old or younger whose neurologic examination is difficult to obtain and interpret. In alert children younger than 2 with minor head injury, a low-risk history, a normal physical examination that includes a normal neurologic and mental status examination appropriate for age, and a scalp hematoma, skull films may be a useful screen.[82] If the skull film is negative for a fracture, a CT scan may be unnecessary. If the skull film shows a fracture, CT imaging is indicated.

In older children, skull films are rarely useful unless a specific lesion is suspected, such as a depressed skull fracture or a penetrating foreign object. Skull fractures are more clinically significant in children than in adults. Fractures, especially complex stellate or multiple injuries, are often seen in abused children, and skull films should be obtained if abuse is suspected. *Ping-pong fractures* occur with concentrated forces that indent the skull. These fractures are unique to infants and appear as multiple indentations in the skull with no significant bone discontinuity. Skull fractures are common in children who have sustained deep scalp lacerations or who have a large scalp hematoma.

Leptomeningeal cysts or *growing skull fractures* are delayed complications of linear skull fractures in infancy. If a tear in the dura accompanies the linear fracture, the meninges may fill with CSF and prolapse through the fracture margins, thus preventing fracture healing.[32] These cysts can grow in size and have the potential to cause a mass effect. If a linear fracture is found by skull radiography, close follow-up is indicated to assess for this delayed complication.

Overall, children who sustain severe head injury have lower mortality and a better neurologic outcome than comparably injured adults.[32,80] This is probably because of the great neuroplasticity of the young brain; however, in children younger than 2 years, the prognosis after severe head injury is poor. Very young children have immature cerebrovascular autoregulation, which increases the risk of cerebral edema formation. The immature brain has increased susceptibility to permanent injury because of incomplete myelination.

The emergency evaluation of children with minor head injury is especially challenging, given their potentially dramatic presentation and the added difficulty of obtaining an accurate neurologic assessment (Box 38-4). In the past few years several practice guidelines have become available for evaluation and management of minor head injury in children.[82,87-89] The guidelines have been advanced for narrowly defined circumstances and are applicable only to children with isolated minor head injury evaluated within 24 hours after trauma. Children with minor head injury outside these parameters may require competent observation and, if symptoms persist or worsen, a CT scan. Disposition of pediatric patients with minor head injury is summarized in Box 38-4. Parents should be educated about the warning signs and symptoms of delayed complications of minor head trauma.

PENETRATING HEAD INJURIES

Epidemiology

Penetrating head injury occurs at a rate of 12 per 100,000 population and can be sustained by missile injuries or impalement.[90] The United States has the highest penetrating head injury rate among developed countries in the world,[3] the most common cause being *gunshot wounds* (GSWs). These dramatic injuries are increasing in frequency, and, unfortunately, the neuroscientific understanding of the complicated cerebral events that occur with penetrating head injury does not yet equal our understanding of the pathophysiology of blunt injuries.

Civilian GSWs to the head account for about 21,000 deaths per year, and up to 66% of all patients who sustain a GSW to the head are dead at the scene.[2,91] Overall, the mortality caused by a GSW to the head is estimated to be 90%.[91,92] If the patient is hemodynamically stable, has not sustained secondary systemic insults such as hypoxia or hypotension, has no expanding mass lesions from the missile injury, and has not ingested intoxicants that may interfere with assessment, prognosis after a GSW to the head can be predicted by the presenting GCS and pupillary responsiveness.[90] If the presenting GCS is less than 5, mortality approaches 100%. If the presenting GCS is greater than 8 and the pupils are reactive, survival approaches 75%.[90] Survivors of GSW to the head tend to do well, with up to 60% returning to their former employment.[91,92]

The treatment of civilian penetrating brain injury (PBI) has not been well studied in the past decade.[93]

Pathophysiology

Missile injuries to the head can result in several different patterns of damage. *Tangential wounds* are caused by an impact that occurs at an oblique angle to the skull. If the missile has high velocity but low energy, it can travel around the skull under the scalp without passing through the skull itself. Intracranial damage, primarily cortical contusions, can occur at the initial site of impact because of pressure waves generated by the impact. In one study, 24% of patients with tangential GSWs also had intracranial hemorrhage, and 16% sustained skull fractures.[91] *Perforating wounds* are usually caused by high-velocity projectiles, which cause through-and-through injuries of the brain with an entrance and an exit wound. This type of injury is largely discussed within the context of military GSWs to the head.[93] In cases of complete traversal (through-and-through) GSW to the head, the entrance wound is usually smaller than the exit wound.

Penetrating missile wounds are produced with moderate- to high-velocity projectiles discharged at close range. The majority of the civilian PBI literature deals with penetrating missile wounds.[93] The penetrating object may travel through the entire skull, bounce off the opposite inner table of the skull and ricochet within the brain, or stop somewhere within the cranial cavity. Bullets that penetrate the skull do not travel in a straight path. The wounding capacity of a firearm is related to the kinetic energy of its missile on impact and how much energy is dissipated in the tissues.[92] Low-velocity missiles tend to be deflected by intracranial structures. The final track is therefore erratic and occasionally bears no relation to the exit or entrance site of the missile. High-velocity missiles can project straight through the tissues and easily fracture bones. Flight stability and the angle at which the bullet strikes its target affect the path through the brain. Within tissue, destabilizing motions include deviation of the longitudinal axis of the bullet from a straight line (yaw), forward rotation of the bullet around its center of mass (tumbling), and oscillatory motion of the bullet axis around its center of mass (rotation).[92] As the bullet passes through the brain, a tissue cavity is created. This cavity can be as much as 10 times the diameter of the missile. A percussion shock wave is also created, lasting 2 milliseconds, but causes little tissue destruction.[92]

The morbidity and mortality from missile injuries to the head depend on the intracranial path, speed of entry, and the size and type of the penetrating object. Projectiles that cross the midline or the geographic center of the brain, pass through the ventricles, or come to rest in the posterior fossa are associated with extremely high mortality.[90] High-velocity wounds are associated with greater mortality than low-velocity injuries. Large missiles or missiles that fragment within the cranial vault are usually fatal. The design of the bullet and its fragmentation potential (capacity to deform or fragment) also contribute to final tissue destruction and patients' morbidity and mortality.[92]

Many GSWs to the head are intentionally self-inflicted injuries. The percentage of penetrating head injuries caused by self-inflicted GSWs ranges from 13% to 88%.[93] Characteristics of self-inflicted GSWs include injury on the dominant side, powder burns at the entrance site, and large stellate scalp lacerations caused by dissection of the subgaleal layer by exploding gases released close to the scalp.[93] In suicide attempts, GSWs to the head tend to traverse the midline in the coronal plane and often involve major vascular structures. If the self-inflicted GSW has an entrance through the mouth, injury to the hard palate may occur with potential upper airway compromise. The careful aim and close range of self-inflicted GSWs to the head make these injuries particularly devastating; mortality is higher than with non–self-inflicted penetrating injuries and odds ratios vary between 1.63 and 5.83.[93]

Clinical Features

Physical assessment of the patient with a missile wound to the head focuses on the presenting GCS and pupillary responsiveness.[94,95] In addition to the physical damage to brain tissue caused by the penetrating injury, other devastating physiologic changes occur immediately after injury. ICP rises, the BBB breaks down, CBF is altered, and cerebral edema develops. Cerebral autoregulation is lost, and CPP may fall.

Management

The emergency department management is directed at reducing the occurrence of the secondary systemic insults of hypoxia and ischemia, with emergent intervention if signs of herniation syndrome develop and the patient is viable. Management should be aggressive until the prognosis can be established by examination and neuroimaging data. When penetration of the cranial vault is established, the patient should be intubated. If the physician waits for coma before intubating the patient, mortality approaches 100%.[96]

Emergency treatment should include IV antibiotics because penetrating missiles are contaminated with skin, bone, and hair. Tissue contamination may be widespread because of the cavitation caused by the missile as it passes through the brain.[97] Seizures typically occur after penetrating head injuries. Anticonvulsants should be given in the acute setting to prevent early posttraumatic seizures in patients with PBI, especially if the patient is to be transported to another institution after acute stabilization.[98] Anticonvulsants should not be given beyond the first week after PBI, as this has not been shown to prevent the development of late seizures.[98]

Skull radiographs are useful in determining the number of penetrating fragments and their track. A CT scan defines the precise location of the missile, its intracranial path, the presence of bone or missile fragments, extraaxial or intracerebral blood collections or other traumatic lesions, and pneumocephalus. CT scanning is the radiologic test of choice for PBI.[99] Pneumocephalus is often associated with missile wounds that penetrate the sinuses but can be caused by free air sucked into the penetration cavity behind the projectile.

When a penetrating head injury is caused by *impalement*, the penetrating object should be left in place to be removed at surgery. A skull radiograph shows the size of the object, the angle of impalement, and the depth of penetration. Angiography may be indicated to better discern location referable to key vascular structures.

COMPLICATIONS AFTER HEAD INJURY

Neurologic Complications

Seizures

Posttraumatic seizures are relatively common in the acute or subacute period. Acute posttraumatic seizures are usually brief and are probably caused by transient mechanical and neurochemical changes within the brain. After the acute seizure, the patient often has no additional seizure activity. In the subacute period, 24 to 48 hours after trauma, seizures are caused by worsening cerebral edema, small hemorrhages, or penetrating injuries. Posttraumatic seizures are common in children and can be precipitated by relatively minor head injury.[80] Acute posttraumatic seizure prophylaxis in the emergency department is recommended for some head-injured patients even if they have not had a seizure (see Box 38-2).[49,51,98] This is especially important in patients who will have neuromuscular blockade to facilitate management or transfer because the clinical manifestations of seizures are lost in these patients. The prevalence of early posttraumatic seizures varies from 4% to 25%.[98] Phenytoin (15 mg/kg) is used as a first-line agent for prophylaxis. The decision to maintain the head-injured patient on long-term anticonvulsant therapy during the recovery period depends on the patient's subsequent course. Long-term seizure prophylaxis is not indicated for all patients who have had posttraumatic seizures in the acute or subacute period.[49,51] The utility of prophylactic anticonvulsants to prevent late posttraumatic seizures has not been proved and their use is not recommended.[49,51,98]

Central Nervous System Infections

Meningitis after Basilar Fractures

Posttraumatic meningitis is caused by a variety of microbes, depending on the portal of bacterial entry. Patients present with typical signs and symptoms of meningitis, including fever, altered mental status, and occasional focal neurologic signs. In patients with a CSF leak after basilar fracture, early meningitis (i.e., within 3 days of injury) is usually caused by pneumococci. Ceftriaxone or cefotaxime is a reasonable antibiotic choice with the addition of vancomycin if a high regional pneumococcal resistance exists. Gram-negative organisms often cause meningitis that develops more than 3 days after trauma.[100] A third-generation cephalosporin, with nafcillin or vancomycin added to ensure coverage of *Staphylococcus aureus,* should be started. In children, posttraumatic meningitis may be caused by *Haemophilus influenzae.* Prophylactic antibiotics are not currently recommended in the acute setting in patients with CSF leaks caused by basilar skull fractures.[100]

Brain Abscess

Brain abscesses develop infrequently after penetrating missile injuries to the head. Abscesses can also develop after open depressed skull fractures, if bone fragments are not removed, or as a postoperative complication. Posttraumatic CSF fistulae and fractures that disrupt air-filled sinuses predispose to the formation of brain abscesses.[100] Clinical manifestations include headaches, nausea, vomiting, declining mental status, signs of increased ICP, or new focal neurologic findings in patients who had been improving after trauma. Occasionally, nuchal rigidity, hemiparesis, or seizures may be present. Systemic signs are often subtle, and CSF leukocytosis may be absent.

Contrast-enhanced CT scanning makes the diagnosis of brain abscess. A ring pattern with a low-density center is characteristic of a brain abscess. The enhanced ring represents surrounding altered vascular permeability and therefore is also seen in the cerebritis stage early in abscess formation. Lumbar puncture is often not helpful and should not be performed in the patient with signs of increased ICP (e.g., headache, vomiting, papilledema).

The treatment of brain abscess is usually operative drainage. The patient with cerebritis may respond to IV antibiotics but requires close monitoring with repeated CT scans. Common organisms isolated from posttraumatic abscesses are S. aureus and gram-negative aerobes.[100]

Cranial Osteomyelitis

Cranial osteomyelitis can occur after penetrating injury to the skull. The clinical manifestations include pain, tenderness, swelling, and warmth at the infected site. More than 50% of cases are obvious on plain skull films.[100] Technetium bone scans can help in the diagnosis when the skull radiographs are negative, but false-positive bone scans occur in patients with previous trauma or craniotomy. Adding a gallium scan helps to differentiate infection from other causes of a positive technetium scan. Patients with posttraumatic cranial osteomyelitis require surgical debridement and removal of the infected bone. Antibiotic choice is determined by culture results. If systemic symptoms are present, an underlying subdural or epidural empyema is often present.

Medical Complications

Disseminated Intravascular Coagulation

The injured brain is a source of tissue thromboplastin that activates the extrinsic clotting system. Disseminated intravascular coagulation (DIC) can develop within hours after any injury disrupting brain tissue. It has been detected in nearly all patients with severe TBI.[101] DIC increases morbidity and mortality after severe head trauma as well as the risks of delayed intracranial hemorrhage. If a stable patient with DIC suddenly deteriorates, a repeated CT scan should be obtained to rule out hemorrhage.

The extent of tissue destruction determines the degree of DIC that develops. The diagnosis is based on abnormalities in international normalized ratio prothrombin and partial thromboplastin times (INR [PT], PTT), platelets, plasma fibrinogen levels, and fibrin degradation products. Patients with coagulopathy or

abnormal platelet function require interventions to correct these.

Neurogenic Pulmonary Edema

Neurogenic pulmonary edema can develop from minutes to days after head trauma. This noncardiac pulmonary edema probably results from altered hydrostatic forces and microvascular permeability directly caused by brain injury. Lowering the ICP appears to reverse the neurogenic stimulation that causes this edema.[102]

Cardiac Dysfunction

A variety of cardiac rhythm, rate, and conduction abnormalities are detected after head injury. These abnormalities can be life threatening and require aggressive therapy. In addition, adequate cardiac output is essential in head-injured patients to ensure cerebral perfusion. Many head-injured patients with cardiac dysfunction have concurrent myocardial injury from underlying disease or from chest injury. However, brain injury can cause primary cardiac dysfunction. Cardiac rhythm abnormalities have been reported in up to 70% of all patients with subarachnoid hemorrhage (SAH) and more than 50% of all patients with intracranial hemorrhage.[34] In SAH, the cardiac dysrhythmias may result from autonomic nervous system dysfunction that subsequently affects ventricular polarization. High levels of circulating catecholamines have been measured in head-injured patients, with increased sympathetic nervous system activation.[34]

The most common cardiac dysrhythmia after head injury is supraventricular tachycardia, but many other rhythms have been observed. Findings on the electrocardiogram include diffuse large upright or inverted T waves, prolonged QT intervals, ST segment depression or elevation, and U waves.[34] The primary goal in the emergency management of cardiac dysfunction after head trauma is ensuring adequate tissue perfusion and avoiding hypoxia. Dysrhythmias in head-injured patients often resolve as ICP is reduced. Standard advanced cardiac life support protocols should then be used because concurrent cardiac injury may also be present in multiply traumatized patients.[34]

SPECIFIC INJURIES

Scalp Wounds

Scalp lacerations are extremely common after head injury and may be a source of significant bleeding because hemostasis may be difficult to achieve. Methods include direct digital compression of the bleeding vessel against the skull, infiltration of the wound edges with lidocaine with epinephrine, and ligation of identified bleeding vessels. If the galea is lacerated, it can be pulled up with a clamp and its edges folded over the lacerated skin edges to tamponade the bleeding vessels. Raney scalp clips applied to the edges of the wound are also effective. In stable patients, quick closure of the wound, after proper debridement and irrigation, is the most effective way to stop a bleeding scalp laceration and prevent the tissue crush injury that may occur if other compressive methods are used for too long.

When hemostasis is obtained, the wound should be irrigated to rinse away any debris. The emissary vessels of the subgaleal layer of the scalp drain directly into the diploë veins of the skull. These in turn drain into the venous sinuses. Contaminated or infected scalp wounds therefore have the potential to cause serious intracranial infections. Blood clots and other debris should be removed and the galea and underlying cranium palpated to detect any remaining debris, disruptions, or bone step-offs. Shear injuries may deposit contaminants at sites distant from the apparent injury. The complexity of stellate lacerations often interferes with thorough inspection and debridement; stellate lacerations are particularly susceptible to infection. Digital exploration of a scalp wound should be carefully performed; if it is done too vigorously, comminuted or depressed bone pieces may be depressed further.

It is easy to confuse a disruption in the galea or a tear in the periosteum with a skull fracture. The base of the laceration should therefore be directly visualized. Clipping away a small area of hair parallel to the edges of the wound may facilitate this. Alternatively, an antibiotic ointment can be applied to the hair immediately surrounding the wound and used to plaster the hair away from the injury site. If the laceration begins on the forehead and extends upward beyond the hairline, surrounding hair should not be removed. Removal obliterates a useful landmark for cosmetic closure and may result in malalignment of the two laceration edges. If hair is accidentally embedded within the repaired laceration, it can delay healing by producing an inflammatory reaction or by serving as a nidus of infection.

Disruption of the galea results in a gaping scalp laceration. Large lacerations of the galea must be closed to prevent the edges of the wound from pulling apart as the muscles within the galea contract. The skin, dermis, and galea can usually be repaired in a single layer with interrupted or vertical mattress sutures of 3-0 nylon or polypropylene.[103] In scalp lacerations in which the galea is not involved, staples can be used in the repair.

Because of the rich blood supply of the scalp, even very large scalp avulsions can survive. If the avulsion remains attached to the rest of the scalp by a tissue bridge, it should be reattached to the surrounding tissue. If the avulsion is completely detached from the scalp, it should be treated as any other amputated part and reimplanted as soon as possible.

Scalp abrasions are often contaminated with pieces of dirt or other debris. The wound should be cleaned as thoroughly as possible and inspected for puncture wounds or other areas that penetrate beyond the superficial layers of the skin to ensure the removal of unsuspected foreign bodies. A careful inspection often reveals a small scalp laceration within the abraded area. Antibiotics are usually not needed for carefully managed scalp wounds because rapid healing is facilitated by the rich blood supply of the scalp.

Skull Fractures

Clinical Assessment and Significance

Skull fractures are local injuries caused by direct impact to the skull. The presence of a skull fracture does not always indicate underlying brain injury. However, the force required to fracture the skull is substantial, and all cases of skull fracture must be carefully evaluated to ensure that no additional injury is present. With increasing severity of head injury the likelihood of skull fracture increases, and the presence of a skull fracture after trauma increases the likelihood of having a TBI.[82,104,105] It is often difficult to predict the presence of a skull fracture by clinical examination, and if this can be done, it is likely that substantial underlying brain injury is also present. The pattern, extent, and type of skull fracture depend on the force of the impact applied and the ratio of the impact force to the impact area. The fracture usually starts at the point of maximum impact.

Clinically significant skull fractures (1) result in intracranial air and pass through an air-filled space (e.g., sinus), (2) are associated with an overlying scalp laceration (open skull fracture), (3) are depressed below the level of the skull's inner table, or (4) overlie a major dural venous sinus or the middle meningeal artery.

The best way to assess for skull fractures is by plain skull radiographs; however, these x-ray films are expensive and time-consuming and should be ordered selectively. The most useful plain radiographs are those that help demonstrate a depressed skull fracture, the depth and extent of a penetrating injury, or the presence of an intracranial foreign body. A CT scan with bone windows also demonstrates these findings, and therefore patients undergoing CT do not require skull radiographs. If the patient is not likely to undergo CT and is at high risk for skull fracture, especially depressed fracture, skull radiographs may prove useful to detect clinically significant fractures. MRI is not useful for detecting skull fractures.

Linear Fractures

A linear skull fracture is a single fracture that goes through the entire thickness of the skull. Linear skull fractures are clinically important if they cross the middle meningeal groove or major venous dural sinuses; they can disrupt these vascular structures and cause the formation of epidural hematomas. Most other linear skull fractures are not clinically significant.

It is sometimes difficult to distinguish linear skull fractures demonstrated on radiographs from cranial sutures. In general, fractures are more lucent than vascular grooves and sutures. Sutures are usually less than 2 mm wide in adults; fractures are often 3 mm or greater in overall width and tend to be widest in the midportion and narrow at each end.[104,105] Linear fractures are most common in the temporoparietal, frontal, and occipital regions of the skull and can usually be visualized on more than one radiographic view. In children, skull fractures heal within 3 to 6 months; in adults, complete healing may take up to 3 years.[104,105]

Sutural diastasis is the traumatic disruption of a cranial suture. In adults, sutural diastasis often involves the coronal or lambdoid sutures. Sutural diastasis usually occurs when a linear fracture extends into the suture line, and it is rare after sutures have undergone bone fusion.[104,105]

Comminuted skull fractures are multiple linear fractures that radiate from the impact site. Usually this injury suggests a more severe blow to the head than that producing a single linear fracture.

A linear *vault* fracture substantially increases the risk of intracranial injury. If any skull fracture is detected, a CT scan should be obtained and the patient should be carefully observed for delayed complications of head trauma.

Depressed Fractures

Depressed skull fractures are clinically important because they predispose to significant underlying brain injury and to complications of head trauma, such as infection and seizures. When a depressed fracture occurs, traumatic impact drives the bone piece below the plane of the skull. The edges of the depressed portion of skull may become locked underneath the adjacent intact bone and fail to rebound into their previous position. As a result, the depressed piece of bone can penetrate tissue and lacerate the dura. Depressed skull fractures are usually caused by direct impact injury with small blunt objects, such as a hammer or a baseball bat. Most depressed skull fractures occur over the parietal or temporal regions. If the free piece of bone is depressed deeper than the adjacent inner table of the skull, most neurosurgeons consider this injury significant enough to require elevation.

On skull radiographs, depressed fractures may be difficult to visualize. The free piece of bone demonstrates increased or double density because it often overlaps the nonfractured bone or it is viewed relatively rotated from the rest of the adjacent cranium. Tangential views of the skull may increase the ability to visualize the fracture.

Depressed skull fractures can often be felt with palpation of the skull beneath a scalp laceration. This examination should be done cautiously to avoid driving a depressed bone fragment deeper into the cranial tissue. The clinical examination for a depressed skull fracture may be misleading. The mobility of the scalp can result in nonalignment of the fracture with an overlying scalp laceration. As a result, the skull underlying the laceration may be normal, with the depressed area several centimeters away. Scalp swelling may also interfere with physical examination findings and hide any palpable bone defects. The signs and symptoms of a depressed skull fracture depend on the depth of depression of the free bone piece. About 25% of patients sustaining a depressed skull fracture report LOC.[104,105] Neurologic deficits may be present, depending on the extent of underlying brain tissue injury.

A CT scan is indicated for patients with a history or physical examination that suggests a depressed skull fracture. The CT scan should include bone windows to determine the depth of depression and the presence of concurrent traumatic intracranial lesions. Patients with depressed skull fractures should be admitted for continued observation.

Depressed skull fractures may increase the risk for developing seizures. Emergency department patients suspected of having a depressed skull fracture warrant prophylaxis for posttraumatic seizures, especially if they have an altered level of consciousness or require chemical paralysis. Depressed skull fractures may also increase the risk for meningitis.[105]

Basilar Fractures

Basilar fractures are linear fractures at the base of the skull. The fracture usually occurs through the temporal bone, with bleeding into the middle ear producing hemotympanum. Often the fracture has caused a dural tear, which produces a communication between the subarachnoid space, the paranasal sinuses, and the middle ear. This offers a route for the introduction of infection into the cranial cavity and is suggested by a CSF leak.[100] As with linear skull fractures, a basilar fracture is not always associated with significant underlying brain injury; these fractures are the result of considerable impact force, however, and TBI must be ruled out.

Basilar fractures can compress and entrap the cranial nerves that pass through the basal foramina, can dislocate the bones of the auricular chain, and can disrupt the otic canal or cavernous sinuses, with subsequent injury to cranial nerves III, IV, and V. Fractures of the sphenoid bone can disrupt the intracavernous internal carotid artery, creating the potential for the formation of pseudoaneurysms or carotid venous fistulae. The diagnosis of a basilar skull fracture is based on associated clinical signs and symptoms (see Box 38-1).

Skull radiographs do not detect basilar fractures well. All patients with clinical evidence suggesting a basilar skull fracture should have a CT scan, to define the fracture and to rule out concurrent intracranial pathology, and should be admitted for observation. Because the basilar skull fracture may afford an entrance for bacteria, antibiotics are often considered. However, most CSF leaks resolve spontaneously with no complications in 1 week, and, in general, antibiotics are not given prophylactically during the first week of CSF rhinorrhea.[100] If a patient with a previously diagnosed CSF leak returns to the emergency department later with fever, the diagnosis of meningitis should be strongly suspected and appropriate workup (i.e., lumbar puncture) and antibiotic treatment initiated immediately.

Open Fractures

A skull fracture is open when a scalp laceration overlies a fracture. If the fracture has disrupted the dura, a communication exists between the external environment and the brain. A fracture that disrupts the paranasal sinuses or the middle ear structures is also considered open. An open skull fracture requires careful irrigation and debridement. Blind probing of the wound should be avoided because it can introduce contaminants into the wound and can further depress comminuted fracture pieces.

Diffuse Axonal Injury

Prolonged traumatic coma not caused by mass lesions, ischemic insult, or nontraumatic causes of coma is thought to result from diffuse axonal injury (DAI). Traditionally, DAI is described as coma beginning immediately at the time of trauma and persisting for at least 6 hours. However, some patients with DAI may recover briefly before lapsing into prolonged coma. No specific acute focal traumatic lesions are noted on a head CT scan. Occasionally, small petechial hemorrhages in proximity to the third ventricle and within the white matter of the corpus callosum or within the internal capsule of the brainstem are detected. DAI is the most common CT finding after severe head trauma, estimated to occur in 50% of all comatose head-injured patients.[106] MRI may be more sensitive in detecting subtle injury in DAI, but it is often not practical to perform MRI on critically injured patients. DAI is probably produced by the same shear and tensile biomechanical forces that produce concussion but with widespread disruption of cortical physiology and microanatomy. Microscopically, axonal fibers are diffusely disrupted in the white matter of the brain and brainstem. Recovery depends on the reversal or correction of structural and physiologic abnormalities.

Because clinical diagnostic studies cannot predict the extent of the axonal damage, the severity of the injury is determined by the clinical course. Patients with *mild* DAI are in coma for 6 to 24 hours. About a third of patients with mild DAI demonstrate decorticate or decerebrate posturing, but by 24 hours they are following commands.[106] The mortality in this group is 15% and is associated with infectious complications or concurrent intracranial injuries. Most patients who recover have mild or no permanent disabilities.

Moderate DAI is the most common clinical picture. Patients with moderate DAI are in coma for longer than 24 hours. Often they are victims of falls or vehicular crashes and have associated basilar skull fractures. Patients may exhibit transient decortication or decerebration but eventually recover purposeful movements. On awakening, patients have prolonged severe posttraumatic amnesia and moderate to severe persistent cognitive deficits. Almost 25% die of complications of prolonged coma.[106]

Severe DAI is almost always caused by vehicular crashes. Patients remain in coma for prolonged periods and demonstrate persistent brainstem dysfunction (posturing) and autonomic dysfunction (e.g., hypertension, hyperpyrexia). Diffuse brain swelling subsequent to injury causes intracranial hypertension. Herniation syndrome can occur if elevated ICP does not respond to medical or surgical intervention. Some patients with severe DAI eventually awaken but are severely disabled. Some patients remain in a persistent vegetative state, but most with severe DAI die from their head injury.[106] All patients with DAI present identically in coma. No early clinical predictor differentiates patients with mild, moderate, or severe DAI.

Contusions

Contusions are bruises on the surface of the brain, usually caused by impact injury. Most often, contusions occur at the poles and the inferior surfaces of the frontal and temporal lobes where the brain comes into contact with bone protuberances in the base of the skull. If the contusion occurs on the same side as the impact injury, it is a *coup injury;* if it occurs on the opposite side, the contusion is a *contrecoup injury.* Contusions also often develop in the brain tissue that underlies a depressed skull fracture. Multiple areas of contused tissue may be produced with a single impact, often in association with other intracranial injuries.

Contusions are produced when parenchymal blood vessels are damaged, resulting in scattered areas of petechial hemorrhage and subsequent edema. Contusions develop in the gray matter on the surface of the brain and taper into the white matter. Often, subarachnoid blood is found overlying the involved gyrus.[7] With time the associated hemorrhages and edema of a contusion can become widespread and serve as a nidus for hemorrhage or swelling, thus producing a local mass effect. Compression of the underlying tissue can cause local areas of ischemia, and tissue infarction is possible if the compression is significant and unrelieved. Eventually these ischemic areas become necrotic, and cystic cavities form within them.

Patients with contusions are frequently delayed in their clinical presentation. They may have sustained only a brief LOC, but the duration of posttraumatic confusion and obtundation may be prolonged. If contusions occur near the sensorimotor cortex, focal neurologic deficits may be present. Many patients with significant contusions make uneventful recoveries, but contusions may cause significant neurologic problems, including increased ICP, posttraumatic seizures, and focal deficits.

Non–contrast-enhanced CT is the best diagnostic test to discover contusions in the early posttraumatic period. These appear heterogeneous and irregular because of mixed regions of hemorrhage, necrosis, and infarction. Often the surrounding edematous tissue appears hypodense. By posttrauma days 3 and 4, the blood located within the contusions has begun to degrade, and MRI becomes more useful.

Epidural Hematoma

Epidural hematomas (EDHs) are blood clots that form between the inner table of the skull and the dura. Most EDHs are caused by direct impact injury that causes a forceful deformity of the skull. Eighty percent are associated with skull fractures across the middle meningeal artery or across a dural sinus and are therefore located in the temporoparietal region.[7] The high arterial pressure of the bleeding vessel dissects the dura away from the skull, permitting the formation of the hematoma. The incidence of skull fractures in children with EDH is lower than in adults because the elasticity of the skull during childhood permits it to spring back to its original position instead of breaking after a significant impact.

An EDH is usually unilateral, and 20% of patients have other intracranial lesions, usually subdural hematomas or contusions.[22] An EDH from arterial bleeding develops rapidly, and at detection minimal underlying brain tissue damage is usually noted. Because of their rapid formation, EDHs from arterial bleeding are usually detected within hours after injury and often earlier in some children. EDHs that develop from a dural sinus tear develop more slowly, and clinical manifestations may be delayed with resultant delays in detection. EDHs are rare in elderly patients, probably because of the close attachment of the dura to the periosteum of the inner table.[7] The dura is also closely attached to the skull in children, and EDHs are rare in children younger than 2 years.[22]

The classical presentation of the EDH is described as head trauma producing a decreased level of consciousness followed by a "lucid" interval. Although the patient's consciousness is less decreased during the lucid interval, a completely normal mental status may not return before a second episode of decreased consciousness occurs. The lucid interval is not pathognomonic for an EDH and occurs in patients who sustain other expanding mass lesions. In fact, only about 30% of patients with EDHs present classically.[107] Patients with an EDH often complain of a severe headache, sleepiness, dizziness, nausea, and vomiting. The development of signs and symptoms depends on how rapidly the EDH is expanding. A small EDH may remain asymptomatic, but this is rare.[107]

Epidural bleeding is present in 0.5% of all head-injured patients and in about 1% of all head-injured patients who present in coma.[22] If the patient is not in coma when the diagnosis is established and if the condition is rapidly treated, the mortality is nearly zero. If the patient is in coma, the mortality from EDH is about 20%. If it is rapidly detected and evacuated, the functional outcome is excellent.

On CT scan an EDH appears hyperdense, biconvex, ovoid, and lenticular. The EDH does not usually extend beyond the dural attachments at the suture lines. The margins are sharply defined, and the hematoma usually bulges inward toward the brain (Figure 38-5). The most common site is the temporal region. EDHs of mixed density on CT may be actively bleeding.

A posterior fossa EDH is the most common traumatic mass lesion of the posterior fossa.[22] Direct occipital trauma resulting in a skull fracture that disrupts a venous sinus is the usual cause, and most patients have external evidence of occipital injury. Most patients become symptomatic within 24 hours after injury, with complaints of headache, nausea, vomiting, and nuchal rigidity. Fewer than 50% of patients have cerebellar signs.[22] Most patients eventually have a decreased level of consciousness. On CT scan a posterior fossa EDH looks similar to other EDHs, but it may cross the

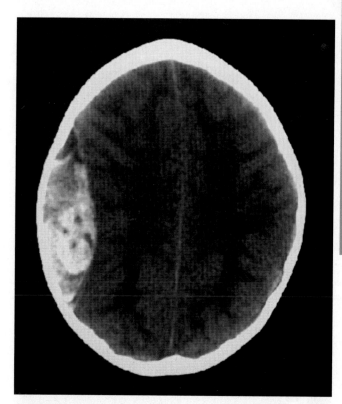

Figure 38-5. Non–contrast-enhanced computed tomography scan of acute epidural hematoma at level of right midconvexity. There is an associated mass effect and moderate midline shift.

midline and extend above the tentorium to the supratentorial compartment (Figure 38-6).

Subdural Hematoma

Subdural hematomas (SDHs) are blood clots that form between the dura and the brain. Usually they are caused by the movement of the brain relative to the skull, as seen in acceleration-deceleration injuries. These hematomas are common in patients with brain atrophy, such as alcoholic or elderly patients. In these patients the superficial bridging vessels traverse greater distances than in patients with no atrophy. As a result, the vessels are more likely to rupture with rapid movement of the head. Once they are ruptured, blood can fill the potential space between the dura and arachnoid.

SDHs are more common than EDHs, occurring in up to 30% of patients with severe head trauma.[22] The slow bleeding of venous structures delays the development of clinical signs and symptoms. As a result, the hematoma compresses the underlying brain tissue for prolonged periods and can cause significant tissue ischemia and damage.

The patient's clinical presentation depends on the amount of brain injury sustained at the time of trauma and the rate of SDH expansion. If the patient with an SDH was rendered unconscious at the time of trauma, the prognosis is poor; these patients often have concurrent DAI.[22] The signs and symptoms after injury that produce a SDH are initially related to the other intracranial injuries that may have been sustained and then to the slow expansion of the SDH.

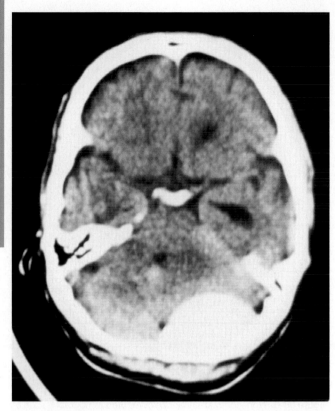

Figure 38-6. Non–contrast-enhanced computed tomography scan of large, left posterior fossa, epidural hematoma. Size of lesion at this high level suggests that it crosses into supratentorial compartment. This lesion is often associated with occipital bone fracture that disrupts transverse sinus.

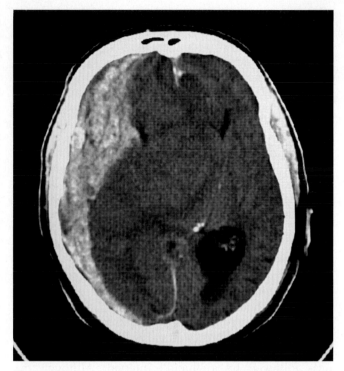

Figure 38-7. Non–contrast-enhanced computed tomography scan of acute right temporal subdural hematoma. There is acute bleeding as well as delayed bleeding, which explains mixed density. Mass effect is large, with midline shift measuring approximately 2.7 cm right to left. Right lateral ventricle has been obliterated.

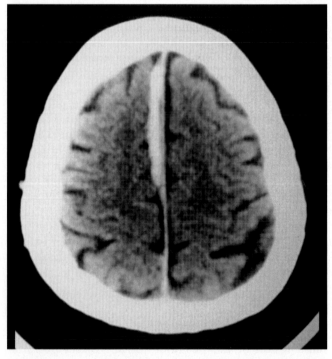

Figure 38-8. Non–contrast-enhanced computed tomography scan of intrahemispheric acute subdural hematoma.

SDHs are classified by the time to clinical presentation. *Acute* SDHs are symptomatic within 24 hours after trauma. Patients with acute SDHs often have a decreased level of consciousness. Between 50% and 70% of patients with SDHs have a lucid interval after injury, followed by declining mental status.[22,29] Pupil inequality, motor deficit, and other signs consistent with increased brain swelling may be present on the initial examination. If the patient is deeply comatose at presentation with flaccidity and without signs of brainstem activity, supportive care should be instituted in the emergency department. Subsequent management decisions should be discussed with the patient's family and the attending neurosurgeon. If the SDH is very small (only a few millimeters thick at its widest point on CT scan), some neurosurgeons may choose careful observation for these patients. Even a small SDH may be accompanied by extensive brain tissue damage that can cause enough increased ICP to precipitate a herniation syndrome. In most patients the optimal treatment for acute SDHs is surgical evacuation. On CT scan an acute SDH appears hyperdense and crescent shaped and lies between the calvaria and the cortex. Unlike EDHs, SDHs often extend beyond the suture lines (Figure 38-7). An SDH may follow the contour of the tentorium and be detected within the interhemispheric fissure (Figure 38-8). Many patients with an acute SDH also show CT evidence of intracerebral lesions contralateral to the SDH.

A *subacute* SDH is symptomatic between 24 hours and 2 weeks after injury. It may appear hypodense or isodense on CT scans. Contrast increases detection of isodense lesions. Patients complain of a headache, altered mental status, muscle weakness, or frank paralysis. Most patients with subacute SDH require surgical evacuation of the lesion.

A *chronic* SDH becomes symptomatic 2 weeks or more after trauma. The signs and symptoms may be very subtle or nonspecific, but up to 45% of patients demonstrate unilateral weakness or hemiparesis.[22] Almost 50% report an altered level of consciousness, but some patients are unable to recall their head injury or describe only a minor injury. Twenty percent of the time chronic subdurals are bilateral.[22] A chronic SDH may have initially been a small asymptomatic SDH that eventually expanded because of a combination of recurrent hemorrhage and escape of plasma into the hematoma. At some point a critical mass is reached, and the chronic SDH becomes symptomatic. On CT scan a chronic SDH may appear isodense or hypodense to brain parenchyma. In these cases, indirect evidence of the lesion includes a midline shift, effacement of the ipsilateral cortical sulci, and ventricular compression. Contrast may increase the likelihood of identifying a chronic SDH that has become isodense. On CT scan, blood of various ages is seen as a mixed-density lesion. On MRI a chronic SDH appears hyperdense. The treatment of chronic SDHs is controversial. If they become symptomatic, chronic SDHs require surgical evacuation. Most patients have a good outcome after surgery. Overall, the mortality from a chronic SDH approaches 10%, with decreased survival in elderly patients.[22]

The prognosis of SDH does not depend on the size of the hematoma but rather depends on the degree of brain injury caused by the pressure of the expanding hematoma on underlying tissue or by other intracranial injury caused by the initial impact itself. The overall survival is 35% to 50%; mortality is highest in older persons, in patients who have a GCS of 8 or less, and in patients with signs of acute herniation syndrome on initial emergency department presentation.[22] Posterior fossa SDHs make up less than 1% of all reported SDHs. They are caused by occipital trauma that tears bridging vessels or venous sinuses. Clinical manifestations of posterior SDH vary but usually include nausea, vomiting, headache, and decreased level of consciousness. Occasionally, cranial nerve palsies may be found, as well as nuchal rigidity, cerebellar signs and symptoms, and papilledema. On a CT scan, a posterior fossa SDH does not cross the midline or extend above the tentorium. The outcome of a posterior SDH is very poor, with less than 5% survival.[22]

In children the presence of an SDH should prompt consideration of child abuse. Many types of injury can produce SDH in children, but the infant who is repeatedly and forcibly shaken is especially susceptible. Infants may have SDH because of birth trauma. In these cases the initial clinical manifestation may be a generalized seizure within the first 6 months of life.[22] On examination, the infant may have a bulging fontanelle or an enlarged head circumference. A careful history may elicit long-standing constitutional symptoms, such as failure to thrive or lethargy.

Subdural Hygroma

A subdural hygroma (SDHG) is a collection of clear, xanthochromic blood-tinged fluid in the dural space. The pathogenesis of an SDHG is not certain. It may result from a tear in the arachnoid that permits CSF to escape into the dural space or effusions from injured vessels through areas of abnormal permeability in the meninges or in the underlying parenchyma. SDHGs are present in as many as 10% of cases of severe head injury.[22] They may accumulate immediately after trauma or in a delayed fashion. Clinically, an SDHG cannot be distinguished from other mass lesions. Most often, patients have a decreased level of consciousness or focal motor deficits. They may complain of headaches, nausea, and vomiting. The ICP can increase because of the mass effect, and signs of increased ICP may be present on examination.

On CT scans, SDHGs appear crescent shaped in the extraaxial space. The CT density is the same as that of CSF. Bilateral SDHGs are common.[22] If SDHGs are asymptomatic, observation is reasonable management. Otherwise, they must be surgically evacuated. Mortality varies from 12% to 28% and appears to depend on the severity of other intracranial injury.[22]

Traumatic Subarachnoid Hemorrhage

Traumatic subarachnoid hemorrhage (TSAH) is defined as blood within the CSF and meningeal intima and probably results from tears of small subarachnoid vessels. TSAH is detected on the first CT scan in up to 33% of patients with severe TBI and has an incidence of 44% in all cases of severe head trauma. It is therefore the most common CT scan abnormality seen after head injury. Data from the National Traumatic Coma Data Bank demonstrate a 60% unfavorable outcome in severely brain-injured patients in the presence of TSAH, compared with a 30% unfavorable outcome if no TSAH occurs.[108] An increased incidence of skull fractures and contusions is found in patients with TSAH compared with patients with no TSAH. The amount of blood within the TSAH correlates directly with the outcome and inversely with the presenting GCS.

Patients may complain of headache and photophobia. A noncontrast CT scan makes the diagnosis, with increased density noted within the basilar cisterns. Blood can also be seen within the interhemispheric fissures and sulci.

TSAH with no other brain injury does not generally carry a poor prognosis. The most serious complication of TSAH is worsening of cerebral vasospasm, which may be severe enough to induce cerebral ischemia. Posttraumatic vasospasm is common, occurring about 48 hours after injury and persisting for up to 2 weeks. Calcium channel blockers (e.g., nimodipine, nicardipine) have been used to prevent or reduce vasospasm after TSAH. Although a radiographic reduction of vasospasm is not consistently seen, the overall outcome of patients treated with these agents seems to be improved compared with no treatment.[109]

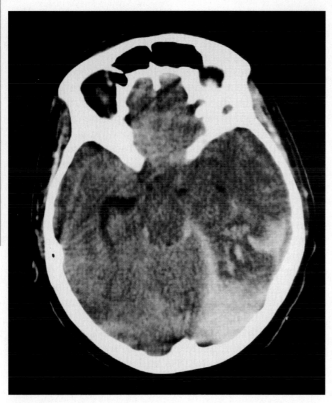

Figure 38-9. Non–contrast-enhanced computed tomography scan of intracerebral hematoma and contusion in left occipital region. Scan also shows layering of tentorial subdural hematoma. Mass effect and early uncal herniation are visible as well.

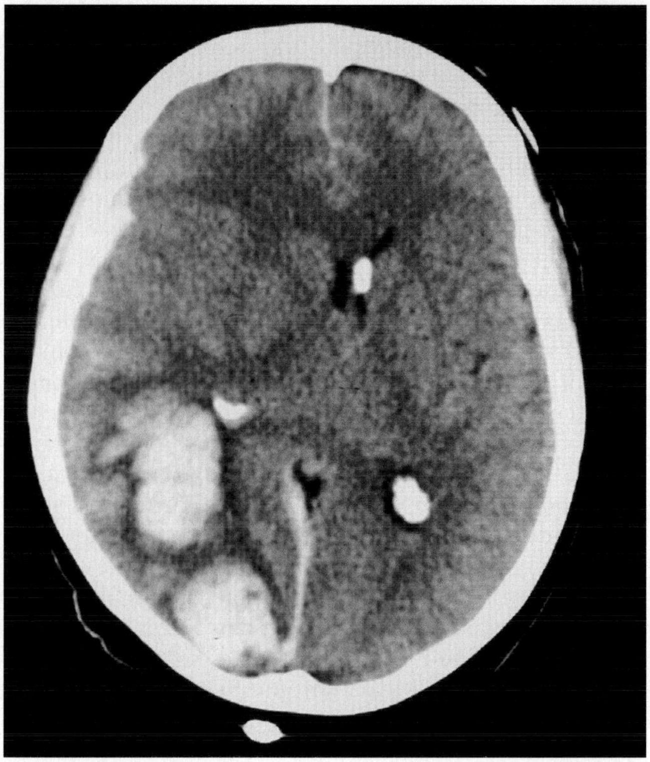

Figure 38-10. Non–contrast-enhanced computed tomography scan of right occipital and temporal intracerebral hematomas, surrounded by mild edema and hemorrhagic contusion. Small intrahemispheric subdural hematoma is visible in posterior interhemispheric fissure. Midline shift is obvious. Ventriculostomy has been placed and is visible as high-density image within ventricles.

Intracerebral Hematoma

Intracerebral hematomas (ICHs) are formed deep within the brain tissue and are usually caused by shearing or tensile forces that mechanically stretch and tear deep small-caliber arterioles as the brain is propelled against irregular surfaces in the cranial vault. Resulting small petechial hemorrhages subsequently coalesce to form ICHs. Almost 85% are in the frontal and temporal lobes. They are often found in the presence of extraaxial hematomas, and in many patients multiple ICHs are present.[107] Isolated ICHs may be detected in as many as 12% of all patients with severe head trauma.

The clinical effects of ICH depend on size, location, and whether the bleeding is continuing. ICHs have been reported with all degrees of severity of head trauma. More than 50% of patients sustain LOC at the time of impact. The patient's subsequent level of consciousness depends on the severity of the impact and coexisting lesions.[107] Combined with contusions, other concurrent lesions, and subsequent perilesion edema, an ICH can produce substantial mass effects and precipitate a herniation syndrome (Figure 38-9).

An ICH may be detected on the first CT scan immediately after injury but often is not seen for several hours or days. Unlike contusions, ICHs are usually deep in the brain tissue and often become well demarcated over time. On CT scan an ICH appears as well-defined hyperdense homogeneous areas of hemorrhage (Figure 38-10).

Many patients with an ICH require emergent intervention or surgery to control elevated ICP. Mortality is low in patients who are conscious before surgery; in unconscious patients, mortality approaches 45%.[110,111] ICHs that bleed into the ventricles or cerebellum also carry a high mortality rate.

Traumatic Intracerebellar Hematoma

Primary traumatic intracerebellar hematomas are rare but can occur after a direct blow to the suboccipital area. Often these patients also have a skull fracture or a posterior fossa SDH. Supratentorial contrecoup hematomas and contusions are also common associated findings.

The clinical presentation of an isolated traumatic cerebellar hematoma is similar to that of other posterior lesions. When other traumatic lesions are present, the picture may be quite confusing. The acute management should first address the most clinically significant lesion. The mortality from isolated traumatic intracerebellar hematoma is very high.[111]

KEY CONCEPTS

Severe and Moderate Head Injuries

- All patients with severe or moderate head injury require serial neurologic examinations while in the emergency department to allow early detection of herniation syndrome related to expanding traumatic mass lesions or increasing cerebral edema.
- Acute herniation syndrome manifested by neurologic deterioration should initially be managed with short-term hyperventilation, to a PCO_2 of 30 to 35 mm Hg, with monitoring and then surgical intervention as soon as possible. Long-term hyperventilation is not indicated. Mannitol should be used only in patients with increasing ICPs or acute neurologic deterioration.
- Secondary systemic insults such as hypoxia and hypotension worsen neurologic outcome after severe and moderate head trauma and should be corrected as soon as detected in the out-of-hospital or emergency department setting.
- For adult patients, hypotension in the presence of isolated severe head injury is a preterminal event. Hypotension usually results from comorbidity, and its cause should be sought and treated.
- The Glasgow Coma Scale is a useful clinical tool for following head-injured patients' neurologic status, but because of its limitations, the initial GCS in the emergency department cannot reliably predict prognosis after acute head injury.
- Head-injured patients who have been chemically paralyzed do not have clinical manifestations of seizures; anticonvulsants should be given prophylactically.
- Most "talk and deteriorate" patients who present with moderate head injury have subdural or epidural hematomas. Early detection, CT scan, and expedient surgical intervention are the keys to a good outcome.

Minor Head Trauma

- Risk stratification of patients with minor head injury into low-risk and high-risk categories can help direct the emergency physician to an appropriate diagnostic workup.
- The decision to perform CT scans on patients with minor head trauma should be individualized but based on consideration of high- and moderate-risk criteria.

- Alcohol can affect the GCS and significantly obscure the neurologic examination. Intoxicated patients should be considered at high risk.
- Most patients with minor head trauma can be discharged from the emergency department after a period of observation but require a competent observer.
- Patients sustaining a concussion are at risk for prolonged and substantial morbidity. Athletes should not be allowed to return immediately to sports activities because of the potential risk of second impact syndrome. All current recommendations for return to play after a sports-related concussion state that players with concussion should not return to play for at least 1 week after they have become asymptomatic. This period is usually increased to at least a symptom-free month if an LOC or prolonged post-traumatic amnesia occurred at the time of concussion.

Pediatric Head Injuries

- Children with severe head trauma have fewer intracranial lesions than adults but more edema. In children, increasing edema alone can cause talk and deteriorate or other significant neurologic decline.
- Skull fractures have more clinical significance in children than in adults.
- In children, unlike adults, hypovolemic hypotension can occur because of head injury, especially those younger than 1 year.
- In very young children, head injury is often caused by nonaccidental causes. Child abuse should be suspected in young children with head trauma, especially those younger than 2 years.

Penetrating Head Injuries

- Tangential gunshot wounds are associated with a high frequency of intracranial traumatic lesions; CT scanning should be performed.
- Anticonvulsant prophylaxis and antibiotics should be given to a patient with penetrating head injuries.
- The clinical outcome after gunshot wounds to the head can be predicted by the initial clinical presentation and the missile path through the brain.

REFERENCES

1. Jager TE, et al: Traumatic brain injuries evaluated in US emergency departments, 1992-1994. *Acad Emerg Med* 7:134, 2000.
2. Adekoya N, et al: Surveillance of traumatic brain injury deaths—United States, 1989-1998. *MMWR Surveill Summ* 51(SS-10):1, 2002.
3. Narayan RK, et al: Clinical trials in head injury. *J Neurotrauma* 19:503, 2002.
4. Sosin DM, Sniezek JE, Waxweiler RJ: Trends in death associated with traumatic brain injury, 1979-1992. *JAMA* 273:1778, 1995.
5. Greenwald BD, et al: Congenital and acquired brain injury. 1. Brain injury: Epidemiology and pathophysiology. *Arch Phys Med Rehabil* 84(Suppl 1):S3, 2003.
6. Carpenter MB: Gross anatomy of the brain. In *Core Text of Neuroanatomy*, 4th ed. Baltimore, Williams & Wilkins, 1991.
7. Rockswold GL: Head injury. In Tintinalli JE, et al (eds): *Emergency Medicine: A Comprehensive Study Guide.* New York, McGraw-Hill, 1996, p 1139.

8. Lenzlinger PH, et al: Overview of basic mechanisms underlying neuropathological consequences of head trauma. In Miller LP, Hayes RL (eds): *Head Trauma: Basic, Preclinical and Clinical Directions*, 1st ed. New York, Wiley-Liss, 2001, pp 4-5.
9. Zwienenberg M , Muizellar JP: Vascular aspects of severe head injury. In Miller LP, Hayes RL (eds): *Head Trauma: Basic, Preclinical and Clinical Directions*, 1st ed. New York, Wiley-Liss, 2001, pp 303-326.
10. Reivech M: Arterial Pco2 and cerebral hemodynamics. *Am J Physiol* 206:25, 1964.
11. Laffey JG, Kavanagh BP: Hypocapnia. *N Engl J Med* 347:43, 2002.
12. Muizelaar JP, et al: Adverse effects of prolonged hyperventilation: A randomized clinical trial. *J Neurosurg* 75:731, 1991.
13. Biros M, Heegaard W: Prehospital and resuscitative care of the head-injured patient. *Curr Opin Crit Care* 7:444, 2001.
14. Conway EE: Nonaccidental head injury in infants: "The shaken baby syndrome" revisited. *Pediatr Ann* 27:677, 1998.

15. Hovda DA, et al: The neurochemical and metabolic cascade following brain injury: Moving from animal models to man. *J Neurotrauma* 12:903, 1995.

16. Doberstein CE, Hovda DA, Becker DP: Clinical considerations in the reduction of secondary brain injury. *Ann Emerg Med* 22:993, 1993.

17. Glass TF, et al: Secondary neurologic injury resulting from non-hypotensive hemorrhage combined with mild traumatic brain injury. *J Neurotrauma* 16:771, 1999.

18. Povlishock JT, Christman CW: The pathology of traumatically induced axonal injury in animals and humans: A review of current thoughts. *J Neurotrauma* 12:555, 1995.

19. Muizelaar JP, Miller LP: Head injury clinical trials: United States. In Miller LP, Hayes RL (eds): *Head Trauma: Basic, Preclinical and Clinical Directions*, 1st ed. New York, Wiley-Liss, 2001, p 417.

20. Wilberger JE: Emergency care and initial evaluation. In Cooper PR, Golfinos JG (eds):*Head Injury*, 4th ed. New York, McGraw-Hill, 2000, p 27.

21. Brain Trauma Foundation, American Association of Neurological Surgeons, Joint Section on Neurotrauma and Critical Care: Guidelines for the management of severe traumatic brain injury. *J Neurotrauma* 17:471, 2000.

22. Greenberg MS: Head trauma. In *Handbook of Neurosurgery*. Lakeland, Fla, Greenberg Graphics, 1997.

23. Graham D, Gennarelli TA: Pathology of brain damage after head injury. In Cooper PR, Golfinos JG (eds): *Head Injury*, 4th ed. New York, McGraw-Hill, 2000, pp 133-155.

24. Greenberg MS: Coma. In *Handbook of Neurosurgery*. Lakeland, Fla, Greenberg Graphics, 1997.

25. Teasdale G, Jennett B: Assessment of coma and impaired consciousness: A practical scale. *Lancet* 2:81, 1974.

26. Brain Trauma Foundation, American Association of Neurological Surgeons, Joint Section on Neurotrauma and Critical Care: Guidelines for the management of severe traumatic brain injury. *J Neurotrauma* 17:563, 2000.

27. Greenberg MS: Spine injuries. In *Handbook of Neurosurgery*. Lakeland, Fla, Greenberg Graphics, 1997.

28. Krause JF: Epidemiology of brain injury. In Cooper PR, Golfinos JG (eds): *Head Injury*, 4th ed. New York, McGraw-Hill, 2000, pp 1-26.

29. Cruz J: Severe acute brain trauma. In Cruz J (ed): *Neurologic and Neurosurgical Emergencies*. Philadelphia, WB Saunders, 1998, pp 405-436.

30. Siegel JH: The effect of associated injuries, blood loss, and oxygen debt on death and disability in blunt traumatic brain injury: The need for early physiologic predictors of severity. *J Neurotrauma* 12:579, 1995.

31. Feickert HJ, Crommer S, Heyer R: Severe head injury in children: Impact of risk factors on outcome. *J Trauma* 47:33, 1999.

32. Weiner HL, Weinberg JS: Head injury in the pediatric age group. In Cooper PR, Golfinos JG (eds): *Head Injury*, 4th ed. McGraw-Hill, New York, 2000, pp 419-456.

33. Brain Trauma Foundation, American Association of Neurological Surgeons, Joint Section on Neurotrauma and Critical Care: Guidelines for the management of severe traumatic brain injury. *J Neurotrauma* 17:573, 2000.

34. Provencio JJ, Bleck TP: Cardiovascular disorders related to neuroemergencies. In Cruz J (ed): *Neurologic and Neurosurgical Emergencies*. Philadelphia, WB Saunders, 1998, pp 39-50.

35. Brain Trauma Foundation: *Guidelines for Prehospital Management of Traumatic Brain Injury*. New York, 2000.

36. Winchell RJ, Hoyt DB: Endotracheal intubation in the field improves survival in patients with severe head injury. *Arch Surg* 132:592, 1997.

37. Bochicchio GV, et al: Endotracheal intubation in the field does not improve outcome in trauma patients who present without an acutely lethal traumatic brain injury. *J Trauma Injury Infect Crit Care* 54:307, 2003.

38. Murray JA, et al: Prehospital intubation in patients with severe head injury. *J Trauma Injury Infect Crit Care* 49:1065, 2000.

39. Davis DP, et al: The effect of paramedic rapid sequence intubation on outcome in patients with severe traumatic brain injury. *J Trauma Injury Infect Crit Care* 54:444, 2003.

40. Modica P, Tempelhoff R: Intracranial pressure during induction of anesthesia and tracheal intubation with etomidate-induced EEG burst suppression. *Can J Anaesth* 39:236, 1992.

41. Brain Trauma Foundation, American Association of Neurological Surgeons, Joint Section on Neurotrauma and Critical Care: Guidelines for the management of severe traumatic brain injury. *J Neurotrauma* 17:591, 2000.

42. Wade CE, et al: Individual patient cohort analysis of the efficacy of hypertonic saline/dextran in patients with severe head trauma and hypotension. *J Trauma* 42(5 Suppl):S61, 1997.

43. Brain Trauma Foundation, American Association of Neurological Surgeons, Joint Section on Neurotrauma and Critical Care: Guidelines for the management of severe traumatic brain injury. *J Neurotrauma* 17:513, 2000.

44. Gaab MR, et al: A comparative analysis of THAM (Trisbuffer) in traumatic brain edema. *Acta Neurochir Suppl (Wien)* 51:320, 1990.

45. Brain Trauma Foundation, American Association of Neurological Surgeons, Joint Section on Neurotrauma and Critical Care: Guidelines for the management of severe traumatic brain injury. *J Neurotrauma* 17:521, 2000.

46. Doyle JA, Davis DP, Hoyt DB: The use of hypertonic saline in the treatment of traumatic brain injury. *J Trauma* 50:367, 2001.

47. Brain Trauma Foundation, American Association of Neurological Surgeons, Joint Section on Neurotrauma and Critical Care: Guidelines for the management of severe traumatic brain injury. *J Neurotrauma* 17:527, 2000.

48. Brain Trauma Foundation, American Association of Neurological Surgeons, Joint Section on Neurotrauma and Critical Care: Guidelines for the management of severe traumatic brain injury. *J Neurotrauma* 17:531, 2000.

49. Treiman DM, et al: A comparison of four treatments for generalized convulsive status epilepticus, Veterans Affairs Status Epilepticus Cooperative Study Group. *N Engl J Med* 339:792, 1998.

50. Schierhout G, Roberts I: Antiepileptic drugs for preventing seizures following acute traumatic brain injury. *Cochrane Database Syst Rev* 4:CD000565, 2001.

51. Chang BS, Lowenstein DH: Practice parameter: Antiepileptic drug prophylaxis in severe traumatic brain injury: Report of the Quality Standards Subcommittee of the American Academy of Neurology. *Neurology* 60:10, 2003.

52. Chestnut RM: Secondary brain insults after head injury: Clinical perspectives. *New Horiz* 3:366, 1995.

53. Britt PM, Heiserman JE: Imaging evaluation. In Cooper PR, Golfinos JG (eds): *Head Injury*, 4th ed. New York, McGraw-Hill, 2000, pp 63-132.

54. Thurman DJ: The epidemiology and economics of head trauma. In Miller LP, Hayes RL (eds): *Head Trauma: Basic, Preclinical and Clinical Directions*, 1st ed. New York, Wiley-Liss, 2001, p 327.

55. Rockswold GL, Pheley PJ: Patients who talk and deteriorate. *Ann Emerg Med* 22:1004, 1993.

56. Colohan ART, Oyesiku NM: Moderate head injury: An overview. *J Neurotrauma* 9:S259, 1992.

57. Stein SC, Ross SE: Moderate head injury: A guide to initial management. *J Neurosurg* 77:562, 1992.

58. Servadei F, Teasdale G, Merry G: Defining acute mild head injury in adults: A proposal based on prognostic factors, diagnosis and management. *J Neurotrauma* 18:657, 2001.

59. Kraus JF, McArthur DL: Epidemiology of brain injury. In Woper PR, Golfinos JC (eds): *Head Injury*, 4th ed. New York, McGraw-Hill, 2000, pp 1-26.

60. Cheung DS, Kharasch M: Evaluation of the patient with closed head trauma: An evidence-based approach. *Emer Med Clin North Am* 17:9, 1999.

61. Arienta C, Caroli M, Balbi S: Management of head injured patients in the ED: A practical approach. *Surg Neurol* 48:213, 1997.

62. Krause JF, et al: Epidemiology of brain injury. In Narayan RK, Wilberger WK, Povlishock JT, (eds): *Neurotrauma*. New York, McGraw-Hill, 1995, p 13.

63. Haydel MJ, et al: Indications for computed tomography in patients with minor head injury. *N Engl J Med* 343:100, 2000.

64. Stiell IG, et al: The Canadian CT head rule for patients with minor head injury. *Lancet* 357:1391, 2001.

65. MacLauren RE, Ghoorahoo HI, Kirby NG: Skull x-rays after head injury: The recommendations of the Royal College of Surgeons Working Party report in practice. *Arch Emerg Med* 10:138, 1993.

66. Wilberger JE: Emergency care and initial evaluation. In Cooper PR, Golfinos JG (eds): *Head Injury*, 4th ed. New York, McGraw-Hill, 2000, pp 27-40.

67. Bergsneider M, et al: Dissociation of cerebral glucose metabolism and level of consciousness during the period of metabolic depression following human traumatic brain injury. *J Neurotrauma* 17:389, 1996.

68. Chen SHA, et al: A study of persistent post-concussion symptoms in mild head trauma using positron emission tomography. *J Neurol Neurosurg Psychiatry* 74:326, 2003.

69. Galbraith S, et al: The relationship between alcohol and head injury and its effect on conscious level. *Br J Surg* 63:128, 1976.

70. Shaw NA: The neurophysiology of concussion. *Prog Neurobiol* 67:281, 2002.

71. Sports-related recurrent brain injuries—United States. *MMWR Morb Mortal Wkly Rep* 46:224, 1997.

72. McCrea M, et al: Acute effects and recovery time following concussion in collegiate football players: The NCAA concussion study. *JAMA* 290:2556, 2003.

73. Guskiewicz KM, et al: Cumulative effects associated with recurrent concussion in collegiate football players: The NCAA concussion study. *JAMA* 290:2549, 2003.

74. McCrory P: Does second impact syndrome exist? *Clin J Sport Med* 11:144, 2001.

75. Harmon KG: Assessment and management of concussion in sports. *Am Fam Physician* 60:887, 1999.

76. de Kruijk JR, et al: Prediction of post-traumatic complaints after mild traumatic brain injury: Early symptoms and biochemical markers. *J Neurol Neurosurg Psychiatry* 73:727, 2002.

77. Dunhaime A, et al: Head injury in very young children: Mechanisms, injury types and ophthalmologic findings in 100 hospitalized patients younger than 2 years of age. *Pediatrics* 90:179, 1992.

78. Mansfield RT: Head injuries in children and adults. *Crit Care Clin* 13:611, 1997.

79. Lobato R, Rivas J, Gomez P: Head-injured patients who talk and deteriorate into coma. *J Neurosurg* 75:256, 1991.

80. Mazzola CA, Adelson PD: Critical care management of head trauma in children. *Crit Care Med* 30(11 Suppl):S393, 2002.

81. Ward JD: Pediatric head injury. In Narayan RK, Wilberger WK, Povlishock JT (eds): *Neurotrauma*. New York, McGraw Hill, 1995, p 859.

82. Schutzman SA, Greene DS: Pediatric minor head trauma. *Ann Emerg Med* 37:65, 2001.

83. Keenan HT, et al: A population-based study of inflicted traumatic brain injury in young children. *JAMA* 290:621, 2003.

84. Greens DS, Schutzman SA: Occult intracranial injury in infants. *Ann Emerg Med* 32:680, 1998.

85. Greenes DS, Schutzman SA: Clinical indicators of intracranial injury in head-injured infants. *Pediatrics* 104:861,1999.

86. Greenes DS, Schutzman SA: Clinical significance of scalp abnormalities in asymptomatic head injured infants. *Pediatr Emerg Care* 17:88, 2000.

87. Palchak, MJ, et al: A decision rule for identifying children at low risk for brain injuries after blunt head trauma. *Ann Emerg Med* 424:492, 2003.

88. American Academy of Pediatrics: The management of minor closed head injury in children. *Pediatrics* 104:1407, 1999.

89. Haydel MJ, Shembekar AD: Prediction of intracranial injury in children aged five years and older with loss of consciousness after minor head injury due to nontrivial mechanisms. *Ann Emerg Med* 42:507, 2003.

90. Kaufman HH, et al: Civilian gunshot wounds to the head. *Neurosurgery* 32:962, 1993.

91. Anglin D, et al: Intracranial hemorrhage associated with tangential gunshot wounds to the head. *Acad Emerg Med* 5:672, 1998.

92. Introduction and methodology: Part 1: Guidelines for the management of penetrating brain injury. *J Trauma* 51(2 Suppl):S3, 2001.

93. Epidemiology. Part 2: Prognosis in penetrating brain injury. *J Trauma* 51(2 Suppl):S53, 2001.

94. Neurologic measures: Level of consciousness and Glasgow Coma Scale. Part 2: Prognosis in penetrating brain injury. *J Trauma* 51(2 Suppl):S64, 2001.

95. Neurologic measures: Pupillary size and light reflex. Part 2: Prognosis in penetrating brain injury. *J Trauma* 51(2 Suppl):S71, 2001.

96. Chestnut RM: Implications of the guidelines for the management of severe head injury for the practicing neurosurgeon. *Surg Neurol* 50:187, 1998.

97. Antibiotic prophylaxis for penetrating brain injury. Part 1: Guidelines for the management of penetrating brain injury. *J Trauma* 51(2 Suppl):S34, 2001.

98. Antiseizure prophylaxis for penetrating brain injury. Part 1: Guidelines for the management of penetrating brain injury. *J Trauma* 51(2 Suppl):S41, 2001.

99. Neuroimaging in the management of penetrating brain injury. Part 1: Guidelines for the management of penetrating brain injury. *J Trauma* 51(2 Suppl):S7, 2001.

100. Lapointe M, et al: Basic principles of antimicrobial therapy of CNS infections. In Cooper PR, Golfinos JG (eds): *Head Injury*, 4th ed. New York, McGraw-Hill, 2000, p 483.

101. Stein SC, et al: Intravascular coagulation: A major secondary insult in nonfatal traumatic brain injury. *J Neurosurg* 97:1373, 2002.

102. Hanson WC: Acute respiratory failure in neuroemergencies. In Cruz J (ed): *Neurologic and Neurosurgical Emergencies*. Philadelphia, WB Saunders, 1998, pp 28-29.

103. Lammers RL: Principles of wound management. In Roberts JR, Hedges JR (eds): *Clinical Procedures in Emergency Medicine*, 3rd ed. Philadelphia, WB Saunders, 1998, pp 560-599.

104. Graham DI: Neuropathology of head injury. In Narayan RK (ed): *Neurotrauma*. New York, McGraw-Hill, 1995, p 43.

105. Cooper PR: Skull fracture and traumatic cerebrospinal fistulas. In Cooper PR (ed): *Head Injury*, 3rd ed. Baltimore, Williams & Wilkins, 1993, pp 117-119.

106. Gennarelli, TA: Cerebral concussion and diffuse brain injury. In Cooper PR (ed): *Head Injury*, 3rd ed. Baltimore, Williams & Wilkins, 1993, pp 144-145.

107. Chiles BW, Cooper PR: Extra-axial hematomas. In Loftus CM (ed): *Neurosurgical Emergencies*. Park Ridge, Ill, AANS Publications, 1994, pp 73-100.

108. Kakarieka A, Braakman R, Schakel EH: Clinical significance of the finding of subarachnoid blood on CT scan after head injury. *Acta Neurochir (Wien)* 129:1, 1994.
109. Barket FG, Ogilvy CS: Efficacy of prophylactic nimodipine for delayed ischemic deficit after SAH: A metaanalysis. *J Neurosurg* 84:405, 1996.
110. Miller JD, Piper IR, Jones PA: Pathophysiology of head injury. In Narayan RK, Wilberger WK, Povlishock JT (eds): *Neurotrauma.* New York, McGraw-Hill, 1995, p 61.
111. Zager EL, Flamm ES: Surgical management of spontaneous intracranial hematomas. In Cruz J (ed): *Neurologic and Neurosurgical Emergencies.* Philadelphia, WB Saunders, 1998, p 243.

39 Facial Trauma

Mary Pat McKay

PERSPECTIVE

This chapter discusses the epidemiology, diagnosis, and treatment of injuries to the skin, soft tissue, and bones of the face. A complex structure vital to the function of the person, the face comprises airway openings; entry to the gastrointestinal tract; and special sensory organs, including eyes, ears, and nose. Facial functioning is essential for eating, speaking, and effective nonverbal communication. The appearance and attractiveness of the face have significant implications for social interactions,[1,2] sexual attraction,[3] and self-esteem.[4]

Apart from immediate threat to the patient's airway and special sense organs, injuries to the face can have serious implications for the patient's mental health[5,6] and future functioning. In one study of predominantly unemployed young African-American and Hispanic men, 25% had symptoms of posttraumatic stress disorder 1 month after being treated emergently for a midface fracture.[7] Although the emergency physician's main goal must be to address life-threatening problems successfully, facial injuries require care aimed at optimizing the patient's cosmetic appearance.

Four main specialties—ophthalmology, plastic surgery, otolaryngology, and oral and maxillofacial surgery —participate in the care of facial injuries. Among teaching hospitals, the specialties of plastic surgery, otolaryngology, and oral and maxillofacial surgery participate in approximately equal proportions.[8] Early consultation with the appropriate specialist can expedite the care of facial injuries.

Epidemiology

In 2002, there were more than 28 million injury-related visits to U.S. emergency departments.[9] Facial injuries account for a significant proportion of these visits and may result from either intentional violence (assaults and attempted suicide) or unintentional trauma (falls, sports, and motor vehicle crashes [MVCs]). Although MVCs previously were the most common cause of facial injuries, windshield improvements, increased use of safety belts, and the prevalence of air bags in vehicles are changing the epidemiology of facial trauma. Dual front impact air bags have been required in all new vehicles since 1999, and safety belts are required for passengers in the front row in 49 states.[10] Seat belts and air bags significantly reduce the incidence and severity of facial injury in adults.[11-16] Because they effectively prevent ejection, safety belts specifically avert the extensive scalp and facial degloving injuries associated with being ejected through the windshield. Alcohol use by the occupant decreases the use of safety belts and independently increases the risk of facial injury in MVCs.[17] As a result of improved safety in motor vehicles, interpersonal violence is increasingly cited as the cause of facial injury, particularly in inner-city populations.[18,19] Falls, dog bites, and flying debris also cause facial injuries.

Because of the lack of external protection, facial injuries are common among injured riders of other motorized vehicles, including all-terrain vehicles and motorcycles. In one series, 21.6% of injured all-terrain vehicle riders had a facial injury, and the presence of a facial injury was associated with increased overall injury severity.[20] In motorcyclists, there is a significant association between facial injury and brain injury.[21] Helmets successfully reduce the risk of brain injury, but may not protect against facial trauma unless they include a face guard.

Among children younger than 17 years old, sports injuries account for 21% of facial and 29% of nasal fractures requiring specialist evaluation.[22] Baseball and football helmets with face guards are successful at preventing childhood facial injury, and their use should be encouraged by emergency physicians.[23] Children younger than age 6 seem to be at significant risk for severe facial injuries from bites sustained from the family dog.[24] Interactions between pet dogs and young children require careful supervision.

Facial injuries are a common acute presentation for victims of domestic violence. In one series, 81% of domestic violence victims presented with maxillofacial injuries, 30% of them with facial fractures. The location of the injury was consistent with the predominance of fisted assaults; left-sided injuries predominated.[25] Women presenting to the emergency department with facial injuries should be interviewed privately to allow an opportunity for disclosure and intervention for domestic violence.

Pediatric facial injury accounts for less than 10% of all facial trauma, and facial injuries are the most common area of trauma in children suspected of being victims of abuse.[26] This fact has been used to suggest that all children with facial injuries are likely to have been the victims of abuse. The epidemiology of facial trauma among children reflects their changing physical abilities and behavioral patterns, however, with a "falling zone" of trauma to the perioral region, nose, and forehead in toddlers who fail to use their arms to prevent facial injury when falling.[27] Younger children are significantly more likely to have minor soft tissue injuries and to have been the recipient of a dog bite. Severe facial injuries in all pediatric age groups are more likely to be the result of a MVC or assault.[28] Care should be taken by the emergency physician to correlate the child's age and behavioral ability with the history of the injury and the physical findings. In particular, injuries to the lips or frenulum in a nonambulatory infant suggest "bottle jamming," and bruises to the cheeks or neck are less common in falls. Although dental fractures in young children are relatively common,[29] facial fractures before age 5 are rare.[30] If there is any question, the appropriate local authorities must be contacted.

Even in high-energy MVCs, appropriate use of child safety restraints protects against many facial injuries. The law in all 50 states requires the use of such restraints for children younger than age 4 and in many beyond that age.[31] For children younger than age 15 who were involved in frontal crashes, children exposed to a deploying frontal impact air bag had a higher incidence of minor facial and chest injuries and severe upper extremity injuries, mostly related to being struck by the bag.[32] As part of preventing facial trauma, parents should be encouraged to ensure that all children ride in the rear seat of the vehicle and are properly restrained.

PRINCIPLES OF DISEASE

Anatomy

The face is a complex hollow space encapsulated by a bony structure overlaid with muscle and skin. It includes several special sensory organs: the eyes, ears, nose, and mouth.

Bones

The posterior portions of the face form the anterior wall of the calvaria, placing the face and its features in an intimate relationship with the structures of the central nervous system. The anterior facial skeleton is composed of the frontal bone, nasal bones, zygomas, maxillary bones, and mandible (Figure 39-1). The sphenoid, ethmoid, lacrimal, vomer, and temporal bones lie deep within the facial structure, providing support and important sites for muscular attachments, including the muscles of mastication, speech, and deglutition. This musculature is innervated by cranial nerves IX and X.

Nerve Supply

The most anterior muscle layer includes the muscles of facial expression that are innervated by the seventh cranial nerve, which exists just inferior to the external auditory canal. The trigeminal nerve (cranial nerve V) supplies sensation to the face through three major divisions (I through III). The ophthalmic division

Figure 39-1. Bones of the facial skeleton.

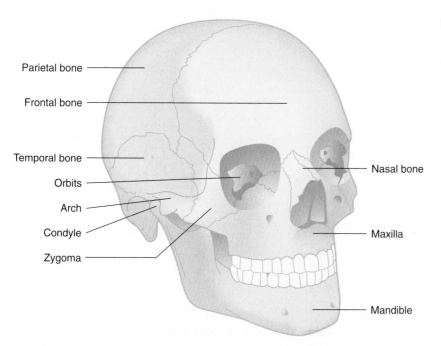

Parietal bone

Frontal bone

Temporal bone

Orbits

Arch

Condyle

Zygoma

Nasal bone

Maxilla

Mandible

(cranial nerve V1) supplies the upper third of the face, including the eye and the nose down to the tip. The maxillary division (cranial nerve V2) provides sensory innervation to the midface and includes the infraorbital nerve. The mandibular division (cranial nerve VIII) supplies sensation to the lower third of the face.

Ears

The ears lie laterally along the sides of the face with the auditory canal exiting through the mastoid process of the temporal bone. The skeleton of the pinna is cartilage covered in closely apposed skin and rolled into a helical shape with a second ridge, the antihelix, defining the inner concha. The external auditory canal, middle ear, cochlea, semicircular canals, and superior origin of the eustachian tube all lie with the temporal bone.

Eye

The structure of the globe and surrounding ocular musculature is discussed in detail in Chapter 70. The bony orbit is composed superiorly of the frontal bone. The zygoma forms the lateral wall and lateral floor of the orbit. The medial floor and anteromedial wall are formed by the maxilla. The lacrimal and ethmoid bones complete the medial wall, where the orbit is at its most delicate. The medial wall of the orbit forms the lateral walls of the intranasal space.

Nose

The nose serves as a major entryway for air and is composed of cartilage and bone covered by skin with mucosa lining the internal surface. Alar cartilage arches over the entrances to the symmetric, mucosa-lined nares, separated by the anterior cartilage of the septum. Superiorly the nasal bones create the bridge of the nose. With the head held in a neutral upright position, the floor of the nose is perpendicular to the ground and leads back into the nasopharynx, passing the turbinates laterally and the bony septum medially. The ethmoid bone lies superiorly and crosses midline, behind the nasal bridge, to form the superior portion of the bony nasal septum and the cribriform plate. The vomer composes the inferior portion of the bony septum, and the palatine process of the maxillary bone forms the posterior floor of the nose and the hard palate.

Air-containing sinuses are structural features unique to the facial skeleton. They serve to warm inhaled air and form chambers that create the unique tone of human voices. These sinuses develop over the period of human growth. At birth, only the ethmoid air cells and the mastoid antrum are aerated. The sphenoid sinus and mastoid air cells become aerated at about age 3. Frontal sinuses form at about age 6, and maxillary sinuses are not fully developed until age 10.

Mouth

The mouth serves as entry to the respiratory and gastrointestinal tracts. In addition, the fine motor movements of the mouth and tongue give humans the ability to communicate through speech. With the mouth in the closed position, the tongue fills the oral cavity. Single rows of teeth lie within the alveolar ridges of the maxilla and the mandible. With the mouth closed, the teeth in normal individuals occlude with the lower row lying just internal to the upper row. The usual occlusion for individuals varies widely, however, and the patient's belief may be the best determinant of whether or not the teeth are meeting as usual. Anterior to the teeth is the vestibule, a fold of mucosa and flexible soft tissue that allows the lips to remain closed while various motor movements occur behind them. The mandible is a U-shaped bone that forms the chin and completes the lower facial skeleton. Containing the lower row of teeth, the body of the mandible meets in midline at the symphysis, which is completely fused by age 2. Posterior to the last molar, the bone turns to form the angle of the jaw and continues upward as the ramus of the mandible. At the most superior point of the ramus is the articular surface of the condyle, separated from the superior surface of the temporomandibular joint (TMJ) by an intervening meniscus of fibrocartilage. Anterior to the condyle lies a thin projection, the coronoid process, which provides the insertion point for the temporal muscle.

The skin of the face is among the thinnest of the body, draping over the underlying musculature. Innervated primarily by the fifth cranial nerve, with age, facial skin falls visibly into predictable creases, following Langer's lines (Figure 39-2). At the mouth, nares, and palpebral fissures, the skin is contiguous with the mucosa lining these structures. The skin of the lips is particularly thin

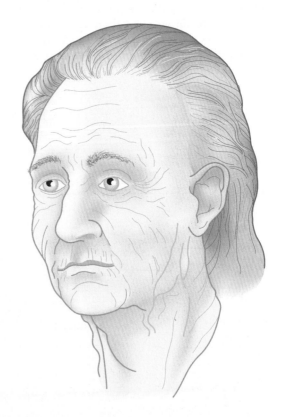

Figure 39-2. Langer's lines: lines of facial expression.

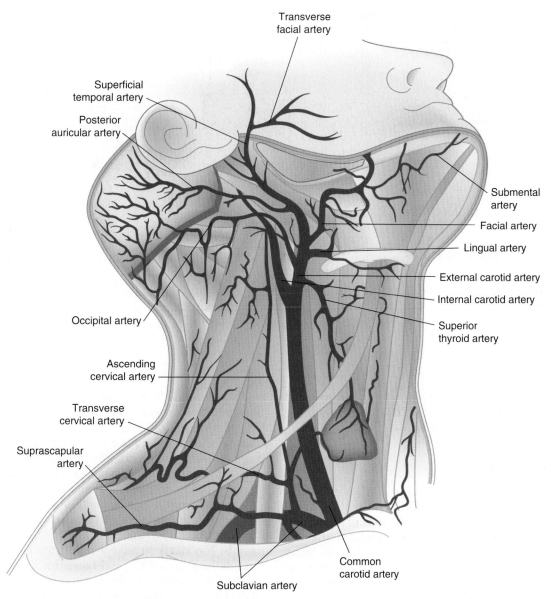

Figure 39-3. Vessels of the face. (Redrawn from *Gray's Anatomy*, 1918.)

Labels in figure:
Transverse facial artery
Superficial temporal artery
Posterior auricular artery
Submental artery
Facial artery
Lingual artery
External carotid artery
Internal carotid artery
Superior thyroid artery
Occipital artery
Ascending cervical artery
Transverse cervical artery
Suprascapular artery
Common carotid artery
Subclavian artery

and lined with vascular papillae, which give the lips their vermilion hue. Lips are particularly important as part of communication; understanding their movement can allow language without sound (lip reading).

The face is a highly vascular structure; this can have grave implications for the treatment of facial injuries. With the exception of the ophthalmic artery, the superficial blood supply comes from the external carotid artery via the facial, superficial temporal, and maxillary arteries (Figure 39-3). Soft tissue injuries and fractures that involve these vessels can lead to significant hematomas or exsanguinations. Because the face has extensive anastomotic connections across the midline and between arterial territories, however, ligation of major branches causes minimal ischemia.

Buried within the structure of the face are a series of named glandular structures and ducts, which are susceptible to injury. In the eye, the lacrimal glands lie within the orbits, superior and lateral to the globes, and secrete tears through ductules into the folds of the conjunctiva. The liquid flows medially into the puncta of the lacrimal canaliculi and drains into the lacrimal sac and then via the nasolacrimal duct into the nasopharynx.

The salivary system consists of the parotid, sublingual, and submandibular glands. The parotid is the largest of these glands, lying just anterior to the ear and wrapping around the mandible. The parotid is superficial to the masseter muscle and drains via Stensen's duct, a 5-cm tube that curves around the anterior edge of the masseter to enter the mouth opposite the second upper molar. In normal subjects, this duct is large enough to be palpated with the masseter clenched (Figure 39-4). The sublingual glands lie entirely within the floor of the mouth and drain into the mouth via ductules. They surround the ducts draining the submandibular glands (Wharton's ducts). The body of the submandibular gland is folded around the mylohyoid muscle so that a portion lies within the floor of the mouth and a portion lies external to it. The sub-

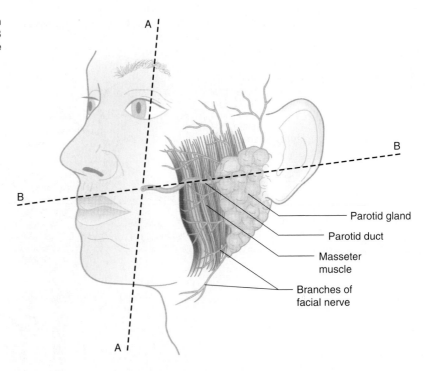

Figure 39-4. Parotid gland and duct (Stensen's) with the surrounding branches of the facial nerve. Line B approximates the course of the duct, which enters the mouth at the junction of lines A and B.

Parotid gland
Parotid duct
Masseter muscle
Branches of facial nerve

mandibular (Wharton's) ducts run from the external portion of the gland to empty into the mouth on either side of the frenulum of the tongue.

Pathophysiology

The basic mechanism of all injury is the transfer of energy, most often kinetic, to the structures of the body. When the energy overcomes the tolerance of the underlying tissue, injury results. Trauma traditionally has been classified as blunt or penetrating, but in many cases the effect is a combination of the two, such as the forehead injury (contusion and complex laceration) resulting from a child's fall against the sharp corner of the coffee table. The likelihood of injury is related to the amount of energy transferred and the condition of the underlying tissue. Significant injury may result when an 80-year-old falls from standing to a carpeted floor, but is more likely to result when the face strikes the steering wheel or dashboard in a high-speed MVC.

The mechanism can be broken down into *low-energy* events, such as a fall from standing or walking into the corner of a piece of furniture, and *high-energy* events, such as a MVC. Understanding the mechanism of injury not only can help predict the severity of the facial injury, but also predict the risk of associated cervical or brain injuries.

Traditional teaching has been that the face actively protects the brain from injury and that patients with facial trauma are less likely to have a significant brain injury. A small and a large study suggesting a significant association between facial and brain injury have now challenged this teaching.[33] In a particular patient, cervical and brain injuries should be considered based on the mechanism of injury and presentation of the patient without allowing the presence or absence of a facial injury to change the level of suspicion.

The association between cervical injury and facial injury is still unclear. The traditional teaching has been that the presence of a facial injury should increase the suspicion of an injury to the cervical spine. This teaching has been challenged. Most of the research supporting this idea are assessments of the incidence of cervical spine injury in patients with facial injury.[34,35] When more sophisticated methods are used to assess for an association between the two and correcting for the mechanism of injury, patients with facial injury may be less likely to have a significant cord injury and no relationship with spinal bony injury.[36,37]

Truly penetrating trauma to the face from gunshots, stab wounds, blast debris, or impalement is often obvious and dramatic (Figure 39-5). The astute emergency physician should search avidly for associated intracranial, spinal, or vascular injuries, which are common in these cases.[38] Facial penetration from pellets (BBs) or small blast debris or shrapnel may be less obvious, and the emergency physician must be alert to the possibility based on the history and carefully search for small skin lesions.[39] More recently, unregulated guns created from plastic pipes and aerosol cans that shoot potatoes have become popular in parts of the United States, mostly among adolescent boys. Significant facial trauma can result from these instruments, which can propel a potato at 200 mph.[40]

CLINICAL FEATURES

History

The history can provide information about the mechanism of the patient's injury. The emergency physician should be alert to limitations of the history, however, when the patient's consciousness is altered by head injury or intoxication, there is an issue of secondary

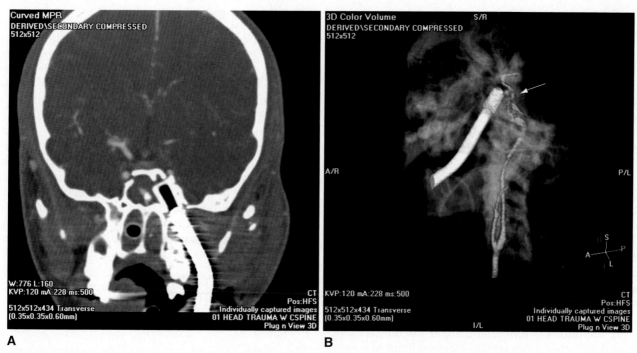

Figure 39-5. Impalement by a turn-signal lever. Computed tomography **(A)** and three-dimensional reconstruction **(B)** from a patient impaled through the face into the cranial cavity by the turn-signal level from his steering column when his vehicle rolled over in a single-car crash. The color three-dimensional reconstruction reveals a significant injury to the facial artery *(arrow)*.

gain, the police are involved, or abuse is suspected. Patients with a clear sensorium are able to describe the events leading up to the injury and localized pain; deficits in motor or sensory function; and abnormalities of vision, hearing, taste, or smell. Although the association between facial trauma and brain or cervical spine injury is unclear, these possibilities should be considered, and the patient should be questioned regarding headache, peripheral weakness, numbness, or paresthesias.

Physical Examination

Many facial injuries can be identified by simple inspection. During the primary assessment, attention is initially on the patient's airway, and inspection of the oropharynx is an essential first step. Airway compromise is often due to intraoral trauma, and the examiner should note excessive bleeding, drooling, dysphonia, swelling of the tongue or posterior pharynx, and the presence of avulsed teeth. When the patient is stabilized, a secondary survey should include a systematic examination of all facial structures and functions. Bony prominences should be palpated for abnormal motion, bony crepitus, tenderness, or step-off. Tenderness and massive swelling associated with facial trauma may preclude reliable palpation of a fracture. Consequently, areas of significant swelling should be imaged radiographically. Assessment of bony integrity includes testing for possible LeFort fracture. The upper incisors are grasped and pulled anteriorly. Movement of the upper alveolar ridge (type I), midface (type II), or entire face (type III) indicates a fracture. Wounds may need to be palpated for underlying bony injury or foreign objects; anesthesia may be required for a thorough

examination within the wound. Complex lacerations involving the cartilage of the nose or ear, eyelids, lacrimal apparatus, eyebrows, or vermilion border of the lips should be identified because their repair requires special techniques.

Eye and Orbit

In addition to looking at lacerations and contusions, the face should be evaluated for symmetry. The appearance of the zygomas may be evaluated by looking at the patient from above. This technique also draws attention to the relative position of the eyeballs. Orbital fractures may result in enophthalmos (sinking of the globe into the orbit), and a large retrobulbar hematoma may cause exophthalmos. The anterior chamber of the globe should be inspected for hyphema or globe rupture. Hyphema is due to bleeding in the anterior chamber and appears as a layer of blood in the dependent portion of the anterior chamber. A complete examination of the eye includes some specific testing. If the patient is able to cooperate, visual acuity should be documented. Contact lenses should be removed. In the event of a significant potential chemical exposure, the pH of the eye may need to be measured. Fluorescein examination of the eye should be performed if there is any concern about corneal abrasion. Victims of MVCs often have particles of glass in the conjunctiva or on the cornea, and these should be sought out and removed. Extraocular motions should be tested. Blowout fractures of the orbit may result in diplopia on upward gaze secondary to entrapment of the inferior rectus muscle or anesthesia of the midface and upper lip in the distribution of second division of the fifth cranial nerve secondary to neurapraxia resulting from fracture through the infraorbital foramen or compression by a local hematoma.

Oropharynx

The integrity of the mouth and nasal complex may be evaluated by listening to the patient's speech. A muffled or overly nasal voice may indicate occlusion of the nose or nasopharynx, whereas dysarthria may indicate a mandibular fracture, tongue injury, or neurologic problem. Oral injury may result in progressive airway compromise, and dysphonia should alert the clinician to the possible need for active airway management. The intraoral examination includes inspection of the palate, teeth, tongue, and gums and palpation with a gloved finger (the latter only if the patient is able to cooperate). The range of motion of the mandible should be determined. If the maximal incisor opening is less than 5 cm, a mandibular fracture may be present. Trismus is likely to indicate a fracture or significant hematoma within the face. If awake, the patient's impression about the normalcy of bite occlusion is a more sensitive determinant of a fracture of the mandible than the physician's impression. Being able to perform tongue blade test (grasping and holding a tongue blade between the teeth while the examiner pulls gently) is associated with greatly reduced probability of mandibular fracture.[41] If the patient is able to crack the tongue blade by biting on both sides of the mouth, the negative predictive value for a mandibular fracture is 95.2%.[42] Injury to the parotid area should raise suspicion of disruption of Stensen's duct. The opening of the duct opposite the second upper molar should be examined for bleeding while the gland is compressed. If blood is expressed from the duct or the severed ends of the duct are identified within a facial wound, specialized repair over a stent is required to prevent formation of a cutaneous fistula.

Ears

Otoscopy is performed to evaluate the integrity of the external canal, look for hemotympanum, and assess for otorrhea. Clear fluid from the ear after trauma should raise the possibility of a leak of cerebrospinal fluid (CSF). At the bedside, a drop of the fluid may be placed onto filter paper. A rapidly advancing halo of clear fluid around red blood defines a positive test. The ear should be inspected for subcutaneous hematomas because these need to be drained.

Nose

The nose is palpated for tenderness, crepitus, or abnormal movement, then each naris is held closed in turn to ensure the patient is able to breathe through either side. The septum should be examined visually to look for septal hematoma, which appears as a large purple mass extending from the septum. If there is any concern about CSF rhinorrhea, the aforementioned filter test may be used.

Neurological Examination

Light touch should be tested for all three branches of the fifth cranial nerve. Motor function (cranial nerve VII) can be examined by having the patient actively wrinkle the forehead, fully open and snug the eyelids shut, smile widely, and bare the teeth. Asymmetry of these movements indicates a potential nerve injury.

The final part of the physical examination is documentation. In one series of complex malar fractures that required operative repair, 30% of patients were involved in litigation.[43] In addition, facial injuries may be evidence of assault, domestic violence, or child abuse. Careful documentation of findings, including photographs or drawings or both, not only communicates initial findings to other practitioners, but also can provide crucial legal evidence.

DIAGNOSTIC STRATEGIES

Imaging

The choice of imaging for facial fractures depends on the patient's stability, the patient's ability to cooperate, and the availability of various options. The two main options are plain x-rays and computed tomography (CT). Fractures are better visualized on CT than magnetic resonance imaging, so magnetic resonance imaging is not an optimal imaging choice. In patients who cannot cooperate with plain x-rays or in whom a serious injury is obvious from the physical examination, CT is the imaging modality of choice.[44] For a complete evaluation, CT scans of the face should include coronal and sagittal reconstructions. Interpreting facial CT scans is an art that requires attention to bones, sinuses, orbital contents, and soft tissue and is best handled by radiology experts. Three-dimensional reconstruction CT scans add significantly to the accuracy of diagnosis and presurgical planning in complex midface fractures (see Figure 39-6B).[45]

In centers where a CT scanner is readily available, and the result can be read by an expert in a timely fashion, CT may be the choice for all patients in whom a midface fracture is a possibility. These criteria are not met in all cases; for patients with low to moderate pretest probability of a midface or maxillary fracture, who are stable and able to cooperate, the current recommendation is for a single screening view (a Water's or occipitomental view), followed by CT if the film is positive for a fracture or air-fluid level in any sinus.[46-48]

The U shape of the mandible and the presence of nearby bony structures make isolating the mandible on flat film impossible. Simple radiographs of the mandible are less sensitive than panorex radiographs and particularly tend to miss fractures of the condyle. Panorex imaging is indicated for isolated mandibular fractures, dental fractures, or fractures of the alveolar ridge. In children, if fracture of the condyle is suspected, coronal CT is more sensitive and specific than panorex studies.[49]

For patients with complex fractures, new imaging techniques may help improve surgical planning and esthetic outcomes. In displaced orbital fractures, using CT data to measure orbital volumes has shown that after repair, an orbital volume greater than 4% larger than the unfractured side is associated with visible postoperative enophthalmos.[50] This method seems to be useful in predicting which patients might benefit from operative repair.[51] In conjunction with more standard two-dimensional facial CT scans, three-dimensional CT seems to improve the diagnosis and aid preoperative planning for patients with complex fractures of the nasoethmoid complex.[52] Three-dimensional CT seems to be more accurate than multi-planar reconstructions and provides information about the relative positioning of fracture lines not appreciable in two-dimensional scans.[53]

Patients with tenderness and swelling isolated to the bony bridge of the nose who do not have a septal hematoma, can breathe through each naris, and have a straight nose do not require nasal bone x-rays because imaging would not alter treatment. If these criteria are not met, there may be an indication for early reduction or referral for surgical intervention, and imaging is indicated. Plain x-rays also may be performed in the setting of legal concerns. If there is concern for a foreign body in a superficial wound, two standard x-ray views (Water's and Caldwell's or occipitofrontal view) are indicated to triangulate the position of observed foreign material.

MANAGEMENT

Management of facial injuries occurs within the overall resuscitation of the patient. Unless the airway is threatened or exsanguination is a concern, treatment of most facial injuries can be deferred until more life-threatening injuries have been stabilized. Care of the patient with penetrating trauma to the face should center on standard trauma care, with initial attention focused on maintaining a patent airway, adequate ventilation, and systemic perfusion.

Prehospital Care

The indications for airway management of a patient with a facial injury are the same as for other patients: Does the patient have a currently patent airway, and if so, can the patient be expected to maintain it without intervention? If the answer to either question is "no," the patient needs to be intubated. If other injuries preclude the patient from ventilating appropriately, intubation also is required.

Patients with expanding hematomas after facial injury present a special dilemma. Injuries to the facial vasculature may cause significant hematomas that can extend into the neck or down to the supraclavicular area. Such hematomas greatly distort the normal anatomy of the pharynx and neck, making intubation and cricothyroidotomy particularly difficult. If the patient has a patent airway, he or she can speak without difficulty and the transport time is expected to be short, no intervention should be performed, and the receiving institution should be notified so that planning can begin for a difficult airway. If intubation must occur in the field, awake orotracheal intubation should be considered. If certified in its use, emergency medical services personnel should be ready to perform a surgical airway as needed. Gunshot wounds to the lower third of the face are particularly likely to require intubation for airway protection, and a significant proportion of these require a surgical airway.[54]

In the setting of significant facial trauma, active bleeding can obscure the view and make intubation considerably more difficult. Double suctioning may be required; this involves an assistant holding one suction catheter in the posterior oropharynx, while the operator uses a second device more anteriorly or inferiorly as needed during the procedure. Conversely, patients with fractures of the mandible may be easier to intubate because increased mobility of the mandible may allow wider opening of the mouth.

Blind nasotracheal intubation is controversial in facial trauma because of concerns about complications.[55] Multiply-injured patients who require intubation may not be breathing actively enough for this method to be of use. Prehospital rapid sequence intubation is associated with a higher success rate and fewer complications in multiply-injured trauma patients.[56] Although reports of intracranial placement of an endotracheal tube in facial trauma are rare, this catastrophic complication is known to occur after blind nasotracheal intubation.[57,58] Any concern about an injury to the skull base or cribriform plate is a contraindication to using this method of intubation.

Control of local bleeding is the other significant prehospital consideration in facial trauma. In many areas, external compression is sufficient to control bleeding during transport. Epistaxis and significant intraoral bleeding can be more difficult to treat. Even in the setting of significant nasal trauma, the soft portions of the nares can be compressed to stop anterior nasal bleeding. In an awake, alert patient with intraoral bleeding, 4 × 4 gauze packing may be placed into the buccal space to provide control. If these maneuvers are insufficient, and the patient's injuries require spinal immobilization, intubation may be a necessary first step to control intraoral or nasopharyngeal bleeding. After intubation, large amounts of gauze can be placed via the mouth into the oropharynx and nasopharynx to obtain control.

If prehospital personnel suspect a ruptured globe, special protection against compression of the eye (eye cup or noncontact shielding) should be provided in the field. Avulsed parts, including ears, the tip of the nose, teeth, or completely avulsed flaps, should be transported with the patient in saline-soaked gauze.

Completely or incompletely avulsed teeth should be removed and carried with the patient in sterile saline during transport. Patients who are not neurologically normal, who are intoxicated, who require cervical spine immobilization, who are nauseated, or who cannot be transported upright should not be transported with avulsed teeth held in the mouth. In such cases, the risk of aspirating the teeth outweighs any other concerns.

General Measures

The initial evaluation in the emergency department should re-address the question of intubation. In the setting of significant distortion of the mouth, oropharynx, or upper neck by avulsion or hematoma, the awake fiberoptic method may optimize the chances of a successful intubation. When there is significant distortion of the oropharynx or larynx, a laryngeal mask airway may not achieve a sufficiently tight fit to allow ventilation. Emergent cricothyroidotomy is the procedure of choice if endotracheal intubation is impossible.

Unless there is life-threatening hemorrhage from the face, after the airway has been secured, facial injuries can be safely left to the secondary survey. The emergency physician should avoid being distracted by a facial injury and search intensively for head, neck, chest, abdominal, pelvic, and extremity injuries. In-depth ocular examinations and other special testing should wait until other serious injuries have been managed emergently.

Significant bleeding often can be controlled by compression. If compression fails, hemostasis can be achieved in the emergency department by ligation of the relevant vessel. Great care should be taken, however, not to clamp or tie structures blindly deep within the face because serious nerve or iatrogenic injury of ductal structures could result. Massive, uncontrollable bleeding from facial fractures occurs rarely and is best treated with arterial embolization, if available.[59,60] In the rare case of a patient acutely exsanguinating from a facial wound, the external carotid artery can be ligated emergently. This ligation is best accomplished with surgical assistance.

Bite wounds, gross contamination, or significant tattooing from foreign bodies should be addressed definitively as soon as possible, given needs of the patient's other injuries. Definitive treatment of simple soft tissue injuries can be left for 24 hours if needed after irrigation and temporary approximation. Ideally, facial fractures are treated early, before significant swelling occurs, or after several days when return of more normal facial contours can aid in the repair. The need for tetanus prophylaxis should be considered in all open wounds. If the injury is an animal bite, the need for rabies prophylaxis should be considered. Because the rabies virus is transmitted to the brain along nerve axons, and symptomatic disease theoretically may occur sooner with wounds of the head, face, and neck, initiating rabies treatment within 5 days of the injury is recommended.

Finally, because lead poisoning has been reported from the ingestion of shotgun pellets in patients with primarily facial injuries, consideration should be given to looking for the presence of pellets in the gastrointestinal tracts of these victims. A plain x-ray of the abdomen suffices. Early endoscopic removal of the pellets should limit future toxicity.[61]

Soft Tissue Injuries

Soft tissue injuries to the face present an acute cosmetic concern for the patient. Areas may be contused, lacerated, abraded, or any combination of the three. When cleaned of any debris, abrasions may be covered in a thin layer of antibiotic ointment and left exposed or covered (as possible given its location). Patients with significant tattooing benefit from topical lidocaine for anesthesia before vigorous scrubbing necessary to remove the embedded material is begun. Careful attention should be placed on removing all of the embedded material as soon as possible because epithelialization requires the creation of a new wound to remove debris later. For contusions, ice and sleeping with the head elevated may limit the degree of swelling anticipated on days 2 and 3. The patient should be cautioned to anticipate the development of periorbital swelling or ecchymosis or both over time as a result of gravity when the primary contusion has been to the brow, forehead, or bridge of the nose.

The most appropriate person to close an open wound may be the emergency physician or a consultant. Decisions about which wounds to close personally and which to ask a consultant to repair are based on the personal judgment of the emergency physician; factors that may enter into the decision include resource availability; the size, shape, depth, and location of the wound; and the time commitment that careful, cosmetic wound closure can entail for the emergency physician in a busy emergency department. The patient's priority with facial lacerations is cosmesis, and a patient may request specialty services for minor wounds out of this concern.[62] Children and patients with behavioral problems may require sedation to allow sufficient control for a cosmetic repair. Repair of facial wounds in uncooperative patients who are acutely intoxicated may be delayed until they become sober enough to cooperate with the procedure.

After anesthesia is obtained, wounds should be explored for depth, foreign bodies, or underlying fractures. Irrigation may not be necessary in simple, clean facial wounds closed within 6 hours.[63] For wounds deeper than the dermis, subcuticular buried sutures using absorbable materials should be placed to close any potential space and relieve any tension on the skin. For skin closure, tissue adhesive is faster and less painful and results in equal cosmetic results in adults and children and can be used to close the skin over deeper sutures.[64-66] Compared with sutures, tissue adhesive has the additional benefit of not requiring later removal, but care must be taken not to glue the eye, naris, or mouth closed unintentionally.

Antibiotics are not required for simple facial wounds, which rarely become infected. Bite wounds, wounds with any evidence of devascularization, wounds through and through the buccal mucosa, wounds involving the cartilage of the ear or nose, and wounds with extensive contamination (particularly with barnyard or fecal matter) are exceptions to this rule.

SPECIAL CONSIDERATIONS BY SITE

Mouth

Lacerations

Lip lacerations are common and require special consideration to maintain the appearance of the lip edge or vermilion border and the natural architecture of the philtrum. Because infiltration of even a small volume of local anesthetic may distort and blanch the soft tissue, marking the vermilion border (with nonpermanent ink or a scratch of a sterile needle) before anesthesia facilitates a cosmetic repair. To minimize any divots and maximize cosmesis and function, wounds that include the muscular layer should be closed in multiple layers. Skin may be closed with nylon or other nonabsorbable suture; the lip itself and mucosa should be closed with gut. Lip lacerations are not amenable to closure with wound adhesives.

Through-and-through lacerations of the mouth should be closed in layers, beginning with the intraoral mucosa and working outward in layers toward the skin. Copious irrigation after closure of the mucosal layer is indicated to remove lingering bacteria that otherwise would be incorporated into the wound. In small case series, prophylactic treatment with penicillin has been shown to decrease the risk of infection after significant oral lacerations.[67] Lacerations that approach the parotid (Stensen's) or submandibular (Wharton's) ducts should be evaluated before intervention for ductal integrity. Saliva milked from the gland should be thin and clear and readily exit the duct. If a duct is involved or there is any doubt, a facial specialist should be consulted for evaluation and repair.

Small lacerations of the tongue or oral mucosa do not require repair. Lacerations that gape, including deep tongue lacerations, collect food and are likely to heal with a significant divot or thick scar that may hinder eating and speaking functions. Deep or gaping lacerations of the tongue or oral mucosa should be closed (in layers if necessary), using absorbable sutures that do not require removal. To facilitate repair, an assistant may be needed to expose the laceration by grasping the tongue between gauze and holding a segment outside of the mouth. Discharge instructions for intraoral lacerations (whether or not repaired) should include gentle cleansing (swish and spit) with a mild antiseptic.

Perioral Burns

Young children use their mouths to explore their environment and may lick electrical outlets or bite electrical cords. The wet oral mucosa provides little electrical resistance, and the current penetrates to deeper structures, often causing a full-thickness burn at the commissure of the lip. These children need a systemic evaluation for other electrical injury (see Chapter 140);

this discussion is limited to the evaluation and treatment of facial wounds. Perioral burns resulting from electrical injury can result in severe cosmetic problems and microstomia. The initial appearance of the wound may be misleadingly trivial; edema and necrosis progress over several days, and even with healing, the defect may become quite disfiguring. Traditionally the main concern has been bleeding from the labial artery when the maturing burn eschar separates from underlying structures 5 to 21 days postburn. Large wounds can cause significant early difficulty with eating, however, and patients may require placement of a nasogastric tube for maintenance of nutrition. Initial emergency department treatment of the wound is aimed at treating discomfort and keeping the area clean.

Treatment of these injuries is controversial; the options include conservative treatment with early oral splinting, immediate surgery aimed at reconstruction, or delayed excision of the burned area.[68] Early involvement of consultants is indicated, even when the burn seems to be trivial. The possibility of abuse or neglect should be considered when a child presents with a perioral burn.

Cheek

Contusions of the cheek should raise concern for an underlying zygomatic or maxillary fracture. Lacerations of the lateral cheek may involve the parotid gland or Stensen's duct; failure to identify and repair ductal injury results in retention of salivary fluid and enlargement of the gland or formation of a cutaneous fistula. Lacerations in the area anterior to the tragus may include injury to the facial nerve, and careful neurologic examination should be carried out before closure. Langer's lines change from mostly horizontal in the superior cheek to diagonal at the nasolabial fold, then curve convexly around the mouth; these changes should be taken into consideration when debridement is required as part of a complex repair.

Nose

Because of its anterior position, soft tissue injuries to the nose are common. Almost any trauma can result in epistaxis. Generally, epistaxis is controllable by pinching the cartilaginous anterior nose closed between two fingers and holding compression for about 10 minutes. If not, anterior packing is indicated. Intranasal inspection is required in any nasal injury to assess for a septal hematoma, which appears as a dark purple or bluish mass against the septum. Hematomas require drainage because they are associated with necrosis of the septum if left untreated. Simple incision and expression of the clot followed by anterior packing is sufficient. Any patient with nasal packing should receive prophylactic antibiotics to cover *Staphylococcus* and *Streptococcus* species to prevent sinusitis and toxic shock syndrome.

Because of its location and structure, fractures of the thin bones of the nasal bridge are common. Patients with contusion or tenderness over the bridge of the nose may be assumed to have fracture of the nasal bones. If the nose is acceptably straight on initial evaluation, there is no septal hematoma, epistaxis is controlled, and the patient is able to breathe out of each naris, no further evaluation is required emergently for isolated nasal injuries. Although still in use, there is no clinical utility to radiographs of the nasal bones.[69-72]

Swelling over the bridge often precludes determination of the acceptability of the appearance at the time of injury; the patient may be provided with a referral for outpatient specialty follow-up in 3 to 5 days if the appearance at that time (when the swelling has improved) is unacceptable. In a series of surgically repaired simple nasal bone fractures, septal fractures were present in more than 50% of cases. CT did not provide any advantage in diagnosing septal fracture.[73]

Children with nasal fractures may have premature closure of sutures and uneven growth, particularly of the vomeroseptal line. In a child, no imaging studies are indicated, but a consultant should evaluate swelling and tenderness over the nose, preferably within 4 days of the injury.[74]

Simple lacerations of the nasal skin may be closed with sutures or tissue adhesive. If needed, anesthesia may be obtained using a nerve block of the infraorbital or supratrochlear nerves. The large pores typically present in the area of the nasal ala increase the likelihood of stitch abscesses after laceration closure in this area. Closure using an absorbable running subcuticular suture may limit the risk of this outcome. If involved, the cartilaginous portions of the ala should be closed in a separate layer. For lacerations through and through the nose, repair should be carried out from the mucosal layer outward, with copious irrigation between layers.

Ears

Blunt trauma to the ear may cause hematoma formation in the subperichondral potential space. Such hematomas are the prelude to the development of a "cauliflower ear" and should be drained by aspiration. Reaccumulation of the hematoma is prevented with a compressive dressing of the ear, but re-examination is crucial, and re-aspiration should be performed as necessary.

Ear lacerations often involve the cartilage. The ear may be anesthetized using a field block: 1% lidocaine *without* epinephrine is injected subcutaneously into the skin around the base of the ear. Simple skin wounds may be closed in a single layer. Lacerations to the underlying cartilage should be repaired using absorbable material. If there is significant degloving or loss of overlying tissue, a consultant should be involved; portions of aural cartilage may be saved temporarily in a distant dermal pocket for later reconstruction. Because cartilage is avascular, chondritis when it occurs requires extensive debridement and is disfiguring. No randomized trials have been performed, but when the cartilage of the pinna requires repair, antibiotic prophylaxis is recommended. Compressive ear dressings (splints) are indicated after any significant repair. Ear injuries occurring before age 1 or injuries to both ears in children are rare and should raise the suspicion of abuse.[75]

Eyes

Simple eyelid lacerations may be repaired in a single layer. Wound adhesives should be used with great caution anywhere near the eye; care must be taken not to glue the eyelids open or shut. Lacerations that involve deeper structures, loss of tissue, or the lid margin should be referred to a consultant. The integrity of the lacrimal apparatus can be assessed by instilling fluorescein into the eye and assessing for dye in the wound. A consultant should handle any injury to the sac or lacrimal duct.

Eyebrow lacerations are common because of the overhanging supraorbital ridge. Careful wound exploration should be performed to assess the integrity of the underlying bony structure. No shaving should be performed because the brow hairs may not regrow, and the hairs are necessary for realignment. If debridement is required, it should be done parallel to the hair follicles (skived) rather than perpendicular to the skin. This approach minimizes the bald area of the scar. Closing the deeper muscular layers preserves the normal expressive function of the brow. Injuries to the globe are discussed in Chapter 70.

FRACTURES AND DISLOCATIONS

For the emergency physician, the key to facial fractures is accurate diagnosis and appropriate referral. Many nondisplaced or minimally displaced facial fractures may be handled on an outpatient basis, with definitive repair or fixation delayed several days. Adult fractures develop firm fibrous union within about 10 to 14 days, however; definitive repair is performed most easily before day 7. Methods for diagnosing fractures were discussed earlier. Fractures to the face of young children are relatively rare and may be incomplete or greenstick fractures. Fibrous union in these cases is rapid; early reduction (within 3 days) is recommended.

Antibiotics are indicated for open fractures and fractures that violate a sinus. Patients with fractures through the nasoethmoid complex that violate the maxillary bones or the floor of the orbit should be cautioned to avoid sneezing and blowing the nose because these activities force air out into the soft tissues of the face.

Surgical repair of simple nasal fractures may be performed closed and the nose splinted internally or packed. Repair of fractures of the floor of the orbit, when necessary, may require the placement of a silicone patch to occlude the opening into the maxillary sinus. Most other fractures of the face that require operative repair are performed using small metal plates (microplates), screws, or wires to stabilize fragments by attaching them to unbroken segments of bone. Efforts are made to return the features to their unfractured locations and to regain facial symmetry, if possible. Complex facial fractures may have to be repaired in a staged fashion, depending on the patient's degree of illness and the amount and quality of the bone remaining. Much of this surgery is best accomplished when the fragments are still freely mobile, but initial swelling has been reduced, on postinjury days 3 to 5.

Specific Considerations by Site

Forehead

Fractures through the superior forehead may occur above the level of the frontal sinus. These are actually skull fractures rather than facial fractures and should be addressed with special attention to risk of injury to the underlying brain. Unlike other skull fractures, frontal skull fractures may require repair for cosmesis alone. More often, fractures in this area involve the anterior portion of the frontal sinus. If even minimally displaced, these fractures require elevation for cosmesis. Fractures through the anterior wall of the frontal sinus are likely to continue through the posterior wall, and a CT scan should be performed to look carefully for this complication; if present, a CSF leak should be assumed until proved otherwise. CSF leaks into the frontal sinus may present in a delayed fashion, days or years after the initial injury.[76]

Orbit

The most common simple fracture of the orbit is blow-out fracture of the orbital floor, often caused by a fisted blow or ball striking the globe, increasing intraorbital pressure enough to force orbital contents through the floor. This injury may happen without other significant bony facial injury. When displaced, the bony fragments sag into the underlying maxillary sinus. If the inferior rectus muscle is entrapped in the defect, the patient is unable to elevate the globe on the affected side, resulting in diplopia on upward gaze. Stretch on the infraorbital nerve, which passes through the floor, may cause anesthesia over the anteromedial cheek and upper lip. Because signs of entrapment may result from contusion and edema and be self-limited, immediate repair is not necessary, but careful follow-up is required. Repair typically is performed 1 to 2 weeks after the injury for persistent enophthalmos or diplopia. Because of the acute limitation in the visual field, discharge instructions for patients with acute diplopia should include patching for comfort and a request not to drive until the diplopia is resolved.

Fractures of the medial orbital wall, through the lamina papyracea, are often associated with nasal injury or more general midface fractures, particularly with telescoping of the midfacial skeleton. Herniation of orbital contents into the ethmoids may occur. In one study, patients with orbital fractures with a medial component were more likely to have ocular signs of diplopia or exophthalmos than patients with fractures that did not involve the medial wall.[77] Fractures involving the superior orbit include the base of the frontal sinus, and all of the concerns about the anterior skull mentioned previously apply. Herniation of orbital structures into the frontal sinus is rare but also can occur.

Many orbital fractures involve more than one wall of the orbit and may present in a constellation with complex midface fractures. One study suggests classification by the number of walls of the orbit involved (one to four) with 53% of fractures involving only one

wall and 5% involving all four,[78] but no classification system is generally accepted.

Injury to the orbit, particularly fractures, can cause a hematoma to form within the orbit, behind the globe. If significant in size, an orbital hematoma can cause acute exophthalmos. Stretch on the retinal artery limiting flow to the retina or neurapraxia of the retinal nerve may cause decreased visual acuity or blindness. Orbital emphysema associated with fractures of the medial wall or floor rarely results in a space-filling lesion with the same effect. This is a true emergency; drainage of the air or blood via lateral canthotomy with cantholysis is indicated to save the patient's vision. Needle aspiration of entrapped air also may be attempted, but this may be best left to a consultant given the proximity of the globe.

Midface

Tripod (or trimalar) fractures are among the simplest fractures of the midface and include fractures of three bones: the lateral orbit, the zygoma, and the maxilla (Figure 39-6). Typically caused by a direct blow, these fractures are often displaced and require operative stabilization. If left untreated, the area may "sink" posteriorly and inferiorly, giving an unacceptable appearance of facial asymmetry emphasized by the inferior position of the orbit and malar flattening. On the initial physical examination, there may be a large contusion over the cheekbone, enophthalmos, or malocclusion of the upper teeth. Fractures through the anterior wall of the maxillary sinus may denervate the maxillary teeth because the dentoalveolar nerves run in tunnels in this area.

More complex fractures of the midface are classified using the Le Fort system, although many complex fractures defy classification with this system. A Le Fort I fracture involves a transverse fracture through the maxilla above the roots of the teeth and may be unilateral or bilateral. Patients may complain of malocclusion, and the maxilla may be mobile when the upper teeth are grasped and rocked. A Le Fort II fracture is typically bilateral and pyramidal in shape. It extends superiorly in the midface to include the fracture of the nasal bridge, maxilla, lacrimal bones, orbital floor, and rim. In these cases, the nasal complex moves as a unit with the maxilla when the teeth are grasped and rocked. In the age of CT scans, a simple Le Fort III fracture is rare, but essentially involves fracturing of the connections between the elements of the skull and the face (craniofacial dysjunction). These fractures start at the bridge of the nose and extend posteriorly along the medial wall of the orbit (ethmoids), along the floor of the orbit (maxilla) and through the lateral orbital wall and finally break through the zygomatic arch. Intranasally, they extend through all the lesser bones to the base of the sphenoid and frequently are associated with a CSF leak.

Significant force to the bridge of the nose may fracture the nasoethmoid complex without creating a formal Le Fort pattern. CT is the initial test of choice in this setting. Fractures to the central portion of the

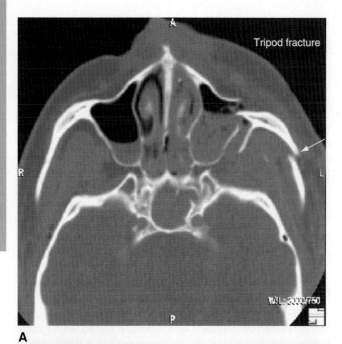

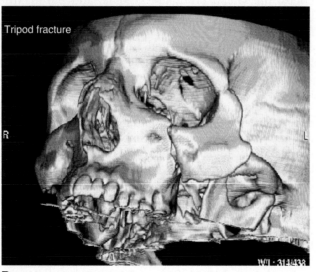

Figure 39-6. Tripod fracture. Computed tomography **(A)** and three-dimensional reconstruction **(B)**.

multiple trauma. Even a 10-cm anterior pack should not reach the skull base in a skeletally mature person. Significant or massive bleeding into the posterior nasopharynx presents a complex problem and occurs in less than 1% of patients with midface fractures. It may be treated with nasal packing and immediate fracture reduction.[37,82] Unless the anatomy is well understood and the skull base known to be intact, however, the use of a long balloon catheter (Foley) should be avoided for control of posterior bleeding. The unintended positioning of these items within the intracranial[83,84] or intraspinal space[85] during blind nasal insertion has been well documented, and when the face is grossly distorted, preinsertion measuring or other methods of preventing this outcome have not been adequately tested. There were no reports of the intracranial placement of commercial catheters designed for posterior epistaxis, but if the midface is significantly distorted or telescoped, they also may be long enough to reach the intracranial space. An alternative method for containing posterior nasal bleeding is to provide compression by packing the area with gauze by hand from the oropharynx after intubation.

Zygoma

Isolated fractures of the zygoma are relatively rare, usually the result of a direct blow, and are often displaced. Because the condyle of the mandible may disturb zygomatic fragments while moving, fractures with significant displacement are likely to result in trismus or discomfort with mouth opening. Surgical repair usually is required to return the cheekbone to an acceptable position.

Mandible

Fractures of the mandible can result from any significant force applied to its U shape. Because of its shape, multiple fractures may result from a single blow, and the fracture sites may be distant from the site of impact. Depending on the location of the fractures, the patient may have trismus (fractures of the coronoid process, neck, or rami), dental malocclusion, swelling, and tenderness intraorally or externally. Anesthesia of the lower lip may occur if there is damage to the inferior dental nerve.

Fractures of the symphysis, body, angle, or rami usually require early splinting, typically by the placement of arch bars to accomplish interdental fixation, commonly known as "wiring the jaw shut." Fixation limits fracture motion, decreases the patient's discomfort, and, if the fracture is minimally displaced, may provide complete fracture care. Impacted and nondisplaced fractures occasionally are treated with only a soft diet, and fractures of the coronoid alone usually require no intervention, but these decisions should be made in consultation with an oral surgeon or other specialist. Arch bars may be placed in the emergency department or operating room and typically are placed by a specialist (Figure 39-7). Fracture reduction may require the extraction of teeth adjacent to the fracture line. Patients with open fractures require antibiotics

ethmoid bone (cribriform plate) are likely to be associated with a CSF leak and commonly result in anosmia.

If possible, patients with CSF leak should have the head elevated 40 to 60 degrees. Head elevation minimizes the intracranial pressure with the idea of decreasing the flow and allowing the leak to seal. Often, these patients are treated with antibiotics; however, this practice is controversial, and most of the studies supporting it involve small, local case series.[79,80] In one meta-analysis, antibiotics did not decrease the rate of meningitis in the setting of CSF leak.[81] Neurosurgeons should be involved in the care of patients with CSF leaks.

Fractures involving the deeper structures of the midface may be associated with significant bleeding into the nose or oropharynx. Anterior nasal packing may be performed safely in the adult patient with

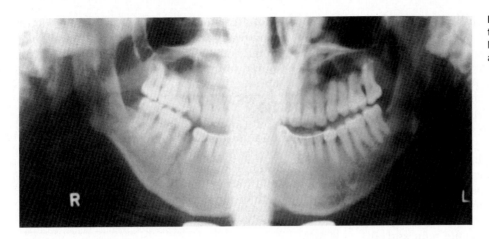

Figure 39-7. Panoramic radiograph of the mandible shows fractures through the left angle and the right body. A dental appliance is in place on the lower incisors.

and usually hospitalization. When the fractures are closed and adequate stabilization can be obtained, elective operative repair can be performed as an outpatient procedure in 3 to 5 days.

In one study, 17% to 22% of pediatric patients 4 to 11 years old developed facial growth disturbances after a fractured mandible and required later orthognathic surgery for correction. Children younger than 4 or older than 11 were much less likely to develop this complication.[86] Because of the frequency of this complication, children in this age group with a blow to the chin and any trismus or tenderness over the TMJ should be assessed carefully with panorex imaging for condylar fracture and referred appropriately.[87]

Dental and Alveolar Trauma

Trauma to the teeth may occur with or without other facial injury. In the setting of caries, tooth fractures may occur with eating relatively soft foods. Tooth fractures are classified by the Ellis system. Class I fractures involve only the enamel of the tooth, are not painful, and can await dental evaluation as an outpatient. Class II fractures expose the yellow dentin and may be painful. These also can await dental care, but may be covered with a dressing of calcium hydroxide and aluminum foil. Class III fractures expose the dental pulp, seen as a red line or dot, and are exquisitely painful. These require early evaluation by dentists or endodontists.

Sufficient energy to the area avulses teeth from their sockets. Multitrauma patients, particularly patients who are intoxicated, required to be supine for cervical spine immobilization, or neurologically impaired, should have avulsed or mostly avulsed teeth removed from the mouth and placed externally in saline as an aspiration precaution. In a critically ill multitrauma patient, avulsed teeth should become among the lowest priorities and replanted only if the care of other injuries would allow it and there is no risk of aspiration if the tooth loosens.

To perform a reimplantation, the physician disturbs the socket as little as possible, gently rinses off the tooth (the root should not be wiped), and places it into the socket where it "clicks" into place. If the tooth is only partially avulsed, extruded, or laterally luxated, it should not be removed; it should be reimplanted or relocated. Intruded teeth should not be manipulated. Reimplantation can be painful and may require local anesthesia. The area of a single socket may be anesthetized by placing approximately 0.5 mL of 1% lidocaine without epinephrine into the buccal sulcus and gum on the outer side of the alveolar ridge. After reimplantation, the tooth requires stabilization with acrylic splint or wiring to the adjacent teeth.

Replanted teeth may or may not "take" acutely, but it can take weeks to assess the final success of reimplantation. The length of time out of the socket seems to play a critical role in the initial success. Among teeth successfully reimplanted in less than 1 hour, more than 66% were radiographically healed and functionally normal after 5 years. For teeth successfully reimplanted after 3 hours, more than 80% had signs of inflammation and bone resorption after the same period of time.[88]

In children, the front maxillary incisors are most commonly avulsed. After reimplantation, these teeth may ankylose and fail to "grow out" normally, requiring later extraction or orthodontic intervention for cosmesis. This situation is most common among children age 6 to 10 with avulsed adult teeth.[89]

Avulsed teeth missing after significant trauma should be carefully sought, including obtaining a chest x-ray. In an acute event, the patient may not recall aspirating a tooth; this is more likely if the patient is intoxicated or neurologically impaired. If the tooth is below the diaphragm on the film, it does not require retrieval. Teeth lodged in a bronchus or the esophagus require bronchoscopic or endoscopic retrieval. Aspirated teeth result in pulmonary abscess formation unless removed.

Fractures through the alveolar ridge may result in a group of teeth being dislodged and out of position, often leaning inward. These teeth require stabilization with wire or acrylic splinting after fracture reduction returns the teeth to their correct location. The involved teeth may or may not survive after such a fracture, and careful follow-up with a dentist or oral surgeon is required.

Temporomandibular Joint

The TMJ is complex, with the condyle of the mandible undergoing rotation and translation anteriorly during normal mouth opening. The function of the joint is preserved by a meniscus, which overlies the condyle. Essentially the joint between the meniscus and the condyle is a hinged joint, allowing rotation, and the joint between the meniscus and the temporal bone is a sliding joint, allowing translation. A formal, thick joint capsule does not exist at the anteromedial portion of the joint; loose, relatively weak synovial tissue is positioned here to allow translation to occur.

Trauma to the TMJ may tear the meniscus or injure the collateral ligaments holding it in a normal position. This injury can cause the meniscus to fail to translate normally, resulting in clicking or popping as it catches up to the condyle or inability to open the mouth fully because the meniscus completely fails to translate. Patients without fracture but with acute pain and difficulty with mouth opening should be placed on soft foods, asked not to yawn or struggle to open their mouths widely, and referred to an oral surgeon with expertise in TMJ pathology. Pediatric patients with posttraumatic internal derangements of the TMJ are prone to asymmetry of facial growth and retrognathia. In one study, 88% of children injured before their ninth birthday had significant facial abnormalities years later.[90]

Because of the anatomy and function of the joint, anterior dislocation of the TMJ can occur after widely yawning, laughing, kissing, singing, or other activities that involve spontaneous, wide opening of the mouth. When the condyle is out, spasm of the muscles of mastication prevents spontaneous reduction. Significant trauma is more likely to cause a fracture-dislocation. Simple dislocation may be unilateral or bilateral, and the patient complains of being unable to close the mouth. In unilateral dislocation, the jaw is rotated laterally away from the affected joint; bilateral dislocation causes significant protrusion of the jaw. The jaws of these patients are often so widely open that they cannot swallow their secretions and are actively drooling. Speech often is garbled by the patient's inability to touch the tongue to the roof of the mouth or the maxillary teeth. There is a depression in the area of the affected TMJ on inspection of the patient's face.

If the mechanism of injury suggests a fracture, the area should be imaged with plain x-ray or panorex before attempting reduction. To reduce simple dislocation, the patient should be seated upright. To maximize leverage, the best position may be seated in a regular chair with the operator standing in front of the patient. As in dislocations of other joints, adequate analgesia and sedation are required for success. Using the thumb or index finger placed into the buccal sulcus on either side of the mouth, the angle of the jaw is pressed downward while rotating the symphysis (chin) upward and backward. Care should be taken not to place fingers along the crowns of the teeth; when relocation occurs, spasm of the muscles of mastication snaps the mouth shut with force. If this is the only location possible for the physician's fingers, gauze wrappings should be placed to protect them.

Panorex or x-rays are suggested after the first episode of dislocation. The patient is discharged with pain medicine, a soft diet for 2 weeks, and outpatient follow-up with an oral surgeon. Patients with an episode of dislocation are predisposed to a recurrence. In patients who are frequently dislocating, interdental fixation may be required for 2 to 3 weeks.

DISPOSITION

The decision to discharge or admit patients with facial trauma depends on their associated injuries, general injury severity, and plans for treatment. Patients with isolated facial trauma that has been repaired or stabilized and with no airway issues are usually discharged.

KEY CONCEPTS

- The face is central to the patient's ability to breathe, eat, and communicate. Injuries to the face can have serious psychological and psychosocial consequences.

- Facial injuries may be prevented by the appropriate use of safety belts, child restraints, air bags, helmets, and face guards.

- The epidemiology of facial injury is changing, with an increasing proportion occurring as a result of interpersonal violence. A careful history is required, and the possibility of abuse should be considered for every patient.

- Shock is rare from facial trauma and results only from obvious external bleeding. Facial injuries should not distract the emergency physician from aggressively searching for other causes of shock.

- Assertive management of the airway is indicated in a patient with significant facial injuries. Surgical management (cricothyroidotomy) may be required, particularly with gunshot wounds.

- Directed facial CT scanning is the best imaging technique in patients with obvious injuries. Patients with low likelihood of clinically significant fractures may be screened with a single Water's view followed by CT only if positive.

- Definitive treatment may be delayed if needed to allow other serious injuries to be addressed.

REFERENCES

1. Rankin M, Borah GL: Perceived functional impact of abnormal facial appearance. *Plast Reconstr Surg* 111:2140, 2003.
2. Langlois JH, et al: Maxims or myths of beauty? A meta-analytic and theoretical review. *Psychol Bull* 126:390, 2000.
3. Pashos A, Niemitz C: Results of an explorative empirical study on human mating in Germany: Handsome men, not high-status men, succeed in courtship. Anthropol Anz 61:331, 2003.
4. Thornton B, Ryckman RM: Relationship between physical attractiveness, physical effectiveness, and self-esteem: A cross-sectional analysis among adolescents. *J Adolesc* 14:85, 1991.
5. Bisson JI, Shepherd JP, Dhutia M: Psychological sequelae of facial trauma. *J Trauma* 43:496, 1997.
6. Shetty V, et al: Psychosocial sequelae and correlates of orofacial injury. *Dent Clin North Am* 47:141, 2003.
7. Glynn SM, et al: The development of acute post-traumatic stress disorder after orofacial injury: A prospective study in a large urban hospital. *J Oral Maxillofac Surg* 61:785, 2003.

8. Le BT, et al: Referral patterns for the treatment of facial trauma in teaching hospitals in the United States. *J Oral Maxillofac Surg* 61:557, 2003.

9. National Center for Injury Prevention and Control, Centers for Disease Control and Prevention: Web-based Injury Statistics Query and Reporting System (WISQARS) 2002. Available at: www.cdc.gov/ncipc/wisqars. Accessed January 5, 2004.

10. Insurance Institute for Highway Safety: Safety belt laws. Available at: http://www.hwysafety.org/safety%5Ffacts/ state%5Flaws/restrain3.htm. Accessed January 6, 2004.

11. Murphy RX, et al: The influence of airbag and restraining devices on the patterns of facial trauma in motor vehicle collisions. *Plast Reconstr Surg* 105:516, 2000.

12. Simoni P, Ostendorf R, Cox AJ 3rd: Effect of air bags and restraining devices on the pattern of facial fractures in motor vehicle crashes. *Arch Facial Plast Surg* 5:113, 2003.

13. Mouzakes J, et al: The impact of airbags and seat belts on the incidence and severity of maxillofacial injuries in automobile accidents in New York State. *Arch Otolaryngol Head Neck Surg* 127:1189, 2001.

14. Duma SM, Jernigan MV: The effects of airbags on orbital fracture patterns in frontal automobile crashes. *Ophthalmol Plast Reconstr Surg* 19:107, 2003.

15. Murphy RX Jr, et al: Influence of restraining devices on patterns of pediatric facial trauma in motor vehicle collisions. *Plast Reconstr Surg* 107:34, 2001.

16. Major MS, MacGregor A, Bumpous JM: Patterns of maxillofacial injuries as a function of automobile restraint use. *Laryngoscope* 110:608, 2000.

17. Shapiro AJ, et al: Facial fractures in a level I trauma centre: The importance of protective devices and alcohol abuse. *Injury* 32:353, 2001.

18. Ogundare BO, Bonnick A, Bayley N: Pattern of mandibular fractures in an urban major trauma center. *J Oral Maxillofac Surg* 61:713, 2003.

19. Leathers R, et al: Orofacial injury in underserved minority populations. *Dent Clin North Am* 47:127, 2003.

20. Touma BJ, et al: Maxillofacial injuries caused by all-terrain vehicle accidents. *Otolaryngol Head Neck Surg* 121:736, 1999.

21. Kraus JF, et al: Facial trauma and the risk of intracranial injury in motorcycle riders. *Ann Emerg Med* 41:18, 2003.

22. Perkins SW, et al: The incidence of sports-related facial trauma in children. *Ear Nose Throat J* 79:632, 2000.

23. Marshall SW, et al: Evaluation of safety balls and faceguards for prevention of injuries in youth baseball. *JAMA* 289:568, 2003.

24. Bernardo LM, et al: A comparison of dog bite injuries in younger and older children treated in a pediatric emergency department. *Pediatr Emerg Care* 18:247, 2002.

25. Le BT, et al: Maxillofacial injuries associated with domestic violence. *J Oral Maxillofac Surg* 59:1277, 2001.

26. Jessee SA: Orofacial manifestations of child abuse and neglect. *Am Fam Physician* 52:1829, 1995.

27. Zerfowski M, Bremerich A: Facial trauma in children and adolescents. *Clin Oral Invest* 2:120, 1998.

28. Shaikh ZS, Worrall SF: Epidemiology of facial trauma in a sample of patients aged 1–18 years. *Injury* 33:669, 2002.

29. Wilson S, et al: Epidemiology of dental trauma treated in an urban pediatric emergency department. *Pediatr Emerg Care* 13:12, 1997.

30. Azevedo AB, Trent RB, Ellis A: Population-based analysis of 10,766 hospitalizations for mandibular fractures in California, 1991 to 1993. *J Trauma* 45:1084, 1998.

31. Insurance Institute for Highway Safety: Child restraint laws. Available at: http://www.hwysafety.org/safety%5Ffacts/ state%5Flaws/restrain2.htm. Accessed January 5, 2004

32. Durbin DR, et al: Risk of injury to restrained children from passenger air bags. *Traffic Inj Prev* 4:58, 2003.

33. Martin RC 2nd, Spain DA, Richardson JD: Do facial fractures protect the brain or are they a marker for severe head injury? *Am Surg* 68:477, 2002.

34. Ardekian L, et al: Incidence and type of cervical spine injuries associated with mandibular fractures. *J Craniomaxillofac Trauma* 3:18, 1997.

35. Hackl W, et al: The incidence of combined facial and cervical spine injuries. *J Trauma* 50:41, 2001.

36. Williams J, et al: Head, facial, and clavicular trauma as a predictor of cervical-spine injury. *Ann Emerg Med* 21:719, 1992.

37. Hills MW, Deane SA: Head injury and facial injury: Is there an increased risk of cervical spine injury? *J Trauma* 34:549, 1993.

38. Demetriades D, et al: Initial evaluation and management of gunshot wounds to the face. *J Trauma* 45:39, 1998.

39. Koren I, et al: Unusual primary and secondary facial blast injuries. *Am J Otolaryngol* 24:75, 2003.

40. Barker-Griffith AE, et al: Potato gun ocular injury. *Ophthalmology* 105:535, 1998.

41. Schwab RA, Genners K, Robinson WA: Clinical predictors of mandibular fractures. *Am J Emerg Med* 16:304, 1998.

42. Alonso LL, Purcell TB: Accuracy of the tongue blade test in patients with suspected mandibular fracture. *J Emerg Med* 13:297, 1995.

43. Koening WJ, Lewis VL Jr: The physician cost of treating maxillofacial trauma. *Plast Reconstr Surg* 91:778, 1993.

44. Sun JK, LeMay DR: Imaging of facial trauma. *Neuroimaging Clin North Am* 12:295, 2002.

45. Remmler D, et al: Role of three-dimensional computed tomography in the assessment of nasoorbitoethmoidal fractures. *Ann Plast Surg* 44:553, 2000.

46. Pogrel MA, Podlesh SW, Goldman KE: Efficacy of a single occipitomental radiograph to screen for midfacial fractures. *J Oral Maxillofac Surg* 58:24, 2000.

47. McGhee A, Guse J: Radiography for midfacial trauma: Is a single OM 15 degrees radiograph as sensitive as OM 15 degrees and OM 30 degrees combined? *Br J Radiol* 73:883, 2000.

48. Goh SH, Low BY: Radiologic screening for midfacial fractures: A single 30-degree occipitomental view is enough. *J Trauma* 52:688, 2002.

49. Chacon GE, et al: A comparative study of 2 imaging techniques for the diagnosis of condylar fractures in children. *J Oral Maxillofac Surg* 61:668, 2003.

50. Dolynchuk KN, Tadjalli HE, Manson PN: Orbital volumetric analysis: Clinical application in orbitozygomatic complex injuries. *J Craniomaxillofac Trauma* 2:56, 1996.

51. Raskin EM, et al: Prediction of late enophthalmos by volumetric analysis of orbital fractures. *Ophthalmol Plast Reconstr Surg* 14:19, 1998.

52. Remmler D, et al: Role of three-dimensional computed tomography in the assessment of nasoorbitoethmoidal fractures. *Ann Plast Surg* 44:553, 2000.

53. Fox LA, et al: Diagnostic performance of CT, MPR and 3DCT imaging in maxillofacial trauma. *Comput Med Imaging Graph* 19:385, 1995.

54. Hollier L, Grantcharova EP, Kattash M: Facial gunshot wounds: A 4-year experience. *J Oral Maxillofac Surg* 59:277, 2001.

55. Rosen CL, et al: Blind nasotracheal intubation in the presence of facial trauma. *J Emerg Med* 15:141, 1997.

56. Walls RM: Blind nasotracheal intubation in the presence of facial trauma: Is it safe? *Emerg Med* 15:243, 1997.

57. Rhee KJ, et al: Does nasotracheal intubation increase complications in patients with skull base fractures? *Ann Emerg Med* 22:1145, 1993.

58. Marlow TJ, Goltra DD Jr, Schabel SI: Intracranial placement of a nasotracheal tube after facial fracture: A rare complication. *J Emerg Med* 15:187, 1997.

59. Shimoyama T, Kaneko T, Horie N: Initial management of massive oral bleeding after midfacial fracture. *J Trauma* 54:332, 2003.

60. Bynoe RP, et al: Maxillofacial injuries and life-threatening hemorrhage: Treatment with transcatheter arterial embolization. *J Trauma* 55:74, 2003.

61. McQuirter JL, et al: Elevated blood lead resulting from maxillofacial gunshot injuries with lead ingestion. *J Oral Maxillofac Surg* 61:593, 2003.

62. Singer AJ, et al: Patient priorities with traumatic lacerations. *Am J Emerg Med* 18:683, 2000.

63. Hollander JE, et al: Irrigation in facial and scalp lacerations: Does it alter outcome? *Ann Emerg Med* 31:73, 1998.

64. Quinn JV, et al: A randomized, controlled trial comparing a tissue adhesive with suturing in the repair of pediatric facial lacerations. *Ann Emerg Med* 22:1130, 1993.

65. Quinn J, et al: A randomized trial comparing octylcyanoacrylate tissue adhesive and sutures in the management of lacerations. *JAMA* 277:1527, 1997.

66. Barnett P, et al: Randomised trial of histoacryl blue tissue adhesive glue versus suturing in the repair of paediatric lacerations. *J Paediatr Child Health* 34:548, 1998.

67. Steele MT, et al: Prophylactic penicillin for intraoral wounds. *Ann Emerg Med* 18:847, 1989.

68. Thomas SS: Electrical burns of the mouth: Still searching for an answer. *Burns* 22:137, 1996.

69. Oluwasanmi AF, Pinto AL: Management of nasal trauma—widespread misuse of radiographs. *Clin Perform Qual Health Care* 8:83, 2000.

70. Logan M, O'Driscoll K, Masterson J: The utility of nasal bone radiographs in nasal trauma. *Clin Radiol* 49:192, 1994.

71. Nigam A, et al: The value of radiographs in the management of the fractured nose. *Arch Emerg Med* 10:293, 1993.

72. Li S, Papsin B, Brown DH: Value of nasal radiographs in nasal trauma management. *J Otolaryngol* 25:162, 1996.

73. Rhee SC, et al: Septal fracture in simple nasal bone fracture. *Plast Reconstr Surg* 113:45, 2004.

74. Haug RH, Foss J: Maxillofacial injuries in the pediatric patient. *Oral Surg Oral Med Oral Pathol Oral Radiol Endod* 90:126, 2000.

75. Steele BD, Brennan PO: A prospective survey of patients with presumed accidental ear injury presenting to a paediatric accident and emergency department. *Emerg Med J* 19:226, 2002.

76. Friedman JA, Ebersold MJ, Quast LM: Post-traumatic cerebrospinal fluid leakage. *World J Surg* 25:1062, 2001.

77. Jank S, et al: Clinical signs of orbital wall fractures as a function of anatomic location. *Oral Surg Oral Med Oral Pathol Oral Radiol Endod* 96:149, 2003.

78. Manolidis S, et al: Classification and surgical management of orbital fractures: Experience with 111 orbital reconstructions. *J Craniofac Surg* 13:726, 2002.

79. Clemenza JW, Kaltman SI, Diamond DL: Craniofacial trauma and cerebrospinal fluid leakage: A retrospective clinical study. *J Oral Maxillofac Surg* 53:1004, 1995.

80. Choi D, Spann R: Traumatic cerebrospinal fluid leakage: Risk factors and the use of prophylactic antibiotics. *Br J Neurosurg* 10:571, 1996.

81. Villalobos T, et al: Antibiotic prophylaxis after basilar skull fractures: A meta-analysis. *Clin Infect Dis* 27:364, 1998.

82. Shimoyama T, Kaneko T, Horie N: Initial management of massive oral bleeding after midfacial fracture. *J Trauma* 54:332, 2003.

83. Pawar SJ, Sharma RR, Lad SD: Intracranial migration of Foley catheter—an unusual complication. *J Clin Neurosci* 10:248, 2003.

84. Engel M, Reif J, Moncrief E: Inadvertent intracranial placement of a Foley catheter: A rare iatrogenic complication of severe frontomaxillary trauma. *Rev Stomatol Chir Maxillofac* 93:333, 1992.

85. Porras LF, et al: Inadvertent intraspinal placement of a Foley catheter in severe craniofacial injury with associated atlanto-occipital dislocation: Case report. *Neurosurgery* 33:310, 1993.

86. Demianczuk AN, Verchere C, Phillips JH: The effect on facial growth of pediatric mandibular fractures. *J Craniofac Surg* 10:323, 1999.

87. Lee CY, et al: Sequelae of unrecognized, untreated mandibular condylar fractures in the pediatric patient. *Ann Dent* 52:5, 1993.

88. Schatz JP, Hausherr C, Joho JP: A retrospective clinical and radiologic study of teeth reimplanted following traumatic avulsion. *Endod Dent Traumatol* 11:235, 1995.

89. Malmgren B, Malmgren O: Rate of infraposition of reimplanted ankylosed incisors related to age and growth in children and adolescents. *Dent Traumatol* 18:28, 2002.

90. Defabianis P: Post-traumatic TMJ internal derangement impact on facial growth (findings in a pediatric age group). *J Clin Pediatr Dent* 27:297, 2003.

CHAPTER

40 Spinal Injuries

Robert S. Hockberger, Amy H. Kaji, and Edward J. Newton

PERSPECTIVE

Background

Prehistoric humans undoubtedly suffered little in the way of significant spinal injury. Their semierect posture combined with well-developed posterior cervical muscles protected the cervical spine against day-to-day trauma. Evolution, however, did much to undo this initial protective state. As humans assumed an upright posture, the shoulders dropped away from the newly elevated head and the hypertrophied paraspinous muscles atrophied. This change increased the head's range of motion but diminished the spine's protection. Although civilization heightened humans' inventiveness, it did little to curb aggressiveness. Automobiles replaced horse-drawn carriages, and fists

Table 40-1. Classification of Spinal Injuries

Mechanisms of Spinal Injury	Stability
Flexion	
Wedge fraction	Stable
Flexion teardrop fracture	Extremely unstable
Clay shoveler's fracture	Stable
Subluxation	Potentially unstable
Bilateral facet dislocation	Always unstable
Atlanto-occipital dislocation	Unstable
Anterior atlantoaxial dislocation with or without fracture	Unstable
Odontoid fracture with lateral displacement fracture	Unstable
Fracture of transverse process	Stable
Flexion-Rotation	
Unilateral facet dislocation	Stable
Rotary atlantoaxial dislocation	Unstable
Extension	
Posterior neural arch fracture (C1)	Unstable
Hangman's fracture (C2)	Unstable
Extension teardrop fracture	Usually stable in flexion; unstable in extension
Posterior atlantoaxial dislocation with or without fracture	Unstable
Vertical Compression	
Bursting fracture of vertebral body	Stable
Jefferson fracture (C1)	Extremely unstable
Isolated fractures of articular pillar and vertebral body	Stable

and clubs gave way to knives and guns, hence making spinal injuries more common in the modern era.

Epidemiology

Statistics from the National Spinal Cord Injury Database show that motor vehicle–related accidents account for 38.5% of all spinal injuries.[1] Speeding, alcohol intoxication, and failure to use restraints are major risk factors. The second largest contributor is intentional acts of human violence, such as gunshot wounds and assaults (24.5%), followed by falls (21.8%) and sports-related injuries (7.2%). Currently, more than 200,000 spinal injury victims are living in the United States, and 11,000 new cases occur each year. Unfortunately, spinal cord injury predominantly afflicts productive young adults, with 55% of cases occurring in those 16 to 30 years of age; 81.6% of patients are male. The total annual cost to society from lifelong medical expenses and lost productivity is estimated at more than $5 billion.[2] The devastating emotional and psychological impact on victims and their families is incalculable.

PRINCIPLES OF DISEASE

Anatomy and Physiology

The human spine consists of 33 bony vertebrae: 7 cervical, 12 thoracic, 5 lumbar, 5 sacral (fused into one), and 4 coccygeal (usually fused into one) (Figure 40-1A and B).[3] These 26 individual units are separated from one another by flexible intervertebral disks and connected to form a single functioning unit by a complex network of ligaments. In addition to providing basic structural support, the vertebral column protects the spinal cord, which extends from the midbrain to the level of the second lumbar vertebra. Nerves that receive and transmit sensory, motor, and autonomic impulses pass to and from the spinal cord through intervertebral foramina.

Fractures involving the first two cervical vertebrae are mechanically unstable because of their relative paucity of ligamentous and muscle support. To assess the stability of spinal injuries below C2, it is helpful to view the spine as consisting of two columns. The anterior column is formed by alternating vertebral bodies and intervertebral disks held in alignment by the anterior and posterior longitudinal ligaments (Figure 40-2A). The posterior column, which contains the spinal canal, is formed by the pedicles, transverse processes, articulating facets, laminae, and spinous processes and is held in alignment by the nuchal ligament complex (supraspinous, interspinous, and infraspinous ligaments), the capsular ligaments, and the ligamentum flavum (Figure 40-2B). If both columns are disrupted, the spine will move as two separate pieces, and it is highly likely that such movement will cause or worsen a spinal cord injury. In contrast, if only one column is disrupted, the other column resists further movement, and the likelihood of a spinal cord injury occurring is much less and depends on the strength of the intact ligaments.

Pathophysiology

Classification of Spinal Column Injuries

Acute spinal injuries are classified according to the mechanism of trauma: flexion, flexion-rotation, extension, and vertical compression (Table 40-1).[4,5]

Flexion

Pure flexion injuries involving the C1-C2 complex can cause unstable *atlanto-occipital* or *atlantoaxial joint dislocation*, with or without an associated fracture of

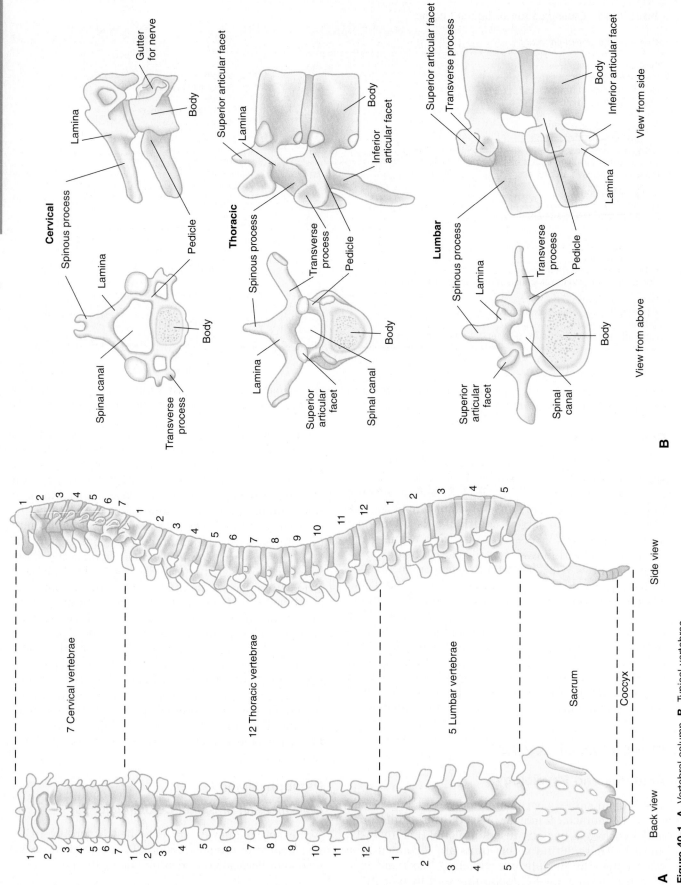

Cervical

Spinous process
Lamina
Gutter for nerve
Body
Pedicle

Lamina
Spinal canal
Body
Transverse process

Thoracic

Superior articular facet
Lamina
Spinous process
Transverse process
Pedicle
Inferior articular facet
Body

Lamina
Superior articular facet
Spinal canal
Body

Lumbar

Superior articular facet
Transverse process
Body
Inferior articular facet
Lamina

Spinous process
Lamina
Transverse process
Pedicle
Superior articular facet
Spinal canal
Body

View from side

View from above

B

7 Cervical vertebrae

12 Thoracic vertebrae

5 Lumbar vertebrae

Sacrum

Coccyx

Side view

Back view

A

Figure 40-1. A, Vertebral column. **B,** Typical vertebrae.

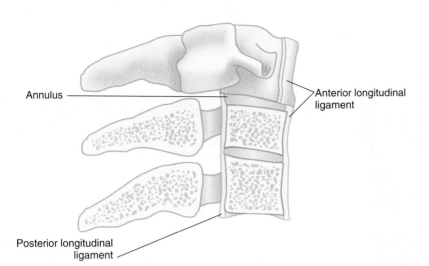

Annulus —

— Anterior longitudinal ligament

Posterior longitudinal ligament —

A

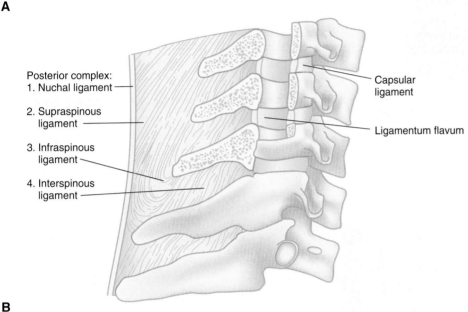

Posterior complex:
1. Nuchal ligament —
2. Supraspinous ligament —
3. Infraspinous ligament —
4. Interspinous ligament —

— Capsular ligament

— Ligamentum flavum

B

the odontoid (Figure 40-3). These injuries are considered unstable because of their location and the relative lack of muscle and ligamentous support. Less commonly, flexion injuries have an additional lateral component resulting in either lateral displacement of the odontoid, which is an unstable injury, or a fracture through the transverse process, which is a stable injury.

In pure flexion injuries below C2, longitudinal pull is exerted on the strong nuchal ligament complex, which usually remains intact. Most of the force is expended on the vertebral body anteriorly, and a *simple wedge fracture* results. Radiographically, there is diminished height and increased concavity of the anterior border of the vertebral body, increased density of the vertebral body as a result of bony impaction, and prevertebral soft tissue swelling (Figure 40-4). Because the posterior column remains intact, this injury is usually stable and rarely accompanied by nervous system damage. However, spinal instability may develop with severe wedge fractures (loss of over half the vertebral height) or multiple adjacent wedge fractures, and such injuries are best treated as being potentially unstable.

A *flexion teardrop fracture* results when flexion forces cause anterior displacement of a wedge-shaped fragment (resembling a teardrop) of the anteroinferior portion of the involved vertebral body (Figure 40-5). Because this injury commonly involves ligamentous disruption, it may be associated with neurologic damage.

A *clay shoveler's fracture* is an oblique fracture of the base of the spinous process of one of the lower cervical segments (Figure 40-6). The injury derives its name from its common occurrence in clay miners in Australia during the 1930s. When a miner lifted a heavy shovelful of clay, abrupt head flexion against the supraspinous ligament resulted in an avulsion fracture of the spinous process. Today, this fracture is more commonly seen after direct trauma to the spinous process and after motor vehicle crashes in which sudden deceleration results in forced neck flexion. Because this injury involves only the spinous process, it is stable and not associated with neurologic involvement.

Pure *spinal subluxation* occurs when the ligamentous complexes rupture without an associated bony injury. This injury begins posteriorly in the nuchal lig-

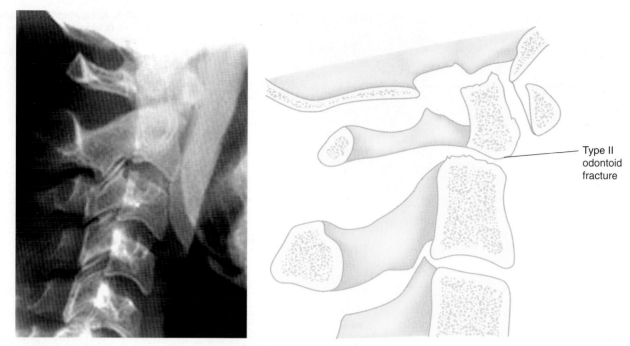

Type II
odontoid
fracture

Figure 40-3. Odontoid fracture with anterior dislocation. Mechanism: flexion with shearing. Stability: unstable. A fracture through the odontoid process is demonstrated along with retropharyngeal swelling.

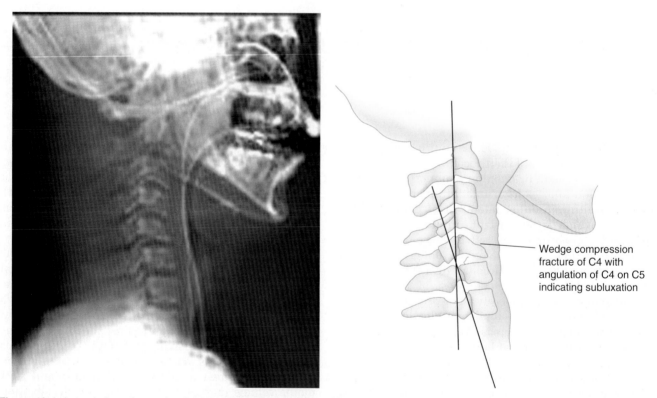

Wedge compression
fracture of C4 with
angulation of C4 on C5
indicating subluxation

Figure 40-4. Lateral view of a wedge fracture of C4 with angulation. Mechanism: flexion. Stability: mechanically stable. Note the anterior wedging of the C4 vertebral body and angulation of C4 on C5.

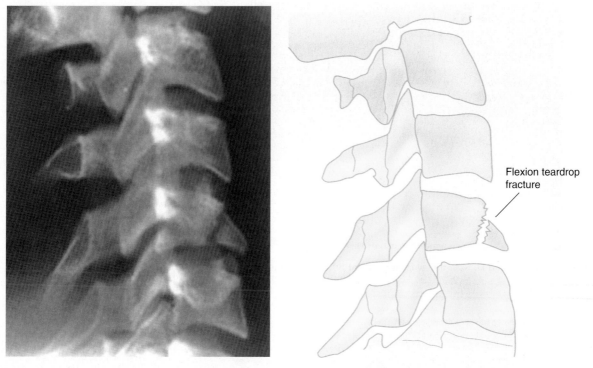

Figure 40-5. Lateral view of a teardrop fracture. Mechanism: flexion. Stability: unstable. The fractured fragment off the C5 body resembles a teardrop.

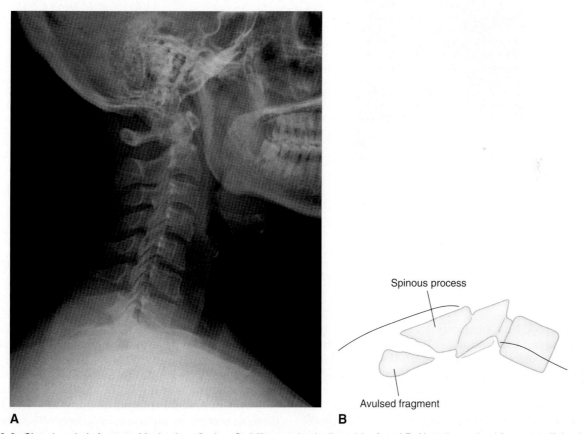

A **B**

Figure 40-6. Clay shoveler's fracture. Mechanism: flexion. Stability: mechanically stable. **A** and **B**, Note the avulsed fragment off the tip of the C7 spinous process in an underpenetrated lateral view.

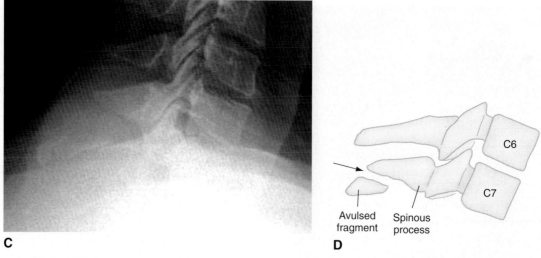

C

D

Avulsed fragment   Spinous process

Figure 40-6.—cont'd. C and **D**, Note the avulsed fragment off the tip of the C7 spinous process in a coned lateral view.

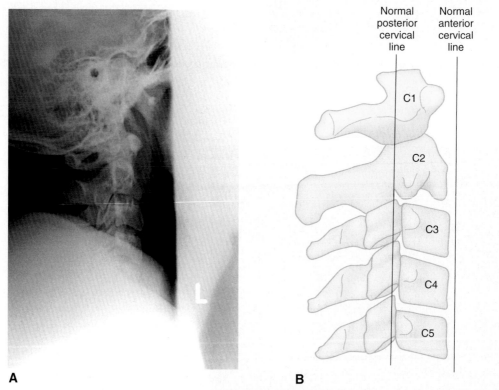

A

B

Figure 40-7. Subluxation with bilateral "perched" facets at C5 and C6. Mechanism: flexion. Stability: unstable. **A** and **B**, Only the first five vertebrae are clearly visible on this cross-table lateral view. No evidence of subluxation is demonstrated.

ament and proceeds anteriorly to involve other ligaments. A lateral radiograph with the neck in neutral position may show widening of both the interspinous and intervertebral spaces posteriorly at the level of injury, and oblique views may demonstrate widening or abnormal alignment of the facets (Figure 40-7A and C). These findings are often subtle and may be missed if flexion and extension views are not obtained. Though rarely associated with neurologic damage, this injury is potentially unstable.

Bilateral facet dislocations occur when a greater force of flexion causes the soft tissue disruption to con-

tinue anteriorly to the annulus fibrosis of the intervertebral disk and the anterior longitudinal ligament; such injury results in an extremely unstable condition. The forward movement of the spine causes the inferior articulating facets of the upper vertebra to pass upward and over the superior facets of the lower vertebra and thereby results in anterior displacement of the spine above the level of injury. Radiographically, the anterior displacement will appear to be greater than half the anteroposterior (AP) diameter of the lower vertebral body with the superior facets anterior to the inferior facets (Figure 40-8).

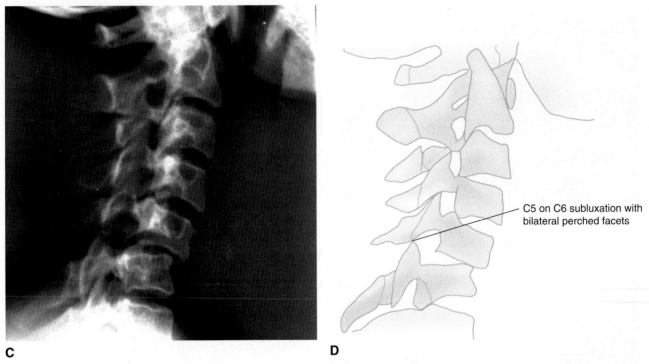

C **D**

Figure 40-7.—cont'd. C and **D,** A repeat lateral view shows severe subluxation of C5 on C6.

C5 on C6 subluxation with bilateral perched facets

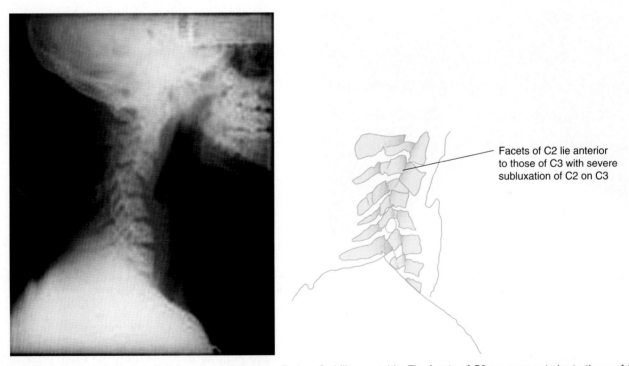

Facets of C2 lie anterior to those of C3 with severe subluxation of C2 on C3

Figure 40-8. A and **B,** Bilateral facet dislocation. Mechanism: flexion. Stability: unstable. The facets of C3 are seen anterior to those of C4, with angulation and subluxation of C3 on C4.

Shear Injury

Trauma to the head directed in an AP direction may result in fracture of the odontoid process above the transverse ligaments (type I) or more commonly at the base of the odontoid process where it attaches to C2 (type II). Slight angulation of the force may result in extension of the fracture into the body of C2 (type III).

Type II odontoid fractures are unstable and often complicated by nonunion. Spinal cord injury is uncommon but can occur (Figure 40-9).

Rotation

Rotary atlantoaxial dislocation is an unstable injury visualized best on open-mouth odontoid radiographs

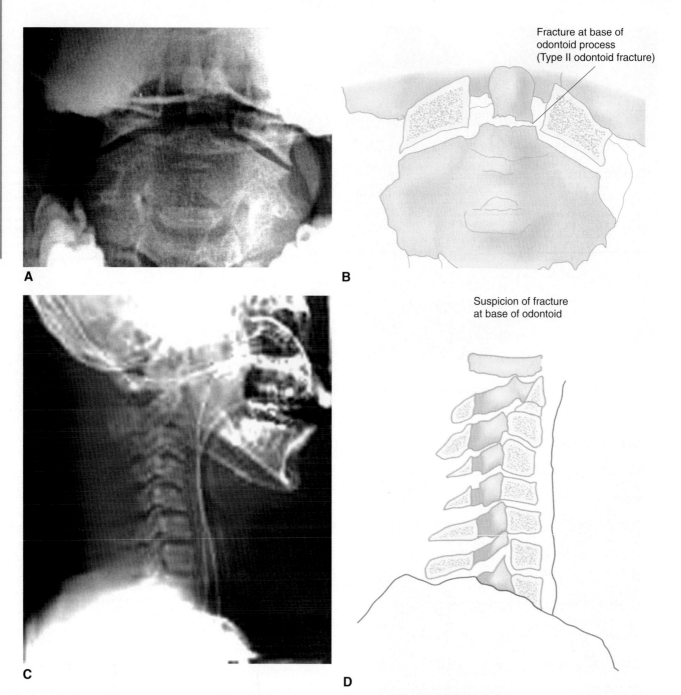

Figure 40-9. **A** and **B**, Odontoid fracture with lateral displacement. Mechanism: flexion. Stability: unstable. The tip of the odontoid process is laterally displaced in this lateral flexion injury. **C** and **D**, Lateral radiograph with suspicion of an odontoid fracture.

(Figure 40-10). The interpretation of odontoid radiographs warrants careful attention. If the skull is shown obliquely, there may be false-positive asymmetry between the odontoid process and the lateral masses of C1. However, when the radiograph reveals symmetrical basilar skull structures, a unilaterally magnified lateral mass confirms C1-C2 dislocation.

A *unilateral facet dislocation* involves both flexion and rotation. The rotational component of this injury occurs around one of the facet joints, which acts as a fulcrum. Simultaneous flexion and rotation cause the contralateral facet joint to dislocate, with the superior facet riding forward and over the tip of the inferior facet and coming to rest within the intervertebral foramen. In this position, the dislocated articular mass is mechanically locked in place, thus making this injury stable although the posterior ligament complex is disrupted. A lateral radiograph shows forward displacement of the dislocated segment on the vertebra below (less than half the AP diameter of this vertebral body) and rotation of the dislocated vertebra and those above it. A frontal radiograph shows that the spinous processes above the level of dislocation are displaced from the midline in the direction of the rotation (Figure 40-11). It may be difficult to differentiate this injury from acute torticollis caused by severe muscle spasm,

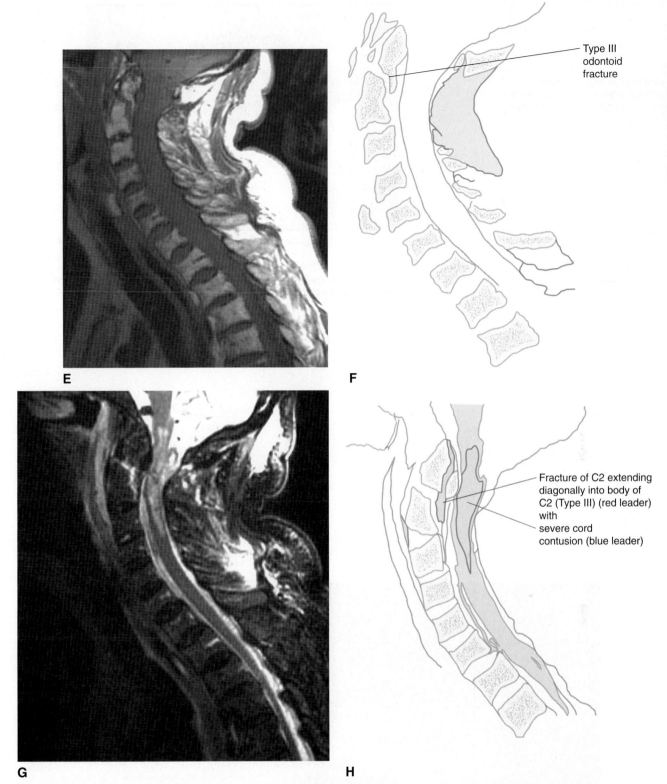

E

F

Type III
odontoid
fracture

G

H

Fracture of C2 extending
diagonally into body of
C2 (Type III) (red leader)
with
severe cord
contusion (blue leader)

Figure 40-9.—cont'd. E and **F**, T1-weighted magnetic resonance imaging (MRI) clearly shows a type III odontoid fracture. **G** and **H**, T2-weighted MRI shows severe spinal cord contusion associated with this fracture.

Figure 40-10. Rotatory subluxation of C1 on C2. Mechanism: rotation. Stability: unstable. **A** and **B**, There is marked asymmetry in the relationship of the lateral masses of C1 to the odontoid process. Rotation causes the right lateral mass to appear slightly larger (farther from the x-ray film) than the left (closer to the x-ray film).

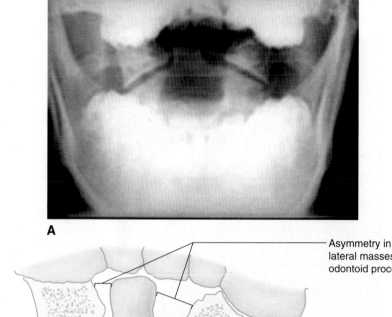

A

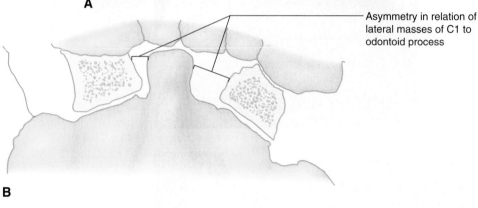

Asymmetry in relation of lateral masses of C1 to odontoid process

B

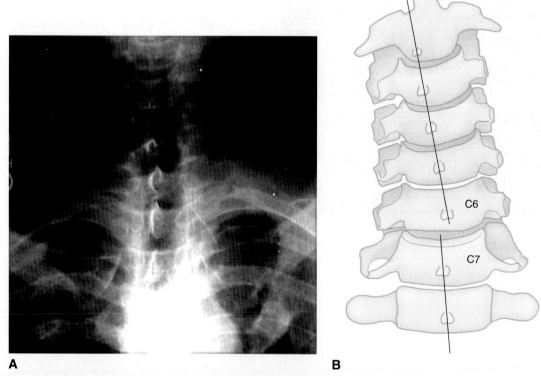

Line bisecting spinous processes

C6

C7

A   **B**

Figure 40-11. Unilateral facet dislocation. Mechanism: flexion and rotation. Stability: stable. **A** and **B**, Anterior view showing the spinous processes of the cervical vertebrae offset in relation to the thoracic vertebrae.

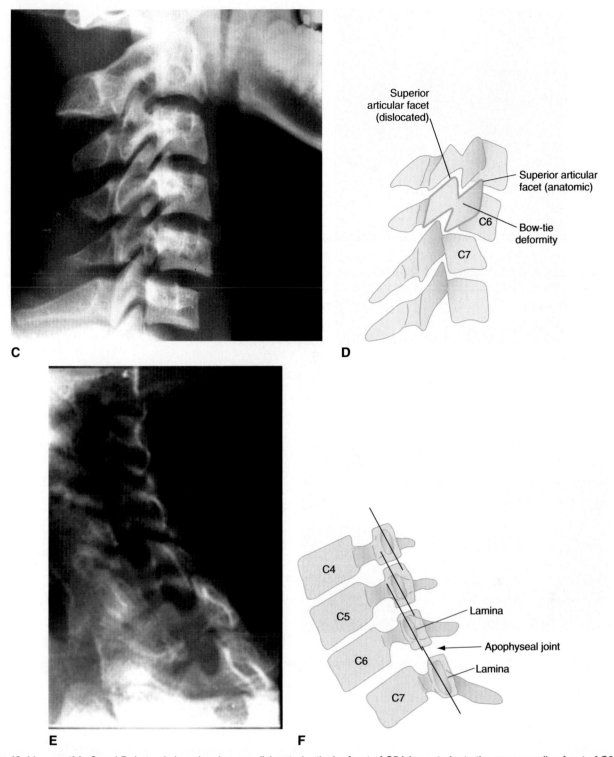

C

D

Superior
articular facet
(dislocated)

Superior articular
facet (anatomic)

C6

Bow-tie
deformity

C7

E

F

C4

C5

C6

C7

Lamina

Apophyseal joint

Lamina

Figure 40-11.—cont'd. C and **D**, Lateral view showing one dislocated articular facet of C5 lying anterior to the corresponding facet of C6 and creating a "bow tie" deformity. The C5 vertebral body is subluxed anteriorly on C6. **E** and **F**, Oblique view of unilateral facet dislocation with the lamina of C6 projecting into the neural foramina.

and oblique projections may be necessary to demonstrate the dislocated facet joint.

Because of the varying shapes of the articular processes, particularly between the cervical and lumbar regions, different types of flexion-rotation injuries can result. In the cervical region, where the articular processes are small, flat, and almost horizontal, unilateral facet dislocations occur as described pre-viously. In the lumbar region, however, where the articular processes are large, curved, and nearly vertical, unilateral facet dislocation is rare. Instead, one or both articular processes fracture, and the upper vertebra swings forward. Commonly seen in the thoracolumbar and lumbar region, this rotation fracture-dislocation is unstable (Figure 40-12).

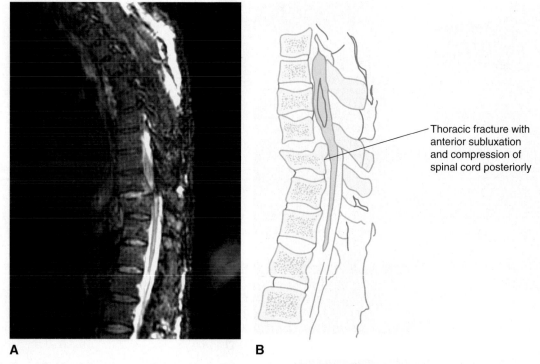

Figure 40-12. A and **B**, Magnetic resonance image showing fracture-dislocation of the thoracic spine.

Thoracic fracture with
anterior subluxation
and compression of
spinal cord posteriorly

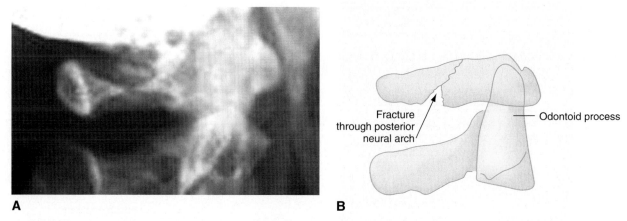

Fracture
through posterior
neural arch

Odontoid process

Figure 40-13. Posterior neural arch fracture of C1. Mechanism: extension. Stability: unstable. **A** and **B**, The fracture line is well visualized.

Extension

A *posterior neural arch fracture* of the atlas (C1) results from compression of the posterior elements between the occiput and the spinous process of the axis (C2) during forced neck extension (Figure 40-13). Though mechanically stable because the anterior arch and the transverse ligament remain intact, this fracture is potentially unstable because of its location.

A *hangman's fracture*, or traumatic spondylolysis of C2, occurs when the cervicocranium (the skull, atlas, and axis functioning as a unit) is thrown into extreme hyperextension as a result of abrupt deceleration. Bilateral fractures of the pedicles of the axis occur with or without dislocation (Figure 40-14). Although this

lesion is unstable, cord damage is often minimal because the AP diameter of the neural canal is greatest at the C2 level and the bilateral pedicular fractures permit the spinal canal to decompress itself. Originally described in victims of hanging injury, today it is most often the result of a head-on automobile crash.

An *extension teardrop fracture* occurs when abrupt extension of the neck causes the anterior longitudinal ligament to pull the anteroinferior corner of a vertebral body away from the remainder of the vertebra; this mechanism produces the classic triangular-shaped fracture. Often occurring in lower cervical vertebrae (C5-C7) as a result of diving accidents, this unstable injury may be associated with a central cord syndrome caused

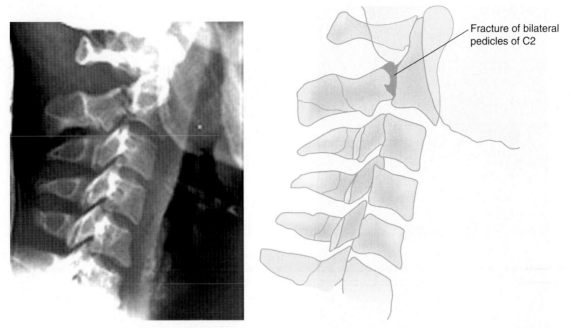

Figure 40-14. Hangman's fracture. Mechanism: extension. Stability: unstable. Fracture lines extending through the pedicles of C2 are well visualized. Retropharyngeal soft tissue swelling is apparent.

Fracture of bilateral pedicles of C2

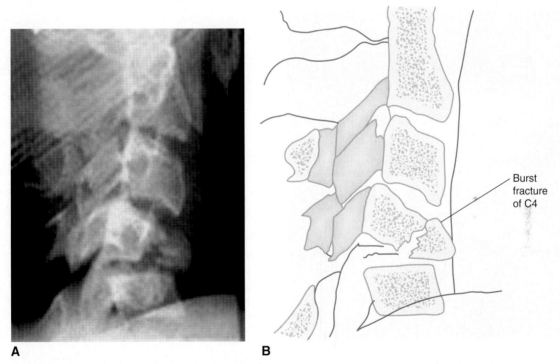

A   **B**

Burst fracture of C4

Figure 40-15. Burst fracture of a vertebral body. Mechanism: vertical compression/flexion. Stability: unstable. **A** and **B**, There is a compression fracture of the C4 vertebral body. During the bursting process the anterior segment of the fracture protrudes anteriorly and its posterior aspect protrudes posteriorly into the spinal canal. Such protrusion is often associated with anterior cord syndrome. The cervical spine is abnormally angulated.

by buckling of the ligamentum flavum into the spinal cord.[6]

Vertical Compression

Vertical compression injuries occur in the cervical and lumbar regions, which are capable of straightening at the time of impact. When force is applied from either above (skull) or below (pelvis or feet), one or more vertebral body end plates may fracture. The nucleus pulposus of the intervertebral disk is forced into the vertebral body, which is shattered outward, and a *burst fracture* results. A lateral radiograph shows an apparent vertebral compression fracture (Figure 40-15). Computed tomography (CT) demonstrates a characteristic

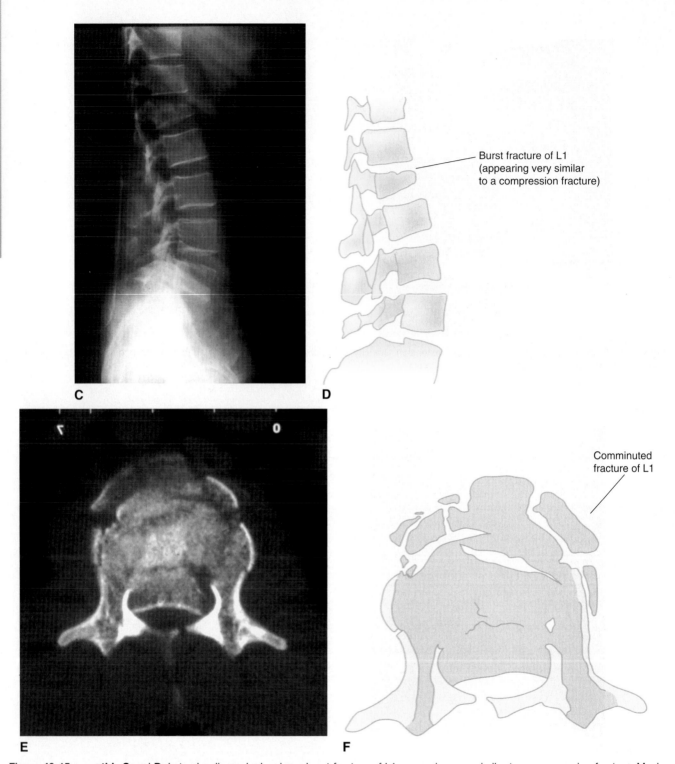

C

D

Burst fracture of L1
(appearing very similar
to a compression fracture)

E

F

Comminuted
fracture of L1

Figure 40-15.—cont'd. C and **D,** Lateral radiograph showing a burst fracture of L1, appearing very similar to a compression fracture. Mechanism: flexion. Stability: usually stable. **E** and **F,** Computed tomographic scan of L1 in the same patient, showing comminution of the fracture and retropulsion of fragments into the spinal canal.

burst fracture of the vertebral body, which helps differentiate it from a simple wedge fracture and a flexion teardrop fracture. This fracture is stable because all the ligaments remain intact. However, fracture fragments may impinge on or penetrate the ventral surface of the spinal cord and cause an anterior cord syndrome.

A *Jefferson fracture* of C1 is an extremely unstable injury that occurs when a vertical compression force is transmitted through the occipital condyles to the superior articular surfaces of the lateral masses of the atlas. This force drives the lateral masses outward and thereby results in fractures of the anterior and posterior arches of the atlas and disruption of the transverse ligament. Because this injury is often associated with prevertebral hemorrhage and retropharyngeal swelling, a lateral film may demonstrate widening of the preden-

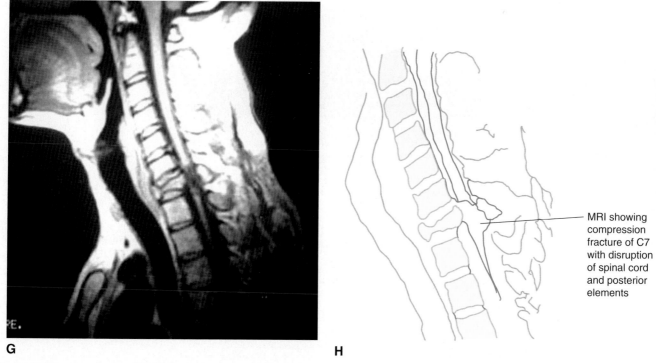

Figure 40-15.—cont'd. G and **H,** Magnetic resonance image showing a burst fracture of C7 with complete spinal cord disruption.

tal space between the anterior arch of C1 and the odontoid, or the dens. A predental space greater than 3 mm in adults and 5 mm in children is abnormal. In a frontal projection the masses of C1 lie lateral to the margins of the articular pillars of C2 (Figure 40-16). When the fragments are minimally displaced, a Jefferson fracture is difficult to recognize, and CT may be necessary.

Vertical compression fractures may rarely result in isolated fractures of the articular pillar or the vertebral body, which display vertical and oblique lines of fracture.

Classification of Spinal Cord Injuries

Primary Spinal Cord Injury
The spinal cord may be injured in a number of ways.[6] First, penetrating trauma or massive blunt trauma with disruption of the vertebral column may result in transection of the neural elements. Because neurons within the central nervous system do not regenerate, such injuries are irreversible. Less severe blunt trauma may produce similar effects from a displaced bony fragment or a herniated disk.

Second, when elderly patients with cervical osteoarthritis and spondylosis are subjected to forcible cervical spine extension, the spinal cord may be compressed between an arthritically enlarged anterior vertebral ridge and a posteriorly located hypertrophic ligamentum flavum (Figure 40-17). This injury frequently results in central cord syndrome.

Primary vascular damage to the spinal cord, a third mechanism of injury, may occur in several ways. The spinal cord may be compressed by an extradural hematoma, particularly in patients who are taking anticoagulants or have bleeding disorders. Vascular injuries should also be suspected in patients with a discrepancy between the clinically apparent neurologic deficit and the known level of spinal injury. For example, a lower cervical dislocation may compress the vertebral arteries as they travel within the spinal foramina of the vertebrae. This compression may result in thrombosis and decreased blood flow through the anterior spinal artery that originates from both vertebral arteries at the level of C1 (Figure 40-18). On physical examination, such an injury may erroneously appear to be localized to the level of C1 or C2. In addition, the great radicular artery of Adamkiewicz, which originates from the aorta and enters the spinal canal at the level of L1, sends branches as cephalad as T4. Therefore, a lumbar fracture or dislocation can produce a neurologic deficit as high as T4.

Secondary Spinal Cord Injury
The maximum neurologic deficit after blunt spinal cord trauma is often not seen immediately and may instead progress over a period of many hours. The histopathology of so-called secondary spinal cord injury has been studied extensively in experimental animal models.[7-9] It is now thought that primary spinal cord injury initiates a complex cascade of events involving free radical–induced lipid peroxidation reactions that result in progressive ischemia of gray and white matter during the postinjury period (Figure 40-19). Other factors such as hypoxia, hypotension, hyperthermia, hypoglycemia, and mishandling by medical personnel also affect the ultimate extent of spinal cord injury.

413

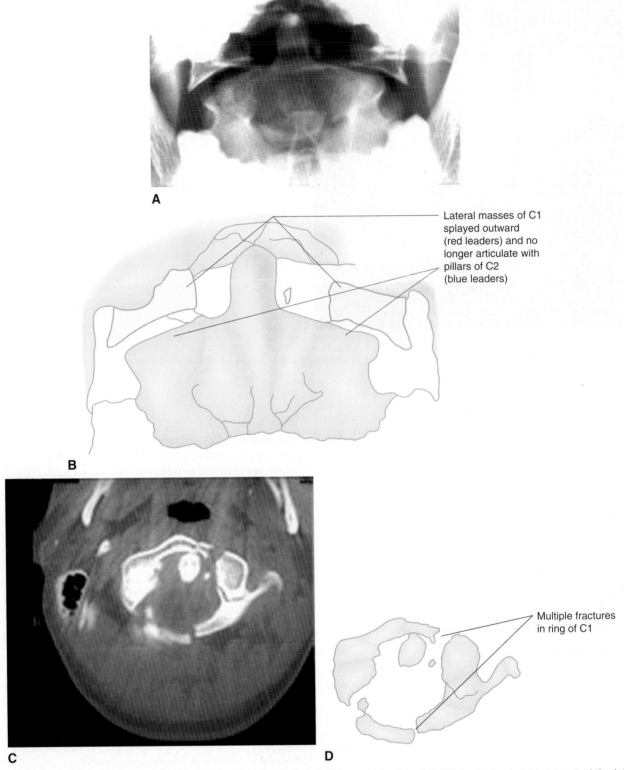

A

Lateral masses of C1
splayed outward
(red leaders) and no
longer articulate with
pillars of C2
(blue leaders)

B

C

D

Multiple fractures
in ring of C1

Figure 40-16. Jefferson fracture. Mechanism: vertical compression. Stability: unstable. **A** and **B**, Bilateral lateral displacement of the lateral masses of C1 with respect to the articular pillars of C2 confirms a Jefferson fracture and differentiates it from fracture of the posterior neural arch of C1 on an anteroposterior view. **C** and **D**, Computed tomographic scan of C1 showing two fracture sites in the ring of C1 with lateral displacement of the lateral mass on the right.

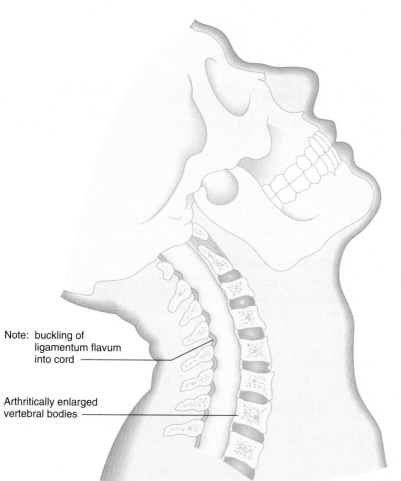

Figure 40-17. Elderly patients subjected to extension forces can sustain cervical spinal cord injury as a result of compression of the spinal cord between the posterior hypertrophic ligamentum flavum and the arthritically enlarged anterior vertebral bodies.

Note: buckling of ligamentum flavum into cord

Arthritically enlarged vertebral bodies

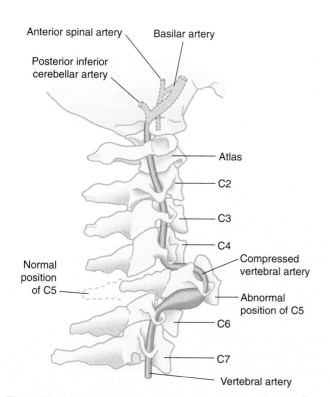

Anterior spinal artery   Basilar artery

Posterior inferior cerebellar artery

Atlas

C2

C3

C4

Normal position of C5

Compressed vertebral artery

Abnormal position of C5

C6

C7

Vertebral artery

Figure 40-18. Mechanism of vascular injury of the spinal cord resulting from cervical vertebral injury.

CLINICAL FEATURES

Neurologic Evaluation

The initial neurologic evaluation of a patient with a suspected spinal injury should begin with simple *observation*. Careful inspection of the patient's entire body, beginning with the head and proceeding downward, may reveal telltale signs of possible spinal involvement. Significant head and facial trauma is associated with a 5% to 10% incidence of cervical spine injury.[10,11] Scapular contusions suggest a rotation or flexion-rotation injury of the thoracic spine. Chest and neck abrasions from automobile shoulder belts and lower abdominal markings from lap belts indicate possible spinal, intrathoracic, and intra-abdominal injuries. As occurs with falls from considerable heights, injuries to the gluteal region, calcaneal fractures, and severe ankle fractures suggest a compression type of spinal injury.

The patient should be observed for the presence and symmetry of both voluntary and involuntary movements. An abnormal breathing pattern may provide an important clue to a cervical injury. The diaphragm is innervated by the phrenic nerve, which originates at the C3-C4 level. The intercostal muscles of the rib cage

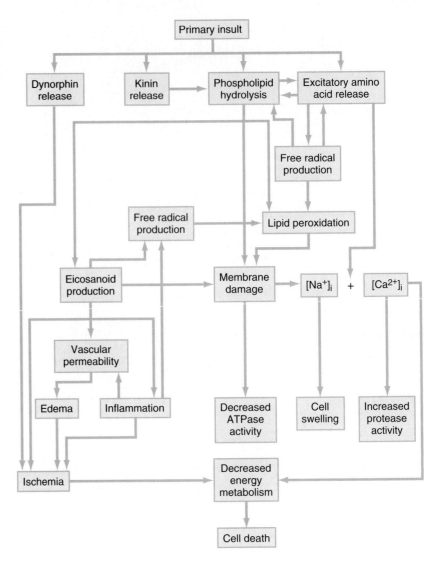

Figure 40-19. Speculative paradigm of secondary pathophysiologic events after primary traumatic injury to the spinal cord. See the text. (From Anderson D, Hall E: Pathophysiology of spinal cord trauma. *Ann Emerg Med* 22:989, 1993.)

are supplied by nerves that originate in the thoracic spine; thus, an abdominal breathing pattern indicates an injury below the C4 level. The presence of Horner's syndrome, characterized by unilateral ptosis, miosis, and anhidrosis, may result from disruption of the cervical sympathetic chain, usually at the level of C7-T2.[5] Priapism may occur with severe spinal cord injury.

The physician should *speak with the patient* during the inspection process. This important part of the patient's assessment should not be overlooked in trauma cases because it provides the patient with reassurance and the physician with valuable information. Patients may experience pain in the sensory dermatome corresponding to the level of the spinal injury. For example, a C2 lesion may cause occipital pain, whereas discomfort in the area of the trapezius muscle, particularly in the absence of signs of local trauma, suggests a C5 injury. The past medical history is important because certain conditions predispose patients to cervical injury. For example, patients with Down syndrome are predisposed to atlanto-occipital dislocation, whereas those with rheumatoid arthritis are prone to rupture of the transverse ligament of C2 with even minor trauma.

Palpation of the entire spine and paraspinal musculature may reveal areas of tenderness, deformity, or muscle spasm. A "gibbus" deformity or step-off may be appreciated with severe subluxation. Widening of an interspinous space indicates a tear in the posterior ligament complex and a potentially unstable spinal injury.

The *motor activity* of the body is complex. Because a single motion is often governed by muscles innervated by multiple spinal segments, localization of a spinal lesion based solely on assessment of motor function is extremely difficult. Testing the presence and strength of the motions outlined in Table 40-2, however, provides a rapid baseline assessment. When a deficit is noted, the motor examination and the remainder of the neurologic examination should be repeated at frequent intervals because progression of dysfunction may occur. If there is apparent total loss of function, every effort should be made to elicit the most minimal of motor responses since any response markedly alters the prognosis for recovery. A slight toe flicker in an otherwise paralyzed individual indicates that the patient may again eventually walk unassisted.

Table 40-2. Spinal Motor Examination

Level of Lesion	Resulting Loss of Function
C4	Spontaneous breathing
C5	Shrugging of shoulders
C6	Flexion at elbow
C7	Extension at elbow
C8-T1	Flexion of fingers
T1-T12	Intercostal and abdominal muscles*
L1-L2	Flexion at hip
L3	Adduction at hip
L4	Abduction at hip
L5	Dorsiflexion of foot
S1-S2	Plantar flexion of foot
S2-S4	Rectal sphincter tone

*Localization of lesions in this area is best accomplished with the sensory examination.

Table 40-3. Spinal Reflex Examination

Level of Lesion (at or above)	Resulting Loss of Reflex
C6	Biceps
C7	Triceps
L4	Patellar
S1	Achilles

Table 40-4. Spinal Sensory Examination

Level of Lesion	Resulting Level of Loss of Sensation
C2	Occiput
C3	Thyroid cartilage
C4	Suprasternal notch
C5	Below clavicle
C6	Thumb
C7	Index finger
C8	Small finger
T4	Nipple line
T10	Umbilicus
L1	Femoral pulse
L2-L3	Medial aspect of thigh
L4	Knee
L5	Lateral aspect of calf
S1	Lateral aspect of foot
S2-S4	Perianal region

The presence of cord-mediated *deep tendon reflexes* can be helpful as a localizing, diagnostic aid (Table 40-3). Classically, muscle paralysis associated with intact deep tendon reflexes indicates an upper motor neuron (spinal cord) lesion, whereas paralysis associated with absent deep tendon reflexes indicates a lower motor neuron (nerve root or cauda equina) lesion. Such differentiation is important since the latter condition is often caused by a surgically correctable lesion. However, because reflexes are typically absent during the phase of spinal shock, examination of reflexes is less useful in the emergency department.

Sensory function can be evaluated quickly by using a structured approach (Table 40-4) or by referring to a graphic representation for comparison (Figure 40-20).

After locating an area of hypoesthesia, one should carefully delineate the area by slowly moving the stimulus from areas of decreased sensation outward rather than the reverse because patients are much more sensitive to the appearance of sensation than to its disappearance. This test should be performed first with a cotton wisp to assess sensitivity to light touch, a posterior column function. A pin should then be used to assess pain sensation, which is an anterior spinothalamic tract function. The presence of islands of preserved sensation within an affected dermatome or below the level of apparent total dysfunction, even in patients with complete motor paralysis, indicates that the patient has a very good chance of functional motor recovery.[12] An accurate baseline sensory examination is imperative because cephalad progression of hypoesthesia is the most sensitive indicator of deterioration. When progression is observed in the cervical region, one should anticipate impending respiratory failure and take steps to ensure airway stabilization.

Complete Spinal Cord Lesions

A complete spinal cord lesion is defined as total loss of motor power and sensation distal to the site of a spinal cord injury. Functional motor recovery is rare in patients with a total cord syndrome that persists for longer than 24 hours after the injury.[5] Before a total cord syndrome is diagnosed, however, two points should be considered. First, any evidence of minimal cord function, such as sacral sparing, excludes the patient from this group. Signs of sacral sparing include perianal sensation, normal rectal sphincter tone, and flexor toe movement. The presence of any of these signs indicates a partial lesion, usually a central cord syndrome, and the patient may have marked functional recovery, including bowel and bladder control and eventual ambulation.

Second, it is important to note that a complete spinal cord lesion may be mimicked by a condition known as *spinal shock*. Spinal shock results from a concussive injury to the spinal cord that causes total neurologic dysfunction distal to the site of injury.[13] Spinal shock usually lasts less than 24 hours, but it may occasionally persist for several days. The end of spinal shock is heralded by return of the bulbocavernosus reflex, which is a normal cord-mediated reflex elicited by placing a gloved finger in the patient's rectum and then squeezing the glans penis or clitoris or by tugging gently on the Foley catheter. An intact reflex results in contraction of the rectal sphincter. Absence of this reflex indicates the presence of spinal shock, during which time the patient's prognosis cannot be accurately assessed. A complete spinal cord lesion will remain unchanged after the cessation of spinal shock.

Incomplete Spinal Cord Lesions

Approximately 90% of incomplete spinal injuries can be classified as one of three clinical syndromes: central cord syndrome, Brown-Séquard syndrome, and anterior cord syndrome.[5] The most common is *central cord syndrome*, which is often seen in patients with degen-

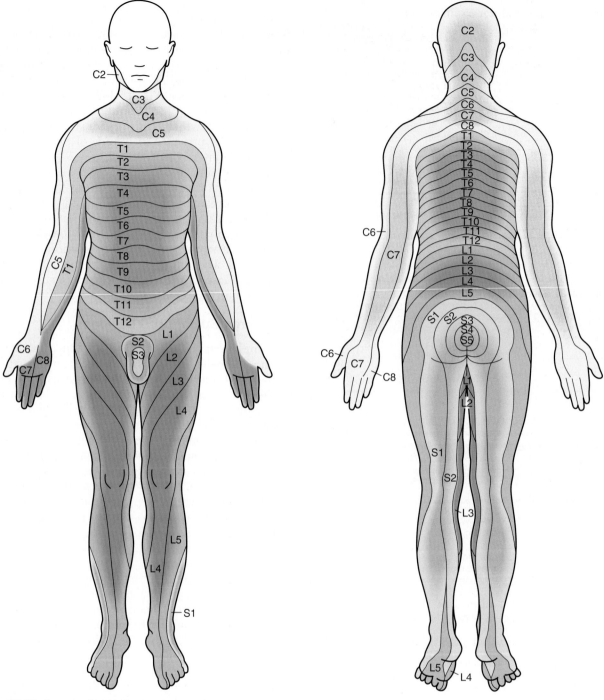

Figure 40-20. Sensory dermatomes.

erative arthritis of the cervical vertebrae when their necks are hyperextended. The ligamentum flavum buckles into the cord, and such impingement results in concussion or contusion of the central portion of the cord, which affects the central gray matter in the most central portions of the pyramidal and spinothalamic tracts (Figure 40-21). Because fibers that innervate distal structures are located in the periphery of the spinal cord, these patients have a greater neurologic deficit in the upper extremities than in the lower extremities. With more severe injuries, patients may appear to be almost completely quadriplegic and have

only minimal evidence of sacral sparing. The prognosis for patients with this syndrome is variable. More than 50% of patients with severe central cord syndrome become ambulatory and regain bowel and bladder control, as well as some hand function.[12]

The *Brown-Séquard syndrome*, or hemisection of the spinal cord, usually results from penetrating trauma but may also be seen after lateral mass fractures of the cervical spine (see Figure 40-21). Patients with this lesion have ipsilateral motor paralysis and contralateral sensory hypoesthesia distal to the level of injury; however, either finding may predominate depending

CROSS SECTION OF CERVICAL SPINAL CORD

Figure 40-21. Incomplete spinal cord syndromes.

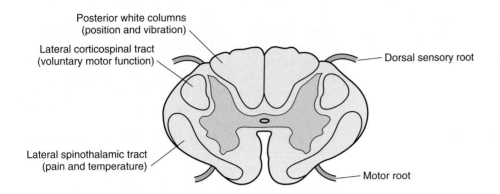

Posterior white columns
(position and vibration)

Lateral corticospinal tract
(voluntary motor function)

Dorsal sensory root

Lateral spinothalamic tract
(pain and temperature)

Motor root

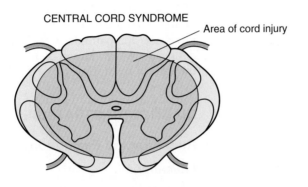

CENTRAL CORD SYNDROME

Area of cord injury

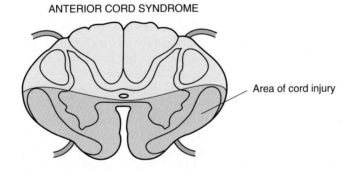

ANTERIOR CORD SYNDROME

Area of cord injury

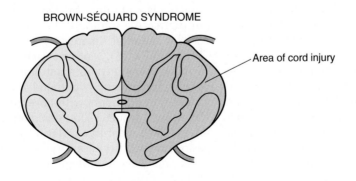

BROWN-SÉQUARD SYNDROME

Area of cord injury

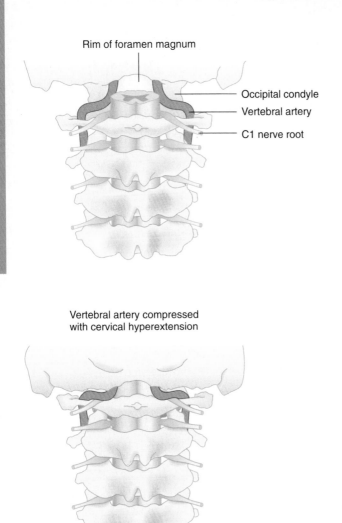

Rim of foramen magnum

Occipital condyle
Vertebral artery
C1 nerve root

Vertebral artery compressed
with cervical hyperextension

Figure 40-22. Mechanism of vertebral artery injury in extension injuries of the cervical spine.

on the exact location and extent of injury. Virtually all patients maintain bowel and bladder function and unilateral motor strength, and most become ambulatory.[5]

The *anterior cord syndrome* usually results from hyperflexion injuries causing cord contusion, by protrusion of a bony fragment or herniated disk into the spinal canal, or by laceration or thrombosis of the anterior spinal artery. This syndrome is characterized by paralysis and hypalgesia below the level of injury with preservation of posterior column functions, including position, touch, and vibratory sensations (see Figure 40-21). Suspicion of an acute anterior cord syndrome warrants immediate neurosurgical consultation because it may be due to a surgically correctable lesion. After surgical intervention, patients have variable degrees of recovery during the first 24 hours but little improvement thereafter.[5]

Several less common spinal cord syndromes may result from direct injury to the cervicomedullary junction and upper cervical segments or from vertebral artery occlusion secondary to severe hyperextension (Figure 40-22).[5] The *posteroinferior cerebellar artery syndrome* may produce dysphagia, dysphonia,

hiccups, nausea, vomiting, dizziness or vertigo, and cerebellar ataxia. The *Dejeune onion skin pattern* of analgesia of the face is caused by damage to the spinal trigeminal tract. *Horner's syndrome* results from damage to the cervical sympathetic chain and is characterized by ipsilateral ptosis, miosis, and anhidrosis. Injuries below the L2 level can result in *acute cauda equina syndrome*, which consists of perineal or bilateral leg pain, bowel or bladder dysfunction, perianal anesthesia, diminished rectal sphincter tone, and lower extremity weakness.

The syndrome of spinal cord injury without radiographic abnormality (SCIWORA) is seen primarily in younger children but may occur in any age group.[14-16] The mechanism is unclear but has been ascribed to the increased ligamentous elasticity seen in the young; such elasticity leads to transient spinal column subluxation, stretching of the spinal cord, and vascular compromise. Patients often experience a brief episode of upper extremity weakness or paresthesia followed by neurologic deficits that appear hours to days later. The prognosis for patients with SCIWORA is variable and depends on the degree of neurologic impairment and the rate of resolution.

DIAGNOSTIC STRATEGIES

Radiographic Evaluation

Indications

Clinicians have historically taken a liberal approach to ordering cervical spine radiographs in the setting of trauma because failure to recognize a spinal cord injury may result in devastating neurologic consequences. However, the incidence of acute fracture or spinal injury in trauma victims is actually less than 1%, and careful review of the literature describing occult cervical injuries reveals that most are case reports in which there was a significant mechanism of injury and patients had either midline neck tenderness, an alteration in mental status, or a painful, distracting injury.[17-26] Numerous subsequent studies have failed to reveal a spinal fracture or dislocation regardless of the mechanism of injury in alert patients without neck pain or distracting injury.[27-35]

The National Emergency X-Radiography Utilization Study (NEXUS), a prospective observational study involving 34,069 trauma patients seen at 21 U.S. emergency departments, validated a decision instrument for identifying patients with an extremely low probability of spinal injury. The decision instrument required patients to meet five criteria to be classified as having a low probability of injury: no midline cervical tenderness, no focal neurologic deficit, normal alertness, no intoxication, and no painful, distracting injury. The decision rule identified all but 8 of the 818 patients who had spinal injuries. Only two of these patients had a clinically significant injury, and only one required surgical stabilization.[34]

A similar decision rule developed in Canada has demonstrated a sensitivity of 100% and greater specificity (42.5% versus 12.9%) than the NEXUS for identifying "clinically important" cervical spine injuries.[34] The Canadian clinical decision rule consists of three questions:

1. Are there any high-risk factors that mandate radiography?
2. Are there any low-risk factors that allow safe assessment of range of motion?
3. Is the patient able to actively rotate the neck 45 degrees to the left and right?

High-risk factors include age older than 65 years, a "dangerous mechanism of injury" (a fall from a height greater than 1 m, an axial loading injury, high-speed motor vehicle crash [over 100 km/hr], rollover, ejection, motorized recreational vehicle or bicycle collision), or the presence of paresthesias. Low-risk factors include simple rear-end vehicle crashes, ability to sit up in the emergency department, ability to ambulate, delayed onset of neck pain, and the absence of midline neck tenderness. Although the NEXUS criteria are more widely used in the United States, both studies support the recommendation that cervical spine radiographs be obtained only for patients in whom spinal injury is suspected based on clinical assessment.

Radiographs should be considered in patients with a minor mechanism of injury (slip and fall injuries or low-velocity motor vehicle crashes) when patient discomfort or palpable neck tenderness is greater than one would normally expect in such instances. Patients with severe osteoporosis, advanced arthritis, and metastatic cancer may sustain spinal injuries as a result of even minor trauma.

Standard Trauma Series

The normal radiographic anatomy of the cervical spine in the AP, lateral, swimmer's, oblique, and odontoid views is presented in Figures 40-23 and 40-24. All vertebrae suspected of being injured must be visualized. Generally, such visualization is easily accomplished, although two problem areas exist. The C7 vertebra may be obscured in large, muscular, or obese patients, as well as in those with spinal lesions that have resulted in paralysis of the muscles that act to depress the shoulders. The paralysis leaves the trapezius muscles, which elevate the shoulders, unopposed. Such lesions are located in the lower cervical region, and thus patients who are most difficult to adequately evaluate radiographically may be those who need an accurate diagnosis immediately. The shoulders can usually be depressed by pulling the patient's hands toward the feet with slow, steady traction. Movement should occur only at the shoulder girdle while the head and neck remain immobilized. If this maneuver is unsuccessful or difficult to perform because of upper extremity injuries, a transaxillary or swimmer's view of the lower cervical vertebrae may be obtained. If the swimmer's view is prohibited because of a concomitant shoulder girdle injury, a CT scan should be obtained. If a CT scan is unavailable, an oblique view with the patient in the supine position can be used to assess bony integrity and alignment.[36,37] The upper three or four thoracic vertebrae are also difficult to visualize on routine lateral views of either the cervical or thoracic spine, and a swimmer's view, an oblique radiograph, or CT is often needed for adequate evaluation.

Although a cross-table lateral view of the cervical spine is the single most helpful radiograph in diagnosing spinal injures, its inadequacy as the sole view is well documented.[38] Because diagnostic yield is significantly increased when the AP and odontoid views are included, all three views of the cervical spine should be evaluated before discontinuation of cervical spine immobilization.[39] NEXUS has shown that a technically adequate three-view trauma series will fail to diagnose spinal injury in only 0.07% of patients with injuries and only 0.008% of patients with unstable injures.[40] These patients invariably have signs or symptoms that lead to further evaluation with CT, magnetic resonance imaging (MRI), or flexion-extension views. Hence, the three-view trauma series is an extremely effective modality for diagnosing cervical spine injury.

Cross-Table Lateral View

Inspection of the lateral cervical spine film should be methodical and complete in every case. To do so, it is helpful to remember the "ABCs" of interpreting a lateral film, in which A stands for alignment, B for bony abnormalities, C for cartilage space assessment, and S for soft tissues.

To check *alignment*, two imaginary lines are drawn that separately connect the anterior and posterior margins of the vertebral bodies, the anterior and posterior contour lines. A third line, the spinolaminal line, connects the bases of the spinous processes extending to the posterior aspect of the foramen magnum (Figure 40-25). All three lines should form a smooth, continuous lordotic curve, and any disruption of these lines suggests a bony or ligamentous injury. An exception to this rule is pseudosubluxation of C2 and C3, which is commonly seen in infants and children. This phenomenon is attributed to their immature muscular development and a hypermobile spine. Thus, if a high cervical injury is suspected in a child, the posterior cervical line, which connects the points bisecting the bases of the spinous processes of C1 and C3, should be used (Figure 40-26). If the base of the spinous process of C2 lies more than 2 mm anterior or posterior to the posterior cervical line, an injury at that level should be suspected. A hangman's fracture should be suspected if the base of the spinous process of C2 lies more than 2 mm behind the posterior cervical line.[41]

On the lateral view, the predental space, which is the distance between the anterior aspect of the odontoid process and the posterior aspect of the anterior ring of C1, should not exceed 3 mm in an adult or 5 mm in a child (see Figure 40-26). Widening of this space usually indicates a Jefferson fracture of C1.

Next, *bony abnormalities* should be assessed. In addition to obvious fractures, subtle changes in bone density should be noted. Areas of decreased density, seen in patients with rheumatoid arthritis, osteoporosis, or metastatic osteolytic lesions, are more apt to

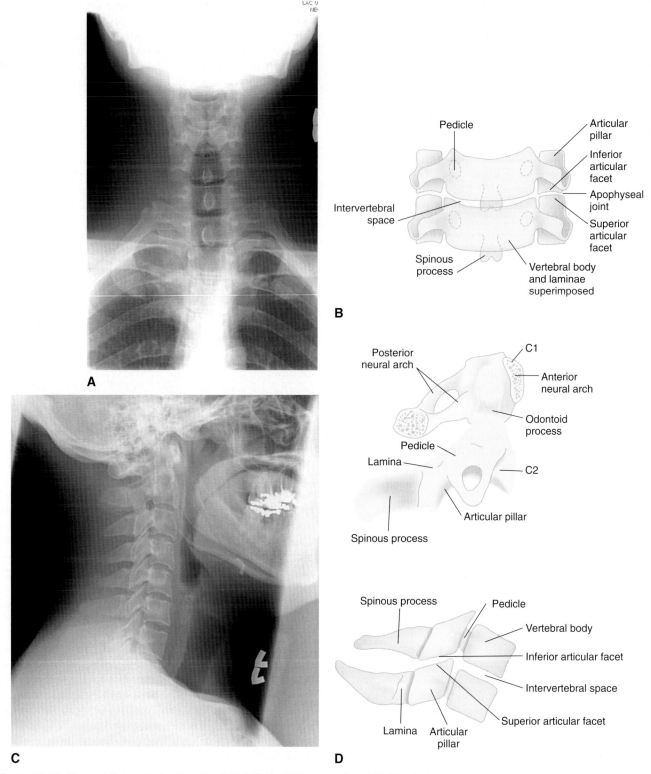

Figure 40-23. Views of the cervical spine. **A** and **B**, Anteroposterior view. **C** and **D**, lateral view.

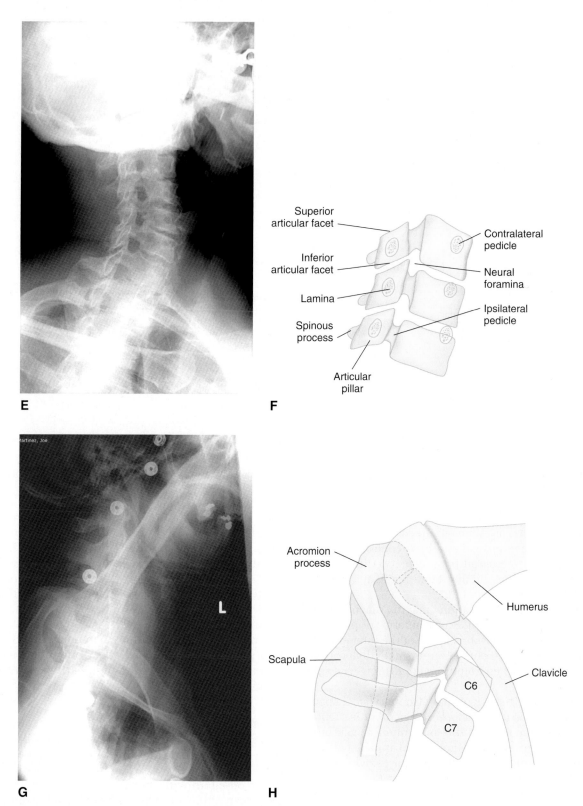

E

F

Superior
articular facet

Contralateral
pedicle

Inferior
articular facet

Neural
foramina

Lamina

Ipsilateral
pedicle

Spinous
process

Articular
pillar

G

H

L

Acromion
process

Humerus

Scapula

Clavicle

C6

C7

Figure 40-23.—cont'd. E and **F,** Oblique view. **G** and **H,** Swimmer's view.

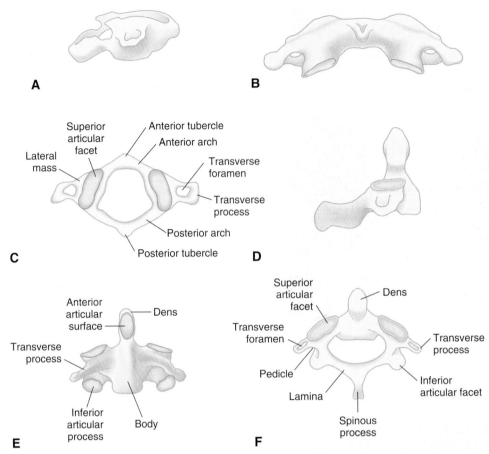

Superior
articular
facet

Anterior tubercle

Lateral
mass

Anterior arch

Transverse
foramen

Transverse
process

Posterior arch

Posterior tubercle

A **B**

C **D**

Anterior
articular
surface

Dens

Transverse
process

Inferior
articular
process

Body

Superior
articular
facet

Dens

Transverse
foramen

Transverse
process

Pedicle

Inferior
articular facet

Lamina

Spinous
process

E **F**

Figure 40-24. Views of C1 and C2. **A,** Atlas in a lateral view. **B,** Atlas in a frontal view. **C,** Atlas in an above view. **D,** Axis in a lateral view. **E,** Axis in a frontal view. **F,** axis in an above view.

succumb under stress. Acute compression fractures of the vertebral bodies and metastatic osteoblastic lesions result in areas of increased bone density. Differentiating new fractures from old may be difficult, and in such cases a CT scan may be helpful.

Subluxations and dislocations may be diagnosed by *cartilage space assessment.* Slight anterior or posterior widening of the intervertebral space or the interspinous space may be the only clue to an unstable dislocation. Oblique views are often helpful in confirming true subluxation.[36,37]

Finally, the *soft tissues* of the retropharyngeal space should be assessed for the presence of prevertebral swelling and hemorrhage; this may often be the only radiographic sign of significant spinal injury, particularly in the case of hyperextension injuries, which may reduce spontaneously immediately after the traumatic event or when the spine is placed in neutral position by paramedical personnel. The retropharyngeal space, measured from the anterior border of the body of C2 to the posterior wall of the pharynx, should not exceed 7 mm in children or adults (Figure 40-27). At the level of C3 and C4, this measurement should not exceed 5 mm or should be less than half the width of the vertebral body at that level. Below the level of C4, the prevertebral soft tissue space is widened by the esophagus and the cricopharyngeal muscle. Here, the retrotracheal space, measured from the anterior border of the body of C6 to the posterior wall of the trachea,

should not exceed 22 mm in adults and 14 mm in children younger than 15 years or should be less than the width of the vertebral body at each level (see Figure 40-27). In children younger than 2 years, the retropharyngeal space may normally appear widened during expiration, and thus inspiratory films should be obtained.[41] Air in the prevertebral space may indicate rupture of the esophagus or some portion of the respiratory tree, and anterior bulging of the prevertebral fat stripe is an excellent sign of an underlying bony or soft tissue injury.

Odontoid View

The second film obtained in the emergency department is an open-mouth or closed-mouth view of the atlas and axis (see Figure 40-24). When fracture or malalignment of the odontoid with the lateral masses of C1 is found, a CT scan of the area should be obtained. Nonfusion of the odontoid in children and congenital anomalies of the odontoid in adults may mimic fractures.

Anteroposterior View

The AP spinal film completes the spinal series. The spinous processes should form a straight line, and the laryngeal and tracheal air shadows should be midline (see Figure 40-27D). The regular outline of the lateral masses should be verified, and the pedicles viewed end-on can be checked for fracture. Widening of the

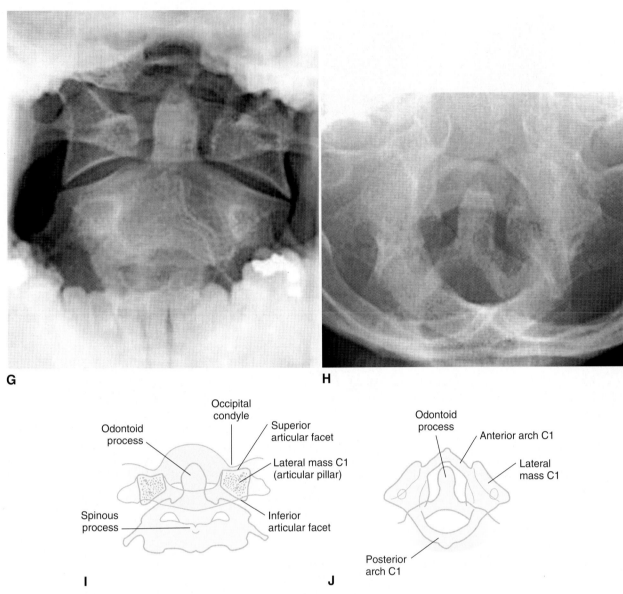

G H

Occipital
condyle
Odontoid   Superior
process   articular facet
                                              Odontoid
                                              process   Anterior arch C1
                            Lateral mass C1
                            (articular pillar)   Lateral
                                                             mass C1
Spinous   Inferior
process   articular facet
                                              Posterior
                                              arch C1

I J

Figure 40-24.—cont'd. G and **H,** Open-mouth view. **I** and **J,** Closed-mouth view.

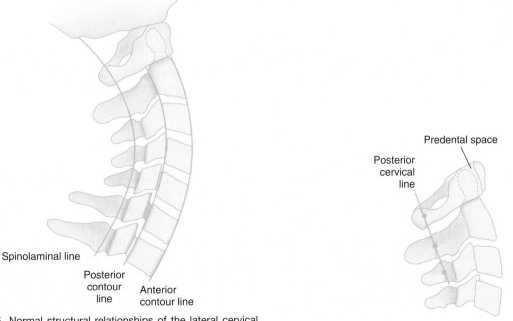

Spinolaminal line

Posterior   Anterior
contour   contour line
line

Figure 40-25. Normal structural relationships of the lateral cervical
spine.

Predental space
Posterior
cervical
line

Figure 40-26. Posterior cervical line of a normal lateral spine.

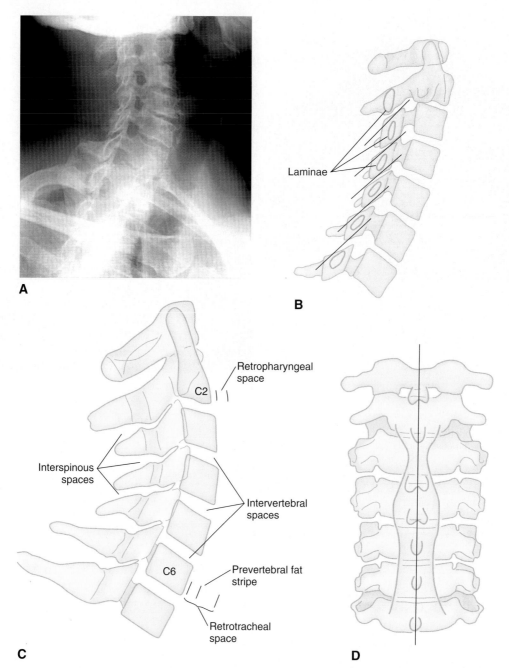

A

B

C

D

Laminae

Retropharyngeal
space

C2

Interspinous
spaces

Intervertebral
spaces

C6

Prevertebral fat
stripe

Retrotracheal
space

Figure 40-27. A and **B**, Normal structural relationships of the cervical spine laminae in an oblique view form a "shingles on a roof" appearance. **C** and **D**, Normal relationship between soft tissues and bony structures of the cervical spine in the lateral and anteroposterior (AP) views. **C**, In the lateral view, the intervertebral spaces and interspinous spaces should be compared with the spaces above and below for asymmetry and important clues in flexion and extension injuries. The retropharyngeal and retrotracheal soft tissues are measured at the C2 and C6 levels for swelling. **D**, In the AP view, the tracheal and laryngeal air shadows should be within the midline. A straight line should connect points bisecting the spinous processes. If such is not the case, rotatory injuries must be suspected.

interpedicular distance in comparison to adjacent vertebrae suggests a burst fracture (Figure 40-28).

In addition to searching for fractures of the vertebral bodies and transverse processes, bulging of the mediastinal stripe may be the only evidence of a thoracic vertebral body fracture. This sign may also be produced by an infection or neoplasm. Fractures of the upper thoracic vertebrae may cause posterior mediastinal hemorrhage of sufficient magnitude to produce mediastinal widening similar to that attributed to traumatic rupture of the aorta. In such instances, CT or angiography is essential.

Oblique Views

Oblique views of the cervical spine may be helpful in certain circumstances.[42] An oblique view may confirm a suspected posterior laminar fracture, a unilateral facet dislocation, or true subluxation. The normal lamina appears as an intact ellipse (see Figure 40-27A and B), and a posterior laminar fracture disrupts the appearance of this ellipse (Figure 40-29). If there is an associated neurologic deficit, surgical decompression is indicated.

On the oblique view, normal overlapping laminae have the appearance of shingles on a roof (see Figure

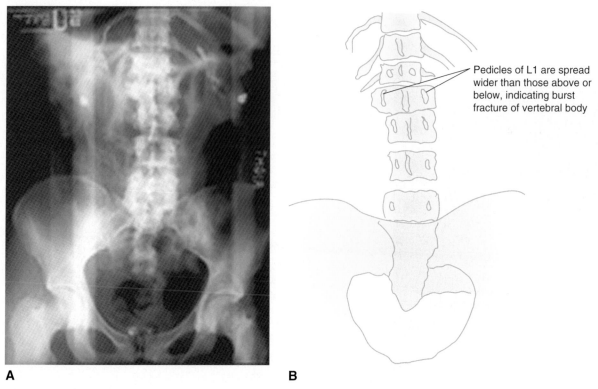

Pedicles of L1 are spread wider than those above or below, indicating burst fracture of vertebral body

A **B**

Figure 40-28. A and **B**, Burst fracture of L1. An anteroposterior radiograph shows increased distance between the pedicles of L1 in comparison to adjacent vertebrae. An intravenous pyelogram showed renal injury on the left.

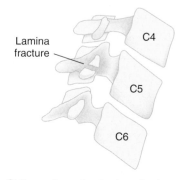

Lamina fracture

C4
C5
C6

Figure 40-29. Oblique view of a laminar fracture. A fracture line extending through the lamina of C5 is well demonstrated on an oblique view.

40-27A). Integrity of these shingles excludes the presence of a unilateral facet dislocation, whereas disruption confirms it (see Figure 40-11G). The normal interlaminar distance, measured from the center points of successive laminar ellipses on an oblique view, should be equidistant. An increased interlaminar distance, which is due to lack of capsular ligamentous integrity, indicates true subluxation (Figure 40-30).

Flexion and Extension Views

Flexion and extension views may identify true subluxation, as suggested on the lateral view but not confirmed by the oblique view. The presence of anterior or posterior subluxation greater than 2 mm on one view and not on the neutral view confirms ligamentous injury.[43] Some authorities advocate the use of flexion-extension radiographs to exclude ligamentous injury in

patients with normal mental status and normal neurologic examination who have a minor malalignment of the cervical spine on routine films or in patients with normal x-ray findings who complain of significant neck pain or spinal tenderness. However, the exact role and timing of the use of flexion-extension views are currently controversial. The NEXUS investigators demonstrated that 86 of the 818 (10.5%) patients ultimately found to have cervical injury underwent flexion-extension testing.[44] Although two patients had bony injuries and four patients had subluxations demonstrated only on flexion-extension views, all six patients had other injuries apparent on routine radiographs. Thus, flexion-extension views appear to add little information in the immediate postinjury period. Because minor subluxations may be masked by concomitant muscle spasm, delayed flexion-extension views obtained a week or two after injury when the spasm has abated may be more helpful. Moreover, other studies such as CT and MRI may be more reasonable adjunctive imaging modalities in patients with severe, localized symptoms who have normal radiographs.

Computed Tomography

Conventional radiographic examination is frequently limited as a result of the nature of equipment, difficulties in positioning, lack of patient cooperation, and the often critical status of patients with associated head, upper extremity, and chest injuries. The incidence of an inadequate lateral cervical view, specifically, visualization of C7 to T1, is reportedly as high as 25%.[45] CT effectively deals with these limitations and in many

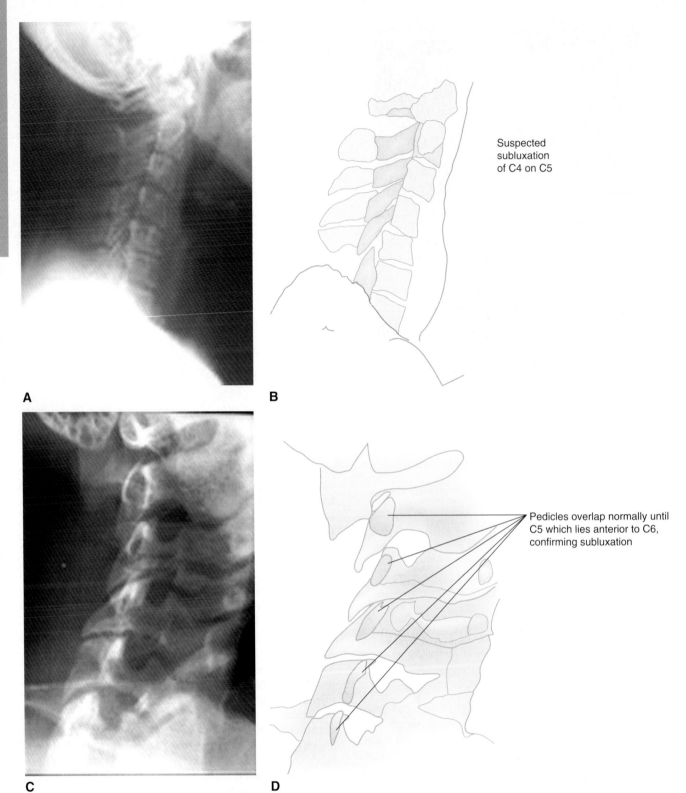

A

B

Suspected
subluxation
of C4 on C5

C

D

Pedicles overlap normally until
C5 which lies anterior to C6,
confirming subluxation

Figure 40-30. A and **B**, True subluxation, lateral view. Anterior subluxation of C5 on C6 is questionable. **C** and **D**, True subluxation, oblique view. The pedicle of C5 lies slightly anterior to that of C6, thus confirming subluxation.

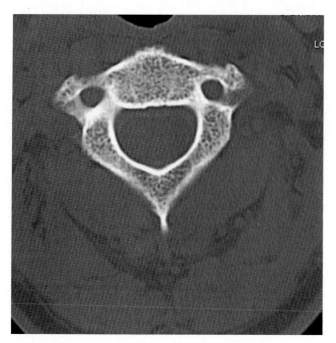

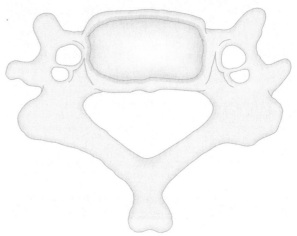

Figure 40-31. Normal axial computed tomographic section of the cervical vertebra.

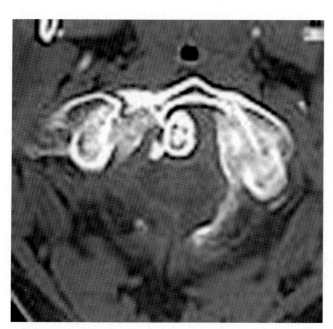

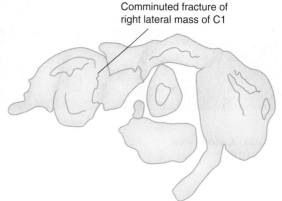

Comminuted fracture of
right lateral mass of C1

Figure 40-32. C1 fracture through the left lateral mass.

cases (Box 40-1) is the technique of choice for definitive evaluation of acute cervical spine trauma.[46-50]

Advantages of CT over plain radiography include
improved fracture detection rates, spinal canal evaluation, and paravertebral soft tissue assessment and
reduced manipulation of the patient and exposure to
radiation. The superiority of CT in detecting fractures
is a critical advantage (Figures 40-31 and 40-32), and
thus unclear fractures or displacements on standard
radiographs should be further evaluated by CT. Because

BOX 40-1. Major Indications for CT Scan in Cervical
Spine Trauma

1. Inadequate plain film survey
2. Suspicious plain film findings
3. Fracture/displacement demonstrated by standard
   radiography
4. High clinical suspicion of injury despite normal plain film
   survey

429

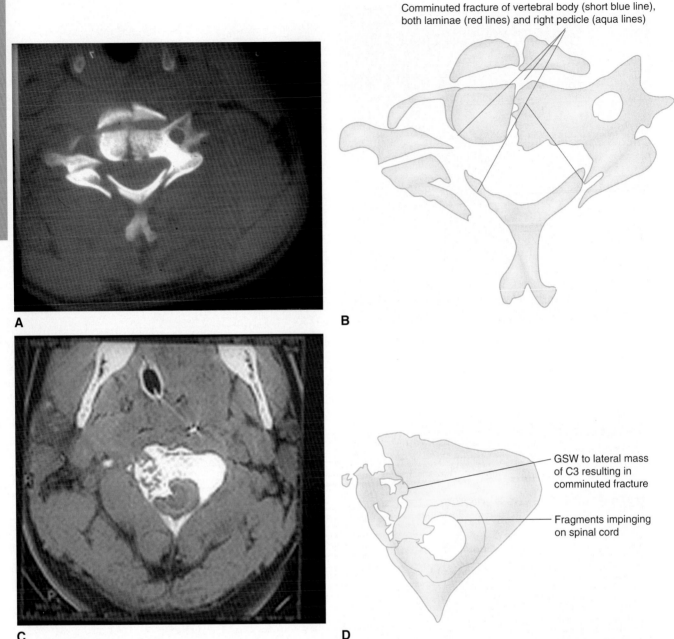

Comminuted fracture of vertebral body (short blue line), both laminae (red lines) and right pedicle (aqua lines)

GSW to lateral mass of C3 resulting in comminuted fracture

Fragments impinging on spinal cord

A **B** **C** **D**

Figure 40-33. **A** and **B**, Axial computed tomography of C5 showing a comminuted vertebral body fracture and bilateral lamina fractures with narrowing of the spinal canal. **C** and **D**, Gunshot wound of the lateral mass with fragments impinging on the spinal cord.

fractures in contiguous vertebrae are fairly common, the area to be scanned should include the vertebrae immediately above and below the level of suspected injury. CT can also identify bony fragments, acute disk herniation, a foreign body, or an extramedullary hematoma that may impinge on the spinal cord or neural foramina (Figure 40-33). Finally, in addition to limiting radiation exposure, CT can assess paravertebral soft tissues and delineate the presence of a paraspinal hematoma; it also permits examination without moving the patient from the supine position and is thus preferable in terms of fracture stabilization, airway control, and other life support measures.

Disadvantages of CT include limited demonstration of vertebral body displacement or subluxation in the sagittal plane and poor visualization of horizontally oriented fractures. These problems have primarily been overcome with the advent of the latest-generation spiral (helical) CT scan, which provides for continuous acquisition of data (volume scan) via a rotating x-ray tube and simultaneous patient movement through the CT gantry (Figure 40-34). Its chief advantage is its ability to reconstruct axial CT data in two-dimensional and three-dimensional formats, which is helpful to nonradiologists who are less accustomed to performing the mental integration of multiplanar images (Figure 40-

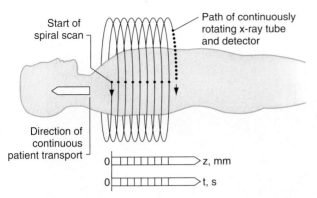

Figure 40-34. Technique for performing a spiral computed tomographic scan.

35). A spiral CT scan can also demonstrate cervical spine injuries not apparent on plain film or axial CT images (Figure 40-36).

Magnetic Resonance Imaging

MRI, with its superior resolution and definition of the spinal canal, multiplanar capabilities, and lack of ionizing radiation, has become the optimal imaging modality for the evaluation of spinal disease. In fact, MRI has become the study of choice for detecting neurologic injury secondary to trauma, even surpassing myelography and postmyelography CT scanning.[51-57]

The primary advantage of MRI is its ability to directly image nonosseous structures, including intramedullary

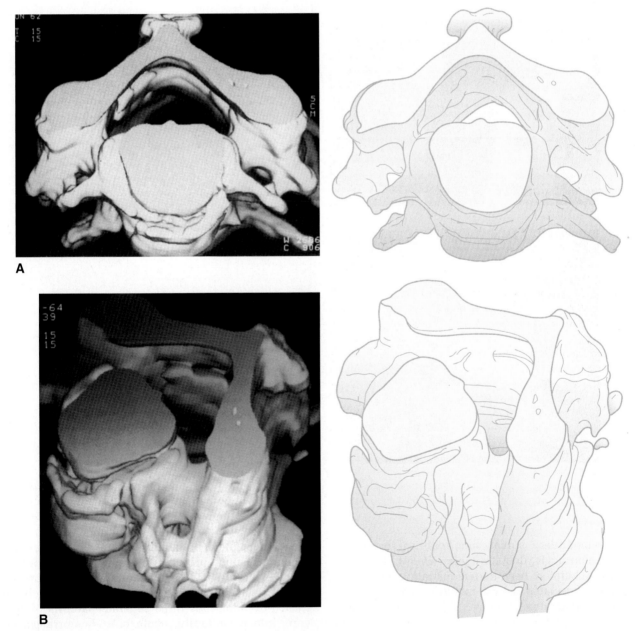

A

B

Figure 40-35. Three-dimensional computed tomography images of the cervical vertebrae. **A,** Superior view. **B,** Oblique view.

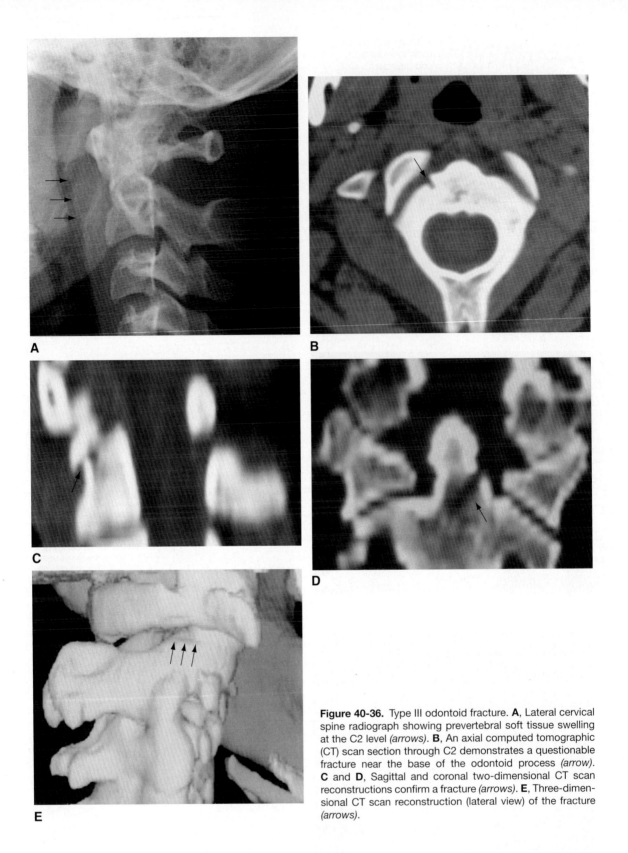

Figure 40-36. Type III odontoid fracture. **A,** Lateral cervical spine radiograph showing prevertebral soft tissue swelling at the C2 level *(arrows)*. **B,** An axial computed tomographic (CT) scan section through C2 demonstrates a questionable fracture near the base of the odontoid process *(arrow)*. **C** and **D,** Sagittal and coronal two-dimensional CT scan reconstructions confirm a fracture *(arrows)*. **E,** Three-dimensional CT scan reconstruction (lateral view) of the fracture *(arrows)*.

and extramedullary spinal abnormalities that could cause a neurologic deficit (Figure 40-37). Its major impact has therefore been in demonstrating potentially surgically correctable lesions, including acute disk herniation, ligamentous injury, bony compression, epidural and subdural hemorrhage, and vertebral artery occlusion (Figure 40-38).

Although plain films and CT can demonstrate bone fragments, blood, disks, and foreign bodies impinging on the spinal cord, the diagnosis of cord injury with these modalities is based on indirect criteria. In contrast, MRI identifies three separate patterns of spinal cord injury, including acute cord hemorrhage, cord edema or contusion, and mixed cord injury. Patients

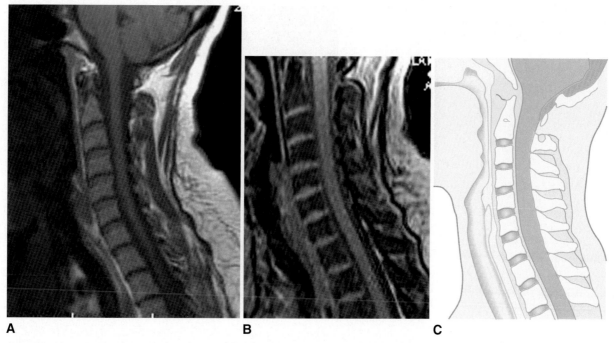

Figure 40-37. Normal sagittal magnetic resonance images of the cervical spine: T1-weighted (**A**) and flip-angle (**B**) scans. **C**, Illustration of the cervical spine.

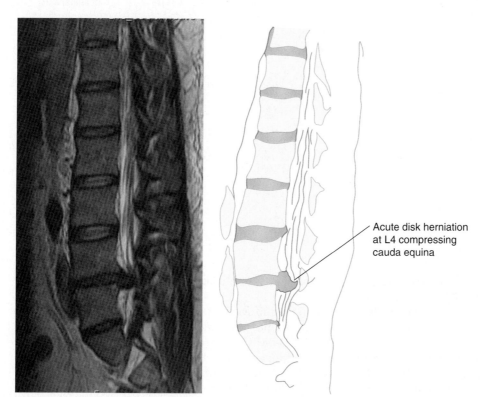

Acute disk herniation
at L4 compressing
cauda equina

Figure 40-38. Magnetic resonance image showing acute L4 disk herniation with compression of the cauda equina.

Figure 40-39. Magnetic resonance image showing a small area of central cord hemorrhage and both anterior and posterior ligamentous disruption.

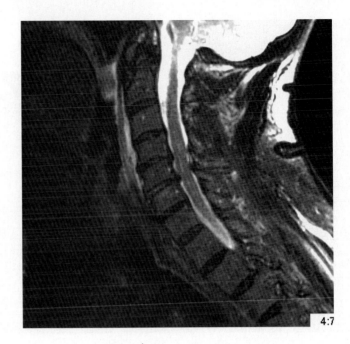

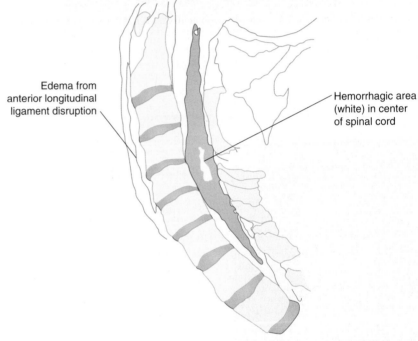

Edema from anterior longitudinal ligament disruption

Hemorrhagic area (white) in center of spinal cord

with cord edema or contusion show significant neurologic improvement, whereas those with cord hemorrhage (Figure 40-39) fare far worse. MRI therefore has diagnostic and prognostic capabilities in the evaluation of cervical spine injury.

Contraindications to the use of MRI include the presence of a pacemaker, cerebral aneurysm clips (MRI-compatible clips are now available), and metallic (ferromagnetic) foreign bodies. In addition, MRI cannot be performed when MRI-incompatible life support equipment, monitoring systems, and cervical traction devices are being used (some MRI-compatible support systems have been developed). Finally, plain films and CT are still superior to MRI in evaluating osseous

anatomy and fractures, particularly posterior element fractures.

The role of MRI in the evaluation of acute cervical spine trauma continues to evolve, and some advocate immediate MRI in patients with clinical signs or plain film evidence suggesting ligamentous injury (Figure 40-40).[57] Patients with a strong clinical suggestion of spine injury who have normal plain radiographs, including those with persistent neck pain or neurologic deficit, should undergo MRI evaluation to exclude occult injuries. MRI is also useful in the evaluation of a previously traumatized spinal cord.[56] Progressive neurologic dysfunction in a patient with a previously stable cord injury may indicate undiagnosed disk or

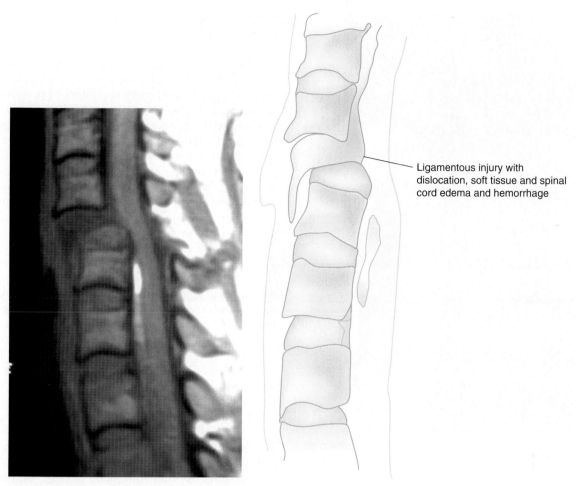

Ligamentous injury with dislocation, soft tissue and spinal cord edema and hemorrhage

Figure 40-40. Anteroposterior longitudinal ligament disruption. A sagittal magnetic resonance image demonstrates ligamentous disruption between C4 and C5 with blood tracking in the anterior spinal canal.

bone impingement on the spinal cord, myelomalacia, a developing intramedullary (posttraumatic) syrinx, or subarachnoid cystic changes (Figure 40-41). These entities can be diagnosed by MRI and, with the exception of myelomalacia, are potentially operable conditions.

MANAGEMENT

A spinal injury should be suspected in all trauma victims with an unknown or suggestive mechanism of injury associated with complaints of neck or back pain, evidence of significant head or facial trauma, spinal tenderness, signs of focal neurologic deficit, impaired consciousness, potentially distracting injuries, or unexplained hypotension. All patients suspected of having a significant spinal injury should be approached in a manner similar to that outlined in Figure 40-42.

Spinal Column Stabilization

Prehospital Care

Paramedical personnel should suspect a spinal injury in any victim of trauma, especially injuries caused by

motor vehicle accidents, assaults, falls, and sports. Because of drug or alcohol intoxication, head trauma, or shock, trauma victims may have an altered state of consciousness that makes cooperation difficult and spinal movement likely, unless steps are taken to immobilize the potentially traumatized spine.

Spinal immobilization should be initiated at the scene and maintained until a spinal injury is excluded in the emergency department. A variety of effective spinal immobilization orthoses are commercially available. The most widely implemented and perhaps the most effective approach involves the use of a combination of a spinal backboard, a rigid cervical collar, and supportive blocks placed on either side of the head and held in place by straps or tape stretched across the patient's forehead.[58-63] Children younger than 8 years have heads that are somewhat large in proportion to their bodies, which results in mild neck flexion when they are placed on a flat backboard. Such flexion can be avoided by using a special backboard with an occipital recess or by placing a rolled sheet under the upper part of the child's back to mildly elevate the thorax.[62] Further prehospital care should be directed at evaluation and stabilization of associated injuries or problems requiring immediate intervention.

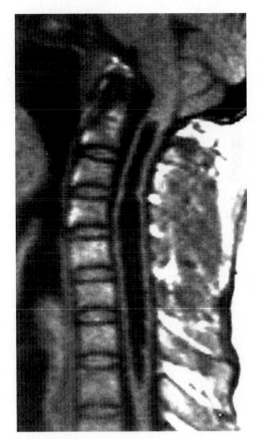

Figure 40-41. Magnetic resonance image showing posttraumatic syrinx of the spinal cord.

Emergency Department

Trauma victims who arrive at the emergency department with their spine immobilized should be quickly assessed by a physician. If the probability of spinal injury is moderate to high, it is advisable to remove the patient's clothes, evaluate any associated injuries, and perform resuscitative maneuvers without removing the immobilization apparatus. When the probability of injury is low, the immobilization device may be removed and the patient carefully assessed before additional tests are ordered.

Patients with probable spinal injury who are conscious and cooperative should be cautioned against attempted movement until radiographic studies have been performed. Patients who are uncooperative because of head injury, drug or alcohol intoxication, hypotension, or the presence of multiple painful injuries require a more aggressive approach. Suspected thoracic and lumbar spinal injuries are best managed by simply keeping the patient supine and immobile. The goal of stabilization in cases of cervical spine trauma is immobilization of both the neck and body because any movement may extend the initial injury. If the patient is not already immobilized on a backboard, the torso should be firmly anchored to the examining table by straps or rolled sheets. Supportive blocks or sandbags can be placed on either side of the head and a piece of 3-inch tape then placed across the forehead and blocks to immobilize the head and neck. A combative patient may require an individual assigned to hold the patient's head in alignment with the longitudinal axis of the body. Sedation, drug-induced paralysis, and intubation may be necessary in patients who pose a danger to themselves because of excessive movement. Spinal precautions should be maintained in patients with an altered sensorium until the presence of an injury can be excluded clinically or radiographically. Suctioning should be immediately available to prevent aspiration, and emergency department personnel must be aware of this ever-present possibility. When vomiting occurs, patients should be immediately placed on their side while maintaining spinal alignment and suctioning then performed.

Airway Management

Airway management problems should be anticipated in patients with cervical spinal injuries. Lesions above the level of C3 may cause immediate respiratory paralysis, and lower lesions that are ascending from the spread of edema may cause delayed phrenic nerve paralysis. Cervical injuries may also be associated with airway obstruction from retropharyngeal hemorrhage or edema or from maxillofacial trauma. In addition to head or chest injuries requiring airway control or respiratory support, acute pulmonary edema has also occurred after cervical spine injuries unassociated with significant head injury.[64]

According to the American College of Surgeons' advanced trauma life support guidelines, the preferred method of airway management for patients with traumatic cardiopulmonary arrest, even with evidence of spinal injury, is rapid sequence intubation with in-line spinal immobilization.[64] Performance of in-line spinal immobilization should not involve axial traction on the head or neck because of the potential for distraction and subluxation of unstable cervical spine injuries.[65] This is also the best approach for patients who are breathing but unconscious and in need of airway control or ventilatory support.[66-72] Cricothyrotomy should be considered in patients with severe maxillofacial injuries and when rapid sequence intubation is contraindicated or if attempts at orotracheal intubation fail.

Because a normal cross-table lateral cervical x-ray examination does not exclude the presence of an unstable bony or ligamentous injury, establishment of a definitive airway should not be delayed to obtain this film if immediate airway management is required.

Spinal Shock

Spinal shock is a clinical syndrome characterized by the loss of neurologic function and autonomic tone below the level of a spinal cord lesion. Patients usually exhibit flaccid paralysis with loss of sensation, deep tendon reflexes, and urinary bladder incontinence, along with bradycardia, hypotension, hypothermia, and intestinal ileus. Though generally lasting less than

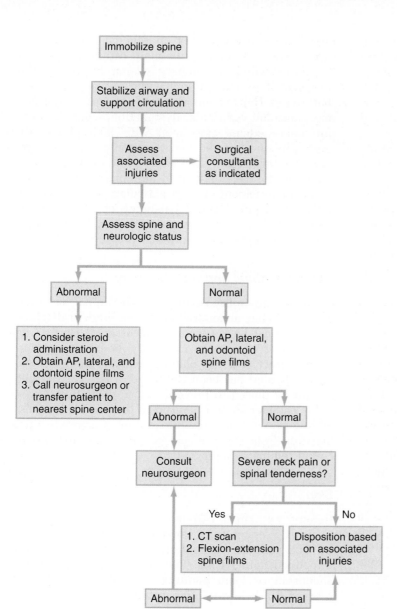

Figure 40-42. Approach to a patient with suspected cervical spine injury.

CHAPTER 40 Spinal Injuries

Immobilize spine

Stabilize airway and support circulation

Assess associated injuries → Surgical consultants as indicated

Assess spine and neurologic status

Abnormal

Normal

1. Consider steroid administration
2. Obtain AP, lateral, and odontoid spine films
3. Call neurosurgeon or transfer patient to nearest spine center

Obtain AP, lateral, and odontoid spine films

Abnormal

Normal

Consult neurosurgeon

Severe neck pain or spinal tenderness?

Yes

No

1. CT scan
2. Flexion-extension spine films

Disposition based on associated injuries

Abnormal

Normal

24 hours, spinal shock may occasionally persist for several days.[13]

Neurogenic hypotension secondary to spinal shock as a result of loss of vasomotor tone and lack of reflex tachycardia from disruption of autonomic ganglia should always be a diagnosis of exclusion in a trauma victim. It should not be considered the cause of hypotension unless the patient is flaccid and areflexic; reflex tachycardia and peripheral vasoconstriction are absent; and most importantly, the possibilities of coexisting hemorrhagic shock, cardiac tamponade, and tension pneumothorax have been eliminated. The absence of vasomotor activity in patients experiencing neurogenic hypotension can mask the usual signs and symptoms of these life-threatening injuries.

Although no consensus in the literature has been reached regarding the most appropriate treatment of neurogenic hypotension, it is prudent to begin resuscitation of all newly arrived, hypotensive trauma victims with crystalloid fluid infusion. Most cases of pure

neurogenic hypotension are mild and will initially respond to this approach. Severe neurogenic hypotension, seen in 20% to 30% of all spinal injuries, occurs most commonly with high cervical injuries associated with total or near-total loss of neurologic function.[13] Fluid resuscitation is often ineffective in such patients and may result in fluid overload if aggressively pursued. As a result, symptomatic neurogenic hypotension should be managed with fluids and vasopressors, based on hemodynamic monitoring, once the diagnosis is established and the coexistence of other causes of traumatic shock is excluded.

Pharmacologic Therapy for Incomplete Cord Injury

The beneficial effects of a number of pharmacologic agents found to improve neurologic outcome in experimentally induced spinal cord injury have been attributed largely to their antioxidant effects.[73,74] Such agents include glucocorticoids, naloxone, thyrotropin-releasing hormone, insulin-like growth factor, dimethyl sulfoxide, calcium channel blockers, tirilazad mesylate, GM_1 ganglioside, and hyperbaric oxygen therapy.[75-82] Of these, only methylprednisolone is currently used routinely for human victims of spinal cord injury, and its use is highly controversial.

The National Acute Spinal Cord Injury Study (NASCIS) group has published several studies showing that early administration of high-dose methylprednisolone improves the neurologic outcome of spinal cord injury victims.[78-81] Methylprednisolone is administered as an initial 30-mg/kg intravenous bolus, followed by an infusion of 5.4 mg/kg/hr. The infusion is maintained for 24 hours in patients who are treated within 3 hours of injury and for 48 hours in patients who are treated within 3 to 8 hours after injury. The administration of steroids resulted in a worse outcome when started after 8 hours.

The NASCIS reports have been criticized for having methodologic flaws and for failing to assess whether the mild neurologic improvement seen in patients treated with methylprednisolone actually resulted in an improvement in day-to-day functioning.[83,84] Moreover, other studies have reported that patients treated with methylprednisolone have a higher rate of respiratory and gastrointestinal complications than placebo-treated patients do.[85] Recent guidelines published jointly by the American Association of Neurological Surgeons and the Congress of Neurological Surgeons state that "treatment with methylprednisolone for either 24 to 48 hours is recommended as an option in the treatment of patients with acute spinal cord injuries only with the knowledge that the evidence suggesting harmful side effects is more consistent than any suggestion of clinical benefit."[86] However, based on an analysis of all randomized trials of steroids for acute spinal cord injury, the Cochrane Database Systematic Review concludes that "high dose methylprednisolone steroid therapy is the only pharmacological therapy shown to have efficacy in a Phase Three randomized trial when it can be administered within 8 hours of injury . . . and that there may be additional benefit by extending the maintenance dose from 24 to 48 hours if treatment is not started until between 3 and 8 hours after injury."[87] Given this conflicting evidence, additional randomized trials will be needed to clarify the role of steroids and other pharmacologic therapies in acute spinal cord injury.

Associated Injuries

Cardiopulmonary

Although deterioration in a trauma victim's cardiopulmonary status is usually the result of hemorrhagic shock or direct injury to the heart or lungs, it may reflect the development of pulmonary edema that occasionally occurs in response to brain or spinal cord injury.[88] Spinal cord trauma may stimulate an intense sympathetic discharge with two subsequent effects.

First, pulmonary capillary endothelial cells are disrupted, which leads to pulmonary capillary leak syndrome in which pulmonary edema occurs in the presence of normal pulmonary artery pressure (less than 18 mm Hg). Second, marked increases in afterload may cause left ventricular dysfunction, which leads to pulmonary edema associated with high pulmonary artery pressure (greater than 18 mm Hg). Volume overload from aggressive fluid resuscitation can also contribute to the development of pulmonary edema. As a result, management of such patients is often complex and may require careful balancing of fluid requirements, afterload-reducing agents, and artificial ventilation with positive end-expiratory pressure.[88]

Gastrointestinal and Genitourinary

If spinal cord injury renders the abdominal examination unreliable, abdominal CT, ultrasound, or diagnostic peritoneal lavage is often necessary.[89] During the acute stages of spinal cord injury, both the gastrointestinal tract and the bladder become atonic. Thus, once a patient has been stabilized, a nasogastric tube should be placed to prevent gastric distention, and a Foley catheter should be used to prevent bladder distention and to monitor fluid output. Gastrointestinal bleeding from stress ulcers occurs in 2% to 20% of spinal trauma patients.[90]

Skin

Denervated skin is extremely susceptible to pressure necrosis. Pressure sores can develop in less than 1 hour in such patients, particularly if they are managed on unpadded spinal carts. Padding pressure areas with sheepskin or foam padding early in the course of therapy can help minimize decubitus ulcers.

Definitive Treatment and Prognosis

The role of immediate surgical intervention in the management of spinal injuries is currently limited to relieving impingement on the spinal cord caused by foreign bodies, herniated disks, bony fracture fragments, or an epidural hematoma.[91,92] Surgery may later be necessary to stabilize severe bony injuries or to reduce spinal dislocations.

Major spinal injuries were once almost uniformly fatal. Most patients died of pulmonary complications or sepsis from skin necrosis or urinary infection. The advent of antibiotic therapy has made long-term survival not only possible but expected. Today, patients with spinal cord injury are best managed by early referral to a regional spine injury center where a team of neurosurgeons, orthopedic surgeons, psychologists, and physical therapists can initiate rehabilitation. Specialized spinal cord injury treatment centers offer patients a chance to return to a productive life within the limits of their disability. Experience has shown that with the exception of patients with high cervical lesions (above C5), most patients attain sufficient independence to live outside a high-level care environment.[93]

DISPOSITION

Minor Ligamentous Injuries

Musculoskeletal injuries of the spine involving only mild to moderate discomfort and no neurologic impairment, no abnormal radiographic findings, and no other injuries requiring hospitalization are best managed on an outpatient basis. Treatment should include analgesics and referral for follow-up evaluation.

Minor Fractures

Most patients with spinal fractures require hospitalization. Patients with isolated cervical vertebral body compression fractures or spinous process fractures may be managed on an outpatient basis if the mechanism of injury is not significant, there is no evidence of neurologic impairment or associated ligamentous instability, and the degree of patient distress is not severe. Appropriate follow-up care should be arranged in all instances because even minor spinal injuries may be associated with prolonged disability as a result of chronic pain.[94-96]

Wedge fractures of the thoracic and lumbar spine are usually best managed in the hospital for several reasons.[97,98] First, patients with these injuries generally have marked discomfort, often requiring parenteral narcotics. Second, significant force is typically required to fracture thoracic or lumbar vertebrae, and associated intrathoracic or abdominal injuries should be considered. Finally, lower thoracic and lumbar fractures are frequently associated with prolonged and occasionally delayed gastrointestinal ileus requiring continuous nasogastric suction.

KEY CONCEPTS

- Victims of motor vehicle crashes, falls from heights, and sports-related injuries should have their entire spines examined for evidence of injury. Spinal radiographs should be obtained in the presence of suggestive signs or when abnormal mental status or distracting injuries hamper clinical assessment.

- To prevent inadvertent movement of the spinal column, spinal precautions should be maintained in patients with altered mentation until the presence of a spinal injury can be excluded either clinically or radiographically.

- Until further randomized clinical trials are performed, the use of high-dose steroids for acute spinal cord trauma will remain controversial. Thus, decisions regarding the use of steroids should be made in conjunction with neurosurgical consultants. Steroids should not be given if they cannot be initiated within 8 hours of injury.

REFERENCES

1. Spinal Cord Information Network: Spinal cord injury: Facts and figures at a glance. Available at www.spinalcord.uab.edu, accessed July 15, 2003.
2. Berkowitz M: Assessing the socioeconomic impact of improved treatment of head and spinal cord injuries. J Emerg Med 11:63, 1993.
3. Snell RS, Smith MS (eds): Clinical Anatomy for Emergency Medicine. St Louis, CV Mosby, 1993.
4. Harris JH, Harris WH (eds): The Radiology of Emergency Medicine, 4th ed. Philadelphia, Lippincott Williams & Wilkins, 2000.
5. Maroon JC, Abla AA: Classification of acute spinal cord injury, neurological evaluation and neurosurgical considerations. Crit Care Med 3:655, 1987.
6. Guthkelch AN, Fleischer AS: Patterns of cervical spine injury and their associated lesions. West J Med 147:428, 1987.
7. Meyer PR, et al: Spinal cord injury. Neurol Clin 9:3, 1991.
8. Anderson DK, Hall ED: Pathophysiology of spinal cord trauma. Ann Emerg Med 22:987, 1993.
9. Young W: Secondary injury mechanisms in acute spinal cord injury. J Emerg Med 11:13, 1993.
10. Sinclair D, et al: A retrospective review of the relationship between facial fractures, head injuries and cervical spine injuries. J Emerg Med 6:109, 1988.
11. Tator CH: Management of associated spine injures in head injured patients. In Narayan RK, Wilberger JE, Poulishock JT (eds): Neurotrauma. New York, McGraw-Hill, 1996.
12. Merriam WF, Taylor TK, Ruff SJ, McPhail MJ: A reappraisal of acute traumatic central cord syndrome. J Bone Joint Surg Br 68:708, 1986.
13. Atkinson PP, Atkinson LD: Spinal shock. Mayo Clin Proc 71:384, 1996.
14. Pang D, Pollack IF: Spinal cord injury without radiographic abnormality in children—the SCIWORA syndrome. Trauma 29:658, 1989.
15. Kokoska ER, et al: Characteristics of pediatric cervical spine injuries. J Pediatr Surg 36:10, 2001.
16. Apuzzo ML: Spinal cord injury without radiographic abnormality. Neurosurgery 50(3):S100, 2002.
17. Dilberti T, Lindsey RW: Evaluation of the cervical spine in the emergency setting: Who does not need an x-ray? Orthopedics 15:179, 1992.
18. Marx JA, Biros MH: Who is at low risk after head and neck trauma? N Engl J Med 343:138, 2000.
19. Thambyrajah K: Fractures of the cervical spine with minimal or no symptoms. Med J Malaya 26:244, 1972.
20. Maull KI, Sachatello CR: Avoiding a pitfall in resuscitation: The painless cervical fracture. South Med J 70:477, 1977.
21. Panacek E, et al: Test performance of the individual NEXUS low-risk clinical screening criteria for cervical spine injury. Ann Emerg Med 38:22, 2001.
22. Webb JK, et al: Hidden flexion injury of the cervical spine. J Bone Joint Surg Br 58:322, 1976.
23. Bresler MJ, Rich GH: Occult cervical spine fracture in an ambulatory patient. Ann Emerg Med 11:440, 1982.
24. Haines JD: Occult cervical spine fractures. Postgrad Med 80:73, 1986.
25. Reid DC, et al: Etiology and clinical course of missed spine fractures. J Trauma 27:980, 1987.
26. Austin P, Hanlon D: Unrecognized pathologic fractures of the cervical spine: Two case reports and review of the literature. J Emerg Med 11:409, 1993.
27. Gbaanador GB, Fruin AH, Taylon C: Role of routine emergency cervical radiography in head trauma. Am J Surg 152:643, 1986.

28. Neifeld GL, et al: Cervical injury in head trauma. *J Emerg Med* 6:203, 1988.

29. Cadoux CG, White JD, Hedberg MC: High-yield roentgenographic criteria for cervical spine injuries. *Ann Emerg Med* 16:738, 1987.

30. Roberge RJ: Selective application of cervical spine radiography in alert victims of blunt trauma: A prospective study. *J Trauma* 28:784, 1988.

31. Ringenberg BJ, et al: Rational ordering of cervical spine radiographs following trauma. *Ann Emerg Med* 17:792, 1988.

32. McNamara RM, et al: Cervical spine injury and radiography in alert, high-risk patients. *J Emerg Med* 8:177, 1990.

33. Roth BJ, et al: Roentgenographic evaluation of the cervical spine—a selective approach. *Arch Surg* 129:643, 1994.

34. Hoffman JR, et al: Validity of a set of clinical criteria to rule out injury to the cervical spine in patients with blunt trauma. *N Engl J Med* 343:94, 2000.

35. Stiell IG, et al: The Canadian C-spine rule for radiography in alert and stable trauma patients. *JAMA* 286:1841, 2001.

36. Juretsky DB, et al: Technique and use of supine oblique views in acute cervical spine trauma. *Ann Emerg Med* 22:685, 1993.

37. Mann FA, et al: Supine oblique views of the cervical spine: A poor proxy for the lateral view. *Emerg Radiol* 2:214, 1995.

38. West OC, et al: Acute cervical spine trauma: Diagnostic performance of single-view versus three-view radiographic screening. *Radiology* 204:819, 1997.

39. Petri R, Gimbel R: Evaluation of the patient with spinal trauma and back pain: An evidence based approach. *Emerg Med Clin North Am* 17:25, 1999.

40. Mower WR, et al: Use of plain radiographs to screen for cervical spine injuries. *Ann Emerg Med* 38:1, 2001.

41. Fesmire FM, Luten RC: The pediatric cervical spine: Developmental anatomy and clinical aspects. *J Emerg Med* 7:133, 1989.

42. Doris PE, Wilson RA: The next logical step in the evaluation of cervical spine trauma: The five-view trauma series. *J Emerg Med* 3:371, 1985.

43. Knopp R, et al: Defining radiographic criteria for flexion-extension studies of the cervical spine. *Ann Emerg Med* 38:31, 2001.

44. Pollack C, et al: Use of flexion-extension radiographs of the cervical spine in blunt trauma. *Ann Emerg Med* 38:8, 2001.

45. Murphy MD, et al: Diagnostic imaging of spinal trauma. *Radiol Clin North Am* 27:855, 1989.

46. Domenicucci M, et al: Three-dimensional computed tomographic imaging in the diagnosis of vertebral column trauma: Experience based on 21 patients and review of the literature. *J Trauma* 42:254, 1997.

47. Acheson MB, et al: High-resolution CT scanning in the evaluation of cervical spine fractures: Comparison with plain film examinations. *Am J Radiol* 148:1179, 1987.

48. Schleehauf K, et al: Computed tomography in the initial evaluation of the cervical spine. *Ann Emerg Med* 18:815, 1989.

49. El-Khoury GY, Kathol MH, Daniel WW: Imaging of acute injuries of the cervical spine: Value of plain radiography, CT and MR imaging. *AJR Am J Roentgenol* 164:43, 1995.

50. Ross SE, et al: Clearing the cervical spine: Initial radiologic evaluation. *J Trauma* 27:1055, 1987.

51. Rietz LA, et al: Acute spinal cord injury: Clinical aspects and magnetic resonance imaging. *Emerg Radiol* 1:221, 1994.

52. Orrison WW, et al: Magnetic resonance imaging evaluation of acute spine trauma. *Emerg Radiol* 2:120, 1995.

53. Nichols JS, et al: Magnetic resonance imaging: Utilization in the management of central nervous system trauma. *J Trauma* 42:520, 1997.

54. Keiper MO, et al: MRI in the assessment of the supportive soft tissue of the cervical spine in acute trauma in children. *Pediatr Neuroradiol* 40:359, 1998.

55. Stucky AV, Potter HG: Use of MRI in spinal trauma: Indications, techniques and utility. *J Am Acad Orthop Surg* 6:134, 1998.

56. Quencer RM, et al: Magnetic resonance imaging of the chronically injured cervical spinal cord. *AJNR Am J Neuroradiol* 7:457, 1986.

57. Apuzzo ML: Radiographic assessment of the cervical spine in symptomatic trauma patients. *Neurosurgery* 50(3):S36, 2002.

58. Graziano A, Scheidel E, Cline JR, Baer LJ: A radiographic comparison of prehospital cervical immobilization methods. *Ann Emerg Med* 6:10, 1987.

59. Solot JA, Winzelberg GG: Clinical and radiographic evaluation of vertebrae extrication collars. *J Emerg Med* 8:79, 1990.

60. Chandler DR, et al: Emergency cervical spine immobilization. *Ann Emerg Med* 21:1185, 1992.

61. Apuzzo ML: Cervical spine immobilization before admission to the hospital. *Neurosurgery* 50(3):S7, 2002.

62. Apuzzo ML: Management of pediatric cervical spine and spinal cord injuries. *Neurosurgery* 50(3):S85, 2002.

63. DeLorenzo RA: A review of spinal immobilization techniques. *J Emerg Med* 14:603, 1996.

64. *Advanced Trauma Life Support Student Course Manual*, 6th ed. Chicago, American College of Surgeons, 1997.

65. Bivins HG, et al: The effect of axial traction during orotracheal intubation of the trauma victim with an unstable cervical spine. *Ann Emerg Med* 17:25, 1988.

66. Aprahamian C, et al: Experimental cervical spine injury model: Evaluation of airway management and splinting techniques. *Ann Emerg Med* 13:584, 1984.

67. Talucci RC, Shaikh KA, Schwab CW: Rapid sequence induction with oral endotracheal intubation in the multiply injured patient. *Am Surg* 54:185, 1988.

68. Holley J, Jorden R: Airway management in patients with unstable cervical spine fractures. *Ann Emerg Med* 18:1237, 1989.

69. Rhee KJ, et al: Oral intubation in the multiply injured patient: The risk of exacerbating spinal cord damage. *Ann Emerg Med* 19:511, 1990.

70. Wright SW, et al: Cervical spine injuries in blunt trauma patients requiring emergent endotracheal intubation. *J Emerg Med* 10:104, 1992.

71. Scannell G, et al: Orotracheal intubation in trauma patients with cervical fractures. *Arch Surg* 128:903, 1993.

72. Rhee KJ, O'Malley RJ: Neuromuscular blockade–assisted oral intubation versus nasotracheal intubation in the prehospital care of injured patients. *Ann Emerg Med* 23:37, 1994.

73. Hall ED: The role of oxygen radicals in traumatic injury: Clinical implications. *J Emerg Med* 11:31, 1993.

74. Bracken MB: Pharmacological treatment of acute spinal cord injury: Current status and future projects. *J Emerg Med* 11:43, 1993.

75. Haghighi SS, Chehragi B: Effect of naloxone in experimental acute spinal cord injury. *Neurosurgery* 20:385, 1987.

76. Geisler FH, et al: Recovery of motor function after spinal cord injury—a randomized, placebo-controlled trial with GM-1 ganglioside. *N Engl J Med* 324:1829, 1991.

77. Geisler FH, et al: Past and current clinical studies with GM-1 ganglioside in acute spinal cord injury. *Ann Emerg Med* 22:1041, 1993.

78. Bracken MB, et al: A randomized, controlled trial of methylprednisolone or naloxone in the treatment of acute spinal cord injury. *N Engl J Med* 322:1405, 1990.

79. Bracken MB, et al: Methylprednisolone or naloxone treatment after acute spinal cord injury: 1 year follow-up data. *J Neurosurg* 76:23, 1992.

80. Bracken MB, et al: Administration of methylprednisolone for 24 or 48 hours or tirilazad mesylate for 48 hours in the treatment of acute spinal cord injury. *JAMA* 277:20, 1997.
81. Bracken MB, et al: Methylprednisolone or tirilazad mesylate administration after acute spinal cord injury: 1-year follow-up—results of the Third National Acute Spinal Cord Injury Randomized Controlled Trial. *J Neurosurg* 89:699, 1998.
82. Luer MS, et al: New pharmacologic strategies for acute neuronal injury. *Pharmacotherapy* 16:830, 1996.
83. Coleman WP, et al: A critical appraisal of the reporting of the National Acute Spinal Cord Injury Studies (II and III) of methylprednisolone in acute spinal cord injury. *J Spinal Disord* 13:185, 2000.
84. Nesathurai S: Steroids and spinal cord injury: Revisiting the NASCIS 2 and NASCIS 3 trials. *J Trauma* 45:1088, 1998.
85. Matusmoto T, et al: Early complications of high-dose methylprednisolone sodium succinate treatment in the follow-up of acute cervical spinal cord injury. *Spine* 26:426, 2001.
86. Apuzzo ML: Pharmacological therapy after acute cervical spinal cord injury. *Neurosurgery* 50(3):S63, 2002.
87. Bracken MB: Steroids for acute spinal cord injury. *Cochrane Database Syst Rev* 3:CD001046, 2002.
88. Lemons VR, Wagner FC: Respiratory complications after cervical spinal cord injury. *Spine* 19:2315, 1994.
89. Soderstrom CA, et al: The diagnosis of intraabdominal injury in patients with cervical cord trauma. *J Trauma* 23:1061, 1983.
90. Matsumura JS, et al: Gastrointestinal tract complications after acute spinal injury. *Arch Surg* 130:751, 1995.
91. Vacarro AR, et al: Neurologic outcome of early versus late surgery for cervical spinal cord injury. *Spine* 22:2609, 1997.
92. Mizra SK, et al: Early versus delayed surgery for acute cervical spinal cord injury. *Clin Orthop* 359:104, 1999.
93. Dollfus P: Rehabilitation following injury to the spinal cord. *J Emerg Med* 11:57, 1993.
94. McNamara RM, et al: Post-traumatic neck pain: A prospective and follow-up study. *Ann Emerg Med* 17:906, 1988.
95. Ditunno JF, Formal CS: Chronic spinal cord injury. *N Engl J Med* 330:550, 1994.
96. Ross PD: Clinical consequences of vertebral fractures. *Am J Med* 103:305, 1997.
97. Savitsky E, Votey S: Emergency department approach to acute thoracolumbar spine injury. *J Emerg Med* 15:49, 1996.
98. Vollmer DG, Gegg C: Classification and acute management of thoracolumbar fractures. *Neurosurg Clin N Am* 8:499, 1997.

CHAPTER

41 Neck

Kim Newton

PERSPECTIVE

Neck trauma can result in a spectrum of injuries and complications ranging from incidental to life threatening, including hemorrhagic shock, acute neurologic injury, and airway obstruction. Vascular and laryngeal injuries can rapidly compromise the airway, challenging the most experienced physician. Stable-appearing patients can harbor insidious injuries associated with high morbidity and mortality if not recognized and treated in a timely fashion. Practicing emergency physicians not only must be familiar with the spectrum of injuries and subtle presentations associated with neck trauma but also should be well versed in neck anatomy, diagnostic evaluation, management controversies, and airway salvage techniques.

Neck trauma is divided into three major mechanisms: blunt, penetrating, and strangulation or near hanging. The injuries caused by these mechanisms can be further categorized into injuries of the airway (laryngotracheal), digestive tract (pharyngoesophageal), vascular system, and neurologic system. Each of these injuries has unique features and is discussed separately.

PRINCIPLES OF DISEASE

Pathophysiology

Penetrating Trauma

The incidence of penetrating neck trauma is reported to be 5% to 10% of all traumatic injuries and typically results from one of three major mechanisms: gunshot wounds (GSWs), stab wounds, and miscellaneous injuries that include impalement and shrapnel wounds.[1] GSWs are further divided into high-velocity and low-velocity injuries. High-velocity missiles include military-style weapons and hunting rifles that can achieve bullet velocities of 2200 to 3200 feet/sec and greater. These missiles can easily penetrate soft tissue or bone; their pathway is generally direct and predictable unless deflected, although they can also cause remote injuries through a blast effect. Bone penetration requires a minimum velocity of 350 feet/sec. Low-velocity injuries (small-caliber handguns and air guns) are caused by missiles that travel at significantly slower velocities (e.g., 300 feet/sec for .22-caliber pistols). Slower moving missiles tend to produce erratic pathways, often demonstrating no direct relationship to the entrance or exit wounds.[2]

2% to 6%, and the leading cause of immediate death is exsanguination.[1,5]

Blunt Trauma

Blunt neck trauma most frequently results from motor vehicle crashes but can occur after assaults, "clothesline" injuries, strangulation, and sports injuries.[6] Blunt vascular injuries are rare but represent some of the most underdiagnosed injuries seen by trauma surgeons.[7] Blunt injuries to the aerodigestive tracts are uncommon compared with penetrating injuries but can cause acute airway compromise and delayed complications.

Anatomy

The neck is a complex, closed anatomic area dense with vital structures and invested with fascia creating several compartments. Because of this close anatomic relationship, vascular injury with hemorrhage either can be tamponaded by fascial planes and neighboring structures or can cause marked anatomic distortion, making evaluation and airway management extremely difficult. Two methods are used to describe the external neck: zones and triangles.[8] Anatomically, the neck has been divided into triangles (anterior and posterior). The *anterior triangle* is laden with vital structures (neurovascular and aerodigestive tracts) and is bordered anteriorly by the midline, posteriorly by the sternocleidomastoid muscle, and superiorly by the lower edge of the mandible. The *posterior triangle* is located within the boundaries of the sternocleidomastoid muscle anteriorly, the clavicle inferiorly, and the anterior border of the trapezius muscle posteriorly. Excluding spinal trauma, injury to this region often has a more favorable prognosis because of the relative paucity of vital structures.

Current trauma literature favors neck division into zones I, II, and III. This division has both anatomic and management implications for penetrating neck trauma.[4] *Zone I* (base of neck) extends superiorly from the sternal notch and clavicles to the cricoid cartilage. It comprises the thoracic outlet below the cricoid cartilage. Injury to this region can affect both neck and mediastinal structures. *Zone II* (midneck) is the area between the cricoid cartilage and the angle of the mandible. Zone II injuries are therapeutically distinct because they lie in the most exposed region of the neck, making these injuries accessible to direct surgical visualization with easier proximal and distal vascular control. *Zone III* (upper neck) extends from the angle of the mandible to the base of the skull. As with zone I injuries, proximal and distal vascular control in this region is difficult to achieve (Box 41-1).

Two fascial layers, the superficial fascia and the deep cervical fascia, cover neck structures. The superficial fascia covers the platysma muscle and is located just below the skin. The deep cervical fascia is divided into three parts: the *investing layer* surrounds the neck and splits to encase the sternocleidomastoid and trapezius muscles, the *pretracheal layer* adheres to the cricoid and thyroid cartilages and travels caudally behind the sternum to insert on the anterior pericardium, and the

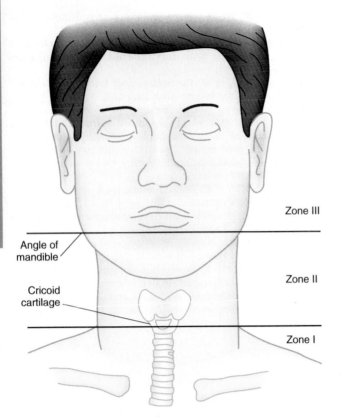

Figure 41-1. Zones of the neck.

Labels on figure: Zone III, Zone II, Zone I, Angle of mandible, Cricoid cartilage

Table 41-1. Incidence of Injuries in Penetrating Neck Trauma

Location	Number (1275 total)	Percentage (%)*
Arterial	320	12.8
Venous	281	11.3
Tracheolaryngeal	253	10.1
Pharyngoesophageal	240	9.6
Spinal cord	76	3
Neurologic, other	85	3.4
Thoracic duct	20	0

*Incidence based on other reported series.
From McConnell DB, Trunkey D: Management of penetrating trauma to the neck. *Adv Surg* 27:97, 1994.

The zone and mechanism of injury should be noted because lower energy injuries (knife, handgun, long-range birdshot or buckshot) cause a 50% lower incidence of clinically significant lesions (Figure 41-1).[3] Zone I and III injuries pose a greater surgical challenge, and clinicians are more likely to order preoperative diagnostic tests to determine the best surgical approach (Table 41-1).[4]

Stab wounds, being of very low velocity compared with missiles and most often limited to one side of the neck, are more amenable to nonsurgical management. Miscellaneous penetrating neck wounds can occur from any object capable of impalement, puncture, or laceration but most often result from glass fragments after motor vehicle crashes or from dog bites. The overall mortality rate for penetrating neck injuries is

BOX 41-1. Vascular and Other Contents in Neck Zones

Zone I
Proximal common carotid artery
Vertebral artery
Subclavian artery
Major vessels of upper mediastinum
Apices of lungs
Esophagus
Trachea
Thyroid
Thoracic duct
Spinal cord

Zone II
Carotid artery
Vertebral artery
Larynx
Trachea
Esophagus
Pharynx
Jugular vein
Vagus nerve
Recurrent laryngeal nerve
Spinal cord

Zone III
Distal carotid artery
Vertebral artery
Distal jugular vein
Salivary and parotid glands
Cranial nerves IX–XII
Spinal cord

BOX 41-2. "Hard" and "Soft" Signs of Penetrating Neck Trauma

Soft Signs
Hemoptysis/hematemesis
Oropharyngeal blood
Dyspnea
Dysphonia/dysphagia
Subcutaneous or mediastinal air
Chest tube air leak
Nonexpanding hematoma
Focal neurologic deficits

Hard Signs
Expanding hematoma
Severe active bleeding
Shock not responding to fluids
Decreased/absent radial pulse
Vascular bruit/thrill
Cerebral ischemia
Airway obstruction

that suggest decompensation in a previously stable patient can include dyspnea, dysphonia, expanding hematoma, bruit, cerebral ischemia, or shock.

DIAGNOSTIC STRATEGIES

The reliability of physical examination in detecting serious neck injury in a stable patient is controversial. A prospective study of 393 patients with penetrating neck injuries determined that 30% of patients with no physical findings subsequently had positive neck explorations.[9] In contrast, another large prospective series of 223 patients with penetrating neck wounds found that physical examination was reliable in determining which patients needed vascular or esophageal diagnostic studies.[10] The literature remains divided between those who do and those who do not believe that physical examination is reliable.[11-14] Stable patients should be evaluated for the presence of "soft" and "hard" signs of aerodigestive or neurovascular injury (Box 41-2). Most patients with hard signs benefit from surgical intervention. Controversy surfaces over the stable patient with soft signs or no signs of injury. Some centers advocate mandatory surgical exploration for these patients, citing the unreliability of physical examination.[15] Others prefer a selective protocol using either diagnostic testing coupled with physical examination or only serial examinations.[10,16]

prevertebral layer envelops the cervical prevertebral muscles and extends to form the axillary sheath, which covers the subclavian artery. The pretracheal layer is clinically important because of its connection from the neck to the anterior mediastinum. Missed aerodigestive injuries can result in mediastinitis because of this anatomic continuity. The carotid sheath is made of portions from all three divisions of the deep cervical fascia. The *platysma muscle*, sandwiched between the superficial and deep cervical fascia, covers the anterolateral neck. It has clinical significance because of its superficial location and proximity to vital structures. If the platysma muscle is violated, injury to these structures should be suspected. Examination of any penetrating neck wound should document the zone or zones of injury and presence of platysma violation (without deep probing).[9]

CLINICAL FEATURES

Patients with neck injury can manifest numerous signs and symptoms, but most are nonspecific. This makes diagnostic strategies difficult, especially in the stable patient. Much debate in the current literature centers on the safest and most cost-effective approach to evaluating patients with possible neck injury. Serial examinations are crucial, watching for evidence of progressive airway or vascular compromise. Features

MANAGEMENT

Stable Patients

Ideally, stable patients with neck injury should be transported to a trauma center. Despite a stable initial appearance, airway compromise can ensue rapidly and intervention is essential at the first sign of airway distress. Prehospital initiation of intravenous access should not delay transport. Necessary procedures should be initiated in most patients during transport to the emergency department rather than at the scene. Wounds should be covered and sufficient compression applied to control bleeding and prevent air embolus without occluding the airway or blood flow to the brain.

Unstable Patients

Airway management must be the highest initial priority in the unstable patient. Cervical spine immobilization is typically unnecessary in penetrating neck trauma unless the patient has coexistent blunt trauma or evidence of a spinal cord injury. Oral intubation using rapid sequence intubation (RSI) is considered safe in most patients with neck trauma.[17] When the airway has been stabilized, breathing assessment is standard, with consideration of the associated risk of hemothorax or pneumothorax, seen primarily with penetrating zone I injuries. Caution is required when bag-valve-mask ventilation is necessary because air can be forced into injured tissue planes, resulting in massive subcutaneous emphysema with airway distortion or, rarely, air embolus. Active bleeding sites or wounds with blood clots should not be probed because massive hemorrhage can ensue. Ideally, bleeding is controlled by direct pressure. Blind clamping of active bleeding sites should be avoided because of the high concentration of neurovascular structures in the neck. If a vascular injury is suspected, mild Trendelenburg's position is recommended to reduce the risk of air embolism. Intravenous access is best placed on the noninjured side, avoiding the ipsilateral neck or upper extremity until vascular injury has been excluded. Cervical collars might obscure neck pathology and preclude adequate examination. Partial removal of the collar while maintaining in-line stabilization may be necessary to perform adequate serial examinations.

The presence of profound shock or cardiopulmonary arrest unresponsive to fluids should prompt the physician to consider venous air embolism (VAE). If this condition is suspected, the patient should be placed in a head-down, left lateral decubitus position to cause intracardiac air to accumulate in the apex of the right ventricle. If this maneuver alone does not improve cardiac output, aspiration of air from the apex of the right ventricle either through an ultrasound-guided pericardiocentesis needle or under direct vision after emergency department thoracotomy may be lifesaving. Evidence of cerebral ischemia, as manifested by profound alteration in consciousness, or stroke-like symptoms suggests injury to the cervical vessels or cerebral arterial air embolism.

Caution is advised in any patient with suspected vascular injury who requires a nasogastric tube (NGT). The retching typically seen with placement can dislodge a hematoma, resulting in immediate hemorrhage. If indicated, an NGT should ideally be placed after the patient is intubated. Conversely, an NGT can be therapeutic (remove gastric contents to prevent aspiration) and diagnostic (bloody aspiration implies visceral injury).

Airway Management

Orotracheal Rapid Sequence Intubation

Although the ideal airway technique for neck trauma patients has been debated over the past decade, orotracheal intubation using RSI has been shown to be safe and effective and is the most commonly used technique. Opponents cite potential complete airway obstruction after administration of neuromuscular blocking agents and movement of an unstable cervical spine fracture as reasons to seek other airway options.[18] Less commonly used airway salvage techniques, however, may diminish the emergency physician's comfort level and prolong the airway stabilization procedure.

The literature supports orotracheal RSI in trauma patients with either blunt or penetrating injuries, and it should be considered the first-line airway technique unless contraindications exist.[17,19,20] Concerns over the possibility of sedative-induced muscle relaxation leading to airway obstruction have not been validated. Orotracheal RSI is often successful even after neck trauma with airway distortion.[21,22] RSI also has been shown to be superior to intubation without neuromuscular blocking agents.[23] However, RSI medications should be used only by an experienced intubator. If the cervical spine must remain immobilized, an assistant should maintain in-line stabilization of the head and neck. Relative contraindications to RSI include massive facial trauma or suspected laryngeal injury. When time allows, an initial inspection of the airway can be made using a laryngoscope in the awake patient. In cases in which orotracheal intubation is expected to be difficult, an attempt to intubate over a nasopharyngoscope may be prudent in patients who do not have massive bleeding into the oropharynx. All emergency physicians must have a thorough knowledge of alternative techniques for intubation in the event that orotracheal RSI fails.[24,25]

However, even some of the usual rescue airway techniques (e.g., laryngeal mask airway) may be inadequate if there is significant bleeding in the oropharynx.

Nasotracheal Intubation

Historically, nasotracheal intubation was recommended for the majority of trauma patients, especially if cervical spine injury was suspected (see Chapter 1). In the past, advanced trauma life support courses also taught that blind nasotracheal intubation (BNTI) was the procedure of choice in patients with neck trauma.[26] BNTI has profound potential complications, including bleeding, vomiting, aspiration, increased intracranial pressure, turbinate damage, and sinusitis.[27] In addition, if cervical spine injury has not been excluded, cervical protection can be difficult to maintain because of the retching and neck movement (procedural discomfort) often seen during BNTI in awake patients. Success rates for BNTI range from 66% to 93%.[28] Nasotracheal intubation is contraindicated in apneic patients and in those with suspected basilar skull fractures or laryngeal injury.

Surgical-Invasive Airways

Cricothyrotomy remains a common airway salvage technique used by many emergency physicians and is a preferred first-line procedure for others.[29] Despite clear descriptions of this technique in the literature,[19,30] it is not always simple to perform. Anterior neck hematoma or potential laryngeal injury should make the intubator consider a different means of securing the airway. Although it appears efficacious, controversy surrounds the safety of prehospital cricothyrotomy when performed by emergency medical services personnel.[31] Percutaneous transtracheal jet insufflation, an effective method of providing a temporizing airway in selected adult or pediatric trauma patients, is fraught with potential complications. These include inadvertent catheter dislodgment resulting in massive subcutaneous emphysema, catheter kinking, perforation of the posterior wall of the trachea and esophagus, pneumothorax, and hypercarbia. Complete upper airway obstruction is considered a relative contraindication because barotrauma can result from inadequate exhalation.[32,33]

Miscellaneous Techniques

Other airway techniques include fiberoptic laryngoscopy and bronchoscopy, which have been used successfully for difficult airways, although excessive bleeding can render these techniques difficult. Others cite lack of experience and time constraints as reasons why these techniques are not preferred in the emergency department.[1,17] Emergency tracheostomy is not a common emergency department procedure because it is technically difficult and time consuming to perform. It should be attempted only in selected cases in which other techniques are contraindicated or not available. Esophageal obturator airway, retrograde intubation, laryngeal mask airway, and awake endotracheal intubation, although reported in the literature, are generally not used as primary procedures or airway salvage techniques in trauma patients.[34-38]

Pediatric Considerations

Airway management in the pediatric trauma patient tends to cause the emergency physician more anxiety, in part because of the different anatomic considerations. Ideally, the approach to the pediatric airway is similar to that to the adult airway, using orotracheal RSI. The incidence of unstable cervical fractures in children is lower than in adults.[39] As in adults, airway salvage techniques may be necessary, but fewer options are available in young children. The airway of the young child and infant is higher and more anterior, with the narrowest region of the airway at the cricoid cartilage.[40] The small cricothyroid membrane and the soft, poorly mineralized pediatric larynx make cricothyrotomy contraindicated in children younger than 10 years. Emergency tracheostomy, which is a difficult procedure in young children, or transtracheal jet insufflation can serve as a salvage technique.[33,41] BNTI in the infant and very young child is also not recom-

mended, in part because the smaller endotracheal tubes are too pliable to be consistently passed.

Cervical Spine

Numerous papers have been written on the safety of orotracheal intubation in patients with known or suspected cervical spine injury.[18,42,43] Despite fear of head movement during intubation generated by cadaver studies, which caused some to abandon the orotracheal route of intubation, RSI with in-line stabilization has not been shown to produce neurologic sequelae in humans.[18,42-44] Fear of delayed neurologic sequelae from cervical spine injury after intubation should not preclude using RSI with in-line stabilization. Neurologically intact patients with unstable cervical fractures secondary to penetrating trauma rarely manifest delayed neurologic sequelae.[5] A greater concern for occult or overt cervical spine injury exists in the patient with blunt neck or multisystem trauma, although cervical spine injuries in this population are not as common as once thought.[20] Armed with this knowledge and barring contraindications, emergency physicians should use the airway technique with which they are most comfortable. Delays in securing an airway because of indecision regarding which technique to use can lead to hypoxic brain injury.

Mandatory versus Selective Exploration

The debate is ongoing in the trauma literature concerning the best way to manage penetrating neck injuries. Before World War II, patients with penetrating neck trauma were treated expectantly rather than aggressively despite unacceptably high mortality rates (18% to 35%).[1] In an attempt to reduce the mortality associated with penetrating neck injuries, the concept of *mandatory surgical exploration of all penetrating neck wounds* was developed.[45] Mandatory surgery drastically reduced mortality rates to only 6%.[7] Wartime experience justified the ongoing utilization of mandatory surgery in victims with penetrating neck injury, and this was widely accepted for decades.[46]

Despite low mortality rates achieved with mandatory surgery, negative neck explorations concurrently increased (40% to 63%) during the middle to later 1900s as many institutions adopted a mandatory surgical approach.[4] As with other traumatic injuries, an effort to reduce the negative exploration rate while maintaining low morbidity and mortality rates led to the concept of *selective surgical management*, which remains institution specific. Selective management offers a spectrum of approaches, ranging from serial physical examinations to an array of diagnostic tests in the stable patient. A selective approach is justified because (1) military injuries were often secondary to high-velocity missiles, as opposed to currently used weapons (e.g., knives, handguns) and animal bites, and (2) improved technology currently allows much greater accuracy in the detection of injuries. A review of zone II penetrating neck trauma cites similar overall mortality rates of 5.85% in the mandatory group and 3.74%

in the selective group.[4] The mandatory versus selective controversy is still unresolved, with compelling literature to support both approaches.[9,13,47,48] Current literature, however, seems to favor the selective approach with the trend in the literature being to minimize invasive procedures.[4]

Transcervical Gunshot Wounds

Transcervical gunshot wounds (TC-GSWs) represent a subset of penetrating neck trauma and are included in the debate between mandatory and selective management schools. TC-GSWs are associated with a twofold increased incidence of injuries compared with GSWs that do not cross the midline (79% versus 31%). The most common injury seen is vascular (48%), followed by spinal cord (24%).[49] Some believe that TC-GSWs are a reliable marker for visceral injuries, and therefore they subject all patients to surgical exploration.[50] Prospective studies, however, suggest that stable patients with TC-GSWs can be safely evaluated using a selective surgical approach with the appropriate diagnostic studies and frequent serial examinations.[49] GSWs in the anterior midline also involve an increased incidence of vascular and visceral injuries, and a more aggressive diagnostic approach should be considered in these patients.[51]

DISPOSITION

Many patients who present to the emergency department with penetrating or blunt neck trauma have predetermined disposition, especially when their condition warrants further diagnostic studies, surgery, or intensive care. Most stable patients should be admitted for observation. All patients with platysma muscle violation should be admitted to the surgical service for ongoing observation, regardless of their stability. Careful observation should be maintained for patients with blunt neck injury because they can manifest delayed signs and symptoms with serious consequences.

Because smaller hospitals may have neither the ancillary support nor the personnel to perform serial bedside examinations, mandatory exploration might be in the patient's best interest in these facilities. Level I trauma centers have sufficient ancillary support and diagnostic tools and are more suited to avoid surgery safely in stable patients. Studies suggest that surgeons with trauma experience tend to perform fewer neck explorations.[52]

SPECIFIC INJURIES

Pharyngoesophageal Trauma

Epidemiology

Esophageal injuries are infrequently reported after penetrating neck trauma, representing only 0.11% of all trauma admissions.[53] Blunt esophageal perforation is even less common, with only 10 case reports in the literature before 1990. Blunt pharyngoesophageal perforation accounts for less than 2% of all perforations in that anatomic region.[54] The low incidence of injury most likely results from the relatively protected position of the esophagus. The cervical esophagus is injured more often than the distal segment. Mortality from esophageal injuries has remained relatively high over the past two decades, with an overall rate of 22%.[53]

Pathophysiology

Early diagnosis of esophageal injury is crucial because spillage of orogastric contents with bacterial contamination leads to florid inflammation, infection (abscess, mediastinitis), and death. Esophageal injuries represent the most frequently missed injuries in the neck[13,55] and may be the leading cause of delayed death resulting from neck trauma.[56]

Clinical Features

Although there are no pathognomonic signs of esophageal injury, soft signs of injury include hematemesis, odynophagia, subcutaneous emphysema, and blood in the saliva or NGT, and the presence of these should increase concern for esophageal injury. Other associated findings include dyspnea, hoarseness, stridor, cough, pain and tenderness in the neck, and resistance to passive neck movement.

Physical examination has been shown to be unreliable in diagnosing esophageal injury, with an accuracy of only 72%.[56] Because timely diagnosis is so important, most believe that sole reliance on physical examination is not warranted in stable patients with soft signs of esophageal injury.[57]

Diagnostic Strategies

Unfortunately, esophageal injuries are difficult to diagnose. To compound this, delays in diagnosis and thus treatment are strongly associated with adverse outcomes.[7,10] Ideally, the diagnosis should be made within 12 hours so that definitive treatment can be initiated.[58]

Diagnosing esophageal injury often depends on more than a high clinical suspicion. Contrast esophagography is considered relatively unreliable for diagnosing esophageal injuries, with a sensitivity of 80% to 89%.[4,56] This study requires adequate views for accurate interpretation and thus requires the patient's cooperation. Flexible endoscopy has been reported as insensitive, primarily missing proximal esophageal injuries because the scope is unable to efface the mucosa in this region as can a rigid endoscope.[7] The combination of rigid esophagoscopy and contrast esophagography is much more sensitive, but the former requires general anesthesia. Currently, the combination of contrast swallow and flexible endoscopy appears to be accurate in diagnosing esophageal injuries, yielding a sensitivity of 100%.[56] Despite the selective management options mentioned, a prospective study suggested that only obtunded or symptomatic patients (hematemesis, painful swallowing, or subcutaneous emphysema) need studies to exclude esophageal injuries.[10] Plain films of the neck and chest radiographs suggest esophageal perforation if pneumomediastinum or retropharyngeal air is present.[3]

With the advent of the higher resolution computed tomography (CT) scan, there has been a controversial suggestion that high-speed, thin-cut CT scanning may increase the sensitivity for penetrating zone II esophageal injuries and either supplement the physical examination in selectively managed patients or negate the need for other diagnostic studies. However, sole reliance on this diagnostic modality is currently not supported by the literature.[59,60]

Management

When esophageal injury is suspected, broad-spectrum antibiotics with anaerobic coverage should be administered, and the patient should receive nothing by mouth pending surgical exploration. Some advocate placement of an NGT preoperatively, with suction to reduce the spillage of gastric contents into the wound.[58]

Laryngotracheal Trauma

Mechanisms of Disease

Laryngotracheal (LT) injuries account for less than 1% of all trauma injuries, with most confined to the cervical trachea. Most LT injuries result from direct blunt force sustained in motor vehicle crashes, where the extended neck strikes the steering wheel or dashboard and the larynx is compressed between the fixed object and the cervical spine. Other mechanisms leading to LT injuries include clothesline injuries, improperly fitting shoulder harnesses, near hanging, assaults, athletic events, attempted strangulation, and iatrogenic wounds.[61] Penetrating LT injuries compose 10% of all penetrating neck trauma.[7] Associated cervical spine injuries should always be considered simultaneously, especially when evaluating a patient with blunt neck trauma.

The cricoid cartilage is the only complete, solid ring in the larynx. Fractures of the cricoid cartilage can lead to death through acute airway obstruction and are the most serious laryngeal injuries.[61] Calcification of the laryngeal cartilages begins during the teenage years, and fractures before this age are much less likely to appear on plain neck films. The degree of airway obstruction after blunt trauma to the larynx is inversely related to the degree of cartilage calcification, putting children at highest risk.

Clinical Features

Bubbling from the wound should signal injury to the respiratory tract. Massive subcutaneous air and bony crepitus over the larynx should alert the clinician to possible LT injury, as should a clothesline mechanism.[62] Other clinical features of LT injury include dysphonia, aphonia, dyspnea, stridor, hemoptysis, subcutaneous emphysema, laryngeal crepitus, neck tenderness or pain over the larynx, visible neck wound, or

loss of anatomic landmarks secondary to hematoma. Pain with tongue movement implies injury to the epiglottis, hyoid bone, or laryngeal cartilage.[1] In one study, dyspnea and stridor were the most common signs of injury in children with LT trauma.[63] Others cite subcutaneous air found by examination or on radiographs and tenderness over the larynx or trachea as the most common findings.[64] One study found that all patients with significant aerodigestive injuries requiring repair had clinical signs or symptoms suggesting injury.[65]

Diagnostic Strategies

Diagnostic evaluation options exist for the stable patient. Missed injuries can lead to long-term sequelae, including voice change, dysphagia, laryngeal stenosis, and chronic pain. Patients with penetrating trauma are managed by a mandatory or selective protocol. Plain radiographs should be evaluated for extraluminal air, edema, foreign bodies, and fracture of the cartilaginous laryngeal structures. Direct laryngoscopy or flexible nasopharyngoscopy allows evaluation of laryngeal integrity. With appropriate local anesthesia, laryngoscopy is well tolerated by most patients who remain in cervical spine immobilization, and it can detect hypopharyngeal tears.[61] Rigid endoscopy is useful to evaluate injury distal to the larynx but requires general anesthesia.[66]

Spiral CT scanning is a valuable adjunct, rapidly providing detailed information about laryngeal integrity and the surrounding region.[59] CT is useful for detecting fractures of the hyoid bone, disrupted laryngeal or tracheal cartilages, significant exolaryngeal or endolaryngeal hematoma, and dislocations of the cricothyroid or cricoarytenoid joints and for assessing vocal cord integrity and airway lumen diameter. Despite these advantages, CT has limitations and should not be relied on to detect mucosal perforations, degloving injuries of the cartilage with denuded mucosa, and certain types of LT separation. CT is not yet routinely utilized in penetrating neck trauma and may be less helpful when evaluating poorly calcified pediatric cartilaginous structures because these fractures can be more difficult to visualize.

Management

Airway compromise in patients with LT trauma can be immediate or delayed. Clinical judgment must be exercised in patients who initially appear to have stable, patent airways if they are to be sent to other departments for further diagnostic testing. Delayed airway occlusion can be rapid and life threatening, and thus these patients require close monitoring. Ongoing airway controversies between orotracheal intubation and tracheostomy related to LT trauma persist.[61] Orotracheal intubation can complete a partial LT separation or create a false passage. Likewise, cricothyroidotomy can further damage an injured larynx. If complete LT separation is present with distal retraction of the trachea, orotracheal intubation is likely to be unsuccessful, and tracheostomy might unknowingly be performed proximal to the tracheal segment. Tracheostomy in these cases is best done at the fourth or fifth tracheal ring to avoid the larynx.[67] Because blunt LT injuries are often seen in association with multisystem trauma, they can be easily overlooked when other overt injuries are present.

Vascular Trauma

The great vessels of concern in the neck include the carotid, subclavian, and vertebral arteries and the internal and external jugular veins. Injury to these vessels can produce morbidity and mortality through exsanguination, hematoma expansion with subsequent airway distortion and compromise, direct vessel injury leading to vascular occlusion, or embolization of a foreign body (e.g., shotgun pellet to brain or heart).[61]

Epidemiology

Penetrating Injury

Historically, blunt trauma appeared responsible for a greater number of cervical vascular injuries; however, with the advent of better imaging studies, penetrating trauma has been found to be responsible for more injuries in some series.[68] Vascular injuries represent 25% of all penetrating neck wounds, and mortality rates range from 10% to 50%.[4,5] GSWs are more likely to be associated with hard signs of vascular injury than are stab wounds.[55] Hard signs of vascular injury include pulsatile bleeding, expanding hematoma, bruit, or focal neurologic deficits consistent with carotid or vertebrobasilar arterial occlusion. Exsanguination from vascular injuries is the most common cause of immediate death after penetrating neck trauma.[69] The jugular vein is the most frequently injured vessel in the neck,[4] although the common carotid artery is the most frequently injured artery (22% of all cervical vascular injuries).[56] The vertebral artery is injured in only 1.3% of all cases.[7] Vertebrobasilar arterial injuries may follow relatively minor trauma such as chiropractic neck manipulation but most commonly occur in association with fractures of the spinal column. They typically arise after a delay of hours to months with signs of posterior circulation embolus or infarction. The prognosis is poor.

Blunt Injury

Three percent to 10% of all carotid injuries result from some form of blunt trauma, but blunt carotid injuries affect only 0.08% to 0.33% of all blunt trauma victims.[70,71] Mortality rates with blunt cervical vascular injuries range from 20% to 40%. Blunt cervical vascular injuries are rare, and until the mid-1990s, only 480 cases were reported in the literature.[71] Because the internal carotid artery is the most frequently injured artery, many studies use blunt vascular and carotid artery injuries synonymously, although the vertebral artery is injured in up to 20% of cases.[72] The actual incidence of blunt vascular injuries may be higher because of asymptomatic cases and difficulties in making the diagnosis.

Pathophysiology

Penetrating Injury

Most cases of penetrating trauma in adults are caused by knife or bullet wounds.[16] Vessel damage most often results from direct injury, although the blast effect can cause intimal injury without directly striking the vessel, making the vascular insult similar to that seen with blunt trauma. Some centers routinely obtain angiographic studies of all significant neck wounds; others restrict angiography to zone I and zone III injuries. Zone I injuries in particular can harbor clinically occult arterial injuries, and routine preoperative arteriography is commonly used to detect injury and facilitate a judicious surgical approach when positive. Likewise, zone III vascular injuries can be exceedingly difficult to approach surgically, and thus many surgeons prefer preoperative angiography followed by exploration for any positive or equivocal findings. Many surgeons believe that preexploratory vascular studies are noncontributory in zone II injuries and may lead to delays in definitive care because these lesions are easily approached surgically.

Blunt Injury

Blunt trauma to the cervical vessels can result in a spectrum of arterial injuries, including intimal tears, thrombosis, dissection, and pseudoaneurysm.[6,72-74] Embolization can occur from a thrombus that develops at the injury site. The most common mechanism for blunt internal carotid artery injury is sudden, forceful hyperextension and lateral rotation of the neck. This mechanism can cause stretching of the carotid artery over the transverse processes of the upper cervical vertebrae, resulting in intimal injury.[72] Other mechanisms responsible for this type of injury include direct blunt force to the side of the neck, intraoral trauma (e.g., children falling on lollipops), and basilar skull fractures, which have rarely been associated with injury to the intracranial portion of the carotid artery. Blunt carotid artery injuries most often result from motor vehicle accidents but have also been reported after fights, athletic events, seat belt injuries, clothesline injuries, and near hangings.[72-74] Seat belt signs on the neck may suggest insidious vascular injury, but an article found that of 131 patients with a seat belt sign at the neck, only 0.76% had a significant vascular injury.[75]

Clinical Features

The debate over whether the physical examination is sensitive enough to detect vascular injuries in stable patients with minimal signs and symptoms is unresolved. Angiographically documented arterial injuries have not been reliably detected by physical examination in some series.[14] Some authors argue that although discrepancies may exist, they are not clinically relevant in the asymptomatic patient and rarely change management, and thus conclude that serial examinations are adequate.[76] Signs and symptoms of vascular injury include pulsatile hematoma, bruits, pulse deficit, hemothorax, airway compromise (from hematoma expansion), shock, and neurologic deficits.

Delayed presentation of a vascular injury is most often neurologic in nature, with symptoms ranging from transient ischemic attack (TIA) to global cerebral ischemia.[74] Horner's syndrome has been associated with vascular injury.[77] Delays in the onset of neurologic sequelae of weeks to years have been reported.[74] TIAs usually result from release of small emboli from the injured vessel, which can herald the onset of a profound deficit. Thus, any focal neurologic abnormality should prompt the emergency physician to include vascular injuries in the differential diagnosis, especially after a normal head CT scan.

Because they are rare or delayed in their presentation, blunt vascular lesions are often not considered initially. Other injuries can divert the emergency physician's attention to more immediately life-threatening wounds. Diagnosis is also often delayed because 17% to 35% of patients do not develop neurologic symptoms for more than 24 hours.[78] Other investigators report that 58% of patients develop the onset of neurologic symptoms by 12 hours.[6] Drugs, alcohol, or head trauma can further obscure or contribute to delays in the diagnosis of blunt vascular injury. Because of the low incidence of blunt vascular injuries, no large prospective study has fully defined the "at risk" patient.

Diagnostic Strategies

There is also controversy about how aggressive the search should be for vascular injuries using surgical exploration or other diagnostic modalities in the patient with minimal symptoms. Blunt cervical injuries represent some of the most underreported injuries because of their insidious presentation yet ultimate association with a catastrophic neurologic outcome.

Arteriography has been used extensively to detect vascular injury in patients with both blunt and penetrating injuries. A four-vessel arteriogram is time consuming and expensive but may be helpful in planning the best surgical approach.[79] The majority of patients require four-vessel studies, although occasionally a two-vessel (ipsilateral carotid and vertebral) arteriogram may be warranted if the injury is isolated to one side of the neck.[1] These contrast studies should include the intracranial portion of the carotid artery with zone III injuries or suspected blunt cervical trauma. Zone I injuries should include the aortic arch with its branches. To date, arteriography remains the "gold standard" for diagnosing vascular injuries,[72] and if the study is negative, many recommend nonsurgical management when aerodigestive injuries have been excluded.[1] Despite a sensitivity and specificity of nearly 100% and a complication rate of less than 2% for arteriography, other, less invasive diagnostic tests have been evaluated for accuracy, speed, cost, and efficacy.[80]

Duplex ultrasonography has been used in combination with or instead of arteriography to exclude cervical vascular injury in patients with both penetrating and blunt trauma.[81] Despite clinical success, limitations of ultrasonography include the risk of missing zone I and III injuries and the lack of 24-hour availability at many centers. Whether duplex scanning can reliably detect pseudoaneurysms or intrathoracic, distal internal carotid, and vertebral artery injuries remains unproved. Also, some patients must remain in cervical spine protection, limiting neck manipulation necessary for optimal views. Many surgeons are not comfortable with serial duplex examinations as a means of detecting traumatic vascular lesions and continue to use arteriography as the mainstay of diagnosis.

Other diagnostic modalities have been used with variable success. With newer generation machines, CT angiography appears to be a popular, promising screening tool.[82] Further benefits of this noninvasive test include easy access at most centers, although CT angiography can potentially miss lethal lesions such as pseudoaneurysms. Magnetic resonance angiography has also been reported to be helpful despite high cost and lack of 24-hour availability.[83] Because none of these studies has shown the arteriogram's high degree of accuracy, they should not be relied on solely to the exclusion of proven diagnostic modalities.

Head CT scans are often ordered in response to vascularly induced neurologic deficits because many suspect closed-head injury initially. When these symptoms result from traumatic occlusion of the carotid artery, the head CT scan is frequently normal because the ischemic changes are often not obvious for more than 24 hours. Any unexplained focal neurologic deficits should prompt the emergency physician to consider vascular injuries.

Plain films, although not indicated in most cases of suspected vascular injury, can occasionally be useful. Anteroposterior and lateral neck films can help determine a bullet trajectory by comparing the entrance wound with the location of the foreign body, if present. Chest radiographs allow evaluation of the mediastinum and identification of hemothorax or pneumothorax.

Management

Blunt Injury

Treatment options for blunt artery injuries depend in part on the mechanism and type of injury and location of the lesion. Treatment modalities include surgery, anticoagulation, and observation. Heparin has been reported to be successful in some blunt vascular injuries[71] but can carry risk because many of these patients have sustained multisystem trauma. Others have not found heparin to be beneficial.[72] Antiplatelet therapy has been suggested for carotid artery dissection to prevent clot propagation.[70] Because of possible complications, none of these treatment modalities should be initiated without appropriate consultation. Surgical procedures include ligation, resection, thrombectomy, and stent placement.[1,72]

Penetrating Injury

The ideal management strategy for injuries of the vascular system resulting from penetrating trauma has not been determined. Because many of these patients are young with anticipated "clean" carotid arteries, some surgeons routinely attempt surgical repair.

Because of concern in patients with profound neurologic deficit that reperfusion might convert an ischemic infarction to a hemorrhagic infarction, others prefer ligation over repair in a selected population of patients.[84]

Venous Air Embolism

VAE is a subset of vascular injuries that can lead to life-threatening complications if not detected. VAE has been reported after blunt, penetrating, and iatrogenic mechanisms. VAE occurs when air enters the injured vessel, usually during inspiration, resulting in distal vascular occlusion.[85] In any patient with a suspected major venous injury, direct pressure should be maintained over the wound while the patient is kept in Trendelenburg's position. Autopsy reports on trauma victims reveal air in both the right side of the heart and the pulmonary artery. When standard treatment fails in a pulseless trauma patient, VAE should be immediately suspected and the right ventricle aspirated for air after the aorta is cross-clamped. Rarely, air embolism has been reported with arterial injuries as well.[1]

Nervous System

When evaluating any patient with neck trauma, the examiner must remember that the brachial plexus, peripheral nerve roots, cervical sympathetic chain, and cranial nerves VII, IX, X, XI, and XII are vulnerable as well as the spinal cord. Neurologic deficit can also result from vascular injury with subsequent cerebral ischemia. Complete cord injury can result in spinal (neurogenic) shock with paraplegia, bradycardia, and hypotension. Brown-Séquard syndrome (hemisection of the spinal cord) arises with ipsilateral hemiplegia and contralateral sensory deficit. Brachial plexus, spinal root, and peripheral nerve injuries have been reported after neck trauma and can result in both sensory and motor deficits. Phrenic nerve injury may compromise spontaneous respiration by causing ipsilateral diaphragmatic paralysis. Hoarseness can result from direct laryngeal trauma, but injury to the recurrent laryngeal nerve, which branches off the vagus nerve (cranial nerve X), should also be suspected, with vocal cord paralysis on the affected side.

Thoracic Duct, Glandular, and Retropharyngeal Injuries

Other, less common injuries have been reported in association with neck trauma with variable signs and symptoms. Thoracic duct injuries are less likely to be apparent initially and are frequently diagnosed intraoperatively or after development of a chylothorax. Glandular wounds, including those of the thyroid, parathyroid, and salivary glands, are reported rarely. Retropharyngeal hematomas are also extremely rare but can result in life-threatening airway compromise.[1,86]

Near Hanging and Strangulation

Epidemiology

Hanging and strangulation represent the second most common form of suicide in the United States after firearm use.[87] The number of deaths from suicidal hanging has been rising.[88] Approximately 5330 strangulation deaths occur annually in the United States.[89]

The terms *hanging* and *strangulation* are often used interchangeably, with hanging being a subset of strangulation. Hanging is categorized as judicial (complete hanging) or nonjudicial (incomplete hanging). *Complete hanging* refers to the presence of a ligature around the victim's neck and a subsequent drop resulting in the victim being freely suspended. In contrast, *incomplete hanging* refers to the partial suspension of the victim's body with some part still in contact with the ground. Judicial hanging victims classically fall at least the height of their body, whereas incomplete hanging is more likely to be seen in confined spaces (e.g., homes, jail cells), where a fall from height resulting in full body suspension is less possible. On the basis of the location of the ligature knot, hanging is further divided into atypical and typical categories. *Typical hanging* refers to the knot being midline directly under the occiput, which leads to a higher likelihood of complete arterial occlusion. *Atypical hanging* refers to all other knot placements.[90]

Manual strangulation and *ligature strangulation* refer to external compression of the neck, usually by hands or ligature, but independent of the weight of the victim. *Postural strangulation*, generally seen in the younger pediatric population, refers to death sustained by the victim's body weight compressing the anterior neck against a firm object.[90]

Pathophysiology

Judicial hanging with adequate fall distance results in forceful distraction of the head from the neck and body. This classically leads to high cervical fractures, complete cord transection, and death.[91] Attempted-suicide hangings frequently occur at inadequate height and therefore tend to mimic nonjudicial strangulation. Cervical fractures in the latter group are rare, and no fractures have been reported in near-hanging victims.[91,92] In essentially all types of nonjudicial strangulation, the ligature or external force initially applied causes venous congestion with stasis of cerebral blood flow leading to unconsciousness. Once the person is limp, the ligature or external force can tighten further, leading to complete arterial occlusion and ultimately to brain injury or death. Vagal reflexes resulting from pressure on the carotid body may contribute to fatal dysrhythmias, as may increased sympathetic tone from pericarotid sinus pressure. Surprisingly, compression of the airway does not play as significant a role in incomplete hanging as vascular occlusion.[90]

Pulmonary sequelae are frequently seen in near-hanging victims and include pulmonary edema, bronchopneumonia, and adult respiratory distress syndrome (ARDS).[93] These complications are responsible for most in-hospital deaths after near hanging. Pulmonary edema occurs from one of two mechanisms. *Neurogenic* pulmonary edema results from centrally mediated, massive sympathetic discharge. Because it is more often seen in association with serious brain injury, neurogenic pulmonary edema has poor prognostic implications. *Postobstructive* pulmonary edema is generally associated with a better neurologic outcome. It is initiated by marked negative intrapleural pressure, which is generated by forceful inspiratory effort against an extrathoracic obstruction. When the obstruction is removed, the onset of pulmonary edema can be rapid and lead to ARDS.[90,94]

Clinical Features

External trauma may or may not be evident, depending on the mechanism of injury. If present, ligature marks appear as indentations around the neck, ranging from mild erythema to leather-like grooves following the course of the ligature. Fingernail scratches, abrasions, and contusions are variably present on the external neck as well. *Tardieu's spots* are highly correlated with asphyxial deaths; these petechial hemorrhages are seen in the conjunctiva, mucous membranes, and skin cephalad to the ligature marks. They occur when the venous pressure rises in response to ligature tightening. Laryngeal injuries are reported in near-hanging victims. Thyroid cartilage fractures are seen in approximately 50% of all nonjudicial hanging deaths, and hyoid bone fractures occur in 20%. Cricoid cartilage fractures are rarely reported. Manual strangulation is responsible for the majority of fractures.[90] Resulting laryngeal fractures are rarely clinically significant in survivors, and standard airway techniques are recommended.

Vascular injury leading to delayed neurologic sequelae after near hanging is rare but reported. It most often results from carotid intimal dissection or thrombus formation, resulting in partial or complete vascular occlusion or embolism.[92] Carotid vascular studies should be considered in patients with unexplained focal or global neurologic deficits.[95]

Management

Frequently, ventilatory support is indicated to maintain adequate oxygenation and ventilation in the comatose patient. The addition of positive end-expiratory pressure is often necessary, especially when pulmonary edema or ARDS develops.[90] Aggressive resuscitation is warranted in the unconscious patient; the initial Glasgow Coma Scale score is generally not predictive of outcome.[96] The altered or comatose patient should be assumed to have cerebral edema with elevated intracranial pressure, and cerebral resuscitation measures need to be actively initiated using standard technique.

Definitive studies providing guidelines on the management of hypoxic brain injury specifically related to near-hanging or strangulation injuries are lacking. Therefore, prudent cerebral protection measures may be interpreted from other data on this topic (and are discussed in detail in Chapter 6).

KEY CONCEPTS

- Neck trauma results from one of three major mechanisms: blunt injury, penetrating injury, or near-hanging/strangulation.
- The leading cause of *immediate* death after neck trauma is exsanguination secondary to vascular injury.
- The leading cause of *delayed* death after neck trauma is esophageal injury. These wounds are rare, frequently insidious, and associated with high mortality rates if missed.
- Neck wounds should never be probed because massive hemorrhage or air embolus can ensue.
- Cervical collars can obscure impending airway disasters (e.g., expanding hematomas) and other signs suggestive of injury if not removed periodically to allow serial examinations.
- Unless a contraindication exists, orotracheal rapid sequence intubation is safe and effective in the hands of an experienced intubator.
- Vascular injuries resulting from blunt trauma represent some of the most underreported injuries because of their propensity for delayed neurologic sequelae.
- Ongoing debate exists as to whether physical examination is sensitive at detecting visceral or vascular injury, and the role of angiography versus serial examination is unresolved.
- Suspicion of venous air embolism should prompt direct wound pressure, occlusive dressings, Trendelenburg's position, and, if the patient is in cardiopulmonary arrest, aspiration of air from the right side of the heart.
- Transcervical gunshot wounds are a subset of injuries with a twofold increased incidence of visceral-vascular injuries compared with injuries that do not cross the midline.
- All near-hanging or strangulation patients who are comatose or have altered consciousness may have elevated intracranial pressure, and appropriate cerebral resuscitation measures should be initiated.
- The leading cause of in-hospital death in this population is pulmonary complications (pneumonia, pulmonary edema, ARDS).

REFERENCES

1. Thal ER, Meyer DM: Penetrating neck trauma. *Curr Probl Surg* 29:10, 1992.
2. Bond SJ, Schnier GC, Miller FB: Air-powered guns: Too much firepower to be a toy. *J Trauma* 4:674, 1996.
3. Biffl WL, et al: Selective management of penetrating neck trauma based on cervical level of injury. *Am J Surg* 174:678, 1997.
4. Asensio JA, et al: Management of penetrating neck injuries: The controversy surrounding zone II injuries. *Surg Clin North Am* 71:267, 1991.
5. Kendall JL, Anglin D, Demetriades D: Penetrating neck trauma. *Emerg Med Clin North Am* 16:85, 1998.
6. Cogbill TH, et al: The spectrum of blunt injury to the carotid artery: A multicenter perspective. *J Trauma* 37:473, 1994.
7. McConnell DB, Trunkey DD: Management of penetrating trauma to the neck. *Adv Surg* 27:97, 1994.
8. Hollinshead WH: *Textbook of Anatomy,* 4th ed. Philadelphia, Harper & Row, 1985.
9. Apfelstaedt JP, Muller R: Results of mandatory exploration for penetrating neck trauma. *World J Surg* 18:917, 1994.

10. Demetriades D, et al: Evaluation of penetrating injuries of the neck: Prospective study of 223 patients. *World J Surg* 21:41, 1997.

11. Rivers SP, et al: Limited role of arteriography in penetrating neck trauma. *J Vasc Surg* 8:112, 1988.

12. Rose SC, Moore EE: Trauma angiography: The use of clinical findings to improve patient selection and case preparation. *J Trauma* 28:240, 1988.

13. Velmahos GC, et al: Selective surgical management in penetrating neck injuries. *Can J Surg* 37:487, 1994.

14. Sclafani SJ, et al: The role of angiography in penetrating neck trauma. *J Trauma* 31:557, 1991.

15. Walsh MS: The management of penetrating injuries of the anterior triangle of the neck. *Injury* 25:393, 1994.

16. Demetriades D, et al: Penetrating injuries of the neck in patients in stable condition. *Arch Surg* 130:971, 1995.

17. Mandavia DP, Qualls S, Rokos I: Emergency airway management in penetrating neck injury. *Ann Emerg Med* 35:221, 2000.

18. Holley J, Jorden RC: Airway management in patients with unstable cervical spine fractures. *Ann Emerg Med* 18:1237, 1989.

19. Walls RM: Airway management. *Emerg Med Clin North Am* 11:53, 1993.

20. Wright SW, Robinson GG, Wright MB: Cervical spine injuries in blunt trauma patients requiring emergent endotracheal intubation. *Am J Emerg Med* 10:104, 1992.

21. Drummond GB: Comparison of sedation with midazolam and ketamine: Effects on airway muscle activity. *Br J Anaesth* 76:663, 1996.

22. Eggen JT, Jorden RC: Airway management, penetrating neck trauma. *J Emerg Med* 11:381, 1993.

23. Li J, et al: Complications of emergency intubation with and without paralysis. *Am J Emerg Med* 17:141, 1999.

24. Blanda M, Gallo UE: Emergency airway management. *Emerg Med Clin North Am* 21:1, 2003.

25. Butler KH: Management of the difficult airway: Alternative airway techniques and adjuncts. *Emerg Med Clin North Am* 21:259, 2003.

26. American College of Surgeons: *Advanced Trauma Life Support Instructor Manual.* Chicago, The College, 1984.

27. Ligier B, et al: The role of anesthetic induction agents and neuromuscular blockage in the endotracheal intubation of trauma victims. *Surg Gynecol Obstet* 173:477, 1991.

28. O'Brien JD, et al: Airway management of aeromedically transported trauma patients. *J Emerg Med* 2:49, 1988.

29. Shearer VE, Giesecke AH: Airway management for patients with penetrating neck trauma: A retrospective study. *Anesth Analg* 77:1135, 1993.

30. Holmes JF, et al: Comparison of 2 cricothyrotomy techniques: Standard method versus rapid 4-step technique. *Ann Emerg Med* 32:442, 1998.

31. Spaite DW, Joseph M: Prehospital cricothyrotomy: An investigation of indications, technique, complications, and patient outcome. *Ann Emerg Med* 19:279, 1990.

32. Toye FJ, Weinstein JD: Clinical experience with percutaneous tracheostomy and cricothyroidotomy in 100 patients. *J Trauma* 26:1034, 1986.

33. Jorden RC: Percutaneous transtracheal ventilation. *Emerg Med Clin North Am* 6:745, 1988.

34. Senthuran S, Lim S, Gunning KE: Life-threatening airway obstruction caused by a retropharyngeal haematoma. *Anaesthesia* 54:674, 1999.

35. McLaughlin J, Iserson KV: Emergency pediatric tracheostomy: A usable technique and model for instruction. *Ann Emerg Med* 15:463, 1986.

36. Hammargren Y, Clinton JE, Ruiz E: A standard comparison of esophageal obturator airway and endotracheal tube ventilation in cardiac arrest. *Ann Emerg Med* 14:953, 1985.

37. Barriot P, Riou B: Retrograde technique for tracheal intubation in the trauma patient. *Crit Care Med* 16:712, 1988.

38. Benumof JL: Laryngeal mask airway and the ASA difficult airway algorithm. *Anesthesiology* 84:686, 1996.

39. Proctor MR: Spinal cord injury. *Crit Care Med* 30(Suppl): S489, 2002.

40. Litman RS, et al: Developmental changes of laryngeal dimensions in unparalyzed, sedated children. *Anesthesiology* 98:41, 2003.

41. Gilmore BB, Mickelson SA: Pediatric tracheostomy. *Otolaryngol Clin North Am* 19:141, 1986.

42. Criswell JC, Parr MJ, Nolan JP: Emergency airway management in patients with cervical spine injuries. *Anaesthesia* 49:900, 1994.

43. Rhee KJ, et al: Oral intubation in the multiply injured patient: The risk of exacerbating spinal cord damage. *Ann Emerg Med* 19:511, 1990.

44. Knopp RK: The safety of orotracheal intubation in patients with suspected cervical-spine injury [editorial]. *Ann Emerg Med* 19:603, 1990.

45. Fogelman ML, Steward RD: Penetrating wounds of the neck. *Am J Surg* 91:581, 1956.

46. McConnell DB, Trunkey DD: Management of penetrating trauma to the neck. *Adv Surg* 27:97, 1994.

47. Wood J, Fabian TC, Mangiante EC: Penetrating trauma of the neck. *J Trauma* 29:602, 1989.

48. Bishara RA, et al: The necessity of mandatory exploration of penetrating zone II neck injuries. *Surgery* 100:655, 1986.

49. Demetriades D, et al: Transcervical gunshot injuries: Mandatory operation is not necessary. *J Trauma* 40:758, 1996.

50. Hirschberg A, et al: Transcervical gunshot injuries. *Am J Surg* 167:309, 1994.

51. Feliciano DV, et al: Combined tracheoesophageal injuries. *Am J Surg* 150:710, 1985.

52. Irish JC, et al: Penetrating and blunt neck trauma: 10-year review of a Canadian experience. *J Crit Care* 40:33, 1997.

53. Asensio JA, et al: Penetrating esophageal injuries: Time interval of safety for preoperative evaluation—how long is safe? *J Trauma* 43:319, 1997.

54. Niezgoda JA, McMenamin P, Graeber GM: Pharyngoesophageal perforation after blunt neck trauma. *Ann Thorac Surg* 50:615, 1990.

55. Demetriades D, et al: Complex problems in penetrating neck trauma. *Surg Clin North Am* 76:661, 1996.

56. Weigelt JA, et al: Diagnosis of penetrating cervical esophageal injuries. *Am J Surg* 154:619, 1987.

57. Asensio JA, et al: Penetrating esophageal injuries: Multicenter study of the American Association for the Surgery of Trauma. *J Trauma* 50:289, 2001

58. Armstrong WB, Detar TR, Stanley RB: Diagnosis and management of external penetrating cervical esophageal injuries. *Ann Otol Rhinol Laryngol* 103:863, 1994.

59. Gonzalez RP, et al: Penetrating zone II neck injury: Does dynamic computed tomographic scan contribute to the diagnostic sensitivity of physical examination for surgically significant injury? A prospective blinded study. *J Trauma* 54:61, 2003.

60. Mazolewski PJ, et al: Computed tomographic scan can be used for surgical decision making in zone II penetrating neck injuries. *J Trauma* 51:315, 2001.

61. Fuhrman GM, Stieg FH, Buerk CA: Blunt laryngeal trauma: Classification and management protocol. *J Trauma* 30:87, 1990.

62. Offiah CJ, Endres D: Isolated laryngotracheal separation following blunt trauma to the neck. *J Laryngol Otol* 111:1079, 1997.

63. Kurien M, Zachariah N: External laryngotracheal trauma in children. *Otorhinolaryngology* 49:115, 1999.

64. Kadish H, Schunk J, Woodward GA: Blunt pediatric laryngotracheal trauma: Case reports and review of the literature. *Am J Emerg Med* 12:207, 1994.

65. Vassiliu P, et al: Aerodigestive injuries of the neck. *Am Surg* 67:75, 2001.

66. Jacobs I, et al: Hypopharyngeal perforation after blunt neck trauma: Case report and review of the literature. *J Trauma* 46:957, 1999.

67. Brent JP, Silver JR, Porubsky ES: Acute laryngeal trauma: A review of 77 patients. *Otolaryngol Head Neck Surg* 109:441, 1993.

68. Nanda A, et al: Management of carotid artery injuries: Louisiana State University Shreveport experience. *Surg Neurol* 59:184, 2003.

69. Rao PM, et al: Cervical vascular injuries: A trauma center experience. *Surgery* 114:527, 1993.

70. Colella JJ, Diamond DL: Blunt carotid injuries: Reassessing the role of anticoagulation. *Am Surg* 62:212, 1996.

71. Fabian TC, et al: Blunt carotid injury: Importance of early diagnosis and anticoagulant therapy. *Ann Surg* 223:514, 1996.

72. Sanzone AG, Torres H, Doundoulakis SH: Blunt trauma to the carotid arteries. *Am J Emerg Med* 13:327, 1995.

73. Eachempati SR, et al: Blunt vascular injuries of the head and neck: Is heparization necessary? *J Trauma* 45:997, 1998.

74. Frykberg ER, Vines FS, Alexander RH: The natural history of clinically occult arterial injuries: A prospective evaluation. *J Trauma* 29:577, 1989.

75. DiPerna CA, et al: Clinical importance of the "seat belt sign" in blunt trauma to the neck. *Am Surg* 68:441, 2002.

76. Brennan JA, Meyers AD, Jafek BW: Penetrating neck trauma: A 5-year review of the literature, 1983-1988. *Am J Otolaryngol* 11:191, 1990.

77. Menawat SS, et al: Are arteriograms necessary in penetrating zone II neck injuries? *J Vasc Surg* 16:397, 1992.

78. Bilbao R, Amoros S, Murube J: Horner syndrome as an isolated manifestation of an intrapetrous internal carotid artery dissection. *Am J Ophthalmol* 123:562, 1997.

79. Fry WR, et al: Duplex scanning replaces arteriography and operative exploration in the diagnosis of potential cervical vascular injury. *Am J Surg* 168:693, 1994.

80. Hessel SJ, Adams DF, Abrams HL: Complications of angiography. *Radiology* 138:273, 1981.

81. Ginzburg E, et al: The use of duplex ultrasonography in penetrating neck trauma. *Arch Surg* 31:691, 1996.

82. McKevitt EC, et al: Blunt vascular neck injuries: Diagnosis and outcomes of extracranial vessel injury. *J Trauma* 53:472, 2002.

83. Bok AP, Peter JC: Carotid and vertebral artery occlusion after blunt cervical injury: The role of MR angiography in early diagnosis. *J Trauma* 40:968, 1996.

84. Demetriades D, et al: Carotid artery injuries: Experience with 124 cases. *J Trauma* 29:91, 1989.

85. Adams VI, Hirsch CS: Venous air embolism from head and neck wounds. *Arch Pathol Lab Med* 113:498, 1989.

86. Kaufman HJ, Ciraulo DL, Burns RP: Traumatic fracture of the hyoid bone: Three case presentations of cardiorespiratory compromise secondary to missed diagnosis. *Am Surg* 65:877, 1999.

87. Pesola GR, Westfal RE: Hanging-induced status epilepticus. *Am J Emerg Med* 17:38, 1999.

88. Suicide among children, adolescents, and young adults— United States, 1980-1992. *JAMA* 274:451, 1995.

89. National Safety Council: *Injury Facts.* Itasca, Ill, The Council, 1999.

90. Kaki A, Crosby ET, Lui AC: Airway and respiratory management following non-lethal hanging. *Can J Anaesth* 44:445, 1997.

91. Vander Krol L, Wolfe R: The emergency department management of near-hanging victims. *J Emerg Med* 12:285, 1994.

92. Maier W, et al: Diagnostic and therapeutic management of bilateral carotid artery occlusion caused by near-suicide hanging. *Ann Otol Rhinol Laryngol* 108:189, 1999.

93. Kaki A, Crosby ET, Lui C: Airway and respiratory management following non-lethal hanging. *Can J Anaesth* 44:445, 1997.

94. Murphy PG, et al: Adult respiratory distress syndrome after attempted strangulation. *Br J Anaesth* 70:583, 1993.

95. Ramadian F, et al: Carotid artery trauma: A review of contemporary trauma center experiences. *J Vasc Surg* 21:46, 1995.

96. Wahlen BM, Thierbach AR: Near-hanging. *Eur J Emerg Med* 9:348, 2002.

CHAPTER

42 Thoracic Trauma

Marc Eckstein and Sean Henderson

PERSPECTIVE: EPIDEMIOLOGY

Thoracic injury directly causes 20% to 25% of deaths resulting from trauma, accounting for more than 16,000 deaths annually in the United States. The most common cause of injuries leading to accidental deaths in the United States is motor vehicle crash (MVC), in which immediate deaths are often due to a rupture of the myocardial wall or the thoracic aorta. Early deaths (within the first 30 minutes to 3 hours) resulting from thoracic trauma are often preventable. Causes of these early deaths include tension pneumothorax, cardiac tamponade, airway obstruction, and continued uncontrolled hemorrhage. Because these problems are often reversible or may be temporized nonoperatively, it is vital that emergency physicians be thoroughly familiar with the pathophysiology, symptoms, and treatment.

Injuries to the lung parenchyma are reported to occur in 25% of patients and include contusion, laceration, and hematoma. Hemothorax and pneumothorax also are common injuries in patients with thoracic trauma. Treatment of these injuries has changed primarily because of advances in diagnostic imaging techniques and an increased understanding of the pathophysiology.

CHEST WALL INJURY

Epidemiology

Among victims sustaining thoracic trauma, approximately 50% have chest wall injury: 10% minor, 35% major, and 5% flail chest injuries.[1] Chest wall injuries are not always obvious and can be overlooked easily during the initial evaluation.

Anatomy and Pathophysiology

An intact chest wall is necessary for normal ventilation. Outward expansion of the thorax by the respiratory muscles with descent of the diaphragm creates negative intrathoracic pressure. This negative pressure causes passive air entry into the lungs during inspiration. Chest trauma, particularly blunt trauma, can severely disturb the physiology of respiration. Most individuals have substantial respiratory reserve and can tolerate significant chest wall injury with adequate support.

Clinical Features

Elderly patients and patients with preexisting pulmonary disease sometimes are unable to compensate for even minor chest wall trauma and require closer attention. It is important to disrobe the patient completely and observe the respiratory rate, adequacy of tidal volume, and respiratory effort. Many chest wall injuries may be detected only by careful palpation of the chest wall, noting any areas of deformity, tenderness, or crepitus.

Rib Fracture

Epidemiology

Simple rib fractures are the most common form of significant chest injury, accounting for more than half of cases of nonpenetrating trauma.[1] The importance of this injury is not the fracture itself, but the associated potential complications, particularly pneumothorax or hemothorax.

Anatomy and Pathophysiology

Ribs usually break at the point of impact or at the posterior angle, which is structurally the weakest area. The fourth through ninth ribs are most commonly involved. Ribs 1 to 3 are relatively protected, and ribs 9 to 12 are more mobile at the anterior end; this confers the "high" and "low" ribs' relative resistance to fracture. Fractures occur more commonly in adults than in children, and this is attributed to the relative inelasticity of the chest wall in adults compared with the more compliant chest wall in children.

The true danger of rib fracture involves not the rib itself, but the potential for penetrating injury to the pleura, lung, liver, or spleen. Fractures of the 9th, 10th, or 11th ribs suggest an associated intra-abdominal injury. Patients with right-sided rib fractures are almost three times more likely to have a hepatic injury, and

patients with left-sided rib fractures are almost four times more likely to have a splenic injury.[2] Fractures of ribs one to three may indicate severe intrathoracic injury. The presence of two or more rib fractures at any level is associated with a higher incidence of internal injuries. Elderly patients with multiple rib fractures have been found to have a fivefold increased incidence of mortality compared with patients younger than 65 years old.[3,4] To prevent a minor injury from developing into a serious complication, rib fractures should be diagnosed rapidly and treated expectantly.

Clinical Features

The diagnosis of a rib fracture can be suspected clinically with tenderness, bony crepitus, ecchymosis, and muscle spasm over the rib being the most common findings. Also, bimanual compression of the thoracic cage remote from the site of injury usually produces pain at the site of fracture.

Diagnostic Strategies

Although clinical impression and physical findings are sensitive, they are not specific and are unreliable in making an accurate diagnosis. Chest x-rays often do not show the presence of rib fractures, but are of greatest value in disclosing significant intrathoracic and mediastinal injuries.[5] Still, x-ray examination is the most effective way to diagnose rib fracture, with the upright posteroanterior chest radiograph having the highest yield in detecting fractures or their complications.[6] Rib series, expiratory, oblique, and coned-down views should not be used routinely. They may be useful if there is suspicion of high (1 to 3) or low (9 to 12) rib fractures for multiple rib fractures, especially in elderly patients (Box 42-1).

Fractures of the first or second ribs used to be called the "hallmark of severe chest trauma." Routine arteriography was recommended in the past to rule out the possibility of aortic injury whenever the first or second rib was fractured because these ribs are short and broad and protected by other parts of the musculoskeletal system, and because the brachial plexus, great vessels, and lungs are in close proximity (Figures 42-1 and 42-2). Numerous studies have shown, however, that unless there is direct evidence of vascular or neurologic trauma, fracture of either or both of the first two ribs is not associated with an increase in morbidity or mortality, and mandatory arteriography is not warranted.[7] Isolated first rib fracture is associated with major vascular injury in only 3% of cases. When first rib fracture

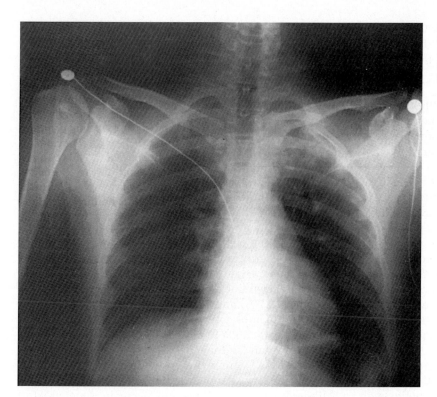

Figure 42-1. First rib fracture *(right)* and displaced second rib fracture *(left)*. Alveolar infiltrate in the left upper lobe is compatible with a pulmonary contusion. There is a lack of clarity of superior mediastinal silhouette.

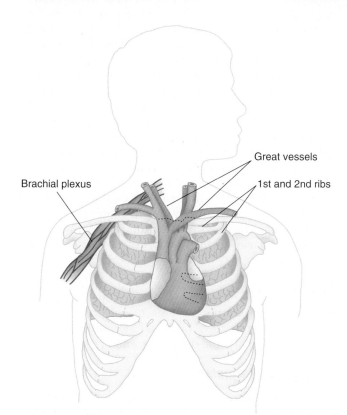

Figure 42-2. Relation of brachial plexus, great vessels, heart, and lungs to the first three ribs.

Brachial plexus

Great vessels

1st and 2nd ribs

occurs in association with major head, thoracic, abdominal, or long bone injury, the incidence of major vascular injury increases to 24%.[7] First and second rib fractures are sometimes difficult to appreciate on routine chest radiographs and are often easier to visualize on the standard anteroposterior cervical spine radiograph. A distinction should be made, however, between the relatively benign isolated first rib fracture and its presence with other rib fractures. When the two classes are evaluated separately, there is a markedly different outcome. The mortality of an isolated first rib fracture is only 1.5%, but when it is associated with other rib fractures, there is a 10-fold increase in mortality.

Helical computed tomography (CT) scans have largely replaced arteriography for the diagnosis of major vascular injuries in the chest and have the added advantage of diagnosing other serious nonvascular injuries. Patients with first or second rib fractures who also have suspected intrathoracic injuries, clinical evidence of distal vascular insufficiency, a widened mediastinum on plain films, large hemothorax or apical hematoma, intercostal artery injury, brachial plexus injury, or significant displacement of the fracture should undergo contrast-enhanced helical chest CT.[8,9]

Clinical Course

Most rib fractures heal uneventfully within 3 to 6 weeks, and patients should expect a gradual decrease in their discomfort during this period. Analgesics are usually necessary during the first 1 to 2 weeks. In addition to the complications associated with hemopneumothorax, atelectasis, and pneumonia, rib fractures can result in posttraumatic neuroma or costochondral separation. These unusual complications are painful and heal slowly.

Management

Treatment of patients with acute rib fractures is based on adequate pain relief and the maintenance of pulmonary function. Oral pain medications are usually sufficient for young and healthy patients. Continuing daily activities and deep breathing should be stressed to ensure ventilation and to prevent atelectasis. For this reason, pain relief should be truly effective, or patients do not maintain activity. Binders, belts, and other restrictive devices should not be used; although they can decrease pain, they also promote hypoventilation with subsequent atelectasis and pneumonia. Older patients are likely to require narcotic preparations, but care should be taken to avoid oversedation. If there is a question about the older patient's ability to cough, breathe deeply, and maintain activity, and particularly if two or more ribs are fractured, it is preferable to admit the patient to the hospital for aggressive pulmonary therapy. Elderly patients with displaced rib fractures may be at higher risk for delayed and profound intercostal artery bleeding, and serial hemoglobin measurements should be done during observation of these patients. As in penetrating chest trauma, patients with displaced rib fractures should be observed for the occurrence of delayed pneumothorax with a repeat chest x-ray at 3 hours.

The presence of more than one rib fracture is associated with significant morbidity and mortality. Intercostal nerve blocks with a long-acting anesthetic, such as bupivacaine with epinephrine, may relieve symptoms for 12 hours with excellent results. This regimen consists of administering 1% or 2% lidocaine or 0.25% bupivacaine along the inferior rib margin several centimeters posterior to the site of the fracture. One rib above and one rib below the most superior and inferior fractured rib also must be blocked to obtain optimal analgesia. An alternative for hospitalized patients is thoracic epidural analgesia.[10]

Sternal Fracture

Epidemiology

Sternal fractures and dislocations are caused primarily by anterior blunt chest trauma, usually from an MVC when the chest strikes the steering wheel. Risk factors for sternal fracture from blunt trauma include types of vehicular passenger restraint systems and patient age. Restrained passengers are more likely than unrestrained passengers to sustain a sternal fracture. The rate of occurrence of sternal fractures has increased threefold since the use of across-the-shoulder seat belts became widespread. The deployment of an air bag during an MVC would be expected to diminish the risk of sternal fracture, although this has not been studied specifically.

Anatomy and Pathophysiology

Sternal fracture usually results from the diagonal strap of a seat belt restraining the upper part of the sternum. During rapid deceleration from a frontal impact, the forward thrust of the body against the fixed seat belt across the sternum results in a fracture at that location. The location of the sternal fracture varies depending on the position of the belt, patient size, magnitude of the impact, and vector of the forces.

Similarly, depending on patient age, the likelihood of sternal fracure varies. In general, sternal fractures are more common in older patients than in younger patients and slightly more common in women than in men. It is believed that the more elastic and pliable chest wall of younger people allows more efficient transmission of kinetic energy to the underlying mediastinum. Although skeletal injury is less likely to occur in younger patients, damage to mediastinal soft tissue structures underneath is greater. In older patients, the energy of impact is dissipated in the sternum, resulting in fewer intrathoracic injuries.

The natural history of sternal fractures is contrary to intuition. It had been thought that the magnitude of the forces required to fracture the sternum must be associated with significant trauma to the mediastinal structures. More recent reports suggest, however, that isolated sternal fractures are relatively benign, with low mortality (0.7%) and low intrathoracic morbidity.[11,12]

Cardiac complications, such as myocardial contusion, occur in 1.5% to 6% of cases. There is no association between sternal fracture and blunt traumatic aortic injury.[11] Spinal fractures are seen in less than 10% of the cases, and rib fractures are seen in 21%.[13] Although sternal fractures may occur in the context of major blunt chest trauma, the presence of a sternal fracture does not imply other major life-threatening conditions. The presence of associated mediastinal injuries should be considered, however.

The accumulation of blood in the mediastinum (mediastinal hematoma) may be due to injury of the proximal great vessels or, less commonly, injury to the esophagus. Thoracic spinal fractures may produce apparent mediastinal widening secondary to paraspinal bleeding. Whether or not related to aortic injuries, mediastinal hematoma can be life-threatening. The dual problems of acute blood loss and sudden alterations in cardiopulmonary physiology can result in hemodynamic deterioration. In addition to circulatory collapse from exsanguination, mediastinal hematomas can cause death from compression of adjacent structures.

Clinical Features

Sternal fractures typically present with anterior chest pain, point tenderness over the sternum, soft tissue swelling, and palpable deformity and crepitus.

Diagnostic Strategies

Most sternal fractures are transverse, and a lateral radiographic view is diagnostic. These fractures are often missed radiographically, however, because a lateral plain chest film usually is not obtained during the initial trauma evaluation. Displaced sternal fractures usually are seen easily on a lateral radiograph; however, undisplaced fractures may be subtle. Associated mediastinal injuries are best diagnosed by CT of the chest. Because of the close proximity of the anterior myocardium to the sternum, patients with sternal fracture should be screened for myocardial contusion with electrocardiogram (ECG) and serum troponin

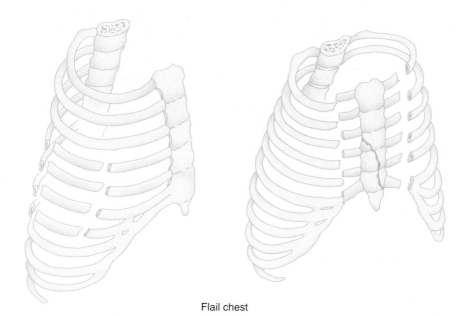

Flail chest

level. If the ECG and troponin level are normal, there is a low probability of a clinically significant myocardial contusion.

Management

Management consists of providing adequate analgesia.[11] In the absence of associated injuries, patients with isolated sternal fractures who can achieve adequate pain control with oral medications can be discharged home safely.

Costochondral Separation

Costochondral separation also may result from blunt anterior chest trauma. The signs and symptoms are similar to those of rib fracture, but because of the poor vascularity of healing cartilage, pain may persist for many weeks. The chest film is usually normal, but there may be a snapping sensation with deep respiration. Similar to patients with sternal fracture, admission to rule out cardiac contusion should be considered in these patients. Outpatient management of these patients is similar to that of patients with rib fractures. Flail chest also can occur from massive costochondral separation, but this is rare.

Flail Chest

Epidemiology

Flail chest is a common injury, found in almost one third of a large series of major trauma patients with major chest injuries.

Anatomy and Pathophysiology

Flail chest results when three or more adjacent ribs are fractured at two points, allowing a freely moving segment of the chest wall to move in paradoxical motion (Figure 42-3). Flail chest is one of the most commonly overlooked injuries resulting from blunt chest trauma. Because of its common association with pulmonary contusion, it is also one of the most serious chest wall injuries.

The physiology of respiration is affected adversely in many ways by flail chest. The paradoxical motion of the chest wall is the hallmark of this condition, with the flail segment paradoxically moving inward with inspiration and outward with expiration. Underlying pulmonary contusion now is considered to be the major cause of respiratory insufficiency with flail chest. In addition, the pain of the injury causes muscular splinting with resultant atelectasis and hypoxemia.

Clinical Features

Flail chest usually is diagnosed by physical examination. This examination requires exposure of the patient's thorax and examination of the chest wall for paradoxical motion. Pain, tenderness, and crepitus can direct the examiner. In addition, the flail segment sometimes can be seen to move separately and in an opposite direction from the rest of the thoracic cage during the respiratory cycle. Endotracheal intubation and positive-pressure ventilation internally splint the chest wall, making the flail segment difficult to detect on physical examination.

Diagnostic Strategies

Multiple rib fractures usually can be identified on chest films. The presence of multiple contiguous rib fractures (i.e., a potential flail segment) on chest x-ray should prompt close re-examination of the chest wall because paradoxical motion of the chest may be clinically subtle. The diagnosis of flail chest is frequently missed; 30% of cases are not appreciated within the first 6 hours of admission.[14,15] CT is much more accurate than plain films in detecting the presence and extent of underlying injury and contusion to the lung parenchyma; in some centers, CT is used for all patients with major chest trauma. The flail segment itself is often more apparent on chest x-ray than on CT scan, however, and all patients with significant blunt chest trauma should undergo routine chest x-ray to identify life-threatening injuries (e.g., pneumothorax) before undergoing CT.

Management

Oxygen should be administered in the field, cardiac and oximetry monitors should be applied if available, and the patient should be observed for signs of an associated injury, such as tension pneumothorax. Because many different physiologic mechanisms have been implicated in flail chest, there is no true consensus about hospital treatment. The cornerstones of therapy include aggressive pulmonary physiotherapy, effective analgesia, selective use of endotracheal intubation and mechanical ventilation, and close observation for respiratory compromise. Prehospital or emergency department stabilization of the flail segment, by positioning the patient with the injured side down or placing a sandbag on the affected segments, has been abandoned. These interventions actually inhibit expansion of the chest and increase atelectasis of the injured lung.

Respiratory decompensation is the primary indication for endotracheal intubation and mechanical ventilation for patients with flail chest. Obvious problems, such as hemopneumothorax, should be managed before intubation and ventilation are presumed necessary. In an awake and cooperative patient, continuous positive airway pressure by mask may obviate the need for intubation. Generally the most conservative methods for maintaining adequate oxygenation and preventing complications should be used.

Patients without respiratory compromise generally do well without ventilatory assistance. Several studies have found that patients treated with intercostal nerve blocks or high segmental epidural analgesia, oxygen, intensive chest physiotherapy, and careful fluid management have shorter hospital courses, fewer complications, and lower mortality rates than patients who require intubation.[16] Avoidance of endotracheal intubation, particularly prolonged intubation, is important in preventing pulmonary morbidity because intubation increases the risk of pneumonia.[17] Despite efforts to maintain ventilation with less invasive means, many patients with pulmonary contusion and flail chest ultimately need to be intubated and ventilated until the contusion shows signs of resolving. Box 42-2 lists some of the generally accepted indications for intubating patients with flail chest and placing them on positive-pressure ventilation.[18] Evidence also suggests that early operative internal fixation of the flail segment resulted in a speedier recovery, decreased complications, and better ultimate cosmetic and functional results and was cost-effective.[19] This is particularly true for patients with flail chest and no pulmonary contusion.[20]

The mortality rate associated with flail chest is 8% to 35% and is directly related to the underlying and associated injuries.[21] Patients who recover may develop

---

BOX 42-2. Indications for Treatment of Flail Chest with Mechanical Ventilation

Respiratory failure manifested by one or more of the following criteria:
Clinical signs of respiratory fatigue
Respiratory rate >35/min or <8/min
PaO_2 <60 mm Hg at FIO_2 ≥0.5
$PaCO_2$ >55 mm Hg at FIO_2 ≥0.5
Alveolar-arterial oxygen gradient >450
Clinical evidence of severe shock
Associated severe head injury with lack of airway control or need to ventilate
Severe associated injury requiring surgery

PaO_2, partial arterial oxygen tension; FIO_2; fraction of inspired oxygen; $PaCO_2$, partial arterial carbon dioxide tension.

---

long-term disability with dyspnea, chronic thoracic pain, and exercise intolerance.

Nonpenetrating Ballistic Injury

Epidemiology

Many law enforcement officers, emergency medical services personnel, and private security guards now don lightweight synthetic body armor for protection against gunshot injury. There also have been numerous reports of armed robbers donning such vests in anticipation of exchanging gunfire with police or security personnel.[22] These vests are "bullet resistant" rather than "bullet proof," depending on the weapon being used against them. They are composed of many different combinations of synthetic fibers, such as Kevlar.

Another type of nonpenetrating ballistic injury is caused by rubber bullets and beanbag shotgun shells. Rubber bullets have been used for many years by police agencies around the world for crowd dispersal and for nonlethal use of force. Beanbag shotgun shells are nylon bags filled with pellets, which are fired from a standard shotgun. Both of these projectiles have the potential to cause serious injury despite their classification as "nonlethal" or "less than lethal" use of force.[23]

Anatomy and Physiology

Although bullet penetration is usually prevented, the heart, liver, spleen, lung, and spinal cord are vulnerable to nonpenetrating ballistic injury that may occur despite innocent-appearing skin lesions.[24] Bullet-resistant vests are usually capable of stopping penetration by the low-velocity missiles of most handguns, but the kinetic energy of the missile can be transmitted through the layers of protective cloth or armor and produce significant injury without penetration.

Clinical Features

Patients who have been shot with "less than lethal projectiles" or with standard bullets while wearing bullet-resistant vests usually present with erythema, ecchymosis, and marked tenderness to palpation over the impacted area. There may be a projectile itself, such as the beanbag, still located in the wound. The area of tenderness and surrounding structures should be palpated carefully to identify any subcutaneous emphysema, crepitus, or bony step-offs.

Diagnostic Strategies

Plain film radiography should be used to identify intrathoracic injuries, any retained foreign bodies, and any fractures or cortical violation of bone. CT should be considered based on the type of projectile and the clinical examination and degree of tenderness and location of the wounds.

Management

It is recommended that all victims of nonpenetrating ballistic injury be observed closely, with consideration for overnight observation. Protective body armor has improved survival rates significantly and has decreased dramatically the need for surgical intervention in people protected by it. In addition, the less than lethal projectiles, such as rubber bullets and beanbag shotgun shells, have offered law enforcement an alternative to conventional weapons that are considered use of deadly force.

Traumatic Asphyxia

Anatomy and Physiology

Traumatic asphyxia is a rare syndrome caused by severe compression of the thorax by a heavy object causing a marked increase in thoracic and superior vena caval pressure, resulting in retrograde flow of blood from the right heart into the great veins of the head and neck. The vena cava and the large veins of the head and neck do not have valves and allow the transmission of pressure to the capillaries of the head and neck, which become engorged with blood.

Clinical Features

Traumatic asphyxia is characterized by a deep violet color of the skin of the head and neck, bilateral subconjunctival hemorrhages, petechiae, and facial edema. Stagnation develops from capillary atony and dilation, and as the blood desaturates, purplish discoloration of the skin occurs. Although the appearance of these patients can be quite dramatic, the condition itself is usually benign and self-limiting.

Diagnostic Strategies

The clinical significance lies with the possibility of intrathoracic injury from the violent force necessary to produce traumatic asphyxia. Chest wall and pulmonary injuries are most common. These patients should undergo CT of the chest to identify any potentially serious intrathoracic injuries.

Disturbance of vision has been attributed to retinal hemorrhage, which is generally a permanent injury, and to retinal edema, which may cause transient changes in vision. One third of these patients lose consciousness, usually at the time of injury. Intracranial hemorrhages are rare, probably because of the shock-absorbing ability of the venous sinuses, but CT of the head should be done in patients with neurologic symptoms or signs. Neurologic manifestations typically clear within 24 to 48 hours, and long-term sequelae are uncommon.[25]

PULMONARY INJURIES

Subcutaneous Emphysema

Anatomy and Physiology

Subcutaneous emphysema in the presence of chest wall trauma usually indicates a more serious thoracic injury. Although the presence of air itself in the tissues is a benign condition, in cases of chest trauma it usually represents serious injury to any air-containing structure within the thorax. Air enters the tissues either extrapleurally or intrapleurally. Extrapleural tears in the tracheobronchial tree allow air to leak into the mediastinum and soft tissues of the anterior neck, producing a pneumomediastinum. Intrapleural lesions usually produce a pneumothorax by allowing air to escape the lung through the visceral pleura into the pleural space and on through the parietal pleura into the thoracic wall. An esophageal tear resulting from penetrating injury also may produce a pneumomediastinum manifested by subcutaneous emphysema over the supraclavicular area and anterior neck, although this finding may be delayed 24 hours.

An additional cause of subcutaneous emphysema, which may or may not indicate intrathoracic injury, is found immediately adjacent to a penetrating wound of the thorax. A small amount of air may be introduced into the adjacent subcutaneous tissues from the outside at the time of penetration. It must be assumed, however, that this air is secondary to a pneumothorax or pneumomediastinum, and appropriate diagnostic and therapeutic maneuvers to rule out or treat the intrathoracic injury should be carried out.

The presence of localized subcutaneous emphysema over the chest wall in the presence of blunt trauma usually indicates the presence of a traumatic pneumothorax, whereas the presence of subcutaneous emphysema over the supraclavicular area and anterior neck usually indicates a pneumomediastinum. Massive swelling of the face and neck from subcutaneous air most often indicates a ruptured bronchus as the source.

Rarely a pneumomediastinum may progress to a tension pneumomediastinum, which may be life-threatening secondary to the presence of a tension pneumopericardium. This situation most often occurs in patients who are undergoing positive-pressure ventilation. The patients also may have a Hamman crunch, which is a crunching sound heard on cardiac auscultation with each heartbeat.

Diagnosis

Palpation of the chest wall and neck may reveal the presence of subcutaneous air as crepitance. Auscultation of the heart may reveal a Hamman crunch. Chest x-ray often reveals air tracking along a tissue plane in the chest and neck or outlining the upper borders of the heart in the case of pneumomediastinum. Air also may outline mediastinal structures, such as the esophagus, extending as a thin vertical lucency from the mediastinum into the neck. Ultrasound has been used to detect pneumomediastinum, in which air appears as an echogenic thickening of the pericardium.

Management

Tension pneumothorax must be considered and treated appropriately. If a tension pneumopericardium is suspected, an immediate pericardiocentesis with aspiration of air from the pericardial space may be lifesaving. Guidance of the needle by portable ultrasound facilitates the procedure and can decrease its complications.

Although subcutaneous emphysema is a benign condition, massive accumulations can be uncomfortable to the patient. The underlying cause, such as pneumothorax, ruptured bronchus, or ruptured esophagus, must be treated appropriately. Benign pneumomediastinum secondary to a Valsalva maneuver is treated with observation and high-flow oxygen to facilitate the reabsorption of nitrogen from tissues.

Pulmonary Contusion

Epidemiology

Pulmonary contusion is reported to be present in 30% to 75% of patients with significant blunt chest trauma, most often from MVCs with rapid deceleration.[1] Pulmonary contusion also can be caused by high-velocity missile wounds and the high-energy shock waves of an explosion in air or water. Pulmonary contusion is the most common significant chest injury in children, and it is most commonly caused by an auto or pedestrian accident.[26]

Anatomy and Pathophysiology

Pulmonary contusion is a direct bruise of the lung parenchyma followed by alveolar edema and hemorrhage but without an accompanying pulmonary laceration, as first described by Morgagni in 1761.[27]

Clinical Features

The clinical manifestations include dyspnea, tachypnea, cyanosis, tachycardia, hypotension, and chest wall bruising. There are no specific signs for pulmonary contusion, but hemoptysis may be present in 50% of patients at some point in their course, and moist rales or diminished breath sounds may be heard on auscultation. Palpation of the chest wall commonly reveals

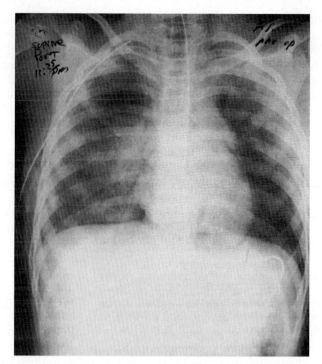

Figure 42-4. Bilateral alveolar infiltrates suggesting pulmonary contusion. Pneumopericardium and pneumomediastinum also are present.

fractured ribs. Pulmonary contusion is a common finding in the presence of flail chest.

Many of the worst contusions occur in patients without rib fractures. It has been theorized that the more elastic chest wall, as in younger individuals, transmits increased force to the thoracic contents. Although isolated pulmonary contusions can exist, they are associated with extrathoracic injuries in 87% of patients.[28]

Diagnostic Strategies

Care must be taken not to focus solely on more dramatic injuries at the expense of failing to recognize the evolving pulmonary contusion. This is particularly true with the initial x-ray studies when overlying rib fracture, pneumothorax, aspiration pneumonitis, or poor radiograph quality may mask the contusion. Typical radiographic findings begin to appear within minutes of injury and range from a patchy, irregular alveolar infiltrate to frank consolidation (Figure 42-4). Usually these changes are present on the initial examination, and they are always present within 6 hours. The rapidity of changes on chest x-ray visualization usually correlates with the severity of the contusion.

CT has been found to be particularly sensitive for detecting the early phase of pulmonary contusion and has proved to be sensitive for identifying many thoracic injuries.[9] CT is particularly valuable to identify a pulmonary contusion in the acute phase after injury because plain chest films have a low sensitivity.[29] Although CT may not be necessary to diagnose a pulmonary contusion that is evident on plain chest radiography, it is often invaluable to define further the extent of the contusion and to identify other thoracic injuries.

Pulmonary contusion should be differentiated from acute respiratory distress syndrome, with which it is often confused. The contusion usually manifests itself within minutes of the initial injury, is localized to a segment or a lobe, is apparent on the initial chest study, and tends to last 48 to 72 hours. Acute respiratory distress syndrome is diffuse, and its development usually is delayed, with onset typically 24 to 72 hours after injury.[30]

Arterial blood gases may be helpful in diagnosing pulmonary contusion because most patients are hypoxemic at the time of admission. A low or dropping partial pressure of oxygen alone may be reason to suspect pulmonary contusion. A widening alveolar-arterial oxygen difference indicates a decreasing pulmonary diffusion capacity of the patient's contused lung, and it is the earliest and most accurate means of assessing the current status, progress, and prognosis.

Management

Management of pulmonary contusion is essentially the same as management of flail chest. When only one lung has been severely contused and has caused significant hypoxemia, intubating and ventilating each lung separately should be considered. This differential lung ventilation uses a double-lumen endotracheal tube and two ventilators. This technique accommodates the different compliance between the injured and normal lung and prevents hyperexpansion of one lung and gradual collapse of the other.[31] As with flail chest, intubation and mechanical ventilation should be avoided if possible because they are associated with an increase in morbidity, including pneumonia, sepsis, pneumothorax, hypercoagulability, and longer hospitalization.

Certain procedures may ameliorate the pulmonary contusion, including the restriction of intravenous fluids to maintain intravascular volume within strict limits and aggressive supportive care consisting of vigorous tracheobronchial toilet, suctioning, and pain relief. These maneuvers may preclude the need for ventilator support and allow a more selective approach to flail chest and pulmonary contusion. Although steroids have been shown to decrease the size of experimental pulmonary contusion, effectiveness in patients has not been proved.[32]

Another area of historical controversy in management of pulmonary contusions is the appropriate use of crystalloid versus colloid solutions in resuscitation of a multiply injured patient with suspected contusion. Because of the potential for colloid sequestration within the pulmonary alveoli owing to capillary leak, colloids are not recommended for use in treating these patients.

Pneumonia is the most common complication of pulmonary contusions, and it significantly worsens the prognosis. Pneumonia develops insidiously, especially in patients treated with prophylactic antibiotics. The use of antibiotics for pulmonary contusion is not recommended and should be reserved for specific organisms of associated pneumonia rather than given prophylactically. Mortality of patients with an isolated pulmonary contusion is only 5% to 16%, whereas the mortality of patients with even one associated extrathoracic injury is significantly greater.[33]

Pulmonary Laceration

The lungs are most often lacerated from penetrating injury, but they also may be injured by the inward projection of a fractured rib or avulsion of a pleural adhesion. These injuries are usually minor and uncommonly life-threatening, and they usually can be treated with observation or tube thoracostomy. Severe lacerations in which hemorrhage does not cease spontaneously are present in only 3% of patients with thoracic trauma and usually are associated with hemopneumothorax, multiple rib fractures, and hemoptysis. Life-threatening lacerations may require thoracotomy with resection to control bleeding.

Pneumothorax

Epidemiology

Pneumothorax, the accumulation of air in the pleural space, is a common complication of chest trauma. It is reported to be present in 15% to 50% of patients with severe chest trauma, and it is invariably present in patients with transpleural penetrating injuries.[1]

Anatomy and Pathophysiology

Pneumothorax can be divided into three classifications, depending on whether air has direct access to the pleural cavity: simple, communicating, and tension. A pneumothorax is considered simple (Figure 42-5) when there is no communication with the atmosphere or any shift of the mediastinum or hemidiaphragm resulting from the accumulation of air. It can be graded according to the degree of collapse as visualized on the chest radiograph. A small pneumothorax occupies 15% or less of the pleural cavity; a moderate pneumothorax, 15% to 60%; and a large pneumothorax, more than 60%. Traumatic pneumothorax is caused most often by a fractured rib that is driven inward,

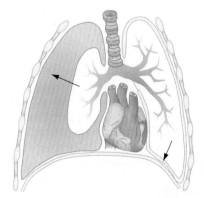

Figure 42-5. Closed pneumothorax. Simple pneumothorax is present in the right lung with air in the pleural cavity and collapse of the right lung.

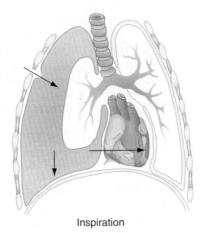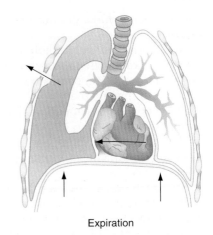

Figure 42-6. Communicating pneumothorax. Collapse of the right lung and air in the pleural cavity are seen, with communication to outside through a defect in the chest wall. In a sucking chest wound, lung volume is greater with expiration.

Inspiration

Expiration

lacerating the pleura. It also may occur without a fracture when the impact is delivered at full inspiration with the glottis closed, leading to a tremendous increase in intra-alveolar pressure and subsequent rupture of the alveoli. A penetrating injury, such as a gunshot or stab wound, also may produce a simple pneumothorax if there is no free communication with the atmosphere.

Communicating Pneumothorax

A communicating pneumothorax (Figure 42-6) is associated with loss of integrity of the chest wall and most commonly occurs in combat injuries. Among civilians, this injury most commonly is secondary to shotgun wounds that produce a large chest wall defect. Air sometimes can be heard flowing sonorously in and out of the defect, prompting the term *sucking chest wound*. The loss of chest wall integrity causes the involved lung paradoxically to collapse on inspiration and expand slightly on expiration, forcing air in and out of the wound. This situation results in a large functional dead space for the normal lung and, together with the loss of ventilation of the involved lung, produces a severe ventilatory disturbance.

Tension Pneumothorax

Tension pneumothorax (Figures 42-7 and 42-8) refers to the progressive accumulation of air under pressure within the pleural cavity, with shift of the mediastinum to the opposite hemithorax and compression of the contralateral lung and great vessels. Tension pneumothorax occurs when the injury acts like a one-way valve, prevents free bilateral communication with the atmosphere, and leads to a progressive increase of intrapleural pressure. Air enters on inspiration, but cannot exit with expiration. The resulting shift of mediastinal contents compresses the vena cava and distorts the cavoatrial junction, leading to decreased diastolic filling of the heart and subsequent decreased cardiac output. These changes result in the rapid onset of hypoxia, acidosis, and shock.

Clinical Features

Shortness of breath and chest pain are the most common presenting complaints of pneumothorax. The

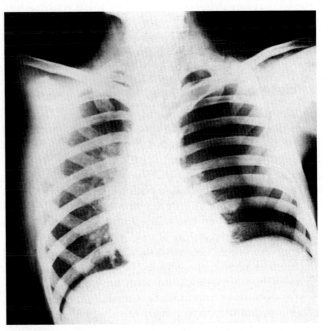

Figure 42-7. Radiograph of tension pneumothorax on the left with shift of mediastinal structures to the right. Subcutaneous emphysema in soft tissues of the neck also is present.

patient's appearance varies, ranging from acutely ill with cyanosis and tachypnea to misleadingly healthy. The signs and symptoms are not always correlated with the degree of pneumothorax. The physical examination may show decreased or absent breath sounds and hyperresonance over the involved side and subcutaneous emphysema, but smaller pneumothoraces may not be detectable on physical examination.

Patients with tension pneumothorax become acutely ill within minutes and develop severe cardiovascular and respiratory distress. They are dyspneic, agitated, restless, cyanotic, tachycardic, and hypotensive and display decreasing mental activity. The cardinal signs of tension pneumothorax are tachycardia, jugular venous distention, and absent breath sounds on the ipsilateral side. Hypotension does not occur as early as hypoxia and may represent a preterminal event.

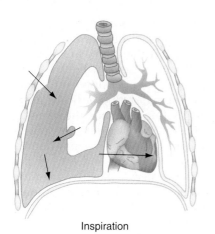
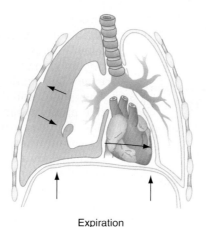

Inspiration   Expiration

Figure 42-8. Tension pneumothorax. Right pneumothorax under tension, total collapse of right lung, and shift of mediastinal structures to the left are seen.

CHAPTER 42 Thoracic Trauma

Diagnostic Strategies

The chest radiograph is the preferred initial study for diagnosing a simple pneumothorax, and it should be obtained as rapidly as possible. Because intrapleural air tends to collect at the apex of the lung, the initial study should be an upright full inspiratory film if the patient's condition permits. An upright film often reveals small pleural effusions that are not visible on supine films, and it allows better visualization of the mediastinum.

If a pneumothorax is suspected but not visualized on the initial inspiratory film, an expiratory film should be obtained because it makes the pneumothorax more apparent by reducing the lung volume. One third of initial chest films do not detect a pneumothorax in trauma patients.[34] Although it is not recommended as a primary method of diagnosing pneumothorax, CT is sensitive in finding a small pneumothorax even in a supine patient. When CT scans are obtained to evaluate the abdomen, it may be helpful to take a few low cuts into the chest to exclude the presence of a small pneumothorax. Bedside ultrasound is a rapid, minimally invasive method for diagnosing pneumothorax, although the sensitivity and specificity have yet to be determined in a large series of patients. Findings suggesting the presence of pneumothorax include absence of the pleural line, absence of "lung sliding" or motion of the lung against the pleura, and the presence of a "lung point" (exclusive horizontal lines).[35,36]

Occult Pneumothorax

A pneumothorax that is absent on initial chest x-ray but is identified on subsequent chest or abdominal CT scan is called an *occult pneumothorax*. CT scan of the chest or abdomen detects approximately twice as many pneumothoraces as chest x-ray. Although some of these patients require tube thoracostomy, in many cases, a minuscule or anterior occult pneumothorax is an incidental finding and can be safely observed until it resolves. Anterolateral occult pneumothorax more commonly requires drainage.[37,38]

The diagnosis and treatment of tension pneumothorax should not be delayed awaiting a chest x-ray or because the patient is normotensive. Although tension pneumothorax usually occurs dramatically, the clinical diagnosis is sometimes obscure, and a chest x-ray may

be required to confirm the diagnosis. The chest film shows near-complete or complete lung collapse and shift of the mediastinum to the opposite side. Ideally the diagnosis and treatment should be completed without a chest x-ray because the delay in obtaining this radiograph may adversely affect patient outcome.

Management

Pneumothorax Absent—Penetrating Trauma

In the setting of penetrating trauma when the patient is asymptomatic and the initial chest x-ray study is negative, the patient can be safely observed and the x-ray repeated. Previously, it was thought that if the patient was still asymptomatic and the radiograph negative after 6 hours, the patient could be discharged. More recent experience indicates that 3 hours is probably sufficient for observation with a repeat normal x-ray before discharge.[39]

Simple Pneumothorax

Treatment of a simple pneumothorax depends on its cause and size. Most authors advocate treating a traumatic pneumothorax with a chest tube to correct any respiratory compromise and because treatment with a chest tube is generally thought to be safer than observation in these patients. Small pneumothoraces, whether spontaneous or traumatic, have been treated with hospitalization and careful observation if the patient is otherwise healthy, is symptom-free, and does not need anesthesia or positive-pressure ventilation, and the size of the pneumothorax is not increasing.

Isolated apical pneumothoraces of less than 25% may be observed in patients with stab wounds.[40] This conservative method seldom has application in multisystem trauma, and a chest tube should be inserted immediately for any signs of deterioration. Some authors suggest that because it is small and lacks symptoms, occult traumatic pneumothorax found only on CT can be observed and does not need treatment. Studies indicate that these injuries can be handled similar to small but initially detectable pneumothoraces with observation in hemodynamically stable patients without symptoms. One third of patients who require positive-pressure ventilation experience progression of

BOX 42-3. Indications for Closed-Tube Thoracostomy

Traumatic cause of pneumothorax
Moderate-to-large pneumothorax
Respiratory symptoms regardless of size of pneumothorax
Increasing size of pneumothorax after initial conservative therapy
Recurrence of pneumothorax after removal of the initial chest tube
Patient requires ventilator support
Patient requires general anesthesia
Associated hemothorax
Bilateral pneumothorax regardless of size
Tension pneumothorax

From Dougall AM, et al: Chest trauma—current morbidity and mortality. *J Trauma* 17:547, 1977.

the pneumothorax, however, and require tube thoracostomy, perhaps under exigent circumstances.[41,42]

Moderate-to-large pneumothoraces should be treated with a chest tube (Box 42-3). The preferred site for insertion is the fourth or fifth intercostal space at the anterior or midaxillary line. If the tube is directed posteriorly and toward the apex, it can remove air and fluid effectively. This lateral placement of the tube is preferred not only because it is more efficient, but also because it does not produce an easily visible cosmetic defect, in contrast to the anterior site at the second interspace at the midclavicular line, a site that should not be entertained in trauma patients. With multisystem trauma, an adequate size chest tube should always be used, particularly in cases of major trauma, when hemothorax is likely to occur.

Care must be taken to be certain the vent holes along the side of the tube all are inside the chest cavity. A radiopaque line along the side of the tube with interruptions at these drainage holes helps greatly when radiographically interpreting tube position. The tube should be attached to a water-seal drainage system that allows re-expansion of the pneumothorax. If there is significant air leak or a large hemothorax, the tube may be connected to a source of constant vacuum at 20 to 30 cm H_2O for more rapid re-expansion. Continuous leak despite these measures may represent tracheobronchial disruption. Tube thoracostomy has some potentially serious complications, including the formation of a hemothorax, pulmonary edema, bronchopleural fistula, pleural leaks, empyema, subcutaneous emphysema, infection, and contralateral pneumothorax. Pneumothoraces that have been present for more than 3 days should be re-expanded gradually without suction to avoid inducing re-expansion pulmonary edema.

Communicating Pneumothorax

For a patient with a communicating (open) pneumothorax in the prehospital setting, the defect should be covered immediately; this helps convert the condition to a closed pneumothorax and eliminates the major physiologic abnormality. An occlusive dressing of petrolatum gauze can be applied, but care should be taken because this can convert the injury to a tension pneumothorax, especially in patients who are intubated and undergoing positive-pressure ventilation. The wound should never be packed because the negative pressure during inspiration can suck the dressing into the chest cavity. These considerations are not as important when the patient is in the emergency department, where endotracheal intubation and tube thoracostomy can be performed. Positive-pressure ventilation can be started without the fear of producing a tension pneumothorax, and the patient can be prepared for definitive surgical repair.

Tension Pneumothorax

When the diagnosis of tension pneumothorax is suspected clinically, the pressure should be relieved immediately with needle thoracostomy, which is performed by inserting a large-bore (16-gauge or 18-gauge) needle through the second or third interspace anteriorly or the fourth or fifth interspace laterally on the involved side. This method can be performed easily in the field or emergency department, allowing vital signs to improve during transport or preparation for a tube thoracostomy in the emergency department.[43] The earliest sign of the development of tension pneumothorax in an intubated patient is an increase in resistance to ventilation. If the patient has vital signs, the blood pressure decreases, and the central venous pressure (CVP) increases. Misplacement of an endotracheal tube into the main stem bronchus does not result in tension pneumothorax, but rather asymmetry of breath sounds.

Hemothorax

Epidemiology

Traumatic hemothorax is the accumulation of blood in the pleural space after blunt or penetrating chest trauma and is a common complication that may produce hypovolemic shock and reduce vital capacity to dangerously low levels. It is commonly associated with pneumothorax (25% of cases) and extrathoracic injuries (73% of cases).

Anatomy and Pathophysiology

Hemorrhage from injured lung parenchyma is the most common cause of hemothorax, but this tends to be self-limiting, particularly after lung expansion via chest tube insertion, unless there is a major laceration. Specific vessels are less often the source of hemorrhage, with intercostal and internal mammary arteries causing hemothorax more often than hilar or great vessels. Bleeding from the intercostal arteries may be brisk, however, because they branch directly from the aorta.

Clinical Features

Depending on the rate and quantity of hemorrhage, varying degrees of hypovolemic shock are manifested. Tactile fremitus is decreased, and breath sounds are diminished or absent on the affected side.

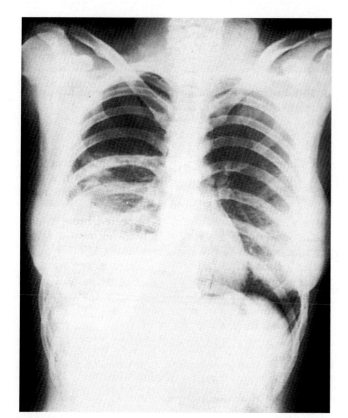
Figure 42-9. Hemopneumothorax is seen on the right side in this erect chest radiograph.

BOX 42-4. Indications for Thoracotomy

Initial thoracostomy tube drainage is >20 mL/kg of blood
Persistent bleeding at a rate >7 mL/kg/hr
Increasing hemothorax seen on chest x-rays
Patient remains hypotensive despite adequate blood replacement, and other sites of blood loss have been ruled out
Patient decompensates after initial response to resuscitation

BOX 42-5. Indications for Emergency Department Thoracotomy

Penetrating Traumatic Cardiac Arrest
Cardiac arrest at any point with initial signs of life in the field
Blood pressure <50 mm Hg systolic after fluid resuscitation
Severe shock with clinical signs of cardiac tamponade

Blunt Trauma
Cardiac arrest in the emergency department

Miscellaneous
Suspected air embolus

Diagnostic Strategies

Clinical features are often sufficient to warrant tube thoracostomy without diagnostic radiography. Blunting of the costophrenic angles on chest radiograph requires at least 200 to 300 mL of fluid in the upright position (Figure 42-9). The supine view chest film is less accurate, and it may be more difficult to diagnose hemothorax with the patient in this position. This is often the only film available because of the patient's unstable condition. In the supine patient, blood layers posteriorly, creating a diffuse haziness that can be subtle, depending on the volume of the hemothorax.

Management

Close monitoring of the initial and ongoing rate of blood loss must be performed to determine the need for thoracotomy. Immediate drainage of more than 1500 mL of blood from the pleural cavity usually is considered an indication for emergency thoracotomy. Perhaps even more predictive of the need for thoracotomy is a continued output of at least 200 mL/hr for 3 hours. General considerations for urgent thoracotomy are outlined in Box 42-4.[44] Criteria for emergency department thoracotomy are listed in Box 42-5.

Treatment of hemothorax consists of restoring the circulating blood volume, controlling the airway as necessary, and evacuating the accumulated blood. Tube thoracostomy allows constant monitoring of the blood loss and re-expansion of the lung. A large-bore tube (36F to 40F) should be inserted preferably in the fifth interspace at the midaxillary line and connected to underwater-seal drainage and suction (20 to 30 cm H_2O). Some experts believe that small hemothoraces may be observed in stable patients, although others maintain that any hemothorax should be drained to avoid the formation of pleural adhesions as the blood reabsorbs. A moderate hemothorax or any hemothorax in an unstable or symptomatic patient clearly requires tube thoracostomy. Severe or persistent hemorrhage requires thoracotomy (see Box 42-4).

Autotransfusion has been successful in recycling autologous blood from the patient via tube thoracostomy. Simplification and commercial availability of the equipment have made autotransfusion feasible in most emergency departments. Autotransfusion also eliminates the risk of incompatibility reactions and transmission of certain diseases, such as hepatitis C. Because most blood loss occurs immediately after tube thoracostomy placement, autotransfusion apparatus must be immediately available in the emergency department. Preparation for autotransfusion should begin as soon as it becomes apparent that a patient with chest trauma may require transfusion or presents with evidence of significant blood loss (falling hemoglobin level, massive hemothorax on chest x-ray or hemorrhagic shock).

Although out of the scope of emergency medicine, thoracoscopy is particularly useful for evaluation and evacuation of retained hemothorax, control of bleeding from intercostal vessels, and diagnosis and repair of diaphragmatic injuries.[45,46] As surgeons gain more experience with the technique, and the sophistication of the equipment improves, thoracoscopy is likely to become more widely used.[47]

Tracheobronchial Injury

Epidemiology

Tracheobronchial injuries may occur with either blunt or penetrating injuries of the neck or chest. Penetrating injuries tend to be more obvious because of their nature, alerting the patient and the physician, whereas blunt injuries can be quite occult. MVCs are the most frequent mechanism causing tracheobronchial injury, accounting for more than half of all cases.[46] Although there has been an increase in the occurrence of tracheobronchial disruption, it is still a relatively rare injury, occurring in fewer than 3% of patients with significant chest injury. The associated mortality rate is reported to be approximately 10%, although mortality rates are significantly affected by associated injuries and the timing of diagnosis and surgical repair.[48,49]

Anatomy and Pathophysiology

Tracheobronchial injuries caused by knife wounds develop almost exclusively from wounds in the cervical trachea, whereas gunshot wounds may damage the tracheobronchial tree at any point. Intrathoracic injury to the tracheobronchial tree occurs most commonly from blunt trauma. These injuries may result from direct blows, shearing stresses, or burst injury. A direct blow to the neck may crush the cervical trachea against the vertebral bodies and transect the tracheal rings or cricoid cartilage. Shear forces on the trachea produce injury at the carina and the cricoid cartilage, which are its relatively fixed points.

Sudden deceleration of the thoracic cage, as occurs in a decelerating MVC, pulls the lungs away from the mediastinum, producing traction on the trachea at the carina. When the elasticity of the tracheobronchial tree is exceeded, it ruptures. It also has been suggested that if the glottis is closed at the time of impact, the sudden increase in intrabronchial pressure ruptures the tracheobronchial tree. Regardless of the mechanism, more than 80% of these injuries occur within 2 cm of the carina.

Clinical Features

Massive air leak, hemoptysis, and subcutaneous emphysema should suggest the diagnosis of major airway damage. Auscultation of the heart may reveal a Hamman crunch. Patients with tracheobronchial disruption have one of two distinct clinical pictures. In the first group, the wound opens into the pleural space, producing a large pneumothorax. A chest tube fails to evacuate the space and re-expand the lung, and there is continuous bubbling of air in the underwater-seal device.

The second group has a complete transection of the tracheobronchial tree but little or no communication with the pleural space. A pneumothorax is not usually present. The peribronchial tissues support the airway enough to maintain respiration, but within 3 weeks granulation tissue obstructs the lumen and produces atelectasis. These patients are relatively symptom-free

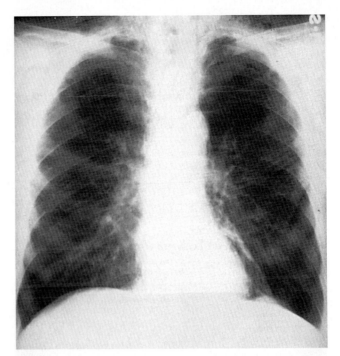

Figure 42-10. Massive subcutaneous emphysema secondary to pneumomediastinum. There is no pneumothorax.

at the time of injury but weeks later have unexplained atelectasis or pneumonia. Radiographic signs in either group of patients may include pneumomediastinum, extensive subcutaneous emphysema (Figure 42-10), pneumothorax, fracture of the upper ribs (first through fifth), air surrounding the bronchus, and obstruction in the course of an air-filled bronchus.

Diagnostic Strategies

When tracheobronchial injury is suspected, bronchoscopy should be performed. Fiberoptic bronchoscopy is the most reliable means of establishing the diagnosis and determining the site and extent of the injury.[50] Bronchopleural fistula is the persistence of a communication between the bronchus and the pleura, which commonly results in a pneumothorax that does not reinflate after tube thoracostomy; this also is called a *persistent air leak*. It can occur as a complication of tracheobronchial disruption and in some cases has been treated successfully via a fiberoptic bronchoscope.

Management

If possible, endotracheal intubation over a bronchoscope should be performed because it allows visualization of the tube as it passes beyond the site of injury. Care must be taken when attempting blind intubation not to place the endotracheal tube through a transected airway into the soft tissue or a false passage or to convert a partial tracheal tear into a complete one. In most cases, thoracotomy with intraoperative tracheostomy and surgical repair of the disrupted airway should be performed as soon as possible. In exigent circumstances, the emergency physician must intubate the patient using standard methods and with as much care as possible.

CARDIOVASCULAR TRAUMA

Blunt Cardiac Trauma

Epidemiology

Blunt cardiac injury usually results from high-speed MVCs, in which the chest wall strikes against the steering wheel. Other causes, such as falls from heights, crushing injuries, blast injuries, and direct blows, are less common. The significance of blunt injuries as a cause of myocardial or cardiac contusion was described in the 1930s by Bright and Beck.[51] Nevertheless, the diagnosis of a blunt injury to the heart remains elusive because of the usual concomitant serious injuries to other body organs and, more important, because there is as yet no "gold standard" for making the diagnosis.

The importance of detecting blunt myocardial injury lies in the recognition of associated potentially fatal complications. Life-threatening dysrhythmias, conduction abnormalities, congestive heart failure, cardiogenic shock, hemopericardium with tamponade, cardiac rupture, valvular rupture, intraventricular thrombi, thromboembolic phenomena, coronary artery occlusion, ventricular aneurysms, and constrictive pericarditis all have been reported as complications.

Anatomy and Pathophysiology

Blunt cardiac trauma may be viewed as part of a continuous spectrum (i.e., myocardial concussion, contusion, infarction, and rupture).[52] *Myocardial concussion* occurs when a blunt injury to the interior chest produces a "stun" response in the myocardium. No permanent cellular injury occurs, but transient clinical effects may result. *Myocardial contusion* is the least severe form of injury that can be shown pathologically. Cellular injury occurs with extravasation of red blood cells into the muscle wall, along with localized myocardial cellular necrosis. Permanent myocardial damage is rare. *Traumatic myocardial infarction* (MI) results from either direct trauma to the coronary arteries or a severe contusion of the myocardium, leading to irreversible cellular injury and ultimately cell death. Direct injury to the coronary arteries via laceration, thrombosis, or spasm is thought to be the most common mechanism for traumatic MI. *Cardiac rupture* is the most severe form of blunt cardiac injury.

Myocardial Concussion

The term *myocardial concussion* or *commotio cordis* is used to describe an acute form of blunt cardiac trauma that usually is produced by a sharp, direct blow to the midanterior chest that stuns the myocardium and results in a brief dysrhythmia, hypotension, and loss of consciousness. If the patient survives the initial dysrhythmia, there are no lasting histopathologic changes, and it is difficult to make the definitive diagnosis of myocardial concussion. Myocardial concussion explains cases of sudden death after a blow to the chest in which no histopathologic changes in the myocardium are shown at autopsy. If prolonged cellular dysfunction occurs, it may result in a nonperfusing rhythm, such as asystole or ventricular fibrillation, and irreversible cardiac arrest. Numerous cases are documented of successful resuscitation with rapid provision of cardiopulmonary resuscitation and the use of an automated external defibrillator.[53]

Myocardial Contusion

Epidemiology

The term *myocardial contusion* describes a poorly understood and nebulous condition. Decades of research and widely varied clinical practice have failed to produce a consensus as to its diagnosis, complication rate, and proper disposition.[54,55] The reported incidence of myocardial contusion varies from 3% to 55% in reported series of severe closed-chest trauma, depending on the criteria used for establishing the diagnosis. Although high-speed deceleration injuries are the most common cause of myocardial contusion, MVCs that occur at slow to moderate speeds also may result in cardiac injury. In one study, an automobile collision speed of only 20 to 35 mph resulted in myocardial contusion in several patients, without external evidence of chest trauma.

Anatomy and Pathophysiology

Several mechanisms have been postulated by which the heart may be injured in cases of nonpenetrating trauma. A direct blow to the chest transmits energy through the ribs to the spine. When a large force is applied to the chest wall over an extended period, the sternum is displaced posteriorly, and the heart is compressed between the sternum and vertebrae or an elevated diaphragm. Either can result in cardiac injury. Increased intrathoracic pressure from a direct blow to the chest may contribute to the injury. In addition, compression of the abdomen and pelvis may displace abdominal viscera upward and result in cardiac injury.

The heart has relatively free movement in the anteroposterior direction within the chest; in cases of sudden deceleration, the heart continues to move forward because of its momentum, striking the sternum with considerable force. Severity of injury is likely related to the phase of the systolic-diastolic cycle during which the trauma occurs. Because a compressible organ is more capable of diffusing energy than a rigid one, injuries that occur during a rigid stage (late diastole and early systole) are more damaging than injuries that occur during the other phases of the cardiac cycle.

Microcellular damage ranges from mild disruption of myofibrils to a complete loss of structure, necrosis, and polymorphonuclear infiltration of the area, as is seen in cases of ischemic MI. An accumulation of edema and cellular infiltrate in the wall of the heart may result in a decrease in ventricular compliance, resulting in cardiac dysfunction.

Vascular damage usually is restricted to the capillaries. Acute thrombus formation may occur, especially in diseased, atheromatous vessels, and result in coronary artery occlusion and MI. A blunt injury may cause a coronary vascular occlusion by arterial spasm, an intimal tear, or compression from adjacent hemorrhage and edema.

Small pericardial effusions occur in more than 50% of cases of contusion, usually during the second week. These probably are caused by pericardial irritation, and they neither imply significant cardiac injury nor increase the risk of tamponade. A fibrinous reaction at the contusion site also may occur, resulting in pain, a friction rub, and adhesion to the pericardium. In a few cases, the reabsorption of the hematoma is accompanied by necrosis of the ventricular wall, which may result in a delayed rupture of the myocardium or a scarred and weakened area with subsequent development of a ventricular aneurysm. If necrosis occurs, it usually is manifested in the second week after injury as rupture of the septum, papillary muscle, or free ventricular wall and is one of the causes of delayed sudden death after blunt trauma to the chest.

Most myocardial contusions heal spontaneously, with resolution of cellular infiltrate and hemorrhage leading to scar formation. Repair in myocardial contusion occurs in a patchy, irregular pattern, whereas more generalized fibrosis occurs in MI caused by coagulation necrosis. High-resolution angiograms and histologic sections have revealed tortuous new capillary vessels in the area of injury, resulting in enhanced circulation to that area; this probably results from the usual patency of the healthy surrounding coronary arteries of a contused heart, in contrast to the diseased vessels found in cases of MI.

Clinical Features

Myocardial contusion presents clinically as a spectrum of injuries of varying severity. Although most patients with myocardial contusion have external signs of thoracic trauma (e.g., contusions, abrasions, palpable crepitus, rib fractures, or visible flail segments), absence of thoracic lesions decreases the suspicion but never excludes cardiac injury. Other associated injuries may include pulmonary contusion, pneumothorax, hemothorax, external fracture, and great vessel injury.[52] The most sensitive but least specific sign of myocardial contusion is sinus tachycardia, which is present in approximately 70% of patients with documented myocardial contusion. Conduction block, particularly right bundle branch block, may occur but is rarely clinically significant. A reduction in cardiac output, which can be clinically insignificant or manifest as pronounced cardiogenic shock, may occur in patients with significant cardiac contusion.

Diagnostic Strategies

Significant controversy exists regarding the importance of establishing the diagnosis of myocardial contusion in otherwise hemodynamically stable patients.[55] Even when the diagnosis of a myocardial contusion is considered, confirming the diagnosis without a true gold standard is problematic. Clinical evidence is often nonspecific, especially in cases of multiple trauma. Patients may have dysrhythmias or ST-T wave changes caused by significant hypoxemia as a result of pulmonary injuries or blood loss, which are reversed when the hypoxemia or blood loss is corrected. Likewise, severe intracranial injury, electrolyte abnormalities, and excessive vagal or sympathetic tone may give rise to dysrhythmias or an abnormal ECG. Under these conditions, ECG abnormalities may not represent true myocardial damage. On the contrary, they may cause one to overlook the potential for traumatic cardiac injury.

Because myocardial contusion cannot be positively identified short of biopsy or autopsy, there is much confusion regarding the role of the various laboratory and imaging studies used to diagnose myocardial injury. Most myocardial contusions probably do not cause clinically significant complications. Based on mechanism alone, the relative risk of a life-threatening dysrhythmia is far too low to warrant routine admission to rule out myocardial contusion in all patients with blunt chest trauma. The usefulness of diagnostic studies is not to diagnose the presence of a myocardial contusion; rather, it is to distinguish patients at low risk who can be discharged safely from the emergency department from patients who require further management.

Diagnostic strategies that have been used to "diagnose" myocardial contusion and assess the risk of complications and the need for admission include ECG, biochemical cardiac markers (serum creatine kinase [CK-MB] isoenzyme levels or troponin I or T concentrations), radionuclide imaging studies, and two-dimensional echocardiography. Use of these tests should be considered in every patient with high-energy force to the anterior chest, particularly patients with anterior rib fractures, sternal fracture, pulmonary contusion, hypotension, or dysrhythmias evident on cardiac monitoring.

Electrocardiogram

The ECG after blunt chest trauma may be normal or may show nonspecific abnormalities. Because of its anterior position in the thorax and proximity to the sternum, the right ventricle is far more likely to be injured than the left ventricle. The standard 12-lead ECG is relatively insensitive to right ventricular damage, as shown by pathologic evidence of cellular damage in patients with normal ECGs. A cardiac contusion usually results in moderate right ventricular damage with only minor electrical changes, which can be missed easily on a standard 12-lead ECG. Right-sided ECGs (the addition of V4R) have not been found to be of any benefit.[56]

To date, little is known of the relative risk of dysrhythmia as a function of the ECG abnormality As such, any new ECG finding warrants consideration of further diagnostic studies or admission for further monitoring. A severely injured right ventricle may cause a right bundle branch block, usually transient. Less commonly, various degrees of atrioventricular block have been documented after blunt chest trauma. In addition, myocardial cell damage produces electrical instability, which may result in a variety of supraventricular or ventricular arrhythmias. Sinus tachycardia and ventricular and atrial extrasystoles are the most frequently reported rhythm disorders. More serious arrhythmias, such as atrial fibrillation, ventricular tachycardia, and ventricular fibrillation, occur less often but may acutely compromise the hemodynamic state or even result in sudden death.[57]

A few cases of delayed life-threatening dysrhythmia have been reported 12 hours after injury, and patients may develop less lethal dysrhythmias 72 hours after injury.[58] The onset of ECG changes may be delayed 48 hours after injury, and all ECG changes usually resolve in 4 to 60 days.[58] The presence of ECG abnormalities is neither specific enough to confirm the diagnosis of myocardial contusion nor reliable enough to predict subsequent complications.

Cardiac Enzymes

Because myocardial contusion is characterized histologically by intramyocardial hemorrhage and necrosis of myocardial muscle cells, similar to in acute MI, cardiac enzymes were the first screening tools used to detect myocardial injury. CK is nonspecifically increased in trauma patients as a result of associated skeletal muscle injury, and CK-MB levels have been found to be falsely elevated and to be a nonspecific finding in multiple-trauma patients. CK-MB levels are of limited utility to screen for myocardial contusion and no longer are recommended.[55,58]

Serum cardiac troponins, troponin I and troponin T, are highly specific for myocardial injury because they are myocardial contractile proteins not found in skeletal muscles. Several studies have shown that troponin I and troponin T are highly sensitive and accurate markers to identify and to rule out myocardial contusion. If troponin I or T concentrations are within normal ranges on initial evaluation in the emergency department, a secondary measurement after 4 to 6 hours should be performed to exclude myocardial injury reliably.[59-61]

Echocardiography

Echocardiography provides a means for direct visualization of cardiac structures and chambers. Because contused myocardium resembles infarcted myocardial tissue histologically and functionally, two-dimensional echocardiography is useful in diagnosing myocardial contusion by evaluating wall motion abnormalities and identifying associated lesions, such as thrombi, pericardial effusion, and valvular disruption.[62,63] Echocardiography offers the practical advantages of being portable, noninvasive, and easy to use at the bedside. It should be considered in patients with positive ECG findings, elevated troponin level, or unexplained hypotension. If patients have painful chest wall injuries, transthoracic echocardiography may be limited. In these cases, transesophageal echocardiography (TEE) is an alternative.[64,65]

Radionuclide Studies

Other tests that have been evaluated to diagnose myocardial contusion include gated radionuclide angiography, which measures left and right ventricular ejection fractions, and thallium-201 myocardial scintigraphy, which detects underperfused areas of the heart. Although abnormal studies strongly suggest an underlying myocardial contusion, little information is available as to the added clinical implications of a positive study, and both are rarely available in the emergency department on a 24-hour basis. Because of the widespread availability of echocardiography, the use of radionuclide studies to facilitate the diagnosis of myocardial contusion has been largely abandoned.

Management

Appropriate workup and treatment of a patient with suspected myocardial contusion begins with accurate prehospital evaluation. Paramedics should observe and relay information to the emergency department concerning mechanism of injury, status of the motor vehicle, steering wheel and dashboard damage, use of seat belts and air bags, speed of the vehicle before the crash, and position of the patient when found. Pertinent clinical data to be recorded include vital signs, level of consciousness, cardiac rhythm, and presence of chest wall trauma.

A wide variety of atrial and ventricular dysrhythmias result from myocardial contusion caused by blunt chest trauma. Significant conduction system defects that result in various bradydysrhythmias and bundle branch blocks may occur. Reduction in cardiac output may manifest in 50% to 75% of patients with significant myocardial contusion because of extensive myocardial muscle injury.[66] Congestive heart failure and cardiogenic shock have been described, and transmural MI caused by blunt coronary artery injury has occurred. Delayed discovery of an aneurysm of the left anterior descending coronary artery in a young patient after blunt chest trauma has been reported. Although rare, cardiac rupture, valvular rupture, and ventricular aneurysm formation have been described as late complications. The formation of intraventricular thrombi with resulting recurrent thromboembolic events also has been reported. Small, insignificant pericardial effusions are common early in a patient's course. Rarely, constrictive pericarditis is found as a late complication.

The value of admitting and carefully monitoring patients with suspected mild cardiac contusions is not supported. More recent studies suggest that troponin I and troponin T are helpful in risk stratification of patients suspected of having myocardial contusion. One strategy is to obtain emergent echocardiography for all severely injured patients who present with hemodynamic instability and are suspected to have structural damage to the heart or great vessels. A similar recommendation exists for severely injured patients with a sternal fracture, although the presence of an isolated sternal fracture is not a sign of cardiac injury.[67]

Increased levels of troponin I or troponin T or ECG abnormalities indicate a higher risk of developing cardiac complications. Further investigation, including echocardiography, serial ECGs, and serial troponin levels, is recommended.[57,58,68] In patients who have chest wall injuries and are otherwise asymptomatic, elevated levels of troponin I or T and minor ECG abnormalities do not indicate a clinically significant myocardial contusion. Few of these patients develop complications. Normal troponin I or T levels (4 to 6 hours after injury) along with normal (or unchanged) ECGs correlate with minimal risk of cardiac complications. In-hospital monitoring may be limited to patients with acute ECG abnormalities, elevated troponin concentrations, or both. Serial ECGs and troponins should be obtained until the troponin results return to normal. Echocardiography has been found to be required rarely in this low-risk subset of patients who have chest wall injuries and are otherwise asymptomatic. If the patient's clinical status deteriorates, or there is inconsistency between the troponins and ECG changes, echocardiography can be useful to rule out structurally significant myocardial injuries.

On admission, treatment of a suspected myocardial contusion should be similar to that of an MI: intravenous line, cardiac monitoring, and administration of oxygen and analgesic agents. Dysrhythmias should be treated with appropriate medications as per current advanced cardiac life support guidelines.[69] No data exist to support prophylactic pharmacologic agents for dysrhythmia suppression. Measures should be taken to treat and prevent any conditions that increase myocardial irritability (e.g., metabolic acidosis). Although general anesthesia is avoided in the setting of acute MI, no complications have been reported in patients with suspected myocardial contusions receiving general anesthesia for necessary operations.[70,71] Thrombolytic agents and aspirin are contraindicated in the setting of acute trauma. In the rare instances of acute MI associated with trauma, angioplasty may be a treatment option.

In the setting of depressed cardiac output caused by myocardial contusion, judicious fluid administration is required. Dobutamine may be useful after optimal preload is ensured. Intra-aortic balloon counterpulsation has been used successfully in refractory cardiogenic shock. The priority is to be certain that the decreased cardiac output is not the result of other undiagnosed injuries, particularly aortic rupture.

Prognosis

The prognosis of a patient with myocardial contusion depends on the character and magnitude of the initial trauma, the size and location of the contusion, the preexisting condition of the coronary arteries, and, most important, any other organ trauma and its complications. Major morbidity and mortality correlate most closely with the number of associated serious injuries. Recovery without complications is the usual course.

Myocardial Rupture

Myocardial rupture refers to an acute traumatic perforation of the ventricles or atria, but it also may include a pericardial rupture or laceration or rupture of the interventricular septum, interatrial septum, chordae, papillary muscles, or valves. A delayed rupture of the heart also may occur weeks after blunt trauma, probably as a result of necrosis of a contused or infarcted area of myocardium.

Epidemiology

High-speed MVCs are responsible for most cases of traumatic myocardial rupture.[52] Myocardial rupture is nearly always immediately fatal and accounts for 15% of fatal thoracic injuries. It has been estimated that blunt cardiac rupture accounts for 5% of the 50,000 annual highway deaths in the United States.[53] In various series, the incidence of cardiac rupture in cases of blunt chest trauma ranges from 0.5% to 2%.[71] The most common cause of death in cases of nonpenetrating cardiac injuries is myocardial rupture. Approximately one third of these patients have multiple chamber rupture, and one fourth have an associated ascending aortic rupture. Bright and Beck[51] reviewed 152 autopsy cases of traumatic cardiac ruptures and found that 20% of patients survived 30 minutes or more, which might have allowed them to reach the operating room had the problem been recognized. The first report of successful repair of blunt cardiac rupture occurred in 1955 in a patient with right atrial rupture.[72]

Anatomy and Pathophysiology

The chambers most commonly involved in cardiac rupture are the ventricles; ruptures occur almost equally on each side. Ruptures of the atria are less common, with right atrium rupture being more common than left. Multiple chamber involvement occurs in 30% of patients.[51] Twenty percent of nonsurvivors have concomitant aortic rupture.[73]

A rupture occurs during closure of the outflow track when there is ventricular compression of blood-filled chambers by a pressure sufficient to rupture the chamber wall, septum, or valve. This is the most likely mechanism for ventricular rupture when injury occurs in diastole or early systole concomitant with maximal ventricular distention. The atria are most susceptible to rupture by sudden compression in late systole when these chambers are maximally distended with venous blood and the atrial ventricular valves are closed. Other proposed mechanisms of rupture include the following: (1) deceleration shearing stresses acting on the "fixed" attachment of the inferior and superior vena cava at the right atrium; (2) upward displacement of blood and abdominal viscera from blunt abdominal injury that causes a sudden increase in intracardiac pressure; (3) direct compression of the heart between the sternum and vertebral bodies; (4) laceration from a fractured rib or sternum; and (5) complications of a myocardial contusion, necrosis, and subsequent cardiac rupture.

Because of the nature of the mechanisms involved in cardiac rupture, associated multisystem injuries are common. More than 70% of reported survivors of myocardial rupture had other major associated injuries, including pulmonary contusions, liver and spleen lacerations, closed-head injuries, and major fractures. Twenty percent of nonsurvivors have concomitant aortic ruptures.[73]

The immediate ability of the patient to survive cardiac rupture depends on the integrity of the pericardium. Two thirds of patients with cardiac rupture have an intact pericardium and are protected from immediate exsanguination. These patients may survive for variable periods but eventually develop significant hemopericardium and pericardial tamponade. One third of patients with cardiac rupture have associated pericardial tears and succumb promptly to exsanguination. A patient occasionally survives if the pericardial tear is small, or the rupture is small enough to seal itself.[71] A small pericardial laceration may allow partial and intermittent release of tamponade while still controlling bleeding. Among the cases of prolonged survival noted in two large autopsy series, 43 of 44 patients died from cardiac tamponade, and 1 patient died from exsanguination.

Clinical Features

The clinical presentation of a patient who has sustained a myocardial rupture is usually that of cardiac tamponade or severe intrathoracic hemorrhage. Rarely, a patient is seen with a large hemothorax, hypotension, and hypovolemia, suggesting rupture with associated pericardial tear. A patient with an intact pericardial sac and developing tamponade displays physical findings of tamponade usually with subsequent clinical deterioration. Initial inspection of the torso may reveal little more than a bruised area over the sternum or no external physical evidence at all. More often, signs of significant chest trauma or other associated injuries are present, however, indicating a mechanism of injury that could result in myocardial rupture. Auscultation may reveal a harsh murmur, known as a *bruit de moulin*, which sounds like a splashing mill wheel and represents a succussion splash with high-pitched "metallic" tinkling secondary to hemopneumopericardium.

In a review of survivors of myocardial rupture, common symptoms and signs included hypotension (100%); elevated CVP (95%); tachycardia (89%); distended neck veins (80%); cyanosis of the head, neck, arms, and upper chest (76%); unresponsiveness (74%); distant heart sounds (61%); and associated chest injuries (50%). The following findings are suggestive of pericardial rupture:

1. Hypotension disproportionate to the suspected injury
2. Hypotension unresponsive to rapid fluid resuscitation
3. Massive hemothorax unresponsive to thoracostomy and fluid resuscitation
4. Persistent metabolic acidosis

5. Presence of pericardial effusion on echocardiography or elevation of CVP and neck veins with continuing hypotension despite fluid resuscitation

Diagnostic Strategies

Early use of emergency department ultrasound may facilitate the early diagnosis of cardiac rupture (and pericardial tamponade).[74] The combination of shock and an elevated CVP in a patient with blunt chest trauma should immediately suggest pericardial tamponade. Other differential considerations of these signs include tension pneumothorax, right ventricular myocardial contusion, superior vena cava obstruction, ruptured tricuspid valve, or preexisting pulmonary disease. Ultrasound visualization of pericardial fluid in this setting mandates emergent thoracotomy.

A chest radiograph should be obtained immediately in all cases of acute, blunt chest injuries. Although this study usually does not help diagnose cases of myocardial rupture, it notes the presence of other intrathoracic injuries (e.g., hemothorax, pneumothorax, and signs of possible blunt traumatic aortic injury). An increase in the size of the cardiac silhouette more commonly reflects preexisting disease or valvular incompetence with chamber enlargement caused by increased filling pressures. ECG changes may occur with myocardial injury, but these are often nonspecific for myocardial rupture. Early use of bedside echocardiography in the emergency department should be performed in any case of suspected cardiac rupture, pericardial tamponade, a previously undiagnosed murmur, or shock unexplained by other etiologies (i.e., exsanguination).

Management

When prehospital care providers evaluate a patient who has sustained blunt chest trauma, they should concentrate on rapid transport and pay attention for any signs of pericardial tamponade. En route to the hospital, the possibility of a tension pneumothorax should be considered as well.

In the emergency department, treatment of patients with a myocardial rupture is directed toward immediate decompression of cardiac tamponade and control of hemorrhage. Pericardiocentesis usually is performed as a diagnostic or temporizing therapeutic procedure until surgical correction can be undertaken. Emergency thoracotomy and pericardiotomy may be required in the emergency department if the patient has rapidly deteriorating vital signs or a cardiac arrest. After emergency thoracotomy and pericardiotomy, the myocardial rupture should be controlled until the patient can be transported to the operating room for definitive repair. Hemorrhage from a ruptured atrium often can be controlled by finger occlusion or application of a vascular clamp. Insertion of a Foley catheter through the defect, followed by inflation of the balloon and traction on the catheter also may control the bleeding. Ventricular rupture usually can be controlled by direct digital pressure or by suturing with nonabsorbable vascular sutures with pledgets. Cardiopulmonary bypass is required in only 10% of successful repairs of myocardial rupture.[71] For patients with suspected myocardial rupture, it is appropriate to undertake emergency thoracotomy in institutions that have qualified surgeons but no immediate access to cardiopulmonary bypass.

Prognosis

Only a few survivors of ventricular rupture have been reported.[71] Most survivors of cardiac rupture are patients with atrial rupture, including one patient with multiple atrial tears. Most undergo surgical repair within 3 to 4 hours of injury.[73] Approximately 60% of successful repairs have been performed more than 60 minutes after injury.[71]

Miscellaneous Cardiac Injuries

The occurrence of intracardiac injuries that result from blunt chest trauma (e.g., septal defects or valvular injuries) is less common. Valve rupture may involve the chordae tendinae, leaflets, or papillary muscles. Involvement of the aortic valve is more common than involvement of the mitral or tricuspid valves. Mitral and tricuspid valve injuries associated with a pericardial laceration have been reported in a survivor of blunt chest trauma. The exact incidence of cardiac valvular injuries and septal defects is unknown. Serial echocardiography, monitoring of ECG changes, and frequent auscultation may aid in earlier diagnosis of these lesions.

Clinical Features

The clinical presentation of patients with intracardiac injuries depends on which valve or septum is involved and whether coincident cardiac injuries are present. A complete rupture of the mitral valve usually results in immediate death. The clinical presentation of an incomplete rupture depends on the hemodynamic state of the patient. Cardiogenic shock is common. Findings of acute mitral insufficiency and rapidly developing pulmonary edema are usually predominant. A loud, harsh diastolic murmur with frank left heart failure suggests acute aortic insufficiency. If the patient is in a low cardiac output state, the associated thrills and murmurs of aortic or mitral insufficiency may not be appreciated. The signs and symptoms of tricuspid insufficiency that follow a rupture of that valve may be less dramatic or even minimal. Examination may reveal only a diastolic murmur and prominent V waves of the jugular venous pulsations.

Patients with isolated septal defects may have minimal symptoms of exertional dyspnea or severe progressive shock and pulmonary edema, depending on the size and location of the defect. Dysrhythmias and conduction defects are rare because the lower muscular septum is principally involved. The typical holosystolic murmur along the left sternal border is an important clue in diagnosing a ventricular septal defect, but it may not appear for days or months after the injury. Serial echocardiography and ultimately cardiac catheterization for valvular and septal defects are necessary for a definitive diagnosis.

Management

The therapy selected depends primarily on how well the patient tolerates the insult. Many years may elapse before operative treatment is required. In cases of ventricular septal defects, a period of observation is valuable because there have been reports of the spontaneous closure of traumatic ventricular septal defects months after the injury when the defects and resultant shunt are small. Medical therapy commonly relieves the symptoms of congestive failure, but intractable or progressive heart failure or the development of pulmonary hypertension usually reflects the need for surgery.

Penetrating Cardiac Injury

Penetrating cardiac injuries are among the leading causes of death in the settings of urban violence. Improvements in emergency medical services systems in recent years along with the emphasis on rapid transport have been responsible for an increasing number of penetrating cardiac injury patients arriving in impending or full cardiopulmonary arrest to busy urban trauma centers. The proportion of gunshot wounds versus stab wounds varies widely in reported case series, depending on the location of the trauma center.

The right ventricle is affected more often (43%) than the left ventricle (34%) owing to its anterior anatomic location. The left or right atrium is affected in 20% of cases.[75] One third of penetrating cardiac wounds affect multiple chambers, and survival is much worse in these cases. In 5% of cases, a coronary artery is lacerated, although these injuries usually involve a distal segment of the artery and rarely produce significant acute MI when they are ligated. More proximal coronary artery lacerations require coronary bypass.[76] Rarely the interventricular septum, a valve, papillary muscle, or chordae tendinae is lacerated, producing an acute shunt or valvular insufficiency. These lesions are poorly tolerated and can produce massive pulmonary edema and cardiogenic shock quickly.

Two conditions may occur after penetrating heart injury: exsanguinating hemorrhage, if the cardiac lesion communicates freely with the pleural cavity, or cardiac tamponade, if the hemorrhage is contained within the pericardium. Patients with exsanguinating wounds frequently die before they reach medical attention or present with rapidly progressive hemorrhagic shock culminating in cardiac arrest.[76,77] This presentation is seen most typically in patients sustaining gunshot wounds of the heart. These patients often require immediate resuscitation by emergency department thoracotomy if they meet the criteria listed in Box 42-5. Cardiac tamponade is itself a life-threatening condition, but seems to offer some degree of protection and increased survival in patients with penetrating cardiac wounds. A third condition can occur rarely in which the tamponade decompresses intermittently as intrapericardial pressure builds up to a threshold, then releases through the wound into the thoracic cavity. These patients may show a waxing and waning hemodynamic course and have improved overall survival.

Acute Pericardial Tamponade

Epidemiology

The reported incidence of acute pericardial tamponade is approximately 2% in patients with penetrating trauma to the chest and upper abdomen; it is rarely seen after blunt chest trauma. It occurs more commonly with stab wounds than gunshot wounds, and 60% to 80% of patients with stab wounds involving the heart develop tamponade.[78] Patients with acute pericardial tamponade can deteriorate in minutes, but many can be saved if proper steps are taken.

Anatomy and Pathophysiology

The primary feature of a pericardial tamponade is an increase in intrapericardial pressure and volume. As the volume of the pericardial fluid encroaches on the capacity of the atria and ventricles to fill adequately, ventricular filling is mechanically limited, and the stroke volume is reduced. This reduction in stroke volume results in decreased cardiac output and ultimately diminished arterial systolic blood pressure and decreased pulse pressure. The clinical picture of tamponade may be produced by 60 to 100 mL of blood and clots in the pericardium. Concomitantly, CVP increases because of the mechanical backup of blood into the vena cava. Coincident hemorrhage from this and other extracardiac injuries may cause the CVP to be normal or low in the face of tamponade.

Several compensatory mechanisms subsequently occur. The heart rate and total peripheral resistance increase in an attempt to maintain adequate cardiac output and blood pressure. A less effective compensatory response, resulting in a greater increase of CVP, is an increase in venomotor tone caused by contractions of the smooth muscles within the wall of the vena cava.

In a normotensive patient, the earliest response to pericardial tamponade is a progressive increase in CVP to a level greater than 15 cm H_2O. An increasing CVP in a hypotensive patient indicates that the normal compensatory responses are unable to maintain an adequate cardiac output. A simultaneous decrease in the CVP and blood pressure, which can occur precipitously and without warning, signals decompensation and imminent cardiac arrest. In animal studies, electromechanical dissociation and sudden bradycardia have been shown to precede the terminal event.

The diagnosis of pericardial tamponade should be suspected in any patient who has sustained a penetrating wound to the thorax or upper abdomen. One cannot be certain of the trajectory of the bullet or the length, force, and direction of a knife thrust. Wounds directly over the precordium and epigastrium are more likely to produce a cardiac injury resulting in tamponade than wounds in the posterior or lateral thorax. Nevertheless, it must be assumed that a penetrating wound, particularly a gunshot wound, anywhere in the thorax or upper abdomen may have injured the heart.[78]

Clinical Features

Patients with cardiac tamponade initially may appear deceptively stable if the rate of bleeding into the pericardial space is slow or if the pericardial wound allows intermittent decompression. Other patients may complain primarily of difficulty breathing, which suggests pulmonary rather than cardiac pathology. The physical findings of pericardial tamponade are hypotension, distended neck veins, and, rarely, distant or muffled heart tones. This so-called Beck's triad is sometimes difficult to show clinically, especially in the midst of a major resuscitation with concomitant hypovolemia.[79] The most reliable signs of pericardial tamponade are an elevated CVP (>15 cm H_2O) in association with hypotension and tachycardia. When this triad is present either before or after adequate volume replacement, the diagnosis of acute pericardial tamponade and tension pneumothorax should be considered.

Acute pericardial tamponade may be seen with three distinct clinical pictures. If the hemorrhage is confined to the pericardial space, the patient is initially normotensive but has a tachycardia and elevated CVP. If untreated, most of these patients go on to develop hypotension.

If significant hemorrhage has occurred outside the pericardial sac, either through a rent in the pericardium or from associated trauma, the clinical picture is that of hypovolemic shock with hypotension, tachycardia, and a low CVP. If the CVP increases to 15 to 20 cm H_2O with volume replacement, and hypotension and tachycardia persist, the presence of a pericardial tamponade must be considered. One also must consider other causes, such as a tension pneumothorax, Valsalva's maneuver, venous air embolus, or pulmonary edema secondary to fluid overload.

The third clinical picture is that of an intermittently decompressing tamponade. In this case, intermittent hemorrhage from the intrapericardial space occurs, decompressing and partially relieving the tamponade. The clinical picture may wax and wane depending on the intrapericardial pressure and volume and total blood loss. In general, this condition is compatible with a longer survival than are the first two clinical presentations.

Pulsus paradoxus is defined as an excessive decline in systolic blood pressure during the inspiratory phase of the normal respiratory cycle. This sign may be an additional clue to the presence of pericardial tamponade, but is often difficult to measure during an intensive resuscitation, particularly if the patient is hypotensive.

Diagnostic Strategies

Ultrasound

Ultrasound, which is becoming more widely available in emergency departments around the world, enables rapid, accurate, and noninvasive diagnosis of pericardial tamponade.[80] Ultrasound can be performed at the bedside in the emergency department during the initial

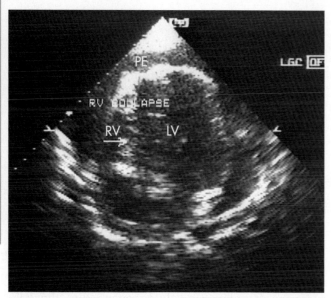

Figure 42-11. Cardiac ultrasound in same patient as in Figure 42-12 shows pericardial effusion without right ventricular collapse. PE, pericardial effusion; RV, right ventricle; LV, left ventricle.

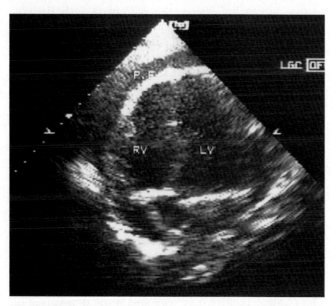

Figure 42-12. Cardiac ultrasound shows pericardial effusion and right ventricular collapse. PE, pericardial effusion; RV, right ventricle; LV, left ventricle.

resuscitation of the patient. Although the sonographic definition of tamponade is the simultaneous presence of pericardial fluid and diastolic collapse of the right ventricle or atrium (Figure 42-11), the presence of pericardial fluid in a patient with chest trauma is highly suggestive of pericardial hemorrhage (Figure 42-12). An indirect sonographic sign of tamponade is the demonstration of a dilated inferior vena cava in a hypotensive patient. Emergency departments performing cardiac ultrasonography using subcostal and long parasternal views have reported a sensitivity of 98.1% and a specificity of 99.9% for the detection of pericardial effusion.[81] Because ultrasound is noninvasive and extremely accurate, its immediate availability in the

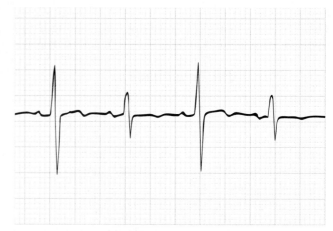

Figure 42-13. Lewis lead ECG revealing total electrical alternans of the QRS complexes. (From Sotolongo RP, Horton JD: Total electrical alternans in pericardial tamponade. *Am Heart J* 101:853, 1981.)

initial phase of a major trauma resuscitation can be helpful because it can detect pericardial fluid before the patient deteriorates hemodynamically.

Electrocardiography

Many ECG changes of pericardial tamponade have been described in the literature, but few are diagnostic, and each is more likely to be seen with chronic rather than acute tamponade. Electrical alternans has been reported to be a highly specific marker of pericardial tamponade. Electrical alternans is an ECG change in which the morphology and amplitude of the P, QRS, and ST-T wave in any single lead alternates in every other beat (Figure 42-13). The postulated cause is the mechanical oscillation of the heart in the pericardial fluid, which is called the "swinging heart" phenomenon. In uncomplicated pericardial effusion, the heart swings back and forth but returns to approximately the same position before the next systole. Electrical alternans does not occur in this situation.

Echocardiographic studies have revealed that when fluid accumulates to a critical extent and cardiac tamponade ensues, the frequency of cardiac oscillation may decrease abruptly to half the heart rate. The cardiac position alternates, with the heart returning to its original position with every other beat, and electrical alternans may be seen. Electrical alternans, when present, is pathognomonic for tamponade. It is much more common in chronic pericardial effusions that evolve into a tamponade, however, and it is rarely seen in acute pericardial tamponade.

Radiography

The radiographic evaluation of the cardiac silhouette in acute pericardial tamponade generally is not helpful, unless a traumatic pneumopericardium is present. Because small volumes of hemopericardium lead to tamponade in the acute setting, the heart typically appears normal; this is in contrast to the "water-bottle" appearance of the heart with chronic pericardial effusion. This latter condition is tolerated for a long period (Figure 42-14).

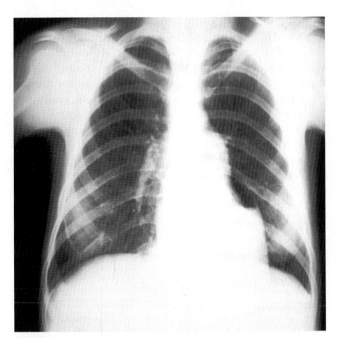

Figure 42-14. Air-fluid level in pericardium immediately after pericardiocentesis.

Management

Prehospital Care

Field treatment for cases of pericardial tamponade is essentially the same as outlined for any victim of major trauma. The diagnosis of tamponade should be suspected by the location of penetrating wounds or by the patient's poor response to vigorous volume resuscitation. Tension pneumothorax, which is much more common, may mimic acute pericardial tamponade. If the patient presents in extremis or the clinical condition rapidly deteriorates, performing a needle thoracostomy should be considered. If the needle thoracostomy is not therapeutic, it suggests pericardial tamponade under the appropriate clinical presentation by virtue of "diagnosis of exclusion." Expedient transport to the nearest trauma center should be of paramount concern in most cases. In certain venues (e.g., prolonged helicopter transport) and if their scope of practice permits, some prehospital providers are authorized to perform pericardiocentesis in the field.

Emergency Department

When the patient arrives in the emergency department, volume expansion with crystalloid solution via two or three large-bore (14-gauge or 16-gauge) catheters should be established immediately. The presence of a pneumothorax or hemothorax, which is often associated with penetrating cardiac trauma, must be treated expeditiously with tube thoracostomy. Bedside echocardiography should be performed as quickly as possible to establish the diagnosis of pericardial tamponade, which then mandates urgent surgical repair.

There is increasing controversy with regard to the role of pericardiocentesis. Earlier literature recommended that pericardiocentesis should be performed for diagnostic and therapeutic reasons. Aspiration of 5 to 10 mL

of blood may result in dramatic clinical improvement. Reducing the total intrapericardial volume to just below the critical level allows compensatory mechanisms to maintain adequate hemodynamics.[82]

Pericardiocentesis is not a benign or invariably successful procedure. Blood in the pericardial space tends to be clotted, and aspiration may not be possible. Possible complications include the production of pericardial tamponade, the laceration of a coronary artery or lung, and induction of cardiac dysrhythmias. Whenever possible, pericardiocentesis should be performed under ultrasound guidance because this approach increases the success rate and decreases the incidence of complications.[83] A catheter, preferably a pig-tailed catheter that can be anchored in the pericardial space, may be introduced for repeated aspirations while preparations are under way to transport the patient quickly to the operating room for definitive therapy. If pericardiocentesis is unsuccessful or the clinical status deteriorates, and if acute pericardial tamponade remains important in the differential diagnosis, thoracotomy should be performed as quickly as possible.[84] Patients with penetrating cardiac injury invariably require surgical repair. The location (operating room versus emergency department) and timing (immediate versus urgent) depends on the patient's clinical status.

Emergency Department Thoracotomy

Emergency department thoracotomy is a drastic, dramatic, and potentially lifesaving procedure in which emergency physicians should be proficient. Although the procedure is not described in detail here, a few technical points merit discussion. A left lateral incision is preferred because it is accomplished rapidly; allows the best exposure of the heart, aorta, and left hilum; and facilitates open cardiac massage and internal defibrillation.[84] With right-sided or multiple injuries, it may be necessary to extend the incision across the sternum and right chest wall, creating a "clamshell" incision. The internal mammary arteries need to be ligated if this maneuver restores effective perfusion. After the heart is sufficiently exposed, the phrenic nerve is identified, and a vertical incision in the pericardium is made anterior to the phrenic nerve. Release of a tamponade may restore cardiac output rapidly. The heart is delivered through the pericardium, and penetrating wounds are identified.

There are several alternatives for repairing cardiac wounds. Small wounds can be compressed by digital pressure to control bleeding en route to the operating room. If the injury is quite large, balloon tamponade can be achieved by applying gentle traction on a Foley catheter inserted into the wound with the balloon inflated with saline. This maneuver can temporarily stop the hemorrhage to allow suture repair of the injury (cardiorrhaphy) or to gain time while the patient is transferred to the operating room for a more definitive surgical procedure. Lacerations of the atria can be controlled temporarily with a vascular clamp.[84]

Suture of cardiac wounds over pledgets is the time-honored and effective technique but is technically more difficult and more time-consuming. Use of a monofilament suture, such as 2-0 polypropylene (Prolene), is recommended. Some trauma surgeons recommend stapling cardiac wounds with standard skin staplers because this technique has been shown to be much quicker and equally effective in closing these wounds.[85] Care must be taken to avoid ligating coronary arteries during the repair. Direct insertion of a large-bore catheter (e.g., a 5F catheter) into the left atrial appendage provides a route for rapid infusion of fluids. If the heart is empty or the patient fails to respond to rapid fluid administration, the aorta is cross-clamped to divert cardiac output to the brain and heart. Prolonged ischemia and severe acidosis often result in postresuscitation myocardial depression with ineffective contraction and diminished cardiac output.

Indications for Emergency Department Thoracotomy. Although it is often tempting to perform emergency department thoracotomy on all traumatic arrest victims presenting to the emergency department, there are cases in which it has virtually no chance of salvaging a neurologically uncompromised patient. Consequently, guidelines have been established for performing emergency department thoracotomy to restrict the procedure to patients with some chance of achieving a neurologically functional outcome (see Box 42-4).[86] Patients with penetrating trauma with signs of life in the field, even if only electrical activity on cardiac monitor or agonal respirations, are candidates for emergency department thoracotomy if transport times are less than 10 minutes.[87,88]

Prognosis

After penetrating wounds to the heart, several factors adversely affect survival, including gunshot wound mechanisms and wounds that involve the left ventricle, multiple cardiac chambers, intrapericardial great vessels, or one or more coronary arteries. Factors favorable to survival include stab wound mechanisms with minor perforations, isolated right ventricular or atrial wounds, a systolic blood pressure greater than 50 mm Hg on arrival at the emergency department, and the presence of cardiac tamponade. Survival rates after emergency department thoracotomy (Table 42-1) have been correlated with the mechanism and location of injury, field and transport times, the duration of arrest, and the physiologic status of the patient in the prehospital and hospital setting.

A meta-analysis of the literature reveals that emergency department thoracotomy had an overall survival rate of 7.4%, with normal neurologic outcomes noted in 92.4% of surviving patients. Survival rates for mechanism of injury were 8.8% for penetrating injuries and 1.4% for blunt injuries. When penetrating injuries were separated further, the survival rates were 16.8% for stab wounds and 4.3% for gunshot wounds. Survival rates based on the anatomic location of injury were 10.7% for thoracic injuries, 4.5% for abdominal injuries, and 0.7% for multiple injuries. Isolated cardiac injuries were associated with the highest reported survival rates (<20%). The presence of pericardial tamponade is a favorable prognostic finding. If signs of life were present on arrival at the hospital, survival rate was 11.5% compared with 2.6% if none were present. Absence of any signs of life in the field yielded a survival rate of 1.2%.[89]

Blunt Traumatic Aortic Injury

Epidemiology

The thoracic aorta is the most common vessel injured by blunt trauma. The mortality rate has increased dramatically from less than 1% in 1947 to 15% in more recent years, suggesting a strong association with high-speed automobile transportation.[90] Many crash victims sustain this injury without dying immediately; 10% to 20% survive, at least temporarily, because of tamponade of aortic blood by the adventitia. The mean age of patients sustaining aortic rupture is 33 years; more than 70% of these patients are men. Because patients who survive to reach the hospital were usually healthy before the trauma, almost 85% survive if diagnosis and surgical intervention are prompt.

Anatomy and Pathophysiology

Eighty percent to 90% of aortic tears occur in the descending aorta at the isthmus, just distal to the left subclavian artery (Figures 42-15 and 42-16). Other, less common sites of involvement are the ascending aorta, the distal descending aorta at the level of the diaphragm, the midthoracic descending aorta, and the origin of the left subclavian artery. Although ruptures of the ascending aorta are much less common than ruptures of the descending aorta, they have a 70% to 80% incidence of associated lethal cardiac injuries. In contrast, ruptures at the isthmus have a 25% incidence of associated cardiac injuries. Lethal cardiac injuries commonly include pericardial tamponade, aortic valve tears, myocardial contusion, and coronary artery injuries. Passenger ejection, pedestrian impact, severe falls, and crush injuries commonly result in ascending thoracic aortic ruptures. Survival long enough to be evaluated in the emergency department is rare among patients who sustain an ascending aortic rupture.

Several theories about the mechanism of blunt traumatic aortic rupture have predominated in the literature. The descending thoracic aorta is relatively fixed and immobile because of its tethering by intercostal arteries and the ligamentum arteriosum. With sudden deceleration, the more mobile aortic arch swings forward, producing a shearing force or "whiplash

Table 42-1. Outcome of Emergency Department Thoracotomy

Condition	Survival (%)
Cardiac arrest in field	0
Cardiac arrest in emergency department	30
Agonal in emergency department	40
Unresponsive shock in emergency department	50

From Brown J, Grover FL: Trauma to the heart. *Chest Surg Clin N Am* 7:325, 1997.

effect" on the aorta at the isthmus. A bending stress at the isthmus, created by sudden lateral oblique chest compression, also may result in rupture by causing flexion of the aortic arch on the left main stem bronchus and the pulmonary artery. It has been suggested that the forces created by the whiplash effect or lateral oblique compression may not be sufficient to provoke aortic tears. It is now postulated that those injuries may be caused by inferior and posterior rotation of anterior thoracic osseous structures (manubrium, first rib, medial clavicles) pinching and shearing the interposed aorta as they strike the vertebral column.

Rupture of the ascending aorta just distal to the aortic valve likely occurs through a different mechanism. At the time of rapid deceleration and chest compression, the heart is displaced into the left posterior chest, which causes a shearing stress just above the aortic valve. A sudden increase in intra-aortic pressure, the "waterhammer effect," also may cause an explosive rupture of the aorta at this location. Involvement of the coronary ostia with coronary artery occlusion may occur in association with tears to the ascending arch. The intraluminal pressure tolerance of the aorta may be exceeded in a high-speed MVC. It is likely that a combination of the preceding mechanisms accounts for the multiple aortic ruptures that have been found in 20% of traffic accident victims examined at autopsy.

Aortic rupture may occur from causes other than high-speed MVC deceleration. Rupture has been documented as a complication of external cardiac massage and has been known to occur after fracture-dislocations of the thoracic spine, presumably as the result of direct shearing force. Vertical deceleration injuries resulting from falls can cause a rupture of the ascending aorta by producing an acute lengthening of the ascending aorta; this is the likely mechanism responsible for aortic rupture in the setting of airplane and elevator accidents. Direct kicks by animals, crush injuries, sudden burial by landslide, and air bag deployment also have been reported as causes of aortic rupture. Direct compression of the compliant thorax has been postulated to contribute to aortic rupture in children. Displaced fractures of the sternum, ribs, and clavicle also have been shown to lacerate the aorta directly.

Clinical Features

The possibility of aortic disruption must be considered in every patient who sustains a severe deceleration injury. This is especially true if the automobile was moving in excess of 45 mph or if evidence of severe

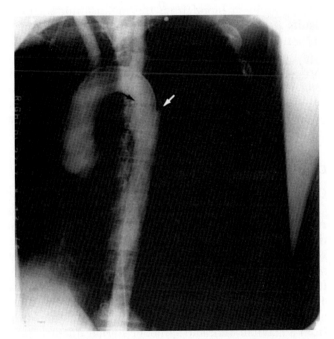

Figure 42-15. Follow-up aortogram shows tear in aorta *(arrows)* at most common location at or just distal to take-off point of left subclavian artery, which is not visualized.

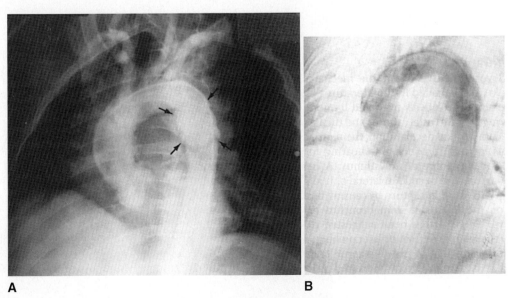

A   **B**

Figure 42-16. A, Follow-up aortogram of patient in Figure 42-15. Arch study with catheter in ascending aorta. Tear in aorta *(arrows)* distal to left subclavian artery is seen with dissection and extravasation of contrast material. **B,** Reverse image.

blunt forces to the chest (e.g., from a damaged steering wheel) exists. In the case of any moderate-speed or high-speed MVC, it is imperative that paramedics carefully evaluate the extent of damage to the vehicle, the complaints of the victims, and the physical manifestations of blunt chest trauma. This information should be relayed promptly to the emergency physician.

Despite the severe nature of the injury, the clinical manifestations of an aortic rupture are often deceptively meager. Associated pulmonary, neurologic, orthopedic, facial, and abdominal injuries are commonly present. Coexisting injuries can mask the signs and symptoms of an aortic injury or divert the physician's attention away from the more lethal aortic rupture. The absence of any external evidence of a chest injury does not eliminate the possibility of an aortic tear. One third to one half of patients reported in the literature have no external signs of chest trauma.

The most common symptom is interscapular or retrosternal pain. It often is found in nontraumatic aortic dissection, but is present in only 25% of patients with blunt traumatic aortic rupture. Other symptoms described in the literature but uncommonly present include dyspnea resulting from tracheal compression and deviation, stridor or hoarseness caused by compression of the laryngeal nerve, dysphagia caused by esophageal compression, and extremity pain caused by ischemia from decreased arterial flow.

Clinical signs are uncommon and nonspecific. Generalized hypertension, when present, is an important clinical sign. Sympathetic afferent nerve fibers, located in the area of the aortic isthmus, are capable of causing reflex hypertension as a response to a stretching stimulus. A mean systolic pressure of 152 mm Hg (range 142 to 198 mm Hg) and a mean diastolic pressure of 98 mm Hg (range 90 to 124 mm Hg) were measured in 72%

of patients with traumatic aortic rupture before fluid or vasoactive drug therapy. A less common clinical finding is the acute onset of upper extremity hypertension, along with absent or diminished femoral pulses. This pseudocoarctation syndrome has been reported to occur in one third of these patients and is attributed to compression of the aortic lumen by a periaortic hematoma.

The presence of a harsh systolic murmur over the precordium or posterior interscapular area may be heard in one third of patients. The murmur is thought to result from the turbulent flow across the area of transection. A less commonly encountered physical finding is a swelling at the base of the neck caused by the extravasation of blood from the mediastinum, which results in an increased neck circumference or a pulsatile neck mass. Other clinical signs suggesting aortic rupture include lower extremity pulse deficit and lower extremity paralysis. Initial chest tube output greater than 750 mL also suggests aortic rupture.[91] The physical examination is neither sensitive nor specific for aortic injury, however, preventing accurate diagnosis without ancillary studies.

Diagnostic Strategies

Chest Radiography

Chest radiography is a valuable tool when aortic rupture is suspected. Many patients have died because the presence and significance of radiographic findings were not appreciated. An increase in the width of the superior mediastinum is the most sensitive sign and is found in 50% to 92% of aortic ruptures (Figure 42-17).[92] Specificity of this radiologic sign is 10%. Mediastinal widening may be caused by venous bleeding from a clavicle, thoracic spine, or sternal fracture; pul-

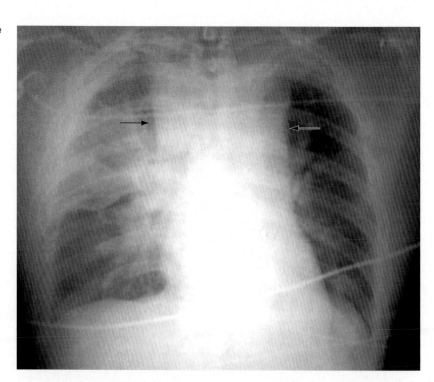

Figure 42-17. Anteroposterior radiograph of the chest showing wide mediastinum (arrows).

monary contusions; a previous mediastinal mass; a misplaced CVP catheter; or magnification caused by the anteroposterior and supine position of a portable chest radiograph. The sign is not pathognomonic for aortic rupture.

Commonly cited guidelines for abnormal mediastinal widening include a mediastinal width greater than 6 cm in the erect posteroanterior film, greater than 8 cm in the supine anteroposterior chest film, or greater than 7.5 cm at the aortic knob or a ratio of mediastinal width to chest width greater than 0.25 at the aortic knob. Disagreement exists regarding the reliability of these parameters in confirming or excluding aortic rupture. A subjective interpretation of mediastinal widening is more reliable than direct measurement of mediastinal width.[93] Positioning of the patient and the degree of inspiration are important factors in assessing the mediastinum. Every effort should be made to obtain a standard upright inspiratory posteroanterior film, if clinically feasible, before a mediastinum is declared abnormal to avoid false-positive interpretations.[94,95]

Current literature is replete with various diagnostic radiologic criteria thought to be sensitive indicators of aortic rupture.[94,95] Several authors have shown that an interpretation of widened mediastinum and an obscured aortic knob are the most sensitive signs of aortic rupture. The opacification of the clear space between the aorta and the pulmonary artery, displaced nasogastric tube, widened paratracheal stripe, and widened right paraspinal interface are thought to provide the most specific evidence for aortic rupture.[95] Other authors believe that deviation of the nasogastric tube to the right combined with depression of the left main stem bronchus below 40 degrees from the horizontal, is the most specific (although relatively insensitive) sign positively associated with the diagnosis.

Other reported radiologic signs of a ruptured aorta include left hemithorax, obliteration of the medial aspect of the left upper lobe apex (left apical pleural cap), deviation of the trachea to the right, and multiple rib fractures.[92] Fractures of the first and second ribs, previously classically described as highly suggestive of aortic injury, do not seem to be associated with increased risk compared with patients without these fractures.[91]

Although previous reports suggested that a negative chest radiograph is highly predictive of a normal aortogram,[94] several more recent studies challenge this widely held belief. The sensitivity of a negative chest radiograph (i.e., normal mediastinum) is limited. Several authors recommend liberal use of helical chest CT in patients with high-speed deceleration mechanisms of injury. Reported rates of false-negative chest x-rays with no mediastinal widening in patients with proven aortic injury vary from 0% to 45%, with most studies finding a 7% to 10% false-negative rate.[96-99]

Chest Computed Tomography

Helical chest CT has largely replaced the need for aortography to detect blunt traumatic aortic rupture.[98,99] All studies that reported poor results in diagnosing aortic rupture used conventional CT. The development of helical CT in the early 1990s has revolutionized trauma radiology with its speed and superior definition, largely obviating the false-negative results obtained with conventional CT. Helical CT has almost 100% sensitivity and specificity for detecting aortic rupture.[9,98] A mediastinal hematoma may be seen, or direct evidence of vascular injury may be confirmed by the presence of a flap in the aortic lumen (Figure 42-18).

Chest CT with intravascular contrast offers many advantages over aortography. CT is noninvasive, pro-

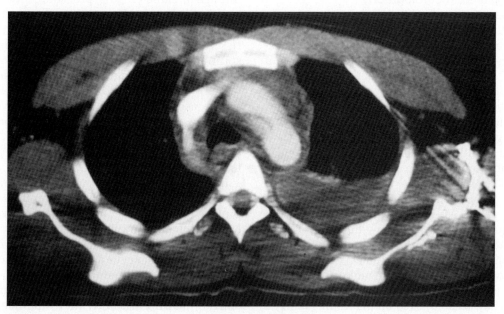

Figure 42-18. Dynamic computed tomography scan of the chest shows periaortic hemorrhage and an intimal flap.

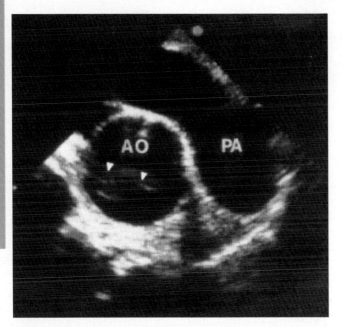

Figure 42-19. Transesophageal echocardiogram shows periaortic hemorrhage and aortic dissection (arrows). AO, aorta; PA, periaortic.

vides significantly more information on other thoracic injuries than chest radiography, and can be performed much more rapidly than angiography. It is able to discern blunt traumatic aortic rupture from simple periaortic hematoma, the latter not requiring operative therapy.[99,100] At most centers, an immediate chest CT scan is readily available. In addition, in patients with a widened mediastinum, CT may be useful in evaluating not only the aorta, but also the spine because spinal fractures may be the cause of a widened mediastinum. It is now recommended that all patients with a mechanism of injury suggesting potential aortic injury should undergo CT evaluation of the mediastinum, regardless of chest x-ray findings.[9]

Transesophageal Echocardiography

TEE is an alternative method to CT or aortography for establishing the diagnosis of aortic rupture. It offers many advantages: It is fast, does not require intravenous contrast administration, provides concomitant evaluation of cardiac function, does not risk allergic contrast reactions or deterioration of renal function, and can be performed in the emergency department.[81] Sedation is necessary to avoid hypertension while inserting the probe.

TEE allows identification of an intimal flap and a periaortic hematoma (Figure 42-19). When only a monoplane TEE is used, the upper portion of the ascending aorta represents a blind zone because of the interposition of the air-filled trachea. Because most injuries are located at the isthmus, however, TEE is highly accurate with a reported sensitivity of 87% to 100% and a specificity of 98% to 100%.[100,101] When the technique is available, TEE offers an alternative to chest CT as a diagnostic screening test for aortic injury. Aortic repair may be predicated on the findings of TEE

alone, but aortography is still needed when TEE results are equivocal, when TEE is not tolerated or contraindicated, or when other suspected vascular injuries require evaluation by arteriography.[102]

Intravascular Ultrasound

Use of intravascular ultrasound has been described to detect subtle injuries to the aorta. This modality involves a small ultrasound probe that is inserted through the femoral artery and guided up the aorta. At present, availability is limited to a few trauma centers because the technique requires sophisticated equipment and is performed in the operating room or angiography suite.[101,103] Preliminary data suggest that intravascular ultrasound is extremely sensitive and specific in detecting blunt aortic injury.[99,102,103]

Aortography

Aortography had long been considered the gold standard for establishing the diagnosis of aortic disruption.[104] The major objective for patients with a ruptured aorta is the early recognition of the lesion before adventitial disruption and exsanguination. Multiple aortic tears occur in 15% to 20% of cases, necessitating precise anatomic localization of these injuries. Before the widespread availability of helical CT scanners, aortography was recommended not only for patients with a widened mediastinum, but also for patients who had sustained significant blunt chest trauma and who had any of the radiologic signs previously mentioned. An aggressive approach is particularly warranted in elderly patients because the risk for aortic injury increases with age as the aorta becomes less elastic and more prone to "fracture." In contrast, aortic injury is rare in children.

Aortography should be delayed in patients with more immediate life-threatening injuries to the abdomen, pelvis, and head. High-quality aortography can be performed with the aid of a rapid film changer by directly injecting the contrast medium into the root of the aorta through a catheter. The procedure involves a risk of further damage to the aorta or other ruptured vessel if the catheter crosses the site of the injury; however, this risk can be reduced by using meticulous technique, a soft-tipped C-curve guidewire, and fluoroscopy. Simultaneous coronary angiography is often indicated, particularly in patients with an aortogram that shows a tear in the ascending aorta, because involvement of the coronary ostia by the dissection or the presence of significant arteriosclerotic disease may warrant coronary artery bypass grafting together with surgical repair of the aorta.

Intravenous digital subtraction angiography is significantly faster and less expensive than conventional biplane angiography, and when intravenous digital subtraction angiography films are of diagnostic quality, they reliably show the presence of traumatic aortic transection and may be as accurate as conventional aortography.[105] The procedure requires intra-arterial injection of contrast material into the aortic arch as in conventional aortography, but it eliminates the need for a conventional biplane imaging system, obtaining preliminary radiographs, and developing and mounting the cut-film sequence procedures needed for conventional angiography. A potential reduction in overall contrast load and the ability to use smaller catheters are additional advantages of this technique.

As surgeons have gained more experience with the diagnostic capabilities of helical CT, the need for preoperative angiography has declined. Aortography now should be reserved for high-risk patients with indeterminate helical chest CT scans.[9,100]

Management

Prehospital

In the prehospital care of any patient who has sustained blunt chest trauma, evaluation for possible aortic rupture should concentrate on identifying a mechanism of injury compatible with aortic rupture and treating hypotension, tension pneumothorax, and pericardial tamponade. Immediate communication of the patient's condition and expeditious transport to a trauma center increase the patient's chance for survival.

Emergency Department

The lesion should be repaired as soon as the diagnosis is made because of the ever-present risk of sudden free rupture and exsanguination. Management of a patient with multiple injuries who has documented rupture of the thoracic aorta depends, however, on the nature of associated injuries. Surgical repair of the aortic rupture should be delayed in the presence of life-threatening intracranial or intra-abdominal injury or profuse retroperitoneal hemorrhage.[77,106,107] Delaying the procedure should be considered in patients at high risk for infection (e.g., patients who have extensive body surface burns, contaminated large open wounds, established sepsis, or severe respiratory insufficiency caused by thoracic trauma).

Careful regulation of blood pressure is mandatory until definitive surgical repair can be performed. If operative repair is delayed, systolic blood pressure should be maintained between 100 and 120 mm Hg. The objective of lowering the blood pressure is to decrease the shearing jet effect of an elevated pulse pressure, decreasing the possibility of continued adventitial dissection and subsequent free rupture.

Esmolol, a short-acting titratable β-blocker, may be ideally suited for this purpose because, in contrast to nitroprusside sodium, it decreases the pulse pressure and minimizes the shearing effect on the intact adventitia of the aorta. If the blood pressure is not adequately controlled, nitroprusside sodium can be added as a second agent when the pulse pressure has been decreased with a short-acting β-blocker.

Surgical Techniques

Many surgical techniques have been described since the first successful repair by Passaro and Pace in 1959.[108] Current therapeutic approaches (Box 42-6) most widely used include simple clamp repair using

---

BOX 42-6. Current Therapeutic Approaches to the Treatment of Blunt Thoracic Aortic Injuries

1. Surgical
   a. Clamp and direct reconstruction with or without an interposition graft
   b. Passive bypass shunts
   c. Pump-assisted bypass
   d. Atriofemoral bypass
2. Nonoperative or delay of surgery with pharmacologic control of hypertension and close radiologic surveillance
3. Endovascular stenting

From Le Maire SA, Mattox KL: Injury to the thoracic great vessels. In Mattox KL, Feliciano DV, Moore EE (eds): *Trauma.* New York, McGraw-Hill, 2004, pp 202-213.

---

pharmacologic means to control upper extremity hypertension, use of heparin-bonded bypass shunts, use of a centrifugal pump with heparin-bonded tubing, and cardiopulmonary bypass.[109] Many surgeons advocate the clamp repair technique, which directly isolates the injury between vascular clamps without use of bypass tubes or pumps.[108,109] These surgeons believe that this new method is advantageous because it decreases clamp time, minimizes aortic dissection, allows rapid control of the aorta, avoids complications from shunt bypass procedures, and avoids heparinization. Overall mortality rates and incidence of paraplegia are thought to be minimized with this procedure. Other surgeons argue that shunting procedures offer better protection against spinal cord ischemia and subsequent neurologic deficits, especially when cross-clamp time is expected to exceed 30 minutes.[110] The use of cardiopulmonary bypass is controversial. Some authors recommend the use of bypass for patients with complex injuries, stating that its use eliminates subsequent paraplegia from prolonged aortic cross-clamp times.[110,111]

The pathologic condition found dictates the type of repair. A synthetic graft often is required because of extensive tension on the vessel walls or jaggedly torn ends of the vessel. Data on successful primary (without use of a graft) repair of aortic disruption are encouraging.[111] The procedure requires less operative time and has a lower potential infection risk, blood loss through a prosthesis is avoided, the possibility of pseudoaneurysm formation is eliminated, and secondary embolism arising from mural thrombosis is avoided. Multiple tears of the descending thoracic aorta have been repaired successfully using the primary suture technique. Direct end-to-end anastomosis seems to be most feasible in patients younger than 30 years of age.

For patients who arrive at the hospital alive but who have descending thoracic aortic injuries, the incidence of mortality during surgery is 20% to 30%, and the paraplegia rate is 5% to 7%.[108-110] Younger patients have the highest survival rate. Mortality is related to the presence or absence of extensive dissection and to the preoperative condition of the patient.

A growing body of evidence shows the safety and efficacy of endovascular repair of traumatic aortic tears. Endovascular repair involves the use of a stent placed through a femoral or iliac artery approach. Preliminary data have shown that success rates and complication rates are comparable if not better than traditional open surgical repairs.[112,113]

Chronic Aneurysms

Chronic thoracic aneurysms are usually asymptomatic and are discovered through chest radiographs obtained for other reasons. Symptomatic patients show signs of mediastinal compression (e.g., dyspnea, back and chest pain, chronic cough, dysphagia, or recurrent laryngeal nerve palsy causing hoarseness). Although acute ruptures produce chronic aneurysms in only 2% to 5% of cases, half of these aneurysms show instability or enlargement during the first several years (or even >5 years) after the injury. Asymptomatic chronic thoracic aneurysms should be surgically corrected.

ESOPHAGEAL PERFORATION

Epidemiology

Perforation of the esophagus has been called the most rapidly fatal perforation of the gastrointestinal tract because death is almost ensured if the diagnosis is delayed more than 24 hours.[114] The classic description of esophageal perforation resulting from forceful vomiting was published in 1724 by Boerhaave, and between 1724 and 1941, the occurrence of Boerhaave's syndrome was almost uniformly fatal.[115] In 1941, the first successful surgical treatment, a drainage procedure, was reported, and in 1947, the first successful closure of a ruptured esophagus was described. Since then, improved surgical techniques, a greater physician awareness leading to a more prompt diagnosis, the availability of more effective antibiotics, and better general supportive measures have reduced the mortality to approximately 30%.[116] Mortality data cited for perforation are affected by several variables, such as location (with perforations of the thoracic segment having the highest mortality rate), mechanism of injury, time elapsed between injury and diagnosis, presence of preexisting esophageal disease, and general health of the patient.

Anatomy and Pathophysiology

The anatomic feature responsible for the prolonged morbidity and high mortality associated with esophageal perforation is the lack of an esophageal serosal covering that allows perforation at any level direct access to the mediastinum. Perforations in the upper or cervical esophagus enter the retropharyngeal space where fascial planes extend from the base of the skull to the bifurcation of the trachea. Perforations in the midesophagus and lower esophagus enter directly

into the mediastinum. Only the thin mediastinal pleura prevents free access to the entire pleural cavity, and this barrier is commonly overcome by continued drainage and the massive exudative inflammatory reaction induced by chemical and bacterial mediastinitis. When the mediastinal pleura is penetrated, the negative pressure generated by respiratory efforts tends to increase the soilage by promoting drainage from the gastrointestinal tract into the mediastinum and pleural space.

When esophageal rupture results from emetic pressure, as in cases of Boerhaave's syndrome, the intrinsic weakness of the left posterior distal esophagus is important. Other areas (including cervical, midthoracic, and infradiaphragmatic sites) have been reported only rarely to rupture secondary to emesis. In addition, the esophagus has three areas of anatomic narrowing[114]—the cricopharyngeal muscle near the esophageal introitus, the level at which the esophagus crosses the left main stem bronchus and the aortic arch, and the gastroesophageal junction. It is unusual, in the absence of a preexisting esophageal disease, such as carcinoma, for a perforation caused by a foreign body to occur anywhere other than these three sites. Foreign bodies may cause perforation by direct penetration, pressure, or chemical necrosis.

Etiology

The most common causes of an esophageal perforation are shown in Box 42-7.

Iatrogenic

Most esophageal perforations are iatrogenic, most commonly as a complication of endoscopy (0.2% to 1% of all esophageal endoscopies).[116] The rigid endoscope is the most common offender, particularly when general anesthesia is used. Although use of the flexible endoscope has made this complication less likely, the total number of perforations has increased as more procedures are performed. Injuries tend to occur either near the esophageal introitus or at the distal esophagus.[117] Endoscopic procedures that are too vigorous in the presence of a corrosive burn or carcinoma also are a common cause of iatrogenic esophageal injury.

Esophageal dilation performed for benign or malignant strictures of the esophagus is the second most common iatrogenic cause of esophageal perforations.[116] A too-rapid increase in the dilator size during these procedures may lead to perforation. The preexisting fibrotic process that resulted in the stricture tends to scar the surrounding mediastinal tissues, however, limiting free access to the mediastinum provided by many other perforations. In the emergency department, nasotracheal or nasogastric intubations are the most common causes of iatrogenic perforations with the perforation usually occurring in the pyriform sinus. In a closed claims analysis published in 1999, esophageal injuries by anesthesiologists were associated overwhelmingly with difficult intubations.[118] Risk factors for a difficult airway include obesity, cervical arthritis, haste, and improper muscle relaxation. Claims involving airways that were classified as nondifficult involved other esophageal instrumentation, such as a nasogastric tube, esophageal dilator, or esophageal stethoscope. In all cases, esophageal injuries were more severe than any other type of airway injury sustained during airway maneuvers.

The use of an esophageal obturator airway also was associated with occasional esophageal trauma, specifically midesophageal perforation. The use of the esophageal obturator airway's most recent successor, the laryngeotracheal Combitube, does not seem to be associated with trauma more severe than occasional esophageal abrasions or contusions.

Several cases of esophageal rupture secondary to compressed air have been reported, including two cases of pharyngoesophageal perforation secondary to gas in carbonated beverages and in tartaric acid–sodium bicarbonate mixtures administered to treat esophageal food impactions. Esophageal perforation also has been caused by placement of a cervical fixation device and secondary to the Heimlich maneuver.

Foreign Bodies

Foreign bodies can cause an esophageal injury by direct laceration, by pressure necrosis, or during endoscopic removal. Foreign bodies account for approximately 10% of esophageal perforations.[117] Small perforations tend to seal without sequelae, but pressure necrosis or lacerating injuries provide ample access to the mediastinum.[114] Foreign bodies usually lodge in the cervical esophagus, but if a distal stricture is present, this too is a common site. In children younger than 4 years old, the cricopharyngeal narrowing is the usual point of foreign body impaction. After the age of 4 years, most objects pass this region and traverse the remaining normal esophagus. In adults, a foreign body impaction, especially in cases of repeated episodes, raises the possibility of a stricture and mandates further investigation.

In elderly patients, foreign bodies commonly enter the esophagus because of a loss of oral tactile sensation resulting from intoxication or a poorly fitting set of dentures.[116] Inadequate dentures also may lead to the swallowing of large pieces of poorly chewed food. Other esophageal foreign bodies include sharp fish or chicken bones and corn chips that may impale the esophageal wall leading to eventual leakage.

Caustic Burns

Caustic burns of the esophagus occur from intentional or accidental ingestion of acid or alkali. There are two peaks of incidence: 1 to 5 years of age, when ingestion is usually of a small amount of material and accidental, and in the teens and 20s, when larger quantities are ingested during suicide attempts. Symptoms include hematemesis, respiratory distress, vomiting, drooling, or the presence of oropharyngeal lesions on physical examination.[119] Perforation usually occurs during the latent granulation stage of the disease, approximately 4 to 14 days after ingestion.

The liquefaction necrosis classically resulting from strong alkali burns (pH >12) is more likely to cause esophageal perforation than the coagulation necrosis resulting from strong acid burns (pH <2). Individuals ingesting alkali substances with a pH less than 11.5 rarely sustain injuries more serious than superficial mucosal burns. Acid ingestions cause damage more frequently in the stomach as opposed to the esophagus.[119]

In treating a patient who has ingested a caustic substance, decontamination should involve only the rinsing of the mouth. Dilution of the substance with milk or water has been suggested; however, further liquid ingestion should be avoided if there is suspicion of perforation. Emesis, gastric lavage, and charcoal should be avoided.

Endoscopy within the first 6 to 18 hours may be used to determine the extent of the injury and to guide therapy. Antibiotics are reserved for patients with evidence of perforation, and steroids are suggested by some authors if the burns are circumferential or transmural. Other authors have shown that in the setting of large alkali ingestions, corticosteroids not only did not prevent the formation of esophageal stenosis, but increased the risk of other complications.[120]

Although admission after significant ingestion is the rule, some authors suggest that in the setting of accidental ingestion in children and in the absence of symptoms, endoscopy and admission may not be indicated.[121] Esophagoscopy is commonly undertaken to ascertain the presence or absence of esophageal injury. Advancing the esophagoscope beyond the first burn in the esophagus increases the risk of perforation and is a common iatrogenic cause of esophageal perforation.

Penetrating and Blunt Trauma

Because of its well-protected position posteriorly, esophageal trauma occurs in approximately 5% of patients with injuries to the neck, but only 1% of blunt trauma victims, and it is usually not an isolated injury.[122] Cervical esophageal injuries are the most common because of a lack of protection by the bony thorax, and the trachea is the most common associated site of injury.[123] In some cases, the esophageal injury may be overlooked initially because of the dramatic presentation of a patient with a tracheal injury.

Typical symptoms seen in cervical esophageal injuries include neck pain, dysphagia, cough, voice changes, and hematemesis. Physical findings may include neck tenderness, resistance to flexion, crepitus, or stridor.[123] In one large series, the most common life-threatening problem in the emergency department was compromise of the airway. Most of these cases were handled using rapid sequence intubation, but a significant number (12%) of patients required cricothyroidotomy.[122]

If the patient's condition is stable, a preoperative esophagogram with a liquid-soluble agent should precede any endoscopy. Although chest and neck radiograph and CT also may be used to diagnose this injury, emergent bedside flexible endoscopy seems to be the test of choice to confirm negative findings on esophagography (especially in the setting of penetrating trauma).[122-124] Operative repair is indicated in most of these injuries (>90%) and should be done as quickly as possible to avoid the development of fistulae, mediastinitis, or abscess formation.

Blunt traumatic injuries to the esophagus occur much less often than penetrating injuries. The pathophysiology and prognosis of blunt injuries to the esophagus are similar to that resulting from spontaneous rupture or emesis. In some cases, rupture of the cervical esophagus has been reported in association with cervical spine fracture.

Spontaneous Rupture

Spontaneous esophageal ruptures, postemetic ruptures, and Boerhaave's syndrome are synonymous terms. This esophageal injury is associated with a poor prognosis because the forces required to rupture the esophagus result in almost instantaneous and massive mediastinal contamination. The distal esophagus is the usual site of injury, with a longitudinal tear occurring in the left posterolateral aspect. More than 80% of these injuries occur in middle-aged men who have ingested alcohol and large meals.

In vitro, a tear similar to that seen in cases of Boerhaave's syndrome requires a force of 3 to 6 psi, which may be generated in vivo by gastric pressure caused by the reverse peristalsis (seen with emesis) pushing against a closed cricopharyngeal muscle.[125] The role of preexisting gastrointestinal disease in spontaneous rupture of the esophagus is unclear. Some authors emphasize its importance, whereas others report that 80% of esophageal ruptures occur in a previously normal esophagus.[125] Less pressure is required to perforate a diseased esophagus. Approximately 25% of patients with Boerhaave's syndrome have no history of emesis.[116] Increases in intra-abdominal pressure resulting from blunt trauma, seizures, childbirth, laughing, straining at stool, and heavy lifting all have been reported to cause this injury.

Diagnostic Findings

The diagnosis of esophageal perforation is aided by consideration of clinical circumstances. In patients with classic Boerhaave's syndrome, emesis is followed by severe chest pain, subcutaneous emphysema, and cardiopulmonary collapse. Development of these

signs and symptoms after instrumentation of the esophagus or removal of an esophageal foreign body is relatively straightforward. One third of cases of perforated esophagus are atypical, however.[116] Only a careful history and physical examination supplemented with appropriate laboratory and diagnostic studies enable the clinician to diagnose a subtle case at an early stage. When considering any of the diagnoses listed in Box 42-8, a perforated esophagus also should be considered.

Clinical Features

The most reliable symptom of an esophageal injury is pleuritic pain localized along the course of the esophagus that is exacerbated by swallowing or neck flexion. Pain may be located in the epigastrium, substernal area, or back; usually worsens over time; and may migrate from the upper abdomen to the chest. As the infectious process worsens, dyspnea usually ensues.

The early physical signs of an esophageal perforation are sparse. As air and caustic contaminated material move through the esophageal tear into the mediastinum and pleural space, and before any subcutaneous air is palpable at the root of the neck, the mediastinal air may impart a nasal quality to the voice.[117] Mediastinal air may surround the heart and produce a systolic crunching sound (Hamman's crunch). As air and fluid move into the pleural space, signs of a hydropneumothorax or an empyema may develop. Eventually the air travels into the subcutaneous tissues, dissecting into the neck, where subcutaneous emphysema first may become evident. This classic sign is present in only about 60% of patients, however, and in the absence of a tracheal injury, it may occur in only 30%.[116] As the infectious and inflammatory process advances, the patient's general appearance and vital signs begin to manifest the signs of cardiopulmonary collapse and sepsis with fever, cyanosis, hypotension, anuria, and eventually death.

Diagnostic Strategies

Laboratory studies provide largely nonspecific findings. If tested, the pleural effusion of esophageal perforation may show a high salivary amylase level and a low pH. The radiographic examination usually suggests

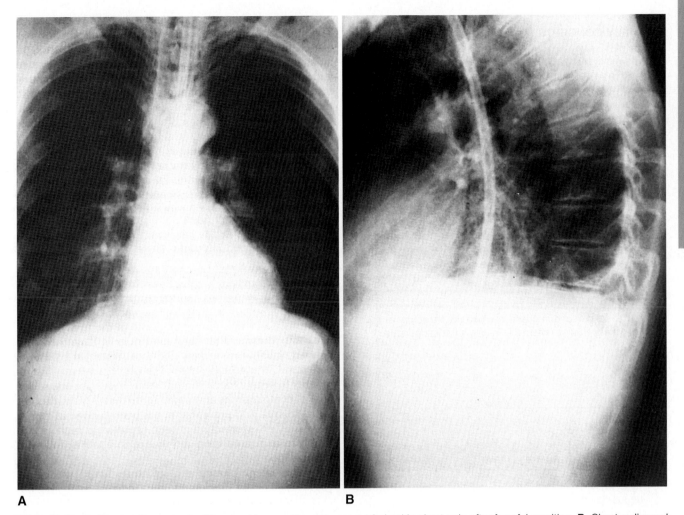

A   **B**

Figure 42-20. A, Chest radiograph of a 36-year-old man with acute onset of pleuritic chest pain after forceful vomiting. **B,** Chest radiograph shows mediastinal and subcutaneous air typical of ruptured esophagus. Mediastinum is not yet widened, and there is no soilage of the pleural cavity.

the diagnosis of an esophageal perforation. The classic chest radiograph findings are as follows:

1. Mediastinal air with or without subcutaneous emphysema
2. Left-sided pleural effusion
3. Pneumothorax
4. Widened mediastinum

Lateral views of the cervical spine may reveal air or fluid in the retropharyngeal area that is characteristic of a cervical esophageal perforation, but also is found when perforations in the lower parts of the esophagus release air or fluid that dissects superiorly (see Figure 42-19). Most patients exhibit one or more of these abnormalities at some point in the course of the illness, but radiographic evidence of the perforation may be absent early on.

The literature is not conclusive on whether insoluble barium contrast medium or water-soluble diatrizoate meglumine (Gastrografin) is the preferred initial study. Gastrografin does not obscure visualization with subsequent endoscopy, and it produces less mediastinal soiling than does barium. It is generally recommended that the initial study use this water-soluble

agent, then if no leak is shown, a barium study may be undertaken to define the mucosal detail better (Figure 42-20).

Endoscopy, similar to contrast studies, is not an infallible aid in establishing the presence or absence of an esophageal perforation. The size and location of the perforation and the skill of the endoscopist are important factors in the low incidence of false-negative studies.[126] If the accuracy of the endoscopy is in doubt, an esophagogram should be performed.

Management

Early diagnosis can best be accomplished if one is aware of the pathophysiology and clinical settings in which esophageal perforations occur. Time is crucial in minimizing the mortality and morbidity of this condition. If the diagnosis is strongly suggested or confirmed, management should include broad-spectrum antibiotics (covering oral flora), volume replacement, and airway maintenance.[119] An emergency surgical consultation should be obtained because prognosis worsens with delays longer than 24 hours.

KEY CONCEPTS

- Even relatively minor chest wall injuries, such as rib fractures, may result in serious complications in elderly patients and patients with preexisting pulmonary disease.

- Children are more susceptible to pulmonary contusion because of greater compliance of the chest wall.

- Unless there are abnormalities on the initial ECG, there is no need to pursue the diagnosis of myocardial contusion with more sophisticated tests.

- Many patients with myocardial rupture or traumatic aortic rupture survive to reach the hospital and can be salvaged with rapid diagnosis and intervention.

- Pericardial tamponade can be diagnosed accurately before hemodynamic decompensation occurs by standard cardiac ultrasound performed by emergency physicians.

- Injury of the esophagus is relatively common with penetrating trauma of the chest or neck. Because the presentation is initially subtle and the potential complications so severe, the diagnosis of esophageal perforation must be actively pursued in cases in which the trajectory of the penetrating wound potentially involves the esophagus.

REFERENCES

1. LoCicero J, Mattox KL: Epidemiology of chest trauma. *Surg Clin North Am* 69:15, 1989.
2. Shweiki E, et al: Assessing the true risk of abdominal solid organ injury in hospitalized rib fracture patients. *J Trauma* 48:684, 2000.
3. Bergeron E, et al: Elderly trauma patients with rib fractures are at greater risk of death and pneumonia. *J Trauma Inj Infect Crit Care* 54:478, 2003.
4. Holcomb JB, et al: Morbidity from rib fractures increases after age 45. *J Am Coll Surg* 196:549, 2003.
5. Thompson BM, et al: Rib radiographs for trauma: Useful or wasteful? *Ann Emerg Med* 15:3, 1986.
6. Kattan KR: What to look for in rib fractures and how. *JAMA* 243:262, 1980.
7. Gupta A, Jamshidi M, Rubin JR: Traumatic first rib fracture: Is angiography necessary? A review of 730 cases. *Cardiovasc Surg* 5:48, 1997.
8. Fabian TC, et al: Prospective study of blunt aortic injury: Helical CT is diagnostic and antihypertensive therapy reduces rupture. *Ann Surg* 227:666, 1998.
9. Nagy K, et al: Guidelines for the diagnosis and management of blunt aortic injury: An EAST Practice Management Guidelines Work Group. *J Trauma* 48:1128, 2000.
10. Worthley LIG: Thoracic epidural in the management of chest trauma: A case study of 161 cases. *Intensive Care Med* 11:312, 1985.
11. Brookes JG, Dunn RJ, Rogers IR: Sternal fractures: A retrospective analysis of 272 cases. *J Trauma* 35:46, 1993.
12. Bar I, et al: Isolated sternal fracture—a benign condition? *Isr Med Assoc J* 5:105, 2003.
13. Roy-Shapiro A, Levi I, Khoda J: Sternal fractures: A red flag or a red herring? *J Trauma* 37:59, 1994.
14. Heare MM, Heare TC, Gillespy T III: Diagnostic imaging of pelvic and chest wall trauma. *Radiol Clin North Am* 27:287, 1989.
15. Van Hise ML, et al: CT in blunt chest trauma: Indications and limitations. *Radiographics* 18:1071, 1998.
16. Barone JE, et al: Indications for intubation in blunt chest trauma. *J Trauma Inj Infect Crit Care* 26:334, 1986.
17. McRitchie DI, Matthews JG, Fink MP: Pneumonia in patients with multiple trauma. *Clin Chest Med* 16:135, 1995.
18. Livingston DH, Hauser CJ: Trauma to the chest wall and lung. In Mattox KL, Feliciano DV, Moore EE (eds): *Trauma.* New York, McGraw-Hill, 2004, pp 507-538.
19. Ahmed Z, Mohyuddin Z: Management of flail chest injury: Internal fixation versus endotracheal intubation and ventilation. *J Thorac Cardiovasc Surg* 110:1676, 1995.
20. Voggenreiter G, et al: Operative chest wall stabilization in flail chest—outcomes of patients with or without pulmonary contusion. *J Am Coll Surg* 187:130, 1998.
21. Clemmer TD, Fairfax WR: Critical care management of chest injury. *Crit Care Clin North Am* 2:759, 1986.
22. Eckstein M, Cowen AR: Scene safety in the face of automatic weapons fire: A new dilemma for EMS? *Prehosp Emerg Care* 2:117, 1998.
23. de Brito D, et al: The injury pattern of a new law enforcement weapon: The police bean bag. *Ann Emerg Med* 38:383, 2001.
24. Carroll AW, Soderstrom CA: A new nonpenetrating ballistic injury. *Ann Surg* 188:753, 1978.
25. Jonegwaard WR, Cogbill TH, Landercasper J: Neurologic consequences of traumatic asphyxia. *J Trauma* 32:28, 1992.
26. Roux P, Fisher RM: Chest injuries in children: An analysis of 100 cases of blunt chest trauma from motor vehicle accidents. *J Pediatr Surg* 27:551, 1992.
27. Morgagni JB: *Epistola.* 54:140, 1761.
28. Hill JW, Deluca SA: Pulmonary contusion. *Am Fam Physician* 38:219, 1988.
29. Hoff SJ, et al: Outcome of isolated pulmonary contusion in blunt trauma patients. *Am Surg* 60:138, 1994.
30. Hoff SJ, Shotts SD, Eddy VA: Outcome of isolated pulmonary contusion in blunt trauma patients. *Am Surg* 60:348, 1994.
31. Adoumie MD, Shennib H, Brown R: Differential lung ventilation. *J Thorac Cardiovasc Surg* 105:229, 1993.
32. Robertson C: A review of the use of corticosteroids in the management of pulmonary injuries and insults. *Arch Emerg Med* 2:59, 1985.
33. Clark GC, Schecter WP, Trunkey DD: Variables affecting outcome in blunt chest trauma: Flail chest vs. pulmonary contusion. *J Trauma* 28:298, 1988.
34. Bridges KG, Welch G, Silver M: CT detection of occult pneumothorax in multiple trauma patients. *J Emerg Med* 11:179, 1993.
35. Beckh S, Bolskei PL, Lessnau KD: Real-time chest ultrasonography: A comprehensive review for the pulmonologist. *Chest* 122:1759, 2002.
36. Chan SS: Emergency bedside ultrasound to detect pneumothorax. *Acad Emerg Med* 10:91, 2003.
37. Wolfman NT, et al: Validity of CT classification on management of occult pneumothorax: A prospective study. *AJR Am J Roentgenol* 171:1317, 1998.
38. Neff MA, et al: Detection of occult pneumothoraces on abdominal computed tomographic scans in trauma patients. *J Trauma* 49:281, 2000.
39. Kiev J, Kerstein M: Role of three hour roentgenogram of the chest in penetrating and non-penetrating injuries. *Surg Gynecol Obstet* 175:249, 1992.
40. Rhea JT, et al: The frequency and significance of thoracic injuries detected on abdominal CT scans of multiple trauma patients. *J Trauma* 29:502, 1989.
41. Enderson BL, Abdulla R, Frame SB: Tube thoracostomy for occult pneumothorax: A prospective randomized study of its use. *J Trauma* 36:726, 1993.
42. Collins JC, Levine G, Waxman K: Occult traumatic pneumothorax: Immediate tube thoracostomy versus expectant management. *Am Surg* 58:743, 1992.
43. Eckstein M, Suyehara D: Prehospital needle thoracostomy. *Prehosp Emerg Care* 2:132, 1998.

44. Richardson JD, Spain DA: Injury to the lung and pleura. In Mattox KL, Feliciano DV, Moore EE (eds): *Trauma. Manual* 4th ed. New York, McGraw-Hill, 2003, pp 188-201.

45. Velmahos GC, et al: Predicting the need for thoracoscopic evacuation of residual traumatic hemothorax: Chest radiograph is insufficient. *J Trauma* 46:65, 1999.

46. Carrillo EH, Richardson JD: Thoracoscopy in the management of hemothorax and retained blood after trauma. *Curr Opin Pulm Med* 4:243, 1998.

47. Sosa JL, et al: Thoracoscopy in the evaluation and management of thoracic trauma. *Int Surg* 83:187, 1998.

48. Kiser AC, O'Brien SM, Detterbeck FC: Blunt tracheobronchial injuries: Treatment and outcomes. *Ann Thorac Surg* 71:2059, 2001.

49. Balci AE, et al: Surgical treatment of post-traumatic tracheobronchial injuries: 14-year experience. *Eur J Cardiothorac Surgery* 22:984, 2002.

50. Hara KS, Prakash UBS: Fiberoptic bronchoscopy in the evaluation of acute chest and upper airway trauma. *Chest* 96:627, 1989.

51. Bright EF, Beck CS: Nonpenetrating wounds of the heart: A clinical and experimental study. *Am Heart J* 10:293, 1935.

52. Fabian TC, et al: Myocardial contusion in blunt trauma: Clinical characteristics, means of diagnosis and implications for patient management. *J Trauma* 29:50, 1988.

53. Maron BJ, et al: Clinical profile and spectrum of commotio cordis. *JAMA* 287:1142, 2002.

54. Lindstaedt M, et al: Acute and long-term clinical significance of myocardial contusion following blunt thoracic trauma: Results of a prospective study. *J Trauma* 52:479, 2002.

55. Sybrandy KC, Cramer MJ, Burgersdijk C: Diagnosing cardiac contusion: Old wisdom and new insights. *Br Heart J* 89:485, 2003.

56. Walsh P, et al: Use of V4R in patients who sustain blunt chest trauma. *J Trauma* 51:60, 2001.

57. Illig KA, et al: A rational screening and treatment strategy based on the electrocardiogram alone for suspected cardiac contusion. *Am J Surg* 162:537, 1991.

58. Nagy KK, et al: Determining which patients require evaluation for blunt cardiac injury following blunt cardiac injury following blunt chest trauma. *World J Surg* 25:108, 2001.

59. Bertinchant JP, et al: Evaluation of incidence, clinical significance, and prognostic value of circulating cardiac troponin I and T elevation in hemodynamically stable patients with suspected myocardial contusion after blunt chest trauma. *J Trauma* 48:924, 2000.

60. Swaanenburg JC, et al: Troponin I, troponin T, CKMB-activity and CKMB-mass as markers for the detection of myocardial contusion in patients who experienced blunt trauma. *Clin Chim Acta* 272:171, 1998.

61. Ferjani M, et al: Circulating cardiac troponin T in myocardial contusion. *Chest* 111:427, 1997.

62. Karalis DG, et al: The role of echocardiography in blunt chest trauma: A transthoracic and transesophageal echocardiographic study. *J Trauma* 36:53, 1994.

63. Hiatt JS, Yeatman LA, Child JS: The value of echocardiography in blunt chest trauma. *J Trauma* 28:914, 1988.

64. Garcia-Fernandez MA, et al: Role of transesophageal echocardiography in the assessment of patients with blunt chest trauma: Correlation of echocardiographic findings with the electrocardiogram and creatine kinase monoclonal antibody measurements. *Am Heart J* 135:476, 1998.

65. Brooks SW, et al: The use of tranesophageal echocardiography in the evaluation of chest trauma. *J Trauma* 32:761, 1992.

66. Sutherland GR, et al: Hemodynamic adaptation to acute myocardial contusion complicating blunt chest injury. *Am J Cardiol* 57:291, 1986.

67. Chui WC, D'Amerlio LF, Hammond JS: Sternal fractures in blunt chest trauma: A practical algorithm for management. *Am J Emerg Med* 15:252, 1997.

68. Adams JE, et al: Improved detection of cardiac contusion with cardiac troponin I. *Am Heart J* 131:308, 1996.

69. American Heart Association: *Guidelines 2000 for Cardiopulmonary Resuscitation and Emergency Cardiovascular Care.* Chicago, American Heart Association, 2000.

70. Flancbaum L, Wright J, Siegel JH: Emergency surgery in patients with post-traumatic myocardial contusion. *J Trauma* 26:795, 1986.

71. Pevec WC, et al: Blunt rupture of the myocardium. *Ann Thorac Surg* 48:139, 1989.

72. DesForges G, Ridder WP, Lenock RJ: Successful suture of ruptured myocardium after nonpenetrating injury. *N Engl J Med* 252:567, 1955.

73. Calhoon JH, et al: Management of blunt rupture of the heart. *J Trauma* 26:495, 1986.

74. Symbas NP, et al: Blunt cardiac rupture: The utility of emergency department ultrasound. *Ann Thorac Surg* 67:1274, 1999.

75. Asensio JA, et al: One hundred five penetrating cardiac injuries: A 2-year prospective evaluation. *J Trauma* 44:1073, 1998.

76. Asensio JA, et al: Penetrating cardiac injuries: A complex challenge. *Injury* 32:533, 2001.

77. Harris DG, et al: Current evaluation of cardiac stab wounds. *Ann Thorac Surg* 68:2119, 1999.

78. Asensio JA, et al: Penetrating thoracoabdominal injuries: Ongoing dilemma—which cavity and when? *World J Surg* 26:539, 2002.

79. Beck CS: Acute and chronic compression of the heart. *Am Heart J* 14:515, 1937.

80. Rozycki GS, et al: The role of surgeon-performed ultrasound in patients with possible cardiac wounds. *Ann Surg* 223:737, 1996.

81. Plumer D: The sensitivity, specificity, and accuracy of ED echocardiography. *Acad Emerg Med* 2:339, 1995.

82. Steward JH, Crane NF, Dietrick JE: Studies of the circulation of pericardial effusion., *Am Heart J* 16:189, 1938.

83. Ma OJ, et al: Prospective analysis of a rapid trauma ultrasound examination performed by emergency physicians. *J Trauma* 38:879, 1995.

84. Asensio JA, et al: Penetrating cardiac injuries. *Surg Clin North Am* 76:685, 1996.

85. Mayrose J, et al: Comparison of staples versus sutures in the repair of penetrating cardiac wounds. *J Trauma* 46:441, 1999.

86. Working Group, Ad Hoc Subcommittee on Outcomes, American College of Surgeons Committee on Trauma: Practice management guidelines for emergency department thoracotomy. Working Group, Ad Hoc Subcommittee on Outcomes, American College of Surgeons Committee on Trauma. *J Am Coll Surg* 193:303, 2001.

87. Rosemurgy AS, et al: Prehospital traumatic arrest: The cost of futility. *J Trauma* 35:468, 1993.

88. Stratton SJ, Brickett K, Crammer T: Prehospital pulseless, unconscious penetrating trauma victims: Field assessments associated with survival. *J Trauma* 45:96, 1998.

89. Rhee PM, et al: Survival after emergency department thoracotomy: Review of published data from the past 25 years. *J Am Coll Surg* 190:288, 2000.

90. Feczko JD, et al: An autopsy case review of 142 nonpenetrating (blunt) injuries of the aorta. *J Trauma* 33:846, 1992.

91. Kram HB, et al: Diagnosis of traumatic aortic rupture: A 10-year retrospective analysis. *Ann Thorac Surg* 47:282, 1989.

92. Lee FT Jr, et al: Reevaluation of plain radiographic findings in the diagnosis of aortic rupture: The role of inspiration and positioning on mediastinal width. *J Emerg Med* 11:289, 1993.

93. Woodring JH, King JG: Determination of normal transverse mediastinal width and mediastinal-width to chest-width ratio in control subjects. *J Trauma* 29:1268, 1989.

94. Mirvis SE, et al: Value of chest radiography in excluding traumatic aortic rupture. *Radiology* 163:47, 1987.

95. Heystraten FN, et al: Chest radiography in acute traumatic rupture of the thoracic aorta. *Acta Radiol* 29:411, 1988.

96. Demetriades D, et al: Routine helical computed tomographic evaluation of the mediastinum in high-risk blunt trauma patients. *Arch Surg* 133:1084, 1998.

97. Vignon P, et al: Routine transesophageal echocardiography for the diagnosis of aortic disruption in trauma patients without enlarged mediastinum. *J Trauma* 40:422, 1996.

98. Fabian TC, et al: Prospective study of blunt aortic injury: Helical CT is diagnostic and antihypertensive therapy reduces rupture. *Ann Surg* 227:666, 1998.

99. Malhotra AK, et al: Minimal aortic injury: A lesion associated with advancing diagnostic techniques. *J Trauma* 51:1042, 2001.

100. Fabian TC, Richardson JD, Croce MA: Prospective study of blunt aortic injury: Multicenter Trial of the American Association for the Surgery of Trauma. *J Trauma* 42:374, 1997.

101. Vignon P, et al: Comparison of multiplane transesophageal echocardiography and contrast-enhanced helical CT in the diagnosis of blunt traumatic cardiovascular injuries. *Anesthesiology* 94:615, 2001.

102. Goarin JP, et al: Evaluation of transesophageal echocardiography for diagnosis of traumatic aortic injury. *Anesthesiology* 93:1373, 2000.

103. Fishman JE: Imaging of blunt aortic and great vessel trauma. 5th ed. *J Thorac Imaging* 15:97, 2000.

104. Patel NH, Hahn D, Comess KA: Blunt chest trauma victims: Role of intravascular ultrasound and transesophageal echocardiography in cases of abnormal thoracic aortogram. *J Trauma* 55:330, 2003.

105. Pozzato C, et al: Acute posttraumatic rupture of the thoracic aorta: The role of angiography in a 7-year review. *Cardiovasc Interv Radiol* 14:338, 1991.

106. Merrill WH, et al: Surgical treatment of acute traumatic tear of the thoracic aorta. *Ann Surg* 206:699, 1988.

107. Hemmila MR, et al: Delayed repair for blunt thoracic aortic injury: Is it really equivalent to early repair? *J Trauma* 56:13, 2004.

108. Passaro E Jr, Pace WC: Traumatic rupture of the aorta. *Surgery* 46:787, 1959.

109. Mattox KL, Wall MJ Jr, Le Maire SA: Injury to the thoracic great vessels. In Mattox KL, Feliciano DV, Moore EE (eds): *Trauma*. 5th ed. New York, McGraw-Hill, 2004, pp 571-591.

110. Razzouk AJ, et al: Repair of traumatic aortic rupture: A 25-year experience. *Arch Surg* 135:913, 2000.

111. Miller PR, et al: Complex blunt aortic injury or repair: Beneficial effects of cardiopulmonary bypass use. *Ann Surg* 237:877, 2003.

112. Carter Y, et al: Anatomical considerations in the surgical management of blunt thoracic aortic injury. *J Vasc Surg* 34:628, 2001.

113. Doss M, et al: Surgical versus endovascular treatment of acute thoracic aortic rupture: A single-center experience. *Ann Thorac Surg* 76:1465, 2003.

114. Marty-Ane CH, et al: Endovascular repair for acute traumatic rupture of the thoracic aorta. *Ann Thorac Surg* 75:1803, 2003.

115. Derbes VS, Mitchell RE Jr: Herman Boerhaave's atrocis, *Ned Descript, Prins Morbi Historia*: First translation of classic care report of the esophagus, with annotations. *Bull Med Libr Assoc* 43:217, 1955.

116. Loop FD, Groves LK: Esophageal perforations: Collective review. *Ann Thorac Surg* 10:571, 1970.

117. White RK, Morris DM: Diagnosis and management of esophageal perforations. *Am Surg* 58:112, 1992.

118. Hatzitheofilou C, Strahlendorf C: Penetrating external injuries of the esophagus and pharynx. *Br J Surg* 80:1147, 1993.

119. Domino KB, et al: Airway injury during anesthesia: A closed claims analysis. *Anesthesiology* 91:1703, 1999.

120. Swann LA, Munter DW: Esophageal emergencies. *Emerg Med Clin North Am* 14:557, 1996.

121. Mamede RCM, De Mello Filho FV: Treatment of caustic ingestion: An analysis of 239 cases. *Dis Esophagus* 15:210, 2002.

122. Lamireau T: Accidental caustic ingestion in children: Is endoscopy always mandatory? *J Pediatr Gastroenterol* 33:81, 2001.

123. Vassiliu P, et al: Aerodigestive injuries of the neck. *Am Surg* 67:75, 2001.

124. Pineau BC, Ott DJ: Isolated proximal esophageal injury from blunt trauma: Endoscopic stricture dilatation. *Dysphagia* 18:263, 2003.

125. Srinivasan R, et al: Role of flexible endoscopy in the evaluation of possible esophageal trauma after penetrating injuries. *Am J Gastroenterol* 95:1725, 2000.

126. Horwitz B, Krevensky B: Endoscopic evolution of esophageal injuries. *Am J Gastroenterol* 88:1249, 1993.

43 Abdominal Trauma

John A. Marx and Jennifer Isenhour

PERSPECTIVE

Background

The management of abdominal trauma should be approached in an organized, vigilant, and knowledgeable manner. Reliance on key clinical features and the timely use of diagnostic procedures tremendously alter morbidity and mortality. Missed or delayed diagnoses remain the most serious pitfalls in the management of abdominal injuries.[1]

Penetrating Abdominal Trauma

Whether by accident or intention, penetrating trauma can result from a wide variety of weapons or instruments, and certain elements of therapy vary accordingly. The management of patients with penetrating trauma has changed dramatically since 1960, when Shaftan introduced the concept of selective laparotomy and serial observations. Before that time, surgery was mandatory. The careful integration of physical examination and certain diagnostic procedures, notably local wound exploration, diagnostic peritoneal lavage, ultrasonography, computed tomography (CT), and laparoscopy, now provides the emergency physician and trauma surgeon with an accurate means of determining whether laparotomy should be undertaken. The approach varies according to the clinical status of the patient, the instrument responsible for injury, and the site of penetration. Nonoperative management has gained favor for both stab wounds and gunshot wounds (GSWs) with the intent to reduce the incidence of and morbidity from nontherapeutic laparotomies.[2,3]

Blunt Abdominal Trauma

Blunt trauma to the abdomen is a supreme challenge to the emergency specialist's clinical acumen. Historical data may be incomplete, absent, or presumptive. The symptoms and signs can be unreliable and obfuscated by head injury, alcohol, or other toxins. The likelihood of extra-abdominal systems trauma adds further complexity, underscoring the need for a carefully organized approach.

Epidemiology

Blunt injuries carry a greater risk of mortality than penetrating injuries because they are more difficult to diagnose and are commonly associated with severe trauma to multiple intraperitoneal organs and extra-abdominal systems.

Penetrating Abdominal Trauma

Wounds from stabbing implements occur nearly three times more often than wounds from firearms, but the latter have a significantly greater mortality rate and are responsible for 90% of penetrating trauma mortality.[4] The small intestine, colon, and liver are, successively, the most likely organs to sustain injury after penetrating trauma.[4] The highest risk of death from penetrating injury occurs among African Americans in the 15- to 34-year-old age range, followed by Hispanic persons in that same age group. The rate for non-Hispanic whites is greatest at 75 years of age and older. The predominant intent is homicide among African Americans and suicide among non-Hispanic whites.[5,6]

The use of firearms in the United States contributes heavily to the morbidity and mortality of trauma. The current U.S. civilian population is the most heavily armed in history. The number of homicides committed with firearms exceeds the number of homicides resulting from all other forms of violence combined. More than 850,000 American civilians have been killed by bullets in this century alone, and GSWs continue to occur with an increasing incidence in major U.S. cities.

Blunt Abdominal Trauma

The spleen is the organ most often injured, and in nearly two thirds of these cases, it is the only damaged intraperitoneal structure. The liver is the second most commonly injured intra-abdominal organ, and the intestine is the most likely hollow viscus to be damaged.

The automobile is the major cause of blunt abdominal trauma. Motor vehicle crashes and auto-pedestrian crashes have been cited as causes in 50% to 75% of cases, blows to the abdomen in approximately 15% of cases, and falls in 6% to 9%.[7]

Pediatrics

Each year in this country, trauma results in approximately 22,000 deaths and accounts for $160 billion of health care expenditures for children to the age of 16 years. Nearly 10% of children admitted to pediatric trauma centers are proven to have abdominal injury, and this category follows only head and thoracic trauma as the cause of injury-related death.[8] Blunt mechanism causes approximately 85% of pediatric injury, although penetrating violence is becoming a greater concern.

As is true with adults, motor vehicle crashes are responsible for most of the morbidity and mortality in cases of trauma in children.[9] Auto-pedestrian accidents and falls out of cars cause a significant percentage of these.

Child abuse continues to gain attention, and deservedly so. It is both common and extremely harmful. Soft tissue, skeletal, and intracranial injuries are most likely, but abdominal injuries occur occasionally and are second only to head injuries as the cause of death. Children in the preverbal stage, generally those younger than 2 years of age, are at greatest risk. The history of trauma is extremely difficult to obtain because of the inability or fear of the child to communicate and the reluctance of parents to divulge information. Injuries inconsistent with the history provided or not in keeping with the child's level of physical maturity should alert the physician to the possibility of child abuse.

PRINCIPLES OF DISEASE

Anatomy and Physiology

The abdominal cavity and its contents can be reached not only through the anterior abdominal wall and lower chest but also through the flank, back, and buttocks. Missiles can also lodge intraperitoneally after traversing proximal extremities. The *anterior abdomen* is defined as that region between the anterior axillary lines from the anterior costal margins to the groin creases. The *low chest* begins at the nipple line or fourth intercostal space anteriorly and the inferior scapular tip or seventh intercostal space posteriorly, and then extends down to the inferior costal margins. The *flank* is between the anterior and posterior axillary lines bilaterally from the inferior scapular tip to the iliac crest. The *back* is between the posterior axillary lines, beginning at the inferior scapular tip and extending down to the iliac crest. The intraperitoneal cavity is vulnerable when penetration occurs as high as the fourth intercostal space anteriorly and the sixth or seventh laterally and posteriorly because the diaphragm can ascend to this level during expiration. Likewise, simultaneous thoracic abdominal penetration has been found in 15% to 46% of cases of abdominal thoracic trauma.[10] Scrutiny of entrance and exit sites, as well as wound tracts, is imperative.

Pathophysiology

Penetrating Abdominal Trauma

The instruments responsible for penetrating injuries of the abdomen are varied. Knives, handguns, rifles, and shotguns are at the fore; but flying glass, scissors, arrows, picket fences, horned animals, and the like, although less common, can cause pronounced morbidity as well. Certain impalement injuries caused by fences, stakes, or similar objects can be treated as stab wounds. Likewise, various propelled missiles from lawn mowers, chain saws, and other machinery or resulting from violent weather should be managed as GSWs.

Fragmentation injuries produced by grenades and bombs are rare in this country, but industrial explo-

sions can produce similar injuries, which are best categorized as shotgun-type wounds. Blunt abdominal trauma from blast effect can coexist in this setting. With more widespread terrorism, an increased number of these injuries can be predicted.

The liver, followed by the small bowel, is the organ most often damaged by stab wounds, in keeping with the surface area each of these structures presents.[11] The frequency of organ injury caused by gunshot wounds is greatest for small bowel, followed by the colon and then the liver.[4] Typically, multiple organ injuries are sustained, notably perforations to bowel. This same pattern is seen in the pediatric patient.

Stab Wounds

Knives are not the sole implement used in stabbings. Ice picks, pens, coat hangers, screwdrivers, and broken bottles, to name a few, have been used by assailants. Stab wounds of the abdomen occur most commonly in the upper quadrants, the left more commonly than the right. They are multiple in 20% of cases and involve the chest in up to 10% of cases. Most stab wounds do not cause an intraperitoneal injury, and the incidence varies with the direction of entry into the peritoneal cavity. Anterior stab wounds penetrate the peritoneum in approximately 70% of cases but inflict a visceral injury in only half of these.[12] Lower chest wounds are associated with a 15% incidence of coincident intraperitoneal damage in addition to the expected high rate of diaphragmatic injuries.[12] Abdominal entries from the flank and back have reported incidences of up to 44% and 15%, respectively.[13,14] The organ injured cannot be well predicted by the site of entry in the abdominal wall. The liver and spleen are the viscera most commonly damaged.

Gunshot Wounds

The science of ballistics is complex, but a few basic principles are helpful in understanding the pathophysiologic processes of these injuries. The magnitude of the injury is proportional to the amount of kinetic energy imparted by the bullet to the victim, according to the following equation:

$$E = \frac{7000\, mv^2}{2\, g}$$

E is the kinetic energy (in foot-pounds), m is the mass of the bullet, v is the velocity of the bullet (in ft/sec), and g is gravitational acceleration (in ft/sec). In other words, the degree of injury depends on the mass of the bullet and the square of its velocity.[15] Additional factors that affect injury created by a missile include the resistance and viscoelastic properties of the tissue through which it passes, as well as the stability of the missile in this medium. Missile velocities are categorized as low (slower than 1100 ft/sec), medium (1100-2000 ft/sec), and high (faster than 2000-2500 ft/sec); the impact velocity is the most important determinant of wounding capability. The impact velocity depends on the distance between the firearm and the victim, the muzzle velocity, and various characteristics of the missile. At medium and high velocities, the missile has an explosive effect and creates a temporary passage in the tissue along its course. The size of this passage is directly proportional to the specific gravity of the penetrated tissue. This sudden formation of a tract displaces nearby organs and vascular structures, and bone and viscera may be fractured or torn without being directly struck by the missile. Several cases of an intraperitoneal injury caused by a bullet that remained extraperitoneal throughout its entire course have been reported.[16] Solid viscera such as the liver and spleen are more vulnerable to this effect.

High-Velocity Missiles. Wounds from high-velocity missiles involve additional problems. First, external contaminants tend to be dragged into the wound. Second, the closure of the tract immediately after the bullet's passage may lead to an underestimation of tissue damage. Finally, high-velocity bullets can fragment internally. In fact, a missile at any velocity can fragment after contact with bone and cause additional multiple trajectories and injuries. Civilian wounds have usually resulted from low-velocity handguns, but unfortunately a trend toward more destructive weapons such as the .38 and .357 may be occurring.

Shotgun Wounds. The shotgun was designed to strike a small, fast-moving target at close range. Because of the ballistic shape of the individual pellets, a rapid falloff in velocity occurs, making this weapon ineffective in producing severe wounds at long distances. An initial muzzle velocity of 1300 ft/sec drops to 950 ft/sec within 20 yards, a decrease of 25%. At close range (<15 yards), however, the shotgun is extremely lethal.

The kinetic energy imparted to the victim depends on the pellet's size, the number of striking pellets, the type and amount of powder, and the barrel choke (constriction). The most important variable is the distance between the shotgun and the victim. At a distance of 10 yards, 19% of the pellets cluster in a 9-inch diameter circle if fired from a full choke (maximum constriction) barrel. At a distance of 20 yards, the circle is approximately double that diameter. Because the kinetic energy is proportional to the square of the velocity, a 25% loss of velocity at 20 yards results in a significant decrease in the damage produced by the blast.

Shotgun wounds have been previously classified in three groups according to the range and pattern of distribution. More recently, classification has been according to the pattern of injury on the victim. Based on distance from the weapon to the victim, type I wounds involve a long range (>7 yards) and a penetration of subcutaneous tissue and deep fascia only. Type II wounds occur at a distance of 3 to 7 yards and may create a large number of perforated structures. Type III wounds occur at point-blank range (<3 yards) and involve a massive destruction of tissue. When categorized by pattern, type I wounds produce a spread greater than 25 cm; type II, 10 to 25 cm; and type III, less than 10 cm, respectively, in diameter.[17] The tissue damage is proportional to the specific gravity and inversely proportional to the elastic properties of the affected organ. Thus, the liver is more vulnerable than

the lungs to this injury. Close-range shotgun wounds, in addition to the shot, force external contaminants (e.g., clothing and parts of the shell wadding) into the wounds. Type III wounds carry a substantial mortality risk.

Blunt Abdominal Trauma

Several pathophysiologic mechanisms have been described to occur in patients with blunt abdominal trauma. First, sudden and pronounced rises in intra-abdominal pressures created by outward forces can cause rupture or burst injury of a hollow organ. Lap-belt restraints produce such a mechanism. Second, the compression of abdominal viscera between the applied force to the anterior wall and the posterior thoracic cage or vertebral column produces a crushing effect. Solid viscera are especially vulnerable to this injury, helping account for the high incidence of liver and spleen injuries in cases of blunt abdominal trauma. Crush injuries are more likely to occur with the lax abdominal wall characteristic of elderly and alcoholic patients. Finally, sharp shearing forces affecting both hollow and solid viscera cause organs and vascular pedicles to tear, especially at relatively fixed points of attachment.

Seatbelt Injuries

Unrestrained front and rear seat passengers are at unequivocally greater risk of intra-abdominal injury than their restrained counterparts.[18] The three-point shoulder-lap belt is the most effective restraining system and is associated with the lowest incidence of abdominal injuries, compared with older systems. However, abdominal injuries are still ascribed to shoulder-lap and lap-belt systems. The shoulder belt component can lead to right-sided and left-sided rib fractures for the driver and front seat passenger, respectively, with potential for injury to underlying abdominal viscera. Improper underarm usage of the shoulder belt increases compressive forces to the upper abdomen, particularly in the event of a front-end crash.

Injuries resulting from solitary lap belts are most often to the abdomen. This is true of nearly half the injuries caused by lap belts. The pathogenesis is usually the compression of bowel between the belt and the vertebral column. Occasionally, an acute short closed-loop obstruction occurs along with perforation secondary to the sudden generation of high intraluminal pressures. The resultant injury is primarily a contusion or perforation of the intestines or a tear of the mesentery.

Clinically, two symptom patterns emerge. Approximately one fourth of these patients develop evidence of a hemoperitoneum secondary to mesenteric lacerations. In the remainder, the intestinal injury most commonly involves the jejunum, and the initial signs and symptoms are often absent or considered insignificant. Subsequent delays in diagnosis of up to 8 weeks have been reported. The "seatbelt sign," contusion or abrasion across the lower abdomen, is found in less than one third of patients with abdominal injuries caused by lap belts. Its presence, however, is highly correlated with intraperitoneal pathologic lesions.[19] Rupture of the diaphragm, an elusive diagnostic problem, can also occur. Rare cases of acute abdominal aortic dissection with incomplete or complete occlusion have also been described, and injuries to the lumbar spine are not uncommon.[20]

Iatrogenic Injuries

Although well intentioned, diagnostic and therapeutic efforts in patient care are not risk-free. Abdominal injuries may be sequelae of various medical procedures and in certain instances are not only extremely difficult to recognize but may contribute to or cause pronounced morbidity or death. Numerous procedures may cause an iatrogenic injury.

Artificial ventilation can lead to gastric distention, particularly in children. Besides compromising ventilation and increasing the risk of vomiting and aspiration, a significant distention may lead to an esophageal or gastric laceration and perforation. These may occur with bag/mask ventilations, an inadvertent esophageal intubation with a nasotracheal or endotracheal tube, or the mistaken connection of the nasogastric tube to oxygen rather than suction. The esophageal obturator airway and similar devices placed in the trachea cause an airway obstruction and the unintended ventilation of the esophagus and stomach. Esophageal, gastroesophageal junction, and gastric lacerations are evidenced by bloody emesis or nasogastric return. If a gastric perforation occurs and positive-pressure breathing is maintained, a tension pneumoperitoneum may ensue with inferior vena cava compression and decreased cardiac output. External cardiac compressions have produced splenic, hepatic, and gastric injuries. Manual thrusts to clear an airway obstruction, as taught in basic life support courses, and the Heimlich maneuver have caused rib fractures with lacerations and the rupture of abdominal viscera. In cases of a cardiac arrest, these injuries may be occult but life-threatening. If hypotension occurs after cardiopulmonary resuscitation, an abdominal injury and hemorrhage must be considered along with cardiogenic shock.[21]

Tube thoracostomy has resulted in injury to the liver and spleen. These injuries may result from an unknown elevation of the diaphragm on the side of the thoracostomy or the placement of the tube too low in the chest with resulting intra-abdominal penetration. Peritoneal lavage, paracentesis, and peritoneal dialysis have caused a series of complications, especially vascular penetration and bowel perforation. Signs of blood loss from a hemoperitoneum in the former case and peritonitis in the latter will evolve.

A liver biopsy can lead to a hemoperitoneum or hemobilia. Endoscopic procedures of the bowel may cause a hollow viscus perforation and peritonitis, particularly when a biopsy is performed.[22] Peritoneoscopy has been reported to cause small bowel perforations and iliac vessel lacerations. Barium enemas have an extremely low incidence of perforation but can be another cause of unexplained peritonitis and pneumoperitoneum.

Pediatrics

Congenital anomalies and intra-abdominal neoplasms may be first discovered after a history of blunt trauma. Coagulopathies (e.g., hemophilia) can contribute to the pathologic condition and complicate therapy after apparent minor trauma to the abdomen.

A child's abdomen has poorly developed musculature and a relatively smaller anteroposterior diameter. These factors increase the vulnerability of abdominal contents to compression between a blunt anterior force and the solid posterior vertebrae. The rib cage is extremely compliant in children and less prone to fractures but nonetheless provides only partial protection against splenic and hepatic injuries.

The liver, spleen, and kidney are the organs most commonly damaged by blunt mechanism of all varieties, and the incidence of injury for each of these three solid viscera is roughly the same. Gastrointestinal tract perforation is not uncommon with blunt trauma, and these injuries may be isolated. In cases of nonaccidental trauma, those injuries seen most commonly are duodenal and small bowel hematomas and perforations, pancreatic contusions, lacerations and pseudocysts, lacerations and rupture of the liver and spleen, and lacerations of mesenteric vessels.

CLINICAL FEATURES

History

The patient's history may be unobtainable, elusive, or temporarily abandoned while resuscitative measures are carried out. When the situation permits and a reliable source is available, certain information is valuable.

The patient's ability to relate the course of events may be compromised by head or spinal cord injury, alcohol intoxication, mental retardation, hysteria, and any number of toxins. At times, the trauma may have preceded the onset of symptoms by days or weeks and may have been forgotten or considered trivial by the patient. Witnesses at the scene, particularly paramedical personnel, often provide the most reliable data.

Knowledge of substance exposure or events that could interfere with the clinical evaluation of the patient is helpful. Alcohol or drug use, a head or spinal cord injury, and psychiatric problems are the most common among these factors. Appreciation of comorbid medical conditions, particularly cardiovascular disease and coagulopathies, optimizes fluid and blood component therapy. Finally, when a prehospital care team or transferring hospital is involved, the vital signs, physical assessment, prehospital course, and response to therapy should be obtained. Clinical records and laboratory and radiologic studies obtained at an outlying hospital should be carefully reviewed. The symptomatology in cases of abdominal trauma is twofold. Volume loss may produce orthostatic or frank dizziness, lightheadedness, and confusion. A hematic, infectious, acidic, or enzymatic irritation of the peritoneum produces pain. The pain may be clearly present at the outset or delayed for hours to days.

The patient's communication may be dulled or ineffectual, or the subjective sensation of pain may be impaired by a spinal cord injury or an underlying medical problem such as diabetes. Occasionally, intense, competing pain at another body site dominates and distracts both the patient and physician away from the abdomen. Abdominal pain can be localized, as it sometimes is in the left upper quadrant with a splenic injury, or diffuse, as in septic peritonitis subsequent to bowel perforation. Referred pain to the right and left shoulder tips or neck can occur with hemoperitoneum, particularly when the patient has been in the Trendelenburg position, allowing the blood to irritate the diaphragm; this most often occurs with hepatic and splenic injuries. Pain referred to the testicle is compatible with a retroperitoneal injury and is seen most commonly with urogenital and duodenal trauma.

Nausea and vomiting can accompany peritoneal irritation or hypovolemia. These can also be caused by an obstruction, as can occur with a duodenal hematoma. Dyspnea sometimes occurs with gastric distention or diaphragmatic irritation or when abdominal contents herniate into the chest, impairing respiratory dynamics.

Penetrating Abdominal Trauma

Stab Wounds

It is helpful to obtain information regarding the mode of injury from the patient, paramedic, or witnesses. The number of stabs inflicted, type and size of the instrument, posture of the victim relative to the direction of assault, estimated blood loss at the scene, time of injury, and response to fluids should be sought. A significant proportion of victims of stab wounds are found under the influence of alcohol or another drug. This state can make obtaining an accurate history a futile effort and further compromise the validity of symptoms and signs.

Gunshot Wounds

As initial stabilization measures are instituted in the emergency department, the emergency physician can elicit certain facts that can contribute greatly to the evaluation of the patient. These include the weapon used, its distance from the victim when shot, the position of the victim in relationship to the weapon when fired, the suspected number of shots, the blood loss at the scene, the amount and type of field fluids administered, and the vital signs during the prehospital course.

Blunt Abdominal Trauma

With blunt injuries, specifically those resulting from vehicular trauma, inquiries should be made regarding the extent of damage to the car; the patient's location within the car; whether the patient struck the steering wheel; whether seat belts were used and, if so, what type; and whether front or side air bags were deployed. The magnitude of injury to pedestrians varies with the speed and size of the striking vehicle. A triad of injuries to the torso, cranium, and lower aspect of the lower extremity has been well described, and pathologic

lesions discovered in two of these sites should prompt careful attention to the third. Motorcycle crashes can be placed in one of four categories: frontal, lateral or angular, ejection, or "laying the bike down." Different pathologic lesions can be projected based on the offending mechanism.

Pediatrics

Assessment and management of abdominal injuries in children are based on the same principles as in adults. The symptoms and signs are similar and in alert, cooperative patients are valuable. Age-related difficulties in communication, fear-induced uncooperative behavior, or a concomitant head injury, however, make the clinical examination less reliable. In cases of unexplained abdominal tenderness or peritonitis, it is important to inquire about vaginal bleeding or discharge and rectal bleeding and to examine the rectum and vagina for foreign bodies. Such objects may be inserted by inquisitive children or by adults during acts of child molestation.

Physical Examination

Abdominal trauma provokes a wide spectrum of presentations that range from seemingly insignificant symptoms and signs to severe shock and coma. Evidence of abdominal tenderness, peritoneal irritation, gastrointestinal hemorrhage, and hypovolemia not attributable to extra-abdominal causes represents most of the signs suggestive of an intraperitoneal injury. These signs may be initially absent or obscure, and careful attention to the abdomen with serial examinations can aid in making an early, accurate diagnosis.

The physical examination of a hemodynamically unstable patient is performed coincident with therapy, but care and thoroughness are not precluded by these circumstances. When an obvious intracranial, thoracic, or orthopedic injury is present, the abdomen must always be considered. Chest trauma itself is a risk factor for coincident intraperitoneal pathology. This is particularly true in cases of suspected multiple blunt trauma accompanied by a head injury, coma, or obtunded mental status resulting from drugs or alcohol.

The abdomen, then, should neither be ignored nor be the sole focus of the emergency physician. All of the patient's clothing must be removed, and a careful inspection of the patient's body should be conducted, to include the scalp, perineum, skin folds, and beneath the hair. Wounds from penetrating trauma can be exceptionally small, difficult to find, and yet lethal.

Hypotension in the acute stage results from hemorrhage that is most often from a solid visceral or vascular injury. Traumatic pancreatitis may produce significant third-space fluid loss, but hours to days are usually required for this to appear, and shock is an uncommon presentation.[23] When hypotension accompanies significant multiple blunt trauma and is unexplained, one should assume the presence of intraperitoneal hemorrhage until it is excluded. However, a known extra-abdominal source of hemorrhage does not mitigate the need to evaluate the peritoneal cavity. A head injury alone does not explain shock except in cases of profound head injury or in the very small infant for whom traumatic intracranial or extracranial (e.g., cephalohematoma) blood may be proportionally substantial.[24]

In cases of penetrating trauma, inspecting the abdomen for entrance and exit wounds may help determine the path of injury. Distention can occur as a result of pneumoperitoneum, gastric dilation, or ileus produced by peritoneal irritation. An ecchymotic discoloration of the flanks (Gray-Turner sign) or umbilicus (Cullen's sign) indicates retroperitoneal hemorrhage, but these signs are usually delayed for 12 hours to several days. Abdominal contusions can result from various implements, and when caused by lap-seat belts, they herald abdominal injuries in one third of cases.

Markedly decreased or absent bowel sounds have traditionally been considered one of the more reliable clinical parameters of intraperitoneal injuries. However, the presence of audible peristalsis, although uncommon, does not rule out ileus or serious injury, and the absence of bowel sounds occurs in up to 20% of patients with a suspected injury from abdominal trauma who prove to have no such injury at laparotomy. In such instances, coexisting electrolyte disturbances or thoracolumbar vertebral body or transverse process fractures may be responsible for the ileus. Auscultation of bowel sounds in the thorax should alert the emergency physician to the presence of a diaphragmatic injury.

Local or generalized tenderness is palpated in approximately 90% of alert patients with an intra-abdominal visceral injury. Local and generalized rebound tenderness and rigidity can be signs of peritoneal irritation and occur less commonly. These signs lack specificity, however, and can be found with lower rib fractures and contusions of the thoracoabdominal wall. These findings or, more important, their absence, are more reliable in alert patients. However, false-positive and false-negative abdominal manifestations have been well demonstrated even in conscious, responsive patients.[25,26]

Rarely, encapsulated bleeding into regions walled off by blood clots or adhesions can form palpable intra-abdominal masses; these usually appear at least several hours later. Severe contusions of the abdominal wall can cause tenderness and voluntary guarding that is localized and usually exacerbated by use of the affected muscle. A palpated mass can represent a rectus hematoma or ventral hernia. Shifting dullness results from a massive hemoperitoneum and is accompanied by signs of shock. A loss of gastric tympany in the left upper quadrant can be found with enlarging splenic injuries. Dullness to percussion over the flank that is not affected by position suggests a retroperitoneal hematoma, but it is not commonly found in such cases.

A rectal examination rarely reveals blood or subcutaneous emphysema, but the presence of either is highly correlated with abdominal injuries. The evaluation of rectal tone is an important part of determining

the patient's spinal cord integrity, and palpation of a high-riding prostate suggests urethral injury.

A nasogastric tube should routinely be placed in the absence of severe maxillofacial trauma to decompress the abdomen, decrease the likelihood of aspiration, and determine whether blood is present. Orogastric placement should be used when a cribriform plate fracture is suspected to prevent intracranial insertion. Foley catheters are useful in unstable patients for following renal output and rapidly obtaining urine samples to search for blood, myoglobin, and toxins.

Thus, a number of signs are valuable in assessing the patient with abdominal trauma. Although the presence of physical findings makes intraperitoneal injury more likely, their absence does not preclude serious pathology, and none is exclusively diagnostic of a specific injury. Extensive observation and the use of certain laboratory procedures greatly help prevent erroneous or missed diagnoses.

Penetrating Abdominal Trauma

Stab Wounds

Serial physical examinations performed by the same observer are gaining acceptance in centers where these have been found useful, particularly with patients who are alert, communicative, and neurologically intact. The presence of intoxicants does not necessarily preclude reliance on examination but may undermine its value. In other series, patients with impressive physical findings after penetrating trauma to the abdomen have undergone exploratory laparotomy, with negative results in 14% to 28% of cases.[27] Moreover, up to one third of patients with significant intra-abdominal injuries have no suggestive physical signs, particularly when a retroperitoneal injury has occurred.[28]

Gunshot Wounds

As with blunt or other modes of penetrating trauma, there is dispute regarding the value of the physical examination of patients with abdominal GSWs. In various series, 20% of patients with a documented intraperitoneal injury had no peritoneal signs before exploration.[29] Moreover, objective physical findings suggestive of intra-abdominal damage have been misleading and falsely positive in 15% of patients in whom laparotomy revealed no injury. Other authors contend that selective management can be undertaken safely when physical examination is the fundamental evaluative measure.[3,30]

Blunt Abdominal Trauma

Overall, the accuracy of the physical examination in patients with blunt abdominal trauma is 55% to 65%.[31] The initial presentation may be exceptionally benign in cases of blunt intra-abdominal injury. The most reliable symptoms and signs in alert patients are pain, tenderness, and peritoneal findings, particularly when risk factors for abdominal injury are present. When altered sensorium intercedes, the physical signs become less reliable. Frequent evaluations by the same examiner are indicated even in alert patients, but especially in sensorium-altered patients, particularly as they clear.

DIAGNOSTIC STRATEGIES

Laboratory

Hematologic and chemical values are of limited use in the management of the acutely traumatized patient.[32] They should be considered adjuncts to diagnosis and not substitutes for clinical assessment.

Hematology

Hematocrit

The hematocrit reflects baseline value, extent of and time from hemorrhage, exogenous fluid administration, and endogenous plasma refill. The last of these is a physiologic compensatory shift of extracellular fluid into the intravascular space, the intent of which is to restore the original blood volume. Based on a study of volunteers sustaining a 10% to 20% blood loss, this restoration proceeds at a rate of only 40 to 90 mL/hr for the first 10 hours and requires 30 to 40 hours for completion.[33] However, patients evidencing hemorrhagic shock with a blood loss of at least 40% demonstrate much faster plasma refill rates, estimated as high as 1500 mL in the first 90 minutes after injury, with significant decreases in hematocrit within this period. Although the hematocrit is an easily acquired measure, it is often a conundrum when viewed in isolation, and serial determinations are more helpful.

White Blood Cell Count

The white blood cell count is of little predictive assistance in cases of abdominal trauma, particularly its acute phase.[32] Leukocytosis with a count of 12,000 to 20,000/mm³ and a moderate left shift may occur within several hours of a major injury and lasts several days. It is attributed to tissue injury, acute hemorrhage, and peritoneal irritation and is partially a result of epinephrine-induced demargination. Intra-abdominal infections and peritonitis can cause a pronounced elevation of the white blood cell count and often produce toxic granulations in the leukocytes.

Chemical

Pancreatic Enzymes

Neither serum amylase nor lipase is useful when obtained in rote fashion. Normal levels do not exclude a major pancreatic injury, and elevated values may be caused by any of an assortment of reasons in addition to an injured pancreas. The use of serum amylase isoenzymes has not appreciably improved accuracy. Nontraumatic causes of hyperamylasemia include several diseases and the use of alcohol, narcotics, and various other drugs. Amylase or lipase may also be elevated with pancreatic ischemia produced by the systemic hypotension that often accompanies trauma. Clearly, these enzymes are neither highly specific nor sensitive for pancreatic injuries. Elevated or rising levels may indicate damage but in themselves are not conclusive.[34]

In these cases, clinical correlation and further investigation are indicated.

Base Deficit

Metabolic acidosis in the setting of trauma can suggest the presence of hemorrhagic shock. This can be witnessed chemically as a decreased serum bicarbonate level, increased base deficit, or elevated serum lactate level. Although normal values do not exclude abdominal injury, substantive abnormalities, such as a base deficit greater than or equal to 6, may be predictive. These findings should be considered in clinical context, because the resolution of the laboratory findings will lag behind the clinical improvement of the patient.

Liver Function Tests

Elevated serum transaminases can result from hepatic trauma but do not distinguish minor contusions from severe injury.[35] Alternatively, these may be symptomatic of alcohol-induced liver damage.

Toxicology Analysis

Screens for ethanol and drugs are often used in trauma centers. Their utility in the management of abdominal trauma per se has not been established, particularly in patients with normal mental status.[36] Positive study findings may prompt the emergency physician to interdict and the patient to decrease the recidivistic use of ethanol or drugs.

Radiology

Radiologic procedures for traumatized patients are not without risk and in a substantial number of patients may be contraindicated. Resuscitation and initial stabilization measures must always precede abdominal radiographic studies. Any potential cervical or thoracic spinal injury must be excluded or presumed as the clinical situation dictates. In patients whose symptoms and signs demonstrate a likely need for exploratory laparotomy, delay to operation because of radiologic diagnostics is permissible only when the patient has been stabilized and only if studies might aid in determining management. Adequate radiographic detail cannot be achieved in an uncooperative patient. Trained personnel must accompany any patient who has potential to deteriorate precipitously. The placement of a patient in the radiology department for even a brief period can have disastrous consequences. Abdominal studies are indicated in a stable patient when findings on the physical examination and other laboratory procedures are inconclusive and the information will guide therapy.

Plain Films

The chest radiograph and anteroposterior pelvic films can be invaluable in cases of penetrating and blunt trauma, respectively. However, although plain abdominal films can demonstrate numerous findings, their place in acute trauma is limited. Because of spinal precautions, hemodynamic instability, or patient discomfort, plain films can be difficult and time-consuming to acquire. In the patient who has sustained blunt trauma, such studies usually contribute little to management and should be reserved for specific indications. The finding of rib, pelvic, vertebral body, or transverse spinous process fractures warrants special consideration for nearby visceral damage.

Although hemoperitoneum can be seen as opacification locally or diffusely on the x-ray film of a supine patient, these findings are mostly of historical interest. Similarly, retroperitoneal accumulations can obscure the psoas shadow or renal shadow and can displace the bladder away from the side of hemorrhage. Injuries to solid viscera can cause intracapsular bleeding and increase the shadow cast by the organ on the chest or abdominal film. This may also cause an indentation or displacement of colonic flexures and the gastric bubble, as is seen in cases of hepatic and splenic trauma.

Very small quantities of readily detectable free intraperitoneal air are present in most patients with gastric, duodenal bulb, and colonic perforations but in fewer than one fourth of those with jejunal and ileal perforation. These are seen more readily on CT than plain films. Free intraperitoneal air can be generated by mediastinal or pulmonary injury, as well as by barotrauma, and thus its presence is not pathognomonic of hollow viscus perforation. Intraperitoneal air is mobile, and to maximize visualization the patient should be kept in the appropriate upright or decubitus position for 10 to 15 minutes, if this is tolerable, before these films are obtained. In upright films, air is located under the diaphragm or the central tendon of the diaphragm anteriorly. In supine films, air tracks under peritoneal attachments, such as the falciform ligament and urachus, up to the anterior abdominal wall. On films in which the patient is in a lateral decubitus position, air is located in the superior flank and outlines the liver edge (Figure 43-1). In cases of gastric perforations, air may be limited to the lesser sac. A rupture of a retroperitoneal hollow viscus can be detected by a stippling pattern outlining the duodenum, kidney, or psoas muscle (Figure 43-2). Extraperitoneal colonic perforations may extravasate air, which outlines the psoas muscle and perinephric region.

Foreign bodies and missiles are easily identified on abdominal films. Therefore, their absence without a known exit wound warrants further search. A ricochet off the spine or pelvis into the chest or proximal extremities can occur. An entry into the vascular system may carry the object toward and into the right side of the heart or peripherally into the arterial tree. It may also find its way into the gastrointestinal tract and either produce obstruction or pass through unnoticed.

Computed Tomography

Over the last 25 years, CT scanning has continued to advance its place among diagnostics for trauma. Evolution to 16- and 64-slice helical and spiral scanners has improved resolution and greatly decreased the time required for the scan itself. However, CT scanning is imperfect, and its use is largely restricted to patients with hemodynamic stability who have sustained trauma caused by blunt mechanism unless penetration of the retroperitoneum or colorectal area is suspected.[37]

Advantages

When CT scanning is compared with other modalities, notably diagnostic peritoneal lavage (DPL), numerous advantages are cited, including the fact it is noninvasive. CT scanning via differential signal absorption between traumatic lesions, hemorrhage, and normal parenchyma has the potential to define the injured organ and the extent of the pathologic condition. It is most accurate for solid visceral pathologic lesions and is often capable of discerning the presence, source, and approximate quantity of intraperitoneal hemorrhage by the use of attenuation coefficients (Figure 43-3). It can

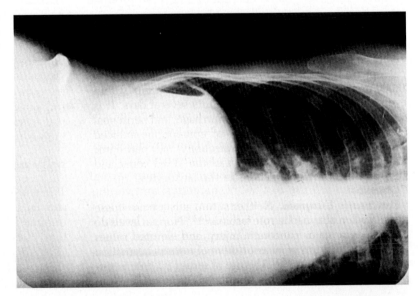

Figure 43-1. Demonstration of free intraperitoneal air on left lateral decubitus film. This is the preferred decubitus position because it avoids confusion with the gastric bubble and splenic flexure.

demonstrate active bleeding from the liver or spleen, which appears as a blush and which may lend itself to therapeutic angiographic embolization.[38] CT scanning coincidentally evaluates the retroperitoneum (Figure 43-4), an area not sampled by DPL, as well as the vertebral column and can be readily extended above or below the abdomen to visualize the thorax or pelvis.[39] It is helpful in the evaluation of hematuria and, if used early enough, in determining renal artery injury.[40] CT scanning is particularly helpful in affecting non-

operative management of solid organ damage.[41] This includes as-needed follow-up studies of convalescing patients with these injuries.[42] It has also proven effective when incorporated in delayed fashion for patients with decreasing hematocrit, increasing base deficit, or subtle examination changes. By minimizing the incidence of nontherapeutic laparotomies for self-limited injury to the liver or spleen, it decreases morbidity and cost attendant to this operation.

Disadvantages

Disadvantages of CT scanning include its suboptimal sensitivity for injury of the pancreas, diaphragm, small bowel, and mesentery.[43] These latter two are particularly worrisome because isolated coincidental hollow viscus injury is not uncommon in patients with blunt trauma, and profound morbidity and death can ensue from delayed and missed diagnoses. Findings on CT scans, including the suspected quantity of hemoperitoneum or the presence of isolated free fluid, are not able to forecast well the need for operative intervention.[44] Complications can result from intravenous contrast administration or uncommonly from contrast material administered orally if it is not used in a cautious manner.[45] Moreover, oral contrast rarely adds to diagnostic accuracy and delays completion of the study.[46,47] The cost of CT scanning is significant, particularly if established indications are not followed. It may be unnecessary in the follow-up evaluation of stable splenic injuries.[41] Finally, the logistic and personnel aspects of CT scanning can pose great hazard to the monitoring of ill trauma patients. The patient's fate should not be jeopardized by ill-advised or poorly supervised studies.

Technique

The technique for CT scanning is reasonably standardized, but certain conventions are debated. The studies

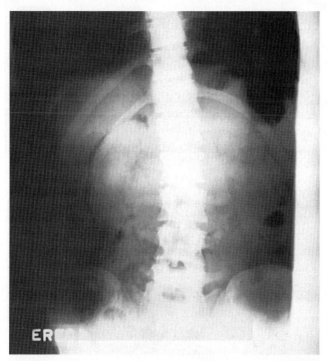

Figure 43-2. Erect film demonstrates the soap bubble appearance of retroperitoneal air outlining the right kidney. Duodenal perforation is the responsible pathologic condition.

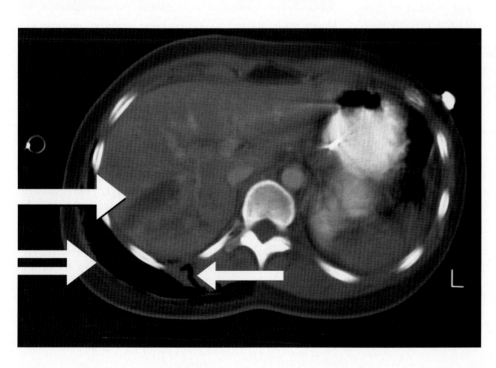

Figure 43-3. Computed tomography scan of the abdomen demonstrating a deep intrahepatic laceration (large solid arrow), pneumothorax (large hollow arrow), and retroperitoneal air (small solid arrow).

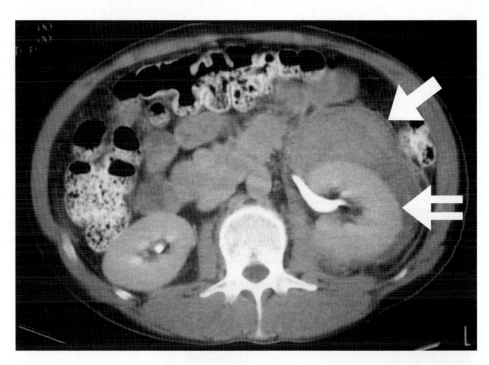

Figure 43-4. Computed tomography scan of the abdomen displays an extensive perirenal hematoma (solid arrow) surrounding the left kidney (hollow arrow).

should begin in the low chest and be taken through the pelvis. "Quick look" but less thorough studies are problematic and should be avoided. Most centers perform enhanced and nonenhanced scans because the latter alone may not demonstrate intraparenchymal hematomas well. Other practitioners believe that the noncontrast portion contributes little other than time to the procedure. Oral contrast delivery to opacify bowel is infrequently useful and often omitted.[46,47]

Ultrasonography

Ultrasonography is rapidly becoming an integral diagnostic component in this nation's trauma centers. Since its first use in the trauma setting in Germany in 1971, ultrasonography has undergone a large number of clinical evaluations in Europe, Asia, and the United States. Its primary role is detecting free intraperitoneal blood after blunt trauma. This is accomplished by a focused examination of Morison's pouch, the splenorenal recess, and the pouch of Douglas, which are dependent portions of the intraperitoneal cavity where blood is likely to accumulate (Figure 43-5). Anechoic areas caused by the presence of blood are best visualized when contrasted against solid organs (e.g., liver, spleen, and kidneys). With penetrating mechanisms, ultrasonography can evaluate the pericardial space and intraperitoneal spaces. It has also been used to inspect thoracoabdominal wound tracts with some success.[48]

Advantages

Ultrasonography carries a host of advantages. It is a portable instrument that can be brought to the bedside in the trauma resuscitation area. Studies of the pericardial and intraperitoneal spaces can be accomplished in less than 5 minutes. Sensitivity in detecting as little as 100 mL and, more typically, 500 mL of intraperitoneal fluid ranges from 60% to 95% in most recent

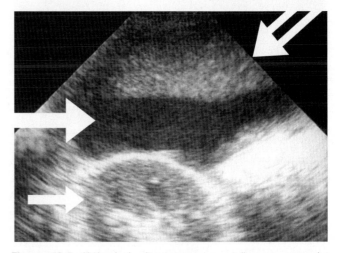

Figure 43-5. Abdominal ultrasonogram revealing an extensive amount of blood in Morison's pouch (large solid arrow) surrounding the liver (large hollow arrow). The right kidney is seen in the bottom of the figure (small solid arrow).

studies and specificity for hemoperitoneum is excellent.[49] Therefore, when time is precious in the critical patient, ultrasonography can enable the emergency physician to rapidly answer the key question in the decision matrix, which is whether hemoperitoneum is present. Unlike DPL, ultrasonography can rapidly gauge the mediastinum, is noninvasive, and can be performed serially and by multiple technicians. Unlike CT scanning, it is not a potential radiation hazard and does not require administration of contrast agents. The skill of performing focused examinations in trauma is not restricted to radiologists, which makes ultrasonography more available in real time in most centers. Accuracy correlates with length of training and experience, but expertise can be readily accomplished in emergency medicine and surgical training programs.[50]

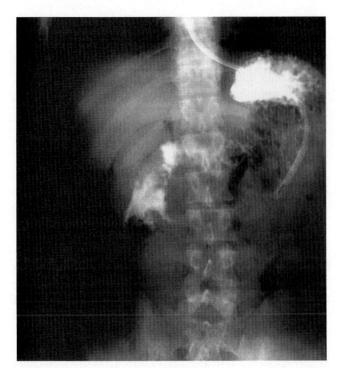

Figure 43-6. Gastrografin study demonstrating rupture of the second portion of the duodenum with extravasation of contrast material.

Overall, ultrasonography can serve as an accurate, rapid, and less expensive diagnostic screening tool than DPL.[51]

Disadvantages

Ultrasonography does not image solid parenchymal damage, the retroperitoneum, or diaphragmatic defects well. It is technically compromised by the uncooperative, agitated patient, as well as by obesity, substantial bowel gas, and subcutaneous air. Indeterminate studies require follow-up attempts or alternative diagnostic tests.[52] It is less sensitive and more operator dependent than DPL in revealing hemoperitoneum and cannot distinguish blood from ascites. Ultrasonography, as well as DPL, will not detect the presence of solid parenchymal damage if free intraperitoneal blood is absent, as in subcapsular splenic injury.[53] For the pediatric patient, studies have been inconsistent but generally have demonstrated lower sensitivity. Ultrasonography appears to be as accurate in the pregnant as in the nonpregnant woman.[54] Finally, ultrasonography is poor at recognizing bowel injury in which hemorrhage tends to be inconsequential, and failure to diagnose hollow viscus perforation in a timely manner can have catastrophic results.[55]

Contrast Studies

Contrast studies with a water-soluble medium (e.g., Gastrografin) can be helpful in cases of suspected gastric, duodenal, and rectal perforations (Figure 43-6). Barium mixtures should be used to visualize intramural duodenal hematomas.[56] A CT scan may be able to discern duodenal hematomas and can distinguish these from perforations.[57]

Magnetic Resonance Imaging

Magnetic resonance imaging scans are usually impractical and sometimes impossible to perform in the acute phase of multiple blunt trauma. Currently, in acutely injured trauma patients, magnetic resonance imaging scanning should be reserved for the evaluation of spinal fractures and elusive diaphragmatic defects.

Angiography

Angiography, a time-consuming procedure, is usually reserved for the unstable patient with blunt trauma and pelvic fracture in whom it can be used to embolize bleeding vessels. It can be a means of staunching solid visceral hemorrhage from blunt trauma, notably of the spleen,[38] and has been used rarely for intraperitoneal and retroperitoneal hemorrhage after trauma by a penetrating mechanism.[58] Angiography can also be used in the further workup of a patient in whom vascular pedicle injury is suspected, particularly of the kidney.

Endoscopic Retrograde Cholangiopancreaticoduodenography

The role of endoscopic retrograde cholangiopancreaticoduodenography is limited to the detailed delineation of pancreatic injury, particularly to the ductal system. CT scanning can supplement this test to reaffirm ductal injury or clarify equivocal results of endoscopic retrograde cholangiopancreaticoduodenography.[59]

Special Procedures

Diagnostic Peritoneal Lavage

In 1964, Root and colleagues[60] introduced DPL and reported 100% accuracy in their series of 28 patients. Although subsequent evaluations have not matched this perfection, DPL continues to be an accurate and important adjunct to the diagnosis of abdominal injuries.

Diagnostic peritoneal lavage comprises two interrelated steps. The first is the attempted aspiration of free peritoneal blood. The recovery of hemoperitoneum is a strong predictor of intraperitoneal injury, and the procedure is then terminated. If aspiration findings are negative, lavage is conducted in which the peritoneal cavity is washed with saline. This fluid is introduced by catheter, recovered by gravity drainage, and analyzed. The sole absolute contraindication to DPL is the established need for laparotomy. Relative contraindications include prior abdominal surgery or infections, coagulopathy, obesity, and second- or third-trimester pregnancy.

Various methods of introducing the catheter into the peritoneal space have been described.[61] These include a closed technique in which the catheter is inserted in a blind percutaneous fashion by the Seldinger technique; a semi-open technique in which sharp and blunt dissection to the rectus fascia is followed by percutaneous delivery of the catheter through the peritoneum into the peritoneal cavity; and an open technique, which extends the semiopen method through the rectus

Table 43-1. Preferred Site of Diagnostic Peritoneal Lavage

Clinical Circumstance	Site	Method
Standard adult	Infraumbilical midline	C or SO
Standard pediatric	Infraumbilical midline	C or SO
Second- and third-trimester pregnancy	Suprauterine	FO
Midline scarring	Left lower quadrant	FO
Pelvic fracture	Supraumbilical	FO
Penetrating trauma	Infraumbilical midline*	C or SO

C, closed (percutaneous Seldinger technique); SO, semi-open; FO, fully open.
*The stab wound or gunshot wound site should be avoided.
From Marx JA: Peritoneal procedures. In Roberts JR, Hedges JR (eds): *Clinical Procedures in Emergency Medicine*, 4th ed. Philadelphia, Saunders, 2004.

Table 43-2. Diagnostic Peritoneal Lavage Red Blood Cell Criteria (per mm³)

	Positive	Indeterminate
Blunt trauma	100,000*	20,000-100,000
Stab wound		
Anterior abdomen	100,000	20,000-100,000
Flank	100,000	20,000-100,000
Back	100,000	20,000-100,000
Low chest	5000-10,000	1000-5000
Gunshot wound	5000-10,000	1000-5000

*In a hemodynamically stable patient with pelvic fracture and positive or equivocal red blood cell count, computed tomography should be obtained to corroborate or refute intraperitoneal injury.

fascia with direct visualization of the peritoneum (Table 43-1).

Advantages

In cases of blunt trauma, DPL's signal virtue is the triage of the patient who is hemodynamically unstable and has multiple injuries. In this complex scenario, DPL can promptly reveal or exclude the presence of intraperitoneal hemorrhage. Positive aspiration findings are a strong indication for laparotomy, whereas a negative study finding allows the clinician to undertake alternate management steps. Peritoneal aspiration and ultrasonography are now competitive for this role. In addition, DPL can be used to discern solid and hollow visceral injury under less critical circumstances. It can be especially valuable in the discovery of potentially lethal bowel perforations in which patients are poor candidates for serial clinical observations, and other instruments are notoriously unreliable.[62]

After a stab wound to the abdomen, low chest, flank, or back, DPL can meet three needs: (1) immediate disclosure of hemoperitoneum, particularly in a patient who may have mediastinal or pulmonary causes of or contributors to hypotension, (2) determination of intraperitoneal organ injury, and (3) detection of isolated diaphragmatic violation. Laparotomy is undertaken more commonly on clinical grounds for gunshot wounds. In these situations, DPL can serve these same tasks, but it is used far less often.[63]

Disadvantages

The morbidity associated with DPL occurs at a low rate and can be categorized as local or systemic infection, intraperitoneal injury, and technical failure. Wound complications, including hematoma and infection, occurred in 0.3% of cases in two large reviews.[64]

Technical failure can result in an inaccurate study and difficulty with fluid collection. A faulty technique with inadequate hemostasis or the insertion of the catheter through an abdominal wall hematoma can create a hemoperitoneum of sufficient magnitude to produce positive results. In addition, DPL is exquisitely sensitive for hemoperitoneum and in a hemodynamically stable patient can lead to unnecessary laparotomy.

False-negative interpretations can result from the failure to recover lavage fluid. This can occur in the following circumstances[61]: (1) inadvertent placement of the catheter into the preperitoneal space, (2) compartmentalization of fluid by adhesions, (3) impedance of fluid egress by obstructing omentum, and (4) large diaphragmatic tears typical of blunt mechanism that permit lavage fluid to move from the intraperitoneal to the intrathoracic cavity.

Results

A battery of hematologic, chemical, enzymatic, and microscopic tests has been applied to peritoneal aspirate and lavage effluent. Gross inspection of the effluent alone is considered neither adequate nor reliable. Little correlation between fluid color and cell count has been found.

In cases of blunt trauma, the aspiration of 10 mL or more of blood has a positive predictive value of greater than 90% for intraperitoneal injury, predictably solid visceral or vascular, and is responsible for approximately 80% of true positive DPL findings in blunt trauma.[64] The red blood cell (RBC) count of the lavage fluid is the next most widely used and accurate parameter (Table 43-2).

In cases of blunt trauma, an RBC count exceeding 100,000/mm³ is considered positive and generally specific for injury. However, while sensitive to the presence of injury, it may detect self-limited pathology for which laparotomy is unnecessary.

In patients with pelvic fractures, there is a well-known association of false-positive peritoneal lavage in the presence of retroperitoneal hematoma associated with pelvic fracture.[64] This is ascribed to tears in the posterior peritoneum, diapedesis of RBCs across the peritoneum into the peritoneal cavity, or dissection of a retroperitoneal hematoma out of the pelvis to the anterior abdominal wall. However, the key aspect in the setting of pelvic fracture is a positive aspiration finding because this presages active intraperitoneal hemorrhage in more than 85% of cases.[65,66] Negative aspiration or refutation of retroperitoneal injury by CT scan steers the clinician away from laparotomy and toward pelvic angiography with possible embolization.[67]

With anterior abdominal stab wounds, the removal of 10 mL of gross blood or the return of lavage fluid with an RBC count greater than $100,000/mm^3$ carries a sensitivity exceeding 90% (see Table 43-2). The incidence of visceral injury with counts less than $100,000/mm^3$ ranges from 1% to 29%. It is recommended that patients with equivocal RBC counts be carefully observed for 12 to 24 hours.[28,68] Most injuries associated with RBC counts less than $100,000/mm^3$ are to hollow viscera, and clinical manifestations of these should develop within this observation period.

With lower chest stab wounds, a positive RBC count of 5000 to $10,000/mm^3$ should be adopted to assist in detecting diaphragmatic injuries. Because of the more serious nature and greater likelihood of an injury with abdominal gunshot wounds, RBC counts of $5000/mm^3$ are advocated as the cutoff, as these will signal peritoneal penetration, if not injury.[69]

White blood cells enter the peritoneal cavity as part of shed blood or in response to an inflammatory stimulus. However, this finding lags after injury by 3 to 6 hours. Initial elevated counts greater than $500/mm^3$ are nonspecific and unhelpful. An elevated level in a lavage more than 4 hours after injury may indicate a perforation, but this finding can be a false-positive.[70]

Elevations in lavage amylase and alkaline phosphatase levels have been demonstrated in the immediate post-injury period following small intestinal injury.[71] These are postulated to result from spillage of hepatobiliary secretions and the release of enzymes from bowel wall. Elevated lavage amylase levels are less specific and sensitive for pancreatic trauma. Rising levels in serial lavages and clinical correlation may provide more suggestive evidence of a pancreatic injury.

Other parameters used in peritoneal lavage have been less extensively investigated. Poor cost-effectiveness argues against the routine use of bile staining and Gram stain of lavage fluid.

Local Wound Exploration

Because stab wounds do not reach the peritoneum in a significant number of cases, local wound exploration (LWE) is useful in determining the depth of penetration. The wound should be infiltrated with a local anesthetic containing epinephrine and thoroughly prepared for exploration. The stab wound may be extended if required and then carefully visualized through each successive layer of tissue. Blind probing with digits, instruments, or cotton-tipped swabs is inaccurate and hazardous. If the peritoneum is violated, further diagnostics are indicated. Likewise, when the end of the wound tract cannot be determined clearly, peritoneal entry must be presumed. When the stab wound is documented to be superficial to the abdominal cavity, the patient can be safely discharged home after appropriate wound care.[72]

Local wound exploration is generally advocated in cases of anterior abdominal stab wounds, but in other areas the decision is less clear. Abdominal, flank, and back wounds have been evaluated with this method, particularly when the entry is more superficial.[13,14] The flesh of obese or heavily muscled patients in particular can present technical problems and decrease the relia-

bility of exploration while increasing its risk. Wound explorations in patients with multiple entrances are not economic, and peritoneal penetration should be assumed. Deep exploration over the thoracic cage is precluded by attendant complications to neurovascular structures and pleura. However, careful inspection of superficial chest wounds (e.g., slash wound) is safe and can provide valuable data. CT, laparoscopy, or thoracoscopy is occasionally used in lieu of local wound exploration.

Laparoscopy

Laparoscopy is another rediscovered diagnostic tool being used in a limited number of centers. This procedure entails placement of a subumbilical or subcostal trocar for introduction of the laparoscope and creation of other ports for clamps, retractors, and other tools necessary for visualization or repair. Insufflation with carbon dioxide generally follows to allow improved visibility. General anesthesia in an operating suite is customary, although local anesthesia in the outpatient setting has been effective as well. This latter approach helps diminish the complications and cost of the procedure.

Laparoscopy has been most useful in assessing penetrating trauma, especially for injury to the diaphragm and intrathoracic abdominal organs.[73] Organs repaired via the laparoscope include the diaphragm, solid intraperitoneal viscera, stomach, and small bowel. Wound tracts have been assessed as accurately as by local wound exploration. Very little experience in blunt trauma has been documented thus far.

Drawbacks of laparoscopy include poor sensitivity for hollow visceral injury, notably to the small bowel, and difficulty in assessing the retroperitoneum and extent of damage to the liver and spleen.[74] Complications can result from trocar misplacement. If the diaphragm has been violated by the original trauma, tension pneumothorax can occur. This consequence and the theoretical risk of gas embolization and cardiovascular compromise can be avoided by using gasless laparoscopy. This technique is based on expanding the peritoneal cavity from without via mechanical retractors, but experience is limited to date.

At this time, the greatest value of laparoscopy is in the management of equivocal penetrating wounds to the thoracoabdominal region of stable patients. This approach can realize a reduced incidence of nontherapeutic laparotomy.[74] However, advancements in miniature optics that will improve resolution and imaging capability are sure to occur. In turn, this will decrease the need for general anesthesia and operating rooms and the resultant cost and complications of these methods.[75]

DIFFERENTIAL CONSIDERATIONS

Trauma versus Medical Condition

Medical and traumatic pathologic conditions can be coincident or lead one to the other. For instance, patients fall off roofs because of hypoglycemia and their altered mental status surmised to be closed-head injury is simply an easily treated metabolic disturbance. Likewise, precipitous anaphylactic, cardiac, or neurologic emergencies can initiate a motor vehicle crash and be partly or wholly responsible for the clinical presentation in the emergency department. Patients with infectious mononucleosis can experience splenic rupture after trivial and remote trauma. Finally, patients with premorbid coagulopathy or compromised immune status are more susceptible to the pathophysiology of solid or hollow organ injury, respectively.

Single versus Multisystem Trauma

Emergency physicians must be wary and not miss the proverbial forest for the trees. For instance, the pedestrian struck by a car who has an alleged isolated tibial-fibular fracture may well harbor significant intra-abdominal pathology, irrespective of a nontender abdomen.

Single versus Multiple Intraperitoneal Organ Injury

There has been an increasing trend toward nonoperative management of known intraperitoneal solid organ injury, specifically of the spleen and liver. It must be remembered, however, that coincident hollow viscus pathologic lesions may exist but not be discernible initially to clinical examination or certain diagnostic studies.[76]

Intraperitoneal Injury versus Necessary Laparotomy

Formerly, suspicion or knowledge of any intraperitoneal injury mandated laparotomy. Now, diagnostic effort is appropriately aimed at determining whether surgery is necessary or whether the injury is self-limited and does not require repair measures.

MANAGEMENT

General Measures

Prehospital

The trauma situation in the field calls for rapid stabilization and evacuation. The initial measures taken vary with the need for active airway management, the presence of concomitant injuries, and the skills of the prehospital personnel. Hemorrhage is the major life threat in cases of penetrating or blunt abdominal trauma, and two large-bore intravenous lines should be inserted in transit when possible. Penetrating wounds and eviscerations in particular should be covered with sterile dressings. Contact should be made with the base-station physician to communicate pertinent matters of the history, vital signs, treatment measures and their effects, and the estimated time of arrival.

Emergency Department

The principles of trauma care apply. The use of diagnostic aids for abdominal trauma should be carefully

restricted according to the patient's stability and the usefulness of the information sought in guiding management. Those patients who do not require immediate laparotomy will likely undergo one or more diagnostic procedures to determine whether abdominal injury exists and, if so, whether operative intervention is necessary.

Thoracotomy

Thoracotomy and subsequent cross-clamping of the descending aorta have been used to stabilize patients with thoracoabdominal injuries and profound hypovolemic shock. However, it is rarely lifesaving in the emergency department.

In a patient with massive abdominal injuries and hypotension secondary to a hemoperitoneum, the primary purpose of aortic cross-clamping is to shunt available blood into the coronary and cerebral circulation during resuscitation. Second, it is helpful in providing proximal bleeding control of certain vascular and parenchymal injuries, although continued bleeding can occur via collateral flow, until direct clamping, packing, or repair is achieved. Third, it can allow direct atrial access for rapid fluid administration. Finally, it has been advocated as a prophylactic measure in the operating room before laparotomy is performed for a massive hemoperitoneum. In certain instances, abdominal decompression, particularly in the face of a vascular injury, may result in worsening shock and death.

Antibiotics

An intestinal perforation and spillage can occur after blunt or, more commonly, penetrating trauma to the abdomen. Anaerobes and coliforms are the predominant organisms found. Antibiotics given prophylactically have been demonstrated to be effective in decreasing the incidence of intra-abdominal sepsis and should be given as soon as such an injury is suspected. A variety of regimens have been recommended.[77]

Penetrating Abdominal Trauma: Stab Wounds

Diagnostic Studies

The purpose of diagnostic studies is to determine whether the peritoneal cavity has been violated or whether there is intraperitoneal injury requiring operative repair. Tests used for the former purpose include plain films, local wound exploration, ultrasonography, and laparoscopy. Those most commonly used with the latter intent are DPL, serial physical examinations, laparoscopy, ultrasonography, and CT scans. These modalities are undertaken only if clinical determinants that would mandate laparotomy do not exist.

Management

Selective management of abdominal stab wounds is now well accepted[71] because of the relatively low incidence of intraperitoneal injuries coupled with the success of various diagnostic strategies. The appropriateness of these strategies is predicated on the site of penetration, the clinical status of the patient, and the experience and preference of an institution and its personnel. Formerly, the goal of mandatory exploration of all stab wounds was to eliminate missed injuries. Currently, selective management has resulted in a tremendous reduction in unnecessary laparotomies and their associated morbidity, with minimal and acceptable loss in sensitivity for significant intraperitoneal injury. Although certain authors promote the relative safety of nontherapeutic operations, others cite considerable immediate and delayed hazards, as well as increased cost.[78] It is generally preferred that the nondiagnostic laparotomy rate be less than 15%.

Anterior Abdomen

In approaching the management of stab wounds to the anterior abdomen, the clinician is faced with three fundamental tasks. The first and most prevailing is to determine whether clinical indications exist that presage with high likelihood the need for laparotomy. The presence of one or more of these indications, particularly in the context of an unstable patient, sets the course to exigent operation. If none is found, however, the clinician may address the second issue of whether the peritoneal cavity has been violated. If it can be definitively demonstrated that it has not, no further diagnostics are required, and the patient can be discharged. If the cavity has been violated, or if it cannot be determined that the cavity has not been violated, the third question is pursued: does injury exist and, if so, is laparotomy required? One general approach to abdominal stab wounds founded on these three queries is summarized in Figure 43-7.[62,72] This algorithm is largely based on clinical indicators of injury, local wound exploration, DPL, CT scan, and other radiologic modalities. Other strategies rely more heavily on other techniques, such as serial abdominal examinations or laparoscopy.

Step I: Clinical Indications for Laparotomy. Seven clinical determinants are used to predict the need for laparotomy after stab wounds to the abdomen (Table 43-3). Although there is consensus regarding the reliability of some of these, each has suboptimal predictive value.

1. *Hemodynamic compromise.* This is the preeminent indication of the need for laparotomy and is the most likely reason that a patient will be taken urgently to the operating room without preliminary diagnostic studies. This is typically an appropriate approach after middle and lower abdominal penetration. However, stab wounds to the upper abdomen and lower chest may produce hemodynamic instability because of intrathoracic hemorrhage, pneumothorax, or pericardial tamponade.

2. *Peritoneal signs.* There is considerable debate over the reliability of peritoneal signs, particularly in the early postinjury period. Among physical examination findings, unequivocal peritoneal signs have the highest positive predictive value, whereas an entirely normal examination even in the presence of mild to moderate intoxication has the greatest negative predictive value for therapeutic laparotomy.[79]

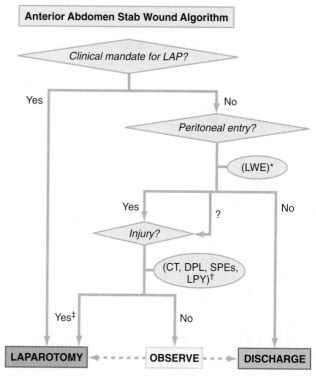

Figure 43-7. Anterior abdomen stab wound algorithm. *Plain films, ultrasonography, laparoscopy (LPY), and computed tomography (CT) can also assess peritoneal entry. †CT, diagnostic peritoneal lavage (DPL), serial physical examinations (SPEs), or LPY can be used in singular or complementary fashion depending on the clinical scenario. ‡Expectant management of injuries is infrequently attempted. LAP, laparotomy; LWE, local wound exploration.

Table 43-3. Clinical Indications for Laparotomy Following Penetrating Trauma

Manifestation	Premise	Pitfall
Hemodynamic instability	Major solid visceral or vascular injury	Thorax or mediastinum, causal or contributory
Peritoneal signs	Intraperitoneal injury	Unreliable, especially immediately post-injury
Evisceration	Additional bowel, other injury	No injury in one fourth to one third of stab wound cases
Diaphragmatic injury	Diaphragm	Rare clinical, radiographic findings
Gastrointestinal hemorrhage	Proximal gut	Uncommon, unknown accuracy
Implement in situ	Vascular impalement	Comorbid disease or pregnancy creates high operative risk
Intraperitoneal air	Hollow viscus perforation	Insensitive; may be caused by intraperitoneal entry only or be due to cardiopulmonary source

Modified from Marx JA: Diagnostic peritoneal lavage. In Ivatury RR, Cayten CG (eds). *The Textbook of Penetrating Trauma.* Baltimore, Williams & Wilkins, 1996.

3. *Evisceration.* With isolated omental evisceration, both a selective and a mandatory operating approach have been espoused. Omentum has been successfully ligated, excised, and restored to the peritoneal cavity. However, patients with viscus or omental evisceration sustain up to an 80% incidence of major intraperitoneal injury, rendering laparotomy a reasonable next step in management.[72,80]

4. *Diaphragmatic injury.* In contradistinction to blunt mechanism, penetrating trauma to the diaphragm produces small tears and evanescent clinical clues to their presence. Thus, clinical examination and plain chest films are rarely diagnostic of injury. Other diagnostic measures, such as DPL or laparoscopy, or a mandatory laparotomy approach, are necessary to discern this pathologic condition.

5. *Gastrointestinal hemorrhage.* Recovery of blood via a nasogastric tube or emesis may reflect a violation of the stomach or duodenum but is an unusual occurrence. Likewise, examination of the rectum or vagina may reveal hemorrhage that is the result of intraperitoneal or retroperitoneal trauma.

6. *Implements in situ.* The conservative and widely held maxim is to remove implements in situ of the torso in the operating room. This is to ensure expeditious control of hemorrhage should the implement reside within a vascular space or highly vascularized organ. Although implements in situ are most safely removed in the operating room, exceptions to this practice exist. These include situations in which emergency department resuscitation is impeded by the presence of the implement or the patient is at high risk of significant morbidity from nontherapeutic laparotomy because of severe comorbid conditions or pregnancy, for example.

7. *Intraperitoneal air.* The presence of free intraperitoneal air is often not sought because of the insensitivity and nonspecificity of this finding. Free intraperitoneal air can impute communication of the knife with the intraperitoneal space or the presence of pulmonary or mediastinal injury. Thus, it does not necessarily indicate hollow visceral perforation and should not be used in isolation as an indicator for operation.

Step II: Peritoneal Violation. If clinical indications for laparotomy are absent, a logical next step is assessing the wound tract itself. The presence of peritoneal violation can be determined by a variety of means. There is great value in establishing that a wound tract is superficial to the peritoneal, retroperitoneal, intrathoracic, and pericardial cavities. In this event, the patient can be discharged from the emergency department after receiving appropriate wound care. If a study is inconclusive, it should be assumed that one or more of these cavities has been violated and other means of assessment are required. The five methods of assessing the intactness of the peritoneum are as follows:

1. *Evisceration.* Evisceration of bowel or omentum is clear evidence of peritoneal entry. These situations are usually handled by mandatory laparotomy. In certain centers, however, these eviscerations are reduced in the emergency department and further diagnostics pursued.[80]

2. *Intraperitoneal air.* A finding of intraperitoneal free air on an upright chest or a lateral decubitus abdominal radiograph generally establishes that the knife has entered the peritoneal cavity and drawn air in with it, has disrupted a hollow viscus, or both. Rarely, a false-positive determination of peritoneal entry can be made when the actual source of intraperitoneal free air is the pulmonary tract. CT has exquisite sensitivity in detecting intraperitoneal free air. However, it can yield a false-positive finding and is an otherwise unnecessary diagnostic study in most cases of abdominal stab wounds.

3. *Local wound exploration.* This has been demonstrated to be an effective tool in determining the depth of the stab wound tract.

4. *Ultrasonography.* Ultrasonography has determined the intactness of the pleura and peritoneum in one small series and could be especially helpful in the case of a vexing wound to the low chest or upper abdomen when the mediastinum and diaphragm are at risk and no diagnostic modality is fail-safe.[48] Experience with ultrasonography for this purpose has been successful but very limited.

5. *Laparoscopy.* This has compared favorably with local wound exploration in assessing the wound tract but requires far more expertise and carries a far greater risk of complications. It is the most invasive and costly means of evaluating the integrity of the peritoneum. However, laparoscopy may also discover and serve as the mode of repair of certain diaphragmatic or organ injuries, or both.

Step III: Injury Requiring Laparotomy. In this algorithm, patients requiring an operation on clinical grounds have proceeded to laparotomy, and those in whom peritoneal, retroperitoneal, intrathoracic, and pericardial cavity violations have been excluded are discharged home. The patients remaining have presumed or known peritoneal violation. The next consideration is whether injury exists that dictates operative repair. In any case, patients who reach this stage of evaluation should be observed for at least 12 to 24 hours.

For the past 25 years, the diagnostic standard to address the issue of intraperitoneal injury has been DPL. It is especially valuable as a rapid means of determining hemoperitoneum in the critical patient and for the discovery of occult hollow viscus perforation and isolated diaphragmatic injury.[64,69,70,81] Ultrasonography may be somewhat less accurate than DPL in establishing the presence or absence of hemoperitoneum, but it can simultaneously ascertain hemopericardium, and in most centers ultrasonography can be accomplished as quickly as or more quickly than peritoneal aspiration. Emphasis on serial examinations with selective use of other studies on an as-needed basis can be successful when an adequate number of experienced clinicians are available.[82] A CT scan has been particularly useful for potential colorectal trauma or further assessment of patients submitted to serial examination alone. However, some centers routinely perform CT in these cases and not simply for possible colorectal trauma. Laparoscopy works best in experienced hands for restricted indications. Although this technique can enable direct visualization and repair of certain injuries, it has suboptimal sensitivity and only moderate specificity in determining the need for operation. Finally, "one-shot" intravenous pyelography prior to laparotomy to ensure two functioning kidneys is unnecessary, because less than 1% of the population have only one kidney.[83]

Thoracoabdominal

Even a single stab wound to the low chest can violate the mediastinum, thoracic cavity, diaphragm, peritoneal cavity, and retroperitoneum. The risk of diaphragmatic penetration from a left thoracoabdominal stab wound has been measured at 17%.[73] Ultrasonography can be extremely useful by quickly assessing for hemopericardium and hemoperitoneum in the marginally stable patient, if thoracotomy or laparotomy is not already clinically indicated.[84] LWE of slash-type wounds may obviate the need for further evaluation. However, the depth of investigation cannot be taken beyond the anterior rib margin to maximize safety and accuracy. Further assessment for intraperitoneal and diaphragmatic injury can be made by DPL. The RBC criterion is lowered to 5000 to 10,000/mm^3 to optimize sensitivity for isolated diaphragmatic injury.[64,69] Laparoscopy or thoracoscopy can visualize and potentially repair the diaphragm and other organs. A very conservative approach to the left lower chest stab wound, in particular, is mandatory exploration. This approach avoids any opportunity for missed diaphragmatic rents and their delayed consequences but results in an exceptionally high incidence of nontherapeutic operation. Rapid slice helical CT or magnetic resonance imaging may provide easier solutions to this vexing concern, but data are limited to date.

Flank and Back

The incidence of retroperitoneal injuries after stab wounds to the flank and back is greater than with injury to the anterior wall. However, risk of intraperitoneal organ injury is significant, ranging from 15% to 40%.[13] Again, local wound exploration can be a useful first step. However, the paraspinal muscles are quite thick, rendering the procedure more difficult. DPL is useful for diaphragmatic and intraperitoneal evaluation and, if it yields negative findings, can be followed by CT.[14] A double-contrast CT scan with prolonged oral contrast administration can assist in determining the depth of injury and the presence of retroperitoneal injury.[85] The addition of CT scan with contrast-enhanced enema is specifically intended for colorectal injuries but can be difficult to perform and is occasionally insensitive. Observation with serial examinations alone has been successfully implemented for stab wounds to the back and flank when the diaphragm is not considered at risk.[86]

Implement In Situ

It is routinely advised that foreign bodies in situ of the torso be removed under operating conditions. This is considered safest in the event that the implement is intravascular or in a highly vascularized organ. Plain films are generally all that is required. A CT scan may be indicated in stable patients if plain films suggest impalement of major vascular structures. Angiography may also be necessary. For pregnant patients or those with severe comorbid illness in whom unnecessary laparotomy should be strictly avoided, a CT scan may be able to discern the depth of entry and extent of injury. In these cases, the foreign body may be removed safely outside of the operating room.

Penetrating Abdominal Trauma: Gunshot Wounds

Diagnostic Studies

Diagnostic studies are used in a fashion similar to that for stab wounds. Moreover, the same diagnostic agents are applied, although in more restricted circumstances. The principal uses of diagnostic studies are to determine whether the missile has entered the peritoneal cavity or whether injury requiring operative intervention has occurred.

Management

Like stab wounds, GSWs typically produce multiple organ injuries and a high incidence of hollow visceral injury. However, the risk of mortality is significantly greater, especially if vascular structures are involved. Missiles striking the low chest commonly penetrate both intrathoracic and abdominal structures, including the diaphragm.

Abdominal GSWs enter the peritoneal cavity in approximately 80% of cases, and in more than 90% of those involving penetration there is intraperitoneal damage.[29] These statistics significantly exceed the figures for stab wounds, and most trauma surgeons adjust their management to a conservative bent accordingly. These authors promote the principle that although selective management is widely accepted for stab wounds, its application in the management of GSWs is more limited, and therefore conservative clinical criteria for mandatory laparotomy should be applied. Other authors argue, however, that although peritoneal penetration and intraperitoneal injury are far more likely to result from GSWs, damage requiring operative repair should be the instrumental concern, and this may be less common than previously stated. More recent series report intra-abdominal injury in only 70% to 80% of cases, supporting the contention that nonoperative management could be appropriate for a substantial percentage of patients.[87]

A prudent approach to GSWs to the abdomen can follow the same sequential three-step algorithm as for stab wounds (Figure 43-8). First and foremost, are there clinical grounds for operation? Second, if none exists, has peritoneal violation occurred? Third, does injury

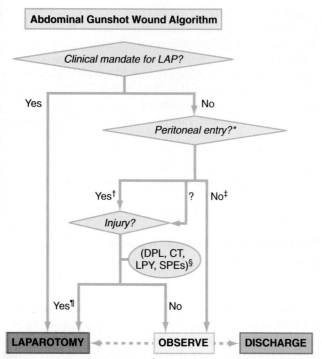

Abdominal Gunshot Wound Algorithm

Clinical mandate for LAP?

Yes — No

Peritoneal entry?*

Yes† — ? — No‡

Injury?

(DPL, CT, LPY, SPEs)§

Yes¶ — No

LAPAROTOMY ◀- - - - ▶ OBSERVE - - - ▶ DISCHARGE

Figure 43-8. Abdominal gunshot wound algorithm. *Can be assessed by missile path, plain films, local wound exploration, ultrasonography, and laparoscopy. †Most centers proceed to laparotomy if peritoneal entry is suspected. ‡Patients with documented superficial and low-velocity injuries can be discharged; unknown-depth or high-velocity injuries require further tests or observation. §Diagnostic peritoneal lavage (DPL), computed tomography (CT), laparoscopy (LPY), or serial physical examinations (SPEs) can be used in singular or complementary fashion depending on the clinical scenario. ¶Expectant management of injuries caused by gunshot wounds is rarely attempted. LAP, laparotomy.

requiring laparotomy exist? Those centers that adhere to the tenet that known or suspected peritoneal violation imputes high likelihood of intraperitoneal injury will proceed to laparotomy if the second question is answered affirmatively. Those who believe that there is a lower incidence of significant organ damage use other diagnostic agents, including serial physical examination, irrespective of whether the peritoneal cavity has been violated.

Step I: Clinical Indications for Laparotomy. These clinical demands are similar to those proposed for stab wounds (see Table 43-3).

Step II: Peritoneal Violation. Six methods are used to determine whether the missile has entered or traversed the peritoneal cavity. This question is most germane for those centers that perform laparotomy based on peritoneal violation alone.

1. *Missile path.* Clear entrance and exit wounds allow for a reasonably reliable estimate of the missile path. However, multiple GSWs ricochet and the tendency of low-velocity missiles to follow fascial planes of lower resistance can render this approach misleading.
2. *Plain films.* An anteroposterior and lateral projection of the abdomen can assist in placing the missile in the peritoneal cavity, but such estimations are

imprecise and are largely unhelpful in patients with through-and-through or multiple GSWs.

3. *Local wound exploration.* Because GSWs produce considerably more tissue damage than stab wounds, local wound exploration is a less useful tool for GSWs of the abdomen, flank, and back. Its role should likely be restricted to low-velocity projectiles with suspected superficial entry. Because of the much greater technical difficulty and hazard in visualizing these extensive missile tracts, there is a tendency to underestimate the degree of damage.
4. *Ultrasonography.* The experience with ultrasonography in coincidentally assessing wound tracts and the mediastinum for low chest and upper abdominal penetration has been successful but very limited.[48]
5. *Laparoscopy.* Laparoscopy is the most invasive and costly means of evaluating the integrity of the peritoneum. However, it may also discover and serve as the mode for repair of certain diaphragmatic or organ injuries or both.
6. *CT.* CT has been helpful when trajectory is indeterminate.[88]

Step III: Injury Requiring Laparotomy. In most institutions, the algorithm terminates after the second step, in which determination or strong suspicion of peritoneal violation presupposes the need for laparotomy. At more liberal centers, these facts are deemed insufficient and additional diagnostics are undertaken.

1. *Serial examinations.* Patients with normal examination findings or localized wound tenderness can be observed only if clinical circumstances and institutional policy allow.[87] Physical examination may be more reliable than previously suspected in the presence of alcohol or illicit drug intoxication.
2. *Diagnostic peritoneal lavage.* Peritoneal lavage has been highly successful in determining or excluding intraperitoneal injury. When DPL is used, all criteria for positivity remain the same with the exception of the RBC count, which is lowered to 5000 to 10,000 RBCs/mm³ to maximize sensitivity.[62,64]
3. *CT.* Higher resolution scanners may augment the ability of CT to identify hollow visceral damage in addition to solid organ and vascular pathologic lesions.[63]
4. *Laparoscopy.* The greatest use for laparoscopy is in the evaluation of the diaphragm in patients with left thoracoabdominal GSWs who do not have indications for standard operative intervention.[89]

Thoracoabdominal

Patients with GSWs to the low chest have intraperitoneal injuries reported in 45% of cases. Clinical indications for laparotomy are unchanged. Diagnostic peritoneal lavage is particularly helpful in these cases to discern diaphragm injury, and the RBC threshold of 5000 to 10,000/mm³ produces excellent sensitivity.

Flank and Back

Operative exploration is generally recommended because of the increased likelihood of a serious injury and the greater fallibility of both the physical examination and DPL in cases of retroperitoneal injuries. As for stab wounds, a triple-contrast CT scan can assist in delineating retroperitoneal pathologic lesions.[37] As with stab wounds, laparoscopy or observation alone can be attempted in selected circumstances.[88]

Shotgun Wounds

Type I injuries can be effectively managed by reserving laparotomy for patients with clear peritoneal signs or progressive abdominal tenderness. Certain authors advocate an expectant approach to type II injuries, stating that small punctures of the bowel cause no wound eversion and no peritoneal leakage and will spontaneously close.[63] A more prudent approach is to perform laparotomy in cases of these penetrating wounds, especially if there are signs of peritonitis. Reconstruction of abdominal wall defects may be required. Type III injuries are commonly associated with multiple organ injuries, shock, and pronounced tissue destruction, requiring hemostasis and extensive debridement.

Blunt Abdominal Trauma

Diagnostic Studies

Most centers assimilate physical examination, ultrasonography, CT, and DPL into a clinical algorithm.[90] Other tests, such as angiography, may be indicated. To reiterate, a clinical assessment of an alert patient that depends on abdominal findings alone is reasonably accurate but is accompanied by both false-positive and false-negative errors.[91] Such an assessment is more hazardous for a patient who is under the influence of a variety of toxins or whose examination is compromised by a head injury, spinal injury, or difficulty in communication resulting from retardation, a language barrier, or age.

The purpose of diagnostic studies in patients with blunt abdominal trauma is twofold (Table 43-4): to discern or eliminate the presence of hemoperitoneum in the patient whose condition is critical and unstable to properly sequence management and, in less urgent circumstances, to demonstrate organ injury that requires operative repair.

Determining Hemoperitoneum

Ultrasonography. Ultrasonography has a safety advantage in that it can be performed rapidly and conducted in the resuscitation suite in the emergency department. In contradistinction to DPL, ultrasonography is hazard free, and serial examinations can be undertaken with ease in any patient. Its record in revealing hemoperitoneum is more checkered than that of DPL, although most recent studies suggest that it is accurate in this regard.[49,92]

Diagnostic Peritoneal Lavage. DPL is exceptionally sensitive in discovering hemoperitoneum, with a false-negative rate of less than 2%. This procedure can be performed in virtually any patient by varying the site and technical method. Aspiration of the peritoneum generally requires less than 5 minutes.[61]

Table 43-4. Diagnostic Studies in Blunt Abdominal Trauma

Scenario	Study Purpose	Primary Study	Alternate/ Compensatory
Hemodynamically Unstable			
General	IPH	US, DPA	—
Pelvic fracture	IPH	US, DPA*	—
Hemodynamically Stable			
General	OI[††]	CT	DPL, SPEs
Nonoperative management[§]	OI	CT[¶]	DPL**, SPEs
CHI	OI, HVI	DPL**, CT[¶]	SPEs[††]
BAI	IPH	DPL, US	CT[‡‡]

BAI, blunt aortic Injury; CHI, closed-head injury; CT, computed tomography; DPA, diagnostic peritoneal aspiration; DPL, diagnostic peritoneal lavage; HVI, hollow viscus injury; IPH, intraperitoneal hemorrhage; OI, organ injury; SPEs, serial physical examinations; US, ultrasonography.
*Positive peritoneal aspirate mandates laparotomy, positive red blood cell count only, warrants attention to pelvic fracture.
[†]To discover fluid/blood suggesting injury.
[‡]US for OI much less reliable than for IPH.
[§]Institutional capability should be carefully considered.
[¶]CT less reliable for HVI than for solid visceral injury.
**Complementary to CT if HVI suspected.
[††]SPEs are unreliable in the patient with CHI.
[‡‡]May be more appropriate if helical CT is primary study for BAD or can be rapidly acquired.

Computed Tomography Scans. Although a CT scan can both visualize and estimate the quantity of hemoperitoneum, the time required to accomplish the procedure, including transport of the patient and setup, can be problematic, depending in part on the location of the scanner. Moreover, the ability to carry out CT scanning in a safe manner depends on the availability and expertise of personnel to monitor the patient while he or she is in the CT scanner.

Demonstrating Organ Injury that Requires Laparotomy

Indications for the respective studies will vary with clinical need and with the experience, resources, and attitudes of individual institutions.

Ultrasonography and Diagnostic Peritoneal Lavage. Ultrasonography or DPL is clearly warranted in the acutely injured and unstable patient with multiple trauma. Even in stable patients, DPL is generally excellent in determining the need for operation after blunt mechanism. However, its value is undermined by a 6% to 12% unnecessary laparotomy rate primarily attributable to minor injuries of liver and spleen that at laparotomy are found to be nonbleeding. It is important to note that certain patients with suspected hepatic or splenic injury who are relegated to nonoperative management will have coincident but occult hollow viscus pathologic conditions. Measurement of amylase and alkaline phosphatase in lavage effluent may be especially helpful in revealing these injuries, particularly in situations in which serial evaluation is compromised (e.g., in the patient with severe head injuries).[55]

The primary value of ultrasonography is in the search for hemoperitoneum. It is far less reliable in specifying organ pathology, with the exception of traumatic pancreatic pseudocysts.

Computed Tomography Scans. A CT scan alone is sufficient and appropriate in the patient who is hemodynamically stable and has no obfuscating clinical factors. The great advantage of the CT scan is its ability to distinguish intraperitoneal organ injury and simultaneously evaluate the retroperitoneum.[93] It is the most capable instrument in diagnosing liver and spleen pathologic lesions, and it allows visualization and semiquantitation of hemoperitoneum. Its track record in visualizing injuries to hollow viscera and the pancreas, diaphragm, and mesentery is less consistent.[94] The finding of free fluid on CT without other organ injury may indicate a hollow viscus pathologic condition. In cases in which DPL has been undertaken, a CT scan can provide useful additional information in the following circumstances: DPL is positive by RBC criteria only in the presence of pelvic fracture or suspected, isolated solid visceral injury; DPL results are equivocal; technical difficulties occurred with DPL; and evaluation of the retroperitoneum is indicated. Complications related to contrast administration, the potential need for sedation and its hazards, and difficulty in providing continuous assessment of the patient must be considered.

Laparoscopy. At this time, the role of laparoscopy in trauma cases is relegated mostly to a penetrating mechanism.

Management

In cases of blunt trauma, it is the exception when a patient undergoes laparotomy based on clinical grounds alone. Far more typically, one or a complementary battery of diagnostic tests are performed. The choice of these tests is influenced by the patient's hemodynamic status, the clinical scenario, and the institution's resources and preferences (Figure 43-9).

Clinical Indications for Laparotomy

Immediate laparotomy after injury from a blunt mechanism is rarely determined solely by clinical parameters. Potential indications are any of the following (Table 43-5):

Figure 43-9. Blunt abdominal trauma (BAT) algorithm. *Determined by unequivocal free intraperitoneal fluid on ultrasonogram (US) or positive peritoneal aspiration on diagnostic peritoneal aspiration (DPA). †Can be unreliable because of closed-head injury, intoxicants, distracting injury, or spinal cord injury. ‡One or more studies may be indicated. §Need for laparotomy is based on clinical scenario, diagnostic studies, and institutional resources. ¶Duration of observation should be 6 to 24 hours depending on whether diagnostic tests have been performed, the results of the tests, and clinical circumstances including the absence of factors rendering the examination unreliable. CT, computed tomography; DPL, diagnostic peritoneal lavage; IP, intraperitoneal; IPH, intraperitoneal hemorrhage; LAP, laparotomy; SPEs, serial physical examinations.

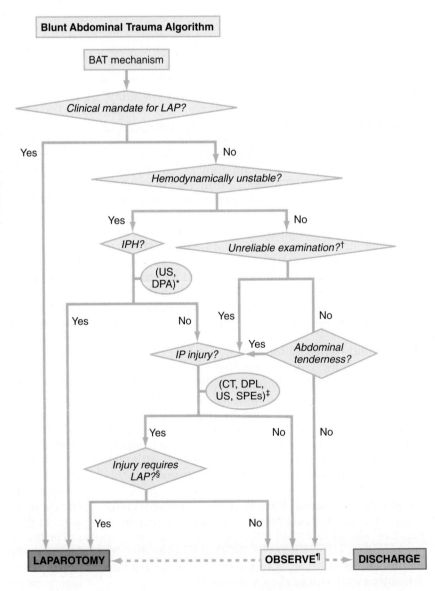

Table 43-5. Clinical Indications for Laparotomy after Blunt Trauma

Manifestation	Pitfall
Unstable vital signs with strongly suspected abdominal injury	Alternate sources shock
Unequivocal peritoneal irritation	Unreliable
Pneumoperitoneum	Insensitive; may be due to cardiopulmonary source or invasive procedures (diagnostic peritoneal lavage, laparoscopy)
Evidence of diaphragmatic injury	Nonspecific
Significant gastrointestinal bleeding	Uncommon, unknown accuracy

1. Unexplained signs of blood loss or hypotension in a patient who cannot be stabilized and in whom intra-abdominal injury is very strongly suspected
2. Clear and persistent signs of peritoneal irritation
3. Radiologic evidence of pneumoperitoneum consistent with a viscus rupture
4. Evidence of a diaphragmatic rupture
5. Persistent, significant gastrointestinal bleeding seen in the nasogastric return or in vomitus

Establishing the need for urgent celiotomy on clinical grounds is particularly problematic in the patient with multiple blunt injuries. Numerous extra-abdominal potential sources of hypotension exist. In addition, there is often coincident head injury or intoxication to further impair the reliability of examination. A nontherapeutic laparotomy may imperil the patient, not so much because of the potential morbidity of the procedure but rather because more vital diagnostic and therapeutic steps are delayed. Where confusion exists, corroborative diagnostic tests are strongly preferred.

Hemodynamically Unstable Patients

In the patient with multiple blunt injuries who is threatened by shock, three cavities are immediately targeted. Chest and pelvic radiographs seek blood loss in the thoracic and retroperitoneal spaces, respectively. Ultrasonography or peritoneal aspiration is undertaken to reveal or exclude the presence of blood in the peritoneal cavity. Hemoperitoneum in a clinically unstable patient is a mandate for laparotomy.

Hemodynamically Stable Patients

In patients who are hemodynamically stable, CT scanning is the widely preferred diagnostic modality because of its ability to specify organ pathology, semiquantitate hemoperitoneum, and study nonabdominal body regions. Its potential drawbacks in certain clinical circumstances must be understood, however. Ultrasonography, DPL, and, very uncommonly, laparoscopy can be used in a complementary or primary mode.

Operative versus Nonoperative Management. Patients with certain intraperitoneal injuries can be watched expectantly and need not be subjected to laparotomy. Specifically, this has been successful with even moderate- to high-grade liver or spleen trauma. Failures, including deaths, have occurred with this approach. Thus, although it is preferable to avoid unnecessary laparotomy, it is imperative to prevent significant morbidity or mortality by waiting too long. The patient with normal sensorium and minor to intermediate severity of mechanism is a superior candidate for expectant management. It is critical that an institution appraise its ability to manage such patients. This includes having experienced nursing staff, trauma surgeons, and radiologists and the ability to take a patient to undergo laparotomy urgently if the need arises.

Several pitfalls in the expectant approach are noteworthy. First, multiple injuries of intraperitoneal organs, including hollow viscera, are common.[76] Operative management of hollow visceral injury is necessary, and delay can have severe consequences.[55] The ability of the CT scan to detect coincident injury to these structures is suboptimal. The patient with multisystem injury and, specifically, closed-head trauma is most vulnerable to having delayed diagnosis of perforated intestinal injury.[95] Second, expectant management may lead to increased use of blood products. Finally, this management approach will fail in those patients whose hemorrhage is not amenable to therapeutic angiography and embolization and will not abate from apparent or misperceived minor injury of solid organs. In such cases, the lag time from injury to operation may increase morbidity and mortality.

Pelvic Fracture. In the setting of pelvic fracture, the clinical triage determinant is the presence or absence of hemoperitoneum (Figure 43-10). In an unstable patient, a positive ultrasonographic finding or grossly bloody peritoneal aspirate predicts active intraperitoneal hemorrhage and the need for emergency laparotomy. In the absence of other nonabdominal sources, negative study findings or a positive DPL finding by RBC count only strongly suggests life-threatening retroperitoneal hemorrhage. In this setting, attention should be turned to pelvis-stabilizing appliances, pelvic angiography, and pelvic embolization.

Multiple System Injury. Management of the abdominal trauma patient with more than one life-threatening injury cannot be dogmatic. It is not unusual to confront intraperitoneal hemorrhage in a patient with apparent closed-head injury or suspected blunt aortic disruption or both. Repair of the abdomen is said to take precedence over that of the head and chest. However, these situations are highly complex, and decision making is influenced by numerous and dynamic variables. The key tenet is that a patient with known hemoperitoneum whose vital signs cannot be stabilized must undergo laparotomy or face imminent exsanguination.

Closed-Head Injury. In general, patients with coincident severe closed-head injury but without lateralizing signs do not have intracranial lesions that require craniotomy.[96] When lateralizing features do exist, the clinician must choose between a rapid prelaparotomy CT scan of the head or preemptive burr holes at lapa-

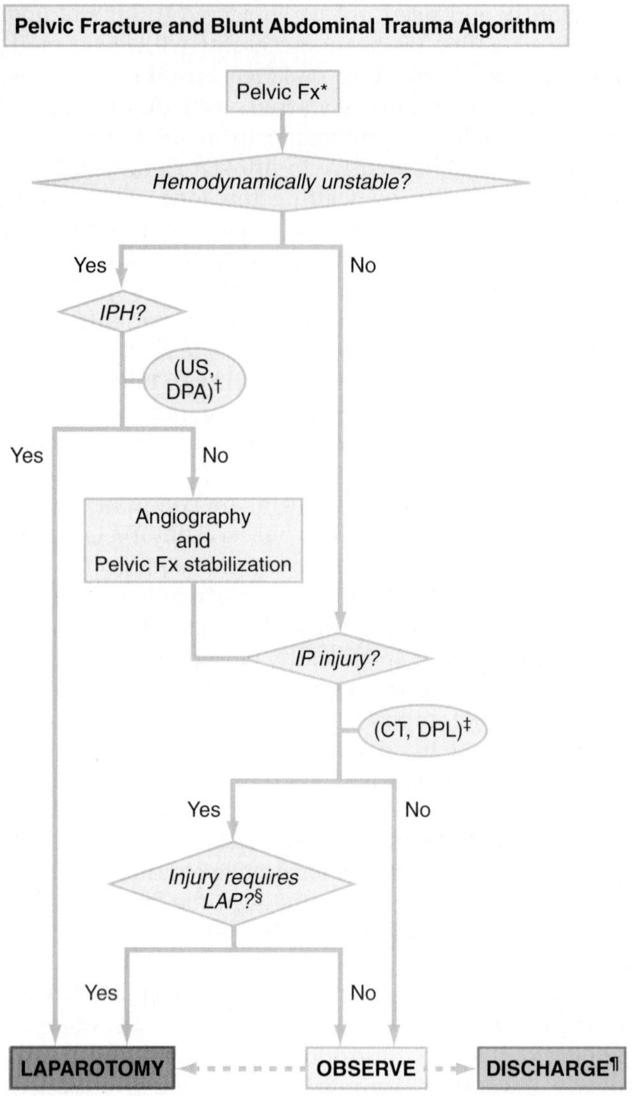

Pelvic Fracture and Blunt Abdominal Trauma Algorithm

Figure 43-10. Pelvic fracture (Fx) and blunt abdominal trauma algorithm. *Certain pelvic fractures are more likely to cause pelvic vascular disruption and subsequent retroperitoneal hemorrhage. †Determined by unequivocal free intraperitoneal fluid on ultrasonogram (US) or positive peritoneal aspiration on diagnostic peritoneal aspiration (DPA). ‡One or more studies may be indicated. Serial physical examinations are generally considered unreliable owing to the presence of pelvic fracture. §Need for laparotomy is based on clinical scenario, diagnostic studies, and institutional resources. ¶Discharge from the perspective of need for further consideration for laparotomy. CT, computed tomography; DPL, diagnostic peritoneal lavage; IP, intraperitoneal; IPH, Intraperitoneal hemorrhage; LAP, laparotomy.

rotomy. This judgment rests mostly on the clinical state of the patient with particular regard to his or her response to resuscitative measures and the timely availability of CT.[97] An approach to this scenario is presented in Figure 43-11.

Blunt Aortic Injury. Clinical or radiographic features that portend great vessel injury, notably a widened mediastinum on a supine anteroposterior chest radiograph, have variable sensitivity and specificity. In addition, although the course of any single aortic lesion is unpredictable, there is more likely than not a lag of at least several hours before rupture. Therefore, exigent laparotomy should precede great vessel diagnostics. Should the patient's condition precipitously deteriorate, left lateral thoracotomy allows aortic cross-clamp with its circulatory benefits and generally affords access to the injured portion of the vessel (Figure 43-12).

Pediatrics

Children are prone to aerophagia, and decompressive nasogastric tubes are particularly important to help prevent compromised lung function and aid in the abdominal examination. Care must be taken in fluid resuscitation and drug administration, with attention being paid to the patient's size, using surface area or body weight as a guide. Because of their size and relatively larger surface area, children are more susceptible to hypothermia resulting from the administration of unwarmed fluids and blood products. The use of overhead heat lamps, blood warmers, and prewarmed intravenous fluids helps obviate this condition.

Children with major injuries may cause fear and anxiety even in the most experienced emergency physician or surgeon. It is imperative to maintain careful vigilance and overcome any tendency to avoid indicated procedures.

For physiologic reasons, the expectant management of blunt hepatic or splenic injury has better success in the child than in the adult patient.[98] If stability exists, nonoperative management can ensue if capable personnel and resources are present. CT scanning is the primary diagnostic agent in both the initial and convalescent periods to define and grade solid organ injury. As for adults, this modality is insensitive for the discovery of hollow viscus and, to a lesser degree, pancreatic pathologic conditions.[99] Ultrasonography has been found to be useful for the detection of free fluid and can be used in triage to send the unstable child with visualized hemoperitoneum for laparotomy.[100] However, ultrasonography appears to have less sensitivity when compared with the adult experience.[101] Therefore, DPL, specifically peritoneal aspiration, can also uncover hemoperitoneum in the initial management of the critical, multiply injured child. Reliance on cell count alone has prompted significant nontherapeutic laparotomy rates.

In the course of expectant treatment, the child should undergo laparotomy if instability develops, transfusion requirements are excessive, peritoneal signs are unequivocal, or observation is not feasible because of associated injuries or lack of institutional resources. Closed-head injury need not preclude nonoperative management of known solid parenchymal injury, but the risk associated with undiscovered and coincident hollow viscus perforation is greatly increased. The diagnostic approach to penetrating trauma in children is the same as that in adults.

Transfer

Trauma patients in rural settings may require a stabilizing damage control laparotomy by a general surgeon prior to being transferred to a trauma center for definitive care.[102]

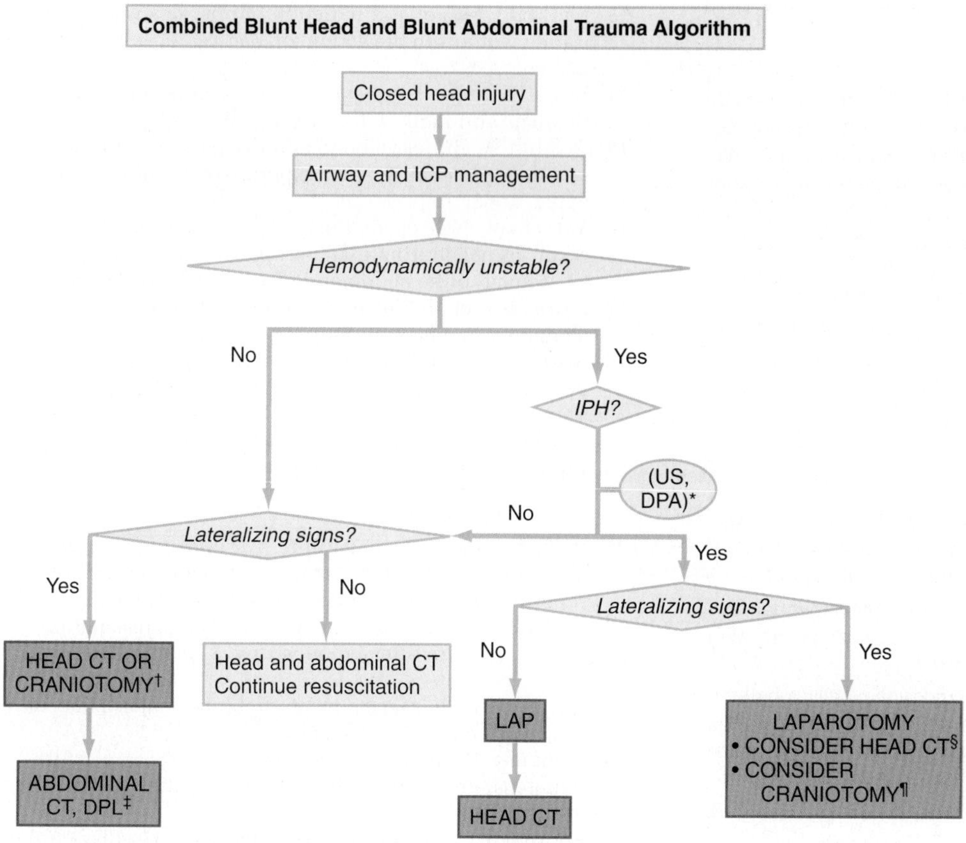

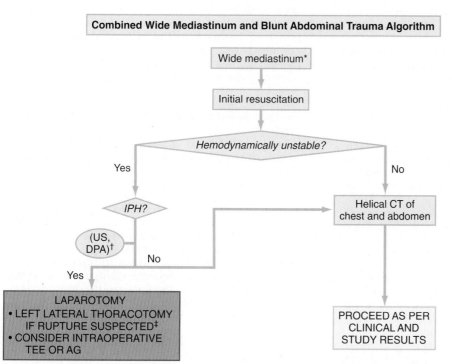

Combined Blunt Head and Blunt Abdominal Trauma Algorithm

Closed head injury

Airway and ICP management

Hemodynamically unstable?

No / Yes

IPH?

(US, DPA)*

No

Yes

Lateralizing signs?

Yes / No

HEAD CT OR CRANIOTOMY†

Head and abdominal CT Continue resuscitation

ABDOMINAL CT, DPL‡

Lateralizing signs?

No / Yes

LAP

LAPAROTOMY
• CONSIDER HEAD CT§
• CONSIDER CRANIOTOMY¶

HEAD CT

Figure 43-11. Combined blunt head and blunt abdominal trauma algorithm. *Determined by unequivocal free intraperitoneal fluid on ultrasonogram (US) or positive peritoneal aspiration on diagnostic peritoneal aspiration (DPA). †Craniotomy or burr holes based on clinical picture and unavailability of computed tomography (CT). ‡Diagnostic peritoneal lavage (DPL) can be complementary to CT in determining hollow viscus injury. §Consider prelaparotomy (LAP) head CT based on clinical picture and availability of CT. ¶Consider craniotomy or burr holes simultaneous with laparotomy. ICP, intracranial pressure; IPH, intraperitoneal hemorrhage.

Combined Wide Mediastinum and Blunt Abdominal Trauma Algorithm

Wide mediastinum*

Initial resuscitation

Hemodynamically unstable?

Yes / No

IPH?

(US, DPA)†

No

Helical CT of chest and abdomen

Yes

LAPAROTOMY
• LEFT LATERAL THORACOTOMY IF RUPTURE SUSPECTED‡
• CONSIDER INTRAOPERATIVE TEE OR AG

PROCEED AS PER CLINICAL AND STUDY RESULTS

Figure 43-12. Combined wide mediastinum and blunt abdominal trauma algorithm. *Preferably based on upright posteroanterior film and mechanism of injury; other radiographic signs or mechanism alone may signal need for evaluation. †Determined by unequivocal free intraperitoneal fluid on ultrasonogram (US) or positive finding on diagnostic peritoneal aspiration (DPA). ‡Allows surgical access to majority of aortic disruption sites. AG, aortogram; CT, computed tomography; IPH, intraperitoneal hemorrhage; TEE, transesophageal echocardiogram.

KEY CONCEPTS

- The accuracy of physical examination is limited in cases of blunt and penetrating trauma. It is rendered less reliable by distracting injury, altered sensorium (e.g., head trauma, alcohol or drug intoxication, mental retardation), and spinal cord injury.

- Implements and missiles frequently violate the lung parenchyma, diaphragm, mediastinum, intraperitoneal cavity, and retroperitoneum in some combination.

- The choice of diagnostic studies for abdominal trauma is based on clinical need first and foremost, as well as study availability and the trustworthiness of that study in a respective center.

- Ultrasonography and peritoneal aspiration are rapid methods of determining or excluding the presence of hemoperitoneum in the critically ill blunt or penetrating trauma patient. DPL is more sensitive but invasive. Ultrasonography is noninvasive and is less sensitive than DPL but can simultaneously evaluate for hemopericardium.

- Clinical indications for laparotomy are more dependable in and more frequently applicable to cases of penetrating trauma than cases of blunt trauma.

- The critical determinant in hemodynamically unstable patients with pelvic fracture is the existence of active intraperitoneal hemorrhage. Discovery of this by ultrasonography or peritoneal aspiration mandates laparotomy, whereas its absence prompts diagnostic and potentially therapeutic angiography.

REFERENCES

1. Prall JA, et al: Early definitive abdominal evaluation in the triage of unconscious normotensive blunt trauma patients. *J Trauma* 37:792, 1994.
2. Velmahos GC, et al: Selective nonoperative management in 1,856 patients with abdominal gunshot wounds: Should routine laparotomy still be the standard of care? *Ann Surg* 234:395, 2001.
3. Conrad MF, et al: Selective management of penetrating truncal injuries: Is emergency department discharge a reasonable goal? *Ann Surg* 69:266, 2003.
4. Nicholas JM, et al: Changing patterns in the management of penetrating abdominal trauma: The more things change, the more they stay the same. *J Trauma* 55:1095, 2003.
5. Kim AN, Trent RB: Firearm-related injury surveillance in California. *Am J Prev Med* 15:31, 1998.
6. Cherry D, et al: Trends in nonfatal and fatal firearm-related injury rates in the United States 1985-1995. *Ann Emerg Med* 32:51, 1998.
7. Davis JJ, Cohn I, Nance FC: Diagnosis and management of blunt abdominal trauma. *Ann Surg* 183:672, 1976.
8. Cooper A, et al: Mortality and thoracoabdominal injury: The pediatric perspective. *J Pediatr Surg* 27:33, 1992.
9. Centers for Disease Control: Childhood injury facts, 1999. Available at http://www.cdc.gov/ncipc/factsheets/childh.htm.
10. Hirshberg A, et al: Double jeopardy: Thoracoabdominal injuries requiring surgical intervention in both chest and abdomen. *J Trauma* 39:229, 1995.
11. Feliciano DV, Rozcyki GS: The management of penetrating abdominal trauma. *Adv Surg* 28:1, 1995.
12. Moss L, Schmidt F, Creech O: Analysis of 550 stab wounds of the abdomen. *Am Surg* 28:483, 1962.
13. McCarthy MC, et al: Prediction of injury caused by penetrating wounds to the abdomen, flank and back. *Arch Surg* 128:962, 1991.
14. Boyle EM, et al: Diagnosis of injuries after stab wounds to the back and flank. *J Trauma* 42:260, 1997.
15. Demuth W: Bullet velocity and design as determinants of wounding capability: An experimental study. *J Trauma* 6:222, 1966.
16. Velitchkov NG, et al: Delayed small bowel injury as a result of penetrating extraperitoneal high-velocity ballistic trauma to the abdomen. *J Trauma* 48:169, 2000.
17. Cairns BA, et al: Management and outcome of abdominal shotgun wounds. *Ann Surg* 221:272, 1995.
18. Rivara FP, et al: Effectiveness of automatic shoulder belt systems in motor vehicle crashes. *JAMA* 283:2826, 2000.
19. Velmahos GD, Tatevossian R, Demetriades D: The use of seat belts is shown to cause a specific pattern of internal injuries. *Am Surg* 65:181, 1999.
20. Prince JS, et al: Unusual seat-belt injuries in children. *J Trauma* 56:420, 2004.
21. Reiger J, et al: Gastric rupture: An uncommon complication after successful cardiopulmonary resuscitation—report of two cases. *Resuscitation* 35:175, 1997.
22. Olshaker JS, Deckleman C: Delayed presentation of splenic rupture after colonoscopy. *J Emerg Med* 17:455, 1999.
23. Lin BC, et al: Management of blunt major pancreatic injury. *J Trauma* 56:774, 2004.
24. Mahoney EJ, et al: Isolated brain injury as a cause of hypotension in the blunt trauma patient. *J Trauma* 55:1065, 2003.
25. Rodriguez A, DuPriest RW, Shatney CH: Recognition of intra-abdominal injury in blunt trauma victims: A prospective study comparing physical examination with peritoneal lavage. *Am Surg* 48:456, 1982.
26. Livingston DH, et al: Admission or observation is not necessary after a negative abdominal computed tomographic scan in patients with suspected blunt abdominal trauma: Results of a prospective, multi-institutional trial. *J Trauma* 44:273, 1998.
27. Thal ER: Evaluation of peritoneal lavage and local exploration in lower chest and abdominal stab wounds. *J Trauma* 17:642, 1977.
28. Moore EE, Marx JA: Penetrating abdominal wounds: Rationale for exploratory laparotomy. *JAMA* 253:2705, 1985.
29. Moore EE, et al: Mandatory laparotomy for gunshot wounds penetrating the abdomen. *Am J Surg* 140:847, 1980.
30. Chmielewski GW, et al: Nonoperative management of gunshot wounds of the abdomen. *Am Surg* 8:665, 1995.
31. Brown CK, Dunn K, Wilson K: Diagnostic evaluation of patients with blunt abdominal trauma: A decision analysis. *Acad Emerg Med* 7:385, 2000.
32. Asimos AW, et al: Value of point-of-care blood testing in emergent trauma management. *J Trauma* 48:1101, 2000.
33. Moore FD: The effects of hemorrhage on body composition. *N Engl J Med* 273:567, 1965.
34. Takishima T, et al: Serum amylase level on admission in the diagnosis of blunt injury to the pancreas: Its significance and limitations. *Ann Surg* 226:70, 1997.
35. Holmes JF, et al: Identification of children with intra-abdominal injuries after blunt trauma. *Ann Emerg Med* 39:500, 2002.
36. Sloan EP, et al: Toxicology screening in urban trauma patients: Drug prevalence and its relationship to trauma severity and management. *J Trauma* 29:1647, 1995.
37. Chiu WC, et al: Determining the need for laparotomy in penetrating torso trauma: A prospective study using triple-contrast enhanced abdominopelvic computed tomography. *J Trauma* 51:860, 2001.

38. Haan JM, et al: Splenic embolization revisited: a multi-center review. *J Trauma* 56:542, 2004.

39. Hauser CJ, et al: Prospective validation of computed tomographic screening of the thoracolumbar spine in trauma. *J Trauma* 55:228, 2003.

40. Peng MY, et al: CT cystography versus conventional cystography in evaluation of bladder injury. *Am J Roentgenol* 173:1269, 1999.

41. Thaemert BC, Cogbill TH, Lambert PJ: Nonoperative management of splenic injury: Are follow-up computed tomographic scans of any value? *J Trauma* 43:748, 1997.

42. Mele TS, et al: Evaluation of a diagnostic protocol using screening diagnostic peritoneal lavage with selective use of abdominal computed tomography in blunt abdominal trauma. *J Trauma* 46:847, 1999.

43. Sivit CJ, Eichelberger MR: CT diagnosis of pancreatic injury in children: Significance of fluid separating the splenic vein and the pancreas. *Am J Roentgenol* 165:921, 1995.

44. Marx JA: So what's a little free fluid? *Acad Emerg Med* 7:383, 2000.

45. Lim-Dunham JE, et al: Aspiration after administration of oral contrast material in children undergoing abdominal CT for trauma. *Am J Roentgenol* 169:1015, 1997.

46. Allen TL, et al: Computed tomographic scanning without oral contrast solution for blunt bowel and mesenteric injuries in abdominal trauma. *J Trauma* 56:314, 2004.

47. Stafford RE, et al: Oral contrast solution and computed tomography for blunt abdominal trauma: A randomized study. *Arch Surg* 134:622, 1999.

48. Fry WR, et al: Ultrasonographic examination of wound tracts. *Arch Surg* 130:605, 1995.

49. Dorlich MO, et al: 2,576 ultrasounds for blunt abdominal trauma. *J Trauma* 50:108, 2001.

50. Smith RS, et al: Institutional learning curve of surgeon-performed trauma ultrasound. *Arch Surg* 133:1254, 1998.

51. Boulanger BR, et al: Prospective evidence of the superiority of a sonography-based algorithm in the assessment of blunt abdominal injury. *J Trauma* 47:632, 1999.

52. Henderson SO, Sung J, Mandavia D: Serial abdominal ultrasound in the setting of trauma. *J Emerg Med* 18:79, 2000.

53. Miller MT, et al: Not so fast. *J Trauma* 54:52, 2003.

54. Goodwin H, et al: Abdominal ultrasound examination in pregnant blunt trauma patients. *J Trauma* 50:689, 2001.

55. Fakhry SM, et al: Relatively short diagnostic delays (<8 hours) produce morbidity and mortality in blunt small bowel injury: An analysis of time to operative intervention in 198 patients from a multicenter experience. *J Trauma* 48:408, 2000.

56. Edney JM, Marx JA: Utility of contrast duodenography in the detection of proximal small bowel injury following blunt trauma. *Ann Emerg Med* 18:481, 1989.

57. Lorente-Ramos RM, et al: Sonographic diagnosis of intramural duodenal hematomas. *J Clin Ultrasound* 27:213, 1999.

58. Velmahos GC, et al: Angiographic embolization for arrest of bleeding after penetrating trauma to the abdomen. *Am J Surg* 178:367, 1999.

59. Harrell DJ, Vitale GC, Larson GM: Selective role for endoscopic retrograde cholangiopancreatography in abdominal trauma. *Surg Endosc* 12:387, 1998.

60. Root HD, et al: Diagnostic peritoneal lavage. *Surgery* 57:633, 1965.

61. Marx JA: Peritoneal procedures. In Hedges JR, Roberts JR (eds): *Clinical Procedures in Emergency Medicine,* 3rd ed. Philadelphia, WB Saunders, 1997.

62. Fang JF, et al: Small bowel perforation: Is urgent surgery necessary? *J Trauma* 47:515, 1999.

63. Brackenridge SC, et al: Detection of intra-abdominal injury using diagnostic peritoneal lavage after shotgun wound to the abdomen. *J Trauma* 54:329, 2003.

64. Henneman PL, et al: Diagnostic peritoneal lavage: Accuracy in predicting necessary laparotomy following blunt and penetrating trauma. *J Trauma* 30:1345, 1990.

65. Radlauer M, Marx JA, Moore EE: Peritoneal aspiration in patients with pelvic fractures [abstract]. *J Emerg Med* 11:372, 1993.

66. Mendez C, Gubler KD, Maier RV: Diagnostic accuracy of peritoneal lavage in patients with pelvic fractures. *Arch Surg* 129:477, 1994.

67. Stephen DJG: Early detection of arterial bleeding in acute pelvic trauma. *J Trauma* 47:638, 1999.

68. Gonzales RP, et al: Abdominal stab wounds: Diagnostic peritoneal lavage criteria for emergency room discharge. *J Trauma* 51:939, 2001.

69. Nagy KK, et al: Experience with over 2500 diagnostic peritoneal lavages. *Injury* 31:479, 2000.

70. Otomo Y, et al: New diagnostic peritoneal lavage criteria for diagnosis of intestinal injury. *J Trauma* 44:991, 1998.

71. Marx JA, et al: Utility of lavage alkaline phosphatase in detection of isolated small intestinal injury. *Ann Emerg Med* 14:10, 1985.

72. Rosemurgy AS, et al: Abdominal stab wound protocol: Prospective study documents applicability for widespread use. *Am Surg* 61:112, 1995.

73. Leppäniemi A, Haapiainen R: Diagnostic laparoscopy in abdominal stab wounds: A prospective, randomized study. *J Trauma* 55:636, 2003.

74. Simon RJ, et al: Impact of increased use of laparoscopy n negative laparotomy rates after penetrating trauma. *J Trauma* 53:297, 2002.

75. Marks JM, Youngelman DF, Berk T: Cost analysis of diagnostic laparoscopy vs. laparotomy in the evaluation of penetrating abdominal trauma. *Surg Endosc* 11:272, 1997.

76. Hackam DJ, et al: Effects of other intra-abdominal injuries on the diagnosis, management, and outcome of small bowel trauma. *J Trauma* 49:606, 2000.

77. Luchette FA, et al: Practice management guidelines for prophylactic antibiotic use in penetrating abdominal trauma: The EAST practice management guidelines work group. *J Trauma* 48:508, 2000.

78. Ross SE, et al: Morbidity of negative coeliotomy in trauma. *Injury* 26:393, 1996.

79. Keleman JJ III, et al: Evaluation of diagnostic peritoneal lavage in stable patients with gunshot wounds to the abdomen. *Arch Surg* 132:909, 1997.

80. Nagy KK, et al: Evisceration after abdominal stab wounds: Is laparotomy required? *J Trauma* 47:622, 1999.

81. Sriussadaporn S, et al: Clinical use of diagnostic peritoneal lavage in stab wounds of the anterior abdomen: A prospective study. *Eur J Surg* 168:490, 2002.

82. Soto JA, et al: Penetrating stab wounds to the abdomen: Use of serial US and contrast-enhanced CT in stable patients. *Emerg Radiol* 220:365, 2001.

83. Nagy KK, et al: Routine preoperative "one-shot" intravenous pyelography is not indicated in all patients with penetrating abdominal trauma. *J Am Coll Surg* 185:530, 1997.

84. Tayal VS, et al: FAST accurate for cardiac and intraperitoneal injury in penetrating chest trauma. *Acad Emerg Med* 7:492, 2000.

85. Kirton OC, et al: Stab wounds to the back and flank in the hemodynamically stable patient: A decision algorithm based on contrast-enhanced computed tomography with colonic opacification. *Am J Surg* 173:189, 1997.

86. Demetriades D, et al: The management of penetrating injuries of the back: A prospective study of 230 patients. *Ann Surg* 207:72, 1988.

87. Demetriades D, et al: Selective nonoperative management of gunshot wounds of the anterior abdomen. *Arch Surg* 132:178, 1997.
88. Carrillo EH, et al: The role of computed tomography in selective management of gunshot wounds to the abdomen and flank. *J Trauma* 45:446, 1998.
89. Sosa JL, et al: Negative laparotomy in abdominal gunshot wounds: Potential impact of laparoscopy. *J Trauma* 38:194, 1995.
90. Branney SW, et al: Ultrasound based key clinical pathway reduces the use of hospital resources for the evaluation of blunt abdominal trauma. *J Trauma* 42:1086, 1997.
91. Ferrera PC, et al: Injuries distracting from intra-abdominal injuries after blunt trauma. *Am J Emerg Med* 16:145, 1998.
92. Chiu WC, et al: Abdominal injuries without hemoperitoneum: A potential limitation of focused abdominal sonography for trauma (FAST). *J Trauma* 42:617, 1997.
93. Myers JG, et al: Blunt splenic injuries: Dedicated trauma surgeons can achieve a high rate of nonoperative success in patients of all ages. *J Trauma* 48:801, 2000.
94. Frick EJ, et al: Small bowel and mesentery injuries in blunt trauma. *J Trauma* 46:920, 1999.
95. Sartorelli KH, et al: Nonoperative management of hepatic, splenic, and renal injuries in adults with multiple injuries. *J Trauma* 49:56, 2000.
96. Thomason M, et al: Head CT scanning versus urgent exploration in the hypotensive blunt trauma patient. *J Trauma* 34:40, 1993.
97. Winchell RJ, Hoyt DB, Simons RK: Use of computed tomography of the head in the hypotensive blunt trauma patient. *Ann Emerg Med* 25:737, 1995.
98. Nwomeh BC, et al: Contrast extravasation predicts the need for operative intervention in children with blunt splenic trauma. *J Trauma* 56:537, 2004.
99. Nadler EP, et al: Management of blunt pancreatic injury in children. *J Trauma* 47:1098, 1999.
100. Patrick DA, et al: Ultrasound is an effective triage tool to evaluate blunt abdominal trauma in the pediatric population. *J Trauma* 46:357, 1999.
101. Patel JC, Tepas JJ III: The efficacy of focused abdominal sonography for trauma (FAST) as a screening tool in the assessment of injured children. *J Pediatr Surg* 34:44, 1999.
102. Weinberg JA, et al: Trauma laparotomy in a rural setting before transfer to a regional center: does it save lives? *J Trauma* 54:823, 2003.

CHAPTER

44 Genitourinary System

Robert E. Schneider

PERSPECTIVE

Despite the advances in the initial management and treatment of the severely injured patient, confusion remains regarding the recognition and subsequent management of genitourinary trauma. Only main renal vein lacerations or a severely shattered kidney, both of which are rare, portend a rapid death. Thus, most genitourinary injuries pale in comparison to the immediate life threats posed by injuries to the chest and abdomen. Hence, the urinary tract as an anatomically injured system is by necessity relegated to a position of secondary importance. Nevertheless, to maintain excellence and expertise in the overall management of all injured patients, it is mandatory for the emergency physician to have a thorough understanding of the global spectrum of genitourinary injury and how it can affect eventual patient outcome.

Genitourinary trauma commonly is a covert entity associated with a wide spectrum of injury. Approximately 10% of all multiply injured patients have some manifestation of genitourinary involvement.[1] Because of its uncommon occurrence and subtle presentation, it is often overlooked in the initial evaluation of the trauma victim. Nevertheless, after the primary survey for life-threatening injuries, Foley catheter placement as part of the secondary survey may disclose the first sign of urinary tract injury.

The urinary tract is unique in that diagnostic evaluation is always done in a retrograde fashion; that is, suspicion and elimination of urethral injury before bladder injury before ureteral or renal injury. Adherence to this axiom will permit discovery of virtually any important urinary tract injury, even during the resuscitation of critically injured patients.

Definitions

For purposes of investigation and staging of urologic injuries, genitourinary trauma is divided into lower tract (i.e., bladder or urethral injury), upper tract (i.e., renal or ureteral injury), and external genitalia (i.e., penile, scrotal, and testicular injury). Each category is further subdivided on the basis of a blunt or penetrating mechanism of injury.

Historical Perspective

The basic tenets of lower urinary tract injury have not changed appreciably in the last 25 years. A thoroughly performed physical examination and the recognition of blood at the urethral meatus or gross hematuria will identify all significant lower urinary tract injuries. Major advances in the identification of significant upper tract genitourinary injuries, their clinical markers, and ultimate staging procedures have come to the forefront over the last 18 years. Before 1985, any trauma patient with any amount of microhematuria was described as "at risk" for genitourinary injury and underwent intravenous pyelography (IVP). This was neither diagnostically definitive nor cost-effective and simply perpetuated the existing confusion and controversy. In 1985, Nicolaisen and colleagues[2] published the first of a series of articles that established guidelines to identify significant upper tract genitourinary injuries, their markers, and the diagnostic studies that would define the exact extent of these injuries and aid in subsequent patient management. In addition, the advent of ultrasonography and computed tomographic (CT) scanning has greatly simplified the diagnosis and management of external genitalia trauma.

CLINICAL FEATURES

Signs and Symptoms

The signs and symptoms of genitourinary trauma are varied and nonspecific. Acutely, these signs may include flank, abdominal, rib, back, or scrotal pain; urinary retention; and penile/urethral bleeding. Renovascular hypertension may be the only finding weeks to months after injury.

Physical Examination

Examination of the torso and pelvis during the secondary survey is the first step in the evaluation for urologic injury. Any evidence of abdominal tenderness should alert the examining physician to the possibility of a bladder rupture in addition to other intra-abdominal injuries. This likelihood increases significantly in the presence of a pelvic fracture. Tenderness elicited by pelvic compression or palpation of the pelvic girdle or pubic symphysis supports the diagnosis of a potential pelvic fracture with possible lower urinary tract injury.

Examination of the genitalia can be informative. The emergency physician should look for evidence of hematoma or ecchymosis of the penile shaft, scrotal skin, or perineum. Gross blood at the urethral meatus is diagnostic of a urethral injury and dictates the need for early retrograde urethrography. In circumstances in which emergency surgical exploration for life-threatening injuries is needed, the retrograde urethrogram can be performed in the operating room or after the operative procedure. A Foley catheter should never be introduced when there is suspected urethral trauma without first ensuring urethral integrity by retrograde urethrography. Failure to do this may convert a partial urethral tear into a complete disruption.

Careful inspection for blood at the vaginal introitus is particularly important in the female patient known to have a pelvic fracture. A thorough vaginal examination will discern vaginal lacerations or urethral disruption caused by displaced bony pelvic fracture fragments. Unlike male urethral injuries, urethrography is not helpful in suspected female urethral injuries because of the urethra's short length. The inability to pass a Foley catheter in a young premenopausal female patient with a pelvic fracture signifies the potential for

urethral injury and subsequent necessity for suprapubic urinary drainage. Successful passage of a Foley catheter in the same type of patient with blood at the vaginal introitus does not exclude urethral injury, and these worrisome physical examination findings must be conveyed to the urologist, who can plan subsequent urethral evaluation.[3] In an older postmenopausal female trauma patient, urethral injury must be distinguished from a superiorly retracted urethral meatus and accompanying meatal stenosis. These preexisting conditions are common in an atrophic vaginal setting, and a 12- or 14-Fr coudé or Foley catheter usually is required for successful bladder access.

Rectal examination evaluates sphincter tone, bowel wall integrity, and most important, the position of the prostate. Normally, the posterior lobe of the prostate is palpable and well defined (Figure 44-1). A pelvic fracture may disrupt the puboprostatic ligaments and the prostatomembranous urethra, resulting in significant retropubic venous bleeding. This may produce a large pelvic hematoma that can displace the prostate superiorly, resulting in a boggy, ill-defined mass on rectal examination (Figure 44-2).

Foley Catheter

In any trauma patient presenting with a major mechanism of injury and the absence of any findings suggestive of urethral injury, a Foley catheter should be passed into the bladder. The initial bladder effluent must be observed by the responsible physician. Because of its importance in dictating subsequent patient evaluation, observation of the initial bladder effluent should optimally not be relegated to any other member of the resuscitation team. Any color to the urine other than clear or yellow must be considered a sign of gross hematuria until proved otherwise. The presence of gross hematuria indicates urologic injury. Rarely, severe rhabdomyolysis produces large quantities of urine myoglobin, the gross appearance of which can be confused with gross hematuria. In these cases, urinalysis will document the absence of red blood cells (RBCs) consistent with myoglobinuria. Most significant lower urinary tract injuries will be accompanied by either the presence of a pelvic fracture with blood at the urethral meatus or gross hematuria on Foley catheter placement.[4] Upper tract trauma, however, tends to be more subtle. It is often coincident with nonurologic organ disruption, the bleeding from which can be life-threatening. These events may dictate rapid volume resuscitation that can clear gross hematuria quickly. Moreover, blunt injury to the renovascular pedicle or penetrating ureteral injury may not produce gross or even microscopic hematuria.

LOWER URINARY TRACT

Urethral Trauma

Anatomy

The urogenital diaphragm divides the anterior (bulbous and pendulous) urethra from the posterior (membra-

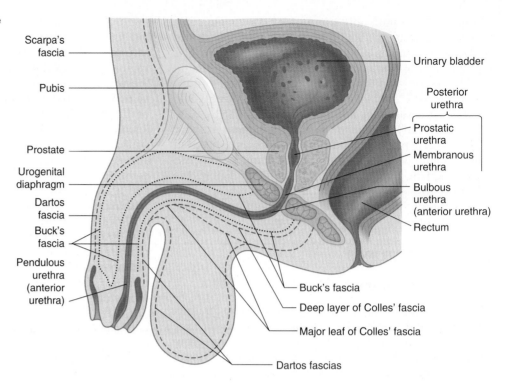

Figure 44-1. Anatomy of male genitalia.

Scarpa's fascia

Pubis

Prostate

Urogenital diaphragm

Dartos fascia

Buck's fascia

Pendulous urethra (anterior urethra)

Urinary bladder

Posterior urethra

Prostatic urethra

Membranous urethra

Bulbous urethra (anterior urethra)

Rectum

Buck's fascia

Deep layer of Colles' fascia

Major leaf of Colles' fascia

Dartos fascias

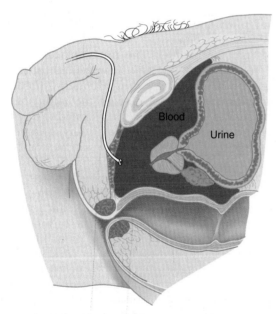

Blood

Urine

Figure 44-2. Injury to the posterior (membranous) urethra. The prostate has been avulsed from the membranous urethra secondary to fracture of the pelvis. Extravasation occurs above the triangular ligament and is periprostatic and perivesical. (From McAninch JW: In Tanagho EA, McAninch JW [eds]: *Smith's General Urology*, 14th ed. Norwalk, Conn, Appleton & Lange, 1995.)

nous and prostatic) urethra. It is a 1.5 cm fascial layer that lies between the ischial rami. It attaches anteriorly to the symphysis, posteriorly to the perineal body and ischial tuberosity, and laterally to the inferior ischial pubic rami. It is traversed by the membranous urethra. The prostatic urethra is contiguous with the urogenital diaphragm and is attached to the posterior symphysis pubis by the puboprostatic ligaments. A fracture of the pelvis with displacement of the symphysis may result in a laceration or avulsion of the prostatic urethra because of the shearing force on the fixed prostatic and membranous urethra. Injuries to the anterior and posterior urethra are caused by different mechanisms, involve different symptoms, and are treated differently.

Pathophysiology

Urethral disruption is the most significant injury that must be identified. Failure to do so may lead to significant morbidity (i.e., converting a partial urethral tear into a complete tear). Urethral manipulation can convert a partial urethral tear into a complete tear, thus precluding accurate assessment of urinary output, and subsequently potentiating the long-term complications of urethral trauma (e.g., urethral stricture formation and urinary incontinence). Pelvic fractures account for most posterior urethral injuries proximal to the urogenital diaphragm (see Figure 44-2).[5] Anterior urethral injuries distal to the urogenital diaphragm are most often caused by straddle injuries, falls, gunshot wounds, and self-instrumentation (Figure 44-3).[6]

Clinical Features

During the secondary survey, examination of the lower abdomen, pelvis, genitalia, and rectum provides both direct and indirect evidence to support or refute urethral injury. Lack of pelvic and suprapubic tenderness; absence of penile, scrotal, or perineal hematoma; and normal findings on rectal examination all support the integrity of the urethra. These physical findings permit the safe passage of a 14- or 16-Fr Foley catheter into the bladder if the patient is unable to void and provide a suitable specimen for evaluation.

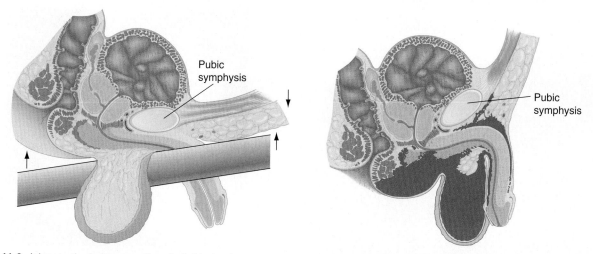

Figure 44-3. Injury to the bulbous urethra. *Left:* Mechanism: usually a perineal blow or fall astride an object; crushing of urethra against inferior edge of pubic symphysis. *Right:* Extravasation of blood and urine enclosed within Colles' fascia. (From McAninch JW: In Tanagho EA, McAninch JW [eds]: *Smith's General Urology,* 14th ed. Norwalk, Conn, Appleton & Lange, 1995.)

Diagnostic Strategies

Catheter Placement

The following technique for catheter placement assumes a normal urethra and includes the use of sterile technique, proper control of the foreskin, the use of copious amounts of lubricating jelly, and the gentle passage of a 14- or 16-Fr Foley or coudé catheter into the bladder. In all uncircumcised patients, continuous foreskin retraction with a folded 4 × 4 inch gauze pad is necessary to control the foreskin during catheter placement (Figure 44-4). Without this maneuver, the foreskin tends to repeatedly reduce itself over the glans penis, which contaminates the field and makes catheterization difficult or impossible. Slight resistance to the advancing catheter should be expected at the urogenital diaphragm secondary to voluntary contraction of the external sphincter. This is more apt to occur in a combative, anxious trauma patient than in a cooperative or unconscious patient. When this occurs, the patient should be reassured and asked to relax the perineum and rectal area while gentle advancing pressure is applied to the catheter. This combined approach allows the catheter to navigate the urogenital diaphragm successfully and pass easily into the bladder. If reassurance and relaxation do not allow easy passage of the catheter, it should be removed and a retrograde urethrogram performed. In all cases, the catheter must be passed to its fullest extent before the balloon can be inflated safely, then withdrawn to the point of catheter balloon approximation with the bladder neck and left to drain. Inflation of the catheter balloon under any other circumstances may result in iatrogenic urethral trauma.

Successful passage of a Foley catheter precludes a complete urethral disruption. Nonetheless, the possibility of a partial urethral injury not manifested by history, mechanism of injury, presence of meatal blood, or other indirect signs on physical examination may exist. If this injury is suspected initially, a retrograde urethrogram should be obtained. The presence of ure-thral extravasation together with contrast material filling the bladder is diagnostic of a partial urethral injury (Figure 44-5).[6] Identification of a partial urethral injury would permit one careful attempt at urethral placement of a 12- or 14-Fr Foley or coudé catheter, depending on the size of the patient. If any difficulty is encountered, the catheter should be removed and a urologist consulted. If a partial urethral tear is suspected subsequent to successful passage of a Foley catheter, a small feeding tube can be placed alongside the urethral catheter and a modified retrograde urethrogram performed.[4] In this circumstance, the urethrogram is for documentation and subsequent management purposes only because appropriate therapy has already been instituted (i.e., Foley catheter drainage). Under no circumstances should a successfully placed Foley catheter be removed to perform standard retrograde urethrography.

Radiology

In all cases of suspected urethral injury, a retrograde urethrogram is the diagnostic procedure of choice.[4,6] Retrograde urethrography is not an emergency and should always follow more critical resuscitative measures.

In a patient with a pelvic fracture, the entire retrograde urethrogram should be conducted with the patient in a supine rather than oblique position. Certain authors recommend oblique films for portions of the retrograde urethrogram to enhance urethral definition.[4,6] These views add little information to a good supine study. More important, pelvic fractures are often associated with significant retropubic venous bleeding and hematoma formation. Maintenance of this stable hematoma can be crucial in the initial hemodynamic resuscitation of the patient. Any patient movement from the supine to the oblique position has the potential to disrupt the organized hematoma with resultant significant and potentially lethal rebleeding. The entire urethral integrity can be defined with the patient in the

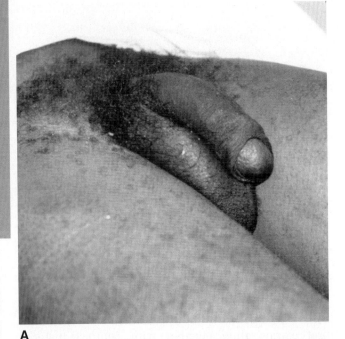

A

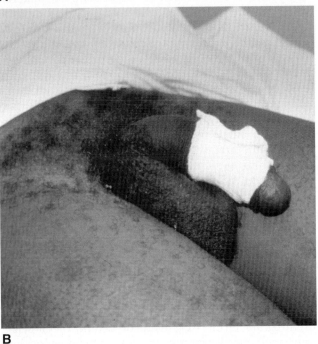

B

Figure 44-4. A, A normal uncircumcised man. **B,** Foreskin has been retracted and a folded 4 × 4 inch gauge sponge wrapped around it to prevent foreskin reduction during instrumentation.

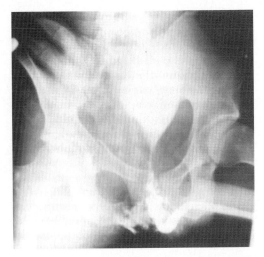

Figure 44-5. Retrograde urethrogram demonstrates a partial urethral disruption. Note the elongation of the posterior urethra with filling of the bladder. (From Spirnak JP: Pelvic fracture and injury to the lower urinary tract. *Surg Clin North Am* 68:1057, 1988.)

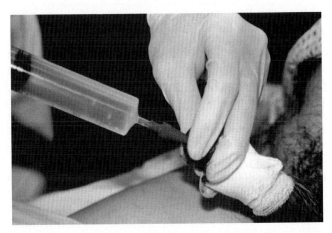

Figure 44-6. Christmas tree adapter on the end of a 60 mL syringe has been gently placed inside the fossa navicularis in preparation for retrograde urethrography.

supine position throughout the examination, aided by oblique stretching of the penis over the left or right thigh to promote necessary urethral unfolding.

A preinjection kidney, ureter, and bladder (KUB) film is first obtained. A simple Christmas tree adapter, a Cooke adapter placed on the end of a 60 mL Toomey syringe, or a Toomey syringe alone is gently passed into the urethral meatus until a snug fit inside the meatus is confirmed (Figure 44-6). Some authors have recommended inflation of a Foley catheter balloon just proximal to the fossa navicularis or the use of other cumbersome adjuncts to facilitate injection of con-

trast media.[4,6] These techniques should be avoided, however, because they promote leakage of contrast material around the penis, which can simulate extravasation on the urethrogram and promote a spurious examination. Next, 60 mL (or 0.6 mL/kg) of full-strength or half-strength iothalamate meglumine (Conray II) is injected over 30 to 60 seconds. A radiograph is taken during the injection of the last 10 mL of contrast material. Retrograde flow through the urethra and into the bladder without extravasation ensures continuity of the urethra and absence of urethral injury (Figure 44-7). Extravasation of contrast material outside the urethra with concomitant evidence of bladder filling distinguishes a partial urethral injury (see Figure 44-5) from a complete urethral disruption in which there will be absence of contrast material inside the bladder (Figure 44-8).[4,5] The latter situation requires immediate urologic consultation for appropriate surgical management. In the interim, if measurement of urinary output is essential, the bladder should be accessed by the suprapubic placement of a peel-

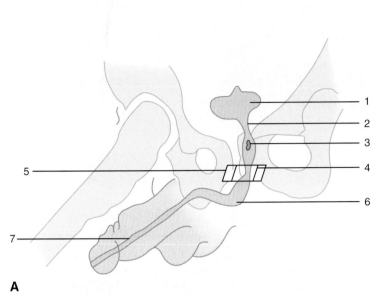

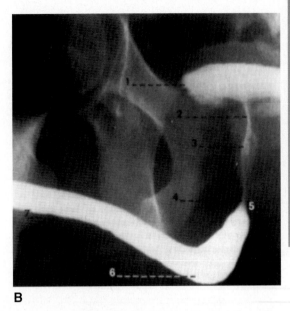

A

B

Figure 44-7. Normal anatomy is demonstrated by a line drawing **(A)** and by dynamic retrograde urethrography **(B)**. Bladder (1), prostatic urethra (2), verumontanum (3), membranous urethra (4), position of the urogenital diaphragm (5), bulbous urethra (6), and penile urethra (7). The penile and bulbous urethra together are considered the anterior urethra; the prostatic and membranous urethra compose the posterior urethra. (Adapted from McCallum RW, Colapinto V: *Urological Radiology of the Adult Male Lower Urinary Tract*. Springfield, Ill, Charles C Thomas, 1976.)

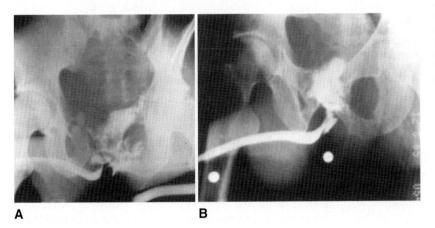

A

B

Figure 44-8. Retrograde urethrograms demonstrates complete urethral disruption. Note the absence of bladder filling, a finding diagnostic of complete disruption. (From Spirnak JP: Pelvic fracture and injury to the lower urinary tract. *Surg Clin North Am* 68:1057, 1988.)

away sheath and Foley catheter using the Seldinger technique (Figure 44-9).

Management

During physical examination, urethral injury is suggested by the presence of a pelvic fracture, blood at the urethral meatus, the presence of a high-riding or absent prostate on rectal examination, or evidence of a perineal, scrotal, or penile hematoma. Any one of these latter three findings necessitates a retrograde urethrogram to disclose the anatomy and integrity of the urethra. If these findings are absent or the urethrogram is normal, the urethra is intact and a Foley catheter can be passed into the bladder. If a partial urethral disruption is identified, one careful attempt to pass a 12- or 14-Fr Foley or coudé catheter can be undertaken. If a complete urethral disruption is identified, consultation with a urology specialist and placement of a suprapubic catheter for urinary drainage are necessary.

Bladder Trauma

Anatomy

When empty, the bladder lies retroperitoneally almost entirely within the bony pelvis. It rests on the pubis and adjacent pelvic floor parts. When full, the bladder can extend up to the level of the umbilicus, where it is most vulnerable to blunt and penetrating trauma. The bladder consists of an inner longitudinal, a middle circular, and an outer longitudinal muscle layer. These three layers constitute the detrusor muscle, which contracts to propel urine out the urethra. Blood is supplied to the bladder by the internal iliac artery and vein. The nerve supply comes from the lumbar and sacral segments of the spinal cord. It includes parasympathetic motor fibers to the detrusor muscle and sensory fibers to the detrusor that give rise to the sensation of fullness and urgency when the detrusor is stretched. The third nerve group, the sympathetic fibers, innervate the blood vessels of the bladder and the bladder neck musculature.

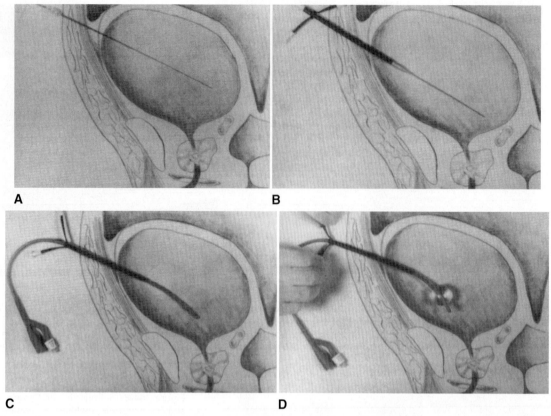

Figure 44-9. Percutaneous placement of a suprapubic tube with peel-away sheath introducer. **A,** An 18-gauge needle is in the bladder. A guidewire is advanced through needle. **B,** A dilator and peel-away sheath are advanced over the guidewire. **C,** The dilator and guidewire are removed. Through the peel-away sheath, an appropriately sized catheter can be introduced into bladder. **D,** The balloon is inflated, and the sheath is pulled back and peeled away. (From O'Brien WM: Percutaneous placement of suprapubic with peel away sheath introducer. *J Urol* 145:1015, 1991.)

The mechanism of injury with bladder trauma is usually severe. This is reflected in the high mortality rate of 22% to 44%.[7] There is a high incidence of associated life-threatening nonurologic injury, the treatment of which always takes precedence. The diagnostic evaluation of the bladder, like the urethra, can be accomplished quickly without elaborate radiographic equipment or can be part of the CT evaluation if other nonurologic injuries are being evaluated.

Pathophysiology

Extraperitoneal bladder perforation, intraperitoneal bladder perforation, and a combination of the two are the significant injuries in bladder trauma. Proper classification is critical because treatment options are completely different.[8] Whereas most ruptures occur singly as extraperitoneal or intraperitoneal, their coexistence is being recognized more often as the mechanism for bladder injury becomes better understood. The time-honored explanation for extraperitoneal rupture has been pelvic fracture with subsequent bladder laceration from an errant bony fracture fragment. It has become apparent, however, that extraperitoneal perforation can result from blunt trauma alone and need not require a lacerating fracture bony fragment.

Intraperitoneal bladder rupture has been ascribed to blunt lower abdominal trauma in a patient with a full bladder. These blunt forces are directed to the dome of

the bladder where the urachus originates during embryonic life. Because of this developmental hiatus, the dome is attenuated and represents the anatomic area most susceptible to rupture from sudden rises in intravesical pressure associated with blunt trauma. The dome also is unique in its isolated peritoneal reflection so that rupture in this area most likely will result in intraperitoneal urinary contamination.

Clinical Features

Lower abdominal or suprapubic pain, the inability to urinate, or the presence of blood at the urethral meatus may alert the physician to the possibility of lower urinary tract trauma.

Diagnostic Strategies

Laboratory

Gross hematuria in the initial bladder effluent is indicative of urologic injury. The literature clearly defines gross hematuria alone or in conjunction with a pelvic fracture as the absolute markers for significant bladder injury.[2,9] Grossly clear bladder urine in a trauma patient without a pelvic fracture virtually eliminates the possibility of bladder rupture.

The overwhelming majority (98%) of patients with bladder rupture have gross hematuria (JW McAninch, personal communication, 1998). The other 2% are rep-

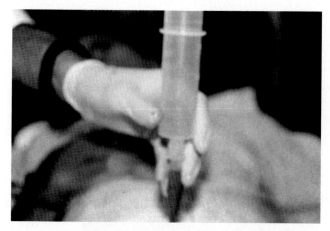

Figure 44-10. Retrograde cystogram. A Toomey syringe without its central piston is connected to the catheter and held by the examiner while gravity-instilled contrast material fills the bladder.

resentative of the select group of patients with a pelvic fracture and only microhematuria. Clinical judgment is required when deciding when these patients need a bladder evaluation.

Radiology

Conventional retrograde cystography or retrograde CT cystography are the diagnostic procedures of choice for suspected bladder injury.[8,10,11] It is key that these studies *not* be done in an antegrade fashion, as such procedures may produce incomplete and spurious findings (e.g., injecting intravenous contrast material, clamping the Foley catheter, and allowing the examination to be dependent on antegrade filling of the bladder from renal excretion of progressively dilute contrast material).

Conventional Retrograde Cystogram. Performance of either conventional or CT retrograde cystography assumes or follows exclusion of urethral trauma and the presence of an indwelling Foley catheter in the bladder. A Toomey syringe alone without its central piston is used for gravity instillation of contrast material (Figure 44-10). Allowing the contrast material to freely infuse from a hanging bottle connected to an indwelling Foley catheter runs the risk of the tubing becoming disconnected with subsequent leakage of contrast material onto the examination table (Figure 44-11A and B). This may promote an inaccurate examination that results in an unnecessary operative procedure (Figure 44-11C). For patients with a pelvic fracture, it is imperative that they remain supine throughout the examination rather than be repositioned obliquely for selected radiographs. This lessens the potential for rebleeding from an organized retropubic hematoma.

A preliminary KUB or scout film is obtained to provide a baseline evaluation of the pelvis, abdomen, and surrounding bony structures. It will become the film of reference for the post-evacuation radiograph obtained after completion of the cystogram. Potential areas of extravasation on the post-evacuation film will be confirmed when compared with the preliminary

KUB film (Figure 44-12). Contrast material should not be instilled into the bladder until the quality and anatomic information on the preliminary KUB film are confirmed.

Full-strength iothalamate meglumine (Conray II) is instilled under gravity filling to one of three endpoints: (1) 100 mL with immediate fluoroscopic evidence of gross extravasation; (2) a total instillation of 300 to 400 mL in any patient 11 years of age or older; in patients younger than 11 years of age, the correct amount of contrast medium is determined by the formula (age in years + 2) × 30; or (3) the instillation of a lesser amount than 100 mL, which initiates a bladder contraction. This will become evident by the retrograde filling of the Toomey syringe with bladder contents. After a few minutes, the original contrast material can again be instilled to the point of stimulating a bladder contraction, at which time an additional 50 mL of full-strength iothalamate meglumine should be injected slowly but forcefully into the bladder. The Foley catheter should be clamped, and an anteroposterior radiograph should be taken of the filled bladder (Figure 44-13A and B). A lateral film may help clarify any areas in question (Figure 44-13C). After the film of the filled bladder meets standards for quality and detail, the bladder should be completely evacuated into a large basin or, preferably, into an available bedside drainage bag. Any spillage of contrast material onto the pelvic genitalia or examination table may lead to false-positive findings on the postevacuation radiograph. The postevacuation film may disclose evidence of posterior bladder wall or extraperitoneal extravasation not seen on the anteroposterior radiograph of the filled bladder (Figure 44-14).

In cases of extraperitoneal bladder perforation, contrast material will be evident in the area of the pubic symphysis and pelvic outlet (Figure 44-15). With intraperitoneal perforation, contrast material outlines intraperitoneal structures (e.g., loops of bowel, the liver, and spleen) (Figure 44-16).

Several studies have documented that false-negative results are associated with the use of less than 300 to 400 mL or an age-appropriate amount of contrast material for cystography.[6,12] This has been seen primarily in penetrating bladder injuries in which the perforation from a small-caliber gunshot wound or a thin blade stab wound can be missed. The anatomically interlacing bladder wall muscle fibers are arranged such that these wounds lend themselves to immediate muscle fiber reapproximation and tenuous sealing of the wound by covering peritoneum and intra-abdominal mesentery. Unless an adequate amount of full-strength contrast material is used to fully distend or even overdistend the bladder, extravasation will not be evident, the injury will be missed, and there will be potential for significant morbidity.

Computed Tomography Retrograde Cystogram. The same anatomic information regarding bladder injury may be obtained using retrograde CT cystography rather than routine plain film radiography.[11] CT cystography is best done in trauma patients who are undergoing CT evaluation for other suspected injuries.

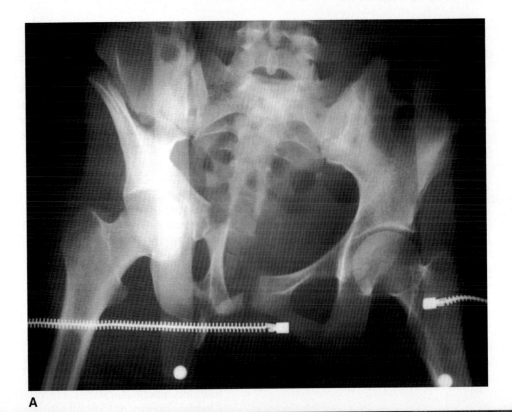

A

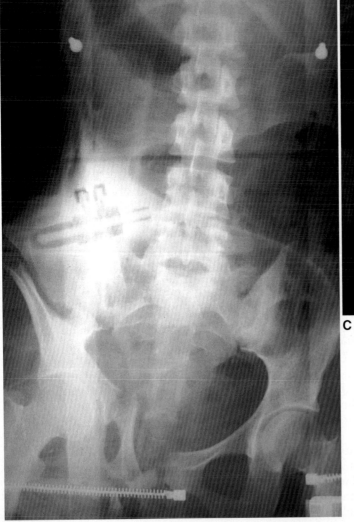

B

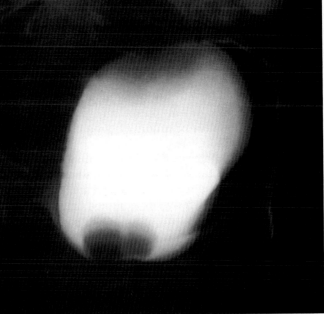

C

Figure 44-11. Spurious retrograde cystogram. This examination resulted when the tubing from the contrast bottle became disconnected from the Foley catheter after both were placed on the examination table, and bladder filling was completed without direct supervision. **A,** Kidney, bladder, ureter (KUB) film. **B,** Postinfusion KUB film interpreted as intraperitoneal bladder perforation. **C,** Intraoperative retrograde cystogram showing no evidence of extravasation.

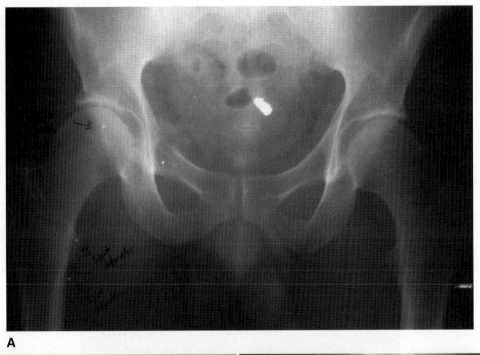

A

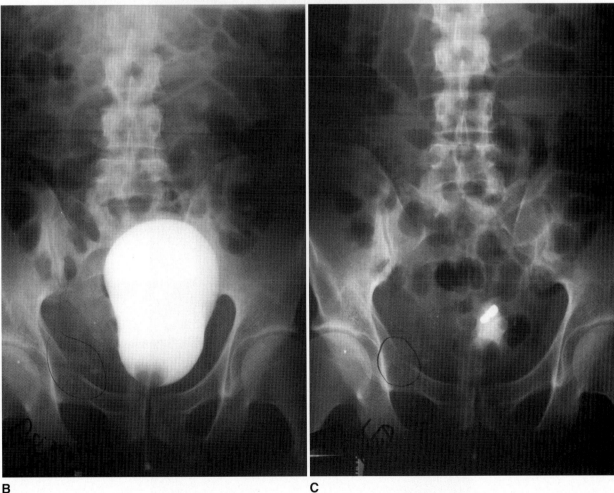

B   C

Figure 44-12. Retrograde cystogram. **A,** Preliminary kidney, bladder, ureter (KUB) film. **B,** Film of filled bladder. **C,** Postevacuation film comparing posterior extravasation with the preliminary KUB film.

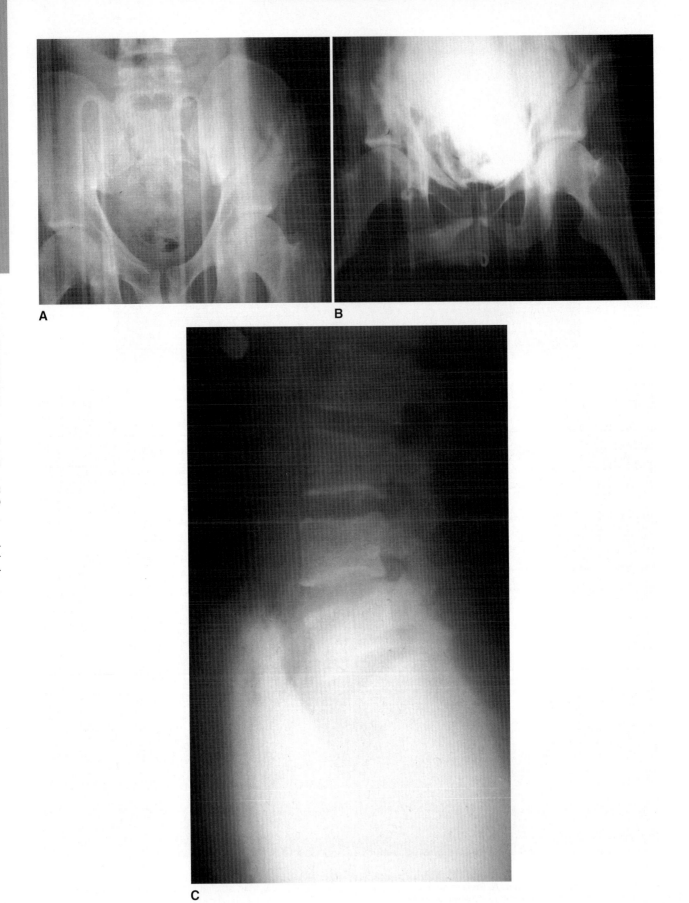

Figure 44-13. Retrograde cystogram. **A,** Preliminary kidney, bladder, ureter (KUB) film. **B,** Film of filled bladder showing extravasation that could be intraperitoneal, as well as extraperitoneal. **C,** Film of patient in a lateral position shows no evidence of intraperitoneal extravasation.

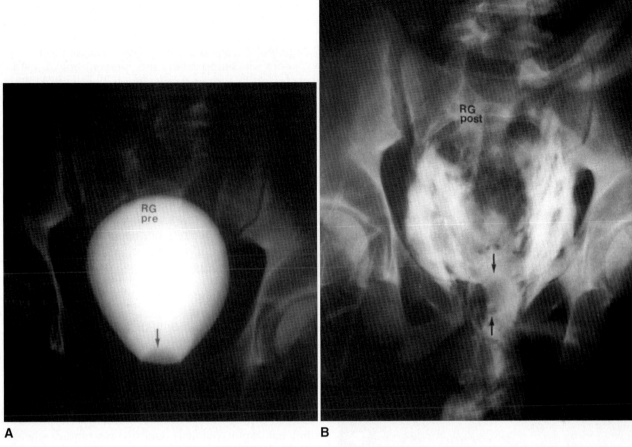

Figure 44-14. Retrograde cystogram. **A,** Film of filled bladder. **B,** Postevacuation film showing extensive extraperitoneal extravasation.

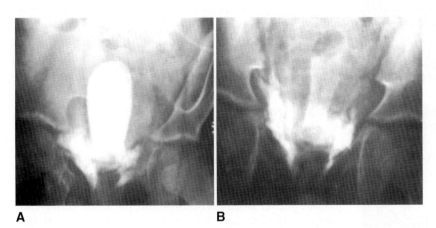

A   **B**

Figure 44-15. Cystographic appearance of extraperitoneal bladder perforation. **A** and **B,** Note the teardrop deformity caused by extrinsic compression by the pelvic hematoma and the flamelike wisps of extravasation confined by the pelvis. The bladder itself is elongated by a collection of perivesicular fluid. (From Spirnak JP: Pelvic fracture and injury to the lower urinary tract. *Surg Clin North Am* 68:1057, 1988.)

In either study, undiluted iothalamate meglumine (Conray II) must first be instilled in a retrograde fashion. Intraperitoneal perforation will be disclosed on helical CT scan by the presence of extravasated contrast material throughout the abdominal cavity (i.e., contrast ascites). Extraperitoneal extravasation will be more difficult to visualize but can be appreciated on images taken through the pelvic area (Figure 44-17A and B).

Management

In cases of superficial mucosal bladder lacerations, bladder contusions, or simple bladder hematomas, there will be no evidence of extravasation on retrograde cystography. For these injuries, expectant management with or without Foley catheter drainage is the standard of care.[4,13]

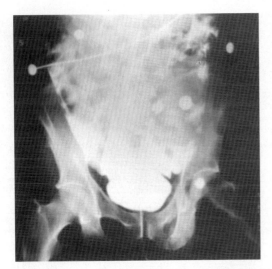

Figure 44-16. Cystographic appearance of intraperitoneal bladder perforation. Cystogram reveals massive intraperitoneal perforation and extravasation. (From Spirnak JP: Pelvic fracture and injury to the lower urinary tract. *Surg Clin North Am* 68:1057, 1988.)

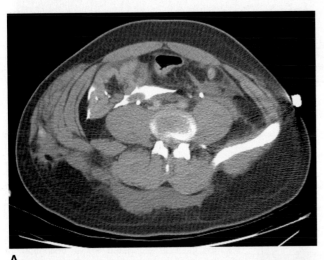

A

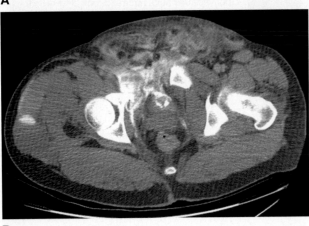

B

Figure 44-17. Bladder rupture. **A,** Intraperitoneal rupture shows contrast material extravasated from the bladder outlining loops of bowel in the lower abdomen. **B,** Extraperitoneal rupture shows contrast material extravasating into the disrupted soft tissue plains of the anterior and left pelvic side wall. (Courtesy of Charlotte Radiology, Emergency Radiology Section, Charlotte, North Carolina.)

Extraperitoneal Bladder Rupture

Extraperitoneal bladder rupture heals spontaneously in most circumstances after simple Foley catheter drainage for 7 to 14 days using a 20-Fr or larger Foley catheter.[4,13] Care must be taken to ensure continuous bladder decompression and prevention of catheter occlusion by clot or debris. In a patient with known or suspected infected urine before the traumatic event, consideration must be given both to Foley or suprapubic catheter drainage and to surgical placement of drains in the perivesical space to prevent subsequent abscess formation. Primary surgical repair of extraperitoneal bladder rupture should be considered in any trauma patient whose bladder injury appears to extend into the bladder neck or proximal urethra.[3,4] This is most important in the female trauma patient because the short length of the female urethra lends itself to a higher incidence of urinary incontinence after injury. This can hopefully be reduced by primary surgical repair. Any patient whose other associated nonurologic injuries dictate abdominal exploration is a candidate for primary surgical repair of the extraperitoneal bladder injury provided the bladder laceration is easily accessible and does not require operative exposure through a large, organized, stable retropubic hematoma.[4,6,13]

Intraperitoneal Bladder Rupture

Larger, gaping intraperitoneal bladder perforations will not heal spontaneously and always require operative repair.[6] Without operative intervention for intraperitoneal injury, lower urinary tract contamination will quickly infect initially sterile urine and promote the development of subsequent bacterial peritonitis. Bladder repairs are never emergencies and normally follow operative repair of more urgent life-threatening injuries.

UPPER TRACT TRAUMA

Renal Trauma

Perspective

Renal trauma is a capricious injury that has no known identifiable markers. Mechanisms responsible for significant renal injury almost never affect the kidney alone, but most often disrupt and perforate other vital organs that can be solely responsible for the patients' death and may demand immediate operative intervention. Significant renal injuries define a small subset of the trauma population at large. This by itself promotes diagnostic uncertainty and causes some of these injuries to be overlooked initially. Renal injuries are graded 1 through 5 according to the Organ Injury Scale Committee Guidelines, which identifies most injuries requiring operative intervention.[14]

Complications

Development of renovascular hypertension occurs in approximately 1% of cases and is the main complication associated with failed arterial repairs or missed

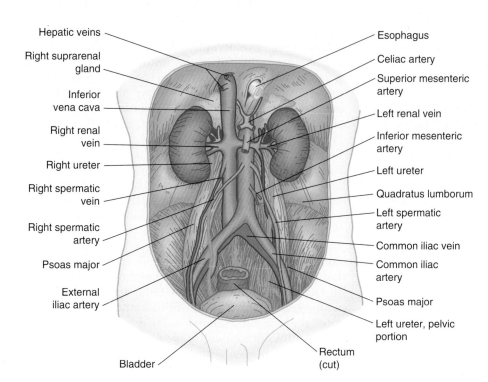

Hepatic veins

Right suprarenal gland

Inferior vena cava

Right renal vein

Right ureter

Right spermatic vein

Right spermatic artery

Psoas major

External iliac artery

Bladder

Esophagus

Celiac artery

Superior mesenteric artery

Left renal vein

Inferior mesenteric artery

Left ureter

Quadratus lumborum

Left spermatic artery

Common iliac vein

Common iliac artery

Psoas major

Left ureter, pelvic portion

Rectum (cut)

Figure 44-18. Dissection of abdomen showing kidneys and ureters and their relationship to other anatomic features in the retroperitoneal space.

pedicle injuries.[14] When associated with elevated renal vein renin levels, nephrectomy is curative. For these reasons, the issue of whether to actively pursue this diagnosis is debated. An isolated pedicle injury in a young, healthy trauma patient would seem to be the ideal circumstance in which an all-out attempt should be made to reconstruct the renal artery or vein.

Anatomy and Physiology

The kidneys are located in the retroperitoneal space, are surrounded by adipose tissue and loose areolar connective tissue, and lie along the lower two thoracic vertebrae and the first four lumbar vertebrae. The left kidney is suspended slightly higher than the right (Figure 44-18). The kidneys are not fixed. They move with the diaphragm and are supported by their renal arteries, veins, and adipose tissue, which is connected to a layer of fibrous tissue called the renal fascia, or Gerota's fascia.

The indented medial border of the kidney is called the *hilum*. The major renal vessels and ureter make up the renal pedicle and enter and exit at the hilum. The longitudinal section of the kidney (Figure 44-19) shows an outer renal cortex and an inner renal medulla with its columns of Bertin. Each column of Bertin forms a papilla that empties into the renal pelvis. The renal pelvis is a funnel-shaped sac with cup-shaped extensions called *calyces*, which receive urine from each papilla and are the important decompression areas for varied rises in intrapelvic pressure.

The kidneys are perfused by 1200 mL of blood per minute, or 20% to 25% of cardiac output. Of this, 90% goes to the cortex and 10% to the medulla. Reduced blood flow to the kidney, whether from blunt or penetrating injury, causes renin to be released from the juxtaglomerular cells. Renin enters the bloodstream and

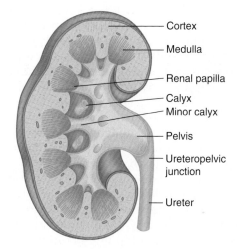

Cortex

Medulla

Renal papilla

Calyx

Minor calyx

Pelvis

Ureteropelvic junction

Ureter

Figure 44-19. Longitudinal section of kidney.

combines with a plasma protein to form angiotensin. Angiotensin raises blood pressure by causing arteriolar vasoconstriction and acting on the adrenal cortex to augment aldosterone secretion. Aldosterone acts on the renal tubules to promote sodium reabsorption. Water follows passively with subsequent increase in blood volume. These changes increase blood flow to the kidney and other organs. The body requires only one third of normal renal function to sustain life. It is unusual in cases of genitourinary trauma to lose total renal function unless the patient's injured kidney is a solitary kidney, which carries a 1 in 1000 to 1 in 5000 incidence.[15]

Epidemiology

Renal trauma represents the most common of all urologic injuries.[2] Blunt renal trauma accounts for 80% to

85% of all renal injuries and is five times more common than penetrating renal trauma.[2] With the increasing prevalence nationwide of gunshot and stab wounds in association with drug-related violence, the proportion of injuries due to penetrating trauma may rise. Blunt mechanisms are seen most often after motor vehicle crashes, domestic violence, and sporting injuries. The pathophysiologic mechanisms include rapid deceleration, displacement, and, rarely, an explosion-type injury of the ureteropelvic junction. Approximately 20% of blunt renal trauma cases are associated with intraperitoneal injury.[2] Penetrating renal trauma is associated with intraperitoneal injury in approximately 80% of cases.[2]

Diagnostic Strategies

Laboratory

No accurate markers for renal injury exist. In all types of renal trauma, the degree of hematuria is not indicative of the severity or extent of injury. Formerly, a trauma patient who exhibited gross or microscopic hematuria was labeled "at risk" for urologic injury and underwent intravenous pyelography. Experience has shown that most of the identifiable injuries were renal contusions that could be managed expectantly. Moreover, in a significant number of severely traumatized patients, vigorous initial fluid resuscitation precluded satisfactory contrast concentration in the kidney, yielding an incomplete, nondiagnostic initial radiographic examination.

In 1989, Mee and associates[16] published the hallmark article that established guidelines for the evaluation and treatment of blunt renal trauma. Their 10-year prospective study clearly established that (1) major renal lacerations represent significant reparable renal injuries; (2) adult patients at risk for having sustained major lacerations have either gross hematuria or microhematuria (≥ 3 to 5 RBCs/hpf) with shock (systolic blood pressure ≤ 90 mm Hg) initially in the field or on arrival at an emergency department, or, rarely but importantly, a history of sudden deceleration without hematuria or shock; and (3) intravenous contrast-enhanced CT scan is the procedure of choice in identifying the full extent of urologic injury.[2,16,17] These guidelines are not applicable for cases of penetrating renal trauma or in children.

Pediatrics. In children, the kidney is the most commonly injured genitourinary organ in blunt abdominal trauma.[18] Additionally, unlike adults, major renal injuries can occur in the presence of microhematuria without shock or even in the presence of a normal urinalysis. Prior meta-analyses defined 50 RBCs/hpf as the microscopic quantity below which imaging could be confidently deleted without missing significant injuries.[19] Current literature supports radiographic investigation based mainly on mechanism of injury and clinical suspicion, because no absolute parameters for excluding significant renal injury exist.[20] As with adults, intravenous contrast-enhanced helical CT scanning is the diagnostic imaging technique of choice.

Radiology

Intravenous Pyelography. Whether simple, routine IVP is ever indicated in the initial evaluation of suspected renal trauma depends on the institution and the radiologist. At a center that does not have 24-hour availability of radiologists and technicians, bolus infusion IVP with nephrotomography rather than simple IVP is the initial study of choice.[16,21] Bolus infusion denotes the rapid injection of 2 mL of contrast material per kilogram of body weight to a maximum of 150 mL after a preliminary KUB film has been obtained.[15] Immediately on completion of the injection, a postinfusion supine film is obtained, followed by 1-, 2-, and 3-minute supine films, specifically tailoring the study to identify both renal outlines and evidence that contrast is extending down the collecting system of the kidney and ureter to the bladder without extravasation. In fact, most authors propose bolus infusion IVP with nephrotomography as the initial study of choice for uncommonly encountered isolated renal injury, which can be difficult to identify prospectively.[16] In the spectrum of experience with bolus infusion IVP as a diagnostic tool for renal injury, most authors find this study adequate only 60% to 85% of the time.[21] Often, abnormal findings are nonspecific and require more sophisticated studies, such as CT scanning, to identify the full extent of the existing renal injuries.

When immediate, life-saving, nonurologic surgical intervention is mandated or an expanding retroperitoneal hematoma with the potential for significant renal injury is encountered in the operating room, a 2 mL/kg intraoperative bolus infusion of contrast and a 10-minute film are recommended to ensure the presence of both kidneys before the retroperitoneum is opened and control of the renal pedicle is attempted. A "single-shot" IVP in the emergency department used as a screening examination before the patient is transported to the operating room is discouraged because of the equally unacceptable incidence of false-positive and false-negative results.[15]

Computed Tomography. An intravenous contrast-enhanced helical CT scan is the diagnostic radiographic procedure of choice in evaluating significant upper tract blunt renal trauma. It is more sensitive and specific than bolus infusion IVP with nephrotomography (Figure 44-20A-E).[21,22]

Management

Blunt Injury

Both an adult blunt trauma patient with microhematuria (≥ 3 to 5 RBCs/hpf) but no shock (systolic blood pressure ≤ 90 mm Hg) in the field or in the emergency department and a pediatric blunt trauma patient with 50 RBCs/hpf or fewer and no other coexisting major organ injuries can be confidently discharged from the emergency department if no other complicating nonurologic injuries are present that would dictate observation or hospital admission. Outpatient follow-up with a urologist until the microhematuria has cleared is mandatory to be certain it does not represent another more serious underlying condition.[23]

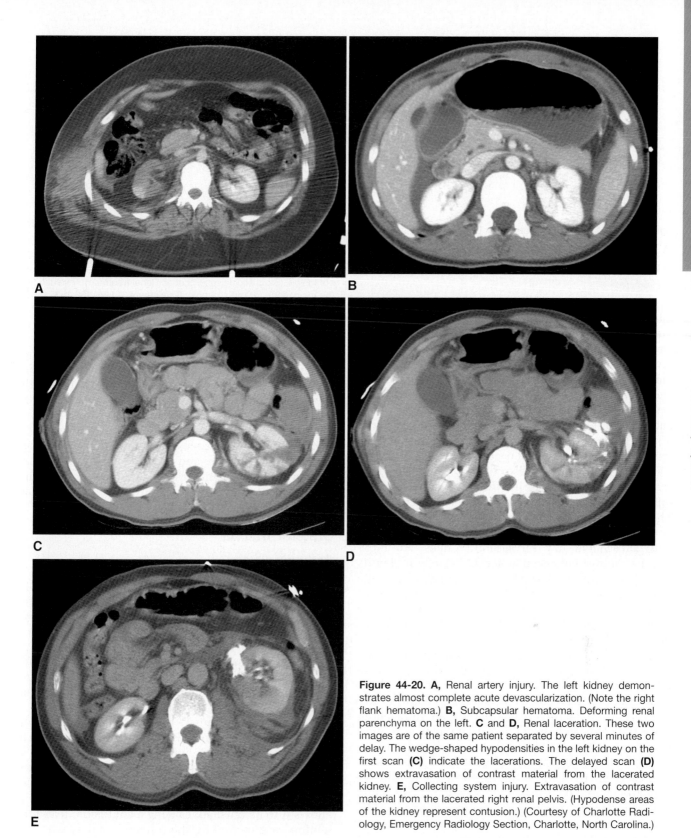

Figure 44-20. A, Renal artery injury. The left kidney demonstrates almost complete acute devascularization. (Note the right flank hematoma.) **B,** Subcapsular hematoma. Deforming renal parenchyma on the left. **C** and **D,** Renal laceration. These two images are of the same patient separated by several minutes of delay. The wedge-shaped hypodensities in the left kidney on the first scan **(C)** indicate the lacerations. The delayed scan **(D)** shows extravasation of contrast material from the lacerated kidney. **E,** Collecting system injury. Extravasation of contrast material from the lacerated right renal pelvis. (Hypodense areas of the kidney represent contusion.) (Courtesy of Charlotte Radiology, Emergency Radiology Section, Charlotte, North Carolina.)

Renal artery avulsions, intimal tears, and renal venous injuries should be considered under the classification of significant injuries. Although only 1% to 2% of all renal injuries involve the renal pedicle, their evaluation and management remain a real dilemma based on the frustrating and dismal experience with pedicle injuries from major centers.[24] Experience has shown that even under the most ideal clinical circumstances (i.e., fortuitous early recognition and prompt surgical repair), the salvage rate at best for a life-sustaining functioning kidney approaches only 15% to 20%.

Renal vein injuries are more common than renal artery avulsions or intimal tears. Both injuries are often associated with rapid deceleration events. Most venous

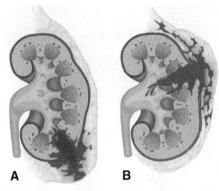

Figure 44-21. Major renal lacerations. **A,** Deep medullary laceration. **B,** Laceration into collecting system. (From Nicolaisen GS, et al: Renal trauma: Re-evaluation of the indications for radiographic assessment. *J Urol* 133:183, 1985.)

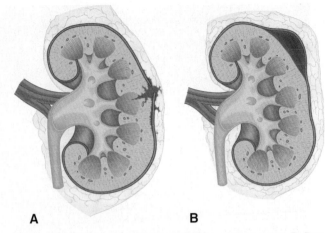

Figure 44-22. Minor renal injuries. **A,** Minor renal laceration. **B,** Renal contusion. (From Nicolaisen GS et al: Renal trauma: Re-evaluation of the indications for radiographic assessment. *J Urol* 133:183, 1985.)

injuries tend to be partial rather than complete tears, or they involve segmental renal vein branches and therefore often occur in the periphery of the vein (i.e., involving contiguous adrenal or gonadal attachments to the left renal vein rather than at the junction of the main renal vein with the vena cava). As expected, a venous injury can potentially contribute more to a patient's unstable hemodynamic status than an arterial injury. The protective secondary vasospasm following arterial disruption does not occur with venous injuries.

Pedicle injuries rarely occur alone. Most often they are associated with other life-threatening, nonurologic injuries that require immediate surgical intervention. This delays their diagnosis and repair for up to 6 to 8 hours, which results in significant warm ischemia time with subsequent low salvageability rates. An intravenous contrast-enhanced helical CT scan will identify most renal artery disruptions, whereas renal vein injuries must be indirectly diagnosed by the presence of a normal-appearing kidney in association with a large hematoma disproportionate to the rest of the radiographic study.

Major renal lacerations represent approximately 2% to 4% of all renal injuries, and by definition are associated with renal fractures extending deep into the renal medulla and collecting system (Figure 44-21). They also are readily diagnosed by an intravenous contrast-enhanced helical CT scan. Immediate surgical treatment of these injuries is controversial and depends on the presence or absence of continued renal bleeding, the hemodynamic status of the patient, and the degree of continued urinary extravasation.[25] This injury is in sharp contrast to minor renal lacerations (8-15%) and renal contusions (85-92%) that do not extend into the renal medulla or collecting system, are not associated with extravasation of urine, and heal spontaneously (Figure 44-22). These latter two injuries can be managed expectantly and rarely, if ever, require initial or subsequent operative intervention.[16]

Penetrating Injury

In cases of penetrating renal trauma, the presence or absence of hematuria is of no consequence in predicting upper urinary tract injury. Rather, the location of the penetrating wound in relation to the urinary tract is the most important determining factor in deciding the need for radiographic investigation. Therefore, the absence of hematuria in a patient with a gunshot or stab wound in proximity to the urinary tract does not eliminate the need for an intravenous contrast-enhanced CT scan as the initial diagnostic examination. Significant injuries to the kidney and ureter occur in penetrating trauma *without* hematuria.[3] The majority of penetrating renal and ureteral injuries require surgical intervention.

Ureteral Trauma

Pathophysiology

Ureteral injuries are rare. Most are traumatic in origin and tend to occur as a result of shootings or stabbings or during various intra-abdominal or retroperitoneal operations.[26] Penetrating ureteral injuries are twice as common as blunt ureteral injuries. Most are localized in the upper third of the ureter.[27] This diagnosis should be considered when patients seen in the emergency department have a recent history of penetrating trauma, fever, and a palpably tender flank mass.

If the ureter is injured by blunt trauma, there are often multiple associated nonurologic injuries. The gastrointestinal tract is injured in more than 50% of cases.[28] In pelvic fractures, the ureter is most likely to be injured as it crosses the pelvic brim. The intimate relationship of the ureter to the pelvis at this point allows it to be crushed, causing a contusion, tear, transection, or puncture by sharp fracture spicules.

Clinical Features

The clinical picture of blunt ureteral injuries includes hematuria, flank pain similar to renal colic, and a flank mass. These classic signs are often overlooked initially because of the striking abdominal findings caused by associated nonurologic injuries.

Hematuria may be present in association with ureteral contusion or partial ureteral tear but is rarely present in cases of complete ureteral transection. Pain in the lower abdomen, a palpable mass containing blood or urine, chills, fever, urgency, frequency, and pyuria are all symptoms of this injury.

Diagnostic Strategies

In a Parkland Memorial Hospital series of 71 penetrating ureteral injuries, 32% of patients had no hematuria, 40% had gross hematuria, and 28% had microscopic hematuria.[29] If the patient survived the original penetrating event, the injury usually manifested itself 10 days later with the appearance of urine at the entrance or exit wounds or on the surgical dressings. If there is no vent for extravasated urine, a retroperitoneal urinoma will develop. If the diaphragm or peritoneum has been violated, the urine may cause an empyema or peritonitis.

Radiology

If a ureteral injury is suspected, a contrast-enhanced helical CT scan with delayed films or bolus infusion IVP with delayed films should be done.[30] The clarity of injury identification depends on renal function and the lapsed time from the injury. If the study is performed soon after the injury, extravasation often has a ground-glass or hazy appearance as a result of contrast dilution from fluid resuscitation. If the injury is near the ureteropelvic junction, the contrast may extend peripherally around the kidney, giving the appearance of a lacerated renal pelvis or kidney. If the initial study of delayed films is inconclusive, retrograde pyelography is indicated to delineate a ureteral laceration or avulsion (Figure 44-23A and B). The more concentrated contrast used in retrograde pyelography compared with that used with routine IVP and the adjunctive use of fluoroscopy promote rapid identification of ureteral injury.

Management

All ureteral injuries must be repaired surgically. If these injuries are diagnosed early, the kidney and ureter can be saved in most cases. In cases of delayed diagnosis, the rate of nephroureterectomies dramatically increases.[31]

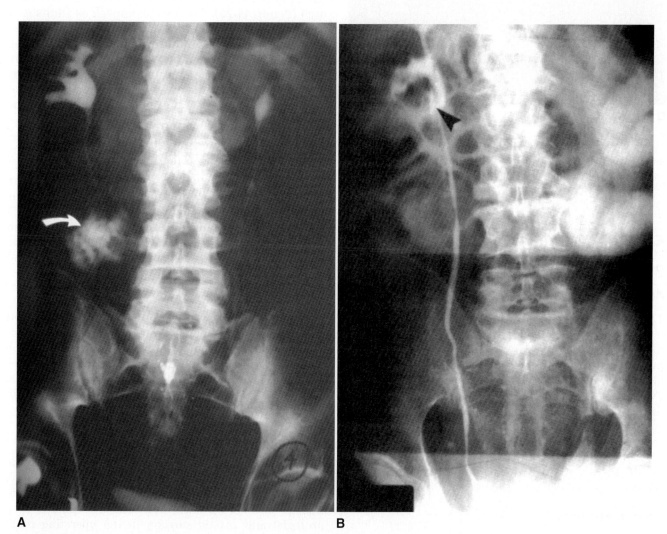

A   **B**

Figure 44-23. Ureteral injuries. **A,** Intravenous pyelography (IVP) of patient with upper ureteral injury demonstrating extravasation (arrow). **B,** Retrograde pyelogram demonstrating extravasation at the ureteropelvic junction (arrow).

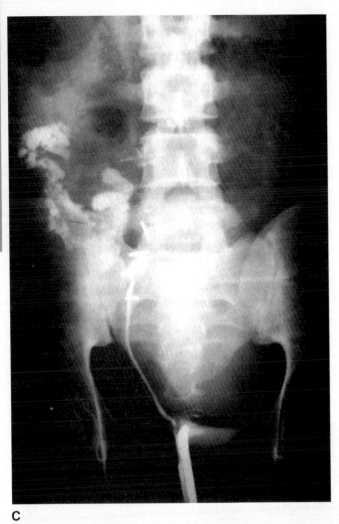

C

Figure 44-23.—cont'd. C, Retrograde pyelogram demonstrating extravasation into a urinoma in a patient with delayed diagnosis. (From Presti JC Jr, Carroll PR, McAninch JW: Ureteral and renal pelvic injuries from external trauma: Diagnosis and management. *J Trauma* 29:370, 1989.)

EXTERNAL GENITALIA TRAUMA

Penile Trauma

Anatomy

The penis contains three masses of erectile tissue (Figure 44-24). The two corpora cavernosa constitute the main bulk of the penis and lie in the center of the penis. The corpus spongiosum is smaller, lies on the ventral surface of the penis, encases the urethra, and expands at the penile tip to form the glans penis. The tunica albuginea is a dense fibrous envelope that surrounds the corpus spongiosum and each corpus cavernosum. Blood is supplied through arteries lying in each of the three erectile masses and two dorsal penile arteries. A single dorsal vein drains most of the penis.

Clinical Features

Injuries to the penis range from small lacerations or contusions to skin degloving or amputation. Strangula-

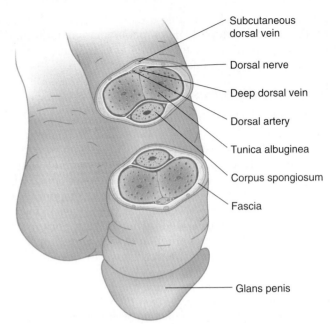

Figure 44-24. Cross-sectional view of the penis.

tion injuries of the penis with string or scalp hair tightly encircling the shaft of the penis are seen in children (Figure 44-25). Adolescents as well as adults may have various objects of penile incarceration such as bottles, washers, and metal rings (Figure 44-26). These objects are often used to facilitate masturbation, prevent detumescence, and heighten sexual pleasure. These constricting devices must be identified and removed, a procedure that can test the ingenuity of the most experienced physician. If the strangulation is prolonged or appears to be associated with necrosis, the constricting object must be removed on an emergency basis. Various creative techniques, using saws, metal cutters, or emery wheels, may be necessary to remove some metal objects. Plastic surgery repair of the penis may eventually be needed but should be delayed until penile tissue viability has clarified. Fortunately, each corpora body has a separate blood supply and may be preserved even though the penile skin may slough and require skin grafting.

Pediatrics

In small children, penile trauma may be associated with possible child abuse, especially when the explanations given for the event do not match the type of injury and objective physical findings. Examples include bruises that look like pinches, cigarette burns, or an injury reportedly caused by a falling toilet seat in a child who is too small to stand unsupported.

Management

Superficial lacerations of penile-scrotal skin may be primarily reapproximated with 4-0 chromic or Vicryl absorbable suture. Patients with degloving penile injuries and scrotal skin loss should be treated by a urologist and plastic surgeon in the operating room with cleansing, debridement, and skin flaps or skin grafts. Traumatic penile amputation can be handled by

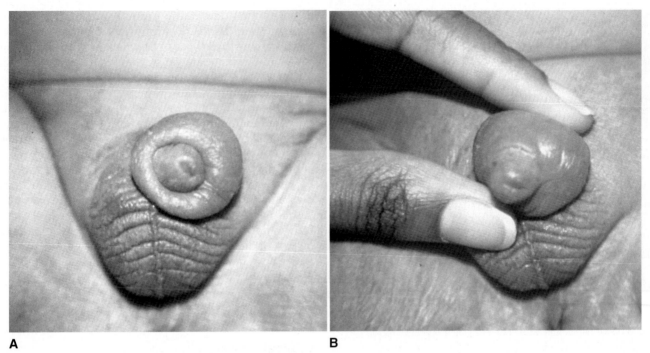

Figure 44-25. Idiopathic foreskin edema. **A,** This is the same picture that can be seen with penile strangulation injuries in children. **B,** The edematous foreskin must be retracted proximally and distally looking for encircling hair, string, or other objects that may lead to vascular compromise.

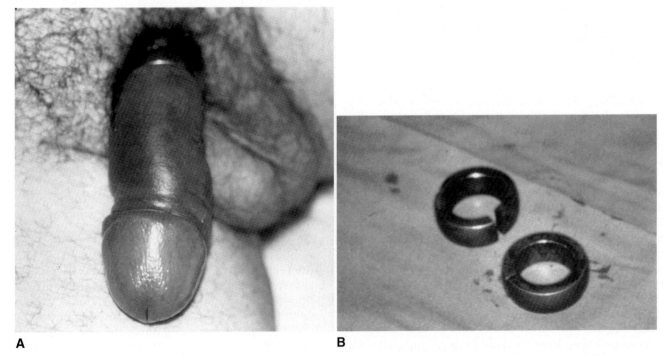

Figure 44-26. A, Self-induced priapism. This patient placed two steel washers **(B)** around the base of his penis to prolong his erection. Subsequent priapism developed and the incarceration necessitated emergency intraoperative removal with a pneumatic orthopedic drill.

primary reanastomosis (replantation) or local reshaping of the amputated penis. A recovered amputated distal penis should be placed in a clean plastic bag then immersed in cold saline if available. If the proximal penile stump is hemorrhaging, direct pressure on the bleeding source may promote hemostasis. A circumferentially placed Penrose drain at the base of the penis can be used acutely to control blood loss but should

not be used for extended periods. Reanastomosis of a severed penis is possible up to 6 hours after amputation. Beyond this period, local reshaping is recommended. Both a urologist and a plastic surgeon should be involved in the patient's management if reimplantation is considered.

Traumatic rupture of the corpus cavernosum, or penile fracture, occurs when the tunica albuginea is

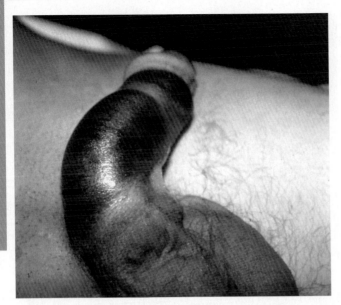

Figure 44-27. Fracture of the penis. Traumatic rupture of the corpus cavernosum, usually associated with sexual activity, results in a profound penile hematoma, most often requiring operative repair.

torn (Figure 44-27). This usually occurs during vigorous sexual intercourse. The patient may hear a snapping sound and experience localized pain, detumescence, and a slowly progressive penile hematoma. Voiding is possible if the urethra is not injured. Ultrasonography is not diagnostically helpful in this setting. Occasional nonoperative management includes bed rest and ice packs for 24 to 48 hours followed by local heat and a pressure dressing. Most injuries are treated surgically. The penile hematoma is evacuated, the torn penile tunica albuginea is sutured, and a pressure dressing is applied. Of patients with a fractured penis, 10% experience a permanent deformity, suboptimal coitus, or impaired erections, especially if managed non-operatively.

Traumatic lymphangitis of the penis is a self-limiting disease usually caused by vigorous or prolonged sexual intercourse or masturbation. It is seen as a translucent, firm, nodular, almost cartilaginous cordlike configuration beginning at the coronal sulcus in the subcutaneous tissue. It may involve one side of the penis or encircle it completely. It is usually not tender and is freely mobile. It is best treated by abstinence from sexual activity and resolves in 2 to 3 weeks. Nonsteroidal anti-inflammatory drugs (NSAIDs) may be of some benefit.

Traumatic lymphangitis should not be confused with Peyronie's disease, which is caused by recurring microtrauma leading to the formation of plaquelike fibrosis in the dorsal aspect of the tunica albuginea between the two corpora cavernosa. This fibrotic area causes decreased penile distensibility with subsequent dorsal curvature of the penis leading to painful erections and difficult or unsuccessful vaginal penetration. Reassurance and daily doses of vitamin E (400 IU) are the initial modes of therapy with subsequent urologic follow-up evaluation.

Thrombosis and thrombophlebitis of the dorsal vein of the penis are usually associated with a history of direct trauma, idiopathic thrombophlebitis, or thromboangiitis obliterans. The physical findings are much more striking than those of traumatic lymphangitis, and the condition is treated symptomatically with heat and NSAIDs.

Most human bites to the penis are acquired during sexual activity and represent a potentially serious polymicrobial infection. With this history and an examination showing localized swelling or generalized edema of the penile shaft with erythema suggestive of cellulitis, an immunocompromised patient should be admitted to the hospital for broad-spectrum intravenous antibiotic coverage that is sensitive to both aerobic and anaerobic organisms. Careful observation for the development of bacteremia or septicemia must be part of the management plan. An immunocompetent patient can be treated as an outpatient with cephalexin, NSAIDs, and re-evaluation within 2 to 3 days.

TESTICULAR TRAUMA

Clinical Features

Testicular injuries are most often caused by a fall or kick, or they are incurred while playing a sport and result in a contusion, laceration, fracture, or dislocation. The symptoms include severe pain, faintness, nausea, vomiting, and occasionally urinary retention secondary to pain. On examination, a tender swollen testicle may be present, but often only a small hematoma is noted. Therefore, anyone with a remote history of testicular trauma should undergo testicular color Doppler ultrasonographic examination, the diagnostic procedure of choice, to evaluate the integrity of the testis.[32] It can disclose testicular disruption, extruded testicular parenchyma, or a fragmented testicle. Loss of the normal homogeneous testicular pattern and the presence of a heterogeneous testicular pattern are diagnostic of testicular injury and require urologic evaluation (Figure 44-28). Benign trauma often acts as the inciting event that discloses testicular torsion or malignancy.

Management

Testicular contusions are treated conservatively with bed rest, ice packs, NSAIDs, and appropriate urologic follow-up evaluation. Testicular dislocation occurs as a result of excessive pressure on the scrotum or thigh. In 80% of cases, the testis lies under the abdominal wall. Associated injuries are common, such as a pelvic fracture, hip dislocation, or cutaneous contusions. On examination, the affected hemiscrotum is swollen and ecchymotic with an absent testis. Operative repair is required for testicular laceration, disruption, or dislocation. Hematoma evacuation, testicular parenchymal debridement, and primary closure of the tunica albuginea are the treatments of choice. Immediate surgery allows earlier resumption of daily activity, a shorter hospital stay, greatly reduced morbidity, and a lower orchiectomy rate.

Infrequent dog bites to the scrotum occur most often in children.[33] Careful examination of the scrotal tunica

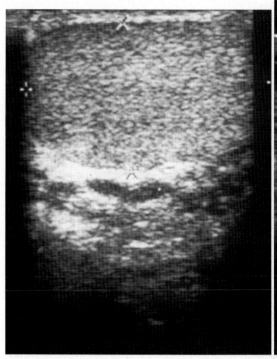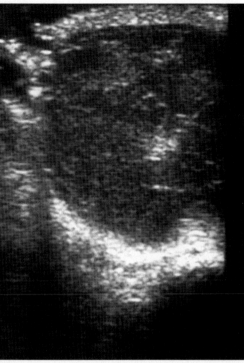

A   **B**

Figure 44-28. Testicular rupture. **A,** Testicular ultrasonogram demonstrates the normal homogeneous testicular pattern. **B,** The heterogeneous pattern of injury, tumor, or disruption.

vaginalis will disclose involvement of the intrascrotal contents that dictates operative evaluation and repair. All other bites can be washed out thoroughly and closed primarily with absorbable suture. Prophylactic antibiotics can be administered based on the extent of the bite, subsequent injury, and the patient's immune status.

 KEY CONCEPTS

- Diagnostic evaluation of the urinary tract is generally undertaken in retrograde fashion. That is, suspicion and elimination of urethral injury before bladder injury before ureteral or renal injury.

- Urethral injury is suggested by the presence of a pelvic fracture, blood at the urethral meatus, the presence of a high-riding or absent prostate on rectal examination, or evidence of a perineal, scrotal, or penile hematoma.

- Gross hematuria alone or in conjunction with a pelvic fracture is the absolute marker for significant bladder injury. Grossly, clear bladder urine in a trauma patient without a pelvic fracture virtually eliminates the possibility of bladder rupture.

- Adult patients at risk for major renal lacerations have gross hematuria or microhematuria (3-5 RBCs/hpf) with shock (systolic blood pressure ≤90 mm Hg) initially in the field or the emergency department, or, rarely, a history of sudden deceleration without hematuria or shock. Pediatric patients can suffer major renal injuries without any hematuria.

- If a ureteral injury is suspected, a contrast-enhanced helical CT scan with delayed films or bolus infusion IVP with delayed films should be done. If the initial study of delayed films is inconclusive, retrograde pyelography is indicated to delineate a ureteral laceration or avulsion.

REFERENCES

1. McAninch JW: Injuries to the genitourinary tract. In Tanagho EA, McAninch JW (eds): *General Urology.* Norwalk, Conn, Appleton & Lange, 1999.
2. Nicolaisen GS, et al: Renal trauma: Re-evaluation of the indications for radiological assessment. *J Urol* 133:183, 1985.
3. Perry MO, Husmann DA: Urethral injuries in female subjects following pelvic fractures. *J Urol* 147:139, 1992.
4. Corriere JN: Trauma to the lower urinary tract. In Gillenwater JY, et al (eds): *Adult and Pediatric Urology,* 4th ed. Philadelphia, Lippincott Williams & Wilkins, 2002.
5. Sandler CM, Goldman SM, Kawashima A: Lower urinary tract trauma. *World J Urol* 16:69, 1998.
6. Spirnak JP: Pelvic fracture and injury to the lower urinary tract. *Surg Clin North Am* 68:1057, 1988.
7. Cass AS, Luxenberg M: Features of 164 bladder ruptures. *J Urol* 138:743, 1987.
8. Vaccaro JP, Brody JM: CT cystography in the evaluation of major bladder trauma. *Radiographics* 20:1373, 2000.
9. Hochberg E, Stone NN: Bladder rupture associated with pelvic fracture due to blunt trauma. *Urology* 41:531, 1993.
10. Schneider RE: Genitourinary trauma. *Emerg Med Clin North Am* 11:137, 1993.
11. Deck AJ, Shaves S, Talner L, Porter JR: Computerized tomography cystography for the diagnosis of traumatic bladder rupture. *J Urol* 164:43, 2000.
12. Corriere JN Jr, Sandler CM: Mechanisms of injury, patterns of extravasation and management of extraperitoneal bladder rupture due to blunt trauma. *J Urol* 139:43, 1988.
13. Corriere JN Jr, Sandler CM: Bladder rupture from external trauma: Diagnosis and management. *World J Urol* 17:84, 1999.
14. Santucci RA, McAninch JW: Diagnosis and management of renal trauma: Past, present, and future. *J Am Coll Surg* 191:443, 2000.
15. Morey AF, et al: Single shot intraoperative excretory urography for the immediate evaluation of renal trauma. *J Urol* 161:1088, 1999.

16. Mee SL, et al: Radiographic assessment of renal trauma: A ten-year prospective study of patient selection. *J Urol* 141:1095, 1989.
17. Bretan PN, et al: Computerized tomographic staging of renal trauma: 85 consecutive cases. *J Urol* 136:561, 1986.
18. Brown SL, Elder JS, Spirnak JP: Are pediatric patients more susceptible to major renal injury from blunt trauma? A comparative study. *J Urol* 160:138, 1998.
19. Morey AF, Bruce JE, McAninch JW: Efficacy of radiographic imaging in pediatric blunt renal trauma. *J Urol* 156:2014, 1996.
20. Nguyen MM, Das S: Pediatric renal trauma. *Urology* 59:762, 2002.
21. Carroll PR, McAninch JW: Staging of renal trauma. *Urol Clin North Am* 16:193, 1989.
22. Goldman SM, Sandler CM: Upper urinary tract trauma: Current concepts. *World J Urol* 16:62, 1998.
23. Hardeman SW, et al: Blunt urinary tract trauma: Identifying those patients who require radiological diagnostic studies. *J Urol* 138:99, 1987.
24. Cass AS, Luxenberg M: Management of renal artery lesions from external trauma. *J Urol* 138:266, 1987.
25. Tong YC, et al: Use of hematoma size on CT and calculated average bleeding rate as indications for immediate surgical intervention in blunt renal trauma. *J Urol* 147:984, 1992.
26. Campbell EW, Filderman PS, Jacobs SC: Ureteral injury due to blunt and penetrating trauma. *Urology* 40:216, 1992.
27. Rober PE, Smith JB, Pierce JM: Gunshot injuries of the ureter. *J Trauma* 30:83, 1990.
28. McAninch JW, Corriere JN Jr: Renal and ureteral injuries. In Gillenwater JY, et al (eds): *Adult and Pediatric Urology,* 4th ed. Philadelphia, Lippincott Williams & Wilkins, 2002.
29. Brandes SB, et al: Ureteral injuries from penetrating trauma. *J Trauma* 36:766, 1994.
30. Presti JC, Carroll PR, McAninch JW: Ureteral and renal pelvic injuries from external trauma: Diagnostic and management. *J Trauma* 29:370, 1989.
31. Palmer LS, et al: Penetrating ureteral trauma at an urban trauma center: 10-year experience. *Urology* 54:34, 1999.
32. Fournier GR Jr, Laing FC, McAninch JW: Scrotal ultrasonography and the management of testicle trauma. *Urol Clin North Am* 16:377, 1989.
33. Cummings JM, Boullier JA: Scrotal dog bites. *J Urol* 164:57, 2000.

CHAPTER

45 Peripheral Vascular Injury

Edward J. Newton

PERSPECTIVE

Injury to major arteries or veins invariably poses a threat to the viability of the affected limb and even to life. Historically, because of rapid blood loss, injury to major vessels was often quickly fatal in the field. Most patients who survived to reach a hospital had relatively minor limb injuries. However, with the advent of modern Emergency Medical Service systems with advanced extrication methods and rapid transport, more patients with major vascular injury reach the hospital alive.[1] In addition, the incidence of penetrating civilian injuries from interpersonal violence and blunt injuries from motor vehicle–related trauma in the United States has increased dramatically over the past 50 years. Consequently, emergency physicians are frequently confronted with critically ill patients harboring overt or occult vascular injuries. Management of vascular injuries has evolved with advances in diagnostic methods and surgical techniques. Treatment of vascular injuries before and during World War II was simple ligation of the peripheral artery or vein involved. This approach resulted in limb amputation rates ranging from 40% for axillary artery injuries to 72% for popliteal artery injuries. During the Korean War, routine attempts to repair injured arteries decreased the amputation rate for popliteal injuries to 32%.[2] During the Vietnam War, repair of axillary and popliteal artery injuries with routine angiography and improved surgical techniques decreased the amputation rate to as low as 5% and 15%, respectively, which approaches the current rate of amputation for civilian injuries.[2,3] However, extrapolation of high-velocity military wound data to low-velocity civilian gunshot wounds may not be valid, and even lower rates might be expected with civilian wounds.

Tremendous progress has been achieved in diagnostic and therapeutic techniques for dealing with peripheral vascular injuries, and several noninvasive diagnostic modalities have emerged as accurate alternatives to surgical exploration or angiography. These techniques are easily used in the emergency department, and the goal of timely detection and repair of serious vascular injuries is achievable in the vast majority of cases.

Epidemiology

Throughout the world, the etiology of peripheral vascular injuries is divided almost equally between blunt and penetrating mechanisms.[4] In the United States, 70% to 90% of these injuries are due to penetrating wounds.[5,6] Penetrating wounds are particularly common in inner-city urban areas, although the incidence of low-velocity gunshot wounds has decreased over the past several years.[7] Because of the increased use of percutaneous endovascular diagnostic and therapeutic procedures, the incidence of iatrogenic vascular injuries has increased and accounts for up to a third of all cases in some series.[8] Major venous injuries are present in 13% to 51% of cases, but more than 80% are associated with arterial injury as well.[9] Approximately 90% of patients with vascular injury are male, and most are younger than 40 years.[5]

PRINCIPLES OF DISEASE

Pathophysiology

Blunt and penetrating types of trauma result in a similar spectrum of vascular injuries, although the mechanisms of injury differ. Even though blunt vascular injuries are less common than penetrating injuries, they are often more severe and more commonly require amputation because of associated injuries to nerves, bone, and soft tissue. Certain mechanisms of injury, such as close-range shotgun wounds and animal bites that crush and lacerate vessels, routinely combine penetrating and blunt mechanisms.

Penetrating Trauma

Penetrating trauma from gunshot wounds results in the formation of a temporary cavity within distensible soft tissues with almost immediate recoil of these tissues. The size of the cavity and hence the degree of soft tissue injury depend directly on the velocity of the missile, as well as the tumble and yaw of the bullet. Consequently, gunshot wounds can cause direct arterial laceration or transection in addition to vascular injury at some distance from the track of the bullet. The latter injuries tend to be tears in the intima of an artery with subsequent thrombosis that may not become apparent for hours to months after the injury.

Stab wounds can cause vascular injury by complete or partial transection of vessels. Partial laceration of an artery may produce few symptoms of arterial insufficiency on initial evaluation but commonly results in delayed complications. The vascular structures at risk can be predicted more reliably with stab wounds than with gunshot wounds by taking into consideration the anatomic location, the depth and direction of the wound, and the implement involved.

Shotgun wounds are less common than gunshot or stab wounds and cause injuries varying from minor soft tissue wounds to massive destruction of soft tissue and bone, depending primarily on the range from which the shotgun was fired. The presence of multiple missiles ranging from 9 or 10 (buckshot) to dozens (birdshot) also complicates the evaluation of these injuries because of the many potential sites for vascular injury to occur. In addition, close-range shotgun wounds can cause significant blunt trauma to blood vessels, as well as a higher rate of bone and nerve injury than occurs with gunshot wounds. Migration of pellets proximally through the venous system to the heart or migration through an artery with subsequent distal occlusion has been reported frequently as a delayed complication.

Blunt Trauma

Blunt injury involves avulsion forces that can stretch vessels beyond their capacity or direct crushing injury that disrupts the vessel wall. Fracture fragments resulting from blunt extremity trauma can lacerate or entrap vessels. Vascular injury can range from small intimal tears to complete avulsion of arteries and nerves. Open avulsion injury of a limb is particularly severe because the skin is the final structure to tear, and once such tearing occurs, it is inevitable that vessels and nerves will be torn as well.[10] Vascular injury must also be suspected in patients with massive soft tissue avulsion or crush injury, displaced long bone fractures, electrical or lightning injuries, and severe burns, as well as in those with compartment syndrome from trauma or prolonged immobilization as a result of stroke, coma, drug overdose, or other causes.[11-13] Dog bites that are inflicted by large animals, such as those used by law enforcement, are particularly prone to the development of arterial injury and wound complications.[11,12] Collateral circulation may continue to perfuse the limb adequately, but injuries that occur proximal to the collateral branch point or that involve both the main trunk and collateral branches will preclude adequate flow.

Distal ischemia results from the inability of tissues to continue aerobic metabolism. Eventually, anaerobic metabolism consumes all substrate, thereby resulting in the accumulation of lactic acid. As ischemia progresses, cellular integrity is lost and irreversible cell death occurs. A vicious cycle of tissue edema and further impairment of the blood supply occurs.

When no specific measures are taken to cool the limb, it is said that the limb is undergoing "warm ischemia" at room temperature. Although individuals may vary, 6 hours of complete warm ischemia is generally considered the point at which irreversible nerve and muscle damage begins to occur. After 6 hours of warm ischemia, 10% of patients will have irreversible damage; by 12 hours, 90% will. Artificially cooling the limb to just higher than freezing temperature will reduce the metabolic demands of unperfused tissues and greatly prolong the tissue's tolerance of ischemia.

Two main types of vascular injury can result from trauma: *occlusive injury* (transection, thrombosis, and reversible spasm), in which all effective perfusion distal to the occlusion is lost, and *nonocclusive injury* (intimal flap, arteriovenous fistula [AVF], and pseudoaneurysm), in which some arterial flow continues past the injury.

Complete Occlusive Injury

Transection
The most common vascular injury is complete transection in which distal flow is effectively eliminated. Cleanly transected arteries will often retract and undergo spasm so that blood loss is minimized. With longitudinal arterial lacerations and venous injuries, blood loss cannot be limited by this means, and such injuries tend to result in greater blood loss. Pulsatile bleeding may lead to exsanguinating hemorrhage and shock.

Thrombosis
Intraluminal thrombosis (Figure 45-1) may occur in an injured artery acutely (within 24 hours) or may be

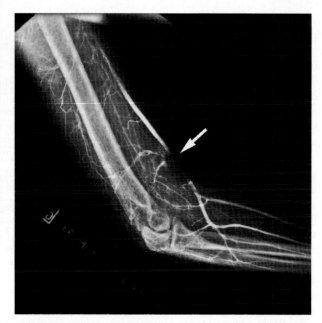

Figure 45-1. Complete thrombosis of the distal brachial artery after reduction of a posterior elbow dislocation. (Courtesy of D. Demetreades, MD.)

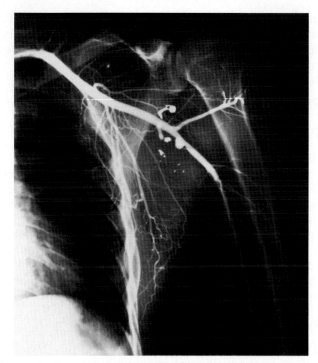

Figure 45-2. Multiple small pseudoaneurysms of the axillary artery after penetrating injury. (Courtesy of D. Demetreades, MD.)

delayed for many months. Acute thrombosis is initiated by stasis resulting from compression of the artery or from a disruption in the intima of an artery that becomes a nidus for thrombus formation. As the thrombus propagates, complete occlusion of the vessel can occur. Delayed thrombosis can occur months to years after injury if the injured vessel heals with stricture formation and decreased blood flow distally, followed by stasis and clot formation.

Reversible Arterial Spasm

The precise cause and incidence of significant reversible arterial spasm after trauma are unknown. In many cases the spasm occurs at some distance from the site of traumatic injury. In response to a traumatic stimulus, segmental narrowing of an artery may occlude the artery and produce distal ischemia. The spasm usually reverses with conservative treatment (topical warm saline or topical nitroglycerin paste), but prolonged spasm may require infusion of vasodilators such as nitroglycerin, lidocaine, or saline.[14] In many series, segmental arterial spasm is the most common arteriographic finding. However, it should never be assumed on clinical grounds that symptoms of ischemia are due to arterial spasm; that diagnosis is based on arteriographic results only.

Nonocclusive Injuries

Intimal Flap

An intimal flap occurs when there is a break in the intima of a vessel, generally from excessive stretch or concussive forces. Although flow is not altered by small flaps and the associated soft tissue wounds often appear benign initially, these intimal flaps may become a nidus for thrombosis that can occur hours to months after the initial injury. However, most intimal flaps heal spontaneously, and asymptomatic injuries that do not disrupt perfusion of the limb can be treated conservatively.

Pseudoaneurysm

A true aneurysm contains all three layers of the vessel wall (intima, media, and adventitia) and rarely is caused by trauma. A pseudoaneurysm is formed when hemorrhage from a vessel is contained by surrounding fascia and the resulting hematoma is gradually encased by a capsule of fibrous tissue, analogous in consistency to the adventitia of a normal vessel (Figure 45-2). Because it is relatively thin walled, rupture of a pseudoaneurysm is a distinct possibility. In addition, because its diameter inevitably expands under arterial pressure over days to months, compression of adjacent tissue may result in neuropathy, venous obstruction with resultant peripheral edema and venous thrombosis, and even erosion into adjacent bone. The cavity of a pseudoaneurysm is in direct communication with the lumen of the vessel, so embolization of mural clots may produce distal arterial occlusion. Patients with pseudoaneurysm are commonly seen months to years later with symptoms of compression neuropathy or peripheral arterial embolism or for investigation of a soft tissue "tumor" that represents the growing aneurysm.

Arteriovenous Fistula

An AVF is formed when both the artery and an adjacent vein are injured. Higher-pressure arterial flow is directed into the lower-pressure vein, thereby diverting the blood supply to distal tissues and engorging the distal veins. Because the aperture of the fistula is often relatively narrow and thus results in turbulent flow, a bruit and palpable thrill are common diagnostic findings. Symptoms are primarily those of distal ischemia, but rarely, high-output congestive heart failure may occur when large central vessels are involved. Symptoms are often delayed for months because it takes time for the fistula to mature.

Compartment Syndrome

Compartment syndrome is most common after crush injury or a long bone fracture but may also be seen after reperfusion of an ischemic limb. Initially, blood flow is diminished and the injury can be considered nonocclusive. Smaller-caliber vessels are compressed first whereas larger vessels remain relatively patent, so pulses may be palpable until late in the course. If allowed to progress, however, all blood flow may end and the injury is then an occlusive one. Progressive edema elevates tissue pressure above capillary pressure, thus ending arterial flow and initiating a cascade of events that results in compartment syndrome. The risk for this complication is increased when ischemia time is prolonged, in the presence of combined arterial and venous injury, after ligation or repair of a major artery or vein, or in the presence of significant soft tissue injury.[5] After restoration of arterial flow to a previously ischemic limb, a cascade of reperfusion injury has been identified that results from release of oxygen free radicals, lipid peroxidation, and influx of intracellular calcium. These mediators give rise to progressive cellular damage, edema, and necrosis, thereby propagating the vicious cycle that increases compartment pressure.[15] Consequently, frequent reexamination of the limb is indicated to assess compartment pressure after arterial repair.

CLINICAL FEATURES

Detection and treatment of vascular injuries must take place within the context of the overall resuscitation of the patient according to established principles of trauma care.[16] If the source of bleeding is readily identifiable, it is compressed with digital pressure. Once control of active bleeding has been achieved in this manner, detection and treatment of other life-threatening injuries can proceed. Peripheral vascular injury can occur coincident with nonvascular life-threatening trauma, which takes higher priority in resuscitating the patient. In other cases, peripheral vascular injury may be the most serious or only injury, and evaluation and management of these injuries can proceed directly. Despite rapid transport to a hospital through a modern Emergency Medical Service, injury to large central arteries and veins is still often fatal, and many of these deaths occur before medical contact. Patients who survive to reach the hospital may have obvious exsanguinating hemorrhage or only very subtle signs of vascular injury. Many patients have no evidence of injury but are considered at risk for vascular injury because of penetrating wounds in close proximity to major neurovascular bundles or because they have sustained high-risk injuries such as posterior knee dislocation. Patients who remain hypotensive after an initial fluid challenge may harbor an occult vascular injury if no other cause is found. In addition, patients with symptoms of intermittent claudication or with unexplained peripheral embolization and a history of previous trauma to the limb should be suspected of having occult arterial injury.

Peripheral vascular injury can be divided into three categories by physical examination: hard findings, soft findings, and asymptomatic high-risk wounds based on the mechanism of injury.

Hard Findings of Vascular Injury

Most patients have the classic "hard" findings of arterial injury, including pulsatile bleeding, an audible bruit or palpable thrill indicative of an AVF, an expanding or pulsatile hematoma, or any combination of the "five P's" of arterial insufficiency: pain on passive extension of the muscle compartment involved, pulselessness, paresthesias, pallor, and paralysis. In addition, cyanosis and decreased temperature are common in a poorly perfused extremity, and massive distention of distal superficial veins may indicate an AVF as arterial flow is directed into distensible veins. The incidence of arterial injury in patients with any hard finding is consistently greater than 90%,[17] and the presence of these findings requires either further investigation by emergency angiography or immediate surgical intervention, depending on the duration of warm ischemia and the overall status of the patient.

Soft Findings of Vascular Injury

An additional group of patients have "soft findings" of vascular injury, including a palpable but diminished pulse in comparison to the uninjured extremity, isolated peripheral nerve injury, or a large nonpulsatile hematoma.[18] The significance of prolonged capillary refill is controversial; some experts find it to be a reliable sign of vascular injury (when combined with a pulse deficit) and consider delayed capillary refill to be a valid soft sign of vascular injury. Others have found this sign to be a nonspecific and unreliable predictor of arterial injury.[2,5] Delayed capillary refill in itself is insufficient to diagnose arterial injury but, in combination with other physical signs, supports the diagnosis.

Isolated penetrating injury to a peripheral nerve is commonly associated with vascular injury because of the close proximity of these structures within the neurovascular bundles. Vascular injury occurs in 8% to 45% of cases of penetrating peripheral nerve injury.[19] Conversely, vascular injuries have associated peripheral nerve injury in almost half the cases.[20] It is sometimes difficult to distinguish whether the pain, paresthesias, or paralysis is due to a primary nerve injury or to an associated vascular injury or compartment syndrome. In general, primary nerve injury occurs immediately at the time of injury, whereas vascular neuropathy occurs over minutes to hours after the injury.[21] Up to 35% of patients with "soft" findings of vascular injury have positive angiographic studies, although only a small proportion of these injuries require emergency repair.[17]

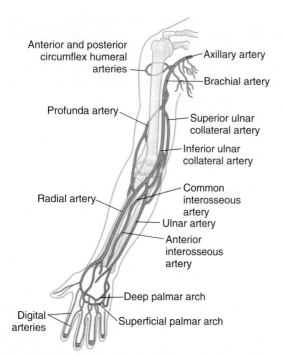

Figure 45-3. Major arteries of the upper limb. (From Snell R, Smith M [eds]: *Clinical Anatomy for Emergency Medicine.* St Louis, CV Mosby, 1993.)

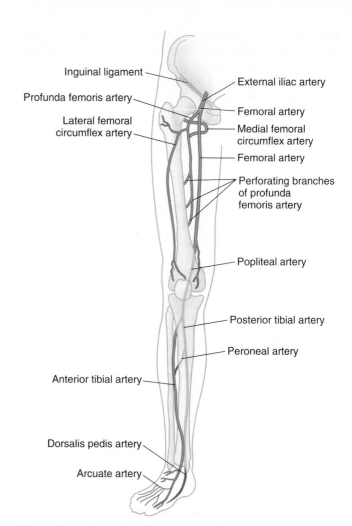

Figure 45-4. Major arteries of the lower limb. (From Snell R, Smith M [eds]: *Clinical Anatomy for Emergency Medicine.* St Louis, CV Mosby, 1993.)

High-Risk Injuries

The proximity of a penetrating wound to a neurovascular bundle is defined imprecisely. Various definitions include 1 cm, 1 inch, or 5 cm as constituting "proximity." Certainly, penetrating wounds that occur within 1 cm of a major neurovascular bundle or whose presumed trajectory has crossed such a bundle ("proximity wounds") are more likely to produce an occult vascular injury. Major neurovascular bundles include large limb arteries proximal to critical branch points, such as the axillary, brachial, common femoral, and popliteal arteries (Figures 45-3 and 45-4).[22] In addition, a substantial minority of patients with high-risk injuries, such as bites from large dogs or other animals, severely displaced fractures, crush injuries, or major joint dislocations (especially knee dislocation), will initially have occult vascular injury that is not detected by physical examination. The risk of missing such injuries is that the traditional 6-hour window of "warm ischemia time" will be exceeded or the patient will experience delayed complications resulting in loss of the limb. For example, patients with intimal flaps may be completely asymptomatic initially but can subsequently be subject to arterial thrombosis. Similarly, pseudoaneurysms progressively enlarge to produce compression of adjacent structures but may be very small and undetectable on initial physical examination. Consequently, many centers routinely perform some ancillary confirmation of arterial patency in these cases.

History

In patients who achieve and maintain hemodynamic stability, a more comprehensive history can be obtained. Important historical points to note include the exact time and mechanism of the injury. The time of injury is important because of the limitations of warm ischemia time noted earlier. The mechanism is of clinical and often forensic importance in that the injury is frequently inflicted during an assault or other violent crime, in the context of domestic violence or physical abuse, or in association with work. Various mechanisms of injury may mandate special reporting and may alter the patient's ultimate disposition. Certain types of injuries, such as crush or bite wounds, are particularly prone to complications. The occupation, avocation, and hand dominance of the patient are pertinent because a more aggressive strategy may be indicated in certain cases. Medical conditions that pose a risk of complications are important to note. Patients who are immunocompromised because of diabetes, acquired immunodeficiency syndrome, asplenia, cancer, or steroid use are at increased risk for infection and impaired wound healing. Patients with previous vascular insufficiency have more tenuous perfusion, are more susceptible to ischemia from elevated compartment pressure, and have a higher incidence of complications.[23] As with most aspects of trauma care, patients whose sensorium is altered by head injury or intoxication, patients with spinal cord injury who cannot perceive pain, and those with significant painful distracting injuries will not reliably be able to report pain or paresthesias suggesting vascular insufficiency, so extra caution must be exercised in these cases.

Physical Examination

Physical examination is directed at discovering evidence of local wound complications and distal ischemia suggestive of vascular injury. Palpation of pulses in the affected extremities is the initial step. A comparison of the strength and quality of the pulses between the injured limb and its uninjured counterpart is then made. Isolated detection of a pulse deficit distal to the site of injury is a finding that merits further investigation rather than immediate surgery because palpation of pulses is a relatively inaccurate means of predicting arterial injury. False-positive findings of a pulse deficit may occur because of shock, in which all pulses are diminished, congenital absence of a pulse in one extremity, preexisting vascular disease, or arterial spasm. A false-positive finding of a pulse deficit occurs in 10% to 27% of cases.[5,17] False-negative findings can occur with transmission of the pulse through a "soft clot," past an intimal flap, or through collateral circulation. Distal pulses can persist in 6% to 42% of patients despite significant arterial injury.[24] Compression of an artery by casts, splints, or dressings may produce a pulseless extremity, and these should be removed if evidence of ischemia occurs.[25] Finally, even though the pulse may be absent, the limb may be well perfused by collateral arterial supply, thus making repair of the arterial injury less compelling. Simultaneous palpation of the injured and unaffected limb can detect relatively small differences in skin temperature that may suggest hypoperfusion. Testing two-point discrimination on the injured and unaffected limbs is similarly an effective means of detecting sensory deficits. Auscultation over the site of injury is an often-ignored examination that may reveal a bruit suggestive of an AVF. A bruit is audible in more than half of patients with an AVF.[26] Repeated examination of the hematoma adjacent to the wound is indicated to determine whether it is expanding or pulsatile.

Despite the limitations just noted, reliance on the history and physical examination to triage patients into immediate surgery, angiography, and observation groups has been found to be relatively dependable, with a sensitivity of 92% and a specificity of 95%.[17]

DIAGNOSTIC STRATEGIES

The diagnostic strategy for detection of peripheral vascular injury must be tailored to the clinical situation. Patients with clearly evident major arterial injury (e.g., pulsatile hemorrhage from a penetrating wound with a cold, pulseless distal end of the extremity) may require emergency operative intervention without the benefit of any ancillary confirmation of their injury. At times, the use of an intraoperative angiogram may be helpful

in delineating the exact location and nature of the injury in patients taken directly to the operating room. However, delaying definitive treatment of an obvious arterial injury that is approaching the 6-hour limit of warm ischemia time to obtain an arteriogram is ill advised.

Plain Radiography

Plain radiographs of the affected extremity are indicated to detect fractures, joint penetration, and foreign bodies. With gunshot wounds, the sum of the number of intact bullets seen on x-ray and the number of wounds in the body must be an even number. Failure to locate a bullet can result in unexpected complications. Rarely, bullets or shotgun pellets can migrate distally and produce vascular occlusion or migrate proximally through the venous system to the heart. These emboli are readily detected on plain radiographs.[27,28] Lead bullets retained within a synovial joint can result in systemic absorption and elevated lead levels and should be removed electively.[29]

Pulse Oximetry

Several relatively simple, noninvasive maneuvers can be performed at the bedside to elicit evidence of arterial injury. The use of pulse oximetry has been suggested as a means of identifying limb ischemia after trauma, but its utility in this setting has not been well studied. Clearly, in the absence of a pulse, no reading can be obtained. As the technology of transcutaneous measurement of physiologic indices advances, measurement of tissue oxygenation by near-infrared spectroscopy to quantify muscle oxyhemoglobin may prove more useful in detecting vascular injury.[30,31]

Hand-Held Doppler

An inability to palpate pulses in an injured extremity should be verified by auscultation with a hand-held Doppler unit. Apart from the absence of any signal, arterial injury may be suggested by a change in the usual triphasic quality of the Doppler pulse to a biphasic or monophasic waveform as the pulse is "damped" by partial occlusion. Though more sensitive, auscultation of the pulse by Doppler is subject to the same types of limitations as is palpation of the pulse.

Ankle-Brachial Index and Arterial Pressure Index

Determination of the ankle-brachial index (ABI) or the arterial pressure index (API) has been well studied and provides somewhat more accurate information than does physical examination alone. Systolic pressure is measured by inflating a standard blood pressure cuff proximal to the injury and recording hand-held Doppler systolic pressure distal to the injury. The process is repeated on the uninjured limb, and a ratio of injured to uninjured systolic pressure is calculated (API). Generally, a ratio less than 0.90 is considered abnormal and is an indication for further investigation. Unfortunately, there is no consensus on the appropriate cutoff ratio to consider abnormal, and figures ranging from 0.85 to 0.99 are cited in various studies.[2,5,32-34] If an API less than 0.90 is used as the cutoff, sensitivity decreases slightly but specificity increases. In one series a cutoff of 0.90 resulted in a false-negative rate of almost 40%. In other studies, an API less than 0.90 yielded a sensitivity of 95%, specificity of 97%, positive predictive value of 100%, and negative predictive value of 96%.[34-36] Using an API cutoff of less than 1 produced a sensitivity of 96% to 100% but included many false-positive results.[33,34] Still, the use of an API ratio less than 0.90 can eliminate a large number of unnecessary angiograms for proximity wounds and increase the diagnostic efficiency of angiography by limiting its use to high-yield cases. Limiting angiography to patients with either an abnormal physical examination (primarily a pulse deficit) or an API less than 0.90 appears to be an effective and safe strategy for detecting arterial injury.[37,38]

Patients with an API of 0.90 to 0.99 merit observation for 12 to 24 hours for repeated physical examination and API measurements to detect evolving injury.

Exclusive reliance on API to screen for arterial injury has significant limitations. Comparisons cannot be made when both limbs are injured or when severe soft tissue mangling precludes placing a blood pressure tourniquet or locating the artery to be measured with the Doppler unit.[39] As with physical examination, the sensitivity of API is limited when an intimal flap allows near-normal flow or when collateral circulation is sufficient to produce near-normal systolic pressure, as in proximal injuries to the subclavian or iliac vessels. Certain arteries (e.g., the profunda femoris, profunda brachii, and peroneal arteries) normally do not produce palpable pulses, and API is of limited utility in these injuries. Shotgun wounds often have normal APIs despite multiple small arterial wounds; angiography is the preferred diagnostic modality in this group. As with angiography, API cannot detect venous injuries.

In spite of the limitations just noted, API has proved effective in screening patients with proximity wounds. The vast majority of injuries missed by API heal spontaneously. Those that do not heal are generally seen within 3 months with hard signs of arterial injury.

Ultrasound

The development of relatively small portable ultrasound (US) units has made possible direct visualization of both arterial and venous flow in major vessels. There are several different types of US that can detect vascular injury, and newer, more accurate techniques are being developed rapidly. B-mode (real-time) ultrasound is the most readily available form of US in portable units. It can easily visualize arterial pulsation in major vessels. Loss of pulsation distal to an obstruction or thrombosis is readily apparent. However, B-mode US cannot visualize certain anatomic areas accurately (subclavian and iliac vessels) because of overlying gas and is unreliable in detecting a fresh, relatively nonechogenic thrombosis or hematoma. As blood liquefies within a hematoma, it becomes echolu-

cent and more readily distinguishable from surrounding tissues.

Doppler US interprets sound moving toward or away from the transducer as flow. Venous flow is heard as a low-pitched hum, whereas arterial flow has a higher-pitched triphasic quality. The combination of B-mode and Doppler US is called duplex US and has enhanced accuracy in examining blood vessels. Duplex scans showing a focal increase in peak systolic velocity suggest partial obstruction of the vessel. However, duplex scanning is slightly less accurate in detecting injuries that do not decrease flow, such as small pseudoaneurysms, AVF, and intimal flaps,[32] and it is technically limited in examining certain anatomic areas such as the profunda femoris and profunda brachii arteries and the iliac and subclavian vessels. Duplex US findings may be subtle, and as with other applications of US, its accuracy is highly operator dependent. Despite these limitations, the sensitivity of duplex US in comparison to angiography ranges from 83% to 100%, with a specificity of 99% to 100% and an accuracy of 96% to 100%.[39-44]

Color flow Doppler converts Doppler echoes into quantitated visual signals. Flow toward the transducer is seen as red, and flow away from the transducer is seen as blue. The intensity of the color (the number of pixels on the screen) is proportional to flow through the vessel. Small prospective studies have indicated a high rate of accuracy in detecting arterial injury.[42] Absence of flow is readily apparent, but more subtle injuries, such as intimal flaps and small pseudoaneurysms, are more difficult to identify.[39] In addition, color flow Doppler is more accurate than standard venography in detecting major venous injuries.[45] The overall sensitivity of color flow Doppler in detecting arterial injury is 50% to 90%, with a specificity of 95% to 99%. The sensitivity for detecting injuries requiring surgical repair is significantly higher.

The use of intravascular US for examination of abdominal aortic aneurysms has been well documented. Though not yet applicable to smaller peripheral vessels, with further reduction in size of the transducers, this technique may eventually be applicable for peripheral vascular injury as well.

Computed Tomography and Magnetic Resonance Imaging

Computed tomography with contrast enhancement has had limited utility in the past, but newer-generation helical computed tomographic angiography scans have proved accurate in several small series, with 100% accuracy when compared with angiography or surgical exploration.[46-48] Magnetic resonance angiography has also been described and is highly accurate, but it has yet to prove clinically useful.[49,50]

Arteriography

The policy of routinely exploring proximity wounds greatly improved the preservation of injured limbs in World War II. With the advent of arteriography, it became apparent that many negative wound explorations could be avoided with routine arteriography. In a study using routine arteriography, the negative surgical exploration rate in patients with "soft signs" of arterial injury or with proximity wounds fell from 84% to 2%.[51] As a result, until recently standard contrast angiography has been the gold standard for diagnosing peripheral arterial injury.

Beginning in the 1980s, the number of civilian penetrating wounds increased tremendously. Because of high cost, limited availability at all hours, and poor reimbursement rates, the policy of routine arteriography for proximity wounds has been questioned. From a practical perspective, the time required to mobilize the angiography team and perform the study may be several hours, thus making this option less desirable when dealing with the time limitations posed by arterial injury. In addition, arteriography has a small, but measurable complication rate, including allergic reactions to contrast media, renal complications, hematoma formation, and false aneurysm formation at the site of cannulation. Finally, the clinical utility of the information provided by arteriography has become increasingly suspect as more of these injuries are being managed expectantly in recent years. Routine "exclusion" arteriography for proximity wounds detects unsuspected arterial injury in 0% to 21% of cases.[18,51,52] However, relatively few of these patients require emergency surgery. In a series of 284 patients who underwent routine angiography for proximity wounds, 17% had unsuspected arterial injury detected, but only 1.8% (5 patients) required emergency surgical repair.[53] In other series reporting on a total of 483 patients who underwent angiography for proximity wounds, only one arterial injury that required emergency repair was discovered.[51-55] In the presence of "soft signs" of injury, the yield for angiograms increases to 29% to 35%, but many of these injuries do not require emergency repair and can be detected by noninvasive means.[53] In addition, angiography results in an approximately 5% false-positive and false-negative rate when compared with surgical exploration. Many of the injuries detected on angiography are due to reversible vasospasm or very small intimal defects that generally heal spontaneously. Consequently, angiography for proximity wounds can detect injury in up to 21% of cases but results in acute surgical intervention in only 0% to 4.4% of cases.[6,32,33,51] Many centers now successfully manage proximity wounds by repeated physical examination over a 24-hour period and reserve angiography for those with abnormal physical findings or an ABI less than 0.9.[33,52,53] Angiography is also limited in that it cannot detect major venous injuries, which are increasingly being repaired surgically. The use of angiography is difficult in children because of the small caliber of their vessels and a propensity for vasospasm induced by angiography. Consequently, physical examination and noninvasive methods are preferred for detection of vascular injury in young children.[54,56]

Digital subtraction angiography (DSA) has been used for detecting vascular injuries as well. DSA has been found to be more accurate than standard angiography for detection of extravasation and has the advantage of requiring the administration of a smaller load of contrast material. However, the field of view is much smaller with DSA than with standard angiography, thus making it technically difficult to study the entire course of a limb artery with DSA. Standard angiography is also more accurate than DSA in detecting intimal flaps and dissection.

Emergency center angiography involves the administration of intra-arterial contrast in a single bolus with a single radiograph as a rapid bedside alternative to formal angiography. Although technical difficulties occasionally limit its usefulness, accuracy approaching that of formal angiography can be achieved.[57,58]

TREATMENT

Initial treatment is directed at ensuring a patent airway and adequate air exchange before assessing the circulation. Once this is accomplished, active hemorrhage is controlled by direct digital pressure. Blind clamping of a bleeding vessel is not recommended because of the risk of crushing adjacent nerves. The use of tourniquets is similarly discouraged because occlusion of veins results in increased compartment pressure and an increased risk for venous thrombosis.[5] In cases in which proximal and distal control cannot be readily achieved in the emergency department, insertion of a Foley catheter into the wound and inflation of the balloon with sterile water can temporarily tamponade the bleeding. Intravenous lines should not be started in the injured extremity because they may be ineffective in delivering resuscitation fluid and because extravasation from an injured vein may increase compartment pressure. Serial hemoglobin determinations may indicate unexpected blood loss from occult vascular injury. Patients with significant blood loss should have blood typed and crossmatched and may require immediate transfusion for stabilization. Patients with significant vascular injury often remain hypotensive despite such infusion and require further volume infusion or blood transfusion. Moribund patients with multiple severe injuries may require urgent amputation as part of their overall stabilization or extrication from wrecked automobiles. Between 50% and 70% of patients with severely mangled limbs require urgent amputation, especially if they have multisystem trauma.

The issue of "hypotensive resuscitation" is controversial with major vascular injuries. A tenuous clot can form in injured arteries and prevent further blood loss as long as the patient remains hypotensive. Once arterial pressure reaches a critical, but variable point, the clot may be expelled and massive blood loss can ensue. Therefore, when the arterial injury is inaccessible for occlusion by direct pressure, the target blood pressure for resuscitation should be lowered to a systolic pressure of approximately 90 mm Hg. Overly aggressive and rapid fluid administration in the field or in the emergency department can produce transient intravascular hypervolemia and may ultimately increase the rate of blood loss. Close monitoring of vital signs and the total volume of fluid infused is indicated in these situations.

Once a vascular injury is identified, a specific diagnostic and therapeutic strategy can be developed that is consistent with the severity of the injury, the presence of other injuries, and the resources available.

Major Vascular Injuries

Major vascular injuries that compromise the viability of a limb must be repaired within 6 hours to avoid irreversible ischemic neuropathy and myonecrosis.[5] If other life-threatening injuries must be repaired first, a temporary polytetrafluoroethylene (PTFE) vascular shunt can be placed in the operating room to restore perfusion to a limb.[59] These temporary PTFE shunts can be left in place for up to 24 hours before thrombosis begins to occur within the shunt. Major arterial transection or thrombosis is ideally repaired by end-to-end reanastomosis if possible without placing undue tension on the suture line. If a larger segment of the artery is destroyed, interposition of a reverse saphenous vein graft is the preferred technique. PTFE grafts are suitable for grafting larger arteries if necessary, but they tend to occlude when used in smaller arteries (e.g., distal to the femoral or brachial arteries). Before completing the reanastomosis, a Fogarty catheter is passed through both ends of the repair to extract any thrombi that may have formed. The distal circulation is flushed with a dilute 1:10 solution of heparin or enoxaparin to prevent early clot formation.[60] Systemic administration of heparin is usually contraindicated in major trauma patients. Pretreatment with mannitol has been shown to reduce compartment pressure and may decrease the risk for compartment syndrome if given preoperatively.[15] Assessment of distal perfusion and, in particular, compartment pressures is indicated frequently after repair and reperfusion of the limb. The use of broad-spectrum antibiotics such as a first-generation cephalosporin is recommended before commencing a vascular repair. A course of hyperbaric oxygen therapy has been shown to increase the rate of primary wound healing in patients with severe crush injuries, but it is not standard clinical practice.[61]

Apart from excision of the affected arterial segment and repair of the vessel, less invasive techniques have been developed to manage pseudoaneurysms. Percutaneous embolization with Silastic beads, gel clot emboli, or thrombogenic coils is often successful.[19,62] Placement of an endovascular sleeve can exclude the aneurysm and is also a successful alternative to open repair.[63] Similarly, repair of an AVF can be undertaken through open surgical ligation of the fistulous connection, by endovascular placement of a sleeve to exclude the fistula, or by percutaneous embolization of the fistulous tract.[62]

Late Complications

Despite timely optimal repair of arterial injuries, approximately 21% of patients experience delayed complications requiring further surgical intervention, even including delayed amputation. The most common of such complications is delayed thrombosis, which often occurs after many months as stenosis at the repair site progresses. Other complications include intermittent claudication, chronic pain or edema of the limb, and aneurysm formation in the graft.[64]

Venous Injuries

Venous injuries may be primarily ligated if the condition of the patient cannot tolerate prolongation of surgery. However, the current trend is to repair major venous injuries if possible, particularly in the lower extremity, because wound healing is improved and the incidence of compartment syndrome, venous thrombosis, pulmonary embolism, and chronic edema is decreased.[65] Extensive venous collaterals in the upper extremity make surgical repair less compelling.

The timing of repair of a vascular injury when associated with complex fractures requiring fixation is controversial. Historically, the fracture was repaired first to give a more accurate measurement of limb length and the length of graft required for vascular repair and because of fear that manipulation of long bones during reduction might damage the vascular repair. However, the need for postoperative fasciotomy is higher in these patients than in those who undergo vascular repair first (80% versus 36%).[66] Currently in most centers, vascular repair is prioritized over orthopedic repair.

Minor Vascular Injuries

Increasingly, minor, nonocclusive vascular injuries are being treated expectantly. Criteria for observation of vascular injuries include low-velocity missile wounds, intact distal circulation, absence of active hemorrhage, and minimal arterial wall disruption on angiography if performed. Angiographic findings meeting these criteria include intimal flaps extending less than 5 mm and pseudoaneurysms smaller than 5 mm in diameter.[5] Follow-up of these injuries with repeat angiography or US reveals that approximately 85% resolve spontaneously.[53] Patients meeting these criteria can be monitored as outpatients for 3 months with repeat physical examination and US to detect delayed complications. Some authors suggest caution with this policy because of multiple cases in which conservative treatment failed after prolonged delay.[67] Others have reported large series demonstrating the safety of this approach.[18,53,68,69] However, almost all pseudoaneurysms ultimately require repair and, once discovered, should be repaired electively. Failure to detect and repair occult arterial injuries in children often results in severe differential limb growth, and thus a more aggressive policy of repairing any arterial injury that causes even a relatively minor decrease in blood flow to a child's growing limb may be justified.

SPECIFIC INJURIES

Upper Extremity

Subclavian Artery and Vein

Subclavian artery injuries represent 1% to 2% of all vascular trauma.[70] Isolated injury to the subclavian vein is more common than isolated arterial injury, but in almost half the cases both the vein and artery are injured.[71] The vast majority (95% to 99%) are penetrating wounds, and because of massive hemorrhage, these injuries are often lethal before arrival at a hospital. Mortality in those who reach the hospital alive averages 15%, but overall mortality as high as 75% has been reported.[72,73] The right subclavian artery arises from the brachiocephalic artery, the left from the arch of the aorta. From their origin, they course posterior and inferior to the clavicles to the outer margins of the first ribs, where they become the axillary artery and vein. The left subclavian rises higher than the right and extends into the root of the neck.[22]

The clinical manifestation is that of hemorrhagic shock in 77% of cases. Occasionally, unsuspected subclavian vascular injury is discovered at thoracotomy for excessive blood loss from a chest tube.[71] Approximately 60% have an associated pneumothorax or hemothorax, and additional injury to mediastinal and spinal structures is relatively common.[70] Symptoms of limb ischemia may be apparent with absent radial and brachial pulses. However, pulses are completely absent in only 33% of cases because collateral flow from the thyrocervical trunk may provide sufficient perfusion to avoid the symptoms and signs of ischemia.[71] Neurologic deficits in the upper extremity occur in more than half the patients. The most severe of these injuries is disruption of the brachial plexus, which occurs in almost 50% of patients.[71]

In a series of 100 cases of subclavian artery injury, the combination of physical examination and chest x-ray findings suggestive of subclavian injury (hemothorax, pneumothorax, apical pleural cap, or wide mediastinum) was 100% sensitive and could have eliminated the need for 69% of the arteriograms obtained.[72] If the patient's clinical condition permits, angiography can provide an accurate diagnosis and can locate the injury precisely. APIs are relatively inaccurate with proximal thoracic outlet injuries because of collateral arterial flow. US techniques are also relatively inaccurate in detecting subclavian injuries because of interference by overlying gas-filled lung tissue. Therefore, in cases in which the clinical diagnosis is equivocal ("soft signs" of injury or proximity wounds), arteriography is required to detect the injury. Immediate proximal and distal control of the subclavian artery is very difficult. An incision along the course of the clavicle is recommended but often needs to be extended to a sternotomy.[74] If primary reanastomosis is not possible, synthetic grafts are usually successful.

Blunt subclavian injuries are often associated with clavicular fracture or dislocation. Isolated first rib fracture is rarely combined with vascular injury unless posterior displacement has occurred. However, first rib fracture in association with other major injuries, a wide mediastinum on chest x-ray, an expanding hematoma, an upper extremity pulse deficit, or a brachial plexus injury is accompanied by arterial injury in 24% of cases and merits investigation by angiography.[75] Several cases of shear injury of the subclavian artery have been reported to result from a loose shoulder restraint of a seat belt during a motor vehicle accident. Overall, blunt subclavian artery injuries are more severe than penetrating injuries because of higher rates of mortality, limb amputation, and associated brachial plexus injury.[70]

Subclavian vein injuries are even more lethal than those to the artery. In addition to massive blood loss, there is a relatively high risk of massive air embolism, which is frequently fatal in association with penetrating subclavian vein injuries.

Axillary Artery and Vein

Injury to the axillary vessels constitutes 3% to 9% of all vascular injuries and is divided nearly equally between penetrating and blunt mechanisms.[3] Forceful reduction of a chronically dislocated shoulder is a common iatrogenic cause of axillary artery injury. The axillary artery courses from the lateral border of the first rib to the inferior border of the teres major muscle, where it becomes the brachial artery. The axillary vein runs medial to the artery. The extensive anastomotic arterial connections around the shoulder joint usually permit good collateral flow,[22,71] and up to half of these patients will have palpable pulses as a result of collateral circulation.[76] Because of the close proximity of the brachial plexus and the axillary vessels, significant denervation of the upper extremity can occur. Near-avulsion injuries resulting in scapulothoracic dissociation invariably produce severe disruption of the brachial plexus and often ultimately result in amputation despite successful vascular repair. There is a high rate of amputation for the combination of axillary vascular and brachial plexus injury, mainly because the presence of a flail limb results in amputation for placement of a prosthesis. In addition, patients with a flail limb have a 40-fold increased rate of suicide.[10]

Brachial Artery

The brachial artery continues from the lower border of the teres major muscle and divides into the radial and ulnar arteries at the level of the proximal aspect of the radial head. The median and ulnar nerves and the basilic vein are in close proximity to the brachial artery. The profunda brachii artery is a major branch that arises soon after the origin of the brachial artery and often contributes good collateral flow if the brachial artery is injured distal to this branch point.[22,71] Brachial artery injuries occur as a result of penetrating trauma, humeral shaft fracture, elbow dislocation, or animal bites. They are the most common major vascular injuries in the upper extremity. In 75% of cases, the radial pulse is absent.[24] Repair is indicated in all cases because the amputation rate is high with ligation.

Forearm Arteries

The radial artery begins in the cubital fossa and runs superficially to the distal end of the radius, where it ultimately joins the deep branch of the ulnar artery to form the deep palmar arch of the hand. The ulnar artery begins in the cubital fossa and runs with the ulnar nerve anterior to the flexor retinaculum, at which point it joins the radial artery to form the superficial palmar arch of the hand.[77]

Injuries detected by arteriography or US that are below the bifurcation of the arterial supply in the upper extremity do not need to be repaired unless there are signs of ischemia in the hand; hard signs of arterial injury such as an expanding hematoma, pseudo-aneurysm, or AVF; or injury to both the radial and ulnar arteries. Some authors recommend repairing all these injuries because of the risk of intermittent claudication or cold intolerance in patients who have one artery ligated. Certain patients are almost exclusively dependent on the ulnar arterial supply to the hand because of an underdeveloped deep palmar arch. These patients clearly must have ulnar artery injuries repaired. Compartment syndrome in the forearm is common after repair of proximal arteries and veins and may require fasciotomy.

Lower Extremity

Iliac Artery and Vein

Given the intra-abdominal course of the iliac vessels, virtually all these injuries have associated trauma to the small or large intestine, bladder, solid viscera, or bony pelvis. The common and external iliac arteries are injured with equal frequency and more often than the internal iliac vessels.[78] In moribund patients, an initial "damage control" laparotomy with temporary vascular shunting of the iliac vessels is often necessary as resuscitation continues. Once the patient has overcome lactic acidosis, hypothermia, and coagulopathy, a second definitive repair can be undertaken. Surprisingly, the incidence of infection of synthetic or autologous grafts is rather low despite the high degree of bacterial contamination associated with perforation of a hollow viscus. Distal ischemic complications occur in about a third of repaired iliac arteries, and subsequent amputations are required in up to 18%.[78]

Femoral Artery and Vein

The external iliac vessels become the common femoral vessels at the inguinal ligament. After giving off the profunda femoris artery in the femoral triangle, the femoral artery continues as the superficial femoral artery almost vertically to the adductor tubercle of the femur and enters the popliteal fossa as the popliteal artery. There are extensive proximal collaterals around the hip joint, including the gluteal, obturator, and pudendal branches of the iliac artery.[22]

Common femoral artery injury occurs as a result of intertrochanteric hip fracture, hip dislocation, and iatrogenic injury from the placement of arterial catheters or from hip replacement surgery. Ligation of the common femoral artery culminates in amputation of the lower extremity in 80% of cases, so repair should be attempted in all cases. Penetrating wounds of the thigh result in femoral artery injury in 6.2% of cases, and up to 40% of these injuries are clinically occult. A medial or anteromedial wound track is present in

virtually all these cases, and many centers routinely perform angiography on these wounds.[79]

Popliteal Artery and Vein

The popliteal artery gives off the genicular branches in the popliteal fossa and then divides into the anterior and posterior tibial arteries at the lower border of the popliteus muscle. The peroneal artery arises from the posterior tibial artery shortly after its origin. The anterior and posterior tibial arteries and the peroneal artery form the trifurcation of the popliteal artery, and each runs with a corresponding vein and nerve in different compartments of the leg.[22]

Popliteal artery injury is relatively common and in most cases is due to blunt trauma. The most common cause is posterior knee dislocation in which bony elements directly lacerate or cause thrombosis of the artery, although displaced fractures of the knee may also result in popliteal artery injury. Anterior knee dislocations may cause excessive stretch on the popliteal vessels that can culminate in arterial thrombosis, but this injury is relatively rare. Overall, knee dislocation results in popliteal artery injury in 25% to 33% of cases.[80] Up to 40% of these injuries may be clinically occult, and diagnosis is delayed in up to 40% of cases,[2] although other series note that more than two hard signs of ischemia occur in 71% to 94%.[4,5] Twenty-five percent of cases have an associated injury to the peroneal and posterior tibial nerves, and in half the cases the knee dislocation may reduce spontaneously so that there may be little evidence of the original trauma, particularly in obtunded patients.[81] Patients showing complete ligamentous disruption of the knee on physical examination should be suspected of having a spontaneously reduced knee dislocation. Hemarthrosis may be absent if the joint capsule is torn because blood can track into the fascial planes of the leg.

No consensus has been reached on the diagnostic approach to detect popliteal artery injury resulting from knee dislocation. There are three possible strategies, and each has proponents and detractors. The first option is to perform routine arteriography on every case of knee dislocation. The second is to perform arteriography on selected cases in which vascular injury is not certain in spite of the combination of physical signs, abnormal ABI measurement, or findings on noninvasive tests such as color flow Doppler, duplex scan, or computed tomographic angiography. The third option is to rely completely on these physical findings and ABI. If both these findings are normal, advocates of this approach claim 100% negative predictive value for vascular injury that requires surgery.[82-86] The choice of these options is institution specific, but most centers continue to use arteriography in selected cases. Abnormal ABI and US (duplex and color flow Doppler) have been found to be very accurate in detecting popliteal injuries, and many centers reserve arteriography for cases in which noninvasive tests result in equivocal findings. As a general rule, high-energy mechanisms of trauma (e.g., auto versus pedestrian, motor vehicle accident) and posterior knee dislocations are more likely to produce popliteal artery injury than low-energy mechanisms are (e.g., sports injuries), and a more aggressive diagnostic approach (i.e., arteriography) may be warranted in such cases. However, patients with *penetrating* trauma and more than one hard sign of popliteal artery injury can be taken directly to the operating room for repair because delaying these cases to obtain an angiogram is "superfluous, unnecessary, costly and potentially dangerous."[87] Patients with *blunt* trauma can have false-positive hard findings generated by soft tissue swelling and external arterial compression, and these patients should undergo diagnostic testing first to confirm arterial injury. The amputation rate for popliteal injuries was as high as 40% in the past but has currently been reduced to zero in some series with modern diagnostic and repair techniques.[5,87] Most amputations are due to blunt trauma with severe mangling of the extremity or delay in repair exceeding 8 hours of warm ischemia time.[81] Because of the high incidence of compartment syndrome with lower leg injuries, fasciotomy is required in 36% to 62% of cases, and some centers routinely perform fasciotomy in all such cases.[88] Approximately two thirds of patients with popliteal artery injury will have persistent deficits caused by peripheral nerve injury, chronic ischemia, or amputation.

Lower Leg Arteries

The popliteal artery divides into three branches, the anterior and posterior tibial and the peroneal arteries at the inferior margin of the popliteal fossa. Injuries below the trifurcation at the knee may need repair if hard signs of arterial injury are apparent in the foot or if two of the three arteries are occluded on angiography.[18] However, vascular injuries in the lower part of the leg are notorious for causing compartment syndrome and need to be monitored closely. Amputation is usually due to a combination of soft tissue, nerve, and bone injuries. If significant injury to all three of these tissues is present, the amputation rate may reach 54%.[18,89] The combination of orthopedic and vascular injury, particularly as a result of crush injury, and shock on initial evaluation culminates in amputation in 35% of cases and should be considered a poor prognostic sign for limb viability.[90]

DISPOSITION

Patients with confirmed injury to major vessels, equivocal findings on diagnostic tests, or symptoms of limb ischemia must be admitted to the hospital for further investigation or observation. Consultation with a vascular surgeon is indicated as soon as vascular injury is confirmed and the need for emergency operative repair established. Patients who are unstable because of vascular or other injuries may undergo further investigation or exploration in the operating room. If the treating hospital is incapable of performing vascular surgery or appropriate investigations, transfer to a trauma center should be initiated. Delaying transfer for angiograms of proximity wounds in centers that are incapable of

acting on positive results is unwise because it often delays definitive care beyond the safe limits of warm ischemia time.

KEY CONCEPTS

- The overall condition of the patient determines the extent of diagnostic study and stabilization in the emergency department. Critical patients may require immediate surgery, which should not be delayed for confirmatory study of obvious vascular injury.

- Arterial injury may be readily apparent or clinically occult. Up to 21% of proximity wounds show arterial injury on angiography. Similarly, various US modalities and abnormal APIs frequently detect clinically inapparent vascular injuries.

- Symptoms of arterial injury may be delayed by hours to months after the initial injury. Late onset of symptoms suggests delayed thrombosis, pseudoaneurysm or AVF formation, compartment syndrome, or intermittent claudication resulting from stenosis or reliance on small-caliber collateral vessels for arterial perfusion.

- Reperfusion injury can occur after restoration of arterial flow and result in compartment syndrome. Frequent reexamination of the reperfused limb is indicated in the postoperative period.

- Compartment syndrome frequently develops in limbs with arterial injury, and fasciotomy is often required.

REFERENCES

1. Wall MJ, et al: Penetrating thoracic vascular injuries. *Surg Clin North Am* 76:749, 1996.
2. Applebaum R, et al: Role of routine arteriography in blunt lower extremity trauma. *Am J Surg* 160:221, 1990.
3. Martinez R, et al: Endovascular management of axillary artery trauma. *J Cardiovasc Surg* 40:413, 1999.
4. Fitridge RA, et al: Upper extremity arterial injuries: Experience at the Royal Adelaide Hospital, 1969 to 1991. *J Vasc Surg* 20:941, 1994.
5. Modrall JG, Weaver FA, Yellin AE: Diagnosis and management of penetrating vascular trauma and the injured extremity. *Emerg Med Clin North Am* 16:129, 1998.
6. Bynoe RP, et al: Noninvasive diagnosis of vascular trauma by duplex ultrasonography. *J Vasc Surg* 14:346, 1991.
7. Cherry D, et al: Trends in nonfatal and fatal firearm-related injury rates in the United States, 1985-95. *Ann Emerg Med* 32:51, 1998.
8. Giswold ME, et al: Iatrogenic arterial injury is an increasingly important cause of arterial trauma. *Am J Surg* 187:590, 2004.
9. Zamir G, et al: Results of reconstruction in major pelvic and extremity venous injuries. *J Vasc Surg* 28:901, 1998.
10. Pretre R, et al: Blunt injury to the subclavian or axillary artery. *J Am Coll Surg* 179:295, 1994.
11. Snyder KB, Pentecost MJ: Clinical and angiographic findings in extremity arterial injuries secondary to dog bites. *Ann Emerg Med* 19:983, 1990.
12. Hutson HR, et al: Law enforcement K-9 dog bites: Injuries, complications, and trends. *Ann Emerg Med* 29:637, 1997.
13. Fish RM: Electrical injury, part II: Specific injuries. *J Emerg Med* 18:27, 2000.
14. Gillespie DL, et al: Role of arteriography for blunt or penetrating injuries in proximity to major vascular structures: An evolution in management. *Ann Vasc Surg* 7:145, 1993.

15. Perry MO: Compartment syndromes and reperfusion injury. *Surg Clin North Am* 68:853, 1988.

16. *Advanced Trauma Life Support*, 6th ed. Chicago, American College of Surgeons, 1997.

17. Gonzalez RP, Falimirski ME: The utility of physical examination in proximity penetrating extremity trauma. *Am Surg* 65:784, 1999.

18. Weaver FA, Papanicolaou G, Yellin AE: Difficult vascular injuries. *Surg Clin North Am* 76:843, 1996.

19. Howlett DC, Holemans JA, Downes MO: Case report: The role of arteriography in patients with isolated neurological deficit following a penetrating upper limb injury. *Br J Radiol* 68:764, 1995.

20. Nichols JS, Lillehei KO: Nerve injury associated with acute vascular trauma. *Surg Clin North Am* 68:837, 1988.

21. Shaw AD, et al: Vascular trauma of the upper limb and associated nerve injuries. *Injury* 26:515, 1995.

22. Snell R, Smith M (eds): *Clinical Anatomy for Emergency Medicine*. St Louis, CV Mosby, 1993.

23. Wilson RF: Pre-existing peripheral arterial disease in trauma. *Crit Care Clin* 10:567, 1994.

24. Fields EF, Latifi R, Ivatury RR: Brachial and forearm vessel injuries. *Surg Clin North Am* 82:105, 2002.

25. Odland MD, et al: Combined orthopedic and vascular injury in the lower extremities: Indications for amputation. *Surgery* 108:660, 1990.

26. Illyevski N, et al: Emergency surgery of acute arteriovenous fistulas. *Cardiovasc Surg* 8:181, 2000.

27. Bongard F, et al: Peripheral arterial shotgun missile emboli: Diagnostic and therapeutic management—case reports. *J Trauma* 31:1426, 1991.

28. Michelassi F, et al: Bullet emboli to the systemic and venous circulation. *Surgery* 107:239, 1990.

29. Meggs WJ, et al: The treatment of lead poisoning from gunshot wounds with succimer (DMSA). *J Toxicol Clin Toxicol* 32:377, 1994.

30. Cohn SM, Crookes BA, Proctor KG: Near-infrared spectroscopy in resuscitation. *J Trauma* 54(5 Suppl):S199, 2003.

31. Velmahos GC, Toutouzas KG: Vascular trauma and compartment syndromes. *Surg Clin North Am* 82:125, 2002.

32. Johansen K, et al: Non-invasive vascular tests reliably exclude occult arterial trauma in injured extremities. *J Trauma* 31:515, 1991.

33. Schwartz MR, et al: Refining the indications for arteriography in penetrating extremity trauma: A prospective analysis. *J Vasc Surg* 17:116, 1993.

34. Hood DB, Weaver FA, Yellin AE: Changing perspectives in the diagnosis of peripheral vascular trauma. *Semin Vasc Surg* 11:255, 1998.

35. Nassoura ZE, et al: A reassessment of Doppler pressure indices in the detection of arterial lesions in proximity penetrating injuries of extremities: A prospective study. *Am J Emerg Med* 14:151, 1996.

36. Lynch K, Johansen K: Can Doppler pressure measurement replace exclusion arteriography in the diagnosis of occult extremity arterial trauma? *Ann Surg* 214:737, 1991.

37. Gahtan V, Bramson RT, Norman J: The role of emergent arteriography in penetrating limb trauma. *Am Surg* 60:123, 1994.

38. Atteberry LR, et al: Changing patterns of arterial injuries associated with fractures and dislocations. *J Am Coll Surg* 183:377, 1996.

39. Bergstein JM, et al: Pitfalls in the use of color-flow duplex ultrasound for screening of suspected arterial injuries in penetrated extremities. *J Trauma* 33:395, 1992.

40. Fry WR, et al: The success of Duplex ultrasonographic scanning in diagnosis of extremity vascular proximity trauma. *Arch Surg* 128:1368, 1993.

41. Kuzniec S, et al: Diagnosis of limbs and neck arterial trauma using duplex ultrasonography. *Cardiovasc Surg* 6:358, 1998.

42. Bynoe RP, et al: Noninvasive diagnosis of vascular trauma by duplex ultrasonography. *J Vasc Surg* 14:346, 1991.

43. Anderson RJ, et al: Reduced dependency on arteriography for penetrating extremity trauma: Influence of wound location and noninvasive vascular studies. *J Trauma* 30:1059, 1990.

44. Knudson MM, et al: The role of duplex ultrasound arterial imaging in patients with penetrating extremity trauma. *Arch Surg* 128:1033, 1993.

45. Gagne PJ, et al: Proximity penetrating extremity trauma: The role of ultrasound in the detection of occult venous injuries. *J Trauma* 39:1157, 1995.

46. Soto JA, et al: Diagnostic performance of helical CT angiography in trauma to large arteries of the extremities. *J Comput Assist Tomogr* 23:188, 1999.

47. Nunez D Jr, et al: Helical CT of traumatic arterial injuries. *AJR Am J Roentgenol* 170:1621, 1998.

48. Busquets AR, et al: Helical computed tomographic angiography for the diagnosis of traumatic arterial injury of the extremities. *J Trauma* 56:625, 2004.

49. James CA: Magnetic resonance angiography in trauma. *Clin Neurosci* 4:137, 1997.

50. Yaquinto JJ, et al: Arterial injury from penetrating trauma: Evaluation with single-acquisition fat-suppressed MR imaging. *AJR Am J Roentgenol* 158:631, 1992.

50. Geuder JW, et al: The role of arteriography in suspected arterial injuries of the extremities. *Am Surg* 51:893, 1985.

51. Reid JDS, et al: Assessment of proximity of a wound to major vascular structures as an indication for arteriography. *Arch Surg* 123:942, 1988.

52. Dennis JW, et al: New perspectives on the management of penetrating trauma in proximity to major limb arteries. *J Vasc Surg* 11:85, 1990.

53. Weaver FA, et al: Is arterial proximity a valid indication for arteriography in penetrating extremity trauma? A prospective analysis. *Arch Surg* 125:1256, 1990.

54. Gillespie DL, et al: Role of arteriography for blunt or penetrating injuries in proximity to major vascular structures: An evolution in management. *Ann Vasc Surg* 7:145, 1993.

55. Rose SC, Moore EE: Trauma angiography: The use of clinical findings to improve patient selection and case preparation. *J Trauma* 28:240, 1988.

56. De Virgilio C, et al: Noniatrogenic pediatric vascular trauma: A ten year experience at a level I trauma center. *Am Surg* 63:781, 1997.

57. Itani KM, et al: Emergency center arteriography. *J Trauma* 32:302, 1992.

58. Itani KM, et al: Emergency center arteriography in the evaluation of suspected peripheral vascular injuries in children. *J Pediatr Surg* 28:677, 1993.

59. Shah DM, et al: Polytetrafluoroethylene grafts in the rapid reconstruction of acute contaminated peripheral vascular injuries. *Am J Surg* 148:229, 1989.

60. Chen LE, et al: Effects of enoxaparin, standard heparin, and streptokinase on the patency of anastomoses in severely crushed arteries. *Microsurgery* 16:661, 1995.

61. Bouachour G, et al: Hyperbaric oxygen therapy in the management of crush injuries: A randomized double-blind placebo-controlled trial. *J Trauma* 41:333, 1996.

62. Naidoo NM, et al: Angiographic embolization in arterial trauma. *Eur J Vasc Surg* 19:77, 2000.

63. Criado E, et al: Endovascular repair of peripheral aneurysms, pseudoaneurysms and arteriovenous fistulas. *Ann Vasc Surg* 11:256, 1997.

64. Rich NM: Complications of vascular injury management. *Surg Clin North Am* 82:143, 2002.

65. Kuralay E, et al: A quantitative approach to lower extremity vein repair. *J Vasc Surg* 36:1213, 2002.

66. McHenry TP, et al: Fractures with major vascular injuries from gunshot wounds: Implications of surgical sequence. *J Trauma* 53:717, 2002.

67. Tufaro A, et al: Adverse outcome of nonoperative management of intimal injuries caused by penetrating trauma. *J Vasc Surg* 20:656, 1994.
68. Frykberg ER, et al: Nonoperative observation of clinically occult arterial injuries: A prospective evaluation. *Surgery* 109:856, 1991.
69. Dennis JW, et al: Validation of nonoperative management of occult vascular injuries and accuracy of physical examination alone in penetrating extremity trauma: 5- to 10-year follow-up. *J Trauma* 44:243, 1998.
70. Cox CS, et al: Blunt versus penetrating subclavian artery injury: Presentation, injury pattern, and outcome. *J Trauma* 46:445, 1999.
71. Demetriades D, et al: Penetrating injuries to the subclavian and axillary vessels. *J Am Coll Surg* 188:290, 1999.
72. Gasparri MG, et al: Physical examination plus chest radiography in penetrating periclavicular trauma: The appropriate trigger for angiography. *J Trauma* 49:1029, 2000.
73. McKinley AG, Carrim ATO, Robbs JV: Management of proximal axillary and subclavian artery injuries. *Br J Surg* 87:175, 2000.
74. Degiannis E, et al: Penetrating injuries of the subclavian vessels. *Br J Surg* 81:5246, 1994.
75. Gupta A, Jamshidi M, Rubin JR: Traumatic first rib fracture: Is angiography necessary? *Cardiovasc Surg* 5:48, 1997.
76. Gonzalez RP, Falimirski ME: The role of angiography in periclavicular penetrating trauma. *Am Surg* 65:711, discussion 714, 1999.
77. Gates JD: Penetrating wounds of the extremities: Methods of identifying arterial injury. *Orthop Rev* 10(Suppl):2, 1994.
78. Woodman G, Croce MA, Fabian TC: Iliac artery ischemia: Analysis of risks for ischemic complications. *Am Surg* 64:833, 1998.
79. Shayne PH, et al: A case-controlled study of risk factors that predict femoral arterial injury in penetrating trauma. *Ann Emerg Med* 24:678, 1994.
80. Trieman GS, et al: Examination of the patient with knee dislocation: The case for selective arteriography. *Arch Surg* 127:1056, 1992.
81. Wascher DC: High-velocity knee dislocation with vascular injury. *Clin Sports Med* 19:457, 2000.
82. Mills WJ, Barei DP, McNair P: The value of ankle-brachial index for diagnosing arterial injury after knee dislocation: A prospective study. *J Trauma* 56:1261, 2004.
83. Abou-Sayed H, Berger DL: Blunt lower-extremity trauma and popliteal injuries: Revisiting the case for selective arteriography. *Arch Surg* 137:585, 2002.
84. Klineberg EO, et al: The role of arteriography in assessing popliteal artery injury in knee dislocations. *J Trauma* 56:786, 2004.
85. Miranda FE, et al: Confirmation of the safety of physical examination in the evaluation of knee dislocation for injury of the popliteal artery: A prospective study. *J Trauma* 52:247, 2002.
86. Stannard JP, et al: Vascular injuries in knee dislocations: The role of physical examination in determining the need for arteriography. *J Bone Joint Surg Am* 86:910, 2004.
87. Frykberg ER: Popliteal vascular injuries. *Surg Clin North Am* 82:67, 2002.
88. Pretre R, et al: Lower limb trauma with injury to the popliteal vessels. *J Trauma* 40:595, 1996.
89. Grossman MD, et al: Gunshot wounds below the popliteal fossa: A contemporary review. *Am Surg* 65:360, 1999.
90. Rowe VL, et al: Shank vessel injuries. *Surg Clin North Am* 82:91, 2002.

Section III **ORTHOPEDIC LESIONS**

CHAPTER
46 General Principles of Orthopedic Injuries
Joel M. Geiderman

MANAGEMENT PRINCIPLES

Patients with orthopedic injuries and nontraumatic musculoskeletal disorders compose a large portion of the more than 100 million patients who present annually to U.S. emergency departments. Although only rarely life-threatening, orthopedic injuries may threaten a limb or its function, and accurate early diagnosis and treatment can avert long-term problems. Many of these injuries can and should be treated definitively by the emergency physician. Consultation with an orthopedist should be sought for the treatment of most long bone fractures, open fractures, and flexor tendon injuries and for follow-up of certain patients initially treated in the emergency department.

Orthopedic injuries often occur as a result of accidents (industrial or otherwise) and frequently involve young, otherwise healthy, working individuals. Accurate initial diagnosis, treatment, and documentation assume great importance medically and economically. Many problems can be avoided if the following 10 general principles are kept in mind:

1. Most orthopedic injuries can be predicted by knowing the chief complaint, the age of the patient, the mechanism of injury, and an estimate of the amount of energy delivered.
2. A careful history and physical examination predict x-ray findings with a high degree of accuracy. Many fractures were accurately described before the advent of roentgenology (Table 46-1).
3. If a fracture is suspected clinically, but x-ray films appear negative, the patient initially should be

Table 46-1. Common Fracture Names and Their Origins

Fracture Eponym	Description	Comment
Aviator's	Vertical fracture of the neck of the talus with subtalar dislocation and backward displacement of the body	First described in flyers during World War I. Arises from forced dorsiflexion of the foot in flying accidents and in traffic accidents after a head-on collision
Barton's	Intra-articular fracture-dislocation of the wrist	Considered complicated and unstable. Requires surgical reduction in most cases. Described by Barton in 1838 before the advent of radiography
Dorsal Barton's	Oblique intra-articular fracture of the dorsal rim of the distal radius with displacement of the carpus along with the fracture fragment	Results from high-velocity impact across the articular surface of the radiocarpal joint, with the wrist in dorsiflexion at the moment of impact
Volar Barton's	Wedge-shaped articular fragment sheared off of volar surface of the radius (volar rim fracture), displaced volarly along with the carpus	Similar mechanism as dorsal Barton's but with wrist in volar flexion at time of injury. Also referred to as a reverse Barton's. Much more rare than dorsal Barton's
Bennett's	Oblique fracture through base of the first metacarpal with dislocation of the radial portion of the articular surface	Usually produced by direct force applied to the end of the metacarpal. Dorsal capsular structures disrupted by the dislocation. Marked tenderness along medial base of thumb
Boxer's	Fracture of the neck of the fourth or fifth metacarpal	Results from striking a clenched fist into an unyielding object, usually during an altercation, or against a wall, out of frustration or anger
Bosworth	Fracture-dislocation of the ankle resulting in the fibula being entrapped behind the tibia	Rare injury, produced by a severe external rotation force applied to the foot. Physical examination reveals foot severely externally rotated in relation to the tibia
Chance's	Vertebral fracture, usually lumbar, involving the posterior spinous process, pedicles, and vertebral body	Caused by simultaneous flexion and distraction forces on the spinal column, usually associated with use of lap seatbelts. Anterior column fails in tension along with the middle and posterior columns. May be misdiagnosed as a compression fracture
Chauffeur's	Solitary fracture of radial styloid	Occurs from tension forces sustained during ulnar deviation and supination of the wrist. Name derives from occurrence in chauffeurs who suffered violent, direct blows to the radius incurred while turning the crank on a car, only to have it snap back, during previous eras
Clay shoveler's	Fracture of the tip of the spinous process of the sixth or seventh cervical vertebra	First described in Australian clay shovelers who sustained a fracture of the spinous process by traction as they lifted heavy loads of clay
Colles'	Fracture of the distal radius with dorsal displacement and volar angulation; with or without an ulnar styloid fracture	Most common wrist fracture in adults, especially in the elderly. Results from fall on an outstretched hand. Also known as silver fork deformity, which accurately describes the gross appearance in the lateral view. First described by Colles in 1814, before the advent of radiography
Cotton's	Trimalleolar fracture	Fracture of the lateral malleolus, the posterior malleolus, and either a fracture of the medial malleolus or a disruption of the deltoid ligament with visible widening of the mortise on ankle radiograph
Dashboard fracture	Fracture of the posterior rim of the acetabulum	Named for mechanism of injury: a seated passenger striking the knee on a dashboard, driving the head of the femur into the acetabulum
Dupuytren's	Fracture-dislocation of the ankle	Results from a similar mechanism as the better known Maisonneuve fracture (i.e., external rotation of the ankle), resulting in either deltoid ligament rupture or medial malleolus fracture, diastasis of the inferior tibiofibular joint, and indirect fracture of the fibular shaft. Maisonneuve was the student of Dupuytren
Essex-Lopresti	Fracture of radial head with dislocation of distal radioulnar joint	Results from longitudinal (axial) compression of the forearm
Galeazzi's	Fracture of the shaft of the radius with dislocation of the distal radioulnar joint. Ligaments of inferior radioulnar joint are ruptured and head of ulna displaced from ulnar notch of the radius	Results from fall on outstretched hand, with the wrist in extension and the forearm forcibly pronated. Inherently unstable with tendency to redisplace after reduction
Hangman's	Fracture-dislocation of atlas and axis, specifically of pars interarticularis of C2 and disruption of C2-3 junction. Separation occurs between second and third vertebral bodies from anterior to posterior side	Results from extreme hyperextension during abrupt deceleration. Most common cause is the forehead striking the windshield of a car during a collision. A bit of a misnomer in that hanging usually produces death by strangulation rather than cord damage
Hume	Fracture of the proximal ulna associated with forward dislocation of the head of the radius	Essentially a high Monteggia injury
Jefferson	Burst fracture of ring of C1, or atlas	Axial loading results in a shattering of the ring of the atlas. Decompressive type of injury. Associated with disruption of transverse ligament; an unstable injury
Jones'	Transverse fracture of the metatarsal base, occurring at least 15 mm distal to the proximal end of the bone, distal to the insertion of the peroneus brevis	Should not be confused with the more common avulsion fracture of fifth metatarsal styloid, produced by avulsion at the insertion of the peroneus brevis. Jones described the fracture that bears his name in 1902, after suffering the injury himself, while dancing

Table 46-1. Common Fracture Names and Their Origins—cont'd

Fracture Eponym	Description	Comment
Le Fort	Maxillary fracture	Types I, II, and III (see Chapter 39)
Le Fort-Wagstaffe	Avulsion fracture of the anterior cortex of the lateral malleolus	Rare pull-off injury of the fibular attachment of the anterior tibiofibular ligament
Lisfranc's	Fracture located around the tarsometatarsal (Lisfranc's) joint, usually associated with dislocation of this joint	Lisfranc, a field surgeon in Napoleon's army, described an amputation performed through the tarsometatarsal joint in a soldier who caught his foot in a stirrup when he fell off his horse. Since then, the joint has borne his name
Maisonneuve	Fracture of proximal third of fibula associated with rupture of the deltoid ligament or fracture of the medial malleolus and disruption of the syndesmosis	Results from external rotation of the ankle with transmission of forces through syndesmosis; proximally the force is relieved by fracture of the fibula. Described experimentally in 1840, before radiography
Malgaigne	Fracture of the ilium near the sacroiliac joint with displacement of the symphysis; or a dislocation of the sacroiliac joint with fracture of both ipsilateral pubic rami	Resultant pelvic injury is unstable. Described by Malgaigne, based on clinical findings, in 1847
March	Fatigue, or stress, fracture of the metatarsal	Arises from long marches or other repetitive use trauma (e.g., marathon running) or less commonly from single stumbling movements
Monteggia's	Fracture of the junction of the proximal and middle thirds of the ulna associated with anterior dislocation of the radial head	Usually caused by fall on outstretched hand along with forced pronation of forearm or by a direct blow on the posterior aspect of the ulna. Reported by Monteggia in 1814
Nightstick	Fracture of either ulna or radius, or both	Name derived from a citizen's attempt to protect himself from a police officer's baton or "nightstick" by offering the forearm
Piedmont fracture	Closed fracture of the radius at the middle third/distal third junction, without associated ulnar fracture	Named for a series of cases presented at the Piedmont Orthopaedic Society of Durham, North Carolina
Pott's	Definitions vary (see comment); most commonly a bimalleolar fracture or a fracture of the distal fibula, 4-7 cm above the lateral malleolus	The exact fracture Pott described in 1769 is uncertain; clearly it referred to a fracture of the lower fibula, usually associated with other fractures or dislocations about the ankle
Rolando's	Intra-articular fracture at base of metacarpal. Frequently Y- or T-shaped, or may be severely comminuted	Produced by an axial load with the metacarpal in partial flexion. Worse prognosis than a Bennett's fracture and, fortunately, more rare
Salter-Harris	An epiphyseal fracture occurring in children or adolescents	Graded I-V, depending on degree of involvement and/or displacement of epiphysis and metaphysis (see text dealing with Salter-Harris fractures and also Figure 46-1)
Stener	Avulsion of the ulnar corner of the base of the proximal phalanx of the thumb	Bony equivalent of rupture of the ulnar collateral ligament, or "gamekeeper's thumb"
Smith's	Extra-articular fracture of the distal radius with volar displacement of distal fragment	Reverse of the Colles' fracture but much more uncommon. Sometimes referred to as a "garden spade" deformity. Usually results from fall with force to back of hand. First described by Smith in 1847
Teardrop	Wedge-shaped fracture of the anteroinferior portion of the vertebral body, displaced anteriorly	Commonly involves a ligamentous injury and may produce neurologic injury
Thurston Holland's fragment	Triangular metaphyseal fragment that accompanies the epiphysis in Salter-Harris type II fractures	Described by Thurston Holland in 1929. Commonly hyphenated, although technically it should not be
Tillaux	Isolated avulsion fracture of the anterolateral aspect of the distal tibial epiphysis	Occurs in older adolescents (12-15 years old) after the medial parts of the epiphyseal plates close, but before the lateral part closes. External rotation force places stress on anterior talofibular ligament. Described by Tillaux in 1872

managed with immobilization as though a fracture were present.

4. Criteria for adequate radiographic studies exist; inadequate studies should not be accepted.

5. X-ray studies should be performed before attempting most reductions except when a delay would be potentially harmful to the patient or in some field situations.

6. Neurovascular competence should be checked and recorded before and after all reductions.

7. Patients must be checked for the ability to ambulate safely before discharge from the emergency department and should not be discharged unless this can be established.

8. Patients should receive explicit aftercare instructions before leaving the emergency department, covering such areas as monitoring for signs of neurovascular compromise or increasing compartment pressure, cast care, weight bearing, crutch use, and an explicit plan and timing for follow-up.

9. In a patient with multiple trauma, noncritical orthopedic injuries should be diagnosed and treated only after other more threatening injuries have been addressed.

BOX 46-1. Fracture Description

Identification
Open versus closed
Exact anatomic location
Direction of fracture line
Simple/comminuted
Position (displacement, alignment)

Additional Modifiers
Complete versus incomplete
Involvement of articular surface (%)
Avulsion
Impaction
    Depression
    Compression

Special Situations
Pathologic
Stress

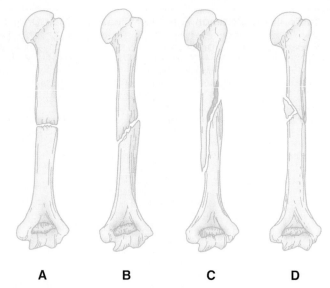

Figure 46-1. Types of fractures. **A,** Transverse. **B,** Oblique. **C,** Spiral. **D,** Comminuted.

10. All orthopedic injuries should be described precisely and according to established conventions.

FRACTURES

Fracture Nomenclature

Describing orthopedic injuries using precise language according to established convention permits relevant information to be communicated clearly to other parties. Terms commonly used to describe a fracture are listed in Box 46-1. A fracture is a break in the continuity of bone or cartilage. Clinically a history of loss of function, pain, tenderness, swelling, abnormal motion, and deformity suggests a fracture. X-ray studies are the mainstay of diagnosis and are usually, although not always, confirmatory. At times, special views, radionucleotide bone scans, computed tomography (CT) scans, or magnetic resonance imaging (MRI) studies are necessary to confirm a clinical suspicion. These studies should be considered when the clinical impression is at odds with the findings of routine radiography.

General Descriptors

Description of a fracture should begin by stating whether the fracture is *closed* or *open* (less desirable terms are *simple* or *compound*). In a closed fracture, the skin and soft tissue overlying the fracture site are intact. The fracture is open if it is exposed to the outside environment in any manner. This exposure may be as obscure as a puncture wound or as gross as splintered bone protruding through the skin. It is sometimes difficult to determine whether a small wound in proximity to a fracture actually communicates with that fracture. Some physicians advocate probing such a wound with a blunt sterile swab to establish a relationship; no study has established the safety, benefit, or accuracy of this maneuver. If doubt exists, an open fracture should be assumed to be present.

The next item that should be noted in the description of a fracture is the exact anatomic location, including the name of the bone, left or right, and standard reference points, for example, the *humeral neck* or *posterior tibial tubercle*. Long bones can be divided into thirds—proximal, middle, or distal—and these thirds or the junction of any two of them (e.g., the junction of the middle and distal third of the tibia) are used to describe fractures. The most descriptive language possible should be used. It is better to say "closed fracture of the right ulnar styloid" than "closed fracture of the right distal ulna" because the former conveys more precise anatomic information.

An additional modifier describes the direction of the fracture line in relation to the long axis of the bone in question. A *transverse* fracture occurs at a right angle to the long axis of the bone (Figure 46-1A), whereas an *oblique* fracture runs oblique to the long axis of the bone (Figure 46-1B). A *spiral* fracture results from a rotational force and encircles the shaft of a long bone in a spiral fashion (Figure 46-1C). A fracture in which there are more than two fragments present is termed *comminuted* (Figure 46-1D).

The position and alignment of the fracture fragments (i.e., their relationship to one another) should be described. Fragments are described relative to their normal position, and any deviation from normal is termed *displacement*. By convention, the position of the distal fragment is described relative to the proximal one. In Figure 46-2, there is a dorsal displacement of the fractured radius, and in Figure 46-3, there is lateral, or valgus, displacement of the distal tibia and fibula.

The terms *valgus* and *varus* are sometimes confusing. *Valgus* denotes a deformity in which the described part is angled away from the midline of the body. Conversely, *varus* denotes a deformity in which the angulation of the part is toward the midline. *Alignment* refers to the relationship of the longitudinal axis of one

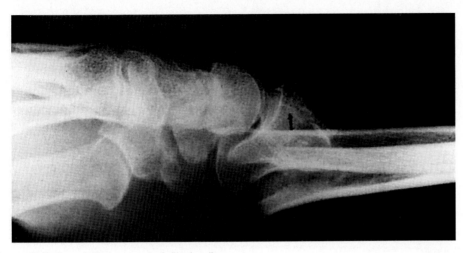

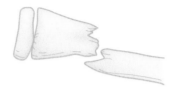

Figure 46-2. Dorsal displacement of distal radius.

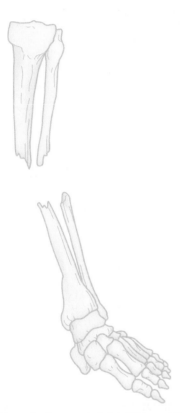

Figure 46-3. Valgus displacement of distal tibia and fibula. The distal segment is angled away from the midline of the body.

fragment to another; deviation from the normal alignment is termed *angulation*. The direction of angulation is determined by the direction of the apex of an angle formed by the two fracture fragments (Figure 46-4). This angle is opposite to the direction of displacement of the distal fragment.

Descriptive Modifiers

A fracture is termed *complete* if it interrupts both cortices of the bone and *incomplete* if it involves only one. It should be noted whether a fracture extends into and involves an *articular surface*. Frequently the percent-age of articular surface that is involved is estimated; in some cases, the percentage that is involved dictates the need to perform a surgical reduction. In general, it is important that the articular surface be restored to anatomic integrity.

Avulsion fracture refers to a bone fragment that is pulled away from its normal position by either the forceful contraction of a muscle (Figure 46-5A) or the resistance of a ligament to a force in the opposite direction (Figure 46-5B). *Impaction* refers to the forceful collapse of one fragment of bone into or onto another. In the proximal humerus, this collapse typically occurs in a telescoping manner, particularly in elderly patients, whose bones are soft and brittle. In the tibial plateau, impaction occurs frequently in the form of a depression (Figure 46-6A and B), and in the vertebral bodies, impaction frequently occurs in the form of compression (Figure 46-6C).

A fracture that occurs through abnormal bone is termed *pathologic*. A pathologic fracture should be suspected whenever a fracture occurs from seemingly trivial trauma. Diseases that cause structural weakness predisposing to injury include primary or metastatic malignancies, cysts, enchondromata, and giant cell tumors. In addition, osteomalacia, osteogenesis imperfecta, scurvy, rickets, and Paget's disease all weaken bones, making them susceptible to fracture. The term *pathologic* also is applied to fractures through osteoporotic bone when the demineralization is a result of disease, as in polio. Fractures through osteoporotic bone of the elderly usually are not described as pathologic. When fractures occur in normal bones and a history of "trivial trauma" is elicited, violence or battering should be suspected. Repeated low-intensity trauma may lead to resorption of normal bone, resulting in a stress fracture. Other names for this condition are *fatigue fracture* and *march fracture* (see Table 46-1). Most stress fractures occur in the lower extremities and commonly affect individuals involved in activities such as running, basketball, aerobics, and dancing. The tibia, fibula, metatarsals, navicular, cuneiform, calcaneus, femoral neck, or femoral shaft may be involved.[1,2]

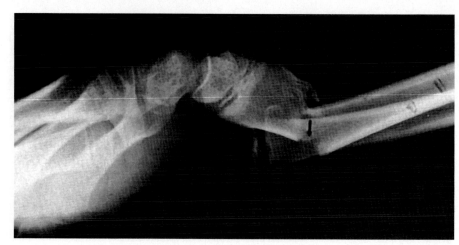

Figure 46-4. Volar angulation of fractured radius.

Figure 46-5. Avulsion fractures.

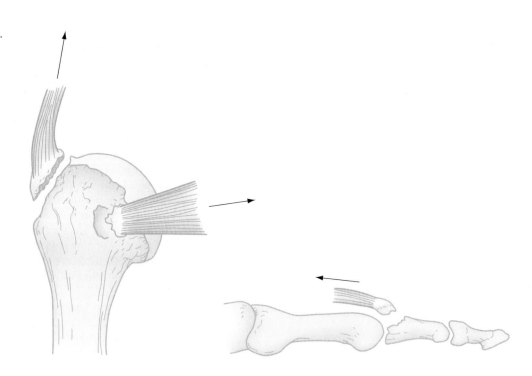

Fracture Eponyms

Many fractures were described before the advent of radiography and are described by an eponym rather than the exact bony injury. These eponyms reflect the rich history of orthopedic care and, despite the objections of some, are still commonly used to describe orthopedic injuries (see Table 46-1).

Fractures in Children

Certain features of children's bones distinguish pediatric fractures from adult fractures. Bones of children are necessarily soft and resilient and sustain numerous incomplete fractures. *Greenstick* fractures are incomplete angulated fractures of long bones. The resultant bowing of the bone causes an appearance resembling a moist, immature branch that breaks in a similar fashion when bent (Figure 46-7A). A *torus* fracture is another form of incomplete fracture, characterized by a wrinkling or buckling of the cortex. In Greek architecture, a torus is a bump at the base of a column, and these fractures, occurring at the end of long bones, take on such an appearance. These fractures may be extremely subtle on radiographs (Figure 46-7B).

Another feature of growing long bones that is a frequent source of trouble and confusion is the presence of epiphyses, cartilaginous centers at or near the ends of bone that give rise to growth of the bone. Figure 46-8 is a schematic review of the anatomy of a growing bone. Because cartilage is radiolucent, the cartilaginous portion of an epiphysis is not visualized on radiographs. A tendency exists to consider only the ossified nucleus and to ignore the cartilaginous structure that bridges to the metaphysis. Cartilage is present even before an ossified nucleus is seen. Because the epiphyseal growth plate is represented by a radiolucent line,

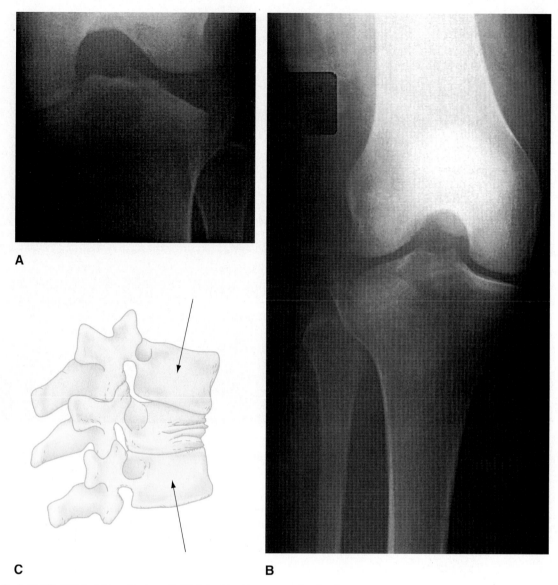

Figure 46-6. A and **B,** Tibial plateau fracture. **C,** Vertebral body compression fracture.

confusion may exist as to whether a fracture line is present. These complexities in interpreting radiographs in children sometimes, but not always, require comparison x-ray views of the noninjured side. Injuries to the epiphyses may result from either compressive or shearing forces. These injuries are relatively common during childhood as opposed to sprains or shaft fractures and must be considered in children with a "sprained ankle" because of the relative weakness of the cartilaginous growth zone, which separates before stronger ligaments and bones are torn or broken. Epiphyseal injuries should be described according to the Salter-Harris classification (Table 46-2).

Type I injuries involve only a slip of the zone of provisional calcification. Comparison radiographs are usually necessary to detect small slips. A child with swelling and tenderness over an epiphysis (e.g., of the lateral ankle) and a negative x-ray should be suspected to have an epiphysis injury, rather than a sprain, because the epiphysis is weaker than the overlying ligaments.

Type II injuries are similar to type I injuries, with a fracture extending into the metaphysis. The triangular metaphyseal fragment sometimes is referred to as the *Thurston Holland sign* (see Table 46-1). Type II injuries account for approximately three fourths of all epiphyseal fractures. Because the germinal layer is not involved, growth disturbance usually does not occur with type I and II injuries.

Type III injuries are composed of a slip of the growth plate plus a fracture through the epiphysis, involving the articular surface. Because this fracture involves the germinal layer, growth may be disrupted. Anatomic reduction does not eliminate the possibility of growth disturbance. Type IV fractures are similar to type III fractures, with the additional involvement of a metaphyseal fracture. Anatomic reduction is essential and usually requires surgery. Growth disturbance occurs in a high proportion of patients.

Type V fractures are crush injuries of the epiphyseal plate, usually produced by a compressive force.[3] This type of injury usually occurs in joints that move in one

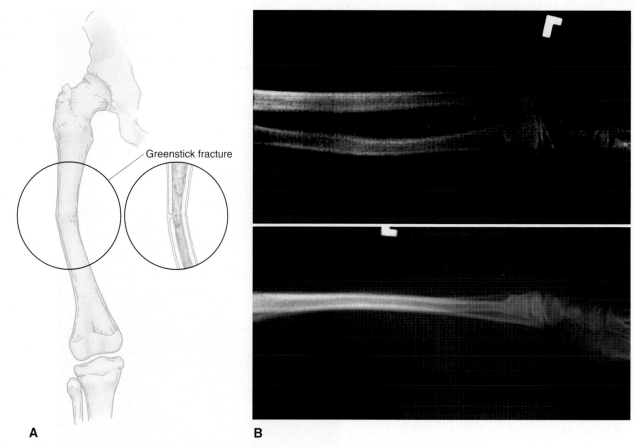

Figure 46-7. A, Greenstick fracture of midshaft of femur. **B,** Torus fracture of distal third of radius.

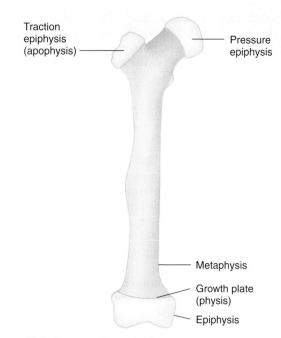

Figure 46-8. Anatomy of growing bone.

plane, most commonly the knee and ankle. Because this injury occurs in a radiolucent area, the injury may be difficult to diagnose on x-ray, but it should be suspected by mechanism of injury and pain over the epiphysis. The diagnosis can be established by MRI if

hemorrhage or a hematoma is identified within the growth plate immediately after injury.[4] Also reported is loss of MRI signal from the cartilage.[5] Growth arrest, manifest by shortening or angulation, is the rule in this injury. Type V injuries are extremely rare.[6]

In a study of 410 fractures in children, 16.3% were torus fractures, and 13.9% were epiphyseal injuries.[6] Dislocations and subluxations were rare (3%), and most involved the radial head or the patella. There were no shoulder dislocations. The most common sites were the bones of the distal forearm and the hands (usually the phalanges), each group accounting for 20% of the total. The clavicle was involved 13% of the time; the elbow, 8%; the ankle, foot, and femur, 7% each; and the midforearm, lower leg, and humerus, 4% to 6% each.

Another study found an incidence of physeal injury of 18% in 2000 bony injuries in children.[7] The peak age at the time of injury was 12 years in boys and 11 years in girls. In this series, the incidence of injury by category was type I, 8.5%; type II, 73%; type III, 6.5%; type IV, 12%; and type V, 0.5%. The sole Salter-Harris type V injury in this series occurred in the proximal tibia. The most frequent sites of Salter-Harris type III fractures are the phalanges and distal tibia, and most type IV fractures occur in the distal humerus and distal tibia. The overall frequency of growth arrest in all injuries is 1.4%, whereas the frequency of serious complications is less than 0.6%. The prognosis depends more on the location of the fracture than the Salter-Harris classifi-

Table 46-2. Salter-Harris Classification

	Description	Diagram
Type I	Fracture extends through the epiphyseal plate, resulting in displacement of the epiphysis (this may appear merely as widening of the radiolucent area representing the growth plate)	
Type II	As above; in addition, a triangular segment of metaphysis is fractured	
Type III	Fracture line runs from the joint surface through epiphyseal plate and epiphysis	
Type IV	Fracture line occurs as in type III, but also passes through adjacent metaphysis	
Type V	This is a crush injury of the epiphysis; it may be difficult to determine by x-ray examination	

cation. The proximal tibia is the most common site for growth disturbance. Because the epiphysis is closer to fusing, the chances of growth disturbance are less; this influences decision making in terms of surgical versus conservative management.

Diagnostic Modalities for Fracture Diagnosis

Plain Radiography

Plain radiography is the mainstay in diagnosing fractures. In addition to confirming or excluding fractures, other pathologic conditions can be identified. With penetrating trauma, foreign bodies, air, and gas also may be detected. With minor trauma, and when good follow-up monitoring is ensured, it is acceptable to delay x-ray films. Delay cannot be permitted, however, when the suspected injury is one that might be made worse by delayed diagnosis, such as a nondisplaced hip fracture.

At least two views perpendicular to each other are mandatory in examining long bones, and an oblique view also is usually obtained. In certain locations, such as the phalanges, oblique views are necessary. If doubt still exists, the clinician should ask for more views in various degrees of obliquity to the other films. A fracture line is most visible when it is parallel to the x-ray beam and is invisible when it is exactly 90 degrees to the beam. *The clinician should never accept a study*

that examines the bone in only one plane. When a long bone is found to be fractured, it is imperative that the bone be viewed radiographically in its entire length.

Each film must be examined to ensure that proper technique is used and that no important area is omitted from the film. Overexposed films may fail to reveal an abnormality. Although there is some loss of fine detail on portable films, these are acceptable in unstable patients, in whom the risk of moving the patient does not outweigh the benefit of the more detailed study. Computed (digital) radiography is now in widespread use. An advantage of this technique is the ability to alter the image-processing parameters based on a specific clinical problem after an exposure has been made.[7] Disadvantages are that the spatial resolution of computed radiographs, and especially of computer monitor formats, is less than that of standard screen-film combinations and that minification is often necessary when larger body parts, such as the thoracic spine, lumbar spine, and pelvis, are being examined. Minification also may contribute to reduced accuracy in the diagnosis of subtle, high-frequency chest abnormalities, such as pneumothorax. Despite these considerations, computed radiography seems to be acceptable and does not seem to diminish reader performance significantly.[8]

Even with good technique, some fractures are not visible initially and do not appear until the margins of the fracture absorb. Absorption widens the radiolucent line, and a defect appears in 7 to 10 days. At that time, new bone produced beneath the periosteum at the margins of the fracture accentuates the fracture. Accordingly, if a fracture is suspected but not visible at the initial visit, the injury should be treated as a fracture and re-examined clinically and radiographically in 7 to 10 days, and the patient should be informed of the rationale for this regimen.

Stress views of joints are used in some instances to evaluate the degree of ligamentous injury. Some authors argue against the use of stress views, citing a risk of injuring further an already traumatized structure, additional radiation exposure to the patient and the technologist, and the possibility that pain may not allow sufficient stress to be applied. For these reasons, stress views should be used judiciously in circumstances when other methods of evaluating ligamentous injuries are not available. *Comparison views* are useful in selected situations, but should not routinely be performed in all pediatric examinations.[9] If a fracture is definitely present on the affected side, the comparison view exposes the child to radiation and adds expense with no benefit. Similarly, an experienced physician generally is able to read a normal film with reasonable certainty. It is rational to use comparison views in instances when radiographs are inconclusive and when the confusion arises specifically out of the need to distinguish between a possible fracture and normal developmental anatomy. Obtaining a wide field of the affected extremity is more useful than routine comparison views for a young child because the child often does not localize the pain well; this is especially true with regard to complaints of knee pain in cases of hip injury or wrist complaints in forearm and elbow injury. Comparison views sometimes are helpful in adults when a question of accessory ossicles or nonfused bones (e.g., bipartite patella) exists because these anomalies are usually bilateral. The bleeding that inevitably accompanies fractures may produce soft tissue swelling and may impinge on or obliterate overlying muscle planes. Fat pads, such as in the elbow, may be displaced. Another useful sign is the fat-fluid level, which may accompany fractures extending into the knee joint. The fat-fluid level is visible, however, only if the cross-table technique is used.

The bones themselves should be examined systematically. Normal adult bones possess a smooth unbroken contour. A distinct angle is highly suggestive of a fracture. In an adult, the typical fracture is represented by a lucent line that interrupts the smooth contour and usually extends to the opposite side. Nutrient arteries may be confused with fractures, but have different radiographic characteristics: They are fine, sharply marginated, extend obliquely through the cortex, and are less radiolucent than fractures. *Pseudofractures* can be created by soft tissue folds, bandages or other overlying material, or a radiographic artifact called the *Mach effect*. If lucencies extend beyond the bones, the line is highly unlikely to represent a fracture. Anomalous bones and calcified soft tissue likewise may be mistaken for fractures. Avulsions and small fracture fragments have an irregular, uncorticated surface, and a defect in the adjacent bone is present, whereas anomalous ossification centers (accessory ossicles) and sesamoids are characterized by smooth cortical margins. Reference texts are useful in identifying and confirming these anomalies because they tend to occur in predictable locations.[10] Compression fractures are represented by increased density rather than a lucency. Finally, "the most commonly missed fracture is the second fracture." One must be diligent in searching for a second fracture after discovering the first fracture on a study. In particular, certain paired fractures, such as the distal tibia and proximal fibula, should be sought out.

Special Imaging Techniques

Radionucleotide Bone Scanning

In the past, radionucleotide bone scanning was used to detect skeletal abnormalities not radiographically evident in children and adults.[11] Occult lesions, especially stress fractures, acute osteomyelitis, and tumors, can be detected on these scans, although there are problems with specificity and sensitivity. This modality has been largely supplanted by CT and MRI and now is seldom used.

Computed Tomography

CT is used to confirm suspicious fractures or to define better displacement, alignment, or fragmentation of fractures. It also is useful in trauma to rule out cervical spine fracture when plain films are equivocal and in noncompressive vertebral fractures to assess the number of fragments and their spatial relationship

to the spinal canal. A CT scan is used frequently to define the integrity of articular surfaces in the acetabulum, knee, wrist, or ankle and in Salter-Harris type IV fractures.[3]

Magnetic Resonance Imaging

MRI constitutes the most advanced noninvasive examination of orthopedic structures, delineating lesions of bone, cartilage, ligaments, and other structures, such as menisci, disks, and epiphyseal structures. MRI is expensive and time-consuming and should be reserved for instances when the diagnosis is in doubt and specific findings would alter the treatment.

Complications of Fractures

Infection (Osteomyelitis)

Open fractures are treated as true orthopedic emergencies because of the risk of infection; the dreadful nature of the complication of osteomyelitis dictates that no time should be wasted in initiating therapy (Box 46-2). Wounds should be covered with sterile dressings, and parenteral antibiotics should be instituted as early as possible. Currently, suggested therapy includes a first-generation cephalosporin, such as cefazolin, for all open fractures, with the addition of an aminoglycoside for types II and III fractures.[12,13] Although the traditional recommendation has been to obtain culture and sensitivity before starting antibiotics, the usefulness of this approach has not been supported by a controlled study.[14] A retrospective analysis of perioperative cultures in open fractures in children failed to show any value in predicting the identity of subsequent infecting pathogens.[15] It is prudent to omit such cultures.[16]

Table 46-3. Blood Loss Associated with Fracture in Adults

Fracture Site	Amount of Blood Loss (mL)
Radius and ulna	150-250
Humerus	250
Tibia and fibula	500
Femur	1000
Pelvis	1500-3000

Table 46-4. Nerve Injuries Accompanying Orthopedic Injuries

Orthopedic Injury	Nerve Injury
Elbow injury	Median or ulnar
Shoulder dislocation	Axillary
Sacral fracture	Cauda equina
Acetabulum fracture	Sciatic
Hip dislocation	Femoral nerve
Femoral shaft fracture	Peroneal
Knee dislocation	Tibial or peroneal
Lateral tibial plateau fracture	Peroneal

Hemorrhage

Because of the rich blood supply to the skeleton, fractures can result in large amounts of blood loss, shock, and death from exsanguination. In particular, certain pelvic fractures can cause great blood loss because adequate tamponade is not possible. In adults, blood loss can range from 100 mL from a forearm fracture to 3 L from a pelvis fracture (Table 46-3).

Vascular Injuries

Vascular injuries characteristically are associated with certain fractures. Fractures and dislocations about the knee result from tremendous force that often injures the popliteal artery. In the extremities, assessment of vascular injuries may be difficult. The initial survey should note the presence or absence of pulses and the state of capillary filling. If an end artery is completely disrupted, the tissue distal to the injury may exhibit the classic five *P*s: pain, pallor, pulselessness, paresthesias, and paralysis. Incomplete and subclinical injuries occasionally occur, however, that initially may be asymptomatic and nondetectable. Likewise, in an unconscious, multiply-injured patient, major vascular injuries may not be obvious. The mechanism of injury and anatomy dictate the need to assess the possibility of an injured vessel. If pulses cannot be palpated, a Doppler stethoscope should be used to listen for blood flow. Even palpable pulses may be misleading, however, because it has been shown that in 10% to 20% of significant arterial injuries, distal pulses may initially be normal. When pulses are present, but the mechanism of injury suggests the possibility of vascular injury, additional diagnostic studies or surgical exploration may be necessary. Late complications of undiagnosed vascular injuries include thrombosis, arteriovenous fistulae, aneurysm, false aneurysm, and tissue ischemia with limb dysfunction.

Nerve Injuries

Nerves can be injured by either blunt or penetrating trauma. *Neurapraxia* is the contusion of a nerve, with disruption of the ability to transmit impulses. Paralysis, if present, is transient, and sensory loss is slight. Normal function usually returns to a neurapraxic nerve in weeks to months. *Axonotmesis* is a more severe crush injury to a nerve. The injury to nerve fibers occurs within their sheaths. Because the Schwann tubes remain in continuity, spontaneous healing is possible but slow. *Neurotmesis* is the severing of a nerve,

usually requiring surgical repair. Because of proximity, specific nerve injuries characteristically accompany certain fractures (Table 46-4).

When the nerve is completely severed, all functions are absent, including superficial sensation to touch, pain, and temperature; deep sensation to muscle and joint movements, position, deep pressure, and vibration; motor supply and deep tendon reflexes (to distally innervated muscle groups); and response to electrical stimulation. For less severe injuries, any subjective change in sensation should be noted. Light touch is a good screening test. Two-point discrimination is a more sensitive examination and should be used routinely in evaluating digital nerves. Two-point discrimination may be of limited value in children in whom a subjective response may be misleading; this is also true in patients with calloused fingertips and in patients who are uncooperative, comatose, in severe pain, or intoxicated. Testing for sympathetic nerve function using the O'Riain wrinkle test may be helpful.[17] Soaking the normally innervated digits in warm saline for 20 minutes causes the digital pulps to wrinkle through a mechanism that is not understood. The presence of wrinkling probably indicates the nerve is intact, whereas absence of wrinkling may be more difficult to interpret. The Ninhydrin test, another sudomotor test used to assess peripheral nerve integrity, is reportedly more reliable than the O'Riain test, but is not practical to perform in the emergency department.

Compartment Syndrome

Compartment syndrome is a serious acute emergency complication that should be considered whenever pain and paresthesias occur in an extremity after a fracture within an enclosed osseofascial space (Table 46-5). The immediate threat is to the viability of nerve and muscle tissue within the involved compartment, but infection, gangrene, myoglobinuria, and renal failure also may ensue. Compartment syndrome is associated most commonly with a closed long bone fracture of the tibia, but it also is well described in the thigh, forearm, arm, hand, and foot.[18-22] In addition, compartment syndrome can occur with soft tissue trauma alone and even with open fractures. It also has been described in a host of unusual situations, including prolonged procedures in the lithotomy position, the tuck position (knees tucked to the chest for lumbar surgery), spontaneous hemor-

Table 46-5. Life-Threatening or Limb-Threatening Emergencies

Condition	Possible Adverse Outcome
Open fracture	Osteomyelitis
Fracture or dislocation with major vascular disruption (especially popliteal)	Amputation
Major pelvic fracture	Exsanguination
Hip dislocation	Avascular necrosis of femoral head
Compartment syndrome	Ischemic contracture; myoglobinuria, renal failure

rhage, use of pneumatic antishock trousers, and the application of excessive traction in treatment of a fracture.[23-25]

Pathophysiology

Increased pressure in a closed nonexpandable compartment essentially represents a mismatch between the volume of that space and its contents. As such, it may arise from one of three circumstances: (1) increased compartment contents, (2) decreased compartment volume, or (3) external pressure (Box 46-3). As tissue pressure increases, so does venous pressure, resulting in compromise of the local circulation and tissue hypoxia; this is believed to occur at pressures that are above normal diastolic pressure but below systemic arterial pressure because of a reduced arteriovenous gradient at the tissue level. The body responds by releasing histamine in an attempt to dilate capillaries and increase blood flow to the affected area. Histamine also increases capillary membrane permeability, resulting in a leak of proteins and fluid into the surrounding tissue, further increasing compartment pressure.

As tissue pressure continues to increase, venous blood flow is impaired as capillary perfusion pressure is exceeded. Finally, arterial capillary blood flow falls to a point where the basic metabolic needs are no longer met, leading to ischemic necrosis of muscles and nerves within the compartment. An important concept in the management of compartment syndrome is that because local venous pressure cannot be significantly below local tissue pressure, and because elevation of a dependent limb decreases local arterial pressure by 0.8 mm Hg for each 1 cm of limb elevation, elevation of a limb with resultant reduction in the local arteriovenous gradient may be counterproductive and may exacerbate compartment syndrome. Vascular spasm seems to play an insignificant or minimal role in the development of compartment syndrome, as evidenced angiographically, where spasm has never been shown, and clinically, where it is observed that distal pulses usually are maintained until late in the course.

Normal compartment pressure is 0 mm Hg. Microcirculation generally is impaired when tissue pressures reach 30 mm Hg or more; however, some patients can tolerate much higher compartment pressures without compartment syndrome developing. Controversy exists over attempts to define compartment syndromes on the

BOX 46-3. Causes of Compartment Syndrome

Increased Compartment Content
Bleeding
  Major vascular injury
  Coagulation disorder
  Anticoagulant therapy
Increased capillary filtration
  Reperfusion after ischemia
    Arterial bypass grafting
    Embolectomy
    Ergotamine ingestion
    Cardiac catheterization
    Lying on limb
  Trauma
    Fracture
    Convulsion
  Intensive use of muscle
    Exercise
    Seizures
    Eclampsia
    Tetany
  Burns
    Thermal
    Electrical
  Intra-arterial drug injection
  Orthopedic surgery
    Tibial osteotomy
    Hauser's procedure
    Reduction and internal fixation of fractures
  Snakebite
Increased capillary pressure
  Intensive use of muscles
  Venous obstruction
    Phlegmasia cerulea dolens (i.e., acute inflammation and edema of the legs)
    Ill-fitting leg brace
    Venous ligation
  Diminished serum osmolarity (i.e., nephritic syndrome)

Decreased Compartment Volume
Closure of fascial defects
Excessive traction on fractured limbs

Miscellaneous
Infiltrated infusion
Pressure transfusion
Leaky dialysis cannula
Muscle hypertrophy
Popliteal cyst

External Pressure
Tight casts, dressings, or air splints
Lying on limb

From Matsen FA III: *Compartmental Syndromes*. New York, Grune & Stratton, 1980.

basis of specific tissue pressure. The tolerance to tissue ischemia varies among individuals because of shock, compensatory hypertension, altered tone in resistance vessels, and other unknown factors. Inadequate perfusion and relative ischemia begin when tissue pressure within a closed compartment increases to within 30 mm Hg of a patient's diastolic pressure.[26] When tissue pressure equals or exceeds the patient's diastolic pressure, tissue perfusion effectively ceases. The development of muscle ischemia depends not only on the magnitude, but also on the duration of elevated pressure. Intracompartmental pressures do not measure muscle and nerve ischemia, but rather suggest the existence of the proper setting for compartment syndrome.[27]

Anatomic Considerations and Risk Factors

Compartment syndrome theoretically can develop in any location where neuromuscular tissue is contained in a limiting envelope. The condition has been reported in the leg, thigh, buttock, arm, forearm, and hand (Box 46-4). By virtue of its location and higher likelihood of sustaining high-energy trauma, the leg, particularly the anterior compartment, is most commonly involved.

In a study of 164 patients treated over an 8-year period in the United Kingdom, a fracture was present in 69%, and half of these involved the tibial shaft.[28] Perhaps more significant is that 31% of patients had only soft tissue injury *without* fracture. Most patients were men younger than age 35. Ten percent of patients either had a bleeding disorder or were taking anticoagulants. Traffic accidents and sports activities were the most common mechanisms of injury.

Clinical Presentation

In a conscious and fully oriented patient, pain that is disproportionate to the injury or physical findings is a hallmark finding in compartment syndrome. Pain often is characterized as deep, burning, and unrelenting and is difficult to localize. The need for increasing amounts of analgesics should not lead the clinician automatically to the conclusion that the patient is drug seeking; rather, it should serve as a prompt to the possibility that a compartment syndrome is developing or is present.

Pain on passive stretching of the muscle groups in the suspect compartment is an important finding. In addition, active flexion of involved muscles may produce pain. Other reliable suggestive signs and symptoms are hypoesthesias and paresthesias in the distribution of nerves crossing the compartment or tenderness, tenseness, or the sensation of tightness of the compartment.

Skin color, temperature, capillary refill, and distal pulses all are unreliable monitors for compartment syndrome because the pressure necessary to produce compartment syndrome is well below arterial pressure. Pallor and loss of pulses are late and ominous signs. Diminished pulses should suggest concomitant pathologic conditions responsible for reduced arterial flow. Although it is still frequently taught that the five *P*s—pain, pallor, pulselessness, paresthesias, and paralysis—are signs and symptoms of compartment syndrome, this is generally not true. Rather they are the signs of acute disruption of arterial flow. Subjective complaints are an important indicator of compartment syndrome. Patients who are not fully alert or cooperative must be assessed with particular care.

Diagnostic Tests

If the history and examination suggest compartment syndrome, compartment pressures should be measured by using any of the commercially available monitors (Figure 46-9). The Stryker device is a hand-held digital

---

BOX 46-4. Reported Anatomic Locations of Compartment Syndromes

Lower Extremity
Leg
    Anterior compartment
    Lateral compartment
    Deep posterior compartment
    Superficial posterior compartment
Thigh
    Quadriceps compartment
Buttock
    Gluteal compartment

Upper Extremity
Hand
    Interosseous compartment
Forearm
    Dorsal compartment
    Volar compartment
Arm
    Deltoid compartment
    Biceps compartment

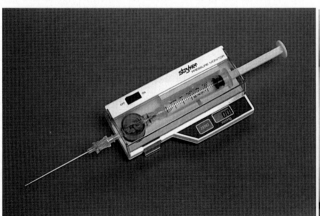
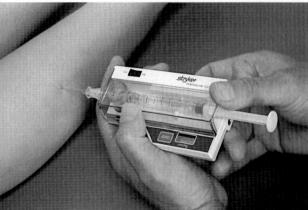

A   **B**

Figure 46-9. **A,** Hand-held device for measuring compartment syndrome. **B,** Insert device perpendicular to skin.

display that is easy to use with minimal training. Care must be taken to zero the monitor in the plane in which it will be inserted to account for the effects of gravity. It is also paramount that the appropriate compartment is measured. Pressures of less than 30 mm Hg generally do not produce compartment syndrome. Pressures exceeding 30 mm Hg or within 30 mm Hg of the patient's mean arterial pressure are an indication for fasciotomy. Serial or continuous pressure measurements should be performed in cases that are not clear-cut. Compartment syndrome can occur at pressures significantly below systemic pressure. Doppler ultrasound is not useful in evaluating these patients because excellent arterial blood flow may be documented even in the presence of a significant compartment syndrome.

Treatment, Complications, and Disposition

Complete fasciotomy is the only treatment that can reliably normalize elevated compartment pressure. Preparation for surgery must be done as quickly as possible. Delaying fasciotomy for more than 12 hours often results in irreversible muscle and nerve damage. While the patient is awaiting definitive treatment, the affected part should not be elevated above the level of the heart because this maneuver does not improve venous outflow and reduces arterial inflow. Slight dependency has been suggested to maximize the pressure head in the extremity.

Rhabdomyolysis, hyperkalemia, and myoglobinuria may occur and should be managed aggressively to avoid renal failure. Lactic acid also is released from necrotic muscle tissue. Other complications include infection and tissue loss. Delayed treatment results in loss of nerve and muscle function and eventual contracture formation. The magnitude of these disasters may be measured by the fact that in 1993, the average indemnity award in cases of missed compartment syndrome was nearly $280,000. For these reasons, when the diagnosis of compartment syndrome is confirmed, fasciotomy should be done without delay. Gulli and Templeman[26] advise, "The functional and cosmetic results are always acceptable if done early. The results of inadequate treatment of compartment syndrome are never satisfactory."

Avascular Necrosis

Because of their blood supply, certain bones may undergo avascular necrosis after fracture, especially if fractures are comminuted and go untreated for any length of time. The femoral head, talus, scaphoid, and capitate are particularly prone to this complication.[29-32]

Complex Regional Pain Syndrome (Reflex Sympathetic Dystrophy and Causalgia)

Definitions

The terms *reflex sympathetic dystrophy* (RSD) and *causalgia* have been used to describe pain syndromes that sometimes follow fractures, orthopedic surgery, soft tissue injuries, and other unrecognized trauma to the limbs and their appendages. Other names previously used for this spectrum of posttraumatic injuries include *Sudeck's atrophy, shoulder-hand syndrome,* and *postinfarction sclerodactyly.* In an attempt to reduce misunderstanding about their etiology and treatment, the International Association for the Study of Pain issued a consensus statement renaming the syndromes formerly called RSD and causalgia.[33,34] *Complex regional pain syndrome type I* (CRPS-I), replacing the term RSD, is a pain syndrome that develops after an initiating noxious event, extends beyond the distribution of a single peripheral nerve, and is usually disproportionate to the inciting event. The site is most often the distal end of the affected extremity, with a distal-to-proximal gradient. It is associated with edema, changes in blood flow to the skin, abnormal sudomotor activity in the region of the pain, allodynia (pain resulting from non-noxious stimulation to the skin), hyperpathia (pain persisting or increasing after mild or light pressure), or hyperalgesia. The presence of a condition that otherwise would explain the degree of pain and dysfunction excludes the diagnosis of CRPS-I. Because so much of the literature still refers to RSD, this chapter still uses the terms RSD and CRPS-I interchangeably. The definition of *CRPS-II* is the same as for CRPS-I except that there is demonstrable peripheral nerve injury. This term replaces *causalgia* under the International Association for the Study of Pain taxonomy.

Pathogenesis and Etiology

The pathogenesis of CRPS-I has not been elucidated. The sympathetic nervous system seems to play a role in the maintenance of the symptoms in some, but not all, patients. Cases of CRPS-I have been reported after fractures and as iatrogenic complications of surgery or after minor procedures, including subcutaneous excision and intravenous injection. Forceful manipulations and tight casts also are alleged to have produced the syndrome. In 10% to 26% of patients, no inciting event is identified.[35,36]

Although malingering and secondary gain are suspected in some patients, they are not the causes in most patients, as evidenced by pathologic tissue changes in patients who actually have CRPS-I.[37] CRPS-I occurs in children and adolescents.[38] Girls are affected three times as often as boys, and the median age is 12 years. The lower limb is affected twice as often as the upper, and history of inciting trauma can be identified in only half the children with the disorder.

Diagnosis

No correlation exists between the severity of the original trauma and the incidence, severity, and cause of the symptoms, making early diagnosis a challenge, especially after trivial injury. Early diagnosis is crucial because the earlier treatment is initiated, the better the response. The diagnosis is not always easy to make, however.

An RSD score consisting of nine criteria has been proposed to aid in the diagnosis of RSD and to enhance comparisons of outcome studies.[39] The criteria are as follows:

1. Allodynia (pain resulting from non-noxious stimulation to the skin) or hyperpathia (pain persisting or increasing after mild or light pressure)
2. Burning pain
3. Edema
4. Color or hair growth changes
5. Sweating changes
6. Temperature changes
7. Radiographic changes (i.e., demineralization)
8. Quantitative measurement of vasomotor/sudomotor disturbance
9. Triple-phase bone scan consistent with RSD

One point is given for each positive criterion, none if absent, and half a point if equivocal. Patients with more than five points are probable RSD patients. Pain that is abolished with temporary selective sympathetic blockade is another test that is highly suggestive of RSD.

Treatment

Treatment of CRPS is controversial. Debate arises because randomized, placebo-controlled studies are lacking; individual response to treatment varies; and experts disagree regarding the pathogenesis of the disease. A multidisciplinary approach, including physical therapy and psychological counseling, is often necessary to treat CRPS.[40] For some patients, definitive treatment involves sympathetic blockade, usually with regional anesthesia and occasionally by surgical sympathectomy.[41] Oral medications, including calcitonin, indomethacin, tricyclic antidepressants, gabapentin, and others, have been used to treat RSD with variable success.[35,42] In one study, vitamin C was shown to reduce the incidence of RSD after wrist fracture.[43]

Fat Embolism Syndrome

Fat embolism refers to the presence of fat globules in the lung parenchyma and peripheral circulation after a long bone fracture or major trauma.[44] The phenomenon of fat embolization is probably common as a subclinical event after long bone fracture. Intravascular fat droplets appear in nearly one of five patients admitted with major trauma, although not all patients are symptomatic or require treatment.

Fat embolism syndrome is a serious manifestation of fat embolism, occurring most commonly after long bone fractures (usually tibia and fibula) in young adults and after hip fractures in elderly patients. Symptoms usually appear 1 to 2 days after an acute injury or after intramedullary nailing. Respiratory distress syndrome is the earliest, most common, and most serious manifestation. Neurologic involvement, manifest as restlessness, confusion, or deteriorating mental status, also is an early sign, as are thrombocytopenia and a petechial rash. Fever, tachycardia, jaundice, retinal changes, and renal involvement may occur. Fat is seen in the urine in 50% of patients within 3 days of the injury. The incidence of full-blown fat embolism syndrome varies from 0.5% to 2% in patients with isolated long bone fractures to 5% to 10% in patients with multiple fractures. Management of fat embolism syndrome is primarily supportive, usually in an intensive care unit. No specific therapy has shown benefit.

Fracture Blisters

Fracture blisters are tense blisters or bullae that accompany high-energy injuries in areas of relatively little skin coverage over a fracture site. The ankle, elbow, foot, and knee (in that order) are the most common sites; all of these contain fewer hair follicles and sweat glands to anchor together the epidermal-dermal junction than do other limb locations.[45] Fracture blisters are believed, in many cases, to occur in the setting of increased underlying tissue pressure and may be a harbinger of compartment syndrome.

Early surgical intervention reduces the incidence of fracture blister formation.[45] In addition, the presence of a fracture blister requires an alteration of the surgical approach or a delay in surgery. Most experts discourage incisions through a fracture blister because such incisions seem to increase infection. Measures to perform early surgery after high-energy injuries and to minimize increases in tissue pressures might reduce the incidence of this complication. Intact blisters should be covered with povidone-iodine solution and a sterile dressing.

Complications of Immobilization

Fractures frequently result in long periods of immobilization. Immobility may lead to multiple medical problems, especially in elderly patients, including pneumonia, deep venous thrombophlebitis, pulmonary embolism, urinary tract infection, wound infection, decubitus ulcers, muscle atrophy, stress ulcers, gastrointestinal hemorrhage, and psychiatric disorders (Box 46-5). Early ambulation is a major goal of optimal orthopedic care.

BOX 46-5. Complications of Fractures and Immobility

Fractures
Hemorrhage
Vascular injuries
Nerve injuries
Compartment syndrome
Volkmann's ischemic contracture
Avascular necrosis
Reflex dystrophy
Fat embolism syndrome

Immobility
Pneumonia
Deep venous thrombosis
Pulmonary embolism
Urinary tract infection
Wound infection
Decubitus ulcers
Muscle atrophy
Stress ulcers

Fracture Healing

Specific fractures are discussed in subsequent chapters. In general, the goal is to realign bony fragments so that healing or union can take place, and normal function is restored. The process from fracture to union begins with a hematoma that bridges the fragments. The hematoma is followed by an inflammatory phase when granulation tissue forms on the fracture surfaces with resorption of the hematoma to provide the first continuity between the fragments. Callus subsequently is formed on the periosteal and endosteal surfaces of the bone, acting as a biologic splint. This area first becomes calcified by deposition of calcium phosphate, then undergoes osseous metaplasia. Callus is resorbed as the original fracture surfaces develop firm bony union. In some bones, such as the skull and the neck of the femur, where periosteum is deficient, there may be virtually no callus formation. The process finally ends with remodeling.

On x-ray studies, at 10 to 14 days, the bone surrounding the fracture line becomes less dense because of localized bone resorption and hyperemia associated with the formation of granulation tissue. As a result, the fracture becomes considerably easier to visualize radiographically about 10 days after injury. After 2 to 3 weeks, soft tissue swelling has regressed, and callus first becomes visible, initially in a mottled pattern and then taking on a dense appearance. The callus undergoes organization, with peripheral margins becoming smooth.

For a healthy adult, the whole process from injury to consolidation takes about 2 months for the humerus and about 4 months for a large bone such as the femur. Oblique fractures tend to heal more quickly than transverse fractures. Healing is quicker in children and slower in the elderly. The rate of fracture healing is affected by many factors, including the type of bone (cancellous bone heals faster than cortical bone); degree of fracture and opposition; and systemic states, such as hyperthyroidism or excess corticosteroidism. Exercise speeds healing, whereas chronic hypoxia has been known to slow repair.

The presence of abundant callus seen on x-ray that is beginning to organize usually is associated with clinical union. If any suggestion of movement at the fracture site is noted on clinical examination, union must be regarded as inadequate. Several terms are used to denote abnormal union. *Delayed union* is union that takes longer than usual for a particular fracture location. *Malunion* occurs when a residual deformity exists. *Nonunion* is the failure of a fracture to unite. When nonunion results in a false joint, it is termed a *pseudarthrosis.*

If the ends of the bone have remained constant on serial films and an adequate surrounding sheath of organizing callus can be seen, it is permissible for the patient to return to limited active use, even if the original fracture remains visible. The final process of consolidation develops later.

SUBLUXATION AND DISLOCATIONS

Nomenclature

Abnormal forces applied to joints may result in the loss of continuity between two articulating surfaces. Partial loss of continuity is termed *subluxation,* and complete loss is termed *dislocation.* In general, dislocations are named for the major joint involved, as in a dislocated shoulder or hip. In three-bone joints, the injury is named for the joint involved if the disturbance involves the two major bones, or, if the lesser bone is involved, the disturbance is named for that bone. Separation of the femur from the tibia is termed *dislocation of the knee,* whereas displacement of the patella from its normal articulation is termed *dislocation of the patella* (Figure 46-10). At the elbow, separation of the olecranon from the humerus is a dislocation of the elbow, whereas separation of the radius from the humerus is termed *radial head dislocation.*

Dislocations and subluxations should be described according to the direction of the distal segment relative to the proximal segment or of the displaced bone relative to the normal structures. The injury shown in Figure 46-11 is termed *dorsal dislocation of the distal interphalangeal joint of the thumb.* Disruption of articulation also may occur in combination with a fracture. The term *fracture-dislocation* is used to describe this combination. If the overlying skin is broken in any way, dislocations, subluxations, or fracture-dislocations are described as open and constitute the same emergency as does an open fracture alone.

Assessment

In most cases of dislocation, severe to excruciating pain exists because the joint capsule is stretched or torn. Movement of the joint exacerbates the pain. This useful sign is lost in an obtunded, intoxicated, or unconscious patient and may lead to failure to diagnose if a careful survey is not performed. Some dislocations, such as anterior shoulder dislocation, have an obvious deformity, whereas others, such as posterior shoulder dislocation, may be subtle. Swelling of soft tissues also may obscure the diagnosis, such as in the tarsal-metatarsal region. Gentle passive testing of range of motion should be performed but never forced. Assessment for neurovascular function is similar to that for fracture. Certain dislocations (e.g., knee) are so commonly associated with vascular injuries that in many institutions arteriography is performed routinely in evaluating these injuries.

Plain x-ray studies detect most dislocations, provided that the correct views are ordered. Radiographs should be performed before and after attempts at reduction of first-time or complicated dislocations to confirm the diagnosis and to ensure that associated fractures are documented before treatment is undertaken.

Treatment

Methods of relocating specific joints are reviewed in subsequent chapters, but a few general principles

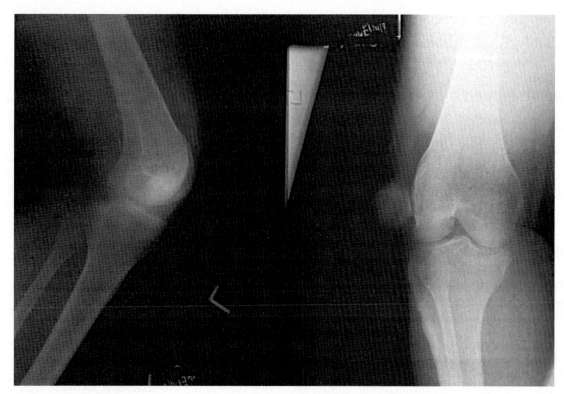

Figure 46-10. Dislocation of the patella.

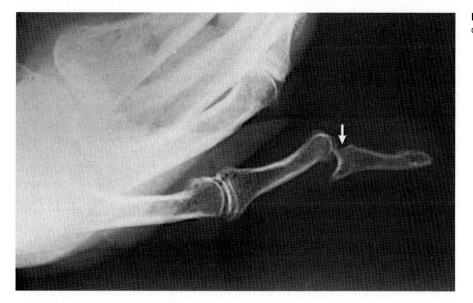

Figure 46-11. Dorsal dislocation of the distal phalanx of the thumb.

apply. In general, the sooner a joint is relocated, the better. Later, swelling and muscle spasm make reduction more difficult. Also, pain is not adequately relieved until the dislocation is reduced. In the hip, early reduction is mandatory to restore vascular supply and to avert the complication of avascular necrosis. Before attempting relocation, adequate analgesia or conscious sedation should be used. Nerve blocks are especially useful on the digits. The general principle of reducing a dislocation is to recreate and reverse the mechanism of injury, pulling the proximal end of the dislocated bone out and away from whatever is trapping it in its final resting place. As this maneuver is accomplished, the disarticulated surface is manipulated back or may snap back spontaneously toward its normal anatomic position. If the reduction is difficult, it should not be forced. A single good attempt is better than repeated attempts in an inadequately relaxed patient. Some joints cannot be reduced in the emergency department because (1) the opposing muscles are contracting too forcefully and general anesthesia is necessary to overcome these forces or (2) mechanical obstruction by a bony fragment or a torn piece of cartilage, tendon, or joint capsule requires surgical removal for reduction to occur.[46,47]

SOFT TISSUE INJURIES

Sprains

Nomenclature

Ligamentous injuries resulting from an abnormal motion of a joint are termed *sprains*. A sprain is defined as injury to the fibers of a supporting ligament of a joint. Sprains may be graded according to the severity of pathologic findings; clinically, however, the grades are often indistinct. *First-degree* sprains are characterized by minor tearing of ligamentous fibers with resultant mild hemorrhage and swelling. Minimal point tenderness can be elicited. Stressing the ligament produces some pain, but there is no opening or abnormal joint motion.

A *second-degree* sprain is a partial tear of a ligament, meaning more fibers are torn than in the first-degree injury. Clinical findings include moderate hemorrhage and swelling, tenderness, painful motion, abnormal motion, and loss of function. There may be a tendency toward persistent instability and recurrence, and prevention of these complications is a major goal of treatment.

A *third-degree* sprain describes the complete tearing of a ligament. Signs include a further exaggeration of the signs mentioned for second-degree sprain. In addition, stressing the joint reveals grossly abnormal joint motion, provided that this is not limited by pain or swelling. Analgesia and the evacuation of a hemarthrosis may be used to allow a more complete diagnosis of these injuries. Chronic joint instability is the rule if severe ligamentous injuries do not heal properly.

Assessment

The clinical presentation of a patient with a sprain of the extremity may be indistinguishable from that of a patient with a fracture. The injury frequently occurs during vigorous athletic activity when forces applied in opposite directions result in a joint being stressed in an abnormal or exaggerated direction. The patient may complain of hearing a "snap" or a "pop" at the moment of injury and conclude that a fracture must be present. Other patients report "seeing stars" or "almost passing out" at the moment the injury occurred and may still be in extreme pain, appearing pale and diaphoretic, if seen shortly after the injury. Analgesia should be provided to these patients. Evaluation should include a careful history of the exact sequence of events at the time of the injury and ascertaining the position of the extremity and the forces applied to it at that moment. A history of any audible sounds at the time of injury should be elicited. Examination of the joint should include stressing it to show abnormal motion. If radiographs are planned to rule out a fracture anyway or if exquisite pain is produced by mild attempts to

apply stress, it is probably better to delay stressing until films have verified the absence of a significant fracture. Plain radiography is indicated in some, but not all, cases to rule out a fracture. It has been well shown that clinical decision rules can reduce the number of studies that are ordered without missing significant fractures.[48-51]

Avulsion fractures may occur concomitantly with sprains. In children, epiphyseal fractures occur more commonly than ligamentous disruption because of the relative ligamentous strength compared with the ease of disrupting the epiphyses. Arthroscopy or MRI is indicated in the follow-up evaluation of some of these injuries (e.g., for suspected cruciate tears) when significant pain or disability is present.[52-54]

Treatment and Disposition

Specific management of sprains varies depending on the location and severity of the injury. In general, initial measures should include the traditional recommendations of ice, elevation, and analgesia. Nonsteroidal anti-inflammatory drugs (NSAIDs) are effective analgesics in many patients, but their anti-inflammatory properties have never been shown to affect the underlying pathophysiology of, or recovery from, a sprain.[55]

Immobilization is used to provide protection and comfort in the initial management of most injuries, using one of the following methods. Because the severity of injury is sometimes difficult to establish at the first visit, it is reasonable to immobilize the affected joint for the first 48 to 72 hours, after which the extent of injury can be better determined. At that time, early mobilization is often desirable, particularly in lateral ankle injuries because this leads to earlier return to work and athletic activities and better preservation of proprioceptive neuromuscular function.[56,57] For lower extremity injuries, protected weight bearing with crutches provides patients with comfort and avoids motion of the impaired part. In elderly patients, safe ambulation sometimes cannot be accomplished, and a short hospitalization or admission to a skilled nursing facility may be necessary.

For complete or nearly complete ligamentous disruption, urgent orthopedic consultation is usually mandatory. Less severe injuries can be followed up 3 to 7 days postinjury when acute swelling has subsided. Copies of x-ray films ordered in the emergency department should be sent with the patient if possible. Physical therapy and rehabilitative exercises sometimes are begun at these visits and carried on for several weeks. Because ligaments are relatively avascular, healing is slow, and patients with significant sprains should be informed of this. Sprains should be diagnosed as precisely as possible and should not be trivialized. Too often, after radiographs have ruled out fracture of an affected extremity, the term *sprain* is applied indiscriminately, or the patient is told that the injury is "only a sprain." The expression "only a sprain" is misleading and should be avoided. Aside from creating false expectations regarding recovery, thoughtless mislabeling of injuries not in evidence may lead to missed occult fractures in adults or epiphyseal injuries in children.

Strains

Nomenclature

A *strain* is an injury to a musculotendinous unit resulting from violent contraction or excessive forcible stretch. The term *pulled muscle* sometimes is used interchangeably with muscle strain. These injuries are graded in a manner similar to sprains.

A *first-degree* strain is a minor tearing of the musculotendinous unit, characterized by swelling, local tenderness, and minor loss of function. Findings increase along a continuum such that in a *second-degree* strain, more fibers are torn, but without complete disruption; swelling, ecchymosis, and loss of strength are more marked. In a *third-degree* strain, the muscle or tendon is completely disrupted, with resultant separation of muscle from muscle, muscle from tendon, or tendon from bone. An accompanying avulsion fracture may be present on radiographs in either second-degree or third-degree injuries.

Assessment

Signs and symptoms include pain, ecchymosis, swelling, and loss of function. A force applied to the muscle, either passive stress or active contraction, produces sharp pain at the site of injury even as the injured muscle may be relatively comfortable at rest. A palpable defect sometimes is present at the site of a complete rupture, which usually involves the region of the muscle tendon junction, or a bunching up of the muscle may be appreciated.[58,59] Among nonathletes, strains commonly are seen in patients who have either overstressed a muscle group or tried to generate excessive force in a nonconditioned muscle. Examples are the weekend gardener or mover who presents on Monday morning with lower back strain, the aerobics student who strains the rectus muscles, and the weightlifter who presents with chest wall pain resulting from pectoralis major strain. These are usually first-degree injuries, and the onset is slow. Rapid acceleration (e.g., in a tennis player) may result in a third-degree gastrocnemius or plantaris tear, whereas pushing off to jump is a common cause of ruptures of the Achilles tendon in a basketball player. A sudden violent attempt at lifting in an older individual can result in a complete biceps brachii disruption. Sudden generation of forces of which the thighs are capable results in second-degree strain of the hamstrings, quadriceps, or thigh abductor muscles.

In athletes, generation of tremendous contraction forces coupled with excessive forcible stretching (while the body may be either accelerating or "planting") results in severe strains. Involvement of almost any muscle group is possible, and the onset of such injuries is usually acute. Immediate removal from activity, application of ice, and rest of the affected limb for 48 to 72 hours usually are advised to prevent further injury. A competitive athlete usually is unable to continue anyway because of the accompanying loss of function. After a brief rest period, however, early mobilization and rehabilitation should be encouraged.

Treatment and Disposition

Treatment depends on the degree of disruption, location, and functional loss. Most first-degree injuries respond in a few days to rest, application of ice, and, for some patients, analgesics. NSAIDs commonly are recommended and prescribed, although their efficacy for other than analgesic purposes is unproven. Second-degree strains are treated similarly, with protection against aggravating activity required for longer periods. Third-degree strains receive similar initial treatment in the emergency department plus early orthopedic consultation. Some of these injuries are amenable to surgical repair, whereas others may be treated with immobilization. The muscle affected and the age, occupation, and activity level of the patient all are factors in deciding whether surgical intervention is appropriate. Many athletes and their trainers believe and it is universally espoused that many strains can be prevented by proper training, warm-up, stretching exercises, and avoidance of overexertion, although limited scientific data exist to support these recommendations.[60,61]

Tendinitis and Tendinosis

Tendinitis is classically described as an inflammatory condition characterized by pain at tendinous insertions into bone, occurring in the setting of overuse.[62,63] It is now believed that the pathophysiology of this condition is more complex than mere overuse, with the roles of load and use affecting cell-matrix interaction.[64] Etiologic factors are believed to include aging, with decreased blood supply and decreased tensile strength; muscle weakness and imbalance; insufficient flexibility; male gender; obesity (in weight-bearing joints); smoking; malalignments; training errors; and improper equipment.[65,66] Additionally, certain systemic diseases, including diabetes mellitus, chronic renal failure, rheumatoid arthritis, and systemic lupus erythematosus; steroids; and occasionally fluoroquinolone use are associated with the development of tendinopathy.[67]

With chronicity, involved tissues are characterized morphologically by signs of chronic rather than acute inflammation (infiltration by macrophages, plasma cells, and lymphocytes rather than leukocytes) and degeneration (cell atrophy). It also has been shown that prostaglandin E_2 levels are normal.[68] This evolving understanding of tendinitis in the future should allow for more logical treatment of these injuries aimed at the underlying pathophysiology. It also has led some authors to propose that chronic painful conditions of the tendon should be referred to as *tendinosis* rather than *tendinitis* or other terms previously used to describe this condition, including *tendonitis, degenerative changes, chronic tendonopathy,* or *partial rupture.*[65,69] In this chapter, *tendinitis* and *tendinosis* are used interchangeably.

Common sites for tendinitis are the rotator cuff of the shoulder, the Achilles tendon, the radial aspect of the wrist (de Quervain's tenosynovitis), and the insertion of the hand extensors on the lateral humeral epicondyle (tennis elbow). Also commonly involved in athletes are the patellar tendon, particularly in athletes engaged in jumping sports; the biceps femoris, semitendinosus, and semimembranosus (hamstring syndrome); posterior tibial tendon (shin splint syndrome); the iliotibial band; and the common wrist flexors (medial epicondylitis) seen in little league pitchers and golfers.[64] In some locations, most commonly the shoulder, calcium deposition occurs along the course of the tendon, resulting in a painful condition termed *calcific tendinitis*. This condition also may occur in the wrist, hand, neck, hip, knee, ankle, or foot.[70]

Physical examination reveals pain with motion and limitation of function and may include point tenderness and palpable crepitus over the involved tendon with motion. In general, a clinical test can be performed by forcible flexion of the involved muscle while keeping the point of insertion fixed or by operating the involved muscle against resistance. Either test should intensify the discomfort. Radiographs are usually negative. A small fleck of bone may suggest an avulsion, or the surface of the bone at the attachment may be roughened, indicating periostitis. As mentioned, there also may be calcium deposits along the course of the tendon, which should not be confused with an avulsion fracture. Ultrasound is sometimes useful in confirming the diagnosis of tendinitis. Although a normal tendon is characterized by a relatively homogeneous pattern, tendinitis is characterized by one or more of the following features: loss of the fibrillar echotexture, focal tendon thickening, diffuse thickening, focal hypoechoic area, irregular or ill-defined borders, or microruptures.[71]

There is little evidence to support any specific treatment for tendinosis. The classic approach consists of rest, ice, and NSAIDs initially, followed by rehabilitation and training and control of force loads to prevent recurrences. Although NSAIDs may be useful for a brief period at the onset of symptoms for their analgesic effects, no evidence exists that they significantly alter the pathophysiology of this condition, and no rationale exists for ordering them in patients at any risk for complications from this class of drugs.[72] Peritendinous local infiltrations of anesthetics and corticosteroids may be useful, but should not be repeated too often because tendon rupture may occur. Injection therapy is especially useful in calcific tendinitis around the shoulder. Injection of steroids directly into the Achilles tendon should be avoided because of reports of partial or complete rupture after even a single injection. Some cases of calcific tendinitis that do not respond to conservative therapy may require either arthroscopic or open surgery.[73,74]

Bursitis

Bursitis is a painful inflammation of the bursa that may be either traumatic or infectious. Commonly involved sites include the olecranon, the greater trochanter of the femur, and the prepatellar and anserine bursae around the knee. Physical findings are tenderness and swelling over the involved bursa, whereas warmth and erythema may signal infection. If infection is suspected, aspiration with Gram stain and culture of the bursal fluid are recommended. Otherwise, treatment may be conservative and is similar to treatment for tendinitis. Most patients can be managed as outpatients.[75]

TREATMENT MODALITIES

Splinting and Bandaging

Fractures or dislocations that are suspected or confirmed should be splinted to avoid damage to muscles, nerves, vessels, and the skin. Splinting also may restore blood flow to ischemic tissue by removing pressure caused by a bone fragment resting against a blood vessel. Finally, splinting relieves pain; conversely, movement of fracture fragments results in severe pain.

Prehospital Care

Splinting should begin in the prehospital setting. Numerous commercial devices are available, and most ambulances carry an assortment of immobilization devices (Figure 46-12). Minimal equipment includes long and short backboards, cervical collars, sandbags, and extremity splints. A half-ring traction splint also is essential. Inflatable air splints are favored by some authors because they are convenient, easy to apply, transparent, and radiolucent and because they tamponade low-pressure bleeding. Other authors prefer to avoid these devices because theoretically they could contribute to the development of a compartment syndrome. If used, inflatable splints should be inflated only by mouth and to the point that still permits indentation by gentle finger pressure.

Field personnel should splint suspected fractures before the patient is moved. Severely angulated long bone fractures should be straightened in the prehospital setting before they are splinted. Splints should be applied in such a way as to immobilize the joints above and below the fracture site to avoid motion of the involved bone. The skin should be padded to avoid local necrosis, and the splint should be secured by a circumferential wrapping material. This material should allow for some expansion and should not be applied in a constricting manner.

Emergency Department Care

In the emergency department, the indications for splinting are the same as in the field. All splints should be checked and, if properly applied, need not be changed. Splinting or other immobilization also is used after diagnosis and treatment of injuries. In some cases, a splint is all that is needed for definitive treatment. Injuries other than sprains and fractures (e.g., inflammatory and infectious processes, bites, burns, and repaired injuries of muscle bellies or tendons) also benefit from immobilization. Splints also can be used to improve function, such as with wristdrop that

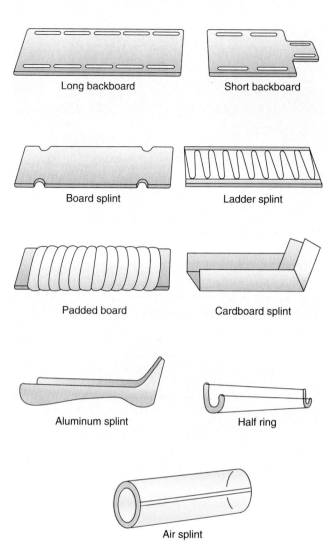

Figure 46-12. Commercial splints.

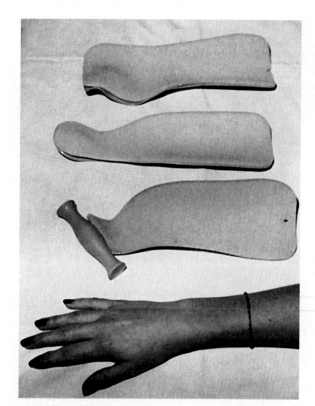

Figure 46-13. Wrist splints.

accompanies radial nerve palsy. When the injury is immobilized, it is important to stress elevation of the affected part to avoid edema formation. Many different devices and materials are available. Some devices that are commonly used are described next.

Upper Extremity

Sling-and-Swathe and Velpeau Bandages
Sling-and-swathe and Velpeau bandages are useful in immobilizing the shoulder, humerus, and elbow. They are commonly used after reduction of dislocated shoulders and to treat impacted fractures of the humeral neck. The axillae should be padded and powdered to avoid skin maceration. A commercial shoulder immobilizer also is available and is useful after reduction of a shoulder dislocation. Its advantages are ease of application and ease of removal and reapplication by the patient for bathing.

Clavicle Splint
Historically, middle one third clavicle fractures routinely were initially treated with a figure-of-eight clavicle strap with or without the addition of a sling. This device is commercially available or can be fashioned from tubular stockinette. If used, a clavicle splint should be applied snugly enough to keep the shoulders back in the "at-attention" position, but not so tight as to compress the axillary artery or brachial plexus. Chafing of the skin can be avoided by padding and powdering the axillae. Superiority of the figure-of-eight clavicle strap over a simple sling has not been shown.

Plaster Splints
Well-fitting, customized plaster splints can be fashioned easily to immobilize the elbow, forearm, wrist, and hand. The advantage of these splints is the ability to mold them to an exact size and shape (e.g., along the ulnar side of the forearm and hand to immobilize a midshaft fourth or fifth metacarpal fracture, the so-called gutter splint). Several commercially available products consist of multiple layers of plaster or fiberglass strips, inside a covering of foam and flannel, on a continuous roll that can be applied to any length. While the splint is still wet, a bandage is wrapped over it, and the splint is molded and held in the desired position as the plaster hardens.

Forearm and Wrist Splints
Numerous preformed splints are available for splinting fractures of the distal forearm and wrist. They are lightweight, neat, and easy to apply and are easily removed and replaced by the patient (Figure 46-13).

Lower Extremity

Femur and Hip
Fractures of the femoral shaft can be immobilized by using a traction device, such as the Hare traction splint

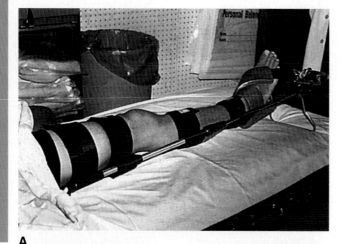

A

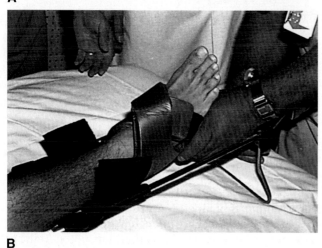

B

Figure 46-14. **A,** Hare traction splint. **B,** This commercial hitch is designed to protect the ankle and heel during traction.

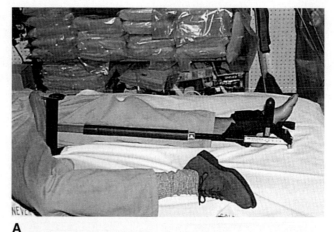

A

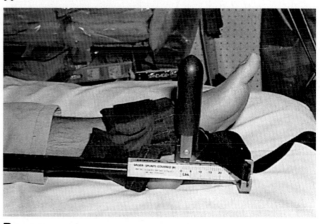

B

Figure 46-15. **A,** Sager splint. **B,** Detail of distal splint end.

or a similar appliance (Figure 46-14). These devices should be applied in the prehospital setting if possible; most ambulances carry them. The principle is that a proximal ring engages the ischial tuberosity for countertraction while the longitudinal traction is applied through the ankle by means of an ankle hitch. A commercial ankle hitch is recommended, but if one is not available, an improvised hitch can be fashioned with a triangular bandage or a wide piece of cloth tied in a Collins hitch. The patient's ankle bones, Achilles tendon, and arch of the foot should be padded, and the circulation should be checked to ensure it is intact. A properly applied splinting device relieves pain from a fracture rather than exacerbating it.

The Sager splint might offer advantages over other appliances in that it is applied to the medial and lateral aspect of the thigh, rather than having a half-ring posteriorly (Figure 46-15). The Sager splint is more acceptable for use in the presence of pelvic fractures and avoids compression of the sciatic nerve. Because the half-ring devices may produce angulation at the fracture site, the Sager device is purported to result in better alignment, although this has never been measured. The Sager splint is shorter and more compact than the Hare traction splint, rendering it more accept-

able for certain transport helicopters and body scanners. Also, the amount of traction is metered at the ankle, and overtraction can be avoided.

Skin traction using a pulley and hanging weights (Buck's traction and others) formerly was recommended for patients awaiting surgery for displaced hip fractures, allegedly to reduce pain and the need for analgesics. Studies have shown no benefit from this treatment, however, while citing risks to skin and soft tissue and noting that it is time-consuming to apply.[76-78] Placing the affected leg in a comfortable position on a pillow provides more comfort.[76]

Knee

Knee immobilizers are commercially available devices that can be used after acute injuries to provide firm but not rigid stabilization of the knee. The device is essentially a foam cylinder with medial and lateral aluminum stays, attached by Velcro straps, and spanning the upper thigh to upper ankle. This device is commonly used after trauma to let the knee "cool off" until a better physical examination or diagnostic study can be performed in a few days.

Another dressing that may be applied at the knee is the Jones "compression" dressing. Some authors believe the word *compression* should not be used here to discourage application that is too tight. The Jones dressing is a bulky dressing that is used by some clinicians in situations when swelling is expected, including internal fixation procedures. The ability to flex and extend at the knee is maintained. The dressing consists of a thick layer of absorbent cotton bandage (Webril) wrapped with an elastic bandage, followed by another layer of cotton bandage, followed by an additional elastic wrap. If more stability is required, slabs of plaster can be placed on the medial and lateral side of the limb, just under the last bandage. Caution must be exercised because burns have been reported with this type of dressing when too many layers of plaster are used. A similar type of bulky dressing may be used for some injuries of the ankle and fractures of the calcaneus. In general, commercial knee immobilizers have replaced the Jones dressing in the treatment of acute knee injuries.

Ankle

Immobilization of the ankle can be accomplished by numerous means. Plaster splints can be used temporarily for the treatment of nondisplaced ankle fractures or for the treatment of severe sprains. These can be fashioned in the same manner as described for the upper extremity. An alternative method is to apply a full circular cast, bivalve it on either side, discard the anterior piece, and affix the posterior mold with an elastic bandage or bias-cut stockinette. Most ankle injuries should be splinted with the patient's ankle in neutral position. Injuries to the Achilles tendon, plantaris muscle, or gastrocnemius muscle initially should be treated with the foot held in slight equinus (plantar flexion) for comfort. The toes should be free to move distal to the metatarsophalangeal joints, and the proximal border should end below the tibial tubercle to avoid pressure on the peroneal nerve.

Adhesive strapping is an alternative method of ankle immobilization that provides good support and limitation of motion. Taping reportedly loses its "protective properties" with cyclic loading and sweating; although this is cited as a disadvantage, it may actually be helpful in encouraging and allowing early mobilization. This method is lightweight and not bulky, and a shoe can be worn over it. Tape is applied in a noncontinuous manner, which allows for swelling and avoids constriction. First, the hair is shaved. Next, strips of tape are measured and torn off; 1½-inch or 2-inch cloth-backed adhesive tape or Elastoplast is used. Elastoplast is an elastic-backed tape, constructed to stretch only in the longitudinal direction; this serves to spring the foot back automatically to a neutral position if the foot is plantar flexed for any reason. The tape should be applied directly to the skin after a skin adherent, such as tincture of benzoin, is applied. The tape should lie flat because wrinkles may damage the skin (Figure 46-16).

A dome-paste bandage, or Unna's boot, is a bandage impregnated with zinc oxide, calamine lotion, glycerin, and gelatin that also is well suited to immobilize an ankle sprain.[79] This combination is gentle to the skin, which is especially important if atrophy or venous incompetence is present. In addition, hair need not be shaved, the bandage is easy to apply, and a shoe can be worn over it. Some patients complain about the sticky sensation against the skin, especially in warm weather. Another disadvantage is that it is applied concentrically, and problems can arise if the bandage is wrapped too tightly. The bandage should be applied directly to the skin, starting at the foot and working upward; it should overlap at each turn approximately half the width of the previous turn and continue up to just below the tibial tubercle. Then the bandage should be covered with either bias-cut stockinette or an elastic bandage. The dome-paste bandage hardens to about the consistency of sturdy cardboard and provides firm support. Removal is best accomplished with bandage scissors.

An increasingly preferred device for moderate to severe lateral ankle sprains is a commercial support composed of molded plastic with Velcro straps (e.g., Air Cast, AirStirrup) (Figure 46-17).[56,80] This product may be worn in the patient's shoe and permits early weight bearing and return to activity. It is designed to permit dorsiflexion and plantar flexion but to limit inversion and eversion, a concept referred to as *functional bracing*. Some authors also find this device useful during athletic activities instead of adhesive taping to prevent recurrences.[81,82] Although these orthoses are relatively expensive, the cost might be more than offset by their ease of application, their reusability, and the benefit derived from earlier return to work.[80]

Severe ankle sprains also may benefit from immobilization in a cam walker, which is a commercial appliance consisting of a layer of padding extending from the tibial tubercle to the metatarsal heads, supported by metal plates along the length of the lower leg. These plates articulate with a molded hard plastic boot at the ankle. The position of the foot can be adjusted as desired, and when set, the ankle is kept firmly immobile. The rounded undersurface of the boot allows for ambulation without movement of the ankle joint.

Casts

Plaster casts perform a function similar to splints in that they provide stability and pain relief. Casts sometimes are used in conjunction with internal stabilizing devices, such as Kirschner wires or Steinmann pins. Casts are not mandatory for all fractures, and in situations in which they are, application is usually not an immediate necessity. Swelling and subsequent pressure under the cast are highest during the first 24 hours after injury.[83] Plaster is applied as strips or rolls of cloth that are impregnated with a hemihydrate of calcium sulfate. When this cloth is dipped in lukewarm water, a creamy paste is formed that can be molded into a cast. An exothermic reaction takes place that causes the plaster to harden and can burn the skin.[84] Factors that have been shown experimentally to increase skin temperatures during plaster application are dip-water temperatures greater than 24° C, cast thickness greater than eight plies, and inadequate ventilation of the newly applied cast.

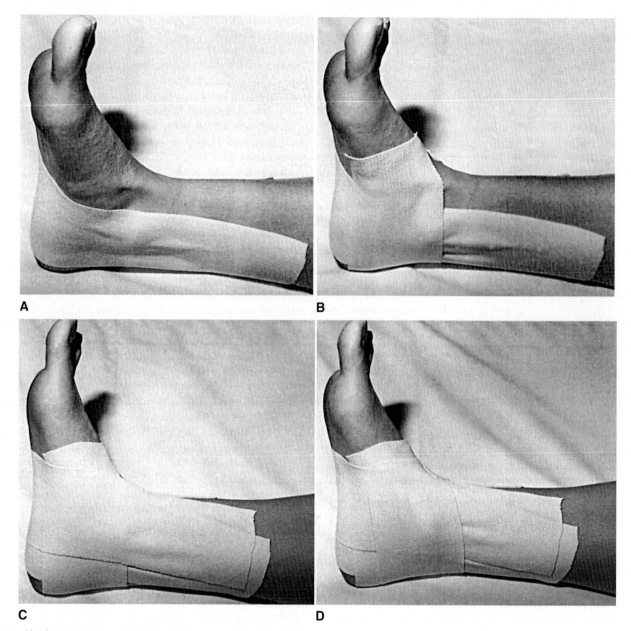

Figure 46-16. Application of adhesive strips to immobilize the ankle.

Immersing the plaster in water for too short a time or squeezing too much water out also may lead to generation of excess heat. To avoid pressure on the skin and over bony prominences, stockinette and layers of cotton sheet wadding (Webril) are snugly applied first. Padding that migrates under a formed cast can be uncomfortable and result in pressure sores. Padding alone does not prevent burns.[85]

Variations of the basic cast exist. A window may be placed in the cast, and the cutout area may be used as access to skin wounds that require care during immobilization. Walking heels may be worked onto a lower extremity cast and should be placed in the center of the foot. Synthetic casts (fiberglass and other materials) are lightweight, durable, and water resistant. In addition, their setting temperatures are significantly lower, and they are less likely to produce burns.[86] They are more expensive and more difficult to apply.

Patients with casts may present to the emergency department for complaints related to their casts; these usually are pain, local irritation, swelling, or numbness of the distal part. A cast that is too tight results in swelling, pain, coolness, and change in skin color of the distal parts. Pain also may be caused by the initial injury or by local pressure, or it may be a result of a developing compartment syndrome or wound infection. The safest thing to do if a patient complains of pain is to bivalve the cast and inspect the extremity. This is done by cutting the plaster and the padding on each side and removing half the cast at a time, using the other half as a mold to keep the extremity immobile. Afterward, the bivalved cast can be held together with bias-cut stockinette or elastic wrap until a new cast is applied. If relieving external pressure does not alleviate symptoms, the diagnosis of compartment syndrome should be seriously considered. Casts may

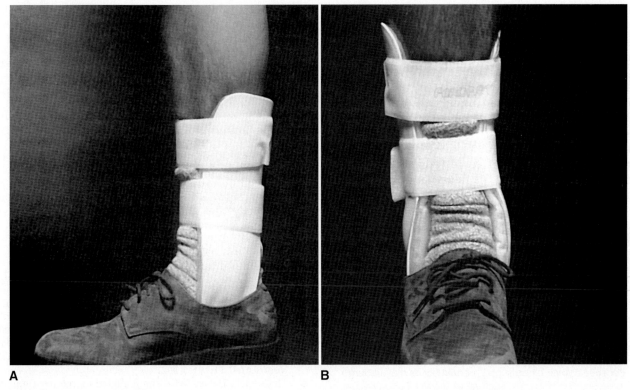

Figure 46-17. Air cast. **A,** Lateral view. **B,** Anteroposterior view.

obscure wound infections, sources of sepsis, and even the source of tetanus. The clinician should not hesitate to bivalve the cast and inspect the extremity.

The need for mandatory routine cast checks 1 day after initial application has been questioned.[87] In a retrospective study of 250 patients, none experienced problems from neurovascular compression, although 24% required some alteration of the cast. In the study, it may be simply that the casts were applied incorrectly in the first place. It is probably advisable to continue routine cast checks if casts are applied in the emergency department.

Thermal Therapy

Some confusion exists as to the role of cryotherapy versus heat therapy in the treatment of acute orthopedic injuries, although the available literature uniformly favors cryotherapy. Part of this confusion arises because heat may be more soothing to the patient. Cryotherapy produces physiologic effects that favor a better prognosis. Cold causes vasoconstriction, limiting blood flow and hemorrhage into the traumatized area. Metabolic requirements are reduced in cooled tissues, as is histamine, and less capillary breakdown occurs as a result. Reduced blood flow also limits edema formation. Lower extravascular fluid pressure allows better lymphatic drainage of injured areas. Cryotherapy produces three, and perhaps four, stages of sensation of which the physician and the patient should be aware. In the first stage, a cold sensation is noted for 1 to 3 minutes. The second stage consists of a burning or aching sensation for 2 to 7 minutes after the appli-

cation of cold. This stage is uncomfortable, but must be endured to receive the benefits of the next two stages. Heat therapy, by contrast, is soothing, and patients are likely to prefer this to the second stage of cryotherapy. The third stage begins 5 to 12 minutes after the application of ice and produces local numbness or anesthesia. The pain-spasm cycle is interrupted. While under this anesthetic effect, passive exercise may be desirable. This exercise helps to prevent atrophy, mobilize edema, clear injury debris, and reduce adhesions.[88-90]

A fourth stage sometimes occurs 12 to 15 minutes after intense cryotherapy is begun, consisting of reflex deep tissue vasodilation without a corresponding increase in metabolism (reminiscent of the situation in rewarming shock). Because of this, a maximum of 15 minutes of cold application per treatment usually is advised.[91,92] An experimental study using triple-contrast bone scans compared the effect of icing times from 5 to 25 minutes on blood flow to the knee. Five minutes produced a measurable decrease in all tissues of the knee, whereas 25 minutes increased this effect fourfold and produced the overall maximal effects. A paradoxical increase in blood flow, perhaps reflecting reflex vasodilation, occurred at 10 minutes, but then reversed.[93] These results suggest that longer icing times than previously recommended may be beneficial. Absolute contraindications to cryotherapy include severe cold allergy (with hives and joint pain) and Raynaud's phenomenon. Relative contraindications include some rheumatoid conditions and paroxysmal cold hemoglobinuria with renal dysfunction and secondary hypertension. Anesthetic skin in a paralyzed or comatose patient is at risk with ice therapy. One case of gangrene has been reported, but in this instance cold was applied for 16 hours a day for 2 months.[94] These contraindications to cryotherapy are rare, especially in the athletic population most at risk for serious injuries. Heat increases blood flow and the inflammatory response and edema. Warm tissues and cells have a higher metabolic rate and increased requirements of nutrients and oxygen. Ice, rather than heat, is the method of choice of most authorities in the acute treatment and rehabilitation of acute orthopedic injuries and should be initiated as soon as possible for maximum benefit.

KEY CONCEPTS

- Compartment syndrome is associated most commonly with a closed long bone fracture of the tibia, but also is well described in the thigh, forearm, arm, hand, and foot and can occur with soft tissue trauma alone. Elevation of a limb with resultant reduction in the local arteriovenous gradient may be counterproductive and may exacerbate compartment syndrome.

- Because of their blood supply, certain bones may undergo avascular necrosis after fracture, especially if fractures are comminuted and go untreated for any length of time. The femoral head, talus, scaphoid, and capitate are particularly prone to this complication.

- Fat embolism syndrome is a serious manifestation of fat embolism, occurring most commonly after long bone fractures in young adults (usually tibia and fibula) and after hip fractures in elderly patients. Respiratory distress syndrome is the earliest, most common, and serious manifestation. Neurologic involvement, manifest as restlessness, confusion, or deteriorating mental status, is also an early sign, as are thrombocytopenia and a petechial rash.

- In children, epiphyseal fractures occur more commonly than ligamentous disruption because of the relative ligamentous strength compared with the ease of disrupting the epiphyses.

REFERENCES

1. Courtenay BG, Bowers DM: Stress fractures: Clinical features and investigation. *Med J Aust* 153:155, 1990.
2. Umans H, Pavlov H: Stress fractures of the lower extremities. *Semin Roentgenol* 29:176, 1994.
3. de Sancis N, Della Corte S, Pempinello C: Orthopaedics distal tibial and fibular epiphyseal fractures in children: Prognostic criteria and long-term results in 158 patients. *J Pediatr Orthop* 9:40, 2000.
4. Rogers LF, Poznanski AK: Imaging of epiphyseal injuries. *Radiology* 91:297, 1994.
5. Jaramillo D, Hoffer FA: Cartilaginous epiphysis and growth plate: Normal and abnormal MR imaging findings. *AJR Am J Roentgenol* 58:1105, 1992.
6. Reed MH: Fractures and dislocations of the extremities in children. *J Trauma* 17:351, 1977.
7. Mizuto T, et al: Statistical analysis of the incidence of physeal injuries. *J Pediatr Orthop* 7:518, 1987.
8. Lund PJ, et al: Comparison of conventional and computed radiography: Assessment of image quality and reader performance in skeletal extremity trauma. *Acad Radiol* 4:570, 1997.

9. Chacon D, et al: Use of comparison radiographs in the diagnosis of traumatic injuries of the elbow. *Ann Emerg Med* 21:895, 1992.
10. Keats TE, Anderson MW: *Atlas of Normal Roentgen Variants That May Simulate Disease,* 7th ed. St Louis, Mosby, 2001.
11. Conway JJ, et al: The role of bone scintigraph in detecting child abuse. *Semin Nucl Med* 23:321, 1993.
12. Sorger JI, et al: Once daily, high dose versus divided, low dose gentamicin for open fractures. *Clin Orthop* 366:197, 1999.
13. Vasenius J: Clindamycin versus cloxacillin in the treatment of 240 open fractures: A randomized prospective study. *Ann Chir Gynaecol* 87:224, 1998.
14. Patzakis MJ, Wilkins J, Moore TM: Considerations in reducing the infection rate in open tibial fractures. *Clin Orthop* 178:36, 1983.
15. Kreder HJ, Armstrong P: The significance of perioperative cultures in open pediatric lower-extremity fractures. *Clin Orthop* 302:206, 1994.
16. Juren CT, Di Stadio AJ: Treatment of grade IIIB and IIIC open tibial fractures. *Orthop Clin North Am* 25:561, 1994.
17. O'Riain S: New and simple test of nerve function in hand. *BMJ* 3:615, 1973.
18. Good LP: Compartment syndrome. *AORN J* 56:904, 1992.
19. Weinstein SM, Herring SA: Nerve problems and compartment syndromes in the hand, wrist, and forearm. *Clin Sports Med* 11:161, 1992.
20. McGee DL, Dalsey WC: The mangled extremity: Compartment syndrome and amputations. *Emerg Med Clin North Am* 10:783, 1992.
21. Myerson M, Manoli A: Compartment syndromes of the foot after calcaneal fractures. *Clin Orthop* 142, 1993, pp 142-150.
22. Kahan JS, et al: Acute bilateral compartment syndrome of the thigh induced by exercise. *J Bone Joint Surg* 76A:1068, 1994.
23. Hastings H II, Misamore G: Compartment syndrome resulting from intravenous regional anesthesia. *J Hand Surg* 12A:559, 1987.
24. Reddy PK, Kaye KW: Deep posterior compartment syndrome: A serious complication of the lithotomy position. *J Urol* 132:144, 1984.
25. Aschoff A, Steiner-Milz H, Steiner HH: Lower limb compartment syndrome following lumbar discectomy in the knee-chest position. *Neurosurg Rev* 13:155, 1990.
26. Gulli B, Templeman D: Compartment syndrome of the lower extremity. *Orthop Clin North Am* 25:677, 1994.
27. Whitesides TE Jr, et al: Tissue pressure measurement as a determinant for the need of fasciotomy. *Clin Orthop* 113:43, 1975.
28. McQueen MM, Gaston P, Court-Brown CM: Acute compartment syndrome: Who is at risk? *J Bone Joint Surg Br* 82:200, 2000.
29. Lu-Yao GL, et al: Outcomes after displaced fractures of the femoral neck: A meta-analysis of one hundred and six published reports. *J Bone Joint Surg* 76:15, 1994.
30. Coombs RR, Thomas RW: Avascular necrosis of the hip. *Br J Hosp Med* 51:275, 1994.
31. Proctor MT: Non-union of the scaphoid: Early and late management. *Injury* 25:15, 1994.
32. Yoo CI, et al: Avascular necrosis after fracture-separation of the distal end of the humerus in children. *Orthopedics* 15:959, 1992.
33. Rowbotham M: Complex regional pain syndrome type I (reflex sympathetic dystrophy): More than a myth. *Neurology* 51:4, 1998.
34. Stanton-Hicks M, Janig W, Hassenbusch S: Reflex sympathetic dystrophy: Changing concepts and taxonomy. *Pain* 63:127, 1995.
35. Rogers JN, Valley MA: Reflex sympathetic dystrophy. *Clin Podiatr Med Surg* 11:73, 1994.

36. Veldman P, Reynan HM, Arntz IE: Signs and symptoms of reflex sympathetic dystrophy: Prospective study of 829 patients. *Lancet* 342:1012, 1993.

37. Van der Laan L, et al: Complex regional pain syndrome type I (RSD): Pathology of skeletal muscle and peripheral nerve. *Neurology* 51:20, 1998.

38. Murray CS, et al: Morbidity in reflex sympathetic dystrophy. *Arch Dis Child* 82:231, 2000.

39. Gibbons JJ, Wilson PR: RSD score: A criterion for the diagnosis of reflex sympathetic dystrophy and causalgia. *Clin J Pain* 8:260, 1992.

40. Oerlemans HM, Oosteodorp RA, de Boo T, Goris RJ: Pain and reduced mobility in complex regional pain syndrome I: Outcome of a prospective randomized, controlled clinical trial of adjuvant physical therapy versus occupational therapy. *Pain* 83:77, 1999.

41. Tountas AA, Noguchi A: Treatment of post-traumatic reflex sympathetic dystrophy (RSDS) with intravenous blocks of a mixture of corticosteroid and lidocaine: A retrospective review of 17 consecutive cases. *J Orthop* 5:412, 1991.

42. Kingery WS: A critical review of controlled clinical trials for peripheral neuropathic pain and complex regional pain syndromes. *Pain* 73:123, 1997.

43. Zolinger PE, et al: Effect of vitamin C on frequency of sympathetic reflex dystrophy in wrist fractures: A randomized trial. *Lancet* 354:2025, 1999.

44. Bulger EM, Smith DG, Maier RV: Fat embolism syndrome: A 10 year review. *Arch Surg* 132:435, 1997.

45. Varela CD, et al: Fracture blisters: Clinical and pathological aspects. *J Orthop Trauma* 7:417, 1993.

46. Rodriguez-Merchan EC: Controversies on the treatment of irreducible elbow dislocations with an associated non-salvageable radial head fracture. *J Orthop Trauma* 9:341, 1995.

47. Sabapathy SR, Bose VC, Rex C: Irreducible dislocation of the interphalangeal joint of the thumb due to sesamoid bone interposition: A case report. *J Hand Surg* 20:487, 1995.

48. Stiell IG, et al: A study to develop clinical decision rules for the use of radiography in acute ankle injuries. *Ann Emerg Med* 21:384, 1992.

49. Stiell IG, et al: Decision rules for the use of radiography in acute ankle injuries: Refinement and prospective validation. *JAMA* 269:1127, 1993.

50. Stiell IG, et al: Implementation of the Ottawa ankle rules. *JAMA* 271:827, 1994.

51. Stiell IG, et al. Implementation of the Ottawa knee rule for the use of radiology in acute knee injuries. *JAMA* 278:2075, 1997.

52. Maffulli N, et al: Acute haemarthrosis of the knee in athletes: A prospective study of 106 cases. *J Bone Joint Surg* 75B:945, 1993.

53. Fanelli GC: Posterior cruciate ligament injuries in trauma patients. *Arthroscopy* 9:291, 1993.

54. Ruwe PA, et al: Can MR imaging effectively replace diagnostic arthroscopy? *Radiology* 183:335, 1992.

55. Dupont M, Beliveau P, Theriault G: The efficacy of antiinflammatory medication in the treatment of the acutely sprained ankle. *Am J Sports Med* 15:41, 1987.

56. Konradsen L, Holmer P, Sanderguard L: Early mobilizing treatment for grade III ankle ligament injuries. *Foot Ankle* 12:69, 1991.

57. Scheuffelen C, et al: Orthotic devices in functional treatment of ankle sprain: Stabilizing effects of real movements. *Int J Sports Med* 14:140, 1993.

58. Safran MR, et al: The role of warmup in muscular injury prevention. *Am J Sports Med* 16:123, 1988.

59. Garrett WE, et al: The effect of muscle architecture on the biochemical failure properties of skeletal muscle under passive extension. *Am J Sports Med* 16:7, 1988.

60. Arrington ED, Miller MD: Skeletal muscle injuries. *Orthop Clin North Am* 26:411, 1995.

61. Worrell TW: Factors associated with hamstring injuries: An approach to treatment and preventative measures. *Sports Med* 17:338, 1994.

62. Guidotti TL: Occupational repetitive strain injury. *Am Fam Physician* 4:585, 1992.

63. Nirschl RP: Elbow tendinosis/tennis elbow. *Clin Sports Med* 11:851, 1992.

64. Leadbetter WB: Cell-matrix response in tendon injury. *Clin Sports Med* 11:533, 1992.

65. Alfredson A, Lorentzon R: Chronic achilles tendinosis: Recommendations for treatment and prevention. *Sports Med* 29:135, 2000.

66. Fenwick SA, Hazleman BL, Graham PR: The vasculature- and its role in the damaged and healing tendon. *Arthritis Res* 4:252, 2002.

67. Zabraniecki L, et al: Fluoroquinolone induced tendinopathy: Report of 6 cases. *J Rheumatol* 23:516, 1996.

68. Alfredson H, et al: In situ microdialysis in tendon tissue: high levels of glutamate but not prostaglandin E2 in chronic Achilles tendon pain. *Knee Sports Surg Traumatol Arthosc* 7:378, 1999.

69. Maffulli N, Wong J, Almekinders LC: Types and epidemiology of tendinopathy. *Clin Sports Med* 22:675, 2003.

70. Holt PD, Keats TE: Calcific tendinitis: A review of the usual and unusual. *Skeletal Radiol* 22:1, 1993.

71. Grassi W: Sonographic imaging of tendons. *Arthritis Rheum* 43:969, 2000.

72. Astrom M, Westlin N: No effect of piroxicam on Achilles tendinopathy: A randomized study of 70 patients. *Acta Orthop Scand* 63:631, 1992.

73. Weiler JM: Medial modifiers of sports injury: The use of nonsteroidal anti-inflammatory drugs in sports soft tissue injury. *Clin Sports Med* 11:625, 1992.

74. Read MTF, Motto SG: Tendo achillis pain: Steroids and outcome. *Br J Sports Med* 26:15, 1992.

75. Stell I: Management of acute bursitis: Outcome study of a structured approach. *J R Soc Med* 92:5216, 1999.

76. Finsen V, et al: Preoperative traction in patients with hip fractures. *Injury* 23:242, 1992.

77. Needoff M, Radford P, Langstaff R: Preoperative traction for hip fractures in the elderly. *Injury* 24:317, 1993.

78. Anderson GH, et al: Preoperative skin traction for fractures of the proximal femur: A randomized prospective trial. *J Bone Joint Surg* 75:794, 1993.

79. Pointer J: Using an Unna's boot in treating ligamentous ankle injuries. *West J Med* 139:257, 1983.

80. De Maio M, Paine R, Dreg D Jr: Chronic lateral ankle instability-inversion sprains: Part I. *Orthopedics* 15:87, 1992.

81. Gross MT, et al: Comparison of support provided by ankle taping and semirigid orthosis. *J Orthop Sports Phys Ther* 9:33, 1987.

82. Rovere GD, et al: Retrospective comparison of taping and ankle stabilizers in preventing ankle injuries. *Am J Sports Med* 16:228, 1988.

83. Patrick JH, Levack B: A study of pressures beneath forearm plasters. *Injury* 13:37, 1987.

84. Kaplan SS: Burns following application of plaster splint dressings. *J Bone Joint Surg* 63:670, 1981.

85. Lavalette R, Pope MH, Dickstein H: Setting temperatures of plaster casts: The influence of technical variables. *J Bone Joint Surg* 64:907, 1982.

86. Pope MH, Callahan G, Lavalette R: Setting temperatures of synthetic casts. *J Bone Joint Surg* 67:262, 1985.

87. Riding G, Edgel M, James M: Plaster checks: A waste of resources? *J Accid Emerg Med* 11:266, 1994.

88. Hocutt JE, et al: Cryotherapy in ankle sprains. *Am J Sports Med* 10:316, 1982.

89. McMaster WC: A literary review on ice therapy in injuries. *Am J Sports Med* 5:124, 1977.

90. Basur RL, Sheperd E, Mouzas GL: A cooling method in the treatment of ankle sprains. *Practitioner* 216:708, 1976.

91. Riverburgh DW: Physical modalities in the treatment of tendon injuries. *Clin Sports Med* 11:645, 1992.
92. Ernot E, Fialka V: Ice freezes pain? A review of the clinical effectiveness of analgesic cold therapy. *J Pain Symptom Manage* 9:56, 1994.
93. Ho SS, et al: Comparison of various icing times in decreasing bone metabolism and blood flow in the knee. *Am J Sports Med* 23:74, 1995.
94. Fye KH, Denkler K: Gangrene as a complication of topical ice therapy [letter]. *J Rheumatol* 20:1808, 1993.

CHAPTER

47 Hand

Everett Lyn and Robert E. Antosia

PERSPECTIVE

The hand is intricate, dynamic, and unique in function. It combines extreme mobility, precision, power, and sensation and is used to express and execute. Because the hands are more exposed to the environment than the rest of the body, they are commonly injured. Function depends on intact relationships between intrinsic structural components, musculotendinous units originating from more proximal areas, and motor and sensory connections with the central nervous system. Restoration of function rather than appearance is the primary goal in management of hand injuries and infections. Early recognition and timely initiation of therapy for limb-threatening conditions are essential to outcome. The fate of the hand largely depends on the physician who initially cares for it. Mismanagement may result in unnecessary functional loss that may not be recoverable, even with the best convalescent care. An understanding of the functional anatomy of the hand is necessary for the appropriate evaluation and management of these disorders.

Epidemiology

Overall, hand injuries are reported to represent 5% to 10% of emergency department visits, and approximately 6% of these patients have deep, significant injuries.[1] Injuries have environmental, occupational, and recreational causes and are seen in all age groups. The spectrum of injury includes infections, lacerations, fractures, crush wounds, amputations, and burns. It is estimated that 10% of all patients with hand injuries require referral to a hand specialist, and most patients referred from emergency departments have fractures.[2] The disability potential of hand injuries is generally high and may result from loss of strength, flexibility, or sensation. Data suggest that hand injuries account for 19% of lost-time injuries and 9% of workers' compensation cases.[3] Approximately 3 to 4 million working days are lost each year as a result of hand injuries.[4] Overall, hand and fingers are the most frequent body parts injured in the workplace and cared for in emergency departments.[5]

PRINCIPLES OF DISEASE, FUNCTIONAL ANATOMY, PHYSIOLOGY, AND EXAMINATION OF THE HAND

Terminology

To avoid confusion, it is important that standard terminology for the surface anatomy of the hand be used (Figure 47-1). The back of the hand and fingers is called the *dorsal surface,* and the palm side is called either the *palmar* or the *volar surface.* The borders of the hand are *radial* and *ulnar.* The five digits often are designated by numerals, but common names are preferable: I (thumb), II (index finger), III (long or middle finger), IV (ring finger), and V (little finger). Each finger has three joints: the metacarpophalangeal (MCP), the proximal interphalangeal (PIP), and the distal interphalangeal (DIP) joints. The thumb has an MCP joint and only one interphalangeal (IP) joint. There are proximal, middle, and distal phalanges in the fingers and only a proximal and a distal phalanx in the thumb. The *thenar mass* or *eminence* refers to the muscular area on the palmar surface overlying the thumb metacarpal. The *hypothenar eminence* is the muscle mass on the palmar surface overlying the little finger metacarpal.

Hand and digit motion is standardized and is illustrated in Figures 47-2 through 47-6. The carpometacarpal (CMC) joint is more mobile in the thumb than in the other fingers and is the key to the grasp and dexterity that characterize the human hand. Motions of this joint include palmar abduction (also called *flexion*), radial abduction, retroposition (extension), adduction, and opposition (see Figure 47-6). The IP joints are essentially hinge joints and are capable of only two motions: flexion and extension.

Structural Framework

Skin Cover

The hand has two skin surfaces, each with differing functions. The skin of the palm is thick compared with the dorsal skin and is stabilized by fibrous connections on its deep surface. The skin creases in the palmar aspect of the hand are largely transverse and represent

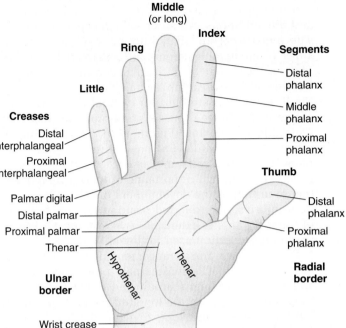

Surface anatomy
(Volar surface)

Middle
(or long)

Ring

Index

Little

Segments

Distal
phalanx

Middle
phalanx

Proximal
phalanx

Creases

Distal
interphalangeal

Proximal
interphalangeal

Palmar digital

Distal palmar

Proximal palmar

Thenar

Hypothenar

Thenar

**Ulnar
border**

Wrist crease

Thumb

Distal
phalanx

Proximal
phalanx

**Radial
border**

Figure 47-1. Surface anatomy of the hand. (From Burton RI, et al: *The Hand: Examination and Diagnosis,* 3rd ed. New York, Churchill Livingstone, 1990, p 6.)

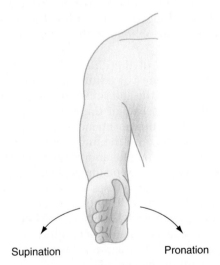

Supination

Pronation

Figure 47-2. Pronation and supination of the hand.

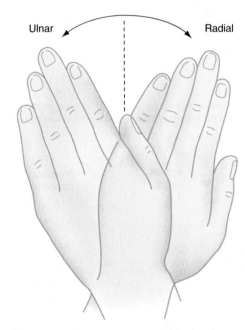

Ulnar

Radial

Figure 47-3. Ulnar and radial deviation of the hand.

adherence between skin and underlying fascia, without intervening adipose tissue. These features facilitate flexion and limit the development of inflammatory edema in the palm.[6] The other noteworthy characteristic of the palmar skin is the unique arrangement of epithelial ridges of the dermis that form cutaneous striations. They have forensic importance in the pulp as "fingerprints" and play an important role in increasing friction when grasping objects.[7]

The dorsal skin is relatively thin and mobile, permitting motion of the various joints. As a path of least resistance, the dorsum of the hand also swells easily after inflammation or trauma and may limit flexion of the MCP joints.[7] In addition, infection in the palmar

aspect of the hand may cause dorsal swelling and can be misleading without a careful physical examination.

Skeleton

The hand and wrist contain 27 bones: 14 phalangeal bones, 5 metacarpal bones, and 8 carpal bones (Figure 47-7). There are eight small carpal bones in the region of the wrist that are strongly united to one another by ligaments. These bones form synovial joints and are

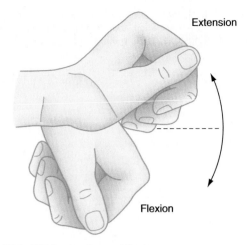

Figure 47-4. Wrist extension and flexion.

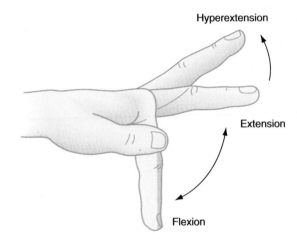

Figure 47-5. Finger flexion is volar and occurs at the metacarpophalangeal joint; extension and hyperextension are as shown.

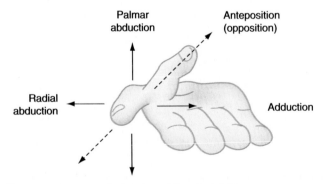

Figure 47-6. Perpendicular view of thumb mobility.

arranged in two rows, proximal and distal, with four bones in each row. Together the bones of the carpus present a concavity on their volar surface, which is bridged by a strong membranous band, the flexor retinaculum. In this way, the bridge and the bones form a tunnel, known as the *carpal tunnel,* through which passes the median nerve and long flexor tendons of the fingers. The IP joints are inherently more stable than the MCP joint, by virtue of their bicondylar configura-

tion, which gives a modified tongue-in-groove appearance (Figure 47-8).

The soft tissue supporting these joints includes the capsular ligamentous structures, which afford stability, and the tendinous structures, which generate mobility. The metacarpal and IP joints are stabilized on both sides by collateral ligaments and anteriorly by a palmar fibrocartilaginous "volar plate." Because of anatomic differences between the metacarpals and phalanges, the IP collaterals are tight throughout the entire range of motion, whereas the collaterals of the MCP joint are tightest in flexion (Figure 47-9). The IP joints are hinges, but the MCP joint has additional side-to-side mobility and rotational movement to facilitate efficient grasp.[7] The clinical importance of these differences is that to minimize the development of contractures after joint injuries, the preferred position of immobilization of the PIP joints is extension, whereas the MCP joints are more properly placed in flexion.

The structure and arrangement of the metacarpals are noteworthy. The metacarpals participate in three arches: the proximal (carpal) and distal (metacarpal) transverse arches and the longitudinal arch (Figure 47-10).[8] The index and long finger metacarpals form a fairly immobile segment because of their ridged articulation with the carpals. The adjacent metacarpals are more mobile. This unique anatomy gives the human palm a longitudinal and transverse concavity when the thumb is alongside the index finger; however, this changes to an oblique gutter when the thumb is extended.

The small bones of the child's hand differ significantly from the bones of adults and from other long bones because of the presence of an epiphysis or growth plate at one end of the bone. The phalangeal epiphyses and the thumb metacarpal epiphysis occur at the proximal end, and the finger metacarpal epiphyses are located at the distal end of the bone (Figure 47-11). In boys, the proximal phalangeal epiphysis appears at 15 to 24 months and fuses at 16 years. In girls, it appears at 10 to 15 months and fuses at 14 years.[9] The time of appearance and fusion are related to skeletal maturity and can be judged accurately until puberty from hand and wrist radiographs because the sequence of development is age specific.[10]

Muscle and Tendon Function

The muscles that power the hand may be divided into extrinsic and intrinsic muscles. The intrinsic muscles have their origins and insertions within the hand. The extrinsic muscles have origins in muscle bellies in the forearm and tendinous insertions on bones in the hand. They are divided further into extrinsic flexor and extensor muscles. The flexors of the digits in the hand lie on the volar surface of the forearm; the extensors are on the dorsal surface.

Intrinsic Musculature

The intrinsic muscles of the hand include the muscles of the thenar and hypothenar eminences, the adductor pollicis, the interossei, and the lumbricals (Figure 47-

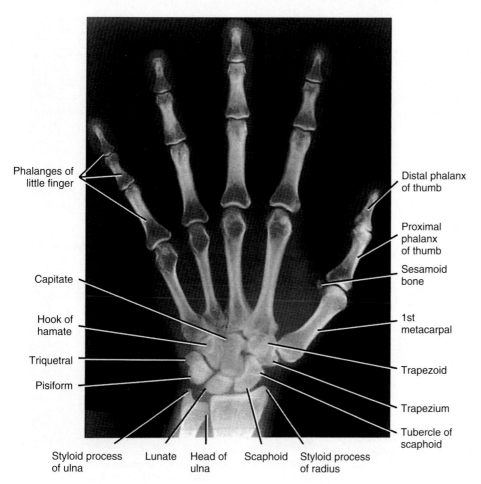

Figure 47-7. Posteroanterior radiograph of the wrist and hand with the forearm pronated. (From Snell RS, Smith MS: *Clinical Anatomy for Emergency Medicine.* St. Louis, Mosby, 1993, p 650.)

Phalanges of little finger

Capite

Hook of hamate

Triquetral

Pisiform

Styloid process of ulna

Lunate

Head of ulna

Scaphoid

Styloid process of radius

Distal phalanx of thumb

Proximal phalanx of thumb

Sesamoid bone

1st metacarpal

Trapezoid

Trapezium

Tubercle of scaphoid

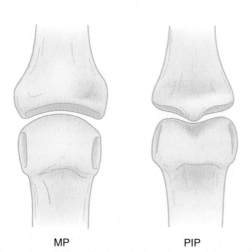

MP

PIP

Figure 47-8. The metacarpophalangeal (MP) and proximal interphalangeal (PIP) joints are quite different structurally. The PIP joint has a bicondylar configuration, making it inherently more stable than the globular MP joint. (From DeLee JC, Drez D Jr: *Orthopedic Sports Medicine: Principles and Practice,* 2nd ed. Philadelphia, Saunders, 2003.)

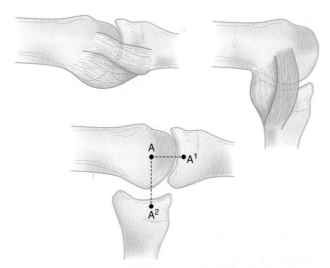

Figure 47-9. The shape of the metacarpal head is eccentric, resulting in a cam effect that makes the collateral ligaments more taut in flexion than in extension. Distance A-A^1 is less than A-A^2. The cam effect is not present in the proximal interphalangeal joint. (From DeLee JC, Drez D Jr: *Orthopedic Sports Medicine: Principles and Practice,* 2nd ed. Philadelphia, Saunders, 2003.)

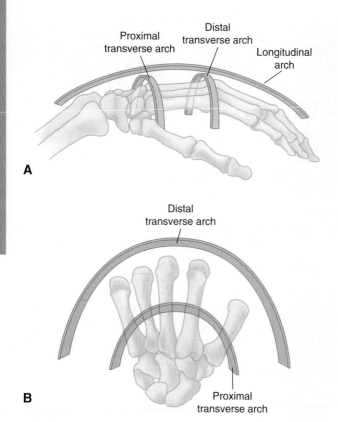

Figure 47-10. The three arches of the metacarpals. **A,** Sagittal view. **B,** Transverse view. (From American Society for Surgery of the Hand: *Regional Review Course in Hand Surgery Syllabus,* 10th ed. Aurora, Colo, ASSH, 1990.)

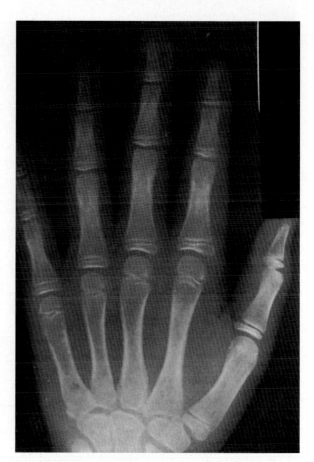

Figure 47-11. Normal location of the epiphysis of the hand. All of the phalangeal epiphyses are located at the proximal end. The metacarpophalangeal epiphyses all are distally situated, however, except for that of the wrist, which is proximal. (From Harris WH, Harris CC: *The Radiology of Emergency Medicine.* Baltimore, Williams & Wilkins, 1993, p 440)

12). The thenar muscles cover the thumb metacarpal. This group includes the abductor pollicis brevis, opponens pollicis, and flexor pollicis brevis. These muscles originate in the flexor retinaculum and on the carpal bones and insert at the base of the first metacarpal and first proximal phalanx. They act in concert with the long flexors and extensors to carry the thumb through its intricate range of motion. The muscles are evaluated by palpating the thenar eminence for contraction as the patient touches the tips of the thumb and little finger. They also can be tested by asking the patient to place the dorsum of the hand on a flat surface and to raise the thumb up straight to form a 90-degree angle with the palm. The thenar muscles usually are innervated by the motor branch of the median nerve. In some cases, they may be partially innervated by the ulnar nerve.

The adductor pollicis arises from the second and third metacarpals and inserts on the first proximal phalanx. This muscle is innervated by the ulnar nerve. Thumb adduction is tested separately by having the patient forcibly hold a piece of paper between the thumb and radial side of the index proximal phalanx. If the adductor pollicis is weak or nonfunctioning, the thumb IP joint flexes with this maneuver (Froment's paper sign).[11] In this evaluation, the two hands should be compared.

The lumbrical muscles arise from the sides of the flexor digitorum profundus (FDP) tendons; the interos-

sei muscles lie between the metacarpal bones and originate from them. Both of these muscle groups insert in the extensor expansions of digits II to V and act on the fingers to flex the MCP joints and extend the IP joints. The radial two lumbricals are innervated by the median nerve, and the ulnar two are innervated by the ulnar nerve. The seven interossei (three palmar and four dorsal) can be considered together. They lie on either side of the finger metacarpals and are innervated by the ulnar nerve. The dorsal interossei muscles abduct the fingers away from the midline; the volar muscles adduct the fingers. For an accurate test that isolates their function from the extrinsic muscles, the patient should place the palm flat on a table, extend the digit, and move it from side to side.

The hypothenar group of intrinsic muscles includes the opponens digiti minimi, the flexor digiti minimi, and the abductor digiti minimi. These muscles arise from the carpal bones and in the flexor retinaculum and insert on the proximal phalanx and metacarpal of the little finger. The flexor and abductor flex the proximal phalanx and abduct the little finger. The three muscles are evaluated as a group by having the patient place the wrist in a neutral position and abduct the little finger (move it away from the other fingers) against resistance.

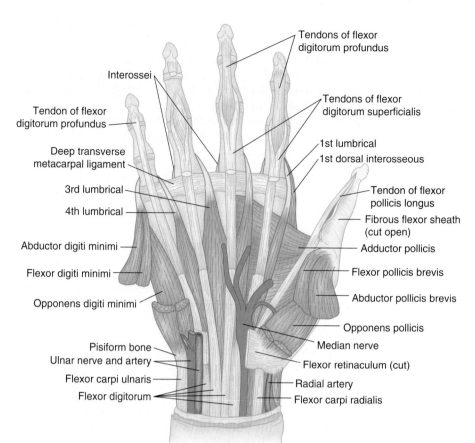

Interossei

Tendon of flexor digitorum profundus

Deep transverse metacarpal ligament

3rd lumbrical

4th lumbrical

Abductor digiti minimi

Flexor digiti minimi

Opponens digiti minimi

Pisiform bone

Ulnar nerve and artery

Flexor carpi ulnaris

Flexor digitorum

Tendons of flexor digitorum profundus

Tendons of flexor digitorum superficialis

1st lumbrical

1st dorsal interosseous

Tendon of flexor pollicis longus

Fibrous flexor sheath (cut open)

Adductor pollicis

Flexor pollicis brevis

Abductor pollicis brevis

Opponens pollicis

Median nerve

Flexor retinaculum (cut)

Radial artery

Flexor carpi radialis

Figure 47-12. Anterior view of the palm of the hand. The palmar aponeurosis and the greater part of the flexor retinaculum have been removed to display the median nerve, the long flexor tendons, and the lumbrical muscles. Segments of the tendons of the flexor digitorum superficialis muscle have been removed to show underlying tendons of the flexor digitorum profundus muscles. (From Snell RS, Smith MS: *Clinical Anatomy for Emergency Medicine*. St. Louis, Mosby, 1993, p 641.)

This muscle mass is palpated at that time, and a dimpling of the hypothenar skin is noted. All the intrinsic muscles of the little finger are innervated by the ulnar nerve.

Extensor Tendons

The extensor tendons are on the dorsal side of the forearm, wrist, and hand. The nine extensor tendons cross the wrist joint dorsal to its axis of rotation, pass under the extensor retinaculum, and are separated on the dorsum of the hand by a series of six fibro-osseous canals or compartments. Figure 47-13 outlines the compartments and their contents. The fibrous roof of these compartments prevents the tendons from bowstringing dorsally during active finger extension, particularly when the wrist also is extended.

The first dorsal wrist compartment contains the tendons of the abductor pollicis longus, which inserts at the dorsal base of the thumb metacarpal, and the extensor pollicis brevis, which inserts on the proximal phalanx of the thumb. The abductor pollicis longus serves to abduct the first ray radially, and the extensor pollicis brevis acts primarily to extend the ray at the MCP joint. These tendons are evaluated by having the patient abduct and extend the thumb with resistance applied to the thumb; they can be palpated on the radial side of the wrist during this maneuver.

Two tendons lie in the second compartment: the extensor carpi radialis longus and brevis. These tendons insert at the dorsal base of the index and middle metacarpals. They act primarily to extend and deviate the wrist radially. These tendons can be palpated by having the patient extend the wrist against resistance while making a fist.

In the third compartment, a single tendon, the extensor pollicis longus, arises from the deep muscles of the midforearm, passes around a bony prominence on the dorsum of the wrist termed *Lister's tubercle,* and inserts on the base of the distal phalanx of the thumb. This tubercle can be palpated just proximal to the wrist joint. The extensor pollicis longus forms the dorsal border of the anatomic snuff-box, and the abductor pollicis longus forms the volar border (Figure 47-14). The floor of this area contains the radial artery and two carpal bones, the scaphoid and trapezium. The extensor pollicis longus functions to extend and adduct the entire first ray and extend and hyperextend the IP joint of the thumb. This muscle is evaluated by placing the hand flat on a table and having the patient lift only the thumb off the surface. Because the abductor pollicis brevis and the adductor pollicis add terminal extension, complete laceration of the extensor pollicis longus tendon may not eliminate the patient's ability to extend the thumb.[12]

The tendons that extend the fingers—the extensor indicis proprius and the extensor digitorum communis—are in the fourth compartment. The extensor digitorum muscle divides into four tendons proximal to the wrist. In the dorsum of the hand, these tendons are connected by juncturae, which help stabilize them to their insertions in the extensor expansions of digits II to V. The tendon to the index finger is joined on its radial side by the tendon of the extensor indicis proprius. The tendon to the little finger is joined on its

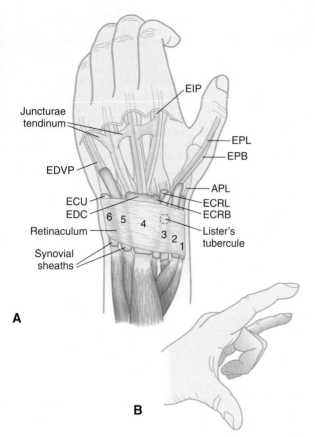

A

B

Figure 47-13. A, The extensor tendons gain entrance to the hand from the forearm through a series of six canals, five fibro-osseous and one fibrous (the sixth dorsal compartment, which contains the extensor digiti quinti proprius [EDQP]). The first compartment contains the abductor pollicis longus (APL) and extensor pollicis brevis (EPB); the second, the radial wrist extensors; the third, the extensor pollicis longus (EPL), which angles around Lister's tubercle; the fourth, the extensor digitorum communis (EDC) to the fingers and the extensor indicis proprius (EIP); the fifth, the EDQP; and the sixth, the extensor carpi ulnaris (ECU). The communis tendons are joined distally near the metacarpophalangeal joints by fibrous connections called *juncturae tendinum.* Beneath the retinaculum, the extensor tendons are covered with a synovial sheath. **B,** The proprius tendons to the index and little fingers are capable of independent extension, and their function may be evaluated as depicted. With the middle and ring fingers flexed into the palm, the proprius tendons can extend the ring and little fingers. ECRB, extensor carpi radialis brevis; ECRL, extensor carpi radialis longus. (From Doyle JR: In Green DP [ed]: *Operative Hand Surgery.* New York, Churchill Livingstone, 1993, p 1927.)

Labels in figure: EIP; Juncturae tendinum; EPL; EPB; EDVP; APL; ECU; ECRL; EDC; ECRB; 6 5 4 3 2 1; Retinaculum; Lister's tubercule; Synovial sheaths

---

all of the fingers. The function of the extensor indicis proprius can be isolated from the common extensors by asking the patient to make a fist and then to point the second digit. The extensor digiti minimi is examined by having the patient straighten the little finger while the hand is closed into a fist.

The extensor mechanism of each digit is a complex interrelationship of muscle tendon units of the long extrinsic extensor tendons and the intrinsic system (Figure 47-15). The extensor expansion divides into a central slip that attaches to the middle phalanx and two lateral bands that join with the tendons of the lumbrical and interosseous muscles and attach to the base of each distal phalanx. The interossei and lumbrical muscles insert in the lateral aspects of the dorsal hood. Most of the power of the common extensors serves to extend the MCP joint. Distal digit extension is provided by continuation of the lateral band mechanism and the oblique retinacular ligament. Because of this complex anatomy, injuries involving the extensor mechanism require meticulous repair.

The sixth compartment contains the extensor carpi ulnaris. This tendon passes distal to the head of the ulna on the ulnar aspect of the wrist and inserts on the base of the little finger metacarpal. The extensor carpi ulnaris functions to extend and deviate the wrist ulnarly. This tendon is evaluated by having the patient extend and push the hand to the ulnar side against resistance; the tendon can be palpated distal to the ulnar styloid process.

Flexor Tendons

The flexor tendons reside on the volar side of the forearm and cross the wrist joint volar to its axis. Generally, 12 tendons function to flex the wrist and digits; 3 of them—the flexor carpi radialis, flexor carpi ulnaris, and palmaris longus—primarily flex the wrist and deviate the wrist radially or ulnarly (Figure 47-16). The remaining tendons pass into the digits through the carpal tunnel. A single tendon, the flexor pollicis longus, inserts on the distal phalanx of the thumb, and two flexor tendons go to each remaining finger. The flexor digitorum superficialis (FDS) tendons bifurcate near the base of the proximal phalanges and surround the tendons of the FDP before inserting on the middle phalanges of digits II to V (Figure 47-17). The FDS flexes all the joints it crosses, including the wrist, PIP joints, and MCP joints. The profundus tendons lie deep to the superficialis tendons over most of their course in the forearm. At the level of the MCP joint, they perforate the superficialis tendon to emerge to a superficial position. They insert at the base of the distal phalanx and act primarily to flex the DIP joint and all joints flexed by the FDS. From the level of the MCP joint distally, the two flexor tendons become enclosed in a fibrous flexor sheath lined by synovium. Regions of thickening in this sheath form pulleys that help prevent bowstringing of the flexor tendons across the joint and assist smooth, effective flexion (Figure 47-18).

After observation, each muscle-tendon unit is tested with a functional examination. The flexor carpi radi-

---

ulnar side by two slips from the extensor digiti minimi. The extensor digiti minimi is contained in the fifth dorsal compartment and lies ulnar to the small finger extensor. The extensor indicis lies ulnar and deep to the index extensor. The dual extensor system for the index and small fingers gives these two digits extension independent of the other digits. The middle finger and especially the ring finger have considerably limited independent extension. The restrictive motion is due to the junctura, which also prevents retraction of the proximal tendon end after distal division of an extensor. Complete division of an extensor proximal to the junctura can be associated with normal MCP joint extension.[7] This extension occurs through the junctura connection. The extensor digitorum communis tendons can be evaluated by asking the patient to straighten out

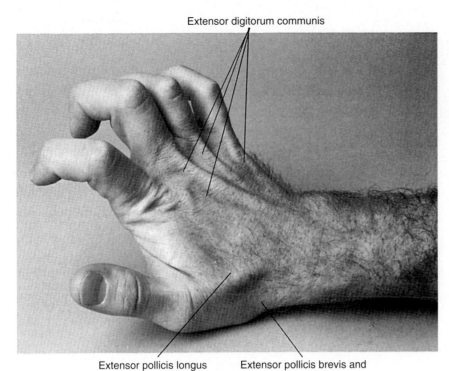

Extensor digitorum communis

Extensor pollicis longus

Extensor pollicis brevis and abductor pollicis longus

Figure 47-14. Surface anatomy of the wrist and hand. The tendons that are palpated with the thumb abducted and extended form an anatomic snuff-box.

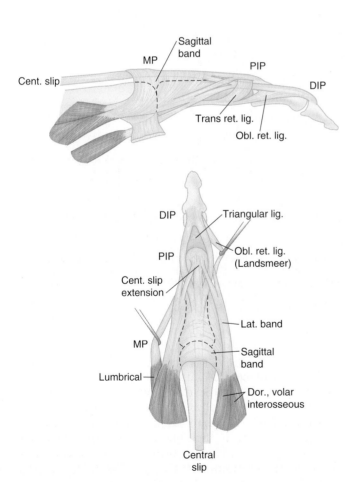

Cent. slip

MP

Sagittal band

PIP

DIP

Trans ret. lig.

Obl. ret. lig.

DIP

PIP

Triangular lig.

Cent. slip extension

Obl. ret. lig. (Landsmeer)

MP

Lat. band

Sagittal band

Lumbrical

Dor., volar interosseous

Central slip

Figure 47-15. The extensor tendon at the metacarpophalangeal (MP) joint level is held in place by the transverse lamina or sagittal band, which tethers and centers the extensor tendons over the joint. This sagittal band arises from the volar plate and the intermetacarpal ligaments at the neck of the metacarpals. Any injury to the extensor hood or expansion may result in subluxation or dislocation of the extensor tendon. The intrinsic tendons from the lumbrical and interosseous muscles join the extensor mechanism at about the level of the proximal and midportion of the proximal phalanx and continue distally to the distal interphalangeal (DIP) joint of the finger. The extensor mechanism at the proximal interphalangeal (PIP) joint is best described as a trifurcation of the extensor tendon into the central slip, which attaches to the dorsal base of the middle phalanx and the two lateral bands. These lateral bands continue distally to insert at the dorsal base of the distal phalanx. The extensor mechanism is maintained in place over the PIP joint by the transverse retinacular ligaments. (From Doyle JR: In Green DP [ed]: *Operative Hand Surgery.* New York, Churchill Livingstone, 1993, p 1928.)

Figure 47-16. Palmaris longus accentuation.

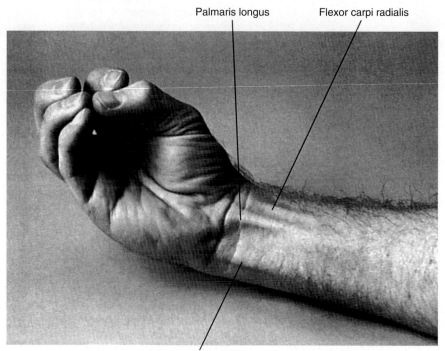

Palmaris longus   Flexor carpi radialis

Flexor carpi ulnaris

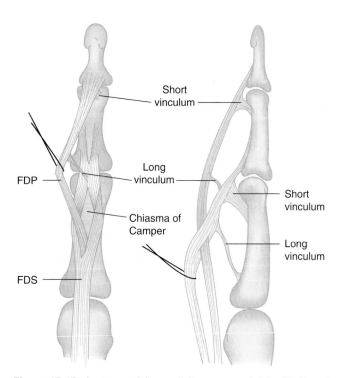

Short
vinculum

Long
vinculum

Short
vinculum

FDP

Chiasma of
Camper

Long
vinculum

FDS

Figure 47-17. Anatomy of flexor digitorum superficialis (FDS) and profundus (FDP) in the finger. (From Schneider LH: *Flexor Tendon Injuries*. Boston, Little, Brown, 1985.)

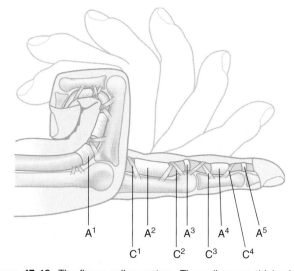

A^1 A^2 A^3 A^4 A^5

C^1 C^2 C^3 C^4

Figure 47-18. The flexor pulley system. The pulleys are thickenings in the fibrous flexor sheath. There are five annular pulleys (transversely oriented fibers) *(A)*. There are four cruciate pulleys (oblique with some crisscrossing fibers) *(C)*. (Courtesy of Kleinert, Kutz and Associates Hand Care Center.)

alis, palmaris longus, and flexor carpi ulnaris are tested together by having the patient flex the wrist against resistance while the examiner palpates the individual tendons. The tendon of the flexor pollicis longus attaches to the base of the distal phalanx of the thumb and flexes the thumb MCP and IP joints. This tendon is tested by having the patient bend the tip of the thumb

against resistance. FDP function can be tested by having the patient flex the distal phalanx of each finger while the PIP is stabilized in extension by the examiner (Figure 47-19). The FDS is tested individually by asking the patient to flex the PIP joint while the other fingers are held in extension to block the flexion produced by the profundus tendons (Figure 47-20). This is a subtle but important distinction because lacerations of the digital creases can easily damage one or more of the tendons or adjacent neurovascular bundles. The FDP is more commonly lacerated in the finger because of its paradoxically superficial position. If movement against resistance is intact but accompanied by pain or diminished strength, the involved tendon may be partially disrupted. Pathologic nodular swelling of one of the long flexor tendons may result in intermittent catching, or "triggering," on a thickened flexor sheath anterior to the MCP joint. This condition, known as *trigger finger,* may cause a palpable and sometimes audible snapping when a patient is asked to flex and extend the fingers.

Synovial Spaces

Bursae are synovial sheaths that cover tendons as they pass through osseofibrous tunnels. They contain synovial fluid and serve two essential functions: They decrease friction during tendon movement, and they help supply nutrients to the relatively avascular tendons (Figure 47-21). These sheaths also can provide pathways for spread of infection. Extensor tendons do

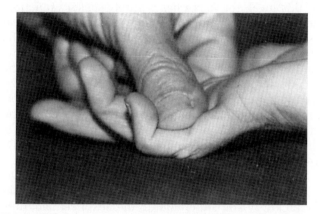

Figure 47-19. To test for an intact profundus tendon, the examiner maintains the digit in extension, while the patient attempts to flex the terminal phalanx.

not lie within definite sheaths and are afforded a greater resistance to infections. The synovial sheaths of the flexors in the index, middle, and ring fingers are enclosed from their insertion to approximately the level of the distal palmar crease. The sheath of the flexor pollicis longus extends from the tip of the thumb to the proximal volar wrist crease, where it communicates with the radial bursa in the palm and carpal tunnel. Similarly the synovial sheath of the little finger communicates with the ulnar bursa. Clinical features of flexor tenosynovitis are caused by inflammation and distention of these synovial sheaths. Kanavel[13] described the classic signs, including a flexed posture of the digits, pain on passive extension of the digits, incomplete flexion, and tenderness of the synovial sheath.

Blood Supply

Arterial System

The hands and the digits have a dual blood supply (Figure 47-22). The major blood supply to the hand is from the radial and ulnar arteries. The radial artery lies on the anterior aspect of the radius in the distal part of the forearm. It continues around the lateral side of the wrist onto the dorsum of the hand by passing deep to the tendons of the abductor pollicis longus and the extensor pollicis brevis. On entering the palm, the radial artery terminates as the deep palmar arch. The ulnar artery enters the hand anterior to the flexor retinaculum on the radial side of the ulnar nerve and pisiform bone. The artery gives off a deep branch, then continues into the palm as the superficial palmar arch. This complex arterial arch system anastomoses and sends branches to the individual digits and the deep palmar spaces. Because of extensive collateralization, the hand usually survives even if both vessels are transected at the wrist.[14] The circulation of the hand is

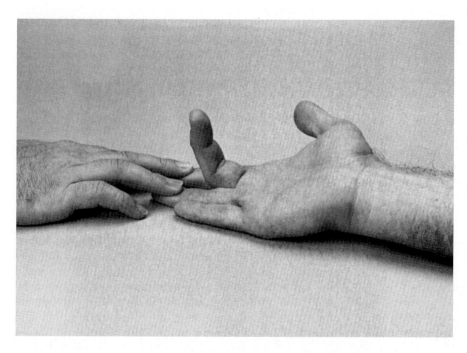

Figure 47-20. Examination to assess function of the flexor digitorum superficialis.

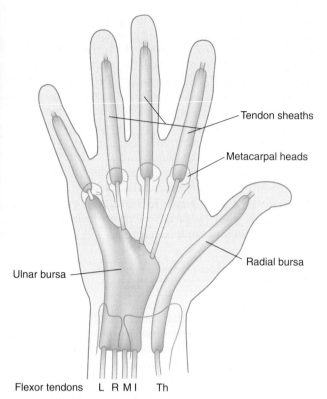

Th Tendon sheaths

Metacarpal heads

Radial bursa

Ulnar bursa

Flexor tendons   L R M I   Th

Figure 47-21. Radial and ulnar bursae and their relation to flexor tendons and to each other. Th, thumb; I, index finger; M, middle finger; R, ring finger; L, little finger. (From Siegel DB, Gelberman RH: Infections of the hand. *Orthop Clin North Am* 19:779, 1988.)

evaluated by palpating the radial and ulnar artery on the volar aspect of the wrist, by noting the color and warmth of the skin, and by noting capillary refill. Because these findings vary among patients, the injured hand should be compared with the normal side.

Although Allen's test is an imperfect predictor of vascular compromise, it is commonly used to determine the patency of the arteries supplying the hand and the contributions to the circulation of the hand derived from each of the major vessels. The radial and ulnar arteries are compressed by the examiner at the wrist (Figure 47-23). The patient opens and closes the hand repeatedly to exsanguinate it, then maintains a relaxed position. The radial artery is released. If the palm and fingers fill immediately with blood, the radial artery is patent with good collateral flow into the ulnar artery system. To evaluate the ulnar artery, the same steps are repeated, but the ulnar artery is released. This method also can be used on a single digit to help evaluate the patency of each digital vessel to that finger. Similar to the hand, the digit usually survives even if both digital vessels are transected at the base of the finger; however, healing of associated injuries may be delayed or may be compromised by excessive scar formation because of associated, although relative, ischemia.[14]

Venous and Lymphatic Systems

The veins generally follow the arterial pattern in the deep system. The abundant dorsal, superficial veins are more extensive than the deep system and drain most of the blood from this region. The lymphatic vessels essentially follow the veins, with most lymph flowing into channels in the dorsal subcutaneous space. This vascular anatomy and the laxity of the dorsal skin account for palmar infections causing swelling on the dorsum rather than the palmar surface of the hand.

Nerve Supply

The nerve supply to the hand comes from the radial, ulnar, and median nerves. All three nerves control movement of the wrist, fingers, and thumb. In the hand, the ulnar and median nerves are mixed motor and sensory nerves, whereas the radial nerve is purely sensory. Each of the three major nerves passes through a muscle in the forearm, and each passes points of potential entrapment en route to the hand.

Motor Innervation

The radial nerve (C6 through C8) passes through the supinator muscle and enters the dorsal aspect of the wrist between the radial styloid and Lister's tubercle. At this level, the nerve has a purely sensory function. Its important motor function is to innervate the dorsal extrinsic muscles in the forearm, which extend the wrist and MCP joints and abduct and extend the thumb. No intrinsic muscles in the hand are innervated by the radial nerve. Motor function in this nerve is tested by having the patient extend the wrist against resistance. Proximal injury to the radial nerve causes a condition known as *wristdrop*: The fingers are held in flexion at the MCP joints, and the thumb is adducted (Figure 47-24A).

The ulnar nerve (C7, C8, and T1) passes through the flexor carpi ulnaris muscle in the forearm and lies ulnar to the artery and superficial to the flexor retinaculum. It enters the hand at the wrist through a tunnel called the *ulnar tunnel* or *Guyon's canal*. The ulnar nerve innervates the hypothenar muscles, the seven interosseous muscles, the lumbrical muscles to the ring and little fingers, and the adductor pollicis. Innervation of the flexor pollicis brevis is variable. In the forearm, the flexor carpi ulnaris and the ulnar half of the FDP also are innervated by the ulnar nerve. Loss of motor function of the ulnar nerve results in inability to pinch a piece of paper tightly between the thumb and the index finger. A late characteristic of distal ulnar damage is Duchenne's sign, manifested by clawing of the ring and little fingers (Figure 47-24B). The ring and little fingers are hyperextended at the MCP joints by the extensor digitorum communis (radial nerve) and flexed at the IP joints by the FDP (intact proximal ulnar nerve). In addition, the interosseous and hypothenar muscles are atrophied.

The median nerve enters the forearm through the pronator teres muscle. At that level, it innervates that muscle, the flexor carpi radialis, the FDS, the radial part of the FDP, the flexor pollicis longus, and the pronator quadratus. The branch of the median nerve that innervates the last three muscles is called the *anterior interosseous nerve*. The median nerve enters the hand through the carpal tunnel accompanied by the nine extrinsic flexor tendons of the digits. The thenar

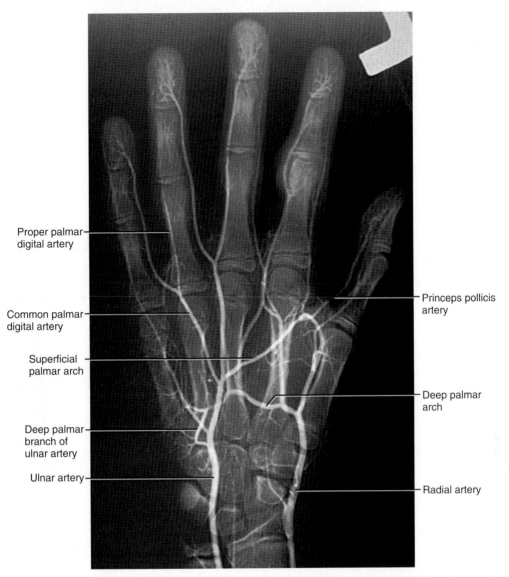

Proper palmar digital artery

Common palmar digital artery

Superficial palmar arch

Deep palmar branch of ulnar artery

Ulnar artery

Princeps pollicis artery

Deep palmar arch

Radial artery

Figure 47-22. Arteriogram of the hand. The ulnar artery is the principal contributor to the superficial palmar arch. (Courtesy of Dr. D. Armstrong, Associate Professor of Radiology, University of Toronto, Ontario, Canada.)

motor branch (recurrent median nerve) innervates the abductor pollicis brevis, the opponens pollicis variably, and the flexor pollicis brevis. Common digital branches innervate the lumbrical muscles to the index and long fingers. Injury to this nerve occurs most commonly at the level at the wrist, by laceration or by compression in the carpal tunnel. Motor function is tested by having the patient oppose the thumb to the index digit. Injury to the median nerve in the upper forearm or at the elbow usually results in weakness or absence of flexion of the index finger distal phalanx, the middle phalanx, and the thumb and weakness of thumb abduction and opposition.[15] With passage of time, the muscles of the thenar eminence atrophy, and the hand looks flattened and "apelike" (Figure 47-24C).

Sensory Innervation

The typical distribution of the sensory nerves to the hand is shown in Figure 47-25. Because some overlap occurs between various sensory nerves, it is preferable to test sensation in the areas least likely to have dual innervation. The anatomic area of least ulnar variation and overlap is the volar tip of the little finger. The median nerve exclusively innervates the volar tip of the index finger. The dorsal first web space is entirely within the radial nerve distribution.

Several methods exist to assess sensation. The preferred method, which is most accurate and objective, is comparative two-point discrimination. An uninjured hand is able to distinguish two points that are 2 to 5 mm apart at the fingertips and 7 to 10 mm apart at the base of the palm. The dorsum of the hand is the least sensitive region, with a normal threshold at 7 to 12 mm. Two-point threshold distances wider than these ranges indicate impaired sensory function.[15] The threshold and two-point discrimination tests may be of limited value in children, patients with heavily calloused fingertips, uncooperative patients, comatose patients, patients in severe pain, or suspected malingerers.

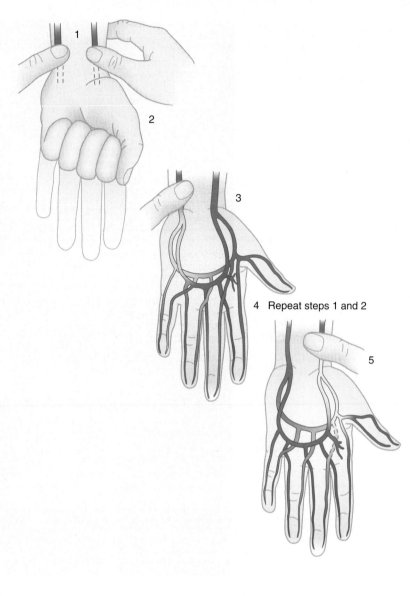

Figure 47-23. Allen's test. (From ASSH: *The Hand: Examination and Diagnosis,* 3rd ed. New York, Churchill Livingstone, 1990, p 46.)

1

2

3

4   Repeat steps 1 and 2

5

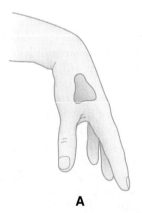

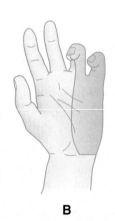

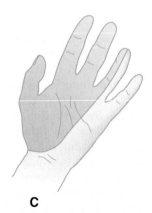

A   **B**   **C**

Figure 47-24. Deformities of the hand. **A,** Radial palsy—wrist drop. **B,** Ulnar nerve palsy—main en griffe (clawhand). **C,** Median nerve palsy—main en singe (monkey hand). The shaded areas represent the usual distribution of anesthesia. (From Ellis H: *Clinical Anatomy: A Revision and Applied Anatomy for Clinical Students,* 7th ed. Oxford, UK, Blackwell Scientific, 1983.)

Fingertip

The fingertip generally is defined as the area distal to the insertion of the flexor profundus and extensor tendons (Figure 47-26). The pulp is the tissue of the fingertip between the volar skin and the distal phalangeal bone. The fingertip is well padded by adipose tissue and is covered by highly innervated skin that is tethered to the distal phalanx by a series of fibrosepta. The dorsal skin is thinner and less vascularized than the volar skin. Sensation is supplied by nerves that travel with arteries bilaterally along the radial and ulnar aspect of the fingers. The arteries branch to form volar anastomoses or arches similar to those in the palm. Dorsal branches supply the nail bed and matrix.

Nail

The nail (or nail plate) consists of compacted scales that originate from cornified epithelial cells. The prox-imal part of the nail is called the *root*; it emerges from a groove in the skin to form the body of the nail, which is exposed. The root of the nail is covered by a fold in the skin called the *proximal nail fold*. A small portion of the epidermis of the nail fold extends out over the proximal body of the nail to form the cuticle, or *eponychium*. The floor of the nail plate or nail bed is composed of tissue known as the *nail matrix*. The distal skin of the nail bed complex is called the *hyponychium*. The skin overlying the nail laterally is called the *perionychium*. The semicircular white crescent region near the nail fold is called the *lunula*.

The nail bed complex on the dorsum of the fingertips is important in providing additional stabilization of the palmar soft tissues against compression and shear forces. The nail grows from the nail matrix along the nail bed and is firmly adherent to the bed. It is now believed that the entire nail bed is active in the generation and migration of the nail. As new nail forms, the nail glides forward over the nail bed at a rate of about 0.5 to 1.2 mm per week (toenails grow much more slowly). The nail itself is a hard, firm, and relatively translucent structure; the underlying vascular tissue showing through gives the nail its pink appearance. A smooth nail bed is essential to normal function. If the nail bed sustains injury that is not repaired accurately, granulation tissue forms scar that impedes normal nail production and growth. The result may be a split or absent nail that is cosmetically unappealing and sometimes functionally debilitating.[16]

CLINICAL FEATURES: SIGNS AND SYMPTOMS

The initial evaluation of an acutely injured hand is crucial because it affords the best opportunity to assess accurately the extent of damage and to restore altered anatomy.[17] Evaluation of any hand injury should begin by obtaining the historical facts of the patient's age, occupation, hand dominance, and previous hand impairment or injury. In traumatic injuries, the time of occurrence, length of elapsed time since the injury,

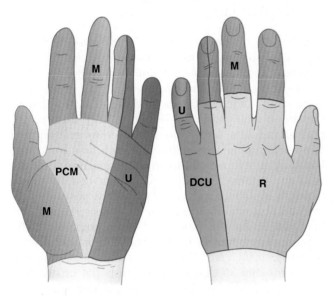

Figure 47-25. The cutaneous nerve supply in the hand. M, median; R, radial; U, ulnar; PCM, palmar cutaneous branch of median nerve; DCU, dorsal cutaneous branch of ulnar nerve. (Courtesy of Kleinert, Kutz and Associates Hand Care Center.)

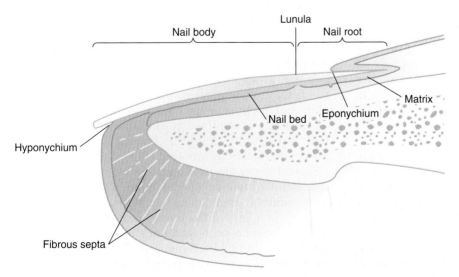

Figure 47-26. Sagittal section of the distal finger. (From Siegel DB, Gelberman RH: Infections of the hand. *Orthop Clin North Am* 19:779, 1988.)

BOX 47-1. General Physical Examination of the Hand

I. General appearance
   A. Active hemorrhage
   B. Amputations or avulsions
   C. Position at rest
II. Skin
   A. Integrity
   B. Moisture
   C. Swelling or edema
   D. Discoloration
   E. Inflammation
   F. Scars
III. Vascular
   A. Color and warmth
   B. Pulses
   C. Capillary refill
   D. Allen's test
IV. Neurologic
   A. Motor function
      1. Ulnar nerve—finger abduction and adduction
      2. Radial nerve—wrist extension
      3. Median nerve—flexion of digits I, II, and III; thumb opposition
   B. Sensory function
      1. Ulnar nerve—tip of digit V
      2. Median nerve—tip of digit II
      3. Radial nerve—dorsal first web space
V. Bone and joint
   A. Deformity
   B. Local tenderness
   C. Pain with axial compression
   D. Joint range of motion
   E. Ligamentous stability: distal interphalangeal, proximal interphalangeal, metacarpophalangeal joints
VI. Musculotendinous
   A. Function of each muscle-tendon group
   B. Strength against resistance
   C. Pain with motion

mechanism of injury, posture of the hand at the time of injury, and treatment before arrival in the emergency department all are useful data. In nontraumatic problems, pain, swelling, sensory change or contracture, timing of symptoms, presence of similar symptoms in other extremities, aggravating or alleviating factors, and functional impairment are useful historical points. A review of the medical history and a review of systems complete the evaluation.

After a detailed history is taken, the entire extremity should be exposed and evaluated when the hand is examined. A system of priorities, based primarily on threat to ultimate function, should direct the sequence of the examination. In order of priority, the examination includes evaluation of vascular and neurologic integrity, skin cover, skeletal stability, and joint and tendon function (Box 47-1). The general appearance of the hand should be noted with focus on its color, presence of swelling or edema, and any abnormal posture or position. In traumatic injuries, the precise area of maximal tenderness should be localized. Rotational, angular, and shortening deformities should be noted

with regard to direction and extent. Angular deformity may be seen best with the fingers in full extension. Rotational deformity is best observed during digital flexion. Digital or wrist block anesthesia may be helpful in some cases to accurately assess fracture deformity and stability during digital motion and, if necessary, stress testing. Open wounds should be assessed with regard to location, relationship to skin creases, direction and viability of skin flaps, extent of skin loss, degree of contamination of the wound, and extent of soft tissue injury. The examiner must have a sterile field, good light, adequate exposure, and a nearly bloodless field for a thorough evaluation. The complete examination also may require an evaluation of active shoulder motion, elbow motion, and pronation and supination of the forearm and assessment of the contralateral hand.

DIAGNOSTIC STRATEGIES: RADIOGRAPHIC EVALUATION

Despite the development of numerous new and sophisticated imaging techniques, the plain radiograph remains the most important imaging modality for the hand and wrist. The standard radiographic series of the hand should include a posteroanterior, a true lateral, and an oblique projection (Figure 47-27). With correct positioning, the bones do not overlap on the film, allowing complete evaluation of each area for visualization of fractures, subluxation, dislocation, deformities, and retained radiopaque foreign bodies.[18] On a hand series, the wrist is not properly positioned for radiographic examination, and vice versa; if the patient has injuries to the hand and wrist, separate radiographic series should be performed. For an adequate posteroanterior view, the forearm and hand should be fully pronated so that the palm rests flat on the film. This view forms the basis of all assessments, but is poor at showing fractures of the articular surface of the metacarpal head. The lateral view is normally a radioulnar projection and is made by positioning the palm and forearm at 90 degrees to the film with the fingers splayed. This view is essential to show displacement of fracture fragments and joint dislocations. If the projection is not a true lateral, joint dislocation, avulsion fractures, or fractures through the articular surface of the base of the phalanx may be missed. The oblique view is made with the hand and forearm pronated at 45 degrees to the film. It is particularly useful for assessing dislocation of the MCP and CMC joints and fractures at the base of the metacarpal bones. When injury is confined to the distal end of a single digit, radiography should be limited to that digit, but the same projections are used (Figure 47-28).

Special views are used to diagnose specific injuries. The standard views of the hand do not give true posteroanterior and lateral projections of the thumb because the plane of the thumb is at 90 degrees to the fingers. Separate posteroanterior and lateral views of the thumb should be requested. The posteroanterior projection of the thumb is taken with the hand and

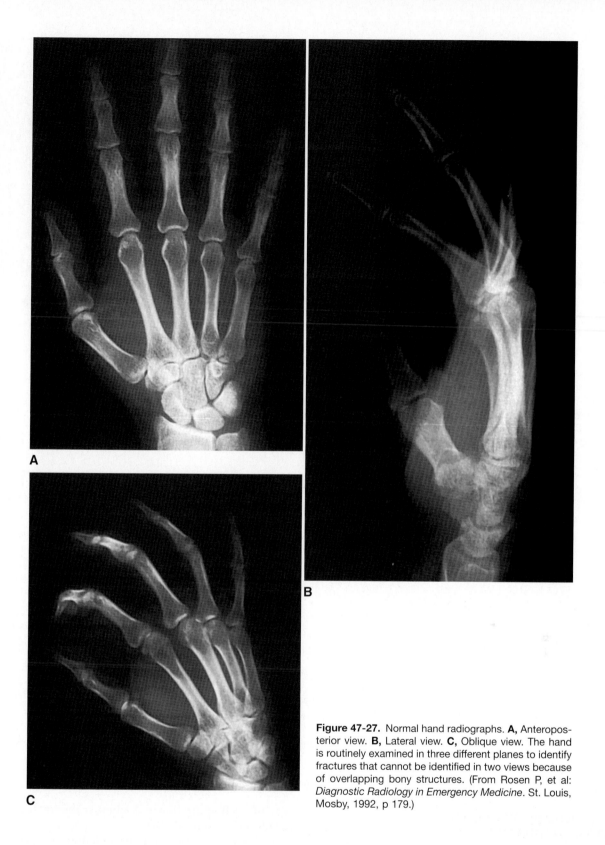

A

B

C

Figure 47-27. Normal hand radiographs. **A,** Anteroposterior view. **B,** Lateral view. **C,** Oblique view. The hand is routinely examined in three different planes to identify fractures that cannot be identified in two views because of overlapping bony structures. (From Rosen P, et al: *Diagnostic Radiology in Emergency Medicine*. St. Louis, Mosby, 1992, p 179.)

forearm hyperpronated so that the dorsal surface of the thumb and first metacarpal rests flat on the film. The lateral view is obtained by pronating the hand and forearm to allow the lateral surface of the thumb to lie on the film. Stress views are used most often to rule out ligamentous injury to the first MCP joint. Localized widening of the joint space or subluxation may indicate a significant collateral ligament injury. Plain films taken in multiple projections can help detect and localize soft tissue foreign bodies. Whether an object is visualized on plain films depends on its composition, configuration, size, and orientation. Many foreign bodies encountered in the emergency department, including almost all glass, are more dense than soft tissue and can be readily seen on plain radiographs.[19]

Figure 47-28. Normal radiographs of the finger.

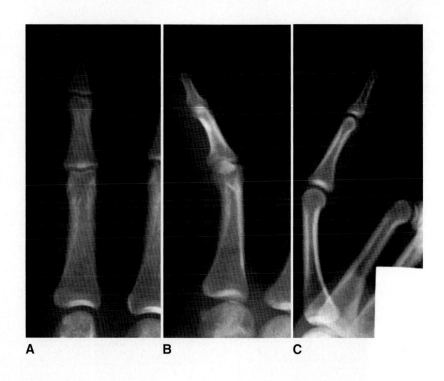

A   B   C

Figure 47-29. Fracture terminology. (From Idler RS, et al [eds]: *The Hand: Examination and Diagnosis,* 3rd ed. New York, American Society for Surgery of the Hand, 1990, p 64.)

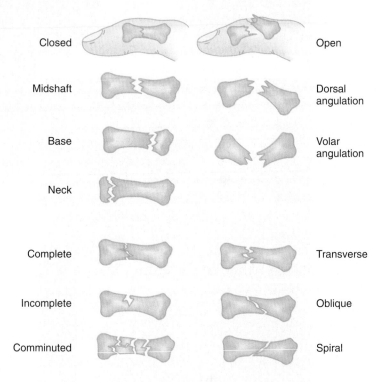

MECHANISMS OF INJURY AND MANAGEMENT

Trauma

The bones of the hand are the most commonly fractured bones in the body. Radiographic evaluation of significant hand injuries is mandatory. Any hand injury that causes swelling should be evaluated radiographically with a minimum of three views. Although the classification of hand fractures is difficult and at times confusing, it is generally done according to the nature and

site of the fracture line and whether the fracture is open or closed (Figure 47-29).

A fracture is unstable if it cannot be reduced or maintained in an anatomic or near-anatomic position without fixation when the hand is placed in the "safe" or functional position. The four principal determinants of fracture stability or instability are (1) fracture configuration, (2) integrity of the periosteal sleeve and surrounding soft tissues, (3) muscle balance or imbalance, and (4) external forces.

In general, transverse fractures have a stable configuration. Spiral, oblique, and comminuted fractures are unstable. The degree of displacement also is an indicator of potential fracture instability. Fractures of unstable configuration may be stable if they are non-displaced or only minimally displaced because the periosteum is undamaged or minimally disrupted. Displacement is defined by the deformity it creates and can result in rotation, angulation, shortening, or a combination of these fractures. Although shortening has an adverse effect on muscle tension, the hand accommodates more easily to this component of deformity than to others.[20]

Definitive management of many hand fractures is controversial and beyond the scope of this text. The emphasis here is on appropriate initial interventions, including proper splinting techniques to minimize morbidity and understanding which fractures may require operative fixation and their potential complications. Most closed injuries may be treated initially in the emergency department. Most open, intra-articular, periarticular, and unstable fractures require operative management by a hand surgeon.[20]

Distal Phalanx Fractures

Pathophysiology and Clinical Features
Fractures of the distal phalanx are the most common fractures of the hand. They occur most often as a result of crush or shearing forces, usually as a sports-related injury in children and adolescents, industrial accidents in adults, or accidental falls in the elderly.[21] Distal phalangeal fractures are classified into extra-articular fractures (longitudinal, transverse, and comminuted) and intra-articular fractures. The most common location for fractures is the distal tuft (Figure 47-30). Because the

mechanism of injury is usually direct trauma, tuft fractures are often comminuted and usually associated with soft tissue injury to the nail, nail bed, and nail matrix.[22] Supporting fibrous septa that radiate from the bone to the skin prevent displacement of fracture fragments and contain soft tissue swelling, contributing to the severe pain that can accompany these fractures. Examination typically reveals tenderness and swelling over the distal phalanx, including the pulp.

Fractures at the base of the distal phalanx may be associated with tendon avulsion. As previously mentioned, the flexor profundus tendon attaches to the volar aspect of digits II through V, and the terminal slip of the extensor tendon attaches on the dorsal surface of the distal phalanx. In the distal phalanx of the thumb, the flexor pollicis longus inserts on the volar base, and the extensor pollicis longus inserts on the dorsal base. These tendons can avulse when subjected to excessive stress. Clinically, loss of function is evident, and radiographically small avulsion fractures along the dorsal or volar surface may be seen. These fractures are considered intra-articular, and their management is considered with other tendon injuries.

Management
Treatment of most fractures of the distal phalanges is directed toward the accompanying soft tissue injury. Closed tuft fractures need only symptomatic treatment with elevation (to reduce swelling) and analgesics. Fracture immobilization is rarely necessary; however, a short volar splint or hairpin splint (Figure 47-31) is recommended for 2 to 3 days to protect the tip of the finger from further trauma and allow swelling without constriction. Immobilization should not include the PIP joint. Transverse shaft fractures with angulation or displacement may be irreducible because of interposition of soft tissue. Closed reduction may be attempted with dorsal traction on the distal fragment followed

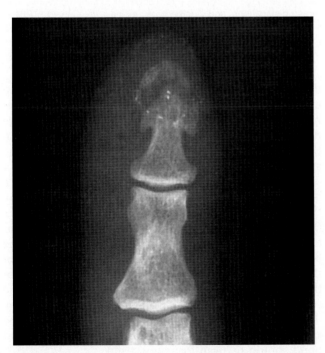

Figure 47-30. Tuft fracture of the distal phalanx of the thumb, antero-posterior view. This radiograph reveals the comminuted displaced fracture fragments and some radiopaque foreign material on the substance of the nail. (From Rosen P, et al: *Diagnostic Radiology in Emergency Medicine*. St. Louis, Mosby, 1992, p 180.)

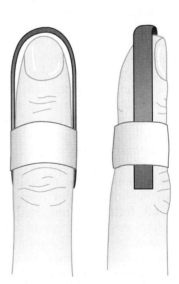

Figure 47-31. The hairpin splint used for distal phalangeal fractures. (From Simon RR, Koenigsknecht SJ: The hand. In Simon RR [ed]: *Emergency Orthopedics: The Extremities*, 2nd ed. Norwalk, Conn, Appleton & Lange, 1995, p 59.)

by immobilization with a volar splint and repeat radiographs for documentation of position. If this approach is unsuccessful, referral to a hand surgeon is indicated for Kirschner wire fixation.[22]

Distal phalangeal fractures associated with nail bed laceration are considered open fractures. This may be obvious if the nail has been avulsed or torn, but the recognition of nail bed laceration is more difficult in closed tuft fractures with an intact nail and a subungual hematoma present. Subungual hematomas are often associated with occult lacerations of the nail bed, and such cases uncommonly may require removal of the nail for accurate assessment and laceration repair.

Complications

Distal phalanx fractures are generally uncomplicated; however, distal phalanx fractures that appear apparently innocuous can result in prolonged morbidity, especially if there is concomitant soft tissue crush injury. In a long-term follow-up series, DaCruz and associates[23] showed that 31% of tuft fractures had not healed radiographically, and 70% of patients had bothersome symptoms at 6 months, including numbness, hyperesthesia, and cold sensitivity. Trauma to the nail bed may result in abnormal nail growth despite exact tissue approximation. Failure to recognize and extricate an entrapped nail bed in the fracture site may result in nonunion of the fracture. Osteomyelitis from open fractures is a rare but potentially serious complication.

Proximal and Middle Phalangeal Fractures

Pathophysiology and Clinical Features

Because the anatomy, mechanism of injury, and treatment of proximal and middle phalangeal fractures are similar, they are discussed together. The proximal phalanx has no tendinous attachments. Fractures in this region have a typical volar angulation resulting from forces exerted from the extensors and the interosseous muscles. The middle phalanx has two important insertions. The tendon of the FDS divides and inserts along nearly the entire volar surface of the phalanx, and the extensor tendon inserts on the proximal dorsal base of the middle phalanx. Because of this alignment, fractures at the base of the middle phalanx usually result in dorsal angulation, and fractures at the neck of the middle phalanx usually result in volar angulation.[24] The mechanism of injury often determines the nature of the fracture; a direct blow is more likely to cause a transverse or comminuted fracture, whereas a twisting injury more often results in an oblique or spiral fracture. Associated injuries may include contusion or transection of digital nerves, vascular disruption, and tendon rupture.

Intra-articular fractures include condylar fractures; comminuted fractures; dorsal, volar, or lateral base fractures; fracture-dislocations; and shaft fractures involving the joint. Extra-articular fractures involve the neck, shaft, or base of the phalanx. Although most phalangeal fractures may be easily seen, condylar fractures and

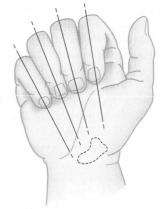

A

Normal flexion of fingers pointing toward region of scaphoid

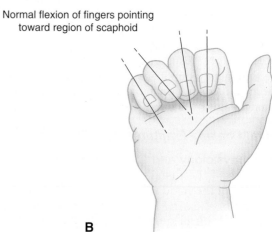

B

Flexion of fingers with malrotation of ring finger

Figure 47-32. Any malrotation of a metacarpal or phalangeal fracture must be corrected. **A,** Normally all fingers point toward the region of the scaphoid when a fist is made. **B,** Malrotation at fracture causes the affected finger to deviate. (From Jobe MT, Calandruccio JH: Fractures, dislocations and ligamentous injuries. In Canale ST (ed): *Campbell's Operative Orthopedics,* 10th ed. St. Louis, Mosby, 2003, p 3484.)

displaced neck fractures are not always apparent on anteroposterior radiographs; oblique views may be needed to identify them.[25] Rotational deformities are difficult to determine by x-ray study but may appear on the lateral view as discrepancies in the diameter of the shaft at the fracture site.

Skeletal alignment can be assessed radiographically, but rotational alignment must be judged clinically by the relationship of the finger to adjacent normal fingers (Figure 47-32). Symmetric flexion of adjacent injured and normal fingers at their MCP and PIP joints is the best possible guide to accurate rotational alignment of the injured segment.[26] Normally, all of the fingers of the closed fist except the thumb should point to the scaphoid. Alternatively, when the fingers are loosely flexed, the nails of opposing digits should lie in the same parallel plane (Figure 47-33). The noninjured hand should be used for comparison.

Management

Similar to metacarpal fractures, phalangeal fractures require precise anatomic alignment to ensure a good

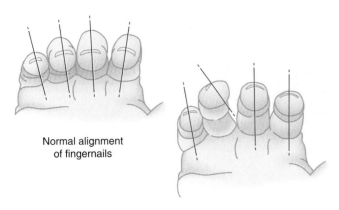

Normal alignment
of fingernails

Alignment of fingernails with
malrotation of ring finger

Figure 47-33. Observing the plane of the fingernails helps detect any malrotation at the fracture. (From Jobe MT, Calandruccio JH: Fractures, dislocations and ligamentous injuries. In Canale ST (ed): *Campbell's Operative Orthopedics,* 10th ed. St. Louis, Mosby, 2003, p 3484.)

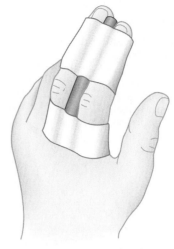

Figure 47-34. The injured finger is splinted to the adjacent normal finger. This splint provides support for the injured digit, while permitting motion of the metacarpophalangeal joint and some motion at the interphalangeal joint. A piece of felt cut to the proper size is inserted between the fingers, and the two digits are taped together as shown. (From Simon RR, Koenigsknecht SJ: The hand. In Simon RR [ed]: *Emergency Orthopedics: The Extremities,* 3rd ed. Norwalk, Conn, Appleton & Lange, 1995, p 518.)

result because of the intimate relationship of the flexor and extensor tendons to the phalanx.[27] Appropriate treatment selection depends on accurate assessment of fracture stability. The angle of the fracture is an important factor in determining this stability. Transverse fractures are usually stable, whereas oblique fractures are inherently unstable. It also is important to ascertain whether the fracture has been impacted or displaced and what deforming forces are acting on it. If there is any question of the fracture's stability, the digit should be anesthetized, and stress should be applied. Reduction of phalangeal fractures is not usually necessary because approximately 75% are stable and nondisplaced.[28] Such fractures should be started on early protected motion as soon as pain subsides (within the first 3 to 5 days). Protection is provided by taping the injured digit to an adjacent normal finger, a form of dynamic splinting. This technique, known as "buddy-taping," encourages the patient to move the finger and use the hand as normally as possible while the fracture heals (Figure 47-34).

If the fracture is displaced or unstable, it is not suitable for dynamic splinting. In general, treatment depends on the type of trauma and the ability to achieve a stable reduction. Phalangeal fractures that are satisfactorily managed by closed reduction can be immobilized by several methods. In such cases, it is advisable to immobilize the wrist and the injured finger. Specific types of immobilization include circular cast, the Böhler method of incorporating a cast with an outrigger, gutter splints, and anterior and posterior splints (Figure 47-35). Immobilization of phalangeal fractures should not exceed 3 weeks to prevent stiffness and to minimize disability. In addition to temporary immobilization, emergency management includes ice for comfort, elevation, analgesics, and follow-up referral. Repeat radiographs in 7 to 10 days are recommended to ensure that there has been no delayed displacement.

Unstable fractures that cannot be reduced by closed manipulation and maintained with external splinting require internal fixation. Midshaft transverse fractures tend not to be amenable to closed reduction; similarly, spiral oblique fractures and intra-articular fractures are inherently unstable and require surgical fixation if a significant portion of the articular surface is involved.[29] Intra-articular fractures of the proximal metaphysis of the middle phalanx that have extreme comminution may require treatment in static or dynamic traction or external fixation with or without ancillary Kirschner wire fixation.[29]

Complications

Malunion is the most common bony complication of phalangeal fractures and may result from malrotation, volar or lateral angulation, or shortening. Malrotation usually is seen after oblique or spiral fractures of the proximal and middle phalanges and may require osteotomy through the phalanx or metacarpal for correction. Volar angulation of proximal phalangeal fractures greater than 25 to 30 degrees results in pseudoclawing. This deformity makes use of the hand awkward and esthetically unacceptable. Other potential complications include diminished motion resulting from tendon adhesions and stiffness of the PIP joint after intra-articular fractures with incongruity.[27]

Metacarpal Fractures

Metacarpal fractures generally are divided into two groups: fractures involving the first metacarpal and fractures involving metacarpals II through V. This distinction is based on the fact that the base of the thumb metacarpal is biomechanically distinct from the remaining metacarpals because of its high degree of

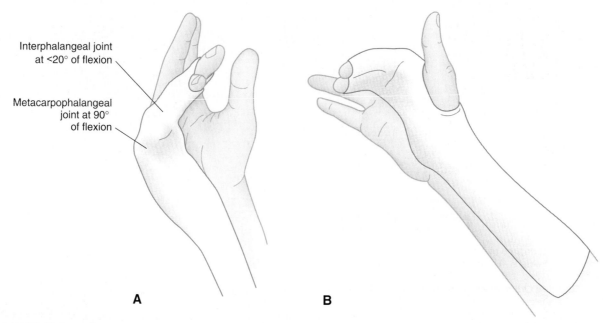

Interpphalangeal joint
at <20° of flexion

Metacarpophalangeal
joint at 90°
of flexion

A   **B**

Figure 47-35. Gutter splints are used for the treatment of phalangeal and metacarpal fractures. **A,** Fractures of the ring and little fingers are immobilized in an ulnar gutter splint. **B,** Fractures involving the index finger and the long finger are immobilized in a radial splint. The splint is made by using plaster sheets cut to the proper size. The measurement should be from the tip of the finger to a point two thirds of the way up the forearm. (From Simon RR, Koenigsknecht SJ: The hand. In Simon RR [ed]: *Emergency Orthopedics: The Extremities,* 3rd ed. Norwalk, Conn, Appleton & Lange, 1995, p 519.)

mobility. For this reason, these two groups are discussed separately.

Metacarpal Fractures of Digits II Through V

The hand can adjust functionally to dorsal angulation in the metacarpal equal to its motion at the CMC joint, plus 10 to 15 degrees in some patients. Because the index and middle fingers are immobile at their CMC joints, they may accommodate 10 to 15 degrees of dorsal angulation. The ring finger usually has 20 to 30 degrees of mobility at its CMC joint and may accommodate 40 to 45 degrees of dorsal angulation. The small finger generally has 30 to 50 degrees of motion at its base and may accommodate 50 to 70 degrees of dorsal angulation. Finger metacarpals may tolerate 10 to 15 degrees of lateral angulation and 3 to 4 mm of shortening. Rotational deformity, most commonly seen in spiral and oblique fractures, is poorly tolerated. A small amount of rotational deformity can translate into a substantial digital overlap when the fingers are closed to form a fist. More than 5 degrees of malrotation may cause overlapping (scissoring) of the fingers during flexion.[20]

Metacarpal Head Fractures

Pathophysiology. Fractures of the metacarpal head are rare. They usually occur secondary to direct trauma or crush injury and typically result in a comminuted fracture.[22] These fractures occur distal to the attachment of the collateral ligaments. Physical examination reveals tenderness and swelling over the involved MCP joint. Pain is increased if axial compression is applied along the extended digit. The presence of lacerations over the metacarpal heads is significant and suggests the possibility of an open fracture or human bite injury.

Diagnostic Strategies: Radiology. Although routine imaging of the injured hand reveals most fractures, the metacarpal heads can be difficult to assess because of overlap on the lateral view. In such cases in which clinical suspicion of a fracture exists and the initial views are normal, the Brewerton "ball-catcher's" view may be helpful.[30] This view is obtained with the digits in 65 degrees of flexion at the MCP joints and the x-ray beam angled 15 degrees radially, projecting the metacarpal heads in profile. Occasionally, computed tomography also may be required to evaluate accurately the degree of displacement of intra-articular fractures at the MCP level.

Management. Emergency management of closed metacarpal head fractures consists of elevation, ice for comfort, analgesics, and immobilization of the hand in the "safe" or functional position, which balances the forces of the intrinsic muscles. In this position, the wrist is extended 20 degrees, the MCP joints are flexed to 90 degrees, and the PIP and the DIP joints are extended (Figure 47-36). Referral to a hand surgeon for management and follow-up evaluation is required in all cases. Because these are intra-articular fractures, displacement greater than 1 to 2 mm predisposes to a poor result; however, there is little consensus as to optimal definitive treatment.[31]

Lacerations or puncture wounds over the dorsum of the MCP joint associated with a metacarpal head fracture should be considered open until proved otherwise. Such injuries often are caused by a clenched-fist injury and are highly contaminated wounds. Emergent consultation with a hand surgeon for operative debridement and irrigation is recommended. Prophylactic coverage with a cephalosporin is routinely recom-

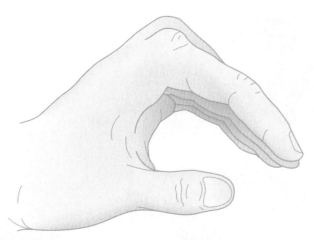

Figure 47-36. The "safe" position described by James. (Modified from Stern PJ: Fractures of the metacarpals and phalanges. In Green DP [ed]: *Green's Operative Hand Surgery,* 4th ed. New York, Churchill Livingstone, 1999.)

mended, although highly contaminated wounds also should receive penicillin and an aminoglycoside. Several studies have found preoperative wound cultures to be of no value in predicting the risk of infection or the nature of the likely pathogen, and some authors have abandoned their use.[32,33]

Complications. Metacarpal head fractures may be associated with debilitating hand complications, including avascular necrosis, rotational malalignment, interosseous muscle fibrosis, extensor tendon injury or fibrosis, and chronic stiffness of the MCP joint. Many of these fractures also may require late arthroplasty.[22]

Metacarpal Neck Fractures

Pathophysiology. Fractures of the metacarpal neck are among the most common fractures in the hand. The mechanism of injury is a direct impaction force (e.g., a punch with a closed fist). A *boxer's fracture* is a fracture of the neck of the fifth metacarpal (Figure 47-37). Most metacarpal neck fractures have a typical apex dorsal angulation (palmar angulation of the distal fragment). They are inherently unstable because of the deforming muscle forces and frequent comminution of the volar cortex. Management generally is difficult because of this instability and the difficulty in maintaining reduction.

Management. For treatment purposes, metacarpal neck fractures are divided into two groups: fractures involving the ring and little finger metacarpals and fractures involving the index and long finger metacarpals. There is considerably more mobility of the metacarpals of the ring and little fingers compared with the index and long fingers. The greater mobility makes them more prone to fracture, and the immobility of the index and long finger metacarpals increases the need for accurate alignment after reduction. Generally less than 15 degrees is allowed in the index and long finger metacarpals; in the ring and little finger metacarpals, 35 degrees and 45 degrees of angulation is allowed. Any rotational malalignment must be completely corrected.

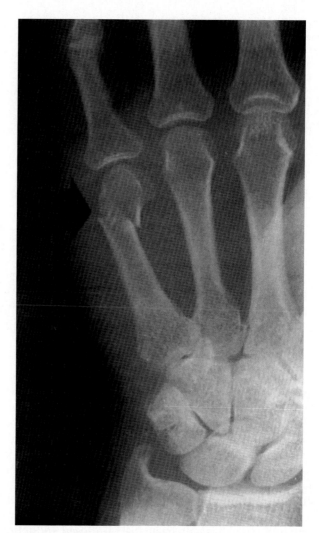

Figure 47-37. Boxer's fracture. (From Harris JH Jr, et al: *The Radiology of Emergency Medicine.* Baltimore, Williams & Wilkins, 1993, p 444.)

Nondisplaced ring and little finger metacarpal fractures without angulation deformity can be treated initially with ice, elevation, analgesia, and immobilization in a gutter splint. Nondisplaced, nonangulated metacarpal fractures of the index and long finger metacarpals are treated similarly. The splint should be in standard position of function and extend from below the elbow up to, but not including, the PIP joint. Generally, it is recommended to begin PIP and DIP motion without delay. Protected MCP motion can begin in 3 to 4 weeks.[22] For isolated fractures of the little finger metacarpal neck, some authors advocate immediate mobilization of fractures regardless of the degree of angulation. These results show excellent function and early return to work and only minor cosmetic deformity. Early follow-up evaluation is advised to exclude residual angulation, rotational deformity, and delayed displacement.[34]

Reducing ring and little finger metacarpal neck fractures with significant angulation or deformity may be attempted in the emergency department. After appropriate anesthesia, usually a hematoma block, traction is

Figure 47-38. The 90-90 method for metacarpal neck fracture reduction.

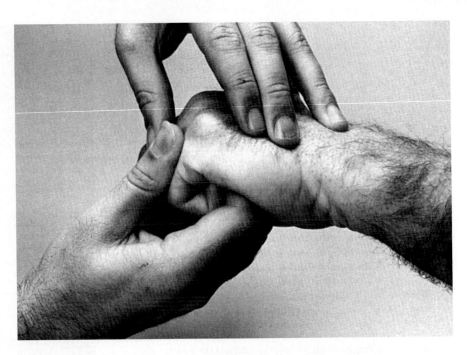

applied on the metacarpal to disimpact the fracture. The MCP joints and IP joints are flexed at 90 degrees, and simultaneous pressure is applied in a volar direction over the metacarpal shaft and in a dorsal direction over the flexed PIP joint (Figure 47-38). This maneuver is termed the *90-90 method* and should complete reduction. A gutter splint in position of function should be applied. Postreduction radiographs should be obtained immediately and after 1 week to ensure that reduction has not been lost. If closed reduction is unable to be achieved or maintained, pin fixation by a hand surgeon is necessary, and early referral is indicated.

Displaced or angulated index or long finger metacarpal neck fractures commonly require anatomic reduction and surgical fixation. Emergency department management consists of ice, elevation, and the application of a volar splint. Prompt referral to a hand surgeon is mandatory.

Complications. Metacarpal neck fractures may have an associated rotational component that can impair function and result in overlapping of the affected finger over an adjacent finger. If excessive angulation is not corrected, the patient may experience forced hyperextension of the MCP joint and flexion of the PIP joint when extending the finger and pain when tightly grasping objects. Other complications include extensor tendon injury and collateral ligament damage. Nonunion is rare after closed metacarpal fractures.

Metacarpal Shaft Fractures

Pathophysiology. There are three types of metacarpal shaft fractures: transverse, oblique or spiral, and comminuted. Transverse and comminuted fractures usually result from a direct blow and commonly exhibit dorsal angulation (Figure 47-39). Indirect trauma or rotational torque applied to the finger may result in a spiral shaft fracture. These fracture fragments tend to shorten and rotate rather than angulate.

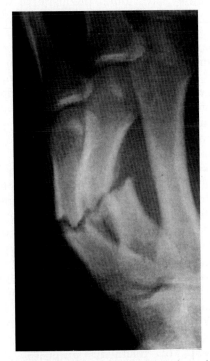

Figure 47-39. X-ray film shows the typical dorsal angulation of fractures of the metacarpal shafts. These fractures are usually the result of a direct blow and generally angulate dorsally because of the interosseous muscles exerting a volar force. (From Green DP, Rowland SA: Fractures and dislocations in the hand. In Rockwood CA Jr, Green DP [eds]: *Fractures in Adults*. Philadelphia, JB Lippincott, 1991, p 490.)

Management. Metacarpal shaft fractures are treated differently than fractures involving the neck because rotational deformity and shortening are more likely, and less angular deformity is acceptable. In general, any rotational deformity must be corrected. Angulation deformities are unacceptable in the index and long finger metacarpals, whereas a small amount of angulation may be compensated for in the ring and little finger metacarpals. Acceptable reduction is less than 10 degrees of angulation in the former and less than 20 degrees in the latter, with less than 3 mm of shortening and normal rotational alignment.[20]

Most metacarpal shaft fractures can be managed initially with ice, elevation, analgesia, and immobilization in a gutter splint. The splint should include the wrist and the entire metacarpal shaft, but not the MCP joint if the fracture is proximal to the neck. Repeat radiographic examination and referral to a hand surgeon are recommended. If manipulative reduction is necessary, operative fixation usually is indicated. Multiple displaced metacarpal shaft fractures, oblique or spiral fractures with rotational deformity, irreducible transverse fractures, and displaced open fractures require internal fixation.[34]

Complications. Complications seen in metacarpal shaft fractures are similar to the complications described for other metacarpal fractures. In addition to malrotation, which can cause a chronic painful grip, limitation of extensor function and interosseous muscle fibrosis may develop.

Metacarpal Base Fractures

Clinical Features. Fractures of the metacarpal base generally are stable and occur infrequently. They may result from either a direct blow over the base of the metacarpal or an axial force or torque applied along the digit. Examination reveals tenderness and swelling at the base of the involved metacarpal, and a significant degree of rotational deformity may be evident. Fractures at the base of the ring or little finger metacarpals may cause injury to the motor branch of the ulnar nerve and result in paralysis of the intrinsic hand muscles. In addition, they may be associated with a carpal bone fracture.

Management. Initial management in the emergency department consists of ice, elevation, analgesia, and immobilization in a bulky compressive dressing or volar splint with referral to a hand surgeon for definitive management.

Complications. Metacarpal base fractures may be associated with extensor or flexor tendon damage and significant rotational malalignment. Chronic CMC joint stiffness is often associated with intra-articular fractures and may necessitate arthrodesis or arthroplasty.

Thumb Metacarpal Fractures

Fractures of the thumb metacarpal are relatively uncommon because of its high degree of mobility. Although the shaft occasionally may be involved, most fractures involve the base of the metacarpal. These fractures are classified into two groups: extra-articular and intra-articular. The two common types of intra-articular fractures of the thumb are Bennett's and Rolando's fractures.

Extra-articular Fractures. Extra-articular fractures are seen more commonly than intra-articular fractures and usually result from direct trauma or impaction. The three types of extra-articular fractures are transverse, oblique, and epiphyseal in children. Examination

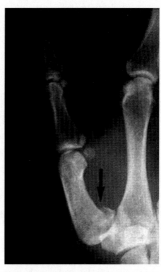

Figure 47-40. Bennett's fracture, anteroposterior view. Avulsion fracture of the articular surface of the first metacarpal with subluxation at the carpometacarpal joint. This fracture must be differentiated from Rolando's fracture and the more common extra-articular varieties. (From Rosen P, et al: *Diagnostic Radiology in Emergency Medicine.* St. Louis, Mosby, 1992, p 181.)

reveals localized pain and swelling over the fracture site.

Mobility of the thumb metacarpal allows 20 to 30 degrees of angular deformity without functional impairment. Extra-articular fractures with a greater degree of angulation should undergo closed reduction, postreduction radiographs, and immobilization of the thumb in abduction with its IP joint extended using a thumb spica cast for 4 weeks. Transverse fractures are usually stable and can be managed with closed reduction and immobilization. If the fracture is oblique, it may require Kirschner wire fixation because of instability and a propensity for rotational deformity.[20]

Intra-articular Fractures

Bennett's Fracture. Bennett's fracture is an intra-articular fracture at the base of the thumb metacarpal combined with a dislocation or subluxation of the CMC joint. The ulnar portion of the metacarpal remains in place, and the larger fragment subluxes dorsally because of the pulling force of the abductor pollicis longus and adductor pollicis muscle (Figure 47-40). There is complete disruption of the ligaments about the CMC joint. Because stability is conferred mostly by the dorsal ligament (posterior oblique CMC ligament), dislocation ensues. The mechanism of injury usually involves an axial force acting on a partially flexed metacarpal (e.g., striking a rigid object with a closed fist). This is the most common fracture of the thumb base.[35]

Bennett's fracture requires an anatomic reduction. Treatment goals are to achieve stability of the CMC joint by rejoining the volar lip fragment to the first metacarpal and to restore articular congruity. Initial management consists of immobilization in a thumb spica splint, ice, elevation, and analgesia. Early referral to a hand surgeon is warranted because although closed reduction can be achieved, the fragments are difficult to hold in position as a result of the pulling forces of the abductor pollicis longus and adductor pollicis muscle. Definitive treatment consists of conservative management, closed reduction with percutaneous pinning, or, less often, open reduction and internal fixation.

Rolando's Fracture. Rolando's fracture is a comminuted fracture of the base of the thumb metacarpal. Various degrees of comminution occur, but the typical configuration is in a Y- or T-shaped pattern. The severity of comminution is often underrepresented on radiographic studies. The mechanism of injury is the same as in Bennett's fracture, but Rolando's fracture occurs much less commonly and generally has a much worse prognosis.

Emergency department management of Rolando's fracture consists of immobilization in a thumb spica splint, ice, elevation, analgesia, and early referral to a hand surgeon for surgical reduction. Definitive treatment is controversial and depends on the severity of comminution of the base of the thumb and the degree of displacement. If open reduction is indicated, a plate is often placed dorsally to maintain the reconstruction; with severe comminution, Kirschner wire fixation, bone graft placement, and external fixation may be used for continued distraction until healing occurs.[35]

Complications. Complications include joint stiffness, degenerative arthritis, and malunion. Malunion is the most common late complication but is usually well tolerated at the thumb CMC joint.[36] Posttraumatic arthritis is more common after Rolando's fracture and may require arthrodesis or resection hemiarthroplasty. Nonunion is rare.

Pediatric Fractures of the Hand

Pathophysiology and Assessment

The hand is the most commonly injured body part in children.[37] In young children, the most common hand fracture involves a crush injury of the fingertip with an open fracture of the distal tuft.[34] The most distinctive feature of the immature skeleton is the presence of epiphyseal growth centers. Although the cartilaginous epiphysis is believed to be a weak link in the immature skeleton, injuries involving this region reportedly account for only 18% of pediatric fractures.[38]

The Salter-Harris classification of epiphyseal fractures is used to direct treatment and predict outcome. The injuries are classified numerically I through V, with higher numbers corresponding to an increased risk for growth disturbance.[39] The most common epiphyseal fracture in the hand is a Salter-Harris type II fracture of the proximal phalanx.[37] It usually results from a twisting or hyperextension mechanism and most often involves the ring and little fingers and the thumb. Although lack of cooperation may make examination difficult, the clinician should look for swelling, ecchymosis, and deformity. In addition, one should palpate for bony tenderness and for tenderness over the collateral ligaments. Persistent limitation of motion in a young child usually implies a significant injury of the bones or joints of the digit.

Radiographic studies should be obtained and should include the same views that are obtained in an adult. In addition, comparison views may be helpful, particularly in subtle fractures. Epiphyseal fractures may be particularly difficult because they appear differently at different ages, and their varied radiographic appearance may be mistaken for a fracture.

Management

Most pediatric hand fractures can be readily treated with either simple splinting or closed reduction, followed by brief immobilization, usually for no longer than 3 weeks. A plaster or fiberglass gutter splint incorporating the adjacent uninjured finger and including the wrist is the best means of immobilizing a child's finger fracture. The previously mentioned safe position still should be used whenever possible. Some authors advocate that even stable injuries that ordinarily would be treated by buddy splinting in an adult should be protected with full splinting for several weeks in children to prevent further injury. Open reduction and surgical fixation may be necessary for displaced intra-articular fractures, displaced Salter-Harris type III or IV fractures, and unstable fractures that cannot be maintained by closed methods.[40]

Complications

Pediatric hand fractures heal more quickly compared with similar injuries in adults. In addition, remodeling allows correction of some step-offs or angular deformities in younger children, but does not correct rotational deformities. The ability of bone to correct angular deformities by remodeling is diminished with age and cannot be relied on in adolescents and adults. Residual deformity is the most commonly reported complication. Other complications, including joint stiffness, tendon adherence, and nonunion, are rarely seen.

Soft Tissue Injuries

Soft tissue injuries of the hand are extremely common, accounting for 82% of hand injuries seen in the emergency department.[41] Trauma accounts for most of these injuries to the tendons, ligaments, and cartilage. Although such injuries are not life-threatening, they may result in potentially disabling complications, including joint laxity, loss of motion, chronic pain, swelling, and deformity.

Dislocations and Ligamentous Injuries

Ligamentous injuries to the hand are common and often missed. Injury may range from mild sprain to complete rupture and may produce varying degrees of joint instability. Purely ligamentous injuries may be "tears in continuity" (grade I), partial tears (grade II), or complete tears (grade III). The disruption of joints may be complete, with the articular surfaces completely separated (a dislocation), or incomplete, leaving the articular surfaces in partial communication (a subluxation).

Because the goal of treatment is to restore functional stability, it is essential to perform a systematic evalua-

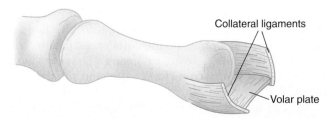

Figure 47-41. The collateral ligaments on either side of the joint and the volar plate form a boxlike support around the joint. (From Simon RR, Koenigsknecht SJ: In Simon RR [ed]: *Emergency Orthopedics: The Extremities,* 3rd ed. Norwalk, Conn, Appleton & Lange, 1995.)

tion of joint stability. Functionally, stability may be determined by using a two-phase test of the IP and MCP joints of the hand. Because range of motion is heavily influenced by pain, accurate assessment generally requires digital or wrist block anesthesia in even the most cooperative patients. Active stability is tested by allowing the patient to move the digit through the normal range of motion. Completion of a full range without displacement indicates that adequate joint stability remains. Passive stability is assessed by applying gentle radial and ulnar stress to each collateral ligament and posteroanterior stress to assess volar plate integrity. Stress testing should be done in extended and moderately flexed positions to avoid the stabilizing effect of the volar plate. Comparisons with the same joint of the uninvolved hand may assist in the diagnosis. Supplemental stress radiographs also may be helpful in evaluating difficult cases.[42]

The diagnosis of incomplete or partial ligamentous injuries is made when the joint is stable to active and passive stress but is significantly swollen, with pain elicited on stress and palpation of the involved ligament systems. The examiner should attempt to ascertain whether the most tender area is over the central slip (dorsal), collateral ligaments (radial and ulnar), or volar plate (volar). Grade I and II injuries exhibit pain with stability on stress testing. Grade III injuries show instability on stress testing. Stability of the joint provides strong evidence that optimal functional recovery would result from short-term immobilization rather than surgical intervention. Because of the three-dimensional boxlike configuration that the collateral ligaments and volar plate form around the joint, wide displacement indicates that at least two components of the ligament-box complex are disrupted (Figure 47-41).[22,41] Joints with demonstrable instability should be immobilized in a gutter splint and referred for assessment by a hand surgeon to determine whether surgical repair is necessary. Immobilization should be done with the IP joints splinted at 30 degrees of flexion and the MCP joints splinted at 45 to 50 degrees of flexion; when the thumb MCP is involved, it should be splinted in 30 degrees of flexion. Because the long-term effects of joint injuries are almost always joint stiffness and loss of flexion rather than persistent instability, immobilization is usually brief (2 to 3 weeks) and should be followed by a gradual procession of active range-of-motion exercises.[22]

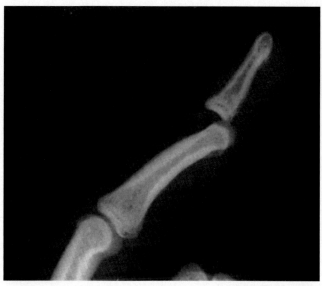

Figure 47-42. Dorsal dislocation of the distal interphalangeal joint without associated fracture. (From Harris JH Jr, et al: *The Radiology of Emergency Medicine.* Baltimore, Williams & Wilkins, 1993, p 446.)

Distal Interphalangeal Joint

The DIP joint structure is analogous to that of the PIP joint. Additional stability is provided by the adjacent insertions of the flexor and extensor tendons, and dislocations are uncommon. Most dislocations are dorsal and usually are associated with an open wound (Figure 47-42). Routine radiographs are used more to rule out associated fractures than to confirm a suspected diagnosis. Treatment consists of closed reduction under digital or wrist block anesthesia, followed by active and passive stability testing. Reduction usually is accomplished easily by longitudinal traction and hyperextension to distract the bayonet-opposed distal phalanx followed by direct application of dorsal pressure to the base of the distal phalanx. Irreducible cases require surgery for open reduction. Irreducible cases may be caused by an avulsion fracture with interposition in the joint, entrapment of the profundus tendon, or buttonhole tear through the volar plate.[43]

If the dislocation is open, the joint is contaminated, and treatment should include debridement and copious wound irrigation. The skin should be sutured and the joint splinted in slight flexion with a dorsal splint for 3 weeks. Most authors recommend prophylactic antibiotics.[43,44]

Proximal Interphalangeal Joint

Dislocations of the PIP joint are the most common ligament injuries in the hand. Stability is derived from the strong conjoined attachments of the paired collateral ligaments and the volar plate. Three types of displacement of the PIP joint may occur: dorsal, lateral, and volar. The mechanism of injury is usually sports related with a high-velocity blow to the end of the finger, which causes an axial load and hyperextension. Simple dorsal dislocations result when the volar plate ruptures and the middle phalanx assumes the position of bayonet opposition. Alternatively a lateral dislocation may result from a radially or ulnarly directed force on the joint that leads to rupture of one collateral ligament and at least partial avulsion of the volar plate from the middle phalanx. In lateral dislocations, the ratio of radial-to-ulnar collateral ligament (UCL) rupture is 6:1, and the digit is usually ulnarly deviated. Volar dislocation of the PIP joint is rare. The most common mechanism of injury is a rotary longitudinal compression force on a semiflexed middle phalanx that results in unilateral disruption of a collateral ligament and partial avulsion of the volar plate. Physical examination reveals swelling and tenderness over the PIP joint and inability to extend the joint. Routine radiographs of the injured digit reveal the type of dislocation and any associated avulsion fractures.

Management. Small bony fragments at attachment sites seen on radiographs are associated with avulsions of minor ligamentous attachment points and do not indicate the need for open repair. Avulsion fractures involving 33% or more of the articular surface are usually unstable and require surgery.[45]

Most closed dorsal and lateral PIP dislocations are treated nonoperatively.[46] Reduction is facilitated by digital nerve block and usually can be accomplished by longitudinal traction and mild hyperextension followed by firm dorsal pressure on the proximal aspect of the middle phalanx. When reduction is achieved, active motion is tested. Reduction is stable if there is no displacement during active range of motion and passive stressing of the joint. More than 20 degrees of deformity and instability with lateral testing indicate a complete ligamentous injury.[47] If there is stability to active range of motion, treatment consists of 3 weeks of immobilization in 20 to 30 degrees of flexion, followed by active exercises. Although stiffness, pain, and swelling are likely to persist for months, the long-term prognosis is good, and subluxation usually does not recur unless the finger is hyperextended again.[20] If the joint is irreducible or there is evidence of complete ligamentous disruption with dislocation on active range of motion, operative repair is required.

The management of volar dislocations of the PIP joint is controversial. The dislocation has been described as irreducible and requiring open reduction; however, some authors state that most volar dislocations can be reduced by a closed technique of applying gentle traction with MCP and PIP joints flexed.[48] A stable reduction with repair of the soft tissue structures and transarticular pinning in the fully extended position also has been recommended.[43]

Metacarpophalangeal Joint of the Fingers

Pathophysiology. MCP dislocations are considerably less common than dislocations of the PIP joint. The MCP joints of the fingers are resistant to ligamentous injury and dislocation because of their inherent ligamentous structure, their surrounding supporting structures, and their protected position at the base of the fingers. Similar to the DIP and PIP joints, each MCP joint has two collateral ligaments and a volar fibrocartilaginous plate; however, the MCP joints are condyloid joints and permit, in addition to flexion and extension,

30 degrees of lateral motion while the joint is extended. Because of the shape of this articulation, the joint is more stable in flexion when the collateral ligaments are stretched than they are in extension. They are most vulnerable to injury from forces directed ulnarly and dorsally.

Isolated injury to the collateral ligaments and volar plate of the MCP joint is rare. These injuries usually occur with hyperextension stress applied to the MCP joint with the finger extended. The patient has ecchymosis and swelling of the joint. Examination reveals tenderness along the joint and varying degrees of instability. Routine radiographs are usually normal, but some authors recommend a Brewerton view to show any evidence of avulsed bone fragments.[49] Treatment for most of these injuries is gentle compression dressing with light plaster reinforcement and early orthopedic referral.

Dislocations of the MCP joints of the fingers are relatively rare injuries and are usually dorsal. The most common digit involved is the index finger, followed by the little finger. These dislocations result from hyperextension forces that rupture the proximal volar plate and are divided into simple and complex types. In the simple dislocation (subluxation), the joint appears to be hyperextended to 60 to 90 degrees, and the articular surfaces are in contact without interposed soft tissue. With complex (complete) dislocations, the MCP joint is in moderate hyperextension and angulated, the metacarpal head is prominent in the palm, and the distended palmar skin is dimpled. Complex dislocations have a less striking presentation but are a more severe injury; the volar plate is interposed in the MCP joint space, and closed reduction is not possible (Figure 47-43). Radiographic examination shows an obvious dislocation in the lateral view. Posteroanterior views reveal widening of the joint space in complex dislocations. In addition, sesamoids may be seen in the joint and are a pathognomonic sign (Figure 47-44).

Management. After appropriate anesthesia, simple dorsal dislocations should be reduced in a way that prevents entrapment of the volar plate in the joint.

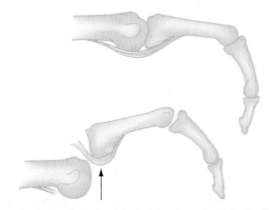

Figure 47-43. The most important element preventing reduction in a complex metacarpophalangeal dislocation is interposition of the volar plate within the joint space. It must be extricated surgically. (From Green DP, Rowland SA: Fractures and dislocations in the hand. In Rockwood CA Jr, Green DP [eds]: *Fractures in Adults*. Philadelphia, JB Lippincott, 1991, p 521.)

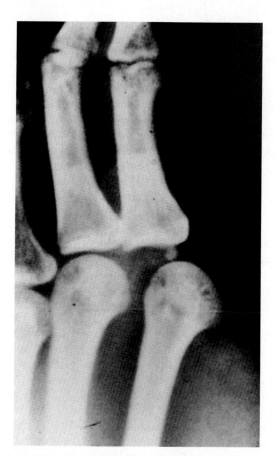

Figure 47-44. A pathognomonic radiographic sign of complex metacarpophalangeal dislocation is the presence of a sesamoid bone in the widened joint space, indicative of interposition of the entrapped volar plate. (From DeLee JC, Drez D Jr, Miller MD: *Orthopedic Sports Medicine: Principles and Practice,* vol 2. 2nd ed. Philadelphia, WB Saunders, 2003, p 1387.)

Reduction is accomplished by flexing the wrist to relax the flexor tendons and applying firm pressure over the dorsum of the proximal phalanx in a distal and volar direction. Excessive hyperextension or longitudinal traction should be avoided. The MCP joints should be splinted in flexion, and referral to a hand surgeon is necessary. Complex dorsal dislocations do not reduce with closed methods and require operative reduction. Volar dislocations are rare and generally require operative reduction.

Carpometacarpal Joints of the Fingers
Pathophysiology. The CMC joints of the digit form the base of the transverse metacarpal arch of the hand. The metacarpal bases articulate with each other and with the distal carpal row in a complex interlocking structural arrangement. The joints are supported by strong dorsal, volar, and interosseous ligaments and are reinforced by the broad insertions of the wrist flexors and extensors (Figure 47-45). Dislocations of the CMC joints are uncommon and often are missed.[50] Overall the most commonly injured CMC joint is the little finger, and most of these injuries are dorsal fracture-dislocations.[51] The injury occurs as a result of motor vehicle accidents, falls, crushes, and closed-fist trauma.

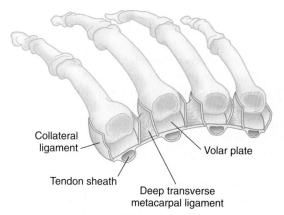

Figure 47-45. The volar plates of four palmar metacarpals are held together firmly by the deep transverse metacarpal ligament, which is continuous with the volar plate. Eaton calls this the intervolar plate ligament. (From Green DP, Rowland SA: Fractures and dislocations in the hand. In Rockwood CA Jr, Green DP [eds]: *Fractures in Adults.* Philadelphia, JB Lippincott, 1991, p 518.)

Clinical Features and Diagnostic Strategies. Clinically the patient has swelling on the dorsum of the hand and tenderness over the involved CMC joints. Routine radiographs must be viewed carefully because fracture lines may be subtle, and the metacarpals may be obscured by superimposition. Other radiographs that may be helpful include multiple oblique, forearm in 30-degree pronation, and Brewerton views.[51]

Management. Initial treatment consists of ice for comfort, elevation, and analgesia. Closed reduction of the dorsal fracture-dislocation may be attempted under adequate regional anesthesia. Traction and flexion with simultaneous longitudinal pressure on the metacarpal base, followed by extension of the metacarpal head when length has been restored, generally results in reduction. Even in cases in which reduction is achieved by closed means, early referral to a hand surgeon is needed because Kirschner wire fixation is advisable to ensure adequate stability. The late sequelae of fracture-dislocations include pain and weakness from traumatic arthritis secondary to imprecise alignment or chronic dislocation of the CMC joints.

Interphalangeal Joint of the Thumb
The IP joint of the thumb is similar to a finger DIP joint except that the phalanges of the thumb are typically larger and stronger than the phalanges of the fingers. Even with the thumb's vulnerable position, IP dislocation is uncommon. Most dislocations are dorsal, and they often are associated with open injuries. Reduction is usually simple after a median nerve block. The joint usually remains stable because the volar plate remains attached to the distal phalanx, and immobilization in mild flexion for 3 weeks usually suffices.

Metacarpophalangeal Joint of the Thumb
The MCP joint of the thumb is a condyloid joint that allows mainly flexion and extension; however, it also permits some degree of abduction, adduction, and rotation. Its volar plate and collateral ligaments are stronger than other MCP joints, but its vulnerable position leads

to frequent traumatic injury. Overall, injury to the MCP joint of the thumb accounts for five times the injuries of all the other MCP joints combined.

Most dislocations of thumb MCP joints are dorsal and result from a hyperextension force that ruptures the volar plate, joint capsule, and at least part of the collateral ligament. Similar to other dorsal MCP dislocations, displacement varies from subluxation of the phalanx to a complex dislocation with the proximal phalanx resting over the metacarpal head. The complex dislocation is not easily reduced because of volar plate entrapment in the joint. Clinically the complex dislocation may show a dimple over the thenar eminence. Radiographic studies confirm the dorsal dislocation and reveal the sesamoids in close proximity to the proximal phalanx.

Management. Closed reduction may be attempted under radial and median nerve wrist block anesthesia. Pressure is directed distally on the base of the proximal phalanx with the metacarpal flexed and adducted. If reduction is difficult, the IP joint and wrist can be flexed to relax the entrapped flexor pollicis longus tendon. When reduction is accomplished, the collateral ligaments should be tested, and reduction should be confirmed by radiography. Stability to active range of motion and stress testing suggest that immobilization in a thumb spica splint with the MCP joint in 20 degrees of flexion for 4 weeks is adequate. Nonreducible (complex) dislocations or dislocations with significant lateral instability require open reduction and operative repair. Hyperextension, instability, and chronic pain on pinching may occur after these injuries.

Ulnar Collateral Ligament Injuries (Gamekeeper's Thumb, Skier's Thumb)

Pathophysiology. Injury to the UCL was first described as an occupational hazard of Scottish gamekeepers who damaged their thumbs by repeatedly twisting the necks of hares.[52] Skiing is now the most common cause of acute and chronic injury to the UCL.[53] *Skier's thumb* is the most common upper extremity injury in skiing and results from interference with release of the pole at the moment of impact. UCL rupture occurs 10 times more often than radial collateral ligament injury.[42] The mechanism of injury is forced radial deviation (abduction), and the subsequent tear usually occurs at the insertion into the proximal phalanx. Stener[54] showed that in nearly two thirds of cases of complete UCL rupture, the adductor pollicis becomes interposed between the superficial proximal portion and the deep distal portion of the ligament (see Figure 47-45). Besides the collateral ligament, associated injuries of the dorsal capsule and volar plate are common.

Clinical Features. Physical examination reveals swelling and localized tenderness over the ulnar border of the joint and weakness of pinch. Complete and partial ruptures usually can be differentiated by clinical examination. Valgus stress testing of the UCLs is required and should be performed in full extension and in 30 degrees of flexion to avoid the stabilizing effect of the volar plate. If examination is accompanied by pain and guarding, the test should be done under median and radial nerve block at the wrist or local infiltration anesthesia. More than 35 degrees of joint laxity or 15 degrees more laxity than is present in the uninjured thumb is consistent with complete UCL rupture.[37] Routine radiographs should be taken before stressing the joint and may reveal a bony avulsion from the insertion of the UCL into the proximal phalanx or an associated condylar fracture. Radiographic findings of proximal phalanx volar subluxation and radial deviation may indicate complete UCL rupture.[37] Because of the difficulty in diagnosing complete rupture, it is commonly misdiagnosed as a simple sprain in the emergency department, resulting in chronic disability.[55]

Management. Acute partial ruptures of the UCL can be treated effectively by a 4-week period of immobilization in a thumb spica cast; full recovery is the rule. Complete ligament tears require surgical repair because a high percentage are associated with soft tissue interposition from the adductor aponeurosis (Stener's lesion) with limited predicted healing potential. Anatomic repair within 3 weeks of injury achieves good or excellent results in 90% of patients.[37] Long-term complications include chronic pain and instability with the loss of pinch strength, which may require arthrodesis.

Radial Collateral Ligament Injuries. Radial collateral ligament injuries of the MCP joint of the thumb are less common but equally debilitating.[56] The usual mechanism is forced adduction with or without hyperextension. Diagnosis and treatment are generally similar; however, anatomic differences between the two sides of the MCP joint do not allow a Stener-like lesion on the radial side, and the role of surgical repair is not well defined.[37]

Carpometacarpal Joint of the Thumb

Injuries of the volar ligament of the thumb CMC joint, similar to in other joints of the hand, may be complete or partial. Complete rupture permits the entire thumb metacarpal to dislocate dorsally.[57] These dislocations are reduced easily but are unstable after reduction. Initial management consists of ice, analgesia, elevation, and application of a thumb spica splint. The patient should be referred to a hand surgeon promptly for possible operative repair of the ligament. If the capsule is allowed to heal with imperfect metacarpal reduction, joint instability may occur with progressive degenerative changes resulting in chronic pain.

Tendon Injuries

Tendon injuries may involve one or more of the extensor or flexor tendons in the hand and encompass a spectrum of abnormalities, ranging from simple stretching of the fibers to complete tendon rupture with or without an associated avulsion fracture. The most common mechanisms of injury of tendons are lacerations, avulsions, and crush injuries. In a normal resting position, the fingers are flexed, with the little finger having the greatest degree of flexion and the index finger having the least. In the resting hand, a finger with greater or lesser degree of flexion than that of the opposite hand often indicates a tendon injury. This observation may be especially useful in an uncooperative patient or child. If the patient can move a joint, but active flexion or extension is limited or painful, a partial tendon laceration may be present. To assess the tendons adequately, motion should be tested against resistance. This testing may cause a partially ruptured tendon to rupture, but identifies a lesion that needs surgical repair. The tendon should be placed in maximal stretch before testing to provide for the greatest strength during contraction. As a general rule, extensor injury causes greater impairment of motion than does a similar flexor injury. Vessels and nerves travel closely with flexor tendons, particularly in the fingers. Damage to one of these structures is likely to be associated with damage to the other two.

The position the hand was in when the injury occurred is important. When trauma occurs while the hand is held in flexion, the flexor tendons may be transected, and the distal stump would lie distal to the wound. If the hand is in the extended position, however, the tendon stumps would lie at wound edges. When the tendons are injured by a direct blow to the hand or the fingers, the closed injury may hide significant tissue damage. Partial tendon lacerations may be associated with small surface wounds. To help exclude injury, wounds and visible tendons should be inspected while the joints are taken through a full range of motion.

Extensor Tendon Injuries

The most common site of tendon injury is the extensors over the dorsum of the hand. The extensors are predisposed to laceration because of their superficial location on the dorsum of the hand and the minimal amount of subcutaneous tissue between the tendon and overlying skin. This anatomic feature also predisposes the extensor mechanism to more complex tendon injuries, including abrasion, crush, and avulsion. Because the extensor tendons are not constrained in tight fibro-osseous canals except in the wrist, they also are easily located and repaired.

Injuries to the extensor tendons have been grouped into anatomic zones for easy understanding and classification. There are different systems for assigning zones, but the most widely accepted is that of Verdan[58] (Figure 47-46). In this system, there are eight zones, from zone I at the DIP joint level to zone VIII at the distal forearm level. The use of zones is convenient for assessing injury patterns, repair techniques, and rehabilitation.

Zone I Injuries

Pathophysiology. Zone I is the area over the distal phalanx and DIP joint. In this region, the conjoint extensor tendon is well defined and dorsally positioned. Injuries that occur here disrupt the terminal extensor tendon; they may be open or closed and may occur with or without a fracture. Complete laceration of the conjoint tendon results in a flexed posture of about 40 degrees at the DIP joint. Partial transection results in a lesser extension lag and a decrease in the

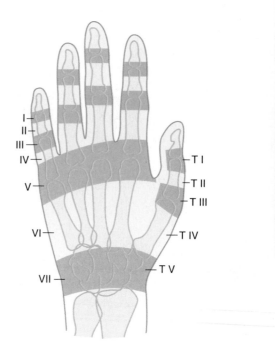

Figure 47-46. Zone classification for extensor tendon injuries. (From Kleinert HE, et al: Flexor tendon injuries. *Surg Clin North Am* 61:267, 1981.)

strength of extension against resistance from a flexed position. The extension lag may increase if the partial injury is not treated appropriately. For this reason, exploration of dorsal lacerations near the DIP joint is important.

Mallet finger is the most common injury in zone I and refers to a closed disruption of the distal extensor apparatus.[22] As a result of loss of extensor tendon continuity to the distal phalanx, there is a flexion deformity of the DIP joint. The injury can be seen in any finger but is seen most commonly in the long, ring, and little fingers. Overall, mallet finger represents the most common tendon injury in the hand seen in athletes.[59] The mechanism of injury is often sudden forceful flexion of an extended finger when an object, such as a ball, strikes the tip of the finger. This mechanism is commonly encountered in athletes and is often described as "jamming" the finger. Other mechanisms include hyperextension with axial compression and direct crush injury at the DIP joint. Three types of injury patterns may occur: type 1 tendon rupture (no fracture), type 2 tendon avulsion with a small bone fragment, and type 3 tendon avulsion with a large bone avulsion (25% to 33% of the articular surface) (Figure 47-47).[60] Fractures of varying size are seen in one fourth to one third of cases (Figure 47-48). Small avulsion fractures are usually the result of hyperflexion injuries, whereas large fracture fragments usually result from a hyperextension mechanism.[61]

Clinical Features. In the acute injury, the patient has swelling, pain, and tenderness over the DIP joint. The distal phalanx is flexed because of the unopposed action of the FDP. There is usually complete passive but incomplete active extension at the DIP joint. Although the diagnosis is easily made, the patient often seeks

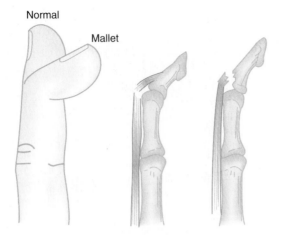

Figure 47-47. Mallet finger occurs with loss of extensor function to the distal phalanx. This may be caused by a tear of the tendon itself or an avulsion fracture of the dorsal base of the distal phalanx.

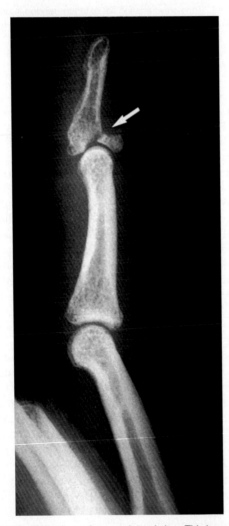

Figure 47-48. Mallet finger fracture, lateral view. This is an intra-articular avulsion of the dorsal surface of the distal phalanx. (From Rosen P, et al: *Diagnostic Radiology in Emergency Medicine*. St. Louis, Mosby, 1992, p 181.)

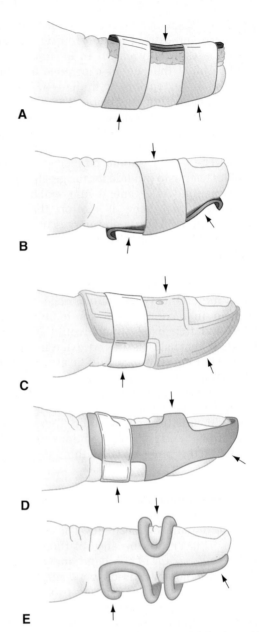

Figure 47-49. Only the distal interphalangeal joint is mobilized in treating mallet fingers. This may be done with a dorsal padded aluminum splint **(A),** a volar unpadded aluminum splint **(B),** a Stack splint **(C),** a modified Stack splint **(D),** or an Abouna splint **(E)**. Each of these splints uses a three-point fixation principle. (From Green DP, Rowland SA: Fractures and dislocations in the hand. In Rockwood CA Jr, Green DP [eds]: *Fractures in Adults*. Philadelphia, JB Lippincott, 1991, p 450.)

treatment late because the functional disability is not great.

Management. The primary goal of treatment is the maintenance of continuous DIP joint extension until tendon healing occurs. Treatment of type 1 and 2 injuries is nonoperative. Immobilization can be accomplished with either a volar or a dorsal splint made from a variety of materials, including aluminum and plastic (Figure 47-49). The DIP joint is immobilized in slight hyperextension for 6 to 8 weeks, but the PIP and MCP joints are allowed to move freely.[22,62] Definitive treatment of a type 3 injury is controversial. Some authors recommend operative repair; others recommend con-

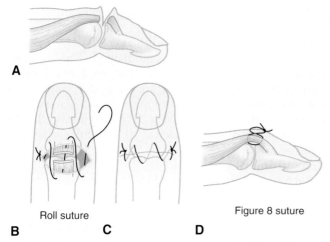

A

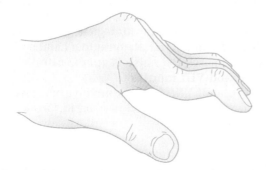

Roll suture   Figure 8 suture

B   **C**   **D**

Figure 47-50. Lacerations of the extensor mechanism over the distal joint with mallet finger deformity **(A)** can be repaired by a roll-type suture, which simultaneously approximates skin and tendon **(B and C)**. A small dressing is applied with a splint to maintain the joint in full extension. Sutures are removed at 10 to 12 days. A figure-of-eight vertical suture **(D)** also may be used, which simultaneously closes the defect in tendon and skin. Splinting is mandatory for 6 weeks. (From Doyle JR: In Green DP [ed]: *Operative Hand Surgery*. New York, Churchill Livingstone, 1993, p 1939.)

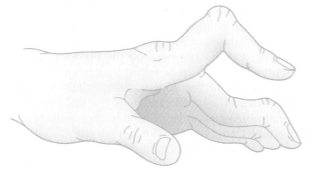

Figure 47-52. Buttonhole (boutonnière) deformity of the index finger with swan neck deformity of other fingers.

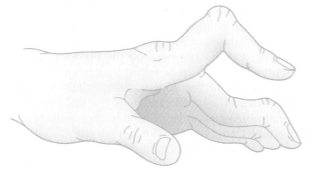

Figure 47-51. Swan neck deformity of the fingers.

servative management with uninterrupted splinting of the digit.[12]

Open zone I injuries that divide the extensor tendon are treated by suturing the cut ends (Figure 47-50). Partial and compete lacerations are repaired with either a roll suture or figure-of-eight stitch using 5-0 nonabsorbable sutures. This repair should be followed by continuous splinting of the DIP joint in full extension for a minimum of 6 weeks.

Prognosis. The results of treatment of mallet fingers are not universally good by any method. Although most patients are improved, only 30% to 40% regain normal function in the DIP joint after treatment.[63] Possible delayed complications include dorsal deformity, cold intolerance, pain, and development of a swan neck deformity (Figure 47-51). This abnormality develops when the lateral bands displace proximally and dorsally, resulting in increased extension forces on the PIP joint. Secondarily, the extensor lag at the DIP joint increases because the force of the FDP tendon is unopposed, and the tendon is functionally increased by the greater distance required to pass over the hyperex-

tended PIP joint. The swan neck deformity is not seen acutely, unless the injured finger has a normally hyperextended PIP joint. Classically, this deformity occurs as a complication of a chronic untreated mallet finger.[63]

Zone II Injuries

Zone II is the area over the middle phalanx. As the lateral bands blend dorsally to form the conjoint tendon, they are thin and oriented around the dorsal half of the middle phalanx. Injuries here are usually the result of simple lacerations that seldom transect all of the dorsal apparatus. Examination reveals a typical mallet deformity. The treatment is identical to that of open zone I injuries.

Zone III Injuries

Pathophysiology. Zone III is the area over the PIP joint. The central tendon is the most commonly injured structure in this zone and represents the second most common closed tendon injury in athletes.[59] The mechanisms for closed rupture include forced flexion of an actively extended finger, a direct blow to the dorsum of the PIP joint, and hyperextension with volar dislocation of the PIP joint. It often results from a "jamming" injury. Lacerations that occur just distal to the PIP joint also may divide the central tendon and readily extend into the joint. Wounds must be carefully explored to define the status of the PIP joint capsule.

Disruption of the central tendon causes an imbalance in the extensor mechanism. The FDS is now unopposed and flexes the PIP joint. The lateral bands displace volarly to the axis of the PIP joint and become flexors of the joint. In addition, the extensor hood retracts proximally, causing extension of the MCP and DIP joints. The resulting tendon imbalance leads to the so-called buttonhole, or *boutonnière*, deformity, with flexion of the PIP joint and hyperextension of the DIP and MP joints (Figure 47-52). Although open injuries of the central tendon may cause an acute boutonnière deformity, this is usually delayed several weeks after a closed athletic injury.

Clinical Features. Early diagnosis of a closed central tendon rupture or avulsion is difficult before the boutonnière deformity has developed. The patient typically has a history of trauma to the involved digit and a painful, swollen PIP joint. The finger is held in slight flexion at the PIP joint and slight extension at the DIP joint. Rupture of the central tendon may be differentiated from the more common injury to the collateral ligament by the location of the maximal area of tenderness of the dorsum rather than sides of the joint and by the patient's inability to extend the PIP joint actively. PIP joint extension can be tested by having the patient attempt to extend the fingers against slight resistance with the hand flat on the table and the PIP joint flexed 90 degrees over an edge of a table (the tabletop test). Radiographs are typically normal but may be diagnostic if an avulsion fracture of the volar base of the middle phalanx is visualized on the lateral view.

Management. Patients with suspected closed central tendon injuries should be treated with splinting of the PIP joint in full extension for 5 to 6 weeks. Only the PIP joint should be immobilized, and passive and active DIP joint flexion is encouraged from the outset. Operative repair may be required for an acute closed boutonnière injury associated with a displaced avulsion fracture and injury with volar PIP joint dislocation. Early referral to a hand surgeon is advised.

When an acute boutonnière deformity is caused by an open injury, exploration of the central slip is mandatory, and a hand surgeon should be consulted. Primary repair of the tendon and Kirschner wire fixation of the PIP joint are often performed. If the joint capsule has been violated, the joint should be thoroughly debrided and irrigated, and the use of prophylactic antibiotics is recommended.

Zone IV Injuries

Zone IV includes the area over the proximal phalanx. The clinical findings are similar to the findings of zone III injury, but are less severe because the PIP joint and lateral bands are intact. The resulting injury is usually partial, and the tendon ends usually do not retract appreciably. These injuries are treated with primary or delayed primary repair and appropriate splinting for 3 to 6 weeks. Simple injuries in this zone can be well approximated with 5-0 nonabsorbable sutures with buried knots. Immobilization should be done with maintenance of the wrist in extension and the MCP joints in about 15 degrees of flexion. Tendon adhesions are common in this zone because of associated damage to the periosteum.

Zone V Injuries

Zone V injuries involve the areas over the MCP joint and should be presumed to be due to a human bite until proved otherwise. These injuries occur most commonly over the MCP joints of the long and ring fingers. Radiographs are mandatory and may include Brewerton views to assess the metacarpal head closely for injury. The clinical findings of injuries to the extensor tendon at this level are flexion of the MCP joint and inability to extend the joint fully.

In an open joint injury caused by a human bite, the potential for mixed aerobic and anaerobic infections is high. Operative exploration, debridement, and irrigation are necessary. A combination of penicillin and antistaphylococcal agent or a single β-lactamase inhibitor drug is recommended empirically for infections related to human bites.[64] The wound is left open and may be closed at 4 to 5 days if free from infection. The resultant tendon injury is usually only a partial lac-

eration and may be treated with primary or delayed primary repair.

For simple lacerations at this level caused by a sharp, clean object, primary repair is indicated. The involved tendon ends do not retract and can be approximated with 4-0 nonabsorbable sutures. Sagittal bands also must be repaired if injured to prevent loss of extension or subluxation. The wrist and MCP joints should be immobilized. Early referral to a hand surgeon is advised.

Zone VI Injuries

Zone VI includes the area of the dorsum of the hand. Although these injuries may have a similar clinical appearance to zone V injuries, the joint is not involved, and these injuries are generally not as severe. Because the extensor tendons are superficial at this level, a relatively trivial-appearing skin laceration may be associated with one or more tendon lacerations. If the injury is proximal to the junctura tendineae, the patient may be able to extend the involved MCP joint because weak extensor forces are transmitted to the junctura from adjacent extensor tendons.

The tendons in this area are round or oval and easily exposed. Primary repair using a modified Kessler stitch with a 4-0 nonabsorbable material or a figure-of-eight stitch with a buried knot on the deep, palmar surface of the tendon suffices. This repair is followed by immobilization of the wrist at 30 degrees of extension and the MCP joint at neutral. Referral to a hand surgeon for delayed primary repair also is appropriate.

Zone VII and VIII Injuries

Zone VII and VIII injuries involve the wrist and forearm. Management follows basic principles for tendon injuries.

Flexor Tendon Injuries

Pathophysiology. Flexor tendon injuries are not as common as injuries to the extensor complex and are often subtle. The most common mechanism of injury is laceration, but closed traumatic disruption also may occur. FDP avulsion is the third most common tendon rupture in the hand in athletes.[59] This injury is usually sports related and involves a hyperextension force applied to an actively flexing digit; the classic example is a football player who grabs the jersey or pants of an opponent who is breaking free from a tackle. Although the reason is not clearly understood, more than 75% of these injuries involve the ring finger.[65] Because of the closed nature of these injuries, the patient may not seek immediate care, or the condition initially may be misdiagnosed.

Clinical Features. Careful assessment is necessary to diagnose flexor tendon disruption and associated neurovascular injury. With the normal hand at rest, there is a cascade of flexion of the digits, beginning with less flexion at the index finger and progressing to more flexion toward the little finger. An injury to a flexor tendon may be evident if the involved finger does not assume a naturally flexed position. Complete disruption of the profundus tendon results in an extended position of the DIP joint as a result of unopposed extensor forces. If the FDS is completely severed, or a partial tendon injury has occurred, the digit rests in less flexion than normal. An abnormal posture of the injured digit may suggest a flexor tendon injury; this is usually confirmed by a functional examination. The FDP and the FDS should be tested separately as previously described. This examination must be observed carefully because the patient may flex the distal tip with an intact profundus, but an injury to the FDS precludes flexion at the PIP joint. Disruption of the FDP tendon leads to loss of flexion at the DIP joint, instability in pinch, and loss of grip strength. Partial flexor tendon lacerations may be clinically occult. Because the tissue is torn and not lacerated, the degree of soft tissue injury and hemorrhage is greater than that seen with a laceration in the same zone. As a result, scarring within the sheath is often significant, and adjacent superficialis tendon may become secondarily involved.[62] Such injuries may be present if the patient complains of subjective weakness or if there is an abnormal position of the hand at rest. Clinically, injuries are associated with pain and weakness with flexion against resistance. Despite these findings, it may not be possible to arrive at a complete and accurate diagnosis until the wound is surgically explored. The palmaris longus, which is not present in approximately 15% of people, is not a functionally significant wrist flexor. Palmaris longus lacerations have tremendous diagnostic significance, however, because most (80% to 90%) have concomitant partial or complete median nerve lacerations. For this reason, all patients with palmaris longus lacerations should be assumed to have median nerve laceration until proved otherwise.[66]

Management. Flexor tendon repairs require the expertise of a hand surgeon. Immediate or delayed primary repair is now advocated for most acute flexor tendon injuries, including avulsions of the FDP and injuries involving the so-called no man's land, which extends from the distal palmar crease to the midportion of the middle phalanx. The advantages of primary repair with surgical reapproximation over secondary grafting for treatment of acute injuries have been well described in the literature.[67] Relative contraindications to immediate primary flexor repair are few and include crush wounds with poor skin coverage or tendon loss greater than 1 cm, possibly contaminated injuries over 12 hours that cannot be converted to clean wounds (human bites are not repaired initially), the presence of inadequate pulleys, an uncooperative patient, and surgical inexperience.[68] In such cases, a delayed primary repair can be performed 10 days after injury. Secondary repair of flexor tendons may be performed 4 weeks after injury but is considered late after that. Generally the results of primary, delayed primary, and early secondary repair are about equal. Treatment of partial flexor tendon lacerations is controversial, but referral to a hand surgeon for further exploration and possible repair is prudent.

If a hand surgeon is not immediately available, open wounds should be copiously irrigated, closed with 5-0 nylon, and splinted with the wrist in 30 degrees of flexion—the MCP joints flexed approximately 70 degrees and the IP joint flexed 10 to 15 degrees. This flexion ensures that no further damage occurs to the tendon and that the tendon will not contract further on movement. The patient also should receive tetanus immunization as indicated, and most authors recommend empiric use of broad-spectrum antibiotics. Most closed tendon injuries require referral to a hand surgeon because of the risk of long-term disability.

Complications. With optimal management, 80% of patients with flexor tendon injuries have good to excellent results.[67] Injuries involving the no man's land may result in poor outcomes and occasionally require tendon grafting. Overall, adhesions remain the most significant problem after operative repair. Other complications include triggering, bowstringing, and intratendinous epidermoid cyst formation.[69]

Mutilating Injuries

Mutilating injuries to the hand are encountered frequently in the emergency department. These are severe multistructural injuries that destroy the anatomy and functional integrity of the hand. Initial evaluation should focus on preservation of vital structures, analgesics, early consultation, wound care with debridement of devitalized tissue, and antibiotics. Evolving over recent years is a more aggressive push with respect to procedure timing regardless of being single stage or multistage.[70] Successful long-term clinical and socioeconomic outcomes have brought focused attention on procedure timing. The concept of early primary reconstruction with fast rehabilitation should be pursued based on case profile.[70] One such type is snowblower-associated or lawnmower-associated hand injuries, which can result in substantial deformity and disability. Snowblower injuries typically occur in clusters and are responsible for approximately 1000 amputations and 5000 emergency department visits annually.[71] The dominant hand is involved approximately 86% of the time, with middle and ring fingers most commonly injured. Phalangeal fractures are the most common type of injury.[72] Snowblower injuries are often managed as open fractures with intravenous antibiotics, irrigation, and debridement, with repair of bone, soft tissue, and nail bed structures.[72] Irreparable devascularization currently is considered the only absolute indication for immediate or early digital amputation after injury.[73] The concept and techniques for reimplantation and revascularization in mutilating injuries in children are similar to those of adults.[74]

Fingertip Injuries

Fingertip injuries may involve any structures distal to the DIP joint, including the skin, volar pulp tissue, distal phalanx, nail, nail bed, and related structures. These are among the most common injuries of the upper extremity and, although usually minor, may be associated with significant long-term consequences. The goals of management are to maintain finger length and achieve good tissue coverage, near-normal sensibility, and early functional recovery.

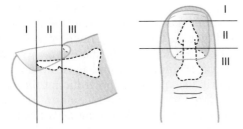

Figure 47-53. Classification of nail bed and fingernail injuries: zone I, distal to the bony phalanx; zone II, distal to lunula (between distal end of lunula and end of phalanx); zone III, proximal to distal end of lunula. (From Rosenthal EA: Treatment of fingertip and nail bed injuries. *Orthop Clin North Am* 14:675, 1983.)

Fingertip Amputations

Classification. Fingertip amputations are the most common type of amputation of the upper extremity. In zone I injuries (Figure 47-53), the proximal two thirds of the nail bed are preserved. In zone II injuries, bone is exposed, and in zone III injuries, the entire nail bed is lost.[75] Radiographic studies are indicated if bony avulsion injury or fracture cannot be excluded. Most of these fingertip injuries can be managed on an outpatient basis.

Management. Treatment of distal fingertip injuries is controversial; consequently, management must be individualized, and few guidelines are available. Generally, most hand surgeons try to maintain length of the thumb by whatever means possible.[75] The index finger is considered next before the other fingers. An intact pulp-to-pulp pinch mechanism is the principal goal. Other factors to consider include the patient's age, health, occupation, and handedness.

In most fingertip amputations distal to the DIP joint, adequate care can be provided with conservative wound management. The simplest and often best method for managing a fingertip amputation is allowing the wound to heal by secondary intention. This method is generally effective and produces good results if the wound is less than 1 cm. Large dorsal wounds also heal well by this method. It is the treatment of choice in childhood fingertip amputations, particularly when no bone is exposed. In cases in which a small protuberance of phalangeal bone (<0.5 cm) is exposed, it may be trimmed back with a rongeur to just below skin level and allowed to heal by secondary intention; if the bone is left exposed without soft tissue coverage, the patient will need an operative procedure. In most cases, the wound heals through a process of granulation, wound contracture, and re-epithelialization within a few weeks. Initial management should include careful and meticulous wound cleansing, a nonadherent dressing, appropriate tetanus prophylaxis, and splinting to protect the tip. Amputations that involve the distal phalanx usually are treated as contaminated open fractures with an initial intravenous dose of a cephalosporin followed by an oral course. Patients should have appropriate follow-up care to ensure adequate healing and recovery.

Fingertip injuries that involve significant soft tissue (especially volar) or bone loss usually require the expertise of a hand surgeon. Surgical management may include primary closure, full-thickness or partial-thickness skin grafts, composite grafts, adjacent flaps, regional flaps from the hand, distant flaps, and reimplantation. Most of these operative techniques are best performed as primary procedures under ideal circumstances or as a delayed procedure when necessary. A flap may be used to cover exposed bone or soft tissue avulsion and to add bulk to the tip. The nail bed tissues should be preserved because the presence of a nail affects the cosmetic result. At least 5 mm of healthy nail bed distal to the lunula is needed for nail adherence. Skin grafting is a common method for treating fingertip amputations with significant avulsed tissue and can provide a functional and an esthetic reconstruction.

Complications. These injuries commonly leave the patient with a painful, cold-intolerant fingertip; this complication occurs after primary closure, coverage with grafts or flaps, and healing by secondary intention. Skin grafting may result in induration, fissuring, and diminished sensibility. Nail deformity is common, particularly if there is considerable volar loss of tissue.[76]

Acute Nail Bed Injuries

Injuries of the nail bed most commonly result from localized trauma to the nail with subsequent compression of the nail bed. The most common type of injury is the simple laceration followed by stellate laceration, crush, and avulsion.[77] The middle and distal thirds of the nail bed are the most common sites of injury, and 50% of injuries involve fractures of the distal phalanx or tuft.[78] Radiographs are required in most cases to show occult fractures and foreign bodies.

Subungual Hematoma. Subungual hematomas result from crush injury or blunt trauma to the nail bed with bleeding from the rich vascular bed. The nail bed is predisposed to injury because it is interposed between the firm nail and the distal phalanx. The injury is manifested by pain and dark red-to-black discoloration of the nail bed and is classified by the percentage of area beneath the nail that is involved. When the fingertip is unstable or the mechanism of injury suggests a significant distal phalanx fracture, a radiograph should be obtained to identify associated fracture.

Management. Small subungual hematomas do not require drainage; the blood is incorporated into the nail and eventually removed with the free edge. Large hematomas cause significant discomfort and should be removed by nail trephination with a heated paperclip or a hot microcautery unit. Some authors recommend a surgical scrub of the finger before perforation of the nail to prevent contamination of the subungual area and the subsequent risk of infection and potential osteomyelitis, but this is generally unnecessary. Anesthesia is not necessary, and pain relief is immediate with decompression. If a significant fracture is present, the digit should be splinted. Although a distal phalangeal fracture with a subungual hematoma is technically an open fracture, such injuries usually heal without problems. Ungual tuft fractures are not associated with osteomyelitis. The risk of infection with an open fracture of the phalanx proper must be considered, and a broad-spectrum antibiotic and close follow-up monitoring are recommended. Patients with significant hematomas should be informed that they may lose the nail.

Simon and Wolgin[79] attempted to correlate the association between subungual hematomas, digital phalanx fractures, and occult nail bed lacerations. In their series, patients with a subungual hematoma greater than half the size of the nail had a 60% incidence of nail bed laceration requiring repair, and if there was an associated fracture of the distal phalanx, the incidence was 95%. If more than 25% to 50% of the visible portion of the nail is undermined by hematoma, many authors recommend removal of the nail, inspection of the nail bed, and repair of injuries.[77] Another study found no notable differences in outcome between nail trephination alone versus formal nail bed repair regardless of hematoma size in cases with an intact nail and nail margins.[80]

Nail Bed Lacerations. Lacerations of the nail bed should be repaired to minimize esthetic deformity and the duration of functional impairment. These injuries generally do well after primary repair, but late reconstruction of the nail bed is unpredictable, and usually little improvement is obtained.

Simple and crushing lacerations should be repaired accurately with 5-0 or 6-0 absorbable suture, ideally under loupe magnification. The results for both should be satisfactory in more than 90% of cases.[80] After the nail bed is accurately approximated, a hole is burned through the nail to allow drainage of serum or hematoma from the subungual area after the nail is reinserted into the nail fold. The avulsed nail may be sutured in place or secured with tape. A single thickness of nail-shaped Adaptic or other nonadherent gauze may be placed in the nail fold if the nail is unavailable. The replaced nail or gauze is used as a temporary splint to help protect the integrity of the underlying nail bed and maintain the fold for new nail growth and help prevent synechiae and subsequent nail deformity. Complete nail growth takes 70 to 160 days, but after the injury the growth pattern often is changed.

Nail bed avulsion commonly leaves fragments of nail bed attached to the undersurface of the avulsed nail.[81] In these cases, it is advisable to replace the nail as accurately as possible onto the avulsion site. Repair should be done using mattress sutures without attempting to separate the nail from the nail bed. If the tissue is not available and the defect is small, effective healing occurs by secondary intention.

Clenched-Fist Injuries

All human bites should be considered serious and at risk for significant complications. Clenched-fist injuries, also called "fight bite," are notorious for being the worst human bites. Inadequate initial management leads to significant morbidity. Misleading history, innocuous wound appearance, intoxication and lack of cooperation of the patient leading to inadequate examination, patient reluctance to admit the nature of the injury, delayed presentation, and inadequate exploration all may lead to mismanagement. Clenched-fist injuries have the highest incidence of complications of any closed-fist injury and of any type of bite wound.[82]

Clinical Features

The classic injury is a bite wound over the third MCP joint, but injury can occur over any joint. Soft tissue injury is apparent with possible extensor tendon injury and violation of the joint capsule. The fist is subsequently opened, and the bacterial innoculum is dragged with the extensor tendon and soft tissue proximally into the dorsum of the hand.[82] Presentation may be acute or delayed. Swelling, limited range of motion, erythema, and pain out of proportion to severity of injury are typical findings. Pain is more severe with range of motion.

Management

Aggressive management should be employed in all cases. Radiographs should be considered in all cases. Immediate consultation with a hand surgeon should be done. Analgesics, tetanus, cultures, intravenous antibiotics, appropriate wound care, elevation, and admission should be considered for all patients. Foreign bodies must be excluded with radiographic studies and possibly exploration. Tendon injuries must be ruled out with careful exploration. The hand should be splinted in the position of function. Pathogens are usually polymicrobial, with *Staphylococcus aureus,* streptococci, and anaerobes the predominant species. Multiple regimens are recommended with amoxicillin/clavulinic acid or penicillin with a first-generation cephalosporin commonly used.

High-Pressure Injection Injuries

Epidemiology

High-pressure injection injuries to the hand are uncommon, and most are occupation related. The usual cause is industrial equipment, with machinery such as grease guns, spray guns, and diesel engine injectors accounting for most of these injuries.[83] A wide variety of materials, including paint, paint thinner, grease, oil, hydraulic fluid, plastic, wax, water, and semifluid cement, have been reported to be injected. Generally, substances that are highly viscous (e.g., grease) require higher forces than do paint, oil, and solvents. The high pressures involved are sufficient to penetrate skin from a distance, and contact of the device with the hand is not a prerequisite for injury to occur. High-pressure injection injuries have been associated with amputation rates of 60% to 80%.[84] Early recognition and intervention is necessary. Even with early intervention, the injury leads to significant impairment. Amputation is more likely if debridement is delayed more than 6 hours.[84]

Pathophysiology

Patient characteristics and injury circumstances are often similar in high-pressure injection injuries. The patient generally has a history of coming into close proximity to the jet stream during cleaning of the nozzle, testing, or operation of the equipment. The patient is usually a young working man, and the non-dominant hand is most commonly involved, with the index finger the most common site. Operator inexperience has been cited as the most common cause of injury.

Tissue injury from high-pressure injection generally depends on physical, chemical, and biologic factors. Of particular importance are the type, amount, and velocity of injected material and the anatomic location. The most important factor is the type of material injected. The material determines the likely tissue inflammatory response and the resulting fibrosis that develops during healing. Paint and paint thinner produce a large, early inflammatory response and result in a high percentage of amputations.[85] In contrast, grease injuries cause a small inflammatory response and have a lower amputation rate, but are associated with oleogranuloma formation, fistulae, scarring, and loss of digit function.[86] The amount of material injected into the confined space of the digits or palm determines the degree of mechanical distention and the potential for vascular compromise. The velocity of the injected material and the site of tissue penetration determine dispersion, which may include the digit, hand, and forearm.

Clinical Features

The patient who seeks treatment early after injury may have minimal symptoms with either an innocuous entrance wound or no visible break in the skin. Fusiform swelling resulting from mechanical distention of the tissue by the injectant usually is apparent. Several hours later, the involved digit or palm becomes extremely painful, swollen, and pale because of vascular compromise and tissue necrosis. Careful examination is necessary to document the extent of injury and associated neurovascular function. Radiographs of the involved hand help determine the spread of material and the amount of debridement necessary because certain injected materials are radiopaque. In addition, they may reveal subcutaneous emphysema.

Management

Initial emergency department management includes splinting, elevation, tetanus prophylaxis, analgesia, and broad-spectrum antibiotics. Digital blocks are contraindicated because of the potential for increased tissue pressure, which may aggravate vascular compromise. Urgent hand surgery consultation is warranted because most cases require early extensive surgical decompression and debridement. The keystone in treatment of these injuries is prompt recognition of the severe nature of the injury and aggressive early debridement. Current treatment methods using irrigation and wide debridement have reduced the amputation rate significantly.[87]

Complications

Early recognition and treatment, including operative decompression and debridement, greatly influence outcome. Early amputation should be considered in cases in which the affected digit is initially cool or poorly perfused.[88] In most other cases, joint stiffness is a late sequela.

Amputations and Ring Avulsion Injuries

Few epidemiologic studies have been done on amputation injuries. Amputations have been reported to constitute 0.1% to 1% of all hand injuries.[2] Amputation may be complete or partial. Injuries with interconnecting tissue between the distal and the proximal portions are considered incomplete, or partial, amputations. Complete amputations are replanted, whereas partial amputations are revascularized. Traumatic amputations most commonly result from local crush injuries and occur infrequently from a sharp guillotine mechanism. Partial and complete amputations reportedly occur with equal frequency. The former are often related to the use of power saws and lawnmowers.

Ring avulsions include a spectrum of injuries from partial degloving of the skin of a finger to loss of the entire digit and entire length of a flexor tendon. These injuries usually occur when a ring on a finger catches on an object during a fall. In addition to neurologic and arterial injuries, there may be complete disruption of the venous return of the finger. Generally, these injuries represent complex management problems, and treatment may range from primary amputation to microvascular repair with reimplantation and free tissue transfer in addition to local flap, pedicle flap, or graft coverage.[89]

The initial care and treatment of the patient who has a body part amputated are the same as care and treatment for any trauma patient. After the initial primary assessment and stabilization of the patient, the injured extremity should be examined carefully with documentation of neurologic, vascular, and musculotendinous function. Subsequent care should be directed toward preservation of the limb and its components. General management goals include the following: provide supportive care, such as control of hemorrhage with direct pressure and elevation; prolong the time that the amputated tissues remain viable; protect wounds from further injury; and arrange expeditious consultation by a surgical subspecialist. With few exceptions, all completely amputated parts should be considered for reimplantation, and all partially amputated parts should be considered for revascularization.

In complete amputations, the proximal stump and the amputated part should be examined for the degree of tissue injury, contamination, and associated injuries. Gross contamination can be removed by irrigation with normal saline. Local antiseptics, especially hydrogen peroxide or alcohol, should not be used because they may damage viable tissues. The wound should not be manipulated, clamped, tagged, or traumatized further in any way. The stump should be covered with a saline-moistened sterile dressing to prevent further contamination and desiccation and elevated to help reduce edema and control bleeding. The amputated part requires minimal handling and should be cooled as soon as possible. After wrapping in saline-moistened gauze, the part is sealed in a dry plastic bag and placed in ice water. Ice should not come in direct contact with the tissue because this can cause local damage. Amputated parts should not be discarded or sent to the pathology department because even if they cannot be replanted, they may serve as a donor source for skin, bone, or vessel grafts. Radiographs of the amputated part and proximal stump should be obtained. The use of analgesic medications may be necessary, and appropriate tetanus prophylaxis may be administered. The use of prophylactic antibiotics is indicated in amputation injuries because significant devitalized tissue is often present. Most authors recommend empiric coverage for *S. aureus* with a combination of penicillin G and an antistaphylococcal antibiotic or first-generation cephalosporin.

Treatment for partial amputations with vascular compromise is the same as that just described. The wound should be cleaned with normal saline irrigation, wrapped in a sterile moist dressing, and splinted to protect it from further injury. Cold packs are applied to the dressings to prevent warm ischemia.

The time that an amputated part can survive before reimplantation has not been determined. As a general rule, the more proximal the amputation, the less ischemia time the amputated part can tolerate. Attempts to extend viability during ischemia have shown that the most important controllable factor is the temperature of the amputated part. Warm ischemia may be tolerated for 6 to 8 hours; cooling the part to 4° C extends this time to approximately 12 to 24 hours with distal amputations. There are reports of successful reimplantation of digits after 30 hours of warm ischemia.[90]

The decision of whether to attempt reimplantation should be made by the surgeon who is responsible for performing the procedure. Patient selection generally is based on the nature and level of the injury and patient age and health-related factors. The classic indications and contraindications for reimplantation are listed in Box 47-2. The thumb is required to preserve the function of opposition, and all such amputations should be considered for microvascular salvage regardless of the level of amputation or mechanism of injury. Loss of the thumb is equivalent to a 40% loss of function of the hand.[91] Similarly, all amputations in children should be considered for reimplantation. In reimplantation of digits amputated distal to the insertion of the FDS between the PIP joint and the DIP joint, good motor and sensory function is often achieved. If the amputated part is crushed, mangled, or amputated at multiple levels, however, reimplantation is usually contraindicated. Digits that cannot be replanted require skin coverage by flaps or ray resection.

Complications

Replanted fingers and hands never regain premorbid function. Replanted and revascularized parts may develop cold intolerance, stiffness, loss of sensation, pain, malunions, and nonunions. Even successful reimplantations may require repeated operative proce-

---

BOX 47-2. Classic Indications and Contraindications for Replantation

Indications
Multiple digits
Thumb
Wrist and forearm
Sharp amputations with minimal to moderate avulsion proximal to the elbow
Single digits amputated between proximal interphalangeal joint and distal interphalangeal joint (distal to flexor digitorum superficialis insertion)
All pediatric amputations

Contraindications
Amputations in unstable patients secondary to other life-threatening injuries
Multiple-level amputations
Self-inflicted amputations
Single-digit amputations proximal to the flexor digitorum superficialis insertion
Serious underlying disease, such as vascular disease, complicated diabetes mellitus, congestive heart failure
Extremes of age

---

dures and involve prolonged disability. Necrosis is an obvious sign of failure.

Vascular Injuries

Significant vascular disorders of the hand are uncommon compared with other problems of the hand. The vascular supply to the hand and digits is duplicated so that isolated arterial injuries to either side seldom result in ischemia. Lacerations of the arteries of the hand may stop bleeding by the time the patient is evaluated; in these situations, a history of pulsatile bleeding is highly suggestive of an arterial injury. Although most arterial injuries are the result of penetrating trauma, blunt trauma to the hand occasionally can result in arterial thrombosis or a false aneurysm.[92] In addition, associated injuries should not be overlooked. Because digital nerves invariably cross with and are superficial to the digital artery, an arterial lesion should raise the possibility of an accompanying nerve injury.

Circulatory status is assessed as previously described by observation for cyanosis or pallor, palpation of radial or ulnar pulses at the wrist, assessment of capillary refill, and the use of Allen's test. Ischemic pain is the most common initial complaint of vascular insufficiency, along with physical manifestations of pallor and gangrene. The presence of a mass, with or without pain and tenderness, is the second most common initial complaint.

Management

Lacerations or amputations of the upper limb rarely cause life-threatening hemorrhage. Even a major vessel that is completely transected usually retracts, constricts, and clots. Major vessels often continue to bleed briskly, however, from partial transections with life-threatening hemorrhage. Usually, hemorrhage can be adequately controlled with direct pressure and eleva-

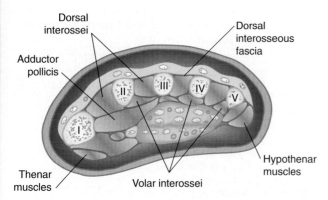

Figure 47-54. Cross section through the palm showing compartments of the hand. (From Rowland SA: In Green DP [ed]: *Operative Hand Surgery,* 3rd ed. New York, Churchill Livingstone, 1993, p 670.)

tion. If necessary, a proximally placed blood pressure cuff inflated to 30 mm Hg above systolic pressure can be used for short periods (<30 minutes) to control severe bleeding. Vascular clamps and hemostats should not be used in the emergency department to control bleeding in the hand because of the danger of inadvertently crushing nerves and tendons. Lacerated arteries should be repaired if symptoms of ischemia are present or if there is an associated nerve injury. Arterial repair is not mandatory in isolated arterial injuries with good distal vascularity because there is a high rate of thrombosis after reanastomosis. If the decision is made not to repair a lacerated artery, both stumps should be ligated to prevent further bleeding. Palmar arch lacerations may be difficult to visualize in the emergency department and usually require surgical exploration to control bleeding.

Compartment Syndrome in the Hand

A compartment syndrome develops when elevated pressure within a closed fascial space reduces perfusion to the point of muscle and nerve dysfunction. In the hand, 10 compartments are visible on cross section through the palm (Figure 47-54). In addition, the fingers are compartmentalized by fascia and skin at flexor creases. Because these compartments are not interconnected, each additional compartment must be surgically decompressed if muscle ischemia is suspected.[93]

Nerve Injuries

Nerve injuries may result from a direct blow, puncture or laceration, crush injury, injection injury, and amputation. These injuries are primarily divided into three groups: neurapraxia, axonotmesis, and neurotmesis. In neurapraxia, there is loss of function of the nerve, but the axon, Schwann's sheath, and endoneurium remain intact. Recovery in these cases is usually complete within days. In axonotmesis, the axon is severed within an intact endoneurial tube. The distal axon degenerates and is absorbed after disruption. The proximal portion of the severed axonal stump can regenerate along the intact endoneurial tube at a rate of approximately 1 to 3 mm/day. Neurotmesis refers to complete disruption of all nerve elements. Regrowth of the proximal axonal

endings does not occur along the endoneurial tubes, unless the severed nerve endings are reapproximated.[94]

Peripheral nerve injuries are diagnosed by physical examination by showing loss of motor or sensory function. Specific nerves at risk should be examined as previously outlined. Injury most commonly involves one of the digital nerves, but also may be localized to the median, radial, or ulnar nerves.[37]

Management

Identification of the injury and proper referral are important aspects in the initial management of patients with nerve injuries in the hand. Patients with closed nerve injuries not associated with compartment syndromes should be referred to a hand specialist for serial examinations. All digits that have lost function as a result of a nerve injury should be splinted to prevent further inadvertent injury. If function does not return within 3 weeks, electromyograms and nerve conduction studies can help differentiate neurotmesis from axonotmesis and determine the need for surgical exploration.[95]

Lacerated nerves require reapproximation by hand surgeons. In general, all motor branches of the ulnar and median nerves should be repaired. Additionally, digital nerve injuries proximal to the DIP crease on the radial aspect of the index finger, the ulnar aspect of the little finger, and both sides of the thumb should be considered for repair.[53] Clean, single-nerve lacerations should be repaired primarily when feasible. Complex nerve injuries may involve wound contamination or extensive tissue damage and are usually managed by delayed repair to allow for improved soft tissue conditions. Although the functional recovery is never complete, a good outcome can result from primary and delayed repair. In general, sensory recovery returns more often than does motor function.

Complications

Complications of nerve injuries include motor and sensory loss, atrophy from denervation, chronic paresthesias, regrowth of painful neuromas, and sympathetic dystrophy.

Infections of the Hand

The unique anatomic structures of the hand affect the nature of infections in this region of the body. In general, hand infections can be divided into infections involving the skin, subcutaneous tissues, fascial spaces, tendon, joint, and bone. Fibrous compartments of the distal fingertips contain the spread of infection, whereas flexor tendon sheaths allow infection to travel considerable distances along the lengths of the tendons from the original site. Infections in the deep spaces of the palm usually manifest on the dorsal surface of the hand.

Paronychia

Pathophysiology

A paronychia is a localized superficial infection or abscess involving the lateral nail fold. It is the most

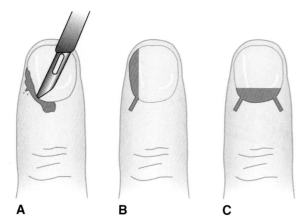

Figure 47-55. Drainage of paronychia. **A,** Eponychial fold is elevated from the nail for a simple paronychia. **B,** Lateral nail is removed if pus tracks under it. A small eponychial incision may be necessary. **C,** Proximal nail is removed if pus tracks under it. Two incisions are needed to remove the proximal nail. (From Moran GJ, Talan DA: Hand infections. *Emerg Med Clin North Am* 11:601, 1993.)

common infection in the hand and is thought to be caused by frequent trauma to the delicate skin around the fingernail and cuticle. Clinically, swelling and tenderness of the soft tissue along one or both sides of the lateral nail fold are evident. A paronychia begins as a cellulitis, but a frank abscess may form, and occasional extension to the overlying proximal nail (termed an *eponychia*) may occur. *S. aureus* is the most common isolate, followed by streptococci.[96] Paronychias in children are often caused by anaerobes, and it is believed that this is the result of finger sucking and nail biting.[97] Atypical mycobacteria and *Candida albicans* should be considered as etiologic agents in chronic cases.[98]

Management

In the early cellulitis phase, management consists of frequent warm soaks, elevation, and administration of an oral antistaphylococcal antibiotic, such as dicloxacillin or cephalexin. When the area becomes fluctuant, drainage is necessary and is usually curative. Adequate drainage often can be obtained by lifting the skin edge off the nail to allow the pus to drain (Figure 47-55). This can be accomplished without anesthesia in selected patients, but drainage for more extensive lesions is best carried out under digital block anesthesia. After softening the eponychium by soaking, a No. 11 blade scalpel or an 18-gauge needle may be advanced parallel to the nail and under the eponychium at the site of maximal swelling.[99] If the infection is more extensive, the lateral one fourth of the nail may be bluntly dissected from the underlying nail bed and germinal matrix and the lateral nail plate excised. After the cavity is irrigated, a small piece of packing gauze may be slipped under the eponychium for 24 hours to provide continual drainage. Cultures are not indicated. Antibiotics are commonly prescribed, although not essential if drainage is complete or if the surrounding area of cellulitis is minimal. Most paronychias resolve in 5 to 10 days, and patients are advised to have primary care follow-up evaluation. A well-known com-

plication of even a properly drained paronychia is osteomyelitis of the distal phalanx. Patients with a chronic, indolent infection of the perionychium seldom respond to emergency department intervention. These patients should be referred to a dermatologist or hand surgeon because of the prolonged treatment required.

Felon

Pathophysiology

A felon is an infection of the pulp of the distal finger or thumb. It differs from other types of subcutaneous abscesses because of the presence of multiple vertical septa that divide the pulp into small fascial compartments. The usual cause is penetrating trauma with secondary bacterial invasion. The most common pathogen is *S. aureus,* although gram-negative organisms also have been described.[98] Although the septa may facilitate an infection in the pulp and inhibit drainage after incomplete surgical decompression, they provide a barrier that protects the joint space and the tendon sheath by limiting the proximal spread of infection. Clinically a felon begins as an area of cellulitis and inflammation that progresses rapidly to severe throbbing, pain, swelling, and pressure in the distal pulp space.

Management

Traditional management of felons emphasizes the need for early and complete incision through the septa to provide adequate drainage and to relieve pressure in septal compartments. Most felons can be drained by a single lateral incision.[100] The incision should be made along the ulnar aspect of digits II to IV and the radial aspects of digits I and V, avoiding pincher surfaces. The incision is begun approximately 0.5 cm distal to the DIP joint crease and dorsal to the neurovascular bundle of the fingertip. The incision is extended to the free edge of the nail (Figure 47-56). The wound should be irrigated, loosely packed with gauze, and splinted. The packing is removed in 48 to 72 hours, and the wound is left to close secondarily. Most felons are treated empirically with an antistaphylococcal oral antibiotic for at least 5 days pending culture results. Some authors recommend draining this abscess where it points, using a volar midline incision that does not cross the distal flexion crease.[100]

Complications

If untreated, the expanding abscess can extend toward the phalanx, producing an osteitis or osteomyelitis, or toward the skin, causing necrosis and a sinus tract on the palmar surface of the digital pulp. Other complications include soft tissue and bony tuft necrosis, osteomyelitis, septic arthritis of the DIP joint, and flexor tenosynovitis from proximal extension. The lateral incision used to drain felons commonly leaves unstable finger pads or may result in painful neuromas or anesthetic fingertips. "Fish-mouth" incisions may destroy the blood supply to the fingertip.[100] Longitudinal midline incisions on the volar surface may leave

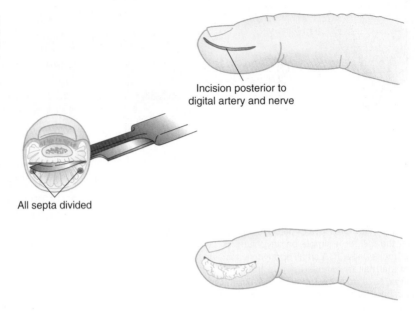

Figure 47-56. Incision and drainage of felon using the unilateral longitudinal approach. Most felons should be drained via this incision. (From Milford L: In Crenshaw AH [ed]: *Campbell's Operative Orthopedics,* 8th ed. St. Louis, Mosby, 1992.)

Incision posterior to digital artery and nerve

All septa divided

scars over an important area for sensation, but do not have the other disadvantages of lateral incisions. Any incision that is made too deeply and proximally can injure the flexor tendon sheath and initiate a tenosynovitis.

Herpetic Whitlow

Epidemiology and Pathophysiology

Herpetic whitlow is a self-limited herpes simplex viral infection of the distal finger. It is the most common viral infection of the hand. Infection by herpes simplex virus type I or II is clinically indistinguishable.[101] Direct inoculation of the virus into an open wound or broken skin is the usual mechanism of primary infection. Herpetic whitlow is commonly reported in adult women with genital herpes and children with coexistent herpetic gingivostomatitis. Health care workers are at increased risk for developing this infection as an occupational hazard secondary to exposure to orotracheal secretions; however, a more recent review of herpes infection in the hand found that only 14% of adult cases are in health care workers.[102] The incidence has decreased probably as a result of heightened awareness of the condition and strict infection control precautions.

Clinical Features

The infection usually involves a single finger and begins with localized pain, pruritus, and swelling, followed by the appearance of clear vesicles. Systemic symptoms are usually absent; however, secondary infection of the vesicles can occur.[103] More typically, the vesicles coalesce over 2 weeks to form an ulcer, which may develop a hemorrhagic base. At this stage, it may be difficult to distinguish herpes simplex infection of the hand from more common bacterial infections, such as felon or paronychia. The distinction is important because drainage of the herpetic lesions is contraindicated and may lead to viral dissemination and secondary bacterial infection. A careful history is important to determine risk of a possible herpetic etiology. On examination, tenderness is present but is noticeably less than that seen with bacterial infections. In addition, the pulp space remains soft and does not become tense, as it does in a bacterial felon.[104]

Diagnostic Strategies

The diagnosis usually is made clinically based on the appearance of the lesion and the history of recurrence or potential sources of inoculation. The diagnosis may be confirmed by viral culture or a Tzanck test showing multinucleated giant cells in a scraping taken from the base of an unroofed vesicle.[105]

Management

Herpetic whitlow usually resolves spontaneously in 3 to 4 weeks. The main goals of treatment are to prevent oral inoculation or transmission of the infection and to provide symptomatic relief. The involved digit should be kept covered with a dry dressing. Oral acyclovir has a role in treatment of immunocompromised patients and patients with frequently recurring infections, but its role in nonimmunocompromised patients is less clear.[105] Topical acyclovir has not been shown to be effective in either the treatment or the prophylaxis of this disorder.

Tenosynovitis

Pathophysiology

Acute synovial space infections in the hand usually involve the flexor tendon sheaths and the radial and ulnar bursae. The tendon sheaths are double walled, with a visceral layer adherent to the tendon and a parietal layer extending from the midpalmar crease to just proximal to the DIP joint. The flexor tendon sheath of the thumb is continuous with the radial bursa of the palm, and the small finger sheath is continuous with the ulnar palmar bursae. The ulnar bursa surrounds the superficial and deep flexor tendons, and the radial bursa surrounds the flexor pollicis longus. These two bursae communicate in 80% of individuals; however, for most individuals, the tenosynovial coverings of digits II, III, and IV do not communicate. Infections in the synovial spaces in the hand tend to spread along the course of the flexor tendon sheaths and may spread to the midpalmar, thenar, and lumbrical compartments. Infections usually are caused by penetrating trauma to the sheath, but they occasionally result from hematogenous spread. The most commonly isolated organism is *S. aureus*.

Clinical Features

Four cardinal signs of acute flexor tenosynovitis are usually present and help differentiate tenosynovitis from other soft tissue infections in the hand: (1) tenderness along the course of the flexor tendon, (2) symmetric swelling of the finger, (3) pain on passive extension, and (4) a flexed posture of the finger.[13] All four signs may not be present early in the course of infection. The third sign may be the most important. Early recognition and treatment are essential because elevated pressure within the enclosure of the flexor tendon sheath can occlude the already tenuous circulation to the tendon, resulting in necrosis and proximal spread.

Management

All patients with flexor tenosynovitis require hospital admission and prompt consultation with a hand surgeon to determine whether open drainage or closed tendon sheath irrigation is indicated. In early cases or uncertain diagnoses, the hand should be splinted in a bulky dressing and elevated, and intravenous antibiotics should be initiated. Infections secondary to penetrating trauma should be treated with a penicillinase-resistant antistaphylococcal penicillin or first-generation cephalosporin. Disseminated gonorrhea must be considered in all sexually active individuals, especially if there is no apparent traumatic etiology of the infection. In such cases, some authors recommend empiric treatment with ceftriaxone until final cultures are available.[106] Surgical treatment is indicated for established cases or when improvement is not evident within 24 hours.

Deep Fascial Space Infections

Anatomy and Pathophysiology

The deep fascial spaces of the hand include the dorsal subaponeurotic space, the subfascial web space, the midpalmar space, and the thenar space (Figure 47-57). The fascial spaces are potential rather than actual spaces in a normal hand.[94] These closed compartments are susceptible to infection from direct penetrating trauma, infection in contiguous compartments, or hematogenous seeding. The most commonly isolated pathogens are *S. aureus,* streptococci, and coliforms.

Clinical Features

The unique anatomic features of the deep fascial spaces lead to characteristic clinical findings when these regions are involved with pyogenic infection. The

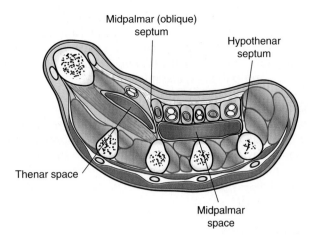

Figure 47-57. Potential midpalmar spaces. (From Neviasser RJ: In Green DP [ed]: *Operative Hand Surgery,* 3rd ed. New York, Churchill Livingstone, 1993, p 1028.)

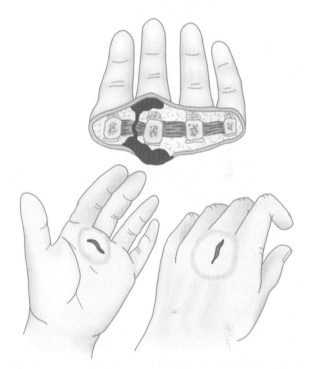

Figure 47-58. Collar-button abscess. The palmar space infection has spread to the dorsum of the hand. (From Lewis RC Jr: Infections of the hand. *Emerg Med Clin North Am* 3:263, 1985.)

dorsal subaponeurotic abscess causes swelling and erythema on the dorsum of the hand. Pain with passive movement of the extensor tendons is often present, but it may be difficult to distinguish clinically from simple cellulitis on the dorsum of the hand. Subfascial web space infections commonly result when palmar blisters become secondarily infected. The infection tends to spread dorsally into the interdigital space and produce a characteristic hourglass configuration, or the so-called collar-button abscess (Figure 47-58). Thenar space infections are characterized by pain and swelling of the thenar eminence and the first web space; the thumb is held in abducted and flexed position.[108] In midpalmar infections, there is loss of the normal hand concavity and tenderness of the central palm;

movement of digits III and IV is painful. Suppurative tenosynovitis of the second digit can rupture proximally into the thenar space and create an abscess. Tenosynovitis of digits III, IV, and V may be responsible for a midpalmar space infection.

Management

Treatment of all deep fascial space infections involves intravenous antibiotics and operative exploration and drainage by experienced surgeons. Most authors recommend broad-spectrum empiric coverage with a β-lactamase–resistant penicillin or a first-generation cephalosporin.

Septic Arthritis

Pathophysiology

Septic arthritis in the hand may involve the IP, MCP, CMC, or radiocarpal joints. These joints usually are infected by direct inoculation of bacteria from penetrating trauma or spread from contiguous infection, such as a felon or tenosynovitis. Hematogenous spread may occur but is less common than in other joints of the body. *S. aureus* is the most common cause; streptococci, *Haemophilus influenzae, Pseudomonas aeruginosa,* and coliforms are involved much less commonly.[109] Monarticular nontraumatic septic arthritis also may be caused by *Neisseria gonorrhoeae.*

Clinical Features

Clinically the involved joint appears red and swollen and is extremely tender; an overlying puncture wound may be visible. The joint is held in a position that maximizes its volume, and passive motion of the joint, however slight, is painful. In contrast to flexor tenosynovitis, tenderness is localized to the involved joint.[110] Pain also may be elicited by axial compression of the joint. The diagnosis is made by arthrocentesis.

Management

Treatment includes parenteral antibiotics with a semisynthetic antistaphylococcal penicillin and emergent drainage of the joint. Most infected joints require open drainage, but some hand surgeons may choose to manage certain cases with closed joint catheter irrigation and repeated aspiration.

Osteomyelitis

Osteomyelitis in the hand occurs most commonly with open fractures or with secondary involvement of bone from soft tissue infections. The incidence of infection in open fractures of the hand is much lower than in open long bone fractures and is reported to be 1% to 11%. McLain and colleagues[111] found that injuries with severe skeletal trauma, gross contamination, and significant soft tissue injury have the highest risks for infection. The presentation of osteomyelitis is seldom rapid and fulminant, unless associated with septic arthritis or other deep space infection of the hand. Physical signs may include fever, localized redness, swelling, warmth, and tenderness. Children with osteomyelitis may have pseudoparalysis, which is refusal of the child to use the affected limb.[112] Radiographs may show bony destruction or periosteal elevation. Treatment includes debridement of infected bone and sequestra and parenteral antibiotics.

Nontraumatic Disorders of the Hand

Stenosing Tenosynovitis

The most common type of stenosing tenosynovitis in the hand involves the flexor tendons at the level of the MCP joint where the tendon passes through the pulley systems. Repetitive strain can result in tendon and pulley hypertrophy with localized tenderness. When there is painful blocking of flexion and extension at the involved joint, the syndrome is called *trigger finger.* The ring and long fingers are the most commonly involved digits. Injection therapy is recommended and works well in most patients. A mixture of 2 mL of lidocaine and 0.5 mL of steroid suspension is given through the web space and over the nodule.[113] After the injection, extension of the finger is usually possible. The finger should be splinted in extension, and referral to a hand surgeon is advised because multiple injections or surgical release may be required.

Ganglion

A ganglion is the most common soft tissue tumor of the hand and consists of a synovial cyst from either a joint or the synovial lining of a tendon that has herniated. Ganglia contain a jelly-like fluid that is secreted by the synovial tissue. They are common in the wrist and the flexor tendon sheaths of the fingers and usually have an insidious onset. A specific traumatic event can be elicited from only 15% of patients, although most give a history of chronic stress.[114] Patients commonly complain of a dull ache or mild pain over the ganglion. Reassurance is important, and the patient should be informed of the benign nature of the lesion. A large or troublesome ganglion can be aspirated. Because of the high rate of recurrence, definitive treatment is operative excision, which is done on an elective basis.

Foreign Bodies in the Hand

Penetrating trauma to the hand may result in a foreign body becoming lodged in the soft tissues. The presence of a foreign body should be considered in any wound regardless of its size. A detailed and accurate history of the injury should be obtained because the mechanism often gives clues to the possibility of a foreign body. The most common foreign bodies are pieces of wood, glass, or metal. Useful signs of occult foreign bodies include sharp pain with deep palpation over a puncture wound, pain associated with a mass, or a wound that fails to heal or continues to cause pain with movement.[115]

Initial examination of hand wounds should include local exploration using sterile technique in a bloodless field. After exploration and removal of easily accessible foreign bodies, radiographs should be taken, using soft tissue technique with multiple views. Radiographs are the best method for detecting radiopaque foreign bodies and detect metals, most glass, many plastics, gravel, and sand.[115] Wooden foreign bodies are difficult to visualize radiographically.[116] Whether an object shows on plain films depends on its composition, configuration, size, and orientation. When a foreign body is clinically suspected and initial radiographic studies are negative, other imaging methods should be considered. The identification of nonmetallic objects such as splinters may be improved by the use of modalities including computed tomography, magnetic resonance imaging, and ultrasound.[115-117]

Management

Removal of embedded foreign bodies can be difficult and time-consuming, and potential damage to tissues caused by the procedure must be weighed against the risk posed by a particular foreign body. Generally, if a foreign body contaminating a wound is clearly visible and easily extracted during local exploration, it should be removed in the emergency department. In some cases, the entrance wound may need to be enlarged with a small skin incision. In general, foreign bodies should be removed only under direct vision. When the object is buried within the intricate anatomy of the hand, this procedure should be referred to a hand specialist.

Decisions regarding the necessity and timeliness of removal of a foreign body are based on the size and the reactivity of the foreign body, proximity to vital structures, degree of wound contamination, and presence or absence of symptoms.[115] Foreign bodies that cause continued pain, interfere with hand function because of their size or their position, or cause local or systemic toxicity (e.g., paints or mercury) should be removed. Foreign bodies associated with fractures require prompt surgical debridement to prevent osteomyelitis.[118] Wounds that are grossly contaminated with soil or organic material require immediate irrigation, debridement, and removal of the foreign body. Foreign bodies near tendons, nerves, and vessels and foreign bodies causing ischemia or hemorrhage require cautious removal under optimal conditions.

Patients who do not require immediate removal of the foreign body may be referred to a hand surgeon for delayed surgical exploration. If the hand specialist plans to remove the object within 3 to 4 days after injury, and there is minimal bacterial contamination, the wound may be closed primarily. Initial treatment also should include tetanus prophylaxis and an appropriate wound dressing. The patient should be informed about the presence of the foreign body and the reason for delayed removal. If no removal is planned, the physician should explain to the patient that the dangers of removal outweigh the benefits.

Complications

Foreign bodies can damage soft tissues, provoke excessive inflammation with granuloma formation, predispose to infection, and cause systemic toxicity.

Iatrogenic damage to tissue can result from blind probing or excessively aggressive searches for foreign bodies and should be avoided, particularly in the hand.

KEY CONCEPTS

- Injuries and infections of the hand are among the most commonly encountered problems in the emergency department.
- An accurate history and carefully performed physical examination of the hand have a central role in evaluation and treatment. Hand radiographs should be obtained if suggestive signs are present. Highly technical diagnostic modalities are rarely indicated.
- The best functional outcomes of hand injuries usually are achieved by accurate initial evaluation and treatment.
- A key factor in the evaluation of hand injuries is determining which entities require specialty referral or urgent consultation.
- Management of the injured hand should focus on restoration of function and minimizing long-term disability.

REFERENCES

1. Overton DT, Uehara DT: Evaluation of the injured hand. *Emerg Med Clin North Am* 11:585, 1993.
2. Atroshi I, Rosenberg H: Epidemiology of amputations and severe injuries of the hand. *Hand Clin* 17, 2001, pp 343-350.
3. Altman RS, Harris GD, Knuth CJ: Initial management of hand injuries in the emergency patient. *Am J Emerg Med* 5:400, 1987.
4. Chung K, Spilson S: The frequency and epidemiology of hand and forearm fractures in the United States. *J Hand Surg* 26A, 2001, pp 1044-1053.
5. Sorock G, et al: *J Occup Environ Med* 44:345, 2002.
6. Snell R, Smith M: The wrist and hand. In: *Clinical Anatomy for Emergency Medicine*. St. Louis, Mosby, 1993, pp 629-675.
7. Belliappa PP, Scheker LR: Functional anatomy of the hand. *Emerg Med Clin North Am* 11:557, 1993.
8. Ashkenaze DM, Ruby LK: Metacarpal fractures and dislocation. *Orthop Clin North Am* 23:19, 1992.
9. Graham TJ, O'Brien ET: Fractures of the hand and wrist region. In Rockwood CA Jr, Wilkins KE, King RE (eds): *Fractures in Children,* 5th ed. Philadelphia, Lippincott-Raven, 2001, p 655.
10. Hodgkinson DW, et al: The hand: ABC of emergency radiology. *BMJ* 308:401, 1994.
11. American Society for Surgery of the Hand: *The Hand: Examination and Diagnosis,* 3rd ed. Edinburgh, Churchill Livingstone, 1990.
12. Doyle JR: Extensor tendons—acute injuries. In Green DP (ed): *Operative Hand Surgery,* 4th ed. New York, Churchill Livingstone, 1999, p 1950.
13. Kanavel AB: *Infections of the Hand,* 6th ed. Philadelphia, Lea & Febiger, 1993.
14. Hentz VR: Functional anatomy of the hand and arm. *Emerg Med Clin North Am* 3:197, 1985.
15. Sloan EP: Nerve injuries in the hand. *Emerg Med Clin North Am* 11:651, 1993.
16. Hart RG, Kleinert HE: Fingertip and nail bed injuries. *Emerg Med Clin North Am* 11:755, 1993.

17. Mark H: Fractures and dislocations in the hand. In Rockwood CA Jr, Green DP (eds): *Fractures in Adults,* 5th ed. Philadelphia, Lippincott-Raven, 2001.

18. Wilson AJ, Mann FA, Gilula CA: Imaging the hand and wrist. *J Hand Surg* 15B:153, 1990.

19. Lammers RL, Magill T: Detection and management of foreign bodies in soft tissue. *Emerg Med Clin North Am* 10:767, 1992.

20. Freeland AE: *Hand Fractures, Repair, Reconstruction, and Rehabilitation.* New York, Churchill Livingstone, 2000.

21. DeJonge JJ, et al: Phalangeal fractures of the hand: An analysis of gender and age-related incidence and aetiology. *J Hand Surg* 19B:168, 1994.

22. Simon RR, Koenigsknecht SJ: *Emergency Orthopedics: The Extremities,* 4th ed. New York, McGraw-Hill, 2001.

23. DaCruz DJ, Slade RJ, Malone W: Fractures of the distal phalanges. *J Hand Surg* 13B:350, 1988.

24. Bowman SH, Simon RR: Metacarpal and phalangeal fractures. *Emerg Med Clin North Am* 11:671, 1993.

25. Wayne PH: Radiology of the occupationally injured hand. *Hand Clin* 2:467, 1986.

26. Agee J: Treatment principles for proximal and middle phalangeal fractures. *Orthop Clin North Am* 23:35, 1992.

27. Green DP: Complications of phalangeal and metacarpal fractures. *Hand Clin* 2:307, 1986.

28. Wilson RL, Carter MS: Management of hand injuries. In Hunter JM, Schneider LH, Mackin EJ (eds): *Rehabilitation of the Hand: Surgery and Therapy.* St. Louis, Mosby, 1990, pp 284-294.

29. Stern PJ, et al: Pilon fractures of the proximal interphalangeal joint. *J Hand Surg* 16A:844, 1991.

30. Margles SW: Intraarticular fractures of the metacarpophalangeal and proximal interphalangeal joints. *Hand Clin* 4:67, 1988.

31. Hastings H, Carroll C: Treatment of closed articular fractures of the metacarpophalangeal and proximal interphalangeal joints. *Hand Clin* 4:503, 1988.

32. Wolfe SW, Dick HM: Articular fractures of the hand: Part I. Guidelines for assessment. *Orthop Rev* 20:27, 1991.

33. McLain RF, Steyers C, Stoddard M: Infections in open fractures of the hand. *J Hand Surg* 16A:108, 1991.

34. Ashkenaze DM, Ruby LK: Metacarpal fractures and dislocations. *Orthop Clin North Am* 23:19, 1992.

35. Pellegrini VDJ: Fractures at the base of the thumb. *Hand Clin* 4:87, 1988.

36. Foster RJ, Hastings H II: Treatment of Bennett, Rolando, and vertical intraarticular trapezial fractures. *Clin Orthop* 214:121, 1987.

37. Graham TJ: Hand. In Beaty JH (ed): *Orthopaedic Knowledge Update 6: Home Study Syllabus.* Rosemont, Ill, American College of Orthopaedic Surgeons, 1999.

38. Della-Guistina K, Della-Guistina DA: Emergency department evaluation and treatment of pediatric orthopedic injuries. *Emerg Med Clin North Am* 17:895, 1999.

39. Salter RB, Harris WR: Injuries involving the epiphyseal plate. *J Bone Joint Surg* 45A:587, 1963.

40. Stahl S, Jupitur JB: Salter-Harris types III and IV epiphyseal fractures in the hand treated with tension-band wiring. *J Pediatr Orthop* 19:233, 1999.

41. Clark DP, Scott RN, Anderson IWR: Hand problems in an accident and emergency department. *J Hand Surg* 10:297, 1985.

42. Hossfeld GE, Uehara DT: Acute joint injuries of the hand. *Emerg Med Clin North Am* 11:781, 1993.

43. Glickel SZ, et al: Dislocations and ligament injuries in the digits. In Green DP (ed): *Operative Hand Surgery,* 4th ed. New York, Churchill Livingstone, 1999, p 772.

44. Thayer D: Distal interphalangeal joint injuries. *Hand Clin* 4:1, 1988.

45. Kahler D, McCue F: Metacarpophalangeal and proximal interphalangeal joint injuries of the hand, including the thumb. *Clin Sports Med* 11:57, 1992.

46. Freiberg A, et al: Management of proximal interphalangeal joint injuries. *J Trauma* 46:523, 1999.

47. Kiefhaber TR, Stern PH, Grood ES: Lateral stability of the proximal interphalangeal joint. *J Hand Surg* 11A:661, 1986.

48. Inoue G, Maeda N: Irreducible palmar dislocation of the proximal interphalangeal joint of the finger. *J Hand Surg* 15A:301, 1990.

49. Wilson RL, Liechty BW: Complications following small joint injuries. *Hand Clin* 2:329, 1986.

50. Henderson JJ, Arafa MAM: Carpometacarpal dislocation: An early missed diagnosis. *J Bone Joint Surg* 69:212, 1987.

51. Gurland M: Carpometacarpal joint injuries of the fingers. *Hand Clin* 8:733, 1992.

52. Campbell CS: Gamekeeper's thumb. *J Bone Joint Surg* 37B:148, 1955.

53. Harrison BP, Hilliard MW: Emergency department evaluation and treatment of hand injuries. *Emerg Med Clin North Am* 17:793, 1999.

54. Stener B: Displacement of the ruptured ulnar collateral ligament of the metacarpophalangeal joint of the thumb. *J Bone Joint Surg* 44:869, 1962.

55. Heyman P: Injuries to the ulnar collateral ligament of the thumb: Metacarpophalangeal joint. *J Am Acad Orthop Surg* 5:224, 1997.

56. Durham JW, Khuri S, Kim MH: Acute and late radial collateral ligament injuries of the thumb metacarpophalangeal joint. *J Hand Surg* 18A:232, 1993.

57. Chen VT: Dislocation of the carpometacarpal joint of the thumb. *J Hand Surg* 12B:246, 1987.

58. Kleinert HE, Smith DJ: Primary and secondary repair of flexor and extensor tendon injuries. In Flynn JE (ed): *Hand Surgery,* 4th ed. Baltimore, Williams & Wilkins, 1991, pp 241-261.

59. Pyne JI, Adams BD: Hand tendon injuries in athletics. *Clin Sports Med* 11:833, 1992.

60. Hart RG, Uehara DT, Kutz JE: Extensor tendon injuries of the hand. *Emerg Med Clin North Am* 11:637, 1993.

61. Blair WF, Steyers CM: Extensor tendon injuries. *Orthop Clin North Am* 23:141, 1992.

62. Perron A, Brady W, Keats T, Hersh R. Orthopedic pitfalls in the emergency department: Closed tendon injuries of the hand. *Am J Emerg Med* 19, 2001, pp 76-80.

63. Stern PJ, Kastrup JJ: Complications and prognosis of treatment of mallet finger. *J Hand Surg* 13A:329, 1988.

64. Moran GJ, Talan DA: Hand infections. *Emerg Med Clin North Am* 11:601, 1993.

65. Steinberg DR: Acute flexor tendon injuries. *Orthop Clin North Am* 23:125, 1992.

66. Ablove RH, Moy OJ, Peimer CA: Pediatric hand disease diagnosis and treatment. *Pediatr Clin North Am* 45:1507, 1998.

67. Strickland JW: Flexor tendons: acute injuries. In Green DP (ed): *Operative Hand Surgery,* 4th ed. New York, Churchill Livingstone, 1999, p 1851.

68. Kleinert HE, Smith DJ: Primary and secondary repairs of flexor and extensor tendon injuries. In Jupiter JB (ed): *Flynn's Hand Surgery,* 4th ed. Baltimore, Williams & Wilkins, 1991, p 241.

69. O'Hara JJ, Stone JH: An intratendinous epidermoid cyst after trauma. *J Hand Surg* 15:477, 1990.

70. Geissler GA, Erdmann D, Germann G: Soft tissue coverage in devastating hand injuries. *Hand Clin* 19:63, 2003.

71. Proano L, Partridge R: Descriptive epidemiology of a cluster of hand injuries from snowblowers. *J Emerg Med* 22, 2002, pp 341-344.

72. Chin G, et al: Snowblower injuries to the hand. *Ann Plast Surg* 41:390, 1998.

73. Arellano A, Wegener E, Freeland A: Mutilating injuries to the hand: Early amputation or repair and reconstruction. *Orthopedics* 22:683, 1999.

74. Buncke G, Buntic R, Romeo O: Pediatric mutilating hand injuries. *Hand Clin* 19:121, 2003.

75. Louis DS, et al: Amputations. In Green DP (ed): *Operative Hand Surgery,* 4th ed. New York, Churchill Livingstone, 1999, p 48.

76. Burkhalter WE: Fingertip injuries. *Emerg Med Clin North Am* 3:245, 1985.

77. Zook EG, Brown RE: The perionychium. In Green DP (ed): *Operative Hand Surgery,* 4th ed. New York, Churchill Livingstone, 1999, p 1353.

78. Guy RJ: The etiologies and mechanisms of nail bed injuries. *Hand Clin* 6:9, 1990.

79. Simon RR, Wolgin M: Subungual hematoma: Association with occult laceration requiring repair. *Am J Emerg Med* 5:302, 1987.

80. Roser SE, Gellman H: Comparison of nail bed repair versus nail trephination for subungual hematomas in children. *J Hand Surg* 24A:1166, 1999.

81. Shepard G: Perionychial grafts in trauma and reconstruction. *Hand Clin* 18:595, 2002.

82. Perron A, Miller M, Brady W: Orthopedic pitfalls in the ED: Fight bite. *Am J Emerg Med* 20:114, 2002.

83. Sirio CA, Smith JS Jr, Graham WP III: High-pressure injection injuries of the hand: A review. *Am Surg* 55:714, 1989.

84. Vasilevski D, Noorbergen M, Depierreux M, Lafontane M: High pressure injections injuries to the hand. *Am J Emerg Med* 18:820, 2000.

85. Neal NC, Burke FD: High-pressure injection injuries. *Injury* 22:467, 1991.

86. Curka PA, Chisholm CD: High-pressure water injection injury to the hand. *Am J Emerg Med* 7:165, 1989.

87. Schnall S, Mirzayan R: High pressure injections to the hand. *Hand Clin* 15:245, 1999.

88. Lewis HG, et al: A 10-year review of high-pressure injection injuries to the hand. *J Hand Surg* 23B:479, 1998.

89. Kay S, Werntz J, Wolff TW: Ring avulsion injuries: Classification and prognosis. *J Hand Surg* 14A:204, 1989.

90. Chiu Y, Chen MT: Revascularization of digits after thirty-three hours of warm ischemia time: A case report. *J Hand Surg* 9A:63, 1984.

91. Neumeister M, Brown R: Mutilating hand injuries: Principles and management. *Hand Clin* 19:1, 2003.

92. Komar LA, et al: Vascular disorders. In Green DP (ed): *Operative Hand Surgery,* 4th ed. New York, Churchill Livingstone, 1999, p 2254.

93. Rowland SA: Fasciotomy: The treatment of compartment syndrome. In Green DP (ed): *Operative Hand Surgery,* 4th ed. New York, Churchill Livingstone, 1999, p 689.

94. Hainline B: Nerve injuries. *Med Clin North Am* 78:327, 1994.

95. Frykman GK, Wolf A, Coyle T: An algorithm for management of peripheral nerve injuries. *Orthop Clin North Am* 12:239, 1986.

96. Canales FL, Newmeyer WL III, Kilgore ES: The treatment of felons and paronychias. *Hand Clin* 5:515, 1989.

97. Brook I: Bacteriologic study of paronychia in children. *Am J Surg* 141:703, 1981.

98. Hausman MR, Lisser SP: Hand infections. *Orthop Clin North Am* 23:171, 1992.

99. Butler KH: Incision and drainage. In Robert JR, Hedges JR (eds): *Clinical Procedures in Emergency Medicine,* 4th ed. Philadelphia, WB Saunders, 2004, p 717.

100. Wright PE: Hand infections. In Canale ST (ed): *Campbell's Operative Orthopaedics,* vol 4, 10th ed. St. Louis, Mosby, 2003.

101. Fowler JR: Viral infections. *Hand Clin* 5:613, 1989.

102. Gill MJ, Arlette J, Buchan K: Herpes simplex virus infection of hand: A profile of 79 cases. *Am J Med* 84:89, 1988.

103. Haedicke GJ, Grossman JAI, Fisher AE: Herpetic whitlow of the digits. *J Hand Surg* 14B:443, 1989.

104. Mann RJ, Hoffeld TA, Farmer CB: Human bites of the hand: Twenty years of experience. *J Hand Surg* 2:97, 1985.

105. Habif TP: *Clinical Dermatology: Diagnosis and Therapy,* 3rd ed. St. Louis, Mosby, 1996.

106. Levy CS: Treating infections of the hand: Identifying the organism and choosing the antibiotic. *Instr Course Lect* 39:533, 1990.

107. Lampe EW: Surgical anatomy of the hand. *Clin Symp* 40:1, 1988.

108. Siegel DB, Gelberman RH: Infections of the hand. *Orthop Clin North Am* 19:779, 1988.

109. Freeland AE, Senter BS: Septic arthritis and osteomyelitis. *Hand Clin* 5:533, 1989.

110. Schurman DJ, Smith RL: Surgical approach to the management of septic arthritis. *Orthop Rev* 16:241, 1987.

111. McLain RF, Steyers C, Stoddard M: Infections in open fractures of the hand. *J Hand Surg* 16A:1108, 1991.

112. Sonnen GM, Henry NK: Pediatric bone and joint infection: Diagnosis and antimicrobial management. *Pediatr Clin North Am* 43:4, 1996.

113. Newport ML, et al: Treatment of trigger finger by steroid injection. *J Hand Surg* 15A:748, 1990.

114. Strickland JW, Rettig AC: *Hand Injuries in Athletes.* Philadelphia, WB Saunders, 1992.

115. Rudnitsky GS, Barnett RC: Soft tissue foreign body removal. In Roberts JR, Hedges JR (eds): *Clinical Procedures in Emergency Medicine.* Philadelphia, WB Saunders, 1998.

116. Russell RC, et al: Detection of foreign bodies in the hand. *J Hand Surg* 16A:2, 1991.

117. Gooding GAW: Sonography of the hand and foot in foreign body detection. *J Ultrasound Med* 6:441, 1987.

118. Stein F: Foreign body injuries of the hand. *Emerg Med Clin North Am* 3:383, 1985.

Wrist and Forearm

Karen G. H. Woolfrey and Mary A. Eisenhauer

WRIST

PERSPECTIVE

The wrist is anatomically and biomechanically complex. This complexity allows for its diverse functional capabilities, but also puts it at risk for injury. Bony and ligamentous injuries are common, and a detailed knowledge of the anatomy and appropriate clinical evaluation and an understanding of mechanism of injury are essential for proper diagnosis and treatment of wrist injuries.[1] Although certain wrist injuries may provide a diagnostic challenge, most are evident on routine wrist views and can be diagnosed and treated by an emergency physician.

Anatomy

By definition, the wrist includes the distal radioulnar joint (DRUJ), the radiocarpal joint, and the midcarpal joints. With these complex articulations, the wrist is capable of flexion, extension, and radial and ulnar deviation. Pronation and supination of the hand occur at the proximal radioulnar joint and DRUJ.

The bones of the wrist joint include the distal articular surfaces of the radius and ulna and the bones of the carpus (Figure 48-1). The distal radius articulates directly with the proximal carpal row, and the articular surface of the ulna is separated from direct contact with the carpus by the triangular fibrocartilage. The carpal bones are divided into two rows: a proximal row consisting of the scaphoid, lunate, triquetrum, and pisiform and a distal row consisting of the trapezium, trapezoid, capitate, and hamate.

The stabilizing ligaments of the wrist joint are divided into two major groups: the extrinsic ligaments and the intrinsic ligaments. The extrinsic ligaments link the carpal bones to the distal radius and ulna and the metacarpals, and the intrinsic ligaments interconnect the individual carpal bones. The extrinsic ligaments are divided further into a volar and a dorsal group. The volar extrinsic ligaments are divided into two V-shaped ligamentous bands called the *proximal* and *distal arcades,* which generally are thicker and stronger than the dorsal extrinsic ligaments and are the most important in providing ligamentous stability to the wrist. Between these volar arcades is an area relatively devoid of ligamentous support called the *space of Poirier.* This space enlarges when the wrist is dorsiflexed, and an injury to the joint capsule in this region can result in significant carpal instability (Figure 48-2). The intrinsic ligaments interconnect adjacent carpal bones within each carpal row. The most important of these ligaments, in terms of maintaining carpal stability, are the scapholunate and lunotriquetral ligaments.[2]

Most structures that cross the wrist joint are contained within individual compartments formed by the deep fascia of the wrist. On the dorsal surface of the wrist, the extensor tendons are divided by the extensor retinaculum into six compartments, each having a separate synovial sheath that extends proximal and distal to the retinaculum. On the volar surface of the wrist, the flexors of the digits and the median nerve are contained within the carpal tunnel, which is formed by the flexor retinaculum and its attachments to the carpal bones. Radial to the carpal tunnel, the flexor carpi radialis tendon crosses the wrist joint in its own compartment.

The vascular supply to the wrist is provided by the radial and ulnar arteries, which join in a series of dorsal and palmar arches to supply the bones of the carpus. The intrinsic blood supply to most carpal bones enters the distal portion of the bone, leaving the proximal portion at risk of devascularization and avascular necrosis when fractured. This is particularly true for the scaphoid, capitate, and lunate because they each receive their blood supply from a single vessel (Figure 48-3).

The innervation of the wrist and hand is via the radial, median, and ulnar nerves. The radial nerve and the dorsal sensory branch of the ulnar nerve cross the dorsum of the wrist near the radial and ulna styloids. The median nerve crosses the volar radial aspect of the wrist within the carpal tunnel, just lateral to the palmaris longus tendon, and the ulnar nerve is within Guyon's canal between the pisiform and the hook of the hamate (see Figure 48-3).

CLINICAL FEATURES

The clinical examination of the wrist begins with a complete history, including the mechanism of injury and the site of maximal pain or tenderness. Most wrist injuries are caused by a fall on the outstretched hand. The physical examination begins with inspection of the wrist, using the opposite noninjured wrist as the "normal" reference, and includes an assessment of the presence of swelling, discoloration or obvious deformity, and the ability of the patient to move the joint through a normal range of motion.

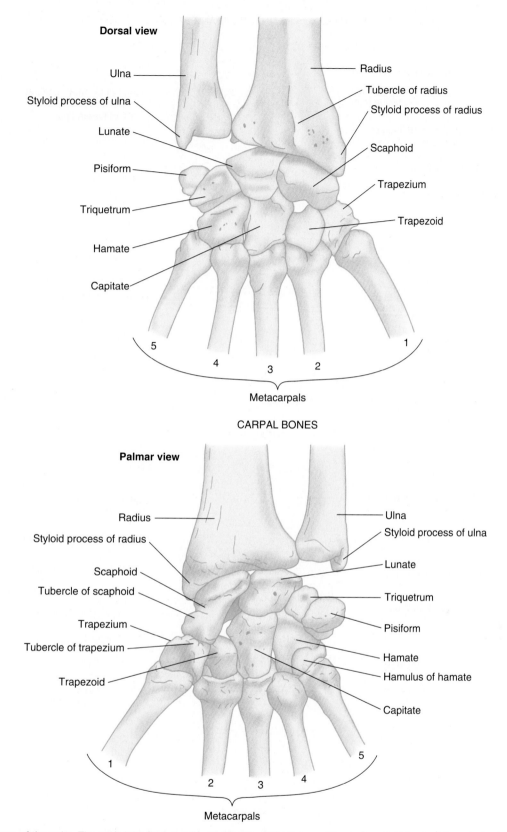

Dorsal view

Ulna

Styloid process of ulna

Lunate

Pisiform

Triquetrum

Hamate

Capitate

Radius

Tubercle of radius

Styloid process of radius

Scaphoid

Trapezium

Trapezoid

5   4   3   2   1

Metacarpals

CARPAL BONES

Palmar view

Radius

Styloid process of radius

Scaphoid

Tubercle of scaphoid

Trapezium

Tubercle of trapezium

Trapezoid

Ulna

Styloid process of ulna

Lunate

Triquetrum

Pisiform

Hamate

Hamulus of hamate

Capitate

1   2   3   4   5

Metacarpals

Figure 48-1. Bones of the wrist. The wrist joint includes the distal articular surfaces of the radius and ulna and the proximal and distal carpal rows. (Redrawn from Netter: Atlas of Human Anatomy, 3rd edition, Icon, 2003.)

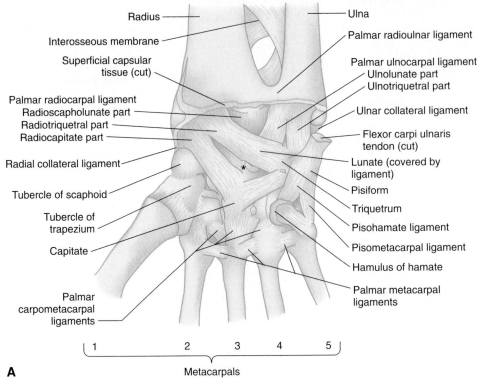

PALMAR VIEW WITH FLEXOR RETINACULUM AND STRUCTURES REMOVED

Radius — — Ulna
Interosseous membrane — — Palmar radioulnar ligament
Superficial capsular tissue (cut) — — Palmar ulnocarpal ligament
— Ulnolunate part
— Ulnotriquetral part
Palmar radiocarpal ligament
Radioscapholunate part — — Ulnar collateral ligament
Radiotriquetral part —
Radiocapitate part — — Flexor carpi ulnaris tendon (cut)
Radial collateral ligament — — Lunate (covered by ligament)
Tubercle of scaphoid — — Pisiform
Tubercle of trapezium — — Triquetrum
Capitate — — Pisohamate ligament
— Pisometacarpal ligament
— Hamulus of hamate
Palmar carpometacarpal ligaments — — Palmar metacarpal ligaments

1   2   3   4   5
Metacarpals

A

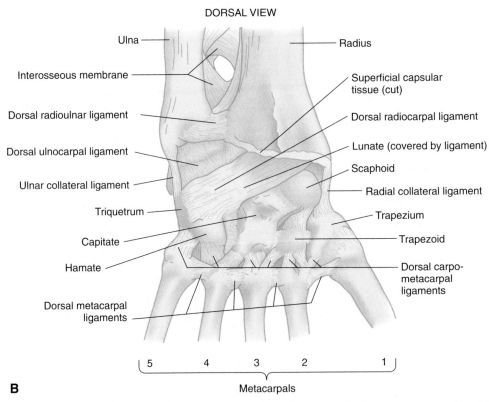

DORSAL VIEW

Ulna — — Radius
Interosseous membrane — — Superficial capsular tissue (cut)
Dorsal radioulnar ligament — — Dorsal radiocarpal ligament
Dorsal ulnocarpal ligament — — Lunate (covered by ligament)
Ulnar collateral ligament — — Scaphoid
Triquetrum — — Radial collateral ligament
Capitate — — Trapezium
Hamate — — Trapezoid
— Dorsal carpo-metacarpal ligaments
Dorsal metacarpal ligaments —

5   4   3   2   1
Metacarpals

B

Figure 48-2. Ligaments of the wrist. **A,** The volar extrinsic ligaments are the most important ligaments in providing stability to the wrist and include the radial collateral ligament, radiocapitate ligament, radioscaphoid ligament, radiotriquetral ligament, ulnotriquetral ligament, capitotriquetral ligament, and ulnar collateral ligament. The space of Poirier (*) is a gap in the volar ligaments and the site of potential weakness. **B,** The intrinsic (intercarpal) ligaments interconnect the individual carpal bones. The most important of these are the scapholunate ligament and the lunotriquetral ligament. (Redrawn from Netter: Atlas of Human Anatomy, 3ʳᵈ edition, Icon, 2003.)

PALMAR VIEW WITH STRUCTURES PASSING THROUGH AND OVER CARPAL TUNNEL

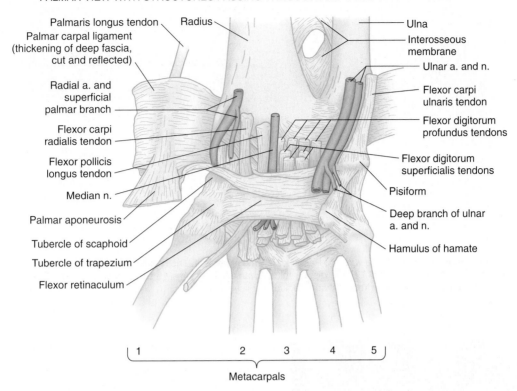

Figure 48-3. Vascular supply to the wrist. Note the relationship of the wrist ligaments to the neurovascular supply to the wrist. (Redrawn from Netter: Atlas of Human Anatomy, 3rd edition, Icon, 2003.)

On palpation, several bony prominences in the wrist act as useful landmarks, and the locations of these are best described in relation to the major reference points in the wrist—the radial and ulnar styloids. Lister's tubercle can be palpated on the dorsum of the wrist just ulnar to the radial styloid. This is an important landmark because just distal to the tubercle lies the scapholunate joint, an important site of ligamentous injury in the wrist. Just distal to the radial styloid is the anatomic snuffbox, bordered radially by the abductor pollicis longus and extensor pollicis brevis tendons and ulnarly by the extensor pollicis longus tendon. The body of the scaphoid is palpable within the snuffbox and is more prominent with the wrist in ulnar deviation.[3] The triquetrum is palpable just distal to the ulnar styloid in the proximal carpal row and can be made more prominent with radial deviation of the wrist. With the wrist in neutral position, the capitate is palpable in a small depression found midway between the base of the third metacarpal and Lister's tubercle. Bringing the wrist into flexion can bring the lunate forward into a palpable position at this same site. On the volar aspect of the wrist, the scaphoid tubercle is palpable just distal and palmar to the radial styloid. It is felt as a rounded prominence at the base of the thenar muscles and is especially prominent when the wrist is extended. On the ulnar border of the wrist, the pisiform is palpable at the base of the hypothenar muscles, just distal to the distal wrist crease. In addition, approximately 1 cm distal and radial to this point, one can palpate the prominence formed by the hook of the hamate.

The clinical examination of the wrist includes an assessment of the neurovascular status. Radial and ulnar pulses are easily palpable on the volar surface of the wrist, and the presence of pulses should be documented in all injuries to the wrist.

DIAGNOSTIC STRATEGIES: RADIOLOGY

Plain radiographs remain the cornerstone of diagnosis of fractures and dislocations of the wrist. Routine radiographic views include the posteroanterior, lateral, and oblique projections, each performed with the wrist in neutral position. Accurate interpretation of these views requires knowledge of the normal appearance and anatomic relationships of the distal radius, ulna, and carpal bones.

On the posteroanterior view of the wrist, the radial styloid process extends beyond the end of the articular surface of the ulna by a normal distance of 9 to 12 mm. This normal difference in length is called the *radial length measurement*. The ulnar slant of the articular surface of the radius is visible on the posteroanterior view and normally should measure 15 to 25 degrees. Both of these measurements are important when assessing the degree of radial shortening seen in association with some fractures of the distal radius (Figure 48-4).[4] The normal appearance of the carpus on the posteroanterior view shows an approximately equal distance (usually 1 to 2 mm) between each of the carpal

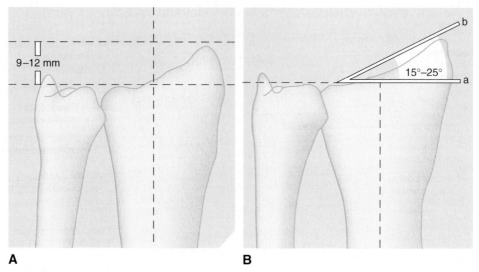

Figure 48-4. Normal posteroanterior view of the wrist. **A,** Radial length measurement. The radial styloid extends 9 to 12 mm beyond the articular surface of the distal ulna. **B,** The ulnar slant of the distal radius noramally measures 15 to 25 degrees. (From Greenspan A: *Orthopedic Radiology: A Practical Approach,* 2nd ed. New York, Gower Medical Publishing, 1992.)

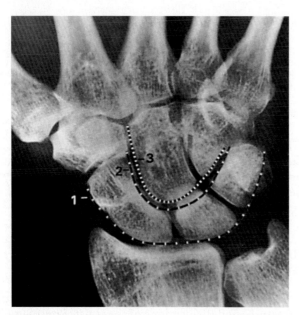

Figure 48-5. Wrist arcs. On the normal posteroanterior view of the carpus, three arcuate lines can be drawn along the carpal articular surfaces. (From Weissman BN, Sledge CB: *Orthopedic Radiology.* Philadelphia, WB Saunders, 1986.)

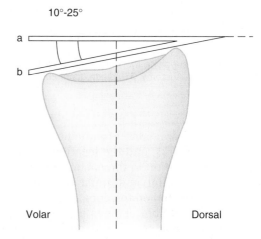

Figure 48-6. Normal lateral view of the wrist. The distal radius has a normal volar tilt of 10 to 25 degrees. (From Greenspan A: *Orthopedic Radiology: A Practical Approach,* 2nd ed. New York, Gower Medical Publishing, 1992.)

bones, and opposing articular surfaces are parallel to one another, known as parallelism. Three smooth curves normally can be drawn along the carpal articular surfaces (Figure 48-5). Disruption of these curves or widening of the carpal spaces is an indication of carpal ligament disruption and carpal instability.[5]

On the lateral view of the wrist, the normal volar tilt of the distal radial articular surface is visible and normally measures between 10 and 25 degrees (Figure 48-6). The normal alignment of the distal radius with the lunate and capitate also is seen on the lateral view and appears as two concentric cups, the cup of the distal radius containing the lunate and the cup of the distal

lunate containing the capitate. Ideally the long axis of the radius, lunate, capitate, and third metacarpal should appear as a straight line on the lateral view, although the "normal" alignment is usually within 10 degrees of this ideal line (Figure 48-7). The carpal alignment on the lateral view is defined further by the scapholunate angle, which normally measures 30 to 60 degrees, and the capitolunate angle, which is normally 0 to 30 degrees (Figure 48-8). Abnormalities in these angles are seen in patients with carpal ligament injuries and carpal instability.

The soft tissues of the wrist also offer valuable clues to the presence of underlying bony injuries. On the lateral view of the wrist, the pronator quadratus line is visible as a linear fat collection in the volar soft tissues just anterior to the distal radius and ulna (Figure 48-9). Fractures of the distal radius or ulna result in volar displacement or complete obliteration of this line.

Additional radiographic views of the wrist include posteroanterior views in ulnar and radial deviation, lateral views in maximal flexion and extension, and the clenched fist anteroposterior view. These views are useful to delineate further abnormal motion of the carpus as a result of carpal ligament injuries. Specific scaphoid views, obtained with the wrist prone and in ulnar deviation, allow for better visualization of the scaphoid along its long axis. The carpal tunnel view is performed with the wrist hyperextended and provides an axial view of the bony margins of the carpal tunnel. This view and the reverse (supinated) oblique view help identify fractures involving the hamate, especially the hook of the hamate, and the pisiform (Table 48-1).[6]

CARPAL INJURIES

Scaphoid Fractures

The scaphoid is the most commonly fractured of the carpal bones and accounts for more than 60% of all carpal fractures.[7] It typically is seen in young adults age 15 to 30 and occurs after a fall on the outstretched hand. Scaphoid fractures in skeletally immature individuals are rare. Fractures of the scaphoid are classi-

fied by the anatomic location of the fracture line and may be divided into three groups: fractures of the tuberosity and distal pole, fractures of the waist, and fractures of the proximal pole. Fractures through the waist of the scaphoid are the most common of these three patterns and account for approximately 70% to 80% of all scaphoid fractures.[8]

Clinically, patients complain of dorsal radial wrist pain just distal to the radial styloid, with limited range of motion of the wrist and thumb. Classically, physical examination reveals tenderness on palpation of the scaphoid and swelling within the anatomic snuffbox, but pain also may be elicited with palpation of the scaphoid tubercle volarly, with axial compression of the thumb metacarpal, or with resisted supination.[9]

Radiographic diagnosis of scaphoid fractures is often difficult, and special scaphoid views should be requested when a fracture is suspected on clinical examination. A visible fracture lucency may be occult, and more subtle findings, such as obliteration or displacement of the scaphoid fat pad, may be the only clue to the presence of a fracture.[10,11] Plain radiographs fail to detect 15% of scaphoid fractures.[12] For this reason, and the associated risk of nonunion when diagnosis

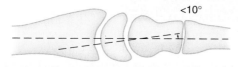

Figure 48-7. Normal relationship of carpal bones on lateral view. Concavity of radius and lunate and convexity of capitate form three C-shaped areas *(stippled)* along a straight line that runs through the central axis of these bones.

Table 48-1. Additional Radiographic Wrist Views

Radiographic View	Benefit
Clenched fist view	Exposes scapholunate ligament injury; pushes capitate into proximal carpal row
Scaphoid view	Elongates scaphoid; exposes waist fractures
Carpal tunnel view	Identifies fractures involving hamate and pisiform; identifies bony encroachment onto the carpal tunnel

Scapholunate angle

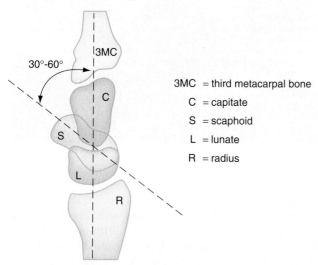

3MC = third metacarpal bone
C = capitate
S = scaphoid
L = lunate
R = radius

A In normal wrist the scapholunate angle is between 30°–60°

Capitolunate angle

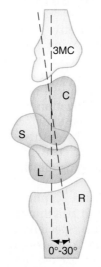

B In normal wrist the capitolunate angle is between 0°–30°

Figure 48-8. A, The normal scapholunate angle is formed by the intersection of the longitudinal axes of the scaphoid and lunate and normally measures 30 to 60 degrees. **B,** The normal capitolunate angle is formed by the intersection of the capitate and lunate central long axes and normally measures 0 to 30 degrees. (From Greenspan A: *Orthopedic Radiology: A Practical Approach,* 2nd ed. New York, Gower Medical Publishing, 1992.)

Figure 48-9. The pronator quadratus is a narrow fat stripe located 1 cm from the volar surface of the radius on the normal lateral wrist view. (From Propp DA, Chin H: Forearm and wrist radiology—Part I. *J Emerg Med* 7:393, 1989.)

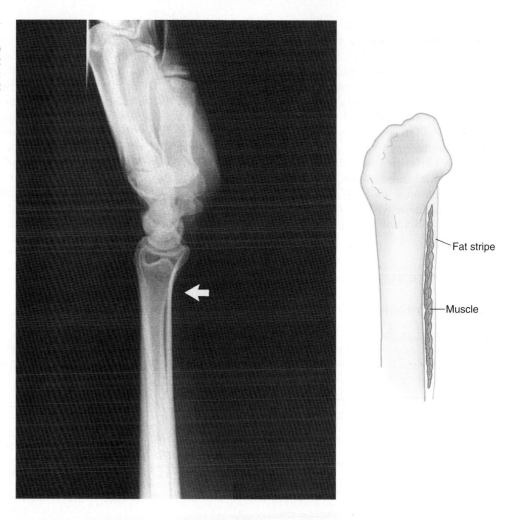

Fat stripe

Muscle

and immobilization are delayed, patients clinically suspected of having a scaphoid fracture are treated with cast immobilization, with repeat radiographs in 10 to 14 days. If a fracture is present, it may be more evident on the repeat radiographs because of resorption associated with fracture healing. If radiographic results remain negative at 10 to 14 days, and clinical examination is still suggestive of fracture, a three-phase technetium bone scan or a computed tomography (CT) scan of the scaphoid should be obtained.[13-18]

More recent studies have shown that a negative bone scan 72 to 96 hours after injury accurately can exclude scaphoid fracture. These studies suggest that a patient can be immobilized for comfort, and a bone scan can be performed within the first few days of injury. A negative bone scan allows much earlier mobilization.[19,20] Magnetic resonance imaging also can be used to detect these radiographically occult fractures, with sensitivities of 100%. High correlation has been shown between bone scan and magnetic resonance imaging of the scaphoid.[21-23]

Treatment of uncomplicated, undisplaced scaphoid fractures involves immobilization in a short arm thumb spica cast (Figure 48-10), although some specialists prefer to use a long arm cast for the first 2 weeks of immobilization, replacing this with a short arm cast for the remainder of the immobilization period. The duration of immobilization varies relative to the location of

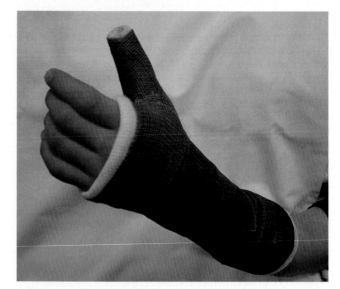

Figure 48-10. Thumb spica cast.

the fracture, but averages 12 weeks, with the more proximal fractures requiring longer immobilization to ensure adequate healing. This variability in healing time is related directly to the pattern of blood supply to the scaphoid, which flows from the distal to proximal portion of the bone through the scaphoid tuberosity. This pattern of blood flow also accounts for the higher incidence of avascular necrosis and fracture nonunion in the more proximal fractures. Overall, avascular necrosis is seen in approximately 3% and nonunion in 5% to 10% of scaphoid fractures, with the risk of complications being greatest in fractures of the proximal pole.[24,25] Any scaphoid fracture that is displaced more than 1 mm or is associated with an increase in the normal scapholunate or capitolunate angles requires prompt orthopedic referral for consideration of operative treatment.

Lunate Fractures

Fractures of the lunate are relatively uncommon, representing fewer than 3% of all carpal fractures. This injury occurs more commonly in individuals with a congenitally short ulna, owing to compromise of the normal triangular fibrocartilage support. The usual mechanism of injury involves a fall on the outstretched hand, causing extreme dorsiflexion, with the resultant force being transmitted from the capitate to the lunate. Patients have pain over the dorsum of the wrist, which is exacerbated by axial loading of the long finger metacarpal. On examination, tenderness may be elicited on palpation over the dorsum of the wrist in the depression felt just distal to Lister's tubercle.

Fractures of the lunate may be difficult to see on plain radiographs because of overlap of the distal radius, ulna, and other carpal bones. For this reason, and because of the risk of avascular necrosis in missed injuries, patients suspected of having a lunate fracture should be immobilized in a short arm cast until a fracture can be confirmed or excluded by CT or technetium bone scan.

Lunate fractures are treated with immobilization in a short arm cast, with orthopedic follow-up evaluation in 1 to 2 weeks. Complications include progression to carpal instability, nonunion, and avascular necrosis. Posttraumatic avascular necrosis is seen in 20% of fractures and is called *Kienbock's disease*. In well-established cases of Kienbock's disease, the lunate appears sclerotic and fragmented on x-ray, and ultimately the bone collapses with resultant proximal migration of the capitate. These changes cause secondary osteoarthritis of the radiocarpal joint and chronic wrist pain. Treatment involves operative intervention, with correction of the articular abnormalities either by lengthening the ulna or by shortening the radius. In more advanced cases, excision and prosthetic replacement of the lunate or arthrodesis may be necessary.[26]

Triquetral Fractures

Fracture of the triquetrum, the second most common fracture of the carpals, usually results either from a direct blow to the bone causing a fracture of the body or from a fall on the outstretched hand. In the latter situation, the mechanism of fracture is believed to be impact of the ulnar styloid against the triquetrum, which results in a dorsal chip fracture.[27,28] Patients have localized tenderness over the dorsum of the wrist just distal to the ulnar styloid. On physical examination,

swelling may be noted in this same area, and wrist motion is limited because of pain. The fracture is best seen on the standard lateral view of the wrist as a small dorsal chip fragment, although a more oblique pronated lateral view may be necessary. Treatment with immobilization in a short arm cast or splint usually results in an uncomplicated course with prompt fracture healing over 4 to 6 weeks.

Pisiform Fractures

The pisiform is a unique carpal bone because it is a sesamoid bone that lies within the flexor carpi ulnaris tendon and articulates on its dorsal surface with the triquetrum. Fractures of the pisiform usually occur from a fall on the outstretched hand, but also may be seen with direct blows to the hypothenar eminence. On clinical examination, there is tenderness over the ulnar aspect of the volar wrist crease, which may be exacerbated with wrist flexion and ulnar deviation.[29] Fractures of the pisiform can impinge on Guyon's canal, resulting in ulnar nerve injury. Paresthesias in the distribution of the ulnar nerve and hand clumsiness from intrinsic muscle dysfunction can occur. Pisiform fractures are poorly seen on routine wrist radiographs, so special views must be requested. A reverse (supinated) oblique view and the carpal tunnel view allow for better visualization of these fractures.[6]

Fractures of the pisiform generally have an excellent prognosis and are treated with immobilization in a short arm cast or splint for 3 to 4 weeks. If evidence of nerve compromise exists, orthopedic consultation for possible urgent surgical decompression is indicated to restore nerve function. Fractures that are complicated by nonunion may require excision of the pisiform to prevent chronic pain.

Hamate Fractures

Hamate fractures are rare and account for approximately 2% of all carpal bone fractures. The hook or hamulus is the most common site of fracture, although fractures through the articular surfaces or body also are seen. Fracture of the hook usually occurs from a fall on the outstretched hand or by a direct blow to the palm of the hand. Commonly, the use of hammers and vibration from equipment also can cause fractures. Patients present with pain over the hypothenar eminence with associated decreased grip strength. Pain may be localized on palpation of the hamate, 1 cm distal and radial to the pisiform. Fractures of the hamate body and articular surface usually are seen on posteroanterior views of the wrist, but fractures of the hook are seen best on the reverse oblique and carpal tunnel views.[6] When these views are inconclusive, plain tomography or a CT scan may allow confirmation of fracture.[30]

Initial treatment is by immobilization in a short arm cast with orthopedic follow-up in 1 to 2 weeks. Fractures of the hook of the hamate often are complicated by associated ulnar nerve injury or progression to nonunion. In both cases, operative intervention with excision of the hook at the fracture site is necessary.[31,32]

Trapezium Fractures

Fractures of the trapezium are uncommon and represent only 1% to 5% of all carpal injuries. There are two main types of fractures: fractures involving the body and fractures involving the trapezial ridge. A direct blow to the adducted thumb causes fracture through the body of the trapezium with the force being transmitted by the base of the thumb metacarpal. Avulsion fractures of the trapezial ridge occur with forceful radial deviation or rotation of the wrist. On examination, patients complain of pain with movement of the thumb and on direct palpation of the trapezium just distal to the scaphoid in the anatomic snuffbox. Fractures are seen best on slightly pronated oblique views of the wrist, although a true anteroposterior view of the trapezium (Roberts' view) or CT scan may be necessary.[33] Patients are treated with immobilization in a thumb spica cast for 6 weeks, unless the fracture is displaced or involves the carpometacarpal joint, in which case referral for open reduction and fixation is indicated.

Capitate Fractures

The capitate lies in a central position in the distal carpal row, and because of this protected location, it is rarely fractured. When fracture does occur, the mechanism is generally a direct blow to the dorsum of the wrist. Fracture also may be seen in association with a perilunate dislocation after a fall on the outstretched dorsiflexed hand. Clinical examination reveals dorsal wrist pain and swelling, with localized tenderness on palpation of the capitate. Fractures usually are visible on the standard posteroanterior view of the wrist, although the lateral view may be helpful in determining the presence of rotation or displacement of the fracture fragment.

Undisplaced isolated fractures of the capitate may be managed with immobilization in a short arm cast for 6 weeks. Any fracture with displacement or associated carpal dislocation requires prompt orthopedic referral for open reduction and fixation. Complications of nonunion and avascular necrosis of the proximal fragment are rare, but do occur because the capitate receives its blood supply through its distal half.[29]

Trapezoid Fractures

The trapezoid rarely is fractured and is said to account for fewer than 1% of all carpal bone fractures.[34] The typical mechanism of injury is a direct blow down the long axis of the index metacarpal, which may result in isolated fracture to the trapezoid or may cause a dorsal fracture-dislocation. On clinical examination, pain and tenderness are localized over the dorsum of the wrist at the base of the second metacarpal. The fracture may be visible on routine posteroanterior views of the wrist; however, oblique views or tomography may be necessary to visualize this injury. Undisplaced fractures are treated with immobilization in a short arm cast for 6 weeks, and fracture-dislocations need prompt orthopedic referral for reduction and fixation.[29]

Carpal Instability

Mayfield and associates[35] described a progressive pattern of carpal ligamentous injury caused by wrist hyperextension, ulnar deviation, and intercarpal supination. Their studies of the pathomechanics of these injuries led to the classification of carpal instability into four distinct stages. Each stage represents a sequential intercarpal injury beginning with scapholunate joint disruption and proceeding around the lunate, creating progressive ligamentous injury and progressive carpal instability (Figure 48-11). Each stage also may be associated with specific bony fractures, which if present should alert the physician to the possibility of an occult perilunate ligamentous injury. These associated fractures include fractures of the radial styloid, scaphoid, capitate, and triquetrum.

A stage I injury, or scapholunate dissociation, results in a characteristic widening of the scapholunate joint on the posteroanterior view, which has been called the "Terry Thomas sign," after the British comedian with a gap between his front teeth.[36] If associated with rotatory subluxation of the scaphoid, the scaphoid is seen end on with the cortex of the distal pole appearing as a ring shadow over the scaphoid; this is called the *signet ring sign* (Figure 48-12). Routine radiographs may appear normal so that when a scapholunate ligament injury is suspected clinically, additional stress views should be obtained. Views taken with a clenched fist and ulnar deviation (the clenched fist anteroposterior view) accentuate widening of the scapholunate joint.

A stage II injury, or perilunate dislocation, is seen best on the lateral view of the wrist. Although the lunate remains in position relative to the distal radius, the capitate is dorsally dislocated. The posteroanterior view shows overlap of the distal and proximal carpal rows and may show an associated scaphoid fracture or subluxation (Figure 48-13).[37]

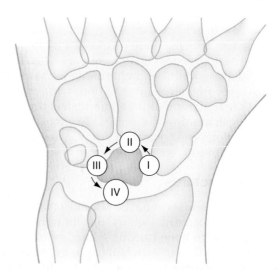

Figure 48-11. Sequential stages of carpal dislocation. Each of four stages represents a sequential intercarpal ligament injury proceeding around the lunate. (From Greenspan A: *Orthopedic Radiology: A Practical Approach,* 2nd ed. New York, Gower Medical Publishing, 1992.)

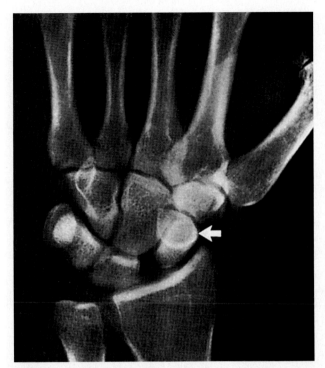

Figure 48-12. Scapholunate dissociation with scaphoid subluxation. Posteroanterior wrist view shows characteristic widening of the scapholunate joint and a ring shadow over the scaphoid *(arrow)*. (From Sonnenberg J: Carpal injuries. *Trauma Q* 1:71, 1985.)

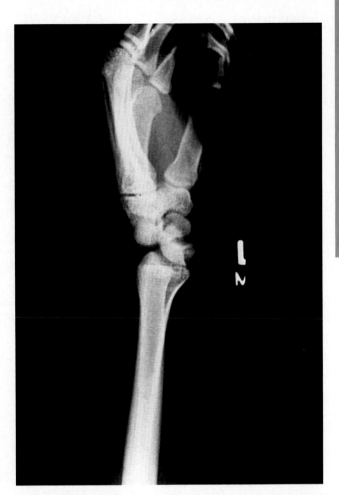

Figure 48-13. Perilunate dislocation. Lateral view shows lunate in normal position and the capitate dorsally dislocated. (From Propp DA, Chin H: Forearm and wrist radiology—Part I. *J Emerg Med* 7:393, 1989.)

A stage III injury appears identical to a stage II injury but includes a dislocation of the triquetrum that is seen best on the posteroanterior view, with overlap of the triquetrum on the lunate or hamate. This injury may be associated with a volar triquetral fracture.

A stage IV injury, or lunate dislocation, results in a characteristic triangular appearance of the lunate on the posteroanterior view because of the rotation of the lunate in a volar direction. This triangular appearance is known as the "piece of pie sign." This rotation also is visible on the lateral view of the wrist, where the lunate looks like a cup tipped forward and spilling its contents into the palm. This latter sign is called the "spilled teacup sign." On the lateral view, the capitate is seen to lie posterior to the lunate and often migrates proximally to contact the distal radius (Figure 48-14).

Patients with these carpal dislocation injuries typically have a history of a fall on the outstretched hand. They complain of pain and swelling over the dorsum of the wrist, with limited range of motion. On physical examination, there is palpable tenderness over the dorsum of the wrist, particularly in the region of the scapholunate ligament. With perilunate and lunate dislocations, visible deformity of the wrist also is present, and diminished two-point sensation is often present in the median nerve distribution. Complications of carpal dislocation injuries include median nerve injury and chronic carpal instability with resultant degenerative arthritis.

Carpal dislocation injuries require orthopedic consultation in the emergency department for reduction and stabilization. Either arthroscopically guided reduc-

tion and pinning or open reduction with ligament repair is now recommended for the optimal management of these acute injuries.

Intercalated Segment Instability

Not all patterns of carpal instability follow the pattern described by Mayfield and associates.[35] Two other common types of carpal instability—dorsal intercalated segment instability (DISI) and volar intercalated segment instability (VISI)—are better understood as a pattern of midcarpal joint collapse (Figure 48-15).[38] These patterns of carpal instability are recognized radiographically by specific deformities on the lateral view of the wrist (Figure 48-16).

With the DISI pattern of instability, there is dorsiflexion of the lunate relative to the capitate, which results in an increase in the scapholunate and capitolunate angles. With the VISI pattern of instability, there is volar flexion of the lunate relative to the capitate, with a decrease in the scapholunate angle and an increase in the capitolunate angle. These angles are best visualized on the lateral view radiograph and appear as if the articular surface of the lunate is tilting dorsally (DISI) or volarly (VISI). DISI is the most common pattern of carpal instability and may be seen after

Figure 48-14. Lunate dislocation. **A,** Posteroanterior view shows the characteristic triangular shape of the lunate (arrow). **B,** Volar displacement of the lunate resembles a spilled teacup on lateral view *(arrow)*, with dorsal displacement of the capitate. (From Propp DA, Chin H: Forearm and wrist radiology—Part I. *J Emerg Med* 7:393, 1989.)

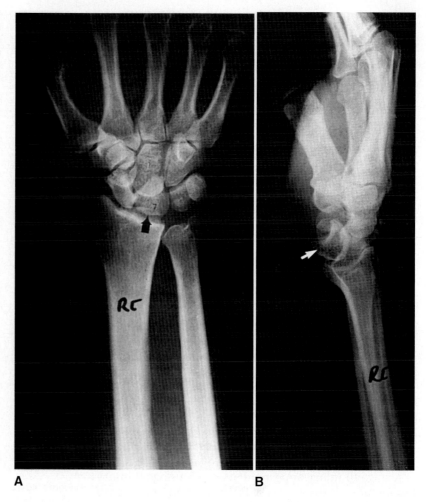

A　　　　　**B**

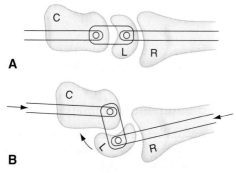

Figure 48-15. The wrist as a link mechanism. **A,** The wrist as a link mechanism in which the distal radius (R), proximal carpal row (represented by the lunate [L]), and distal carpal row (represented by the capitate [C]) compose the individual links. **B,** With axial compression *(arrows)*, carpal collapse occurs in a zigzag pattern if there is loss of the carpal longitudinal supports (the scaphoid and ligamentous attachments). (From Green DP: *Operative Hand Surgery,* vol 1, 3rd ed. New York, Churchill Livingstone, 1993.)

scapholunate dissociation or with scaphoid fractures with or without associated perilunate dislocation. VISI patterns of instability occur after lunotriquetral or triquetrohamate joint disruption. Either pattern may be seen in association with radiocarpal joint malalignment, as is seen in lunate collapse with Kienbock's disease, rheumatoid arthritis, or congenital carpal ligamentous laxity.[38,39]

Clinically, patients have chronic pain, weakness, and limited range of motion of the wrist and may complain of the wrist clicking with ulnar deviation. On physical examination, there is point tenderness over the area of primary injury, usually the scapholunate or lunotriquetral joints. Gross deformity of the wrist, resulting from subluxation, also may be apparent compared with the unaffected "normal" wrist. Patients should be referred to an orthopedic surgeon for definitive treatment of these injuries. Operative treatment involves reduction and stabilization, with ligamentous reconstruction or repair.

DISTAL RADIUS AND ULNA INJURIES

Colles' Fracture

Colles' fracture, first described in 1814, is the most common wrist fracture seen in adults.[40] It is a transverse fracture of the distal radial metaphysis, which is dorsally displaced and angulated. The fracture usually is located within 2 cm of the radial articular surface and may be associated with intra-articular extension into the radiocarpal or radioulnar joints. There is commonly an associated fracture of the ulnar styloid.

Clinically, patients have a history of a fall on the outstretched hand and complain of immediate pain and swelling over the dorsum of the wrist. On examination,

DISI AND VISI DEFORMITIES

DISI

Dorsal intercalated segment instability
(Dorsiflexion Carpal Instability)

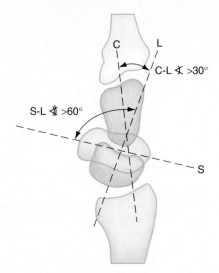

A
1. Dorsal tilt of lunate
2. Volar tilt of scaphoid

VISI

Volar intercalated segment instability
(Volarflexion Carpal Instability)

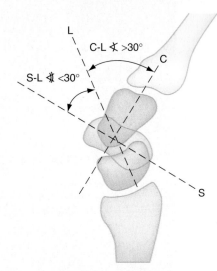

B
1. Volar tilt of lunate
2. Dorsal tilt of capitate

Figure 48-16. A, Dorsal intercalated segment instability (DISI). In this pattern of carpal instability, the scapholunate angle measures more than 60 degrees, and the capitolunate angle measures more than 30 degrees. **B,** Volar intercalated segment instability (VISI). In this pattern of carpal instability, the scapholunate angle measures less than 30 degrees, and the capitolunate angle measures more than 30 degrees. (From Propp DA, Chin H: Forearm and wrist radiology—Part I. *J Emerg Med* 7:393, 1989.)

there is an obvious "dinner fork" deformity of the wrist caused by the dorsal displacement and angulation of the fracture. A neurovascular examination should be performed to exclude an associated median nerve injury or vascular compromise caused by this deformity.

The posteroanterior and lateral views of the wrist show the fracture through the radial metaphysis. The posteroanterior view may show extension of the fracture into the radioulnar or radiocarpal joints and shows the amount of radial shortening present. The degree of dorsal displacement and angulation is seen best on the lateral view, with loss of the normal volar tilt of the distal radial articular surface (Figure 48-17).

Colles' fracture requires prompt anatomic reduction in the emergency department, with full restoration of radial length and correction of the dorsal angulation either to a neutral position or ideally to the normal volar tilt position. Closed reduction, using local or regional anesthesia, with cast immobilization is successful in most cases (Figure 48-18). An effective method of anesthesia is placing a 22-gauge needle in the dorsum of the distal radius, withdrawing until a hematoma is encountered, then instilling 5 to 10 mL of 2% lidocaine (Xylocaine) (Figure 48-19). Finger traps also are an effective means of obtaining the reduction and allow positioning for casting (Figure 48-20). The more comminuted and displaced the fracture, the more likely operative reduction will be necessary. Complicated fractures with significant displacement (>20 degrees of dorsal angulation), marked dorsal comminution, or intra-articular extension should be followed closely by an orthopedic specialist because loss of reduction often occurs and mandates early operative reduction with internal or external fixation. Immediate referral to an orthopedic surgeon should be considered if initial attempts at closed reduction are unsuccessful, if there is associated neurovascular compromise, or if the fracture is open.

Complications of Colles' fracture are seen most often in elderly patients and in patients with inadequate fracture reduction.[41,42] Median nerve injury may be seen acutely either because of traction from the original fracture displacement or because of direct injury to the nerve by fracture fragments. Injury to the median nerve also has been described after closed reduction because of traction on the nerve, direct pressure from the cast or position of immobilization, or swelling causing compression in the carpal tunnel. Treatment is repositioning, decreasing the splint pressure, or occasionally carpal tunnel release. For this reason, it is important to document neurologic function before and after fracture reduction. A more common complication is malunion of the fracture, resulting in chronic wrist pain and limited range of motion. This complication is more likely to occur in cases of fracture involving the radiocarpal joint.

Smith's Fracture

Smith's fracture is a transverse fracture of the metaphysis of the distal radius, with associated volar displacement and volar angulation. In some cases, the fracture may extend into the radiocarpal joint. Because the resultant deformity is opposite to that seen in Colles' fracture, Smith's fracture is often called a *reverse Colles' fracture*. The typical mechanism of injury involves a direct blow to the dorsum of the wrist or fall onto the dorsum of the hand, resulting in

Figure 48-17. Colles' fracture. **A,** Posteroanterior view shows fracture and shortening of radius. **B,** Lateral view shows typical dorsal displacement and angulation of radial fracture. (From Propp DA, Chin H: Forearm and wrist radiology—Part I. *J Emerg Med* 7:393, 1989.)

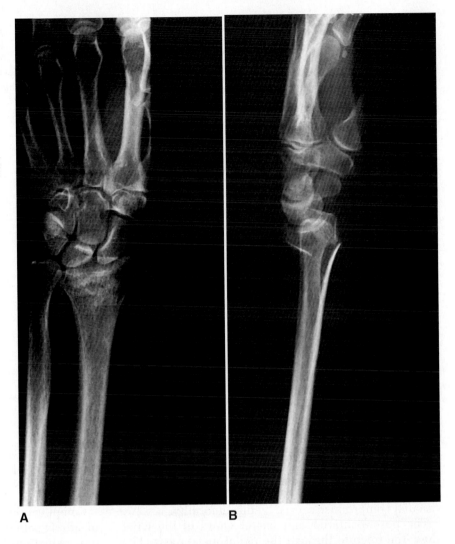

A **B**

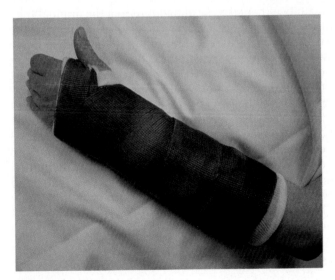

Figure 48-18. Short arm cast.

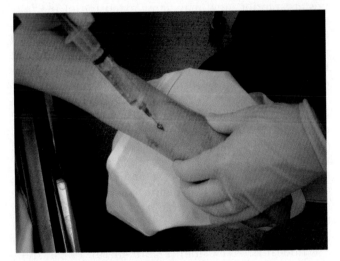

Figure 48-19. Hematoma block.

extreme palmar flexion. The fracture also may be seen after a fall backward on an outstretched hand with the forearm in supination. The patient has a swollen, painful wrist, which is deformed with fullness visible on the volar aspect. The fracture is visible on pos-

teroanterior and lateral radiographs of the wrist, but the lateral view best shows the degree of volar displacement and angulation (Figure 48-21).

Treatment of this fracture involves closed reduction with cast immobilization for 6 to 8 weeks; however, molding of the cast to maintain the reduction can lead to median nerve compression. Orthopedic consultation

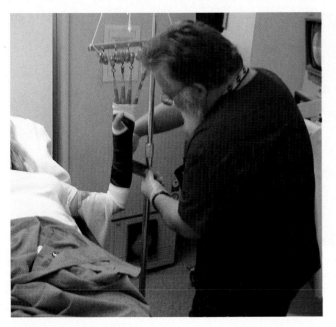

Figure 48-20. Finger traps.

is recommended because open reduction and internal fixation may be required. Complications include median nerve injury, malunion, and posttraumatic arthritis, especially in fractures with significant displacement or intra-articular extension. As with Colles' fracture, prognosis is most favorable in patients with successful reduction, with restoration of the normal radial length and volar tilt.[43]

Barton's Fracture

Barton's fracture is an oblique intra-articular fracture of the rim of the distal radius, with displacement of the carpus along with the fracture fragment. The fracture may involve the dorsal rim of the radius with dorsal carpal subluxation (Barton's fracture), or it may involve the volar rim with volar carpal subluxation (volar Barton's fracture). These fractures are rare and account for only 1.2% to 4.2% of all distal radius fractures.[44] The volar-anterior margin fracture is seen more often than the dorsal-posterior margin fracture.

The mechanism of injury for these fractures involves a high-velocity impact across the articular surface of the radiocarpal joint, with the wrist in either volar flexion (causing a volar rim fracture) or dorsiflexion (causing a

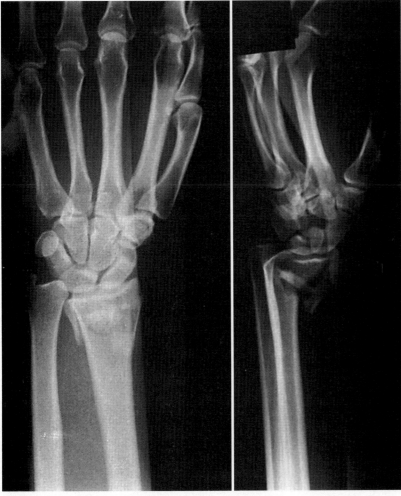

Figure 48-21. Smith's fracture. **A,** Posteroanterior view shows a metaphyseal fracture of the radius with shortening. **B,** Lateral view shows volar displacement of the distal fracture fragment along with the carpus. (From Propp DA, Chin H: Forearm and wrist radiology—Part I. *J Emerg Med* 7:393, 1989.)

A   **B**

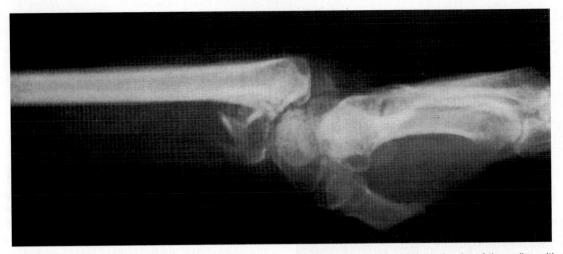

Figure 48-22. Volar Barton's fracture. Lateral view shows typical oblique intra-articular fracture of the volar rim of the radius with associated volar displacement of the distal radial fragment along with the carpus. (From Harris JH, et al: *The Radiology of Emergency Medicine,* 3rd ed. Baltimore, Williams & Wilkins, 1993.)

dorsal rim fracture). Volar and dorsal rim fractures are easily visible on posteroanterior and lateral wrist radiographs; however, the lateral view best shows the degree of articular surface involvement and the amount of associated fracture displacement (Figure 48-22).

Treatment of these fractures requires orthopedic consultation for reduction and stabilization. Closed reduction occasionally may be successful. Most authors now advocate early operative management, however, with either closed reduction under fluoroscopy followed by percutaneous pinning or open reduction and internal fixation to restore accurately the articular surface of the radius and stabilize the carpus.[44] Complications include posttraumatic arthritis of the radiocarpal joint and delayed carpal instability. Both complications are seen more commonly when reduction fails to achieve or maintain anatomic realignment of the radiocarpal joint surface.

Hutchinson's Fracture

Hutchinson's fracture, or chauffeur's fracture, is an intra-articular fracture of the radial styloid. The mechanism of injury is usually a direct blow or fall resulting in trauma to the radial side of the wrist. The term *chauffeur's fracture* originated from the era of hand-cranked automobiles, when this injury occurred because of direct trauma to the radial side of the wrist from the recoil of the crank. The fracture is seen best on the posteroanterior view of the wrist, as a transverse fracture of the radial metaphysis with extension through the radial styloid into the radiocarpal joint (Figure 48-23).

Nondisplaced fractures may be immobilized in a short arm cast for 4 to 6 weeks; however, displaced fractures require open/closed reduction and fixation. Because the radial styloid is the primary site of attachment for many of the ligaments of the wrist, accurate fracture reduction and union are crucial.[45] Complications of radial styloid fracture include associated

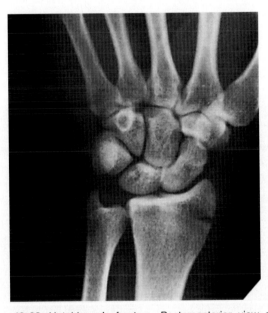

Figure 48-23. Hutchinson's fracture. Posteroanterior view shows intra-articular fracture of the radial styloid. (From Greenspan A: *Orthopedic Radiology: A Practical Approach,* 2nd ed. New York, Gower Medical Publishing, 1992.)

scapholunate ligament disruption and posttraumatic arthritis, both of which are more likely when there is fracture displacement.

Radioulnar Joint Disruption

Dislocation of the DRUJ may be seen in association with distal radial fractures and Galeazzi's fractures. It also may be seen as an isolated injury without fracture. Diagnosis is often difficult because plain radiographs commonly are reported as normal, so a careful clinical examination looking for certain characteristic findings may be the only clue to the presence of this injury.

The typical mechanism of injury is a fall on the out-stretched hand with either hyperpronation, resulting in dorsal dislocation, or hypersupination, causing volar dislocation of the ulna. Another mechanism known to cause DRUJ dislocation occurs when the hand is caught in rotating machinery, resulting in the same forcible hyperpronation or supination. This forcible rotation of the wrist causes disruption of the triangular fibrocartilage complex, the major stabilizer of the DRUJ, and may result in an associated avulsion fracture of the ulnar styloid.

Patients with this injury have a history of sudden onset of pain with a "snapping" sensation in the wrist, swelling, and limited range of motion. On examination, there is tenderness over the ulnar aspect of the wrist, with palpable crepitus on supination and pronation. With a dorsal dislocation of the ulna, the ulnar styloid appears more prominent than on the unaffected side, and there is significant pain and limitation of movement on supination of the wrist. With a volar dislocation of the ulna, there is loss of the normal ulnar styloid prominence, with pain and limitation of movement on pronation. These characteristic clinical findings should alert the physician to the possibility of DRUJ disruption and prompt the appropriate investigations to confirm the presence or absence of this injury.

Plain radiographs of the wrist may show the presence of DRUJ dislocation, but pain and inability of the patient to rotate the wrist fully may cause a false-negative result because a true lateral view cannot be obtained. It also is important to assess for radial head fractures because these fractures commonly are associated with DRUJ disruption. If there is significant clinical suspicion of injury and plain radiographs appear normal, a CT scan of the DRUJ is recommended.[46,47]

Treatment of these acute injuries requires orthopedic consultation for reduction and stabilization. Closed reduction with the forearm in supination and a long arm cast is often successful. Alternatively, open reduction is often necessary with volar dislocations because the ulnar head often is locked on the volar distal radius. Operative reduction also is necessary in dorsal dislocations to repair the associated injury to the triangular fibrocartilage complex. Immobilization in a long arm cast usually is maintained for 6 weeks.

Pediatric Fractures of the Distal Radius

Fractures of the distal radius in children may be divided into two types: fractures involving the distal radial metaphysis and fractures involving the growth plate. They usually occur as a result of a fall on an outstretched hand with the wrist forcibly dorsiflexed. Fractures of the radial metaphysis are of three types: torus fractures, greenstick fractures, and complete fractures. The torus fracture is the most common of these fractures and results in a buckling of the radial cortex, which, because of the strong periosteum, is seen without significant displacement (Figure 48-24). These fractures are treated with immobilization in a short arm cast with orthopedic follow-up. Healing usually occurs over 2 to 3 weeks, and complications are rarely seen.[48] Greenstick fractures also are incomplete metaphyseal fractures, with disruption of the cortex on one side and angulation or bowing on the opposite side. By definition, these fractures are displaced and require reduction with regional or general anesthesia if angulated more than 10 degrees. Angulations of less than 10 degrees usually remodel. Short arm well-molded cast

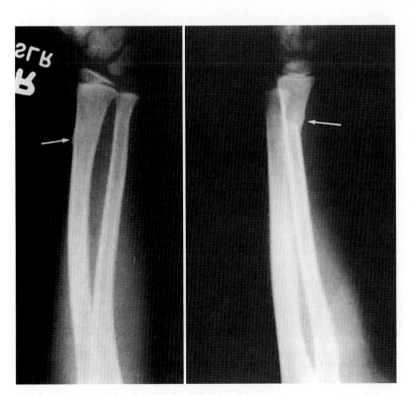

Figure 48-24. Torus fracture of the distal radius. Antero-posterior and lateral views of a radial torus fracture with buckling of the radial cortex. (From Dvorkin ML: *Office Orthopaedics.* Norwalk, Conn, Appleton & Lange, 1993.)

Table 48-2. Salter-Harris Classification

Salter-Harris Type	Radiographic Finding	Complication
I	Epiphyseal and metaphyseal separation. No fracture on x-ray	None
II	Fracture through metaphysis and physis (Thurston Holland sign)	Usually none
III	Fracture through epiphysis to physis	Concern with anatomic alignment. High rate of displacement while casted
IV	Fracture from epiphysis through physis to metaphysis	Early partial growth arrest. Surgical management recommended
V	Severe crush force through epiphysis to an area of the physis. Initial x-rays are normal	Severe growth arrest with progressive shortening or angular deformity. Premature or uneven physeal fusion
VI (Rang)	Peripheral bruise or injury to the perichondrial ring or periosteum at the edge of the physis	Severe growth arrest, angular deformity, or osseous bridge formation between physis and metaphysis. Osteochondroma formation

immobilization is recommended, with close orthopedic follow-up to ensure maintenance of reduction. Complete fractures of the radial metaphysis involve complete disruption of both cortices of bone and usually result in significant displacement and angulation. These fractures also may be associated with a fracture of the distal ulna. Closed reduction by an orthopedic surgeon with regional or general anesthesia may be successful, but if alignment is unsatisfactory or if the fracture is unstable, open reduction with internal fixation may be necessary.[49]

In 1963, Salter and Harris classified growth plate injuries in children (Table 48-2). Growth plate or physeal fractures of the distal radius are usually Salter-Harris type I or type II. Although these injuries result in disruption of the growth plate, they rarely result in growth disturbance.[50] Type I injuries cause pain and palpable tenderness over the distal radial physis, with the only radiographic abnormality being volar displacement of the pronator quadratus fat pad. These injuries may be treated with a short arm cast or splint immobilization for 3 to 4 weeks; orthopedic follow-up is suggested within 1 week of the injury. Type II injuries involve a fracture through the radial metaphysis and the physis and are visible on routine wrist radiographs as a triangular metaphyseal fragment on the dorsal surface of the radius (Figure 48-25). These fractures may be complicated by displacement of the radial epiphysis or by an associated fracture of the distal ulna.

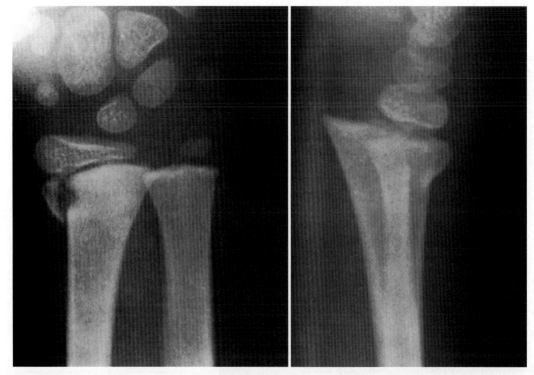

Figure 48-25. Salter-Harris type II distal radial fracture showing typical triangular metaphyseal fracture fragment, with associated epiphyseal fracture displacement. (From Harris JH, et al: *The Radiology of Emergency Medicine*, 3rd ed. Baltimore, Williams & Wilkins, 1993.)

If displaced, these injuries require orthopedic referral for closed reduction under general anesthesia and immobilization in a short arm cast for 6 weeks. Operative fixation may be necessary if adequate alignment can-not be achieved or maintained with closed reduction and casting.

SOFT TISSUE INJURIES OF THE WRIST

Carpal Tunnel Syndrome

Carpal tunnel syndrome is a neuropathy of the median nerve at the wrist that occurs as a result of compression of the median nerve within the carpal tunnel. The transverse carpal ligament and the volar surfaces of the carpal bones form the carpal tunnel. It is a rigid compartment that contains nine flexor tendons (the flexor pollicis longus tendon, four flexor digitorum superficialis tendons, and four flexor digitorum profundus tendons) and the median nerve. Any process (local or systemic) that results in an increase in pressure within this compartment may produce carpal tunnel syndrome.

The most common causes of carpal tunnel syndrome are distal radius fractures and repetitive strain. Carpal tunnel syndrome also can be associated with rheumatoid arthritis, hypothyroidism, diabetes mellitus, and collagen vascular diseases. Each of these systemic diseases is thought to produce an increase in pressure within the carpal tunnel from thickening of the flexor synovia or transverse carpal ligament. Hormonal changes associated with pregnancy and menopause also are known to cause carpal tunnel syndrome, probably by retention of fluid in the soft tissues about the wrist.[51]

The classic symptoms include a gradual onset of numbness, paresthesia, and pain in the thumb, index finger, and long finger. These symptoms are often bilateral and are worse during the night and after strenuous activities. Typically, patients report numbness and paresthesias on awakening that improves when the hands are shaken or held in a dependent position.

On physical examination, the most sensitive provocative test is the wrist flexion test, or Phalen's test (sensitivity 76%, specificity 80%) (Figure 48-26).[52] This test is performed by asking the patient to flex the wrists fully for 60 seconds while the forearms are held in a vertical position. The test is positive if paresthesias or numbness develops in the median nerve distribution. Another test, Tinel's sign, is positive if light tapping or percussion over the median nerve at the wrist produces pain or paresthesias in the median nerve distribution. Analysis of the literature suggests, however, that Tinel's sign (sensitivity 64%, specificity 55%) is not as powerful a test as Phalen's test in detecting median nerve compression, although neither is 100% sensitive. Given that neither Phalen's test nor Tinel's sign is completely reliable in making the diagnosis of carpal tunnel syndrome, nerve conduction studies have been

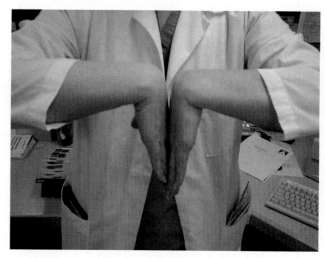

Figure 48-26. Phalen's test.

used to confirm the diagnosis, with reports of 90% sensitivity.[53] Conservative treatment for carpal tunnel syndrome has varying results. Treatment includes splinting the wrist in a neutral position and cortisone injections in the carpal tunnel. Splinting initially may be prescribed full-time for 3 or 4 weeks, then reduced to splinting at night only. Nonsteroidal anti-inflammatory drugs have proved to be of little benefit. Surgical release of the flexor retinaculum to unroof the carpal tunnel is indicated when nonoperative management fails.[53,54]

FOREARM

PERSPECTIVE

Accurate evaluation of forearm injuries requires a thorough knowledge of the complex anatomic relationships between the radius and ulna. The ulna may be thought of as a stable structure around which the radius rotates, allowing supination and pronation to occur. With any injury to the forearm, the clinician should suspect an associated injury involving the elbow or wrist joints. The clinical and radiologic evaluation of forearm injuries should include the wrist and elbow. The biomechanical interdependence of the radius and ulna means that accurate reduction and fixation of forearm fractures is essential to maintain full pronation and supination.[55]

Anatomy

The bones of the forearm consist of the radius and ulna, which articulate at each end at the proximal radioulnar joint and DRUJ. The capsule of the elbow joint and the annular ligament provide soft tissue support at the proximal articulation. Distally the anterior and posterior radioulnar ligaments and the triangular fibrocarti-

Table 48-3. Compartments of the Forearm

	Muscles	Nerves	Vessels
Volar compartment			
Superficial layer	Pronator teres Flexor carpi radialis Palmaris longus Flexor carpi ulnaris	Median nerve (except flexor carpi ulnaris supplied by ulnar nerve)	Ulnar and radial arteries
Deep layer	Flexor digitorum superficialis Flexor pollicis longus Pronator quadratus Flexor digitorum profundus	Median nerve (except medial half of flexor digitorum profundus supplied by ulnar nerve)	Ulnar and radial arteries
Dorsal compartment			
Superficial layer	Brachioradialis Extensor carpi radialis longus Extensor carpi radialis brevis Extensor digitorum Extensor digiti minimi Extensor carpi ulnaris	Radial nerve	Ulnar artery
Deep layer	Supinator Abductor pollicis longus Extensor pollicis brevis Extensor pollicis longus Extensor indicis proprius	Radial nerve	Ulnar artery

lage complex support the radioulnar joint. Of all these soft tissue supports, the triangular fibrocartilage complex acts as the major stabilizer of the DRUJ. The interosseous membrane and the supinator, pronator teres, and pronator quadratus muscles join the shafts of the radius and ulna. These muscles act as important supports to the radial and ulnar shafts and are responsible for the significant bony displacement seen with some forearm fractures.

The forearm is divided into two compartments, one volar to the forearm bones and interosseous membrane and one dorsal, and the antebrachial fascia encloses each compartment. The volar compartment contains the flexors and pronators of the wrist and hand, and the dorsal compartment contains the extensor muscles of the wrist and hand. The muscles of each compartment are divided further into a superficial and deep layer. The nerves and vessels of each compartment lie between the superficial and deep muscle layers (Table 48-3).

CLINICAL FEATURES

The clinical assessment of forearm injuries begins with a detailed history of the mechanism of injury. The physical examination includes inspection of the injured forearm, taking note of any deformity or discoloration or lacerations of the overlying skin. Observation of the patient's attempts at range of motion at the wrist and elbow joints is important, and results can be compared with range of motion of the "normal" uninjured side. The site of maximal tenderness should be determined by palpation along the entire length of the radius and ulna and by palpation of the soft tissues over the dorsal and volar surfaces of the forearm. The neu-

rovascular examination of the forearm should include evaluation of the brachial artery pulse proximally and the radial and ulnar pulses distally and an assessment of distal radial, median, and ulnar nerve function.

DIAGNOSTIC STRATEGIES: RADIOLOGY

The routine radiographic views of the forearm are anteroposterior and lateral views and should include the wrist and elbow joints. The inclusion of the joint above and below the forearm is crucial because a fracture or dislocation at one end may be associated with a similar abnormality at the opposite end. The normal anatomic relationships between the distal radius and ulna, including the radial length measurement, the normal volar tilt of the radius, and the ulnar slant of the distal radial articular surface, have been described in the section on radiology of the wrist (see Figure 48-4). These same relationships are visible on the anteroposterior view of the forearm. The normal proximal radial alignment is seen best on the lateral view of the forearm, when a line drawn through the proximal radial shaft and radial head should intersect the capitellum (Figure 48-27). This alignment is particularly important to assess when looking for the presence of a radial head dislocation.

Observing the orientation of several bony projections of the radius and ulna assesses normal alignment of the radial and ulnar shafts. On the normal anteroposterior view, the radial styloid should point in a radial direction, and the biceps tuberosity of the proximal radius should point in an ulnar direction. On the normal lateral view, the ulnar styloid should point dorsally, and the coronoid process of the proximal ulna should point volarly. Any alteration in these normal relationships implies an abnormal rotational or axial deformity (Figure 48-28).

FOREARM FRACTURES

Shaft Fractures of Radius and Ulna

Fracture of the radial and ulnar shafts usually occurs as a result of a direct blow to the forearm, but may be

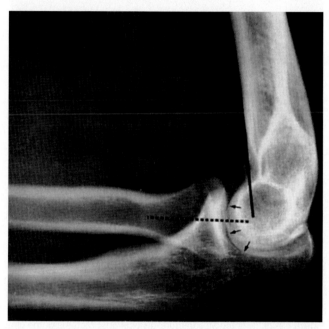

Figure 48-27. Normal lateral view of elbow. A line *(dashed)* bisecting the proximal radial shaft bisects the capitellum. (From Weissman BN, Sledge CB: *Orthopedic Radiology*. Philadelphia, WB Saunders, 1986.)

seen after a fall on the outstretched hand. In either case, the degree of force required to fracture both bones usually results in fracture displacement. Clinically, patients have obvious deformity of the forearm and pain and swelling at the fracture site. All movements of the forearm and hand are resisted because of pain. A neurovascular examination must be done to exclude associated neurologic impairment or early compartment syndrome. Anteroposterior and lateral radiographs of the forearm must include elbow and wrist joints to exclude an associated dislocation or articular fracture. Although these fractures are usually obvious on clinical examination, radiographs allow an accurate means of determining the amount of fracture displacement and comminution.

Undisplaced fractures are rare in adults, but when they do occur, they are treated conservatively with immobilization in a long arm cast for a minimum of 8 weeks. Prompt orthopedic follow-up and repeat radiographs should be arranged within 1 week of injury to ensure that displacement does not occur after casting.[56,57] Displaced fractures of the radial and ulnar shafts are treated surgically and should be splinted, and an orthopedic consultation should be obtained for open reduction and internal fixation. Fracture healing is usually complete in 6 months. Nonunion and malunion may occur in 3% to 5% of cases.[58] The most significant complication of this fracture is a compartment syndrome, which may result from the initial trauma or occur after surgery.

Ulnar Shaft Fractures

Isolated ulnar shaft fractures, or nightstick fractures, are relatively common and usually are caused by a direct blow to the forearm. Patients have localized pain

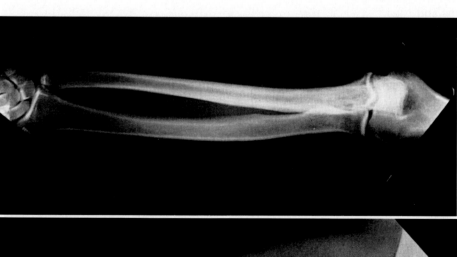

Figure 48-28. Normal anteroposterior and lateral views of the forearm. Both bones should be visible their entire length and should include the wrist and elbow joints. (From Propp DA, Chin H: Forearm and wrist radiology—Part I. *J Emerg Med* 7:393, 1989.)

and swelling over the site of the fracture. Radiographs of the forearm show this fracture and depict the degree of fracture displacement if present.

Undisplaced fractures of the distal third of the ulna may be treated with immobilization in a short arm cast for 6 to 8 weeks. Fractures of the middle or proximal third of the ulna require long arm cast immobilization. Weekly follow-up monitoring is recommended to confirm continued lack of displacement during the period of fracture healing. If loss of fracture position occurs, open reduction and internal fixation are necessary.

Displaced fractures of the ulna are defined as fractures with greater than 10 degrees of angulation or fractures with displacement greater than 50% of the diameter of the ulna.[59] Whenever significant displacement is present, radiographs should be examined carefully to rule out an associated dislocation of the radial head (Monteggia's fracture). Isolated displaced ulnar shaft fractures should be referred to an orthopedic surgeon for open reduction and internal fixation. Most fractures heal uneventfully with excellent results. Fractures of the middle third of the shaft may be complicated by nonunion if reduction is not adequately achieved or maintained.[59]

Monteggia's Fracture

In 1814, Monteggia described a fracture at the junction of the proximal and middle thirds of the ulna associated with anterior dislocation of the proximal radial head. This original description accounts for only 60% to 65% of proximal ulnar fractures with associated radial head dislocation. The entire spectrum of fracture-dislocations has since been classified by Bado[60] into four types of *Monteggia lesions,* depending on the site of the proximal ulnar fracture and the direction of fracture angulation and associated radial head dislocation. Overall, this injury is rare and accounts for only 7% of all fractures of the radius and ulna.[61]

The mechanism of injury of Monteggia's fracture is forced pronation of the forearm during a fall on the outstretched hand or a direct blow to the posterior aspect of the ulna. On clinical examination, pain and tenderness are present at the fracture site, and range of motion is limited at the elbow joint. The forearm may appear shortened compared with the unaffected side, and the radial head dislocation may be palpable in the antecubital fossa. A complete neurovascular examination is essential to rule out an associated radial nerve injury, which may be present in 17% of cases.

The proximal ulnar fracture is readily seen on anteroposterior and lateral radiographs of the forearm, but the elbow joint must be examined carefully to avoid missing the associated radial head dislocation (Figure 48-29). This dislocation is commonly missed, and delayed diagnosis has been reported in 24% of cases.[62] To avoid missing the associated radial head dislocation, the alignment should be confirmed on anteroposterior and lateral radiographs. A line drawn through the radial shaft and head normally should intersect the capitellum on all views.

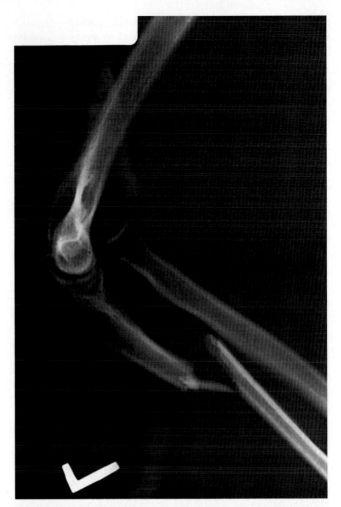

Figure 48-29. Monteggia's fracture-dislocation. Fractures of the ulna diaphysis with anterior angulation and associated anterior dislocation of the radial head. (From Propp DA, Chin H: Forearm and wrist radiology—Part I. *J Emerg Med* 7:393, 1989.)

Treatment of Monteggia's fracture is surgical, and immediate orthopedic referral should be arranged for definitive open reduction and internal fixation. An exception may be made in a pediatric patient, in whom closed reduction followed by a long arm cast may be effective. Casts should be in a flexed and supinated position to maintain fracture position. Flexion should be as close to 90 degrees as possible while ensuring the maintenance of a good radial pulse. Common complications include malunion or nonunion of the ulna fracture with redislocation or subluxation of the radial head. These complications are more likely to occur when the diagnosis has been delayed or when fracture fixation has been inadequate.[62]

Galeazzi's Fracture

Galeazzi's fracture involves the junction of the middle and distal thirds of the radius, with an associated dislocation or subluxation of the DRUJ. This rare injury accounts for only 7% of all fractures of

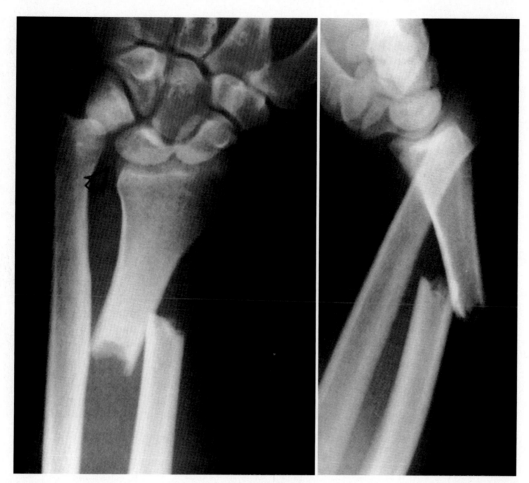

Figure 49-30. Galeazzi's fracture-dislocation. An obvious fracture of the distal third of the radius with severe displacement and an associated dislocation of the distal radioulnar joint *(open arrow).* (From Harris JH, et al: *The Radiology of Emergency Medicine,* 3rd ed. Baltimore, Williams & Wilkins, 1993.)

the forearm. This injury occurs as a result of a fall on the outstretched hand, with the wrist in extension and the forearm forcibly pronated. Another less common but well-described mechanism of injury is a direct blow to the dorsoradial aspect of the wrist. Clinical examination is often the key to diagnosis because disruption of the DRUJ may not otherwise be apparent. The radial fracture causes obvious swelling and deformity on the radial side of the forearm, and pain is localized over the fracture site. In addition, the DRUJ is swollen and painful on palpation, and the ulnar head appears prominent compared with the unaffected wrist.

On the anteroposterior radiograph, a transverse or short oblique fracture of the radius is visible at the junction of the middle and distal thirds of the radius. The radius appears shortened, and an increase in joint space may be visible between the distal radius and ulna. The lateral view shows dorsal angulation of the radial fracture, and the head of the ulna is displaced dorsally (Figure 48-30). An associated ulnar styloid fracture is seen in approximately 60% of cases and should alert the physician to the presence of disruption of the DRUJ.[63]

Galeazzi's fractures are inherently unstable. Occasionally, if the radial fracture is distal, a closed reduction of the radius and reduction of the DRUJ in supination with a long arm cast can be successful. These fractures often require operative fixation, however. The instability is the result of several factors, including the distracting pull of the brachioradialis and pronator quadratus muscles and the associated disruption of the DRUJ. Operative treatment involves open reduction and internal fixation of the radial shaft fracture, with immobilization of the forearm in supination to maintain reduction of the DRUJ. Reports have suggested that failure of closed reduction of the DRUJ in some patients is due to soft tissue interposition, and in these cases open reduction and fixation of the DRUJ is recommended.[66]

Complications of Galeazzi's fracture include malunion and nonunion of the radial fracture and recurrent subluxation or dislocation of the DRUJ. These complications result in chronic pain, with significant limitation of pronation and supination, and are thought to be largely avoidable with appropriate open anatomic reduction and rigid internal fixation of the fracture.[65]

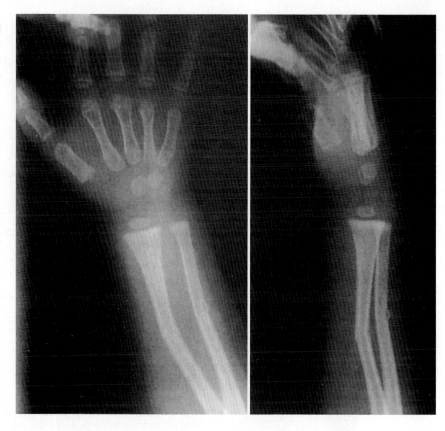

Figure 48-31. Pediatric forearm fracture. Anteroposterior and lateral views of radial and ulnar shaft fractures with dorsal angulation. (From Dvorkin ML: *Office Orthopaedics.* Norwalk, Conn, Appleton & Lange, 1993.)

Pediatric Forearm Fractures

Shaft Fractures of Radius and Ulna

In children, fractures to both bones of the forearm usually occur as a result of a fall on the outstretched hand. Fractures generally are classified into three types: buckle, or torus, fractures; incomplete, or greenstick, fractures; and complete fractures. The forearm fracture is usually obvious clinically, with significant pain, swelling, and visible deformity at the fracture site. Anteroposterior and lateral radiographs of the forearm distinguish whether fractures are complete or incomplete and show the degree of angulation and rotational deformity (Figure 48-31).

The objective of successful treatment of forearm fractures in children does not differ significantly from treatment in adults; the goal is successful reduction of fracture deformity. Nevertheless, in children, there is the potential for spontaneous correction of residual fracture angulation with bone remodeling. The younger the child (especially <10 years old), and the closer the fracture is to the growth plate, the greater the potential for remodeling. These principles govern the acceptability of fracture reduction, and generally angulations of less than 10 degrees are considered acceptable.[67]

Greenstick and complete forearm fractures require orthopedic referral for closed reduction under deep procedural sedation or general anesthesia. Results are usually excellent if correction of angular and rotational deformity is achieved and maintained. Immobilization in a long arm cast is usually necessary for 7 to 8 weeks. Open reduction and internal fixation are occasionally necessary if closed reduction is unsuccessful or cannot be maintained with casting. Complications of malunion and nonunion are rarely seen because of rapid healing and a tremendous capacity for remodeling.[49]

Plastic Deformation

The occurrence of plastic deformation of bone is unique to children and refers to a bending of the bone without overt fracture. Plastic deformation may be seen as an isolated injury to the radius or ulna, or it may be seen in one bone in combination with a fracture of the other bone. Clinically, this injury produces localized pain and deformity of the forearm, and radiographically it appears as a fixed curvature of the bone shaft (Figure 48-32). If significant curvature is present, the deformity is obvious, and pronation and supination are significantly restricted. Treatment requires orthopedic referral for closed reduction under general anesthesia and immobilization in a long arm cast for 6 to 8 weeks.[68]

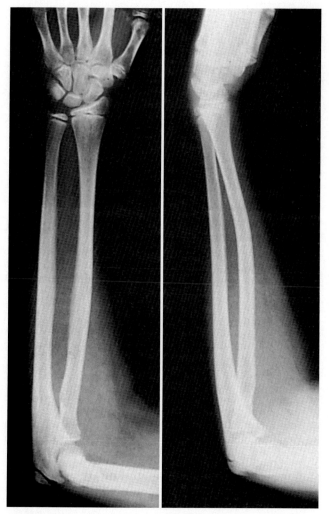

Figure 48-32. Acute plastic bowing fracture of the forearm. Anteroposterior and lateral views show broad volar bowing of the radial shaft with no visible fracture lucency. (From Komara JS, et al: Acute plastic bowing fractures in children. *Ann Emerg Med* 15:585, 1986.)

 KEY CONCEPTS

- Plain radiographs fail to detect 15% of scaphoid fractures. For this reason, and the associated risk of nonunion when diagnosis and immobilization are delayed, patients clinically suspected of having a scaphoid fracture should be placed in a short arm thumb spica cast with repeat x-rays in 10 to 14 days.

- Triquetral fracture is best seen on the standard lateral view of the wrist as a small dorsal chip fragment, although a more oblique pronated lateral view may be necessary.

- Lunate dislocation results in a characteristic triangular appearance of the lunate on the posteroanterior view (piece of pie sign) because of the rotation of the lunate in a volar direction. This rotation also is visible on the lateral view of the wrist, where the lunate looks like a cup tipped forward and spilling its contents into the palm (spilled teacup sign).

- In carpal dislocations, the articular surfaces on the posteroanterior view form three parallel arcs. The articular surfaces between carpal bones are parallel and 1 to 2 mm apart (parallelism).

- Colles' fracture requires prompt anatomic reduction in the emergency department, with full restoration of radial length and correction of the dorsal angulation either to a neutral position or ideally to the normal volar tilt position. Closed reduction, using local or regional anesthesia, with cast immobilization is successful in most cases.

- Anteroposterior and lateral views of the forearm must include the wrist and elbow joints because radial and ulnar forearm fractures may be associated with proximal, radial, or DRUJ dislocations.

REFERENCES

1. Larsen CF, Lauristen J: Epidemiology of acute wrist trauma. *Int J Epidemiol* 22:911, 1993.
2. Bednar JM, Osterman AL: Carpal instability: Evaluation and treatment. *J Am Acad Orthop Surg* 1:10, 1993.
3. Watson HK, Weinzweig J: Physical examination of the wrist. *Hand Clin* 13:17, 1997.
4. Greenspan A: *Orthopedic Radiology: A Practical Approach,* 2nd ed. New York, Gower Medical Publishing, 1992.
5. Schreibman KL, et al: Imaging of the hand and wrist. *Orthop Clin North Am* 28:537, 1997.
6. Lacey JD, Hodge JC: Pisiform and hamulus fractures: Easily missed wrist fractures diagnosed on a reverse oblique radiograph. *J Emerg Med* 16:445, 1998.
7. Amadio PC, Taleisnik J: Fractures of the carpal bones. In Green DP (ed): *Operative Hand Surgery,* vol 1. New York, Churchill Livingstone, 1993, 799.
8. Cooney WP, Linscheid RL, Robyns JH: Fractures and dislocations of the wrist. In Rockwood CA, Green DP, Bucholz RW (eds): *Fractures in Adults,* vol 1, 4th ed. Philadelphia, Lippincott-Raven, 1996, pp 563-678.
9. Parvizi J, et al: Combining the clinical signs improves diagnosis of scaphoid fractures: A prospective study with follow-up. *J Hand Surg* 23B:324, 1998.
10. Kirk M, Orlinsky M, Goldberg R: The validity and variability of the navicular fat stripe as a screening test for the detection of navicular fractures. *Ann Emerg Med* 19:1371, 1990.
11. Mehta M, Brautigan MW: Fracture of the carpal navicular: Efficacy of clinical findings and improved diagnosis with six view radiography. *Ann Emerg Med* 19:255, 1990.
12. Tiel van Buul MMC, et al: The value of radiographs and bone scintigraphy in suspected scaphoid fracture. *J Hand Surg* 18B:403, 1993.
13. Shewring DJ, Savage R, Thomas G: Experience of the early use of technetium 99 bone scintigraphy in wrist injury. *J Hand Surg* 19B:114, 1994.
14. Murphy DG, Eisenhauer MA: The utility of a bone scan in the diagnosis of clinical scaphoid fracture. *J Emerg Med* 12:709, 1994.
15. Tiel van Buul MMC, et al: Significance of a hot spot on the bone scan after carpal injury: Evaluation by computed tomography. *Eur J Nucl Med* 20:159, 1993.
16. Jonsson K, et al: CT of the wrist in suspected scaphoid fracture. *Acta Radiol* 33:500, 1992.
17. Bain GI, et al: Longitudinal computed tomography of the scaphoid: A new technique. *Skeletal Radiol* 24:271, 1995.
18. Kukla C, et al: Occult fractures of the scaphoid. *J Hand Surg* 22B:810, 1997.

19. Murphy DG, et al: Clincial scaphoid fracture: Can day four bone scans accurately predict the presence or absence of scaphoid fracture? *Ann Emerg Med* 26:434, 1995.

20. Woolfrey K, et al: Accuracy of day four bone scans and efficacy of clinical findings in the assessment of patient with clinical scaphoid fractures. *Ann Emerg Med* 34:544, 1999.

21. Breitenseher MJ, et al: Radiographically occult scaphoid fractures: Value of MR imaging in detection. *Radiology* 203:245, 1997.

22. Hunter JC, et al: MR imaging of clinically suspected scaphoid fractures. *AJR Am J Roentgenol* 168:1287, 1997.

23. Fowler C, Sullivan B, Williams LA: A comparison of bone scintigraphy and MRI in the early diagnosis of the occult scaphoid waist fracture. *Skeletal Radiol* 28:683, 1998.

24. Kerluke L, McCabe SJ: Non-union of the scaphoid: A critical analysis of recent natural history studies. *J Hand Surg* 18A:1, 1993.

25. Duppe H, et al: Long term results of fracture of the scaphoid. *J Bone Joint Surg* 76A:249, 1994.

26. Salmon J, Stanley JK, Trail IA: Kienbock's disease: Conservative management versus radial shortening. *J Bone Joint Surg Br* 82:820, 2003.

27. Cohen MS: Fractures of the carpal bones. *Hand Clin* 13:587, 1997.

28. Hocker K, Menshik A: Chip fractures of the triquetrum: Mechanism, classification and results. *J Hand Surg* 19B:584, 1994.

29. Chin HW, Visotsky J: Wrist fractures. *Emerg Med Clin North Am* 11:703, 1993.

30. Andresen R, et al: Imaging of hamate bone fractures in conventional x-rays and high resolution computed tomography. *Invest Radiol* 34:46, 1999.

31. Whalen JL, Bishop AT, Linscheid RL: Nonoperative treatment of acute hamate hook fractures. *J Hand Surg* 17A:507, 1992.

32. Carroll RE, Lakin JF: Fracture of the hook of the hamate: Acute treatment. *J Trauma* 34:803, 1993.

33. Inston N, Pimpalnerkar AL, Avafa MA: Isolated fracture of the trapezium: An easily missed injury. *Injury* 28:485, 1997.

34. Yasuwaki Y, et al: Fracture of the trapezoid bone: A case report. *J Hand Surg* 19A:457, 1994.

35. Mayfield JK, Johnson RP, Kilcoyne RK: Carpal dislocations: Pathomechanics and progressive perilunar instability. *J Hand Surg* 5A:226, 1980.

36. Frankel VH: The Terry Thomas sign. *Clin Orthop* 135:311, 1978.

37. Herzberg G, et al: Perilunate dislocations and fracture-dislocations: A multicenter study. *J Hand Surg* 18A:768, 1993.

38. O'Heeghan CJ, et al: The natural history of an untreated isolated scapholunate interosseous ligament injury. *J Hand Surg* 28B:307, 2003.

39. Watson HK, Weinzweig J, Zeppieri J: The natural progression of scaphoid instability. *Hand Clin* 13:29, 1997.

40. Colles A: On the fracture of the carpal extremity of the radius. *Edinb Med Surg J* 10:182, 1814.

41. Aro HT, Koivunen T: Minor axial shortening of the radius affects outcome of Colles' fracture treatment. *J Hand Surg* 16A:392, 1991.

42. Trumble TE, Schmitt SR, Vedder NB: Factors affecting functional outcome of displaced intra-articular distal radius fractures. *J Hand Surg* 19A:325, 1993.

43. Mehta JA, Bain GI: An overview of distal radius fractures. *Aust J Rural Health* 7:121, 1999.

44. Mehara AK, et al: Classification and treatment of volar Barton fractures. *Injury* 24:55, 1993.

45. Leibovic SJ, Geissler WB: Treatment of complex intra-articular distal radius fractures. *Orthop Clin North Am* 25:685, 1994.

46. Bruckner JD, Alexander AH, Lichtman DM: Acute dislocations of the distal radioulnar joint. *Instr Course Lect* 45:27, 1996.

47. Burk DL Jr, Kavasick D, Wechsler RJ: Imaging of the distal radioulnar joint. *Hand Clin* 7:263, 1991.

48. Dicke TE, Nunley JA: Distal forearm fractures in children. *Orthop Clin North Am* 24:333, 1993.

49. Wilkins KE, O'Brien ET: Fractures of the shafts of the radius and ulna. In Rockwood CA, Wilkins KE, Beaty JH (eds): *Fractures in Children,* vol 3, 4th ed. Philadelphia, Lippincott-Raven, 1996, pp 415-508.

50. Salter RB, Harris WR: Injuries involving the epiphyseal plate. *J Bone Joint Surg* 45A:587, 1963.

51. Skandalakis JE, et al: The carpal tunnel syndrome: Part I. *Am Surg* 58:72, 1992.

52. Kushner SH, et al: Tinel's sign and Phalen's test in carpal tunnel syndrome. *Orthopedics* 15:1297, 1992.

53. Slater RR, Bynum DK: Diagnosis and treatment of carpal tunnel syndrome. *Orthop Rev* 22:1095, 1993.

54. Jimenez DF, Gibbs SR, Clapper AT: Endoscopic treatment of carpal tunnel syndrome: A critical review. *J Neurosurg* 88:817, 1998.

55. Graham TJ, et al: Disorders of the forearm axis. *Hand Clin* 14:305, 1998.

56. Griggs SM, Weiss AC: Bony injuries of the wrist, forearm, and elbow. *Clin Sports Med* 15:373, 1996.

57. Schemitsch EH, Richards RR: The effect of malunion on functional outcome after plate fixation of fractures of both bones of the forearm in adults. *J Bone Joint Surg* 74A:1068, 1992.

58. Richards RR, Corley FG: Fractures of the shafts of the radius and ulna: Part II. In Rockwood CA, Green DP, Bucholz RW (eds): *Fractures in Adults,* vol 1, 4th ed. Philadelphia, Lippincott-Raven, 1996, p 869.

59. Villarin LA, Belk KE, Freid R: Emergency department evaluation and treatment of elbow and forearm injuries. *Emerg Med Clin North Am* 17:843, 1999.

60. Bado JL: The Monteggia lesion. *Clin Orthop* 50:71, 1967.

61. Boyd HB, Boals JC: The Monteggia lesion: A review of 159 cases. *Clin Orthop* 66:94, 1969.

62. Ring D, Jupiter JB, Simpson NS: Monteggia fractures in adults. *J Bone Joint Surg* 80A:1733, 1998.

63. Bruckner JD, Lichtman DM, Alexander AH: Complex dislocations of the distal radioulnar joint. *Clin Orthop* 275:90, 1992.

64. Perron AD, et al: Orthopaedic pitfalls in the ED: Galeazzi and Monteggia fracture-dislocation. *Am J Emerg Med* 19:225, 2001.

65. Beneyto FM, et al: Treatment of Galeazzi fracture-dislocations. *J Trauma* 36:352, 1994.

66. Budgeon A, et al: Irreducible Galeazzi injury. *Arch Orthop Trauma Surg* 118:176, 1998.

67. Price CT: Fractures of the shafts of the radius and ulna: Part II. In Rockwood CA, Wilkins KE, Beaty JH (eds): *Fractures in Children,* vol 3, 4th ed. Philadelphia, Lippincott-Raven, 1996, p 443.

68. Komara JS, Kottamasu L, Kottamasu SR: Acute plastic bowing fractures in children. *Ann Emerg Med* 15:585, 1986.

49 Humerus and Elbow

Joel M. Geiderman

PERSPECTIVE

Injuries in the region of the elbow have a high potential for complications and residual disability. Early recognition of neurovascular and soft tissue complications has a salutary effect on the outcome in many of these injuries.

Anatomy

The humerus is a long bone that articulates proximally, at the shoulder, with the glenoid of the scapula to form the glenohumeral joint and distally with the radius and ulna to form the three-way elbow joint. The upper end of the humerus, the humeral head, is shaped like a near-hemisphere. Adjacent to the humeral head are two bony prominences, the greater and lesser tuberosities. Between these, on the anterolateral aspect of the humerus, runs the bicipital groove. The shaft of the humerus extends from the upper border of the insertion of the pectoralis major muscle superiorly to the supracondylar ridges inferiorly. The shaft is cylindrical on cross section in the upper half and tends to become flat in the distal portion in an anteroposterior direction. Three surfaces are described. The anterolateral surface presents the deltoid tuberosity for the insertion of the deltoid muscle, and below this is the radial soleus, which transmits the radial nerve and profunda artery. The anteromedial surface forms the floor of the intertubercular groove, but it normally has no outstanding surface markings. An exception is when the supracondylar process is present. The posterior surface is the origin for the triceps and contains the spiral groove.

The bony anatomy of the distal humerus and elbow is diagrammed in Figure 49-1. The distal end of the humerus tapers into two columns of bone, the medial and lateral condyles. Between the condyles, the bone thins, and the recess created is the coronoid fossa. The more proximal nonarticular portions of the condyles are the epicondyles. Just proximal to the epicondyles, the supracondylar ridges run up each side of the humerus. Collectively, these areas serve as points of origin for the muscles of the forearm. The wrist flexors originate from the medial epicondyle, and the wrist extensors originate from the lateral epicondyle. Fractures of the distal humerus often result in fragment displacement because of the pull of these strong forearm muscles on attachment sites.

The bony anatomy of the elbow allows for two complex motions: flexion-extension and pronation-supination. The elbow is composed of three articula-

tions within a common joint cavity. The trochlea is the articular surface of the medial condyle and articulates with the deep trochlear notch of the ulna formed by the olecranon inferiorly and posteriorly and by the coronoid process anteriorly. This articulation permits hinged flexion and extension at the elbow. The articular surface of the lateral condyle is the capitellum, which permits the radius to hinge on the elbow. The proximal radius consists of a disklike head supported by the smooth narrow radial neck. The radial head articulates with the capitellum of the humerus and with the radial notch of the ulna.

Four ligamentous structures are important in evaluating elbow injuries (Figure 49-2). The radial head is held in place by the annular ligament and the radial collateral ligament. Rotation of the radial head within the annular ligament permits pronation and supination. In addition, the ulnar collateral ligament and anterior capsule add stability to the joint. These structures

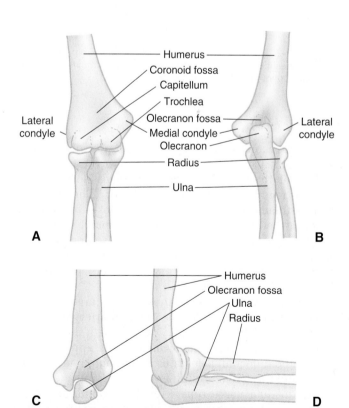

Figure 49-1. Bony anatomy of distal humerus and elbow region. **A,** Anterior view. **B,** Posterior view. **C,** Posterior view, 90 degrees flexion. **D,** Lateral view. Right elbow is shown. (Modified from Connolly JF: *DePalma's Management of Fractures and Dislocations.* Philadelphia, WB Saunders, 1981.)

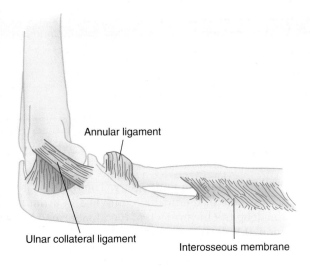

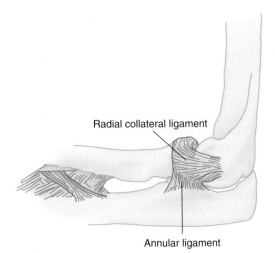

Figure 49-2. Ligamentous structures of elbow. (From Simon R, Koenigsknecht S: *Emergency Orthopaedics: The Extremities,* 2nd ed. Norwalk, Conn, Appleton & Lange, 1987.)

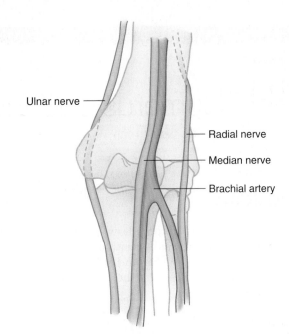

Figure 49-3. Neurovascular structures of elbow region. Volar surface of left elbow is shown.

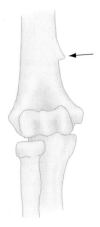

Figure 49-4. Supracondylar process of the humerus *(arrow).* Volar surface of right elbow is shown.

may be severely damaged with fracture or dislocation of the joint.

The soft tissues of the upper arm are divided into two compartments, anterior and posterior. The anterior compartment contains three muscles—the biceps brachii, the brachialis, and the coracobrachialis—and the brachial artery, median nerve, musculocutaneous nerve, and ulnar nerve. The only two structures contained in the posterior compartment are the triceps brachii muscle and the radial nerve.

The neurovascular structures of this area are diagrammed in Figure 49-3. The brachial artery, the continuation of the axillary artery, travels with the median nerve in the anterior compartment of the upper arm. It enters the antecubital fossa as diagrammed and bifurcates into the radial and ulnar arteries.

The median nerve runs with the brachial artery as diagrammed. One important anatomic variation is the presence of a supracondylar process just proximal to the medial epicondyle (Figure 49-4). When present, the median nerve and brachial artery must traverse behind this process, then forward between a fibrous band con-

necting the process to the epicondyle. Median nerve symptoms may develop if this process is fractured or if an injury causes swelling in the vicinity of the supracondylar process.

The radial nerve leaves the axilla and spirals posteriorly around the humerus between the heads of the triceps in the radial groove. It reenters the anterior compartment of the arm laterally, crossing the elbow anterior to the lateral epicondyle, to innervate the extensors of the wrist and fingers. Because of its close relationship to the shaft of the humerus, the radial nerve is particularly susceptible to injury with fractures of the midshaft of the humerus. Fixed in position by the intermuscular septum, the nerve may become trapped between fracture fragments, particularly when reduction is attempted.

The ulnar nerve runs parallel to the median nerve. Halfway down the arm, it penetrates the intermuscular septum to run along the medial aspect of the triceps muscle in the posterior compartment. It enters the forearm by passing behind the medial condyle. Fractures in the vicinity of the medial condyle place this nerve at considerable risk for injury.

Three elbow bursae are clinically important. The olecranon bursa is located between the olecranon and the skin posterior to the joint. This bursa provides protective padding and allows smooth movement of the skin over the olecranon. Because of its position, it is often a site of traumatic or infectious bursitis. The radio-humeral bursa provides for smooth movement over the radial head with supination and pronation. A third bursa cushions the biceps tendon from the radius during flexion of the elbow. As evident by the descriptions of these structures, all are vulnerable when significant skeletal injury occurs in this region.

CLINICAL FEATURES

History

A history detailing musculoskeletal complaints includes a description of any pain in terms of quality, duration, location, palliative and provocative activities, severity, and radiation. Past medical history and occupational features are important in chronic problems. For traumatic injuries, a complete account of the incident is important because it provides information as to the mechanism of injury and some estimate of the energy delivered. Subjective complaints of numbness or weakness distal to the injury are important clues to possible neurovascular injury. In dealing with injuries in children, the possibility of child abuse must be considered.

Physical Examination

Inspection of the upper extremity is important, but manipulation of the painful extremity should be minimized and postponed to the end of the examination when possible. This is especially important with children. A great deal of useful information can be gathered by simple inspection. The position in which the extremity is held should be noted. Children with extension-type supracondylar fractures present with the arm held at the side with a characteristic S-shape configuration, whereas with flexion-type supracondylar fractures, the forearm is supported with the opposite hand with the elbow flexed to 90 degrees. Patients with radial head subluxation have the elbow only slightly flexed and hold the forearm in pronation.

Deformity is evidence not only of significant injury, but also of the type of injury. Increased prominence of the olecranon suggests a posterior dislocation of the elbow or extension supracondylar fracture, whereas loss of the normal olecranon prominence indicates anterior dislocation or flexion supracondylar fracture. The extremity also should be inspected for wounds that may indicate an open fracture, evidence of swelling, and change in color of the distal extremity.

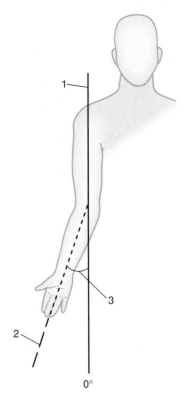

Figure 49-5. Carrying angle (3) is formed by intersection of lines drawn parallel to long axis of humerus (1) and ulna (2). (Modified from Ruiz E, Cicero J: *Emergency Management of Skeletal Injuries*. St Louis, Mosby, 1995.)

One special aspect of the elbow examination is the determination of the carrying angle, the normal outward angulation of the extended forearm at the elbow. This angle allows the long axes of the humerus and forearm to become superimposed when the elbow is flexed (Figure 49-5). This angle varies from 5 to 20 degrees in adults, with men having less angulation than women. Measurement of the carrying angle is helpful in assessing subtle supracondylar fractures in children. As shown in Figure 49-6, lines drawn parallel to the shafts of the humerus and ulna intersect to form an angle with a mean measurement in children of 13 degrees, although this angle varies widely.[1] A difference in carrying angles of greater than 12 degrees (from one side to the other for a particular individual) is associated with fractures.

The vascular status of the extremity is of highest priority. Brachial, radial, and ulnar pulses should be palpated and documented. The ulnar pulse is not palpable in some normal people. Although brisk capillary refill suggests adequate tissue perfusion, a hand-held Doppler device often is required to evaluate major vessel flow if significant swelling is present or if the pulses are not palpable. Any suspicion of arterial injury requires immediate investigation. Poor perfusion may result from direct arterial injury, compression or kinking in the instance of significant displacement from a fracture or dislocation, or a compartment syndrome. Passive extension of the fingers produces severe pain in the forearm in the presence of flexor (volar)

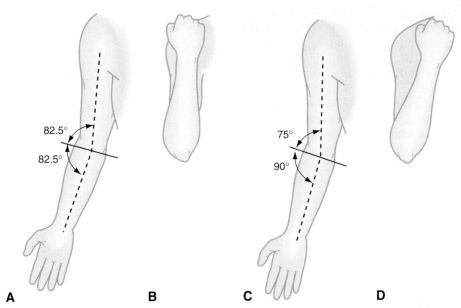

Figure 49-6. A, The axis of the elbow joint bisects the angle formed by the long axes of the humerus and forearm. **B,** This allows these axes to become superimposed when the elbow is flexed. **C,** If the axis of the elbow joint was perpendicular to the long axis of the forearm, the respective axes would diverge when the elbow was flexed, as shown in **D.**

compartment ischemia. Of the five *P*s associated with arterial occlusion (pain, paresthesia, pallor, pulselessness, and paralysis), pain is the only dependable early sign of compartment syndrome. Orthopedic consultation and measurement of compartment pressures should be considered for patients who have pain disproportionate to their injury. Other modalities used to evaluate vascular status before calling in the orthopedist include measurement of the ankle-brachial index and color flow Doppler (see Chapter 45 for further details).

Neurologic evaluation includes assessment of the radial, median, and ulnar nerves. After evaluation of neurovascular function, all bony prominences are palpated, and areas of tenderness are noted carefully and documented. Crepitus and bony deformities are highly suggestive of fracture or dislocation. The radial head specifically should be palpated for tenderness, and if present, an effusion should be noted.

The range of motion of the elbow in all planes (i.e., flexion-extension and pronation-supination) should be determined and documented. With the forearm supinated, the normal range of motion is 0 degrees in full extension to 150 degrees in full flexion. A mild degree of hyperextension is found in some normal individuals and should be symmetrical. With the elbow flexed at 90 degrees and the thumb facing up, the forearm normally supinates and pronates 90 degrees. Range-of-motion testing may be impossible with severe injuries and can be postponed until after radiographic evaluation, avoiding manipulating fractures and dislocations. Any manipulation of the extremity must be followed by re-examination because neurovascular injury has been reported with nearly every therapeutic procedure.

Radiographic Findings

It is not necessary to take x-ray films in all cases. Although clinical decision rules for the elbow have not been validated, it is reasonable to perform radiography when there is significant limitation in range of motion, obvious deformity, joint effusion, or significant tenderness over any of the bony prominences or the radial head. In the absence of these, it seems appropriate to omit radiography.

Routine views of the elbow include at least the anteroposterior and lateral views, with consideration given to obtaining oblique views for certain injuries. Anteroposterior and oblique views are taken with the elbow extended. The lateral view is taken with the elbow in 90 degrees of flexion and the thumb pointing upward. Positioning of the elbow is important because anything but a true lateral view makes accurate interpretation of soft tissue findings and alignment difficult. Corresponding views of the opposite extremity may be helpful, especially for children, but should not be ordered routinely.

Many fractures in the elbow region are obvious on x-ray film, with cortical disruption, angulation, or displacement of fragments. Minor fractures can be subtle and may be missed. Special attention to the contour of the radial head and the fat pads reduces the risk of missing fractures. The normal cortex of the radius is smooth and has a gentle continuous concave sweep. If consistent with history and physical findings, any disruption of this smooth arc is considered evidence of fracture. Abnormalities within the soft tissues on elbow films are particularly important and may be the only radiographic sign of a fracture. Normally, fat surrounding the proximal elbow joint is hidden in the con-

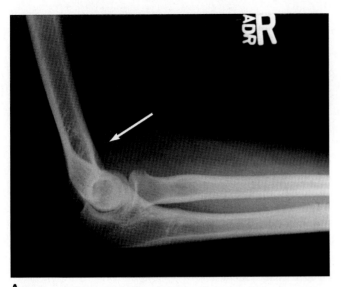

A

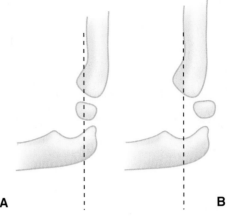

A　　　　　　　　　　　　**B**

Figure 49-8. A, A line drawn down anterior surface of humerus on lateral film should transect the middle of the capitellum. **B,** With extension supracondylar fracture, the line passes more anteriorly. (From Simon R, Koenigsknecht S: *Emergency Orthopaedics: The Extremities,* 2nd ed. Norwalk, Conn, Appleton & Lange, 1987.)

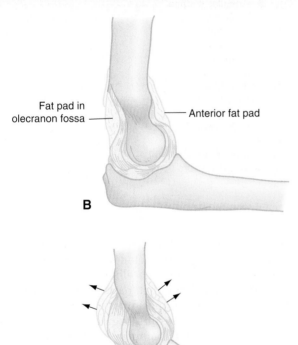

Fat pad in olecranon fossa —　　— Anterior fat pad

B

C

Figure 49-7. A, Anterior fat pad sign on lateral study (*arrow*). **B,** The anterior fat pad is normally a thin radiolucent stripe; the posterior fat pad is now seen. **C,** An effusion displaces both fat pads. This posterior fat pad is now visible.

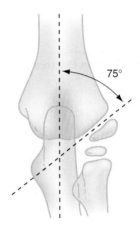

75°

Figure 49-9. Worlock P: Baumann's angle as measured on antero-posterior film. (From Supracondylar fractures of the humerus. *J Bone Joint Surg* 68B:755, 1986.)

cavity of the olecranon and coronoid fossae. The radiographically normal elbow has only a narrow strip of lucency anteriorly (the anterior fat pad), and a posterior fat pad is not visible. Injuries that produce intra-articular hemorrhage cause distention of the synovium and displace the fat out of the fossa, making the posterior fat pad visible on lateral x-ray views. The anterior fat pad also is altered by this swelling, becoming more prominent and taking the shape of a spinnaker sail from a boat (Figure 49-7). In the setting of trauma, more than 90% of patients with the "posterior fat pad" sign have intra-articular skeletal injury. These soft tissue findings occur even with subtle fractures, and

when present in the setting of trauma, an occult fracture is considered to be present even when not visible on the x-ray. In adults, a radial head fracture is implied, whereas in children, a supracondylar fracture is the probable underlying injury. In the absence of trauma, the presence of a fat pad suggests other causes of effusion (e.g., gout, infection, bursitis). The fat pad sign may be absent with a fracture if the injury is severe enough to have ruptured the capsule.

The anterior humeral line is a line drawn on a lateral radiograph along the anterior surface of the humerus through the elbow. Normally this line transects the middle third of the capitellum (Figure 49-8). With an extension supracondylar fracture, this line either transects the anterior third of the capitellum or passes entirely anterior to it. The abnormal relationship between the anterior-humeral line and capitellum may be the only evidence of a minimally displaced supracondylar fracture.

Another diagnostic aid in evaluating radiographs of suspected supracondylar fractures in children is the determination of Baumann's angle. As shown in Figure 49-9, the intersection of a line drawn on the antero-

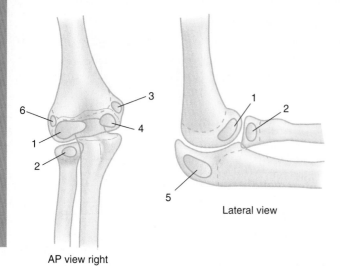

Figure 49-10. Secondary growth centers of the elbow. 1, Capitellum; 2, radial head; 3, medial epicondyle; 4, trochlea; 5, olecranon; 6, lateral epicondyle. (From Townsend DJ, Bassett GS: Common elbow fractures in children. *Am Fam Physician* 53:2031, 1996.)

AP view right

Lateral view

Table 49-1. Ossification Centers of the Elbow: CRITOE

Ossification Centers	Age of Appearance
Capitellum	1-2
Radial head	4-5
Internal (medial) epicondyle	4-5
Trochlea	8-10
Olecranon	8-9
External (lateral) epicondyle	10-11

BOX 49-1. Classification of Fractures

I. Humerus fractures
  A. Shaft of the humerus fractures
  B. Distal humerus fractures
    1. Supracondylar
      a. Extension
      b. Flexion
    2. Transcondylar
      a. Extension
      b. Flexion
    3. Intercondylar
      a. Nondisplaced
      b. Separated
      c. Separated and rotated
      d. Combination with articular surfaces
    4. Condylar
      a. Medial
      b. Lateral
    5. Articular surface
      a. Capitellum
      b. Trochlea
    6. Epicondylar
      a. Medial
      b. Lateral
II. Radial head fracture
  A. Nondisplaced
  B. Displaced
  C. Comminuted
III. Ulnar fracture
  A. Olecranon fracture
  B. Coronoid fracture

posterior film through the midshaft of the humerus and the growth plate of the capitellum defines an angle of approximately 75 degrees. In normal children, Baumann's angle is the same in both elbows, and it has been suggested that a comparison between the injured and uninjured sides be used to assess the accuracy of reduction. An increase in Baumann's angle indicates medial tilting of the distal fragment. Alteration in Baumann's angle is thought to predict the final carrying angle when the fracture heals, although there is controversy regarding its reliability.[2]

Radiographic evaluation of the elbow in children is difficult because of the presence of multiple ossification centers (Figure 49-10). Table 49-1 lists the typical age of first appearance and fusion of ossification centers. Comparison views of the uninjured elbow are often helpful in distinguishing fractures from the normal epiphyses and ossification centers.

Management

General management principles for humerus and elbow injuries are similar to management principles for other orthopedic injuries. Limb-threatening conditions, such as vascular injury, must be addressed immediately by reduction of fractures or surgical exploration. The limb should be splinted in a position of comfort, and appropriate analgesia should be provided. Antibiotics are administered for suspected open fractures. Prolonged immobilization of the elbow frequently results in stiffness of the joint that requires extensive physiotherapy to restore normal function. For this reason, range-of-motion exercises are begun early in the convalescent period, often before a fracture has healed completely.

FRACTURES

Injuries in the region of the shaft of the humerus and about the elbow fall into several categories (Box 49-1). Emergency department management varies with location and type of fracture or dislocation.

Fractures of the Shaft of the Humerus

Pathophysiology

Fractures of the humeral shaft most often result from a direct blow to the arm, such as occurs during a fall or motor vehicle crash. Occasionally, severe twisting of the arm or a fall on an outstretched hand produces this type of fracture. Fractures produced by violent muscle contraction also are reported, such as when throwing a javelin or baseball.[3] Motion of the humerus is controlled by several muscle groups. These same muscle groups also influence the fracture pattern of the

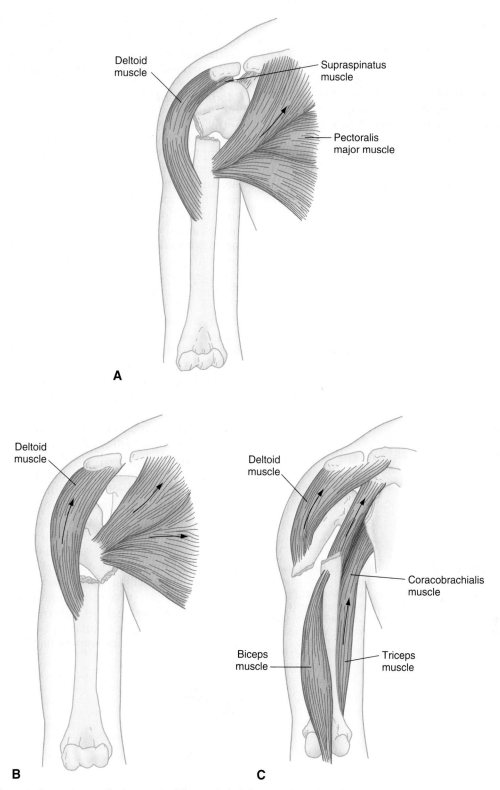

Figure 49-11. Influence of muscles on displacement of humeral shaft fractures based on fracture location (see text).

humeral shaft. If the fracture is located proximal to the attachment of the pectoralis major, the proximal fragment of the humerus abducts and rotates internally owing to the action of the rotator cuff, whereas the distal fragment is displaced medially by the pectoralis major (Figure 49-11A). If the fracture occurs below the pectoralis major insertion but above the deltoid insertion, the distal fragment is displaced laterally by the deltoid muscle, and the proximal fragment is displaced medially by the pull of the pectoralis major, latissimus dorsi, and teres major muscles (Figure 49-11B). In fractures occurring distal to the deltoid insertion, the proximal fragment is abducted by the deltoid, and the distal fragment is proximally displaced (Figure 49-11C). The shaft of the humerus most commonly fractures in the middle third in a transverse fashion.

Clinical Features

The patient complains of localized pain. The arm is visibly swollen and cannot be used. When a fracture is complete, bony crepitus is felt in the shaft of the humerus with any manipulation of the arm. The arm may be shortened or rotated, depending on the displacement of the fracture fragments. When the fracture is incomplete, the skeleton is tender to palpation and swollen, but not otherwise deformed. A complete neurovascular examination is indicated. Attention should be directed to radial nerve function because injury to this nerve is the most common complication associated with humeral shaft fractures.

X-ray findings are confirmatory. Studies routinely should include the shoulder and elbow joints. The humerus is a common site for benign tumors, unicameral cysts, and primary bone malignancies. The humeral shaft also is a common site for metastatic disease. Thinning of the cortex and abnormal osteoblastic or osteoclastic activity are evidence of a pathologic fracture. These fractures do not heal without concomitant treatment of the underlying pathologic condition.

Management

Closed fractures that are isolated injuries are treated conservatively with a high degree of success. Elaborate attempts at fracture reduction and external immobilization are unnecessary and sometimes detrimental to healing. Humeral shaft fractures remain surrounded by a richly vascularized envelope of muscle so that fracture reduction is accomplished most easily with the aid of gravity and muscle balance. Fractures that are nondisplaced or minimally displaced are immobilized by adding a coaptation, or "sugar-tong" splint, to the sling and swathe (Figure 49-12). This is accomplished by first padding the extremity, then carrying a long plaster splint from the lateral side of the shoulder, down the lateral aspect of the upper arm, around the elbow with the elbow flexed, and then up the inner aspect of the arm to the axilla. The sugar tong is wrapped in an elastic bandage, and a sling is used to support the arm in 90 degrees or less of flexion. The weight of the splint aided by gravity applies traction at the same time it immobilizes the fracture. Some authorities use the coaptation splint for only the first 10 to 14 days of treatment followed by a functional brace.

If the fracture is grossly displaced or comminuted, the hanging cast technique sometimes is used. This technique is especially effective with spiral fractures. The cast is lightweight, applied at least 1 inch proximal to the fracture site, and extends to the distal palmar crease of the hand. The elbow is flexed 90 degrees, and the wrist is placed in the neutral position. The sling is attached through a loop at the wrist. Angulation is corrected by placing the plaster loop on the dorsal aspect of the cast (to reduce lateral angulation) or on the volar side of the cast (to reduce medial angulation). Anterior or posterior angulation is corrected by altering the length of the sling apparatus (Figure 49-13). Care

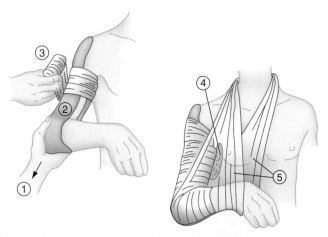

Figure 49-12. Sugar-tong splint for humeral shaft fractures. Gentle traction is applied (1) as the splint is placed (2) from over the deltoid laterally, under the elbow, and up into the axilla. An Ace wrap holds the splint in place (3). The axilla must be padded (4), and a sling is used (5). (Modified from Connolly JF: *DePalma's Management of Fractures and Dislocations.* Philadelphia, WB Saunders, 1981.)

Figure 49-13. Hanging cast technique.

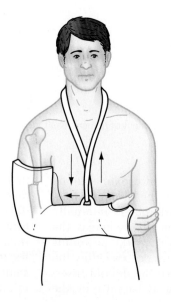
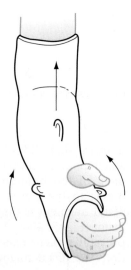

must be taken not to make the cast too heavy because this would distract fracture fragments. The hanging cast has the disadvantage of requiring gravity for traction and requires that the patient remain upright at all times, including during sleep, a situation that many patients find intolerable. Neurovascular examination is repeated after the application of any splint or cast. Loss of nerve function from entrapment of the nerve between fragments can occur after these interventions.

Open reduction and internal fixation is necessary in certain circumstances, including open fractures, presence of multiple injuries that preclude mobilization, bilateral fractures, poor reduction, poor patient compliance, failure of closed treatment, and fractures through pathologic bone.[4,5] Isolated radial nerve palsy usually is assumed to be a neurapraxia and is managed nonoperatively. Exploration and internal fixation are indicated, however, if the radial nerve palsy develops after manipulation because this is highly suggestive of nerve entrapment.[4]

All patients with humeral shaft fractures should be referred to an orthopedic surgeon for close follow-up monitoring. When dependency casting is used, follow-up evaluation within 24 to 48 hours is recommended to be certain that the alignment has been maintained. Emergent referral to an orthopedist is recommended for patients with evidence of radial nerve injury, severely displaced or comminuted fractures, open fractures, or fractures associated with forearm fractures in the same extremity.

Complications

The most common complication, radial nerve injury, occurs in 20% of humerus fractures. This nerve injury is most often a benign neurapraxia that resolves spontaneously in most patients, although recovery may take several months. Radial nerve injuries associated with penetrating trauma or open fractures are likely to be permanent and usually warrant operative exploration. Median and ulnar nerve injuries are rarely seen, usually in the presence of penetrating trauma. Injuries to the brachial artery occur rarely and, if suspected, angiography or other vascular studies should be considered.

Fractures of the Distal Humerus

Supracondylar Fractures

Distal humerus fractures that occur proximal to the epicondyles are called *supracondylar fractures*. This fracture is almost exclusively an injury of the immature skeleton. The peak incidence is in children 5 to 10 years old; the average age in a large combined series was 6.7 years.[6] This injury occurs rarely after age 15. In children, the tensile strength of the collateral ligaments and joint capsule of the elbow is greater than that of bone. In adults, the reverse is true, and a posterior elbow dislocation is sustained instead. Supracondylar fractures are classified as either extension or flexion fractures, depending on the mechanism of injury and the displacement of the distal fragment. Of these injuries, 98% are of the extension type.

Extension Supracondylar Fractures

Pathophysiology. Extension supracondylar fractures occur as a consequence of a fall on the outstretched arm, when the elbow is either fully extended or hyperextended. The elbow is likely to be in the latter position at the time of the fall because ligamentous laxity, with hyperextension of the joints, is a normal phenomenon in younger children. With the forearm acting as a lever, the ground reaction produces a moment of force at the elbow (Figure 49-14).[7] Ultimately the distal humerus fails anteriorly in the supracondylar area. The strong action of the triceps tends to pull and displace the distal fragment in a posterior and proximal direction. There may be anterior angulation of the sharp distal end of the proximal fragment into the antecubital fossa, endangering the brachial artery and median nerve (Figure 49-15). In most cases, however, the brachialis muscle protects the anterior neurovascular structures from injury.

Clinical Features. A child with a complete fracture comes to the emergency department holding the upper extremity immobile in extension to the side, with a typical S-shaped configuration and tenderness and swelling in the region of the elbow. Prominence of the olecranon attached to the posteriorly displaced distal fragment is similar to that seen with posterior dislocation of the elbow. When an incomplete supracondylar fracture exists, the diagnosis may be less obvious, with an elbow effusion as the only clinical sign. A careful neurovascular examination is essential. Although palpation is useful in determining the site of injury, the examining physician should avoid manipulation of the injury to elicit crepitus because movement can cause further neurovascular damage. Alleviating pain often facilitates the examination.

Diagnostic Strategies. On x-ray examination, the distal fragment is often displaced on the lateral view. This displacement is most likely to occur with a complete fracture wherein the muscle activity results in proximal migration of the distal fragment. Because this fracture occurs in children, 25% of supracondylar fractures are of the greenstick variety with the posterior cortex remaining intact. Subtle changes (e.g., the presence of a posterior fat pad or an abnormal anterior humeral line) may be the only radiographic clues to the presence of a fracture. In displaced fractures on the anteroposterior view, the distal fragments may be displaced either medially or laterally in relationship to the humerus. Often, with minimally displaced fractures, the fracture line is transverse and not visible on the anteroposterior view. Based on radiographic findings, extension supracondylar fractures are classified into three types: type I, minimal or no displacement; type II, displaced fracture, posterior cortex intact; and type III, totally displaced fracture, anterior and posterior cortex disrupted.

Management. Nondisplaced fractures (type I) are immobilized primarily for comfort and protection because they are inherently stable. They are treated in a splint or cast flexed to 90 degrees with the forearm in neutral rotation. Protected active range of motion is begun in approximately 3 weeks. Even without definite

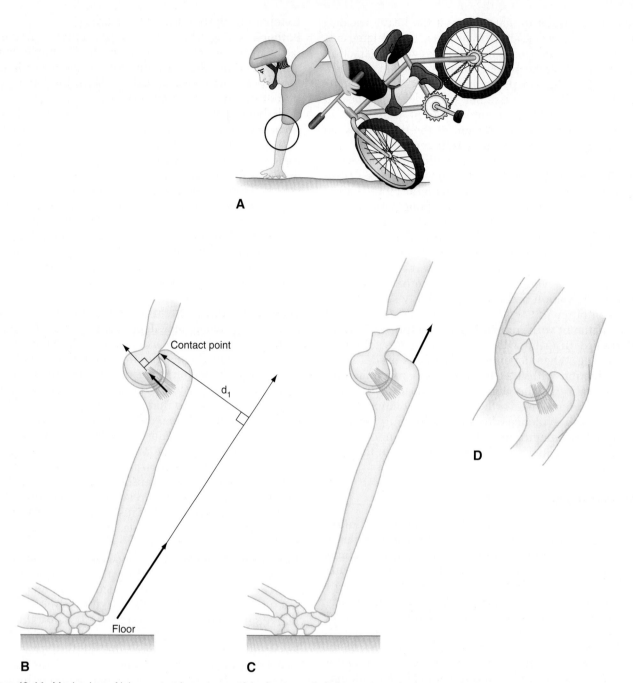

Figure 49-14. Mechanism of injury, extension supracondylar fractures. **A,** Fall on outstretched arm produces hyperextension of elbow. **B,** Ulna levers against distal humerus. **C,** Humerus fails, triceps exerts unopposed force. **D,** Distal fragment displaces.

radiographic findings, a child with localized tenderness consistent with a supracondylar fracture should be splinted and referred for follow-up examination. An x-ray study performed a few weeks after the injury may reveal periosteal new bone formation in the supracondylar region.

Minimally displaced (type II) fractures that are stable after reduction can be treated with splinting or casting with the elbow flexed. Some authors recommend flexion to 110 to 120 degrees for this injury.[6,8,9] This position uses the intact posterior periosteum as a tension band to hold the reduction; however, if swelling

or circulatory obstruction prevents this much flexion, it cannot and should not be used. The greater the flexion at the elbow, the greater the chance of vascular impairment. When swelling peaks at 24 to 48 hours, the risks of vascular obstruction and compartment syndrome are the greatest. Occasionally, these injuries must be pinned percutaneously to maintain stability, especially if a significant rotational component is present. Percutaneous pinning of a fracture after reduction has grown in popularity in recent years.[10]

Type III totally displaced fractures generally are the result of more severe injuries that produce more

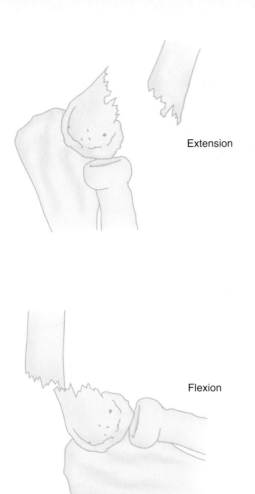

Extension

Flexion

Figure 49-15. Supracondylar fractures, extension and flexion. (Adapted from Simon R, Koenigsknecht S: *Emergency Orthopaedics: The Extremities,* 2nd ed. Norwalk, Conn, Appleton & Lange, 1987.)

swelling than type I or type II injuries. Displacement necessitates the re-establishment of length, increases the chance of varus deformity, and increases the chances of interposed soft tissues and neurovascular injury. For all these reasons, type III fractures require immediate orthopedic consultation.

The general principles that must be adhered to in treating these injuries are (1) achieving adequate reduction, (2) properly assessing reduction, and (3) maintaining the reduction. Closed reduction is attempted with the patient under anesthesia. If closed reduction is not possible or if the brachial artery seems to be trapped in the fracture site, open reduction may be necessary. When adequate reduction has been achieved, most authorities recommend percutaneous pin fixation to maintain the reduction.[7,11-13]

Reduction in the emergency department is indicated only when the displaced fracture is associated with vascular compromise that threatens the viability of the extremity. Under these conditions, closed reduction should be attempted. After appropriate conscious sedation, an assistant fixes the arm of the patient. The physician grasps the patient's wrist and applies steady, firm traction in line with the long axis of the limb (Figure

49-16A). The forearm is kept in the neutral, thumb-up position. While traction is maintained, correction of any medial or lateral displacement is accomplished with the other hand at the elbow (Figure 49-16B). If the distal fragment is displaced laterally, it is pushed inward; if it is displaced medially, it is pushed outward.

After length is restored and the angular deformity is corrected, the thumb of the free hand is placed over the anterior surface of the proximal fragment and the fingers behind the olecranon. While traction is maintained, the elbow is gently flexed to just beyond 90 degrees (Figure 49-16C). Angulation is corrected to a normal carrying angle.

Medially displaced supracondylar fractures are most prone to tilt into cubitus varus and are immobilized with the forearm pronated to tighten the brachioradialis and common extensor muscles. This procedure closes the fracture laterally. The less common laterally displaced fracture is immobilized in supination to close the fracture medially.

Only one attempt should be made at manipulation. Multiple attempts increase the likelihood of neurovascular injury and swelling. If reduction is unsuccessful, simple traction on the extended elbow may restore vascular supply. When reduction is performed, follow-up radiographs are obtained to ensure adequate reduction. Neurovascular function is checked at frequent intervals. Cylinder casts are not applied initially because they increase the risk of forearm ischemia; a posterior plaster splint provides safe and adequate immobilization.

Patients with type I fractures can be discharged safely from the emergency department with instructions to elevate the extremity and apply ice and have a follow-up evaluation in 1 to 2 days. Fractures that require manipulation usually warrant admission to the hospital to ensure compliance and for neurovascular monitoring.

Complications. Ten percent of children lose the radial pulse temporarily, most often as a result of swelling and not direct brachial artery injury. Reducing the fracture, avoiding flexing the elbow more than 90 degrees, and elevating the arm help prevent secondary obstruction to arterial flow. Compartment syndrome, or Volkmann's ischemic contracture as a result of prolonged ischemia of the forearm, is a dreaded complication but is rare in this era (reported incidence <0.5%).[10]

The most common complication is the loss of the carrying angle, resulting in a cubitus varus or "gunstock" deformity. Measurement of Baumann's angle postreduction is predictive of the final carrying angle. Cubitus varus has been reported previously in 25% to 60% of patients, depending on the management used.[2,14] This incidence has decreased significantly (<10%), with the use of percutaneous pinning. The distal humerus has little capacity to remodel because only 20% of the growth of the bone derives from the distal physis. A small amount of extension or flexion deformity produces little disability, has the greatest chance of remodeling, and is not a major cosmetic concern. Valgus or

Figure 49-16. A-C, Steps in reduction of displaced supra-condylar fracture (see text).

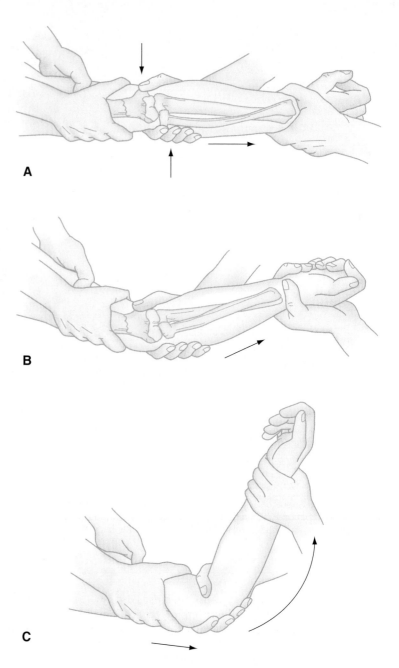

varus deformities, being in the coronal plane, have little or no chance of remodeling. Although cubitus varus is not a significant functional disability, it presents a significant cosmetic problem. In most cases, this complication can be corrected at a later time by an osteotomy.[15]

Nerve injuries occurred in 7% of 4520 fractures compiled from 31 major reported series. The radial, median, and ulnar nerves all are commonly involved. Most deficits seen at the time of injury are neurapraxias that resolve with conservative management. Motor function returns within 7 to 12 weeks, whereas recovery of sensation may take more than 6 months.[16]

Flexion Supracondylar Fractures

Pathophysiology. Flexion-type injuries are much less common, with a reported frequency of 1% to 10%; they account for 2% of all supracondylar fractures in a large pooled series of 7212 patients. The mechanism of injury is a direct blow to the flexed elbow. Energy is

transferred from the posterior aspect of the proximal ulna to the distal humerus, resulting in a supracondylar fracture with anterior displacement of the distal fragment. As the fragment displaces, the periosteum is torn posteriorly.

Clinical and Radiographic Features. The elbow is usually held in flexion rather than the extremity presenting in the S-shaped configuration seen in extension-type injuries. In displaced fractures, the normal olecranon process is not palpable, in contrast to the increased prominence of the olecranon seen with extension injuries.

Radiographically, these injuries can be classified into three types, similar to extension injuries:

- Type I fracture—undisplaced or minimally displaced
- Type II fracture—incomplete fracture; anterior cortex intact
- Type III fracture—completely displaced; distal fragment migrates proximally and anteriorly

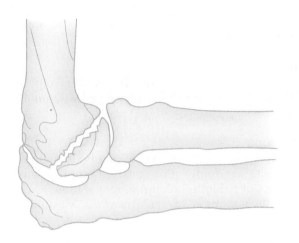

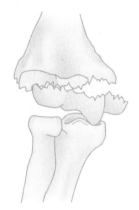

Figure 49-17. Transcondylar fracture of distal humerus. (*Left* from Ruiz E, Cicero J: *Emergency Management of Skeletal Injuries.* St Louis, Mosby, 1995. *Right* modified from Simon R, Koenigsknecht S: *Emergency Orthopaedics: The Extremities,* 2nd ed. Norwalk, Conn, Appleton & Lange, 1987.)

X-ray films may reveal a simple increase in the anterior angulation of the distal supracondylar fragment or gross displacement of the distal fragment proximal and anterior to the distal end of the proximal fragment. In the latter case, the distal end of the proximal fragment protrudes posteriorly. A line down the anterior humeral shaft intersects the capitellum either normally or posteriorly in these fractures, depending on whether there is anterior displacement.

Management. When the posterior periosteum is torn, the anterior periosteum functions as a tension band with the arm in extension. In type I fracture, the periosteum is minimally displaced. These injuries do not need to be immobilized in extension. The elbow can be comfortably flexed and should be immobilized in a splint as with extension injuries. Type II and III injuries should be referred to an orthopedist emergently. Type II injuries are manipulated into extension, then held either in a long arm cast or with percutaneous pins. Type III injuries often require open reduction.

Complications. The most common complication is injury to the ulnar nerve by the proximal fragment. The radial and median nerves are rarely injured. Stiffness of the elbow also may occur, especially after open reduction. Cubitus valgus may occur, but is not as cosmetically problematic as cubitus varus.

Transcondylar Fractures

Transcondylar (or dicondylar) fractures have a fracture line, either transverse or crescent-shaped, that passes through both condyles within the joint capsule just proximal to the articular surface (Figure 49-17). As with supracondylar fractures, two types have been described, extension and flexion, based on the position of the elbow when fractured, and extension types are the most common. The mechanism of injury is similar to that for supracondylar injuries. In contrast to supracondylar fractures, however, the injury is more common in elderly individuals with fragile, osteoporotic bone. These fractures generally are difficult to treat because the small distal fragment possesses little extra-articular bone, and only a small amount of bone contact is available for union.[17] During healing, excessive callus may form in the olecranon or coronoid

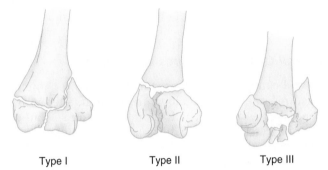

Figure 49-18. Intercondylar T fractures, types I, II, and III. (From Connolly JF: *DePalma's Management of Fractures and Dislocations.* Philadelphia, WB Saunders, 1981.)

fossae with residual loss of motion. Orthopedic consultation should be obtained for these injuries.

Intercondylar Fractures

Intercondylar fractures are usually T-shaped or Y-shaped fractures with variable degrees of separation of the condyles from each other and from the proximal humerus fragment (Figure 49-18). The distal portion of the fracture extends to the articular surface of the distal humerus. These injuries are rare and generally are seen in adults in their 50s and 60s.[18] The usual mechanism of injury is direct trauma to the elbow that drives the olecranon against the humeral articular surface and splits the distal end.

Clinical and Radiographic Features

Patients with intercondylar fractures complain of pain at the elbow, which on examination is tender to palpation. Good-quality anteroposterior and lateral x-rays are essential in evaluating fracture displacement and comminution. A computed tomography scan may be used to delineate fracture patterns further. Neurovascular complications are not common with these injuries.

Management

Intercondylar fractures are notoriously difficult and complicated to treat.[19,20] The goal of treatment is to reestablish articular congruity and alignment and to begin active motion as soon as possible. Open reduction with rigid internal fixation is usually preferred. Closed treatment has been recommended for elderly patients, for patients with medical conditions that prohibit surgery, and historically for patients with nondisplaced fractures. These injuries all should be referred to an orthopedic surgeon emergently. Similar to supracondylar fractures, manipulation should be avoided, unless limb-threatening ischemia is present. Traction across the elbow with the arm extended is helpful in restoring blood flow to an ischemic forearm.

Complications

Historically, loss of elbow joint function is the most common complication reported, although this now can be largely avoided with optimal surgical technique.[21] Any method of treatment that requires prolonged immobilization is likely to result in fibrosis or ankylosis of the joint. Neurovascular complications are rare.

Lateral Condyle Fractures in Children

Lateral condyle fractures are the second most common fractures involving the elbow in children, after supracondylar fractures.[22] The fracture occurs after a fall on the outstretched hand, with a varus stress applied to the extended arm.

Clinical and Radiographic Features

Tenderness and swelling are noted over the lateral aspect of the elbow. Generally, there is less swelling than with supracondylar fractures, and neurovascular compromise is uncommon. Diagnosis usually can be made on standard anteroposterior and lateral views, although an oblique view also may be helpful.

Management

Fractures with less than 2 mm displacement can be treated closed in a cast, whereas fractures with greater displacement require either open or closed reduction with pin fixation for 3 to 4 weeks.[22]

Complications

Fractures diagnosed and treated in a timely manner should have few complications, although historically, nonunion, valgus deformity, and avascular necrosis all have been reported.

Medial Condyle Fractures in Children

Medial condyle fractures are rare, comprising 1% to 2% of pediatric elbow fractures.[23] These fractures are type IV Salter injuries with physeal injury a possible outcome. The mechanism of injury is believed to be a valgus force on the extended elbow.

Clinical and Radiographic Features

The patient presents with tenderness and swelling over the medial aspect of the elbow. Anteroposterior, lateral, and oblique films may show the fracture in older children, but in children younger than age 9 the trochlea does not ossify until this time. Magnetic resonance

imaging (MRI) may be necessary to confirm the diagnosis in these patients.

Management

Operative treatment is indicated if displacement is greater than 2 mm; otherwise, conservative treatment is sufficient.

Complications

A study of 21 patients with medial condyle fractures revealed a 33% complication rate.[23] Complications included loss of reduction requiring reoperation, avascular necrosis, nonunion, and cubitus varus. Most minimally displaced fractures healed uneventfully.

Condylar Fractures in Adults

Condylar fractures are rare in adults and typically involve the articular surface and the nonarticular portion of the distal humerus, including the epicondyle (Figure 49-19). The lateral trochlear ridge is the key to analyzing humeral condyle fractures. It may be involved with either medial or lateral condylar fractures and, when incorporated into the distal fragment, is far more likely to result in instability.

Pathophysiology

Lateral condylar fractures are uncommon, although more common than medial condylar fractures. The mechanism of injury is either a direct blow to the lateral aspect of the flexed elbow or a force that results in adduction and hyperextension with avulsion of the lateral condyle. Medial condylar fractures are rare and result from either a direct blow to the apex of the flexed elbow or a fall on the outstretched arm with the elbow forced into varus.

Clinical and Radiographic Features

The presentation of condylar fractures is similar to that of other distal humerus fractures, with swelling, tenderness, and crepitus localized over either the medial or the lateral elbow. On palpation, independent motion of the involved condyle may be appreciated. In lateral condylar fractures, findings may be accentuated with movement of the radius. On radiographic examination, lateral condylar fractures show a widening of the intercondylar distance. The distal fragment is often displaced, most commonly posteriorly and inferiorly. Because of the location of the ulnar nerve, it is imperative to test its function when this fracture is present. Medial condylar fractures are associated with tenderness over the medial condyle and pain with flexion of the wrist against resistance. On x-ray examination, displaced distal fragments tend to be anterior and inferior because of the pull of the forearm flexors.

Management

Immediate treatment depends on x-ray findings. For undisplaced or minimally displaced condylar fractures, immobilization of the flexed elbow in a long arm posterior plaster splint is sufficient. For lateral condylar fractures, the forearm should be supinated and the wrist extended to relieve the tension on the extensor

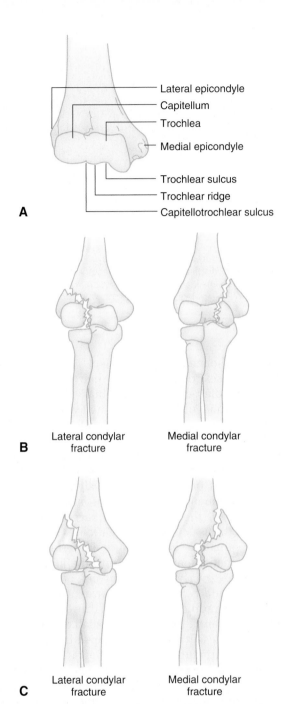

A

Lateral epicondyle
Capitellum
Trochlea
Medial epicondyle
Trochlear sulcus
Trochlear ridge
Capitellotrochlear sulcus

B

Lateral condylar
fracture

Medial condylar
fracture

C

Lateral condylar
fracture

Medial condylar
fracture

Figure 49-19. Condylar fractures. **A,** Normal anatomy. **B,** Lateral trochlear ridge not in fracture fragment (stable). **C,** Lateral trochlear ridge included with fracture fragment (unstable). (Modified from Simon R, Koenigsknecht S: *Emergency Orthopaedics: The Extremities,* 2nd ed. Norwalk, Conn, Appleton & Lange, 1987.)

muscle attachments. For medial condylar fractures, the reverse is true (i.e., the forearm should be pronated and the wrist flexed). For fractures displaced greater than 3 mm, surgical fixation is required.

Complications

Complications include nonunion, restricted range of motion, joint instability, cubitus valgus or varus deformity, arthritis, and ulnar neuropathy. Because of the high rate of complications, all condylar fractures should have orthopedic consultation.

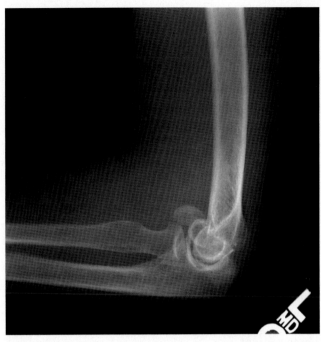

Figure 49-20. Fracture of the capitellum.

Articular Surface Fractures

Capitellum Fractures

Pathophysiology

Although fractures of the capitellum and trochlea do occur as isolated injuries, more often they occur as a result of posterior dislocation of the elbow. Injury to the capitellum occurs when the patient falls on an outstretched hand, jamming the radial head upward, similar to a piston, shearing off the capitellum into the radial fossa. Because the capitellum has no muscular attachments, the fragment may remain nondisplaced. More often, the fragment is displaced (usually anteriorly, but occasionally posteriorly). Because of this mechanism, a radial head fracture also may be present.

Clinical and Radiographic Features

The development of significant signs and symptoms may be delayed with capitellum fractures. Eventually, swelling within the capsule results in severe pain that manifests as well-localized tenderness on examination. Flexion of the elbow increases pain. A true lateral x-ray film usually shows the fragment lying anterior and proximal to the main portion of the capitellum (Figure 49-20).

Management

Treatment begins in the emergency department with a posterior splint, ice packs, elevation, compression, and analgesia. Accurate anatomic alignment, rigid internal fixation, and early mobilization are prerequisites for a good functional result.[24] Fractures of the articular surfaces can be treated nonsurgically only if x-rays show perfect anatomic alignment.

Complications

Complications include posttraumatic arthritis, avascular necrosis of the fracture fragment, and restricted range of motion.

Trochlea Fractures

Pathophysiology

Isolated fractures of the trochlea are exceedingly rare because of the structure's protected position deep within the elbow joint. The shearing force of the ulna against the trochlea is associated more commonly with posterior elbow dislocation.

Clinical Features

The elbow is painful, with an effusion and limited range of motion because this is an intra-articular injury. On x-ray, a fragment is seen lying on the medial side of the joint, just distal to the medial epicondyle, and signs of joint effusion are visible. The fracture may extend into the distal portion of the medial epicondyle.

Management

Nondisplaced fractures may be treated with a posterior splint for 3 weeks followed by early range-of-motion exercises. Displaced fractures should be treated operatively; fragments that can be internally fixed are repaired, whereas small fragments are excised. Immobilization should be minimized to 10 to 14 days.[25,26]

Epicondyle Fractures

Most epicondylar fractures involve the medial epicondyle. Medial epicondyle fractures are most common in children and adolescents and often involve the apophysis, which is the last ossification center to fuse in the distal humerus, usually after age 15. Fractures through this ossification center usually occur in adolescence and compose 11% of pediatric elbow fractures.[27] These are not Salter injuries because the apophysis is involved rather than the physis. Because the lateral epicondyle is almost level with the flattened outer surface of the lateral condyle, it has only minimal exposure to a direct blow, and fracture is extremely rare.

Pathophysiology

Medial epicondyle injuries occur from a variety of mechanisms. First, avulsion fractures are associated with posterior elbow dislocations in patients younger than 20 years old.[28] Second, repetitive valgus stress (as with throwing a ball) results in eventual avulsion fracture of the epicondyle (little leaguer's elbow). Another reported cause of fracture separation of the medial epicondyle, usually in adolescent boys, is from arm wrestling.[29] Violent muscular forces associated with a shifting center of gravity during this activity seem to produce an avulsion just before closure of the epiphyseal plate. Finally, a direct blow to the medial epicondyle can cause this injury.

Clinical and Radiographic Features

The elbow is held in flexion, and any movement is resisted. Isolated fractures are associated with focal ten-

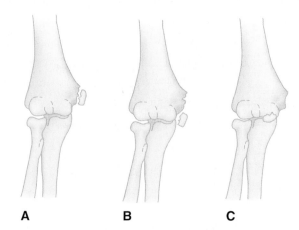

Figure 49-21. Fractures of medial epicondyle. **A,** Minimal displacement. **B,** Marked displacement. **C,** Displacement into joint. (From Connolly JF: *DePalma's Management of Fractures and Dislocations.* Philadelphia, WB Saunders, 1981.)

derness over the medial epicondyle. Use of the forearm flexors increases pain because their attachment is along the medial epicondyle. Ulnar nerve function should be evaluated. When associated with a posterior dislocation, the examination reveals a prominent olecranon.

Simple fractures of the medial epicondyle are extra-articular injuries with limited soft tissue injury.[22] They generally do not produce a fat pad sign on the lateral x-ray view of the elbow. A posterior fat pad or significant swelling of the joint should suggest concurrent injuries, such as elbow dislocation. Careful radiographic evaluation is especially important because fracture fragments may migrate into the joint space. If the fragment is overlying the joint line on x-ray examination, it should be considered intra-articular (Figure 49-21). Radiographic detection of the intra-articular fragment is often difficult.[28] Associated ulnar nerve palsy may be present with an entrapped fragment. Fragments may be difficult to see on radiographs, and a true anteroposterior view is difficult to obtain because of severe pain on extension. In an adolescent patient, there is a tendency to confuse the normal radiolucent epiphyseal growth plate with a fracture. Comparison films of the uninjured elbow may be useful. If dislocation is present, repeat radiographs taken after reduction should be evaluated for fragment location.

Management

If the fracture fragment is minimally displaced, treatment with a posterior splint is appropriate. To minimize distraction of the fragment by the forearm flexors, the elbow and wrist are flexed with the forearm pronated.

Treatment of displaced fractures is controversial.[30] In the past, the amount of displacement often dictated the need for surgery. Results of operative and nonoperative treatment seem to be good, however, regardless of the degree of displacement.[30] Some experts advocate surgery for patients who participate in high-performance athletic activities that involve the injured extremity,

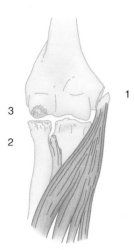

Figure 49-22. Little Leaguer's elbow. Avulsion fracture of medial epicondyle (1). Compression fractures of the radial head (2) and capitellum (3). (From Connolly JF: *DePalma's Management of Fractures and Dislocations.* Philadelphia, WB Saunders, 1981.)

but controlled studies are lacking. Immediate orthopedic consultation should be sought for these injuries. Intra-articular fragments that cannot be removed from the joint by manipulation are an indication for surgery.[30] Treatment of the rare lateral epicondylar fracture in an adult involves simple immobilization until pain resolves.[31]

Little Leaguer's Elbow

Little leaguer's elbow warrants special mention. An adolescent pitcher traumatizes immature epiphyses by repetitive throwing. Throwing the curve ball or breaking ball has been implicated as a particular culprit, although the most important factor is probably the number of innings pitched.[32] It has been shown in a group of highly competitive young baseball players that this injury also is common in catchers and fielders.[33] The adolescent bone structure cannot withstand the extreme loading produced by repetitive hard throwing. Avulsion of the medial epicondyle or compression fracture of the subchondral bone of the lateral condyle or radial head may result (Figure 49-22). This diagnosis should be sought in an athletic adolescent with medial epicondyle or radial head pain in the absence of acute injury by history. Adolescents with this condition should be forced to rest the elbow if throwing causes pain. After healing occurs, the amount of throwing and technique should be monitored carefully.

Olecranon Fractures

Pathophysiology

Fractures of the olecranon may result from one of several mechanisms. Most commonly, a direct blow as a result of a fall, a motor vehicle or motorcycle crash, or an assault produces this injury. Such injuries are frequently comminuted. Less commonly, indirect force applied by forceful contraction of the triceps while the elbow is flexed during a fall can cause a transverse or

oblique fracture through the olecranon. A combination of direct and indirect forces is believed also to cause some of these fractures. Olecranon fractures occur in adults and less commonly in children.[34] The anatomic integrity of the olecranon is essential for triceps strength and normal function of the elbow, similar to the way intact patellar function is necessary for extension of the knee.

Clinical Features

Physical findings may include tenderness and pain over the olecranon, a palpable separation at the fracture site, or the inability to extend the elbow against force. This last finding indicates complete discontinuity of the pulling mechanism and the consequent failure of triceps function. The neurovascular status should be examined, with special attention given to the ulnar nerve distribution because this structure is most vulnerable to injury in this location. Loss of sensation over the palmar aspect of the fifth digit and hypothenar eminence or motor weakness in the interossei muscles of the hand suggests ulnar nerve injury.

Diagnostic Strategies

Lateral x-ray views are most helpful. In addition to noting the fracture, the degree of comminution, the extent of articular surface disruption, and the amount of displacement in the 90-degree flexion position should be noted. Nondisplacement in this position indicates that the triceps aponeurosis is intact, and prolonged immobilization is unnecessary. Displacement of more than 2 mm is considered an indication for surgery. A fracture line that increases in separation with flexion of the elbow also is considered a displaced fracture. When this fracture is associated with elbow dislocation, the plane of instability is located through the fracture site and the radiohumeral joint, resulting in posterior displacement of the proximal fragment of the ulna and anterior dislocation of the radius and ulna as a unit.

Management

Undisplaced fractures can be treated conservatively on an outpatient basis with ice, compression, immobilization in 45 to 90 degrees of flexion, and analgesia. Follow-up films should be done at frequent intervals to ensure that subsequent displacement does not occur. Range-of-motion exercises can be started within 3 weeks in many cases.

Displaced fractures or fracture-dislocations require open reduction and internal fixation and should be referred immediately to an orthopedic consultant. Displaced fractures in elderly patients sometimes are treated conservatively, but this should be left to the discretion of the consultant. Orthopedic referral also is necessary when ulnar nerve symptoms are present. These symptoms occur in 10% of patients, and in most cases the injury is an ulnar contusion that resolves spontaneously. The long-term outcome of treated olecranon fractures in adults is usually favorable with a low incidence of subsequent arthritis.[35]

Radial Head and Neck Fractures

Pathophysiology

Radial head and neck fractures generally are produced by an indirect mechanism, typically a fall on an outstretched hand. The radius transmits the force upward, drives the radial head against the capitellum, and results in fracture of the weaker radial head or neck. Although the fracture of the radial head may be the only radiographic finding, damage to the articular surface of the capitellum and injury to the collateral ligament commonly occur. Displacement of the radial head fragment suggests considerable force and significant soft tissue injury. This injury is characterized by localized tenderness over the radial head or pain with passive rotation of the forearm.

Diagnostic Strategies

Radiographic findings range from a subtle disruption of the usual gradual sweep of the radial neck/head surface to an obvious displaced or comminuted fracture. Undisplaced fractures are notoriously difficult to see on radiographs. Tenderness coupled with a positive fat pad sign on x-ray should be treated as a radial head fracture even in the absence of a visible fracture. Radial head fractures are classified into four types:

- Type I—undisplaced fractures
- Type II—marginal fractures (involving <30% of the articular surface) with displacement, including impaction or angulation
- Type III—comminuted fractures of the entire radial head
- Type IV—any of the above with elbow dislocation

Management

Type I nondisplaced fractures are treated symptomatically by a brief period of sling support and early range-of-motion exercises (within 24 to 48 hours). Aspiration of the hemarthrosis and injection of 0.5% bupivacaine into the joint space may give dramatic relief of pain and improve the range of motion.[36] Most patients with this injury recover well in 2 to 3 months. A few do poorly, however, with long-term pain, contracture, or inflammation.

Type II injuries usually are treated similarly, with aspiration, instillation of bupivacaine, and immobilization in the emergency department, followed by a trial period of range of motion. In these cases, aspiration of the joint and instillation of bupivacaine not only improve pain, but also allow testing of the range of motion to identify entrapped fragments. Radial head excision sometimes is performed later if the patient fails to improve. Early excision is advised for type II fractures when a mechanical block is present and for most type III fractures. Long-term functional results after radial head excision are acceptable in most patients, although a few have some functional disability after this procedure.[37,38] Type IV injuries are treated for the elbow dislocation as described next and for the specific radial head lesion that is present.

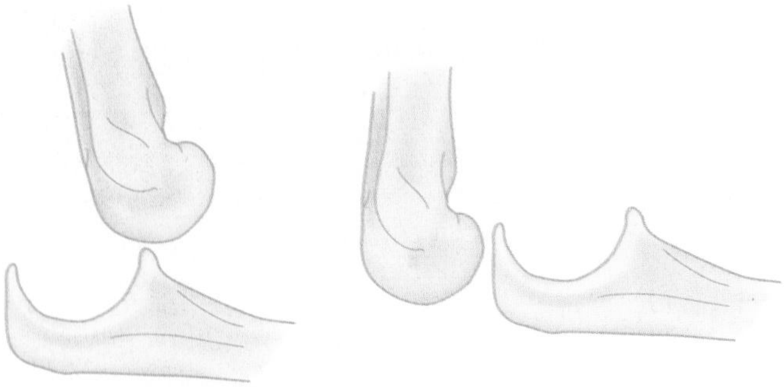

Figure 49-23. Elbow dislocation, posterior and anterior. (Modified from Simon R, Koenigsknecht S: *Emergency Orthopaedics: The Extremities,* 2nd ed. Norwalk, Conn, Appleton & Lange, 1987.)

DISLOCATION AND SUBLUXATION

Elbow Dislocation

Because of its anatomic structure, the elbow is inherently subject to mechanical instability, and dislocations are common. The elbow is second only to the shoulder as the most commonly dislocated large joint. *Elbow dislocation* is a term usually used to describe a disruption of the relationship between the humerus and the olecranon. Generally the radius and ulna, bound together firmly by the annular ligament and interosseous membrane, displace as a unit. Most classifications refer to the abnormal position of the ulna relative to the humerus. The elbow most often dislocates posteriorly, although it may dislocate anteriorly, medially, or laterally (Figure 49-23). A dislocation also may occur between the radius and ulna, and such dislocations rarely occur concurrently with the ulnohumeral type. The latter are termed *divergent* dislocations.

Dislocation of the elbow requires considerable energy, and it is not surprising that a significant number of dislocations are associated with fractures of adjacent bony structures. Immediate reduction of these dislocations is imperative to relieve pain and to prevent circulatory embarrassment or cartilaginous damage.

Posterior Elbow Dislocation

Pathophysiology

The mechanism of injury is a fall on the outstretched hand or wrist, the elbow being either extended or hyperextended at the time of impact. A valgus stress usually also occurs. The resultant forces lever the ulna from the trochlea and produce the dislocation.

Clinical and Radiographic Features

Patients hold the elbow in flexion at approximately 45 degrees and have marked prominence of the olecranon. Some elbow dislocations reduce before examination in the emergency department, presenting a confusing picture. In any case, significant diffuse tenderness and swelling are present. Neurovascular status must be checked because brachial artery and median nerve

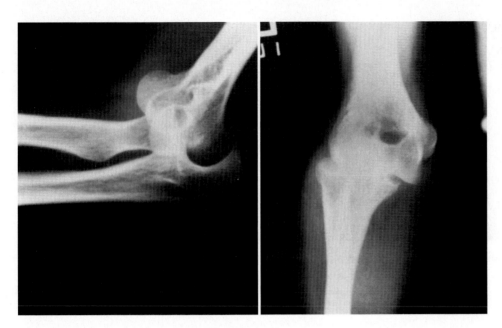

Figure 49-24. Posterior dislocation of elbow. Ligaments and joint capsules are disrupted to the point that lateral displacement also is present.

injuries have been described. Neurovascular injury may occur from numerous mechanisms, including the initial traction, local swelling, and entrapment during reduction.[39] Repeat examinations are mandatory.

A radiographic example of elbow dislocation is provided in Figure 49-24. X-ray evaluation is crucial before manipulation to rule out fractures that can mimic dislocation on examination. Also, several fractures commonly occur in conjunction with dislocation, and these need to be identified and treated when present. These include fractures of the distal humerus, radial head, and coronoid process.

Management

Orthopedic consultation is usually not necessary to proceed. Reduction should be attempted immediately if there is vascular compromise. Conscious sedation is helpful in most cases. Regional blocks are useful in selected cases, and general anesthesia is rarely needed. Posterior dislocations are reduced with an assistant immobilizing the humerus while traction is applied distally at the wrist. The elbow is brought into flexion as steady countertraction is applied to the anterior surface of the distal humerus. When the capitellum slides over the coronoid process, a coupling sound occurs as the articular surfaces mesh. The joint is gently moved through its normal range of motion to check stability. If stable, the elbow is flexed to approximately 90 degrees and immobilized with posterior plaster mold. The neurovascular status should be rechecked. Postreduction radiographs are important to avoid missing concomitant fractures of the coronoid process or radial head or, in children, separation of the medial epicondylar apophysis.

Postreduction management includes immobilization in a posterior splint with the elbow in as much flexion as circulation allows. The arm is suspended in a sling. Circular casting should be avoided initially. Patients can be discharged with instructions to apply ice, elevate, and watch for signs of vascular impairment.

Patients should not be discharged until and unless they can follow such instructions. If the elbow is stable after reduction, gentle range-of-motion exercises may be initiated in 3 to 5 days. Unstable joints may require either prolonged immobilization in the presence of ligamentous instability or internal fixation for instability associated with fracture.[40]

Complications

The most serious complication of elbow dislocation is vascular compromise. Severe disruption results in injury to the brachial artery in 8% of cases.[41] This injury should be sought when a wide opening between the tip of the olecranon and the distal humerus is palpated or seen on a radiograph. The presence of distal pulses is not proof of an intact artery, and if a question of vascular compromise exists, emergent vascular studies or consultation are indicated. Median nerve traction injuries and entrapment also have been reported. Loss of median nerve function after reduction should prompt immediate orthopedic consultation. Recurrent dislocation of the elbow is rare.

Medial and Lateral Dislocations

Medial and lateral elbow dislocations are produced by a similar mechanism as in posterior dislocations with a vector of force displacing the ulna and radius as a unit either medially or laterally. The anteroposterior view is the key to determining these dislocations. Reduction is carried out with the arm in slight extension, but otherwise is similar to that for posterior dislocation. Care must be taken not to convert these to posterior dislocations during reduction. Complications and aftercare are the same as for posterior dislocations.

Anterior Elbow Dislocation

Pathophysiology

Anterior dislocations are rare and occur as a result of a blow from behind to the olecranon while the elbow is

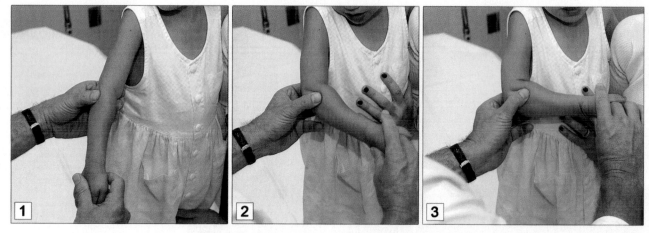

Figure 49-25. Subluxation of the radial head. Method of reduction: (1) Apply pressure to radial head, (2) supinate the forearm, and (3) flex elbow, in one continuous motion.

in the flexed position. Severe associated soft tissue trauma is present, including avulsion of the triceps mechanism or vascular disruption. These dislocations are frequently open.

Clinical Features

The upper arm appears shortened and the forearm elongated. The elbow is fully extended, and the forearm is supinated. The olecranon fossa is palpable posteriorly.

Management

Reduction of closed injuries is performed with distal traction of the wrist and a backward pressure on the forearm, while grasping the distal humerus. A click usually indicates that reduction has been achieved. These injuries have a higher incidence of vascular impairment than the more common posterior dislocation, but ulnar nerve injuries are unusual.[42] Emergent orthopedic referral is advised and is mandatory for open injuries or when vascular disruption is suspected.

Radial Head Subluxation

Pathophysiology

Subluxation of the radial head is a common injury, representing more than 20% of upper extremity injuries in children. Children age 1 to 3 years are most often affected, although cases have been reported in children 6 months to 15 years of age. Girls are affected more commonly than boys. This injury is called *nursemaid's elbow* or *pulled elbow* because it results from a sudden longitudinal pull on the forearm while the child's arm is in pronation. Stretching of the annular ligament allows fibers to slip between the capitellum and the head of the radius, resulting in an inability of the child to supinate the arm. There is a recurrence rate of about 20% for this injury.[43]

Clinical and Radiographic Features

Clinically the arm is in passive pronation, with slight flexion at the elbow. The child is unable or unwilling to move the arm. Resistance to supination and tenderness on direct palpation over the head of the radius are present. Swelling, ecchymosis, and deformity are absent.

X-rays are not required when the history suggests this injury. If there is swelling or deformity, if there is an uncharacteristic history, if the child does not resume use of the arm after reduction, or if there is a suspicion of child abuse, appropriate x-ray studies should be obtained. If palpation of the forearm, wrist, or humerus away from the elbow elicits reproducible tenderness, radiographs should be taken to exclude other diagnoses.

Management

Radial head subluxations usually can be reduced by supination of the forearm while slight pressure on the radial head is applied with the examiner's thumb. In one continuous motion, the elbow is supinated and flexed. A click often, but not always, is felt as the radial head reduces (Figure 49-25). If this method is unsuccessful, supination with extension also has been recommended.

Many patients are asymptomatic within 5 to 10 minutes; 90% of patients regain use of the arm within 30 minutes. Hearing or palpating a click is associated with success. It is a good idea for the physician to leave the room and for parents to distract the child to show return of normal function. A fearful child often does not use even the successfully reduced limb. If function does not return within 24 hours, the patient should be re-evaluated. Immobilization after successful reduction is not necessary. A sling is often recommended, but most children do not keep it in place. Most of these injuries are unintentional on the part of the caregiver, but inflicted injury should be considered in suspicious cases.

SOFT TISSUE DISORDERS

Epicondylitis (Tennis Elbow)

Pathophysiology

Tennis elbow is a term first introduced in the 1880s to describe an inflammatory process that involves the radiohumeral joint or lateral epicondyle of the humerus. It is a common exercise-related syndrome, and the mechanism is thought to be repetitive pronation and supination of the forearm. The actual pathologic nature of this syndrome is unclear. Radiohumeral bursitis or synovitis, tendinitis of the common extensor tendon, periostitis of the lateral epicondyle, and entrapment by scar tissue of the radial nerve all have been suggested as culprits in this syndrome. Histologically the abnormality has been described as *angiofibroblastic hyperplasia,* a term subsequently modified to *angiofibroblastic tendinosis.* The cause has been theorized to be a degenerative process because of the paucity of acute inflammatory cells seen histologically.[44] Medial tennis elbow and posterior tennis elbow have been reported, the former involving the pronator teres and flexor carpi radialis insertions and the latter involving the triceps tendon. The following discussion pertains to lateral tennis elbow.

Clinical and Radiographic Features

Whatever the cause, the onset is usually gradual. Patients have complaints of dull pain over the lateral aspect of the elbow, increased by grasping or twisting motions. Tenderness is located over the lateral epicondyle or radiohumeral joint. Supination and pronation against resistance may be painful. Pain can be shown by stretching the wrist extensors. To test this, the elbow is extended, the forearm pronated, and the wrist fully dorsiflexed.

X-ray findings may be normal, although with chronicity, calcifications may be present over the lateral epicondyle. Characteristic MRI findings also have been described, although MRI is not indicated and generally not available in the emergency department.[45]

Management

Traditional treatment includes protection, rest, ice, compression, elevation, and medication. Initial therapy includes avoidance of the inciting activity and immobilization with a sling. Nonsteroidal anti-inflammatory drugs are often used, but their efficacy probably is limited to their analgesic rather than their anti-inflammatory properties.[46] Injection of a corticosteroid at the point of tenderness provides some relief of pain in most patients.[47-49] Because corticosteroids weaken collagen, premature resumption of heavy loading of the tendon at the lesion should be avoided, as should injection directly into the tendon.[50] Patients with pain that persists despite treatment and a rehabilitation program should be referred for possible surgery.[51] Modification of athletic technique is recommended after the symptoms subside.

Olecranon Bursitis

Pathophysiology

Although several bursae are located in the elbow region, the olecranon bursa is the one most often involved in an isolated pathologic process. Olecranon bursitis commonly is caused by repetitive minor trauma, such as leaning on the elbow during work activities. It also may result from an inflammatory process, such as gout or an infectious process within the bursa (septic bursitis). Septic olecranon bursitis also occurs most commonly in patients engaged in work that predisposes to repetitive trauma to the elbow, such as gardening or plumbing.

Clinical Features

Patients usually have progressive pain, tenderness, and swelling over the olecranon. Some patients with septic bursitis have an abrupt onset instead, with a rapid increase in pain over a few hours. On examination, the septic bursa is typically swollen, hot, erythematous, and tender. Flexion often is limited by pain brought on by tightening of the skin over the inflamed bursa. Minor breaks in the skin, frank abrasions, or healing lacerations over the bursa may be present. In one small series, 7 of 20 patients with septic olecranon bursitis were febrile (38.5° C to 40.3° C), 75% had cellulitis, and 25% had regional adenopathy. Noninfectious bursitis usually presents with less warmth and erythema. The skin is intact, and swelling may be the only finding. The most important aspect of evaluation is the differentiation of a septic process from a benign inflammatory process. This differentiation may be difficult on clinical grounds because considerable overlap exists in the histories and physical findings.

Diagnostic Strategies

If doubt exists, aspiration of the bursa should be performed and the aspirate sent for crystals, white blood cell count, Gram stain, and cultures. Unless it is frankly bloody, traumatic nonseptic olecranon bursitis usually has a leukocyte count of less than 1000 cells/mm^3, whereas septic bursal fluid usually has greater than 10,000 white blood cells/mm^3.

Management

Aspiration is diagnostic and therapeutic because relief of pressure relieves some of the pain. In cases of purulent bursitis, the bursa should be drained, and appropriate penicillinase-resistant antibiotics should be begun in the emergency department. Bursitis refractory to aspiration and penicillinase-resistant antibiotics may require incision and drainage. Noninfectious bursitis can be managed with a compression dressing, ice, nonsteroidal anti-inflammatory medications, and avoidance of the inciting activity. Patients who have had their bursa aspirated should be rechecked within 24 hours to verify culture results and monitor their response to treatment.

Biceps Tendon Rupture

Pathophysiology

Biceps tendon rupture occurs most commonly in the proximal portion of the long head of the biceps. It is most common in middle-aged athletes or physical laborers who sustain repetitive microtrauma to the tendon. Patients experience a snapping sound and pain in the anterior shoulder during strenuous activities that produce rapid loading of the muscle. Rupture also occurs distally, usually as an avulsion from the insertion on the radial tuberosity, although ruptures at the musculotendinous junction occasionally occur. Rupture of the distal biceps tendon occurs almost exclusively in men, most commonly between the ages of 40 and 60 and most often involving the dominant arm.[52] The inciting event is usually an unexpected extension force applied to the arm flexed at 90 degrees. The pathophysiology of tendon rupture is poorly understood, although tendon rupture generally occurs in the setting of underlying tendinosis. Diabetes, chronic renal failure, systemic lupus erythematosus, rheumatoid arthritis, and steroid or fluoroquinolone therapy all may result in tendinosis. Smoking has been shown to be strongly associated with distal biceps tendon rupture.[53]

Clinical Features

The diagnosis is usually obvious. In proximal tendon rupture, the patient usually has a visible defect at the top of the bicipital groove with bunching of the muscle distally. Flexing of the elbow produces pain at the proximal insertion. Flexion remains intact, however, because the short head of the biceps usually maintains its integrity. With distal ruptures, the patient complains of pain and tearing in the antecubital region. There is a visible deformity and palpable defect of the biceps muscle belly with weakness of elbow flexion and supination. If the tendon is completely ruptured, there is a bunching up of the muscle, and this effect is accentuated when the patient attempts flexion. X-rays are not revealing and usually not necessary. MRI may be useful when a partial rupture is suspected.

Management

All patients require urgent referral to an orthopedist. Early anatomic repair of complete ruptures usually is recommended. Partial ruptures occasionally respond to conservative treatment, but also may require surgical repair. Patients should be splinted and advised to apply ice and be given analgesics while awaiting orthopedic consultation.

KEY CONCEPTS

- Clinical decision rules for the elbow joint have not been validated. It is reasonable to perform x-rays when there is significant limitation in range of motion, obvious deformity, joint effusion, or significant tenderness over any of the bony prominences or the radial head. In the absence of these, it would seem appropriate to omit x-rays.

- In the setting of trauma, more than 90% of patients with the posterior fat pad sign of the elbow have intra-articular skeletal injury. In adults, a radial head fracture is implied, whereas in children, a supracondylar fracture is the probable underlying injury. In the absence of trauma, other causes of effusion (e.g., gout, infection, or bursitis) should be considered.

- The most common complication, radial nerve injury, occurs in 20% of humerus fractures. This is most often a benign neurapraxia that resolves spontaneously in most patients, although recovery may take several months. Radial nerve injuries associated with penetrating trauma or open fractures are likely to be permanent and usually warrant operative exploration.

- Generally the radius and ulna, bound together firmly by the annular ligament and interosseous membrane, displace as a unit and typically dislocate posteriorly, although anterior, medial, or lateral dislocations may occur.

- X-ray studies are not required when the history suggests radial head dislocation (nursemaid's elbow). If there is swelling or deformity, if there is an uncharacteristic history, if the child does not resume use of the arm after reduction, or if there is a suspicion of child abuse, appropriate x-ray studies should be obtained.

- Biceps tendon rupture occurs almost exclusively in men, most commonly age 40 to 60, most often involving the dominant arm and usually subsequent to an unexpected extension force applied to the arm flexed at 90 degrees. Smoking, diabetes, chronic renal failure, systemic lupus erythematosus, rheumatoid arthritis, and steroid or fluoroquinolone therapy may predispose to this injury.

REFERENCES

1. Paraskevass G, et al: Study of the carrying angle of the human elbow joint in full extension: A morphometric analysis. *Surg Radiol Anat* 26:19, 2004.
2. Mohammad S, Rymaszewski LA, Runciman J: The Baumann angle in supracondylar fractures of the distal humerus in children. *J Pediatr Orthop* 19:65, 1999.
3. Branch T, et al: Spontaneous fractures of the humerus during pitching. *Am J Sports Med* 20:468, 1992.
4. Vander Griend R, et al: Open reduction and internal fixation of humeral shaft fractures. *J Bone Joint Surg* 68A:430, 1986.
5. Chiu FY, et al: Closed humeral shaft fractures: A prospective evaluation of surgical treatment. *J Trauma* 43:947, 1997.
6. Wilkins KE: Fractures and dislocations of the elbow region. In Rockwood CA, Wilkins KE, King RE (eds): *Fractures in Children*, 4th ed. Philadelphia, JB Lippincott, 1996, p 653.
7. Mikowitz B, Busch MT: Supracondylar humerus fractures. *Orthop Clin North Am* 25:581, 1994.
8. Williamson DM, Cole WG: Treatment of selected extension supracondylar fractures by manipulation and strapping in flexion. *Injury* 24:249, 1993.
9. Wilkins KE: Supracondylar fractures: What's new? *J Pediatr Orthop* 6:110, 1997.

10. Harris IE: Supracondylar fractures of the humerus in children. *Orthopedics* 15:811, 1992.
11. Mehserle WL, Mechan PL: Treatment of displaced supracondylar fracture of the humerus (Type III) with closed reduction and percutaneous cross-pin fixation. *J Pediatr Orthop* 11:705, 1991.
12. Pirone AM, Graham HK, Krajbich JI: Management of displaced extension-type supracondylar fractures of the humerus in children. *J Bone Joint Surg* 70A:641, 1988.
13. Boyd DW, Aronson DD: Supracondylar fracture of the humerus: A prospective study of percutaneous pinning. *J Pediatr Orthop* 12:789, 1992.
14. Weiland AJ, et al: Surgical treatment of displaced supracondylar fractures of the humerus in children: An analysis of fifty-two cases followed up for 5 to 15 years. *J Bone Joint Surg* 60A:657, 1978.
15. Gaddy BC, et al: Distal humeral osteotomy for correction of post-traumatic cubitus varus. *J Pediatr Orthop* 15:419, 1995.
16. Brown IC, Zinar D: Traumatic and iatrogenic neurological complications after supracondylar humerus fractures in children. *J Pediatr Orthop* 15:440, 1995.
17. Perry CR, Gibson CT, Kowalski MF: Transcondylar fractures of the distal humerus. *J Orthop Trauma* 3:98, 1989.
18. Gupta R: Intercondylar fractures of the distal humerus in adults. *Injury* 27:569, 1996.
19. Hotchkiss RN, Green DP: Fractures and dislocations of the elbow. In Rockwood CA, Wilkins KE, King RE (eds): *Fractures,* 4th ed. Philadelphia, JB Lippincott, 1996, p 929.
20. Safran O: Surgical treatment of intercondylar fractures of the humerus in adults. *Am J Orthop* 28:659, 1999.
21. Gupta R, Khanchandani P: Intercondylar fractures of the distal humerus in adults: A critical analysis of 55 cases. *Int J Care Injured* 33:511, 2002.
22. Skaggs D, Pershad J: Pediatric elbow trauma. *Pediatr Emerg Care* 13:425, 1997.
23. Leet AI, Young C, Hoffer M: Medial condyle fractures of the humerus in children. *J Pediatr Orthop* 22:2, 2002.
24. McKee MG: Fractures of the capitellum and trochlea. *Orthop Clin North Am* 31:115, 2000.
25. Wang KC, et al: Intercondylar fractures of the distal humerus: Routine anterior subcutaneous transposition of the ulna nerve in a posterior operative approach. *J Trauma* 36:770, 1994.
26. Foulk DA, Robertson PA, Timmerman LA: Fracture of the trochlea. *J Orthop Trauma* 9:530, 1995.
27. Case SL, Hennrikus WL: Surgical treatment of displaced medial epicondyle fractures in adolescent athletes. *Am J Sports Med* 25:682, 1997.
28. Fowles JV, Slimane N, Kasseb MT: Elbow dislocation with avulsion of the medial humeral epicondyle. *J Bone Joint Surg* 72B:102, 1990.
29. Ogawa K, Ui M: Fracture-separation of the medial humeral epicondyle caused by arm wrestling. *J Trauma* 41:494, 1996.
30. Farsetti P, et al: Long-term results of treatment of fractures of the medial humeral epicondyle in children. *J Bone Joint Surg* 83A:12299, 2001.
31. Kobayashi Y, Oka Y, Munesada S: Avulsion fractures of the medial and lateral epicondyles of the humerus. *J Shoulder Elbow Surg* 9:59, 2000.
32. Green CP: The curve ball and the elbow. In Zarins B, Andres JR, Carson WG (eds): *Injuries to the Throwing Arm.* Philadelphia, WB Saunders, 1985.
33. Hang DW, Chao, CM, Hang YS: A clinical and roentgenographic study of little league elbow. *Am J Sports Med* 32:79, 2004.
34. Evans MC, Graham HK: Olecranon fractures in children: Part 1. A clinical review. Part 2. A new classification and management scheme. *J Pediatr Orthop* 19:559, 1999.
35. Karlsson MK, et al: Fractures of the olecranon: A 15 to 24 year follow up of 73 patients. *Clin Orthop* 403:205, 2002.
36. Dooley JF, Angus PD: The importance of elbow aspiration when treating radial head fractures. *Arch Emerg Med* 8:117, 1991.
37. Coleman DA, Blair WF, Shurr D: Resection of the radial head for fracture of the radial head. *J Bone Joint Surg* 69A:385, 1987.
38. Goldberg I, Peylan J, Yosipovitch Z: Late results of excision of the radial head for an isolated closed fracture. *J Bone Joint Surg* 68A:675, 1986.
39. Platz A, et al: Posterior elbow dislocation with associated vascular injury after blunt trauma. *J Trauma* 46:948, 1999.
40. Phillips CS, Segalman KA: Diagnosis and treatment of post-traumatic medial and lateral elbow ligament incompetence. *Hand Clin* 18:149, 2002.
41. Rao SB, Crawford AH: Median nerve entrapment after dislocation of the elbow in children: A report of two cases and review of the literature. *Clin Orthop* 312:232, 1995.
42. Skaggs D, Pershad J: Pediatric elbow trauma. *Pediatr Emerg Care* 13:425, 1997.
43. Teach SJ, Schutzman SA: Prospective study of recurrent radial head subluxation. *Arch Pediatr Adolesc Med* 150:164, 1996.
44. Nirschl RP: Elbow tendinosis/tennis elbow. *Clin Sports Med* 11:851, 1992.
45. Martin CE, Scweitzer ME: MR imaging of epicondylitis. *Skeletal Radiol* 27:133, 1998.
46. Labelle H, Guibert R: Efficacy of diclofenac in lateral epicondylitis of the elbow also treated with immobilization. *Arch Fam Med* 6:257, 1997.
47. Hay E, Paterson SM, Lewis M: Pragmatic randomized controlled trial of local corticosteroid injection and naproxen for treatment of lateral epicondylitis of elbow in primary care. *BMJ* 319:964, 1999.
48. Guidotti TC: Occupational repetitive strain injury. *Am Fam Physician* 45:585, 1992.
49. Hay EM, et al: Pragmatic randomized controlled trial of local corticosteroid injection and naproxen for treatment of lateral epicondylitis of elbow in primary care. *BMJ* 319:964, 1999.
50. Sperryn PN: Overuse injury in sport. *BMJ* 308:1430, 1994.
51. Field LD, Savoie FH: Common elbow injuries in sport. *Sports Med* 26:193, 1998.
52. Ramsey ML: Distal biceps tendon injuries: Diagnosis and management. *J Am Acad Orthop Surg* 7:199, 1999.
53. Safran M, Graham SM: Distal biceps tendon rupture: Incidence, demographics and the effect of smoking. *Clin Orthop* 404:275, 2002.

PERSPECTIVE

The shoulder joint is a unique and complex articulation unit. It has the largest range of motion of any appendicular joint in the body and can be moved through a space that exceeds a hemisphere. The wide range of motion also predisposes the joint to instability and injury; this was depicted in 3000 B.C. in wall paintings of Egyptian tombs, which show accurate drawings of manipulations (similar to the Kocher technique) used to reduce shoulder dislocations.[1] Hippocrates may have been the first to outline extensively the diagnosis and treatment of shoulder dislocations.[2]

Shoulder injuries are commonly encountered in emergency medicine. Statistical studies show that 8% to 13% of all athletic injuries involve the shoulder and that shoulder dislocations account for more than 50% of all major joint dislocations seen in the emergency department. Almost every major sport or athletic activity involves use of the shoulder joint in one way or another. The shoulder can be injured by trauma (indirect or direct) or by overuse. Traumatic injuries tend to occur in football and ice hockey, whereas overuse injuries (impingement syndromes) are more common in swimming and baseball. Shoulder injuries also are common in wrestling, tennis, volleyball, and javelin throwing.[3]

In general, children are vulnerable to the same injuries as adults; however, the presence of the epiphysis and its growth plate changes the pattern of injuries.[4] The strength of the joint capsule and its ligaments is two to five times greater than that of the epiphyseal plate. An injury that produces a sprain or dislocation in an adult often causes a fracture through the hypertrophic zone of the growth plate in a child. The shoulder girdle has epiphyseal plates at the acromion process, proximal humeral head, coracoid process, glenoid cavity, and medial end of the clavicle. Complete or greenstick fractures of the clavicle and fractures of the proximal humeral epiphysis are encountered more commonly in the pediatric population. Most shoulder injuries in children can be treated conservatively with a good prognosis for full return of function.[4]

PRINCIPLES OF DISEASE

Anatomy

The shoulder girdle connects the upper extremity to the axial skeleton (Figure 50-1). It consists of three bones (clavicle, humerus, and scapula), three joints (acromio-clavicular, glenohumeral, and sternoclavicular), and one articulation (scapulothoracic). The clavicle is an S-shaped bone that acts as a strut to support the upper extremity and keep it away from the chest wall. The clavicle articulates medially with the sternum and laterally with the acromion process. The sternoclavicular joint (SCJ) represents the only true articulation between the upper extremity and the axial skeleton. The large articular surface of the sternal end of the clavicle fits poorly with the sloping narrow clavicular notch on the manubrium sterni. A circular flat fibrocartilaginous disk helps reduce the discrepancy between the two articular surfaces (Figure 50-2). The stability of the joint largely depends on associated ligaments. A loose fibrous capsule whose expansions form the anterior and posterior sternoclavicular ligaments envelops the joint.[5] The interclavicular and costoclavicular ligaments are two additional structures that stabilize the joint. The costoclavicular ligament opposes the pull of the sternocleidomastoid and is the most important stabilizing ligament.[5] The SCJ participates in all movements of the upper extremity and is the most moved joint in the body.[6] The superior mediastinum with its great vessels, trachea, esophagus, and other important structures are immediately posterior to the joint.

The tubular clavicle flattens laterally to provide attachment sites for the coracoclavicular and acromioclavicular ligaments (Figure 50-3). The clavicle also protects the subclavian neurovascular bundle and provides the neck with an acceptable cosmetic appearance. The middle third of the clavicle, which is the most commonly fractured segment, is thin and untethered by any ligamentous structures.[7] Rotation around the long axis of the clavicle increases the range of motion of the glenohumeral joint and improves the strength of the arm-trunk mechanism.[7]

The acromioclavicular joint (ACJ) connects the lateral end of the clavicle with the medial aspect of the acromion process (see Figure 50-3). The bony configuration of the joint varies considerably and provides little or no stability.[8] Stability is a function of associated ligaments and muscles. The joint capsule is strengthened on all sides to form the relatively weak anterior, posterior, superior, and inferior acromioclavicular ligaments. The clavicular and acromial attachments of the deltoid and trapezius muscles provide additional static and dynamic support for the superior aspect of the joint. The powerful coracoclavicular ligament, which is the primary suspensory ligament of the upper extremity, also stabilizes the joint. The coracoclavicular ligament is composed of two parts—the

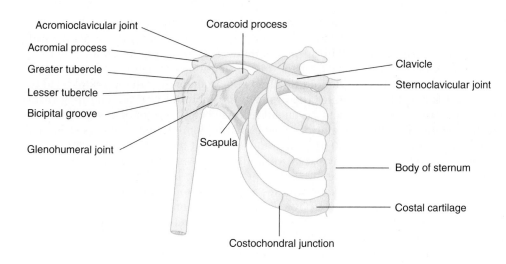

Acromioclavicular joint
Acromial process
Greater tubercle
Lesser tubercle
Bicipital groove
Glenohumeral joint
Coracoid process
Scapula
Clavicle
Sternoclavicular joint
Body of sternum
Costal cartilage
Costochondral junction

Figure 50-1. Anatomy of the shoulder girdle. (From Roy S, Irwin R: *Sports Medicine: Prevention, Evaluation, Management and Rehabilitation.* Englewood, NJ, Prentice Hall, 1983.)

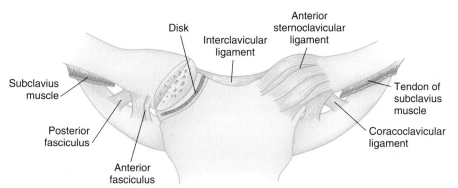

Disk
Interclavicular ligament
Anterior sternoclavicular ligament
Subclavius muscle
Posterior fasciculus
Anterior fasciculus
Tendon of subclavius muscle
Coracoclavicular ligament

Figure 50-2. Ligaments and the interarticular disk of the sternoclavicular joint. (Redrawn from DePalma AF: *Surgery of the Shoulder,* 3rd ed. Philadelphia, JB Lippincott, 1983.)

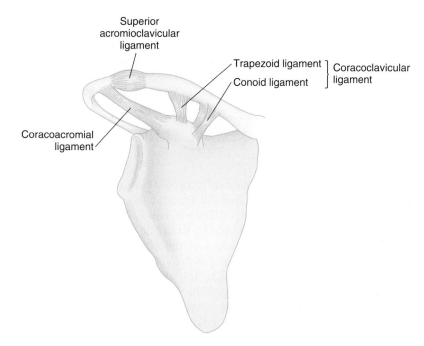

Superior acromioclavicular ligament
Trapezoid ligament
Conoid ligament
Coracoclavicular ligament
Coracoacromial ligament

Figure 50-3. Ligaments of the acromioclavicular joint. (Redrawn from DePalma AF: *Surgery of the Shoulder,* 3rd ed. Philadelphia, JB Lippincott, 1983.)

trapezoid and conoid ligaments.[8] The trapezoid ligament arises from the shaft of the coracoid process and runs superiorly to insert onto the inferior surface of the lateral clavicle. The conoid ligament arises from the base of the coracoid process and inserts more medially on the inferior surface of the distal clavicle. The distance from the clavicle to the coracoid process varies from 1.1 to 1.3 cm in the standing adult. Although the ACJ itself has only 5 to 8 degrees of movement, it allows for 40 to 50 degrees of clavicular rotation. The latter is required to achieve a full range of motion at the glenohumeral joint.

The scapula is a flat triangular bone that forms the posterior aspect of the shoulder girdle. The thin body of the scapula lies flat against the posterior thorax and widens laterally to form the glenoid fossa. A stable base from which glenohumeral motion can occur is provided by 18 muscular origins and insertions on the scapula.[9]

The flat anterior surface of the scapula gives rise to the subscapularis muscle, whereas the serratus anterior muscle inserts onto its thickened medial border. Posteriorly the surface is divided into two parts by the scapular spine. The areas superior and inferior to the spine give rise to the supraspinatus and infraspinatus muscles. The teres minor and major muscles originate from the posterior aspect of the lateral border of the scapula. The thickened posteromedial border serves as the attachment site for the rhomboid and levator scapulae muscles.

The superior border of the scapula gives rise to an anterior projection, the coracoid process (see Figure 50-1). As discussed, the coracoid provides attachment for numerous important ligaments and muscles that help stabilize the glenohumeral joint. The acromion, in conjunction with the strong coracoacromial ligament, forms the coracoacromial arch (see Figure 50-3). Muscles attached to the coracoid process include the short head of the biceps, coracobrachialis, and pectoralis minor. The neurovascular bundle is located beneath the coracoacromial arch, immediately posterior to the coracoid process.

The glenohumeral articulation is a ball-and-socket–type joint (Figure 50-4). The glenoid fossa is deepened by a rim of fibrocartilage (glenoid labrum) and provides a bearing surface for only half of the humeral head at any one time. The absence of congruent surfaces makes the bony joint mechanically unstable. The stability of the joint primarily depends on associated muscles and ligaments. A negative intracapsular pressure completes the stabilization mechanism.[10,11] The absence of bony stability permits a range of motion, however, that is greater than that of any other joint in the body.

A synovial membrane extends from the glenoid fossa to the humeral head. The membrane is large and redundant inferiorly to accommodate the extensive range of movement. The synovial membrane extends medially to form the subscapularis bursa and laterally to envelop the long head of the biceps. Overlying the synovial membrane is a loose and redundant fibrous capsule (see Figure 50-4). Anteriorly the capsule is thickened to form the superior, middle, and inferior glenohumeral ligaments. The inferior glenohumeral ligament is subdivided further into an anterior band, a posterior band, and an interposing pouch. The anterior band of the inferior glenohumeral ligament is the most important restraint to anterior glenohumeral dislocations.[10,11] Superiorly the acromial process and the coracohumeral ligament (see Figure 50-4) protect the capsule.

The proximal humerus articulates with the glenoid fossa and provides for the attachment of many important muscles. The supraspinatus, infraspinatus, and teres minor insert onto facets of the greater tuberosity, whereas the subscapularis inserts onto the lesser tuberosity. Together, this group of muscles forms the rotator cuff, which helps stabilize the humeral head within the glenohumeral joint (Figure 50-5). The long head of the biceps tendon originates from the supraglenoid tubercle and ascends over the humeral head to enter the arm via the bicipital groove. The long head acts as an additional stabilizer for the superior and anterior aspect of the glenohumeral joint (see Figure 50-5). Long muscles that cross the articulation are involved primarily in movements of the glenohumeral joint. The pectoralis major, latissimus dorsi, and teres major muscles all insert into the humeral intertubercular groove. Displacements encountered with fractures of the humerus usually reflect the pull of these attached muscle groups. The proximal humerus is composed primarily of trabecular bone with a thin cortical shell. Changes in bone density with age (osteoporosis) greatly increase the risk of fractures in this area.[7]

The blood supply of the articular surface of the humerus is derived from vessels contained in the rotator cuff tendons and from the anastomosis of the anterior and posterior circumflex humeral arteries. The neurovascular bundle runs anteriorly, and the axillary nerve is in close proximity to the inferior aspect of the joint. Movements of the glenohumeral joint include flexion, extension, abduction, adduction, internal rotation, external rotation, and circumduction.

Four nerves supply most of the shoulder muscles. The axillary nerve supplies the deltoid and teres minor muscles; the suprascapular nerve, the supraspinatus and infraspinatus muscles; the subscapular nerve, the teres major and subscapularis muscles; and the musculocutaneous nerve, the proximal arm muscles. These nerves represent the final branches of the upper bracial plexus (nerve roots C5-8), and injuries to the brachial plexus invariably result in significant shoulder dysfunction.

CLINICAL FEATURES

History

Most complaints usually involve some combination of pain, stiffness, instability, and weakness. Pain can result from many different conditions extrinsic and intrinsic to the shoulder. Extrinsic sources of shoulder pain include disorders of the cervical spine, thoracic outlet syndromes, and Pancoast's tumors. In addition, pain can be referred to the shoulder from myocardial processes, diaphragmatic irritation (e.g., subphrenic abscess, lower lobe pneumonia, splenic hematoma, ruptured ectopic pregnancy, gallbladder disease), and gastric or pancreatic diseases.

Acute intrinsic pain usually is associated with a traumatic event. The most important factors to determine are the time and mechanism of injury, its precise location, and the intensity of the pain. Occasionally the patient may have acute pain in the absence of associated trauma (e.g., calcific tendinitis). Shoulder pain also can present in an insidious manner, unrelated to any precipitating factor. In these instances, the duration,

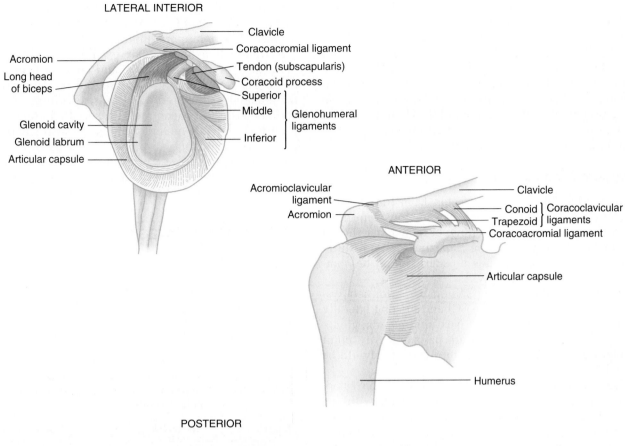

LATERAL INTERIOR

Clavicle
Acromion
Coracoacromial ligament
Long head of biceps
Tendon (subscapularis)
Coracoid process
Superior
Middle — Glenohumeral ligaments
Glenoid cavity
Glenoid labrum
Inferior
Articular capsule

ANTERIOR

Acromioclavicular ligament
Clavicle
Acromion
Conoid — Coracoclavicular ligaments
Trapezoid
Coracoacromial ligament
Articular capsule
Humerus

POSTERIOR

Coracoid process
Coracohumeral ligament
Acromion
Articular capsule
Inferior transverse scapular ligament
Humerus

Figure 50-4. Anatomy of the glenohumeral joint.

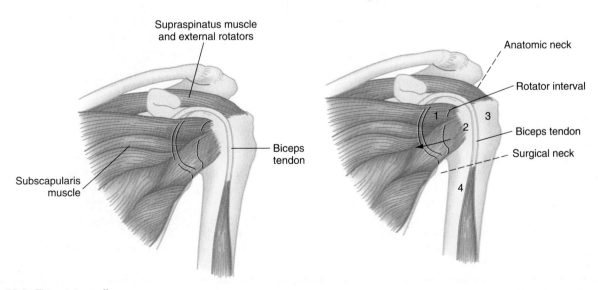

Supraspinatus muscle and external rotators
Biceps tendon
Subscapularis muscle

Anatomic neck
Rotator interval
Biceps tendon
Surgical neck

Figure 50-5. The rotator cuff.

location, character, and aggravating and alleviating factors of the pain should be noted. Intrinsic shoulder pain in general does not radiate past the elbow.

Stiffness usually signifies a restricted range of motion resulting from an underlying painful condition of the shoulder. Instability can be seen in the form of an obvious subluxation or dislocation. Alternatively the patient may relate the sensation of the shoulder almost going out. A rotator cuff tear or an underlying nerve lesion usually causes significant shoulder weakness.

Physical Examination

The shoulder should be inspected from the anterior, posterior, and lateral positions. Any obvious deformity, ecchymosis, laceration, swelling, or hematoma should be noted. The masses of the trapezius, deltoid, infraspinatus, and supraspinatus muscles should be compared to detect any atrophy.

Palpation of the shoulder should be performed systematically, beginning at the SCJ and moving laterally along the clavicle to the ACJ. Next the scapula, glenohumeral joint, and humerus are palpated. Any point tenderness, crepitus, swelling, or deformity should be noted.

Active and passive ranges of motion should be tested. Active range of motion is best determined with the patient in the sitting position, which eliminates the contributions of the lumbar spine and lower extremity joints. Passive range of motion is best evaluated with the patient in the supine position. The degrees of abduction, forward flexion, extension, and internal and external rotation should be recorded and compared with the unaffected extremity. In addition, the motion of the scapulothoracic articulation should be observed

carefully in all cases. After 45 degrees of abduction, the scapula moves approximately 1 degree for every 2 degrees of glenohumeral motion.

A thorough neurovascular examination should be performed in all cases before and after all manipulations. The vascular status is checked by determining the brachial, radial, and ulnar pulses with the arms in various positions. A complete sensory (light touch and pinprick) and full motor examination also should be performed. The brachial plexus can be tested by evaluating the myotomes and dermatomes pertinent to each nerve root (Table 50-1). In addition, the deep tendon reflexes should be evaluated in both upper extremities.

DIAGNOSTIC STRATEGIES

Radiology

The initial assessment of traumatic injuries includes a three-view series of radiographs consisting of true anteroposterior (45-degree lateral), transscapular lateral, and axillary lateral views (Figures 50-6 and

Table 50-1. Sensory and Motor Components of the Brachial Plexus

Level	Sensory Area	Muscle
C2-4	—	Trapezius
C5	Lateral arm	Deltoid
C6	Lateral forearm	Biceps
C7	Index fingertip	Thumb extensors
C8	Little fingertip	Finger flexors
T1	Medial forearm	Interossei

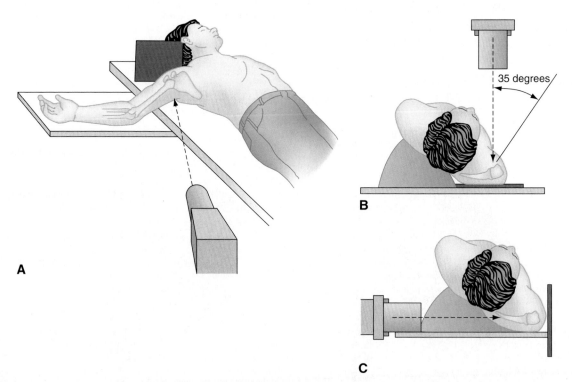

Figure 50-6. Positions for the trauma series of shoulder radiographs. **A,** Axillary view. **B,** True anteroposterior (35-degree oblique) view. **C,** Transscapular lateral view.

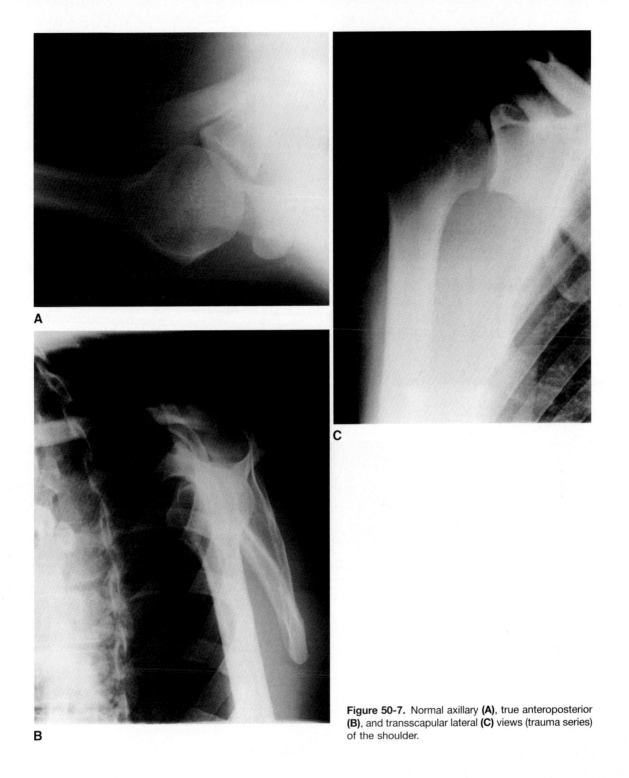

A

B

C

Figure 50-7. Normal axillary **(A)**, true anteroposterior **(B)**, and transscapular lateral **(C)** views (trauma series) of the shoulder.

50-7). The true anteroposterior view (see Figure 50-7B) is preferred over standard anteroposterior views because it projects the glenohumeral joint without any bony overlap. Standard anteroposterior views taken in internal and external rotation profile the lesser and greater tuberosity and are more useful in the evaluation of soft tissue conditions.

Acceptable orthogonal views include the axillary lateral, transscapular lateral, and apical oblique.[12] The preferred view is the axillary lateral (see Figure 50-7A), which projects the glenohumeral joint in a cephalo-caudal plane. This view is particularly useful for defin-

ing the relationship of the humeral head with the glenoid fossa and in identifying lesions of the coracoid process, humeral head, and glenoid rim.[13] Some degree of abduction is required to obtain the axillary view. Because this may not be possible with some injuries, a reverse projection or a modified axillary view (Figure 50-8) may be considered. The difficulty in obtaining the axillary view has led to the popularity of the transscapular view (see Figure 50-7C). Advantages of this projection include its simplicity and reproducibility and the clear delineation of anatomic structures. In this view, the scapula is projected as a *Y,* with the body

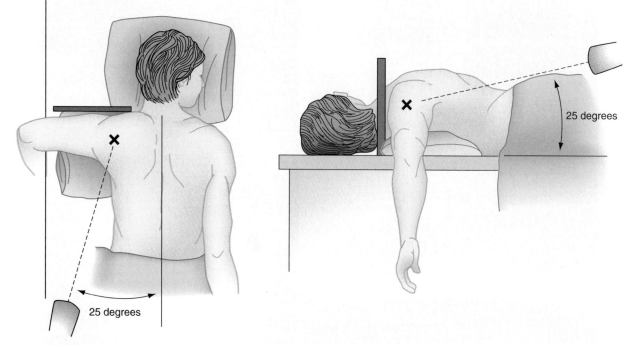

Figure 50-8. Modified axillary view of the shoulder.

Figure 50-9. Displaced midclavicular fracture.

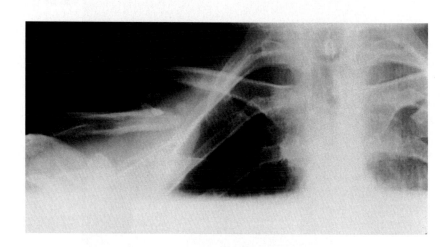

forming the lower limb and the coracoid and acromion processes forming the upper limbs. The humeral head is normally superimposed over the glenoid, which is located at the junction of the three limbs. This view is particularly useful in identifying anterior and posterior glenohumeral dislocations. The apical oblique film (obtained by placing the injured shoulder in a 45-degree oblique position and angling the central ray 45 degrees caudally) provides a unique coronal view of the glenohumeral joint. The view can be obtained easily and painlessly and has been found to be more sensitive than the transscapular view for detecting bone and joint abnormalities in the injured shoulder.[14] Plain radiographs are the mainstay of the radiologic examination in the emergency department, but in selected circumstances, additional bone and soft tissue details may be obtained using computed tomography (CT) or magnetic resonance imaging (MRI).[15]

SPECIFIC INJURIES

Fractures

Clavicle

Pathophysiology

The clavicle accounts for 5% of all fractures and is the most commonly fractured bone in children. Epidemiologic studies in adults have documented an annual incidence rate of 30 to 50 per 100,000 population, with a 2 : 1 male-to-female ratio.[16,17] Clavicular fractures are classified anatomically and mechanistically into three types. Fractures of the medial third are uncommon (5%) and occur as a result of a direct blow to the anterior chest. Fractures of the middle third are the most frequent (Figure 50-9), accounting for 80% of all injuries. The usual mechanism of injury involves a

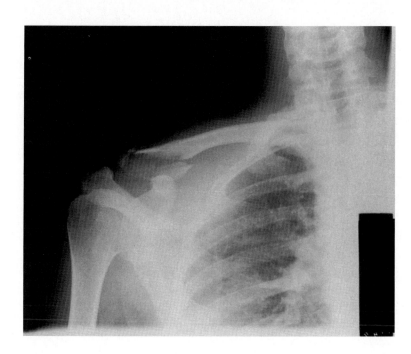

direct force applied to the lateral aspect of the shoulder as a result of a fall, sporting injury, or motor vehicle accident. Fractures of the lateral third (15%) result from a direct blow to the top of the shoulder and are classified further into three subtypes.[18] Type I fractures are stable and occur lateral to the coracoclavicular ligaments. Type II fractures are medial to the coracoclavicular ligaments and have a tendency to displace because the proximal fragment lacks any stabilizing ligaments. Type III injuries involve the articular surface (Figure 50-10).[18]

Clinical Features

The patient has pain over the fracture site, and the affected extremity is held close to the body. With fractures of the middle third, the shoulder typically is slumped downward, forward, and inward. This is a result of the effect of gravity and the pull of the pectoralis major and latissimus dorsi on the distal fragment. The proximal fragment is often displaced upward by the action of the sternocleidomastoid. The head is often tilted toward the injured side in an attempt to relax the effects of these displacing muscular forces. Ecchymosis, crepitus, and a palpable or visible deformity may be present over the fracture site. Although associated neurovascular injury is rare, the close proximity of the subclavian vessels and brachial plexus demands a thorough assessment. Rarely, injury to the dome of the pleura may result in an associated pneumothorax.

Management

Principles of initial management include pain control, immobilization, and proper follow-up. Fractures of the clavicle can be immobilized with supportive devices, such as a simple sling or sling and swathe (Figure 50-11). Another immobilization technique for midclavicular fractures still recommended in the orthopedic literature is the clavicular (figure-of-eight) splint (Figure 50-12). This splint is applied after closed reduction of the fracture, which is accomplished by pulling the shoulders up and back. Such reductions are difficult to maintain and may be associated with increased discomfort at the fracture site. Clavicular splints can lead to skin irritation and compression of the neurovascular bundle in the axilla. Because malunion and shortening are associated with an acceptable functional and cosmetic outcome, treatment with a simple sling is a valid and appropriate alternative to the clavicular splint in the emergency department.[19,20]

Disposition

Immediate orthopedic consultation should be sought for open fractures or fractures associated with neurovascular injuries, skin tenting, or interposition of soft tissues. More urgent orthopedic consultation (before 72 hours) is recommended for type II lateral clavicle fractures because these fractures have a 30% incidence of nonunion and may require surgical repair.[18] Severely comminuted or displaced fractures of the middle third (defined as >20 mm of initial shortening) also may benefit from early orthopedic referral because these have been associated with a higher incidence of nonunion.[21] Greenstick fractures of the midclavicle are common in children (Figure 50-13). Most of these fractures are nondisplaced and heal uneventfully. Initial radiographs may appear normal despite suggestive clinical findings. In these instances, the arm should be immobilized in a simple sling and the radiographs repeated in 7 to 10 days if symptoms persist.

Most fractures of the clavicle heal uneventfully and can be followed by a primary care physician. A sling should be worn until repeat radiographs show callus formation and healing across the fracture site. Passive shoulder range-of-motion exercises (Figure 50-14) are encouraged to reduce the risk of adhesive capsulitis. Younger children generally require shorter periods of

Figure 50-11. Shoulder immobilization. **A,** Sling over swathe. **B,** Velpeau sling immobilization.

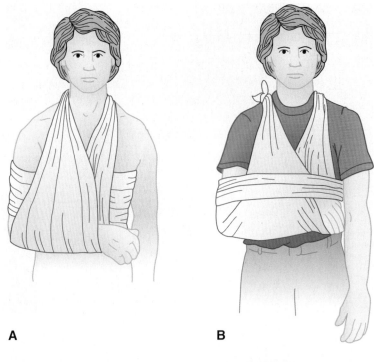

A   B

Figure 50-12. Clavicular or figure-of-eight splint.

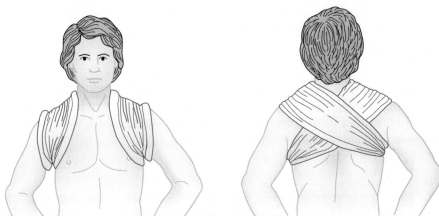

Figure 50-13. Greenstick fracture of the clavicle *(arrow)*.

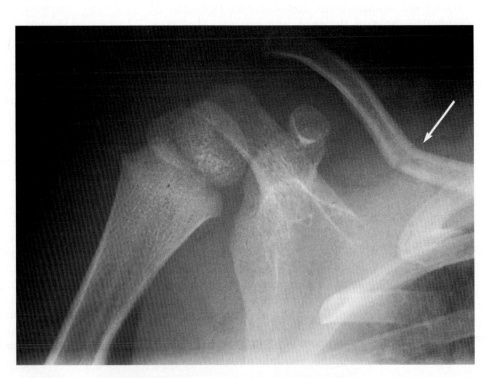

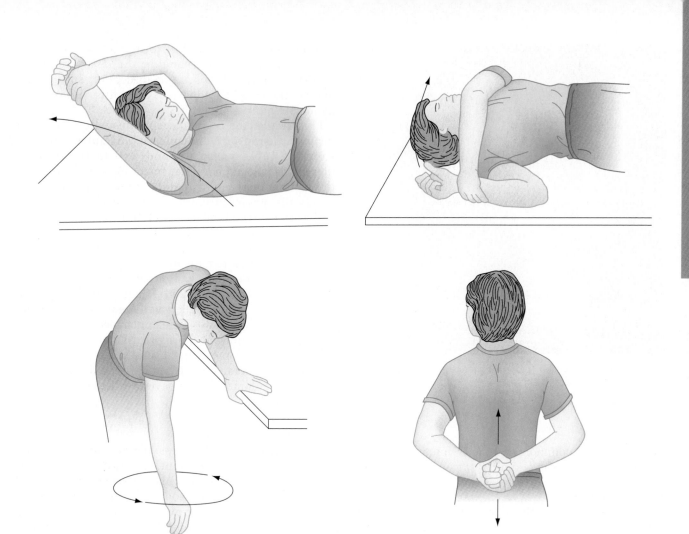

Figure 50-14. Pendular shoulder exercises.

immobilization (2 to 4 weeks) than adolescents and adults (4 to 8 weeks). Vigorous competitive play should be avoided until the bone healing is solid.

Complications

Complications are unusual, with the most common ones being delayed union or nonunion.[16-18] Complications after fractures of the medial third resemble complications associated with posterior sternoclavicular dislocations. Fractures of the middle third have been associated with injuries to the neurovascular bundle and the pleural dome. Articular surface injuries (type III lateral clavicle fractures) can lead to subsequent osteoarthritis of the ACJ.

Scapula

Pathophysiology

Fractures of the scapula are rare injuries, with an annual incidence of 10 to 12 per 100,000 population.[22,23] They account for 1% of all fractures and occur primarily in men 30 to 40 years old.[9] A thick muscle coat and the ability to recoil along the chest wall protect the scapula from direct and indirect trauma. In general, considerable force and energy are required to

fracture the scapula. Most fractures result from high-speed vehicular accidents, falls from heights, or crush injuries.[24] Coracoid process fractures are usually avulsive, and glenoid rim fractures are commonly associated with anterior glenohumeral dislocations. An acromial process fracture usually results from a direct blow applied to the top of the shoulder.

The most important aspect of scapular fractures is the high incidence (75% to 98%) of associated injuries to the ipsilateral lung, chest wall, and shoulder girdle complex.[9,25,26] The most common associated orthopedic injuries are fractures of the ribs, proximal humerus, and clavicle. Associated lung injuries include pneumothorax, hemothorax, and pulmonary contusion; these may be seen in a delayed fashion, 2 to 3 days after the initial injury. Associated injuries of the head, spinal cord, brachial plexus, and subclavian or axillary vessels are more significant but less common.[9,25,26]

Fractures of the scapula can be classified according to their anatomic location. In the system proposed by Ada and Miller,[25] type I fractures involve the acromion process, scapular spine, or coracoid process. Type II fractures involve the scapular neck, and type III injuries are intra-articular fractures of the glenoid fossa (Figure

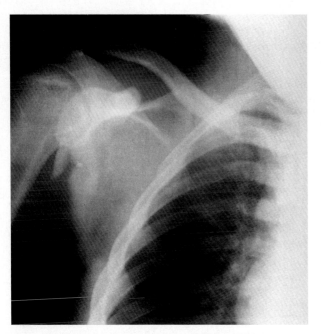

Figure 50-15. Comminuted type III fracture of the scapular. (Courtesy of David Nelson, MD.)

50-15). The most common are type IV fractures, which involve the body of the scapula.[25]

Clinical Features

In a conscious patient, the shoulder is adducted, and the arm is held close to the body. Any attempts at movement result in significant pain. There may be associated tenderness, crepitus, or hematoma over the fracture site. The clinical findings occasionally mimic those seen with a rotator cuff tear. Hemorrhage into the rotator cuff associated with the scapula fracture can result in spasm and a temporary reflex inhibition of function (pseudorupture).[25] The presence of a scapula fracture mandates a thorough search for associated thoracic, intracranial, orthopedic, and neurovascular injuries.

Diagnostic Strategies

The trauma series of shoulder radiographs identifies most fractures, as does careful examination of the scapula on the trauma chest radiograph. The axillary lateral view is especially useful in evaluating fractures of the glenoid fossa and the acromion or coracoid processes.[9] The os acromiale (unfused acromial process epiphysis) is present in 3% of the population and should not be confused with a fracture of the acromion.[7] A comparison film can be useful because the abnormality is present bilaterally in 60% of cases. In many patients, fractures of the scapula initially are overlooked because of the life-threatening nature of the associated injuries.[9]

Management

Most fractures, including fractures with severe comminution and displacement, heal rapidly with conservative therapy.[9,24,25] Initial therapy consists of analgesia and immobilization in a sling to support the ipsilateral upper extremity. Passive shoulder exercises (see Figure 50-14) are initiated as soon as discomfort subsides to reduce the risk of adhesive capsulitis. In general, patients require a sling for 2 to 4 weeks.[24]

Fractures of the body and spine usually require no further therapy. Nondisplaced fractures of the acromion process also respond well to conservative therapy. Displaced acromial fractures that impinge on the glenohumeral joint require surgical management. Rarely the acromion is fractured as part of a superior dislocation of the humeral head. In these instances, an accompanying tear of the rotator cuff is invariably present and requires surgical repair. If the coracoclavicular ligaments remain intact, fractures of the coracoid process respond well to conservative therapy. Severely displaced coracoid fractures with ruptured coracoclavicular ligaments usually require open reduction and internal fixation.[6] Scapular neck and glenoid fossa fractures present the most difficult management issues. Although most of these injuries do well with conservative therapy, open reduction and internal fixation are recommended for severely displaced or angulated fractures.[24,25]

Complications

Associated injuries of the ipsilateral lung, chest wall, and shoulder girdle account for most complications after fractures of the scapula. A shear-type brachial plexus injury has been associated with fractures of the acromion process. Neurovascular (brachial plexus, axillary artery) injuries also have been reported with fractures of the coracoid process.[6] Scapular neck, body, or spine fractures that extend into the suprascapular notch can injure the suprascapular nerve.[6] Delayed complications include adhesive capsulitis and rotator cuff dysfunction.[24]

Proximal Humerus

Pathophysiology

Fractures of the proximal humerus are common and account for 4% of all fractures.[27] A prospective Swedish study reported an incidence of 114 per 100,000 with a mean age of 67 years and a female-to-male ratio of 3 : 1.[28] These fractures occur primarily in the older population, in whom structural changes associated with aging (osteoporosis) weaken the proximal humerus, predisposing it to injury. Although most of these injuries are minimally displaced and do well with conservative therapy, significantly displaced fractures may require operative intervention.

Fractures of the proximal humerus separate along old epiphyseal lines, producing four distinct segments consisting of the articular surface (anatomic neck), greater tuberosity, lesser tuberosity, and humeral shaft (surgical neck). The Neer classification system (Figure 50-16) is based on the relationship of these fracture fragments.[29,30] In this system, a segment is considered displaced if it is angled greater than 45 degrees or separated more than 1 cm from the neighboring segment. Because this classification system considers

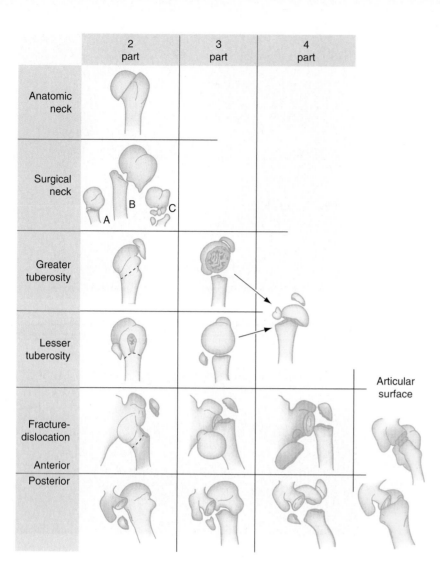

	2 part	3 part	4 part
Anatomic neck			
Surgical neck	A B C		
Greater tuberosity			
Lesser tuberosity			
Fracture-dislocation Anterior Posterior			Articular surface

Figure 50-16. Neer's classification of proximal humeral fractures. (From Neer CS: Displaced proximal humeral fractures: Part 1. Classification and evaluation. *J Bone Joint Surg Am* 52:1077, 1979.)

only displacement, the number of fracture lines is irrelevant. There are four major categories of fracture: minimal displacement (Figure 50-17), two-part displacement (Figure 50-18), three-part displacement, and four-part displacement. When present, anterior and posterior dislocations are included as part of the classification. Impaction and head-splitting fractures are classified separately.

The classic mechanism of injury involves a fall on an outstretched abducted arm. Concurrent pronation limits further abduction and levers the humerus against the acromial process; this produces a fracture or dislocation, depending on the tensile strengths of the bone and surrounding ligaments. Older patients are prone to fracture, whereas younger individuals are apt to dislocate. The combined injury (fracture and dislocation) may be seen in middle-aged individuals. Proximal humerus fractures also may result from a direct blow to the lateral side of the arm or from an axial load transmitted through the elbow. High-energy mechanisms and polytrauma are more common in younger individuals.

Clinical Features

The affected arm is held close to the body, and all movements are restricted by pain. Tenderness,

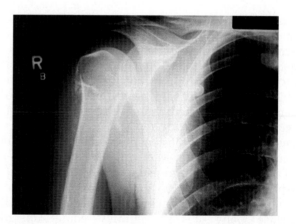

Figure 50-17. Three-part minimally displaced fracture of the proximal humerus.

hematoma, ecchymosis, deformity, or crepitus may be present over the fracture site. Although usually normal, a thorough neurovascular examination helps identify associated injuries of the axillary nerve, brachial plexus, or axillary artery.

Management

Minimally displaced fractures (see Figure 50-17) constitute 80% to 85% of all cases. No displacement

Figure 50-18. Anteroposterior **(A)** and axillary **(B)** views of a two-part displaced fracture of the proximal humerus. The degree of displacement often is visualized better on the axillary view. (Courtesy of David Nelson, MD.)

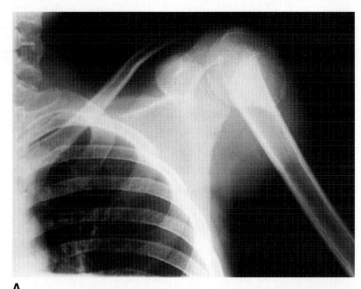

A

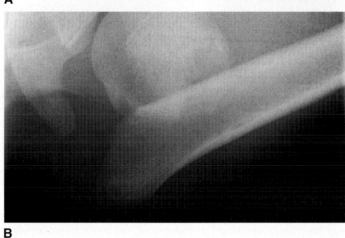

B

or angulation is present, and the fracture segments are held together by the capsule, periosteum, and surrounding muscles. Initial treatment consists of adequate analgesia and immobilization with a sling and swathe device. As soon as clinical union is achieved (head and shaft move together), functional exercises are initiated. Initial passive exercises (see Figure 50-14) are slowly replaced by more active and resistive exercises. Most nondisplaced fractures heal over 4 to 6 weeks.

The treatment of two-part, three-part, and four-part displaced fractures is beyond the scope of this discussion. An orthopedic surgeon should be consulted because many of these injuries require operative repair.[30] Fracture-dislocation injuries also may require an orthopedic surgeon. Care must be used because reductions of these injuries in the emergency department are often unsuccessful and can cause separation of previously undisplaced segments. Closed reduction under x-ray control and general anesthesia may be preferable.[31]

Posterior glenohumeral dislocations usually are associated with anteromedial impression fractures of the articular surface. A similar fracture of the posterolateral aspect of the humeral head is present with anterior dislocations (Hill-Sachs deformity). Impression frac-

tures involving less than 20% of the articular surface are usually stable. With more than 20% involvement, the reduction is usually unstable and requires surgical repair.

Complications

The most common complication of proximal humeral fractures is adhesive capsulitis ("frozen or stiff shoulder"). This complication can be prevented by the early initiation of a thorough rehabilitation program. Two-part fractures of the articular surface and four-part fractures have a high incidence of avascular necrosis of the humeral head. Repeated forceful attempts at reduction of fracture-dislocations may be associated with subsequent heterotopic bone formation (myositis ossificans). Neurovascular injuries (axillary nerve, brachial plexus, and axillary artery) may be encountered with displaced surgical neck fractures and fracture-dislocations.

Proximal Humeral Epiphysis

Pathophysiology

Fractures of the proximal humeral epiphysis are uncommon and account for 10% of all shoulder fractures in children.[32] The injury can occur at any age

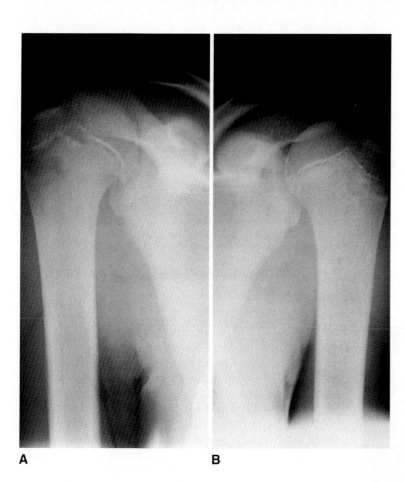

Figure 50-19. A, Salter I injury of the right proximal humeral epiphysis. **B,** Normal left side is included for comparison.

A   B

while the epiphysis remains open but is most common in boys 11 to 17 years old.[33] The most common mechanism of injury involves a fall onto the outstretched hand, and the fracture typically occurs through the zone of hypertrophy in the epiphyseal plate. Injuries can be classified according to their location (Salter system), stability, and degree of displacement.[6]

Clinical Features

The patient has the injured arm held tightly against the body by the opposite hand. The area over the proximal humerus is swollen and extremely tender to palpation. Radiographs obtained at 90 degrees to each other confirm the diagnosis. Comparison views may be helpful with minimally displaced fractures.[33]

Management

Fractures of the proximal humeral epiphysis should not be taken lightly because the potential for growth disturbance exists even under the most ideal conditions. The active healing process at the site of an epiphyseal injury makes delayed reduction extremely difficult. Early orthopedic consultation should be obtained for all such injuries. Children younger than 6 years old usually have Salter I epiphyseal injuries (Figure 50-19) and can be treated conservatively with sling and swathe immobilization and analgesic agents. Children older than age 6 usually have a Salter II epiphyseal injury. Salter II injuries with greater than 20 degrees of angulation should be reduced.[34] Closed reduction is accomplished by reversing the mechanism

of injury. Imperfect reductions are often acceptable because growth and remodeling correct the deformity with time. After reduction, unstable injuries should be immobilized in a shoulder spica cast, whereas stable lesions can be immobilized with a sling and swathe. Fractures of the proximal humeral epiphyses generally heal in 3 to 5 weeks.[34]

Complications

Complications are rare and include malunion, growth plate disturbances, and injuries to the neurovascular bundle. Markedly displaced or angulated fractures are more likely to result in a residual loss of mobility.[32]

Dislocations

Sternoclavicular

Pathophysiology

The SCJ is the least commonly dislocated major joint in the body. Significant forces are required to disrupt the strong ligamentous stabilizers of this joint. The most common causes are motor vehicle accidents and injuries sustained in contact sports, such as rugby or football. The SCJ can dislocate in an anterior or posterior direction. Anterior dislocations, which result from indirect forces, are more common (9 : 1 ratio).[5] The usual mechanism of injury (Figure 50-20) involves an anterolateral force to the shoulder, followed by backward rolling, which levers the medial clavicle out of its articulation. Posterior dislocations (Figure 50-21) can

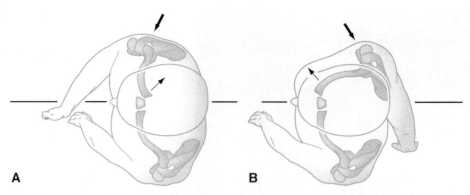

A   B

Figure 50-20. Mechanisms that produce anterior and posterior displacements of the sternoclavicular joint. **A,** When the patient is lying on the ground and a compression force is applied to the posterolateral aspect of the shoulder, the medial end of the clavicle is displaced posteriorly. **B,** When the lateral compression force is directed from the anterior position, the medial end of the clavicle is dislocated anteriorly. The same mechanism could apply with any type of lateral compression injury of the shoulder. (From Neer CS, Rockwood CA: Fracture and dislocations of the shoulder. In Rockwood CA, Green DP [eds]: *Fractures in Adults,* 4th ed. Philadelphia, JB Lippincott, 1984.)

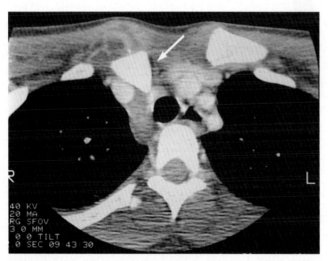

Figure 50-21. CT scan shows posterior dislocation of the right sternoclavicular *(arrow)* joint with compression of the superior mediastinum. (Courtesy of Donald Sauser, MD.)

result from a direct blow to the medial clavicle (30%) or from a posterolateral force to the shoulder followed by inward rolling (70%). Posterior dislocations can be associated with life-threatening injuries within the superior mediastinum. Injuries to the SCJ can be graded into three types.[5] A grade I injury is a mild sprain secondary to stretching of the sternoclavicular and costoclavicular ligaments. A grade II injury is associated with subluxation of the joint (anterior or posterior) secondary to rupture of the sternoclavicular ligament. The costoclavicular ligament remains intact. Complete rupture of the sternoclavicular and costoclavicular ligaments results in a grade III injury (dislocation). In patients younger than age 25, these actually represent Salter Type I injuries because the medial epiphysis of the clavicle has not yet fused.[35]

Clinical Features

Clinical suspicion is the most important factor in diagnosing these injuries, and prompt diagnosis is vital because it is associated with a better prognosis. Patients

have the injured extremity foreshortened and supported across the trunk by the opposite arm. There is pain with any movement of the upper extremity or lateral compression of the shoulders. The SCJ is mildly swollen and tender to palpation. With an anterior dislocation, the displaced medial end of the clavicle may be palpable. Posterior dislocations are associated with more severe pain, and the neck is often flexed toward the injured side.[5] The clavicular notch of the sternum may be palpable, and there may be complaints of hoarseness, dysphagia, dyspnea, and weakness or paresthesias in the upper extremities. Rarely, airway complications can occur. These patients should be examined thoroughly to identify any injuries to superior mediastinal or intrathoracic structures. When necessary, appropriate consultation should be obtained immediately.

Diagnostic Strategies: Radiology

Although the diagnosis of sternoclavicular dislocations can be made clinically, it should be confirmed radiologically. Standard anteroposterior, oblique, and specialized (40-degree cephalic tilt) views are often difficult to interpret because of overlapping rib, sternum, and vertebral shadows. CT is best to visualize these dislocations and associated injuries (see Figure 50-21) or MRI.[15] Ultrasound also may be a useful adjunct in some circumstances.[5]

Management

Treatment of grade I injuries includes immobilization (simple sling), adequate analgesia, and primary care follow-up. Immobilization generally is maintained (1 to 2 weeks) until full painless motion is restored. Grade II injuries should be immobilized with a sling or soft clavicular (figure-of-eight) splint and referred for orthopedic follow-up. The figure-of-eight splint is preferred because it maintains the clavicle in a more anatomic position. Grade II injuries require a longer course of immobilization (3 to 6 weeks) and are more likely to be associated with persistent pain.[5,6] All grade III injuries should be managed by closed reduction. Anterior dislocations may be reduced in the emergency department

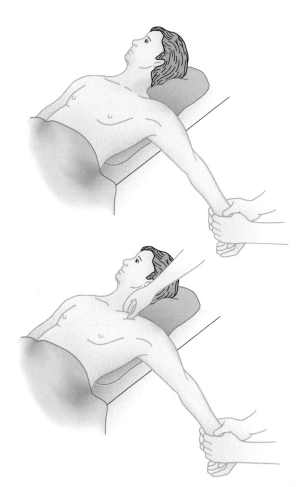

Figure 50-22. Reduction of dislocated sternoclavicular joints. (From Simon RR, Koenigsknecht SJ: *Emergency Orthopedics: The Extremities*, 2nd ed. Norwalk, Conn, Appleton & Lange, 1987.)

after orthopedic consultation and intravenous analgesia (Figure 50-22). A rolled sheet is placed posteriorly between the shoulder blades to elevate both shoulders approximately 5 cm above the table. Traction is applied to the arm in an extended (10- to 15-degree) and abducted (90-degree) position. If reduction does not occur, an assistant can add inward pressure on the medial end of the clavicle. Stable reductions should be maintained in a clavicular splint and referred for orthopedic follow-up.[5,6] Most reductions are unstable. Because the deformity is primarily cosmetic and not functional, the current treatment of choice for recurrent anterior dislocations is benign neglect.

Posterior dislocations are true orthopedic emergencies and should be reduced expeditiously.[5] Ideally, reduction of posterior dislocations should be attempted in the operating room under general anesthesia, although it can be attempted in the emergency department under conscious sedation. Emergency reduction may be required for patients with airway obstruction or vascular compromise. The patient is positioned as described previously, and traction is applied in an extended and abducted position. If traction alone does not reduce the dislocation, concurrent clavicular manipulation may be helpful. The skin is sterilely prepared, and the clavicle shaft is grasped with a sterile towel clip and pulled out anterolaterally. When

reduced, these injuries are generally stable and can be immobilized with a clavicular splint. Buckerfield and Castle[36] described an alternate method of reduction for posterior dislocations. In this technique, traction is applied to the adducted arm while both shoulders simultaneously are forced posteriorly using direct pressure. This technique levers the clavicle into place and requires much less force than the traditional abduction-extension method.

Complications

Complications of anterior injuries are primarily cosmetic. Twenty-five percent of posterior dislocations may be complicated by life-threatening injuries to intrathoracic and superior mediastinal structures. A potential long-term complication of both is degenerative osteoarthritis.

Acromioclavicular Joint

Pathophysiology

Injuries of the ACJ occur primarily in men and account for 25% of all dislocations about the shoulder girdle.[28] The annual incidence is 15 per 100,000, and most injuries result from participation in contact sports, such as football, rugby, ice hockey, and wrestling.[28] A small percentage of injuries are caused by motor vehicle accidents and falls.

The most common mechanism of injury involves a fall or direct blow to the point of the shoulder with the arm adducted. The resultant force drives the scapula downward and medially to produce the injury. The weak acromioclavicular ligaments rupture first. With increasing force, the coracoclavicular ligament ruptures, and the attachments of the deltoid and trapezius muscles are torn from the distal clavicle. The ACJ also can be injured after a fall onto the outstretched hand. In this instance, the force is transmitted to the acromioclavicular ligaments only, and the coracoclavicular ligament, which is relaxed, remains uninjured.[37]

The three-part Tossy and Allman classification system is based on the degree of damage sustained by the acromioclavicular and coracoclavicular ligaments (Figure 50-23).[8] Type I injuries are sprains of the acromioclavicular ligaments. Type II injuries are associated with disruption of the acromioclavicular ligaments. The joint space is widened, and the clavicle displaces slightly upward. There are minor tears in the attachments of the deltoid and trapezius muscles, but the coracoclavicular ligament remains intact, and the coracoclavicular distance is maintained. A type III injury is characterized by complete disruption of the acromioclavicular ligaments, coracoclavicular ligament, and muscle attachments. The joint space is widened, and the coracoclavicular distance is increased. The clavicle is displaced upward by the pull of the trapezius, and the shoulder is displaced downward by the effect of gravity. Rockwood modified this three-part classification system by describing three additional types (IV, V, and VI) of ACJ injuries.[35] In type IV and V injuries, the ligamentous and muscle disruptions are similar to the disruptions encountered in type

Figure 50-23. Mechanism of injury and classification of acromioclavicular joint injuries. **A,** The direct force is applied to the point of the shoulder *(1)*; the scapula and attached clavicle are forced downward and medially; the clavicle approaches the first rib *(2)*. If the force continues, the first rib abuts the clavicle, producing a counterforce *(3)*. Depending on the magnitude of the force, a grade I, II, or III sprain may occur. **B,** Grade I sprain. A few fibers of the acromioclavicular ligament stretch, and a few tear *(1)*; the acromioclavicular joint is stable *(2)*; the coracoclavicular ligament is intact *(3)*. **C,** Grade II sprain (subluxation). The capsule and the acromioclavicular ligament rupture *(1)*; the joint is lax and unstable *(2)*; the end of the clavicle rides upward, usually less than half of the width of the end of the clavicle *(3)*; the coracoclavicular ligament remains intact *(4)*; the attachments to the trapezius and deltoid remain intact. **D,** Grade III sprain (dislocation). The capsule and acromioclavicular ligaments rupture *(1)*; the coracoclavicular ligament ruptures *(2)*; the insertions of the trapezius and deltoid tear away *(3)*; the clavicle rides upward *(4)*; the interval between the clavicle and the coracoid process is greatly increased *(5)*. (From DePalma AF: *Surgery of the Shoulder,* 3rd ed. Philadelphia, JB Lippincott, 1983.)

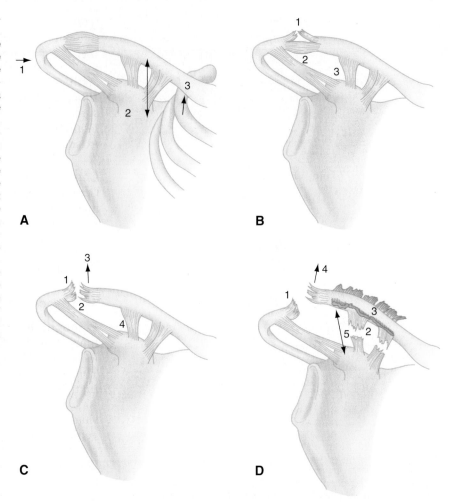

III injuries, but the clavicle displaces either posteriorly into the trapezius (type IV) or superiorly in an exaggerated fashion (type V). In the rare type VI injury, the clavicle displaces inferiorly.

Clinical Features

Patients should be examined while they are in the sitting or standing position because the supine position can mask ACJ instability. Type I injuries are associated with mild tenderness and swelling over the ACJ margin. No deformity occurs, and a full range of motion is usually possible, although painful. Type II injuries produce moderate pain, and the distal end of the clavicle may lie slightly superior or posterior to the acromion. Patients with type III, IV, V, and VI injuries usually have severe pain and hold the arm tightly adducted to reduce traction stress across the joint. In type III injuries, the shoulder hangs downward, and the clavicle rides high, producing a visible clinical deformity. In type IV injuries, the clavicle may be palpable posteriorly, and in type V injuries, the clavicle may be palpable subcutaneously above the acromion. In type VI injuries, the shoulder assumes a flattened clinical appearance.

Diagnostic Strategies: Radiology

The energy settings used for the radiographic trauma series overpenetrate the ACJ. Specific ACJ views that use one third to two thirds less intensity should be ordered. The recommended projections include an anteroposterior view of both joints on a single wide film, an axillary lateral view, and a 15-degree cephalic tilt view.[8,35] The axillary lateral view is useful for identifying associated fractures and posterior dislocation of the clavicle. The normal coracoclavicular distance varies between 11 and 13 mm. A difference of more than 5 mm between the injured and uninjured sides is diagnostic of a complete coracoclavicular disruption. Type I injuries have essentially normal radiographs. Type II injuries show widening of the joint and a slight upward or posterior displacement of the clavicle but a normal coracoclavicular distance. Type III, IV, and V injuries have a widened joint, an increased coracoclavicular distance, and either superior or posterior displacement of the clavicle (Figure 50-24). Historically, stress views of the ACJ have been recommended to differentiate between type II and III injuries. Such views lack efficacy for this purpose, and their routine use is unnecessary.[38]

Management

Type I and II injuries should be immobilized in a sling for comfort and to protect against further injury. These patients should be referred for follow-up with their primary care physician. When pain has subsided (1 to 3 weeks), the patient can begin range-of-motion and

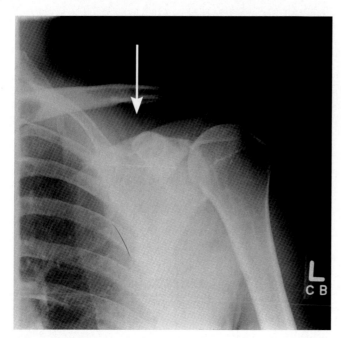

Figure 50-24. Third-degree sprain of the acromioclavicular joint. The coracoclavicular distance measures 18 mm *(arrow)*. (Courtesy of David Nelson, MD.)

strengthening exercises with a return to sports when pain-free function has been achieved.[8] Type IV, V, and VI injuries require early surgical treatment. The management of type III injuries has changed dramatically since the 1980s. Most studies have concluded that conservative treatment provides equal or, in some cases, better functional results than surgical intervention. In addition, surgical patients have longer recovery times and higher complication rates.[8] The main complications of conservative therapy are the persistence of nuisance symptoms (clicking or pain) and a cosmetic deformity. Selected patients who are young, have severe displacement (>2 cm), and perform repetitive overhead activities may be candidates for surgical intervention.[8] Treatment of type III injuries in the emergency department should consist of sling immobilization and early (<72 hours) orthopedic referral. The initial therapy in all cases should include adequate analgesia.

Complications

The most common concurrent injuries are associated fractures of the clavicle and coracoid process. Osteoarthritis of the ACJ is a potential long-term complication of an acute injury.[8] Acromioclavicular arthritis typically presents as an impingement syndrome with shoulder pain between 120 and 180 degrees of abduction.

Glenohumeral Dislocations

Perspective

The glenohumeral joint is the most commonly dislocated major joint in the body. The lack of intrinsic bony stability in conjunction with its wide range of motion predisposes the joint to dislocations. The annual incidence is 17 per 100,000, and there are two distinct age peaks. The first is in men age 20 to 30 years, and the second is in women age 61 to 80 years.[39] The glenohumeral joint can dislocate anteriorly, posteriorly, inferiorly, or superiorly. Anterior dislocations account for 95% to 97% of all glenohumeral dislocations. Posterior dislocations account for most of the remainder, whereas inferior and superior dislocations are rare.

Anterior Dislocations

Pathophysiology. Anterior dislocations can result from indirect or direct forces. The most common mechanism of injury consists of an indirect force transferred to the anterior capsule from a combination of abduction, extension, and external rotation. In younger individuals, the injury usually is sustained during athletic activities. In older patients, a fall onto the outstretched arm is more common.[28] Rarely a direct force applied to the posterolateral aspect of the shoulder can force the humeral head out of the glenoid fossa anteriorly.

Anterior dislocations can be classified according to their etiology (traumatic or nontraumatic), frequency (primary or recurrent), and the anatomic position of the dislocated humeral head.[39] After dislocation, the humeral head can assume a subcoracoid, subglenoid, subclavicular, or intrathoracic position (Figure 50-25). The subcoracoid is the most common type of anterior dislocation. The head is displaced anteriorly and rests on the scapular neck inferior to the coracoid process. The next most common type is the subglenoid dislocation, in which the head is anterior and inferior to the glenoid fossa. Together the subcoracoid and subglenoid types account for 99% of all anterior dislocations. Subclavicular and intrathoracic dislocations are extremely rare and involve the addition of strong lateral to medial forces that push the humeral head medially.

Clinical Features. The patient is in severe pain with the dislocated arm held in slight abduction and external rotation by the opposite extremity. The lateral edge of the acromion process is prominent, and the normally rounded shoulder assumes a "squared-off" appearance. The coracoid process is indistinct, and the anterior shoulder appears full. The patient leans away from the injured side and cannot adduct or internally rotate the shoulder even slightly without severe pain. A neurovascular examination is performed to identify associated injuries of the brachial plexus, axillary nerve, radial nerve, or axillary artery. The reported incidence of axillary nerve injuries after anterior glenohumeral dislocation ranges from 5% to 54%.[40,41] Axillary nerve function can be assessed by testing for sensation over the lateral aspect of the shoulder and by testing motor function of the teres minor and deltoid muscles. Deltoid function is tested by having the patient attempt shoulder abduction while the examiner feels for muscle contraction. Motor testing is more accurate because sensory testing can be misleading owing to the presence of overlapping cutaneous nerve root dermatomes. Axillary nerve injuries occur more frequently in patients older than age 50 years.[41]

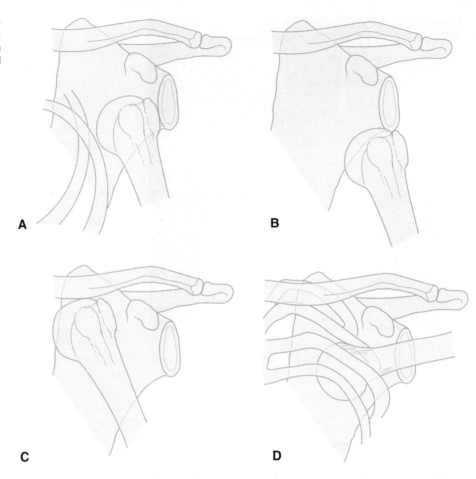

Figure 50-25. Types of anterior dislocation. **A,** Subcoracoid. **B,** Subglenoid. **C,** Subclavicular. **D,** Intrathoracic. (From DePalma AF: *Surgery of the Shoulder*, 3rd ed. Philadelphia, JB Lippincott, 1983.)

Diagnostic Strategies: Radiology. The trauma series of radiographs confirms the clinical diagnosis and identifies the position of the humeral head (Figure 50-26). Associated fractures may be present in 50% of cases. The most common of these is a compression fracture of the posterolateral aspect of the humeral head caused by forceful impingement against the anterior rim of the glenoid fossa. This defect in the humeral head, or Hill-Sachs deformity (see Figure 50-26), is reported to be present in 11% to 50% of all anterior dislocations. The actual incidence is probably much higher because minor compression fractures are difficult to visualize on plain radiographs. The defect is best visualized on an internal rotation anteroposterior view of the glenohumeral joint. A corresponding fracture of the anterior glenoid rim (Bankart's fracture) is present in approximately 5% of cases.[10] Avulsion fractures of the greater tuberosity are present in 10% to 15% of cases.[10,40]

Management. Closed reduction of the dislocation should be accomplished expeditiously because the incidence of neurovascular complications increases with time.[41] Radiographic documentation of the type of dislocation and any associated fractures should be obtained *before* attempting reduction. Reduction can be accomplished using various techniques, most of which involve traction, leverage, or scapular manipulation principles.[42] There are no good comparative studies of one reduction technique over another.[42] The ideal method should be simple, quick, and effective; require little assistance; and cause no additional injury to the

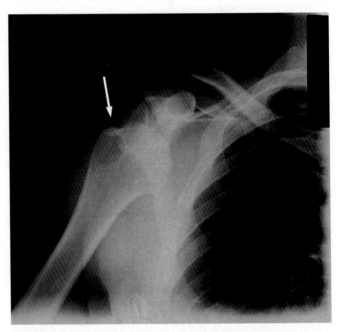

Figure 50-26. Recurrent anterior subcoracoid dislocation with Hill-Sachs deformity of the humeral head *(arrow).*

shoulder. It is wise to be familiar with several techniques of reduction because none is uniformly successful.

Good muscle relaxation is the key to a successful reduction in most settings. Muscle relaxation can be

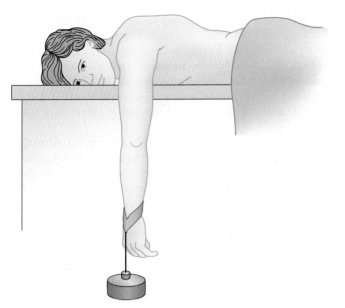

Figure 50-27. Stimson or hanging weight method of reduction for anterior dislocations.

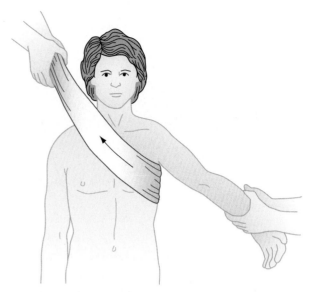

Figure 50-28. Traction-countertraction method for reducing anterior shoulder dislocations.

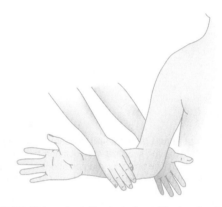

Figure 50-29. External rotation technique. The involved arm is slowly adducted to the patient's side, and the elbow is flexed 90 degrees. Gentle external rotation is applied to the forearm to achieve reduction. (From Simon RR, Koenigsknecht SJ: *Emergency Orthopedics: The Extremities,* 2nd ed. Norwalk, Conn, Appleton & Lange, 1987.)

achieved using conscious sedation or interscalene, supraclavicular, or suprascapular nerve blocks.[43] Occasionally, reductions can be accomplished without the use of any analgesia, especially if the time from injury to reduction is short or if the dislocation is a recurrent one. Muscle relaxation and analgesia also can be provided through intra-articular injection of a local anesthetic agent.[43,44] This technique is especially useful when conscious sedation is contraindicated and is associated with a shorter length of stay in the emergency department after reduction.[44] The joint is entered under sterile technique 2 cm inferior to the lateral edge of the acromion using an 18-gauge or 20-gauge needle. Any associated hemarthrosis is aspirated, then 20 mL of 1% lidocaine is injected over 30 seconds. The patient is allowed to relax for 15 minutes before reduction is attempted.

Gentle traction in various directions (forward flexion, abduction, overhead, lateral) is used to overcome the muscle spasm that holds the humeral head in its dislocated position.[42] In the Stimson or hanging weight technique (Figure 50-27), the patient is placed prone with the dislocated arm hanging over the edge of the examining table. A 10- or 15-lb weight attached to the wrist or lower forearm provides traction in forward flexion. Reduction usually occurs over 20 to 30 minutes. In the traction-countertraction method (Figure 50-28), traction is applied along the abducted arm while an assistant using a folded sheet wrapped across the chest applies countertraction. The forward elevation maneuver of Cooper and Milch is also simple and safe. The arm is initially elevated 10 to 20 degrees in forward flexion and slight abduction. Forward flexion is continued until the arm is directly overhead. Abduction is increased, and outward traction is applied to complete the reduction.[45]

Another simple and effective traction technique is the Snowbird technique.[46] In this method, the patient is seated in a chair, and the affected arm is supported by the patient's unaffected extremity. A 3-foot loop of 4-inch cast stockinet is placed along the proximal forearm of the involved extremity with the elbow at 90 degrees. The patient is assisted or instructed to sit up, and the physician's foot is placed in the stockinet loop to provide firm downward traction. The physician's hands remain free to apply any gentle external pressure or rotation as needed until reduction is accomplished.

The most commonly recommended leverage technique is the external rotation method of Liedelmeyer.[47] With the patient in the supine position, the involved arm is slowly and gently adducted to the side. The elbow is flexed to 90 degrees, and slow, gentle external rotation is applied to achieve reduction (Figure 50-29).

Scapular manipulation accomplishes reduction by repositioning the glenoid fossa rather than the humeral head. The patient is placed in the prone position with the affected arm hanging off the table as for the Stimson

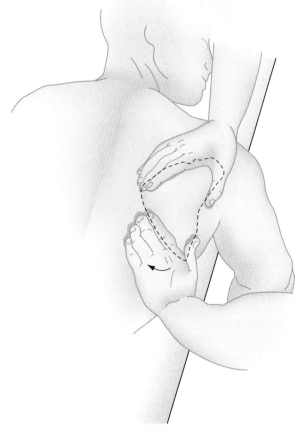

Figure 50-30. Proper hand position and direction of rotation during shoulder relocation using the scapular manipulation technique. (From Kothari RU, Dronen SC: The scapular manipulation technique for the reduction of acute anterior shoulder dislocations. *J Emerg Med* 8:625, 1990.)

technique. After the application of downward traction (manual or hanging weights), the scapula is manipulated by rotating the inferior tip medially (Figure 50-30), while stabilizing the superior and medial edges with the opposite hand.[48] McNamara[49] also described a seated modification of the scapular method in which traction is applied in the forward horizontal position while an assistant manipulates the scapula. Scapular manipulation can be difficult in heavyset individuals, in whom it is difficult to palpate and grasp the inferior tip of the scapula. More traditional techniques, such as the Hippocratic method (traction with the foot in the axilla) and the Kocher maneuver (leverage, adduction, and internal rotation), are no longer recommended because of a high incidence of associated complications (axillary nerve injury, humeral shaft and neck fractures, capsular damage).

The neurovascular examination must be repeated after any attempt at reduction. It also is generally recommended that radiographs be repeated to confirm reduction and to identify any associated fractures not apparent on prereduction films. More recent studies have questioned the need and cost-effectiveness of routine postreduction radiographs.[50-52] The authors of these studies did not find any new clinically significant fractures on postreduction radiographs and argued that in most instances a successful reduction can be determined clinically by the presence of a palpable clunk, decrease in pain, and improvement in the range of motion. These findings must be confirmed in larger prospective studies before they are adopted as a standard of care.

After reduction, the affected extremity is immobilized using a sling and swathe bandage or a Velpeau sling (see Figure 50-11). Patients should be discharged with adequate analgesia and appropriate follow-up. Primary dislocations and complicated cases (associated fracture, rotator cuff tear, axillary nerve injury) should receive orthopedic follow-up. In uncomplicated cases, the shoulder is immobilized for 3 to 6 weeks in younger patients and 1 to 2 weeks in older (>40 years old) individuals.[10] The traditional position of immobilization is with the shoulder in internal rotation. Studies suggest that this positioning may delay healing and is associated with a higher recurrence rate.[53] In a randomized clinical trial, Itoi and coworkers[54] found that 3 weeks of immobilization in 10 degrees of external rotation was associated with a zero recurrence rate at 13 to 15 months compared with a 30% recurrence rate with sling immobilization in internal rotation. If these preliminary findings are confirmed by additional trials, sling immobilization may be replaced by external rotation splints. Regardless of the immobilization technique, early initiation of shoulder exercises (see Figure 50-14) helps reduce the risk of adhesive capsulitis. A meticulous rehabilitation program aimed at restoring the static and dynamic stabilizers of the glenohumeral joint follows the period of immobilization.[10]

Complications. Complications include the aforementioned fractures and neurovascular injuries. Most axillary nerve injuries are neurapraxic, and the prognosis for recovery of function is good.[41] Rotator cuff tears may be present in 10% to 15% of cases.[55] Rotator cuff tears are especially common in primary dislocations in patients older than age 40. In this setting, failure to abduct the arm often is misdiagnosed initially as an axillary nerve injury. Most of these individuals require tendon and capsular repair to restore shoulder stability.[55] Recurrence also is a common complication after anterior dislocation, and patients younger than age 30 have a reported recurrence rate of 79% to 100%.[39] A Hill-Sachs deformity or glenoid rim fracture is associated with increased risk of recurrence.[10] Studies suggest that the traditional method of treatment (immobilization followed by physical therapy) is ineffective in preventing redislocation in young, highly athletic individuals. Arthroscopic studies of primary anterior dislocations in young, highly athletic individuals have detected a high incidence of anterior-inferior capsulolabral avulsions (Perthes-Bankart lesion) from the glenoid rim. This avulsion is believed to be the primary predisposing factor for recurrence, and these individuals seem to benefit from early arthroscopic repair of the lesion.[56] Recurrence rates decline with increasing age and in the presence of a greater tuberosity fracture.[10]

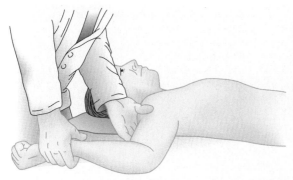

Figure 50-31. Technique for performing the shoulder apprehension test. (From Simon RR, Koenigsknecht SJ: *Emergency Orthopedics: The Extremities,* 2nd ed. Norwalk, Conn, Appleton & Lange, 1987.)

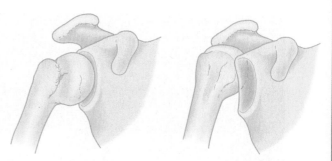

Figure 50-32. Overlap of the glenoid rim associated with posterior dislocation.

Anterior Subluxation

Transient anterior subluxation of the shoulder is encountered often in young athletic adults. The patient complains of sudden sharp shoulder pain and weakness (dead arm syndrome) while performing an abduction and external rotation maneuver. The patient also may relate a sensation of the shoulder slipping in and out. Radiographs are usually normal, and a positive apprehension sign confirms the diagnosis. The latter is performed by gently reproducing the injury motion, abduction, and external rotation of the arm while applying an anterior force to the posterior shoulder (Figure 50-31). This maneuver increases the pain and may cause anterior displacement of the humeral head. A lax or redundant anterior capsule is thought to be responsible for this syndrome, and recurrent episodes are common. These patients should be referred for orthopedic follow-up because definitive therapy (capsulorrhaphy) is surgical.[57]

Posterior Dislocation

Pathophysiology. Posterior dislocations are rare and account for 2% of all glenohumeral dislocations.[58] This rarity is explained partly by anatomy of the shoulder girdle. The 45-degree angulation of the scapula on the thoracic cage positions the glenoid fossa posterior to the humeral head and serves as a partial buttress against posterior dislocation. Greater than 50% of posterior dislocations are missed on initial evaluation, and many remain unrecognized ("locked posterior dislocations") for weeks and months.[59,60]

A posterior dislocation can result from several distinct mechanisms of injury. Convulsive seizures (epileptic or after electrical shock) often are associated with unilateral or bilateral posterior dislocations. In this instance, the larger and stronger internal rotator muscles (latissimus dorsi, pectoralis major, teres major, subscapularis) overpower the weaker external rotators (teres minor, infraspinatus) to produce the injury.[59] A posterior dislocation also can occur after a fall onto the outstretched hand with the arm held in flexion, adduction, and internal rotation or after a direct blow to the anterior aspect of the shoulder. Acute posterior dislocations are classified into three types (subacromial, subglenoid, subspinous) based on the final resting position of the humeral head. The subacromial variety accounts for 98% of all posterior dislocations.[58]

Clinical Features. Early diagnosis is essential to prevent long-term functional and therapeutic complications. As mentioned, the initial examining physician misses the diagnosis with some regularity, in part because of an overreliance on radiologic findings and an underreliance on the clinical examination. The most common misdiagnosis is adhesive capsulitis.[58,60] The patient holds the affected arm across the chest in adduction and internal rotation. Although usually painful, the injury can be relatively painless.[59] The normal shoulder contour is replaced by a flat, squared-off appearance, and the coracoid process is prominent and easily palpated. The humeral head may be palpable posteriorly beneath the acromion process. Abduction is severely limited, and external rotation is completely blocked.

Diagnostic Strategies: Radiology. Standard anteroposterior radiographs can appear deceptively normal with posterior dislocations. The common inability to diagnose posterior dislocation in the frontal plane has led to the description of several characteristic radiographic findings. Standard anteroposterior films show loss of the half-moon elliptical overlap of the humeral head and glenoid fossa. In addition, the distance between the anterior glenoid rim and the articular surface of the humeral head is increased ("rim sign"). The humeral head is profiled in internal rotation and takes on a "light bulb" or "drumstick" appearance. A true anteroposterior film shows abnormal overlap of the glenoid fossa with the humeral head (Figure 50-32). Finally, an impaction fracture of the anteromedial humeral head (reverse Hill-Sachs deformity) is invariably present (Figure 50-33). This fracture may produce a curvilinear density on the frontal projection parallel to the articular cortex of the humeral head ("trough sign"). An orthogonal view, such as an axillary lateral, transscapular, or apical oblique, confirms the diagnosis. The axillary lateral view or apical oblique view also identifies associated fractures of the humeral head and posterior glenoid rim. CT may be helpful in some instances.[61]

Management. Orthopedic consultation should be obtained for all patients with posterior dislocations. Closed reduction may be attempted in the emergency department under conscious sedation. The technique of reduction incorporates axial traction in line with the

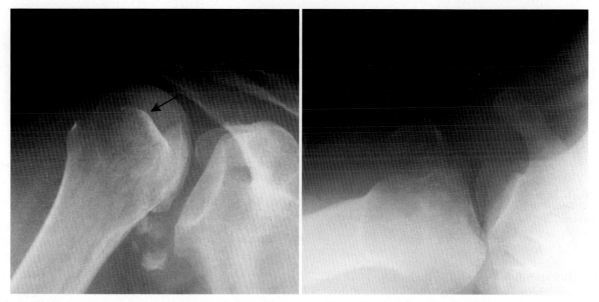

Figure 50-33. Anteroposterior and axillary views of a posterior glenohumeral dislocation. Note the widened joint space (rim sign), anteromedial impaction fracture of the humeral head, and curvilinear density parallel *(arrow)* to the articular surface (trough sign). (Courtesy of Donald Sauser, MD.)

Figure 50-34. Luxatio erecta. **A,** The mechanism by which this injury occurs in hyperabduction. **B,** This is always accompanied by disruption of the rotator cuff and tear through the inferior capsule. (From Simon RR, Koenigsknecht SJ: *Emergency Orthopedics: The Extremities,* 2nd ed. Norwalk, Conn, Appleton & Lange, 1987.)

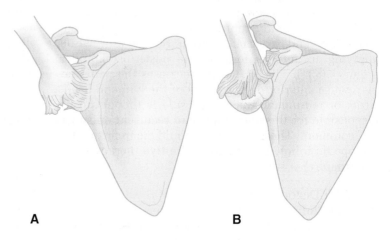

A   B

humerus, gentle pressure on the posteriorly displaced head, and slow external rotation. If this technique fails, reduction with the patient under general anesthesia is indicated. After reduction, the shoulder should be immobilized in external rotation with slight abduction.[60] Cases that were missed initially and present as a chronic or locked posterior dislocation should be referred to the orthopedist for follow-up. Locked posterior dislocations usually require open reduction and internal fixation or arthroplasty.[60,61]

Complications. Fractures of the glenoid rim, greater tuberosity, lesser tuberosity, and humeral head account for most associated injuries. Rarely the subscapularis muscle may be avulsed from its insertion site on the lesser tuberosity. Neurovascular injuries are uncommon because the anterior location of the neurovascular bundle protects it from injury. Recurrent posterior dislocations occur in 30% of patients and predispose the joint to degenerative changes.

Inferior Glenohumeral Dislocation (Luxatio Erecta)

Pathophysiology. Luxatio erecta is a rare type of glenohumeral dislocation in which the superior aspect of the humeral head is forced below the inferior rim of the glenoid fossa. It is estimated that 0.5% of all shoulder dislocations are of this variety. The mechanism of injury involves either direct or indirect forces.[62,63] Application of a direct axial load to an abducted shoulder can disrupt the weak inferior glenohumeral ligament and drive the humeral head downward. Most inferior dislocations result from indirect forces, however, that hyperabduct the affected extremity[62]; this causes impingement of the humeral head against the acromion process. Further levering of the humeral shaft against the acromion ruptures the capsule and dislocates the head inferiorly (Figure 50-34).

Clinical Features. Clinically the patient has the arm locked overhead in 110 to 160 degrees of abduction.

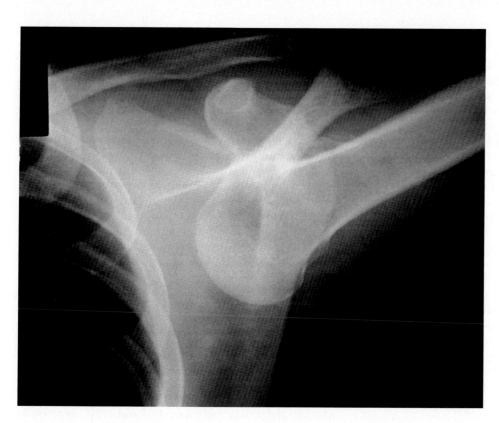

Figure 50-35. Anteroposterior view of an inferior glenohumeral dislocation. The humeral shaft lies parallel to the spine of the scapula.

The elbow is usually flexed, and the forearm typically rests on top of the head. The shoulder is fixed in this position, and any attempts at movement result in significant pain. The inferiorly displaced humeral head may be palpable along the lateral chest wall. A thorough neurovascular examination is essential.

Diagnostic Strategies: Radiology. Many cases of luxatio erecta are mistakenly diagnosed and treated as subglenoid anterior dislocations because the radiographic features of these two clinical entities are remarkably similar. Standard anteroposterior radiographs show the superior articular surface inferior to the glenoid fossa (Figure 50-35). In addition, the humeral shaft characteristically lies parallel to the spine of the scapula on the anteroposterior view.[63] This radiographic feature is useful in distinguishing luxatio erecta from a subglenoid anterior dislocation because in the latter, the humeral shaft lies parallel to the chest wall. Associated fractures of the acromion, coracoid, clavicle, greater tuberosity, humeral head, and glenoid rim are common.

Management. If possible, orthopedic consultation should be obtained before attempting closed reduction under conscious sedation in the emergency department. Reduction usually can be accomplished using traction-countertraction maneuvers. Traction is applied in line with the humeral shaft, while an assistant applies countertraction across the shoulder (Figure 50-36). Gentle abduction usually reduces the dislocation, and the arm is brought down into an adducted position. In rare instances, buttonholing of the capsule prevents closed reduction, necessitating open reduction.

Complications. Neurapraxic lesions of the brachial plexus are common, and thrombosis of the axillary artery has been associated with luxatio erecta.[62] Tears of the rotator cuff almost always accompany luxatio erecta and may require surgical repair. Adhesive capsulitis is a common long-term complication of luxatio erecta.

Scapulothoracic Dislocation

Scapulothoracic dissociation is a rare and severe injury characterized by complete disruption of the scapulothoracic articulation. The mechanism of injury involves a strong traction force applied to the upper extremity (e.g., motorcyclist hangs onto the handlebars while body is forced away). Massive local soft tissue swelling associated with lateral displacement of the scapula is seen on the chest radiograph. Additional osseous injuries include acromioclavicular separation, displaced fractures of the clavicle, and dislocations of the SCJ. Associated neurovascular (subclavian or axillary vessels, brachial plexus) injuries are common and account for the poor functional outcomes associated with this injury.[64]

Soft Tissue Conditions

Subacromial Syndromes and Impingement (Rotator Cuff Tendinitis, Subdeltoid/Subacromial Bursitis)

Pathophysiology

Rotator cuff tendinitis and subacromial bursitis can be considered part of a pathophysiologic continuum whose endpoint is represented by complete rupture of the rotator cuff. These two conditions are common causes of shoulder pain and have similar clinical presentations.[65] A key feature of their clinical presentation is the presence of an impingement or painful arc syndrome (Figure 50-37).

The subacromial space is the area between the coracoacromial arch and the greater tuberosity of the humerus. This space, which is only a few millimeters wide, contains the long head of the biceps, the rotator cuff, and the subacromial bursa. The last-mentioned acts as the gliding mechanism between the musculotendinous cuff and the coracoacromial arch. The functional arc of shoulder elevation is forward, which normally leads to impingement of the cuff and bursa under the anterior third of the coracoacromial arch. Similar impingement also occurs between 60 and 120 degrees of abduction and with the extremes of adduction. The critical wear from impingement is centered on the supraspinatus tendon, near its insertion on the greater tuberosity.[66] Micro-opaque injection studies also have shown a relative avascularity within this "critical" area. The hypovascularity in conjunction with repeated wear and age-related degenerative changes ultimately results in rotator cuff tendinitis. Narrowing of the subacromial space (anatomic variants of anterior acromion) and occupations that require

excessive overhead activity accelerate the entire process. With time, the inflammatory reaction spreads to involve the adjacent bursa. This inflammation leads to edema, thickening, and fibrosis, further narrowing the subacromial space (secondary impingement); this is eventually followed by attritional changes within the rotator cuff. Because the rotator cuff is a primary humeral head depressor, loss of function adds to the secondary impingement process.[65]

The impingement process also may involve the long head of the biceps. If so, bicipital tenosynovitis, degeneration, or rupture may be present. In some cases, osteoarthritis of the ACJ can narrow the subacromial space and accelerate the pathologic process. Impingement in this context occurs between 120 and 180 degrees of abduction (see Figure 50-37).

Clinical Features

Neer[66] classified the progressive pathologic processes underlying subacromial syndromes into three stages (Table 50-2). The impingement sign (Figure 50-38) is positive in all three stages. Patients in stage 1 complain of a dull ache around the deltoid area after strenuous activity. On examination, tenderness is present over the supraspinatus and anterior acromion. A painful arc of abduction between 60 and 120 degrees is characteristic.

Stage 2 is characterized by more persistent pain that is particularly severe at night. The inflammatory process within the bursa and tendons leads to the formation of minor adhesions. Disruption of these adhesions is thought to account for the nighttime pain. Physical findings are similar to those of stage 1. In addition, bursal thickening leads to increased soft tissue crepitus within the glenohumeral joint.

The hallmark of stage 3 is significant tendon degeneration after a prolonged history of tendinitis and bursitis. Findings in this stage are discussed in the section on tears of the rotator cuff. Radiographs are usually normal in stages 1 and 2. Findings in stage 3 are similar to those seen with complete tears of the rotator cuff.

The differential diagnosis of subacromial syndromes is extensive and includes intrinsic and extrinsic causes of shoulder pain. Extrinsic sources include the cervical spine, lung, heart, and diaphragm. Intrinsic conditions include acromioclavicular arthritis, adhesive capsulitis, calcific tendinitis, and traumatic anterior subluxation. A positive impingement sign may be present in many of these conditions. Relief of pain after the subacromial injection of 10 mL of 1% lidocaine (impingement test [see Figure 50-38]) helps localize the condition to the subacromial space.

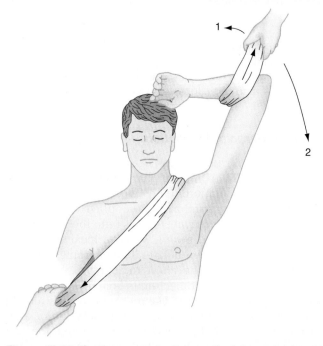

Figure 50-36. Traction-countertraction method for reduction of luxatio erecta humeri. The initial maneuver (1) includes steady axial traction in line with the humeral shaft position followed by gentle abduction. This reduces the glenohumeral dislocation. At this point (2), the arm is brought down to a position of adduction and internal rotation. (From Davids JR, Talbott RD: Luxatio erecta humeri. *Clin Orthop* 252:144, 1990.)

Table 50-2. Three Progressive Stages of Impingement Lesions

Stage	Pathology	Age (yr)	Course	Treatment
I	Edema, hemorrhage	<25	Reversible	Conservative
II	Fibrosis, tendinitis	25-40	Recurrent pain with activity	Conservative, surgical
III	Bone spurs, tendon rupture	>40	Progressive disability	Surgical

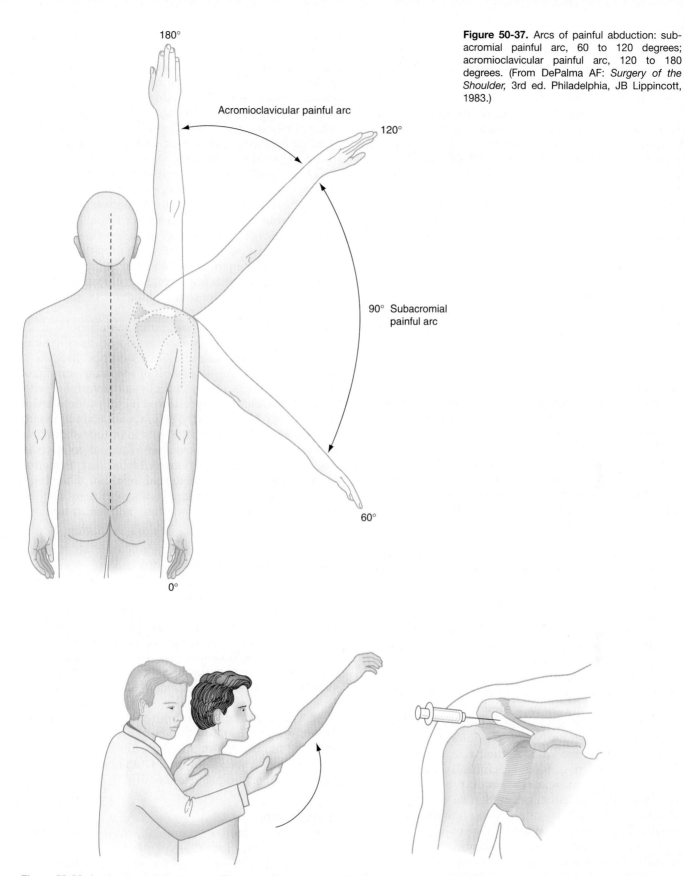

Figure 50-37. Arcs of painful abduction: subacromial painful arc, 60 to 120 degrees; acromioclavicular painful arc, 120 to 180 degrees. (From DePalma AF: *Surgery of the Shoulder,* 3rd ed. Philadelphia, JB Lippincott, 1983.)

180°

Acromioclavicular painful arc

120°

90° Subacromial painful arc

60°

0°

Figure 50-38. Impingement injection test. The impingement sign is elicited with the patient seated and the examiner standing. Scapular rotation is prevented with one hand, while the other hand raises the arm in forced forward elevation, causing the greater tuberosity to impinge against the acromion. This maneuver produces pain in patients with impingement lesions of all stages. It also causes pain in many other shoulder conditions. In the case of impingement lesions, the pain caused by this maneuver is relieved by the injection of 10 mL of 1% lidocaine beneath the anterior acromion. This test is useful in separating impingement lesions of all stages from other causes of shoulder pain. (Redrawn from Neer CS: Impingement lesions. *Clin Orthop* 173:70, 1983.)

Management

Initial treatment in stage 1 is conservative and consists of rest, nonsteroidal anti-inflammatory drugs (NSAIDs), and modification of activities that produce impingement. In stage 2, emphasis is on maintaining flexibility and range of motion through physiotherapy and rotator cuff strengthening exercises. Patients with stage 1 and 2 disease who present to the emergency department reporting treatment failure with NSAIDs may benefit from a subacromial injection of corticosteroids. Refractory stage 2 and some stage 3 patients may require decompression surgery to control pain. Patients with stage 2 and 3 disease may benefit from referral to an orthopedist for more detailed evaluation and treatment.

Rotator Cuff Tears

Pathophysiology

The rotator cuff acts as a dynamic stabilizer of the glenohumeral joint.[67] Its primary function is to hold the humeral head in place throughout the full range of motion (see Figure 50-5). In addition, it contributes power in all directions and is responsible for specific movements. The infraspinatus and teres minor act as external rotators, whereas the subscapularis is an internal rotator. The supraspinatus is essential for the first 30 degrees of shoulder abduction.

The tenuous blood supply of the rotator cuff, abusive tensile overload, and chronic wear under the coracoacromial arch predispose it to age-related degenerative changes. The advanced stage of this process is characterized by complete rupture of the rotator cuff.

The role of impingement in the development of rotator cuff tears is controversial. Primary impingement (e.g., acromial variance) is uncommon, but when present accelerates the degenerative process. More often, weakening or rupture of the cuff with age allows for superior migration of the humeral head, which results in secondary impingement. This impingement produces secondary changes within the subacromial space and symptoms characteristic of the painful arc syndrome.[68]

Most tears involve the dominant arm and occur in men older than age 40 years. The occupational history is significant for strenuous work requiring overhead activity. Most tears occur near the attachment of the supraspinatus and can extend anteriorly into the subscapularis or posteriorly into the infraspinatus. Tears can be classified according to their size, completeness, pattern location, or duration. A clinically useful system is to divide tears into acute or chronic types. *Acute tears* (10%) usually are associated with a specific traumatic event. Often no history of previous shoulder problems exists. The most common mechanism of injury is forced abduction associated with significant resistance; this usually occurs when the patient attempts to break a fall with an outstretched hand. Alternatively the tendon rupture may occur while lifting a heavy object or after falling directly onto an immovable object.[69]

Clinical Features

The patient complains of a sudden tearing sensation in the shoulder followed by severe pain that radiates into the arm. Pain and secondary muscle spasm limit shoulder motion. Physical findings depend on the completeness, size, and location of the tear. Point tenderness is usually present over the site of rupture (greater tuberosity). A palpable defect also may be present. Subacromial injection of 10 mL of 1% lidocaine eliminates pain and allows for proper evaluation of motor function. The patient with a large tear cannot initiate shoulder abduction. A discrepancy between active and passive range of motion is highly suggestive of a rotator cuff tear.[69] The drop-arm test, performed by passively abducting the arm to 90 degrees and asking the patient to hold the arm in this position, is positive with significant tears. Slight pressure on the distal forearm or wrist causes the patient to drop the arm suddenly. The acute pain resulting from hemorrhage and spasm subsides over a few days. Repeat examination at this point confirms the loss of function in significant tears.

Chronic tears account for approximately 90% of all lesions. Chronic tears are attritional and more insidious in their presentation. Early findings include a painful arc syndrome as a result of secondary impingement. The pain is worse at night and interferes with sleep. Worsening pain is followed by the gradual onset of weakness in the arm. Flexion and abduction are affected first. The patient attempts to initiate abduction using scapulothoracic movement. Internal rotation is weakened by anterior extension of the tear. Posterior extension compromises external rotation. The drop-arm test is positive with large tears, and there may be atrophy of the supraspinatus and infraspinatus muscles.

Diagnostic Strategies: Radiology

Radiographs may be normal in acute and chronic tears, but more often they show evidence of nonspecific degenerative changes within the glenohumeral joint and subacromial space. The greater tuberosity can have a sclerotic or cystic appearance. Osteophytic spurs and sclerosis of the undersurface of the acromion may narrow the subacromial space. The hallmark of a complete tear is superior displacement of the humeral head. This displacement is best seen on an external rotation view. The normal distance from the superior aspect of the humerus to the undersurface of the acromion varies from 7 to 14 mm. A distance of less than 6 mm is highly suggestive of a complete tear. Outpatient MRI, ultrasound, or an arthrogram can confirm the diagnosis.

Management

Acute tears should be immobilized in a sling and referred promptly for orthopedic follow-up. Early surgical repair (<3 weeks) is preferred in these instances, especially for a young or active individual. The management of chronic tears includes pain control and a shoulder rehabilitation program. Painful arc symptoms may respond to the subacromial injection of a corticosteroid preparation. Orthopedic follow-up is essential because patients with persistent pain and weakness may require surgical repair.

Lesions of the Biceps Muscle

The biceps is composed of two heads. The long head originates from the supraglenoid tubercle and glenoid labrum and ascends over the humeral head to enter the arm via the bicipital groove. The long head is covered by a synovial sheath and is held in place within the groove by the coracohumeral and transverse humeral ligaments. The short head of the biceps originates from the coracoid process and inserts with the long head onto the tuberosity of the radius. The biceps is responsible for flexion and supination at the elbow.

Bicipital Tenosynovitis

Pathophysiology. Anatomically the long head of the biceps is subject to the same stresses as the rotator cuff within the subacromial space. Irritation and microtrauma as a result of repetitive elevation or abduction of the shoulder produce an inflammatory reaction within the synovial sheath. Bicipital tenosynovitis usually is associated with other acromial arch impingement conditions (e.g., subacromial bursitis and rotator cuff tendinitis).[70]

The typical patient is middle-aged and involved in an occupation or recreational activity that requires overhead movement. The patient complains of pain in the anterior part of the shoulder that radiates into the upper arm. The pain usually is initiated by some minor traumatic event involving forceful contraction of the biceps. Pain increases with activity and decreases with rest. Abduction and external rotation in particular are painful. Pain increases at night and interferes with sleep.

Clinical Features. On examination, tenderness is present over the biceps tendon as it passes through the bicipital groove. This is best shown with the arm in abduction and external rotation. Active range of motion is limited by pain, but the passive range remains intact. Supination against resistance (Yergason's test) with the arm adducted and the elbow flexed to 90 degrees reproduces the pain (Figure 50-39). The biceps resistance test in which forward flexion of the shoulder (elbow extended and forearm supinated) is carried out against resistance also produces pain in the bicipital groove.

Diagnostic Strategies: Radiology. Radiographs may show evidence of subacromial space impingement by associated acromioclavicular arthritis, inferior subluxation of the clavicle, and inferior acromial osteophytes.

Management. Emergency treatment consists of immobilization in a sling and anti-inflammatory medication. Gentle stretching exercises are encouraged, and refractory or progressive cases should be referred to an orthopedic surgeon. Although the bicipital sheath can be injected with a corticosteroid preparation, the procedure is technically difficult. Subacromial decompressive surgery and biceps tenodesis may be necessary in patients who fail to respond to conservative therapy.[71]

Ruptures of the Biceps Tendon

Pathophysiology. Ruptures of the biceps tendon can be classified into proximal and distal types. Distal rup-

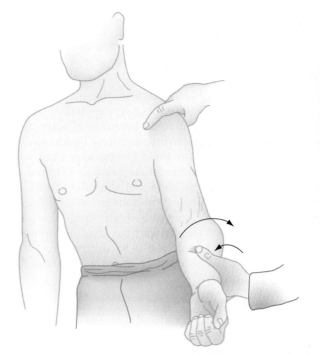

Figure 50-39. Yergason's test. Flexion of the elbow and supination of the forearm against resistance causes pain in the anterior and inner aspect of the shoulder. (From DePalma AF: *Surgery of the Shoulder,* 3rd ed. Philadelphia, JB Lippincott, 1983.)

tures are rare and are not discussed. Proximally, microtears and other age-related attritional changes within the long head predispose it to rupture.[69] The rupture can be spontaneous or may follow a traumatic event involving either forced extension or resisted supination and flexion.

Clinical Features. The classic history of an acute rupture is that of a sudden snap or pop, followed by pain and ecchymosis in the region of the bicipital groove. The tendon usually ruptures at its weakest point, which is just distal to the exit from the glenohumeral joint cavity. With a complete rupture, distal retraction of the muscle results in a "Popeye" appearance of the arm. A difference in muscle contour (Ludington's test) also may be seen when both arms are placed behind the head and the biceps muscles are contracted.[72] Functionally, forearm supination is weakened, but elbow flexion stays strong because the coracobrachialis and short head of the biceps remain intact. Most ruptures also are associated with a rotator cuff tear.

Diagnostic Strategies: Radiology. Radiographs are usually unremarkable, and the confirmatory test of choice is MRI.

Management. The injured arm should be immobilized in a sling with the elbow in 90 degrees of flexion. The local application of ice may provide temporary relief. Analgesia should be provided, and the patient should be referred to an orthopedic surgeon within 72 hours for further evaluation and treatment. Surgical repair is a consideration in young, active individuals. In older individuals, conservative therapy (range-of-motion and strengthening exercise) is preferred because the cosmetic deformity is minimal, and the mild functional loss is usually acceptable.

Subluxation and Dislocations of the Biceps Tendon

Subluxations and dislocations of the biceps tendon usually are associated with a congenitally shallow bicipital groove or atraumatic (attritional) tears of the coracohumeral and transverse humeral ligaments. The patient complains of a snapping sensation in the upper arm with abduction and external rotation. External and internal rotation of the abducted shoulder shows dislocation and relocation of the tendon. With complete dislocation, the arm may reflexively drop to relocate the tendon. These conditions may require operative repair and should be referred to an orthopedist.

Calcific Tendinitis

Pathophysiology

Rotator cuff calcific tendinitis is encountered frequently in the emergency department. The condition occurs in the 40s and 50s and is rare in individuals younger than age 30 or older than age 60. Calcific deposits occur primarily in the supraspinatus tendon near its attachment to the greater tuberosity. Deposits also may involve the infraspinatus, teres minor, or subscapularis tendons. Initially the tendon undergoes fibrocartilaginous transformation. The precipitating factors for this change are unclear and may involve hypoxia or stress-related degenerative changes within the tendon.[73] Calcium crystals are deposited and coalesce within the matrix of the tendon. Subsequent invasion of vascular channels into the deposit allows for the influx of neutrophils and macrophages (inflammatory response), which remove the calcification through phagocytosis. Finally, fibroblasts migrate into the area to create a postcalcification scar.[74]

Clinical Features

The clinical presentation can be divided into silent, subacute, and acute phases based on the physical characteristics of the calcific deposits and the nature of the inflammatory response within the tendon and subacromial bursa. The silent phase consists of a dry powdery deposit with no surrounding inflammatory reaction. It is usually an incidental diagnosis when shoulder radiographs are obtained for other purposes. The deposits may remain painless and eventually reabsorb.

The painful arc syndrome is a hallmark of the subacute phase. Enlargement and softening of the deposit narrows the subacromial space, resulting in impingement under the acromial arch. Pain between 60 and 120 degrees of abduction (see Figure 50-37) is characteristic.

A severe inflammatory reaction within and around the deposit produces the acute phase. The deposit becomes milky and has the appearance of an acute abscess. The patient has severe pain with the arm held close to the chest. Active and passive range of motion is severely limited. The shoulder is warm and extremely tender to the touch. Severe pain is related to increased intratendinous pressure, and spontaneous rupture of the deposit into the subacromial bursa can provide dramatic relief of symptoms.

Diagnostic Strategies: Radiology

Radiographs show calcific deposits in the involved tendon. For the supraspinatus, calcific deposits are best seen on the internal and external rotation anteroposterior views. The axillary view is useful for showing calcification within the other tendons of the rotator cuff.

Management

Subacute symptoms usually respond to NSAIDs and measures to limit any offending activity. The acute phase should be treated with sling immobilization, NSAIDs, and analgesia. Subacromial injection of a local anesthetic may provide dramatic temporary relief. Needle lavage (puncturing of the calcific deposits to decrease intratendinous pressure) also has been described as an effective treatment.[73] The subacromial injection of corticosteroids for impingement symptoms is controversial because these agents may delay the process of calcium resorption and interfere with the natural course of the condition. Patients with chronic symptoms may benefit from extracorporeal shock wave therapy or surgical removal of the calcific deposit.[75] Early shoulder range-of-motion exercises should be encouraged in all patients to minimize the risk of adhesive capsulitis. All symptomatic patients should receive orthopedic follow-up.

Adhesive Capsulitis

Pathophysiology

Adhesive capsulitis is a specific diagnostic entity characterized by an inflammatory reaction within the capsule and synovium of the glenohumeral joint. This inflammatory reaction results in the formation of adhesions within the capsule and inferior axillary fold. Adhesive capsulitis must be differentiated from other, more common causes of the painful stiff shoulder; this is important because any painful condition of the shoulder (e.g., calcific tendinitis, rotator cuff tear, osteoarthritis, or trauma) may be associated with decreased range of motion.[76] Although the cause of adhesive capsulitis is unknown, any condition associated with prolonged dependency of the arm can result in capsular contraction, including voluntary immobilization after calcific tendinitis, rotator cuff injury, mastectomy, or a distal upper extremity injury (Colles' fracture).

Clinical Features

The typical patient is a woman between 40 and 60 years old. The nondominant arm is usually affected, and the patient has trouble with the activities of daily living. The pain is often severe at night and localized over the deltoid area. There is uniform limitation of all glenohumeral movement, especially abduction and internal and external rotation. On passive testing, a sense of mechanical restriction of joint motion is present. The shoulder radiographs are usually normal if there is no associated condition.

Table 50-3. Potency, Duration of Action, and Dose of Commonly Used Corticosteroid Preparations

Preparation (Trade Name)	Relative Potency	Duration of Action	Preparation (Suspension) (mg/mL)	Subacromial Dose (mg)
Hydrocortisone acetate (Hydrocortone)	1	Short	50 mg/mL	25-37.5
Betamethasone sodium phosphate and acetate (Celestone Soluspan)	25	Short/long	6	6
Methylprednisolone acetate (Depo-Medrol)	5	Long	40	40-80
Triamcinolone acetonide (Kenalog-10)	5	Long	10 mg/mL	10-20
Triamcinolone hexacetonide (Aristospan)	5	Long	20 mg/mL	20
Triamcinolone diacetate (Aristocort)	5	Long	25	25
Dexamethasone acetate (Decadron-LA)	25	Long	8	4-16

Management

The best form of therapy is preventive. Prolonged immobilization must be avoided, and early motion of the shoulder should be encouraged in all instances (see Figure 50-14). Treatment of adhesive capsulitis in the emergency department consists of NSAIDs and referral to an orthopedic surgeon. The diagnosis usually is confirmed by an arthrogram, which shows obliteration of the axillary fold and a reduction in the joint volume. Initial therapy is usually conservative and consists of a gentle assisted exercise program. Some patients require shoulder manipulation under anesthesia to improve the range of motion.

Injection Therapy

The local injection of corticosteroid preparations can be useful in many painful conditions that affect the shoulder, including rotator cuff tendinitis and subacromial bursitis. Evidence-based research that supports or refutes the use of injection corticosteroid therapy is limited.[77] Although useful for relieving the inflammatory reaction, corticosteroid injections in general do not alter the underlying disease process. Corticosteroids inhibit all phases of the inflammatory response, including leukocyte migration, edema formation, mediator release, vascular permeability, collagen deposition, and fibroblast proliferation. Systemic complications are rare after local injection therapy. Site-specific complications include articular cartilage damage and subcutaneous atrophy. The incidence of local complications correlates with the injection technique, dose used, and frequency of administration. Direct tendon injection must be avoided at all times, and the frequency of injections should be limited to four injections per year.[78]

Numerous corticosteroid preparations are available on the market (Table 50-3). Injection of a long-acting agent or a combination of a short-acting and long-acting agent is preferred. The dose used depends on the size of the joint or bursa and the response of the individual. Concurrent use of a local anesthetic agent may provide acute pain relief and allow for better diffusion of the steroid preparation.

After injection, the shoulder should be immobilized, and activity should be limited for several days to protect against further injury. Improvement usually begins within 1 to 7 days and can last weeks to months, depending on the preparation and underlying condi-

tion. Local anesthetic injection may result in a dramatic temporary improvement in symptoms.

KEY CONCEPTS

- The most important aspect of scapular fractures is the high incidence of associated injuries to the ipsilateral lung, chest wall, and shoulder girdle complex.
- Posterior SCJ dislocations can be associated with life-threatening injuries within the superior mediastinum, and the preferred imaging technique is a CT scan.
- If the coracoclavicular distance exceeds 10 to 13 mm, or there is a difference of more than 5 mm in this distance between the injured and the uninjured sides, a grade III ACJ dislocation should be suspected.
- Most studies have concluded that conservative treatment of type III ACJ dislocations provides equal or, in some cases, better functional results than surgical intervention.
- A compression fracture of the posterolateral aspect of the humeral head (Hill-Sachs deformity) is present in a large percentage of anterior glenohumeral dislocations.
- Good muscle relaxation is the key to success in the reduction of anterior glenohumeral dislocations.
- Axillary nerve function is best evaluated by motor function of the deltoid muscle.
- Recurrence is a common complication after anterior dislocation, especially in patients younger than age 30 years, and such individuals may benefit from arthroscopic repair.
- A posterior dislocation should be suspected in any individual who complains of shoulder pain after a convulsive episode.
- It is important to evaluate the relationship between the spine of the scapula and the longitudinal axis of the humerus to avoid missing an inferior glenohumeral dislocation.
- Early initiation of passive shoulder range-of-motion exercises helps reduce the risk of adhesive capsulitis.

REFERENCES

1. Hussein MK: Kocher's method is 3,000 years old. *J Bone Joint Surg Br* 50:669, 1968.
2. Rowe CR: Historical development of shoulder care. *Clin Sports Med* 2:231, 1983.
3. Simon RR, Koenigsknecht SJ: *Emergency Orthopedics: The Extremities,* 4th ed. Norwalk, Conn, McGraw-Hill, 2001.
4. Tibone JE: Shoulder problems of adolescents: How they differ from those of adults. *Clin Sports Med* 2:423, 1983.

5. Yeh GL, Williams GR: Conservative management of sternoclavicular injuries. *Orthop Clin North Am* 31:189, 2000.

6. Neer CS, Rockwood CA: Fracture and dislocations of the shoulder. In Rockwood CA, Green DP (eds): *Fractures in Adults,* 4th ed. Philadelphia, JB Lippincott, 1996.

7. McKoy BE, Bensen CV, Hartsock LA: Fractures about the shoulder: Conservative management. *Orthop Clin North Am* 31:205, 2000.

8. Clarke HD, McCann PD: Acromioclavicular joint injuries. *Orthop Clin North Am* 31:177, 2000.

9. Cole PA: Scapular fractures. *Orthop Clin North Am* 33:1, 2002.

10. Wen DY: Current concepts in the treatment of anterior shoulder dislocations. *Am J Emerg Med* 17:410, 1999.

11. Cleeman E, Flatow EL: Shoulder dislocation in the young patient. *Orthop Clin North Am* 31:217, 2000.

12. Brems-Dalgaard E, Davidsen E, Sloth C: Radiographic examination of the acute shoulder. *Eur J Radiol* 11:10, 1990.

13. De Smet AA: Axillary projection in radiography of the nontraumatized shoulder. *AJR Am J Roentgenol* 134:511, 1980.

14. Kornguth PL, Salazar AM: The apical oblique view of the shoulder: Its usefulness in acute trauma. *AJR Am J Roentgenol* 149:113, 1987.

15. Ernberg LA, Potter HG: Radiographic evaluation of the acromioclavicular and sternoclavicular joints. *Clin Sports Med* 22:255, 2003.

16. Robinson CM: Fractures of the clavicle in the adult: Epidemiology and classification. *J Bone Joint Surg Br* 80:476, 1998.

17. Nowak J, Mallmin H, Larsson S: The etiology and epidemiology of clavicular fractures: A prospective study during a two-year period in Uppsala, Sweden. *Injury* 31:353, 2000.

18. Anderson K: Evaluation and treatment of distal clavicle fractures. *Clin Sports Med* 22:319, 2003.

19. Andersen K, Jensen PO, Lauritzen J: Treatment of clavicular fractures. *Acta Orthop Scand* 57:71, 1987.

20. Nordqvist A, et al: Shortening of the clavicle after fracture: Incidence and clinical significance, a 5-year follow-up of 85 patients. *Acta Orthop Scand* 68:349, 1997.

21. Hill JM, McGuire MH, Crosby LA: Closed treatment of displaced middle-third fractures of the clavicle gives poor results. *J Bone Joint Surg Br* 79:537, 1997.

22. Nordqvist A, Petersson CJ: Incidence and causes of shoulder girdle injuries in an urban population. *J Shoulder Elbow Surg* 4:107, 1995.

23. Ideberg R, Grevesten S, Larsson S: Epidemiology of scapular fractures: Incidence and classification of 338 fractures. *Acta Orthop Scand* 66:395, 1995.

24. Zuckerman JD, Koval KJ, Cuomo F: Fractures of the scapula. *Instr Course Lect* 42:271, 1993.

25. Ada JR, Miller ME: Scapular fractures: Analysis of 113 cases. *Clin Orthop* 269:174, 1991.

26. Stephens NG, et al: Significance of scapular fracture in the blunt trauma patient. *Ann Emerg Med* 26:439, 1995.

27. Court-Brown CM, Garf A, McQueen MM: The epidemiology of proximal humeral fractures. *Acta Orthop Scand* 72:365, 2001.

28. Nordqvist A, Petersson CJ: Incidence and causes of shoulder girdle injuries in an urban population. *J Shoulder Elbow Surg* 4:107, 1995.

29. Neer CS: Displaced proximal humeral fractures: Part 1. Classification and evaluation. *J Bone Joint Surg Am* 52:1077, 1979.

30. Williams GR, Wong KL: Two-part and three-part fractures: Open reduction and internal fixation versus closed reduction and percutaneous pinning. *Orthop Clin North Am* 31:1, 2000.

31. Ferkel RD, Hedley AK, Eckardt JJ: Anterior fracture-dislocation of the shoulder: Pitfalls in treatment. *J Trauma* 24:363, 1984.

32. Burgos Flores J, et al: Fractures of the proximal humeral epiphysis. *Int Orthop* 17:16, 1993.

33. Williams DJ: The mechanisms producing fracture-separation of the proximal humeral epiphysis. *J Bone Joint Surg Br* 63:102, 1981.

34. DePalma AF: *Surgery of the Shoulder,* 3rd ed. Philadelphia, JB Lippincott, 1983.

35. Garretson RB, Williams GR: Clinical evaluation of injuries to the acromioclavicular and sternoclavicular joints. *Clin Sports Med* 22:239, 2003.

36. Buckerfield CT, Castle ME: Acute traumatic retrosternal dislocation of the clavicle. *J Bone Joint Surg Am* 66:379, 1984.

37. Richards R: Acromioclavicular joint injuries. *Instr Course Lect* 42:259, 1993.

38. Bossart PJ, et al: Lack of efficacy of weighted radiographs in diagnosing acute acromioclavicular separation. *Ann Emerg Med* 17:20, 1988.

39. Kroner K, Lind T, Jensen J: The epidemiology of shoulder dislocations. *Arch Orthop Trauma Surg* 108:288, 1989.

40. Perron AD, et al: Acute complications associated with shoulder dislocation at an academic emergency department. *J Emerg Med* 24:141, 2003.

41. Perlmutter GS: Axillary nerve injury. *Clin Orthop* 368:28, 1999.

42. Riebel GD, McCabe JB: Anterior shoulder dislocations: A review of reduction techniques. *Am J Emerg Med* 9:180, 1991.

43. Gleeson AP, et al: Comparison of intra-articular lignocaine and a suprascapular nerve block for acute anterior shoulder dislocation. *Injury* 28:141, 1997.

44. Matthews DE, Roberts T: Intraarticular lidocaine versus intravenous analgesia for the reduction of acute anterior shoulder dislocations: A prospective randomized study. *Am J Sports Med* 23:54, 1995.

45. Janecki CJ, Shahcheragh GH: The forward elevation maneuver for reduction of anterior dislocation of the shoulder. *Clin Orthop* 164:177, 1982.

46. Westin CD, et al: Anterior shoulder dislocation: A simple and rapid method for reduction. *Am J Sports Med* 23:369, 1995.

47. Danzl DF, et al: Closed reduction of anterior subcoracoid shoulder dislocation: Evaluation of an external rotation method. *Orthop Rev* 15:311, 1986.

48. Kothari RU, Dronen SC: The scapular manipulation technique for the reduction of acute anterior shoulder dislocations. *J Emerg Med* 8:625, 1990.

49. McNamara RM: Reduction of anterior shoulder dislocations by scapular manipulation. *Ann Emerg Med* 22:1140, 1993.

50. Harvey RA, Trabulsy ME, Roe L: Are postreduction anteroposterior and scapula Y views useful in anterior shoulder dislocations? *Am J Emerg Med* 10:149, 1992.

51. Hendey GW, Kinlaw K: Clinically significant abnormalities in postreduction radiographs after anterior shoulder dislocation. *Ann Emerg Med* 28:399, 1996.

52. Hendey GW: Necessity of radiographs in the emergency department management of shoulder dislocations. *Ann Emerg Med* 36:108, 2000.

53. Murrell GC: Treatment of shoulder dislocation: Is a sling appropriate? *Med J Aust* 179:370, 2003.

54. Itoi E, et al: A new method of immobilization after traumatic anterior dislocation of the shoulder: A preliminary study. *J Shoulder Elbow Surg* 12:413, 2003.

55. Neviaser RJ, Neviaser TJ, Neviaser JS: Anterior dislocation of the shoulder and rotator cuff rupture. *Clin Orthop* 291:103, 1993.

56. Taylor DC, Arciero RA: Pathological changes associated with shoulder dislocations: Arthroscopic and physical

PART TWO TRAUMA • Section III Orthopedic Lesions

exam findings in first-time traumatic anterior dislocations. *Am J Sports Med* 25:306, 1997.

57. Rowe CR: Recurrent transient anterior dislocation of the shoulder. *Orthop Clin North Am* 19:767, 1988.

58. Heller KD, et al: Posterior dislocation of the shoulder: Recommendation for a classification. *Arch Orthop Trauma Surg* 113:228, 1994.

59. Perrenoud A, Imhoff AB: Locked posterior dislocation of the shoulder. *Bull Hosp Joint Dis* 54:165, 1996.

60. Perron AD, Jones RL: Posterior shoulder dislocation: Avoiding a missed diagnosis. *Am J Emerg Med* 18:189, 2000.

61. Wadlington VR, Hendrix RW, Rogers LF: Computed tomography of posterior fracture-dislocations of the shoulder: Case reports. *J Trauma* 32:113, 1992.

62. Grate I Jr: Luxatio erecta: A rarely seen, but often missed shoulder dislocation. *Am J Emerg Med* 18:317, 2000.

63. Davids JR, Talbott RD: Luxatio erecta humeri. *Clin Orthop* 252:144, 1990.

64. Althausen PL, et al: Scapulothoracic dissociation. *Clin Orthop* 416:237, 2003.

65. Morrison DS, Greenbaum BS, Einhorn A: Shoulder impingement. *Orthop Clin North Am* 31:285, 2000.

66. Neer CS: Impingement lesions. *Clin Orthop* 173:70, 1983.

67. SooHoo NF, Rosen P: Diagnosis and treatment of rotator cuff tears in the emergency department. *J Emerg Med* 14:309, 1996.

68. Nirschl RP: Rotator cuff surgery. *Instr Course Lect* 38:447, 1989.

69. Brunelli MP, Gill TJ: Fractures and tendon injuries of the athletic shoulder. *Orthop Clin North Am* 33:497, 2002.

70. Neviaser TJ, Neviaser RJ: Lesions of long head of biceps tendon. *Instr Course Lect* 30:250, 1981.

71. Curtis AS, Snyder SJ: Evaluation and treatment of biceps tendon pathology. *Orthop Clin North Am* 24:33, 1993.

72. Travis RD, Doane R, Burkhead WZ: Tendon ruptures about the shoulder. *Orthop Clin North Am* 31:313, 2000.

73. Hurt G, Baker CL Jr: Calcific tendinitis of the shoulder. *Orthop Clin North Am* 34:567, 2003.

74. Re LP, Karzel RP: Management of rotator cuff calcifications. *Orthop Clin North Am* 24:125, 1993.

75. Gerdesmeyer L, et al: Extracorporeal shock wave therapy for the treatment of chronic calcifying tendonitis of the rotator cuff. *JAMA* 290:2573, 2003.

76. Neviaser RJ, Neviaser TJ: The frozen shoulder: Diagnosis and management. *Clin Orthop* 223:59, 1987.

77. Buchbinder R, Green S, Youd JM: Corticosteroid injections for shoulder pain. *Cochrane Database Syst Rev* 1:CD004016, 2003.

78. Cardone DA, Tallia AF: Joint and soft tissue injections. *Am Fam Physician* 66:290, 2002.

CHAPTER

51 Musculoskeletal Back Pain

Michelle Lin

LOW BACK PAIN

PERSPECTIVE

Background

Approximately 70% to 90% of adults during their lifetime experience *acute low back pain,* defined as pain lasting less than 6 weeks in duration.[1,2] Frustrating for the medical practitioner and the patient, 85% of these patients have an unknown etiology for their pain.[3] These patients frequently are diagnosed with "acute lumbosacral strain," "lumbago," or "mechanical back pain." These nonspecific, catch-all terms reflect the diagnostic challenge and lack of pathognomonic tests for low back pain. More accurately, these patients should be diagnosed with "idiopathic low back pain." Regardless, most of these cases resolve spontaneously within 6 weeks. Based on more recent studies regarding the management of acute low back pain, the most significant discovery, contradictory to traditional teaching from the 1980s, is to avoid bed rest for these patients, including patients with sciatica symptoms.[4,5] Management recommendations for chronic back pain remain controversial, however, and the condition accounts for a significant proportion of costs to the health care system.

Epidemiology

In the ambulatory care setting, the medical complaint of back pain is the fifth most common reason for a visit to a physician's office, with 15 million annual visits in the United States.[6] Low back pain primarily affects adults 30 to 60 years old and has a tremendous impact on the economy and workforce productivity. Approximately 14% of all Americans take at least 1 day off of work secondary to back pain. For people younger than age 45 years, persistent chronic back pain ranks as the leading cause of disability among chronic ailments. For people age 45 to 64, it ranks third behind coronary disease and arthritis.[7] Patients with back pain generate an estimated $24 billion in annual medical expenses and $50 billion to $100 billion in total direct and indirect costs in the United States.[1,2,8,9]

The natural history of most cases of low back pain follows a benign and self-limited course. Approximately 70% to 90% of patients have complete resolution of pain within 6 weeks.[10] If the pain does not resolve within 3 months, however, it is unlikely to resolve after 12 months. The recurrence rate for pain is 66% to 84% within the first 12 months.[11]

Risk factors for low back pain are continually being investigated. Data so far have been elusive and often contradictory.[12,13] It seems that the most consistent risk factor for future back problems is a previous history of back problems. Heavy lifting, pushing and pulling, or vibration at work; poor job satisfaction; smoking; and family history all seem to predispose to future back problems, whether causal or merely linked.[1,8,14-16] There also is early evidence of a genetic predisposition to lumbar disk disease.[17] Multiple other factors have been investigated, including body habitus, various occupations, and psychological profile, with conflicting results.[12,18,19]

PRINCIPLES OF DISEASE

Anatomy and Physiology

The lumbosacral spine consists of five lumbar vertebrae and the sacrum. Moving from anterior to posterior, each vertebra can be divided into the cylindrical vertebral body, two pedicles, two transverse processes, two overarching laminae, and a spinous process. These structures surround the neural canal, which houses the spinal cord and nerve roots and has a midsagittal anteroposterior diameter of 15 to 23 mm. The paired superior and inferior articulating processes join the articulating processes one vertebral level above and below. Each articulation site is called a *facet joint.* An intervertebral disk interposes between each vertebral body, providing elasticity and stability to the vertebral column. Each disk consists of an inner colloidal gelatinous substance, the *nucleus pulposus,* and an outer capsule, the *annulus fibrosus,* which is thinner posteriorly than anteriorly (Figure 51-1).

Various ligaments and musculature also provide stability to the lumbosacral spine. The anterior and posterior longitudinal ligaments course along the anterior and posterior surfaces of the vertebral bodies. The posterior longitudinal ligament forms a border between the intervertebral disks and the neural canal. As

expected, because this ligament thins as it runs inferiorly from L1 to S1, 95% of lumbar disk herniations occur at the L4-5 and L5-S1 levels, causing pain and neurologic deficit in the L5 and S1 distribution. Most herniations extrude posterolaterally to impinge a nerve root asymmetrically.[20] The ligamentum flavum courses just anteriorly to the laminae within the neural canal. With age, this ligament can thicken and cause spinal stenosis.

The spinal cord ends at the L1-2 interspace and the lower cauda equina nerve roots extend inferiorly, exiting the sacral foramina as peripheral nerves to the lower extremity. Pain fibers supplying structures in the lumbosacral region primarily arise from the posterior rami and sinuvertebral nerves at each lumbar vertebral level. Uniquely the nucleus pulposus and inner annular fibers of the intervertebral disk lack any pain fibers.[21] This lack of pain fibers correlates consistently with magnetic resonance imaging (MRI) findings of disk pathology in 20% to 30% of asymptomatic patients. The significance of these findings is unclear.[8,22,23]

Pathophysiology

Most conditions of low back pain have no proven cause. It is estimated that 85% of patients have no definitive diagnosis and are presumed to have pain originating from the soft tissue, including the muscles and ligaments.[8,20] The other 15% of patients with a known etiology have pain at the site of the *(1) nerve root, (2) articular facets,* or *(3) bone itself.*

First, a spinal nerve root can become inflamed and painful with external impingement. Disk herniation, usually at the L4-5 and L5-S1 level, is the most common cause of sciatica (i.e., pain radiating down the posterior leg from sciatic nerve root irritation). As the disk starts to desiccate and degenerate, starting in the 30s, patients are more at risk for outward herniation of the nucleus pulposus and consequently nerve root impingement. With further aging, these disks progressively shrink in size. This corresponds to the finding

Figure 51-1. Lateral and axial views of lumbar vertebral anatomy.

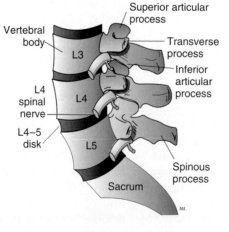

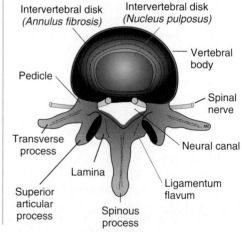

LATERAL VIEW   AXIAL VIEW

that disk herniations typically are found in patients 30 to 50 years old. Local nerve ischemia from physical compression also may contribute to the inflammation and pain. Studies also show that the nucleus pulposus, when exposed during disk herniation, may directly cause local neural inflammation, leading to pain.[24] Nerve root impingement also can occur with spinal stenosis, a narrowing of the neural canal from congenital narrowing or, more often, from degenerative or hypertrophic changes of the disks, vertebrae, facet joints, and ligamentum flavum.[25]

The two most emergent conditions causing nerve irritation are the cauda equina syndrome and a spinal epidural abscess. Cauda equina syndrome is a massive central disk herniation usually compressing multiple, bilateral nerve roots, causing back pain radiating to both legs, saddle anesthesia, and impaired bowel and bladder function. Emergent surgical decompression is indicated to preserve neurologic function. An epidural abscess similarly results in nerve root impingement, causing significant back pain. These rare infections develop most commonly from the hematogenous spread of *Staphylococcus aureus*.[20]

Congenital and developmental spinal abnormalities also may cause back pain by nerve root inflammation in some cases, but much less frequently than was thought previously. Conditions such as kyphosis and scoliosis usually do not cause pain unless the degree of vertebral column misalignment is pronounced.[26] Similarly, spondylolisthesis (slippage of one vertebral body on another) does not usually cause pain if the slippage is less than 25% of the vertebral body depth. Even patients with higher grades of anterior slippage (anterolisthesis) rarely develop severe back pain. Although it is much less common, backward slippage (retrolisthesis) is almost always associated with back pain. Spondylolisthesis occurs most often at the L5-S1 level (82.1%), followed by the L4-5 level (11.3%) and the L3-4 level (0.5%).[27] Multifactorial causes of spondylolisthesis include degenerative changes and trauma. Spondylolisthesis is often associated with bilateral pars interarticularis defects in the affected vertebra (spondylolysis).

Second, similar to any other joint in the body, degenerative changes of the synovial articular facets in the lumbosacral spine occur with age. The exact role of articular facet joints in back pain is unclear, however.

Third, direct irritation of the vertebral bone and its periosteum can cause back pain. The causes for spondylitis (osteomyelitis of the axial skeleton) can range from a slowly progressing tuberculosis infection (Pott's disease) to a more acute bacterial infection. Typically, bacteria seed the bone from a hematogenous source, such as from a skin wound, urinary tract infection, or directly from intravenous drug use. The most common bacterial culprit is *S. aureus.*

Primary and metastatic bone neoplasms can cause back pain from tumor infiltration into the bone. Primary bone tumors, such as multiple myeloma, are 25 times less frequent than metastatic disease.[28] Of the neoplasms, breast, lung, prostate, thyroid, lymphoma, and kidney are the most likely to metastasize to bone.

Inflammatory conditions, such as ankylosing spondylitis and other arthropathies, and osteoporosis also can cause back pain. For osteoporosis, the generalized decrease in bone mineralization can cause pain from microfractures of the vertebral column.

Referred pain, most commonly from intraperitoneal and retroperitoneal abdominal pathology, plays a significant role in back pain. Functional processes play a substantial role in back pain, especially for prolonged symptoms lasting more than 4 to 6 weeks. Functional causes range from fear, depression, and personality disorders to financial motivation. In such cases, there is no anatomic or pathophysiologic correlation with the reported pain.

Chronic back pain is complex and multifactorial. Not only are the structural causes unclear,[29] but also the nonphysical factors are variable and difficult to determine. It is likely that many of these patients do have some kind of chronic pain. What is unknown is why chronic pain triggers depression, drug dependence, and malingering in some people but not others. One difference may be the degree of disruption that the condition causes in the patient's lifestyle. A normally active and athletic person who is incapacitated is more profoundly affected than someone who is normally sedentary. Psychological factors and compensation play a large role in the behavior of many patients with chronic back pain.[30,31]

Pediatric back pain results in a diagnosis more often than adult pain.[32,33] Children complaining of back pain must be investigated. They may turn out to have spondylolysis with varying degrees of spondylolisthesis, Scheuermann's disease (kyphosis and osteochondritis of the vertebral end plates), infectious diseases, or neoplastic etiologies. Disk herniation in children is comparatively rare, but when it does occur, the presentation is similar to that seen in adults.[32]

CLINICAL FEATURES

Signs and Symptoms

A thorough history and physical examination are crucial in evaluating all patients with acute low back pain. The classic historical (Table 51-1) and physical findings for various low back pain etiologies are reviewed in this section. Although most etiologies are benign, there are four that the Agency for Health Care Policy and Research has identified as "cannot miss" or "red flag" diagnoses—spinal fracture, cauda equina syndrome, spinal infection, and malignancy.[34] A methodical and focused approach to the history and physical examination can help assess the patient's pretest probability for each of these disease entities and determine whether further tests should be ordered.

Uncomplicated Musculoskeletal Back Pain

Most patients with back pain can be classified in the category of uncomplicated musculoskeletal back pain after excluding worrisome disease processes. Often,

Table 51-1. Historical Clues for the Etiology of Low Back Pain

Questions for Patient	Potential Diagnosis
Does the back pain radiate down past the knees?	Radiculopathy and likely a herniated disk
Is the pain worse with walking and better with bending forward and sitting?	Spinal stenosis
Do you have morning back stiffness that improves with exercise?	Ankylosing spondylitis
Are you >50 years old?	Osteoporotic fracture, spinal malignancy
Has there been any recent history of blunt trauma?	Fracture
Do you take long-term corticosteroids?	Fracture, spinal infection
Do you have a history of cancer?	Spinal metastatic malignancy
Does your pain persist at rest?	Spinal malignancy, spinal infection
Has there been persistent pain for >6 weeks?	Spinal malignancy
Has there been unexplained weight loss?	Spinal malignancy
Is the pain worse at night?	Spinal malignancy, spinal infection
Are you immunocompromised? (HIV, alcoholic, diabetes)	Spinal infection
Have you had fevers or chills?	Spinal infection
Do you have pain, weakness, or numbness in both legs?	Cauda equina syndrome
Do you have bladder or bowel control problems?	Cauda equina syndrome

HIV, human immunodeficiency virus.

patients are unable to recall an inciting incident. The pain usually is characterized as an "ache" or "spasm" and is localized asymmetrically in the lumbar paraspinous muscle with radiation to the buttock or posterior thigh proximal to the knee. Movement exacerbates the pain, and rest relieves it. There is no associated deficit in sensation, strength, or bowel/bladder sphincter tone by history or examination. The only physical finding may be regional lumbosacral tenderness and a limited range of motion of the lower back. This diagnosis of exclusion is made only after ruling out the more worrisome causes of back pain.

Radiculopathy

Approximately 1% of all low back pain patients exhibit signs of lumbar radiculopathy (i.e., nerve root irritation).[35] The most common etiology is a herniated lumbar disk; other causes include spinal stenosis, malignancy, and infection. The most common type of lumbar radiculopathy is sciatica—an L5 or S1 radiculopathy. Patients with sciatica describe their pain as radiating from the low back to the legs, distal to the knee. Such pain is characterized as "shooting," "lancing," "sharp," or "burning." Associated symptoms include focal numbness or weakness in one of the lower extremities. Exacerbating triggers include sitting, bending, coughing, and straining; relieving factors include lying supine and still.

On physical examination, the patient frequently is tender in the sciatic notch. The straight leg raise (SLR) test is a fairly sensitive assessment tool to determine if the patient has sciatica. The SLR test is done with the patient supine and the legs extended. The symptomatic leg is passively raised, while keeping the knee straight. The presence of back pain, which radiates past the knee while the leg is elevated 30 to 70 degrees, suggests an L5 or S1 radiculopathy. If the SLR test results in isolated low back pain without radiation symptoms to the legs, however, it is considered to be a *negative* finding. A positive SLR test has a sensitivity of 80% but a low specificity of 40%, meaning that a negative result is

fairly accurate in ruling out sciatica. Corroborative tests for sciatica include the "bowstring sign" (reproduction of pain with deep palpation in the midline popliteal fossa) and Lasègue's sign (reproduction of pain with foot dorsiflexion while the leg is elevated just short of the pain threshold during the SLR test). As an alternative to the SLR test, with the patient in a seated position, the knee can be extended ("flip test"), which also should stretch the sciatic nerve. Reproduction of the pain often causes the patient to lean backward reflexively from the pain, almost "flipping" back into a supine position.

A crossed SLR test is done by passively raising the patient's asymptomatic leg, while keeping the knee straight. The presence of pain radiating from the back to the opposite affected leg has a sensitivity of only 25% but a high specificity of 90% for sciatica, meaning that a positive crossed SLR result is almost pathognomonic for sciatica, whereas a negative result is nondiagnostic.[20]

A reverse SLR test is performed to detect L3 or L4 radiculopathy. With the patient prone, each hip is passively extended. If there is irritation of the L3 or L4 nerve root, pain is elicited.

In addition to stressing lumbar nerve roots, a thorough examination of the lower extremities detects subtle findings associated with radiculopathies. This examination includes mapping the distribution of pain and assessing individual nerve root function, specifically strength, sensation, and reflexes. For the sensory examination, the earliest deficit can be detected by examining the most distal aspect of the dermatome. Specifically, light touch and pinprick sensation should be tested in the medial foot (L4), the area between the great and second toe (L5), and the lateral foot (S1) (Figure 51-2).

Herniated Disk

Patients with herniated lumbar disks are usually 30 to 50 years old and often have a long history of recurrent nonradicular low back pain, theoretically from irrita-

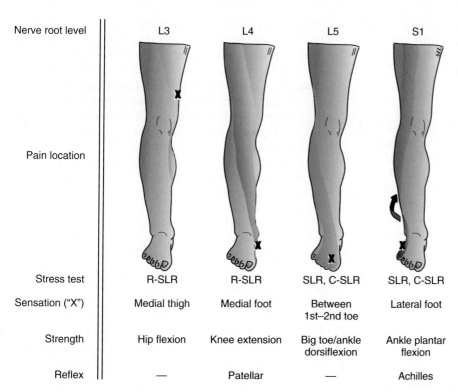

Nerve root level	L3	L4	L5	S1
Pain location				
Stress test	R-SLR	R-SLR	SLR, C-SLR	SLR, C-SLR
Sensation ("X")	Medial thigh	Medial foot	Between 1st–2nd toe	Lateral foot
Strength	Hip flexion	Knee extension	Big toe/ankle dorsiflexion	Ankle plantar flexion
Reflex	—	Patellar	—	Achilles

Figure 51-2. Physical examination findings for L3-S1 radiculopathy. The "X" marks the ideal location to test for sensation for each nerve root. C-SLR, crossed straight leg raise; R-SLR, reverse straight leg raise; SLR, straight leg raise.

tion of the outer annular fibers of the disk. When the nucleus pulposus of the disk prolapses through the annulus fibrosus, local nerve root inflammation and radiculopathy result. Coughing, sitting, and any movement in general exacerbate the patient's pain and radiculopathy symptoms. The severity of leg pain from radiculopathy often overshadows the back pain. Sciatica findings have a sensitivity of 95% for lumbar disk herniation, meaning that herniation is extremely unlikely in the absence of sciatica.[20]

The physical examination should focus on lower extremity neurologic function and signs of radiculopathy. Weakness of ankle dorsiflexion, great toe extension, ankle plantar flexion, and knee extension have respective specificities of 70%, 70%, 95%, and 99% for lumbar disk herniation.

Spinal Stenosis

Patients with spinal stenosis are typically older (mean age 55 years) and constitute only 3% of all low back pain patients.[3,36] The classic history, found in 60% to 75% of patients with spinal stenosis, is one of subacute or chronic pain and lower extremity radiculopathy, which occurs with walking and is relieved with rest and, uniquely, leaning forward.[37] Because these symptoms mimic peripheral vascular claudication symptoms, pain from spinal stenosis is termed *pseudoclaudication*. Typically, vascular claudication lasts 5 minutes after resting, while pseudoclaudication lasts 10 to 15 minutes.[38] Patients with spinal stenosis have symptom relief with spine flexion and leaning forward because it increases spinal canal diameter and reduces spinal cord tension. Sitting improves the symptoms, in contrast to patients with herniated disks.

A typical history involves a patient who walks uphill without pain but develops pain while walking downhill because the back is extended.

On physical examination, most patients have a lumbar radiculopathy at one or multiple levels and increased back pain with extension.[37] Classically, patients with spinal stenosis walk with a slight bent-forward position. To help distinguish spinal stenosis from vascular claudication, peripheral pedal pulses and ankle-brachial indices should be checked.

Degenerative Spondylolisthesis

Most cases of spondylolisthesis, forward displacement of one vertebral body over another, are caused by degenerative changes. This condition is most prevalent in adults older than age 40 and occurs most commonly at the L4-5 and L5-S1 junction. Two thirds of patients with radiographically documented degenerative spondylolisthesis are asymptomatic.[39] For patients with pain, bending, twisting, and lifting activities aggravate the symptoms. Radiculopathies, spinal stenosis symptoms, or both may coexist. On physical examination, patients may have a loss of lumbar lordosis, a step-off along the midline spine if the spondylolisthesis is severe, tight hamstrings, or a radiculopathy.

Arthropathies

Inflammatory arthropathies, such as ankylosing spondylitis, rheumatoid arthritis, and psoriatic arthritis, all are associated with subacute and chronic low back pain. All of these patients exhibit a decreased range of spinal flexibility. Commonly with ankylosing spondylitis, patients complain of morning back stiffness and pain relief with exercise. On physical examination, these patients may have nonspecific findings, such as decreased spinal mobility, sacroiliac joint tenderness, and decreased chest expansion.

Red Flag Diagnosis: Fracture

In all patients with significant blunt trauma to the back or with minimal trauma in the setting of osteoporosis, fractures of the spinal column must be considered. For patients taking long-term corticosteroids, who are predisposed to early osteoporosis, back pain had a specificity of 99.5% for a spinal fracture in one series.[20] This subpopulation of patients must be assessed for a fracture despite the absence of trauma. On examination, tenderness along the midline spine and paraspinous muscles from concurrent muscle spasm usually can be elicited.

Red Flag Diagnosis: Cauda Equina Syndrome

Cauda equina syndrome results from a sudden compression of multiple lumbar and sacral nerve roots. Although it is an extremely rare presentation of back pain, it is a neurosurgical emergency. Usually caused by a massive central disk herniation, other etiologies include a spinal epidural abscess, hematoma, trauma, and malignancy. Patients with cauda equina syndrome present with back pain and multiple-level radiculopathies, often involving both legs. Patients may have difficulty with bladder or bowel function. Diagnostic dilemmas arise because patients can present atypically with equivocal neurologic compromise and only mild-to-moderate pain.

The most consistent examination finding in cauda equina syndrome is urinary retention. With a high sensitivity of 90%, it is highly unlikely to have this disease process if the patient's postvoid residual urine volume is less than 100 to 200 mL. Saddle anesthesia, sensory deficit over the buttocks, upper posterior thighs, and perineal area, is frequently an associated finding with a sensitivity of 75%. In 60% to 80% of cases, the rectal examination reveals a decreased sphincter tone.[20]

Red Flag Diagnosis: Spinal Infection

Epidural abscess and spondylitis (osteomyelitis of the vertebral bone) are two types of dangerous spinal infections. Patients at higher risk include injection drug users, alcoholics, immunocompromised patients (e.g., patients with human immunodeficiency virus, diabetes mellitus, chronic renal failure, long-term corticosteroid use), the elderly, patients recently sustaining blunt trauma to the back, patients with an indwelling catheter, and patients with a recent bacterial infection. For epidural abscesses, approximately 20% of patients have no comorbidities or risk factors. The most common bacterial culprit is *S. aureus,* spreading hematogenously from a remote site or from direct extension of a local infection, such as spondylitis or disk space infection. Less common culprits are streptococci strains and enteric gram-negative bacilli.

Patient history reveals back pain even at rest and subjective fevers. On physical examination, midline spinal tenderness to percussion at the site of abscess is commonly present. What makes a spinal epidural abscess a diagnostic challenge is the fact that about 50% of the patients have no neurologic deficits, and 50% may be afebrile on initial presentation.[40] Nevertheless, it is essential to diagnose this neurosurgical emergency that entails a mortality as high as 23%.[40-42]

For spondylitis, infection often begins as a subtle hematogenous seeding of the disk space, causing diskitis. Subsequent contiguous spread of the disk space infection causes vertebral end plate erosion, leading to spondylitis. Similar to an epidural abscess, the most common bacterial culprit is *S. aureus.* Less commonly, enteric gram-negative bacilli and *Mycobacterium tuberculosis* (Pott's disease) are the infectious organisms. Injection drug users also are at risk for *Pseudomonas* spondylitis. Patient history typically reveals a more indolent course of back pain with subjective fevers. The physical examination findings can range from nonspecific tenderness of the spine to radiculopathy and cauda equina syndrome. Similarly nondiagnostic, the presence of fever has a sensitivity of only 27% to 50% for spondylitis.[20]

Red Flag Diagnosis: Malignancy

Vertebral infiltration with a tumor can be caused by either a primary or, more commonly, a metastatic malignancy. These patients are generally older than age 50 and often complain of subacute or chronic back pain, which is worse at night. Risk factors include a history of known cancer (98% specificity), unexplained weight loss (94% specificity), persistent pain despite bed rest (90% specificity), and pain lasting more than 1 month (specificity 81%).[43] On examination, these patients typically have mild-to-moderate spinal tenderness. Examination of the organs most likely to metastasize to bone, including breast, prostate, and lung, may be indicated.

Referred Back Pain

Referred pain is often difficult to differentiate from pain originating from the lumbosacral structures. It is vital, however, to make the distinction. A sudden onset of severe, tearing back pain is classically an aortic dissection. Abdominal pain radiating to the back could be a ruptured abdominal aortic aneurysm in an elderly patient with atherosclerotic disease. Alternatively, abdominal pain radiating to the back could be pancreatitis in a chronic alcoholic. Unilateral paraspinal pain associated with fever and nausea in a young woman could be pyelonephritis. In all such cases, a thorough examination of the abdomen, genitourinary system, and cardiovascular system is essential. Distinguishing the primary cause of the pain radically alters the therapy for the patient.

Functional Back Pain

Distinguishing functional pain from "real" pain is often difficult, but several clues can be elicited from the history. A prolonged history of nonanatomic pain complaints, vague pain descriptions without localization, multiple lawsuits over similar problems, and lack of coordinated care for a problem that otherwise seems to dominate the patient's life all suggest that a search for a physical cause would be fruitless. These patients are often thought to have secondary gains for their complaints.

On physical examination, maneuvers can be performed to try to detect functional back pain, if a psychological overlay is suspected. The first is performing the SLR test from the sitting instead of the supine position. Seemingly focused on the knee examination, the physician extends the patient's knee; this physiologically reproduces the SLR by stretching the L5 and S1 nerve roots. A positive response includes reproduction of the patient's pain and extension of the back while seated to decrease traction on the sciatic nerve. A positive supine SLR test but a negative sitting SLR test suggests a nonphysiologic cause for the pain.

A second sign involves superficial tenderness. Some patients, to impress the physician with their degree of pain, respond dramatically to superficial palpation. This response is atypical for patients with genuine back pain. Nondermatomal sensory loss and widespread nondermatomal pain complaints also are unlikely to be caused by physiologic processes.

Third, back pain should not be elicited by pushing down on the patient's scalp against the cervical spine. This maneuver axially loads only the cervical and not the lumbar spine.

Fourth, a patient who generally overreacts during the examination is probably not giving a true reflection of the actual discomfort. All of these signs are believed to correlate well with psychopathology but have poor prognostic value. They are suggestive of malingering and functional complaints, but are neither sensitive nor specific enough to rule out organic pathology.[44,45]

Back Pain in the Elderly

When the elderly experience back pain, musculoskeletal back pain and disk herniation are less likely the underlying etiology. Instead, spinal stenosis and degenerative spondylolisthesis should be considered. Also, the incidence of more worrisome diagnoses, such as an osteoporotic fracture, spinal infection, and malignancy, is much greater in this patient population. Consequently in these cases, the threshold for further investigation should be much lower.

Back Pain in Children

The likelihood of congenital etiologies for back pain, such as leg-length discrepancy and spondylolisthesis, is greater for children compared with adults. Spondylolisthesis is diagnosed most often in patients older than age 10 years, who are involved heavily in sports and complain of low back pain worsened with activity. A history suggesting infection or malignancy in children is similar to that of adults. Radicular symptoms are relatively rare in children. Functional processes are

suggested when the pain is present only with certain undesired activities, such as housework or chores.

DIAGNOSTIC STRATEGIES

Laboratory Evaluation

In the absence of historical and physical findings suggesting "red flag" diagnoses for low back pain, laboratory evaluation is unnecessary. When a patient presents with back pain suggesting a spinal infection or malignancy, however, laboratory studies may help with risk stratification. Specifically, a complete blood cell count, erythrocyte sedimentation rate (ESR), and urinalysis should be obtained. Additional laboratory studies should be tailored to the patient's history and physical examination. Liver function tests and amylase/lipase level may need to be checked for abdominal complaints.

For a spinal infection, the ESR usually is elevated (>20 mm/hr), whereas the serum white blood cell (WBC) count may or may not be elevated.[46] In one study, 13 of 40 (32%) patients with an epidural abscess had a falsely reassuring WBC count less than 11,000/μL.[41] When patients are diagnosed with a spinal infection, blood cultures should be drawn because a single strain, most commonly *S. aureus,* can be isolated in 50% to 90% of the cases.[41,47] Performing a lumbar puncture to evaluate the cerebrospinal fluid is unnecessary and is relatively contraindicated because of the risk of seeding the cerebrospinal fluid with bacteria.

For a bony malignancy, the ESR also usually is elevated, whereas the WBC may be equivocal. The hematocrit may be low secondary to anemia of chronic disease. Other additional helpful laboratory tests include alkaline phosphatase, prostate-specific antigen concentrations, and serum immunoelectrophoresis and urine testing for light chains (for multiple myeloma).

Radiology

Plain Radiograph

The utility of "screening" lumbosacral plain radiographs for all patients with acute low back pain is extremely low. Plain radiographs contribute little to patient management in the absence of concerning red flag findings and needlessly expose the patient to irradiation.[48] Most patients with back pain do not need radiographs. Most films are normal, but they also may have incidental findings, which may not be the true cause of the patient's pain. These findings include spondylolisthesis, abnormal spinal curvature, disk space wedging, and degenerative changes.[8] Current indications for radiographs in back pain patients are listed in Box 51-1.

Patients with radiculopathy findings suggesting a herniated disk do not require radiographs. In addition to being radiographically undetectable on plain films, disk herniations resolve with conservative management in most cases.

If radiographs are obtained, anteroposterior and lateral views are usually sufficient in the emergency department, although many centers also prefer a coned-down lateral sacral view. Oblique films are not necessary except in children, in whom spondylolysis and spondylolisthesis may be more prevalent.[49]

On plain radiographs, spondylolisthesis, vertebral osteomyelitis, and vertebral metastatic disease have classic appearances. Spondylolisthesis (Figure 51-3) is classified into grade 1 through grade 4 based on the severity of the anterior slippage of one vertebral body over another. Grade 1, which is often asymptomatic, involves less than 25% slippage. Grade 2 through grade 4 involve 25% to 50%, 50% to 75%, and at least 75% slippage, respectively.

Spondylitis (Figure 51-4) is characterized by erosion of contiguous vertebral endplates and a shortened disk space height, as best seen on the lateral view. Because the anterior subchondral vertebral bone and disk space are highly vascular, it follows that spondylitis has a predilection in these areas because of the hematogenous spread of infection. With more advanced disease, vertebral bony erosion and collapse may occur.

Vertebral metastatic disease (Figure 51-5) can present either as a blastic (hyperdense) or lytic (hypodense) lesion and has a predilection for the vertebral body and pedicles. In contrast to osteomyelitis, the intervertebral disk space is spared.

BOX 51-1. Indications for Plain Lumbosacral Films in Patients with Low Back Pain

- Age younger than 18 or older than 50 years
- Any history of malignancy or unexplained weight loss
- Any history of fever, immunocompromise, or injection drug use
- Recent trauma, other than simple lifting
- Progressive neurologic deficits or other findings consistent with cauda equina syndrome
- Prolonged duration of symptoms greater than 4 to 6 weeks

If a red flag diagnosis is of concern, a plain radiograph may rule out a fracture but may not be adequate to rule out other pathologies, such as cauda equina syndrome, spinal infection, and malignancy. For cauda equina syndrome, patients more often have normal or nonspecific plain film findings because the most common etiology is a central disk herniation. For spinal infection and vertebral malignancy, the sensitivity of a plain radiograph is only fair at 82% and 60%.[48] In these cases, the patient subsequently should undergo MRI if there is a high clinical suspicion.

Computed Tomography and Magnetic Resonance Imaging

For fractures and bony abnormalities of the vertebral column, computed tomography (CT) is superior to MRI. In the case of a fracture, CT helps to elucidate the integrity of the spinal canal and the risk for spinal cord impingement. For all other red flag diagnoses—cauda equina, spinal infection, and malignancy—MRI is the gold standard test. Its superior tissue resolution, especially of the spinal cord and intervertebral disks, and its ability to perform more accurate sagittal reconstructions make MRI the ideal imaging modality. MRI is able to differentiate subtle soft tissue pathology, such as a spinal epidural abscess (Figure 51-6). There is no radiation with MRI, whereas CT exposes the patient to about 4 years' worth of natural background radiation.[50]

Although disk herniation is easily visualized on MRI, patients with findings consistent with an uncomplicated disk herniation (i.e., without objective neurologic findings on examination) should not routinely undergo MRI imaging because of the self-limited nature of the disease in most cases. Overimaging patients with lumbar radiculopathy may lead to an overdiagnosis of disk herniations because incidental MRI-documented herniations have been shown to occur in 20% to 30% of asymptomatic individuals. The result may be unnecessary surgical interventions.[8,51]

Special Investigations

Unless there is suspicion of a process other than uncomplicated back pain or disk herniation, other

---

Figure 51-3. Lateral plain radiograph and schematic diagram of grade 2 anterior spondylolisthesis of L5 on S1. Grading is based on the percentage of slippage with 0% to 25%, 25% to 50%, 50% to 75%, and greater than 75% corresponding to grades 1 to 4, respectively.

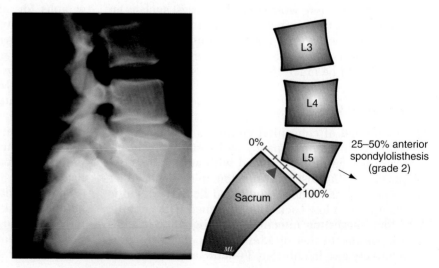

investigations are not required. MRI is the definitive test for most conditions. Radionuclide scans have been used for locating suspected malignancy, infectious foci, and occult fractures as in spondylolysis. Nuclear medicine scans are regarded as sensitive but nonspecific.

DIFFERENTIAL CONSIDERATIONS

Nonspecific low back pain is in many ways a diagnosis of exclusion. In a typical patient, within the 18- to 50-year age range with acute low back pain and with no radiculopathy, prior malignancy, weight loss, or fever, the diagnosis is almost certainly uncomplicated musculoskeletal back pain. When the patient falls outside of the aforementioned parameters, a wide variety of differential diagnoses must be entertained.

Almost anything can cause low back pain. Box 51-2 contains an extensive list of possible diagnoses, but it is useful to look at the most common and most serious causes of low back pain other than musculoskeletal lumbosacral pain. One of the most life-threatening causes of referred back pain is a leaking or ruptured abdominal aortic aneurysm. See appropriate chapters for further discussion of specific problems.

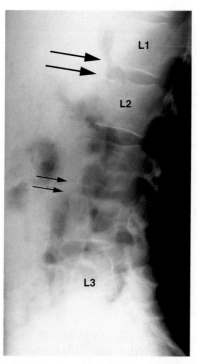

Figure 51-4. Lateral plain radiograph shows *Staphylococcus aureus* spondylitis of L3 and L4. There is narrowing of the L3-4 disk space and erosion of the vertebral end plates of L3 and L4 *(small arrows)*. Notice the distinct vertebral end plate margins in unaffected areas *(large arrows)*.

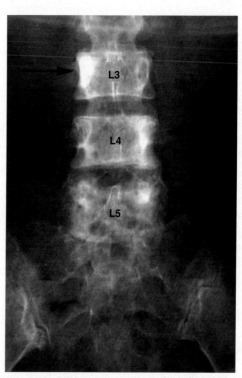

Figure 51-5. Anteroposterior plain radiograph shows blastic infiltration of metastatic breast cancer to the pedicles of L3-5 *(arrows)*.

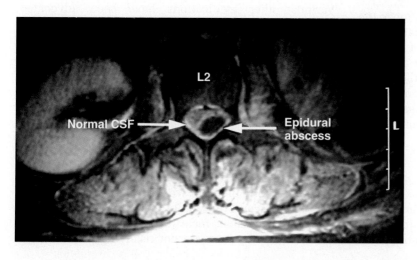

Figure 51-6. Axial T2-weighted magnetic resonance imaging of *Staphylococcus aureus* L2 epidural abscess impinging the dorsolateral aspect of the spinal canal. CSF, cerebrospinal fluid. (Image contributed by Dr. Stephen Bretz.)

BOX 51-2. Differential Diagnosis for Low Back Pain

Localized/Common
Uncomplicated musculoskeletal back pain
Intervertebral disk herniation
Spinal stenosis
Spondylolisthesis
Osteoarthritis
Fracture

Localized/Uncommon Infection
Spondylitis
Epidural abscess
Diskitis
Herpes zoster

Malignancy
Metastatic
   Breast
   Lung
   Prostate
   Kidney, thyroid, colon (less common)
Primary
   Multiple myeloma
   Lymphoma
   Leukemia
   Primary cord/extradural tumors
   Osteoid osteoma
   Other primary bone tumors

Pediatric
Spondylolisthesis/spondylolysis
Severe scoliosis
Scheuermann's disease

Rheumatologic
Ankylosing spondylitis
Psoriatic arthritis
Polymyalgia rheumatica
Reiter's syndrome

Vascular
Arteriovenous malformation of spinal cord
Epidural hematoma

Life-Threatening Referred Pain
Abdominal aortic aneurysm

Gastrointestinal System
Biliary pathology
Pancreatitis
Peptic ulcer disease
Diverticulitis

Genitourinary System
Renal colic
Pyelonephritis
Prostatitis
Cystitis

Gynecologic System
Menstrual cramps
Spontaneous abortion
Labor
Ectopic pregnancy
Pelvic inflammatory disease
Endometriosis
Ovarian cyst
Ovarian torsion

Hematologic System
Sickle cell crisis

Functional
Somatization disorder
Depression
Fibrositis
Malingering

MANAGEMENT

Because most patients with acute low back pain have symptomatic resolution within 4 to 6 weeks, only conservative management is needed. In general, MRI and surgery are reserved for the few patients who have concerning systemic signs and patients with refractory, debilitating back pain. Over the past few decades, the accepted practice has shifted 180 degrees from an overaggressive recommendation for invasive surgical intervention to the minimalistic recommendation of symptomatic pain control and early return to activity. The role of the physician in back pain management is to obtain a correct diagnosis, rule out significant pathology, avoid excessive investigation, provide analgesia, and educate the patient.[52] The management of various etiologies for low back pain is summarized in Figure 51-7. For fractures and referred pain, refer to the appropriate chapters.

Uncomplicated Musculoskeletal Back Pain

Besides a thorough history and physical examination, no further investigations are required for uncomplicated low back pain. Only pain control and patient edu-

cation are indicated. Aside from an initial parenteral opioid or nonsteroidal anti-inflammatory drug, most patients can be managed with oral nonsteroidal medications.[52] Ibuprofen is an ideal choice because it is inexpensive, and various nonsteroidal anti-inflammatory drugs have been shown to have the same efficacy. It is unclear whether ibuprofen is superior to acetaminophen.[53] Short-term opioids also occasionally are needed for break-through pain in the acute setting. Various other medications have been advocated, including benzodiazepines and other muscle relaxants. Based on the current conflicting literature, these medications probably do not provide a significant added benefit, but they do increase the incidence of side effects such as drowsiness and drug dependence.[54] There is no role for corticosteroids in the treatment of uncomplicated low back pain.

In terms of patient education, one of the outdated practices of back pain management was that physicians convinced patients that they were sick. This was done by overinvestigating, overtreating, putting patients to bed, and taking them off work. It now has been shown convincingly and repeatedly that all of those interventions are excessive. Instead, patients should be educated as to why they are not receiving plain films of

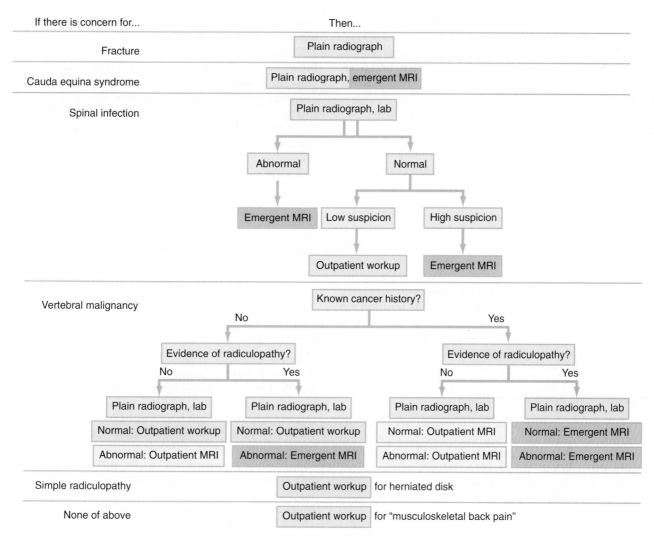

Figure 51-7. Algorithm for management of low back pain. The patient's history may be concerning for more than one red flag diagnosis.

their lumbosacral spine or laboratory tests and reassured on the likely benign course of the pain. Most patients can be convinced by education and an explanation of radiation dosing. A typical lumbosacral spine series involves as much gonadal radiation as a chest x-ray every day for 5 or 6 years.[55] Patients also are discouraged from the outdated recommendation of strict bed rest. Compared with patients who are prescribed strict bed rest, patients experience earlier resolution of pain and return to work sooner if they remain active.[4] Patients should be made aware, however, that the back pain has a 66% to 84% likelihood of recurring within 12 months.[11]

Other supplemental treatment modalities have been shown to be of debatable efficacy in the management of acute and chronic low back pain. These include acupuncture, physiotherapy, chiropractic manipulation, massage, ultrasound, traction, and transcutaneous nerve stimulation.[8,10,56-59]

Lumbar Disk Herniation

Similar to patients with uncomplicated low back pain, patients with disk herniations and radiculopathy do not benefit from strict bed rest.[5] In the acute setting, these patients should receive analgesics, but further investigation with laboratory tests and radiographs is not necessary. Most of these patients have symptomatic resolution within 6 weeks with conservative, nonsurgical management.[60,61]

Corticosteroid injections into the epidural space have been advocated for sciatica in the belief that this helped relieve some of the inflammation associated with disk herniation. Although this treatment may offer some initial symptom improvement, there is no long-term benefit or reduction in the need for later surgery.[62] The use of systemic steroids in back pain and disk herniation remains controversial. It is difficult to argue their benefit in nonspecific low back pain, but the anti-inflammatory effects make empiric sense in the context of radiculopathy. A large retrospective review showed no definite benefit of systemic steroids in either setting, but the definitive trial is yet to be done.[54]

When the pain from disk herniation persists for longer than 4 to 6 weeks, outpatient MRI is indicated. With a documented herniation, these patients benefit from surgical diskectomy. Other indications for surgery include intractable pain and worsening motor or sensory deficit. Although surgical patients tend to have earlier relief of pain compared with nonsurgical patients, the 4- and 10-year results are the same. Microsurgery techniques and laser therapy have not been shown to confer any advantage over conventional techniques.[63]

Spinal Stenosis

Patients with spinal stenosis should be managed conservatively with pain medications. In the absence of alarming red flag findings, these patients do not require laboratory or radiographic studies in the emergency department. These patients may be candidates for surgery if they show any of the following conditions: progressive neurologic deficit, progressive reduction in ability to walk secondary to pseudoclaudication, evidence of cauda equina syndrome, or intractable pain. Elective surgical decompression is more controversial. A 10-year longitudinal study showed that no findings predicted which patients would benefit more from surgery versus conservative management.[64] The benefits of surgery also must be weighed against the risks of surgery itself because these patients are usually elderly.

Degenerative Spondylolisthesis

Patients with symptomatic degenerative spondylolisthesis are managed conservatively with analgesia and lifestyle changes, which include the avoidance of repetitive bending, heavy lifting, and twisting at the waist. For refractory and severe back pain, patients should undergo outpatient MRI and receive neurosurgical follow-up for possible operative decompression.

Red Flag Diagnosis: Fracture

See Chapter 40, Spinal Injuries.

Red Flag Diagnosis: Cauda Equina Syndrome

Cauda equina syndrome is a neurosurgical emergency that requires urgent operative decompression to help preserve distal neurologic function. All patients with concerning findings, such as saddle anesthesia or a large postvoid residual volume, require emergent MRI. On average, these patients may have an improved outcome if decompression takes place within 24 hours.[65] Early evidence exists, however, that shows delayed operative decompression under a more controlled setting may be performed without any adverse effects, particularly for patients who have overflow urinary incontinence.[66]

Red Flag Diagnosis: Spinal Infection

If a patient's history or physical examination is worrisome for a spinal infection, further investigation is paramount. With a low index of suspicion, a normal serum WBC count, ESR, and lumbosacral plain film can safely rule out infection. If any of these tests are abnormal or if the patient has a moderate to high pretest probability for a spinal infection, the next step is to obtain emergent MRI.

Pyogenic spinal infections should be treated with broad-spectrum intravenous antibiotics that cover at least for *S. aureus* and gram-negative bacilli until blood culture results return. Vancomycin should be added if the patient is at risk for methicillin-resistant *S. aureus*. For injection drug users, antibiotic coverage for *Pseudomonas* is necessary. For almost all epidural abscesses, treatment also requires neurosurgical drainage and decompression.

Red Flag Diagnosis: Malignancy

An algorithmic guideline to the management of back pain, which is worrisome for malignancy, involves subdividing patients into two categories—patients with and patients without a history of prior cancer. Of cancer patients, 20% to 85% develop spinal metastasis.[67,68] These patients are subdivided further into patients with and patients without evidence of a radiculopathy.

Most patients fall into the classification of back pain without a history of cancer and without a radiculopathy. They have a history only suggestive of a malignancy, such as unexplained weight loss or back pain that is worse at night. These patients require further risk stratification with plain radiographs and laboratory tests, including a complete blood cell count and ESR. With normal results, these patients can be referred to their primary care physician for further workup. The physician should not feel completely reassured that malignancy has been ruled out, however, because plain films have a false-negative rate of 10% to 17% for vertebral bone metastasis. This false-negative rate is likely due to the fact that a cancer needs to erode at least 50% of the bone before becoming radiographically apparent.[69] With abnormal results, such as a bony lesion or extremely elevated ESR level (>100 mm/hr), these patients should receive urgent MRI as an outpatient within the next 3 to 7 days.

For patients with no known history of cancer but with signs of radiculopathy, the workup also includes a plain radiograph, complete blood cell count, and ESR. If the test results are normal, the patients should be referred to their primary care physician for further evaluation for malignancy and other etiologies for radiculopathy, including spinal stenosis and disk herniation. If the workup shows a bony lesion on plain film or an extremely elevated ESR level (>100 mm/hr), these patients should undergo emergent MRI because (1) the presence of radiculopathy may be an early harbinger of impending spinal cord compression from a mass effect, and (2) it is often difficult to distinguish between a neoplasm from early spondylitis (especially tuberculous osteomyelitis) and an osteoporotic fracture causing a vertebral collapse on plain film.[70]

For patients with a history of prior cancer and low back pain, all require MRI either emergently or urgently within 3 to 7 days. In the absence of radiculopathy findings, these patients should undergo outpatient MRI regardless of plain film and laboratory results. Plain radiography is too insensitive to rule out a vertebral neoplastic process definitively. If radiculopathy is present, however, these patients require emergent MRI regardless of plain radiography findings because of the concern for spinal cord compression. According to one study of known cancer patients with back pain and radiculopathy, the risk of epidural spinal cord compression was 25% despite normal films and 88% with films showing vertebral metastasis.[71]

For all patients undergoing emergent MRI to evaluate for vertebral malignancy and cauda equina syndrome, dexamethasone should be administered to reduce the potential mass effect. In addition to high-dose corticosteroids, patients with a vertebral neoplasm also may benefit from radiation therapy.

Pediatric Back Pain

Management of back pain in children is similar to management for adults and depends on the etiology. Spondylolisthesis is managed by observation, with only 4% to 5% of cases worsening. Progression usually stops as skeletal maturity is achieved in the late teens. Current recommendations are for limited contact sports in children with less than 30% to 50% slippage and surgical stabilization for children with slippage greater than 30% to 50%. Treatment becomes more aggressive if the child is symptomatic.[72]

Chronic Back Pain

Patients with chronic back pain often are regarded as the most challenging of back pain patients. The cause of chronic back pain is complex and multifactorial and usually requires a multidisciplinary approach for the greatest chance for success. There is little doubt that psychosocial factors, including depression, drug dependence, and financial gain, play a significant role in the behavior of many of these patients, making proper assessment and treatment impossible for the emergency physician.

After the emergency physician has made sure that no red flag condition exists, emergency management involves analgesia and follow-up. The main decision usually centers on the use of narcotics, which becomes an individual decision for the physician to make. Patients showing drug-seeking behavior classically are from out of town, have a physician who cannot be contacted, or are "allergic" to all nonopioid medications.

DISPOSITION

Almost all patients with uncomplicated back pain can be discharged from the emergency department. In rare circumstances, severe pain or an unacceptable social situation may preclude discharge. For patients who have a red flag diagnosis of cauda equina syndrome or epidural abscess, an immediate neurosurgical consultation is required for emergent surgical decompression. For spondylitis, patients require hospital admission for intravenous antibiotics. For vertebral malignancy, the decision to hospitalize a patient for pain control, high-dose corticosteroids, and radiation therapy should be made in conjunction with a neurosurgeon, oncologist, and radiation therapist.

One of the most important aspects in the management of patients with low back pain is the discharge instruction. Not only are clear and simple instructions useful to the patient, but they are also a medicolegal necessity for the physician. Physicians must avoid using medical terms. The discharge instructions should include the following:
1. *Diagnosis:* Distinguish between uncomplicated (musculoskeletal) back pain and diskogenic radiculopathy.
2. *Activity:* Recommend maintaining active mobility as limited only by pain, avoiding heavy lifting until symptoms resolve, and getting back to work early.
3. *Reassurance:* Educate patients on the likely benign etiology for the pain.
4. *Warnings:* Instruct patients to return to the emergency department immediately if they have a fever; lose bladder or bowel control; have numbness or tingling around their anus, vagina, or penis; or have new pain or weakness down one or both legs.

Pediatric back pain is subject to the same discharge instructions as that of adults. In patients with pain secondary to spondylolisthesis, activity restrictions should be made in conjunction with an orthopedic surgeon. Emergency department disposition for a patient with chronic back pain is relatively simple: pain management with nonopioids, when possible, and follow-up with a primary care provider. The prognosis is guarded because patients who are off of work for 6 months are usually still off of work after 2 years.[30]

KEY CONCEPTS

- The key to differentiating between benign and serious pathology in low back pain is a focused and thorough history and physical examination.
- The absence of sciatica findings practically rules out a lumbar disk herniation.
- Screening laboratory tests and plain radiographs are not indicated for patients with uncomplicated low back pain or a simple disk herniation.
- The best treatment for uncomplicated back pain and disk herniation is analgesia and resumption of normal activities—not bed rest.
- Age younger than 18 or older than 50 years, fever, injection drug use, immunocompromised status, symptoms lasting more than 4 to 6 weeks, night pain, and prior malignancy all are red flag warnings of potentially serious causes of back pain and should be heeded and evaluated accordingly.
- Bilateral leg pain or weakness, bowel or bladder sphincter problems (especially urinary retention), and saddle anesthesia are worrisome for a cauda equina syndrome—a neurosurgical emergency.

UPPER BACK PAIN

PERSPECTIVE

Background

Thoracic pain is far less common than low back pain. Thoracic pain usually has a musculoskeletal origin, but other more emergent causes must be considered first, including thoracic aortic dissection, pulmonary embolism, and esophageal disease. Compared with lumbar disk herniation, which is fairly common, thoracic disk disease is extremely rare, difficult to diagnose, and difficult to treat.

Epidemiology

The actual incidence of thoracic pain is unknown. The incidence of symptomatic thoracic disk disease is low, with estimates at 1 in 1 million.[73] The average age is in the 40s with equal gender distribution. Surgery for thoracic disks comprises less than 4% of all disk operations.[74] Metastases are more common in the thoracic spine than lumbar spine, with 60% to 70% of spinal metastases localizing there.[8,75]

PRINCIPLES OF DISEASE

Anatomy and Physiology

The thoracic vertebral column can be regarded as an extension of the cervical column with the addition of ribs. There are 12 thoracic vertebrae, connected by the anterior and posterior longitudinal ligaments and the ligamentum flavum, similar to the lumbar vertebrae. Also similarly, intervertebral disks provide elasticity and stability to the thoracic column. The spinal canal diameter remains unchanged through the thoracic and lumbar levels, but at the thoracic level, the space around the spinal cord is smaller compared with the lumbar level. Because lumbar nerve fibers have not yet branched off from the spinal cord, the thoracic cord is thicker than the lumbar cord. Significant neurologic findings may result from minimal spinal canal impingement at the thoracic level.

Pathophysiology

Common thoracic soft tissue pain is likely a combination of sprain and muscle inflammation. Similar to the lower back, innervation of the paravertebral area is provided by the sinuvertebral nerve, and any anatomic disruption of surrounding structures results in nonspecific pain. Thoracic disk herniations, which most commonly occur in the midthoracic to lower thoracic spine, cause pain and neurologic symptoms in much the same way as lumbar disks. It is not clear why their presentation is so varied, although a possible cause is a higher number of centrally herniated disks, resulting in much more frequent myelopathic symptoms.[74]

CLINICAL FEATURES

Symptoms and Signs

History

Nondiskogenic thoracic back pain usually presents with paraspinal discomfort. There may or may not be a history of trauma or recent unusual activity preceding the onset of pain. Complaints with thoracic disk herniations are variable at best, but usually are associated with long-standing pain, neurologic symptoms, or both. Pain may be localized to one part of the thoracic vertebrae, it may radiate down to the sacrum, or it may have a radicular component along the ribs. Central disk herniation can present as diffuse abdominal and back pain or burning sensation in the lower extremities. Associated findings may include mild weakness, spasticity, gait disturbance, bowel or bladder dysfunction, or paraplegia. These usually progress until the condition is diagnosed. The average patient with thoracic disk disease is not diagnosed until 20 months after first presentation. Pain from other causes should be sought in the initial assessment. A history of trauma, fever, previous malignancy, cardiovascular disease, or gastrointestinal problems may indicate problems originating outside the thoracic spine and may warrant further investigation.

Physical Examination

Patients with benign musculoskeletal pain have an unremarkable examination. They may exhibit mild to moderate paraspinal tenderness, pain with motion, and even discomfort from chest wall expansion with respirations, but objective findings are minimal.

The physical examination for patients with thoracic disk herniations varies with the location and degree of herniation. Objective findings may range from a normal examination to a loss of posterior column function (position, touch, vibration) or unilateral or bilateral weakness. Gait and sensory abnormalities are common. Hypotonic abdominal reflexes may be present with distal hyperreflexia. A Babinski response may be present. Myelopathy may result in urinary retention. Muscle wasting may be present with chronic symptoms. The possibility of other pathologic conditions should be kept in mind during the physical examination, with appropriate assessment tailored to the presentation and clinical suspicion.

DIAGNOSTIC STRATEGIES

Laboratory Evaluation

In the face of an unremarkable history and physical examination, the likelihood of useful laboratory results is extremely small. In appropriate clinical circumstances, assessment for malignancy, infection, and inflammation should be undertaken.

BOX 51-3. Differential Diagnosis for Thoracic Back Pain

- Uncomplicated musculoskeletal back pain
- Spinal cord and nerve root pathology (e.g., disk herniation, tumor, hematoma)
- Vertebral column disease (e.g., primary and metastatic malignancy and osteomyelitis)
- Disk infection
- Primary neurologic disease
- Degenerative and autoimmune arthropathies
- Herpes zoster
- Vascular disease (e.g., thoracic aortic dissection, acute coronary syndrome, pulmonary embolism)
- Thoracic cavity pathology (e.g., pleuritis, pericarditis, pneumonia, esophageal pathology)
- Intraperitoneal and retroperitoneal abdominal pathology (e.g., peptic ulcer disease, pancreatitis, hepatobiliary disease)

Radiology

The usefulness of a radiograph is dubious in a patient with atraumatic acute thoracic back pain who has no other preexisting illness or neurologic findings. As a general guide, however, suspicion of other conditions; unexplainable symptoms; extremes of age; concern for trauma, tumor, infection, gastrointestinal pathology, or vascular pathology; or prolonged symptoms should prompt basic radiologic studies and appropriate further investigations. Similar to patients with lower back pain, patients with a history of cancer and upper back pain should undergo plain radiography and possibly MRI to assess for vertebral metastatic disease, especially because metastases have a predilection for the thoracic spine.

MRI has become the modality of choice for evaluating a herniated thoracic disk. The incidence of asymptomatic disk herniations seen on MRI is 37%. Most herniated thoracic disks, whether symptomatic or not, have been seen to recede spontaneously.[73]

DIFFERENTIAL CONSIDERATIONS

Although muscular back pain is extremely common, Box 51-3 lists the expansive differential diagnosis for thoracic back pain.

MANAGEMENT

Commonly, thoracic musculoskeletal pain is managed with analgesia. No studies show that there should be any difference in management compared with musculoskeletal low back pain.

Thoracic disk disease is difficult to diagnose and manage. Symptomatic pain management and outpatient follow-up are recommended. Given the limited space in the spinal canal at the thoracic level compared with the lumbar level, spinal cord compression from a herniated disk is more likely at the thoracic level. Any herniated disk that precipitates an acute neurologic deficit warrants MRI and early neurosurgical evaluation.

DISPOSITION

Patients with benign back pain in any part of the thoracic vertebral column can be discharged with follow-up by the primary care physician. Patients with a suspected thoracic disk require close outpatient follow-up. Most cases of subjective discomfort resulting from thoracic disks without objective neurologic findings resolve on their own, with one study showing a 77% improvement rate.[73] Although there are no clear guidelines as to when emergent neurosurgical consultation is required for thoracic disk herniation, patients with significant pain or neurologic compromise should be assessed rapidly. Radicular symptoms seem to respond better to surgery than nonradicular findings.

KEY CONCEPTS

- Although thoracic disk herniation can result in significant upper back pain, other, more dangerous etiologies must be considered first, such as an aortic dissection, pulmonary embolism, and acute coronary syndrome.
- The associated neurologic examination with thoracic disk herniations can be extremely variable, ranging from non-specific paresthesias to significant upper motor neuron weakness.
- The incidence of vertebral metastatic malignancy is higher in the thoracic spine compared with the lumbar spine.

REFERENCES

1. Frymoyer J, Cats-Baril W: An overview of the incidence and costs of low back pain. *Orthop Clin North Am* 22:263, 1991.
2. Deyo RA, Cherkin D, Conrad D, Volinn E: Cost, controversy, crisis: Low back pain and the health of the public. *Annu Rev Public Health* 12:141, 1991.
3. Deyo RA, Weinstein JN: Low back pain. *N Engl J Med* 344:363, 2001.
4. Malmivaara A, et al: The treatment of acute low back pain: Bed rest, exercises, or ordinary activity? *N Engl J Med* 332:351, 1995.
5. Vroomen PC, et al: Lack of effectiveness of bed rest for sciatica. *N Engl J Med* 340:418, 1999.
6. Hart LG, Deyo RA, Cherkin DC: Physician office visits for low back pain: Frequency, clinical evaluation, and treatment patterns from a U.S. national survey. *Spine* 20:11, 1995.
7. Cunningham LS, Kelsey JL: Epidemiology of musculoskeletal impairments and associated disability. *Am J Public Health* 74:574, 1984.
8. Wipf JE, Deyo RA: Low back pain. *Med Clin North Am* 79:231, 1995.
9. Luo X, et al: Estimates and patterns of direct health care expenditures among individuals with back pain in the United States. *Spine* 29:79, 2004.
10. Nordin M, Campello M: Physical therapy: Exercises and the modalities: When, what and why? *Neurol Clin North Am* 17:759, 1999.
11. Pengel LH, Herbert RD, Maher CG, Refshauge KM: Acute low back pain: Systematic review of its prognosis. *BMJ* 327:323, 2003.

12. Adams MA, Mannion AF, Dolan D: Personal risk factors for first-time low back pain. *Spine* 24:2497, 1999.
13. Videman T, Battie MC: The influence of occupation on lumbar degeneration. *Spine* 24:1164, 1999.
14. Matsui H, et al: Familial predisposition for lumbar degenerative disk disease: A case control study. *Spine* 23:1029, 1998.
15. Feldman DE, Rossignol M, Shrier I, Abenhaim L: Smoking: A risk factor for development of low back pain in adolescents. *Spine* 24:2492, 1999.
16. Leboeuf-Yde C: Smoking and low back pain: A systematic literature review of 41 journal articles reporting 47 epidemiologic studies. *Spine* 24:1463, 1999.
17. Paassilta P, et al: Identification of a novel common genetic risk factor for lumbar disk disease. *JAMA* 285:1843, 2001.
18. Haldorsen EMH, Indahl A, Ursin H: Patients with low back pain not returning to work: A twelve month follow-up study. *Spine* 23:1202, 1998.
19. Croft PR, et al: Short-term physical risk factors for new episodes of low back pain: Prospective evidence from the South Manchester Back Pain Study. *Spine* 24:1556, 1999.
20. Deyo RA, Rainville J, Kent DL: What can the history and physical examination tell us about low back pain? *JAMA* 268:760, 1992.
21. Bogduk N: The lumbar disk and low back pain. *Neurosurg Clin N Am* 2:791, 1991.
22. Paajanen H, et al: Magnetic resonance study of disk degeneration in young low-back pain patients. *Spine* 14:982, 1989.
23. Jensen M, et al: Magnetic resonance imaging of the lumbar spine in people without back pain. *N Engl J Med* 331:69, 1994.
24. Olmarker K: Radicular pain—recent pathophysiologic concepts and therapeutic implications. *Schmerz* 15:425, 2001.
25. Thomas SA: Spinal stenosis: History and physical examination. *Phys Med Rehabil Clin N Am* 14:29, 2003.
26. Ramirez N, Johnston CE, Browne RH: The prevalence of back pain in children who have idiopathic scoliosis. *J Bone Joint Surg Am* 79:364, 1997.
27. Nachemson AL: Newest knowledge of low back pain: A critical look. *Clin Orthop* 279:8, 1992.
28. McGowin PR, Borenstein D, Wiesel SW: The current approach to the medical diagnosis of low back pain. *Orthop Clin North Am* 22:315, 1991.
29. Mayer TG: Rehabilitation: What do we do with the chronic patient? *Neurol Clin North Am* 17:131, 1999.
30. Andersson GB: Epidemiological features of chronic low-back pain. *Lancet* 354:581, 1999.
31. Gatchel RJ, Gardea MA: Psychosocial issues. *Neurol Clin North Am* 17:149, 1999.
32. King HA: Back pain in children. *Orthop Clin North Am* 30:467, 1999.
33. Mason DE: Back pain in children. *Pediatr Ann* 28:727, 1999.
34. Bigos S: Acute Low Back Problems in Adults. Clinical Practice Guideline No. 14 (AHCPR Publication No. 95-0642). Rockville, Md, Agency for Health Care Policy and Research, Public Health Service, U.S. Department of Health and Human Services, 1994.
35. Frymoyer JD: Back pain and sciatica. *N Engl J Med* 318:291, 1998.
36. Turner JA, Ersek M, Herron L, Deyo R: Surgery for lumbar spinal stenosis: Attempted meta-analysis of the literature. *Spine* 17:1, 1992.
37. Radu AS, Menkes CJ: Update on lumbar spinal stenosis: Retrospective study of 62 patients and review of the literature. *Rev Rhum Engl Educ* 65:337, 1998.
38. Hawkes CH, Roberts GM: Neurogenic and vascular claudication. *J Neurol Sci* 38:337, 1978.
39. Kauppila LI, et al: Degenerative displacement of lumbar vertebrae: A 25-year follow-up study in Framingham. *Spine* 23:1868, 1998.
40. Joshi SM, Hatfield RH, Martin J, Taylor W: Spinal epidural abscess: A diagnostic challenge. *Br J Neurosurg* 17:160, 2003.
41. Hlavin M, Kaminski HJ, Ross JS, Ganz E: Spinal epidural abscess: A ten-year perspective. *Neurosurgery* 27:177, 1990.
42. Darouiche R, et al: Bacterial spinal epidural abscess: Review of 43 cases and literature survey. *Medicine* 71:369, 1992.
43. Deyo RA, Diehl AK: Cancer as a cause of back pain: Frequency, clinical presentation, and diagnostic strategies. *J Gen Intern Med* 3:230, 1998.
44. Polatin PB, Cox B, Gatchel RJ, Mayer TG: A prospective study of Waddell signs in patients with chronic low back pain: When they may not be predictive. *Spine* 22:1618, 1997.
45. Main CJ, Waddell G: Behavioral responses to examination: A reappraisal of the interpretation of "nonorganic signs." *Spine* 23:2367, 1998.
46. Martin R, Yuan H: Neurosurgical care of spinal epidural, subdural, and intramedullary abscesses and arachnoiditis. *Orthop Clin North Am* 27:125, 1996.
47. Nussbaum ES, et al: Spinal epidural abscess: A report of 40 cases and review. *Surg Neurol* 38:225, 1992.
48. Jarvik JG, Deyo RA: Diagnostic evaluation of low back pain with emphasis on imaging. *Ann Intern Med* 137:586, 2002.
49. Boos N, Hodler J: What help and what confusion can imaging provide? *Baillieres Clin Rheumatol* 12:115, 1998.
50. Dixon AK: Imaging the bad back: Increasing reliance on MRI. *Hosp Med* 49:496, 1998.
51. Jarvik JG, et al: Rapid magnetic resonance imaging vs radiographs for patients with low back pain: A randomized controlled trial. *JAMA* 289:2810, 2003.
52. Burton AK, Waddell G: Clinical guidelines in the management of low back pain. *Clin Rheumatol* 12:17, 1998.
53. Van Tulder MW, Scholten RJ, Koes BW, Deyao RA: Nonsteroidal anti-inflammatory drugs for low back pain: A systematic review within the framework of the Cochrane Collaboration Back Review Group. *Spine* 25:2501, 2000.
54. Deyo R: Drug therapy for back pain: Which drugs help which patients. *Spine* 21:2840, 1996.
55. Frazier LM, et al: Selective criteria may increase lumbosacral spine roentgenogram use in acute low-back pain. *Arch Intern Med* 149:47, 1989.
56. Koes BW, et al: Physiotherapy exercises and back pain: A blinded review. *BMJ* 302:1572, 1991.
57. Cherkin DC, et al: A comparison of physical therapy, chiropractic manipulation, and provision of an educational booklet for the treatment of patients with low back pain. *N Engl J Med* 339:1021, 1998.
58. Bronfort G: Spinal manipulation: Current state of research and its indications. *Neurol Clin* 17:91, 1999.
59. Van Tulder MW, et al: The effectiveness of acupuncture in the management of acute and chronic low back pain: A systematic review within the framework of the Cochrane Collaboration Back Review Group. *Spine* 24:1113, 1999.
60. Vroomen PC, de Krom MC, Slofstra PD, Knottnerus JA: Conservative treatment of sciatica: A systematic review. *J Spinal Disord* 13:463, 2000.
61. Benoist M: The natural history of lumbar disc herniation and radiculopathy. *Joint Bone Spine* 69:155, 2002.
62. Carette S, et al: Epidural corticosteroid injections for sciatica due to herniated nucleus pulposus. *N Engl J Med* 336:1634, 1997.
63. Gibson JN, Grant IC, Waddell G: The Cochrane review of surgery for lumbar disc prolapse and degenerative lumbar spondylosis. *Spine* 24:1820, 1999.

64. Amundsen T, et al: Lumbar spinal stenosis: Conservative or surgical management? A prospective 10-year study. *Spine* 25:1425, 2000.
65. Shapiro S: Cauda equina syndrome secondary to lumbar disk herniation. *Neurosurgery* 32:743, 1993.
66. Gleave JR, Macfarlane R: Cauda equina syndrome: What is the relationship between timing of surgery and outcome? *Br J Neurosurg* 16:325, 2002.
67. Weigel B, et al: Surgical management of symptomatic spinal metastases. *Spine* 24:2240, 1999.
68. Antunes NL, De Angelis LM: Neurologic consultations in children with systemic cancer. *Pediatr Neurol* 20:121, 1999.
69. Schiff D: Spinal cord compression. *Neurol Clin* 21:67, 2003.
70. Laredo JD, el Quessar A, Bossard P, Vuillemin-Bodaghi V: Vertebral tumors and pseudotumors. *Radiol Clin North Am* 39:137, 2001.
71. Byrne T: Spinal cord compression from epidural metastases. *N Engl J Med* 327:614, 1992.
72. Lonstein JE: Spondylolisthesis in children: Cause, natural history and management. *Spine* 24:2640, 1999.
73. Wood KB, et al: The natural history of asymptomatic thoracic disk herniations. *Spine* 22:525, 1997.
74. Stillerman CB, et al: Experience in the surgical management of 82 symptomatic herniated thoracic disks and review of the literature. *J Neurosurg* 88:623, 1998.
75. Jennis LG, Dunn EJ, An HS: Metastatic disease of the cervical spine. *Clin Orthop* 359:89, 1999.

CHAPTER

52 Pelvis

A. Adam Cwinn

PERSPECTIVE

In evaluating a trauma patient, a pelvic fracture or dislocation indicates the profound magnitude of disruptive energy at the time of injury. Significant pelvic injury alerts the physician to the likelihood of major injury to other body systems, and the pelvic injury itself poses diagnostic and therapeutic challenges.

Epidemiology

Mechanisms of injury in pelvic fractures include motor vehicle crash in 57% to 71% of patients, collisions with pedestrians in 13% to 18%, motorcycle crashes in 5% to 9%, falls in 4% to 9%, and crushing forces in 4% to 5%.[1,2] Depending on the size of the study group, the types of pelvic fractures included in the study, and the associated trauma to other body systems, reported mortality figures for pelvic injuries range from 8% to 13% in studies totaling 4621 patients with heterogeneous mechanisms of injury.[2-4] The subsets of patients with high-energy pelvic injuries or open pelvic fracture from these studies have a much higher mortality rate. Pedestrians who are struck by motor vehicles and sustain pelvic trauma have a mortality rate of 23%.[5] Mortality in patients with blunt trauma who have the combination of pelvic ring fractures and hemorrhagic shock is approximately 50%.[6-8] This chapter reviews the pertinent anatomic and radiologic anatomy and discusses pelvic trauma in three broad categories: (1) injury to the pelvic viscera and soft tissues, (2) bony injury, and (3) related hemorrhage. The term *pelvic fracture* includes fractures and dislocations.

Anatomy

The bony pelvis is composed of the right and left innominate bones, the sacrum, and the coccyx (Figure 52-1). The innominate bone is formed by three bones that fuse at the acetabulum: the ilium, the ischium, and the pubis. The bony pelvis provides protection for its visceral contents, serves as attachment points for muscles, and transmits weight from the trunk to the lower limbs. Strong posterior ligaments—the sacrospinous, sacrotuberous, iliolumbar, and anterior and posterior sacroiliac (SI) ligaments—provide considerable mechanical support, and disruption of these ligaments is the major cause of pelvic instability after injury.

The main weight-bearing forces are transmitted through the posterior wall of the pelvis, called the *posterior arch,* which is composed of thick bone and ligaments. The rich network of major arteries, veins, and nerves that course adjacent to the anterior wall of the posterior arch may be injured concomitantly with forces causing bony injuries of this arch.

Vascular Anatomy and Pathophysiology

Most of the blood supply to the pelvis comes from the left and right internal iliac arteries. The internal iliac arteries course at the level of the SI joints. The various arteries that derive from the internal iliac arteries initially run in close proximity to the posterior pelvic arch and eventually anastomose extensively with each other, forming a rich collateral network. The superior gluteal artery is the largest branch. Because it originates at right angles from the internal iliac artery and has

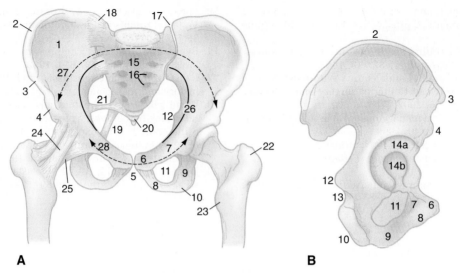

Figure 52-1. Pelvic anatomy. **A,** Anterior view of pelvis. **B,** Lateral view of right innominate bone. 1, Iliac fossa; 2, iliac crest; 3, anterior superior iliac spine; 4, anterior inferior iliac spine; 5, symphysis pubis; 6, body of pubis; 7, superior ramus of pubis; 8, inferior ramus of pubis; 9, ramus of ischium; 10, ischial tuberosity; 11, obturator foramen; 12, ischial spine; 13, lesser sciatic notch; 14, acetabulum (14a, articular surface; 14b, fossa); 15, sacrum; 16, anterior sacral foramina; 17, sacroiliac joint; 18, anterior sacroiliac ligament; 19, sacrotuberous ligament (sacrum to ischial tuberosity); 20, coccyx; 21, sacrospinous ligament; 22, greater trochanter of femur; 23, lesser trochanter of femur; 24, iliofemoral ligament; 25, pubofemoral ligament; 26, arcuate line; 27, posterior or femorosacral arch, through which main weight-bearing forces are transmitted; 28, anterior arch.

little muscular protection, the superior gluteal artery is commonly injured in fractures of the posterior pelvic arch. The obturator and internal pudendal branches are often injured in fractures involving the pubic rami.[9]

The venous system also has many collateral branches and is without valves, allowing bidirectional flow. The veins are arranged in a plexus that adheres closely to the pelvic walls. Because these veins are thin walled, they do not have the ability to constrict in response to damage.[9] This anatomic arrangement of the arteries and veins accounts for the hemorrhage seen with pelvic fractures. Without performing angiography, it is impossible to know clinically if a retroperitoneal hematoma is caused by disruption of major arteries or veins or smaller, unnamed blood vessels. Most pelvic hematomas are venous in origin, however, and are contained and tamponaded retroperitoneally by the intact peritoneum. Normal hemostatic mechanisms contain many hematomas, but some continue to enlarge, producing hemorrhagic shock. The hematoma also may dissect anteriorly to invade the anterior abdominal wall—to the chagrin of the unwary clinician who introduces a scalpel or peritoneal dialysis catheter. A retroperitoneal hematoma also may rupture through the peritoneum into the abdominal cavity, causing a loss of the tamponade effect.

Hemorrhage from pelvic fractures results from lacerations of the rich vascular network supplying the pelvis and collects in the retroperitoneal space, but considerable bleeding also may occur from the marrow at the fracture sites.[9] Coagulopathy is another cause of persistent retroperitoneal bleeding and should be considered when the patient does not respond to fluid and blood replacement.

Neurologic Anatomy and Pathophysiology

The cauda equina course through the sacral spinal canal and exit through the sacral neural foramina to form the lumbar and sacral plexus. Injury to the posterior bony pelvis and sacrum may result in neurologic deficits in the lower extremities and autonomic dysfunction involving the bowel, bladder, and genitalia.

CLINICAL FEATURES

Prehospital Care

Paramedics should recognize mechanisms of injury that may result in severe trauma to the pelvis, such as an automobile striking the pelvis of a pedestrian or heavy objects crushing the pelvis. On-scene times should be kept as short as possible in cases of severe pelvis injury. Paramedics should consider immobilizing the fractured pelvis using commercial pelvic binding devices or by wrapping the pelvis with a sheet and binding the legs together in cases of prolonged transit times of patients in shock with severe pelvis injury.[10]

History and Physical Examination

As priorities permit, the emergency physician should obtain the following history: the mechanism of injury, location and radiation of pain, whether gross hematuria was present if voiding occurred after the injury, last menstrual period, and possibility of pregnancy. On inspection, rotation of the iliac crests indicates a serious pelvic fracture. Leg-length discrepancy may suggest a hip injury or cephalad migration of an unstable hemipelvis.

The presence of tenderness on palpation of the sacrum and SI joints in patients with a Glasgow Coma Scale score of 12 or more is an important and reliable sign of injury to the posterior pelvis ring.[11] The integrity of the pelvic ring can be tested clinically by gentle lateral compression and distraction of the iliac crests and gentle inward compression of the symphysis pubis. Extensive movement of fracture fragments should be avoided when any instability is detected. Pain with axial percussion through the bottom of the foot may localize a hip injury or pelvic fracture site. Care must be exercised so that fractures are not displaced further by these maneuvers, which potentially could exacerbate pelvic fracture–related hemorrhage. Careful inspection of the skin and skin folds is necessary to identify open fractures. Perineal ecchymosis or hematoma may be observed, and in cases when many hours have elapsed since the injury, ecchymosis on the abdomen (Cullen's sign) or flanks (Grey Turner's sign) from retroperitoneal hemorrhage may be present.

The penis should be milked to examine for blood at the meatus. The digital rectal examination should evaluate sensation, sphincter tone, position and consistency of the prostate, presence of a presacral hematoma, bony contour of the sacrum and coccyx, mucosal penetration of bony spicules, and presence of frank or occult blood. In the setting of a pelvic fracture, female patients should undergo a vaginal examination to diagnose an open fracture. Digital rectal and vaginal examinations must be performed carefully, especially in an unconscious patient who cannot localize pain, because it is possible to create an open fracture iatrogenically through the vaginal or rectal wall. The examiner should be mindful when performing these examinations that bony spicules can cause injury to self. Extravasated urine may be detected in the scrotum or the subcutaneous tissues of the penis, vulva, or abdominal wall. The presence and quality of pulses in the lower limb should be assessed, as should sensation, strength, and deep tendon reflexes.

Visceral and Soft Tissue Injuries

Open Pelvic Fractures and Deep Perineal Laceration

An open pelvic fracture is present when there is direct communication between the fracture site and a skin, rectal, or vaginal wound.[12] These are potentially lethal injuries, especially if the open nature is not recognized, with early mortality resulting from hemorrhage in the acute phase and sepsis and multiorgan failure in the delayed phase.[13] Even after introduction of an aggressive patient treatment protocol, the overall mortality rate of open pelvic fractures is 30% in several series and 78% in the subgroup of patients older than age 40.[14,15]

The patient must be rolled on his or her side and the skin over the posterior pelvis and gluteal area inspected carefully for wounds. Some fractures are open only by virtue of a bone spicule penetrating the vagina or rectum, but these must be identified by careful digital rectal and vaginal examinations. Hemorrhage from a large open laceration may be treated by external packing and application of a pressure dressing or packing followed by application of the pneumatic anti-shock garment.[13,16] A perineal laceration should be inspected but not probed, for fear of disturbing hemostasis and introducing infection. The perineal wounds require aggressive operative debridement and irrigation, and in cases in which the rectum is violated, a diverting colostomy is required.[14,17]

Urologic Injury

The overall incidence of bladder or urethral disruption associated with pelvic fracture ranges from 7% to 25%. More than 80% of patients with lower urinary tract injury after blunt trauma have a pelvic fracture, however.[18] The length and tethered anatomy of the male urethra make it vulnerable to rupture in association with high-energy pelvic injuries. Urethral rupture in women with pelvic fractures is less common, but does occur.[19]

Although there does not seem to be a significant relationship between the type of pelvic fracture and the type of bladder injury, fractures adjacent to or involving the symphysis pubis are associated most often with urologic injuries.[20] In 103 patients with pelvic fractures in whom cystography was performed, all patients with bladder rupture had fractures of the anterior pelvic arch.[21]

It formerly was recommended that a pelvic fracture associated with gross or microscopic hematuria mandated cystourethrography; however, several studies show that microscopic hematuria is not associated with significant urologic injury in these patients.[21-23] Urethrography and cystography are unnecessary in the absence of gross hematuria or clinical suspicion of bladder or urethral rupture.[21-23] Blood at the urethral meatus necessitates a retrograde urethrogram followed by a cystogram. Gross hematuria is investigated by a combination of urethrography, intravenous pyelography, cystography, and computed tomography (CT). The sequence and types of examinations are individualized for each patient.

Male sexual dysfunction is a recognized complication of pelvic trauma. The incidence of impotence associated with urethral rupture is significant. In the absence of urethral injury, impotence still may occur secondary to neurovascular disruption associated with the pelvic fracture.[24]

Neurologic Injury

Neurologic injury occurs commonly in patients with pelvic ring fractures that have vertical sacral fractures as a component and with transverse fractures at or above the S3 level. Among patients with vertical fractures that involve the foramina, 28% have associated neurologic deficits. In patients with fractures medial to the foramina involving the spinal canal, 56% have neurologic deficits.[25] Autopsy and clinical studies performed on patients with pelvic fractures have documented disruptions by traction and compressive forces at many levels along the neural pathway: within the sacral spinal canal, within the neural foramina, distally in the roots and divisions that form the sacral and lumbar plexus, and to the various nerves derived from these plexus.[25]

Cauda equina syndrome and various plexopathies and radiculopathies may occur as follows. Injury to the L5 root may cause weakness of muscles in the anterior tibial compartment and sensory deficits in the dorsum of the foot and lateral calf. Injury to S1 and S2 roots may cause weakness of hip extension, knee flexion, and plantar flexion and sensory deficits on the posterior aspect of the leg, sole and lateral foot, and genitalia. Injury to S2-5 roots and distal afferent, efferent, and autonomic fibers causes sensory deficits in the perineum, sexual dysfunction, and bowel and bladder dysfunction. Cauda equina syndrome may be fully or partially present with sacral fractures: There is hyperesthesia and later anesthesia in a saddle-shaped distribution in the groin; weakness of ankle plantar flexion, hamstrings, and gluteus muscles; and decreased or absent ankle jerk. With involvement of the lower sacral roots, a neurogenic bladder with overflow incontinence, motor and sensory deficits in the lower extremities, anal sphincter dysfunction, and sexual dysfunction may occur. All patients with neurologic deficits from sacral fractures require orthopedic or neurosurgical consultation.

Gynecologic Injury

Vaginal bleeding may result from uterine or vaginal wall laceration secondary to deceleration forces or crush injury or, in a pregnant woman, secondary to abruptio placentae or uterine perforation. Most gynecologic injuries associated with pelvic fracture occur in pregnant patients; however, the nongravid uterus and the fallopian tube or ovary also may be injured.[26,27] Dyspareunia may occur as a late sequela of pelvic fracture.[28] Sexual dysfunction in women also is reported as a sequela of pelvic fracture.[29] Gynecologic consultation is indicated when there is injury to the female reproductive tract in association with a pelvic fracture.

Thoracic Aorta

There is a well-documented association between pelvic fracture and injury to the thoracic aorta.[30] This is presumably the result of the enormous forces required to produce either injury. In particular, anteroposterior compression fractures are associated with an eight times greater incidence of aortic rupture than is seen in the overall blunt trauma population.[30]

Penetrating Pelvic Trauma

Because of the complex anatomy of the viscera, blood vessels, and nerves within the pelvis, penetrating trauma to this area presents a major challenge to the physician. Overall mortality in this group of patients has been reported to be 6% to 12%, but the mortality of patients in shock is 50%.[31,32] At surgery, vascular injuries singly and in combination were found to involve the aorta; common iliac artery; and external, internal, and common iliac veins. Injuries to genitourinary structures and hollow viscera were common, and a particular concern was fecal contamination from colorectal injury. When present, the finding of blood on digital rectal examination is an important clue that rectal injury has occurred. Emergent surgical consultation is required in all cases of penetrating pelvic trauma.

DIAGNOSTIC STRATEGIES

Radiology

Routine radiographs of the pelvis are not necessary in asymptomatic, awake, alert blunt trauma patients who have a normal physical examination of the pelvis.[33-35] The physician should obtain an anteroposterior plain radiograph of the pelvis early in the resuscitation phase, however, on all victims of severe blunt trauma who are symptomatic or have a compromised ability to perceive pain. Some sacral fractures and SI joint disruptions may not be well visualized on the anteroposterior view. In hemodynamically stable patients, two additional views—the inlet and outlet (tangential) projections—are often necessary to show these injuries. The anteroposterior, inlet, and outlet views identify virtually all clinically important bony injuries.[36]

Anteroposterior View

The anteroposterior view of the pelvis identifies most pelvic fractures and dislocations but often does not show the degree of bony displacement. On the anteroposterior view, the symphysis pubis is normally no more than 5 mm wide, and a small (1 or 2 mm) vertical offset of the left and right pubic rami is normal.[37] Overlapping at the symphysis pubis is abnormal and is the result of a severe crushing injury. Normally the SI joint is approximately 2 to 4 mm wide.[37]

On the anteroposterior view, the physician may judge the degree of pelvic rotation caused by technique and positioning by the presence of asymmetry in the size and shape of the left and right obturator foramina and iliac wings. Diastasis of the SI joint also causes an asymmetric appearance of the obturator foramina and the iliac wings: If there is displacement into external rotation, the affected iliac wing appears broader, and the anterior iliac spine appears more prominent.[37] Avulsion fracture of the fifth lumbar transverse process by the iliolumbar ligament often accompanies an SI joint disruption or a vertical sacral fracture and is a valuable clue to posterior arch injuries.[37]

Inlet View

The inlet projection is obtained with the x-ray beam angled from the head toward the feet at 60 degrees to

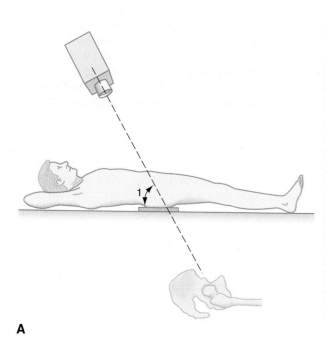

A

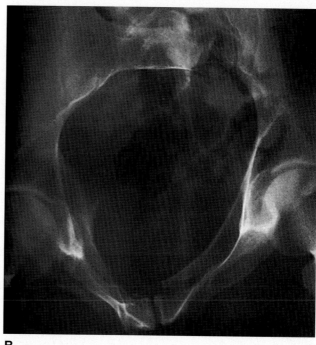

B

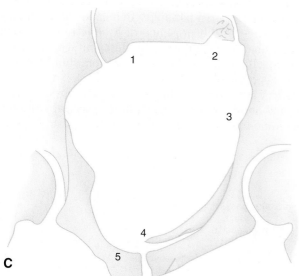

C

Figure 52-2. The inlet view. **A,** Inlet x-ray projection of pelvis. 1, Beam is angled 60 degrees to plate. This view is possible with a portable machine. **B** and **C,** Inlet of pelvis is well shown in this radiograph of a unilateral vertical shear fracture with cephalad and posterior displacement of the left hemipelvis (Tile type C1). 1, Normal sacral ala on the right side; 2, left sacral ala is indistinct because of a vertical fracture, and the cephalad and posterior displacement of this hemipelvis is shown by this inlet projection; 3, ischial spine on the left is partially obscured by bowel gas, but it is located more cephalad compared with the right spine because of cephalad displacement of the left hemipelvis; 4, fractured left superior pubic ramus with displacement cephalad; 5, on the inlet view, we are looking through the superior and inferior pubic rami, which are superimposed so that the obturator foramina are not seen.

the plate such that it is perpendicular to the pelvic inlet (Figure 52-2).[16] This view shows posterior and cephalic displacement of the fractures of the posterior arch, widening of the SI joint, and inward displacement of the anterior arch.

Outlet View

The opposite view is the outlet projection, in which the beam is at 30 degrees of cephalic angulation to the plate and is roughly perpendicular to the long axis of the sacrum. It is useful for showing sacral fractures and disruptions of the SI joints.[16] The inlet and outlet projections are performed by angling the beam, and they do not require the patient to be moved.

Computed Tomography

Although anteroposterior, inlet, and outlet series detect most pelvic fractures and provide the necessary details for accurate classification,[36] CT has an important role in the planning of orthopedic treatment and the diagnosis of associated visceral injuries and hemorrhage. CT shows whether injuries to the posterior arch are impacted or unstable, or whether there is rotational deformity. CT has the added advantage of rapidly acquiring detailed information on the pelvic fracture and can be reconstructed from other studies, such as abdominopelvic CT scan. Because CT provides detailed information on injury to abdominal and pelvic visceral structures as well as the pelvic fracture, in many centers it has largely replaced plain radiography for suspected pelvic fracture in a hemodynamically stable patient.

Evaluation of Hemorrhage

A high percentage of patients with retroperitoneal hemorrhage from pelvic fracture also have active intraperitoneal hemorrhage from coincident organ injury. In a hypovolemic patient with pelvic fracture, it is important to establish early on whether there is hemorrhage within the abdominal cavity necessitating laparotomy. Diagnostic strategies for evaluation of pelvic fracture–associated hemorrhage include diagnostic peritoneal lavage, ultrasound, and CT. Regardless of the modality of evaluation, it is crucial to avoid unnecessary laparotomy because of the higher mortality rate for hemodynamically unstable patients with pelvic fractures who undergo a negative abdominal exploration.

Diagnostic Peritoneal Lavage

Diagnostic peritoneal lavage (DPL) is a widely accepted, rapid, and accurate means of establishing the presence of intra-abdominal hemorrhage. It has been largely supplanted in many centers by ultrasound, which is less invasive, and with CT in stable patients. Nevertheless, DPL is an important and effective tool to assist with difficult triage decisions in the trauma patient.[38] A pelvic fracture presents a special situation for DPL and requires an alteration in the technique and an understanding of the variables that can confound the result. DPL is safe and accurate in the presence of a

pelvic fracture, provided that the fully open technique is employed (i.e., the peritoneum is entered under direct visual control).[39] If this requirement is met, the false-positive and false-negative rates are each 0.7%, which is comparable to the rates reported for DPL in patients without pelvic fractures.[39] Using the fully open technique prevents the operator from blindly entering a retroperitoneal hematoma that may have dissected into the anterior abdominal wall. The DPL may be performed in the infraumbilical location in most patients; however, the supraumbilical location should be employed if any of the following conditions are present: prior abdominal scars, time delay since the injury of more than 1 hour, or a hematoma encountered during the procedure.[39] DPL is useful in establishing the priorities for laparotomy, external fixation, and angiography in a hemodynamically unstable patient with major pelvic fractures, depending on whether the aspirate is negative or positive (Figure 52-3).

A negative peritoneal aspirate indicates that the peritoneal cavity is not a major source of bleeding or a significant contributor to hemorrhagic shock. Assuming that external and thoracic sources of blood loss have been eliminated as causes of hemodynamic instability, a negative DPL in a patient with a major pelvic fracture is evidence of the presence of a large retroperitoneal hematoma. Angiography with therapeutic embolization and mechanical fracture stabilization should be pursued aggressively.

Gross aspiration of blood indicates possible major intra-abdominal hemorrhage. Immediate laparotomy is recommended for hemodynamically unstable patients

Figure 52-3. Algorithm for initial management of hemodynamically unstable pelvic fractures.[10,45] *Note:* Ultrasound is in wide use in this setting, but its accuracy specifically in the presence of pelvic fracture–related hemorrhage has not been studied.

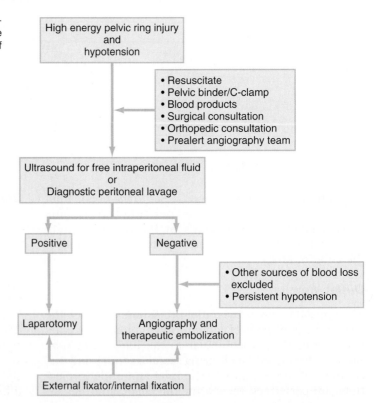

with pelvic fractures.[39,40] The lavage that is positive by cell count criteria alone is a special situation. If these patients are hemodynamically unstable, angiography with therapeutic embolization and external pelvis fixation should be performed before laparotomy.[39-41]

Ultrasound (FAST)

Focused assessment with sonography for trauma (FAST) is widely used to identify free intraperitoneal fluid rapidly in the trauma patient. The accuracy and safety of the FAST technique in evaluating patients with serious pelvic fractures who are hemodynamically unstable have not been published. Nevertheless, a positive FAST study that shows free fluid is widely used as a triage point to decide on laparotomy in a hemodynamically unstable patient with pelvic fracture. Important caveats relating to FAST in patients with pelvic fractures should be kept in mind. First, it is impossible to evaluate the retroperitoneum with diagnostic ultrasound. Second, there is a significant incidence of false-negative diagnostic ultrasound in patients with pelvic fractures.[42]

Computed Tomography

If the patient is hemodynamically stable, CT of the abdomen may be undertaken to evaluate intraperitoneal and retroperitoneal injury. Additional cuts through the pelvis show the degree of displacement and rotation at the sites of pelvic fracture. CT scan with intravenous contrast often can distinguish a stable hematoma from ongoing bleeding from pelvic arteries.[43] The presence or absence of extravasated intravenous contrast material on CT scan of the pelvis is useful in predicting which patients will require therapeutic angiography.[44,45] These comments on CT apply to a hemodynamically stable patient with pelvic injury; however, in a critically ill unstable patient, the value of FAST or DPL in quickly establishing treatment priorities should not be underestimated.

MANAGEMENT

General Management

Attempts should be made to stabilize the patient hemodynamically with crystalloid infusion. Transfusion of blood products should be initiated without delay in the presence of hypotension and a severe pelvic fracture.[10] Lower limb intravenous sites should be avoided in patients with severe pelvic fractures because the infused products may be delivered to the retroperitoneal space.[41] Wrapping the pelvis tightly with a sheet and securing this with towel clips or the use of a pelvic binder to splint the fracture temporarily and tamponade pelvic bleeding is recommended.[8,10,46] Because many patients with severe pelvic fractures have concomitant injuries to other body systems, the potential need for and timing of laparotomy, angiography, and skeletal fixation must be considered early in the course

BOX 52-1. Tile's Classification of Pelvic Fractures

Type A—Stable pelvic ring injury
  A1—Avulsion fractures of the innominate bone
  A2—Stable iliac wing fractures or stable minimally displaced ring fractures
  A3—Transverse fractures of the coccyx and sacrum
Type B—Partially stable pelvic ring injury (rotationally unstable, vertically stable)
  B1—Open book injury—unilateral
  B2—Lateral compression injury
  B3—Bilateral type B injuries
Type C—Unstable pelvic ring injury (vertical shear) (rotationally and vertically unstable)
  C1—Unilateral
  C2—Bilateral, one side type B, one side type C
  C3—Bilateral type C lesions

From Tile M: *Fractures of the Pelvis and Acetabulum*, 2nd ed., Baltimore, Williams & Wilkins, 1995.

of resuscitation. Figure 52-3 is an algorithmic representation of the investigation and resuscitation of a patient with pelvic injury.

Injury to Bone

Classification

Multiple classification schemes for pelvic fractures have been proposed. This chapter uses Tile's classification (Box 52-1).[16] Tile's classification is based on the concepts of high-energy and low-energy forces, the mechanism of injury, and the biomechanical factors that together determine the need for external and internal fixation and predict the likelihood of serious hemorrhage and associated injuries. The biomechanical factors include the direction of forces applied to the pelvis, the concepts of rotational instability and vertical instability, and the importance of injury to the strong posterior ligaments of the pelvis.[16,47] Fractures of the acetabulum are classified separately from other pelvic injuries. The terms *unstable fracture* (referring to mechanical stability) and *unstable patient* (referring to hemodynamic status) should not be confused, although a cause-and-effect relationship often exists.

Low-Energy Fractures (Tile Type A)

Stable Pelvic Ring Injury

Fractures of individual bones without involvement of the pelvic ring represent one third of all pelvic fractures. In general, these are stable injuries that heal well with rest and analgesic drugs for pain control (Figure 52-4).[16]

Avulsion Fractures—Tile Type A1. Avulsion fractures (see Figure 52-4) usually occur during athletic activities and are the result of a sudden, forceful muscular contraction or excessive muscle stretch. They are seen

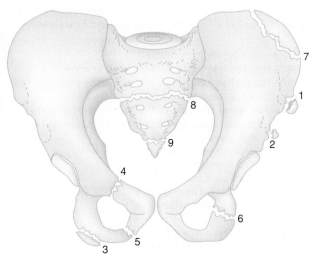

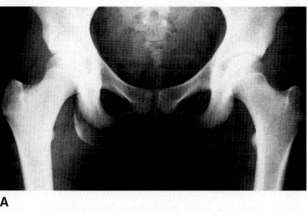

A

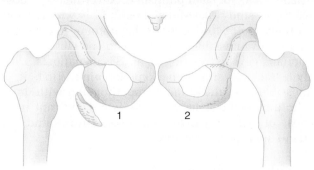

B

Figure 52-4. Fractures of individual pelvic bones. 1, Avulsion of anterosuperior iliac spine; 2, avulsion of anteroinferior iliac spine; 3, avulsion of ischial tuberosity; 4, fracture of superior pubic ramus; 5, fracture of inferior pubic ramus; 6, fracture of ischial ramus; 7, fracture of iliac wing; 8, transverse fracture of sacrum; 9, fracture of coccyx.

Figure 52-5. A and **B,** Radiograph and interpretive drawing. 1, Avulsion of ischial tuberosity through epiphysis; 2, normal ischial epiphysis.

more commonly in older children and teenagers before closure of the corresponding physis occurs; adults may have the same symptoms from ligamentous injury at these sites without radiographic abnormality.

The ischial tuberosity may be avulsed during strenuous contraction of the hamstrings (Figure 52-5). There is pain on palpation of the involved tuberosity, and this pain is increased by flexion of the hip with the knee in extension (hamstrings stretched), but not with the knee flexed (hamstrings relaxed). Ischial tuberosity avulsion also may cause chronic discomfort with no history of acute injury.

A portion of the iliac crest epiphysis may be avulsed by contraction of the abdominal muscles. Similarly, the anterior superior iliac spine may be avulsed by forcible contraction of the sartorius muscle. Forceful contraction of the rectus femoris (as in kicking a ball) can result in the less common injury of anterior inferior iliac spine avulsion; however, this radiographic finding must be distinguished from a normal variant, the os acetabuli, which is a secondary center of ossification at the superolateral margin of the acetabulum.[37] Clinical examination is similar in these injuries and reveals local pain, swelling, and limitation of motion.

The conservative treatment of all these avulsion injuries is analgesia and bed rest in a position that avoids tension on the affected muscles. Orthopedic consultation is advised for follow-up care. Surgical treatment rarely is required.[48]

Stable, Minimally Displaced Fractures of the Pelvic Ring—Tile Type A2

The normal pelvis is not totally rigid because of the slight mobility at the SI joints and symphysis pubis and the inherent elasticity of bone. A single break in the ring is possible. Nevertheless, the pelvis is not totally forgiving, and identification of a single break in the ring should prompt a search for a second disruption.

Iliac Wing Fracture—Tile Type A2-1. Isolated fracture of the iliac wing was described by Duverney in 1751 and now bears his name. It is caused by direct trauma to the iliac crest, usually by lateral compression forces. Although displacement is usually minimal because of the arrangement of the muscle attachments of the abdominal wall, orthopedic consultation is recommended. The fracture may extend into the acetabulum, altering the treatment and prognosis. Severely displaced fractures of the iliac wing require open reduction and internal fixation.[16]

Stable Undisplaced or Minimally Displaced Fractures of the Pelvic Ring—Tile Type A2-2. An isolated fracture of the superior or inferior pubic ramus is the most common pelvic fracture. These fractures are stable and do not displace. They are common fractures in elderly people after a fall and must be considered in the evaluation of an acutely painful hip. Fracture of the body of the ischium is a rare injury that may result from a fall in the sitting position. These fractures around the obturator foramen are treated conservatively with bed rest, analgesia, and early mobilization.

Fracture of the superior and inferior pubic rami on the same side is a commonly encountered injury after a fall or vehicular crash. These are generally stable fractures and are treated conservatively. The presence of significant displacement at the fracture site is an important finding and always indicates a second disruption elsewhere in the pelvic ring that must be diagnosed. Even in the absence of displacement, fractures of both rami on the same side may be associated with an unrecognized impaction fracture of the posterior pelvis. If the patient complains of pain in the posterior pelvis or if the radiograph is at all suspicious, further imaging is required.

After a ramus fracture, some patients may complain of hip or SI pain despite plain radiographs of these areas that appear normal; these patients subsequently may develop symptoms and request re-evaluation. A study of patients who sustained apparently isolated pubic ramus fractures from simple falls showed increased uptake of radionuclides on bone scans in the acetabulum and SI joint, suggesting that occult bony or ligamentous injury accounted for the complaints of pain.[49] When such patients are evaluated, repeat plain radiographs should be performed. If radiographs are normal, symptomatic treatment, rest, and close follow-up can be prescribed. Radionuclide bone scan can be considered if confirmation of occult posterior injury is required.

Stress fractures of the pelvis rarely have been reported with vigorous athletic or military training and in the last trimester of pregnancy.[48,50] Pathologic fracture related to neoplasm, Paget's disease, or dietary osteomalacia is included in the differential diagnosis. Diagnosis of stress fractures is based on the clinical evaluation and can be confirmed by radionuclide bone scan if necessary.

Four-Pillar Anterior Ring Injuries—Tile Type A2-3. Also termed a *straddle fracture,* four-pillar injuries refer to fractures of both pubic rami on both sides of the symphysis pubis, causing the so-called butterfly segment (Figure 52-6). The injury is produced by a direct blow with a straddle mechanism. Four-pillar injuries also commonly are associated with lateral compression or vertical shear forces, in which case there are concomitant injuries to the posterior pelvic arch, and the injury would be classified as a Tile type B or C. A CT scan of the pelvis is required in cases of four-pillar injuries to detect and classify precisely the posterior arch injury and plan orthopedic treatment.[16] The genitourinary tract frequently is injured concomitantly with this type of pelvic fracture and must be evaluated carefully (see Figure 52-6).

Transverse Fractures of the Coccyx and Sacrum—Tile Type A3
Coccygeal Fracture—Tile Type A3-1. Patients may present to the emergency department for evaluation of pain after direct trauma to the coccyx. The mechanism of injury is frequently a fall in the sitting position or a kick. Fracture and injury also may occur during parturition. Physical examination reveals local tenderness to palpation in the gluteal crease, with pain and, sometimes, abnormal motion of the coccyx during palpation on digital rectal examination. Normally the tip of the coccyx moves 30 degrees anteriorly and 1 cm laterally.[51] Displacement also is diagnosed on rectal examination, but attempts at reduction are not recommended.

Radiographic confirmation of a coccygeal fracture is not always necessary. Displaced fractures often are seen on the lateral view, but the diagnosis is evident on rectal examination. Undisplaced fractures may be difficult to show radiographically. The physician must decide whether the knowledge gleaned from x-ray studies would alter the therapy to a degree that warrants radiation exposure to the pelvis, especially considering that most of these fractures occur in women.

Treatment of coccygeal fracture consists of bed rest, stool softeners, analgesia, and sitz baths to relieve muscle spasm. As activity is increased, maneuvers that may minimize discomfort include using an inflatable rubber donut cushion, alternate sitting on the side of each buttock, slouching to displace body weight more proximally, and sitting on a hard chair rather than a soft one (sinking into a soft chair may distribute weight onto the coccyx).[51] Because of muscle action on the fragment, healing is slow and patients must be cautioned that discomfort may be prolonged. In the case of persistent severe disability, an orthopedic consultation is indicated for considerations of local steroid injection or possible coccygectomy.[52] Other causes of coccydynia (besides fracture) include trauma during parturition; faulty posture; midline disk herniations (caused by nonsegmental referral of pain from irritation of the dura); lumbar facet arthropathy; compression of the first, fourth, and fifth sacral roots; neuralgia from sacral plexopathy or sacrococcygeal neuropathy; infections; and local tumors.[51]

Sacral Fractures

Several classification systems have been proposed for fractures of the sacrum and share a distinction between transverse and vertical fractures: The transverse fractures do not involve the pelvic ring, but vertical fractures of the sacrum do.[25,53] The neurologic complication rate secondary to vertical sacral fractures and transverse fractures above the S4 level has been reported to be 21% to 34%[25,53,54]; however, transverse fractures at or below S4 are unlikely to be accompanied by neurologic injury.[53] Orthopedic or neurosurgical consultation is warranted in all cases of sacral fracture.

Transverse Sacral Fracture—Tile Type A3-2 (Undisplaced), A3-3 (Displaced). An upper sacral transverse fracture is the result of a flexion injury, such as being struck on the lower back by a heavy load while bending over, or by direct forces to the sacrum, as in a fall from a great height.[53] The patient complains of pain in the buttocks, perirectal area, and posterior thighs. There may be local pain, swelling, and bruising overlying the sacrum, and on gentle bimanual rectal examination, severe pain, abnormal motion, and palpable hematoma may be elicited. Radiographically the fracture may be difficult to visualize on anteroposterior and lateral projections, in which case an outlet view may be helpful. Neurologic injuries also are common, with upper transverse sacral fractures necessitating careful clinical evaluation of sacral nerve root function. A lower sacral transverse fracture results from direct trauma to the area. Nerve injury is uncommon with this type of fracture.[53] The comments on general physical findings for upper transverse fracture are applicable here.

Attempts at reduction of displaced sacral fractures bimanually through the rectum are discouraged because the injury may be converted to a contaminated open

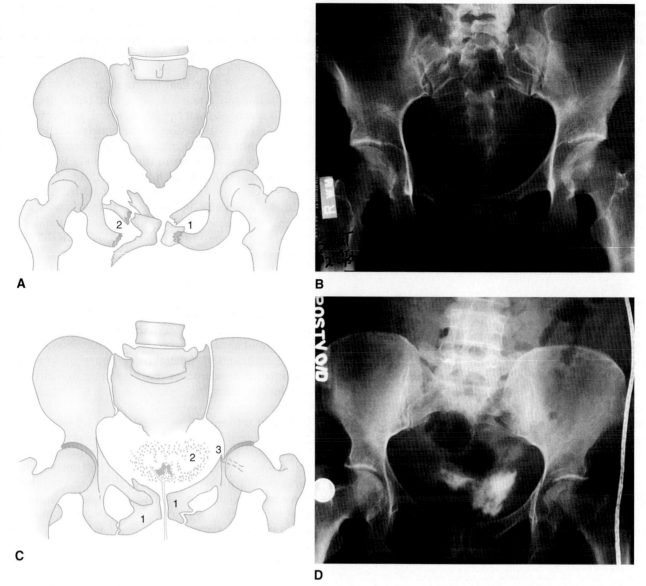

Figure 52-6. Four-pillar (straddle) fracture (Tile type A2-3). **A** and **B,** Partial inlet view of pelvis shows straddle fracture. 1 and 2, Marked comminution of left pubic bone and comminuted right superior and inferior rami. This partial inlet projection shows displacement of fragments into the pelvis, which is not evident on the anteroposterior view of the same patient in **C** and **D**. A true inlet projection and computed tomography scan (not available) would provide further information about the posterior arch, which is injured frequently in straddle fractures and always should be imaged (see text). **C** and **D,** Postvoid cystogram of the same patient with anteroposterior pelvis. 1, Fractures of pubic rami are seen again, but do not appear to be as displaced compared with **A** and **B** because this projection is an anteroposterior view: Even minor degrees of angulation of the x-ray beam can change the appearance of pelvic fracture displacement; 2, extravascular contrast indicates bladder rupture; 3, left acetabular fracture is seen in this projection but not in **B** because of the difference in projection. The acetabular fracture disrupts the ilioischial line (see also Figure 52-10) and is a posterior column fracture.

fracture, or an existing presacral hematoma may be enlarged. Surgery is commonly necessary for fractures associated with neurologic dysfunction.[25,53] Simple lower transverse fractures with no associated injury are managed with bed rest and analgesia.

Vertical Sacral Fracture—Tile Type C1-3. Vertical sacral fractures are seen only as a component of high-energy fractures. Vertical fractures are classified further into three groups according to whether the fracture line extends lateral to the sacral foramina, through the foramina, or medial to them, involving the central spinal canal.[25] The diagnosis of this fracture on radiographs hinges on careful examination of the symmetrical cortical lines that are normally present at the

superior margins of the sacral foramina on the anteroposterior view. Disruption, distortion, or asymmetry of these lines is an important marker of sacral fractures.[37]

High-Energy Fractures (Tile Types B and C)

Transmission of high-energy forces to the pelvis causes injury to the posterior, weight-bearing arch resulting in double breaks in the pelvic ring. These are mechanically unstable fractures by definition, although the degree of instability varies with the pattern of the fractures. Because of the large amount of force required to produce these injuries, they commonly are associated with intraperitoneal injuries, retroperitoneal hemorrhage, and injuries to other body systems. A patient with a double break in the pelvic ring must be considered to be critically injured.

Malgaigne first described these serious double-break fractures in 1859, defining the pattern of multiple fractures that included both pubic rami plus a constellation of posterior arch injuries on the same side. The term *Malgaigne fracture* is mentioned for its historical relevance; the newer classification allows for more precise descriptions of the injuries.

The following discussion of high-energy injuries uses the Tile classification, which is based on the biomechanical concept that stability of the pelvis depends on an intact posterior weight-bearing arch whose tensile strength derives from the thick SI, sacrotuberous, and sacrospinous ligaments.[16] Important radiographic clues to the presence of serious posterior arch fractures are listed in Box 52-2.

Tile Type B: Partially Stable Pelvic Ring Injury (Rotationally Unstable but Vertically Stable)

Open-Book—Tile Type B1 (Unilateral) and B3 (Bilateral). Severe anteroposterior compression forces result in disruption at or near the symphysis pubis. As the forces continue in the anteroposterior vector, external rotation of the hemipelvis occurs, and the anterior SI ligament and sacrospinous ligaments rupture. The SI joint rotates open as a hinge supported by the intact posterior SI ligament, and the resulting injury is aptly described as an open-book fracture.[16] The other ligaments also remain intact; the injury is rotationally unstable but vertically stable.[16] When diastasis of the pubic symphysis is greater than 2.5 cm on the anteroposterior radiograph, the posterior injury is usually evident (most often SI diastasis, but occasionally sacral or iliac fracture) (Figure 52-7).[16] CT of open-book fractures shows the anterior part of the SI joint to be widened, but the posterior portion to be normal; however, if the injurious forces continue, they may separate the hemipelvis, and the SI joint is seen as widely separated on the plain anteroposterior radiograph and the CT scan.[16] The anteroposterior radiograph may be misleading in suggesting a pure open-book fracture in cases with symphysis disruptions greater than 2.5 cm. These cases commonly are associated with severe type C vertical shear fractures, and careful clinical and CT assessment for vertical instability is essential to classify the fracture properly and plan treatment.[16]

These same forces also may injure the neurologic and vascular structures at the posterior arch; the overall volume of the pelvis is increased in the open-book injury, allowing the expansion of a retroperitoneal hematoma. In several studies of patients with major pelvic ring disruptions, patients with severe grades of anteroposterior compression injuries have the highest crystalloid and blood requirements.[1,55]

Lateral Compression Injury—Tile Type B2. Severe forces applied sideways through the pelvis cause inward rotation of the hemipelvis and reduce the pelvic volume by causing the following lesions. In the anterior arch, the possibilities are double rami fractures on the same side as the posterior injury (Tile type B2-1); double rami fractures on the opposite side of the posterior injury, the so-called bucket-handle fracture (Tile type B2-2); or an overriding symphysis pubis. In the posterior arch, the possibilities are impacted vertical fracture through the sacrum, anterior crush of the SI joint with intact posterior ligaments, or an impacted posterior complex with disrupted posterior ligaments and severe rotational instability (Figure 52-8).[16] Compared with anteroposterior compression and vertical shear fractures, lateral compression fractures are associated with the least requirement for fluid replacement in general.[55]

Tile Type C: Unstable Pelvic Ring Injury (Rotationally Unstable and Vertically Unstable)

Vertical Shear. The forces transmitted through the pelvis causing the injury in type C fractures have sheared through the posterior ligamentous complex, tearing them completely, and across the bony trabecular pattern, causing that hemipelvis to displace posteriorly and possibly cephalad.[47] This is a mechanically unstable pelvic injury and doubly so if vertical shear occurs on each side of the sacrum (Figure 52-9). Type C fractures may be unilateral (C1), bilateral (C3), or a combination of a type C on one side and a type B on the other (classified as C2). Anteriorly the symphysis pubis or two to four pubic rami may be disrupted. Posteriorly there is gross displacement and instability through the sacrum, the SI joint, or the ileum.[16,47]

Avulsion of the ischial spine, the lower lateral lip of the sacrum, or the transverse process of the fifth lumbar vertebra (sites of insertion of ligaments) (see Figure 52-9 and Box 52-2) are important clues to the presence of vertical shear fractures.[47] The vertical shearing forces that act on the bone also act on the rich vascular network and nerve plexus that are directly adjacent to the bone. This activity accounts for the major hemorrhage and neurologic injuries associated with vertical shear fractures.

Implications of High-Energy Pelvic Injuries

The implications of these injuries reach far beyond the issue of mechanical stability of the pelvis. The mortality rate for patients with vertical shear fractures was 25% and for anteroposterior compression fractures was 14% to 26% in a series totaling almost 2900 patients.[1,4]

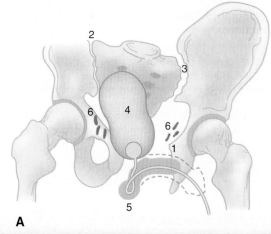

Figure 52-7. A and **B,** Interpretive drawing and radiograph. Severe unilateral open-book fracture (Tile type B1) from anteroposterior compression forces that is also open (compound). 1, Separated pubic symphysis with asymmetry of hemipelvis; 2, normal sacroiliac joint; 3, separated sacroiliac joint; 4, cystogram with displacement and abnormally elongated shape of bladder caused by retroperitoneal hematoma associated with separated left sacroiliac joint, which has pushed the bladder to the right; 5, extravasated contrast into perineum from urethral rupture; 6, soft tissue air indicating an open fracture.

A

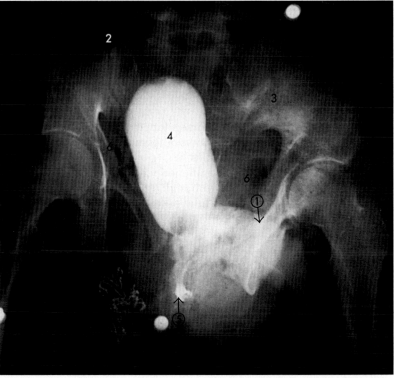

B

High-energy fractures also are associated with major blood transfusion requirements, with one series reporting an average of 14.8 U in the anteroposterior compression group, 9.2 U in the vertical shear group, and 3.6 U in the lateral compression group.[55] These serious fractures attest to the large magnitude of force at the time of injury. They mandate an aggressive search for associated trauma to other body regions and a timely use of blood products, especially in elderly patients. Orthopedic consultation should be obtained early in the care of these patients because surgical stabilization of the pelvis can reduce the amount of retroperitoneal bleeding and late sequelae.

Acetabular Fractures

Many pelvic fractures in adults involve the acetabulum. The force of injury can be transmitted to the

---

BOX 52-3. Acetabular Fractures

- Posterior lip fracture
- Central or transverse fracture
- Anterior column fracture
- Posterior column fracture

---

acetabulum through the femur (e.g., striking the dashboard in an automobile crash) or laterally through the side of the hip. On physical examination, hip pain with reproduction of these forces (percussing the sole of the foot and the greater trochanter) is a helpful finding.

Tile has a widely accepted separate classification for acetabular fractures (Box 52-3). These four types may occur in combination with each other or in association

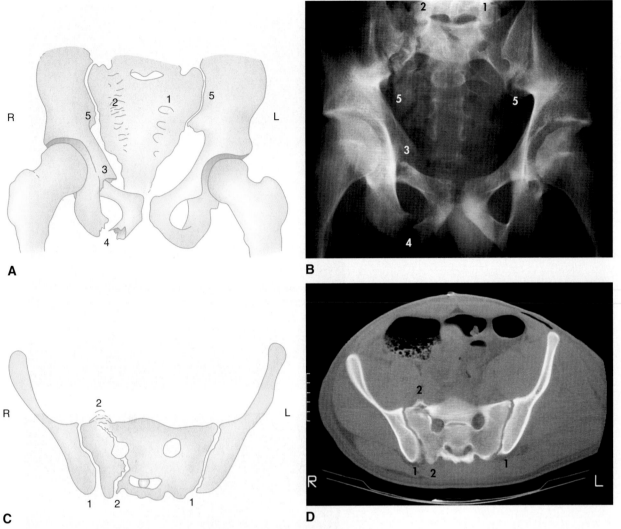

Figure 52-8. Lateral compression fracture (Tile type B2). **A** and **B,** Anteroposterior view of the pelvis. 1, Normal sacral foraminal lines on the left; 2, sacral foraminal lines on the right are indistinct and do not mirror the normal side, indicating the subtle second break in the pelvic ring; 3 and 4, fractures of the superior and inferior pubic rami are overriding and displaced, indicating the lateral compression forces (there must be a second break in the pelvic ring); 5, normal sacroiliac joints. **C** and **D,** Computed tomography scan of same pelvis. 1, Normal sacroiliac joints; 2, compression fracture of the sacrum through the foramen corresponding to the loss of definition of the foraminal lines in **A** and **B**.

with a femoral head dislocation or fractures of the pelvic ring. The radiographic anatomy of the acetabulum is explained in Figure 52-10.

The posterior lip fracture is the first and the most common form of acetabular fracture and usually is associated with posterior dislocation of the femoral head.[16] The second fracture is the central or transverse fracture. On the anteroposterior view of the pelvis, the fracture line crosses the acetabulum horizontally or obliquely and usually is seen clearly (see Figure 52-6D). Three separate centers of ossification join within the acetabulum to form the innominate bone. This junction, called the *triradiate cartilage,* is seen as a Y-shaped lucency in the acetabulum until solid bony union occurs around age 20. On radiographs, this normal anatomic feature may be mistaken for a central fracture, although true fractures also can occur through the triradiate cartilage. Comparison views with the uninjured side may be helpful in difficult cases.

The third fracture type involves the anterior, or iliopubic, column, which is formed by bone extending from the ilium to the pubis. The fracture disrupts the arcuate line, and the iliopubic column and radiographic U are usually displaced medially, but the ilioischial line remains intact (Figure 52-11; see Figure 52-10). In the case of central dislocation, the femoral head also is displaced medially.

The fourth fracture type involves the posterior or ilioischial column, which is the bone extending from the ilium to the ischium. The entire posterior column becomes separated from the pelvis: The fracture line begins at the sciatic notch, traverses the acetabulum, and ends near the ischiopubic junction. In cases in which the acetabular component is not displaced, it may be difficult to diagnose a posterior column fracture on the anteroposterior radiograph. Two helpful radiographic clues are discontinuity of the ilioischial line and separation of the ilioischial line from the radi-

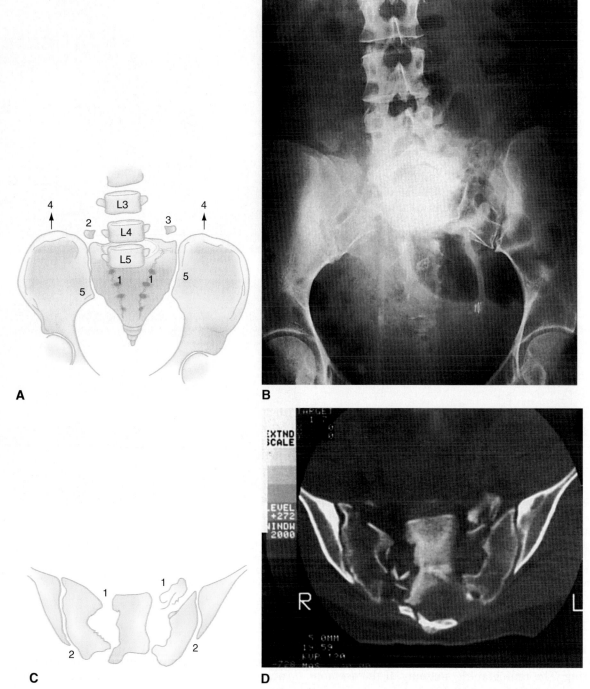

A

B

C

D

Figure 52-9. A and **B,** Vertical shear fractures bilaterally (Tile type C3). At first glance, the pelvis appears normal because of the smooth, uninterrupted arcuate line, but careful interpretation reveals the extremely critical nature of the injuries: 1, Fractures through the sacrum—note loss of definition and symmetry of sacral foramina indicating vertical fractures through both sides of the sacrum (see computed tomography scan in **D**). 2, Transverse process fragment from right L5 (iliolumbar ligament attachment) is pathognomonic for a vertical shear fracture through the right sacrum. 3, Transverse process fragment from left L5, pathognomonic for a vertical shear fracture through the left sacrum. 4, Both hemipelves are dislocated cephalad because of the double-ring fractures through each side of the sacrum. This dislocation explains why the L5 transverse processes appear so close to the iliac crests (the body of L5 is obscured because of rotational dislocation of the central free sacral fragment posteriorly and because of technique). 5, Normal sacroiliac joints. **C** and **D,** Computed tomography scan of same pelvis. 1, Bilateral comminuted fractures of sacrum with lateral displacement of both hemipelves; 2, normal sacroiliac joints.

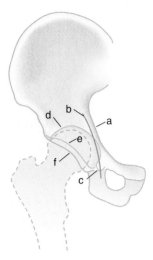

Figure 52-10. Schematic drawing of radiographic anatomy of acetabulum in anteroposterior pelvis projection. a, Arcuate (iliopubic) line. b, Ilioischial line. c, Radiographic U or teardrop caused by superimposition of parasagittal surface of ileum onto anteroinferior portion of acetabulum. d, Acetabular roof. e, Anterior lip of acetabulum. f, Posterior lip of acetabulum. (Redrawn from Rogers LF, Novy SB, Harris NF: Occult central fractures of the acetabulum. *AJR Am J Roentgenol* 124:98, 1975.)

ographic U. CT scan of the acetabulum is the most sensitive imaging modality for further delineation of an acetabular fracture. If CT is not readily available, the external and internal plain film oblique views, also called the *Judet views,* are useful for imaging the acetabulum and both columns.

After a fall, some patients may complain of extreme hip pain and inability to bear weight despite normal anteroposterior pelvis and lateral hip radiographs. An occult acetabular fracture should be considered in this situation, and further imaging should be pursued.

Hemorrhage

Mortality in patients with blunt trauma who have the combination of pelvic ring fractures and hemorrhagic shock is approximately 50%.[6-8] In the emergency department phase of the care of patients with pelvic fractures, the goals in terms of hemorrhage are as indicated in Box 52-4. Blood transfusion is essential treatment, particularly for a patient with anteroposterior compression or vertical shear fracture who is hypotensive and has not responded well to crystalloid infusion. Either of the following simple findings on the anteroposterior view of the pelvis is predictive of the need for major blood transfusions: (1) an open-book fracture or (2) displacement of 0.5 cm or more at any fracture site in the pelvic ring.[56]

In addition to blood transfusion, two important therapeutic modalities for control of hemorrhage are mechanical stabilization of the pelvis and angiographic embolization. There has been some debate as to which of these modalities should take precedence, and this has been predicated on institutional availability. As a general rule, angiography with therapeutic emboliza-tion of bleeding arteries is more effective than and takes precedence over external fixation.[10,45]

Mechanical Stabilization

External Fixation

Acute application of an external fixator has not been proved to decrease morbidity or mortality in a prospective study; however, there is evidence that this technique improves clinical outcome by limiting hemorrhage and restoring mechanical integrity.[57] Many experts believe that this is the preferred method of stabilizing the anterior arch of the pelvis to prevent movement at pelvic fracture sites and attendant bleeding.[16] Application of the fixator is time-consuming, however, and should not delay more definitive treatment of pelvic or other injuries. In many centers with a multispecialty trauma service, indications for and rapid access to external fixation are predetermined by protocol, which mandates orthopedic consultation as soon as a high-energy pelvic injury is identified. From a mechanical point of view, lower grades of anteroposterior and lateral compression fractures can be treated definitively by the external fixator.[16] In vertically unstable fractures and anteroposterior compression fractures with unstable posterior elements, the external fixator can assist in the correction of external or internal rotation, but does not provide definitive stabilization of the important vertical displacement. Its use in these injuries is as a temporizing measure initially or as an adjunct to traction or open reduction and internal fixation.[16,58] The external fixator must be constructed and applied with consideration of the biomechanical properties of the fracture. Most fixators can be constructed to allow convenient surgical access to the abdomen and groin. The antishock pelvic clamp is a device that can be applied rapidly by the orthopedic surgeon in the emergency department to externally stabilize the posterior pelvic arch on an emergency basis.[57-60] The mechanical design of this and similar devices and standards of practice in the use of these devices are evolving.

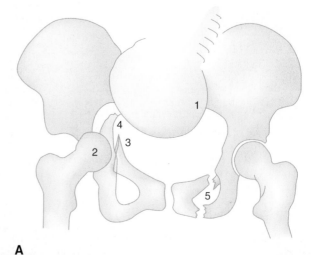

Figure 52-11. A and **B,** Interpretive drawing and radiograph. Acetabular fracture from lateral compression forces in the third trimester. 1, The fetus (cranium punctured by acetabular bone); 2, medial dislocation of femoral head with acetabular fracture; 3, arcuate line (see Figure 52-10) disrupted with medial displacement of anterior (iliopubic) column; 4, ilioischial column fragment; 5, left superior and inferior pubic rami fractures. *Note:* Fetal assessment and management would take precedence in this case over maternal mechanical skeletal dysfunction.

A

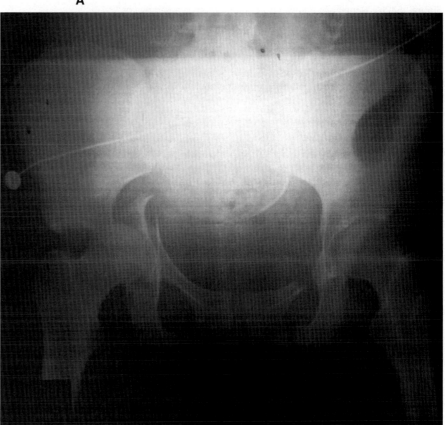

B

Open Reduction and Internal Fixation

Indications and modalities of open reduction and internal fixation, either acute or delayed, vary depending on the patient's other injuries, the timing of other surgeries, and the surgeon's preference.[16,61]

Angiography and Embolization

The techniques of arteriography and venography have been investigated for their usefulness in managing hemorrhage associated with pelvic fractures. Most commonly, the source of retroperitoneal hemorrhage

with pelvic fractures is the venous plexus or smaller veins; however, venography is not useful in managing these patients because even when venous bleeding points are localized, embolization is ineffective because of the extensive anastomoses and valveless collateral flow. In contrast, arteriography is a major diagnostic and therapeutic modality for a patient with severe pelvic hemorrhage from arterial sources.

The arteriogram is performed with the contrast material injected through the femoral artery on the least-injured side or via the upper extremity. The examination starts above the level of the aortic bifur-

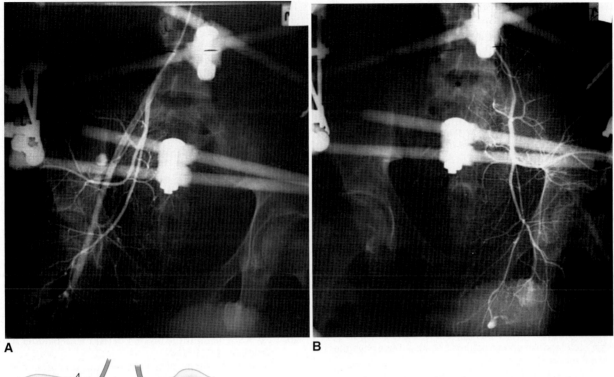

A   B

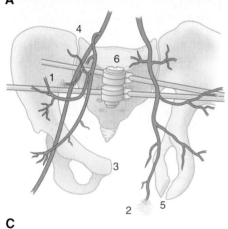

C

Figure 52-12. Unilateral open-book fracture (Tile type B1) from anteroposterior compression forces—pre-embolization angiograms. Despite external fixation and control of nonpelvic sources of bleeding, this patient required ongoing blood transfusion. **A** and **B,** Angiography showed bleeding from a branch of the right ili-olumbar artery (1). Extravasated dye reflects bleeding only at the instant of photograph; actual hematoma would be quite large. After embolizing this artery, the opposite side was examined (**B** and **C**). On this side, arterial hemorrhage from the left internal pudendal artery (2) was identified and embolized (postembolization films are not included because of space considerations). 3, Marked diastasis of symphysis pubis; 4, right sacroiliac joint diastasis; 5, fracture of inferior pubic ramus; 6, external fixator. (Angiograms courtesy of R.L. Desmarais, MD, and P. Rasuli, MD.)

cation and proceeds to selective branches of the internal iliac (hypogastric) artery.[7]

Transcatheter embolization using thrombogenic coils, foam, or spherules is employed to stop the hemorrhage from the branches of the internal iliac artery (Figure 52-12). In one study, the average blood requirement per patient in the 48 hours or less before embolization was 32 U, but it decreased to 5 U in the 48 hours after embolization.[62]

Angiography is indicated when hypovolemia persists in a patient with a major pelvic fracture, despite control of hemorrhage from other sources. Recommended criteria for angiography are (1) more than 4 U of blood transfused for pelvic bleeding in less than 24 hours, (2) more than 6 U of blood transfused for pelvic bleeding in less than 48 hours, (3) large pelvic hematoma seen on CT scan, (4) hemodynamic instability and negative

DPL or negative FAST, and (5) large and expanding retroperitoneal hematoma seen at the time of laparotomy.[63] Additionally, extravasated contrast blush at the time of contrast-enhanced CT is a marker of the need for angiography.[44,45]

The timing of angiography is individualized for each patient depending on priorities for treatment of concomitant injuries. While setting these priorities, physicians should remember that posterior arch disruptions are associated with the most severe hemorrhage; angiography should be considered at an early stage for these patients. Some patients require surgery for treatment of other injuries before undergoing angiography; others proceed directly to the angiography suite from the emergency department. A logistical delay often occurs in mobilizing the angiography team, so this intervention must be anticipated as early as possible.

The transfer of the patient to the angiography suite also requires orchestrating the necessary personnel and equipment to care for the critically injured patient there.

KEY CONCEPTS

- The most serious high-energy pelvic injuries are antero-posterior compression fractures (open book) and vertical shear fractures.
- High-energy pelvic injuries can be diagnosed using antero-posterior, inlet, and outlet views.
- When the patient is hemodynamically stable, a CT scan should be obtained to identify associated injuries to viscera, to identify a retroperitoneal hematoma, and to plan definitive orthopedic care.
- The emergency physician should anticipate the need for large amounts of blood products.
- Concomitant injuries to the aortic arch, diaphragm, solid viscera, and genitourinary tract are common.
- Careful examination of the skin in the perineum and buttocks and digital rectal and vaginal examinations are necessary to diagnose open fractures because these have the highest mortality rates.
- Trauma hospitals should have institutional guidelines and mechanisms to access angiography and external fixation.
- The combination of posterior arch fracture plus a hypotensive patient is potentially lethal, with a mortality rate of approximately 50%. Aggressive resuscitation with blood products is recommended. Decisions regarding the need for angiographic transcatheter embolization and external pelvic fixation must be made early in the course of care.
- Open-book fractures and displacement at any fracture site of more than 0.5 cm are predictors for major blood transfusion requirements.

REFERENCES

1. Dalal SA, et al: Pelvic fracture in multiple trauma: Classification by mechanism is key to pattern of organ injury, resuscitative requirements and outcome. *J Trauma* 29:981, 1989.
2. Poole GV, Ward EF: Causes of mortality in patients with pelvic fractures. *Orthopedics* 17:691, 1994.
3. Pohlemann T, et al: Pelvic fractures: Epidemiology, therapy and long term outcome: Overview of the multicenter study of the pelvis study group. *Unfallchirurg* 99:160, 1996.
4. Gansslen A, et al: Epidemiology of pelvic ring injuries. *Injury* 27(Suppl 1):S-A13, 1996.
5. Eastridge BJ, Burgess AR: Pedestrian pelvic fractures: 5 year experience of a major urban trauma center. *J Trauma* 42:695, 1997.
6. Eastridge BJ, et al: The importance of fracture pattern in guiding therapeutic decision making in patients with hemorrhagic shock and pelvic ring disruptions. *J Trauma* 53:446, 2002.
7. O'Neill PA, et al: Angiographic findings in pelvic fractures. *Clin Orthop* 329:60, 1996.
8. Starr AJ, et al: Pelvic ring disruptions: Prediction of associated injuries, transfusion requirement, pelvic arteriography, complications and mortality. *J Orthop Trauma* 16:553, 2002.
9. Maull KL, Sachatello CR: Current management of pelvic fractures: A combined surgical-angiographic approach to hemorrhage. *South Med J* 69:1285, 1976.
10. Biffl WL, et al: Evolution of a multidisciplinary clinical pathway for the management of unstable patients with pelvic fractures. *Ann Surg* 233:843, 2001.
11. McCormick JP, Morgan SJ, Smith WD: Clinical effectiveness of the physical examination in diagnosis of posterior pelvic ring injuries. *J Orthop Trauma* 17:257, 2003.
12. Brenneman FD, et al: Long-term outcomes in open pelvic fractures. *J Trauma* 42:773, 1997.
13. Jones AL, et al: Open pelvic fractures: A multicenter retrospective analysis. *Orthop Clin North Am* 28:345, 1997.
14. Birolini D, et al: Open pelviperineal trauma. *J Trauma* 30:492, 1990.
15. Hanson P, Milne J, Chapman M: Open fractures of the pelvis. *J Bone Joint Surg* 73B:325, 1991.
16. Tile M: *Fractures of the Pelvis and Acetabulum,* 2nd ed. Baltimore, Williams & Wilkins, 1995.
17. Davidson BS, et al: Pelvic fractures associated with open perineal wounds: A survivable injury. *J Trauma* 35:36, 1993.
18. Watnik NF, Coburn M, Goldberger M: Urologic injuries in pelvic ring disruptions. *Clin Orthop* 329:37, 1996.
19. Diekmann-Guiroy B, Young D: Female urethral injury secondary to blunt pelvic trauma. *Ann Emerg Med* 20:1376, 1991.
20. Cass AS: The multiple injured patient with bladder trauma. *J Trauma* 24:731, 1984.
21. Hochberg E, Stone NN: Bladder rupture associated with pelvic fracture due to blunt trauma. *Urology* 41:531, 1993.
22. Fallon B, Wendt JC, Hawtrey CE: Urological injury and assessment in patients with fractured pelvis. *J Urol* 131:712, 1984.
23. Antoci JP: Bladder and urethral injuries in patients with pelvic fractures. *J Urol* 128:25, 1982.
24. Ellison M, Timberlake GA, Kerstein MD: Impotence following pelvic fracture. *J Trauma* 28:695, 1988.
25. Denis F, Davis S, Comfort T: Sacral fractures: An important problem. *Clin Orthop* 227:67, 1988.
26. Smith J: Avulsion of the nongravid uterus due to pelvic fracture. *South Med J* 82:70, 1989.
27. Doman AN, Hoekstra DV: Pelvic fracture associated with severe intra-abdominal gynecologic injury. *J Trauma* 28:118, 1988.
28. Wilkes RA, Seymour N: Dyspareunia due to exostosis formation after pelvic fracture. *Br J Obstet Gynaecol* 100:1050, 1993.
29. Kiely N, Williams N: Sexual dysfunction in women following pelvic fractures with sacro-iliac disruption. *Injury* 27:45, 1996.
30. Ochsner MG, et al: Associated aortic rupture-pelvic fracture: An alert for orthopedic and general surgeons. *J Trauma* 33:429, 1992.
31. Duncan AO, et al: Management of transpelvic gunshot wounds. *J Trauma* 29:1335, 1989.
32. Malangoni MA, et al: The management of penetrating pelvic trauma. *Am Surg* 56:61, 1990.
33. Civil ID, et al: Routine pelvic radiography in severe blunt trauma: Is it necessary? *Ann Emerg Med* 17:488, 1988.
34. Salvino SK, et al: Routine pelvic x-ray studies in awake blunt trauma patients: A sensible policy? *J Trauma* 33:413, 1992.
35. Koury HI, Peschiera JL, Welling RE: Selective use of pelvic roentgenograms in blunt trauma patients. *J Trauma* 34:236, 1993.
36. Resnick CS, et al: Diagnosis of pelvic fractures in patients with acute pelvic trauma: Efficacy of plain radiographs. *AJR Am J Roentgenol* 158:109, 1992.
37. Rogers LF, Bradd FJ, Kennedy W: *Radiology of Skeletal Trauma.* New York, Churchill Livingstone, 1992.
38. Nagy KK, et al: Experience with over 2500 diagnostic peritoneal lavages. *Injury* 31:479, 2000.

39. Mendez C, Gubler KD, Maier RV: Diagnostic accuracy of peritoneal lavage in patients with pelvic fractures. *Arch Surg* 129:477, 1994.
40. Moreno C, et al: Hemorrhage associated with major pelvic fracture: A multispecialty challenge. *J Trauma* 26:987, 1986.
41. Mucha P, Welch TJ: Hemorrhage in major pelvic fractures. *Surg Clin North Am* 68:757, 1988.
42. Ballard RB, et al: An algorithm to reduce the incidence of false-negative FAST examinations in patients at high risk for occult injury. *J Am Coll Surg* 189:145, 1999.
43. Cerva DS, et al: Detection of bleeding in patients with major pelvic fractures: Value of contrast enhanced CT. *AJR Am J Roentgenol* 166:131, 1996.
44. Stephen DJ, et al: Early detection of arterial bleeding in acute pelvic trauma. *J Trauma* 47:638, 1999.
45. Miller PR, et al: External fixation or arteriogram in bleeding pelvic fracture. *J Trauma* 54:437, 2003.
46. Routt MLC, et al: Circumferential pelvic antishock sheeting: A temporary resuscitation aid. *J Orthop Trauma* 16:45, 2002.
47. Tile M: Pelvic ring fractures: Should they be fixed? *J Bone Joint Surg* 70B:1, 1988.
48. Lynch SA, Renstrom AFH: Groin injuries in sport: Treatment strategies. *Sports Med* 28:137, 1999.
49. Gertzbein SD, Chenoweth DR: Occult injuries of the pelvic ring. *Clin Orthop* 128:202, 1977.
50. Pavlov H: Roentgen examination of groin and hip pain in the athlete. *Clin Sports Med* 6:829, 1987.
51. Traycoff RB, Crayton H, Dodson R: Sacrococcygeal pain syndromes: Diagnosis and treatment. *Orthopedics* 12:1373, 1989.
52. Wray CC, Easom S, Hoskinson J: Coccydynia: Aetiology and treatment. *J Bone Joint Surg* 73B:335, 1991.
53. Gibbons KJ, Soloniuk DS, Razazk N: Neurologic injury and patterns of sacral fractures. *J Neurosurg* 72:889, 1990.
54. Schied DK, Tile M, Kellam JF: Open reduction internal fixation of pelvic ring fractures. *J Orthop Trauma* 5:226, 1991.
55. Burgess AR, et al: Pelvic ring disruptions: Effective classification system and treatment protocols. *J Trauma* 30:848, 1990.
56. Cryer HM, et al: Pelvic fracture classification: Correlation with hemorrhage. *J Trauma* 28:973, 1988.
57. Wolinsky PR: Assessment and management of pelvic fracture in the hemodynamically unstable patient. *Orthop Clin North Am* 28:321, 1997.
58. Kellam JF: The role of external fixation in pelvic disruptions. *Clin Orthop* 241:66, 1989.
59. Ganz R, Krushell RJ, Jakob RP: The antishock pelvic clamp. *Clin Orthop* 267:71, 1991.
60. Heini PF, Witt J, Ganz R: The pelvic C-clamp for the emergency treatment of unstable pelvic ring injuries: A report on clinical experience of 30 cases. *Injury* 27(Suppl 1):S-A38, 1996.
61. Gruen GS, et al: The acute management of hemodynamically unstable multiple trauma patients with pelvic ring fractures. *J Trauma* 36:706, 1994.
62. Matalon TSA, et al: Hemorrhage with pelvic fractures: Efficacy of transcatheter embolization. *AJR Am J Roentgenol* 133:859, 1979.
63. Henry SM, Tornetta P, Scalea TM: Damage control for devastating pelvic and extremity injuries. *Surg Clin North Am* 77:879, 1997.

CHAPTER 53 Femur and Hip

Michael A. Gibbs, Edward J. Newton, and James F. Fiechtl

PERSPECTIVE

Background

Ancient Egyptian and Greek drawings depict a lame person afflicted with hip deformities ambulating with a cane. The first available written description of a hip fracture was by the 16th century French surgeon Ambroise Paré.[1] In 1850, Von Langenbeck was the first to attempt repair of a hip fracture with a nail for internal fixation. Later, Davis used ordinary wood screws in an attempt to aid the healing of femoral neck fractures.[2] With the advent of radiography in the 19th century, the types of fractures and dislocations became easily identifiable, thus allowing discussion and investigation of management strategies, classification systems, and prognosis.

Epidemiology

Both age and gender are important predisposing factors for specific injury patterns and pathologic conditions occurring in the hip, femur, and thigh.

As a whole, the elderly segment of society almost universally suffers from some type of hip pathology. Osteoarthritis of the hip may severely limit one's ability to perform activities of daily living. Approximately 6 million women in the United States suffer from osteoporosis, and an additional 17 million have osteopenia, both of which predispose to hip fracture.[3] During the late 1990s, approximately 250,000 patients a year sought treatment in emergency departments after sustaining a hip fracture.[4] As baby boomers mature, the number of hip fractures is expected to reach half a million a year by 2050.[5] Eighty percent of femoral neck fractures occur in men. The average age of patients with

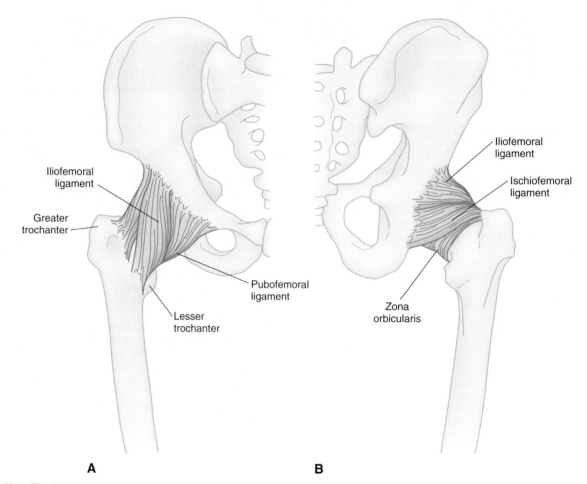

A   B

Figure 53-1. The ligaments of the hip combine to form a tough joint capsule as seen in both anterior (**A**) and posterior (**B**) views.

femoral neck fractures is 72 years for men and 77 years for women.[6] On average, intertrochanteric fractures occur 10 to 12 years later than those of the femoral neck, and women are afflicted eight times more often than men.[7] Overall, three quarters of all hip fractures occur in postmenopausal women older than 50 years.[3]

Perthes' disease (avascular necrosis [AVN] of the femoral head) is four times more common in boys than girls and occurs between 3 and 12 years of age. Slipped capital femoral epiphysis (SCFE) is twice as common in boys and peaks at 13 years of age for boys and 11 years for girls in association with the onset of puberty.

PRINCIPLES OF DISEASE

Anatomy of the Hip and Femur

Skeletal Anatomy

The femoral head is firmly seated in the acetabulum, which is reinforced by labral cartilage. The well-developed capsule, overlying ligaments, and proximal musculature of the lower extremity add strength to the joint (Figure 53-1). The nearly spherical femoral head articulates with the acetabular cup in a variation of the "ball-and-socket" joint.

The femur is the longest and strongest bone in the human body and is routinely subjected to substantial

forces produced during powerful muscle contraction and weight transmission. In an anatomic position, the two femurs extend obliquely from the pelvis medially to the knee and bring the legs closer to the midline, where they can best support the body. Structurally, the femoral neck serves as an oblique strut between the pelvis (the horizontal beam) and the shaft of the femur (the vertical beam) (Figure 53-2). The length, angle, and narrow circumference of the femoral neck permit substantial range of motion at the hip, but these same characteristics subject the neck to incredible shearing forces. A fracture results when these forces exceed the strength of the bone. The intertrochanteric line, an oblique line connecting the greater and lesser trochanter, marks the junction of the femoral neck and its shaft.

The bone in the femoral head, neck, and intertrochanteric region is predominantly cancellous. This type of structural bone is less resistant to forces produced by torsion than is solid bone. Distal to the intertrochanteric region, the femur is composed predominantly of cortical bone. The subtrochanteric region extends from the superior aspect of the lesser trochanter distally to the center of the isthmus of the femoral shaft. The shaft is a nearly cylindrical tubular structure that flares posteriorly along the *linea aspera* (rough line) where the fascia inserts. The shaft becomes predominantly cortical and requires greater force to cause failure. The distal metaphysis widens into the condyles at the knee. As the cortex widens and thins, the stress forces increase at the supracondylar region.

Musculature

The musculature of the hip and thigh is the largest and most powerful in the human body. The muscles in this region of the body are located within three different compartments, each containing associated nerves and vessels (Table 53-1). The muscles are also grouped according to their primary action at the hip. Knowledge of the major muscle actions offers insight into the injury patterns and deformities commonly seen (Figure 53-3).

Vascular Anatomy

Arterial Supply

The arterial supply to the femoral head arises from three sources (Figure 53-4). The major source is the ascending cervical arteries as they branch off the extracapsular ring and run along the femoral neck beneath the synovium. Some blood is supplied to the femoral head from the second source, which is within the marrow spaces as intraosseous cervical vessels. A third and dubious source is from the foveal artery as it lies within the ligamentum teres.

As the external iliac artery passes beneath the inguinal ligament, it forms the common femoral artery.[8] At this point the artery is located midway between the anterior superior spine of the ilium and the symphysis pubis. Approximately 3 to 4 cm distal to the inguinal

ligament, the common femoral artery branches to form the superficial and deep femoral arteries. The larger superficial femoral artery passes along the anteromedial aspect of the thigh and terminates at the junction of the middle and lower thirds of the thigh. Here, the superficial femoral artery passes through the adductor hiatus and forms the popliteal artery. The deep femoral artery runs posterolateral to the superficial femoral artery, supplies the hamstrings, and terminates in the distal third of the thigh as small branches piercing the belly of the adductor magnus. These perforating branches are an additional site of potential injury. The abundant blood supply of the thigh aids in healing fractures of the femoral shaft.

Venous System

In the proximal two thirds of the thigh, the common and superficial femoral veins lie adjacent to the common and superficial femoral arteries. At the inguinal ligament, the common femoral vein is posterior and medial to the common femoral artery and moves to the lateral position as it passes distally. The deep femoral vein and the greater saphenous vein are the two main tributaries to the common and superficial femoral veins. The deep femoral vein and artery run parallel as the vein joins the superficial femoral vein just distal to the inguinal ligament. The greater saphenous vein arises in the dorsum of the foot and ascends anterior to the medial malleolus. This vein is relatively superficial as it passes up the medial aspect of the leg to join the common femoral vein distal to the inguinal ligament.[8]

Nerves

The femoral and sciatic nerves are the major nerves within the thigh. The femoral nerve is the largest branch of the lumbar plexus; it passes under the inguinal ligament lateral to the femoral artery and divides into anterior and posterior branches soon after entering the thigh. The sensory divisions of the anterior branch, the intermediate and medial cutaneous nerves, supply sensation to the anteromedial aspect of the thigh. The motor division of the anterior branch innervates the pectineus and sartorius muscles. The posterior femoral branch forms the saphenous nerve, which supplies sensation to the skin along the medial aspect of the lower part of the leg. The posterior branch also supplies motor function to the muscles of the quadriceps femoris group.[8]

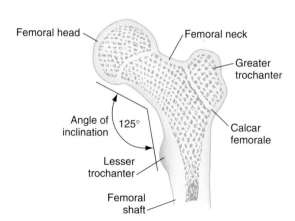

Figure 53-2. Bony architecture of proximal end of the femur.

Table 53-1. Contents Found within the Compartments of the Thigh

Compartment	Muscles	Nerves	Vessels
Anterior	Quadriceps femoris, sartorius, iliacus, psoas, pectineus	Lateral femoral cutaneous	Femoral artery and vein
Medial	Gracilis, adductor longus and magnus, obturator externus	Obturator	Profundus femoris artery, obturator artery and vein
Posterior	Biceps femoris, semitendinosus, semimembranosus, adductor magnus	Sciatic, posterior femoral cutaneous	Profundus femoris branches

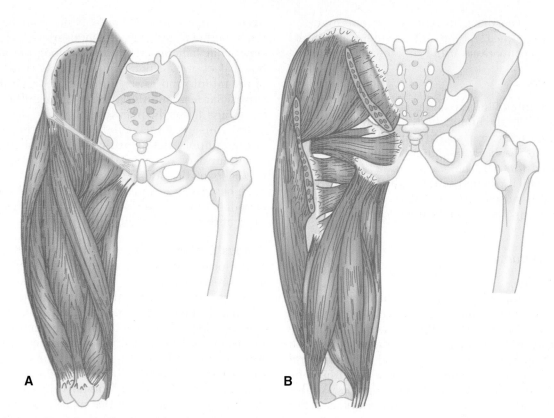

Figure 53-3. A and **B**, Anatomic illustration of the major muscles acting about the hip and thigh.

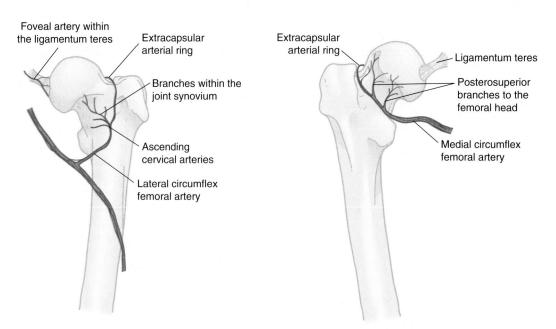

Figure 53-4. The arterial blood supply of the femoral neck and head is provided to varying degrees by three sources: the ascending cervical arteries, the arterial branches within the marrow (not illustrated), and the dubious foveal artery within the ligamentum teres.

The sciatic nerve is the largest peripheral nerve in the body. It arises from the sacral plexus, the fourth and fifth lumbar nerve roots, and the first, second, and third sacral nerve roots. The sciatic nerve exits the pelvis through the greater sciatic foramen and travels through the posterior of the thigh; it extends from the inferior border of the piriformis to the distal third of the thigh. The sciatic nerve gives off articular branches that supply the hip joint. In the thigh, muscular branches innervate the adductor magnus and hamstring muscles. Just proximal to the popliteal fossa, the sciatic nerve divides and forms the tibial and common peroneal nerves.[8]

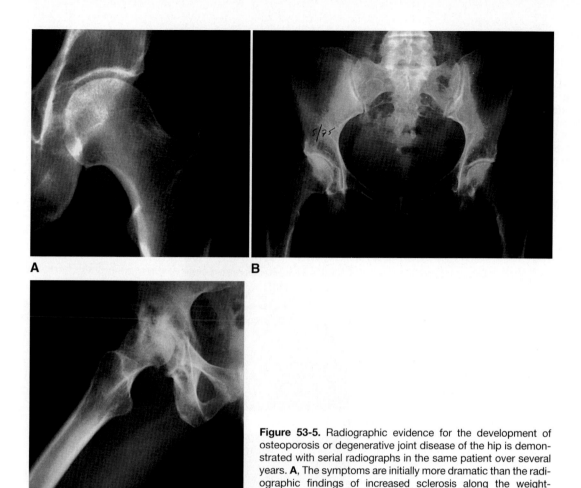

A **B**

C

Figure 53-5. Radiographic evidence for the development of osteoporosis or degenerative joint disease of the hip is demonstrated with serial radiographs in the same patient over several years. **A,** The symptoms are initially more dramatic than the radiographic findings of increased sclerosis along the weight-bearing surface of the superior acetabulum. **B,** The joint space is lost. **C,** Erosion of the head and acetabular surfaces and reactive bony cystic changes develop.

Pathophysiology

Fractures of the Femur and Hip

The pathophysiology of femur and hip fractures is discussed in the description of individual fractures. The vast majority of hip fractures occur in elderly patients with preexisting bone disease after relatively low-energy trauma, usually a ground-level fall. Major trauma such as motor vehicle crashes or falls from significant heights is responsible for the majority of fractures in young, otherwise healthy individuals.

Osteoarthritis of the Hip and Osteoporosis of the Femur

As the population ages, a greater percentage of the population will suffer with the chronic pain associated with degenerative osteoarthritis of the hip. Disability often results from persistent pain and limited physical mobility. The progression of osteoarthritis can be demonstrated with serial radiographs of the affected hip (Figure 53-5).

Osteoporosis is the leading cause of hip fracture. The pathophysiology of osteoporosis is not completely understood, but there are strong associations with hormonal changes related to aging, genetic predisposition, vitamin D deficiency, lack of physical activity, and smoking.[9] Severe osteoporosis and hip fractures are most common in elderly white women. Radiography of the head of the femur can quantify the degree of osteoporosis, even in the nonfractured hip. The trabeculae of the femoral head and neck strengthen the bone and support the large mechanical forces produced across the hip joint. Singh and colleagues introduced a grading system involving the trabecular patterns of the proximal end of the femur that is useful in evaluating the degree of osteoporosis (Figure 53-6).[10] The Singh score for the degree of osteoporosis uses five trabecular groups found within the head, neck, and proximal end of the femur of nondiseased bone. A healthy femur has all five of these groups represented on a plain anteroposterior (AP) radiograph. As osteoporosis begins and then progresses, the groups disappear one at a time in a predictable pattern.

Avascular Necrosis

Epidemiology and Pathophysiology

When a patient has an increasingly painful hip, buttocks, thigh, or knee and no history of recent trauma, AVN of the femoral head should be considered. AVN has been referred to as aseptic necrosis, ischemic necrosis, and osteonecrosis. It is the result of ischemic bone death of the femoral head after compromise of its blood

Figure 53-6. Singh score used to quantify the degree of osteoporosis as it develops. Six grades are differentiated by the presence or absence of trabecular groups. **A**, Grade VI. All normal trabecular groups are visible, and the upper end of the femur is occupied by cancellous bone. **B**, Grade V. The structures of the principal tensile and principal compressive trabeculae are accentuated. Ward's triangle appears prominent. **C**, Grade IV. The principal tensile trabeculae are markedly reduced but can still be traced from the lateral cortex to the upper part of the femoral neck.

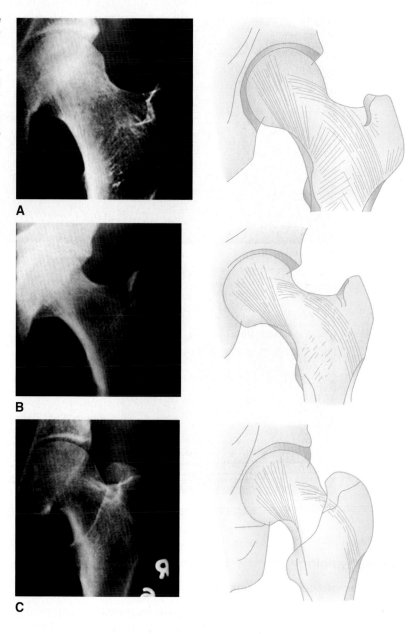

supply. AVN occurs bilaterally in 52% of patients. It is common in relatively young patients, the mean age being 37 years.[11] Although the specific cause is unknown in 20% of cases, known atraumatic causes include chronic corticosteroid therapy, chronic alcoholism, hemoglobinopathy (e.g., sickle cell anemia), dysbarism, and chronic pancreatitis.[11] Traumatic AVN is a subacute manifestation after hip dislocation or femoral neck fracture. It is more common in males and African Americans.

The incidence of AVN as a subacute complication of hip dislocation can reach 40%. Its development is clearly related to both the initial degree of trauma and the amount of time that the femoral head remains out of joint. Reduction of the hip within 6 to 12 hours after dislocation significantly decreases the incidence of AVN.[12] For this reason, hip dislocation should be considered one of the few orthopedic emergencies. The emergency physician must be able to reduce the hip if there is any delay in orthopedic consultation.

Even with optimal treatment, femoral neck fractures are complicated by AVN in 11% to 19% of cases (Figure 53-7). Apart from direct injury to the key arteries supplying the femoral head, a second factor contributing to the development of AVN is its location within a joint. For all practical purposes, femoral neck fractures are effectively intra-articular fractures. Acutely, bleeding from the fracture site may cause high intracapsular pressure and a tamponade effect on the femoral head, thus further impairing the blood supply.[13] In addition, if the bony fragments are not impacted, synovial fluid will lyse the blood clot. Such lysis prevents the development of capillary buds and the scaffolding needed for osseous repair. These factors all contribute to make AVN of the femoral head a common complication.

Intertrochanteric fractures are located in an area of rich blood supply provided by an extracapsular arterial supply. AVN therefore rarely complicates these fractures.

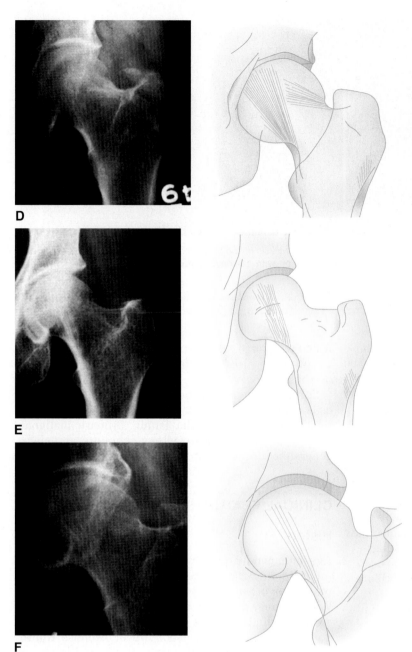

D

E

F

Figure 53-6.—cont'd D, Grade III. A break in the continuity of the principal tensile trabeculae opposite the greater trochanter indicates definite osteoporosis. **E**, Grade II. Only the principal compressive trabeculae are prominent; the others have been completely resorbed. **F**, Grade I. Even the principal compressive trabeculae are markedly reduced in number and are not prominent. (From Singh M, Nagrath AR, Maini PS: Changes in trabecular patterns of the upper end of the femur as an index of osteoporosis. *J Bone Joint Surg Am* 52:457, 1970.)

Classification

Four stages are used in classifying the progression of AVN. Ischemia of the femoral head, regardless of cause, produces an increase in intramedullary pressure and results in bone death. Reactive bone growth, edema, and fibrosis result (Box 53-1).

Calcifying Lesions of the Femur and Hip

Myositis Ossificans

Epidemiology and Pathophysiology. Myositis ossificans (heterotrophic ossification) is pathologic bone formation at a site where bone is not normally found. Traumatic myositis ossificans results from a direct blow or occurs after a fracture. The thigh and hip muscles are most commonly involved. The incidence of myosi-

---

BOX 53-1. Classification of Avascular Necrosis of the Femoral Head

Stage I: Ischemia causes increased pressure, edema, and fibrosis. New bone formation masks changes on plain film; computed tomography is required.

Stage II: Additional bone growth appears as mottled density and lucency. The femoral head maintains its normal contour.

Stage III: Structural collapse of the head. "The crescent sign" is present.

Stage IV: Severe collapse of the femoral head, irregular densities.

From Harris JH, Harris WH, Novelline RA: *The Radiology of Emergency Medicine*, 3rd ed. Baltimore, Williams & Wilkins, 1993.

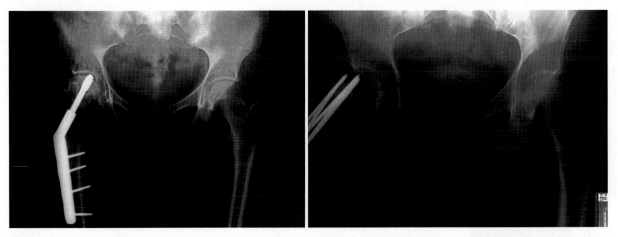

Figure 53-7. Even with optimum treatment of femoral neck fractures, avascular necrosis of the femoral head still may occur as happened in the patient shown. The fracture was treated by open reduction and internal fixation with a sliding compression screw and plate to maintain alignment of the fracture while allowing loading across the site.

tis ossificans is approximately 2% after closed treatment of hip dislocation but rises to 34% when open reduction is required. These lesions are clinically significant in only 10% to 20% of cases.[14]

Bleeding into the muscle after trauma produces a local hematoma with subsequent new bone formation within the hematoma. This inappropriate response may also result from repeated minor trauma for unknown reasons. Within a few weeks, a firm and often painful mass develops in the affected muscles. This lesion matures over a 12-month period.[15]

Radiographically, myositis ossificans appears as irregularly shaped masses of heterogeneous bone in the soft tissues around the joint or along fascial planes. Its appearance may simulate primary bone neoplasm, especially when the periosteum is involved. Osteosarcoma and periosteal osteogenic sarcoma should be considered in the differential diagnosis.

The ossific mass is often palpable and may limit motion, depending on its location. Operative removal of a mature lesion may be indicated if the lesion is near a joint or is causing permanent impairment (Figure 53-8).

Calcifying Peritendinitis and Bursitis
Calcification surrounding tendons and bursae or occurring in the joint capsule is referred to as calcific bursitis or calcifying peritendinitis. The cause of these lesions is unknown but may be similar to that of myositis ossificans. There is no relationship between the radiographic findings and acute symptoms. Calcific bursitis is uncommon, but when it does occur, it most frequently affects the trochanteric bursa of the hip (Figure 53-9). The bursal calcification is seen on radiographs as an amorphous, poorly marginated line that is clearly separate from the cortex of the femur.

Neoplastic Disease in the Hip
Benign neoplasms of the femur may produce pain severe enough to justify a visit to the emergency department. The most common of these neoplasms is osteoid osteoma. A solitary osteochondroma may be manifested as a large, bothersome mass. Primary malignant neoplasm is also common in the femur and may be osteoblastic or osteolytic.

Solitary osteochondroma (Figure 53-10), osteoid osteoma (Figure 53-11), and metastatic lesions are relatively frequent in the femur. Primary malignant neoplasms may be localized (e.g., chondrosarcoma) or generalized (e.g., multiple myeloma).

CLINICAL FEATURES

History

Age and gender are predisposing factors for certain injuries. A detailed description of any antecedent trauma or other precipitating events is often helpful. With trauma, details of the mechanism of injury may aid in predicting injury patterns. With stress fractures, an alteration in physical activity or exercise routine provides a clue to the diagnosis. Systemic illnesses or known metabolic disorders should be noted. Any past steroid use is important to know because it predisposes patients to AVN in the femoral head. There is a linear relationship between the cumulative steroid dose and the incidence and severity of osteoporosis and hip fracture.[16] Past cancer, irradiation, and chemotherapy are clues to pathologic fractures.

A review of systems should include information that may help in ascertaining the cause of atypical groin pain. Pain here may be the result of nephrolithiasis, pelvic inflammation, infection or tumor, inguinal and femoral hernia, or adenopathy from genital or cutaneous infection. A history of low back pain may suggest radiculopathy as the cause of the patient's pain. Elderly patients with a hip fracture sustained in a fall at home may be unable to summon help for hours to days. They often have severe dehydration, electrolyte abnormalities, rhabdomyolysis, and renal insufficiency and require a thorough evaluation of these metabolic pa-

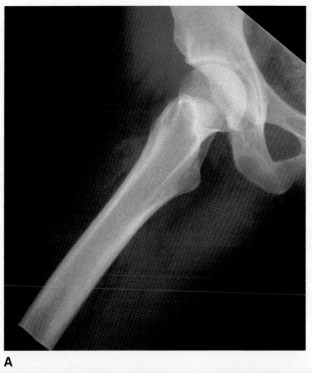

A

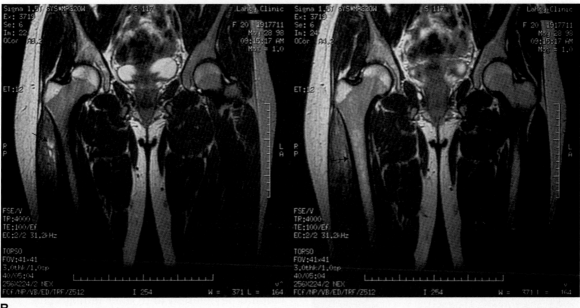

B

Figure 53-8. Myositis ossificans of the proximal end of the femur. **A**, Lesion seen along the lateral cortex of the proximal femoral shaft. **B**, Sagittal magnetic resonance imaging (MRI) views identify calcification within the lateral musculature of the proximal end of the femur.

rameters before considering surgery.[17] In addition, the reason for the fall should be determined if possible because it may reveal other comorbid conditions (e.g., syncope, cardiac dysrhythmias, polypharmacy, alcoholism). Elderly patients may have additional painful injuries sustained in a fall, most commonly fracture of a vertebral body or wrist. A high suspicion for cervical spine and intracranial injuries must also be maintained. Young patients with a hip fracture as a result of high-energy mechanisms have concomitant injuries in 40% to 75% of cases.[12]

Physical Examination

Management principles for injuries of the hip and femur are the same as those for trauma elsewhere.

Hypotension is a problem commonly encountered during the initial resuscitation of a multitrauma patient; however, hemorrhagic shock from an isolated femoral fracture must be a diagnosis of exclusion. Although up to 3 L of blood may be lost into the thigh with a femoral shaft fracture and subsequent hypotension may result, cardiac, pulmonary, intra-abdominal,

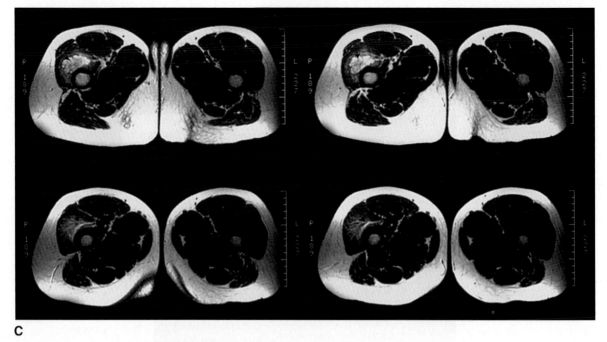

C

Figure 53-8, cont'd C, Same lesion on an MRI axial view demonstrating the extent of the lesion.

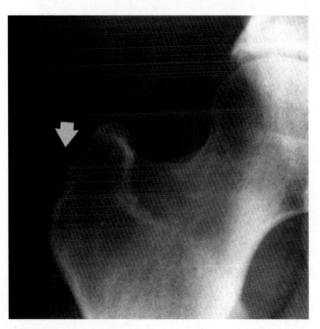

Figure 53-9. Calcific trochanteric bursitis. Faint calcification *(arrow)* in the region of the trochanteric bursa is noted along the lateral cortex of the greater trochanter. (From Harris JH, Harris WH, Novelline RA: *The Radiology of Emergency Medicine,* 3rd ed. Baltimore, Williams & Wilkins, 1993.)

and pelvic trauma must first be considered and excluded. Hypotension, neurovascular compromise, or suspicion of multiple injury requires transfer to a trauma center after the patient has initially been stabilized in the emergency department.

After other life-threatening conditions have been addressed, the injured extremity should be carefully evaluated. Visual inspection will reveal any pallor,

ecchymosis, asymmetry, or deformity. Abrasions, lacerations, or open wounds are critical because their presence alters the management of concomitant fractures. The position that the leg assumes offers a clue to what may be found radiographically. In the presence of a displaced femoral neck fracture, the leg classically assumes the position of external rotation, abduction, and slight shortening. In intertrochanteric fractures, the leg is found in internal rotation with mild shortening. Shortening or a limb length discrepancy is found with fractures, dislocations, and osteoarthritis. Undisplaced fractures, including stress fractures, will not produce limb shortening or rotation but will be painful on passive range of motion, particularly internal and external rotation. These fractures will also prevent the patient from being able to perform a straight leg raise. In patients with obvious deformities, range of motion should be deferred until after radiographs.

Systematic examination will reveal any tenderness or warmth. Active and passive range of motion and muscle strength, though offering important information, are often limited by pain. Detailed neurovascular assessment is vital. Femoral nerve and arterial injury often occurs with subtrochanteric and femoral shaft fractures or anterior hip dislocation. The sciatic nerve can be injured with a hip fracture or posterior hip dislocation. Neurologic examination includes light touch and pinprick sensation. Femoral, popliteal, dorsalis pedis, and posterior tibial pulses are assessed. Comparative blood pressures obtained by Doppler examination in the injured and uninjured extremities may be useful in diagnosing occult femoral arterial injuries. The ankle-brachial index offers useful information regarding arterial injury or insufficiency. An index less than 0.9 strongly suggests arterial injury or stenosis.[18]

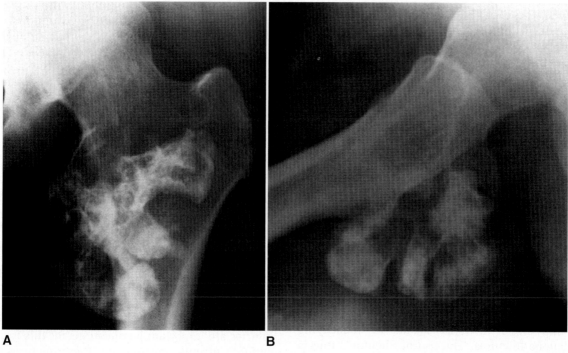

A **B**

Figure 53-10. Classic radiographic appearance of a solitary osteochondroma of the femur as seen in the anteroposterior (**A**) and frog-leg lateral (**B**) views. This lesion is a cartilage-capped bony excrescence typically arising from the cortex of long tubular bones. (From Harris JH, Harris WH, Novelline RA: *The Radiology of Emergency Medicine,* 3rd ed. Baltimore, Williams & Wilkins, 1993.)

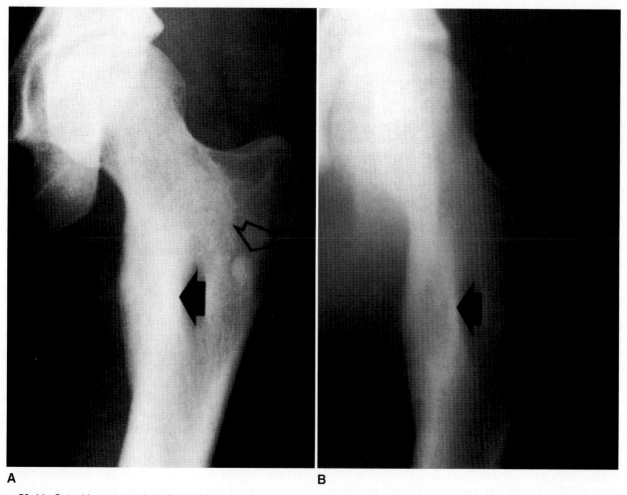

A **B**

Figure 53-11. Osteoid osteoma of the femur *(closed arrow)*. **A**, A large focal area of greater density than that of the surrounding femur represents both cortical and endosteal proliferation. The new cortical bone is smooth and sharply delineated, indicative of a nonaggressive process. The *open arrow* represents a bone island. **B**, A frontal tomogram demonstrates an oval central radiolucent nidus *(closed arrow)*. (From Harris JH, Harris WH, Novelline RA: *The Radiology of Emergency Medicine,* 3rd ed. Baltimore, Williams & Wilkins, 1993.)

DIAGNOSTIC STRATEGIES

Radiographic Anatomy and Evaluation

The normal radiographic and skeletal anatomy is familiar to emergency medicine physicians (Figure 53-12). One common inaccuracy merits clarification: the soft tissue linear radiolucencies superolateral and inferomedial to the femoral head and neck do not represent the hip capsule as is commonly believed. Instead, they represent the fat within the fascial plane covering the gluteus minimus superiorly and the tendon of the iliopsoas muscle inferiorly.[19] Comparison of these lines on the symptomatic side with those on the unaffected side should not be used to determine whether an effusion of the hip is present.

True AP and lateral radiographs of the femur are usually adequate for the evaluation of potential fractures. The femur should be in as much internal rotation as possible. The fracture line may be very subtle, particularly with femoral neck fractures. The authors have found three methods useful in identifying inconspicuous fractures. The use of Shenton's line is described in the section on hip dislocations (see Figure 53-24). Lowell[20] described a second method, which is illustrated in Figure 53-16. When searching for a fracture of the femoral neck, both the medial and lateral cortical margins of the femoral head and neck must be carefully examined for the normal S and reverse S curves found on nonfractured hips. The convex outline of a normal femoral head smoothly joins the concave outline of the femoral neck when in anatomic position. This produces an S and reverse S curve regardless of the angle of the x-ray. A fracture produces a tangential or sharp angle indicative of disruption of the normal anatomic relationship. A third method, useful in the evaluation of seemingly unremarkable hip films, is to trace the trabecular groups as they pass from the femoral shaft to the femoral head. These lines will be disrupted as they pass through the fracture site, and such disruption often provides the only subtle clue. If a fracture is found, radiographs of the knee should be taken as well. It is a basic orthopedic principle to image the joint above and below any fracture.[18]

Occult Hip Fracture

If radiographs do not show a fracture, the patient must be observed while ambulating. An inability to ambulate heightens the suspicion of occult fracture. Approximately 5% of all hip fractures are radiographically "occult" on plain films. Failure to detect these injuries results in increased mortality, risk of subsequent displacement of the fracture, and a higher incidence of AVN.[21] It also affects patients' disposition, in keeping with the admonition "If they can't walk, they can't go home." When a painful hip prevents ambulation and plain films do not reveal a fracture, magnetic resonance imaging (MRI) should be performed.[22] In addition, elderly patients with unexplained chronic hip pain for more than 3 weeks may harbor an occult fracture even if they continue to ambulate. T1-weighted MRI reveals a fracture that was imperceptible at the time of injury with 100% accuracy and has been found to be cost-effective when compared with other strategies.[21] Its use allows either earlier operative repair or physical therapy and immediate mobilization.

Bone scans have been useful in these patients, yet such scans lack adequate sensitivity. To identify most occult fractures, the scan must be delayed 72 hours after the injury. These 3 days of bed rest and hospitalization while awaiting a bone scan are costly and not without risk (e.g., formation of deep venous thrombosis) (Figure 53-13).

MANAGEMENT

Patients with traumatic fracture of the hip or femur should have blood typed and crossmatched for administration of at least 2 U of blood. Hemodynamic instability may result from dehydration and blood loss of up to 3 U into the fracture site. The potential for significant blood loss and the multiple common associated injuries are important justifications for this recommendation. Currently, treatment of these fractures is hemiarthroplasty or open reduction and internal fixation for femoral neck fractures. Internal fixation with a sliding compression screw is generally used to treat intertrochanteric fractures. The goal is to promote immediate postoperative mobilization. It has become widely accepted that the risks of surgery in elderly patients are minimal when compared with the risks of prolonged bed rest, deep venous thrombosis, pulmonary embolism, pneumonia, and urosepsis from an indwelling Foley catheter. If possible, the repair is conducted under spinal anesthesia to decrease the operative risk. Care of an elderly patient with a hip fracture is a multidisciplinary effort and often requires coordination between the emergency physician, orthopedist, internist, neurologist, and cardiologist to stabilize the patient before surgery. Operative repair should be performed as soon as possible after the patient is resuscitated and is in optimal preoperative condition.

Traction and Immobilization

Prehospital personnel often place a Hare splint or similar device that applies traction to the leg before transport if they suspect a femoral fracture. Although such management may provide pain relief and limit blood loss, great care must be given to the proper use of these devices. Prolonged traction during the assessment and management of other injuries can cause or worsen serious neurovascular injury in the thigh. The traction used in the field for transport will produce potentially damaging tension on the nerve and artery. The femoral and sciatic nerves are much more likely to be injured from traction or during surgery than they are from a femoral fracture.[23] Maintaining the leg in flexion at the hip reduces intracapsular pressure, whereas extension of the leg increases pressure and potential for ischemic necrosis of the femoral head. For these reasons, traction should be discontinued once the patient arrives in the emergency department.

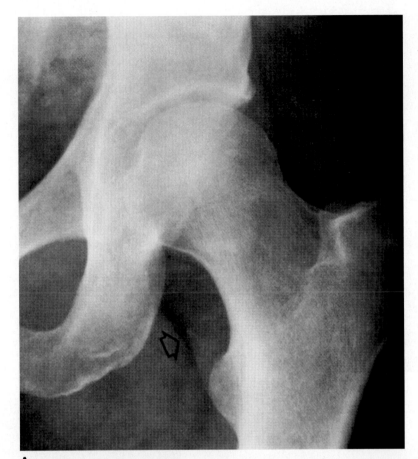

A

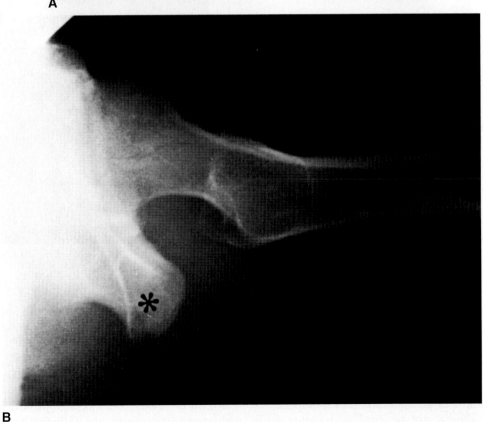

B

Figure 53-12. A, Normal adult hip. The *superior arrow* indicates fatty tissue covering the gluteus minimus; the *inferior arrow* indicates the edge of the iliopsoas muscle shadow. These muscles lie immediately on the capsule of the hip joint. The small concavity in the center of the femoral head is for the attachment of the ligamentum teres. **B**, Cross-table lateral view of the hip demonstrating the normal relationship of the femoral head to the neck. The *asterisk* indicates the ischial tuberosity. (From Harris JH, Harris WH, Novelline RA: *The Radiology of Emergency Medicine,* 3rd ed. Baltimore, Williams & Wilkins, 1993.)

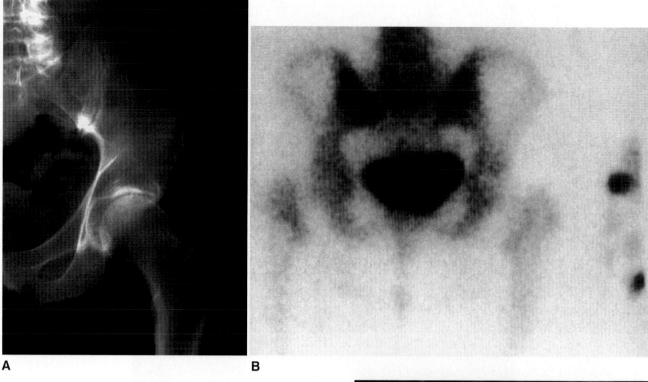

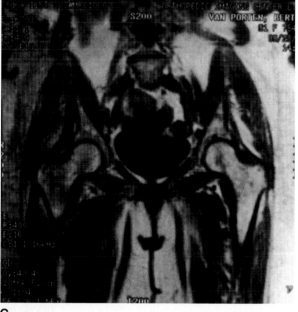

Figure 53-13. A, The patient complained of hip pain and could not ambulate. Initial radiographs failed to demonstrate a fracture. **B**, A radionuclide bone scan 72 hours after the fall provided no evidence of a fracture. **C**, A magnetic resonance image obtained 24 hours after the fall shows an altered signal in the intertrochanteric area, indicative of an acute fracture. (**B** and **C**, From Rockwood JC Jr, Green DP, Bucholz RW [eds]: *Rockwood and Green's Fractures in Adults,* vol 2, 4th ed. Philadelphia, JB Lippincott, 1996).

There are some contraindications to the use of traction. Providers should be instructed that traction should not be applied to any open fracture that has exposed bone. Such reduction pulls grossly contaminated bone fragments back into the wound before adequate debridement can be undertaken in the operating room. Traction should not be used in patients with any suggestion of neurologic involvement because it may worsen the injury. The injured extremity should be immobilized without traction when moving the patient. The leg may be supported in a position of comfort with a pillow placed under the thigh.

Open Fracture Care

By definition, an open fracture is any in which a break in the integrity of the skin and soft tissue allows communication with the fracture and its hematoma. Any wound or break in the skin in proximity must be considered to communicate with the fracture. Open fractures are divided into the three categories (Table 53-2), the third of which may be subdivided according to the amount of nerve, arterial, or periosteal injury present. A bone piercing from the inside outward often causes only a small wound. The contaminated bone tip then

Table 53-2. Classification of Open Fractures

	Type I	Type II	Type III*
Wound size	<1 cm	>1 cm and <10 cm	>10 cm
Soft tissue damage	Minimal, if any	Moderate, without nerve, arterial, or periosteal stripping	Extensive muscle devitalization. Nerve and arterial involvement often classified as type IIIb
Mechanism of injury	Bone edge pierces outward	Variable	High-energy shotgun, high-velocity gunshots

Type I: endosteal or periosteal callus without a definite fracture line on plain radiographs; type II: a definite fracture is identified on plain radiographs, but no displacement; type III: the fracture is displaced.
*Any shotgun wound, high-velocity gunshot wound, segmental fracture, farmyard injury, vascular injury, or crush injury is classified as type III, regardless of wound size.
From Morris JM, Blickenstaff LP: *Fatigue Fractures.* Springfield, Ill, Charles C Thomas, 1967.

slips deceptively back into the soft tissue; therefore, any break in the integrity of the skin makes the fracture an open one. Open wounds should be irrigated and then covered with sterile saline-moistened gauze.

For all type I open fractures, a first-generation cephalosporin should be administered intravenously. Types II and III require additional gram-negative coverage because of the amount of devitalized tissue and increased gram-negative skin flora found in the groin.[24] This additional coverage could be provided by an aminoglycoside such as gentamicin or tobramycin. The use of perioperative first-generation cephalosporins has been shown to reduce postoperative infection even in closed fractures that are to undergo surgery.[18]

Great care should be taken to identify tetanus-prone wounds so that appropriate prophylaxis can be provided with penicillin and tetanus immune globulin when indicated.

Compartment Syndrome

Because of its larger volume, compartment syndrome within the thigh is far less common than in the lower part of the leg. A large amount of bleeding into the compartment is required before the pressure rises above capillary perfusion pressure. It is difficult to clinically differentiate the expected swelling after an injury from early compartment syndrome. Clinical examination and the use of direct compartment pressure measurements can detect the development of compartment syndrome at an early stage.

Pain Management

Systemic Analgesia

It is well known that control of pain in emergency departments is often inadequate.[25] There may be greater reluctance to administer adequate doses of analgesics in the elderly because of possible respiratory depression. Nevertheless, pain control should be a high priority during the initial management period.

Femoral Nerve Block

Femoral nerve blocks have been used to treat femoral shaft fractures for more than 50 years.[26] Despite proven effectiveness and a low complication rate, this technique has not been widely embraced by emergency physicians or surgeons.[27] Femoral nerve block is invaluable as an adjunct or alternative to systemic analgesics in those at risk for hypotensive side effects. For obvious reasons, careful neurovascular examination and consultation with the orthopedic surgeon involved should be carried out and documented before performing the procedure.

If a long-acting anesthetic such as bupivacaine is used, the expected onset of analgesia is 15 to 30 minutes, and its duration is 6 to 8 hours.[28]

Hip Arthroplasty

Background and Epidemiology

Sir John Charnley first described the modern form of total hip arthroplasty (THA) in 1961. Despite many changes in both the design and materials used, Charnley's essential design has been established as the standard.[29] The incidence of THA in the United States rose from 65,000 per year in 1982 to more than 120,000 per year by the mid-1990s.[30] Women account for 62% of THA in the United States. The most common indication for THA is joint failure resulting from severe osteoarthritis. Other indications include rheumatoid arthritis, certain types of hip fracture, AVN, and certain tumors. Arthritis associated with Paget's disease, trauma, ankylosing spondylitis, and juvenile rheumatoid arthritis are also relative indications for total or partial hip arthroplasty.

Outcomes and Complications

THA provides an immediate, substantial improvement in pain, functional ability, and overall quality of life. A 10-year follow-up of patient outcomes, including gait, perception of pain, physical mobility, sleep patterns, and energy scores, showed positive results in more than 90% of cases.[31] Despite the tremendous success of THA, there are numerous complications, aseptic loosening of the prosthesis being the most common. Other complications include component wear, infection, surrounding femoral fractures, and deep venous thrombosis. Postoperative dislocation of the femoral component occurs in 3% of patients. Generally, flexion past 90 degrees, adduction, and internal rotation place the hip at risk for dislocation. This combination can occur when patients bend at the waist (e.g., to sit on a normal

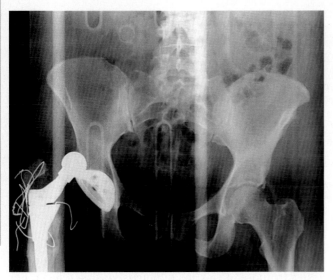

Figure 53-14. Dislocation of the femoral prosthesis in a patient with a total hip arthroplasty. The femoral head often becomes caught on the rim of the acetabular cup, thereby preventing reduction. Reduction may disrupt or dislocate the acetabular cup.

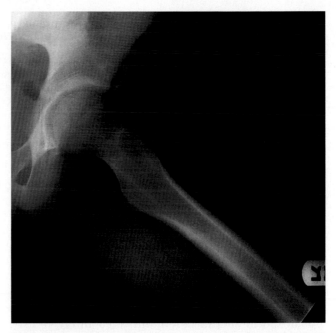

Figure 53-15. Avulsion of the anterior inferior iliac spine by the rectus femoris produced a fracture.

low toilet or to get out of a chair) or cross their legs (Figure 53-14).[32]

SPECIFIC INJURY PATTERNS

Fractures of the Hip and Femur

Avulsion Fractures

The pain of avulsion injuries of the hip may be manifested as referred pain to the thigh and is most common in adolescents and young adult athletes. The muscular origin of this type of injury commonly involves the pelvic apophyses. Avulsion at the site of the growth plate is the result of sudden, maximal muscular exertion. It may occur with rapid acceleration or sudden changes in speed or direction. The athlete classically experiences a sudden piercing pain at the site of injury, describes a "snapping" or "popping" feeling, and frequently falls to the ground because of the intensity of this pain. Avulsion at the anterior superior iliac spine involves the separation of a thin piece of bone as the sartorius muscle suddenly contracts. The anterior inferior spine is avulsed by the rectus femoris, and the hamstring group may pull off the ischial tuberosity (Figure 53-15).

Proximal Femoral Fractures

Classification Systems

Fractures of the proximal end of the femur have been classified on the basis of their relationship to the hip capsule (e.g., intracapsular and extracapsular), geographic location (neck, trochanteric, intertrochanteric, subtrochanteric, and shaft fractures), and degree of displacement. A working knowledge of the classification system allows the emergency physician to communicate with the consulting orthopedist regarding the fracture's pattern, stability, and treatment options.

Femoral Neck Fractures

Pathophysiology. Many now refer to femoral neck fractures as *insufficiency fractures* in acknowledgment of the major role played by osteoporosis. Age-related bone loss is believed to be the most important factor in determining the incidence of femoral neck fractures.[33] The theory that these fractures result from primary skeletal pathology is supported by the fact that minimal or no injury is associated with most of these fractures. Pathologic fractures from metastatic carcinoma are well described.

Classification. Fractures of the femoral neck were originally divided by location into either subcapital or transcervical types. The subcapital fracture line lies just under the dome of the femoral head's articular surface. Although several classification systems were used to describe these fractures, they have been abandoned because of poor inter-rater reliability and limited clinical utility. Currently, femoral neck fractures should be classified as either nondisplaced or displaced fractures.

Fifteen percent to 20% of all femoral neck fractures are *nondisplaced fractures*. The fracture line may often be very subtle. Techniques described for detection of subtle fracture lines may be useful for this reason. Evaluation of the continuity of the subcapital cortical lines, search for an indistinct broad band of increased subcapital density, and identification of the S and reverse S curves (Figure 53-16) will lead to the correct diagnosis in most cases. In impacted femoral neck fractures, the neck cortex is driven into the cancellous femoral head. Bony impaction lends a certain inherent stability (Figure 53-17). Because of this inherent stability, two different approaches have been advocated: early ambulation and internal fixation. AVN, the most common complication, occurs in 20% of patients regardless of

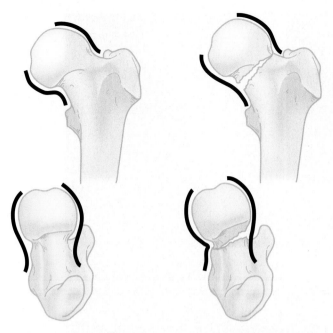

Figure 53-16. Lowell[20] described the normal anatomic x-ray appearance of the femoral head as a smooth S and reverse S lines drawn above. The concave outline of the femoral neck meets the convex outline of the femoral head in all views. Any tangential angle suggests a fracture.

the type of management.[23] The prognosis for nondisplaced fractures is excellent; 96% of patients heal without complication. Without impaction, a nondisplaced femoral neck fracture possesses no inherent stability and will become displaced without internal fixation.

On initial evaluation, a patient with a *displaced fracture* of the femoral neck lies with the limb externally rotated, abducted, and slightly shortened. The diagnosis is confirmed with plain hip films (Figure 53-18). To avoid further disruption of the blood supply to the femoral head, range of motion should be deferred unless radiographs fail to reveal a fracture. In all displaced femoral neck fractures, the femoral head is rendered largely avascular, and subsequent signs of AVN and collapse may occur over the ensuing several years.

Treatment of these displaced fractures is either open reduction with internal fixation or hemiarthroplasty (Box 53-2).

Outcome and Complications. The mortality rate during the first year after a femoral neck fracture is 14%, as compared with 9% for the control population. Factors affecting mortality include age, male sex, psychiatric illness, end-stage renal disease, and congestive heart failure.[34] Institutionalized patients have a death

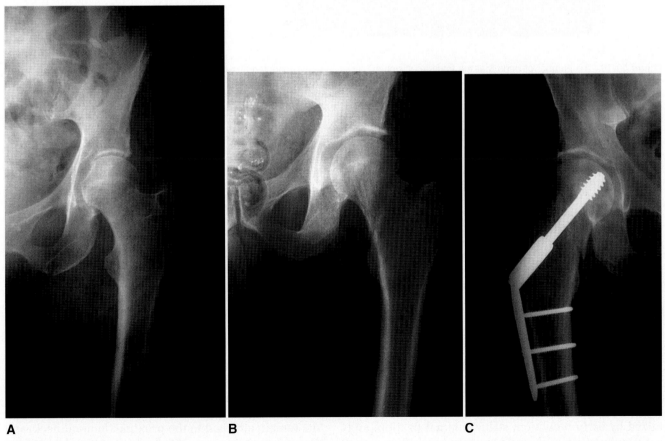

A   **B**   **C**

Figure 53-17. A, Subtle nondisplaced impacted femoral neck fracture (Garden type I). Use of Lowell's S curves aids in identification. **B**, A nondisplaced femoral neck fracture (Garden type II) possesses no stability without impaction. **C**, The same fracture after treatment with a sliding compression screw and side plate.

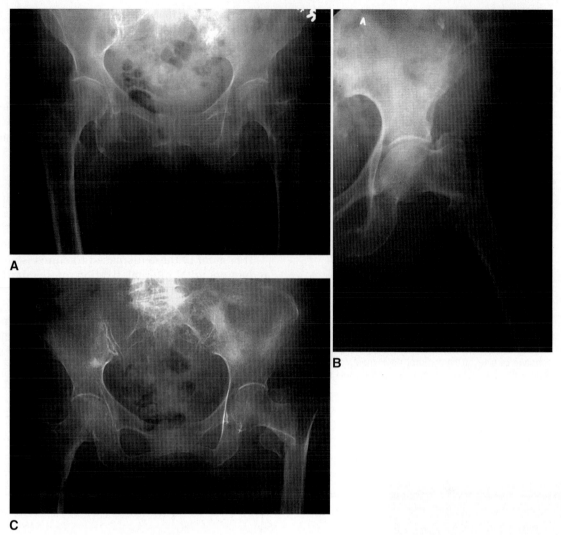

Figure 53-18. The number of parts that the fracture produced classifies intertrochanteric fractures. **A,** Two-part fractures have one part connected to the femoral head and a second part attached to the shaft. **B,** The greater or lesser trochanter is also fractured with three-part fractures. A greater degree of instability is produced because the attached muscles continue to act on the fractured trochanter. **C,** Four-part intertrochanteric fractures involve both trochanters.

BOX 53-2. Relative Indications for Hemiarthroplasty as Treatment of Displaced Femoral Neck Fractures

Parkinson's disease
Hemiplegia or other neurologic disease
Pathologic fracture or Paget's disease
Older than 70 (physiologic age)
Blindness
Severe osteopenia
Poor health that would prevent a second operation

From Rockwood JL Jr, Green DP, Bucholz RW (eds): *Rockwood and Green's Fractures in Adults*, vol 2, 4th ed. Philadelphia JB Lippincott, 1996.

---

rate three times higher.[35] Complications can be minimized by early reduction, stable internal fixation, and early ambulation. AVN and nonunion are the two major complications of femoral neck fractures. AVN is the most common complication, despite optimal treatment,

because of the complex arterial anatomy. Deep infection in the form of osteomyelitis or septic arthritis is more common with femoral neck fractures because the fracture line extends into the joint. The rate of infection has been dramatically reduced with the use of perioperative antibiotics. Pulmonary embolism is another significant complication and is the leading cause of death 7 days after fracture in all orthopedic patients.

Intertrochanteric Fracture

Anatomy

The fracture line of intertrochanteric fractures extends between the greater and lesser trochanter of the femur. They are considered extracapsular fractures. The fracture line extends through cancellous bone and has an excellent blood supply. The hip's short external rotators remain attached to the proximal femoral neck, and the internal rotators are attached to the distal end of the femur, thus explaining the position that the leg assumes with this fracture.

Pathophysiology

An intertrochanteric fracture in younger adults is usually the result of high-speed accidents or high-energy trauma, such as falls from heights. The elderly may sustain this injury during a fall from any height. The fracture lines are the result of both direct and indirect forces. The direct forces act along the axis of the femur and on the greater trochanter as it strikes the ground. Indirect forces are produced as the iliopsoas pulls the lesser trochanter and the abductors pull the greater trochanter; these forces often cause fractures at the site of insertion.

Classification

A large number of classification systems for intertrochanteric fractures have been proposed to predict the possibility of achieving and maintaining stable reduction.[36] An oft-used system, and one sufficient for our use, designates the fracture according to the number of separate bone fragments produced (see Figure 53-18).

Management

Intertrochanteric fractures carry particular pitfalls for the emergency physician. Great care must be taken to address the entire patient and not focus on the fracture alone. Hemodynamic instability may result from dehydration and blood loss of up to 3 U into the fracture site.[37] Poor nutrition before the fall, chronic diuretic use, and decreased oral intake in patients who have to wait until they are found contribute to the level of dehydration. Up to 70% of these patients are under-resuscitated.[17] Associated distal radial, proximal humeral, and rib fractures and compression fractures of the lumbar and thoracic spine are often overlooked because the femoral fracture distracts the attention of both the patient and physician. Spinal compression fractures most commonly involve T12 and L1.

A substantial majority of intertrochanteric fractures require some type of internal fixation. Such fixation allows rapid mobilization, decreased hospital length of stay, reduced mortality, and improved function.[18] The procedure should be performed on an urgent, not an emergency basis. Although the patient's other medical conditions are unlikely to improve significantly, mortality is increased when the patient is taken to the operating room on the day of injury. If delayed longer than 48 hours, however, a 10-fold increase in mortality has been reported.

Outcomes

Intertrochanteric fractures have an associated mortality rate of 10% to 30% in the first year. Life expectancy returns to normal in those who survive that year. Survival is most commonly related to the patient's age and preexisting medical conditions. Additional risks associated with operative treatment include mechanical failure (1% to 16%), implant migration (2% to 10%), and infection (2% to 8%).[38,39] Mechanical failure and nonunion are much more common in unstable fractures and those that were not adequately reduced. Approximately only half of patients sustaining these fractures

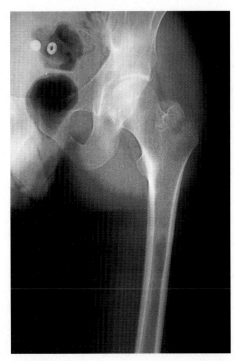

Figure 53-19. Isolated fracture of the greater trochanter. Note that the trochanter is displaced in the typical posterior and superior direction.

are able to eventually regain their original level of ambulation.

Pathologic Intertrochanteric Fractures

Aggressive treatment of patients who have pathologic intertrochanteric fractures or impending fractures is indicated if their life expectancy is more than a few months. Such treatment with subsequent radiation therapy improves the patient's quality of life, decreases pain, and improves mobility.

Isolated Fracture of the Greater or Lesser Trochanter

Fractures of the greater or lesser trochanter are rare. They occur in women more than in men and are the result of a fall directly onto the trochanter or avulsion by the iliopsoas muscle. There may be a comminuted fracture involving only part of the greater trochanter or more subtle impaction of the lateral cortex. If avulsed, the fragments are displaced superiorly and posteriorly (Figure 53-19).[18]

Treatment consists of pain control and early mobilization with crutches; weight bearing is allowed as tolerated by pain. Outpatient management of this injury is possible with a satisfactory social situation. The prognosis is good, and healing is generally excellent.

Subtrochanteric Fracture

Anatomy and Pathophysiology

Subtrochanteric fractures occur between the lesser trochanter and the proximal 5 cm of the femoral shaft. They may accompany intertrochanteric fractures. The subtrochanteric region is composed almost entirely of cortical bone, which lacks the vascularity important to new bone growth and repair. When fractured, it is more likely to be comminuted than bone with a higher cancellous content. Additionally, the majority of the biomechanical forces of the femur are transmitted down the curved medial cortex of the femoral shaft. If this cortex is disrupted, the metal hardware undergoes the majority of the stress. This mechanism accounts for the increased incidence of hardware failure when the medial cortex is largely involved.

These fractures are characteristically deformed because of the unbalanced muscle forces. The attachments of the iliopsoas, gluteal, and external rotator muscles consistently produce flexion, abduction, and external rotation of the proximal fragment.

Epidemiology

Subtrochanteric fractures account for 11% of all fractures of the proximal end of the femur. Although 10% of these fractures are caused by gunshots, the mechanism of injury is usually direct blunt trauma.[40] They occur in a bimodal distribution. The first group consists of elderly patients after a fall. The fracture occurs through an area of weakened cortical bone. Pathologic fractures from metastatic lesions, Paget's disease, renal osteodystrophy, osteogenesis imperfecta, and osteomalacia are well recognized in this area. A second distribution of these fractures occurs in victims of extreme high-energy trauma. In this group of patients, the subtrochanteric fracture is rarely an isolated injury because of the tremendous force required to produce it. Associated thoracic and abdominal injuries are common and must be aggressively sought to adequately manage the patient. Thirty percent to 50% of patients with sub-

trochanteric fractures have associated fractures of the pelvis, spine, or other long bones. Stress fractures can occur in this region but are extremely uncommon.

Classification

A variety of classification systems for these fractures have been proposed, although none are widely accepted.[36] From a practical standpoint, it is best to define and describe these fractures by location *(proximal or distal)*, angle *(transverse, oblique)*, and the presence of comminution (Figure 53-20).

Management

Hemodynamic instability may result from blood loss of up to 3 U into the fracture site.[37] Although such blood loss can lead to hypovolemic shock, other causes of hypotension in a trauma patient must be investigated. Open fractures are rare and, when present, accompany significant soft tissue injury. Vascular and neurologic injuries are also uncommon.

Definitive management of subtrochanteric fractures is a complex issue. Maintaining limb length and controlling rotation are difficult. Open reduction with internal fixation is generally the treatment of choice. However, in the rare case with severe comminution or an open, grossly contaminated fracture, nonoperative management may be preferable.[41] Children younger than 10 years may also be treated nonoperatively. The amount of remodeling and growth stimulation that occurs in children of this age usually ensures good results without internal fixation.

Outcomes

The bone in the subtrochanteric region is largely cortical and relatively avascular when compared with the

Figure 53-20. Variants of subtrochanteric fractures. **A,** Short oblique fracture. **B,** Short oblique fracture with comminution. **C,** Long oblique fracture. **D,** Long oblique fracture with comminution. **E,** High transverse fracture. **F,** Low transverse fracture.

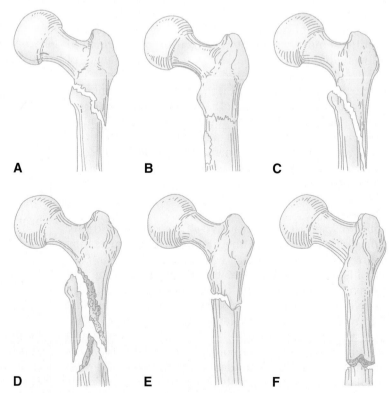

A   B   C

D   E   F

cancellous intertrochanteric region. It logically follows that healing is comparatively slow. Comminution is common and increases the likelihood of nonunion. Because of ample muscle coverage in this area, delayed union, nonunion, and hardware failure are rare. Comminuted and distal subtrochanteric fractures have a worse prognosis.

Complications include fat embolism and the adverse effects of prolonged immobilization in the elderly. The reported mortality rate from subtrochanteric fractures ranges from 12.2% to 20.8%.[42] The violent force and common associated injuries contribute to the high mortality of patients who sustain these fractures.

Femoral Shaft Fractures

Pathophysiology
Femoral shaft fractures are common injuries in young adults after high-energy trauma. As is the case with other femoral cortical fractures, considerable violent force is required to produce a fracture in a normal shaft. Automobile and motorcycle accidents, falls, and pedestrian accidents account for the majority of femoral shaft fractures. The femoral shaft usually fails under tensile strain, and a transverse fracture results. Higher forces produce varying degrees of segmentation or comminution. Open fractures of the femoral shaft are less frequent and are often the result of a gunshot wound. Pathologic fractures occur from a torsional stress that produces a spiral fracture.[43]

Classification
There is no commonly accepted or easily remembered classification for femoral shaft fractures. Location and geometry of the fracture line should be used to describe these fractures. *Transverse*, *oblique*, *spiral*, *wedge*, and *comminuted* are useful terms for describing these fractures.

Clinical Features
Patients often arrive in the emergency department with the injured extremity immobilized by traction devices, which should be removed while maintaining immobilization of the limb. Neurovascular injuries are rarely associated with closed femoral shaft fractures.[44] Significant hemorrhage into the thigh can occur with a femoral shaft fracture, just as it can with intertrochanteric and subtrochanteric fractures. Injuries commonly occurring in the presence of femoral shaft fractures include hip fractures, fracture-dislocations, femoral neck fractures, supracondylar femoral fractures, and patellar fractures.[45] Almost half of femoral shaft fractures have associated ligamentous damage in the knee. If the patient has a femoral fracture, pain often prevents adequate evaluation of knee stability. Any attempt to evaluate the stability of the knee acutely will result in additional pain and hemorrhage without providing useful reliable information.

Management
Internal fixation with intramedullary rods has been demonstrated to shorten both hospitalization and total disability time with most femoral shaft fractures. The vast majority of femoral shaft fractures heal well in time, regardless of the mode of treatment. Severely comminuted fractures are more likely to be treated by closed reduction.

Fractures with Minimal or No Trauma
Most patients who arrive in the emergency department with hip or thigh pain will provide a clear history of a traumatic event. Hip or knee pain in the young, in athletes, and in the elderly deserves investigation, even when minimal or no trauma has been reported. This patient population commonly has occult hip pathology and occasionally femoral pathology. Although senile osteoporosis is the leading cause of femoral neck fractures after minor trauma, pathologic fractures of the femur may result from metastatic, metabolic, or endocrinologic disease.[46] The incidence of fracture in patients with hyperthyroidism is 12%.[47]

Outcomes
Patients sustaining a femoral shaft fracture have close to a 100% union rate, and most are able to return to work after approximately 6 months. Nonunion is relatively uncommon and occurs in about 1% of patients. Even a minor degree of limb shortening or malalignment leads to posttraumatic arthritis.[48] Refracture is a rare occurrence that occurs at two times during the healing process. The leg can refracture during early healing and callus formation or during the brief period after the hardware is removed. After the hardware is removed, the unsupported bone is required to bear the entire weight of axial loading and is at risk for refracture.

Stress Fractures

Biomechanics
Stress fracture of the femoral neck was first reported in 1905 by Blecher.[49] Stress fractures occur when normal bone is repeatedly subject to submaximal forces. This recurring stress stimulates the bones to remodel and strengthen. In a stress fracture, osteoblasts are unable to lay down new bone and remodel fast enough, so the bone fails. Stress fractures can also occur in diseased bone when it is subjected to repeated minimal stress.[50]

Clinical Features
The symptoms of a stress fracture of the femoral neck are often so subtle that they may be mistaken for muscle strain or an overuse injury. Early symptoms frequently include morning stiffness and aching in the hip on the first steps after a period of rest. The pain gradually increases during prolonged exercise and may reach the point at which bearing weight becomes impossible. Pain is felt in the groin or along the medial aspect of the thigh toward the knee.

On examination, an obvious, painful limp is present. This painful or *antalgic* gait is characterized by shortening of the stance phase of the injured extremity. There is no obvious external rotation or shortening of the leg, only minor discomfort with active or passive motion, except at the extremes of flexion and internal rotation. Tenderness is minimal because of the large amount of soft tissue coverage at the femoral neck.

Diagnostic Strategies

Radiographs are helpful if they demonstrate a fracture, but they are often negative until 10 to 14 days after the injury.[18] Endosteal or subperiosteal callus develops during this period and indicates the fracture site. In addition to the standard AP and lateral views of the hip, oblique views may delineate the fracture line. Close attention should be paid to the trabecular fibers of the femoral neck. Often, a stress fracture can be identified as an isolated disruption of either the compressive (medial aspect of the femoral neck) or the tensile (lateral aspect of the femoral neck) trabecular fibers. If a fracture is suspected clinically, negative radiographs should be followed by MRI or computed tomography (CT).[22] If a fracture is found, the other hip should be extensively evaluated because of the significant incidence of bilateral stress fractures.

Classification and Management

Stress fractures are commonly separated into three classes. This division is used to guide management of stress fractures of the femoral shaft. A type I stress fracture is treated in the hospital with strict bed rest until the pain has subsided and the hip has full range of motion. Because of the tremendous disability associated with displaced fractures, types II and III are internally fixed.[5]

Other Causes of Pain

Other considerations in the diagnosis of atraumatic pain of the hip and thigh are listed in Box 53-3.

Dislocations and Fracture-Dislocations of the Hip and Femur

Injury Patterns

Epidemiologists have identified injury patterns in victims according to the mechanism of injury.[51] Pedestrians who are struck by a car have head, chest, pelvic, arm, and femur injuries. Motorcyclists tend to sustain pelvic and ipsilateral leg injuries. A person who stumbles and falls seldom has major associated injuries. Each will be discussed in the following sections.

Hip Dislocations

Dislocations and fracture-dislocations of the hip are two of the few true orthopedic emergencies. The hip joint possesses impressive inherent strength and stability; thus, considerable force is required to produce these injuries. With this understanding, a hip dislocation serves as a "red flag" for multisystem injury and should prompt a diligent search for other occult injuries. Serious associated injuries are found in up to 95% of patients with a dislocated hip.[52,53] Knee fractures, ligamentous injuries, and dislocations are present in up to 30% of patients sustaining a hip dislocation.[54] It is highly recommended that in the presence of this type of injury, patients be evaluated as major trauma victims.

Mechanism and Biomechanics. Traumatic hip dislocations occur primarily in patients sustaining severe multisystem trauma, most often as a result of high-speed motor vehicle crashes. Failure to use seat belts is a significant risk factor. Other less common mechanisms include falls, sports injuries, and pedestrians struck by automobiles.

Posterior dislocations are almost always the result of motor vehicle crashes. A seated vehicle occupant typically has the hip adducted, flexed, and internally rotated at the time of impact. As the knee strikes the dashboard, the force is transmitted through the femoral shaft to the femoral head. With sufficient force, the femoral head dislocates posteriorly. Anterior dislocations result from forceful extension, abduction, and external rotation of the femoral head. These forces lever the head up out of the acetabular cup. Such dislocation most often occurs after a motor vehicle crash when the occupant has the hip abducted and externally rotated at the time of impact. It may also result from a fall or sports injury when the hip is forcefully hyperextended.

Classification. The relationship of the femoral head to the acetabulum is used to classify dislocations into anterior, posterior, central, and inferior types. A fracture-dislocation refers to an associated fracture of the acetabulum or femoral head. Posterior dislocations (Figure 53-21) account for 80% to 90% of cases. Anterior dislocations (Figure 53-22) are seen in 10% to 15% of patients. In anterior dislocations, the femoral head may dislocate medially toward the obturator foramen (obturator dislocation) (Figure 53-23) or laterally toward the pubis (pubic dislocation). Central dislocations, which occur in 2% to 4% of cases, are not true dislocations because the entire femoral head is forced centrally through a comminuted fracture of the acetabulum. Inferior dislocation (luxatio erecta) of the hip is a very rare condition that occurs almost exclusively in children younger than 7 years.

Clinical Features. The position of the injured extremity may provide valuable clues when evaluating a hip dislocation. A patient with a posterior dislocation typ-

---

BOX 53-3. Differential Diagnosis of a Painful Hip without Fracture

Referred pain (lumbar spine, hip, or knee)
Avascular necrosis of the femoral head
Degenerative joint disease or osteoarthritis
Herniation of a lumbar disk
Diskitis
Toxic synovitis of the hip
Septic arthritis
Bursitis
Tendonitis
Ligamentous injuries of the knee or hip
Occult fracture
Slipped capital femoral epiphysis
Perthes' disease
Tumor (lymphoma)
Deep venous thrombosis
Arterial insufficiency
Osteomyelitis

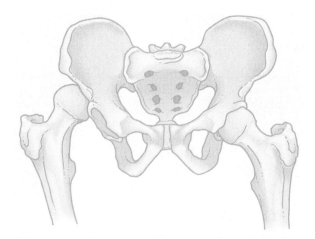

Figure 53-21. In a posterior dislocation the hip is internally rotated and the lesser trochanter is superimposed on the femoral shaft. Failure to visualize the lesser trochanter on the anteroposterior projection identifies a posterior dislocation.

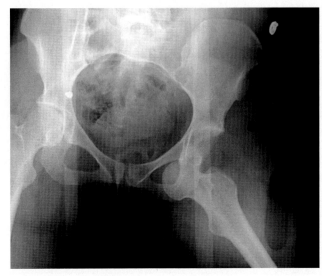

Figure 53-23. Radiograph of obturator dislocation.

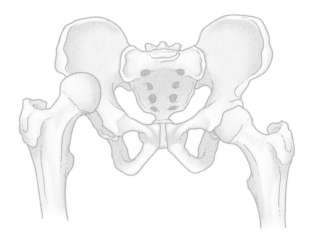

Figure 53-22. In an anterior dislocation the hip is externally rotated, and the lesser trochanter appears in profile. The hip is further from the x-ray cassette than the unaffected side and may appear larger because of the beam's projection.

ically holds the hip flexed, adducted, and internally rotated. The knee of the affected extremity rests on the opposite thigh. The extremity is generally shortened, and the greater trochanter and buttock may be unusually prominent. In contrast, a patient with an anterior dislocation holds the hip in abduction, slight flexion, and external rotation. However, these physical findings may be absent in patients with an associated ipsilateral femoral shaft fracture.

The neurovascular examination should focus on the sciatic nerve and femoral vessels. Sciatic palsy is present in about 10% of patients with hip dislocation and most commonly involves the peroneal nerve branch. The femoral vessels and nerve are particularly prone to injury after an anterior dislocation.

Diagnostic Strategies. Radiologic investigation begins with an AP view of the pelvis. This view alone will identify the majority of hip dislocations. An AP pelvis film should be obtained in all trauma patients with the aforementioned deformities. The AP radiograph should include the entire pelvis and the proximal third of the femur to allow comparison of both hips. When a dislocation is found or suspected, a lateral view of the hip will provide additional definition of the injury.

Although most hip dislocations are seen clearly with these two views, several more subtle radiographic signs may assist physicians in making a confident diagnosis. The first indicator involves the position of the lesser trochanter. Because a posteriorly dislocated hip is internally rotated, the lesser trochanter is superimposed on the femoral shaft and is not seen on the AP projection. In contrast, an anteriorly dislocated hip is externally rotated and the lesser trochanter appears in profile. The second clue is found in the size of the femoral head. Because a posteriorly dislocated hip is closer to the x-ray cassette than the unaffected side is, it appears smaller. The converse is true in anterior dislocations, where the hip is farther from the x-ray cassette than the contralateral side is and thus appears larger. The third finding relates to the integrity of Shenton's line (Figure 53-24). This line is a smooth, curved line drawn along the superior border of the obturator foramen and medial aspect of the femoral metaphysis. Disruption of this line should raise suspicion of a femoral neck fracture or hip dislocation.[55,56]

An obvious dislocation may distract the physician from a search for concomitant fractures. Examination of the trabecular pattern can identify associated fractures of the acetabulum and femoral head, neck, or shaft. It is especially important to identify acetabular fractures before closed reduction is attempted because intra-articular bone fragments may interfere with effective reduction. Oblique radiographs (Judet views) or CT will help visualize the acetabulum and precisely define the injury.[57]

Management. Hip dislocations are true orthopedic emergencies, and reduction should be performed as soon as possible. The earlier the reduction, the better the results. The incidence of AVN, traumatic arthritis, permanent sciatic nerve palsy, and joint instability logarithmically increases with the length of time that the

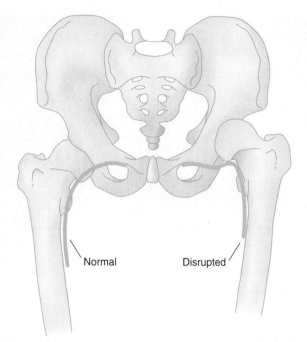

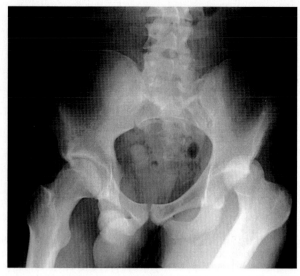

Figure 53-25. Radiograph of posterior dislocation identified by loss of the lesser trochanter on the anteroposterior view.

Figure 53-24. Shenton's line is a smooth curved line drawn along the superior border of the obturator foramen and medial aspect of the femoral metaphysis. Disruption of this line should raise suspicion of a femoral neck fracture or hip dislocation.

hip remains dislocated[58,59]; therefore, prompt anatomic reduction should be attempted.

The timing and method of reduction are dependent on the overall condition of the patient, the type of dislocation, and the presence or absence of associated fractures. In cases of simple dislocation, closed reduction should be attempted first. Although some physicians recommend that this procedure be performed under general anesthesia, this delay and its associated increase in the rate of AVN are not warranted when conscious sedation in the emergency department is readily available. If the emergency physician chooses to attempt closed reduction, the principles of conscious sedation and monitoring should be followed. The primary contraindication to closed reduction is the presence of a femoral neck fracture. Other relative contraindications include coexistent fractures in the dislocated extremity because of an inability to apply traction to the limb. Techniques of closed reduction are described in the next section.

Reduction Techniques. The Stimson technique and the Allis technique are the methods most commonly used for reduction of posterior hip dislocations (Figure 53-25).[18] The Stimson technique (Figure 53-26) uses the weight of the limb and the force of gravity to reduce the dislocation and is relatively atraumatic. Although the Stimson technique is generally effective, placing an acutely and often multiply injured trauma patient in the prone position to perform the procedure may be a challenge. Adequate radiographic clearance of the spine has usually not yet been accomplished, and the administration of sedatives and analgesics in a prone patient has inherent risks. The Stimson technique is performed as follows:

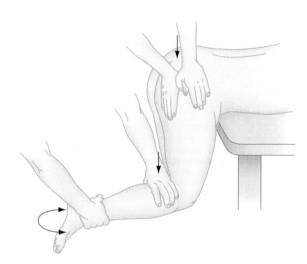

Figure 53-26. Stimson's technique for hip reduction. See the text for a description of this method.

- The patient is placed prone with the leg hanging over the edge of the bed. The hip and knee are flexed at 90 degrees.
- An assistant stabilizes the pelvis.
- The operator applies steady downward traction in line with the femur.
- The femoral head is gently rotated and the assistant pushes the greater trochanter anteriorly toward the acetabulum.
- Once reduction is achieved, the hip is brought to the extended position while traction is maintained.

In a patient who cannot assume the prone position, the Allis technique should be used (Figure 53-27). This technique is usually effective for obturator dislocations. It is perhaps the most commonly used method for hip reductions in the emergency department and is performed as follows:

- The patient is placed in the supine position, and the pelvis is stabilized by an assistant.

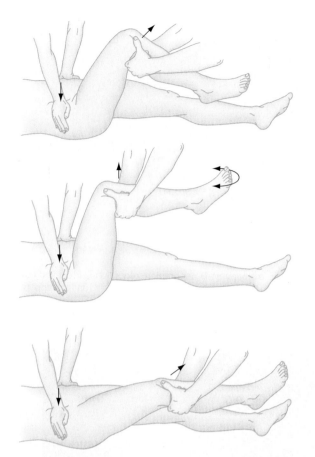

Figure 53-27. The Allis technique for hip reduction. See the text for a description of this method.

- With the knee flexed, the operator applies steady traction in line with the deformity.
- The hip is slowly brought to 90 degrees of flexion while steady upward traction and gentle rotation are applied.
- The assistant pushes the greater trochanter forward toward the acetabulum.
- Once reduction is achieved, the hip is brought to the extended position while traction is maintained.

Other recently described techniques for closed reduction of posterior hip dislocations include the Rochester method[60] and the traction-countertraction technique.[61]

Closed reduction of a pubic dislocation can be quite difficult. The anterior position of the femoral head will resist flexion and thus makes the Allis technique impossible. We recommend reduction with the following maneuvers:

- The patient is placed in the supine position.
- Longitudinal traction is applied in line with the deformity.
- The hip is hyperextended and internally rotated as an assistant applies downward pressure on the femoral head.

Although prompt anatomic reduction is clearly desirable, multiple attempts at reduction in the emergency department should be avoided. Difficulty with reduction is usually the result of incarceration of a tendon, capsular structure, or an unrecognized osteochondral fragment that is blocking reduction. In the case of an irreducible dislocation, closed reduction under general anesthesia or open reduction is often required.

Postreduction Management. After closed reduction, the hip should be tested for stability, which is accomplished by gently placing it through a full range of motion to see whether it will redislocate. An AP radiograph of the pelvis should be obtained to verify the adequacy of reduction. The radiograph should be carefully inspected to verify that the femoral head is in the acetabulum, the shaft of the femur is in neutral position, Shenton's line is intact, and the profile of the lesser trochanter is well visualized. The intra-articular space should be symmetrical and, when measured, the same depth as the unaffected joint. Asymmetry signals an entrapped intra-articular fragment and is an indication for CT scanning (Figure 53-28).

In general, fracture-dislocations should be reduced by closed reduction under general anesthesia or by open reduction. Attempted closed reduction of a fracture-dislocation by an emergency physician is not recommended in view of the rate of complications and associated medicolegal risk.

Outcomes. The precarious blood supply to the femoral head is particularly important with regard to the long-term consequence of hip dislocations. The development of AVN of the femoral head has been reported in 1% to 17% of dislocations. Reduction after 24 hours is correlated with a higher incidence of AVN of the femoral head and posttraumatic arthritis.[58] Other risk factors for the development of AVN include the total dislocation time, the severity of the injury, the number of reduction attempts, and patient comorbid conditions.

Fracture-Dislocation of the Femoral Head

Epidemiology and Mechanism. A small subset of hip dislocations are associated with fractures of the femoral head (Figure 53-29A). Femoral head fracture occurs in 22% to 77% of anterior hip dislocations and in 10% to 16% of posterior hip dislocations.[62] These injuries are almost always the result of high-speed vehicular trauma. Because of the tremendous force required to produce this injury pattern, coexistent multisystem trauma is the rule.

When a femoral head fracture and hip dislocation coexist, patients assume the position typical of the dislocation. Hip mobility is markedly reduced and pain is usually severe. After initial stabilization, the involved extremity should be carefully examined for associated fractures of the femoral shaft and knee. The neurovascular examination should assess for femoral or sciatic injury. Radiographs should be evaluated carefully for any femoral head fracture in all patients with hip dislocations. The fracture of the femoral head can be subtle. These fractures may be detected by following the curve of the dislocated head and the acetabular cup to search for a small fragment that may otherwise be overlooked. Known or suspected injuries can be further defined by CT or MRI.[62]

In most cases, satisfactory results can be obtained by closed reduction (see Figure 53-29B).[57] Several authors

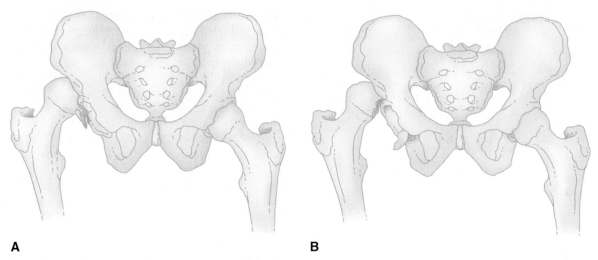

Figure 53-28. **A**, A fracture through the femoral head is seen with this anterior hip dislocation. **B**, Incomplete reduction is identified by examination of the joint space. This space should be the same width as the unaffected joint. Asymmetry signals an entrapped intra-articular fragment, which should be verified by computed tomography.

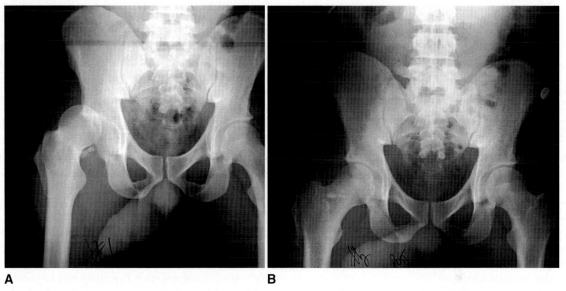

Figure 53-29. **A**, Anterior hip dislocation is identified as the lesser trochanter is brought into profile. Note a fracture of the lateral aspect of the greater trochanter. **B**, A postreduction radiograph demonstrates adequate reduction with symmetrical joint spaces.

recommend obtaining a CT scan of the hip before closed reduction to further define the injury and locate fracture fragments.[57] If the hip cannot be reduced by manipulation or if there is an unsatisfactory reduction of the femoral head fragment, open reduction will be required.

Dislocation of Hip Prosthetics

An increasing number of patients have undergone hip arthroplasty. In addition to those performed as treatment of femoral neck fractures, nearly 200,000 patients undergo elective primary THA each year.[63] Postoperative dislocation of the prosthesis is a common complication that occurs in 1.5% to 3% of patients.[29,32,53,64] Although most dislocations take place within 3 months of surgery, "late dislocations" have been reported up to 10 years after the operative procedure; such disloca-

tions can result from major trauma or from trivial events (e.g., rising from a seated position). Posterior dislocations account for 75% to 90% of cases (see Figure 53-14).[53] Reduction techniques for prosthetic hip dislocations are identical to those described earlier. Consultation with an orthopedic surgeon is essential for safe reduction and development of a long-term treatment plan for the patient. Reduction of the prosthesis does not carry the same urgency as reduction of a dislocated hip because there is no risk for the development of AVN once the femoral head has been replaced. However, traction on the sciatic nerve can occur and makes early reduction more compelling. In addition, the reduction itself carries the unique dangers of loosening of the components, fracturing of the surrounding bone, and movement of the acetabular cup; reduction is best deferred to an orthopedic consultant.

Soft Tissue Injuries

Soft tissues may be subject to muscle or tendon strain or contusions from misuse, overuse, or accidental trauma. Rupture, hemorrhage, or myositis ossificans may develop in muscles.[65]

Muscular Injury

Strenuous exercise in a poorly conditioned person, sudden exertion, and direct trauma may all traumatize soft tissues. Cold temperature, vascular or infectious disease, fatigue, and poor training are known predisposing conditions for this injury.[66] Infectious predisposing diseases include trichinosis, tuberculosis, and typhoid fever.

A detailed classification system of muscular injuries has been devised, but it is of little clinical significance for the emergency physician. Classification of complete and partial tears is reasonable and of greater clinical utility. Partial tears are reversible injuries that are aggravated by movement or tension. Mild spasm, swelling, ecchymosis, and tenderness cause minor loss of function and strength. Complete tears produce a palpable depression, and the torn muscle edge is also often palpable. Severe spasm, swelling, ecchymosis, tenderness, and loss of muscle function occur. In significant muscle strains, radiographs are needed to evaluate the possibility of an accompanying bony avulsion injury.

Initial management of incomplete tears traditionally includes the local application of ice for the first 48 hours, followed by heat.

Compressive wraps cause distal venostasis with the potential for distal venous clot formation and do not significantly decrease recovery time. Nonsteroidal anti-inflammatory agents and sufficient analgesics are important for recovery and patient satisfaction. Muscle relaxants may be useful when the injury is accompanied by muscular spasm. In general, complete rest of the affected muscle should be maintained with the recommendation of "weight bearing as pain tolerated." This progressive muscle loading can be started within 3 to 5 days. Any significant injury should be referred for physical therapy.

A complete muscle tear is a serious condition. Consultation plus follow-up with an orthopedic surgeon or sports medicine specialist is vital for these patients.

Sports Injury Patterns

Athletes commonly experience muscular injury from accidents and overtraining. The two most common injuries involve the hamstrings and the quadriceps.

The Hamstrings. Hamstring muscle strains are common in sports involving running and sudden acceleration. The injury is accompanied by sudden, intense pain in the posterior of the thigh. Any active or passive motion at the hip is poorly tolerated because of the intense pain that movement causes. Crutches and toe-touch weight bearing are recommended until the patient is evaluated by a physician trained in sports medicine. *Toe-touch weight bearing* refers to walking with crutches while the toes of the injured extremity rest on the ground without placing any weight on

it. Appropriate weight-training programs have been shown to speed rehabilitation of this injury.[65] Complete recovery from a hamstring muscle strain may take weeks to months.

The Quadriceps. The quadriceps is the most common muscular group to sustain complete tears. This injury occurs when the muscles are contracted suddenly against the body's weight, such as may occur when an athlete slips or stumbles and attempts to avoid a fall. Ambulation is significantly affected. There is pain with active and passive knee extension. In significant tears, the patient is able to neither actively extend the knee nor maintain its extension against gravity. A depression just proximal to the superior pole of the patella suggests a complete tear. A complete tear of the quadriceps most often requires surgical repair and extensive rehabilitation.

Iliopsoas Strain. Gymnasts and dancers are the most likely group of athletes to experience an injury to the iliopsoas as a result of sudden forceful hip flexion against resistance. Severe pain is often experienced in the groin, thigh, or low back region. Severe intra-abdominal pain is common at the muscle origin and may dominate the clinical picture. Examination reveals groin tenderness and pain with active hip flexion. Radiographs of the femur should be obtained to identify an avulsion fracture of the lesser trochanter. CT will frequently demonstrate a large hematoma. Bed rest with partial flexion at the knee and hip is generally required for 7 to 10 days. With severe strains, symptoms may persist for 2 to 3 months.

Hip Adductor Strain. Injury to the hip adductors occurs as the thigh is forcefully abducted, such as in a straddle injury. The patient complains of pain in the groin, the pubic region, and the medial proximal aspect of the thigh. Abduction and adduction are often limited because of pain. Swelling and skin discoloration confirm the tear. If the tear is complete, a defect in the muscle may be felt along the medial aspect of the thigh near the groin.

Gluteus Muscle Strain. The gluteus muscles may be injured with vigorous or forced hip extension as is seen in track-and-field jumping events. The pain is typically less severe than that associated with injuries to other muscle groups. The hip is tender when extended or abducted.

Tendon Injuries. Clinically, tendon strains tend to have a more insidious onset than muscle strains do. These strains may occur at the attachment of the muscles to the superior or inferior pubic ramus, the pubic symphysis, the ischium, and the femur.

A *groin pull* is the layman's term referring to an injury to the tendons of the hip adductors. The injury usually involves only the adductor longus, yet the adductor magnus and brevis and the pectineus are often involved as well.[66] It commonly occurs in skaters and cross-country skiers when an accidental stress abducts the thigh during a powerful contraction of the adductors. These muscles may also be injured from overuse in an unconditioned patient. Local pain is noted at the inferior pubic ramus and the ischial tuberosity. Extension, abduction, and adduction of the hip are painful. The pain may radiate to the back of the thigh.

Pain over the greater trochanter may represent tendon strain of the attachments of the gluteus medius, gluteus minimus, tensor fasciae latae, or piriformis. Pain is aggravated by resisted abduction. Tenderness in the groin and painful hip movement suggest a strain of the iliopsoas tendon at its attachment to the lesser trochanter. Trochanteric bursitis, peritendinitis, AVN, neoplasm, and other causes should be considered.

Treatment of a tendon strain is similar to that for other soft tissue injuries. The use of crutches with weight bearing as tolerated by pain is helpful for the first 2 weeks. Opioid analgesics and a short course of anti-inflammatory agents should be given. Complete tendon disruption frequently requires surgical repair.

Vascular Injuries

Hip dislocations and the various types of femoral fractures may have an associated arterial injury. The vessel may be partially lacerated, completely severed, or thrombosed. Lack of distal arterial flow may also represent a stretched vessel in spasm. The superficial femoral artery is most commonly injured with trauma to the hip and thigh. The common and the deep femoral arteries are less frequently injured. In the acute setting, penetrating trauma is the usual mechanism of injury.

Arterial injury with femoral shaft fractures is rare and occurs in less than 2% of the cases reported.[67] Anterior- and superior-type dislocations may produce femoral artery injury.[18]

Comparative examination of blood pressure, the ankle-brachial index, and Doppler pulses in the injured and uninjured extremity is critical if arterial injury is suspected. The need for ancillary studies in the evaluation of extremity trauma for vascular injury is somewhat controversial and dependent on the institution.[68]

Diagnostic evaluation must not delay surgical exploration when clinical signs and symptoms of vascular injury are obvious.[69] Early restoration of blood flow is essential to prevent ischemic damage to the leg.

Neurologic Injury

Trauma, infectious agents, and degenerative disease may all injure peripheral nerves. In trauma, nerves may be injured by a blunt object that causes a contusion, by a sharp penetrating object that produces a partial or complete tear, or by the stretch of a missile as it passes in proximity. Nerves are particularly vulnerable to prolonged ischemia, which can lead to necrosis. Compression of the nerve from a hematoma or a dislocated femoral head may also appear as a neurapraxia manifested by transient loss of conductivity. The femoral and sciatic nerves are rarely injured with femoral shaft fractures because they are encased in muscles throughout the length of the thigh.

Treatment of neurovascular compromise and a hip dislocation or a displaced femoral fracture is immediate reduction to ensure limb viability. Reduction should be accomplished before transfer to another facility whenever possible.

Femoral Nerve

When the femoral nerve is injured, the iliac and femoral arteries are commonly involved because of their anatomic proximity. If injured, the femoral nerve is most often traumatized in penetrating trauma of the pelvis, groin, or thigh. Femoral neuropathy can occasionally result from compression by a hematoma within the abdominal wall or the iliopsoas as a complication of hemophilia, anticoagulant therapy, or trauma.[70]

The motor deficit in complete femoral neuropathy is manifested as marked weakness of knee extension. The patient is able to walk on level ground, yet has extreme difficulty walking up stairs or an incline. Patients cannot rise from a sitting position because of significant proximal muscle weakness. The sensory deficit varies, but is localized along the anterior aspect of the thigh and medial lower aspect of the leg. The most reliable spot for testing a sensory deficit is just superior and medial to the patella. The deep tendon reflex of the knee will be diminished or absent.

If a traumatic neuropathy is suspected, immediate orthopedic consultation should be obtained. Nerve exploration and repair are generally preferred for penetrating trauma and when direct impingement on the nerve by bone fragments or hematoma is suspected. Surgical exploration and drainage of a hematoma that is impinging on the femoral nerve are appropriate.

Progressive nontraumatic neuropathies require urgent neurologic consultation. When a chronic neuropathy exists, atrophy of the anterior aspect of the thigh will already have developed. The motor deficits have been discussed previously.

Sciatic Nerve

Sciatic injury is rare with femoral fractures, but it may develop as a result of the traction used to stabilize the fracture during the initial management period. Complete traumatic injury may result from a deep penetrating wound in the hip, thigh, or buttock. Sciatic nerve palsy from both inadvertent injection into the nerve and intraneural or extraneural hemorrhage in patients taking anticoagulants has been described. Posterior hip dislocations and fracture-dislocations produce sciatic neurapraxia in 10% to 14% of these injuries.[18,71] Patients with complete sciatic neuropathy have paralysis of the hamstring muscles and all muscles below the knee. With partial injury, a peroneal palsy with weakness of the extensor hallucis longus muscle is the most sensitive clinical sign. There is sensory loss below the knee and along the posterior of the thigh. The deep tendon reflex at the ankle is absent or diminished.

Sciatic injury from posterior dislocations often consists of only transient loss of conductivity, particularly in its motor fibers. Unfortunately, the other injury patterns to the sciatic nerve carry the worst prognosis of all peripheral nerve injuries. The prognosis is poorest when the injury is proximal and complete. Even with optimal repair, recovery is often inadequate. Sciatic neuropathy is a disabling problem. Obvious atrophy of the lower part of the leg and foot develops, followed by

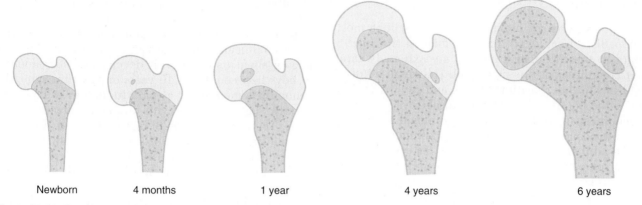

Newborn   4 months   1 year   4 years   6 years

Figure 53-30. Development of the femoral head and neck with its growth plates and two primary ossification centers.

ulceration of the sole of the foot and infection. A below-the-knee amputation is frequently necessary in these cases.

SPECIAL PEDIATRIC CONSIDERATIONS

Anatomy

Development of the femoral head and neck with its growth plates and two primary ossification centers is illustrated in Figure 53-30. A significant proportion of the pediatric hip is radiopaque cartilage and developing new bone. For this reason, almost any type of trauma in this location carries the potential for premature growth arrest. Understanding that large portions of the pediatric hip are radiolucent will dissuade the tendency to focus attention on the ossified elements.

Hip Dislocation

The incidence of hip fractures and dislocations is increasing in young patients, often as a result of high-energy trauma. Up to 50% of children with a hip dislocation will also have fractures elsewhere. In small children, dislocation of the hip is more common than femoral neck fractures. The force required to dislocate a pediatric hip is much less than that required in an adult because the acetabulum is less completely developed than in adults. Seemingly negligible trauma, such as tripping or a minor fall, may dislocate the femoral head in a young child. In a school-age child, athletic injuries are the major cause of traumatic hip dislocation. In the teenage years, motor vehicle accidents predominate as the cause of hip dislocations.

Femoral Fractures

Unlike adults, the vast majority of pediatric hip fractures do not result from high-energy violent trauma. These fractures are usually the result of falling from heights, jumping out of a swing, being struck by a car, or having a bicycle accident. Child abuse must also be considered. Whereas a car commonly strikes an adult at the tibial level, a smaller child is most often hit at the level of the hip, which results in a fracture there.

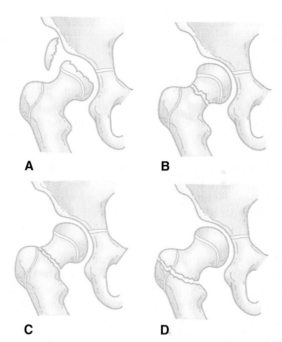

A   **B**

C   **D**

Figure 53-31. Pediatric proximal femoral fractures are classified by a system that separates fractures in the physis (**A**) the transcervical area (**B**), the cervicotrochanteric area (**C**), and the intertrochanteric region (**D**). (From Canale ST, Beaty JH: Fractures of the pelvis. In Rockwood JC Jr, Green DP, Bucholz RW [eds]: *Rockwood and Green's Fractures in Children,* vol 3, 5th ed. Philadelphia, JB Lippincott, 2001, pp 883-911.)

The classic Salter-Harris division of fractures in the pediatric population is not used in the hip. The Delbet classification is a well-accepted system used for pediatric femoral fractures.[72] This system separates fractures through the physis and the transcervical, cervicotrochanteric, and intertrochanteric regions (Figure 53-31).

Spiral Shaft Fractures

If seemingly trivial trauma has resulted in a spiral femoral shaft fracture in a child, child abuse and pathologic fracture must be considered.[73,74] Common causes of pathologic fracture include unicameral bone cysts, fibrous dysplasia, osteogenesis imperfecta, and malignancy.[74,75]

Management

Femoral fractures in children are so rare that most orthopedists treat only three or four in a career.[72] Although these pediatric injuries are extremely rare, their complications are significant. Unlike an adult, a child's femur has growth potential, and any disruption carries the possibility of lifetime disability. Treatment of femoral shaft fractures in adults is aimed at prevention of the complications of prolonged immobilization. Unlike adults, children tolerate bed rest well, which allows more treatment options. The primary goal in children is prevention of the many complications common with femoral fractures. Premature closure of the physeal plate results in a valgus deformity of the hip. AVN, malunion, nonunion, and limb length discrepancy are all complications frequently seen with pediatric femoral fractures. For all these reasons, referral to a pediatric orthopedist is recommended.[72]

The Child with a Limp

A child who comes to the emergency department with a limp is a diagnostic challenge. Both life-threatening and benign disease processes can produce a limp. When the child is too young to give an adequate history, the etiology becomes more elusive. The attending physician should inquire about the chronology of the symptoms, the child's development (i.e., social milestones, weight gain, physical development), and diet. Associated illness and a family history may be helpful. Though challenging, the history and physical examination, combined with appropriate diagnostic modalities, will allow discovery of the cause in most patients. An important point to remember in the pediatric population is that the knee is a common site for referred hip pain. Proper follow-up is crucial to avoid additional morbidity in these children.

Evaluation of the Child's Gait

Gait is a learned, complex combination of motions produced through coordination of the musculoskeletal, peripheral, and central nervous systems. A limp is produced by anything that alters this process and can be divided into categories according to the underlying abnormality. Pain, muscle weakness, structural alteration, peripheral sensory deficit, and cerebellar or vestibular imbalance are major categories. A limp caused by pain is referred to as an "antalgic" gait. Conditions that disturb the biomechanics of the hip or cause the child pain may affect any of the elements of gait. Other conditions such as cerebellar pathology or disease of the knee or foot are discussed in their appropriate sections.

Etiology of the Limp

Inflammation and Infection

Inflammation of the articular surface, the intra-articular synovium, or the joint capsule creates pain. Weight bearing increases the pain. The child limps in an attempt to limit the proportion of time that the affected hip bears the body's weight.

Toxic synovitis is a common nonbacterial inflammatory clinical entity that can cause a limp. Little is known about its etiology. It develops most frequently in boys between 3 and 10 years of age. Clinically, the synovitis is manifested as pain in the hip or knee. An antalgic gait is present with minimal systemic symptoms. There is restriction of hip motion and associated muscle spasm, and the child will often refuse to bear weight on the hip. As the disease progresses, the joint capsule is increasingly stretched and intra-articular pressure rises. The potential volume of the joint capsule is largest with the hip flexed, abducted, and externally rotated. The child prefers to lie in this position as the capsule begins to bulge to minimize the tension and intra-articular pressure.

The diagnosis of toxic synovitis must be one of exclusion of more serious diseases that mimic it. Acute joint inflammation and pain may be associated with juvenile rheumatic arthritis, systemic lupus erythematosus, Perthes' disease, septic arthritis, and tuberculous arthritis. Ultrasound of the hip joint will detect an effusion in 78% of cases of toxic synovitis but cannot distinguish this condition from septic arthritis.[76] Joint aspiration may be required when the diagnosis is in doubt.

Distinguishing between toxic synovitis and septic arthritis can be a diagnostic dilemma. Recent work has illustrated four key predictors: temperature higher than 38.5° C in the preceding week, non–weight bearing (refusal or inability to bear weight even with support), erythrocyte sedimentation rate higher than 40 mm/hr, and a white blood cell count greater than 12,000 cells/mL. These four predictors were developed in a retrospective study and then validated in a prospective study.[77,78] Based on the validation study, the probability of septic arthritis was 2% for zero predictors, 9.5% for one predictor, 35% for two predictors, 73% for three predictors, and 93% for four predictors.[79] These predictors should be used in conjunction with clinical assessment.

Acute bacterial infections of the hip and femur require early identification and intervention to minimize their subsequent morbidity and disability.[79] Unfortunately, the diagnosis is often missed initially because the child may appear relatively nontoxic in the early phases of infection. Signs and symptoms of systemic illness usually accompany infection of the femur or hip. Fever, malaise, decreased oral intake, a limp, or refusal to bear any weight is common.[80] Whereas osteomyelitis most commonly develops in the metaphysis in adults, the physeal region is often the infected site in children. Pyarthrosis (septic arthritis) may result from hematogenous seeding or direct extension of osteomyelitis. The hip and the knee are the most common infected joints.

The causative agent in osteomyelitis and pyarthrosis is nearly always a gram-positive organism, usually *Staphylococcus*. The incidence of *Haemophilus influenzae* infection has fallen as a direct result of its

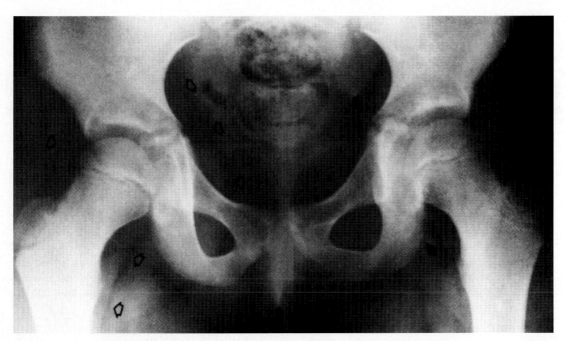

Figure 53-32. Prominence of the soft tissue shadows about the right hip, including bulging of the obturator internus muscle and its aponeurosis *(open arrows)*, indicates distention of the joint capsule. The opposite hip shows the normal soft tissue shadows indicated by the *closed arrows*. (From Harris JH, Harris WH, Novelline RA: *The Radiology of Emergency Medicine,* 3rd ed. Baltimore, Williams & Wilkins, 1993.)

addition to the childhood immunization regimen. Neonates, asplenic children, and children with sickle cell anemia are at risk for infection with gram-negative organisms. *Salmonella* is also more often seen in sickle cell patients with osteomyelitis. Viral and rickettsial diseases (e.g., Lyme disease) have been known to be present in subacute cases.[81]

Radiographic Evaluation

Identification of acute osteomyelitis by plain radiographs is difficult until 2 to 3 weeks after infection. Pyarthrosis may be manifested by widening of the space between the femoral head and the acetabular roof and bulging of the joint capsule and surrounding soft tissues. This is seen as a change in the contour of the gluteus minimus and iliopsoas fat stripes (Figure 53-32). Care should be taken to distinguish the normal shadow of the muscles and the joint capsule as described earlier in this chapter (see Figure 53-12). Plain radiographs are seldom useful in the initial identification of infection because visualization of a joint effusion has low sensitivity for pyarthrosis. Bone scan, MRI, CT, and ultrasound-guided joint aspiration are appropriate to diagnose a septic joint.

The inflammatory process involved in the immune system's attempt to eradicate the intruder also begins to destroy the body's own articular surface. Even with treatment, most children experience some arthritic disability.[82]

Slipped Capital Femoral Epiphysis

Anatomy

The capital femoral epiphysis appears during the first year of life. The epiphysis of the greater trochanter

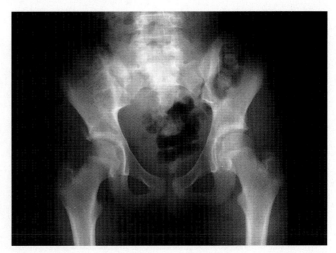

Figure 53-33. An anteroposterior radiograph of a 10-year-old boy demonstrates the normal anatomic relationship of the capital femoral epiphysis, the proximal physis, the apophysis of the lesser trochanter, and the triradiate synchondrosis.

appears by the age of 5 and the lesser trochanter during the 13th year of life. All these structures unite during the 18th through 20th years. The anatomic relationship has been compared with a scoop of ice cream sitting on a cone. This relationship remains symmetrical on both AP and lateral radiographs (Figure 53-33). Asymmetry in any view represents either SCFE or a subcapital fracture (Figures 53-34 and 53-35).

Epidemiology and Pathophysiology

SCFE occurs in approximately 5 people per 100,000 population per year. Twenty-five percent of cases are bilateral.[83] SCFE occurs twice as frequently in boys as

Figure 53-34. Frank slipped capital femoral epiphysis. The capital femoral epiphysis is displaced medially, inferiorly, and posteriorly. The inhomogeneity of the femoral neck is consistent with early avascular necrosis. (From Harris JH, Harris WH, Novelline RA: *The Radiology of Emergency Medicine,* 3rd ed. Baltimore, Williams & Wilkins, 1993.)

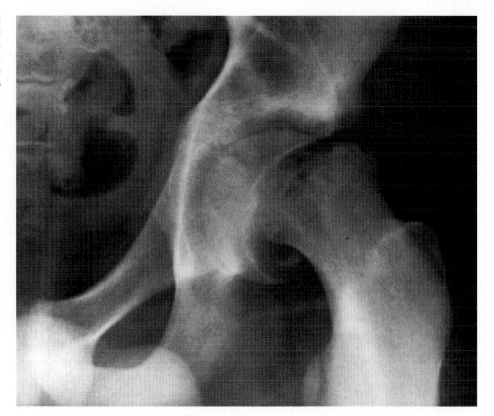

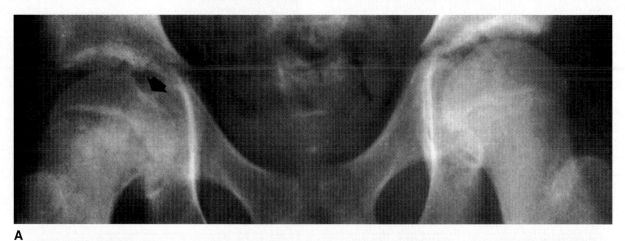

A

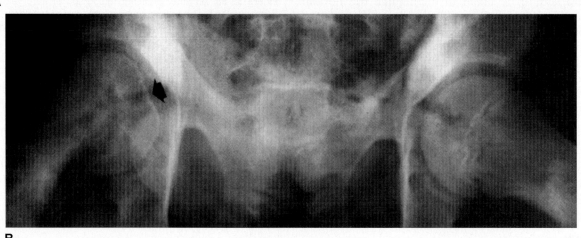

B

Figure 53-35. Right slipped capital femoral epiphysis. **A,** The slippage appears minimal and may be overlooked; however, medial displacement of the capital femoral epiphysis with respect to the metaphysis results in the lateral cortex of the femoral neck and the epiphysis being in the same plane *(open arrow)*. The capital femoral epiphysis is flattened *(arrow)*, and the right hip joint space is widened. **B,** Medial and posterior displacement of the capital femoral epiphysis *(arrow)*. (From Harris JH, Harris WH, Novelline RA: *The Radiology of Emergency Medicine,* 3rd ed. Baltimore, Williams & Wilkins, 1993.)

in girls, with the respective peak incidence being 13 and 11 years old.

Epidemiologic data have provided clues to the pathophysiology of this injury. SCFE is associated with the onset of puberty and rarely occurs before 10 years of age. It most commonly develops in boys 10 to 17 years of age during their period of rapid growth. It is believed to be the result of a structural weakness in physeal cartilage at the onset of pubescence.[84]

The specific cause is not well understood. That SCFE occurs more frequently in male African Americans than in the white population supports the presence of a genetic element in the pathophysiology of this disease.[84] Other risk factors identified are obesity, previous irradiation or chemotherapy, renal osteodystrophy, hypothyroidism, and neglected septic arthritis.[85]

Clinical Features

SCFE is usually an insidious process extending over a period of several weeks to months. Initially, there may be only slight discomfort in the groin, thigh, or knee after activity. Eventually, as slippage progresses, the pain occurs at rest as well. Referred pain to the knee is a classic manifestation. Frequently, the ectopic nature of the pain leads to delayed diagnosis, increased displacement, and a worsened prognosis.[86] As the epiphysis continues to slip, the pain increases. Parents often bring the child in for medical evaluation when they notice the child beginning to limp. Physical examination may reveal hip tenderness, decreased hip range of motion, and an abducted, externally rotated thigh.

Diagnostic Strategies

Children with unexplained hip or knee pain merit clinical as well as radiographic evaluation. Initially, AP, lateral, and frog-leg lateral radiographs of the hip should be obtained. The frog-leg lateral projection shows the hip in a plane midway between the AP and lateral views. The earliest radiographic findings are subtle, with the abnormality visualized on only one projection. The most reliable initial finding of SCFE is asymmetry of the femoral epiphysis in relation to the neck. Small amounts of slippage can be detected by examining the epiphyseal edge as it becomes flush with the superior border of the femoral neck. This can be thought of as "the scoop slipping off the ice cream cone." The dome of the epiphysis may be flattened. A line drawn along the medial aspect of the femoral shaft (Klein's line) should intersect some part of the normal femoral head. Failure of this line to intersect the head indicates medial and posterior movement of the head on the epiphysis.[83] Comparative views of the two hips are indicated if initial radiographs are equivocal. If occult fracture is suspected, MRI or CT should be performed.[20,87] Surgery is required to anchor the epiphysis and prevent further slippage.

Perthes' Disease

Perthes' disease is the name given to AVN of the pediatric femoral head. It has also been called Legg-

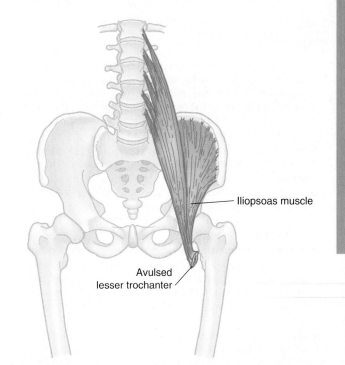

Figure 53-36. Forceful contraction of the iliopsoas muscle results in avulsion of the lesser trochanter.

Calvé-Perthes and Calvé-Perthes disease. It occurs at a younger age than SCFE does—between the ages of 2 and 10. Its peak incidence is at 6 years, and it occurs five times more often in boys than girls. The disease affects both hips in 15% of patients.[88]

Isolated Fracture of the Greater or Lesser Trochanter in Children

An isolated fracture of the greater trochanter is a rare injury. In children, a fracture occurs as the entire greater trochanteric epiphysis is avulsed from the femur. This type of fracture occurs in children and adolescents between 7 and 17 years of age. The mechanism of injury is generally a powerful muscular contraction of the lateral rotators of the hip joint during a twisting fall. If the fragment is large and displaced by more than 1 cm, open reduction and internal fixation may be indicated.

An isolated fracture of the lesser trochanter occurs as a forceful contraction of the iliopsoas muscle avulses the lesser trochanter from the physis during sudden hip flexion (Figure 53-36). Eighty-five percent of all cases occur in patients younger than 20 years, with a peak incidence between 12 and 16 years.[89] Marked tenderness in the femoral triangle is present, and hip flexion against resistance is painful. Clinically, a seated patient is unable to lift the foot of the affected leg from the floor.

Treatment of an isolated lesser trochanter avulsion fracture usually involves bed rest and early mobilization. Painless active hip motion is achieved within 3 weeks.

KEY CONCEPTS

- *Hip dislocation:* Hip dislocation is one of the few orthopedic emergencies. The likelihood of its complication, AVN, is related to both the initial degree of trauma and the amount of time that the femoral head remains out of joint. Reduction of the hip within 6 hours after dislocation significantly decreases the incidence of AVN.

- *Hip fracture:* When a painful hip prevents ambulation and plain films do not reveal a fracture, magnetic resonance imaging should be performed.

- *Intertrochanteric fractures:* Hemodynamic instability may result from dehydration and blood loss of up to 3 U into the fracture site. Up to 70% of these patients are under-resuscitated.

- *Acetabular fractures:* It is especially important to identify acetabular fractures before closed reduction is attempted because intra-articular bone fragments may interfere with effective reduction. Oblique radiographs (Judet views) or CT will help visualize the acetabulum and precisely define the injury.

- *Slipped capital femoral epiphysis:* This condition is most commonly seen in African American boys 10 to 17 years of age; 25% of cases are bilateral. The most reliable initial finding of SCFE is asymmetry of the femoral epiphysis in relation to the neck wherein small amounts of slippage give the appearance of "the scoop slipping off the ice cream cone."

REFERENCES

1. Pare A: The work of that famous chirurgeon, Ambrose Pare, translated out of Latin and compared with the French by Tho Johnson, Book XV. London, T Cotes & R Young, 1634.
2. Von Langenbeck B: Verhandl d, deutch, p 92. Gesellsch F, Chir 1878. As found in Davis GG: The operative treatment of intracapsular fracture of the neck of the femur. *Am J Orthop Surg* 6:481-483, 1908-1909.
3. Gourlay M, Richy F, Reginster JV: Strategies for the prevention of hip fracture. *Am J Med* 115:309, 2003.
4. Koval KJ, Zuckerman JD: Functional recovery after fracture of the hip. *J Bone Joint Surg Am* 77:751, 1994.
5. AAOS Bulletin: *Femoral Neck Fracture (Adult).* Chicago, American Academy of Orthopaedic Surgeons, 1989, pp 11-12.
6. Sernbo I, Johnell O: Changes in bone mass and fracture type in patients with hip fractures. *Clin Orthop* 238:139, 1989.
7. Wadsworth CT: *Manual Examination and Treatment of the Spine and Extremities.* Baltimore, Williams & Wilkins, 1988.
8. Gray H: *Anatomy, Descriptive and Surgical,* revised from English 17th ed. New York, Bounty Books, 1997.
9. Brunner LC, Eshilian-Oates L: Hip fractures in adults. *Am Fam Physician* 67:537, 2003.
10. Singh M, Nagrath AR, Maini PS: Changes in trabecular patterns of the upper end of the femur as an index of osteoporosis. *J Bone Joint Surg Am* 52:457, 1970.
11. Learmonth ID, Maloon S, Dall G: Core compression of early atraumatic osteonecrosis of the femoral head. *J Bone Joint Surg Br* 72:287, 1990.
12. Sahin V, et al: Traumatic dislocation and fracture dislocation of the hip: A long-term follow-up study. *J Trauma* 54:520, 2003.
13. Bachiller FGC, Caballer AP, Portal LF: Avascular necrosis of the femoral head after femoral neck fracture. *Clin Orthop* 399:87, 2002.
14. Garland DE: A clinical perspective on common forms of acquired heterotrophic ossification. *Clin Orthop* 263:13, 1991.
15. Booth DW, Westers BM: The management of athletes with myositis ossificans traumatica. *Can J Sport Sci* 14:10, 1989.
16. Vestergaard P, et al: Corticosteroid use and risk of hip fracture: A population-based case-controlled study in Denmark. *J Intern Med* 254:486, 2003.
17. Koval K, et al: Clinical pathway for hip fractures in the elderly. *Clin Orthop* 425:72, 2004.
18. DeLee JC: Fractures and dislocations of the hip. In Rockwood JC Jr, Green DP, Bucholz RW (eds): *Rockwood and Green's Fractures in Adults,* vol 2, 4th ed. Philadelphia, JB Lippincott, 1996.
19. Harris JH, Harris WH, Novelline RA: *The Radiology of Emergency Medicine,* 3rd ed. Baltimore, Williams & Wilkins, 1993.
20. Rizzo PF, Gould ES, Lyden JP, Asnis SE: Diagnosis of occult fractures about the hip: Magnetic resonance imaging compared with bone scanning. *J Bone Joint Surg Am* 73:395, 1993.
21. Perron AD, Miller MD, Brady WJ: Orthopedic pitfalls in the emergency department: Radiographically-occult hip fracture. *Am J Emerg Med* 20:234, 2002.
22. Guanche CA, et al: The use of MRI in the diagnosis of occult hip fractures in the elderly: A preliminary review. *Orthopedics* 17:327, 1994.
23. Needoff M, Radford P, Langstaff R: Preoperative traction for hip fractures in the elderly: A clinical trial. *Injury* 24:317, 1993.
24. Brillman J, Quenzer RW: *Infectious Disease in Emergency Medicine,* 2nd ed. Philadelphia, Lippincott-Raven, 1998.
25. Jones JS, Johnson K, McNinch M: Age as a risk factor for inadequate emergency department analgesia. *Am J Emerg Med* 14:157, 1996.
26. Ronchi L, et al: Femoral nerve blockade in children using bupivacaine. *Anesthesiology* 70:622, 1989.
27. Fletcher AK, Rigby AS, Heyes FLP: Three-in-one femoral nerve block as analgesia for fractured neck of the femur in the emergency department: A randomized controlled trial. *Ann Emerg Med* 41:227, 2003.
28. Dean E, Orlinsky M: Nerve blocks of the thorax and extremities. In Roberts J, Hedges J (eds): *Clinical Procedures in Emergency Medicine,* 3rd ed. Philadelphia, WB Saunders, 1998.
29. Harkness JW: Arthroplasty of the hip. In Canale ST (ed): *Campbell's Operative Orthopaedics,* 9th ed. St Louis, CV Mosby, 1998.
30. Cushner F, Friedman RJ: Economic impact of total hip arthroplasty. *South Med J* 81:1379, 1988.
31. Thomas BJ, Saa J, Lane JM: Total hip arthroplasty. *Curr Opin Rheumatol* 8:148, 1996.
32. Shaw JA, Greer RB: Complications of total hip replacement. In Epps CH Jr (ed): *Complications in Orthopedic Surgery,* 3rd ed. Philadelphia, JB Lippincott, 1994.
33. Birge SJ: Osteoporosis and hip fracture. *Clin Geriatr Med* 9:69, 1993.
34. Clayer MT, Bauze RJ: Morbidity and mortality following fractures of the femoral neck and trochanteric region: Analysis of risk factors. *J Trauma* 29:1673, 1989.
35. Ahmad LA, Eckhof DG, Kramer AM: Outcome studies of hip fractures: A functional viewpoint. *Orthop Rev* 23:19, 1994.
36. De Boeck H: Classification of hip fractures. *Acta Orthop Belg* 60(Suppl 1):106, 1994.
37. Kovall KJ, Zuckerman JD: Hip fractures II: Evaluation and treatment of intertrochanteric fractures. *J Am Acad Orthop Surg* 2:150, 1994.
38. Sernbo I, et al: Unstable trochanteric fractures of the hip: Treatment with Ender pins, compared with a compression hip-screw. *J Bone Joint Surg Am* 70:1297, 1988.

39. Davis TRC, et al: Intertrochanteric femoral fractures: Mechanical failure after internal fixation. *J Bone Joint Surg Br* 72:26, 1990.

40. Russell TA, Taylor JC: Subtrochanteric fractures of the femur. In Browner BD, et al (eds): *Skeletal Trauma.* Philadelphia, WB Saunders, 1992.

41. Bajaj HN, Kumar B, Chacko V: Subtrochanteric fractures of the femur—an analysis of results of operative and non-operative management. *Injury* 19:169, 1988.

42. Velasco RU, Comfort TH: Analysis of treatment problems in subtrochanteric fractures. *J Trauma* 18:513, 1978.

43. Arneson TJ, et al: Epidemiology of diaphyseal and distal femoral fractures in Rochester, Minnesota, 1965-1984. Clin Orthop 234:188, 1988.

44. Kluger Y, et al: Blunt vascular injury associated with closed mid-shaft femur fracture: A plea for concern. *J Trauma* 36:222, 1994.

45. Taylor MT, Banerjee B, Alpar EK: Injuries associated with a fractured shaft of the femur. *Injury* 25:185, 1994.

46. Hofeldt F: Proximal femoral fractures. *Clin Orthop* 218:12, 1987.

47. Chalmers J, Irvine GB: Fractures of the femoral neck in elderly patients. *Clin Orthop* 229:125, 1988.

48. Bucholz RW, Brumback RJ: Fractures of the shaft of the femur. In Rockwood JC Jr, Green DP, Bucholz RW (eds): *Rockwood and Green's Fractures in Adults,* vol 2, 4th ed. Philadelphia, JB Lippincott, 1996.

49. Blecher A: Über den Einfluß des Parademarsches auf der Entstehung der Fußgeschwulst. *Med Klin* 1:305, 1905.

50. Clement DB, et al: Exercise-induced stress injuries to the femur. *Int J Sports Med* 14:347, 1993.

51. Leung KS, et al: Treatment of ipsilateral femoral shaft fractures and hip fractures. *Injury* 24:41, 1993.

52. Hak DJ, Goulet JA: Severity of injuries associated with traumatic hip dislocation as a result of motor vehicle collisions. *J Trauma* 47:60, 1999.

53. Morey BF: Instability after total hip arthroplasty. *Orthop Clin North Am* 23:237, 1992.

54. Ferguson KL, Harris V: Inferior hip dislocation in an adult: Does a rare injury now have a common mechanism? *Am J Emerg Med* 16:117, 2000.

55. Sanville P, Nicholson DA, Driscoll PA: The hip: ABC of emergency radiology. *BMJ* 308:524, 1994.

56. Bassett LW, Gold RH, Epstein HC: Anterior hip dislocation: Atypical superolateral displacement of the femoral head. *AJR Am J Roentgenol* 141:385, 1983.

57. Hougaard K, Thomsen PB: Traumatic posterior fracture-dislocation of the hip with fracture of the femoral head or neck, or both. *J Bone Joint Surg Am* 70:233, 1988.

58. Dreinhofer KE, et al: Isolated traumatic dislocation of the hip. *J Bone Joint Surg Br* 76:6, 1994.

59. Hillyard RF, Fox J: Sciatic nerve injuries associated with traumatic posterior hip dislocation. *Am J Emerg Med* 21:545, 2003.

60. Stefanich RJ: Closed reduction of posterior hip dislocation: The Rochester method. *Am J Orthop* 28:401, 1999.

61. Dahner LE, Hundley JD: Reduction of posterior hip dislocations in the lateral position using traction-countertraction: Safer for the surgeon? *J Orthop Trauma* 13:373, 1999.

62. Potter HG, et al: MR imaging of acetabular fractures: Value of detecting femoral head injury, intraarticular fragments, and sciatic nerve injury. *AJR Am J Roentgenol* 163:881, 1994.

63. National Institutes of Health: Total hip replacement. NIH consensus statement online, 12:1, 1999.

64. Yuan L, Shih C: Dislocation after total hip arthroplasty. *Arch Orthop Trauma Surg* 119:263, 1999.

65. Young JL, Laskowski ER, Rock MG: Thigh injuries in athletes. *Mayo Clin Proc* 68:1099, 1993.

66. Renstrom AFH: Tendon and muscle injuries in the groin area. *Clin Sports Med* 11:815, 1992.

67. Barr H, Santes G, Stephenson I: Occult femoral artery injury in relation to fractures of the femoral shaft. *J Cardiovasc Surg* 28:193, 1987.

68. Austin OMB, et al: Vascular trauma—a review. *J Am Coll Surg* 181:91, 1995.

69. Frykberg ER, et al: The reliability of physical examination in the evaluation of penetrating extremity trauma for vascular injury: Results at one year. *J Trauma* 31:502, 1991.

70. D'Amelio LF, Musser DJ, Rhodes M: Bilateral femoral nerve neuropathy following blunt trauma. *J Neurosurg* 73:630, 1990.

71. Sunderland S, et al: Repair of a transected sciatic nerve. *J Bone Joint Surg Am* 75:911, 1993.

72. Rockwood JC Jr, Green DP, Bucholz RW (eds): *Rockwood and Green's Fractures in Children,* vol 3, 4th ed. Philadelphia, JB Lippincott, 1996.

73. Dalton HJ, et al: Undiagnosed abuse in children younger than 3 years with femoral fracture. *Am J Dis Child* 144:875, 1990.

74. Azouz EM, et al: Types and complications of femoral neck fractures in children. *Pediatr Radiol* 23:415, 1993.

75. Hughes LO, Beaty JH: Fractures of the head and neck of the femur in children. *J Bone Joint Surg Am* 76:283, 1994.

76. Kermond S, et al: A randomized clinical trial: Should the child with transient synovitis of the hip be treated with non-steroidal anti-inflammatory drugs? *Ann Emerg Med* 40:294, 2002.

77. Kocher MS, Zurakowski D, Kasser JR: Differentiating between septic arthritis and transient synovitis of the hip in children: An evidence-based clinical prediction algorithm. *J Bone Joint Surg Am* 81:1662, 1999.

78. Kocher MS, et al: Validation of a clinical prediction rule for the differentiation between septic arthritis and transient synovitis of the hip in children. *J Bone Joint Surg Am* 86:1629, 2004.

79. Dabney KW, Lipton G: Evaluation of limp in children. *Curr Opin Pediatr* 7:88, 1995.

80. Dressler F: Infectious diseases affecting the musculoskeletal system in children and adolescents. *Curr Opin Rheumatol* 5:651, 1993.

81. Dagan R: Management of acute hematogenous osteomyelitis and septic arthritis in the pediatric patient. *Pediatr Infect Dis J* 12:88, 1993.

82. Betz RR, et al: Late sequelae of septic arthritis of the hip in infancy and childhood. *J Pediatr Orthop* 10:365, 1990.

83. Perron AD, Miller MD, Brady WJ: Orthopedic pitfalls in the emergency department: Slipped capital femoral epiphysis. *Am J Emerg Med* 20:484, 2002.

84. Kelsey JL: The incidence of slipped capital femoral epiphysis in Connecticut. *J Chronic Dis* 23:567, 1997.

85. Canale ST, King RE: Fractures of the hip. In Rockwood CA Jr, Wilkins KE, King RE (eds): *Rockwood and Green's Fractures in Children,* vol 3, 3rd ed. Philadelphia, JB Lippincott, 1991.

86. Ankarath S, et al: Delay in the diagnosis of slipped capital femoral epiphysis *J R Soc Med* 95:356, 2002.

87. Lang P, Genant HK, Jergesen HE: Imaging of the hip joint: Computed tomography versus magnetic resonance imaging. *Clin Orthop* 274:135, 1992.

88. McErlean MA: The child with a limp. In Graff J (ed): *Critical Decisions in Emergency Medicine.* Irving, Tex, ACEP, 2004, 18:1-10.

89. Poston HL: Traction fracture of the lesser trochanter of the femur. *Br J Surg* 9:256, 1921-1922.

54 Knee and Lower Leg

Everett Lyn, Daniel Pallin, and Robert E. Antosia

KNEE

PERSPECTIVE

More than 1 million patients are seen annually in North American emergency departments with complaints of acute knee injuries.[1] Injuries range from simple contusions to complete dislocations, which are true limb-threatening emergencies. The knee is the largest and most complicated joint in the body. Motion at the knee is a complex interaction of flexion, extension, rotation, gliding, and rolling. The knee joins the two longest mechanical levers in the body, the thigh and lower leg. The knee is subject to high forces during ambulation, sports, and blunt trauma and is a frequent site of acute or chronic injury. The knee joint also comprises an enormous synovial space and is frequently involved in infectious or autoimmune inflammatory conditions, ranging from septic arthritis to serum sickness.

PRINCIPLES OF DISEASE: ANATOMY AND PATHOPHYSIOLOGY

The knee is a modified-hinge diarthrodial synovial joint that consists of the tibiofemoral and patellofemoral joints. The distal femur, proximal tibia, and patella compose the bony articulation. The head of the fibula, although not part of this articulation, is closely approximated laterally and provides a site for the attachment of muscles and ligaments. Joint stability is provided by the capsule, ligaments, and surrounding muscles; however, the stability mainly depends on the integrity of the ligamentous structures (Figure 54-1).

The distal femur terminates in the medial and lateral condyles. The V-shaped femoral trochlea between them articulates with the patella. Small protuberances arise from each of the condyles and are called *epicondyles*. The medial and lateral epicondyles serve as important sites of origin for the medial collateral ligament (MCL) and lateral collateral ligament (LCL). The femoral condyles articulate with the superior surface of the tibia and the corresponding medial and lateral tibial condyles. Within the joint, medial and lateral menisci are interposed between the femoral and tibial condyles, providing a form of shock absorption. The cruciate ligaments are located in the intercondylar notch.

Functionally the knee joint can be divided into three compartments: patellofemoral, medial tibiofemoral,

and lateral tibiofemoral. These compartments, defined anatomically by the articulation of the bones, are contained within the same joint capsule. The patellofemoral compartment, located anteriorly, contains the quadriceps tendon, which envelops the patella, continues inferiorly as the patellar tendon, and terminates on the tibial tubercle. The fibers of the medial and lateral retinacula are found on either side of the patella, originating from the vastus medialis and vastus lateralis. The medial and lateral patella retinacula also are called *extensor retinacula*. Normally the patella glides in a rotational manner that increases the mechanical advantage of the quadriceps tendon. The quadriceps tendon is a continuation of the quadriceps femoris muscle, which consists of the rectus femoris, vastus medialis, vastus lateralis, and vastus intermedius, comprising the important extensor structures of the knee. Improper function or weakness may lead to patellar malalignment, which may manifest clinically by the development of chondromalacia patella and peripatellar pain.[2]

The medial tibiofemoral compartment is located on the medial aspect of the knee and consists of the medial femoral condyle, concave medial tibial condyle (plateau), medial meniscus, MCL, adductor tubercle, and pes anserinus. The *pes anserinus* (meaning "goose foot") is a three-pronged tendinous structure that is the conjoined insertion of the sartorius, semitendinosus, and gracilis muscles. The lateral tibiofemoral compartment encompasses the lateral half of the knee joint and includes the lateral femoral condyle and epicondyle, lateral tibial condyle (plateau), LCL, lateral meniscus, and popliteus tendon. The fibular head can be palpated posterolaterally and inferiorly to the joint line but is not usually considered a structure of the lateral tibiofemoral compartment.

There is no complete, independent fibrous capsule uniting the bone. Instead a thick ligamentous sheath constructed largely of tendons or expansions from them surrounds the knee joint. The capsule of the knee joint is reinforced at multiple sites: anteriorly, by the ligamentum patella; medially and laterally, by the medial and lateral patellar retinacula; and posterolaterally, by a combination of structures referred to as the *posterolateral corner*. The posterolateral corner includes the iliotibial band, biceps femoris, fibular collateral ligament, popliteus complex (tendon, tibial attachment, popliteofibular ligament, lateral meniscal attachments), arcuate complex, fabellofibular ligament, capsular ligament, and joint capsule. The popliteofibular ligament has been identified as an important contributor to pos-

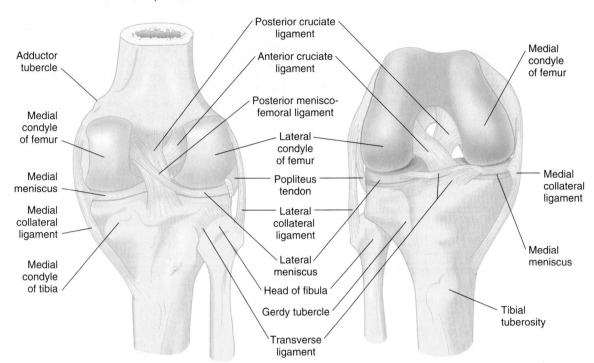

In extension: posterior view

In flexion: anterior view

Figure 54-1. Anterior and posterior views of the right knee.

terolateral stability. The synovial capsule of the knee works in unison with the ligamentous structures in strengthening the knee. The capsule communicates with the suprapatellar bursa, which expands in conditions that cause knee effusion. Although the prepatellar bursa does not communicate with the joint space, prepatellar bursitis frequently is confused with a septic knee joint.

The popliteal fossa is a rhomboid hollow in the posterior aspect of the knee. It is bounded by the biceps femoris laterally, the semimembranosus and semitendinosus muscles medially, and the two heads of the gastrocnemius muscle inferiorly. Found within the popliteal space are the popliteal artery, the popliteal vein, and the peroneal and tibial nerves. Pathologic conditions localized to this area include popliteal cysts and traumatic injuries to the neurovascular structures within the fossa.

The popliteal artery is found deep within the popliteal fossa and represents the direct continuation of the femoral artery beyond the adductor hiatus. The popliteal artery descends across the posterior aspect of the knee joint and terminates at the level of the tibial tubercle, where it divides into the anterior and posterior tibial arteries. The popliteal artery is anchored firmly at the proximal and distal ends of the popliteal fossa, which explains the high incidence of arterial injury with knee dislocations. Blood supply to the knee joint comes from the popliteal artery via the geniculate arteries. Branches of the geniculate arteries interconnect with other vessels, forming a complex anastomosis around the knee. The circumflex fibular artery is a branch from the anterior tibial artery and is the main

blood supply to the head of the fibula. Blood supply to the head of the tibia is derived in part from two branches of the anterior tibial artery: the anterior and posterior recurrent tibial arteries.

The tibial nerve, along with one of its branches, the common peroneal nerve, is responsible for innervation of the knee. The tibial nerve joins the artery and vein in the popliteal fossa. It is not tethered proximally and seems to be injured less often than the popliteal artery. The common peroneal nerve wraps around the head of the fibula and continues inferiorly as the deep and superficial peroneal nerves. Common peroneal nerve injury may occur in association with injury to the fibula head or due to prolonged compression of the lateral aspect of the knee joint. This causes footdrop, in which dorsiflexion strength at the ankle is reduced.

Knee and leg fractures are commonly treated with immobilization. A 19% risk of deep venous thrombosis has been seen with immobilization. Prophylactic treatment with low-molecular-weight heparin reduced this risk to 9%.[3]

CLINICAL FEATURES

Presentation

When a patient complains of a painful knee, the differential diagnosis must include the hip and lumbar nerve roots. This is especially true in children, in whom problems such as a septic hip or slipped capital femoral epiphysis commonly present as knee pain. A swollen knee may result from infection, hemarthrosis, or inflammatory arthritis, and arthrocentesis is commonly required for diagnosis.

In the case of traumatic knee injury, mechanism of injury is more important than any other single piece of information in arriving at a correct diagnosis.[4] By noting the position of the body at the time of injury and the likely forces, predictable patterns of injury are found. High-energy trauma without knee swelling should raise the suspicion of disruption of the joint capsule with expulsion of joint fluid and hemorrhage into the thigh or lower leg. Lower energy injuries are more commonly associated with meniscal tears, patella dislocations, and less severe ligament injuries; in particular, activities with twisting and turning are associated with anterior cruciate tears and meniscal pathology. Immediate deformity, hemarthrosis, or instability suggests intra-articular fracture, major ligamentous injury, or vascular injury. In contrast, a torn meniscus may cause an acutely locked knee, but more commonly has delayed onset of swelling over 12 to 24 hours and intermittent locking associated with joint line pain.

Locking of the knee is a symptom in which there is inability to extend the joint fully. It typically results from either a meniscal tear or a loose body catching in the joint and preventing full extension. A complaint of "giving way" may indicate instability or involuntary muscle inhibition secondary to pain. This is a nonspecific symptom and may be reported in association with arthritis or patellofemoral disorders when inhibition of quadriceps function occurs in association with episodic pain. Although pain remains a helpful indicator of injury, its absence should not be interpreted as proof that only minor injury is present. Partial ligamentous tears may be painful, whereas complete tears may not be because the completely disrupted ligament has no tension across the injured fibers.

Physical Examination

Proper examination of the knee requires the patient to be supine on a stretcher with both legs exposed. The evaluation should begin with an assessment of the neurovascular integrity of the foot. The question of whether knee pain might be the result of hip or spine pathology should be raised early. Examination of the knee begins with visual inspection (Box 54-1). Any obvious deformity, swelling, effusion, or ecchymosis should be noted. Localized swelling must be distinguished from the presence of a joint effusion, which may obliterate the normal contour of the knee. If a large effusion is present, the patella is elevated from the femur by the fluid; ballottement of the patella against the femur is possible by direct pressure on the patella. An effusion also may be shown by tapping the lateral retinaculum with a palpable fluid wave appreciated on the medial side. Loss of the medial peripatellar concavity may be the only sign of a small effusion. A small effusion may be shown by milking the suprapatellar pouch inferiorly to force fluid into the knee joint.

Precise localization of pain helps define the pathology. Palpation is most helpful in localizing the site of

BOX 54-1. Examination of the Knee

1. Outline areas of tenderness.
2. Note whether any effusion is present.
3. Check for range of motion, valgus stress at 0 and 30 degrees of flexion, and varus stress at 0 and 30 degrees of flexion.
4. Evaluate the patellar and extensor mechanism of the knee (quadriceps and patella tendons).
5. Perform Lachman's, anterior drawer, posterior drawer, and pivot shift tests to check for anterolateral rotatory instability and further delineate possible injury to the anterior cruciate ligament.
6. Perform meniscal examination with McMurray's and Apley's tests.

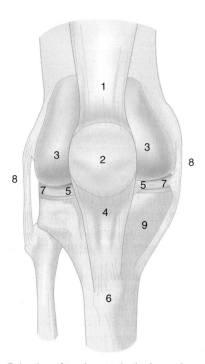

Figure 54-2. Palpation of tenderness in the knee. *1,* quadriceps tendinitis; *2,* prepatella bursitis, patella pain; *3,* retinacular pain after patella subluxation; *4,* patella tendinitis; *5,* fat pad tenderness; *6,* Osgood-Schlatter disease (tibial tubercle pain); *7,* meniscus pain; *8,* collateral ligament pain; *9,* pes anserine tendinitis bursitis. (Adapted from Cailliet R: Knee pain. In *Soft Tissue Pain and Disability*, 3rd ed. Philadelphia, FA Davis, 1976, p 411.)

maximal tenderness (Figure 54-2). In general, it is best to palpate areas of tenderness last because provocation of pain early in the examination may cause anxiety, and the patient may be unable to relax and cooperate fully. In the acute setting, the examination may be limited by the presence of muscle spasm, guarding, and effusion. The patella and the extensor mechanism should be palpated with attention to the superior pole. In the absence of trauma, tenderness localized here is consistent with quadriceps tendinitis. Warmth, erythema, and swelling over the anterior patella may result from prepatellar bursitis. Tenderness along the inferior pole of the patella is seen with peripatellar tendinitis. The insertion of the patellar tendon onto the tibial tubercle should be palpated. Pain at this location in an adolescent is the hallmark of Osgood-Schlatter disease. In an adolescent, pain along the femoral or tibial epiphysis after trauma may represent a nondisplaced fracture through the physis. The joint line should be palpated carefully. Pain along the joint line may indicate meniscal pathology. The posterior aspect of the knee should be examined for fullness, which may indicate a popliteal cyst or popliteal artery pseudoaneursym. Tenderness over the medial or lateral heads of the gastrocnemius may indicate tendinitis or muscle strain.

The range of motion of the knee should be assessed. The knee can be viewed as a hinged joint, with range of motion from slight hyperextension to approximately 135 degrees of flexion. In addition to flexion and extension, complete knee function requires anterior and posterior motion and internal and external rotation. The anatomic arrangement of the knee normally allows the tibia to glide posteriorly and internally rotate about 15 to 30 degrees with knee flexion and move anteriorly and externally rotate with extension. In the extended position, tautness of the ligaments prevents rotary motion. At 90 degrees of flexion, rotation to 40 degrees is possible. Inward rotation is always greater than outward rotation. When range of motion is determined, stability or stress testing should be carried out. Generally the cruciate ligaments provide anteroposterior stability, and medial and lateral stability relies on the joint capsule and collateral ligaments. Range-of-motion evaluation of the knee should include active straight leg raising. Loss of active extension of the knee and inability to maintain the passively extended knee against gravity are the hallmarks of quadriceps and patellar tendon rupture, which otherwise may be clinically occult.

Stability Testing

Stability testing seeks to identify disruption of the connective tissues supporting the knee joint. A progressive decrease in laxity occurs with age.[5] Comparison testing with the opposite knee is necessary because side-to-side differences are more important than absolute laxity. Stability to anterior stress means that the tibia cannot be moved anteriorly relative to the femur, and stability to posterior stress means the opposite. Stability to valgus stress means that the tibia cannot be bent laterally relative to the femur, and stability to varus stress means that the tibia cannot be bent medially. As noted earlier, specific diagnosis of ligamentous or meniscal injury is difficult in the acute setting, and the diagnosis ultimately is made later, during orthopedic follow-up. Nonetheless, familiarity with the standard diagnostic maneuvers is essential.

Anterior Drawer Test

The anterior drawer test is a test for disruption of the anterior cruciate ligament (ACL). A positive test is defined as the ability of the tibia to move forward relative to the femur compared with the other knee. The test is performed with the patient in a supine position,

the hip flexed at 45 degrees, and the knee flexed at 90 degrees. Foot and leg positions are stabilized by sitting on the foot. The examiner determines the amount of step-off between the femoral condyle and the tibial plateau by placing the thumbs over the joint line while exerting a smooth, gentle pull anteriorly on the tibia. The amount of forward displacement is compared with the normal side. The anterior drawer test is not reliable and is of little value in diagnosing acute ACL injuries. It is of more value in a chronic ACL-deficient knee.[6] False-negative findings may occur from an effusion preventing knee flexion to 90 degrees, hamstring muscle spasm caused by pain, or insufficient force applied during performance of the test. A false-positive test can be caused by posterior cruciate ligament (PCL) insufficiency, which allows the tibia to slip back on the femur, showing an abnormal amount of displacement when pulled forward.[7]

Lachman's Test

Since the 1970s, Lachman's test has gained popularity in diagnosing ACL injury; before this, the anterior drawer test was used most often.[8] Lachman's test is currently the best clinical test for determining the integrity of the ACL and one of the only reliably performed tests for a patient with an acute hemarthrosis.[9] Accuracy in diagnosing ACL injury increases from 70% to 99% using Lachman's test rather than the anterior drawer test.[10] The test is especially useful for acute injuries, in which muscle spasm and the presence of an effusion often limit knee flexion. It also minimizes the blocking effect of the posterior horns of the menisci.

Lachman's test is done with the knee flexed 20 to 30 degrees with one hand grasping the thigh and stabilizing it. The tibia is pulled forward with an anteriorly directed force, and the examiner notes tibial excursion. The examiner records "firmness" or a "soft endpoint." The endpoint can be graded as 1+ (0 to 5 mm more displacement than the normal side), 2+ (5 to 10 mm), or 3+ (>10 mm). The tibiofemoral joint should be in a neutral position before manipulation, and the PCL must be intact for the test to be valid. In an acute injury, any difference in translation or the feeling of a soft or indistinct endpoint may indicate a ligament tear. A PCL injury results in a false-positive test as the knee is pulled forward. Potential causes of false-negative tests include hamstring spasm, meniscal tears, and third-degree MCL tears with posterior medial extension. Specific limitations of Lachman's test include difficulty quantitating the amount of anterior translation and inability to limit motion of the femur. In addition, the detection of partial tears of the ACL is problematic and less reliable.[8] Lachman's test also may be difficult to perform if the examiner's hands are small relative to the patient's thigh.

Posterior Drawer Test

The posterior drawer test remains the "gold standard" for evaluating PCL injury. The posterior drawer test can be accomplished with the patient's knee flexed at 90 degrees and the foot stabilized by the examiner's thigh.

A smooth backward force is applied to the tibia. Posterior displacement of the tibia more than 5 mm, or a "soft" endpoint, indicates injury to the PCL. A normal knee should exhibit no significant posterior excursion. The posterior drawer test may be positive in only 85% of patients with PCL insufficiency documented operatively. The phenomenon of an absent or inconclusive posterior drawer test is believed to occur when the mechanism of injury does not stress, strain, or tear the posterolateral corner ligaments (arcuate complex).[11]

Posterior Sag Sign

The posterior sag sign test is a second method of determining PCL integrity. The test can be done as follows. The patient is placed in a supine position, and a pillow is placed under the distal thigh for support while the heel rests on the stretcher. The knee is flexed to either 45 or 90 degrees, depending on which position provides the greatest muscle relaxation. If the tibia sags backward, the test is positive, indicating PCL insufficiency. If the posterior sag sign is not appreciated before the different drawer tests are performed, a false-positive anterior drawer test is misinterpreted as an ACL injury.[7] Posterior sag also may be shown by passive elevation of the leg in a fully extended position, with the examiner applying the elevating force at the ankle. As the leg is elevated, the tibia may fall back on the femur if the PCL is ruptured.

McMurray's Test

McMurray's test is used to identify meniscal tears. The patient is placed in a supine position with the knee hyperflexed. The examiner grasps the lower leg, flexing and extending the knee while simultaneously internally and externally rotating the tibia on the femur with a smooth, firm, controlled movement. A positive test occurs when, with the other hand, a "clicking" sensation is felt along the joint line or the patient experiences pain during internal and external rotation. By twisting the leg into internal rotation, the posterior segment of the lateral meniscus is tested. External rotation tests the posterior segment of the medial meniscus. In the acute setting, limitation of range of motion may not allow sufficient hyperflexion to perform McMurray's test, and the test may be falsely negative.

Apley's Test

Apley's test also aids in diagnosing meniscal tears. With the patient prone, the knee is flexed 90 degrees, and the leg is internally and externally rotated with pressure applied to the heel. Downward pressure eliciting pain suggests meniscal pathology. The pain should be relieved with distraction of the knee and rotation of the leg back to a neutral position.

Pivot Shift

The pivot shift test, also called *subluxation provocation* or the "jerk" test, is performed to detect anterolateral rotatory instability associated with an injury to the ACL or lateral capsular structure. This test must be done carefully, if at all, in the acutely injured knee because the test maneuvers can exacerbate the initial injury. The pivot shift test is performed with the patient supine. The knee is examined in full extension. The tibia is internally rotated with one hand grasping the foot and the other hand applying a mild valgus stress at the level of the knee joint. Then, with flexion of the knee to approximately 20 to 30 degrees, a jerk is suddenly experienced at the anterolateral corner of the proximal tibia. In a positive test, the tibia subluxes when the knee is extended and relocates when it is flexed to 20 to 30 degrees. Grading of the relocation event is as follows: absent (0), rolling (1+), moderate (2+), or momentary locking (3+). Because of pain or spasm, the pivot shift test is unreliable without anesthesia.[6]

Collateral Ligament Stress Test

The collateral ligament stress test is used to test the integrity of the MCL and LCL. The test is performed as follows. With the patient lying supine, the examiner applies varus and valgus stress with the knee at 0 and 30 degrees of flexion. Joint line opening is the amount of movement produced between the tibia and the femur; this can be palpated and estimated in millimeters. The normal knee should be subjected to the same amount of valgus and varus stress and joint line opening compared with the injured knee. Laxity in full extension implies complete collateral ligament tear, with injury to the secondary restraints, such as the ACL, PCL, and posteromedial or posterolateral corners. When the knee is flexed to 30 degrees, the stability provided by the cruciate ligaments to valgus and varus stress is removed. If the knee is stable to valgus stress with the knee in full extension but lax at 30 degrees of flexion, injury is limited to the superficial and deep MCLs. Varus stress at 0 degrees of flexion producing no instability but laxity present at 30 degrees indicates that at least part of the LCL and lateral stability complex has been injured. Laxity may be graded as follows: grade I, some laxity; grade II, marked laxity; and grade III, total laxity.

Instrument Testing

More recent developments have seen the advent of instrument testing to evaluate ACL injury. The arthrometer gives numeric quantitative comparison of ACL laxity of the knee. Studies using commercially available arthrometers indicate that a side-to-side difference exceeding 3 mm anterior displacement at 20 lb is predictive of ACL with 94% accuracy.[12] Reports also indicate that quantitative laxity determination with such instruments can yield prognostic information and may aid clinicians in determining how aggressively to treat ACL injuries. However practical and useful such instruments may be, they have not gained widespread usage or acceptance at present.

DIAGNOSTIC STRATEGIES

Radiographic Evaluation

Plain Radiographs

The traditional standard of care was to obtain antero-posterior and lateral radiographs of the knee in all cases of acute knee trauma. More recent work has led to validation of clinical decision rules that help decrease unnecessary radiography.[13-15] The Ottawa Knee Rule states that radiography is necessary only if any one of five conditions is present: (1) age older than 55 years, (2) inability to transfer weight from one foot to the next four times at the time of injury and in the emergency department, (3) inability to flex the knee to 90 degrees, (4) patellar tenderness with no other bony tenderness, or (5) tenderness of the fibular head. Initial tests found that this rule detected 100% of fractures, while allowing significantly fewer radiographs to be done.[14,16] Similarly the Pittsburgh Knee Rule was found to be 100% sensitive.[17] The Pittsburgh Knee Rule states that radiography is necessary only if the patient fell or sustained blunt trauma to the knee, and either of two conditions is present: (1) age younger than 12 or older than 50 or (2) inability to walk four full weight-bearing steps in the emergency department.

One study compared these two decision rules and found that both had good sensitivity, but that the Pittsburgh rule was more specific, allowing fewer radiographs to be done without sacrificing sensitivity; in this study, the sensitivity of the Ottawa rule was 97% (95% confidence interval, 90% to 99%), and the sensitivity of the Pittsburgh rule was 99% (95% confidence interval, 94% to 100%).[13] Until further work determines the optimal approach, either rule may be used, but patients should be told that there is about a 1% chance of a missed fracture, and they should seek re-evaluation in the event of persistent or progressive symptoms.

One study validated the Ottawa Knee Rule in children older than age 5, finding a sensitivity of 100%. The Ottawa Knee Rule permitted a 31% reduction in the number of radiographic evaluations.[18] In another pediatric study, of 13 fractures, 1 was missed, implying a sensitivity of only 92%, so application of the rule in children still requires clinical judgment.[19]

In another approach, Verma and colleagues[20] recognized that fears of malpractice might limit implementation of decision rules and instead asked whether a single lateral x-ray could replace the traditional three-view "knee series" (anteroposterior, lateral, and tunnel views). These investigators found that a single lateral view could detect 100% of fractures identifiable on the full series.[20] Some clinicians may prefer this more conservative approach until the decision rules are validated further.

Joint space narrowing, as seen in osteoarthritis, is easily discernible on erect standard views. Lateral views may reveal an abnormally low-riding or high-riding patella. Tangential, "sunrise," or "skyline" views are especially good for delineating the patellofemoral joint.[21] Tangential views are useful to assess patella tracking or subluxation. Oblique x-ray studies are particularly useful when tibial plateau fractures are suspected but not seen on routine views.[22] "Tunnel" views, which image the intercondylar notch, are used to detect tibial spine fractures and loose bodies within the notch. Although most ligamentous injuries cannot be diagnosed by plain films, avulsion of the attachment site can be seen occasionally and provides indirect evidence of ligament disruption. Stress radiographs may aid in the diagnosis of collateral ligament disruption but generally are not used in the initial evaluation.

Computed Tomography

Computed tomography (CT) is most useful in detecting and classifying tibial plateau fractures and usually is done when the diagnosis is unclear, or operative intervention is considered.

Ultrasound

Ultrasound is useful in diagnosing several pathologic conditions of the knee. It has gained wide acceptance in the diagnosis of clinically suspected popliteal cyst, which appears as a nonechogenic mass with smooth walls lying medially within the popliteal fossa.[23] Small cysts can lead to false-negative ultrasound results. The popliteal artery is the most common site for peripheral aneurysms, yet the clinical diagnosis can be difficult.[21] Typically the aneurysm occurs just distal to the adductor hiatus in the proximal segment and midsegment of the artery and is bilateral in 50% of cases.[23] Real-time ultrasound is an excellent modality for diagnosing popliteal artery aneurysm and can differentiate aneurysm from cyst.[21]

Contrast Arteriography and Color-Flow Doppler

Contrast arteriography and color-flow Doppler ultrasonography are used to evaluate the arteries of the knee and leg. Traditionally, arteriography was deemed mandatory in all cases of tibiofemoral knee dislocation and in all cases of penetrating trauma in close proximity to major arteries. More recently, serial examination and Doppler scanning have been studied and found to be acceptable alternatives to arteriography in patients with normal distal neurovascular examinations and low-risk mechanisms.[24]

Radionuclide Bone Scan

A radionuclide bone scan can be used to detect osteomyelitis or occult bony injuries, such as stress fractures, osteochondritis dissecans, and avascular necrosis.

Magnetic Resonance Imaging

Double-contrast arthrograms are of primarily historical interest because they have been largely replaced by magnetic resonance imaging (MRI).[21] Arthrography may be performed after prosthetic replacement of the knee to detect loosening. It also may be used if there is a contraindication to MRI, or if MRI is not available.

MRI can be helpful to identify associated injuries to the menisci and articular cartilage when the clinical examination is limited because of pain and swelling. The diagnostic accuracy of MRI in detecting meniscal and capsuloligamentous injuries of the knee is well documented.[25] Although the sensitivity of MRI in identifying ACL injury may be high (90% to 98%), its specificity, particularly in differentiating partial from complete tears, is low (<50% in some series).[26] MRI is extremely sensitive for determining PCL injury; however, the diagnosis usually can be established by history and physical examination. Images with T1 and T2 weighting are required for optimal assessment. Sagittal images are best for evaluating menisci, cruciate ligaments, and articular surfaces; coronal images enable optimal assessment of the collateral ligaments. MRI has proved superior to other imaging modalities in the evaluation of osteonecrosis, osteochondritis dissecans, occult fractures, and bone contusion.[21] Advantages of MRI in evaluating soft tissue injury are that it is noninvasive and painless, and it does not require the use of ionizing radiation. Although MRI is a useful diagnostic tool, because of its high cost and limited availability, it should be used selectively, depending on the specific clinical situation and information desired.

Arthroscopy

The most commonly performed orthopedic surgical procedure in the United States is arthroscopy of the knee.[27] It is useful in diagnosis and treatment of knee injuries, including injuries of the meniscus, cruciate ligaments, articular cartilage, capsule, and synovium. The superior diagnostic accuracy of arthroscopy compared with the clinical knee examination has been well documented. In particular, arthroscopy has increased the accuracy of diagnosis of ACL injuries and small capsular tears. It is especially helpful for children, in whom diagnoses can be difficult because of developing skeletal changes. Difficulties in visualization arise when the capsular structures are tight and when meniscal tears are situated posteriorly. Indications for arthroscopy are situation specific and include drainage of tense hemarthrosis, removal of osteochondral fragments (loose bodies), repair of meniscal tears, and reconstruction of ACLs or PCLs. Rapid rehabilitation and cost savings are two significant advantages over open-knee surgery.

Arthrocentesis

Aspiration of fluid from the knee joint can be diagnostic and therapeutic, although there is no evidence-based support for therapeutic value.[28] Arthrocentesis should be performed if the injured knee is greatly distended with a tight effusion, and when the cause of the joint effusion is unknown. Aspiration of the joint and subsequent analysis can distinguish among hemarthrosis, sympathetic effusion, and septic arthritis. Joint aspiration is diagnostic of fracture if fat globules are present.

Intra-articular injection of morphine and bupivacaine has been used for analgesia after traumatic knee injuries and elective knee arthroscopy. Several studies have shown that although both drugs reduce the need for systemic analgesia, morphine is more effective and can provide relief for 24 hours.[29] The typical dose is 1 to 5 mg (1 mg/mL diluted in normal saline solution to a total volume of 30 mL). Evidence suggests that analgesia is mediated by local action within the joint.

MECHANISMS OF INJURY AND MANAGEMENT

Distal Femur Fractures

Anatomy and Pathophysiology

Distal femur fractures compose approximately 4% of all femoral fractures.[30] The mechanism of injury is often related to motor vehicle accidents or significant falls in which the force of impact is severe. An isolated fracture of the femoral condyle may occur, or the fracture may extend in a T or Y pattern to include the intercondylar or supracondylar region of the femur. Condylar fractures are intra-articular and may result in knee joint incongruity.

Clinical Features

Patients with condylar or intercondylar fractures have pain and swelling in the distal femur and suprapatella region and are often unable to bear weight. Examination may reveal shortening, rotation, and angulation of the extremity and tenderness to palpation along the medial or lateral joint line. Acute hemarthrosis is common and may be secondary to intra-articular extension of the fracture or associated ligamentous injury. Careful assessment of the circulation and motor function of the limb should be documented. Any soft tissue defect in the region of the fracture is considered to be an open fracture until proved otherwise.

Diagnostic Strategies

The diagnosis of a distal femoral fracture is made from radiographs. Routine anteroposterior and lateral radiographs should be obtained and usually show the fracture pattern and any significant displacement of fragments. In high-energy injuries, radiographs of the ipsilateral hip and tibia are required to exclude associated fractures. Occasionally, CT or MRI may be required to diagnose a nondisplaced fracture. If signs of vascular impairment are present, an arteriogram should be obtained promptly when surgical exploration is not being considered.

Management

After the initial examination, the leg should be splinted to prevent excessive motion of the fracture site. Early orthopedic consultation is prudent. In a stable patient with an uncomplicated fracture, reduction may be done with skeletal traction followed by immobilization with a hinged fracture brace. If any degree of joint incongruity is detected on radiographs, the fracture should be treated with open reduction and internal fixation. Fractures of the distal femur are often difficult to fix securely because they must withstand forces from weight bearing and knee motion. Operative techniques include use of multiple fixation screws or a sliding compression screw with side plate, depending on the clinical circumstances and the preference of the orthopedic surgeon. Distal femoral fractures may be associated with several significant complications, including thrombophlebitis; fat embolus syndrome; delayed union or malunion if reduction is incomplete or not maintained; intra-articular or quadriceps adhesions if the fracture is intra-articular; angulation deformities; and osteoarthritis, particularly affecting the patellofemoral articulation.

Proximal Intra-articular Tibial Fractures

Proximal intra-articular tibial fractures include condylar or plateau injuries, epiphyseal fractures, and fractures of the tibial spine. Extra-articular fractures are discussed in the section on the lower leg.

Tibial Plateau Fractures

Anatomy and Pathophysiology

The proximal end of the tibia is expanded into the medial and lateral condyles, the former having the greater surface of the two. Together they make up approximately three quarters of the proximal tibial surface, and their integrity is important for normal knee alignment, stability, and motion. The plateau normally slopes 10 degrees from anterior to posterior; on a straight anteroposterior view, the anterior and posterior portions of the plateau may not appear to be at the same level. In addition, the lateral plateau is slightly convex upward, whereas the medial is slightly concave upward.[22]

Tibial plateau fractures represent 1% of all fractures and 8% of fractures in the elderly.[30] Tibial plateau fractures are intra-articular and result in loss of joint congruity. The forces that normally act on the tibial condyles include axial compression and rotation. The most common mechanism of injury is a strong valgus force with axial loading.[30] Severe high-energy tibial plateau fractures occur primarily in younger age groups and are often the result of motor vehicle accidents or falls from heights.[30] These fractures occur in concert with many other injuries and may be open. Fatigue stress fractures of the tibial plateau occur mostly in elderly persons. These low-energy fractures are the result of compression forces in osteoporotic bones.

Tibial plateau fractures encompass many differing degrees of articular depression and displacement. Because the initial injury is usually a valgus stress with an abduction force on the leg, 55% to 70% of condylar fractures involve the lateral plateau. Medial plateau fractures typically result from adduction forces on the distal leg and account for 10% to 23% of these frac-

tures; both plateaus are involved 11% to 31% of the time.[30] If the knee is extended at the time of injury, the fracture tends to be anterior. Posterior condylar fractures usually occur when the knee is flexed at the time of impact.

The Segond fracture represents a bony avulsion of the lateral tibial plateau. The avulsion occurs at the site of attachment of the lateral capsular ligament. It appears as an oval-shaped fragment adjacent to the lateral tibial plateau and must be differentiated from an avulsion from the adjacent fibular styloid. The Segond fracture is an important marker of ACL disruption and anterolateral rotary instability.[31] Most Segond fractures are caused by sports injuries, and the mechanism is almost always knee flexion with excessive internal rotation and varus stress. Segond fractures can be detected on radiographs (lateral capsule sign) and, when seen, must be regarded as a strong indication that ligament rupture has occurred, and surgical repair may be needed (Figure 54-3).[31]

Clinical Features

Clinical signs of knee fractures are the presence of an effusion, inability to bear weight, severe joint line tenderness, ecchymosis, and localized soft tissue swelling and pain. Acute hemarthrosis, presenting with decreased range of motion, is the most sensitive pre-

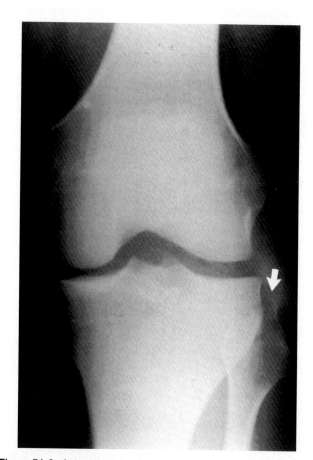

Figure 54-3. Anteroposterior view of the left knee shows lateral curvilinear avulsion fracture *(arrow)* and joint effusion. (From Kerr HD: Segond fracture, hemarthrosis, and anterior cruciate ligament disruption. *J Emerg Med* 8:29, 1990.)

dictor of a knee fracture.[32,33] These findings are not specific for fracture, however, because they are often seen with ligament tears. Tenderness is present over the fracture, but also may be found near torn collateral ligaments. A valgus or varus limb deformity may be present and usually indicates a depressed fracture or concomitant ipsilateral leg fracture. The most important aspect of the initial examination is the neurovascular status. Tibial plateau fractures produce a high percentage of vascular complications. The popliteal artery is immobile in this region and branches into the anterior and posterior tibial artery at the upper edge of the interosseous membrane. The popliteal artery may be injured by fragments from bicondylar or comminuted fractures involving the subcondylar area. Vascular impairment may result in distal circulatory compromise. Displaced fractures of the lateral condyle may produce peroneal nerve paralysis in addition to injury to the anterior tibial artery. Stretch of the peroneal nerve is the usual cause of injury.

Soft tissue injuries also may involve the capsuloligamentous structures of the knee. Ligamentous injuries accompany tibial plateau fractures in 20% to 25% of cases, most often involving the ACL and MCL.[34,35] Although ligament injuries can occur with any type of tibial plateau fracture, they occur more commonly with local compression and split compression fractures (Figure 54-4).[35]

Treatment of ligament injuries associated with tibial plateau fractures is controversial. There is no general consensus that the repair of associated ligament injuries at the time of fracture fixation is necessary or improves late instability after these fractures. Cruciate ligament injuries associated with tibial plateau fractures have an increased incidence of late traumatic arthritis and a poor prognosis.[35] Regardless of the type of treatment, operative or nonoperative, tibial plateau fractures with significant residual laxity fare poorly compared with stable fractures.[35]

Most authors agree that four factors determine the prognosis of tibial plateau fractures: (1) degree of articular depression, (2) extent and separation of the condylar fracture lines, (3) diaphyseal-metaphyseal comminution and dissociation, and (4) integrity of the soft tissue envelope (i.e., open versus closed). Fractures of the tibial plateau generally have a good prognosis, with good to excellent results having been found in 90% of patients more than 20 years after injury; however, high-energy tibial plateau fractures generally have a more guarded prognosis.[36] In high-energy fractures, a large degree of articular depression, multiple displaced condylar fracture lines, and diaphyseal-metaphyseal extension and comminution in association with open injuries or an extensive internal degloving injury may occur and are poor prognostic signs.[37]

Diagnostic Strategies

A plateau fracture is usually evident on routine anteroposterior and lateral radiographs. At times, however, the fracture itself may be difficult to identify on routine radiographs. In such cases, the presence of a fat-fluid

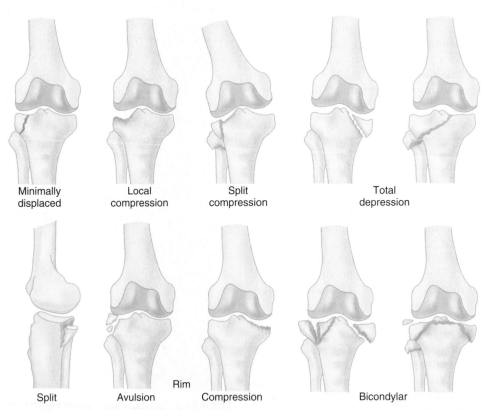

Figure 54-4. Hohl's revised classification of tibial plateau fractures: minimally displaced (22%), local compression (28%), split compression (18%), total compression (13%), split (3%), rim avulsion or compression (5%), and bicondylar (11%). (Modified from Watson JT, Wiss AA: Fractures of the proximal tibia and fibula. In Rockwood CA Jr, Green DP [eds]: *Fractures,* vol 3, 5th ed. Philadelphia, JB Lippincott, 2001.)

level on a "cross-table" lateral radiograph is highly suggestive of an occult fracture; it is believed that the observed fat originates from the bone marrow. Because of the normal contour of the tibial plateau, oblique films usually are required to see a subtle fracture line and for more complete assessment of obvious fractures. All knee radiographs should be examined closely for bony avulsion fragments from the fibular head, femoral condyles, and intercondylar eminence because these may indicate ligamentous injury. Widened joint spaces associated with a fracture of the opposite condyle also may indicate concomitant ligamentous injury.

Tomograms, CT, or MRI may be required in certain clinical situations, particularly nondisplaced or severely comminuted fractures. These studies are more sensitive than plain radiographs, help localize occult lesions, and help quantify the amount of depression in displaced fractures and the extent of articular surface involvement in comminuted fractures.[38] Bone scans also may help detect occult compression fractures.

Several classification systems have been proposed. Most classification systems depend on the mechanism of injury (i.e., the location and force with which the femoral condyle is driven into the plateau). The revised Hohl classification is in common, although not universal, use.[30] As shown in Figure 54-4, this system divides the plateau fractures into two categories: minimally displaced (<4 mm depression or displacement) and displaced. Displaced fractures are subdivided into six distinct types: local compression, split compression, total depression, splint, rim, and bicondylar.

Management

As a rule, accurate reduction and prolonged non–weight bearing are the guidelines to be followed in tibial condylar fractures. The four most common treatment modalities are compression dressing, closed reduction and casting, skeletal traction, and open reduction with internal fixation. Regardless of which treatment is selected, the therapeutic goals include precise reconstruction of the articular surfaces, stable fragment fixation, and early knee motion to prevent stiffness. Weight bearing is generally delayed until healing is complete, usually 6 to 8 weeks.

Consensus on the treatment of tibial plateau fractures is not completely uniform. Conservative treatment is acceptable in stable nondisplaced and stable bicondylar fractures. If displacement is minimal, and there is no significant disruption of the articular surface, initial management with a long leg cast or immobilizer is acceptable. In general, with more severely depressed fractures, operative treatment has better results than nonoperative therapy; however, no universal agreement exists on the acceptable amount of articular depression. Ranges from 4 to 10 mm have been described as tolerable. A long-term study with more than 20 years' follow-up indicates a lack of correlation between residual osseous depression of the joint surface and the development of arthrosis.[37] If the joint deformity or depression is significant enough to

produce joint instability, it is predictive of a poor result.[30] All authors agree that a depressed intra-articular surface will not reconstitute itself if treated by traction alone. Significantly depressed plateau surfaces require surgical elevation and support with bone graft.

Early complications of tibial plateau fractures include wound infection, loss of reduction, and development of compartment syndrome. Compartment syndromes most commonly occur with high-energy fractures, typically within the first 24 to 48 hours after injury. Deep vein thrombosis also may occur. The most common late complication is the development of osteoarthritis in the affected compartment.

Fractures of the Intercondylar Eminence (Tibial Spine)

Anatomy and Pathophysiology

The intercondylar eminence, or tibial spine, is the central portion of the proximal tibial surface. The spine has two prominences: the medial and lateral tubercles. The medial tubercle is larger and located more anteriorly than the lateral tubercle. The ACL and the anterior horns of the medial and the lateral menisci attach in the anterior intercondylar fossa. The PCL and the posterior horns of the menisci attach in the posterior intercondylar fossa.

Fractures of the intercondylar eminence (tibial spine) are commonly seen in children and adolescents, but a study suggests that these fractures occur more commonly in adults than previously thought.[38] Of cases previously reported in the literature, 40% of tibial spine fractures occurred in adults, and 60% occurred in children.[39] The injury is more common in children than adults because the ligaments are stronger than the adjacent physeal plates in the immature skeleton. A fracture of the anterior tibial spine in children is the equivalent of an ACL rupture in adults.

Most tibial spine and intercondylar eminence fractures occur as the result of violent knee twisting, hyperflexion, hyperextension, or valgus-varus forces generated during motor vehicle accidents or athletic activities. The tibial spines are fractured by twisting knee movements, whereas hyperextension or hyperflexion forces may cause avulsion of the intercondylar eminence or of the cruciate ligaments from their tibial attachments.[40]

Clinical Features

After tibial spine or intercondylar eminence fracture, the patient complains of pain and swelling of the knee and may be unable to bear weight on the affected extremity. Examination confirms acute hemarthrosis and may reveal a block to full knee extension. Tense effusion may limit range of motion, hinder physical examination, and mask ligament disruption. Definite ACL laxity is associated with this injury, and patients may exhibit an anterior drawer sign, positive Lachman's test, or other signs of ligamentous laxity. In the presence of open physes, tibial spine fractures are usually isolated injuries. Adults are more likely to have

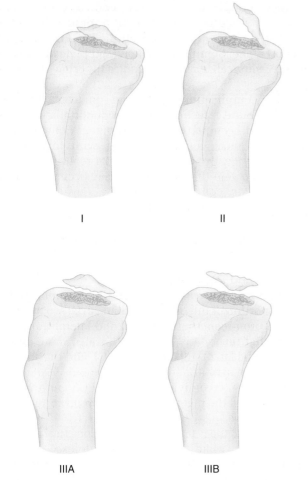

Figure 54-5. Tibial eminence fracture classification. Type I, fracture elevated anteriorly only slightly; type II, anterior fracture fragment elevated with only minimal posterior attachment; type IIIA, fracture fragment completely separated from tibia; type IIIB, fracture fragment completely separated and rotated. (Modified from Meyers M, McKeever F: Fractures of the intercondylar eminence of the tibia. *J Bone Joint Surg* 41:209, 1959.)

an associated tear of the MCL or associated intra-articular fracture and have a worse prognosis.[38]

Diagnostic Strategies

Radiographic evaluation should include standard anteroposterior and lateral views, but a tunnel view provides a clearer look at the intercondylar area and may be necessary to confirm the diagnosis.[22] Joint margins should be examined closely for evidence of collateral or capsular bony avulsions. Tomograms or CT scans sometimes are required to show the location and displacement of the fracture. The fabella is an inconsistent sesamoid bone located in the lateral head of the gastrocnemius muscle. It should not be mistaken for an intra-articular loose body or fracture fragment. The classification of tibial spine fractures is based on the degree of displacement (Figure 54-5). Type I involves incomplete avulsion of the tibial spine without displacement. In type II, there is an incomplete avulsion with minimal displacement of the anterior third of the fracture fragment, but the posterior portion remains adherent. Type III is characterized by complete separa-

tion of the fragment from its fracture bed and has a higher associated rate of collateral ligament injuries and peripheral meniscal tears.[39] Type III may be subdivided into type IIIA, fractures with complete displacement, and type IIIB, fractures with displacement and rotation (see Figure 54-5).

Arthroscopy is useful for diagnosis and treatment of tibial spine fractures. Arthroscopy allows drainage of tense hemarthrosis and enables precise diagnosis and classification, especially for children, in whom the diagnosis can be difficult because of developing skeletal changes.

Management

Conservative treatment is effective for all type I injuries. Nondisplaced or incomplete tibial spine fractures generally heal well when treated with cast immobilization in full extension for approximately 6 weeks. Type I and II fractures may require arthroscopy for lavage and accurate classification. If satisfactory closed reduction cannot be obtained or there is associated ligamentous injury, open or arthroscopic reduction and internal fixation should be performed. To restore normal function of the ACL, displaced or rotated fragments must be reduced. Type III fractures usually require arthroscopic or open reduction; screws and tension band wiring techniques have yielded excellent results.[30] Most uncomplicated fractures of the tibial spine have good results when the fracture heals and restores function to the avulsed ACL. A poor outcome, with residual pain and instability, may be associated with additional intra-articular fractures and damage to the MCL.[40]

Epiphyseal Fractures

Anatomy and Pathophysiology

The physes, which occur at the end of the long bones, are primarily responsible for longitudinal growth through the process of endochondral ossification. The proximal tibia and distal femoral epiphyses are examples of pressure epiphyses and are the largest two in the body. From birth to skeletal maturity, the distal femoral growth plate contributes 70% of the growth of the femur and 37% of the growth of the lower extremity.[41] Likewise, the upper tibial epiphysis accounts for most of the long growth of the tibia.

Biomechanical data and clinical studies in children and adolescents have confirmed that the ligaments and articular capsule are firmer than the bone and epiphyseal plate.[42] As a result, trauma to this region of the maturing skeleton usually injures the cartilaginous epiphyseal plate. In this way, the physis protects the joint surface from the grossly comminuted fractures seen in adults.

Despite data showing that the physis is the weakest link in the immature skeletal unit, only 15% to 20% of all fractures in children occur through the growth plate.[43] The physes of the upper extremities are reported to be involved more often than the physes of the lower extremity, in a ratio of 3:1.[44] Epiphyseal fractures about the knee are even less common, with distal femur epiphyseal separations accounting for only 9% and proximal tibial epiphyseal fractures only 4% of lower extremity epiphyseal fractures.[45]

The proximal tibial physis is far more resistant than other physes as a result of the unique anatomic features of this site.[41] The proximal tibial physis has no significant attachments to the collateral ligaments of the knee. The LCL inserts into the head of the fibula and has no tibial attachment, and the MCL has only a minor attachment to the epiphysis. The major portion of this ligament is attached to the tibial shaft well below the epiphysis. Varus or valgus stress is more likely to injure the distal femoral physis or the tibial metaphysis. Fracture-separation of the distal femoral growth plate and proximal tibial epiphysis is most often caused by an indirect mechanism, commonly related to athletic injuries.[41] The Salter and Harris classification of epiphyseal injuries is described in Chapter 46.

Clinical Features

Epiphyseal injuries should be suspected in a child or adolescent who has juxta-articular (growth plate) tenderness, limps, or refuses to or cannot bear weight. The degree of pain varies, but it is often severe. Depending on the mechanism of injury, the overlying soft tissue may be abraded or lacerated. Swelling is usual in the overlying soft tissue, and an effusion may be present. If the separation is displaced, there may be an angular deformity.

Epiphyseal growth plate fractures in the lower extremity have a high incidence of associated injury. Physeal fractures in the region of the knee may be associated with ligament injuries, especially to the ACL and MCL in half of patients. The most serious injury associated with a proximal tibial physis fracture is neurovascular trauma. In particular, popliteal artery injuries have been associated with these fractures, especially when there is posterolateral or posteromedial displacement. Peroneal nerve injury also has been reported and may range from neurapraxia to complete disruption.[41]

Diagnostic Strategies

Plain radiography remains the primary means for evaluating epiphyseal injuries. Diagnosis is based on epiphyseal displacement, widening of the physis, and obliteration or haziness of the normal sharply defined, fine, sclerotic opposing margins of the metaphysis and epiphysis. The latter may result from angulation at one or both sites. Oblique views may be required to show nondisplaced fractures of the epiphysis. CT or MRI can evaluate more fully or classify injuries that already are established on the basis of plain radiography.

Management

The most common complication of fractures through the proximal tibial physis is growth disturbance.[42] When growth arrest occurs (approximately 1% of cases), it is usually partial and results from a bridge of bone forming from the metaphysis to the epiphysis, crossing the growth plate. Although shortening or deformity is less well tolerated in the lower extremity

because of weight bearing, many of the growth disturbances do not prove clinically significant because of the ability of the immature skeleton to remodel; only 2% or less are reported to be sufficient to interfere with function.[43]

With regard to treatment, important differences exist between fractures in children and fractures in adults. In general, fractures in children heal rapidly. The younger the child, the more rapidly the fracture heals. In newborn infants, callus forms within 1 week after a birth injury. During the first year, callus is established within 2 weeks; callus takes slightly longer to form in toddlers. Fracture modeling also is more extensive in younger children and when the fracture is closer to the end of the bone. Modeling is less perfect in fractures of the mid-diaphysis in older children. Reduction of fractures near the proximal or distal end of the bone need not be perfect.

If a child has juxta-articular tenderness with a negative radiograph, a growth plate injury (Salter-Harris type I) should be assumed. If there is difficulty in deciding whether a line on the radiograph is an epiphyseal line or fracture, a comparison view should be obtained. Because epiphyseal growth centers ossify at different times, this technique of comparing the uninvolved limb is often of great assistance in confirming a suspected physeal injury. In such cases when a physeal injury is suspected, the extremity should be immobilized for approximately 2 weeks and re-evaluated with radiographic study, looking for periosteal new bone or physeal thickening. Generally, emergency management of most epiphyseal fractures of the distal femur or proximal tibia includes ice, elevation, immobilization with a long leg posterior splint, and early orthopedic consultation. Anatomic reduction is desirable for displaced fractures of the distal femur and proximal tibial epiphysis. Open reduction usually is required only for patients in whom closed reduction fails.

Late complications include angular deformity, leg-length discrepancy, stiffness, quadriceps atrophy, and persistent instability of the knee. Delayed union or nonunion is almost never a problem except in a patient with an underlying neuropathy.[41] Because growth inhibition may follow even nondisplaced physeal fractures, long-term orthopedic follow-up is advisable.

Bone Bruise

Bone bruise is a radiographic diagnosis, involving areas of cancellous bone with high signal intensity on MRI fat-suppression sequences. Bone bruise may be present in about half of acutely injured knees.[46] A high proportion of patients with bone bruise have significant soft tissue injury. Nearly all bone bruises resolve after 1 year.[46]

Osteochondritis Dissecans

Osteochondritis dissecans is a rare orthopedic disorder of unknown etiology. The disorder is found mainly in adolescents and results in a segment of articular cartilage and subchondral bone becoming partially or totally separated from the underlying bone. A male predominance (2:1) is reported.[47] It is commonly unilateral, involving the non–weight-bearing lateral aspect of the medial femoral condyle, and it is thought to be related to acute or chronic trauma.[2] Occasionally the lateral femoral condyle or inferior patella pole is involved. Patients often have pain, swelling, and giving-way episodes without a history of trauma. Localized tenderness of the condyle is often the only physical finding. Routine radiographs are usually diagnostic, but occasionally a tunnel view may be needed. The osteochondral fragment appears separated from the condyle by a thin radiolucent line. Tomography may aid in determining the exact location and extent of the osteochondrotic lesion. Bone scanning may be useful in detecting a very early lesion.

The management of these patients is based on the stability of the osteochondral fragment and the maturity of the skeleton.[48] If the epiphyses are open, conservative treatment with protective weight bearing usually results in healing of the lesion. When the epiphyses are closed, the prognosis for healing is guarded. If the fragments are detached, the loose fragments require surgery for removal or fixation. Protected range of motion with non–weight-bearing activity for 6 to 10 weeks is generally advised.

Osteonecrosis

Osteonecrosis occurs when disruption of the blood supply to the bone causes infarction. The knee is a common site of involvement, particularly the weight-bearing surface of the medial femoral condyle.[21] Spontaneous osteonecrosis usually affects middle-aged and elderly patients, whereas secondary osteonecrosis may occur in younger patients related to steroid therapy or in association with sickle cell disease, lupus, or renal transplantation, among many other risk factors.[49] The exact etiology is unknown. The patient often has spontaneous onset of severe localized knee pain that may be accompanied by an effusion and loss of joint motion. The physical examination reveals point tenderness over the involved femoral condyle or tibial compartment. Radiographs performed at the onset of symptoms are usually normal, and the diagnosis is confirmed with technetium bone scanning, with increased activity noted. MRI also is diagnostic of acute osteonecrosis. Subchondral marrow signal abnormality is the earliest change of osteonecrosis; subchondral collapse and fracture may be seen in more advanced cases.[26]

Initially, most patients should be treated conservatively with rest, protected weight bearing, and nonsteroidal anti-inflammatory drugs (NSAIDs). The outcome depends on the percentage of the weight-bearing surface involved with the process. If the lesion is small, no surgical treatment is required. Over the long term, degenerative changes develop in most patients, but initially the changes are not severe. For more advanced stages of femoral osteonecrosis, various surgical treatments have been proposed, including arthroscopic debridement, proximal tibial osteotomy, prosthetic replacement, and allografting.[49]

Extensor Mechanism Injuries

Anatomy and Pathophysiology

The extensor mechanism consists of the quadriceps muscles, quadriceps tendon, medial and lateral retinacula, patella, patellar tendon, and tibial tubercle (Figure 54-6). Passive and dynamic stabilization of the patella are aided by the surrounding soft tissue. Although this anatomic complex encompasses the most superficial aspect of the knee, ruptures of the extensor mechanism are infrequent injuries relative to other types of injuries of the knee joint. Disruptions of the extensor mechanism may occur at any level from the quadriceps muscle to the insertion on the tibial tubercle. Injury generally occurs as a result of sudden vigorous contraction of the quadriceps muscle with the knee in a flexed position, laceration, or a direct blow. Rupture of the quadriceps tendon usually occurs at or just proximal to the patellar insertion. Occasionally the rupture may extend into the vastus intermedius tendon or transversely into the retinaculum. Most patellar tendon ruptures occur at the site of origin on the inferior pole of the patella.

Tendons of the extensor mechanism are extremely resistant to tensile loads and do not rupture under normal physiologic conditions, even with significant degrees of stress. Chronic systemic conditions, including rheumatoid arthritis, gout, systemic lupus erythematosus, hyperparathyroidism, and iatrogenic immunosuppression of organ recipients, may render the tendon vulnerable to rupture.[50] Several studies have implicated steroid use in tendon rupture.[51] Age also seems to be a factor, with quadriceps tendon rupture usually occurring in patients age 40 or older and patellar tendon rupture occurring in patients younger than 40. Overall, patellar tendon rupture is reported to occur one third as often as quadriceps tendon disruption.[52] In the pediatric population, quadriceps and patellar tendon ruptures are rare, and muscle tears seem to predominate.[2] In adolescents, patellofemoral dysplasia, chronic tendinitis, and the use of steroids seem to be predisposing factors. Dysplasia may cause extensor mechanism injury by repetitive tensile overloading, and corticosteroids seem to weaken collagen ultrastructure and impair the reparative process.

Clinical Features

Clinical evaluation can elicit the correct diagnosis in most cases of complete disruption of the extensor mechanism.[52] Patients with extensor disruption may have the following signs and symptoms: (1) acute onset of pain, swelling, and ecchymoses over the anterior aspect of the knee and a palpable defect in the patella, quadriceps tendon, or patella tendon; (2) loss or limited ability for active leg extension (extension lag usually is seen when the last 10 degrees of extension are performed haltingly or with difficulty); (3) high-riding patella (patella alta) with patellar tendon rupture and superior retraction; and (4) low-riding patella (patella baja) with quadriceps tendon rupture and inferior

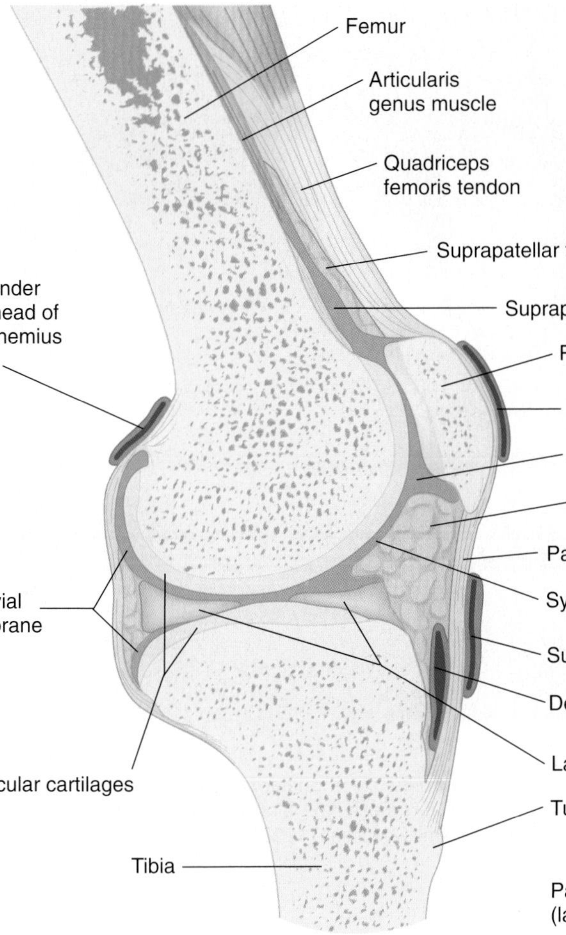

Figure 54-6. Parasagittal section (lateral to midline) of the knee showing extensor mechanisms.

Labels on figure:
- Femur
- Articularis genus muscle
- Quadriceps femoris tendon
- Suprapatellar fat body
- Suprapatellar synovial bursa
- Patella
- Subcutaneous prepatellar bursa
- Articular cavity
- Infrapatellar fat body
- Patellar ligament
- Synovial membrane
- Subcutaneous infrapatellar bursa
- Deep (subtendinous) infrapatellar bursa
- Lateral meniscus
- Tuberosity of tibia
- Bursa under lateral head of gastrocnemius muscle
- Synovial membrane
- Articular cartilages
- Tibia
- Parasagittal section (lateral to midline)

retraction. Partial disruptions may be difficult to diagnose on clinical examination and may require imaging for confirmation.

Diagnostic Strategies

Standard anteroposterior and lateral radiographs should be obtained and may reveal characteristic findings, possibly including obliteration of the quadriceps or patella tendon, a poorly defined suprapatellar or infrapatellar soft tissue mass, soft tissue calcific densities, or a displaced patella (Figure 54-7). Patella alta may be sought on the lateral radiograph using a ratio of patellar tendon length to patellar length. If this ratio is greater than 1:2, patella alta is present.[53] The degree of flexion should not affect this ratio, which relies on the inelasticity of the patellar tendon. In patients with quadriceps rupture, there is commonly degenerative spurring of the patella evident on tangential views (tooth sign). Obliteration of the extensor tendons may be caused by a frayed tendon and surrounding hematoma. A soft tissue mass represents proximal or distal retraction of the torn tendon. Calcific densities may represent avulsed bone fragments of the patella or tibial tubercle or dystrophic calcifications in the substance of the tendons. Despite these multiple radiographic signs, the correct diagnosis is infrequently made by plain radiography in cases of complete quadriceps tendon rupture. MRI scan shows the entire exten-

sor mechanism and is the best imaging modality for diagnosing pathology in this system, even in the acute phase. MRI usually is reserved for patients with possible incomplete disruption or patients with a complication of intra-articular derangements.

Management

Treatment of acute extensor mechanism injuries produces a much better clinical outcome if instituted early, within 2 to 6 weeks of the initial injury. Accurate diagnosis at the time of injury is essential. Patients with delayed diagnosis of patellar tendon rupture may experience significant retraction of the patella proximally and subsequent development of quadriceps contractures or adhesions. If the tear is only partial, immobilization in full extension for 4 to 6 weeks is the treatment of choice.[54] Surgical intervention is required for reattachment of complete tendon ruptures and should be performed as soon as possible after injury to obtain the best results. Numerous techniques have been described for early and late repairs. The choice of repair depends on several factors, including location of the tear, lag time between injury and repair, and presence or absence of adhesions. After primary repair, the knee is immobilized in full extension with a long leg cast until healing is complete. Gradual active and passive range-of-motion exercises must follow to yield optimal results.

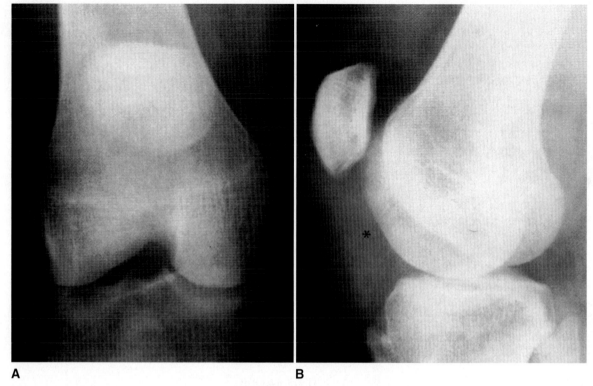

Figure 54-7. Rupture of the infrapatellar tendon, resulting in the high-riding patella in frontal **(A)** and lateral **(B)** projections. In the lateral projection **(B)**, the normally lucent infrapatellar portion of the joint space is dense *(asterisk)*, representing blood within the anterior compartment. (From Harris JH, et al: *The Radiology of Emergency Medicine,* 3rd ed. Baltimore, Williams & Wilkins, 1993.)

Patellar Fractures

Anatomy and Pathophysiology

The patella is the largest sesamoid bone in the body. It is held in place by the quadriceps tendon, the patellar ligament, and the medial and lateral retinacula. As an integral part of the extensor mechanism, the patella increases the effective lever arm of the quadriceps by providing anterior displacement of the quadriceps tendon.[30] Fractures of the patella, except for small avulsion fractures of the rim, are all intra-articular.

Patellar fractures constitute approximately 1% of all skeletal injuries and occur in all age groups.[55] Patellar fractures are classified as transverse, stellate, or comminuted; longitudinal or marginal; proximal pole or distal pole; and rarely osteochondral. They may be either displaced or nondisplaced and occur either from direct or indirect forces or from dislocation. The most common fracture pattern is the transverse fracture (50% to 80%).[55] This type often is seen in young adults and usually results from a powerful contractile force transmitted from the quadriceps tendon. This force may pull the superior portion of the patella upward, leading to wide displacement. In such cases, the medial and lateral retinacula are usually disrupted, resulting in significant functional disability; active extension is impossible. Nondisplaced transverse patellar fractures usually are caused by a direct blow to the anterior aspect of the patella (e.g., a fall on the knee or a direct blow sustained in vehicular trauma). The retinaculum and extensor mechanism usually remain intact, and

patients retain limited functional ability for active extension. Stellate and comminuted fractures account for 30% to 35% of all patellar fractures and commonly result from a direct impact.[55] The fracture elements often appear as separated fragments on plain radiography, but they are held in place and supported by the medial and lateral retinacula and the overlying soft tissues. Small proximal fragments are at risk for avascular necrosis because the patellar blood supply is central and inferior. Longitudinal or marginal vertical fractures constitute 12% to 17%, are usually the result of direct injury, and involve the lateral facet.[56]

Clinical Features

On physical examination, pain, swelling, and ecchymosis over the patella and prepatellar bursa are present. Active extension may be limited or absent, depending on the fracture pattern and amount of fragment displacement. Associated injuries may include fractures of the femoral neck, dislocation of the hip, and acetabulum fractures.

Diagnostic Strategies

Radiologic evaluation of patellar fractures should include standard anteroposterior, lateral, and sunrise views. Most patellar fractures are obvious on plain radiographs, but vertical marginal fractures may be difficult to identify; they are obscured by the femur on the anteroposterior view and not seen at all on the lateral view.[57] Close examination of sunrise (or equivalent)

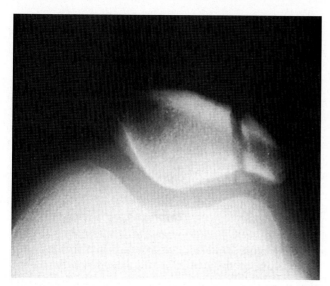

Figure 54-8. Patellar fracture, sunrise view. The sharp nonsclerotic margins identify this as an acute fracture and not a congenital finding. (From Rosen P, et al: *Diagnostic Radiology in Emergency Medicine.* St. Louis, Mosby, 1992, p 196.)

views may reveal an osteochondral avulsion fragment or marginal fracture (Figure 54-8). Bipartite and multipartite patellas are common normal variants and should not be confused with fractures. Ossification centers are found at the upper outer quadrant of the patella and have smooth cortical margins. Comparison radiographs may be helpful because these anatomic anomalies are often bilateral. In some cases, MRI or arthroscopy may be needed to identify occult marginal fractures or free osteochondral fragments.

Management

If the patient can actively extend the knee without displacing the fracture, the retinaculum is intact, and the patient may be treated nonoperatively. Nondisplaced patellar fractures are usually treated with a long leg cast for 4 to 6 weeks and have uniformly good results. Casting the knee in full extension relieves the patella of almost all stress and allows ample time to heal. In the initial management, a knee immobilizer may be used. Patients should be instructed to use crutches with partial weight bearing as tolerated and orthopedic or primary care follow-up.

For widely displaced transverse fractures, open reduction and internal fixation are necessary for optimal results. Although operative techniques vary among surgeons, tension band wire and suturing of the retinaculum are often used. A knee immobilizer or long leg posterior splint can be used initially to immobilize the extremity before definitive care. Treatment options for displaced comminuted fractures include open reduction and internal fixation and partial or complete patellectomy. With the patella removed, the patellar ligament is pulled upward and sutured to the quadriceps femoris tendon, and the retinaculum is repaired. After partial or complete patellectomy, patients generally experience good functional results, although with reduced active knee motion and isokinetic strength.[58]

Fracture fragment separation and dehiscence of the fracture repair are uncommon. They generally result from inadequate internal fixation or, in some cases, an inadequate period of immobilization. Avascular necrosis is rare. Range of motion is generally good after all procedures. Persistent patellofemoral pain and osteoarthritic symptoms are reported as late sequelae of patellar fractures in 56% of patients.[55]

Patellar Dislocation

Anatomy and Pathophysiology

Traumatic patellar dislocation is a relatively common knee injury and can lead to recurrent patellar subluxation and dislocation. It is more common in children than in adults. In adults, patellar dislocation occurs almost exclusively in the setting of patellofemoral dysplasia.[59] Most cases are lateral extra-articular dislocations, and the mechanism of injury is usually a direct blow to the anterior or medial surface of the patella.[2] It may occur from an athletic injury caused by a valgus stress combined with flexion and external rotation. In nearly all cases, there is disruption or sprain in the medial patellar retinaculum caused by stretching of this structure as the patella subluxes laterally; subluxation usually indicates a stretched medial retinaculum, and dislocation suggests a tear. Although extra-articular patella dislocations are common, intra-articular dislocations are rare occurrences that must be considered in any patient with a locked knee. Intra-articular dislocations are usually vertical or horizontal, according to the axis of rotation.[60] Risk factors for partial or complete dislocations are listed in Box 54-2.

The quadriceps angle (Q angle) is measured with the quadriceps contracted. The angle is formed by lines drawn from the tibial tubercle to the center of the patella and from the center of the patella to the anterior superior iliac spine. Normally this angle is 10 degrees or less in men; it may be 15 degrees in women. A Q angle exceeding these dimensions may predispose to patellofemoral problems.

Clinical Features

Patients may complain of the knee giving out accompanied by pain and swelling. Inability to bear weight and inability to flex the knee are common complaints.

There may be a history of previous dislocation. Examination reveals a defect anteriorly with the patella deviated laterally. Tenderness along the medial joint line usually can be elicited by palpation. An effusion also may be present. Acute hemarthrosis is seen most commonly if there is an associated osteochondral fracture. Osteochondral fractures typically occur on the articular surface of the patella and may involve only cartilage (chondral fractures) or include a piece of underlying cortical bone. Patellar dislocations may reduce spontaneously, or the patient may self-reduce the dislocation, usually followed by formation of a large effusion.

The patellar apprehension test is used to aid the clinical identification of patients at risk for patellar dislocation or subluxation. The *apprehension sign* refers to the anxiety the patient exhibits when the examiner attempts to slide the nondisplaced patella laterally. When the patella is displaced laterally, the patient may experience pain and forcefully contract the quadriceps femoris muscle. This is a positive apprehension sign and indicates a tendency for patellar subluxation or dislocation. The test has no value and is not necessary in a patient with acute patellar dislocation, but it may be useful in establishing the diagnosis in patients who report an "event" that occurred and resolved spontaneously.

Diagnostic Strategies

Standard anteroposterior and lateral views are used and are usually adequate. A sunrise (skyline) view usually is not possible because of pain and inability to flex the knee. Radiographic findings show the patella deviated laterally out of the trochlear groove, and an effusion is usually evident. Radiographs should be examined for evidence of avulsion fractures.

Management

After dislocation is diagnosed, closed reduction should be attempted. Force or pressure should be directed anteromedially on the lateral patellar margin, while simultaneously attempting gentle extension of the leg. Postreduction radiographs are mandatory and should reveal the patella in the trochlear grove. Osteochondral avulsion fragments may be visualized radiographically, and postreduction radiographs should be examined carefully for their presence. Radiologically evident intra-articular loose bodies may require arthroscopic removal.

Occasionally, patellar reduction may be difficult. Several cases have been reported in which the conventional method of reducing a laterally dislocated patella either has failed or has proved difficult.[61] In nearly all cases, there has been the suggestion of locking of the medial facet onto the lateral femoral condyle with internal rotation of the patella. Closed reduction can be achieved by applying downward pressure to the lateral aspect of the patella, creating an external rotational force that unlocks the medial patellar facet.[61] Typically, traumatic patellar dislocations occur with disruption of the medial retinaculum but an intact lateral retinaculum, preventing internal rotation. Dislocations that are irreducible by conventional methods may have significant internal rotation and lateral retinaculum pathology.

After successful reduction, the knee should be immobilized in full extension for 3 to 6 weeks to allow adequate time for the medial retinaculum to heal. Ice, elevation, non–weight bearing, and analgesia provide additional benefit in the acute setting. The patient can be discharged with orthopedic or primary care follow-up within 2 weeks. Although the incidence of recurrence may be decreased with appropriate therapy and proper patient selection, at least 30% to 50% of all patients having sustained a primary patellar dislocation continue to have symptoms of instability or anterior knee pain.

Recurrent patellar dislocations reportedly have a 15% incidence and may require surgical intervention, including release of the lateral retinaculum, reconstruction of the medial retinaculum, or tibial tuberosity transfer medially to decrease the Q angle. The most common surgical procedure is arthroscopic release of the lateral retinaculum. Incision of the lateral retinaculum results in decreased pull on the patella. If this is unsuccessful, other operative techniques include shortening of the medial patella retinaculum and tibial tuberosity transfer.

Patellofemoral Pain Syndrome

Anatomy and Pathophysiology

The patellofemoral pain syndrome refers to the clinical presentation of anterior knee pain related to changes in the patellofemoral articulation. Most authors refer to symptoms that result from pathologic changes on the surface of the patella as *chondromalacia patellae*. The term *chondromalacia* has been used imprecisely to define the syndrome of patellofemoral pain.[62] Chondromalacia is a pathologic term that refers to softening of the articular cartilage. Correlating pathologic changes on the surface of the patella and clinical symptoms has been difficult, and the pain mechanism has not been precisely defined.

Clinical Features

Patellofemoral pain is the most common symptom complex in the knee joint. Patients are generally 10 to 20 years old and often have difficulty describing their symptoms clearly. A typical presentation is nonspecific anterior knee discomfort that is nonradiating and occurs in a teenage girl. The pain usually begins gradually and commonly is not related to trauma. One knee is usually more affected than the other. The knee is more painful with prolonged flexion, and the discomfort typically is accentuated by stair climbing and kneeling. The patient may have instability related to patellar subluxation or dislocation. The syndrome also may occur in athletes with patellofemoral pain induced by overactivity. At times, elderly patients may have arthritis affecting the patellofemoral joint. When arthritis is isolated to the patellofemoral joint, the symptoms are identical to symptoms in patients with patellofemoral syndrome pain; however, the response to treatment and prognosis are different. The differential diagnosis includes tears of the menisci, plica syndrome, inflammatory or degenerative arthritis, ligament injuries, and overuse syndromes (e.g., prepatella bursitis and patella tendinitis).

The physical examination should begin with observation. The patient may ambulate with an antalgic gait. Any referred pain syndromes from hip or disk disease should be excluded. Direct knee examination should include documentation of the size of any effusion, palpation of the patella facets for any evidence of tenderness, and compression testing of the patella for apprehension to medial or lateral subluxation.

Diagnostic Strategies

Radiographic examination of the patellofemoral joint is of limited value and relies for the most part on lateral and sunrise axial projections. The axial view can be obtained with the patient prone or supine. Merchant's projection is the most popular axial projection for the evaluation of patellofemoral congruency.[63] It is obtained with the knee flexed 45 degrees. Plain radiography helps rule out arthritic involvement and visualize any malalignment. Further evaluation may be undertaken with CT or MRI. MRI and the combination of CT and arthrography are sensitive in detecting abnormalities of the articular surface of the patella.[63]

Management

Most patients, regardless of the cause of their condition, respond to a rehabilitation program. Conservative treatment for patellofemoral pain is usually effective, with most patients responding to one or more of four types of treatment, including (1) exercises to strengthen the quadriceps, (2) brace support of the patellofemoral mechanism, (3) activity modification limiting flexion, and (4) medications such as NSAIDs for pain. The initial goal is to reduce pain and improve function, with emphasis placed on strengthening the vastus medialis oblique muscle. The patient should receive appropriate referral to ensure that an appropriate rehabilitative scheme is designed.

Tibial Femoral Knee Dislocation

Anatomy and Pathophysiology

Tibial femoral knee dislocation is a severe injury and a limb-threatening emergency. This is a rare injury, but should be considered when an appropriate injury mechanism was present because half of all knee dislocations spontaneously reduce or are reduced in the field by emergency personnel.[64] Patients presenting with knee dislocations that have been reduced have similar risk of injury and coexisting trauma as patients who present with a dislocated knee.[65] Two thirds of all knee dislocations result from motor vehicle crashes, with the remainder occurring from falls, sports injuries, and industrial injuries. Of all knee dislocations, 50% to 60% are anterior.[1]

Epidemiologic data show a peak incidence in the teens and 20s, with a male predominance of 3:1.[65] Dislocations invariably are associated with significant soft tissue and ligamentous injury. There is disruption of the joint capsule with accompanying trauma to the muscles and tendons. Vascular injury to the popliteal artery is the most severe complication and is the major cause of morbidity and limb loss.

The neurovascular bundle, which is composed of the popliteal artery, popliteal vein, and common peroneal nerve, runs posteriorly behind all bony and ligamentous structures in the popliteal fossa. The popliteal artery is fixed in the fibrous tunnel of the adductor magnus hiatus proximally and traverses the fibrous arch of the soleus and interosseous membrane distally. In essence, it is tethered to the femur and the tibia, and its inherent immobility renders it susceptible to injury during dislocation. At that time, the popliteal artery may be stretched, lacerated, or contused. Because of the parallel course of the popliteal vein and peroneal nerve, they are vulnerable to a similar injury.

Traumatic dislocation of the knee can be characterized by the mechanism of injury and the type of dislocation. The injury is most commonly sustained in high-velocity accidents, such as motor vehicle and motorcycle crashes, or in severe crush injuries.[24] Accidents associated with athletic activity (e.g., water skiing) also have produced dislocation. Anatomically, dislocations are described based on the relative displacement of the tibia with respect to the femur. They are classified into five types: anterior, posterior, medial, lateral, and rotary. Anterior dislocation is reported to be the most common type and usually is caused by hyperextension of the knee.[24] Posterior dislocations are the second most common type and usually result from high-velocity direct trauma to the flexed knee, often in association with vehicular trauma (dashboard-type injury). The remaining dislocations are lateral, medial, or rotary dislocations and result from direct or indirect trauma producing valgus, varus, or rotary forces.

Clinical Features

The diagnosis of knee dislocation is based on the mechanism of injury and clinical and radiographic findings. Clinical deformity should be easily palpable when a dislocation is present. Swelling may be absent, however, because of the associated tearing of the capsular structures and dissipation of the acute hemarthrosis into the adjacent soft tissue. The initial evaluation may not reveal an obvious gross deformity because of the variable occurrence of spontaneous reduction. Some authors have advocated expanding the definition of knee dislocation to include patients who have a bicruciate (ACL and PCL) ligament injury, even when the knee is reduced on initial presentation.[65] For this reason, patients with grossly unstable knees but no proven dislocation and patients who have a bicruciate (ACL and PCL) ligament injury should be evaluated for concomitant injuries, similarly to patients with proven dislocation.[66]

Regardless of the type of dislocation, patients usually have associated trauma with high injury severity, most commonly ipsilateral or contralateral lower extremity fractures.[65] Other injuries may include pelvic fractures, multiple rib fractures, skull fractures, and posterior dislocation of the hip.

Vascular injury is a potential catastrophic complication of knee dislocation, and popliteal artery injury is reported in 14% to 65% of these patients.[64] Anterior dislocations usually lead to a severe stretch injury with damage to the long segment of the artery, whereas posterior dislocations produce an isolated transection of the artery.[64] The risk of vascular injury seems to be less when the dislocation is the result of relatively low-energy trauma (except with hyperextension), as might be encountered on the athletic field (5% to 50% in various series), than with high-energy trauma (20% to 50%).[9] The collateral geniculate arteries around the knee also may be damaged directly or secondarily compressed by hematoma formation after the dislocation. Direct arterial injury, decreased collateral circulation, and elevated compartment pressures all may compromise limb perfusion. In addition to being clinically occult, vascular injury in blunt trauma is more difficult to manage because of associated soft tissue injury and edema.

Evaluation of the limb vascular status is the most important part of the initial physical examination of knee dislocation. All knee dislocations probably warrant surgical consultation, but the so-called hard signs of vascular injury mandate immediate surgical consultation.[67] These signs include absence of pulse, limb ischemia, rapidly expanding hematoma, pulsatile bleeding, and bruit or thrill over the wound, especially in penetrating injuries. When repair is delayed beyond 8 hours, the amputation rate may be 86%.[68] The posterior tibial and dorsal pedal pulses should be evaluated. Doppler pressure measurements and peripheral pulse determinations have been found to be highly predictive of major arterial trauma when diminished or absent, but normal values do not rule out vascular injury.[1] In all cases of extremity trauma with vascular injury, approximately 10% are associated with a normal pedal pulse.[69] Even in low-velocity dislocations, the possibility of vascular injury should not be overlooked. Vascular injury also should be sought in patients with ligamentous disruption only. There is no significant difference between patients with documented knee dislocation and patients with severe ligamentous disruption regarding the frequency of major (22% versus 18%) or minor (38% versus 36%) vascular abnormalities.[1] The treatment of minor vascular injuries is controversial. Intimal flap tears are undetectable by a physical examination and are identified by arteriography. Injuries to small branches of the popliteal artery can be managed by observation and serial examinations.[64,70] These "minor" injuries may place the limb at risk if significant bleeding occurs predisposing to compartment syndrome. Any such injury mandates immediate vascular surgical consultation.

Neurologic integrity in the limb also should be assessed because peripheral nerve injury may be associated with all types of dislocation. Peroneal nerve injury is the most common major neurologic problem associated with knee dislocation; some degree of dysfunction occurs in 40% of patients and is permanent in 78% of these.[1] The peroneal nerve should be evaluated by determining sensation of the dorsum of the foot and by having the patient dorsiflex the ankle. Less commonly, the posterior tibial nerve may be injured, manifesting as diminished plantar sensation and plantar flexion of the foot. The exact mechanism is unclear, but is thought to involve traction during displacement. Complete nerve palsy in the acute setting has been associated with a poor prognosis for recovery.[1]

Knee dislocation may involve damage to other structures around the knee joint, including the cruciate ligaments, collateral ligaments, and menisci. Ligament injury is predictable as soon as the displacement exceeds 10% to 25% of the ligament resting length.[52] Classically, complete dislocation of the knee joint has been associated with complete tears of the ACL and PCL, resulting in complete disruption of the tibial femoral articulation. Most accounts of complete knee dislocation in the literature suggest that disruption of both cruciate ligaments is sufficient and necessary to make the diagnosis of knee dislocation; however, knee dislocation without disruption of both cruciate ligaments has been reported.[71,72] No firm assumptions regarding the degree of associated ligamentous injury should be made.

Diagnostic Strategies

Radiographic examination usually confirms the clinical findings (Figure 54-9). In rare posterolateral and rotary dislocations, radiographic interpretation may be more difficult. Radiographic examination also serves to document associated fractures.

There is a high incidence of popliteal artery injury with knee dislocations, and the longer repair is delayed, the more likely it is that amputation will be necessary. Contrast arteriography generally has been considered the standard of care.[73-75] More recently, however, there has been debate in the trauma literature as to whether all patients with knee dislocations require arteriography. Some studies have found that serial examinations can detect all clinically significant injuries, whereas others have emphasized the occasional occurrence of an occult arterial injury.[9,24,76-78,132] A meta-analysis found that absence of normal pulses had only 79% sensitivity for a surgical popliteal artery injury after knee dislocation, suggesting that the default still should be to obtain angiography on these patients.[1,78] Color-flow Doppler ultrasonography is gaining acceptance as an alternative to arteriography in some centers, but it may not be as readily available during off hours.

Management

The dislocated knee should be reduced immediately by longitudinal traction using appropriate analgesia and sedation. Radiologic confirmation is not required before reduction. The neurovascular status should

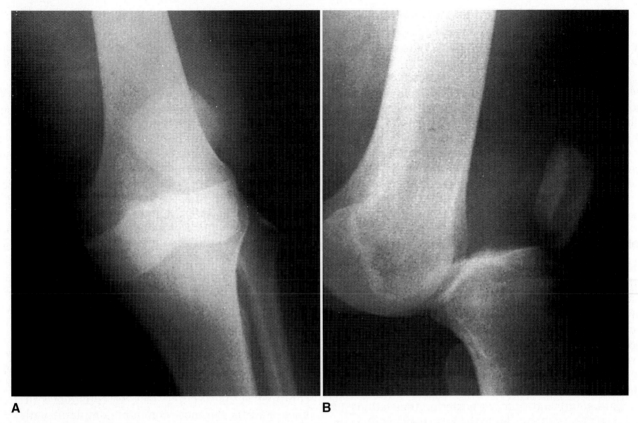

Figure 54-9. Anterior dislocation of the knee. **A,** Anteroposterior view shows overlap of the femur and tibia, which is never seen under normal circumstances. The anteriorly dislocated tibia is magnified. **B,** Lateral view shows anterior dislocation of the tibia in relation to the femur. The patella also is anteriorly dislocated. (From Rosen P, et al: *Diagnostic Radiology in Emergency Medicine*. St. Louis, Mosby, 1992, p 194.)

be checked before and after reduction is achieved. Reduction usually can be accomplished with simple traction-countertraction, preferably using intravenous conscious sedation; general anesthesia is rarely necessary. The limb should be immobilized in a long leg posterior splint with 15 to 20 degrees of flexion. Circumferential casting is avoided in the acute setting. When there is any suspicion for vascular injury or if immediate exploration is not planned, an arteriogram should be obtained. Current indications for immediate surgery include obvious vascular injury with a cool, cyanotic ischemic lower extremity and irreducible or open dislocations. Arthroscopy is contraindicated in the acute setting because of the risk of fluid extravasation secondary to capsular deficiencies.

Prompt and accurate diagnosis of vascular trauma is essential to successful management and limb salvage. Early revascularization also is crucial because delay of more than 6 hours increases the risk of compartment syndrome and amputation. Rates of limb salvage have improved dramatically with widespread application of modern techniques of vascular repair.[72] A large prospective study of limb-threatening injuries (not limited to dislocations) cast doubt, however, on the superiority of reconstruction over amputation, finding equivalent long-term functional outcomes for patients treated with amputation and reconstruction, even though the amputation patients had more severe initial injuries.[79] In the specific case of dislocation, early operative intervention does seem to confer an advantage.[80]

Loss and disability are minimized by expedient revascularization and primary arterial repair, local heparinization when not contraindicated, repair of popliteal venous injury, aggressive wound debridement, and early soft tissue coverage. Four-compartment fasciotomies are done routinely or selectively in various centers to minimize the consequences of reperfusion edema in patients who undergo vascular repair.[9]

If the neurovascular structures remain intact after dislocation, the knee joint is reduced and allowed to rest for 2 to 3 days before reconstruction of the torn ligaments is considered. Although the management of ligament injuries secondary to knee dislocation is controversial, the long-term results of surgical repair of ligaments damaged during dislocations have been good. In follow-up studies, clinical instability is generally not a problem, but chronic pain and discomfort are present in almost half of patients. Loss of motion is a common complication, and extensive damage to the articular surfaces at the time of injury increases the risk of early osteoarthritis.

Inability to achieve a closed reduction is uncommon; however, it may occur as a result of concomitant ligamentous injuries or femoral condyle herniation through a large capsular defect.[81] Complications associated with traumatic knee dislocations include the development of deep vein thrombosis, compartment syndrome, pseudoaneurysms, and arterial thrombosis. Compartment syndromes generally occur within 24 to 48 hours of the initial injury. Pseudoaneurysm formation may occur several hours to months after an undiagnosed acute popliteal artery injury. A review of the literature reveals the civilian incidence of post-traumatic pseudoaneurysms to be rare, accounting for only 0% to 3.5% of all popliteal aneurysms.[82] Heterotopic ossification is a poorly-understood syndrome of calcification of the soft tissues of the knee. It has been observed in uninjured knees of patients who sustained major trauma. In its severest form, heterotopic ossification can cause dramatic decreases in knee mobility. Almost half of dislocated knees go on to have heterotopic ossification, although the most function-limiting form may be limited to patients with severe trauma.[83]

Soft Tissue Injuries

The knee is the most commonly injured joint in the human body, and the ligaments sustain damage in most cases. The incidence of knee ligament injuries in the United States has increased since the 1980s, possibly because of increased activity levels in middle-aged people and increased participation at all levels in a variety of sports.[9] The ligaments of the knee are the MCL, LCL, ACL, and PCL. They function in conjunction with the joint capsule to limit varus-valgus (medial-lateral) and anterior-posterior translations of the knee. Ligament injuries to the knee may involve any or all of the ligaments and may range from mild sprain to complete tears. Collateral ligament injury usually causes tenderness and pain along the joint line. Cruciate injuries pose more of a diagnostic dilemma because they are intra-articular structures.

Cruciate Ligament Injuries

The cruciate ligaments are the primary stabilizers for anterior and posterior displacement of the tibia on the femur. They are so named because they cross each other between their attachments. They form the keystone of the "four-bar cruciate linkage."[84] The ACL extends obliquely upward, medially, and backward from the anterior intercondylar area of the tibia to the medial side of the lateral femoral condyle. The ACL prevents excessive anterior displacement of the tibia on the femur and helps control rotation and hyperextension of the knee during cutting, twisting, and turning activities. It is the most commonly injured major ligament of the knee, with more than 200,000 new ACL tears occurring in the United States annually.[7] The PCL passes upward, laterally, and forward medial to the ACL from the posterior intercondylar area of the tibia to the lateral side of the medial condyle of the femur. The PCL prevents excessive posterior displacement of the tibia on the femur, especially during flexion. The PCL is extremely strong, and injuries are relatively uncommon. Isolated PCL injury accounts for 3.4% to 10% of all knee injuries.[85]

The ACL is commonly injured in association with sporting activities, particularly skiing and football.[86] Numerous mechanisms of injury produce ACL disruption. Although ACL injuries can be caused by contact, they are more common in noncontact sports, with the plant-and-pivot or stop-and-jump mechanisms the predominant injuries.[9] A direct blow to the flexed knee, as might occur in motor vehicle crashes (dashboard), and turf injuries with the knee flexed and the ankle plantar flexed also can result in an ACL injury.

Approximately 50% of patients with ACL injuries have associated meniscal tears.[9] The lateral menicus is torn more commonly than the medial meniscus in acute ACL injuries, but in chronic ACL tears, the medial meniscus is more commonly involved. Several studies suggest that the classically described "unhappy triad" of ACL, MCL, and medial meniscus injury is less common than the association of torn ACL, torn MCL, and torn lateral meniscus.[9]

Acute or chronic ACL insufficiency is uncommon in children younger than age 14 years old with open epiphyses.[87] ACL insufficiency secondary to trauma in this age group most often is associated with avulsion of the intercondylar eminence of the tibia. Nonpathologic ligament laxity or congenital absence of the ACL must be considered in the differential diagnosis in children with suspected ligamentous injury.

The diagnosis of ACL injury often can be made from the history alone. Most patients with acute ACL injury give a history of immediate disability and inability to continue activity, citing lack of confidence in their knee. Pain is the most common complaint with ACL rupture and is usually immediate and often accompanied by acute hemarthrosis. A history of audible "pop" at the time of injury is an important clue and occurs in about 70% of patients with ACL rupture. Reports of the knee giving out suggest ACL rupture or tear; giving out is reported in 17% to 65% of cases.[88] Patients also may complain of the knee buckling, locking, or collapsing and inability to bear weight. In one study of 40 patients with ACL, 86% complained of the knee giving way with strenuous activities.[88] Giving way is commonly associated with activities such as cutting and twisting maneuvers and rapid deceleration, but it may occur with daily activities. Patients with an ACL-deficient knee usually complain of repetitive episodes of buckling with activities.

The diagnostic limitations of clinical knee examination compared with arthroscopy have been well documented. Although the diagnosis of collateral ligament injuries is usually made clinically, reports concerning ACL injury reveal much disparity in accuracy, ranging from 38% to 95%.[9] In the largest prospective study to date, the diagnostic accuracy of the clinical examination for intra-articular injuries of the knee compared with arthroscopy was 56%.[89] The lesions most difficult to diagnose were chondral fractures, tears in the ACL, loose bodies, and fibrotic fat pads.

Immediate swelling and the presence of hemarthrosis indicate an ACL tear or other internal derangement of the knee. Acute hemarthrosis is a common and significant sign with acute ACL injury and occurs in approximately 70% of patients.[90] It is defined as rapid extravasation of blood into the joint and is an indication of significant intra-articular injury. Acute hemarthrosis also occurs in 10% to 15% of patellar subluxations or dislocations, 10% of peripheral meniscal tears, 2% to 5% of osteochondral fractures, and 5% of capsular tears and PCL injuries. The appearance of hemarthrosis of the knee in children usually signifies a serious knee injury and should be treated with the same importance as in adults.[91]

The PCL is less commonly injured than the ACL and generally is injured more often outside of sporting activities.[9] Mechanisms of PCL injury include a fall onto the ground with the foot plantar flexed (striking the tibial tubercle), a direct posterior blow to a flexed knee (e.g., a dashboard injury), hyperflexion, hyperextension, severe varus or valgus loads after failure of the collaterals, and knee dislocations. Ninety-five percent of all PCL injuries are associated with other ligament injuries, including concurrent injuries of the MCL, ACL, or posterolateral complex.[11] PCL injuries are classified as partial (grade I or II) or complete (grade III) tears. Pain and swelling are common complaints with isolated PCL tears and with PCL tears having combined capsuloligamentous disruption. Popping or tearing sensations are infrequently noted, and instability usually is not immediately appreciated. Later the patient may complain of the femur falling off the tibia. The posterior drawer test is commonly done to assess for the integrity of the PCL. Careful inspection also may reveal a posterior sag sign.

Collateral Ligament Injuries

The medial stabilizers of the knee are the joint capsule and the MCL. The semimembranosus and pes anserinus are medial dynamic stabilizers. These structures resist valgus laxity and medial rotary instability. The MCL is a two-part structure with a long superficial and a deep capsular component that attaches to the medial meniscus and acts as a stabilizer for this structure. The MCL usually is injured by a direct blow or impact to the lateral aspect of the knee, which imposes a valgus stress. Overall, MCL injury is the most common isolated knee ligament injury, and it is the injury most commonly associated with ACL injury. MCL injury does not require surgical treatment in most patients.[9]

The lateral stabilizers of the knee are the LCL and the lateral joint capsule. Secondary contributors to lateral stability are supplied by the iliotibial band, biceps tendon, and popliteal arcuate complex in the posterolateral corner of the knee. Resistance to varus stress is provided mainly by the LCL. Fibers descend from the lateral femoral condyle and insert at the fibula head. The lateral ligaments are under tension during standing and walking, when they are at or near maximal extension. The LCL usually is injured by a mechanism of hyperextension with varus stress commonly accompanied by a direct blow or rotation. Injuries to the LCL are less common but more disabling than injuries of the medial side. The lower incidence of injury is attributed to the greater mobility of the LCL and overall greater stability of the lateral compartment. Varus injury is uncommon because the inner aspect of the knee is protected by the opposite leg. The forces necessary to produce LCL injury are usually greater than the forces required for medial injury, which partially

explains the high frequency of associated injuries accompanying LCL injury. The tendon of the biceps femoris muscle attaches to the head of the fibula. Just below this juncture, the common peroneal nerve is close to the head of the fibula. Because of this relationship, common peroneal nerve injury and biceps femoris tendon injury must be considered in patients with LCL injury.

The knee should be examined as soon as possible after an injury to exclude ligamentous damage. Focal tenderness at the origin or insertion sites suggests collateral ligament trauma, but also can occur with muscular injury, osseous pathology, or meniscal tear. Range of motion should be documented and stability testing done to assess ligamentous injury as outlined previously.

Diagnostic Strategies

Plain radiography may be used in cases of suspected ligamentous injury before stress testing to rule out the possibility of an associated fracture. Although patients with isolated collateral ligament strain rarely show acute osseous pathology, the yield increases in cases with traumatic effusions and cases with suspected cruciate ligament injury. The initial radiographic evaluation should include anteroposterior, lateral, intercondylar notch, and sunrise views. Each radiograph should be evaluated for possible osteochondral injuries, loose bodies, or avulsion injuries at the attachment sites of ligaments. The lateral capsular sign (Segond fracture) is highly suggestive of injury to the ACL and is seen in approximately 6% of injuries.[31] Fracture of the posterior aspect of the lateral tibial plateau may represent another indirect radiographic sign of ACL tear.[92] The fracture may represent an injury at the capsular insertion analogous to the Segond fracture.

MRI is an excellent modality for determining the status of the cruciate and collateral ligaments. MRI has been shown in a more recent study to be cost-effective by reducing the number of diagnostic arthroscopies.[93] In other cases, it may aid the orthopedic surgeon in planning therapeutic arthroscopy if a clinically significant, surgically correctable lesion is found. MRI is highly accurate for diagnosing ACL rupture, with reported sensitivity and specificity exceeding 90%.[94] The diagnosis is difficult when the ACL is incompletely torn and in chronic cases, when the ligament may scar down in near-anatomic position. MRI consistently shows the thick PCL and is reportedly 90% sensitive for documenting a PCL injury. Arthroscopy is unquestionably the best method for ascertaining the integrity of the ACL.[52] Arthroscopic observation of the PCL is more difficult, however, and probably not as reliable as MRI. Arthroscopy has the advantage of allowing simultaneous therapy via cruciate ligament debridement or reconstruction.

Management

There is consensus that isolated grade I and II collateral ligament injuries should be managed conservatively, provided that the ACL is intact. The nonoperative approach should focus on pain control, restoring range of motion, regaining muscle strength, and protecting the knee from further injury. Appropriate initial therapy includes ice pack application, NSAIDs, and symptomatic immobilization with a knee immobilizer if necessary. Patients may be placed on a regimen of partial weight bearing or non–weight bearing using crutches. Orthopedic or primary care follow-up is advised, and a rehabilitative exercise program for quadriceps and hamstring strengthening may be instituted when the acute injury resolves. In isolated grade III collateral ligament injuries, nonoperative treatment also is the preferred method of treatment. Generally a completely torn LCL does not lead to significant instability or loss of function, unless associated with an ACL tear. Nonsurgical treatment of all degrees of isolated MCL injury is well established.[9] In cases in which there is a concomitant tear of the ACL and the MCL, the treatment plan may change from conservative management to operative repair.[95]

Management of an ACL tear is controversial because of the variability of patient impairment after an ACL injury and the lack of documentation that operative repair prevents degenerative arthritis. The outcome for a patient with ACL disruption is most closely related to the level of activity. Most young patients with a complete ACL tear who are active in sports require reconstructive surgery to stabilize the knee. Usually surgery is performed arthroscopically after a delay of 2 to 3 weeks to allow swelling to subside. Older patients and patients who do not participate in active sports may be treated conservatively with muscle-strength training. If recurrent functional instability subsequently develops, reconstruction may be considered at a later date.

The natural history of patients with isolated PCL varies. Instability is a less frequent complaint after isolated PCL injuries than after isolated ACL injuries. Isolated PCL injuries are more frequently associated with pain than instability. Some patients function relatively well with a good rehabilitative program that includes quadriceps strengthening and functional bracing. Over time (10 to 20 years), many patients develop disability related to degenerative changes of the articular surface with stiffness and pain. Although some controversy surrounds the natural history and treatment of true isolated PCL injuries, these injuries are usually partial tears and do not require surgery.[9] Nonsurgical treatment should focus on quadriceps rehabilitation. There is general agreement that PCL injuries with combined ligamentous injuries, especially injuries involving the posterolateral corner, should be treated operatively within 2 weeks.[9]

Meniscal Injuries

Anatomy and Pathophysiology

The menisci are of great clinical importance to the normal function and integrity of the knee joint. The medial and lateral menisci are crescent-shaped, semilunar fibrocartilaginous structures that sit on the superior articular surface of the tibia and provide a gliding surface for the femoral condyles. In this interposed position between the femur and tibia, they function as shock absorbers and aid in the distribution of stress across the joint surface by providing a larger area of contact. They also act as secondary stabilizers by deepening the tibial plateau. Normal tibial femoral articulation and function depend on meniscal integrity; damage or loss is associated with degenerative changes within the knee and the accelerated development of osteoarthritis. The medial meniscus is semilunar and firmly attached anteriorly and posteriorly to the joint capsule. The lateral meniscus is less firmly attached to the capsule and more mobile. During flexion and extension, the menisci migrate slightly forward with extension and backward with flexion. Because of the greater mobility, the lateral meniscus is less vulnerable to injury. The meniscus is avascular except at the peripheral one third, which has tremendous clinical importance in that it is this area that has the greatest potential to heal after injury.

Injury to the menisci may be from a single traumatic episode, a degenerative process, or a combination. The mechanism usually involves a twisting maneuver on a weight-bearing knee. The force required sometimes can be as slight as that produced when a middle-aged person arises from a chair and turns to reach for an object. The associated compression and rotation of the knee joint can lead to abnormal shear forces that result in damage to the meniscus. The triad of meniscal tears comprises joint line pain, swelling, and "clicking" or locking of the knee. True locking may occur immediately after the injury, with the knee held at 30 degrees of flexion; this is primarily associated with a displaced meniscal fragment. In general, knee locking that occurs the day after injury is usually the result of "pseudolocking," whereby full range of motion is limited by effusion, pain, and muscle spasm rather than a displaced meniscal fragment.

Meniscal tears can be classified based on their description and orientation. They include radial, horizontal, longitudinal, and complex tears. Radial tears are tears that occur from the inner edge of the meniscus to the peripheral margin. The so-called bucket-handle tears are vertical longitudinal tears typically seen in younger patients in association with ACL insufficiency.[52] The bucket-handle tears are three times as common in the medial compared with the lateral meniscus and can displace into the knee, resulting in a "locked" knee. Complex meniscal injuries are the most common of all meniscal lesions and usually are seen in older individuals without associated ligamentous instability.

Meniscal tears also can be classified based on their location and peripheral and central surface appearances.[96] *Red-red tears* are peripheral detachments that have a functional blood supply and the best prognosis for healing. *Red-white tears* have an active peripheral blood supply that is sufficient for healing if adequately repaired. The last category is the *white-white tear*, which is within the inner two thirds of the meniscus, has no true vascularity, and has minimal to no healing ability.

Clinical Features

Meniscal injuries are unusual in children but become increasingly more common in adolescents and adults. An isolated meniscal tear should be suspected in a patient with a history of intermittent locking, effusion, giving way, and pain and physical examination findings of joint line tenderness and a positive McMurray's test.[97] Cruciate tears invariably result in immediate hemarthrosis; meniscal tears usually result in an effusion forming over 12 to 24 hours. A second, more common presentation is a patient with an unstable knee who has chronic ACL insufficiency and similar history and physical findings. The cardinal sign of a meniscal tear is local pain and tenderness along the joint line. Joint line pain and tenderness are especially apparent with extremes of flexion and extension. Specific joint line tenderness is helpful diagnostically, particularly in the posterior half of the menisci, because 81% of meniscal tears are located posteriorly.[96] Not all tears of the menisci are symptomatic. Degenerative lesions of the posterior horn are relatively common in middle age and later and may be asymptomatic. The differential diagnosis of a torn meniscus is extensive and includes loose bodies, osteochondrotic lesion, tibial spine fractures, patellofemoral pain syndrome, popliteal tendinitis, plica syndromes, inflammatory arthritis, and discoid menisci with or without a concurrent tear.

Much evidence correlates an increased incidence of meniscal pathology with ACL rupture, with an overall incidence of meniscal tears with ACL rupture of 52%. Isolated medial meniscal tears are present in 22%, isolated lateral tears are present in 23%, and a combined meniscal lesion is present in 9% of cases.[98] PCL tears are uncommonly reported in association with meniscal pathology.

The accuracy of clinical diagnosis for meniscal lesions has been well described in the literature.[99] The diagnosis can be made through a careful history and physical examination in 90% of patients.[9] No one specific test is predictive, however, and physical findings suggesting meniscal lesions have decreased reliability in patients with associated ACL tears.[99]

Diagnostic Strategies

Although routine knee radiographs do not reveal direct evidence of injury to the cartilaginous menisci, they should be obtained to rule out other associated osseous injuries. The diagnosis of a meniscal injury may be confirmed by MRI or arthroscopy. The reported sensitivity of MRI for meniscal tears ranges from 87% to 97%, with specificity ranging from 91% to 95%.[100,101] The negative predictive value of MRI for meniscal tears is approximately 95%. Arthroscopy is generally considered the gold standard for diagnosis with which other modalities are compared. It has the advantage of allowing direct visualization with diagnostic accuracy of 97% and can be therapeutic.

Management

Definitive treatment of a meniscal injury is not an urgent concern. Unless the knee is locked and cannot be extended or flexed, a patient with a suspected torn meniscus should be treated initially with NSAIDs for analgesia, knee immobilization, ice, non–weight bearing, and orthopedic or primary care referral. Further management of a meniscal tear may include a conservative, nonoperative approach. Surgical treatment can be done with arthroscopic or open technique and may range from meniscal repair to partial meniscectomy. Current recommendations emphasize preserving as much normal meniscus as possible to decrease the risk of progressive osteoarthritis. The use of meniscal allograft tissue to reconstruct the knee has elicited a great deal of interest in recent years. The indications for meniscal allograft transplantation are currently being defined.[9] The lack of uniformity in patient selection, surgical technique, and follow-up criteria has made the results of clinical studies difficult to interpret, however.

The management of meniscal lesions in a patient with ACL injury is generally influenced by the subsequent treatment of the ligament injury. ACL deficiency of the knee greatly increases the risk of meniscal repair failure. This failure can be obviated by concomitant repair of the ACL.

Overuse Injuries

All overuse syndromes are associated with the development of inflammation. The common mechanism of injury is repetitive microtrauma to tissue, whereby the innate ability of the tissue to repair itself is outpaced by the repetition of the insult. Repetitive stress injury occurs commonly in sports, fitness, and training activities, but it is less commonly seen in free-play activities. These injuries have become more common in children and adolescents with the trend toward increased participation in organized sports. In general, the goal of treatment is to reduce inflammation through rest, activity modification, and medications.

The typical complaint is knee pain, often localized to one of three particular areas: the medial aspect, the lateral aspect, or the peripatella region. Medial knee pain may be caused by subluxation of the patella, a stress fracture of the upper third of the tibia, pes anserine bursitis or tendinitis, and MCL strain related to excessive foot pronation. Lateral knee pain may be caused by iliotibial or popliteal tendinitis, LCL strain, or stress fracture of the fibula. Anterior pain is typical of lateral patellar compression syndrome, peripatellar tendinitis, and patellofemoral syndrome.

Iliotibial Band Syndrome

The iliotibial band syndrome is the result of inflammation secondary to overuse and is most often described in high-mileage runners.[102] The iliotibial band is a thickened strip of fascia lata that extends from the iliac crest to the lateral tibial tubercle. This band serves as a ligament between the lateral femoral condyle and the lateral tibia and functions to stabilize the knee joint in extension.

The irritation associated with overuse can cause inflammation of a bursa underlying the iliotibial band at the lateral femoral epicondyle. Symptoms generally include pain aggravated by repetitive knee movement associated with running or cycling. Discomfort typically appears after a consistent distance is covered. There is usually no history of direct trauma. Physical findings include localized tenderness to palpation of the lateral femoral epicondyle but an otherwise negative knee examination. Knee radiographs are normal. The differential diagnosis includes early degenerative joint disease, cystic or torn lateral meniscus, lateral capsular strain, lateral tibial or femoral condyle osteonecrosis, stress reactions, chondromalacia, and popliteus tendinitis. Treatment consists of rest or decreased distance, shoe changes, modification of exercise technique, anti-inflammatory medications, steroid injections, and stretching. Surgery is generally not required.[102]

Peripatellar Tendinitis

Peripatellar tendinitis, or jumper's knee, refers to a spectrum of patellar tendon and extensor mechanism abnormalities that result from chronic repetitive stress.[103] The condition is commonly seen in athletes, especially athletes involved in some type of repetitive jumping, running, or cutting. The repetitive acceleration and deceleration that occur with jumping activities lead to overload on the extensor mechanism and microtears within the tendon matrix. In children and adolescents, biomechanical stresses are concentrated at the growth plates, which represent the weakest link in a closed system. In Sinding-Larsen-Johansson disease, stress concentrates at the accessory ossification center at the inferior pole of the patella and leads to a traction tendinitis and eventual fragmentation. Traction at the tibial tubercle and proximal tibial physis can result in the insidious development of an Osgood-Schlatter lesion or in an acute avulsion fracture of the tibial tubercle.

The patient may have insidious onset of chronic, well-localized pain in the region of the patellar or quadriceps tendon before, during, or after participation. Complaints of weakness or giving way are common, although true locking, clicking, or effusion is rarely seen. Tenderness over the quadriceps tendon at the upper pole of the patella or the patellar tendon at the lower pole or at the tibial tuberosity is the hallmark of peripatellar tendinitis. The remainder of the examination usually reveals no additional findings. Radiographic changes have been documented but are rare before 6 months of symptoms. At that time, a radiolucency or elongation of the involved pole of the patella may be seen. Bone scans may show localization of tracer activity in the region of inflammation. Conservative therapy is the treatment of choice in the early stages. NSAIDs, rest, and activity modifications all have been successful. Local steroid injections have not proved to be of any long-lasting benefit, increase the risk of tendon rupture, and are not recommended.[103] For highly competitive athletes or for patients who fail conservative treatment, surgery with debridement of abnormal tissue may be performed.

Lateral Patellar Compression Syndrome

Lateral compression of the patella is a clinical radiographic diagnosis characterized by knee pain and patellar tilt.[104] The syndrome usually becomes manifest during the growth period of adolescence. As body weight increases and growth occurs, the lateral stress on the patella increases, and lateral retinacular strain and lateral patella tilt may occur. Several theories have been proposed to explain the mechanism for pain, including subchondral microfractures, marginal synovitis, and excessive tension in the lateral retinacular structures.[104] The pain is classically anterior and is noticed with prolonged knee flexion, ascending or descending stairs, or athletics. The patient also may complain of giving way of the knee, crepitance, and intermittent swelling. Presentation may be similar to patellar subluxation.[104] Physical findings may reveal a slight effusion, marked tenderness on the articular surface of the patella, and crepitation in the patellofemoral joint. The diagnosis may be confirmed by an axial radiograph or a CT scan that reveals patellofemoral malalignment and abnormal patellar tilt. If the lateral compression forces are allowed to continue unabated, articular cartilage degeneration and subsequent patellofemoral osteoarthritis may occur. Nonoperative treatment consists of weight reduction, quadriceps strengthening, and oral anti-inflammatory medications. Surgical treatment involving lateral retinacular release is reserved for refractory cases.

Plica Syndrome

The plica syndrome is an uncommon pathologic condition with symptoms that can be indistinguishable from symptoms of other internal derangements of the knee. Redundant folds of synovium, or plicae, found within the knee joint represent normal embryologic septa that persist into the adult knee. For reasons that are unclear, some plicae become symptomatic, and others remain quiescent. Repetitive bouts of synovitis within the plica may result in a tight, inelastic band and interfere mechanically with knee motion.[105]

The constellation of symptoms seen in plica syndrome are generally nonspecific. Patients typically complain of pain over the region of the medial femoral condyle brought on by activity, but also occurring after sitting for prolonged periods. A snapping sensation is another commonly reported symptom as the plica sweeps across the femoral condyle. Other nonspecific symptoms supporting the diagnosis include intermittent swelling, locking, weakness, and stiffness. The physical examination often elicits tenderness over the medial femoral condyle but not the medial joint line, which is more typical of a medial meniscal lesion. An effusion, crepitus, loss of motion, quadriceps atrophy, and positive McMurray's test may be present as well.

The diagnosis of plica syndrome can be made from the history alone and is supported by the physical examination. Plain radiographs are necessary to eliminate other causes of knee pain, but are of no value in diagnosing plica syndrome. Arthroscopy is most accurate in the diagnosis of this syndrome; however, the mere presence of a plica does not warrant intervention. Most plicae are incidental arthroscopic findings unrelated to underlying knee pathology.[105] Medial patella pain is more likely to be related to patellofemoral maltracking than to plica syndrome. Likewise, anteromedial joint line tenderness is more likely to be related to a meniscal tear than to a pathologic plica.

Treatment is conservative, with a regimen including rest and NSAIDs. When the acute symptoms have resolved, a rehabilitation program is instituted to emphasize quadriceps strengthening and stretching. Arthroscopic excision of pathologic plica may be necessary if conservative treatment fails.

Popliteus Tendinitis

Popliteus tendinitis is an uncommon and often misdiagnosed injury of the posterior aspect of the knee. The popliteus forms part of the floor of the popliteal fossa. It is a small, flat muscle that passes beneath the lateral head of the gastrocnemius and inserts onto the posterior aspect of the proximal tibia. This tendon is surrounded by a synovial bursa that separates it from the fibular collateral ligament, femoral condyle, and capsule. The popliteus muscle has two primary functions. First, it functions to internally rotate the tibia. Second, it acts to withdraw the meniscus during flexion to prevent impingement between the femur and the tibia. A third function, along with the quadriceps and PCL, is to stabilize the knee by preventing forward displacement of the femur on the tibia.

Overuse injuries involving the popliteus are generally the result of quadriceps overuse. The condition usually occurs in athletes and often causes localized pain over the posterior or posterolateral aspect of the knee.[106] Running and walking downhill often initiate and later exacerbate symptoms caused by the excessive eccentric quadriceps load that occurs with this activity. Usually there is no history of recurrent effusions, locking, or buckling.

On physical examination, point tenderness is noted along the lateral joint line on either side of the LCL or at the insertion point of the muscle. Because of its close relationship to other soft tissue structures, the diagnosis may be difficult. The Webb test is a specific provocation test to aid in the diagnosis.[107] This test is performed with the patient supine and the knee flexed 90 degrees. The leg is internally rotated, and the patient is asked to resist the examiner's attempt to externally rotate the leg. Such a maneuver reproduces symptoms and is the most reliable method to diagnose this condition.

The differential diagnosis for popliteus tendinitis includes disorders involving structures of the popliteal fossa. Injuries of the iliotibial band, biceps femoris, and lateral head of the gastrocnemius may mimic popliteus tendinitis. In addition, injuries involving the lateral meniscus must be considered in the differential diagnosis; meniscoid pathology generally is associated with a history of locking, recurrent effusion, or recurrent episodes of giving way.

Because popliteus tendinitis is almost always a result of quadriceps overuse, treatment requires relative rest and intensive quadriceps rehabilitation. NSAIDs, ice, and physical therapy may be useful adjuncts to treatment. A good response is the rule, and the athlete may return to activity gradually in 10 to 14 days.[106]

Bursitis of the Knee

There are numerous bursae about the knee, some of which bear clinical significance. These function to decrease friction between adjacent moving structures. They are usually thin, but with repeated stress may become thickened and fluid filled. The anserine bursa separates the pes anserinus from the distal portion of the MCL and the medial tibial condyle. The prepatellar bursa is located between the patella and the overlying subcutaneous tissues. The superficial infrapatellar bursa is located between the tibial tubercle and the overlying skin. The deep infrapatellar bursa is located between the posterior margin of the distal part of the patellar tendon and the anterior aspect of the tibia. The suprapatellar bursa is not a true bursa, but is an extension of the synovial joint capsule.

Bursae usually become inflamed or swollen as a result of repeated stress or infection, but inflammation may occur with local trauma, with crystal deposition, or in association with a systemic inflammatory arthropathy. Its presence must be differentiated from a knee effusion. Prepatellar bursitis is characterized by swelling with effusion of the superficial bursa overlying the lower pole of the patella. Passive motion usually is fully preserved, and the pain is generally mild. The disorder is usually caused by pressure from repetitive kneeling on a firm surface (housemaid's knee).[108] The prepatellar bursa is also a common site of septic bursitis. Suprapatellar bursitis usually is associated with synovitis of the knees. This may be traumatic in origin or may be associated with an inflammatory arthropathy. The superficial infrapatellar bursa is not a common site for bursitis, but may uncommonly follow direct trauma. Anserine bursitis occurs most commonly in obese women in association with osteoarthritis of the knee, but also may occur from overuse, especially in runners. It is characterized by a relatively abrupt onset of knee pain with localized tenderness and a puffy sensation on the anteromedial side of the knee. It may mimic a medial meniscal tear or injury of the MCL.

Radiographic studies are usually normal. Ultrasound examination may be useful for the detection of a small fluid collection. MRI may be helpful if the diagnosis remains unclear. These lesions represent encapsulated fluid collections and exhibit low signal intensity on T1-weighted images and high signal intensity on T2-weighted images because of their high content of free water.[109] If there is any uncertainty regarding the possibility of infection, the bursa fluid should be aspirated, and a Gram stain and culture should be performed.

Aseptic bursitis is self-limited and can be treated with usual nonoperative modalities, such as ice, rest, and anti-inflammatory medications. Local intrasynovial injection of lidocaine or corticosteroid preparations can be used as an adjunct in the management program to overcome refractory pain.[110] Contraindications to injection therapy are relative and include infections, either local or in the vicinity of the site of involvement, and hypersensitivity to any preparation or substance that might be injected. In septic bursitis, operative drainage may be required in addition to antibiotic therapy.

Osteoarthritis

Osteoarthritis is the result of degenerative changes within the joint. The incidence increases with advancing age, obesity, and antecedent trauma. Knee injuries that most commonly cause early arthritic changes in the knee are ACL tears, meniscal damage, and direct injuries of the hyaline cartilage. Removal of the medial meniscus (meniscectomy) increases the risk of osteoarthritis fourfold.[27] Persistent or recurrent episodes of joint instability caused by ligamentous or bony abnormalities commonly result in accelerated arthritis of the knee.

Pain is usually the initial complaint and often is aggravated by activity and relieved by rest. Associated complaints of locking, giving way, and a sensation of instability are often present. The physical examination may reveal a gross angular deformity—either genu valgum (knock-knee) or genu varum (bowed legs)—and an antalgic gait may be present. Pain is usually present at the joint line of the involved compartment. Osteoarthritis may involve one or all compartments of the knee.

Standard anteroposterior weight-bearing radiographs may reveal narrowing of the joint spaces, peripheral osteophyte formation, subchondral sclerosis, and cyst formation; they also may show angular deformity of the knee. Lateral and oblique films may show the presence of peripheral osteophytes and loose bodies. Tangential sunrise views are needed to evaluate the patellofemoral joint for osteophytes, sclerosis, and maltracking.

The treatment options for early arthritis in young patients are limited. Initial treatment consists of restricting activities, providing NSAIDs, bracing, and strengthening quadriceps and hamstrings. Ambulatory assistance with a cane may be helpful to unload the affected extremity and provide symptomatic relief. If the patient is obese, weight reduction is recommended. Surgical treatment is used for advanced cases and may involve high-tibial osteotomy, hemiarthroplasty, or total knee arthroplasty in selected cases. Currently, total knee replacement is contraindicated in persons younger than age 40 except for patients with rheumatoid arthritis.[27] Total knee replacement may provide excellent pain relief and improved range of motion but does not allow the patient to return to sports or heavy working activities because these contribute to early

loosening and failure of the prosthesis.[111] Overall, longevity of the prosthesis is a major limitation, with most lasting only 10 to 15 years. Research has identified cartilage transplantation and use of biosynthetic cartilage as future options in degenerative knee arthritis, but more work is needed.

Septic Arthritis

The most common joint affected with septic arthritis is the knee. The knee is involved 40% to 50% of the time, followed by the hip (20% to 25%) and the shoulder (10% to 15%).[112] Hematogenous seeding is the most common route of spread. The incidence of septic arthritis is higher in individuals with a history of trauma to the joint, especially individuals with penetrating injuries. Bacterial spread usually affects the vascular synovial membrane, then extends into the joint. Although *Neisseria gonorrhoeae* has been reported to be the most common organism causing septic arthritis, a study has suggested that *Staphylococcus* infection may occur more often.[113] Nongonococcal arthritis is more common at the extremes of age, often in an immunocompromised host. Gonococcal arthritis commonly affects young, sexually active adults, especially women.[114]

Popliteal (Baker's) Cyst

A Baker's, or popliteal, cyst also may be considered in the differential diagnosis of pain in the popliteal region. This lesion of the posterior aspect of the knee is a herniation of the synovial membrane through the posterior aspect of the capsule of the knee, or it may occur through escape of fluid via the normal communication of an anatomic bursa adjoining the semimembranosus or gastrocnemius (Figure 54-10). It is usually the result of an internal knee derangement with recurrent synovitis caused by a torn meniscus, loose body, instability, degenerative change, or other factors. This condition generally causes a mass of varying size occupying the posteromedial corner of the knee and often produces pressure, pain, and limitation of range of motion. Rupture of the bursa with resultant escape of fluid into the calf may produce a clinical picture similar to thrombophlebitis. Although a popliteal cyst can be treated by aspiration or even surgical excision, spontaneous disappearance is common, and no treatment is usually required. Differentiation from other clinical entities may require aspiration, ultrasound, or MRI. Management must be directed at the basic underlying intra-articular pathology to prevent recurrence.

LOWER LEG

PERSPECTIVE

Bony and soft tissue injuries of the lower leg are common. The lower leg's vulnerable position to injury, in combination with specific anatomic features unique

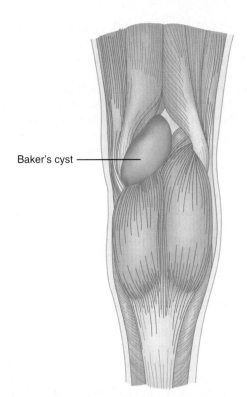

Baker's cyst

Figure 54-10. Baker's cyst is an extension of the semimembranosus bursa posteriorly. This bursa often is connected with a joint cavity.

to the leg, results in various conditions, some of which occur acutely. Other conditions occur some interval of time after the injury itself.

PRINCIPLES OF DISEASE

Anatomy and Pathophysiology

The bony structure of the lower leg is relatively simple, consisting of the tibia and fibula. The tibia is the only weight-bearing bone. The shaft of the tibia is triangular in cross section and poorly covered with soft tissue over its anteromedial aspect. Given its subcutaneous course, it is not surprising that the tibia is the most common long bone to be fractured and to sustain open fracture. In addition, the lack of overlying musculature results in a tenuous blood supply, which increases the rate of osteomyelitis and contributes to the commonly observed delayed union and nonunion after tibial fractures.

The distal end of the tibia is expanded and bears an additional surface, the fibula notch, for the lower tibiofibular joint. The medial malleolus projects from the distal medial aspect of the bone and is grooved posteriorly by the tibialis posterior tendon. The lower inferior surface of the distal tibia is covered with articular cartilage and forms the tibial plafond, the upper anterior surface of the ankle joint. The fibula, in contrast to the tibia, is well covered throughout most of its length except at the ankle, where it is subcutaneous and easily palpable. The fibula is composed of the head with a styloid process, the neck, the shaft, and the lower end or lateral malleolus of the ankle joint.

The tibia and fibula are connected by a superior and inferior tibiofibular joint and an interosseous membrane. The latter is a fibrous band that has particular importance at the distal portion of the lower leg, where it is responsible for keeping the tibia and fibula closely approximated to provide a stable ankle mortise. Disruption of this membrane may have clinical significance because it may cause a widening of the distance between the tibia and the fibula and result in disrupted ankle joint function.

The lower leg is divided into anterior, lateral, superficial posterior, and deep posterior compartments by deep partitions of the investing crural fascia. The anterior compartment contains the tibialis anterior, the long toe extensor muscles, the deep peroneal nerve, and the anterior tibial artery. The deep peroneal nerve supplies sensation to the first web space of the foot. The lateral compartment contains two muscles that evert the foot, the peroneus longus and brevis. No major arteries are contained in this compartment. The superficial peroneal nerve supplies sensation to the dorsum of the foot. The posterior compartment of the leg is divided into superficial and deep divisions. The superficial posterior compartment contains the strong plantar flexors of the ankle, the gastrocnemius, plantaris, and soleus muscles. The sural nerve passes through the superficial compartment for a variable distance before piercing the fascia to supply the lateral side of the foot and distal calf. The deep posterior compartment contains the tibialis posterior muscle, the long toe flexor muscles, the posterior tibial and peroneal arteries, and the tibial nerve, which supplies sensory function to the plantar aspect of the foot. Each compartment has a sensory nerve that runs through it, an anatomic fact that can be used to help diagnose an incipient compartment syndrome.

The vascular supply of the lower leg develops from the popliteal artery, which trifurcates to form three branches: the anterior tibial artery, which passes into the anterior compartment; the posterior tibial artery; and the peroneal artery. The anterior tibial artery can be assessed by palpating the dorsalis pedis artery pulse over the dorsum of the foot, and the posterior tibial artery pulse can be palpated posterior to the medial malleolus.

MECHANISMS OF INJURY AND MANAGEMENT

Proximal Extra-articular Tibial Fractures

Subcondylar Tibial Fractures

Isolated subcondylar fractures are not seen often, and most are associated with tibial plateau fractures, especially bicondylar fractures.[30] Subcondylar fractures involve the proximal tibial metaphysis and are typically transverse or oblique. The mechanism of injury involves a rotational or angular stress accompanied by vertical compression. Examination reveals tenderness and swelling of the involved area. A hemarthrosis may indicate extension of the fracture line into the joint or associated ligamentous injury. Routine radiographs are usually adequate in showing the fracture line. Subcondylar fractures are commonly associated with tibial plateau fractures and are subject to similar complications. Emergency department management includes ice and immobilization with a long leg posterior splint. Stable extra-articular nondisplaced transverse fractures usually are treated conservatively with a long leg splint followed by cylinder casting. Comminuted fractures or fractures associated with an intra-articular (condylar) component require open reduction and internal fixation or may be treated with traction.

Tibial Tubercle Fractures

Anatomy and Pathophysiology

Anatomically the tubercle of the tibia is at the proximal anterior border of the shaft and gives attachment to the ligamentum patella. The anterior aspect of this tubercle is subcutaneous except for the infrapatella bursa immediately in front of it. The proximal tibial epiphysis and the tibial tuberosity develop from two separate ossification centers that coalesce during adolescence. Epiphyseal ossification terminates in late adolescence.

Avulsion fractures of the tibial tubercle are uncommon. They occur predominantly in adolescent boys, most commonly at age 15 or 16 years.[115] The injury typically occurs near the end of growth, when endochondral ossification of the physeal cartilage of the tibial tubercle occurs. Avulsion fractures mainly occur as an indirect injury during sporting activities or active play.[115] The mechanism of injury has been described as a violent flexion of the knee against a tightly contracted quadriceps muscle, and the injury may be a surrogate patellar tendon rupture. An avulsion fracture occurs when the tensile force brought about by the contraction of the quadriceps complex overcomes the cohesive force within the apophyseal cartilage. Watson-Jones described three grades of injury depending on the extent of displacement (Figure 54-11). In type I injuries, the tubercle is hinged upward without displacement from the proximal base. The type II injury has a small portion of the tubercle avulsed, but it is retracted proximally. The articular surface is not involved. Type III fractures are more severe and extend across the articular surface. There is displacement of the fragment and often comminution.

Clinical Features

Physical examination reveals acute tenderness and swelling at the anterior aspect of the knee and proximal tibia. Depending on the type of injury, there is functional disability ranging from extensor lag to complete loss of active extension. Hemarthrosis is evident with type III injury because of intra-articular fracture extension across the proximal epiphysis.

Diagnostic Strategies

Plain radiographs generally confirm the clinical diagnosis. The lateral view shows the avulsion fracture, number of fragments, and amount of displacement. Swelling of the overlying soft tissue is evident. Comparison views may be necessary when a type I injury is suspected. The only differential diagnosis that may lead to confusion with avulsion fractures of the tibial tuberosity is Osgood-Schlatter disease; however, significant clinical and radiographic differences exist to distinguish the two pathologic conditions. Osgood-Schlatter disease typically is associated with chronic pain in the anterior tibial tuberosity in adolescents participating intensively in sports. Functional disability is never complete, and Osgood-Schlatter disease is never accompanied by hemarthrosis. Active extension of the knee is possible, although painful. Radiographs may show an irregularity or fragmentation of the tibial apophysis.

Type I: Incomplete avulsion

Type II: Complete avulsion extraarticular

Type III: Complete avulsion intraarticular

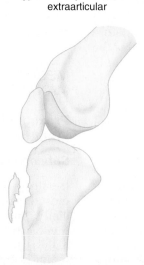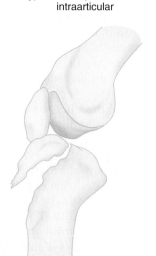

Figure 54-11. Tibial tuberosity fractures.

Management

Treatment depends on the degree of displacement and the presence of joint involvement. Nondisplaced, type I avulsions are treated with cast immobilization with the knee in extension until healing results. Such treatment has consistently provided good results. Minimally displaced, type II avulsions may be treated similarly if the displacement can be reduced by external manual maneuvers. Displaced, type III fractures are treated by open reduction and internal fixation to restore proper biomechanics and joint congruity. Fixation screw and tension band wiring techniques have yielded excellent results. After a period of immobilization and progressive rehabilitation, most patients are able to return to full activity.

Complications of tibial tubercle fractures include genu recurvatum, patella alta, meniscal tears, failure of surgical fixation, and subsequent heterotopic ossification and osteonecrosis of the tubercle.[2] Because the involved growth plates are closing at the time of injury, premature physeal closure rarely results in a significant recurvatum deformity.

Osgood-Schlatter Disease

Anatomy and Pathophysiology

Tibial tubercle apophysitis was first described by Osgood and Schlatter in 1903.[116,117] Trauma was postulated to be the cause of this condition. Seventy years later, Ogden provided histologic support for a traumatic etiology. His work revealed evidence of repetitive microtrauma and subsequent healing of the developing tibial tubercle. It is now believed that Osgood-Schlatter disease is an apophysitis caused by repeated traction to the anterior portion of the developing ossification center of the tibial tuberosity.

This traction apophysitis affects pubescent children in the midst of the adolescent growth spurt. Organized sporting activities commonly are associated with the onset of symptoms, with a fivefold increase in the incidence of Osgood-Schlatter disease in athletically active boys compared with the incidence in nonathletic controls.[118] Past reports have suggested a large male predominance for the development of Osgood-Schlatter disease. As more girls and young women have joined competitive sports, however, no significant sex differences have been found.[118] The development of this disorder seems to depend on the degree of skeletal maturity and activity level rather than gender.

Clinical Features

The disease is characterized by painful swelling over the tibial tubercle, which is exacerbated by activity, is relieved by rest, and is usually of several months' duration. The tubercle may appear abnormally prominent, often on both sides. There is pain on resisted extension of the flexed knee and occasionally an extensor lag. Tenderness is most noticeable at the insertion of the patellar tendon. Bilateral involvement is noted in 20% to 30% of patients.

Diagnostic Strategies

The diagnosis of Osgood-Schlatter disease is based on clinical signs and symptoms. Radiographs of the knee may be useful to exclude other pathologic entities (e.g., tumors, infection, and avulsion fractures), but generally are not required. They typically reveal pretibial soft tissue edema or prominence of the tubercle. Fragmentation of the ossification center is an unreliable sign because ossification patterns of the tubercle are highly variable.

Management

Treatment varies according to the acuteness of the symptoms and the skeletal age of the patient. Initially, rest, ice, and analgesics are the mainstays of therapy. As symptoms subside, a rehabilitation program that stretches and strengthens the quadriceps muscle unit should be instituted. Knee orthoses are used to dampen the pull of the extensor mechanism on the weakened tibial apophysis. Immobilization is reserved for the unreliable patient who will not or cannot comply with the program of relative rest in which aggravating activities are avoided. For children with severe symptoms, immobilization for 2 to 3 weeks may be used. Despite conservative management, some children continue to experience symptoms referable to the tibial tubercle. Surgery may be required if the conservative treatment fails, but it cannot be implemented until the epiphysis is closed, at which time the problem usually is resolved.

Tibial Shaft Fractures

Anatomy and Pathophysiology

Because the tibia and fibula run parallel and are tightly bound to each other, a displaced fracture of one bone typically is associated with an obligatory fracture or ligamentous injury of the other bone. The fibula remains intact in only 15% to 25% of tibial shaft fractures.[119] Similar to tibia plateau fractures, tibial shaft fractures can affect knee alignment, stability, and strength. Compared with other fractures, these are associated with a high incidence of infection, delayed union, nonunion, and malunion.

Tibial diaphyseal fractures may result from either direct or indirect trauma and may be secondary to low-energy or high-energy mechanisms. Direct trauma, as seen with vehicular accidents and certain types of skiing injuries, is the most common mechanism of injury.[120] This typically results in transverse or comminuted fractures and reflects high-energy injury, particularly when the fracture is greatly displaced, severely comminuted, or associated with a fibular fracture. Indirect trauma is associated with low-energy rotatory and compressive forces, such as from skiing, a fall, or child abuse, and usually results in a spiral or oblique fracture.[120]

Tibial fractures also may occur without antecedent trauma. Pathologic fractures are uncommon in the tibia but should be suspected when there is no significant mechanism of injury. Pathologic fractures may be caused by metabolic bone disease; osteomalacia; or benign, metastatic, or primary bone neoplasms. Stress fractures occur most commonly in the tibial shaft. Periosteal reaction is often delayed in such cases, and repeat radiography, bone scans, or tomography may be required to establish the diagnosis. A toddler's fracture is an often subtle, nondisplaced spiral fracture of the distal tibia in 9-month-old to 3-year-old children.[121] Children may have acute onset of a limp or refusal to bear weight. The classic distal fracture often relates to accidental trauma as opposed to a midshaft fracture, which correlates with nonaccidental trauma.

Orthopedic differences in children revolve around two basic features in the immature or growing musculoskeletal system: the potential for growth and the greater elasticity of bone, cartilage, and soft tissue.[119] A child's bone is more porous than an adult's, permitting the bone to bend, buckle, and sustain a greenstick fracture, all of which are unknown in adults. Buckle fractures usually occur in the metaphysis of long bones, such as the tibia or fibula. Radiographically, they manifest as an often subtle buckling without angulation in contrast to the smooth line formed by the normal cortex. A greenstick fracture is a bending fracture, with a break in the periosteum and cortex of the convex side of the angulated bone. These fractures are stable with an intact periosteum so that swelling, crepitance, and mobility at the fracture site are minimal.

Clinical Features

Tibial shaft fractures cause pain, swelling, and deformity of the leg, usually angulation or rotation of the foot. After visual inspection of the injured leg, determination of vascular integrity remains the highest priority. Distal dorsalis pedis and posterior tibial pulses should be assessed. Severe lower limb fractures complicated by vascular injuries are uncommon, with an incidence estimated at 0.1%.[122] Anterior compartment syndromes may follow tibial fractures and usually occur within the first 24 to 48 hours. A careful neurologic examination also must be documented because it serves as a baseline against which subsequent examinations can be compared. Because the peroneal nerve is commonly damaged in lower extremity injuries, its function must be assessed. Motor function of the peroneal nerve is checked by testing active ankle and toe dorsiflexion (deep peroneal nerve function) and active foot eversion (superficial peroneal nerve function). Sensory function of the peroneal nerve is documented by testing sensation in the first dorsal web space in the foot (deep peroneal nerve distribution) and sensation of the dorsal lateral foot (superficial peroneal nerve distribution). Integrity of the posterior tibial nerve is assessed by the presence or absence of plantar sensation. Significant soft tissue damage also may accompany tibial shaft fractures. One study finds a 22% incidence of injury to at least one ligament of the knee.[123] A thorough examination of knee stability is

indicated after fracture stabilization, especially in high-energy injuries.

Diagnostic Strategies

Anteroposterior and lateral x-ray studies are mandatory to document the fracture, define the fracture pattern, and identify any associated bone loss (Figure 54-12). The knee and ankle must be included in both views, and additional x-ray studies of the pelvis and ipsilateral femur may be required to assess for associated injuries. Postreduction views should be taken after any manipulation of the extremity and should include the knee and ankle joints so that alignment of the proximal and distal joint surfaces can be determined.

Management

Open tibial fracture usually is encountered in a multiply injured patient. Unstable high-energy fractures usually are associated with injuries of multiple organ systems and often occur in conjunction with multiple fractures. Open fractures may seem to be associated with more complications than closed fractures; however, closed fractures may be associated with more soft tissue damage. Classification of a tibial fracture as closed or open does not indicate its severity. One of the most prognostically important distinctions is between fractures produced from high-energy forces and fractures from low-energy forces. In all studies of tibial shaft fractures, the fractures that result from high-energy trauma always have a poorer prognosis than the fractures that result from low-energy trauma.

After life-threatening injuries have been evaluated, fracture management should follow. The initial management of closed tibial shaft fractures consists of immobilization in a long leg posterior splint with 10 to 20 degrees of knee flexion. This may require analgesia and sedation. Generally, after fractures are immobilized, the pain decreases. If the patient complains of continued severe pain after immobilization, a complication such as nerve root compression or limb ischemia should be considered, and additional injuries should be sought. A circumferential cast should be avoided in the acute setting because of the risk of compartment syndrome. Initial hospitalization is indicated for most patients with significant tibial shaft fractures for pain control, observation for compartment syndrome, long leg casting, and instruction in crutch walking.

Emergency department treatment of open tibial shaft fractures should be directed at four interventions. First, open fractures should be covered with a sterile dressing. Second, a long leg posterior splint should be applied. Third, if tetanus immunization is not current, appropriate tetanus prophylaxis should be given. Fourth, most authors also recommend empiric antibiotics for open fractures. Intravenous antibiotic prophylaxis using a first-generation cephalosporin is recommended. In tibial fractures caused by high-velocity injuries that have extensive soft tissue defects and significant wound contamination, a loading dose

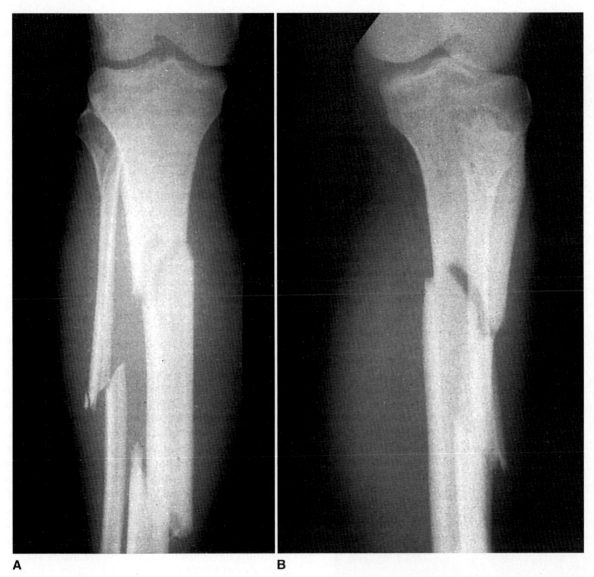

Figure 54-12. Tibiofibular fracture. **A,** Anteroposterior view. Comminuted fractures of the tibial and fibular shafts are present. Note the obliteration of the normal soft tissue planes because of edema or hemorrhage. **B,** Lateral view. (From Rosen P, et al: *Diagnostic Radiology in Emergency Medicine*. St. Louis, Mosby, 1992, p 198.)

of an aminoglycoside may be given in addition to the first-generation cephalosporin.

Emergency operative debridement with external or internal fixation is recommended as soon as possible for open tibial fractures with significant soft tissue disruption. The incidence of osteomyelitis is related in part to the time between contamination and definitive debridement and stabilization of the open fracture site. Open tibial fractures have a fivefold increased risk of developing osteomyelitis, and the incidence of infection correlates directly with the extent of soft tissue damage and classification.

In general, tibial fractures are slow to heal. Delayed union is generally applied to fracture segments that have not united after 20 weeks. The average time to union is approximately 20 weeks for stable tibial shaft fractures caused by a low-energy mechanism and more than 30 weeks for unstable fractures caused by a high-energy mechanism.[124] At times, nonunion may occur. Nonunion is a radiographic diagnosis, with a finding of

rounded, well-corticated edges of the major fracture fragments. It is much more common in adult long bone fractures than childhood fractures, which generally are characterized by rapid healing. Delayed vascular injuries also may occur as a complication of tibial shaft fractures, including pseudoaneurysm, arteriovenous fistula, and deep vein thrombosis. Fat embolism also may occur. Additional late complications include malrotation of the leg, re-fracture, and reflex sympathetic dystrophy.

Proximal Fibula Fractures

Anatomy and Pathophysiology

Isolated proximal fibula and fibula shaft fractures are uncommon, and fibula fracture is usually seen in association with a tibial fracture. Clinically, fibula fractures are relatively unimportant because no significant weight is supported by the fibula. The mechanism of injury is usually a direct blow to the lateral aspect of

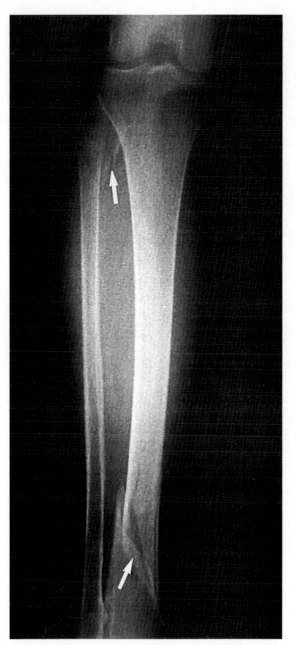

Figure 54-13. Maisonneuve's fracture, anteroposterior view. The rotatory force involved in this injury has caused fractures of the distal tibia and the proximal fibula *(arrows)*. (From Rosen P, et al: *Diagnostic Radiology in Emergency Medicine*. St. Louis, Mosby, 1992, p 197.)

the leg or an indirect varus stress to the knee. An exception to this is Maisonneuve fracture, which is a proximal fibula fracture with an associated ankle fracture or deltoid ligament tear (Figure 54-13). The mechanism resulting in Maisonneuve fracture is often an external rotatory force applied to the ankle that results in partial or complete syndesmotic disruption.

Clinical Features

Isolated fibula shaft fractures cause lateral leg pain that is exacerbated by walking. Local pain, swelling, and tenderness at the fracture site may be elicited. Palpation of the proximal fibula should be performed whenever significant ankle injury is present to assess for a

Maisonneuve fracture. A thorough evaluation should be done to exclude serious associated occult neurovascular or ligamentous injuries. The common peroneal nerve courses around the proximal neck of the fibula and may be contused or lacerated at the time of injury. The LCL may be ruptured or strained in association with the fracture, and anterior tibial artery injury with thrombosis may occur.

Diagnostic Strategies

Radiographic evaluation should be undertaken in cases of suspected proximal fibula fracture. Anteroposterior and lateral radiographs should include the knee and ankle joints and confirm the fracture pattern. A bone scan may be required for diagnosis if a fibular stress fracture is in question.

Management

Isolated uncomplicated fibula shaft fractures are treated symptomatically with ice, analgesia, and non–weight bearing. Immobilization in a long leg cast is rarely done but may provide symptomatic relief beginning 2 days after the acute injury. The patient should remain non–weight bearing until a small amount of weight can be tolerated. Weight bearing may be advanced progressively as tolerated. Patients with nondisplaced or minimally displaced fractures may have little pain and tolerate crutch walking without casting well. In general, isolated fibula shaft fractures can be managed on an outpatient basis and heal without complication.

For severely displaced fibula shaft fractures or fractures with associated peroneal nerve deficit such as footdrop, orthopedic consultation is indicated. Cast immobilization is not recommended in cases with concomitant nerve damage, and follow-up is scheduled at a shorter interval from injury. Elective surgical repair may be indicated if function does not return. Maisonneuve fracture is associated with partial or complete syndesmotic diastasis and may result in an unstable ankle mortise. Stress radiographs are necessary, and operative repair may be indicated.

Proximal Tibiofibular Joint Dislocations

Anatomy and Pathophysiology

The proximal tibiofibular joint is a small synovial joint between a circular or oval facet on the head of the fibula and a similar facet on the inferior aspect of the lateral tibial condyle. The proximal tibiofibular joint is stabilized by the joint capsule and the anterior and posterior tibiofibular ligaments. Dislocation of the proximal tibiofibular joint is rare, occurring most commonly in adolescents and young adults because of its association with motor vehicle accidents and sporting injuries.[125] Several types of dislocations of the joint have been described; anterolateral dislocation is the most common and usually is caused by a fall on a flexed, abducted leg.[126] Posterior medial dislocation generally is caused by a direct blow to the flexed knee and is more often associated with peroneal nerve injury.

Superior dislocation is associated with ankle diastasis and typically occurs simultaneously with an ankle fracture.

Clinical Features

The patient may complain that the knee feels out of place, or if the problem is chronic, the knee may lock or give way periodically. Physical examination reveals tenderness and fusiform swelling over the proximal fibula and tibiofibular joint. In the absence of associated injury, the knee examination is normal, with full range of motion and no joint line tenderness or effusion.

Diagnostic Strategies

Plain radiography may confirm the diagnosis. On the anteroposterior view, the fibula head is displaced laterally, and the interosseous space is widened. Comparison views of the uninjured knee may be necessary to appreciate these findings. If the diagnosis is still suspected but not confirmed by plain radiography, an axial CT scan may be obtained.

Management

Traumatic proximal tibiofibular dislocation is treated initially with closed reduction. If the patient seeks treatment within a few days of injury, reduction of an anterior lateral dislocation can be accomplished in the emergency department by flexing the knee to 90 degrees, everting the ankle, and applying direct pressure to the head of the fibula.[126] Immobilization of the knee for a minimum of 3 to 6 weeks is necessary after reduction. Failure of closed reduction may require open reduction, with repair of the torn capsule ligaments and pinning. Recurrent cases or cases that do not respond to initial treatment may be treated with resection of the proximal fibula or arthrodesis.

Stress Fractures

Anatomy and Pathophysiology

Stress fractures are common skeletal lesions, and most involve the lower limbs. The specific anatomic sites vary depending on the athletic activity. The most common site of stress fracture in the athlete is the tibia, accounting for 50% of stress fractures in some series.[127] Usually the stress fracture occurs on the tibial shaft. Fractures are typically horizontal or oblique, with only 10% reported to be longitudinal.[128] Other sites include the femur, fibula, tarsal navicular, and metatarsal. Stress fractures result from repetitive cyclic and prolonged muscle force on bone and have been well described as overuse injuries in military recruits and athletes.[129] Fatigue fractures occur in normal bone because of abnormally increased stress and commonly are related to activities such as running, jumping, marching, or ballet dancing. Insufficiency fractures occur when normal stresses are applied to bone deficient in mineral content or abnormally inelastic bone. These injuries typically occur in postmenopausal, osteoporotic women, but also are found in patients with osteopenia of any cause, including renal osteodystrophy, rheumatoid arthritis, and diabetes mellitus. Stress fractures are distinguished from pathologic fractures, which occur through bone weakened by tumor.

The incidence of stress fractures in the general population has not been studied. Most studies on stress fractures have concentrated on specific populations that are predisposed to their occurrence, particularly military recruits and athletes. These fractures may constitute 10% of all sports injuries and account for 5% to 15% of all running injuries.[129]

Several factors have been associated with the development of stress fractures. Military recruits typically undergo a vigorous training program over a short period that does not allow sufficient time for proper bone remodeling. Women have been reported to have a higher incidence of stress fractures, which may be related to differences in bone mass, body mass, body habitus, musculoskeletal fitness, or endocrine factors.[130] Race also may play a role in the development of stress fractures. Several reports indicate a higher incidence of stress fractures in whites compared with African Americans. This difference has been attributed to the greater average bone mass in African Americans.

Clinical Features

Clinically the patient exhibits bone pain and tenderness without a history of direct trauma. The diagnosis of stress fractures can be difficult because of limited presenting signs and minimal or no initial radiographic findings. The most important historical information includes a recent increase in physical activity, training on hard surfaces, and inadequate footwear. The pain is usually insidious in onset and progressive but may be sudden. Classically a patient with a stress fracture describes pain associated with a particular activity that is relieved with rest and worsened with continued activity. The relationship between bone pain and stress fractures has been studied using nuclear scintigraphy, and it seems that stress fractures may be present even when pain is poorly localized or absent. The differential diagnosis of lower leg pain also includes shin splints, exercise-induced compartment syndrome, contusion, muscle strains, tendinitis, periostitis, and interosseous membrane strains. The physical examination may reveal localized bony tenderness and swelling of the overlying soft tissues. Usually there is no muscle atrophy, weakness, or restriction of joint range of motion.

Diagnostic Strategies

The radiographic findings vary depending on the location of the fracture and the stage in the repair process at which the radiograph is taken. Only 30% of stress fractures are evident radiographically at the time of initial diagnosis, whereas approximately 50% of treated stress fractures are associated with radiographic findings after 2 to 6 weeks. The radiographic findings are often subtle and may include periosteal new bone, sclerosis, and a lucent line perpendicular to the cortex.

If a stress fracture of the lower extremity is suspected and initial plain radiography is unremarkable, a follow-up in 10 days to 2 weeks may detect radiographic signs of fracture after a period of inactivity. Evidence of healing in response to treatment usually suffices to confirm the diagnosis. If the patient cannot comply with a prescription of rest or if an urgent definitive diagnosis is needed, additional diagnostic studies may be done. Technetium diphosphate bone scintigraphy may be positive 3 days after the onset of symptoms of a stress fracture and has a sensitivity that approaches 100%. Typically, bone scans show a focal area of increased radiotracer uptake on the delayed images in the region of the stress fracture. Bone scintigraphy cannot distinguish fracture from infection or neoplasm and is less specific than plain radiography.

The roles of plain tomography, CT scan, and MRI are uncertain at this time. These studies may be used to gain added specificity in cases that remain indeterminate on prior radiographic studies. Early detection and treatment of stress fractures before the development of cortical disruption prevent increased morbidity and possible disabling sequelae.

Management

Most tibial and fibula stress fractures can be treated nonoperatively. Generally activities should be decreased for 3 to 6 weeks to allow for healing, and serial radiographs should be obtained. In rare instances in which walking causes pain, a cast and non–weight bearing may be required. Serial radiographs are used to evaluate healing. Surgery is reserved for rare patients with tibial stress fractures who have failed nonoperative treatment and have developed characteristic radiographic findings of nonunion.[129]

Compartment Syndrome in the Lower Leg

Compartment syndrome is generally defined as the necrosis of muscle and nerve secondary to increased tissue pressure within an osteofascial compartment and is discussed in Chapter 46.

Soft Tissue Injuries Involving the Lower Leg

Strains

Gastrocnemius Strain

In the lower extremity, the medial head of the gastrocnemius muscle is especially prone to strain injury. A sudden push-off can tear the gastrocnemius muscle or musculotendinous junction, resulting in the so-called tennis leg. The mechanism of injury seems to be a sudden ankle dorsiflexion in the involved leg in which the knee has been previously extended and the ankle plantar flexed. This position is commonly encountered in the back leg of an athlete during the follow-through of a tennis serve. Predisposing factors include increasing age, inadequate stretching, fatigue, and previous muscle injury. The athlete experiences a sudden, intense pain in the posterior and medial aspect of the calf, swelling, diffuse tenderness, and variable loss of function. On physical examination, a palpable gap may be identified in the substance of the muscle, and point tenderness may be elicited in the medial and inferior borders of the muscle belly. Any attempted active or passive ankle dorsiflexion elicits severe pain.

Gastrocnemius strain or rupture may be confused with rupture of the plantaris tendon, which causes tenderness, swelling, and ecchymosis in the proximal calf; rupture of a Baker's cyst, which may result in the escape of fluid into the calf, mimicking thrombophlebitis; and Achilles tendon rupture, which typically results in a palpable gap just proximal to the os calcaneus. If the diagnosis of a soft tissue injury is in doubt, imaging may be useful. Plain radiography is of no help except to exclude an avulsion fracture. MRI is superior to plain radiography and CT as an imaging modality for muscle strain injury.

A mild partial rupture of the medial head of the gastrocnemius can be treated with rest and non–weight bearing for several days. Treatment for an incomplete rupture is casting in equinus position for 8 weeks. For a complete tear, most orthopedists recommend surgical repair to restore normal length and tensile strength. Acute compartment syndrome has been reported as a complication of gastrocnemius strain.[131]

Plantaris Strain and Rupture

The plantaris is a small, variable, pencil-sized muscle that originates at the lateral condyle of the femur and passes beneath the soleus to attach on the Achilles tendon. It is a feeble flexor of the knee and plantar flexor of the ankle joint with little functional significance. Rupture may occur at the myotendinous junction with or without an associated partial tear of the medial head of the gastrocnemius muscle. A strain of the more proximal plantaris muscle also may occur as an isolated injury or in conjunction with injury to the ACL.[132] The patient may complain of a sudden sharp snap in the posterior calf followed by a duller deep ache, which may be disabling. Tenderness is greatest just lateral to the midline of the posterior calf. Repair is not needed here; only symptomatic treatment is indicated.[120]

Shin Splints

The term *shin splints* refers to nonspecific, anterior lower leg pain, usually during or after exercise. The most common causes are a tibial stress reaction or periostitis. Tibial stress reactions are microfractures caused by stress placed on the tibia. The clinical spectrum may range from mild exertional lower leg pain to severe debilitating pain localized to the anterior tibia. The history is important in making the diagnosis of this overuse injury; it occurs most commonly in runners and is often bilateral. Bilateral symptoms are usually seen with chondromalacia, Osgood-Schlatter disease, and anterior tibialis syndrome. Other injuries, such as plantar fasciitis and Achilles tendinitis, are usually unilateral. Shin splints also can be confused with stress fractures.

The physical examination reveals direct localized tenderness over the tibia or medial tibial crest, usually at the junction of the middle and lower thirds of the tibia. Radiographic studies are not helpful in the diagnosis of shin splints but may help exclude a tibial stress fracture. Shin splints, similar to other overuse injuries, are associated with the development of inflammation. The goal of treatment is to reduce inflammation through rest, use of NSAIDs, and alteration of activities. The duration of rest varies with the spectrum of the disease; however, several weeks is usually sufficient.

Foreign Bodies

Soft tissue foreign bodies are a common cause of emergency department visits and may account for 4% of liability claims against emergency physicians.[133,134] Early detection can be challenging, especially if a foreign body is small and radiolucent. Wood and plastic pieces can be elusive on plain films. Plain radiographs are 95% to 100% sensitive in detecting radiopaque objects but not as helpful in detecting radiolucent foreign bodies.[133,134] Foreign bodies to the lower extremity are especially prevalent in children and adolescents. Missed retained foreign bodies to the lower leg can lead to devastating consequences, such as cellulitis, abscess formation, myonecrosis, necrotizing fasciitis, and gangrene. Plain films remain the standard, but when plain films are inconclusive, other modalities, such as ultrasound or CT, must be employed. Surgical exploration remains the diagnostic and therapeutic modality of choice.

KEY CONCEPTS

- Knee injuries are the most common orthopedic injury seen in the emergency department.

- Most knee injuries are ligamentous. The most common injury is to the MCL; however, the most serious injury is to the ACL. Approximately 50% of patients with ACL injury have a concomitant meniscal tear.

- Knee dislocation is a true orthopedic emergency with the potential for vascular injury to the popliteal artery. Immediate attention must be directed to the vascular status of the injured limb. The presence of a distal pulse does not preclude vascular injury, and an arteriogram may be required to exclude significant injury. Early revascularization is crucial because a delay of more than 6 hours increases the risk of compartment syndrome and amputation.

- The most common long bone fracture is that of the tibial diaphysis, and compartment syndrome is an infrequent but serious complication.

ACKNOWLEDGMENT

This chapter would never have been completed without the efforts of Janelle Smith. We are grateful for her endurance through revisions of the chapter and for her patience and meticulous attention to detail.

REFERENCES

1. Roberts DM, Stallard TC: Emergency department evaluation and treatment of knee and leg injuries. *Emerg Med Clin North Am* 18:67, 2000.
2. Thabit G III, Micheli LJ: Patellofemoral pain in the pediatric patient. *Orthop Clin North Am* 3:567, 1992.
3. Lassen MR, Borris LC, Nakov RL: Use of low-molecular-weight heparin reviparin to prevent deep-vein thrombosis after leg injury requiring immobilization. *N Engl J Med* 347:726, 2002.
4. Terry GC: Office evaluation and management of the symptomatic knee. *Orthop Clin North Am* 19:699, 1988.
5. Baxter MP: Assessment of normal pediatric knee ligament laxity using the genucom. *J Pediatr Orthop* 8:546, 1988.
6. Sandberg R, et al: Stability tests in knee ligament injuries. *Arch Orthop Trauma Surg* 106:5, 1986.
7. Müller W, et al: OAK knee evaluation, a new way to assess knee ligament injuries. *Clin Orthop* 232:37, 1988.
8. Wroble RR, Lindenfeld TN: The stabilized Lachman test. *Clin Orthop* 237:209, 1988.
9. Beaty JH: *Orthopedic Knowledge Update 6: Home Study Syllabus.* Rosemont, Ill, American Academy of Orthopedic Surgeons, 1999.
10. Sonzogni JJ: Examining the injured knee. *Emerg Med* 28:76, 1996.
11. Harrner CD, Höher J: Evaluation and treatment of posterior cruciate ligament injuries. *Am J Sports Med* 26:471, 1998.
12. Bach BR Jr, et al: Arthrometric evaluation of knees that have a torn anterior cruciate ligament. *J Bone Joint Surg Am* 72:1299, 1990.
13. Seaburg DC, et al: Multicenter comparison of two clinical decision rules for the use of radiography in acute, high-risk knee injuries. *Ann Emerg Med* 32:8, 1998.
14. Stiell IG, et al: Prospective validation of a decision rule for the use of radiography in acute knee injuries. *JAMA* 275:611, 1996.
15. Stiell IG, et al: Implementation of the Ottawa knee rule for the use of radiography in acute knee injuries. *JAMA* 278:2075, 1997.
16. Ketelslegers E, et al: Validation of the Ottawa knee rules in an emergency teaching center. *Eur Radiol* 12:1218, 2002.
17. Seaberg DC, Jackson R: Clinical decision rule for knee radiographs. *Am J Emerg Med* 12:541, 1994.
18. Bulloch B, et al: Validation of the Ottawa Knee Rule in children: A multicenter study. *Ann Emerg Med* 42:48, 2003.
19. Khine H, Dorfman DH, Avner JR: Applicability of Ottawa knee rule for knee injury in children. *Pediatr Emerg Care* 17:404, 2001.
20. Verma A, et al: A screening method for knee trauma. *Acad Radiol* 8:392, 2001.
21. Langer JE, Meyer SJ, Dalinka MK: Imaging of the knee. *Radiol Clin North Am* 28:975, 1990.
22. Manaster BJ, Andrew CL: Fractures and dislocations of the knee and proximal tibia and fibula. *Semin Roentgenol* 29:113, 1994.
23. Pathria MN, et al: Ultrasonography of the popliteal fossa and lower extremity. *Radiol Clin North Am* 26:77, 1988.
24. Merrill KD: Knee dislocation with vascular injuries. *Orthop Clin North Am* 25:707, 1994.
25. Mink JH, Levy T, Crues JV: Tears of the anterior cruciate ligament and menisci of the knee: MR imaging evaluation. *Radiology* 167:769, 1988.
26. Adalberth T, et al: Magnetic resonance imaging, scintigraphy, and arthroscopic evaluation of traumatic hemarthrosis of the knee. *Am J Sports Med* 25:231, 1997.

27. Schenck RC Jr, Heckman JD: Injuries of the knee. *Clin Symp* 45:1, 1993.

28. Wallman P, Curley S: Aspiration of acute traumatic knee haemarthrosis. *Emerg Med J* 19:50, 2002.

29. VanNess SA, Gittins ME: Comparison of intra-articular morphine and bupivacaine following knee arthroscopy. *Orthop Rev* 23:743, 1994.

30. Wiss DA, Watson JT, Johnson EE: Fractures of the knee. In Rockwood CA Jr, Green DP (eds): *Fractures in Adults,* 4th ed. Philadelphia, Lippincott-Raven, 1996, p 1919.

31. Kerr HD: Segond fracture, hemarthrosis, and anterior cruciate ligament disruption. *J Emerg Med* 8:29, 1990.

32. Kaufman D, Leung J: Evidence based emergency medicine: Evaluation and diagnostic testing. *Emerg Med Clin North Am* 17:77, 1999.

33. Fagan DJR, Davies S: The clinical indications for plain radiography in acute knee trauma. *Int J Care Injured* 31:723, 2000.

34. Hess T, et al: Lateral tibial avulsion fractures and disruptions to the anterior cruciate ligament. *Clin Orthop* 303:193, 1994.

35. Delamarter RB, et al: Ligament injuries associated with tibial plateau fractures. *Clin Orthop* 250:226, 1990.

36. Lansinger O, et al: Tibial condylar fractures: A 20 year follow-up. *J Bone Joint Surg Am* 68:13, 1986.

37. Watson JT: High-energy fractures of the tibial plateau. *Orthop Clin North Am* 25:723, 1994.

38. Kode L, et al: Evaluation of tibial plateau fractures: Efficacy of MR imaging compared with CT. *AJR Am J Roentgenol* 163:141, 1994.

39. Kendall NS, Hsu SY, Chan KM: Fracture of the tibial spine in adults and children. *J Bone Joint Surg Br* 74:848, 1992.

40. Keys GW, Walters J: Nonunion of intercondylar eminence fracture of the tibia. *J Trauma* 28:870, 1988.

41. Schenck RC Jr: Injuries of the knee. In Rockwood CA Jr, Green DP (eds): *Fractures in Adults,* 5th ed. Philadelphia, Lippincott-Raven, 2001, p 1843.

42. Sponseller P, Beaty JH: Fractures and dislocations about the knee. In Rockwood CA Jr, Green DP (eds): *Fractures in Children,* 4th ed. Philadelphia, Lippincott-Raven, 1996, p 1233-1329.

43. Ogden JA: *Skeletal Injury in the Child,* 2nd ed. Philadelphia, WB Saunders, 1990.

44. Mizuta T, Benson WM, Foster BK: Statistical analysis of the incidence of physical injuries. *J Pediatr Orthop* 7:518, 1987.

45. Mann DC, Rajmaira S: Distribution of physeal and non-physeal fractures in 2,650 long-bone fractures in children age 0-16 years. *J Pediatr Orthop* 10:713, 1990.

46. Bretlau T, et al: Bone bruise in the acutely injured knee. *Knee Surg Sports Traumatol Arthrosc* 10:96, 2002.

47. Schenck RC Jr, Goodnight JM: Osteochondritis dissecans. *J Bone Joint Surg Am* 78:439, 1996.

48. Garrett JC: Osteochondritis dissecans. *Clin Sports Med* 10:569, 1991.

49. Lotke PA, Ecker ML: Osteonecrosis of the knee. *J Bone Joint Surg Am* 70:470, 1988.

50. Agarwal S, Owen R: Tendinitis and tendon ruptures in successful renal transplant recipients. *Clin Orthop* 252:270, 1990.

51. Rougraff BT, Reeck CC, Essenmacher J: Complete quadriceps tendon ruptures. *Orthopedics* 19:509, 1996.

52. Scuderi GR, et al: Injuries of the knee. In Rockwood CA Jr, Green DP (eds): *Fractures in Adults,* 4th ed. Philadelphia, Lippincott-Raven, 1996, pp 2001-2126.

53. Ghelman B, Hodge J: Imaging of the patellofemoral joint. *Orthop Clin North Am* 23:523, 1992.

54. Karlsson J, et al: Partial rupture of the patellar ligament. *Am J Sports Med* 20:390, 1992.

55. Wiss DA, Watson JT, Johnson EE: *Injuries of the Knee: Part II. Fractures of the Patella,* 4th ed. Philadelphia, Lippincott-Raven, 1996.

56. Carpenter JE, et al: Fractures of the patella. *J Bone Joint Surg Am* 75:1550, 1993.

57. Miller MD: Commonly missed orthopedic problems. *Emerg Med Clin North Am* 10:151, 1992.

58. Saltzman CL, et al: Results of treatment of displaced patellar fractures by partial patellectomy. *J Bone Joint Surg Am* 72:1279, 1990.

59. Merchant AC: Extensor mechanism injuries: Classification and diagnosis. In Scott WN (ed): *Ligament and Extensor Mechanism Injuries of the Knee: Diagnosis and Treatment.* St. Louis, Mosby, 1991, p 173.

60. Garner JP, Pike JM, George CD, et al: Intra-articular dislocation of the patella: Two cases and literature review. *J Trauma* 47:780, 1999.

61. Roger DJ, Williamson SC, Uhl RL: Difficult reductions in traumatic patellar dislocation. *Orthop Rev* 21:1333, 1992.

62. Kelly MA, Insall JN: Historical perspectives of chondromalacia patellae. *Orthop Clin North Am* 23:517, 1992.

63. Ghelman B, Hodge JC: Imaging of the patellofemoral joint. *Orthop Clin North Am* 23:523, 1992.

64. Wascher D: The dislocated knee. *Clin Sports Med* 19:457, 2000.

65. Wascher DC, et al: Knee dislocation: Initial assessment and implications for treatment. *J Orthop Trauma* 11:525, 1997.

66. Varnell RM, et al: Arterial injury complicating knee disruptions. *Am J Surg* 55:699, 1989.

67. Soto JA, et al: Focal arterial injuries of the proximal extremities: Helical CT arteriography as the initial method of diagnosis. *Radiology* 218:188, 2001.

68. Green NE, Allen BL: Vascular injuries associated with dislocation of the knee. *J Bone Joint Surg Am* 59:236, 1977.

69. Bandyk DF: Vascular injury associated with extremity trauma. *Clin Orthop* 318:117, 1995.

70. Stain SC, et al: Selective management of nonocclusive arterial injuries. *Arch Surg* 124:1136, 1989.

71. Cooper DE, et al: Complete knee dislocation without posterior cruciate ligament disruption: A report of four cases and review of the literature. *Clin Orthop* 284:228, 1992.

72. Wagner WH, et al: Blunt popliteal artery trauma: One hundred consecutive injuries. *J Vasc Surg* 7:736, 1988.

73. Welling RE, Kakkasseril J, Cranley JJ: Complete dislocations of the knee with popliteal vascular injury. *J Trauma* 21:450, 1981.

74. McCabe CJ, Ferguson CM, Ottinger LW: Improved limb salvage in popliteal artery injuries. *J Trauma* 23:982, 1983.

75. Alberty RE, Goodfried G, Boyden AM: Popliteal artery injury with fracture dislocation of the knee. *Am J Surg* 142:36, 1981.

76. Abou-Sayed H, Berger D: Blunt lower extremity trauma and popliteal artery injuries. *Arch Surg* 137:585, 2002.

77. Miranda FE, et al: Confirmation of the safety and accuracy of physical examination in the evaluation of knee dislocation for injury of the popliteal artery: A prospective study. *J Trauma* 52:247, 2002.

78. Barnes CJ, Pietrobon R, Higgins LD: Does the pulse examination in patients with traumatic knee dislocation predict a surgical arterial injury? A meta-analysis. *J Trauma* 53:1109, 2002.

79. Bosse MJ, et al: An analysis of outcomes of reconstruction or amputation after leg threatening injuries. *N Engl J Med* 347:1924, 2002.

80. Rios A, et al: Results after treatment of traumatic knee dislocations: A report of 26 cases. *J Trauma* 55:489, 2003.

81. Nystrom M, Samimi S, Ha'Eri GB: Two cases of irreducible knee dislocation occurring simultaneously in two patients and a review of the literature. *Clin Orthop* 277:197, 1992.

82. Gillespie DL, Cantelmo NL: Traumatic popliteal artery pseudoaneurysms: Case report and review of the literature. *J Trauma* 31:412, 1991.

83. Mills WJ, Tejwani N: Heterotopic ossification after knee dislocation: The predictive value of the injury severity score. *J Orthop Trauma* 17:338, 2003.

84. Yeh WL, et al: Knee dislocation: Treatment of high-velocity knee dislocation. *J Trauma* 46:693, 1999.

85. Andres JR, Edwards JC, Satterwhite YE: Isolated posterior cruciate ligament injuries. *Clin Sports Med* 13:519, 1994.

86. Johnson DL, Warner JP: Diagnosis for anterior cruciate ligament surgery. *Clin Sports Med* 12:671, 1993.

87. Nottage WM, Matsuura PA: Management of complete traumatic anterior cruciate ligament tears in the skeletally immature patient: Current concepts and review of the literature. *Arthroscopy* 10:569, 1994.

88. Caborn DNM, Johnson BM: The natural history of the anterior cruciate ligament-deficient knee. *Clin Sports Med* 12:625, 1993.

89. Oberlander MA, Shalvoy RM, Hughston JC: The accuracy of the clinical knee examination documented by arthroscopy. *Am J Sports Med* 21:773, 1993.

90. Baker CL: Acute hemarthrosis of the knee. *J Med Assoc Ga* 81:301, 1992.

91. Stanitski CL, Harvell JC, Fu F: Observations on acute knee hemarthrosis in children and adolescents. *J Pediatr Orthop* 13:506, 1993.

92. Stallenberg B, et al: Fracture of the posterior aspect of the lateral tibial plateau: Radiographic sign of anterior cruciate ligament tear. *Radiology* 187:821, 1993.

93. Ruwe PA, Wright J, Randall RL: Can MR imaging effectively replace diagnostic arthroscopy? *Radiology* 183:335, 1992.

94. Tung GA, et al: Tears of the anterior cruciate ligament: Primary and secondary signs at MR imaging. *Radiology* 188:661, 1993.

95. Cameron JC, Saha S: Management of medial collateral ligament laxity. *Orthop Clin North Am* 25:527, 1994.

96. Hardin GT, Farr J, Bach BR Jr: Meniscal tears: Diagnosis, evaluation, and treatment. *Orthop Rev* 21:1311, 1992.

97. Diment MT, DeHaven KE, Sebastianelli WJ: Current concepts in meniscal repair. *Orthopedics* 16:973, 1993.

98. Thompson WO, Fu FH: The meniscus in the cruciate deficient knee. *Clin Sports Med* 12:771, 1993.

99. Fowler PJ, Lubliner JA: The predictive value of five clinical signs in the evaluation of meniscal pathology. *J Arthrosc Rel Surg* 5:184, 1989.

100. Crues JV Jr, Ryu R, Morgan FW: Meniscal pathology: The expanding role of magnetic resonance imaging. *Clin Orthop* 252:80, 1990.

101. Crues JV Jr, et al: Meniscal tears of the knee: Accuracy of MR imaging. *Radiology* 164:445, 1987.

102. Barber FA, Sutker AN: Iliotibial band syndrome. *Sports Med* 14:144, 1992.

103. Colosimo AJ, Bassett FH: Jumper's knee: Diagnosis and treatment. *Orthop Rev* 19:139, 1990.

104. Fu FH, Maday MG: Arthroscopic lateral release and the lateral patellar compression syndrome. *Orthop Clin North Am* 23:601, 1992.

105. Dupont JY: Synovial plicae of the knee: Controversies and review. *Clin Sports Med* 16:87, 1997.

106. Hunter SC, Poole RM: The chronically inflamed tendon. *Clin Sports Med* 6:371, 1987.

107. Garrick JG, Webb DR: *Sports Injuries: Diagnosis and Management.* Philadelphia, WB Saunders, 1990.

108. Myllym Adaki T, et al: Carpet layer's knee: An ultrasonographic study. *Acta Radiol* 34:496, 1993.

109. Janzen DL, et al: Cystic lesions around the knee joint: MR imaging findings. *AJR Am J Roentgenol* 163:155, 1994.

110. Neustadt DH: Injection therapy of bursitis and tendinitis. In Roberts JR, Hedges JR (eds): *Clinical Procedures in Emergency Medicine,* 3rd ed. Philadelphia, WB Saunders, 1997, p 1020.

111. Kaplan J, Wilson RW: Orthopedic prostheses. *Emerg Med Clin North Am* 12:849, 1994.

112. Donatto KC: Orthopedic management of septic arthritis. *Rheum Dis Clin North Am* 24:275, 1998.

113. Esterhai JL, Gelb I: Adult septic arthritis. *Orthop Clin North Am* 22:503, 1991.

114. Scopelitis E, Martinez-Osuna P: Gonococcal arthritis. *Rheum Dis Clin North Am* 19:363, 1993.

115. Balmat P, Vichard P, Pem R: The treatment of avulsion fractures of the tibial tuberosity in adolescent athletes. *Sports Med* 9:311, 1990.

116. Osgood RB: Lesions of the tibial tubercle occurring during adolescence. *Boston Med Surg J* 148:114, 1903.

117. Schlatter C: Verletzungen des schnabelformigen fortsatzes der oberen tibiaepiphyse. *Beitr Klin Chir* 38:874, 1903.

118. Kujala UM, Kvist M, Heinonen O: Osgood-Schlatter's disease in adolescent athletes: Retrospective study of incidence and duration. *Am J Sports Med* 13:236, 1985.

119. Böstman O, Kyrö A: Delayed union of fibular fractures accompanying fractures of the tibial shaft. *J Trauma* 31:99, 1991.

120. Simon RR, Koenigsknecht SJ: *Emergency Orthopedics: The Extremities,* 4th ed. New York, McGraw-Hill, 2001.

121. Tenenbein M, Reed MH, Black GB: The toddler's fracture revisited. *Am J Emerg Med* 8:208, 1990.

122. Howard PW, Making GS: Lower limb fractures with associated vascular injury. *J Bone Joint Surg Br* 72:116, 1990.

123. Templeman DC, Marder RA: Injuries of the knee associated with fractures of the tibial shaft: Detection by examination under anesthesia: A prospective study. *J Bone Joint Surg Am* 71:1392, 1989.

124. Oni OOA, Hui A, Gregg PJ: The healing of closed tibial shaft fractures: The natural history of union with closed treatment. *J Bone Joint Surg Br* 70:787, 1988.

125. Halbrecht JL, Jackson DW: Recurrent dislocation of the proximal tibiofibular joint. *Orthop Rev* 20:957, 1991.

126. Love JN: Isolated anterolateral proximal fibular head dislocation. *Ann Emerg Med* 21:757, 1992.

127. Monteleone GP Jr: Stress fracture in the athlete. *Orthop Clin North Am* 26:423, 1995.

128. Umans H, Pavlov H: Stress fractures of the lower extremities. *Semin Roentgenol* 29:176, 1994.

129. Meyer SA, Saltzman CL, Albright JP: Stress fractures of the foot and leg. *Clin Sports Med* 12:395, 1993.

130. Markey KL: Stress fractures. *Clin Sports Med* 6:405, 1987.

131. Jarolem KL, et al: Tennis leg leading to acute compartment syndrome. *Orthopedics* 17:721, 1994.

132. Helms CA, Fritz RC, Garvin GJ: Plantaris muscle injury: Evaluation with MR imaging. *Radiology* 195:201, 1995.

133. Yanay O, Vaughan DJ, Diab M, et al: Retained wooden foreign body in a child's thigh complicated by severe necrotizing fasciitis: A case report and discussion of imaging modalities for early diagnosis. *Pediatr Emerg Care* 17:354, 2001.

134. Manthey DE, Storrow AB, Milbourn JM, Wagner BJ: Ultrasound versus radiography in the detection of soft-tissue foreign bodies. *Ann Emerg Med* 28:7, 1996.

To him whose feet hurt, everything hurts.

Socrates

The ankle and foot are highly evolved structures designed to support the body's weight and to facilitate locomotion over varied terrain. Findings related to ankle and foot injuries are often subtle, and diagnosis may be delayed or missed, particularly in cases of multiple trauma.

The ankle and foot are best approached clinically as a single functional unit. Although they are discussed sequentially in this chapter, their mechanisms of injury overlap, and a pathologic condition in one location may accompany an associated pathologic condition in another.

ANKLE

PRINCIPLES OF DISEASE

Anatomy

The ankle joint is the articulation of the tibia and fibula with the talus. The dome of the talus fits securely into the "mortise" formed by the medial malleolus, the horizontal articular surface of the tibia (the plafond), and the lateral malleolus. The stability of the ankle depends on the bony and ligamentous integrity of the mortise. The calcaneus is also important to the motion and stability of the ankle.

The ankle comprises three primary articulations: the inner surface of the medial malleolus with the medial surface of the talus; the distal tibial plafond with the talar dome; and the medial surface of the lateral malleolus with the lateral process of the talus. These three articular surfaces are contiguous, lined with cartilage, and enclosed by a single joint capsule. The distal tibia also articulates with the distal fibula just proximal to the talus, forming the distal tibiofibular joint. Collectively, these articulations are called the *talocrural joints.*

Three sets of ligaments—the syndesmotic ligaments, the lateral collateral ligaments, and the medial collateral ligaments—support the ankle joint and are essential to its stability (Figures 55-1 and 55-2).

Tendons course through the ankle in four geographic groups. The flexor retinaculum tethers the tendons of the tibialis posterior, the flexor digitorum longus, and the flexor hallucis muscles behind the medial malleo-

lus. The peroneal retinaculum and tendon sheath fasten the peroneus longus and brevis tendons behind the lateral malleolus. The extensor retinaculum aligns the tendons of the tibialis anterior, extensor digitorum longus, extensor hallucis longus, and peroneus tertius over the anterior aspect of the ankle. Posteriorly, in the midline, lie the Achilles and plantaris tendons.

Pathophysiology

Ankle movements are complex, often involving more than one joint. It is best to consider the group of joints about the ankle as one unit, the ankle joint complex. This complex, which is made up of the talocrural joints and the talocalcaneal joints, or the subtalar joints, allows movements along several axes of motion.[1] Dorsiflexion (extension) and plantar flexion (flexion) of the ankle joint complex occur primarily at the talocrural joints, rotating about the horizontal axis that passes through the medial and lateral malleoli (Figure 55-3). Motions of the ankle joint complex in conjunction with the midtarsal joints include inversion and eversion, which are rotational movements about the oblique subtalar axis involving the subtalar joint (see Figure 55-3A), and abduction (external rotation) and adduction (internal rotation), which are rotational movements about the longitudinal axis of the tibia (see Figure 55-3B).

The components providing stability to the ankle are best conceptualized as a ringlike structure surrounding the talus (Figure 55-4).[2] Disruption of one element of this ring does not, by itself, induce instability. However, injury to one ring element should prompt careful scrutiny for a second injury. Any disruption of two or more elements causes ankle instability and can significantly affect the proper functioning of the joint.[2]

Clinical Features

The presence of immediate swelling and severe pain suggests serious ligament disruption, hemarthrosis, or fracture. Inability to bear weight immediately after an injury often implies a significant pathologic condition.[3] Patient recollection of a "pop" sound mandates consideration of ligament, tendon, or retinacular rupture but does not necessarily increase the possibility of a fracture. Rapid progression of symptoms may represent more severe injury.

The patient with a subacute or chronic ankle problem may be unable to correlate symptom onset with a particular traumatic event. Inquiry should elicit the type and extent of physical activities and whether the ankle

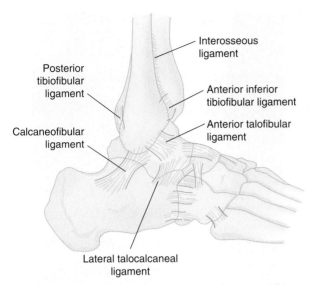

Figure 55-1. Anatomy of the lateral collateral ligaments and the syndesmotic ligaments of the ankle. (From Nicholas JA, Hershman EB [eds]: *The Lower Extremity and Spine in Sports Medicine*, 2nd ed. St Louis, Mosby, 1994.)

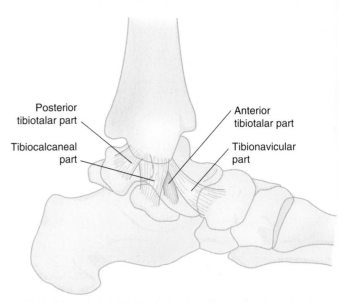

Figure 55-2. Anatomy of the medial collateral ligaments of the ankle. (From Nicholas JA, Hershman EB [eds]: *The Lower Extremity and Spine in Sports Medicine*, 2nd ed. St Louis, Mosby, 1994.)

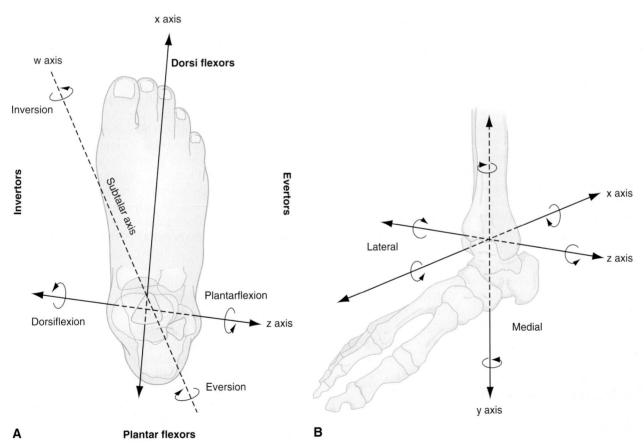

Figure 55-3. Four axes of the ankle joint complex. **A,** The horizontal axis passing through the two malleoli (z axis); the longitudinal axis of the foot (x axis); the oblique subtalar axis (w axis). (From the American Academy of Orthopedic Surgeons: *Atlas of Orthotics*. St. Louis, Mosby, 1975.) **B,** The longitudinal axis of the tibia (y axis) and two additional views of the x and z axes. (Modified from the Department of Orthopedics, Mayo Clinic and Mayo Foundation, Rochester, Minn. Reproduced in Storment, et al: *Am J Sports Med* 13:296, 1985.)

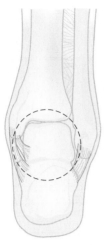

Figure 55-4. The ring structure surrounding the talus is made up of the tibial plafond, medial malleolus, deltoid ligaments, calcaneus, lateral collateral ligaments, and syndesmotic ligaments. The integrity of this ring determines the stability of the ankle. (From Simon RR, Koenigsknecht SJ: *Emergency Orthopedics: The Extremities*, 2nd ed. Norwalk, Conn, Appleton & Lange, 1987.)

gave way. Finally, acute ankle injuries or fractures in elderly patients may present as subacute problems and may reflect neglect by the patient or caregiver.

Physical Examination

Examination of the ankle starts with an assessment of deformity, ecchymosis, edema, and perfusion, followed by active and passive range of motion. Assessment of point tenderness may localize ligament, bone, or tendon injury, particularly when the patient is seen early after injury. Palpation should include the medial and lateral collateral ligaments, the syndesmotic ligaments, the inferior and posterior edges of the medial and lateral malleoli, the whole length of the fibula and tibia, the anterior plafond, the medial and lateral dome of the talus (palpable with the ankle in plantar flexion), the base of the fifth metatarsal, the calcaneus, the Achilles tendon, and the peroneal tendons behind the lateral malleolus. Stress testing of the ankle joint, which will be discussed later in the chapter, should not be performed until a fracture has been excluded. An evaluation of weight-bearing ability should proceed only if clinical suspicion of a fracture is low, the locations of tenderness do not indicate the need for plain radiography, or radiographs have ruled out a fracture.[3]

DIAGNOSTIC STRATEGIES

Radiology

The anteroposterior, lateral, and mortise views make up the standard radiographic series of the ankle. The anteroposterior view identifies fractures of the malleoli, distal tibia or fibula, plafond, talar dome, the body and lateral process of the talus, and the calcaneus. The lateral view identifies fractures of the anterior and posterior tibial margins, talar neck, posterior talar

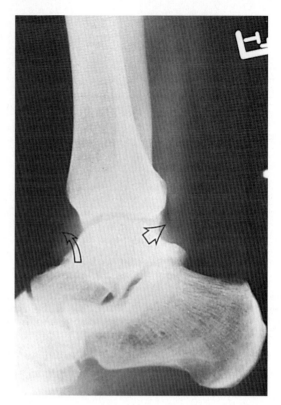

Figure 55-5. Lateral radiograph showing an ankle effusion. The arrows depict the distention of the joint capsule anteriorly *(curved arrow)* and posteriorly *(straight arrow)*. (From Nicholas JA, Hershman EB [eds]: *The Lower Extremity and Spine in Sports Medicine*, 2nd ed. St. Louis, Mosby, 1994.)

process, and calcaneus, and any anterior or posterior displacement of the talus. On this view, any incongruity of the articular space between the talar dome and the distal tibia suggests ankle instability, particularly if narrowing of the anterior joint space is present. The lateral view is also useful in identifying an ankle effusion, which appears as a teardrop-shaped density displacing the normal fat adjacent to the anterior or posterior margin of the joint capsule (Figure 55-5). Its presence suggests the possibility of a subtle intra-articular injury, such as an osteochondral fracture of the talar dome.[4]

The mortise view, which is taken with the ankle in 15 to 25 degrees of internal rotation, is most important for evaluating the congruity of the articular surface between the dome of the talus and the mortise. The lines formed between the articular surfaces should be parallel throughout the tibiotalar and talofibular components of the joint, and the medial clear space should not exceed 4 mm (Figure 55-6).[5]

In most cases of acute and isolated ankle injuries, the Ottawa Ankle Rules (OAR) should be used as a screening tool to determine whether ankle or foot radiographs are necessary.[3,6] The OAR state that an ankle radiographic series is required if there is pain in the malleolar region and any of the following findings:
1. Bone tenderness is present at the posterior edge of the distal 6 cm or the tip of the lateral malleolus, or
2. Bone tenderness is present at the posterior edge of the distal 6 cm or the tip of the medial malleolus, or

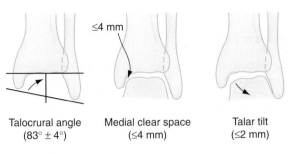

Syndesmosis radiographic criteria
Mortise view

Talocrural angle
(83° ± 4°)

Medial clear space
(≤4 mm)

Talar tilt
(≤2 mm)

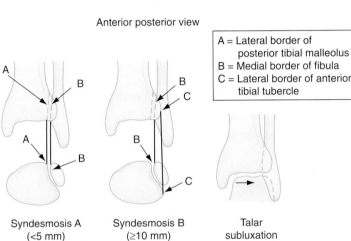

Anterior posterior view

A = Lateral border of
    posterior tibial malleolus
B = Medial border of fibula
C = Lateral border of anterior
    tibial tubercle

Syndesmosis A
(<5 mm)

Syndesmosis B
(≥10 mm)

Talar
subluxation

Figure 55-6. Radiologic criteria for evaluating syndesmosis. (From Stiehl JB: Ankle fractures with diasthesis. In Green WB [ed]: *Instructional Course Lectures*, vol 39, III. Easton, Pa, American Academy of Orthopedic Surgeons, 1990.)

3. The patient is unable to bear weight for at least four steps both immediately after the injury and at the time of evaluation

The OAR further state that a foot radiographic series is required if there is pain in the midfoot region and any of the following findings are present:

1. Bone tenderness is present at the navicular bone, or
2. Bone tenderness is present at the base of the fifth metatarsal, or
3. The patient is unable to bear weight for at least four steps both immediately after the injury and at the time of evaluation

The OAR have a sensitivity approaching 100% in detecting malleolar zone ankle fractures and midfoot zone fractures.[3,6] The OAR do not apply for subacute or chronic injuries. The use of OAR in pediatric patients is encouraging but still uncertain.[7] The decision rules for foot radiography, although applicable to blunt ankle trauma, apply only to the midfoot zone and only to the mechanism of injury defined by the studies. The OAR were not designed to be general guidelines for foot radiography and certainly do not apply to the hindfoot or forefoot. Finally, the OAR are not applicable to intoxicated patients or those who are difficult to assess because of head injuries, multiple injuries, or diminished sensation related to neurologic deficits.

Other Imaging Techniques

Plain radiography can miss subtle ankle fractures, osteochondral fractures, or ligamentous injuries. When unexplained symptoms persist after negative plain radiography, other imaging modalities or orthopedic consultation may be advisable on an elective basis. Radionuclide imaging (bone scanning) can detect soft tissue injuries (e.g., distal syndesmotic disruption) and subtle bony abnormalities (e.g., stress fractures and osteochondral fractures).[8] Computed tomography (CT) scanning provides superior imaging of bones and soft tissues, facilitates surgical planning, and diagnoses subtle fractures and ligamentous injuries.[9] Magnetic resonance imaging (MRI) scanning provides unprecedented clarity in the imaging of soft tissue structures, including ligaments, tendons, and muscles.[10] Arthroscopy of the ankle is useful both diagnostically and therapeutically in cases of subacute or chronic ankle pain, ankle instability, or joint locking or popping. Indications for arthroscopy include the removal of intraarticular foreign bodies, soft tissue or osseous impingements, or osteophytes as well as the treatment of osteochondral defects.[11]

ANKLE FRACTURES

Pathophysiology

Fractures occur when a deforming force is sufficient to overcome the structural strength of a bone. A bone under tension breaks transversely along the axis of the deforming force (Figure 55-7).[12] Alternatively, ligament rupture or a chip avulsion fracture can occur at either end of the stressed ligament.

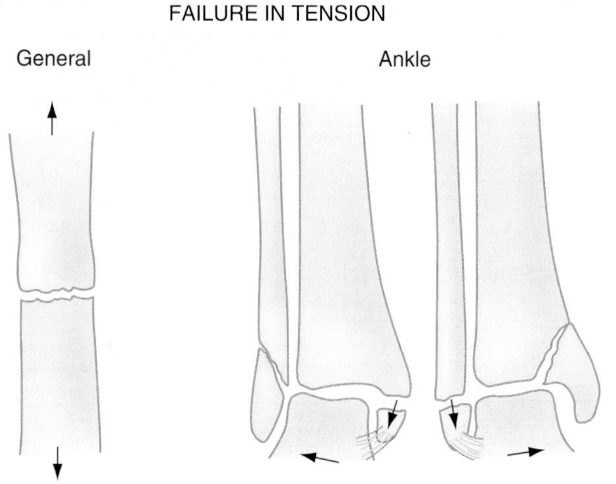

FAILURE IN TENSION

General   Ankle

Figure 55-7. The mechanics of bone failure in tension and types of tension ankle fractures. (From Dahners LE: The pathogenesis and treatment of bimalleolar ankle fractures. In Green WB [ed]: *Instructional Course Lectures*, vol 39, III. Easton, Pa, American Academy of Orthopedic Surgeons, 1990, pp 85-94.)

Management

Management of ankle fractures consists of identification, assessment of stability, immediate reduction of fracture-dislocations that threaten neurovascular or soft tissue viability, and specific treatment and disposition.

The injured ankle should be immobilized, elevated, and iced promptly to minimize swelling and further soft tissue damage. The presence of gross deformity with neurovascular compromise or skin tenting necessitates immediate intervention.[13] Plain radiography before reduction can be helpful but should not be allowed to delay reduction in injuries with vascular compromise.

Appropriate analgesia and sedation techniques should be used during reduction. The underlying principle of closed reduction is to reverse the deforming forces. For example, a fracture dislocation caused by an adduction injury would require an abduction force to reduce. The initial application of a distraction force is often helpful. After reduction, neurovascular status should be reassessed, the lower leg should be immobilized and elevated, and postreduction radiographs should be obtained. The central goal in the definitive treatment of ankle fractures is to achieve perfect reduction.

Disposition

In general, all displaced or potentially unstable ankle fractures require orthopedic consultation in the emergency department (Box 55-1). These injuries include all bimalleolar and trimalleolar fractures and unimalleolar fractures with contralateral ligamentous injuries (e.g., a lateral malleolar fracture with deltoid ligament disruption or a medial malleolar fracture with lateral collateral ligament disruption).[14] Also, all intraarticular fractures, especially those with step deformity of the articular surface, require early orthopedic involvement.

BOX 55-1. Ankle Fractures for which Orthopedic Consultation in the Emergency Department is Recommended

Unimalleolar Fractures
Displaced medial malleolar fracture
Medial malleolar fracture with lateral collateral ligament rupture
Displaced lateral malleolar fracture
Lateral malleolar fracture with deltoid ligament rupture
Lateral malleolar fracture with widened medial clear space
Unimalleolar fracture with syndesmotic diastasis
Fibula fracture at or proximal to the tibiotalar joint line
Displaced posterior malleolar fracture
Posterior malleolar fracture involving more than 25% of joint surface

All Bimalleolar Fractures

All Trimalleolar Fractures

All Intraarticular Fractures with Step Deformity

All Open Fractures

All Pilon Fractures

Extraarticular fractures that disrupt only one ring element generally can be treated with casting for 6 to 8 weeks. Orthopedic follow-up on an outpatient basis within 1 to 2 weeks of the injury would be ideal in the event that any intervention might be required. The presence of any abnormal measurement on the mortise view (see Figure 55-6) suggests instability and the need for orthopedic consultation in the emergency department. Chip avulsion fractures that are less than 3 mm and minimally displaced can be treated as an ankle sprain.

UNIMALLEOLAR FRACTURES

Lateral Malleolar Fractures

The stability of an isolated lateral malleolar fracture depends on the location of the fracture in relation to the level of the tibiotalar joint (Figure 55-8). Fractures below the tibiotalar joint rarely disrupt other bony or ligamentous structures (a Danis-Weber type A1 injury). In the absence of medial injury, lateral malleolar fractures are unlikely to affect the dynamic congruity of the ankle joint.[14] The management of uncomplicated lateral malleolar fractures involves casting for 6 to 8 weeks, with at least the first 3 weeks non-weight-bearing and follow-up to ensure proper healing. Concomitant tenderness over the deltoid ligament, which suggests a biomechanical disruption of both malleoli, an associated fracture of the medial malleolus (a Danis-Weber type A2 injury), or an associated fracture of the posterior malleolus (a Danis-Weber type A3 injury) warrants orthopedic consultation in the emergency department, especially if the medial clear space on the mortise view is widened (see Figure 55-6).[14]

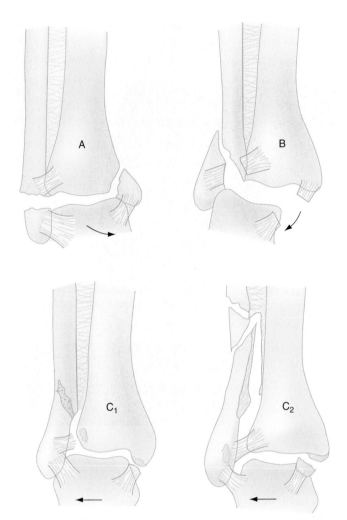

Figure 55-8. The Danis-Weber classification of ankle fractures focuses on the location of the fibular fracture in relation to the tibiotalar joint. See text for explanation. (From Wilson FC: The pathogenesis and treatment of ankle fractures: classification. In Green WB [ed]: *Instructional Course Lectures*, vol 39, III. Easton, Pa, American Academy of Orthopedic Surgeons, 1990, pp 79-83.)

Fibular fractures proximal to the tibiotalar joint line (a Danis-Weber type C injury; see Figure 55-8) frequently, but not always, disrupt the distal tibiotalar syndesmosis and the medial structures[15] and commonly require orthopedic consultation in the emergency department. Treatment of an isolated fracture at the level of the tibiotalar joint (a type B Danis-Weber injury; see Figure 55-8) is controversial because 50% of these have an associated injury to the distal tibiofibular syndesmosis.[16] Tenderness on palpation of the syndesmotic ligament or a widening of the medial joint space on the mortise view adds further support to the need for emergency consultation.

Medial Malleolar Fractures

Medial malleolar fractures usually occur from eversion or external rotation.[16] These two forces exert tension on the deltoid ligament, causing an avulsion of the tip of the medial malleolus or a rupture of the deltoid ligament. Although they can occur in isolation, medial malleolar fractures are commonly associated with lateral or posterior malleolar disruption. Because of

this association, the identification of a medial malleolar fracture demands a careful examination of the entire length of the fibula for tenderness, the presence of which warrants radiographic evaluation to rule out a proximal fibular fracture (Figure 55-9).

An isolated nondisplaced medial malleolar fracture can be treated with casting for 6 to 8 weeks, including non-weight-bearing for at least the first 3 weeks, with close orthopedic follow-up. Any displacement or concomitant disruption of the lateral components of the ankle warrants orthopedic consultation in the emergency department for consideration of operative management.[14]

Posterior Malleolar Fractures

Isolated fractures of the posterior malleolus are rare and imply an avulsion of the posterior tibiofibular ligament. These injuries can be associated with proximal fibular fractures and medial and lateral collateral ligament sprains. Treatment usually consists of casting for 6 weeks, provided no associated injury or ankle instability is present.[17] Fractures involving more than 25% of the posterior tibial surface usually require open reduction and internal fixation.[14]

BIMALLEOLAR FRACTURES

Bimalleolar fractures involve the disruption of at least two elements of the ankle ring and therefore are unstable. These fractures result from adduction or abduction forces, although the latter is more common.[12] Rotational injuries also can cause bimalleolar fractures as well as trimalleolar fractures if the posterior malleolus is involved.

The mechanism of injury can often be deduced from the appearance of the fractures.[12] An abduction injury exerts tension on the medial malleolus, causing a horizontal fracture, and bends the lateral malleolus, causing an oblique shear or a comminuted fracture (see Figure 55-7). An adduction injury causes the reverse, leading to a horizontal fracture of the fibula and an oblique shear fracture of the medial malleolus. A rotational injury causes oblique or spiral fractures of the fibula or medial malleolus. Associated damage to other soft tissue structures (e.g., the syndesmosis) is common with bimalleolar fractures.

Controversy exists about whether such injuries should be treated closed or surgically.[12,18]

Trimalleolar Fractures

Trimalleolar fractures involve fractures of the medial, lateral, and posterior malleoli. Closed treatment of trimalleolar fractures often leads to unsatisfactory results, so operative reduction and internal fixation is the treatment of choice.[19]

OPEN FRACTURES

Open ankle fractures usually occur with severe isolated ankle injuries or multiple trauma and require immedi-

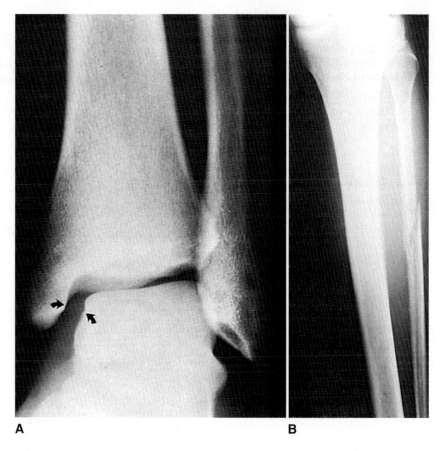

Figure 55-9. Maisonneuve fracture. **A,** Antero-posterior view shows a slight widening of the ankle mortise and the medial clear space. **B,** Lateral view shows an oblique fracture at the proximal shaft of the fibula. (From Nicholas JA, Hershman EB [eds]: *The Lower Extremity and Spine in Sports Medicine*, 2nd ed. St. Louis, Mosby, 1994.)

A   B

ate orthopedic consultation. After documentation of the neurovascular status and the extent of soft tissue trauma, the injured leg should be splinted and saline-soaked sterile gauze applied to the wound.[13] Swabbing the open wound for bacterial culture is unnecessary. If gross deformity is present (which indicates a fracture dislocation), immediate reduction is necessary before splinting.[13] Tetanus immunization should be administered as appropriate. All open fractures are contaminated with bacteria and the patient should receive intravenous antibiotics.[20] For low-energy injuries with mild to moderate contamination, a broad-spectrum cephalosporin is usually sufficient.[13,20] Heavily contaminated wounds require the addition of an aminoglycoside for gram-negative bacterial coverage.[20] Adding penicillin G as a third antibiotic is necessary for farm- or soil-related crush injuries, where contamination with *Clostridium perfringens* is significant.[20] In addition to the ankle, radiographs of the foot, tibia, and fibula should be obtained.

All open fractures benefit from early surgical intervention for debridement and thorough irrigation.[13] Therefore, identification is crucial and emergency orthopedic consultation must be sought for such injuries.

Complications

Early operative complications of closed and open ankle fractures include pin site infection, delayed skin necro-

sis, skin graft rejection, and osteomyelitis. Delayed complications of both operative and nonoperative treatment include malunion, nonunion, osteopenia, traumatic arthritis, chronic instability, ossification of the interosseous membrane, and reflex sympathetic dystrophy.[2,21]

PILON FRACTURES

Pilon fractures involve the distal tibial metaphysis and are usually a result of high-energy mechanisms such as falls from a significant height. These injuries are often comminuted and associated with significant soft tissue trauma, devastation of joint architecture, and leg shortening (Figure 5-10).

Pathophysiology

Destot first coined the term *hammer fracture* to describe the way the head of the talus drives itself into the tibial plafond and causes a pilon fracture. The primary deforming force is one of axial compression, and the position of the foot at the time of injury determines the fracture location and pattern (Figure 55-11).[22] Secondary rotational or shear forces may cause increased comminution and fragment displacement with more extensive soft tissue injuries. Twenty to 25% of pilon fractures are open, and associated injuries include fractures of the calcaneus, tibial plateau, femoral neck, acetabulum, or lumbar vertebrae.

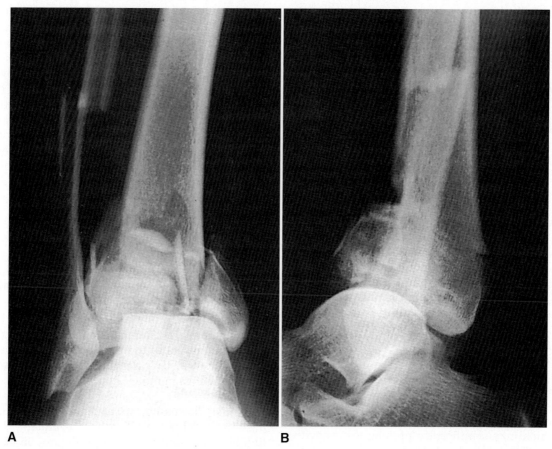

Figure 55-10. Anteroposterior **(A)** and lateral **(B)** radiographs showing a pilon fracture. (From Gustilo RB, et al [eds]: *Fractures and Dislocations*. St. Louis, Mosby, 1993.)

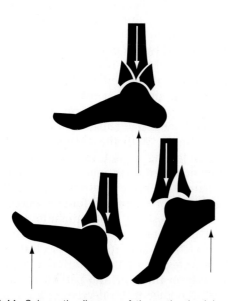

Figure 55-11. Schematic diagram of the pathophysiology of pilon fractures. The position of the foot at the time of impact determines the fracture pattern. (From Gustilo RB, et al [eds]: *Fractures and Dislocations*. St. Louis, Mosby, 1993.)

Management

Radiography should include the entire tibia and fibula, as well as the ankle. The emergency management principles for open fractures, as previously discussed, should be applied. Treatment involves restoration of the articular surface and fibular length, combined with meticulous management of soft tissue injuries.[22,23]

Complications

Although prompt open reduction and internal fixation usually lead to satisfactory outcome for less severe pilon fractures, results for the severe types are discouraging.[23] Complications of pilon fractures are common. Early complications include wound infection, skin sloughing, pin site infection, and wound dehiscence. Delayed and late complications include malunion, nonunion, leg shortening, posttraumatic arthritis, avascular necrosis, and protracted pain. Some patients with severe pilon fractures ultimately require arthrodesis.[23]

SOFT TISSUE INJURIES

Ligament Injuries

Ankle sprains are a common presenting complaint in the emergency department. The term *ankle sprain* refers to a potpourri of ligamentous and nonligamentous injuries.[24] Even when ligamentous injury is certain, the ideal treatment approach remains controversial.

Pathophysiology

Most ankle sprains occur from extreme inversion and plantarflexion. Usually the anterior talofibular ligament is injured first, followed by the calcaneofibular ligament if the deforming forces are sufficiently great. Approximately two thirds of ankle sprains are isolated anterior talofibular ligament injuries, whereas 20% involve both anterior talofibular and calcaneofibular ligament injuries. In addition, the lateral talocalcaneal ligament may be stressed with an inversion injury, leading to avulsion fractures at either end of the attachment sites.[25] Isolated calcaneofibular or posterior talofibular ligament injuries are rare.

Isolated injury of the deltoid ligament occurs in fewer than 5% of ankle sprains. Rupture of this ligament occurs most commonly in conjunction with malleolar fractures, especially when an external rotational force is involved.

Injuries of the distal tibiofibular syndesmotic ligaments are uncommon; the estimated incidence is approximately 1%.[26] Dorsiflexion and external rotation forces are usually responsible for this injury, the presence of which may significantly prolong the recovery time of lateral collateral ligament sprains.[26]

Ligamentous injuries are classified into three grades, based on functional and presumed pathologic findings. A grade I injury involves ligamentous stretching without grossly evident tearing or joint instability. A grade II injury involves a partial tear of the ligament with moderate joint instability, often accompanied by significant localized swelling and pain. A grade III injury involves a complete tear of the ligament with marked joint instability and severe edema and ecchymosis. This classification system, although commonly used, fails to characterize ankle injuries involving two or more ligaments, and it does not consider nonligamentous injuries. This has led to the proposal of other, more comprehensive classification systems.[25]

Clinical Features

Although desirable, an accurate history of ankle position and injury mechanism is often unavailable. Inversion followed by external rotation of the ankle suggests the potential for deltoid or syndesmotic injury. Forced dorsiflexion with snapping may indicate peroneal tendon displacement. Previous injuries to the same ankle, or symptoms of recurrent ankle instability or pain, suggest the presence of subacute or chronic pathology.

On physical examination, the presence of edema, ecchymosis, and point tenderness over the medial or lateral collateral ligaments or the syndesmotic ligaments suggests a ligamentous injury. With inversion injuries, point tenderness may also be present along the distal fibula, the lateral aspect of the talus, the lateral aspect or anterior process of the calcaneus, or the base

of the fifth metatarsal. Deltoid ligament tenderness demands palpation of the full length of the fibula to rule out a proximal fibular fracture (a type C Danis-Weber or Maisonneuve's fracture; see Figures 55-8 and 55-9). The fibular compression test, also known as the squeeze test, reveals fibular and syndesmotic injuries.[26] To perform this test, the examiner places the fingers over the fibula and the thumb over the tibia at midcalf and squeezes the two bones. The precipitation of pain anywhere along the length of the fibula suggests a fibular fracture or an interosseous membrane or syndesmotic ligament disruption at that location.[26] Finally, the Achilles tendon should be assessed.

Diagnostic Strategies: Radiology

Standard ankle radiographs are useful to exclude fractures and to detect instability by the measurement of joint spaces (see earlier discussion and Figure 55-6).[5] Avulsion fractures, which can be located at the bases of the malleoli, the lateral process of the talus, the lateral aspect of the calcaneus, the posterior malleolus, the lateral aspect of the distal tibia, or the base of the fifth metatarsal, provide important clues regarding the location of ligamentous injuries.

In addition to the standard mortise measurements previously discussed, two measurements on the anteroposterior radiograph further evaluate the distal tibiofibular syndesmosis (see Figure 55-6).[5] At the distal overlap between the fibula and the tibia, the distance between the posterior edge of the lateral tibial groove and the medial fibular cortex (syndesmosis A) should not exceed 5 mm.[5] Furthermore, the amount of tibiofibular bony overlap (syndesmosis B) should be at least 10 mm.[5] Measurements outside of these values suggest a syndesmotic diastasis.

Stress testing is the application of a deforming force to assess joint motion beyond the physiologic range, the presence of which suggests ligament disruption or mechanical instability. Indications for stress testing are few and may include an acute and severe ankle injury in which rupture of two or more ligaments is suspected; a fracture suspected to be isolated in which the presence of an additional ligament rupture would influence management; the possibility of a concomitant syndesmotic injury; the follow-up of an acute ankle injury after pain and swelling subside; and a chronically symptomatic ankle. With the exception of these scenarios, stress testing is not indicated because it is painful and does not alter management. The normal ranges for stress tests are controversial, so the uninjured side should be examined for comparison.

Common ankle stress tests include the anterior drawer test, the inversion stress test, and the external rotation test. The anterior drawer test primarily assesses the integrity of the anterior talofibular ligament. To perform this test, the patient is comfortably seated, with the knee in 90 degrees of flexion and the ankle in a neutral position or 10 degrees of plantar flexion. The examiner then pulls on the heel with one hand and pushes the leg posteriorly with the other. Anterior displacement of the talus, the perception of a

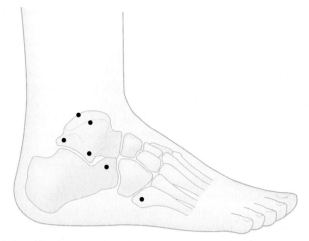

BOX 55-2. Differential Diagnosis of a Presumed Ankle Sprain

Lateral collateral ligament sprain
Peroneal tendon dislocation
Osteochondral fracture of the talar dome
Fracture of the posterior process of the talus
Fracture of the lateral process of the talus
Fracture of the anterior process of the calcaneus
Midtarsal joint injury
Fracture of the base of the fifth metatarsal

Figure 55-12. Differential diagnosis of a presumed ankle sprain: potential locations of bony fractures. (From Gustilo RB, et al [eds]: *Fractures and Dislocations*. St. Louis, Mosby, 1993.)

"clunk," and the induction of a sulcus anteromedially over the joint indicate partial or complete tear of the ligament.

The inversion stress test, or talar tilt test, evaluates both the anterior talofibular ligament and the calcaneofibular ligament. It is performed by inverting the heel with the knee in 90 degrees of flexion and the ankle in neutral position. The palpation of the head of the talus laterally or increased laxity compared with the uninjured side suggests partial or complete tear of these ligaments.

The external rotation stress test is indicated when injury to the distal tibiofibular syndesmotic ligaments is suspected. It is done by externally rotating the foot with the knee in 90 degrees flexion and the ankle in a neutral position. Pain at the syndesmosis or the sensation of lateral talar motion suggests partial or complete tear of the ligaments.

Stress radiographs, which are radiographs taken with the ankle under stress testing, generally do not influence the emergency management of ankle sprains and are not recommended.[27]

Many conditions can masquerade as ankle sprains.[24] Box 55-2 and Figure 55-12 present those conditions.

Management

Most ligament sprains, regardless of severity, heal well and have a satisfactory outcome. Therefore, most patients with acute sprains of the ankle should start with nonoperative, functional treatments.[28] For the minority who fail to respond, delayed operative repair of ruptured ligaments, sometimes years after the injury, has been shown to yield results equivalent to those of primary repair.[28,29]

Functional treatment starts in the emergency department with RICE therapy (rest, ice, compression, elevation).[25,30] For grade I or II injuries, short-term protection with laced-up supports, tensor, tape, bandage, cam walker, or brace and the optional use of crutches for a few days are appropriate.[28,30] Rarely, in cases of severe grade II or grade III injuries, plaster splinting or casting for up to 3 weeks might be necessary. Acutely, splinting is preferred to accommodate edema that peaks at 48 hours. Casting at the initial visit may result in elevated compartment pressure as the leg continues to swell and later, a loose ineffective cast as the swelling subsides. However, there is no evidence that immobilization leads to a more favorable outcome compared to func-

tional treatment in most cases, which involve the use of laced-up supports or air casts that permit some ankle motion.[28,31] Such patients should also use crutches to avoid weight bearing until they can stand and walk a few steps on the injured ankle without pain. How long the crutches will be required varies significantly, ranging from a few days to 2 or 3 weeks. Follow-up with the patient's primary physician within the first 2 weeks is appropriate for minor sprains, whereas orthopedic referral on an outpatient basis is prudent for severe sprains. Short-term use of analgesics may be required for ankle sprains, particularly on the day of injury and in the early days of recovery.

The next two phases of functional treatment occur outside the emergency department. Phase two, which begins after swelling has subsided and the patient is able to bear weight easily, involves strengthening the peroneal and dorsiflexor muscles by isometric, concentric, and eccentric exercises. The final phase begins when full range of motion is reestablished and the patient can exercise painlessly. This begins with exercises to rebuild motor coordination, recondition the muscles, and increase endurance. The patient uses an ankle tilt board or disk to develop coordination and performs increasingly demanding functional activities (e.g., brisk walking, running, and figure-of-eight running to hopping, jumping, and cutting) to build up the muscle groups. In cases of severe sprains, the patient may benefit from the use of splints, air casts, or braces during the latter two phases of functional treatment. The entire treatment program usually lasts 4 to 6 weeks, depending on the injury's severity.[25,30,32]

Disposition

Rarely, orthopedic consultation in the emergency department is indicated for an acute ligament sprain. Primary surgical repair of acute ligament rupture is controversial, and possible indications include sprains with displaced osteochondral fractures, complete tears of both the anterior talofibular and the calcaneofibular ligaments in a young athlete, a ligament sprain associated with a fracture causing instability (e.g., a deltoid ligament rupture with a lateral malleolar fracture), and an acute severe sprain in a patient with a history of recurrent and severe sprains.[25] Failure of nonoperative treatment is also an indication for surgical repair; however, an orthopedic referral on an outpatient basis is adequate.[29]

Small avulsion fractures of the fibula with minimal or no displacement can be treated as an ankle sprain. If the chip fragment is larger than 3 mm or significantly displaced, splinting and orthopedic follow-up on an outpatient basis are justified.

Despite appropriate treatment, approximately 10% to 30% of patients with ankle sprains develop chronic problems.[30] These include functional instability, mechanical instability, chronic pain, stiffness, and recurrent swelling.

Functional instability refers to the patient's subjective sensation that the ankle gives way during activity. Although this may be a minor nuisance for some, it can be devastating and debilitating for those whose activities demand a high degree of ankle stability. Mechanical instability results from ligamentous laxity, which allows ankle joint movements beyond the physiologic range. In contrast to functional instability, mechanical instability can often be demonstrated clinically by the anterior drawer or talar tilt test and stress radiographs.[25]

Soft tissue abnormalities that cause chronic pain include synovial impingement, peroneal tendon subluxation or dislocation, loose bodies, anterior tibiofibular syndesmotic ligament injuries, and degenerative arthritis. Bony causes of chronic pain include osteochondral fractures, fractures of the anterior process of the calcaneus, fractures of the lateral process of the talus, and anterior and posterior impingement.[24,33]

Patients with any of these chronic conditions should have orthopedic follow-up because they may require further imaging or orthoscopy for diagnosis or definitive treatment.

Tendon Injuries

Achilles Tendon Rupture

Achilles tendon rupture usually occurs in middle-aged persons during sporadic or intermittent involvement in recreational sports.[34] This condition has been misdiagnosed in up to 25% of cases, leading to delay in therapy and a worse prognosis.

Achilles tendon rupture occurs from direct trauma or indirectly transmitted forces, including sudden unexpected dorsiflexion, forced dorsiflexion of a plantarflexed foot, and strong push-off of the foot with simultaneous knee extension and calf contraction (e.g., a runner accelerating from the starting position). Factors predisposing to Achilles tendon rupture include rheumatoid arthritis, systemic lupus erythematosus, gout, hyperparathyroidism, chronic renal failure, steroid use or injection, and fluoroquinolone antibiotic therapy.[35,36]

The diagnosis of an Achilles tendon rupture is primarily clinical. Patients usually describe a sudden onset of pain at the back of the ankle associated with an audible "pop" or "snap." Although the pain can resolve rapidly, weakness in plantar flexion persists. On examination, a visible and palpable tendon defect is usually present 2 to 6 cm proximal to the calcaneal insertion.[34] In delayed presentations, this defect may be less apparent because of hematoma or edema. Even in cases of complete Achilles tendon rupture, weak plantar flexion may still be present because of the actions of the tibialis posterior, toe flexors, and peroneal muscles. This finding often leads to the misdiagnosis of ruptures as strains or partial tears.

The classic maneuver to assess the integrity of the Achilles tendon is the Thompson test.[37] This is performed with the patient prone and the knee flexed at 90 degrees. Alternatively, the patient kneels on a chair with both knees flexed at 90 degrees and the feet dangling over the edge. Squeezing the calf muscles in these two positions should cause passive plantar flexion of the foot. Absence of this motion or a weakened response compared with the uninjured side suggests complete rupture. Another diagnostic test involves wrapping a sphygmomanometer cuff around the calf while the patient is prone. With the knee flexed to 90 degrees and the foot relaxed, the cuff is inflated to 100 mm Hg. Dorsiflexion of the foot by the examiner should cause an increase in pressure to approximately 140 mm Hg. Failure to induce a rise in pressure or a significant diminution compared with the uninjured side suggests rupture.[38]

Lateral radiographs of the ankle may confirm rupture by showing opacification of the triangular fatty tissue-filled space anterior to the Achilles tendon (Kager's triangle) or an irregular contour and thickening of the tendon. Ultrasonography or an MRI scan can also demonstrate partial or complete tendon ruptures.[39]

The choice of operative versus nonoperative management is controversial. Surgical repair has a lower incidence of rerupture (1.4% versus 13.4% in nonoperative management), less muscle atrophy, and earlier resumption of activities.[40] Nonoperative therapy, which involves a series of casts changed in 2- to 4-week intervals, avoids operative complications and decreases hospitalization and sick leave time. Achilles tendon rerupture after initial nonoperative treatment usually requires surgical repair. Emergency orthopedic referral of patients with Achilles tendon rupture is recommended.

Peroneal Tendon Dislocation or Tear

The peroneal muscles are the primary evertors and pronators of the foot and also participate in plantar flexion. The peroneus longus and brevis tendons use the posterior peroneal sulcus (the fibular groove), located behind and underneath the lateral malleolus, as a pulley for their midfoot insertions. The peroneus brevis tendon inserts onto the tuberosity of the fifth metatarsal, and the peroneus longus tendon courses beneath the cuboid to insert onto the medial cuneiform and base of the first metatarsal. The superior peroneal retinaculum (Figure 55-13), a fibrous structure running from the distal fibula to the posterolateral aspect of the

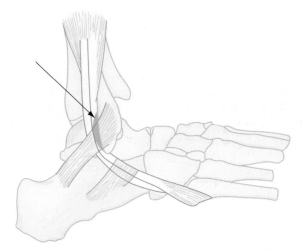

Figure 55-13. The locations of the superior *(arrow)* and inferior peroneal retinaculum in relation to the fibula and the peroneal tendons. (From Arrowsmith SR, et al: Traumatic dislocations of the peroneal tendons. *Am J Sports Med* 11:142, 1983.)

calcaneus, maintains the peroneal tendons against the fibular groove.

Anterior subluxation or dislocation of the peroneal tendons occurs as a result of a tear of the superior peroneal retinaculum attachment from the fibula.[41] These injuries are commonly misdiagnosed as ankle sprains and can occur in isolation or concomitant with other sprains or fractures. The mechanism of injury is usually forced dorsiflexion with reflex contraction of the peroneal muscles. This results in anterior displacement of the peroneal tendons and strips the retinacular attachment from the fibula.[41] Plantar flexion and eversion may also lead to peroneal tendon dislocation.

The patient with a peroneal tendon dislocation complains of sudden pain and a snapping sensation over the posterolateral ankle.[41] Although the pain subsides, weakness of eversion persists. Tenderness and swelling over the lateral retromalleolar area (a location not typically involved in ankle sprains) are present. The dislocated tendons may also be palpable near the inferior tip of the lateral malleolus. In a delayed presentation, the entire lateral malleolar area may be edematous, preventing palpation of the dislocated tendons. Inability to evert the foot actively when it is held in dorsiflexion or frank subluxation of the tendons with this maneuver confirms the diagnosis.[41,42] Clicking and anterior displacement of the tendons behind the lateral malleolus during circular rolling of the foot may also be present. Plain radiography is often normal; however, 15% to 50% of patients have an avulsion fracture of the lateral ridge of the distal fibula. A CT or MRI scan can be helpful in confirming the diagnosis.

All patients with a suspected or confirmed peroneal tendon dislocation should have orthopedic referral. Untreated cases rarely heal spontaneously, and chronic ankle instability and pain often ensue.[42] The treatment of acute peroneal tendon dislocations is controversial.[43] Conservative treatment consists of 6 weeks of cast immobilization. The cast should be well molded over the lateral malleolus, and the foot should be maintained in slight plantar flexion.[43] Surgical management involves either deepening the fibular sulcus or reconstructing the soft tissue tunnel formed by the superior peroneal retinaculum.[43] Both operative and nonoperative management are followed by ankle rehabilitation with strength and proprioceptive training.[43] Patients failing nonoperative management or those with chronic subluxation usually require surgical repair.[42]

Peroneal tendons can also tear longitudinally.[43] During inversion and plantar flexion, the two peroneal tendons are pressed against the sharp edge of the distal fibula, which can lead to tearing.[44] With such an injury, the ankle appears normal at rest but the patient describes recurrent lateral retromalleolar pain and swelling during activities. Symptoms often are accentuated by running on uneven terrain or with "cutting" maneuvers.[44] Localized tenderness is present at the lateral retromalleolar area, and a popping sensation without frank dislocation may occur during active rotation of the foot.

All patients with suspected longitudinal peroneal tears should have orthopedic referral. Conservative treatment with physical therapy is usually unhelpful, and surgical repair of these tears is often necessary.[43,44]

Tibialis Posterior Tendon Rupture

The tibialis posterior is primarily responsible for plantar flexion and inversion along the subtalar joint.[45] Its tendon uses the posteroinferior surface of the medial malleolus as a pulley and inserts onto the navicular, the medial cuneiforms, and the bases of the second through fifth metatarsals. The peroneus brevis opposes the action of the tibialis posterior. With rupture of the tibialis posterior tendon, the peroneus brevis becomes unopposed and the medial longitudinal arch loses its muscular support, leading to valgus deformity of the hindfoot and a unilateral flatfoot. Tibialis posterior tendon ruptures usually occur spontaneously in patients with chronic inflammatory conditions. Acute rupture resulting from trauma is rare in the absence of chronic inflammation or tendinitis. Factors predisposing to tendinitis include trauma, overuse, inflammatory disorders, degenerative tendon disease, infection, and steroid injections.[42]

The mechanism of traumatic tibialis posterior rupture involves pronation and external rotation.[42] This injury may occur simultaneously with malleolar fractures.[42] In addition to a unilateral flatfoot, pain and swelling on the medial aspect of the ankle are also present.[45] Only half of these patients recall a history of an ankle sprain.[45] Tenderness is present over the navicular, and the patient cannot perform a toe raise on the affected side.[42] In addition, the patient cannot invert the foot when it is in plantar flexion and eversion.[45] With a unilateral flatfoot, an observer standing behind the patient can see "more toes" on the lateral aspect of the affected side—a classic sign.[46] Weight-bearing radiography may demonstrate loss of the medial longitudinal arch or a medial displacement of the talus from the navicular.

Orthopedic consultation in the emergency department is necessary for acute tibialis posterior tendon ruptures, whereas outpatient referral is acceptable for subacute or chronic ruptures. Conservative treatment consists of instep orthoses for arch support; however, surgical repair is often necessary.[42,45]

Other Tendon Injuries

The tibialis anterior is the primary dorsiflexor of the foot. Its tendon courses under the superior extensor retinaculum and inserts onto the navicular, the medial cuneiform, and the base of the first metatarsal. Tenosynovitis of the tibialis anterior tendon is associated with overuse and characterized by swelling, tenderness, and crepitus along the tendon. Treatment involves RICE therapy, analgesia, and close follow-up. Rupture of the tibialis anterior is rare and often misdiagnosed as lumbosacral radiculopathy or peroneal palsy because of the footdrop it produces. This condition requires orthopedic consultation in the emergency department because surgical repair is usually necessary.

The flexor hallucis longus is responsible for flexion of the great toe and participates in plantar flexion of the foot. Its tendon courses behind the medial malleolus through a fibro-osseous canal and inserts onto the distal phalanx of the great toe. Flexor hallucis longus tendinitis, also called dancer's tendinitis, most often occurs at the fibro-osseous canal.[42] On examination, tenderness and edema are present posterior to the medial malleolus, and passive extension of the first metatarsophalangeal joint causes significant pain when the foot is in neutral position. Initial treatment involves rest, nonsteroidal anti-inflammatory drugs, and a short course of immobilization. Orthopedic follow-up on an outpatient basis should be arranged to ensure proper resolution. Rarely, surgical intervention may be necessary.[42]

Ankle Dislocation without Fracture

Ankle dislocations are described according to the direction of displacement of the talus and foot in relation to the tibia.[47] Thus, dislocation may be upward, posterior, medial, lateral, posteromedial, or anterior. Medial dislocation is the most common.[47]

Dislocation of the talus from the ankle mortise without an accompanying fracture is rare.[47] The mechanism in all dislocations begins with axial loading of a plantar flexed foot, which forces the talus either anteriorly or posteriorly. The eventual position of the dislocation depends on the position of the foot at the time of injury and the direction of the displacing force. Ankle dislocations can be closed or open and occur most commonly from significant falls, motor vehicle collisions, or high-speed sports. The neurovascular supply to the foot is usually intact but may be compromised in open dislocations.[48] Emergency management involves the assessment of neurovascular status and tendon function, followed by rapid reduction. Radiographs are helpful but should not delay reduction in obvious cases or when neurovascular compromise or skin tenting is present.

Reduction should be performed without delay. After appropriate analgesia or conscious sedation technique, the patient is placed supine and the knee is flexed to 90 degrees. Distraction of the foot, followed by a gentle force to reverse the direction of the dislocation, usually accomplishes the reduction.[49] Splint immobilization, elevation of the ankle, reassessment of the neurovascular status, and postreduction radiography should follow. Open dislocations require the same management as previously discussed.

The prognosis of an ankle dislocation is usually good, although open fractures have an increased incidence of complications.[48,49]

FOOT

PRINCIPLES OF DISEASE

Anatomy

The foot is composed of 28 bones and 57 articulations (Figure 55-14). It can be divided into three anatomic and functional regions: the hindfoot, which contains the talus and calcaneus; the midfoot, which contains the navicular, cuboid, and cuneiforms; and the forefoot, which contains the metatarsals, phalanges, and sesamoids. The midtarsal joints (Chopart's joint) join the hindfoot and midfoot, and the tarsometatarsal joints (Lisfranc's joint) join the midfoot and forefoot. The inferior aspect of the talus has three articulations with the calcaneus that are collectively known as the *subtalar joint.*

The foot's bones interlock in a manner that is often likened to the blocks and keystones of a bridge, forming

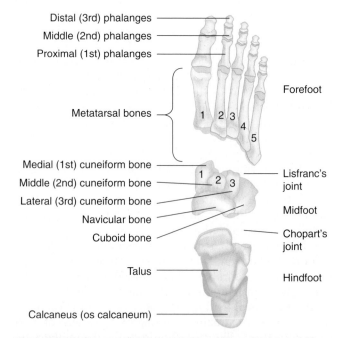

Figure 55-14. Bones and joints of the foot. (From Rockwood CA, et al [eds]: *Rockwood and Green's Fractures in Adults,* 3rd ed. New York, JB Lippincott, 1991.)

a complex system of arches and beams tethered by ligaments and intrinsic muscles. Extrinsic muscles, originating in the leg, are responsible for most of the foot's movements as well as for maintenance of the arch and beam structure. The course and insertion of these extrinsic muscles are important in their actions and in their association with specific avulsions and injuries. The arterial supply to the foot is from the anterior and posterior tibial arteries and the peroneal artery, a proximal branch of the posterior tibial artery. Motor and sensory innervation are from branches of the deep and superficial peroneal, posterior tibial, saphenous, and sural nerves.

The foot is capable of numerous weight-bearing and non-weight-bearing motions (see Figure 55-3), which vary at each articulation. Inversion and eversion of the hindfoot occur primarily through the subtalar joint, adduction and abduction of the forefoot through the midtarsal joints, and flexion and extension through the metatarsophalangeal (MTP) and interphalangeal (IP) joints. The relative importance of specific bones in supporting the body's weight varies from the static to mobile state. The biomechanics of walking and running are extremely complex, and significant forces are imparted to the foot's structures during these precisely coordinated activities.[50]

Clinical Features

An accurate history is essential in the setting of foot trauma because many mechanisms are associated with specific injury patterns. Mechanisms can be broadly divided into direct and indirect (torsional) forces. Falls, twisting injuries, dropped objects, overuse injuries, burns, and penetrating wounds each suggest different potential pathologic conditions. Patient complaints involve any combination of pain, swelling, deformity, reduced function, or altered sensation. The location of pain, along with a description of its quality, duration, and precipitants, focuses the differential diagnosis. The combination of increasing pain with decreasing sensation is particularly compelling because this may indicate neurovascular compromise requiring immediate intervention. Along with general information, the patient should be questioned about underlying pertinent medical conditions, medications, and previous foot problems.

The structures of the foot are uniquely accessible to palpation and assessment. A directed examination, specific for the patient's complaint, is most useful in the emergency department.[51]

If the patient is ambulatory, observation of the gait provides information on the degree of disability and pain and the potential for serious injury. Formal examination begins with observation of the foot in its position of rest, normally one of slight plantar flexion and inversion. Swelling, deformity, ecchymosis, open wounds, color, and temperature should be noted. The use of ecchymosis to localize injuries can be misleading because of blood tracking through tissue planes and pooling in dependent areas. All patients should have a neurovascular examination with assessment of the dor-

salis pedis and posterior tibial pulses, sensation, and motor function. Precise localization of pain or crepitus, when not precluded by swelling, is extremely valuable and facilitates appropriate use of further diagnostic tools. The entire foot should be gently palpated over both the dorsal and plantar surfaces, methodically progressing from the heel to the toes. Particular attention should be paid to areas where injuries commonly occur, such as the base of the fifth metatarsal.

In some situations, an evaluation of range of motion is indicated. This begins with an assessment of active motion with the foot dependent. Next, if active motion is well tolerated, passive motion is assessed, beginning with the subtalar joint in the hindfoot and moving distally to the midtarsal and forefoot joints. Subtalar motion is evaluated by holding the lower leg with one hand and the heel with the other. Then, with the foot in neutral position, the heel is inverted and everted. Normally, there should be at least 25 degrees of mobility in each direction. Midtarsal motion is evaluated by stabilizing the heel with one hand while the other hand grasps the forefoot at the bases of the metatarsals. The forefoot can then be pronated, supinated, abducted, and adducted. Normally, there should be at least 20 degrees of adduction and 10 degrees of abduction. Forefoot motion is evaluated by flexing and extending the MTP and IP joints individually. The first MTP joint has a particularly wide passive range of motion, with 45 degrees of flexion and 70 to 90 degrees of extension. Throughout the physical examination, findings can be compared with the opposite foot.

Diagnostic Strategies: Radiology

Plain radiography of the foot may be indicated by history, physical examination, or both. Standard three-view radiographs of the foot consist of anteroposterior, lateral, and 45-degree internal oblique projections.[52,53] The lateral projection gives the best imaging of the hindfoot and soft tissues, whereas the anteroposterior and oblique projections give the best imaging of the midfoot and forefoot. The numerous overlapping bones of the foot demand this complete radiographic series in all patients for whom radiographs are indicated. Injuries to the hindfoot also warrant the addition of standard ankle projections and, when indicated, calcaneus views.[54]

Foot radiographs are difficult to read.[55] Moreover, foot fractures are often minimally displaced, or nondisplaced, increasing the challenge of radiographic diagnosis. Several additional views improve the imaging of specific areas of the foot. Coned views, weight-bearing radiographs, or a 45-degree external oblique projection can be useful, particularly for midfoot and forefoot pathology. The most commonly obtained atypical views are the Harris (axial) view for the calcaneus and subtalar joints and the tangential view of the sesamoids. Special magnification radiographs or stress radiographs may also be useful in selected cases.

Interpretation of plain radiographs can be complicated by the numerous accessory centers of ossification and sesamoid bones (unipartite and multipartite) that

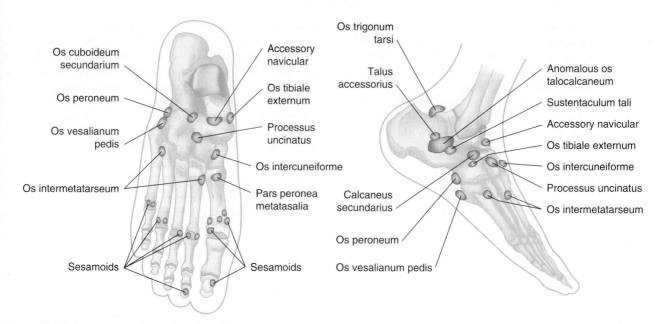

Figure 55-15. Accessory ossicles of the foot. (From Berquist TH [ed]: *Radiology of the Foot and Ankle*. New York, Raven Press, 1989.)

exist as normal variants in up to 30% of the population (Figure 55-15). The most commonly seen accessory bones are the os trigonum, os tibiale externum (also called an accessory navicular bone), os peroneum, and os vesalianum.[54] These can be differentiated from fractures by their smooth corticated surfaces. Comparison radiographs of the opposite foot may be helpful, although such variants are not inevitably bilateral. Accessory bones themselves can also fracture or cause pain syndromes.[56]

Because of the limitations of plain radiography, other imaging techniques have gained importance for specific foot injuries. Radionuclide imaging (bone scanning) is useful for evaluating unexplained foot pain or pain in athletic injuries. In the setting of acute foot trauma, this modality can often demonstrate subtle fractures not visible with plain radiography. More than 80% of such fractures are visible on bone scan within 24 hours of injury. Bone scanning is the imaging modality of choice for the diagnosis of stress fractures.[57]

Plain film tomography or CT scan of the foot can be valuable when complex articulations and overlapping bones make standard radiographs difficult to interpret, particularly in the midfoot and hindfoot.[53] The CT scan is an excellent modality for imaging complex anatomy, including the subtalar joint, the calcaneus, and the tarsometatarsal (Lisfranc) joint complex.

The MRI scan has been applied to many of the same fractures and dislocations as CT scans.[58] As in the ankle, however, the most significant role of the MRI scan is in soft tissue conditions, such as athletic injuries and tendon ruptures, where it has become the imaging modality of choice.

SPECIFIC CONDITIONS

This section covers the major fractures and dislocations seen in the foot, progressing anatomically from the hindfoot through to the forefoot. This corresponds with the sequence of physical examination in patients with foot trauma. Any of these fractures or dislocations may be open, necessitating appropriate wound management.

Hindfoot

The hindfoot is commonly involved in foot injuries and is a difficult area to image. Fractures or dislocations in this region can masquerade as ankle sprains and, if not considered, can be missed.

Talar Fractures

Principles of Disease: Anatomy

The word *talus* comes from the Latin *taxillus,* meaning "dice" and dates to the Roman Empire when soldiers made dice out of the ankle bones of horses. An appreciation of the unique anatomy of the talus is crucial to understanding the pathophysiology and treatment of talar fractures and dislocations.

The talus is the second largest tarsal bone and has seven articulations making up 60% of its surface.[59] It is divided into three regions: the head, which articulates with the navicular and calcaneus; the body, which articulates with the tibia, fibula, and calcaneus; and the neck, which joins the head and body and is the only portion of the talus that is predominantly extraarticular. The talus is the only bone in the lower extremity with no muscular attachments and is held in position by the malleoli and ligamentous attachments. The anterior width of the talus is greater than the posterior, causing it to be less stable and more prone to dislocation when the foot is plantar flexed.

The blood supply to the talus is from a vascular ring formed by branches of the anterior and posterior tibial arteries and the perforating branch of the peroneal artery. Vessels enter the talus from three main sites, any or all of which can be disrupted by fractures or dislo-

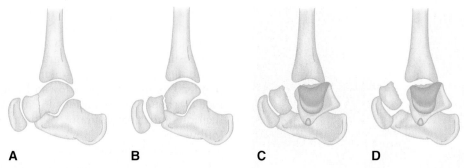

Figure 55-16. **A, B,** and **C,** Hawkins' types 1, 2, and 3 fractures. **D,** Canale and Kelly's type 4 fracture of the talar neck. (From Gustilo RB, et al [eds]: *Fractures and Dislocations*. St. Louis, Mosby, 1993.)

cations. Because of the tenuous nature of these vessels and the inconsistency of collateral circulation, the risk of avascular necrosis is significant with many talar fractures.

Pathophysiology

Talar fractures are the second most common tarsal fracture after the calcaneus.[54] They are best grouped into minor and major fractures, with minor fractures being the more common. Stress fractures of the talus can also occur. Minor talar fractures include chip and avulsion fractures of the superior neck and head, and the lateral, medial, and posterior aspects of the body. These fractures often involve the same mechanism as ankle sprains (see Figure 55-12 and Box 55-2): a combination of plantar flexion or dorsiflexion and an inversion force. Lateral process fractures, a previously uncommon injury, are highly associated with snowboarding and can be occult on plain radiography.[60] Osteochondral fractures of the talar dome also fall into the minor fracture category. Major talar fractures are usually produced by significant forces and occur in the head, neck, or body.

Talar head fractures are uncommon, making up 5% to 10% of all talar fractures.[59] Their mechanism is a compressive force applied on a plantar flexed foot and transmitted up through the talonavicular joint. Comminution is common, and associated navicular fractures can occur, further disrupting the talonavicular articulation.[54]

Talar neck fractures account for 50% of major talar injuries. Their mechanism is usually an extreme dorsiflexion force, as seen in falls or motor vehicle collisions. Associated fractures are common; the most common is an oblique or vertical fracture of the medial malleolus, which is seen in up to 28% of cases. Other associated injuries include calcaneal fractures and vertebral compression fractures. Hawkins classified talar neck fractures into three categories (Figure 55-16). Type 1 fractures are nondisplaced; type 2 fractures show subtalar subluxation; and type 3 fractures, 50% of which are open, involve a dislocation of the talar body from the ankle and subtalar joint. A fourth type that has been added to this classification involves the additional distraction of the talonavicular joint. This classification is important descriptively and because the type of fracture influences both treatment and outcome. Complications are more common with increasing displacement of talar neck fractures.

Talar body fractures account for up to 23% of all talar fractures and include many of the minor talar fractures previously listed.[61] Major talar body fractures are uncommon and usually result from falls with axial compression of the talus between the tibial plafond and the calcaneus.

Clinical Features

Talar fractures range from obvious open fractures to subtle fractures requiring special imaging techniques to diagnose. Typically, a history of a twisting injury, fall, or high-energy impact is present. Dorsal swelling and tenderness over the talus are usually found. Although ankle motion may be preserved, inversion and eversion of the hindfoot are often painful.

Diagnostic Strategies: Radiology

With minor talar fractures, radiographs can be misinterpreted as normal. Despite supplemental views, other fractures may be occult on plain radiography and require a CT or MRI scan for visualization.[62] Standard foot and ankle radiographs usually demonstrate major talar fractures (Figures 55-17 and 55-18), with the anterior and oblique projections showing talar alignment within the mortise, and the lateral projection showing the talar neck and alignment of the posterior aspect of the subtalar joint. Normal variants, such as an os trigonum or os supratalare (see Figure 55-15), must occasionally be differentiated from fractures. Specialized imaging by tomography, CT scan, or MRI scan is often required for complete assessment of talar fractures.[53]

Management

Major talar fractures require precise reduction because more weight per unit area is borne by the superior surface of the talus than by any other bone. Most talar fractures involve multiple articular surfaces, and open reduction and internal fixation are often required. Many minor talar fractures heal with casting, and the initial treatment should be with a non-weight-bearing below-knee cast or posterior slab. Fragments larger than 5 mm in diameter may require excision.[2] Other minor

823

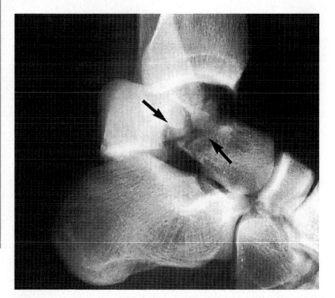

Figure 55-17. Comminuted fracture of the talar body *(arrows)*. (From Rosen P, et al [eds]: *Diagnostic Radiology in Emergency Medicine*. St. Louis, 1990, Mosby.)

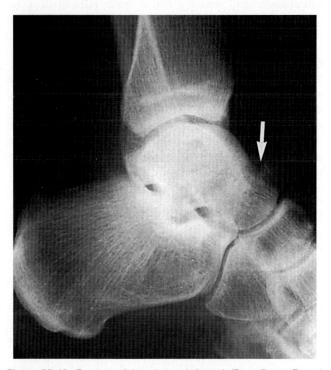

Figure 55-18. Fracture of the talar neck *(arrow)*. (From Rosen P, et al [eds]: *Diagnostic Radiology in Emergency Medicine*. St. Louis, Mosby, 1990.)

fractures, such as displaced lateral process fractures, require operative fixation because of their articular involvement.

The treatment of major talar fractures is controversial. Any significantly displaced fracture, particularly if associated with neurovascular or cutaneous compromise, should have an early attempt at closed reduction in the emergency department. Even if nonoperative reduction is impossible, as is common in type 3 and type 4 neck fractures with an intact medial malleolus, alignment can often be improved. With neurovascular

or cutaneous compromise, reduction should not be delayed by waiting for radiography or consultation. After appropriate analgesia or conscious sedation, reduction is performed by grasping the hindfoot and midfoot and applying longitudinal traction with plantar flexion. This is followed by realignment of the foot as reduction is achieved. Posterior slab immobilization and postreduction radiographs should then follow.

Displaced talar head fractures or those involving more than 50% of the articular surface usually require open reduction and internal fixation followed by non-weight-bearing casting. Smaller fragments may require excision. Type 1 fractures of the talar neck are usually treated with non-weight-bearing casting for 8 to 12 weeks. Most type 2, and all type 3 and type 4 fractures, require open reduction and internal fixation. The management of talar body fractures varies with location.

Disposition

All patients with talar fractures require orthopedic consultation in the emergency department or early orthopedic follow-up on an outpatient basis. Most minor talar fractures are suitable for outpatient follow-up.

Although most minor talar fractures heal well, some result in posttraumatic arthritis. Major talar fractures have a high incidence of complications, the most significant of which is avascular necrosis. Outcome depends on the degree of anatomic reduction and preservation of the vascular supply. The risk of avascular necrosis increases with increasing talar displacement, ranging from 10% for type 1 neck fractures to 70% or more for type 3 neck fractures. Major fractures of the talar body are also prone to avascular necrosis, the risk of which doubles if an associated dislocation is present. Other potential complications include skin infection, skin necrosis, posttraumatic arthritis, malunion, delayed union, nonunion, and predisposition to peroneal tendon dislocation. The incidence of each complication varies with the type of fracture and the aggressiveness of emergency department and operative management.

Osteochondral Fractures of the Talar Dome

Osteochondral fractures of the talar dome account for 1% of talar fractures. These injuries involve both the cartilage and subchondral bone and have many synonyms, including *transchondral fracture*, *dome fracture of the talus*, and *chip* or *flake fracture*.[63] Mechanisms identical to those causing ankle sprains are the most common cause; however, a significant number cannot be ascribed to an acute traumatic event.

An osteochondral fracture should be considered in any patient with ligamentous ankle injury accompanied by gross edema and an effusion on plain radiographs.[4] The diagnosis is often missed initially and not made until the patient returns with chronic ankle discomfort. Physical findings are usually nonspecific, although localized tenderness over the posteromedial side of the talus and increasing pain with exertion, weight bearing, or passive plantar flexion may be present. Standard radiographs are commonly normal or show subtle and easily overlooked abnormalities (Figure 55-19). Bone scanning or plain film tomography is useful in identifying talar dome abnormalities. CT or MRI scans are often required for further evaluation and classification.

When an osteochondral fracture is diagnosed or suspected, outpatient orthopedic referral is advised. The natural history of osteochondral fractures is poorly defined; however, chronic ankle discomfort and osteoarthritis can develop. Osteochondritis dissecans, a subacute or chronic talar dome defect, may occur from a partially treated or untreated osteochondral fracture.[64] However, with appropriate treatment, either by cast immobilization for up to 6 weeks or by excision,

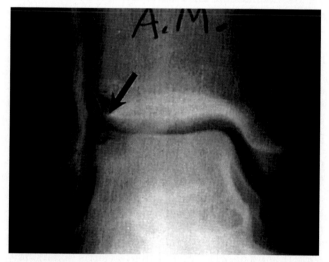

Figure 55-19. Anteroposterior view of an ankle showing an osteochondral fracture over the lateral dome of the talus (arrow). (From Baxter DE [ed]: *The Foot and Ankle in Sport.* St. Louis, Mosby, 1994.)

the prognosis usually is good, particularly if treatment begins within 12 months of symptom onset. The benefit of excision, often done arthroscopically, varies with the type of lesion and its location.[65] The previous discussion underscores the necessity of orthopedic evaluation when a patient is seen with persistent unexplained ankle pain after a previous "sprain."

Subtalar Dislocations

Principles of Disease: Pathophysiology

Subtalar dislocation, also called *peritalar dislocation*, is the simultaneous disruption of both talocalcaneal and talonavicular joints without disruption of the tibiotalar joint (Figure 55-20). This occurs when the talonavicular and talocalcaneal ligaments rupture, while the stronger calcaneonavicular ligament remains intact.[66] Subtalar dislocations are rare and are classified by the direction the foot takes in relation to the talus. Anterior and posterior dislocations occasionally occur; however, most subtalar dislocations are either medial or lateral, with medial dislocations accounting for 80% of these cases. Dislocation of the calcaneus is an exceptionally rare event that is distinct from subtalar dislocation and involves disruption of the talocalcaneal and calcaneocuboid articulations.

Subtalar dislocations are caused by severe torsional forces such as those occurring in motor vehicle crashes or falls. Medial dislocations result from inversion and plantar flexion, whereas lateral dislocations arise from the combination of eversion and plantar flexion. Ten percent of subtalar dislocations are open, and associated fractures are present in half of cases, particularly with lateral dislocations.

Clinical Features

Obvious deformity is typically present, often with tension of the skin on the side opposite the direction of dislocation.[67] Neurovascular status should be care-

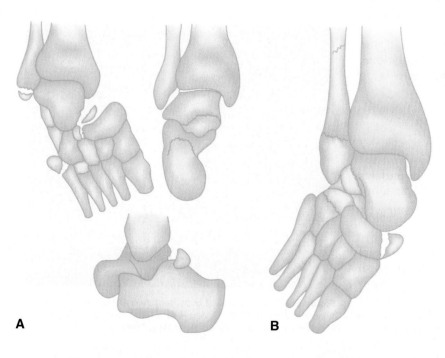

Figure 55-20. Subtalar dislocations with associated fractures. **A,** Medial subtalar dislocation resulting from an inversion force. **B,** Lateral subtalar dislocation resulting from an eversion force. (From McGlamry ED, et al [eds]: *Comprehensive Textbook of Foot Surgery,* vol 2, 2nd ed. Baltimore, Williams & Wilkins, 1992.)

A   **B**

fully assessed, although it is rarely compromised. Swelling can mask the diagnosis, which can be further delayed or missed if only ankle radiographs are obtained.

Diagnostic Strategies: Radiology
Although standard foot radiographs are diagnostic, these may be difficult to obtain because of deformity. Inadequate films can delay diagnosis and treatment. The single most helpful radiograph is an anteroposterior view of the foot, which will demonstrate the talonavicular dislocation.

Management
Subtalar dislocations require expeditious reduction. More than 80% of closed subtalar dislocations can be treated with closed reduction, either under conscious sedation in the emergency department or under general anesthesia. Closed reduction is performed by flexing the knee and applying longitudinal traction to the foot with initial accentuation, followed by reversal of the deformity (using eversion for medial dislocations and inversion for lateral dislocations). Sometimes direct pressure over the head of the talus aids in reduction. Closed reduction may be impossible because of buttonholing of the talus through the extensor retinaculum, entrapment in the peroneal tendons, or associated fractures. After reduction, immobilization in a below-knee cast for 4 to 6 weeks is indicated.

Disposition
Urgent emergency department orthopedic consultation is indicated for subtalar dislocations. Although serious complications are uncommon in cases of closed subtalar dislocation, most patients have limitation of subtalar motion that can affect gait. Avascular necrosis is uncommon.

Total Talar Dislocation
Total talar dislocation is an extremely rare and devastating injury requiring emergency orthopedic consultation. In these injuries, which are the end result of the same forces that produce subtalar dislocation, the entire talus is distracted from all of its articulations. Most are open, and infection and avascular necrosis are common complications.

Calcaneal Fractures

Principles of Disease: Anatomy
The calcaneus is the largest bone in the foot and the most commonly fractured tarsal bone.[68] It articulates with the talus superiorly (forming the subtalar joint) and with the cuboid anterolaterally.

Pathophysiology
Falls with direct axial compression cause most calcaneal fractures. Because of this high-energy mechanism, associated injuries are common: 7% of calcaneal fractures are bilateral, 25% are associated with other lower extremity injuries, and 10% are associated with spinal injuries, typically vertebral compression fractures.[54]

Numerous classification schemes have been developed for calcaneal fractures. Perhaps the most intuitive is to simply categorize the fracture as either extraarticular or intraarticular. Extraarticular fractures usually involve the addition of a rotational mechanism and include fractures of the sustentaculum tali, the tuberosity, and oblique fractures of the body. Avulsion fractures of the anterior process by the bifurcate ligament (which joins the calcaneus, navicular, and cuboid) are also included in this category. Up to 75% of calcaneal fractures are intraarticular, ranging from nondisplaced single fractures to severely crushed, comminuted fractures. Because of the cancellous nature of the calcaneus, fractures are frequently comminuted. Calcaneal stress fractures also occur.

Clinical Features
Typically, the patient has a history of a fall resulting in a direct impact on the heel or heels. Physical examination reveals pain, swelling, and tenderness over the affected heel, and weight bearing on the hindfoot is usually impossible. In cases of significant fracture, the heel may be deformed when viewed from behind, appearing short, wide, and tilted. Ecchymoses may extend over the entire sole, a finding not seen in isolated malleolar fractures. The presence of compartment syndrome or associated injuries such as vertebral compression fractures should be considered.

Diagnostic Strategies: Radiology
Standard foot and ankle radiographs should be obtained. The anteroposterior view of the foot shows the calcaneocuboid joint and the anterosuperior calcaneus, whereas the lateral view shows the posterior facet and can demonstrate compression of the calcaneal body (Figure 55-21).[69] In addition, a Harris (axial) view, when not precluded by pain, should be obtained to image the calcaneal tuberosity, subtalar joint, and sustentaculotalar joints. Anterior process fractures require

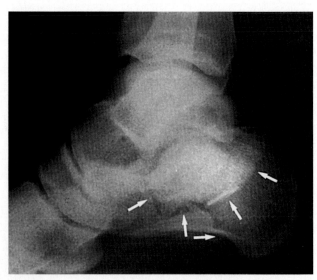

Figure 55-21. Comminuted body fracture of the calcaneus with subtalar involvement. (From Rosen P, et al [eds]: *Diagnostic Radiology in Emergency Medicine*. St. Louis, Mosby, 1990.)

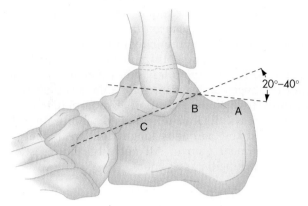

Figure 55-22. Boehler's angle is obtained by drawing two lines, one between the posterior tuberosity (A) and the apex of the posterior facet (B), and the other between the apex of the posterior facet (B) and the apex of the anterior process (C). A value less than 20 degrees suggests a calcaneal compression fracture. (From Rosen P, et al [eds]: *Diagnostic Radiology in Emergency Medicine.* St. Louis, Mosby, 1990.)

differentiation from a calcaneus secundarius (see Figure 55-15).[70]

Two assessments are critical to the management of calcaneal fractures: whether the fracture involves the subtalar joint and the degree of depression of the posterior facet. Compression fractures are not always obvious, and measurement of Boehler's angle (Figure 55-22) can be helpful. Boehler's angle is measured on the lateral view as the angle between two lines, one between the posterior tuberosity and the apex of the posterior facet, and the other between the apex of the posterior facet and the apex of the anterior process. Although several ranges for this measurement have been cited, 20 to 40 degrees gives the best diagnostic performance for fracture detection.[71] An angle of less than 20 degrees suggests a compression fracture, and comparison measurement of the uninjured side is helpful in questionable cases.

Imaging of the calcaneus can be difficult given the complex three-dimensional nature of its articulations. Plain radiography can underestimate injury severity, and the CT scan has revolutionized the assessment of calcaneal fractures and correlates well with outcome. The MRI scan is also an excellent imaging modality for the hindfoot and has a role in selected calcaneal fractures.

Management

The management of intraarticular or displaced calcaneal fractures is controversial, with many operative and nonoperative approaches.[72] If operative fixation is performed, reduction must be as precise as possible to obtain results superior to those obtained with nonoperative treatment. The treatment of nondisplaced extraarticular fractures usually involves casting for 6 to 8 weeks.

Disposition

Intraarticular or displaced calcaneal fractures require orthopedic consultation in the emergency department.

Outpatient orthopedic follow-up can be arranged for more innocuous injuries, provided this is consistent with local practice and there are no associated injuries that warrant hospitalization. When considering outpatient follow-up, it is important to bear in mind that the extent and severity of calcaneal fractures are often significantly underestimated from plain radiographs. Minor extraarticular fractures usually heal uneventfully; however, significant calcaneal fractures frequently have complications, including compartment syndrome. In both conservatively and surgically treated patients, the incidence of long-term pain, loss of joint mobility, and functional disability approaches 50%.

Midtarsal Joint Injuries

The midtarsal joint (Chopart's joint) is composed of the talonavicular and calcaneocuboid joints. Injury in this area, although rare, can occur with any ankle, hindfoot, or midfoot trauma. Midtarsal joint injuries usually result from forced dorsiflexion and are often associated with other significant fractures. Sprains, fracture subluxations and dislocations, or isolated "swivel dislocations" (a variant of a subtalar dislocation) can all occur at the midtarsal joint. Pain, swelling, inability to bear weight, and tenderness over the midtarsal joints are usually found. Although standard radiographs are often abnormal, the diagnosis is frequently overlooked or delayed and symptoms ascribed to an ankle sprain (see Figure 55-12 and Box 55-2). The possibility of a midtarsal joint injury should be considered with any isolated midfoot fracture, particularly those of the navicular tuberosity. Undisplaced injuries may heal with casting, but operative fixation is often required. Complications are common and include persistent pain, arthritis, and long-term disability.

Midfoot

The midfoot is an inherently stable region of the foot and is uncommonly injured. Fractures and relationships of the midfoot tarsals are often difficult to visualize with standard radiographs because of underpenetration and the oblique orientation of the bones and joints. This is compounded by the fact that midfoot injuries often have ill-defined and poorly localized pain. Delay in diagnosis frequently occurs with midfoot injuries. Although isolated fractures of the midfoot tarsals occur, associated injuries, including significant sprains, subluxations, and spontaneously reduced dislocations, are often present.

Navicular Fractures

Principles of Disease: Anatomy

The navicular has a curved shape, hence the derivation of its name from the Latin *navis,* meaning "a ship." Because of the navicular's extensive articular surface, its blood supply can only enter through a small waist of cortex, and the middle third is relatively avascular. As a result, avascular necrosis of the navicular can occur after fractures, analogous to the situation found in the scaphoid bone of the wrist.

Pathophysiology

Navicular fractures, although relatively rare, are the most common midfoot fracture and are classified into dorsal avulsion fractures, tuberosity fractures, and body fractures. Dorsal avulsion fractures account for half of navicular fractures and usually occur when an eversion stress causes bony avulsion from either the talonavicular capsule or the deltoid ligament. These usually do not involve a significant amount of articular surface. Tuberosity fractures also occur from eversion forces, leading to an avulsion at the insertion of the posterior tibial tendon. A tuberosity fracture may be the only clue of a midtarsal joint injury. Body fractures are uncommon and result from an axial loading mechanism.[73] They are often comminuted, intraarticular, and associated with other midtarsal pathologic conditions. Stress fractures of the navicular can also occur.

Clinical Features

Navicular fractures cause localized tenderness over the dorsal and medial aspect of the midfoot. The navicular tuberosity may be tender and is located by first identifying the sustentaculum tali, a shelf of bone on the medial side of the ankle about 2.5 cm below the tip of the medial malleolus. The tuberosity is then easily palpable just anterior to this landmark. In the case of tuberosity fractures, pain may be exacerbated by passive eversion or active inversion of the foot.

Diagnostic Strategies: Radiology

Standard foot radiographs usually demonstrate navicular fractures; however, tomograms or radionuclide bone scans may be required. Care must be taken not to confuse the commonly occurring os tibiale externum, also called an accessory navicular bone, with an acute fracture (see Figure 55-15).

Management

Dorsal avulsion and tuberosity fractures not involving a significant amount of articular surface are usually treated with a walking cast for 4 to 6 weeks. Body fractures and displaced fractures involving more than 20% of the articular surface often require operative fixation.[54,68]

Disposition

Most navicular fractures are suitable for outpatient orthopedic follow-up; however, significant fractures, particularly if intraarticular, should warrant orthopedic consultation in the emergency department. Navicular tuberosity fractures can be complicated by nonunion. Avascular necrosis and arthritis also occur, particularly in body or other intraarticular fractures.

Cuboid Fractures

Isolated cuboid fractures are uncommon and usually result from lateral subluxation of the midtarsal joint in a Lisfranc injury.[74] This has been termed a *nutcracker fracture* because the cuboid is crushed between the bases of the fourth and fifth metatarsals and the anterior calcaneus. Cuboid fractures are also associated with fractures of the posterior malleolus. The cuboid is best evaluated by the oblique view of a standard foot radiographic series because this demonstrates both the calcaneocuboid and the cuboid-metatarsal relationship. The possibility of a Lisfranc injury should be considered with any cuboid fracture. Treatment of isolated injuries ranges from casting for minor nondisplaced fractures to operative fixation. Extraarticular cuboid fractures may still lead to serious disability from dysfunction of the peroneus longus tendon at the level of the peroneal groove. All cuboid fractures should warrant orthopedic assessment.

Cuneiform Fractures

Fractures of the cuneiforms are extremely uncommon and usually result from direct trauma. As with cuboid fractures, the patient should be assessed carefully for the presence of a Lisfranc injury. Treatment is usually by casting; however, displaced fractures require orthopedic assessment.

Dislocations of the Navicular, Cuboid, and Cuneiforms

Isolated dislocations of each of the midfoot bones have been described. These are uncommon injuries that often require open reduction. Orthopedic consultation in the emergency department is required for any of these injuries.

Lisfranc (Tarsometatarsal) Fractures and Dislocations

Principles of Disease: Anatomy

The tarsometatarsal joints (see Figure 55-14) are commonly called Lisfranc's joint. Any injury to this area, whether dislocation or fracture-dislocation, is termed a Lisfranc injury. Knowledge of the anatomy of the Lisfranc joint complex is central to understanding these injuries.

The Lisfranc joint is made up of the articulations of the bases of the first three metatarsals with their respective cuneiforms and the fourth and fifth metatarsals with the cuboid. In concert, the tarsometatarsal joints act to allow supination and pronation of the forefoot. The intrinsic stability of Lisfranc's joint is provided by the bony architecture and associated ligaments. When viewed end-on, the metatarsals have a trapezoidal shape and combine to form a transverse arch with the second metatarsal acting as the "keystone." The second metatarsal is essential for the stability of the entire complex and is further buttressed by its snug articulation in a recess created by the three cuneiforms. Strong transverse intermetatarsal ligaments join the bases of the second through fifth metatarsals, and Lisfranc's ligament joins the medial cuneiform with the second metatarsal base (Figure 55-23). Lisfranc's joint is further supported by dorsal and plantar ligaments, the plantar fascia, and the insertions of the tibialis anterior and peroneus longus tendons at the first metatarsal base.

Pathophysiology

Lisfranc injuries are uncommon because tremendous energy is required to disrupt this complex. Such

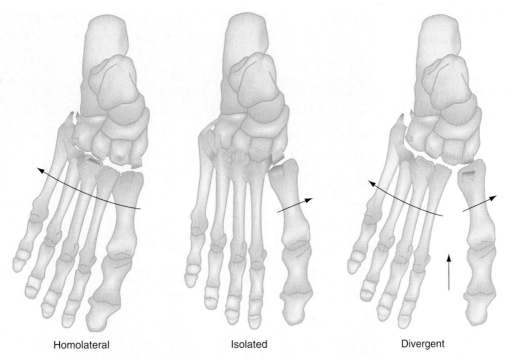

Homolateral   Isolated   Divergent

Figure 55-23. Classification of Lisfranc injuries. The ligamentous anatomy of the Lisfranc complex is also depicted. (From Hardcastle PH, et al: Injuries to the tarsometatarsal joint: Incidence, classification and treatment. *J Bone Joint Surg Br* 64:349, 1982.)

injuries arise from three mechanisms: rotational forces, where the body twists around a fixed forefoot; axial loads, where the weight of the body drives the hindfoot into the bases of the metatarsals; and crush injuries. Because of the mechanisms involved, associated injuries, such as MTP joint dislocations, can occur. Most Lisfranc injuries occur from motor vehicle crashes. Sports involving fixation of the forefoot (e.g., equestrian activities and windsurfing) are also associated with these injuries. Notably, one third of Lisfranc injuries arise from seemingly trivial mechanisms such as stumbles or falls.[75] Most Lisfranc injuries are closed.

Lisfranc injuries are classified by the direction of the dislocation in the horizontal plane (see Figure 55-23). In homolateral injuries, all five metatarsals are displaced in the same direction. In isolated injuries, one or more metatarsals are displaced away from the others. In divergent injuries, the metatarsals are splayed outward in both the medial and the lateral directions. These usually occur between the first and second metatarsals because of their lack of an intermetatarsal connection. A component of dorsal displacement is also commonly present in Lisfranc injuries, whereas plantar displacement is uncommon because of the bony structure and strength of the plantar ligaments and fascia.[76]

Because of ligamentous attachments, Lisfranc injuries almost invariably involve associated metatarsal fractures, usually of the second metatarsal base. Fractures of the cuboid, cuneiforms, and navicular are also common, occurring in 39% of cases.[75] Lisfranc injuries may be complicated by vascular injury because a critical branch of the dorsalis pedis artery dives between the first and second metatarsals to form the plantar arch. Trauma to this vessel can cause significant hemorrhage and, uncommonly, vascular compromise.

Clinical Features
Most Lisfranc injuries are obvious; however, subtle injuries occur and the true extent of the pathologic condition can easily be missed or misdiagnosed.[77] Apparently trivial fractures, if viewed in isolation, fail to reflect the serious soft tissue disruption that can be present.

The clinical presentation varies with the extent of injury and displacement. Severe pain in the midfoot and inability to bear weight, particularly on the toes, usually occur. Paresthesias are occasionally present, and examination usually reveals edema and ecchymosis. In severe injuries, obvious deformity with forefoot abduction, equinus, and prominence of the medial tarsal area can be present. In addition, anteroposterior shortening and transverse broadening may be found. The dorsalis pedis pulse can be absent, or evidence of vascular compromise of the forefoot may be present. Typically, tenderness along the affected tarsometatarsal joints and pain with passive abduction and pronation of the forefoot are present, sometimes with pathologic mobility.

Diagnostic Strategies: Radiology
Standard foot radiographs are usually sufficient to diagnose injuries to the Lisfranc complex (Figure 55-24). The anteroposterior view identifies fractures and alignment, with the oblique view greatly aiding this assessment by eliminating overlap at the metatarsal bases. The lateral view shows the soft tissues and identifies any dorsal or plantar displacement. When possible,

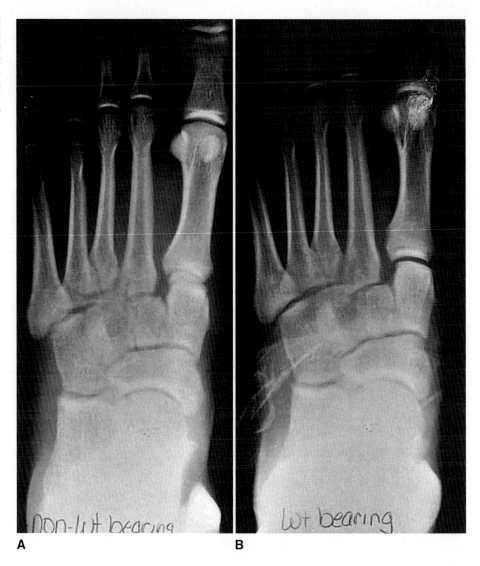

Figure 55-24. Lisfranc injury diagnosed by step-off at the base of the second metatarsal and middle cuneiform and widening between the bases of the first and second metatarsals. **A,** Non-weight-bearing radiograph. **B,** Weight-bearing radiograph (note increase in step-off). (From Baxter DE [ed]: *The Foot and Ankle in Sport*. St. Louis, Mosby, 1994.)

weight-bearing lateral radiographs may be useful to look for flattening of the longitudinal arch in subtle injuries.[78] Comparison views are extremely helpful and a 30-degree oblique view, in addition to the standard 45-degree oblique view, may also be of value. Difficult cases sometimes require plain film tomography or a CT scan for diagnosis.

An appreciation of normal radiographic anatomy is essential to assess Lisfranc injuries. Radiographs should be methodically examined, with assessment of alignment, bones, and soft tissues. The first four metatarsals should each line up with their respective tarsal articulation along their medial edge on antero-posterior and oblique radiographs. The most consistent relationship is the alignment of the medial edge of the base of the second metatarsal with the medial edge of the middle cuneiform. Dorsal alignment of the tarsals with their respective metatarsals should be assessed on the lateral radiograph.

Findings suggestive of a Lisfranc injury include widening between the first and second or second and third metatarsal bases or any fracture around the Lisfranc joint. Fractures of the second metatarsal base (called a *fleck sign*), cuboid fractures, and cuneiform

fractures are particularly common. A fracture of the second metatarsal base is virtually pathognomonic of occult tarsometatarsal joint disruption.

If a suspicious fracture is present and alignment appears normal, a spontaneously reduced dislocation may be present. In addition, plain radiographs may be normal in the setting of a typical history and tenderness over the tarsometatarsal joints, suggesting a sprain of the Lisfranc complex. In either case, stress radiographs may be diagnostic.

Management

Lisfranc injuries are usually treated with closed reduction and internal fixation with percutaneous Kirschner wires. This is followed by non-weight-bearing casting for 12 weeks and an orthotic for 1 year. The Lisfranc "sprain" is a relatively new concept. Treatment is usually immobilization for 6 weeks in a below-knee walking cast.

Disposition

Any obvious or suspected Lisfranc injury requires orthopedic consultation. Patients suspected of having a Lisfranc sprain require casting and orthopedic assessment on an outpatient basis. The incidence of complications with Lisfranc injuries depends on the timing of diagnosis and the degree of anatomic reduction achieved. Aggressive surgical management clearly improves outcome. Degenerative arthritis is a common complication of Lisfranc injuries. Other potential complications include compartment syndrome, residual pain, unequal metatarsal pressure, loss of the metatarsal arch, and reflex sympathetic dystrophy. Because of their instability, Lisfranc sprains can result in biomechanical problems if untreated.

Forefoot

Traumatic forefoot conditions are commonly underdiagnosed and often consist of more than one fracture or dislocation occurring simultaneously. As occurs elsewhere in the foot, forefoot trauma may lead to prolonged disability and dysfunction.[79]

Metatarsal Fractures

Metatarsal fractures are common, accounting for 35% of foot fractures.[80] The best approach is to first anatomically classify the injury as occurring in the shaft, the head and neck, or the base. Management is then dictated by the metatarsal involved, the specific location and type of fracture, and the nature of any associated injuries.

Metatarsal Shaft Fractures

Principles of Disease: Pathophysiology

Metatarsal shaft fractures arise from either direct trauma (e.g., a crush injury from a heavy object) or indirect trauma (e.g., a twisting force applied to a fixed forefoot). Because of these mechanisms, associated phalangeal fractures often occur. Direct trauma may be highly disruptive, resulting in multiple metatarsal fractures and severe complications. The third metatarsal is the most commonly fractured, and metatarsal shaft stress fractures are common.

Biomechanics are an important consideration when approaching metatarsal shaft fractures. During stance, weight is distributed equally between the heel and forefoot, where it is spread across the metatarsals, with the first metatarsal carrying twice its share of the load. Great toe metatarsal fractures, although uncommon, require more aggressive management because of this load-bearing function. Alignment of fractured metatarsals is important because dorsal or plantar displacement can lead to pain or functional disability by altering the transverse arch and load distribution. Dorsal angulation commonly occurs at the site of metatarsal fractures from the action of intrinsic muscles and toe flexors. Medial or lateral displacement, although less critical, can lead to painful bony prominences or neuromas.

Clinical Features

Metatarsal shaft fractures cause weight-bearing difficulty and tenderness, which is usually maximal on the plantar surface and can be difficult to localize if swelling is significant. Axial compression of the involved toe is often painful, and ecchymosis usually occurs within 12 hours of injury. Rotational alignment should be assessed by evaluating the position and plane of the involved digit.

Diagnostic Strategies: Radiology

Standard radiographs are sufficient to diagnose most metatarsal shaft fractures; however, radiographs are usually exposed for the talar bones, and the forefoot may be overpenetrated. Adjustment of penetration or coned views may be required for visualization of subtle fractures. Displacement and angulation, both in the sagittal and mediolateral planes, should be assessed.

Management

Most undisplaced metatarsal shaft fractures of the second through fifth metatarsals are treated with a below-knee walking cast for 2 to 4 weeks. Early casted ambulation may be beneficial to healing and reduce the incidence of reflex sympathetic dystrophy. Although some practitioners recommend a non-weight-bearing cast for 4 to 6 weeks for these fractures, others suggest that a metatarsal pad, stiff shoes, and crutches, if needed, are sufficient. These various approaches attest to the fact that most nondisplaced metatarsal shaft fractures heal well regardless of the treatment.

The great toe metatarsal requires more aggressive management because of its biomechanical role and the stresses imposed on it during gait. Nondisplaced first metatarsal fractures should be treated with casting for 4 to 6 weeks. At least the first 3 weeks of this immobilization, if not the entire period, should be non-weight-bearing.[81]

Reduction should be considered in any metatarsal shaft fracture with more than 3 mm of displacement or 10 degrees of angulation. Closed reduction, with toe traps and countertraction at the ankle, is often successful. Non-weight-bearing casting for 4 to 6 weeks should follow. The indications for open reduction are controversial but generally include the presence of compartment syndrome, unstable fractures, open fractures, fractures that have failed closed reduction, or multiple fractures. These are treated with either Kirschner wires or plates.[80] In particular, displaced first and fifth metatarsal shaft fractures are commonly treated operatively. Major forefoot trauma, with crushing and multiple open metatarsal fractures, requires an aggressive approach with staged operative management.

Disposition

Most undisplaced metatarsal shaft fractures are suitable for management without orthopedic referral. Orthopedic consultation in the emergency department should be obtained for patients with multiple or displaced fractures. Complications are rare in nondisplaced or minimally displaced metatarsal shaft fractures. Reflex sympathetic dystrophy can occur and may be related to the unnecessary use of non-weight-bearing casting.[68] Inadequate reduction, particularly in the sagittal plane, can lead to biomechanical problems and painful callosities or metatarsalgia. Malunion in the mediolateral plane, particularly if involving the first or fifth metatarsal, can lead to pressure points, neuromas, or biomechanical problems. Delayed union, nonunion, compartment syndrome, and soft tissue complications occur uncommonly.

Metatarsal Head and Neck Fractures

Metatarsal head and neck fractures, although similar in their pathophysiology and assessment to shaft fractures, are commonly multiple and often result from direct trauma. Nondisplaced fractures may be treated with a walking cast for 4 to 6 weeks. Often these fractures are displaced, with the distal fragment pulled in a plantar and lateral direction by the flexor tendons, a finding best appreciated on oblique and lateral radiographs. Precise realignment of neck and head fractures is important to maintain the transverse arch. Although reduction may be successful with toe traps, instability is common and operative fixation is more commonly required than with shaft fractures. Most of these fractures should warrant orthopedic consultation in the emergency department, particularly if they are displaced or intraarticular. Complications are similar to those seen with shaft fractures.

Metatarsal Base Fractures

Principles of Disease: Pathophysiology

Isolated fractures of the first through fourth metatarsal bases are uncommon. Most are nondisplaced transverse fractures within 1 cm of the tarsometatarsal articulation and arise as a result of direct trauma. An indirect mechanism is more suggestive of the presence of an occult Lisfranc injury. The most commonly encountered metatarsal base fractures occur at the fifth metatarsal.

Fifth Metatarsal

Jones fracture is a term often erroneously applied to any fracture of the fifth metatarsal base. The eponym is in reference to Jones, who, in 1902, described a fracture he sustained while dancing and a series of similar injuries. In reality, two distinct fractures can occur in the region of the fifth metatarsal base, and debate continues regarding which one Jones actually described.[82] More important than the terminology, these two fractures differ dramatically in their mechanism, treatment, and prognosis.[83]

The more common, and benign, fracture at the fifth metatarsal base is of the tuberosity. Also called the *styloid*, the tuberosity is the bulge of the fifth metatarsal that is easily palpated over the lateral edge of the foot. It is fractured by a sudden inversion of a plantar flexed foot that for decades was thought to be caused by an avulsion at the insertion of the peroneus brevis tendon. Cadaveric studies, however, have implicated the lateral band of the plantar aponeurosis as the actual cause for the location and nature of this fracture. Tuberosity fractures range from tiny flecks to lesions involving the entire tuberosity and are usually extraarticular, although they may extend into the cubometatarsal joint. Often these injuries masquerade as ankle sprains

(see Figure 55-12 and Box 55-2), making the fifth metatarsal base an important area to palpate in any twisting injury.

The more serious acute fracture at the base of the fifth metatarsal is a transverse fracture occurring at least 15 mm distal to the proximal end of the bone.[83] This diaphyseal fracture is probably a true Jones fracture and involves the fourth and fifth intermetatarsal articulations but not the cubometatarsal articulation. Diaphyseal fractures occur as the result of a complex combination of forces occurring when a load is applied to the lateral forefoot in the absence of inversion.[83] Typically, these occur in running and jumping sports. Further subclassification of proximal diaphyseal fractures has been done and can be helpful in determining management.

Clinical Features

The assessment of metatarsal base fractures is similar to that described for the metatarsal shaft. Pain is often diffuse and difficult to localize in these injuries, with the exception of the easily palpable fifth metatarsal tuberosity. Passive inversion may also be painful with a fifth metatarsal base fracture.

Diagnostic Strategies: Radiology

Standard radiography easily demonstrates most metatarsal base fractures. Radiographs should be carefully assessed for fracture angulation, displacement, and articular extension. If the fracture is intraarticular, an estimation of the percentage of articular surface involved is essential in determining management. In difficult cases, plain film tomography may be helpful.

With fractures of the first through fourth metatarsal bases, it is important to search for other radiologic clues of a Lisfranc injury. A fracture of the second metatarsal base is virtually pathognomonic of occult tarsometatarsal joint disruption. When assessing a fifth metatarsal base fracture, differentiation between the tuberosity and diaphysis is essential (Figure 55-25). Care should be taken not to misinterpret an os vesalianum or os peroneum for a fifth metatarsal base fracture (see Fig. 55-15). Standard ankle radiographs also demonstrate the fifth metatarsal base, and this area should be routinely scrutinized.

Management

Nondisplaced extraarticular fractures of the first through fourth metatarsal bases are usually managed with a below-knee cast. Displaced fractures should be reduced and often require fixation. Intraarticular fractures, especially those of the first metatarsal, often lead to complications. Operative fixation may be required, even in nondisplaced intraarticular first metatarsal base fractures, if more than 25% of the articular surface is involved.[81]

The management of fifth metatarsal base fractures depends on the type of fracture. Extraarticular tuberosity fractures, regardless of their size or degree of displacement, heal well and are managed symptomatically with a walking cast for 2 to 3 weeks, compression wrap, or stiff shoes.[82] Intraarticular tuberosity fractures

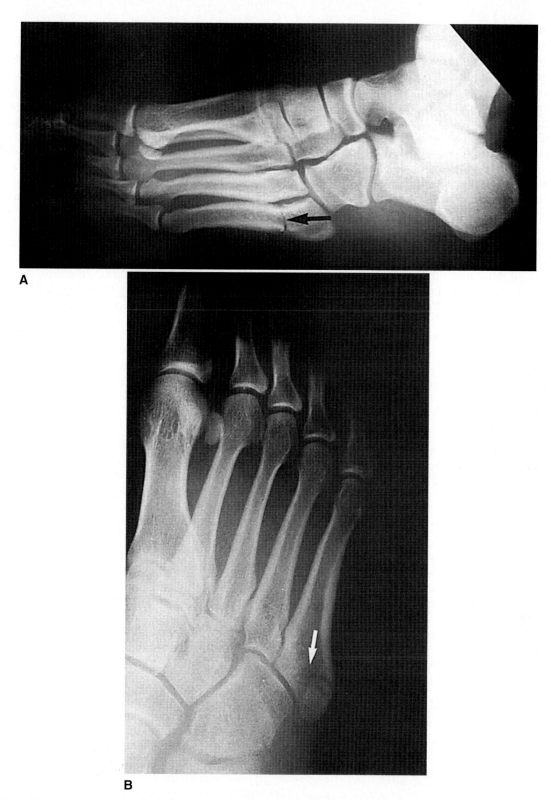

Figure 55-25. A, Diaphyseal fracture of the fifth metatarsal *(arrow)*. This is the more serious of the two fractures occurring at the fifth metatarsal base. (From Rosen P, et al [eds]: *Diagnostic Radiology in Emergency Medicine.* St. Louis, Mosby, 1990.) **B,** Tuberosity fracture of the fifth metatarsal base *(arrow)*. This is the more benign of the two fractures occurring at the fifth metatarsal base.

involving more than 30% of the articular surface, or with more than 2 mm of displacement, may require fixation.[82] Nondisplaced intraarticular fractures are usually treated initially with non-weight-bearing casting for 6 to 8 weeks, followed by repeat radiographic

assessment.[82] Immobilization for up to 6 months may be required for complete healing, and immediate fixation may be advisable in athletes.[83] Displaced fifth metatarsal diaphyseal fractures are usually managed operatively, and lengthy treatment may be necessary.

Disposition

Because they are rare and treatment varies, most first through fourth metatarsal base fractures require orthopedic assessment. Nondisplaced extraarticular fractures of the first through fourth metatarsal bases are suitable for orthopedic follow-up on an outpatient basis. Orthopedic consultation in the emergency department should be obtained in any other first through fourth metatarsal base fracture or if a Lisfranc injury is suspected. Significant or displaced intraarticular fifth metatarsal tuberosity fractures or diaphyseal fractures should also warrant orthopedic evaluation in the emergency department.

Intraarticular metatarsal base fractures involving the first through fourth metatarsals can lead to posttraumatic arthritis requiring arthrodesis. Complications are rare in cases of fifth metatarsal tuberosity fractures, although fibrous nonunion of the fracture fragment can occur. Fifth metatarsal diaphyseal fractures are often complicated by delayed union, nonunion, or recurrence resulting from disruption of the metatarsal vascular supply. These complications occur in more than 50% of patients treated conservatively and often require aggressive surgical therapy and lengthy healing times.

Phalangeal Fractures

Principles of Disease: Pathophysiology

Phalangeal fractures are the most common forefoot fracture. They usually arise from direct trauma, often the result of dropped heavy objects or stubbing of the toe. Less commonly, indirect mechanisms involving twisting of the forefoot can lead to phalangeal fractures. Proximal phalanges are more commonly fractured than middle or distal phalanges, and the proximal phalanx of the fifth toe is most commonly injured.[79] Fractures of the hallux are often displaced, whereas fractures of the lesser phalanges are often comminuted but less commonly displaced.

Clinical Features

Although phalangeal fractures are generally considered minor injuries, they can lead to disabling sequelae and deserve careful assessment.[84] The patient with a phalangeal fracture has acute pain and swelling of the affected toe, often with difficulty ambulating or wearing shoes. Tenderness, crepitus, and reduced range of motion may be found. A subungual hematoma is often present if the distal phalanx is involved, and open fractures are common.

Diagnostic Strategies: Radiology

Standard radiographs are usually sufficient to demonstrate phalangeal fractures, with the lateral view being most sensitive. Often the uninjured toes must be positioned to obtain adequate radiographs, and magnification radiographs are occasionally required. Angulation and joint involvement should be assessed.

Management

Most phalangeal fractures are easily managed and heal well. A subungual hematoma should be evacuated, and nail bed repair may occasionally be required. Nondisplaced lesser phalangeal fractures should be stabilized by "buddy taping," splinting the injured toe to an adjacent toe with adhesive tape. Gauze placement between the splinted toes is advisable to prevent skin maceration. Phalangeal fractures often remain painful for 2 to 3 weeks until stabilized by callus.

If significant displacement or angulation is present, reduction should be performed with manual traction or toe traps after digital block anesthesia. Moderate persistent angulation or displacement is acceptable if the clinical appearance of the toe remains satisfactory. Rarely, operative fixation of lesser phalangeal fractures is indicated, particularly in cases with severe rotatory deformity or in open fractures requiring debridement.

Nondisplaced phalangeal fractures involving the hallux are treated by buddy taping but may require a walking cast for 2 to 3 weeks if painful. Displaced phalangeal fractures of the hallux require reduction. If the reduction is inadequate or unstable, operative fixation may be indicated. Unless completely nondisplaced, most intraarticular fractures involving the hallux are treated with operative fixation, although this is an area of controversy.

Disposition

Most phalangeal fractures do not require orthopedic evaluation; however, if displacement is persistent or causes concern, consultation is advised. Orthopedic consultation in the emergency department is advised for poorly reduced or intraarticular hallux fractures.

Complications of phalangeal fractures are uncommon. Intraarticular phalangeal fractures, particularly those involving the hallux, may lead to arthritis or fragments requiring operative removal. Symptomatic angular malunion and osseous deformity can occur with phalangeal fractures, and exostectomy is sometimes required.

Sesamoid Fractures

Principles of Disease: Anatomy

The sesamoids are two flat oval bones found within the tendon of the flexor hallucis brevis, under the head of the first metatarsal. Their name comes from the Greek word *sesamoeides,* meaning "resembling a sesame seed." Ten percent of the population has sesamoid bones under the fifth metatarsal head and, uncommonly, sesamoids are found under the second, third, or fourth metatarsal (see Figure 55-15). The sesamoids elevate the first metatarsal head, act as shock absorbers, and are a fulcrum for tendons. The medial sesamoid is more directly located under the metatarsal and bears up to three times the body weight during gait.

Pathophysiology

Sesamoid fractures are uncommon and are usually caused by direct trauma from falls. Hyperextension of the great toe can indirectly lead to a sesamoid fracture.[85] Sesamoid fractures can also be found in association with MTP dislocations. The medial sesamoid is more commonly fractured than the lateral, probably because its location leads to a more direct transmission of forces. Stress fractures of the sesamoids also occur.

Clinical Features

Sesamoid fractures produce pain that is maximal during the toe-off phase of gait. Point tenderness and pain with passive hyperextension of the first MTP joint are generally found.

Diagnostic Strategies: Radiology

Most sesamoid fractures are transverse and easily visualized on standard anteroposterior or lateral radiographs. Special tangential views are occasionally required. Radiographic interpretation is complicated by the fact that up to 33% of the population has partition of the sesamoids, particularly the medial sesamoid. Comparison radiographs are helpful; however, 15% of these variants are unilateral. Careful examination, similar to that described for accessory ossification centers, usually differentiates multipartite sesamoids from acute fractures. Occasionally, bipartite sesamoids become symptomatic because of movement of adjacent parts against each other or fibrocartilage union fracture.

Management

Treatment of nondisplaced sesamoid fractures depends on the severity of symptoms. Arch supports may be sufficient, but sesamoid fractures generally require a below-knee walking cast for 3 to 4 weeks. Orthotic metatarsal supports may be necessary after cast removal because symptoms occasionally take up to 6 months to resolve.

Disposition

Most sesamoid fractures heal without complications and do not require orthopedic consultation. Occasionally, degenerative changes of the first MTP joint, aseptic necrosis, nonunion, or continued pain occur. Rarely, if physiotherapy or steroid injections are not sufficient, sesamoid excision may be required.

Metatarsophalangeal Dislocations

Principles of Disease: Pathophysiology

Dislocations of the MTP are uncommon injuries because of the protection footwear provides and the inherent stability of MTP and IP joints. MTP dislocations can occur in any joint and in any direction. First MTP dislocations require large forces and usually result from motor vehicle collisions. These injuries are often open and typically involve dorsal dislocations of the distal component caused by hyperextension of the MTP joint. Associated sesamoid fractures may be present. Complex dislocations, in which the sesamoids or local tendons prevent closed reduction, can occur. Second through fifth MTP dislocations are usually medial or lateral displacements that occur when the toe strikes or hooks an object. The most common is a lateral dislocation of the fifth MTP joint.

Clinical Features

Dislocations of the MTP cause pain, swelling, and difficulty bearing weight on the ball of the foot. First MTP dislocations are usually obvious on clinical examination because the toe is angled upward with dorsal and proximal displacement of the proximal phalanx. This leads to a striking prominence of the metatarsal head over the plantar surface. Skin tenting or a dimple may be present. Rarely, the sesamoids are palpable dorsal to the metatarsal, indicating a complex dislocation. Dislocations of the lesser toes are often more subtle, and comparison with the uninjured foot may be helpful. Neurovascular compromise is rare.

Diagnostic Strategies: Radiology

Dislocations of the MTP are well visualized on standard foot radiographs. In first MTP dislocations, a double density is often present, caused by the base of the proximal phalanx superimposed over the metatarsal head. Radiographs should be scrutinized for signs suggesting complex dislocation, such as the sesamoids lying between the two articular surfaces or dorsal to the metatarsal head.

Management

Most MTP dislocations, particularly of the lesser toes, are easily reduced with longitudinal traction. Appropriate analgesia or local anesthesia should be administered before attempting reduction. Dorsal dislocations of the first MTP joint can be more challenging and may require initial accentuation of the deformity during reduction. Joint stability should be assessed and repeat radiographs obtained after reduction of an MTP dislocation. After reduction, a walking cast with a toe plate is indicated for 3 weeks, followed by physiotherapy to ensure adequate range of motion. Alternatively, buddy taping and an aluminum splint can be used for immobilization.

Disposition

Most MTP dislocations can be managed without orthopedic consultation. If crepitus or obvious instability is present or postreduction radiographs show joint incongruity or an intraarticular fracture, orthopedic consultation should be obtained for possible fixation. First MTP dislocations that are open, show radiographic evidence of complexity, or do not easily reduce require orthopedic consultation in the emergency department because open reduction may be required. Very rarely, MTP dislocations of the lesser toes require open reduction.

Complications are uncommon after MTP dislocations. Arthritis and reduced range of motion, particularly of the hallux, may occur. Dislocations that are delayed in diagnosis for more than 3 weeks are often not amenable to closed reduction and may require metatarsal head excision.

Interphalangeal Dislocations

Interphalangeal dislocations are much less common than MTP dislocations and are sometimes overlooked.

Most IP dislocations occur in the great toe and are a result of axial loading. IP dislocations usually involve dorsal displacement of the distal component and are easily managed without orthopedic consultation. Reduction is performed with longitudinal traction after digital block anesthesia. Initial accentuation of the deformity may be necessary if reduction is unsuccessful with simple traction. If the dislocation involves the great toe, a walking cast with a toe plate for 3 weeks is indicated after reduction. Lesser toes require only buddy taping. As with the MTP joint, complex dislocations involving the first IP joint can occur, and orthopedic consultation in the emergency department for open reduction may be necessary. Very rarely, lesser toe IP dislocations are irreducible with closed methods and require open reduction.

FOOT PAIN

Perspective

Foot pain, particularly in the absence of obvious trauma, poses a diagnostic and therapeutic challenge. Plain radiographs are commonly normal, making history and physical examination assume increased importance. Although definitive diagnosis is often difficult in the emergency department, a structured approach aids in appropriate patient management and disposition. Most causes of foot pain are minor and self-limited, but the possibility of serious pathologic conditions (e.g., infection, arthritis, or tumor) must be considered.[86] Although orthopedic consultation in the emergency department is rarely required, orthopedic follow-up on an outpatient basis is indicated for selected cases.

Foot pain can be classified as acute, acute on chronic, or chronic and is best approached anatomically by localizing symptoms to the hindfoot, midfoot, or forefoot. Three conditions warrant specific mention.

Reflex sympathetic dystrophy is a syndrome of pain in the presence of trophic changes and vasomotor instability from inappropriate sympathetic nervous system activity. Reflex sympathetic dystrophy occurs months after trauma, which may be major, as in a Lisfranc injury, or relatively innocuous. It has many synonyms, including *causalgia* and *Sudeck's atrophy*, and produces pain of a diffuse burning, aching, or searing nature together with evidence of vasomotor instability. Reflex sympathetic dystrophy should always be considered in the differential diagnosis of foot pain after trauma.

Another important consideration in patients with previous penetrating trauma is a *retained foreign body*. Foreign bodies can be a source of chronic drainage or chronic pain. The inciting trauma can occur years previously, and a history of the event may be difficult to extract or may be unknown to the patient.

Finally, *stress fractures* are an important consideration in the differential diagnosis of foot pain, particularly in athletes.

Hindfoot Pain

Hindfoot pain is a common complaint that is usually the result of overuse rather than acute trauma.[87] Bony hindfoot pain necessitates consideration of talar or calcaneal stress fractures. A calcaneal stress fracture may be suspected when pain is elicited on squeezing the calcaneus mediolaterally. Another cause of bony pain is impingement by an os trigonum (see Figure 55-15) or prominent lateral posterior talar process. The "os trigonum syndrome" involves pain during plantar flexion of the foot and is particularly common in ballet dancers. A bone scan may be required for diagnosis, and treatment is surgical.

Most patients with hindfoot pain describe subcalcaneal heel pain, a complaint with an extensive differential diagnosis.[88] The literature on this topic is conflicting and fraught with inconsistent terminology. The most common causes of subcalcaneal pain are plantar fasciitis, subcalcaneal bursitis, acute rupture of the plantar fascia, and nerve compression.

The plantar fascia is a tough layer of the sole that is functionally significant during foot strike and the early stance phase of walking.[89] Plantar fasciitis, an overuse injury of insidious onset, usually begins with pain on first weight bearing in the morning or after prolonged sitting. This progresses to persistent pain during gait. Pain and tenderness are localized to the medial aspect of the heel. Plantar fasciitis accounts for 9% of running injuries and is particularly common in cavus feet.[89] Plain radiography is not diagnostic but shows a calcaneal spur in 50% of patients with plantar fasciitis. This is a stress-related ossification that has a 16% incidence in asymptomatic individuals and is not considered the primary cause of pain in plantar fasciitis. Rarely, fascial ossification (an os subcalcis) may be seen.

Plantar fasciitis is distinct from subcalcaneal bursitis, a condition with an identical presentation in which the pain is localized to the bursa directly below the calcaneus. Differentiating these two conditions can be difficult and is usually academic because initial treatment is identical: a combination of avoiding precipitating conditions, rest, padding, orthotics, and nonsteroidal anti-inflammatory drugs. Very rarely, surgical release of the plantar fascia is required, a therapy that can be beneficial in either condition.

Plantar fascial rupture is a tear of the origin of the plantar fascia at the calcaneus. This usually occurs during the push-off phase of gait. Swelling may be found, and typically pain occurs with passive dorsiflexion of the hallux. Treatment is nonsurgical, often with a period of cast immobilization for symptomatic relief.

Compression of either the abductor digiti quinti nerve or the posterior tibial nerve (the "tarsal tunnel syndrome") can cause subcalcaneal heel pain. Diagnosis of these conditions is difficult and is sometimes facilitated by assessing the impact of selective nerve block with local anesthesia. Initial treatment of these conditions is similar to that for plantar fasciitis, although local steroid injections or surgical release may be required. Other nerve entrapments can also occur in the hindfoot area.[90]

Many tendons course through the hindfoot, particularly the anteromedial aspect, and tendinitis can occur. Other tendon pathologic conditions (e.g., ruptures, dislocations, and retinacular injuries) must be considered because they can result in significant functional disability.

Midfoot Pain

Isolated midfoot pain is less common than forefoot or hindfoot pain. Stress fractures are uncommon in the midfoot and most commonly involve the navicular. Other causes of midfoot pain include symptomatic accessory bones, particularly the os tibiale externum or os peroneum (see Figure 55-15). An os tibiale externum is present in up to 14% of the normal population, most of whom are asymptomatic. This accessory bone can produce debilitating pain on the medial aspect of the midfoot. A bone scan facilitates diagnosis, and surgical excision may be necessary. A painful os peroneum is one of several conditions that can cause lateral plantar pain in the midfoot region. Localization of tenderness is aided by resisted plantar flexion, and treatment ranges from immobilization to surgical excision.

Forefoot Pain

The forefoot is the site for myriad painful problems. Bunions, painful bursae, blisters, corns, calluses, hammertoes, and ingrown toenails are all diagnostically obvious but can pose therapeutic challenges. Many are the result of poor footwear or a biomechanical problem with the foot and respond to appropriate padding, avoidance of precipitants, and occasionally surgical intervention.

Metatarsalgia is an often used, although loosely defined, term referring to pain in the region of the metatarsal heads.[91] This is a common presenting complaint with many causes. Metatarsal stress fractures are extremely common and must be considered in the differential diagnosis of any unexplained forefoot pain. Flexor or extensor tendinitis can also produce metatarsal area pain and is suggested when plain radiographs show areas of tendinous calcification. Arthritis, sesamoiditis, or a sesamoid stress fracture should be considered when pain occurs in the area of the hallux. "Turf toe" is an MTP joint inflammation of the hallux resulting from repeated hyperextension stress. It usually responds to symptomatic measures.[92]

An important cause of unilateral metatarsalgia is a perineural fibrosis of the intermetatarsal plantar digital nerve, more commonly known as a Morton's neuroma. This neuropathy of unknown cause was first described in 1876 and usually involves the second-third or third-fourth interspace, causing lancinating pain with weight bearing. The pain may be associated with paresthesias and can radiate into the toes. In addition, "afterburn" pain can persist during rest. The pain of a Morton's neuroma is reproduced when the affected interspace is pinched or when the metatarsal heads are compressed together. Hence, pain may occur intermittently with tight-fitting footwear (e.g., rock climbing shoes or ski boots). Crepitus or a nodule may be palpable. Treatment usually involves surgical excision or neurolysis.[93] Freiberg's disease is an osteochondrosis of the metatarsal head, usually involving the second metatarsal, and is another cause of pain in this area. Ingrown toenails are a common affliction that can occur in any toe, most commonly the hallux. Often they are perpetuated by short nail trimming, which allows a spicule of nail the opportunity to grow under the nail fold.[94] Allowing the nail to grow out and providing local care usually resolve the condition. Antibiotics are indicated if infection is present. Chronic or recurring ingrown nails require partial or complete nail excision and germinal ablation.[94]

SPECIAL CONSIDERATIONS

Stress Fractures

Principles of Disease: Pathophysiology

Stress fractures can occur anywhere in the appendicular skeleton but are particularly common in the lower extremity. Athletic activities, particularly running, account for most stress fractures. Predisposing factors include training errors, poor footwear, a previous period of inactivity, or a change in running surface. Anatomic variations may play a role, with cavus feet being more prone to stress fractures than flat feet.

Pedal stress fractures may occur anywhere but are most common in the second or third metatarsal shaft. It is not generally appreciated that calcaneal stress fractures occur almost as often as metatarsal stress fractures. Midfoot stress fractures are uncommon and usually occur in the navicular. The type of sport or activity is related to the location of stress fractures, with navicular stress fractures most often seen in basketball, metatarsal shaft stress fractures in running, and fifth metatarsal diaphyseal stress fractures in football.

Clinical Features

Although the history is variable, most stress fractures produce localized pain of insidious onset, usually with aching over a period of weeks.[95] The pain may be anywhere in the hindfoot, midfoot, or forefoot but is most common along a metatarsal. Initially symptoms occur after athletic activities, but later they limit such activities. Often a predisposing factor, such as a training regimen change, is present. A menstrual history should be obtained in female patients because amenorrhea, often a result of training, can predispose to stress fractures.[57]

Physical examination may reveal swelling, point tenderness, or percussion tenderness. In most patients, however, these findings are absent, and the diagnosis must be suspected by history alone.

Diagnostic Strategies: Radiology

Initial plain radiographs are commonly normal because bone reaction in stress fractures depends on the length of time from symptom onset. Radiographic abnormalities in the metaphyses can take up to 4 weeks to develop, and those in the diaphyses can take 6 weeks.[95] Although plain radiographs have low sensitivity for stress fractures, their specificity is high. The three important findings are periosteal new bone, endosteal thickening, or a radiolucent line. Radiographic findings vary with location: Metatarsal fractures usually show callus or periosteal reaction, whereas navicular fractures show a lucent line, and calcaneal fractures show curvilinear sclerosis.

The diagnosis of a stress fracture is easily missed because only 50% of patients develop plain radiographic abnormalities.[96] Radionuclide bone scanning is the imaging modality of choice for stress fractures and should be obtained in any patient with normal radiographs in whom the diagnosis is considered. Bone scans are nonspecific but extremely sensitive for stress fractures, usually showing abnormal uptake within 24 hours of injury. Rarely, a bone scan may be falsely negative if pain occurs before the onset of a demonstrable pathologic condition. A repeat bone scan, a CT scan, or an MRI scan may be necessary in selected patients.[95]

Management

Athletic stress fractures are overuse injuries and necessitate an evaluation of training habits, equipment, and techniques. Most pedal stress fractures resolve in 4 to 6 weeks simply with limitation of impact activities and do not require immobilization unless symptoms are severe. Two locations, however, are unique and deserve specific discussion.

Navicular stress fractures are uncommon and often delayed in diagnosis. Healing is hampered by the relative avascularity of the middle third of the bone, and initial treatment is with non-weight-bearing casting for 6 to 8 weeks. Stress fractures of the fifth metatarsal base are also problematic. Fifth metatarsal diaphyseal stress fractures (also called chronic Jones fractures) are usually initially treated with non-weight-bearing and casting. Similar to acute diaphyseal fractures, delayed healing is common, and casting for up to 20 weeks may be required.[82]

Disposition

Any patient diagnosed with or suspected of having a stress fracture should have orthopedic follow-up on an outpatient basis. Delayed union or nonunion can occur with stress fractures, particularly those of the navicular or fifth metatarsal base. Bone grafting or hardware fixation may be required. Most other pedal stress fractures heal without complications.

Contusions and Sprains

Contusions of the foot, usually from dropped objects, are a common injury. Sprains can occur in the foot, particularly with athletic injuries. The calcaneocuboid and intermetatarsal ligaments are common sites of injury. Localizing such injuries is difficult, and these are often diagnoses of exclusion made after appropriate clinical and radiographic assessment. Both contusions and sprains usually respond rapidly to symptomatic therapy. Sprains of the Lisfranc joint complex are unique and require orthopedic consultation in the emergency department.

Tendon Injuries

Acute tendon ruptures in the foot, apart from the Achilles and posterior tibial tendons, are rare. Although isolated ruptures of the flexor hallucis longus and anterior tibial tendons have been described, most tendon transections are the result of lacerations. These typically arise from one of two mechanisms: penetrating wounds to the sole of the foot or major trauma from such sources as dropped objects, lawn mowers, or motor vehicle crashes. Plantar penetrating trauma usually results in flexor tendon injuries, whereas most major mechanisms involve extensor tendons.

Orthopedic or plastic surgical consultation in the emergency department is indicated for any patient known or suspected to have a tendon injury in the foot. It is clear that flexor and extensor hallucis longus tendons should be repaired primarily; however, the need to repair other tendons is controversial. In general, an attempt should be made to repair any tendon transection because apparently minor injuries can lead to complications such as claw deformity. Tendon injuries associated with innocuous lacerations are easily missed if not carefully sought. Splinting for 2 to 6 weeks is required after tendon repair.

Crush Injuries, Amputations, and Major Vascular Injuries

Rapid assessment, stabilization, and immediate consultation are priorities in the emergency department management of a major crush injury, amputation, or vascular injury of the foot. The injured limb must be handled gently and can be irrigated with sterile saline solution to remove debris. Other irrigating solutions, exploration, or debridement are contraindicated.[97] Antibiotics should be administered, as with any open fracture. Compartment syndrome must always be considered. Many factors enter into surgical decision making with such patients, and objective measures such as the "mangled extremity score" have been developed to predict the need for amputation.[98] Local crush injuries often heal better than diffuse crush injuries.[97] A surgical goal is preservation of as much length as possible to maintain a longitudinal arch. In the presence of a major vascular injury, the likelihood of permanent disability is high.

Compartment Syndrome

Principles of Disease: Pathophysiology

Compartment syndrome is defined as an increase in pressure within a confined osseofascial space that impedes neurovascular function, resulting in tissue damage.[97] Compartment syndrome in the foot, as elsewhere in the body, is a medical emergency. Classically, four foot compartments are described: medial, central, lateral, and interosseous,[99] although studies using dye injection have suggested that there may be as many as nine foot compartments.[97]

Pedal compartment syndrome is most commonly caused by significant crush injuries, fractures, or dislocations. Other causes include bleeding disorders, burns, postischemic swelling after arterial injury or thrombosis, drug or alcohol overdose, exercise, and venous obstruction. Damage is related to the duration and magnitude of compartment pressure rise and the arteriovenous gradient. Compartment syndrome can occur anywhere from 2 hours to 6 days after an insult, although the peak incidence is 15 to 30 hours.

Clinical Features

Compartment syndrome typically causes pain out of proportion to that expected for the injury. The pain is not decreased by immobilization and can be described as a feeling of tautness within the foot.[99] In the case of calcaneal fractures, the pain is often a relentless burning involving the entire foot. Physical examination may reveal tense swelling and sensory deficits. Pain is exacerbated by any movement (active or passive) that stretches the muscles of the involved compartment. Passive dorsiflexion of the toes is often painful. Peripheral pulses and capillary refill are usually normal in compartment syndrome and thus offer no reassurance when present. Open wounds do not guarantee that all compartments are decompressed.

Diagnostic Strategies: Special Procedures

The only way to diagnose a compartment syndrome is to measure intracompartmental pressure. The decision to perform this maneuver relies on appropriate clinical suspicion. Techniques of pressure measurement are well described, with a pressure greater than 35 mm Hg generally considered diagnostic.[99,100] Compartment syndrome can occur at lower pressures in hypotensive patients. The needle localization and distinguishing of foot compartments is challenging because of their small size. For this reason and because of its importance in surgical decision making, measurement of pedal compartment pressures should usually be left to an orthopedic surgeon.

Management

Early identification and prevention of further tissue damage are important considerations in any patient with a mechanism consistent with the development of compartment syndrome. Circumferential bandages and casts should be avoided during the early management of such patients. In diagnosed or suspected cases of compartment syndrome, the limb should be positioned at the level of the heart. Limb elevation is contraindicated because it decreases arterial flow, thus narrowing the arterial-venous pressure gradient.

Disposition

If compartment syndrome is suspected, immediate orthopedic consultation is indicated because the only treatment is decompressive fasciotomy.

KEY CONCEPTS

- Ankle dislocations with skin tenting or neurovascular compromise should be reduced promptly, before radiographs are obtained.
- The entire fibula should be examined if an isolated medial malleolar fracture is present to rule out a proximal fibular (Danis-Weber type C or Maisonneuve's) fracture.
- Before diagnosing an ankle sprain, one should carefully consider whether an injury could be present that mimics an ankle sprain.
- Patients with Achilles tendon rupture can still perform weak plantar flexion. The Thompson test should always be performed if an Achilles tendon rupture is suspected.
- One should remember to think of accessory ossicles when unexpected radiologic lesions in the foot are encountered.
- The possibility of a Lisfranc injury should always be considered with any fracture or dislocation in the tarsometatarsal region, particularly fractures of the second metatarsal base.
- The tuberosity should be carefully differentiated from the diaphysis in all fifth metatarsal base fractures.
- The possibility of a stress fracture should always be considered in patients with long-standing foot pain, particularly if symptoms are in the metatarsal region.
- Compartment syndrome of the foot can occur and lead to devastating results if it is not diagnosed early.

REFERENCES

1. Grimston SK, et al: Differences in ankle joint complex range of motion as a function of age. *Foot Ankle Int* 14:215, 1993.
2. Simon RR, Koenigsknecht SJ (eds): *Emergency Orthopedics: The Extremities,* 2nd ed. Norwalk, Conn, Appleton & Lange, 1987.
3. Stiell IG, et al: Implementation of the Ottawa Ankle Rules. *JAMA* 271:827, 1994.
4. Ho K, et al: Using tomography to diagnose occult ankle fractures. *Ann Emerg Med* 27:600, 1996.
5. Stiehl JB: Ankle fractures with diastasis. In Greene WB (ed): *Instructional Course Lectures,* vol 39. Easton, Pa, American Academy of Orthopaedic Surgeons, 1990, 95-103.
6. Bachmann LM, et al: Accuracy of Ottawa Ankle Rules to exclude fractures of the ankle and mid foot: Systematic review. *BMJ* 326:1, 2003.
7. Clark KD, et al: Evaluation of the Ottawa Ankle Rules in children. *Ped Emerg Care* 19:73, 2003.
8. Martire JR: The role of nuclear medicine bone scans in evaluating pain in athlete injuries. *Clin Sports Med* 6:713, 1987.
9. Oloff-Solomon J, Solomon MA: Computed tomographic scanning of the foot and ankle. *Clin Podiatr Med Surg* 5:931, 1988.
10. Kerr R, Forrester DM, Kingston S: Magnetic resonance imaging of foot and ankle trauma. *Orthop Clin North Am* 21:591, 1990.

11. Ferkel RD, Nuys V, Scranton PEJ: Arthroscopy of the ankle and foot. *J Bone Joint Surg Am* 75:1233, 1993.

12. Dahners LE: The pathogenesis and treatment of bimalleolar ankle fractures. In Greene WB (ed): *Instructional Course Lectures,* vol 39. Easton, Pa, American Academy of Orthopaedic Surgeons, 1990, pp 85-94.

13. Stiehl JB: Open fractures of the ankle joint. In Greene WB (ed): *Instructional Course Lectures,* vol 39. Easton, Pa, American Academy of Orthopaedic Surgeons, 1990, pp 113-117.

14. Michelson JD: Fractures about the ankle. *J Bone Joint Surg Am* 77:142, 1995.

15. Harris IA, Jones HP: The fate of the syndesmosis in type C ankle fractures: A cadaveric study. *Injury* 28:275, 1997.

16. Walling AK: Classification of ankle fractures: Which system to use? In Bassett FH (ed): *Instructional Course Lectures,* vol 37. Easton, Pa, American Academy of Orthopaedic Surgeons, 1988, pp 251-256.

17. Nugent JF, Gale BD: Isolated posterior malleolar ankle fractures. *J Foot Ankle Surg* 29:80, 1990.

18. Wei SY, et al: Nonoperatively treated displaced bimalleolar and trimalleolar fractures: A 20-year follow-up. *Foot Ankle Int* 20:404, 1999.

19. Grantham SA: Trimalleolar ankle fractures and open ankle fractures. In Greene WB (ed): *Instructional Course Lectures,* vol 39. Easton, Pa, American Academy of Orthopaedic Surgeons, 1990, pp 105-111.

20. Sanders R, et al: The management of fractures with soft-tissue disruptions. *J Bone Joint Surg Am* 75:778, 1993.

21. Hoiness P, Stromsoe K: Early complications of surgically managed ankle fractures related to the AO classification: A review of 118 ankle fractures treated with open reduction and internal fixation. *Arch Orthop Trauma Surg* 119:276, 1999.

22. Mast JW, Spiegel PG, Pappas JN: Fractures of the tibial pilon. *Clin Orthop* 230:68, 1988.

23. Brennan MJ: Tibial pilon fractures. In Greene WB (ed): *Instructional Course Lectures,* vol 39. Easton, Pa, American Academy of Orthopaedic Surgeons, 1990, pp 167-170.

24. Fallat L, Grimm DJ, Saracco JA: Sprained ankle syndrome: Prevalence and analysis of 639 acute injuries. *J Foot Ankle Surg* 37:280, 1998.

25. Trevino SG, Davis P, Hecht PJ: Management of acute and chronic lateral ligament injuries of the ankle. *Orthop Clin North Am* 25:1, 1994.

26. Hopkinson WJ, et al: Syndesmosis sprains of the ankle. *Foot Ankle Int* 10:325, 1990.

27. Frost SC, Amendola A: Is stress radiography necessary in the diagnosis of acute or chronic ankle instability? *Clin J Sport Med* 9:40, 1999.

28. Kerkhoffs GMMJ, et al: Functional treatments for acute ruptures of the lateral ankle ligament: A systematic review. *Acta Orthop Scand* 74:69, 2003.

29. Janis LR, Kittleson RS, Cox DG: Chronic lateral ankle instability: Assessment of subjective outcomes following delayed primary repair and a new secondary construction. *J Foot Ankle Surg* 37:369, 1998.

30. Wedmore IS, Charette J: Emergency department evaluation and treatment of ankle and foot injuries. *Emerg Med Clin North Am* 18:85, 2000.

31. Kerkhoffs GMMJ, et al: Immobilisation for acute ankle sprain: A systematic review. *Arch Orthop Trauma Surg* 121:462, 2001.

32. Karlsson J, Eriksson BI, Sward L: Early functional treatment for acute ligament injuries of the ankle joint. *Scand J Med Sci Sports* 6:341, 1996.

33. Sadowski E, et al: Radiologic case study: Fractures of the foot masquerading as ankle injuries. *Orthopedics* 22:363, 1999.

34. Jozsa L, et al: The role of recreational sport activity in Achilles tendon rupture. *Am J Sports Med* 17:338, 1989.

35. Kao NL, Moy JN, Richmond GW: Achilles tendon rupture: An underrated complication of corticosteroid treatment. *Thorax* 47:484, 1992.

36. Hudson KA: Achilles tendinitis and tendon rupture due to fluoroquinolone antibiotics. *N Engl J Med* 331:748, 1994.

37. Thompson TC, Doherty JH: Spontaneous rupture of tendon of Achilles: A new clinical diagnostic test. *J Trauma* 2:126, 1962.

38. Copeland SA: Rupture of the Achilles tendon: A new clinical test. *Ann R Coll Surg Engl* 72:270, 1990.

39. Kalebo P, et al: Soft-tissue radiography, computed tomography and ultrasonography of partial Achilles tendon ruptures. *Acta Radiol* 31:565, 1990.

40. Cetti R, et al: Operative versus nonoperative treatment of Achilles tendon rupture: A prospective randomized study and review of the literature. *Am J Sports Med* 21:791, 1993.

41. Arrowsmith SR, Fleming LL, Allman FL: Traumatic dislocations of the peroneal tendons. *Am J Sports Med* 11:142, 1983.

42. Trevino S, Baumhauer JF: Tendon injuries of the foot and ankle. *Clin Sports Med* 11:727, 1992.

43. Sammarco GJ: Peroneal tendon injuries. *Orthop Clin North Am* 25:135, 1994.

44. Bassett FH III, Speer KP: Longitudinal rupture of the peroneal tendons. *Am J Sports Med* 21:354, 1993.

45. Mann RA: Part III: Rupture of tibialis posterior tendon. In Murray JA (ed): *Instructional Course Lectures,* vol 33. Easton, Pa, American Academy of Orthopaedic Surgeons, 1984, pp 302-309.

46. Funk DA, Cass JR, Johnson KA: Quiet flat foot secondary to posterior tibial tendon pathology. *J Bone Joint Surg Am* 68:95, 1986.

47. Leitner B: The mechanism of total dislocation of the talus. *J Bone Joint Surg Am* 37:89, 1955.

48. Toohey JS, Worsing RA Jr: A long-term follow-up study of tibiotalar dislocations without associated fractures. *Clin Orthop* 239:207, 1987.

49. Wroble RR, Nepola JV, Malvitz TA: Ankle dislocation without fracture. *Foot Ankle Int* 9:64, 1988.

50. Ounpuu S: The biomechanics of walking and running. *Clin Sports Med* 13:843, 1994.

51. Hoppenfeld S: Physical examination of the foot by complaint. In Jahss MH (ed): *Disorders of the Foot and Ankle: Medical and Surgical Management.* Philadelphia, WB Saunders, 1991.

52. De Smett AA, et al: Are oblique views needed for trauma radiology of the distal extremities? *Am J Roentgenol* 172:1561, 1999.

53. Berquist TH, et al: The foot and ankle. In Berquist TH (ed): *Imaging of Orthopedic Trauma,* 2nd ed. New York, Raven Press, 1992.

54. Heckman JD: Fractures and dislocations of the foot. In Rockwood CA, Green DP, Bucholz RW (eds): *Rockwood and Green's Fractures in Adults,* 3rd ed. Philadelphia, JB Lippincott, 1991, p 2267.

55. Gratton MC, Salomone JA, Watson WA: Clinically significant radiograph misinterpretations at an emergency medicine residency program. *Ann Emerg Med* 19:497, 1990.

56. Maffulli N, Lepore L, Francobandiera C: Traumatic lesions of some accessory bones of the foot in sports activity. *J Am Podiatr Med Assoc* 80:86, 1990.

57. Hershman EB, Mailly T: Stress fractures. *Clin Sports Med* 9:183, 1990.

58. Golimbu CN: Ankle and foot. In Firooznia H, et al (eds): *MRI and CT of the Musculoskeletal System.* St. Louis, Mosby, 1992.

59. Adelaar RS: Fractures of the talus. In Greene WB (ed): *Instructional Course Lectures*. vol 39. Easton, Pa, American Academy of Orthopaedic Surgeons, 1990, pp 147-156.

60. Chan GM, Yoshida D: Fracture of the lateral process of the talus associated with snowboarding. *Ann Emerg Med* 41:854, 2003.

61. Abrahams TG, Gallup L, Avery FL: Nondisplaced shearing-type talar body fractures. *Ann Emerg Med* 23:891, 1994.

62. Frankel J, Turf R, Miller GA: Occult fractures of the talus. *J Foot Ankle Surg* 31:538, 1992.

63. Shea MP, Manoli A II: Osteochondral lesions of the talar dome. *Foot Ankle Int* 14:48, 1993.

64. Dickson KF, Sartoris DJ: Injuries to the talus: Neck fractures and osteochondral lesions (osteochondritis dissecans). *J Foot Ankle Surg* 30:310, 1991.

65. Kelberine F, Frank A: Arthroscopic treatment of osteochondral lesions of the talar dome: A retrospective study of 48 cases. *Arthroscopy* 15:77, 1999.

66. Brennan MJ: Subtalar dislocations. In Greene WB (ed): *Instructional Course Lectures*. vol 39. Easton, Pa, American Academy of Orthopaedic Surgeons, 1990, pp 157-159.

67. Love JN, Dhindsa HS, Hayden DK: Subtalar dislocation: Evaluation and management in the emergency department. *J Emerg Med* 13:787, 1995.

68. deSouza LJ: Fractures and dislocations of the foot. In Gustilo RB, Kyle RF, Templeman DC (eds): *Fractures and Dislocations*. St. Louis, Mosby, 1993, p 1119.

69. Koval KJ, Sanders R: The radiologic evaluation of calcaneal fractures. *Clin Orthop* 290:41, 1993.

70. Hodje JC: Anterior process fracture or calcaneus secondarius: A case report. *J Emerg Med* 17:305, 1999.

71. Chen MY, Bohrer SP, Kelley TF: Boehler's angle: A reappraisal. *Ann Emerg Med* 20:122, 1991.

72. Paley D, Hall H: Calcaneal fracture controversies: Can we put Humpty Dumpty back together again? *Orthop Clin North Am* 20:665, 1989.

73. Nyska M, et al: Fractures of the body of the tarsal navicular bone: Case reports and literature review. *J Trauma* 29:1448, 1989.

74. Jahn H, Freund KG: Isolated fractures of the cuboid bone: Two case reports with review of the literature. *J Foot Ankle Surg* 28:512, 1989.

75. Vuori J, Aro HT: Lisfranc joint injuries: Trauma mechanisms and associated injuries. *J Trauma* 35:40, 1993.

76. Adelaar RS: The treatment of tarsometatarsal fracture-dislocation. In Greene WB (ed): *Instructional Course Lectures*, vol 39. Easton, Pa, American Academy of Orthopaedic Surgeons, 1990, pp 141.

77. Englanoff G, Anglin D, Hutson HR: Lisfranc fracture-dislocation: A frequently missed diagnosis in the emergency department. *Ann Emerg Med* 26:229, 1995.

78. Faciszewski T, Burks RT, Manaster BJ: Subtle injuries of the Lisfranc joint. *J Bone Joint Surg Am* 72:1519, 1990.

79. Shereff MJ: Fractures of the forefoot. In Greene WB (ed): *Instructional Course Lectures*, vol 39. Easton, Pa, American Academy of Orthopaedic Surgeons, 1990, pp 133-140.

80. Kirchwehm WW, et al: Fractures of the internal metatarsals. In Scurran BL (ed): *Foot and Ankle Trauma*. New York, Churchill Livingstone, 1989.

81. La Porta G: Fractures of the first metatarsal. In Scurran BL (ed): *Foot and Ankle Trauma*. New York, Churchill Livingstone, 1989.

82. Lawrence SJ, Botte MJ: Jones' fractures and related fractures of the proximal fifth metatarsal. *Foot Ankle Int* 14:358, 1993.

83. Sammarco GJ: The Jones fracture. In Heckman JD (ed): *Instructional Course Lectures*, vol 42. Easton, Pa, American Academy of Orthopedics, 1993, pp 201-205.

84. Schnaue-Constantouris EM, et al: Digital foot trauma: Emergency diagnosis and treatment. *J Emerg Med* 22:163, 2001.

85. Vilke GM: Great toe pain. *J Emerg Med* 24:59, 2003.

86. Saxena A: Unusual foot pathologies mimicking common sports injuries. *J Foot Ankle Surg* 32:53, 1993.

87. Lutter LD: Hindfoot problems. In Heckman JD (ed): *Instructional Course Lectures*, vol 42. Easton, Pa, American Academy of Orthopaedic Surgeons, 1993, pp 195-200.

88. Karr SD: Subcalcaneal heel pain. *Orthop Clin North Am* 25:161, 1994.

89. McBryde AM: Plantar fasciitis. In Murray JA (ed): *Instructional Course Lectures*, vol 33. Easton, Pa, American Academy of Orthopaedic Surgeons, 1984, pp 278-282.

90. Baxter DE: Functional nerve disorders in the athlete's foot, ankle, and leg. In Heckman JD (ed): *Instructional Course Lectures*, vol 42. Easton, Pa, American Academy of Orthopaedic Surgeons, 1993, pp 185-194.

91. Gould JS: Metatarsalgia. *Orthop Clin North Am* 20:553, 1989.

92. Sammarco GJ: Turf toe. In Heckman JD (ed): *Instructional Course Lectures*, vol 42. Easton, Pa, American Academy of Orthopaedic Surgeons, 1993, pp 207-212.

93. Dellon AL: Treatment of Morton's neuroma as a nerve compression: The role of neurolysis. *J Am Podiatr Med Assoc* 82:399, 1992.

94. Eisele SA: Conditions of the toenails. *Orthop Clin North Am* 25:183, 1994.

95. Eisele SA, Sammarco GJ: Fatigue fractures of the foot and ankle in the athlete. In Heckman JD (ed): *Instructional Course Lectures*, vol 42. Easton, Pa, American Academy of Orthopaedic Surgeons, 1993, pp 175-183.

96. Riddervold HO: Easily missed fractures. *Radiol Clin North Am* 30:475, 1992.

97. McGee DL, Dalsey WC: The mangled extremity: Compartment syndrome and amputations. *Emerg Med Clin North Am* 10:783, 1992.

98. Johansen K, et al: Objective criteria accurately predict amputation following lower extremity trauma. *J Trauma* 30:568, 1990.

99. Shereff MJ: Compartment syndromes of the foot. In Green WB (ed): *Instructional Course Lectures*, vol 39. Easton, Pa, American Academy of Orthopaedic Surgeons, 1990, pp 127-132.

100. Smith GH: Measurement of the intracompartmental pressures of the foot. *J Foot Ankle Surg* 29:589, 1990.

CHAPTER

56 Wound Management Principles

Barry Simon and H. Gene Hern, Jr.

PERSPECTIVE

The goals of emergency wound treatment are to restore function, repair tissue integrity with strength and optimal cosmetic appearance, and minimize risk of infection. Risk of infection depends on the location, mechanism, host, and care. The risk in a clean facial wound produced by incision is less than 1%, whereas a dirty crush injury to the foot may have more than a 20% risk. Wound infection generally results in delayed healing, decreased strength, and a poor cosmetic result. These facts highlight the need for high-quality wound care. Understanding the biology of wound healing and the technical aspects of wound treatment facilitates emergency management of these patients.

Emergency physicians also must be aware of the medicolegal risk associated with soft tissue injuries. Including injuries to the hand, wound-related complaints are the fourth most common cause of malpractice claims against emergency physicians. Missed foreign body, wound infection, and missed tendon or nerve injury are the most common complications leading to these claims.

PRINCIPLES OF DISEASE

Anatomy of Skin and Fascia

Understanding of skin anatomy leads to better appreciation of wound closure concepts and techniques. The skin is a complex organ that protects the body against bacterial invasion and ensures thermoregulation. The skin also helps to regulate water content and register sensory stimuli.

The skin and fascia vary in thickness from 1 to 4 mm, depending on the part of the body. The *epidermis,* the outermost layer, is several cell layers thick. The most important parts of the epidermis are the *stratum germinativum* (basal layer), the location where new cells originate, and the *stratum corneum,* the outermost cell layer that gives the skin its cosmetic appearance. The layer of skin directly beneath the epidermis is the *dermis.* The much thicker dermis is primarily composed of connective tissue. The dermis is the key layer for the ultimate healing of skin wounds. Optimal healing and minimal scar formation depend on the removal of debris and devitalized tissue from the dermis. The dermis also functions to anchor suture placed percutaneously or subcutaneously.[1]

The *superficial fascia* lies directly beneath the dermis and encloses the subcutaneous fat. This space must be irrigated and debrided to decrease the risk of infection. The *deep fascia* lies beneath the fat and is a strong, off-white sheath that covers and protects the underlying muscles and helps prevent superficial infection from spreading to deeper tissues. The deep fascia must be closed to maintain its protective role.

Wound Biology

Normal wound healing is a well-choreographed sequence of biologic events. It is described as an orderly process, but actually represents multiple phenomena that seem to occur simultaneously. These events include coagulation, inflammation, collagen metabolism, wound contraction, and epithelialization.[1,2] Maintaining the balance of these events is crucial for normal healing. Delaying any of the stages may result in a weak closure and dehiscence. Prolonging segments of the process may affect the ultimate scar appearance.

Soon after tissue integrity is altered, the process of *coagulation* begins. Platelet release factors initiate and enhance a response from inflammatory cells. Capillary permeability increases to allow white blood cells to migrate into the wound. Neutrophils and monocytes act as scavengers to rid the wound of debris and bacteria. Monocytes transform into macrophages, which seem to have a major role in subsequent healing phenomena. In addition to providing wound defense, macrophages release chemotactic substances, calling on other monocytes to stimulate fibroblast replication and trigger neovascularization.[1]

Collagen is the principal structural protein of most tissues of the body. Normal tissue repair depends on collagen synthesis, deposition, and cross-linking. Fibroblasts synthesize and deposit collagen compounds 48 hours after injury. Immature collagen is highly disorganized because it exists in a gel-like consistency.

After a series of enzymatic processes, characteristic fibrils are produced. Subsequent intermolecular cross links are responsible for a major portion of the strength of the collagen fibril. The entire process depends on tissue lactate and ascorbic acid and is directly related to tissue arterial carbon dioxide partial pressure. In the absence of vitamin C, prolyl and lysyl hydroxylase do not activate, and oxygen is not transferred to proline or lysine. Underhydroxylated collagen is produced, and characteristic collagen fibers are unable to form. Wound healing is poor, and capillaries are fragile. Without oxygen to hydroxylate proline and lysine, a local condition resembling scurvy tends to occur.

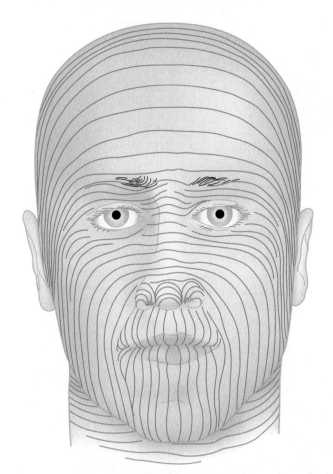

Figure 56-1. Skin tension lines of the face. Incisions or lacerations parallel to these lines are less likely to create widened scars than those that are perpendicular to these lines. (Modified from Simon R, Brenner B: *Procedures and Techniques in Emergency Medicine.* Baltimore, Williams & Wilkins, 1982; as published in Trott A: *Wounds and Lacerations: Emergency Care and Closure,* 2nd ed. St Louis, Mosby, 1997.)

Under normal conditions, collagen synthesis peaks by day 7, coincident with rapid increases in tensile strength. The healing wound has the greatest mass at 3 weeks, but remodels itself over the next 6 to 12 months. Despite these impressive figures, the wound achieves less than 15% to 20% of its ultimate strength by 3 weeks and only 60% by 4 months.[3]

Wound contraction is the movement of whole-thickness skin toward the center of the skin defect. Immediately after injury, the wound edges retract and increase the size of the defect. Normal skin tension along the lines of minimal tension produces this retraction (Figures 56-1 and 56-2). Wounds perpendicular to these lines are under greater tension and result in a larger scar.[1,4]

Over the next 3 to 4 days, the wound size shrinks as its edges move toward the center. This phenomenon is independent of epithelialization, and the presence of collagen is not necessary for it to occur. This process is considered beneficial to healing and should not be confused with contracture that results from scar shortening.[1,3]

Contracture becomes more apparent when the normal healing process is prolonged. The effect is a disfiguring hypertrophic scar. Optimizing the duration of the inflammatory phase and minimizing wound tension help to produce a more "appealing" scar.

Epithelialization is a mechanism in the healing process whereby epithelial cells migrate across the wound. Mitosis appears at the wound edge near the basal cell layer within hours of injury. Eschar or other debris impedes this process. When a wound is properly cleansed and debrided and kept moist and protected, epithelialization proceeds at a maximum rate.[3]

In a surgically repaired laceration, epithelialization bridges the defect by 48 hours. The new tissue proceeds to thicken and grow downward, beginning to resemble the layered structural characteristics of uninjured epidermis within 5 days. Simultaneously, keratin formation loosens the overlying scab.

Biomechanical Properties of Skin

Various forces (lines of tension) exist as a result of skin elasticity from collagen fibers. These static forces may vary more than fivefold with the respective area of body skin surface, but the static tension of a given area of skin remains constant. These static forces are shown clinically by the gaping of wounds after incision. The magnitude of static skin tension is directly related to ultimate scar width.[1,4]

Uneven, jagged wounds have greater surface area than do linear lacerations. The skin tension is distributed over a greater area and is less per unit length of tissue. Meticulous reapproximation of the jagged edges results in a more appealing scar. Sharp debridement, converting a jagged wound to a linear laceration, is often unwise because it may cause too much tissue loss and produce a wider, more visible scar.[4]

Skin forces produced by muscular contraction and movements of flexion and extension influence healing and scar size. These dynamic forces are greatest where skin elasticity is necessary for function. Lacerations parallel to skin folds, lines of expression, and joints do not impair function or produce unattractive scars. Wounds that traverse the skin lines heal with conspicuous scars and may impair function.[4] Knowledge of these lines and forces is necessary for optimal wound repair. In addition, the patient should be educated about wound healing and scarring potential.

CLINICAL FEATURES AND DIAGNOSTIC STRATEGIES

History

A detailed history should be obtained as part of routine wound evaluation. Serious complications can result when basic information is not obtained. If the patient has significant peripheral vascular disease, is immunocompromised, or has a high risk of retained foreign body, wound care decisions may be changed. Essential historical information includes medical history, mechanism and setting of injury, and tetanus status.

Figure 56-2. Skin tension lines of the body surface. (Modified from Simon R, Brenner B: *Procedures and Techniques in Emergency Medicine.* Baltimore, Williams & Wilkins, 1982; as published in Trott A: *Wounds and Lacerations: Emergency Care and Closure,* 2nd ed. St Louis, Mosby, 1997.)

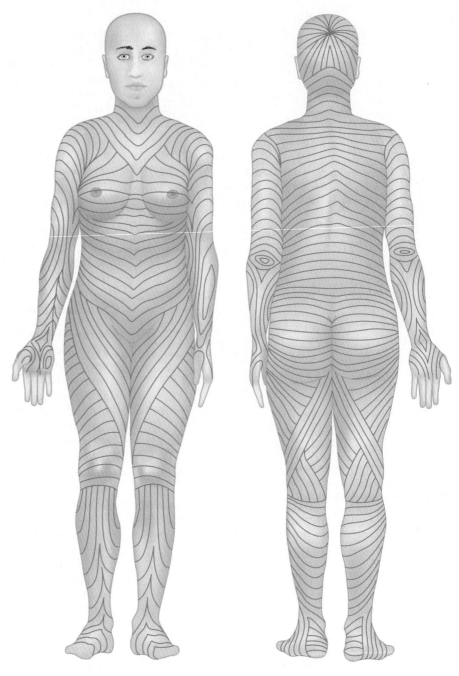

Risk Factors

Risk factors for wound morbidity include prolonged time since injury; crush mechanism; deep penetrating wounds; high-velocity missiles; and contamination with saliva, feces, soil, or other foreign matter (Box 56-1).[1,4,5] Three hours after acute trauma, bacteria proliferate to a level that may result in infection. The risk of infectious complications can be greatly reduced by closing wounds within 8 to 12 hours after injury. Lacerations produced by fine cutting forces resist infection better than crush injuries. Reduction of blood flow to wound edges in the latter may increase the infective

BOX 56-1. Risk Factors for Wound Infection

1. Injury >4 to 8 hours old
2. Location: foot and lower extremity, then hand, then scalp, then face
3. Contamination with devitalized tissue, foreign matter, saliva, or stool
4. Blunt (crush) mechanism
5. Presence of subcutaneous sutures
6. Whether repair is with sutures, staples, or tape
7. Anesthesia with epinephrine
8. High-velocity missile injuries

concentration of bacteria by 100-fold.[4] High-velocity missile injuries produce damage remote from the missile tract. The extent of injury may not be apparent for several days.

Wounds contaminated by foreign matter are at high risk of infection, despite adequate therapeutic intervention. Saliva and feces are composed of a concentration of bacteria (about 10^{11} per gram wet weight) that greatly exceeds the numbers needed to produce infection ($\geq 10^6$ bacteria per gram tissue).[4]

The presence of any foreign matter in the wound decreases resistance to infection. Soil fractions, which include organic components and inorganic clay particles, damage host defenses with adverse interactions between charged soil particles and white blood cells. The presence of these soil fractions greatly increases the infective potential of bacteria.[4]

Optimal physical assessment of wounds requires patience, diligence, and an organized approach. Wound closure decisions must be individualized for each laceration. Sharp, clean lacerations of the face may be safe to close regardless of the time from injury, whereas highly contaminated blunt injuries to the feet should never be closed primarily. When the distal neurovascular evaluation is completed, the examination may proceed. All of these risk factors have to do with the injury; there are three additional areas of concern: (1) immunocompetence of the host, (2) physical characteristics of the host (e.g., peripheral vascular disease), and (3) structural defects that invite bacterial seeding (e.g., damaged or prosthetic heart valves).

Physical Examination

Physical examination errors are minimized with optimal visualization and anesthesia. When the injury occurs on an extremity, use of a sphygmomanometer may help to ensure a bloodless field. The blood pressure cuff is placed proximal to the injury, and the arm is elevated above the heart for at least 1 minute. Exsanguinating the extremity may be hastened by wrapping the limb tightly with an Ace bandage, beginning distally and ending at the base of the cuff. The sphygmomanometer is inflated to a pressure greater than the systolic pressure of the patient. Although this process causes the patient significant discomfort after 1 minute, the cuff can safely remain inflated for 2 hours. A Bier block should be used if prolonged inflation is contemplated.

A thorough examination of the wound requires that the tissues be adequately anesthetized. Subcutaneous tissues quickly reapproximate after injury, giving the appearance of a shallow wound. In addition, significant subcutaneous swelling lends to this appearance and renders examination of the laceration more difficult, as in wounds of the scalp and face. Careful probing and examination are needed to avoid missing damage to structures deep to the skin and subcutaneous tissue. This warning becomes more crucial with wounds on the distal aspects of upper and lower extremities. Finger lacerations are rarely gaping, but crucial structures (e.g., tendons, nerves, vessels) are often damaged. The examiner must pry the wound margins apart, ensure a blood-free field, and examine the tissues as the digit or extremity is placed through range of motion. The injured section of tendon may have been in a different state of tension and in a more proximal or distal location at the time of injury. Wounds that cannot be explored adequately and wounds with probable trauma to underlying tissues or with foreign matter require additional studies. It may be appropriate to extend the laceration to enable improved visualization of wound depth and extent.

Sterile gloves may not be a necessary part of wound closure. Although data are limited, one study found that the use of sterile gloves makes no difference with respect to the incidence of infection.[6] Clean nonsterile gloves should be worn to offer some protection for the patient and perhaps more importantly for the provider.

Foreign Body Assessment

No single method can guarantee the identification and removal of all foreign matter from wounds. The key is to document all efforts and to explain to the patient the possibility of a foreign body. Good follow-up can protect the patient.

Attempts to visualize foreign matter by standard radiography are not as helpful as might be expected. The radiodensity of an object depends on the density of the matter and the adjacent tissue. Pieces of glass greater than 1 mm thick are visible when appropriate views are ordered.[7] Many organic substances, such as wood, are not visible on plain films. A radiolucent shadow may be seen on close inspection because the foreign substance displaces tissue in its path. Xerograms are better than plain radiography but still miss some plastics and organic matter. A computed tomography (CT) scan is excellent for identifying all foreign substances but is expensive and results in significant exposure to radiation. Ultrasonography is a good technique, but the small size of many foreign bodies and pockets of air, edema, pus, and some calcifications may produce confusing echoes, limiting its clinical utility.[8,9] When simpler, standard methods fail to locate a foreign body that is likely or definitely present, ultrasonography or a CT scan should be considered.

MANAGEMENT

Anesthesia

After an appropriate neurovascular examination is documented, the involved tissue should be anesthetized. Careful physical examination and thorough cleansing, irrigation, and debridement require that the patient be free of pain. Regional anesthesia may be preferable for wounds innervated by one superficial nerve. Injections at the wound site produce swelling and further distortion of landmarks. In addition, experimental evidence suggests that anesthetic agents administered at the wound site may delay healing.[10,11] With a regional block, more than one laceration may be repaired in the same nerve distribution without additional anesthesia. Lacerations on the face, hands, fingers, feet, and toes and in the mouth are often well suited for regional anesthesia.

Anesthetic Agents

Lidocaine (Xylocaine) is the most common agent used for local and regional anesthesia. It is safe and fast acting. Onset of action for direct infiltration occurs within seconds and seems to last 20 to 60 minutes. When lidocaine is administered as a regional nerve block, onset occurs in 4 to 6 minutes and generally lasts 75 minutes, although it may remain effective 120 minutes. A 1% lidocaine solution contains 10 mg/mL. It is safe to use 3 to 5 mg/kg, not exceeding 300 mg at a single injection. More volume can be added safely every 30 minutes. When epinephrine is added, the resulting vasoconstriction prolongs the duration of action and increases the safe dose to 5 to 7 mg/kg. The addition of epinephrine has been shown, however, to delay healing and lower resistance to infection. Lidocaine with epinephrine should be avoided in wounds with higher risks of infection and when tissue viability is of concern.[11] Vasoconstrictors should be avoided in most wounds but can be used to prolong the effect of regional blocks (not in fingers or toes) and to decrease bleeding. Digital artery vasospasm, accidentally induced by local injection of epinephrine, can be reversed successfully with a local injection of 0.5-2 mg of subcutaneous phentolamine.[12]

Bupivacaine (Marcaine) provides anesthesia that is equal to that of lidocaine. Onset of action is slightly slower than lidocaine, but the duration of anesthesia is four to eight times longer.[13] These benefits suggest that bupivacaine is the preferred local anesthetic agent for the care of most wounds. In adults, the maximal reported safe dose is about 2.5 mg/kg without epinephrine and 3.5 mg/kg with epinephrine.[1] The dose can be repeated every 3 hours, not exceeding a total of more than 400 mg in a 24-hour period. The maximal intraoral dose is 90 mg.

Local injection of lidocaine should be done with a 27-gauge needle; the slower the injection, the less pain produced.[1] The rate of injection through a 30-gauge needle is far too slow, and the thin needle is difficult to control. A 25-gauge needle is acceptable, but the more rapid injection can result in greater patient discomfort. The needle should be introduced through the cut margin to minimize the pain of the injection. Concerns of spreading bacteria into the adjacent uninvolved tissue and increasing the frequency and severity of wound infections are unfounded. The pain of injecting lidocaine can be ameliorated with the addition of bicarbonate to buffer the solution.[14] The shelf life of the lidocaine-bicarbonate mixture decreases but remains effective for 1 week at room temperature and for 2 weeks if refrigerated. Adding sodium bicarbonate in a 1 : 10 volume ratio to lidocaine (1 mL bicarbonate and 10 mL lidocaine) decreases the pain of injection

without compromising the quality of anesthesia. A much smaller dose of bicarbonate must be added to bupivacaine because the alkalinization results in precipitation. A 1 : 100 volume ratio (0.1 mL of bicarbonate and 10 mL of bupivacaine) has been found to be effective.[15] Warming the anesthetic solution is also an effective means of decreasing the pain of injection.[16]

Topical anesthesia may be an effective painless alternative. Studies show that a combination of tetracaine, adrenaline (epinephrine), and cocaine (TAC) (0.5% tetracaine, 1 : 2000 adrenaline, 11.8% cocaine) can function effectively on skin lacerations. The solution is administered by soaking a cotton ball with 5 mL of the combined drugs (25 mg of tetracaine, 25 mg of adrenaline, 590 mg of cocaine) and applying it to the wound for 10 to 20 minutes. TAC is similar to infiltrative lidocaine in all respects, including risk of complications. It is more effective on the face and scalp than on extremities.[17] Data suggest that half-strength TAC solution is effective and may reduce the potential for toxicity.[18] The tetracaine component may be superfluous and can be eliminated without compromising the quality of anesthesia.[19] By using a topical combination, time to repair is reduced, patient acceptance improves, and landmarks are left undisturbed. Although experimental studies show that TAC increases the infection rate in contaminated wounds, this is not the case with routine wound care.[11] The proven benefits and enhanced patient compliance, especially in pediatric patients, make TAC an excellent medication to use alone or in conjunction with another local anesthetic. The potential toxicity from TAC has been documented by (1) measurable plasma cocaine levels,[20] and (2) a case report of a child's death from exposure to TAC.[21] The child's wound was on the upper lip between the vermilion border and the nares. The solution apparently dripped onto the nasal and oral mucosa, increasing the systemic absorption of the drugs. Until further studies are done, TAC should be avoided in the repair of highly contaminated wounds and in lacerations near mucous membranes. In children, a half-strength solution can be used to reduce potential toxicity.

The potential serious adverse effects of TAC have led to the increasing use of other topically applied anesthetic combinations. A mixture of lidocaine (1% to 4%), epinephrine (1 : 1000 to 1 : 2000), and tetracaine (0.5% to 2%) has been used successfully in place of TAC. This mixture avoids the untoward side effects of cocaine.[22] EMLA (eutectic mixture of local anesthetics) is a cream used to produce anesthesia of wounds. Although the onset of anesthesia is longer than for the other mixtures (1 hour versus about 30 minutes), one study showed that the need for supplemental local anesthesia was reduced.[23] Because the time to onset is greatly delayed with EMLA, its utility may vary with emergency department patient volume.

Allergy

Allergy to local anesthetics is uncommon. Two distinct groups of "caine" anesthetics exist. The esters include procaine, tetracaine, and benzocaine. The second group, including lidocaine and bupivacaine, belong to the amide family. Allergy to the esters is uncommon. True allergy to agents in the amide family is rare. Good history taking is the best way of documenting a true allergic reaction.[24] Many patients labeled as allergic have suffered uncomfortable drug effects or autonomic responses to the pain and the overall setting.

The subject of allergy is complicated further because multidose vials contain the preservative methylparaben, an ester related structurally to anesthetics in the ester family. Apparent allergic reaction to lidocaine or bupivacaine may be a reaction to the methylparaben. Cardiac lidocaine does not contain preservatives, is a standard drug in the emergency department, and can be used for wound anesthesia when concern over potential allergic reactions exists.

When allergy to a local anesthetic is known or strongly suspected, alternatives are available. No cross-reactivity occurs between the amide and ester families, so an agent from a different group may be chosen. Single-dose vials of lidocaine or cardiac lidocaine are not mixed with methylparaben and may be used.[25] A test dose of 0.1 mL may be administered intradermally before proceeding. The patient should be observed for 30 minutes, and as with any allergy testing, the emergency physician should be prepared to treat all complications. Aqueous diphenhydramine (1%) also has been shown to provide effective local anesthesia.[26]

Skin Preparation

Disinfection of the skin (not the wound itself) may be accomplished with several different agents. The ideal agent is fast acting, has a broad spectrum of antimicrobial activity, and has a long shelf life. Povidone-iodine (Betadine) and chlorhexidine (Hibiclens) satisfy all three characteristics. Although excellent as skin disinfectants, both products are toxic to wound defenses and may increase the incidence of wound infection. Povidone-iodine is effective against gram-positive and gram-negative bacteria, fungi, and viruses. Chlorhexidine is less effective against gram-negative bacteria, and its efficacy against viruses is unknown. Care must be taken to avoid spilling these substances into the wound. Exposure of the eye to these agents can be disastrous. Chlorhexidine has been shown experimentally and in case reports to produce serious permanent corneal opacification.[27]

Body, facial, and head hair usually is removed to clean and examine the wound, although this is not necessary to diminish the risk of wound infection. Removal of the hair makes it easier for the patient to keep the area clean and ultimately facilitates suture removal. Exceptions are parts of the body where hairlines provide important landmarks for the accurate reapproximation of tissue margins, most notably the eyebrow. Reports of inconsistent or absent eyebrow hair regrowth suggest that eyebrow hair should not be shaved.

Surgical studies show that hair removal with a razor is three to nine times more likely to result in a wound infection than is clipping the hair. It seems that the razor damages the infundibulum of the hair follicle.[28] The wounded follicle provides access for bacterial invasion and ultimately infection. It is recommended that routine hair removal be accomplished using a razor with a recessed blade. For wounds considered to be at high risk of infection, clipping may be done with electronic shears or scissors because close shaving is not necessary. Another option is to apply a petroleum-based product to the hair adjacent to the wound margins, allowing the provider to keep the hair away from the surgical field.

Wound Preparation

Debridement

Debridement is the removal of foreign matter and devitalized tissue from the wound. With respect to ultimate wound healing and risk of infection, debridement is the most important consideration in wound care.[29] The presence of any devitalized tissue in the wound delays healing and significantly increases the risk of infection. The benefits of debridement have to be weighed, however, against the consequences of producing a larger tissue defect. The resultant closure is exposed to higher tension and results in a wider scar. Skin edges that are clearly devitalized must be debrided before wound closure. On the trunk, where there is little concern for specialized tissue, wide excision and debridement are feasible. On the face and hands, where all tissue must be saved if possible, the process is more difficult. Meticulous sharp excision of small fragments of nonviable tissue should be performed only by experienced physicians. When the viability of large areas of skin or muscle is a significant concern, the wound should be prepared for delayed primary closure.

Wound Cleansing

An ideal wound cleanser has broad antimicrobial activity with a rapid onset. It is nontoxic to the tissue and does not reduce tissue resistance to infection, delay healing, or decrease the tensile strength of the healing wound. Innumerable antiseptic solutions have been used clinically and studied in great detail (Table 56-1). Much debate exists over which agent comes closest to possessing these qualities. Povidone-iodine in various concentrations, saline, and, more recently, tap water have received the most attention.[30-32]

Free iodine, although possessing broad, rapid antimicrobial activity, is too toxic to tissue and its defenses to have therapeutic value in the open wound. An iodophor is a complex of iodine with a carrier to increase its solubility and decrease availability of free iodine. The most widely used iodophor is povidone-iodine, in which the carrier molecule is povidone (formerly polyvinylpyrrolidone). It is generally available in a 10% solution, which is 1% free iodine. The clinical benefit of this complex is a solution that maintains broad antimicrobial activity and eliminates most local and systemic toxicity. It is well documented that even a 5% povidone-iodine solution is toxic to polymorphonuclear neutrophil leukocyte activity and may

Table 56-1. Antiseptic Solutions

Agents	Antimicrobial Activity	Mechanisms of Action	Tissue Toxicity	Indications and Contraindications
Povidone-iodine solution (iodine complexes) (Betadine)	Available as a 10% solution with polyvinylpyrolidine (povidone) containing 1% free iodine with broad rapid-onset antimicrobial activity	Potent germicide in low concentrations	Decreases PMN migration and life span at concentration >1% May cause systemic toxicity at higher concentrations; questionable toxicity at 1% concentration	Probably a safe and effective wound cleanser at a 1% concentration 10% solution is effective to prepare skin around the wound
Povidone-iodine surgical scrub	Same as the solution	Same	Toxic to open wounds	Best as a hand cleanser; never use in open wounds
Nonionic detergents Pluronic F-68 Shur Clens	Ethylene oxide is 80% of its molecular weight No antimicrobial activity	Wound cleanser	No toxicity to open wounds, eyes, or IV solutions	Appears to be an effective, safe wound cleanser
Hydrogen perxoide	3% solution in water has brief germicidal activity	Oxidizing agent that denatures protein	Toxic to open wounds	Should not be used on wounds after initial cleaning; may be used to clean intact skin
Hexachlorophene (polychlorinated bisphenol) (pHisoHex)	Bacteriostatic (2% to 5%) Greater activity against gram-positive organisms	Interruption of bacterial electron transport and disruption of membrane-bound enzymes	Little skin toxicity; the scrub form is damaging to open wounds	Never use scrub solution in open wounds Very good preoperative hand preparation
Alcohols	Low-potency antimicrobial most effective as a 70% ethyl and 70% isopropyl alcohol solution	Denatures protein	Kills irreversibly and functions as a fixative	No role in routine care
Phenols	Bacteriostatic >0.2% Bactericidal >1% Fungicidal 1.3%	Denatures protein	Extensive tissue necrosis and systemic toxicity	Never use >2% aqueous phenol or >4% phenol plus glycerol

IV, intravenous; PMN, polymorphonuclear neutrophil leukocyte.

increase infection rate. A 1% solution is safe and effective with little or no toxicity.[27,33] Evidence suggests that a 0.9% normal saline solution or tap water may be just as effective when used with high-pressure syringe irrigation.[34] Detergent-containing cleansers, such as *povidone-iodine scrub,* may be excellent for skin preparation but are toxic to tissue defenses and should never be allowed to contaminate open wounds.

Saline is the traditional wound irrigating fluid of choice. Tap water has consistently produced equivalent rates of infection and cosmetic outcomes, however. Tap water irrigation allows a large volume of irrigation rapidly and inexpensively and is especially suited to upper extremity injuries.

Although many different irrigation solutions may be beneficial, it seems that the key to cleansing is high-pressure irrigation rather than the type of solution used. Tap water irrigation soon may become the preferred method of irrigation because it is safe, effective, easier to prepare, and less expensive. Wounds close to the eye, where pressure irrigation may be impossible, may be cleaned with a sponge with fine pore cells and a surfactant, such as poloxamer 188.

Irrigation

The quality of mechanical cleansing is one of the most important determinants of wound prognosis. The most effective form of wound cleansing is high-pressure irrigation. Irrigating with pressures greater than 7 pounds per square inch (psi) significantly decreases the number of bacteria and the incidence of infection.[35,36] Although several commercial devices are available, attaching a 19-gauge needle to a 35-mL syringe yields a force of 7 to 8 psi. High pressures of 50 to 70 psi may be obtained by using a commercial water pick. These pressures may cause some tissue damage, but the beneficial effect of ridding the wound of bacteria and debris outweighs this risk. Simply soaking the wound in an antiseptic solution is not beneficial. Scrubbing the wound with a sponge with large-pore cells inflicts tissue trauma and impairs the ability to resist infection. Tissue damage can be decreased by using a sponge with a fine size of pore cell. Adding a surfactant further minimizes the mechanical trauma inflicted by the sponge. Flooding the wound under low pressure using a bulb syringe or gravity alone does not reduce the incidence of infection, regardless of the agent used.

At least one study has shown little benefit to any irrigation in facial and scalp lacerations. This study prospectively compared outcomes of almost 2000 immunocompetent patients. Infection rates and cosmetic outcomes were similar in the irrigation and the nonirrigation groups.[35]

Wound Closure

Decision Making

The first determination required is whether the wound should be treated open or closed. Each wound, patient, and clinical circumstance must be handled individually. Certain lacerations, such as a fine linear laceration to the face, can be closed primarily 24 hours or more after injury. Other injuries may necessitate open management, regardless of the extent of delay.[36] A large stellate laceration to the foot produced by blunt force and contaminated with dirt and grease should not be closed primarily; in addition, human and animal bites to the hand should not be closed primarily. Physician judgment is often the best method for deciding when it is safe to close a wound. In one study in which hand wounds were described as dirty, 22% became infected. When the injury was documented to be clean, the incidence of infection was 7.1%.[37]

Three wound closure options are available. The wound may be (1) closed primarily in traditional fashion, (2) closed in 4 or 5 days (delayed primary closure), or (3) left open and allowed to heal on its own. *Delayed primary closure* is a safe alternative to traditional primary closure.[2,35,38] Overall healing time is not affected, and the risk of infection is greatly decreased if proper technique is used. When a wound is slated for delayed primary closure, it must be prepared, debrided, and irrigated in the same manner as for immediate closure. The wound should be packed to prevent it from closing on its own. If the wound is on an extremity, the injury should be splinted and dressed, and appropriate wound care instructions should be given. The patient should return for a wound check and packing change in 24 hours and instructed to follow up in another 72 hours for definitive repair, with wound closure 96 to 120 hours after injury. No studies offer guidelines for prophylactic antibiotic use when delayed primary closure is the treatment option. Extrapolation from other wound studies strongly suggests that antibiotics offer no benefit.

Individuals who do not seek medical care after an injury select the option of leaving a wound open to heal on its own. Most patients who present to an emergency department with a laceration undergo some form of wound closure. Not closing a wound should be considered an option to save the patient the discomfort associated with wound closure and to save time for the physician. One study that looked at hand lacerations less than 2 cm long followed patients for 3 months and found that there was no significant difference in cosmetic appearance, and there was no difference in time to resume activities of daily living.[39]

Closing a wound loosely is occasionally discussed as an option in the treatment of contaminated wounds. This choice should never be considered. The loosely closed wound approximates the tissue margins enough to allow the wound to seal itself completely within 48 hours. The infection risk when using this method is the same as when closing the wound traditionally.

Wound Tension

The goal of wound closure is optimal anatomic and functional reapproximation of tissue with minimal risk of complication. Consideration must be given to the wound's size, shape, location, depth, and degree of tension. Wounds with high static and dynamic tension that require meticulous closure cannot be closed with tape or staples. Delicate approximation of wound edges under tension can be accomplished only with suture.

Several techniques may be used to reduce wound tension. Deep sutures may be placed in subcutaneous tissue to help bring the wound margins closer together. In this manner, forces on the skin are reduced, and potential dead space can be closed. Care should be taken to avoid suturing adipose tissue because it may become necrotic and increase the likelihood of infection. The number of dermal sutures depends on the characteristics of the wound. Generally the number should be kept to a minimum because suture material acts as foreign matter in the wound and can increase the risk of infection. Subcutaneous sutures should never be placed in the hand or foot because of the major structures that reside near the surface. Another method of ameliorating static tension from cut edges of the wound is to undermine at the lacerated margin. Undermining helps free the dermis from its deeper attachments, allowing the skin edges to be approximated with less force. Care must be taken to preserve the blood supply to the wound margins and not increase dead space in the process.

Suture Technique

Careful surgical technique is important to optimize the ultimate repair. If possible, pickups, hemostats, or forceps should not be used, especially on wound margins. Blind clamping in a wound can damage a nerve, artery, or tendon. Wound margins should be everted and the sutures tied just tightly enough to allow the edges to approximate lightly. The edges can be everted by ensuring that the needle enters and exits perpendicular to the skin. Wounds with opposing margins of different thickness can be difficult to close. If this difference is not considered and corrected, the ultimate scar has uneven margins that cast a shadow on the skin and is unsightly. To close these wounds, the needle should be pulled through the cut margin of one side before entering the opposite edge. This method gives the emergency physician the best opportunity to take an equivalent amount of tissue on both sides of the wound. Viable edges of a jagged wound must be meticulously reapproximated. Because of the greater surface area and the ultimate contraction of the wound, preserving the jagged edges results in a more "natural" scar.

Most lacerations are closed with running or interrupted percutaneous suture. The running technique is appropriate for linear lacerations under minimal tension when there is low risk of infection. This technique is more rapid, requires less suture material, and yields equivalent cosmetic results. Curvilinear or jagged wounds are best closed with interrupted sutures to distribute tension properly. Because tensile strength of interrupted sutures may be superior, wound edges subjected to higher levels of tension should be closed with interrupted sutures.[40]

Basic and Advanced Techniques

Simple Sutures

Wound closure with simple interrupted sutures is the most common method of laceration repair in emergency departments. The placement of simple sutures yields excellent cosmesis and a low infection rate.

Procedure. The needle is placed to one side of the laceration margin and enters the skin at approximately 90 degrees. To pass the needle through the tissue, the clinician's wrist is supinated and guides the needle deep but parallel to the skin surface. Wrist supination is extended as the needle exits the skin on the opposite side perpendicular to the surface. Proper technique produces wound edges that are slightly everted and are lightly touching. Care should be taken not to secure the suture too tightly because necrosis of the wound margin tissue seriously compromises healing.

Intradermal (Buried) Sutures

Placing cutaneous sutures in wounds under tension can lead to ischemia of the wound margin and an unsightly scar. Proper placement of buried intradermal sutures helps to approximate dermal margins and reduce wound edge tension. Buried sutures should not be used in contaminated wounds because they increase the risk of wound infection. Sutures through adipose tissue also increase infection and do not relieve skin tension.

Procedure. Placement of buried sutures differs from traditional suturing because of the need to bury the knot deep to the skin. Failure to do this can interfere with dermal healing and can leave a small lump under the surface of the skin. The needle is introduced deep in the wound in the subcutaneous tissue and emerges from the dermis below the skin surface. The needle is reintroduced in the dermis on the opposite wound margin and emerges from the subcutaneous tissue at the same level on the opposite side. The knot is secured and remains buried deep below the skin surface.

Scalp Laceration Repair

In contrast to small lacerations elsewhere on the body, most scalp lacerations require repair because of the propensity to bleed profusely. The dense connective tissue beneath the skin tends to hold vessels open and delay hemostasis. Frontal scalp lacerations in young men should be considered to be a cosmetically significant wound. Although the scalp laceration currently may be well hidden by hair, most men experience some balding. Care must be taken to explore the laceration thoroughly to look for a defect in the galea, an injury that requires repair with deep sutures. Staples may be ideal for the skin closure of simple linear scalp lacerations. Hair is less of a problem when placing staples,

staples can be placed more quickly than traditional suture, and staples are easier to see and can be removed 1 to 3 days earlier than traditional sutures. Staples may produce artifact on CT scan, but useful information still may be obtained if CT is necessary. Staples may move during magnetic resonance imaging and should not be placed if this imaging modality is being considered. Lightweight stapling devices are available. Most devices come preloaded with five or more staples and are easy to use.

Traditional sutures are used to repair most scalp lacerations, usually with standard nylon suture. Absorbable chromic gut can be used in children and in adults who may not return for suture removal.

Procedure. Anesthesia with epinephrine is recommended to help control bleeding. Hair removal is necessary only if the hair makes closure difficult. A defect in the galea is closed with 3-0 or 4-0 absorbable suture. Failure to repair the galea can lead to a cosmetic deformity related to frontalis muscle function. Linear superficial scalp lacerations that do not require deep sutures can be closed with staples or with monofilament nylon sutures applied using a simple interrupted or running technique. Jagged or macerated lacerations may require some debridement and horizontal mattress sutures. When one chooses to staple a scalp laceration, the adjacent skin margins are pinched together with forceps to evert wound margins. The "mouth" of the stapler is placed gently on the skin surface, taking care not to indent the skin. The handle of the stapler is squeezed carefully to eject the staple into the tissue. Ideally, the staple closely approximates the wound margins without indenting the surface of the skin. To release the staple, the wrist must be pulled back to disengage itself from the last staple.

Staple removal is simple, especially if the patient kept the wound clean and free of dried secretions. The dual prongs on the disposable staple remover slide under the staple crossbar. As the handle is squeezed and the horizontal aspect of the staple is depressed, the sharp edges are eased out of the tissue for removal.

Vertical Mattress Sutures

Vertical mattress sutures improve wound edge eversion. They also are used for the closure of gaping wounds and deep lacerations that may need more than simple sutures to close potential dead space. Areas of lax skin tension, generally where maximal skin mobility is needed, such as over joint surfaces, may need assistance to ensure eversion of the wound margins. Vertical mattress sutures may be ideal to accomplish both tasks.

Procedure. A vertical mattress suture is a combination of deep and superficial components. The needle is introduced at a 90-degree angle about 1 cm from the wound margin. The needle courses through the depth of the wound and emerges on the opposite side, 1 cm from the laceration margin at a 90-degree angle. The needle is reintroduced 1 to 2 mm from the epidermal edge for final approximation of the wound.

Horizontal Mattress Sutures

Horizontal mattress sutures are useful to help disperse excess skin tension and to evert wound edges. The scalp, where there is minimal skin mobility, is one area where gaping lacerations may benefit from this tension reduction method. Horizontal mattress sutures also may be beneficial in thin, fragile skin of elderly persons and lacerations that have lost tissue from the injury or debridement.

Procedure. The initial step is to pass the needle as for a simple interrupted stitch. On exiting the skin, however, the needle is reintroduced about 0.5 cm adjacent to the exit point. This second "bite" re-emerges 0.5 cm adjacent to the initial insertion point and is tied. In contrast to the vertical mattress, each bite always is the same distance from the wound margin.

Dog-Ear Deformity Repair

Some redundant tissue may result on one side of the repair as the closure nears completion, especially in the closure of curvilinear lacerations. This redundant tissue generally can be avoided by placing the initial suture in the middle of a curvilinear wound. If the clinician has limited experience, excising and undermining tissue are likely to result in complications and should not be attempted.

Procedure. The laceration repair begins in a traditional manner and continues to about the final 1 cm of the wound. A short incision (about 1 cm) is made from the end of the laceration at a 45-degree angle. The angle is cut toward the side of the redundant, bunched tissue. In most cases, the subcutaneous tissue from the start of the dog-ear defect to the newly created end of the wound must be gently undermined to mobilize the skin. The next step, and final step before suturing, is the most important. The work that has just been completed leaves a small triangular piece of excess tissue. The redundant piece is gently lifted with the tissue forceps and excised in a line parallel to the incision made above. The wound now can be closed with simple interrupted suture technique. Poor technique can result in a more unsightly repair. If too much tissue is undermined, the edge of the skin can lose its blood supply and necrose.

Corner Stitch
(Half-Buried Horizontal Mattress Sutures)

Jagged and triangular-shaped wounds create corners that can be difficult to repair. The clinician must avoid placing the suture directly in the tip of the flap. This practice may "stretch" the tissue and further compromise blood flow to the wound margin. The corner stitch allows optimal tissue approximation with minimal tension.

Procedure. The needle is introduced percutaneously through the nonflap side of the wound a few millimeters from the corner of the wound. The needle is passed horizontally through the dermis of the flap. The final step is to pass the needle into the dermis of the nonflap aspect of the wound a few millimeters from the opposite side of the corner. The suture is led out through the epidermis and tied. This technique also can be used to encompass multiple flaps either individually or simultaneously if the tips are adjacent to one another. The most difficult yet important aspect of the corner stitch is to take bites of equal depth with each pass of the needle. Failure to take equal bites of tissue results in a wound with opposing sides that do not lie flat; this leads to a more obvious scar. When the corner has been repaired, the remaining two sides of the wound may be closed with simple interrupted or running suture technique.

V-Y Wound Closure

The V-Y closure is indicated for the repair of V-shaped wounds with tissue loss or with nonviable margins that must be trimmed. The tissue loss is such that the adjacent mobile tissue is not sufficient to close the remaining defect.

Procedure. Nonviable tissue is trimmed with fine iris scissors. The long V-shaped portion of the wound is sutured with simple interrupted percutaneous stitches. This first step brings the tip of the flap closer to the newly created corner of the wound. A corner stitch is used to secure the tip of the flap. The remaining limbs of the Y can be repaired with simple interrupted stitches. Some degree of undermining is likely to be needed to mobilize tissue to close the defect. Debridement of too much tissue can make the final repair more difficult and can distort adjacent anatomy.

Materials

In the Middle Ages and earlier, materials used to close wounds included flax, hemp, fascia, hair, linen strips, pigs' bristles, reeds, grasses, and even the mouth parts of the pincher ant. In the early 1900s, natural organic protein products, including silk, cotton, and catgut, were the only available substances. Polyester (Dacron) and nylon were the first synthetic materials available in the 1940s. Since then, a host of other synthetic materials have become available.

Suture

The ideal suture is inert to metabolism, is resistant to infection, has great tensile strength, does not tear tissue, is easy to work with and tie, and is available in convenient colors with a variety of cutting and non-cutting needles (Table 56-2). A common classification of suture material relies on relative *absorbability*. In general, the materials that maintain their tensile strength for more than 60 days after implantation have been defined as *nonabsorbable*.[41] Materials that undergo rapid degradation in tissue and lose their strength in less than 60 days are considered *absorbable*. A second classification considers the source and nature of the material. *Biologic* substances, which include catgut, collagen, silk, linen, and cotton, generally produce the greatest tissue reaction and have the lowest relative tensile strength but have good knot security. These characteristics are in contrast to *synthetic* materials, such as polyester (Dacron), polyamide (nylon),

Table 56-2. Suture Materials for Wound Closure

Type	Description	Security	Strength	Reaction	Workability	Infection	Comment
Nonabsorbables							
Silk		++++	+	++++	++++	++	Suitable around mouth, nose, or nipples, but too reactive and weak to be used universally
Mersilene	Braided synthetic	++++	++	+++	++++		Good tensile strength; some prefer for fascia repairs
Nylon	Monofilament	++	+++	++	++	+++	Good strength; decreased infection rate; but knots tend to skip, especially the first "throw"
Polypropylene (Prolene)	Monofilament	+	++++	+	+	++++	Good resistance on infection; often difficult to work with; requires an extra throw
Ethibond	Braided coated polyester	+++	++++	++$^{1}/_{2}$	+++	+++	Costly
Stainless steel wire	Monofilament	++++	++++	+	+	+	Hard to use; painful to patient; some prefer for tendons
Absorbables							
Gut (plain)	From sheep intima	+	++	+++		+	Loses strength rapidly and quickly absorbed; rarely used today
Chromic (gut)	Plain gut treated with chromic salts	++	++	+++		+	Similar to plain gut; often used to close intraoral lacerations
Dexon	Braided copolymer of glycolic acid	++++	++++	+		++++	Braiding may cause it to "hang up" when tying knots
Vicryl	Braided polymer of lactide and glycolide	+++	++++	+		+++	Low reactivity with good strength; suitable for subcutaneous healing; good in mucous membranes
Polydioxanone	Monofilament	++++	++++	+	Excellent	Unavailable	First available monofilament synthetic absorbable sutures; appears to be excellent

From Swanson NA, Tromovitch TA: *Int J Dermatol* 21:373, 1982.

polypropylene (Prolene), polyglycolide and polylactide polymers (Dexon, Vicryl), polydioxanone (PDS), and steel, which usually have less tissue reactivity, greater strength, and less knot security.[42,43]

Knotting properties and handling characteristics tend to vary inversely. Knot security is of particular importance in maintaining wound closure and the patient's confidence in the physician. Sutures with smooth or slippery surfaces produce little friction and glide effortlessly through tissue and are easy to tie. Smoother materials are more difficult to handle and more likely to untie spontaneously. Certain monofilament synthetic materials tend to return or spring back to their original shape. To overcome this suture memory, the first part of the tie should be a "double throw" pulled tightly enough to approximate the tissue, taking care not to strangulate the margins. The second throw is to lock the tension of the first part into position. A third throw is used for added security. If done properly, additional knotting is not needed after the third throw.

The presence of any suture material in a wound increases the likelihood of infection. Subcutaneous sutures bear the greatest risk.[42] The degree of risk depends on characteristics of the substances used. Braided multifilament materials, such as the polyesters, polyamides, polyglycolides, and silk, yield the highest infection rates, whereas monofilament synthetic substances have the lowest risk of infection. There are several nonabsorbable monofilament synthetic sutures and one absorbable monofilament (PDS). The degree of infectivity of PDS compares well with similar materials having low rates of infectivity.[43]

Consideration of patient comfort in suture selection is important. Although silk is highly reactive, it ties well, is easy to handle, and is comfortable for the patient. It is an excellent choice in and around the lips, where comfort is a major concern. PDS is a comfortable absorbable suture and can be left in intraoral mucosa to be absorbed, with apparently low risks of infection, or it can be removed in 5 to 7 days. Staples or metallic sutures are excellent when strength is needed but may be uncomfortable for the patient. Nylon and polypropylene, which are the most common sutures used on skin, produce little tissue reaction and offer good tensile strength. They tend to be stiff, produce discomfort near the lips, have poor knot security, and may be difficult to work with. A braided, coated polyester nonabsorbable material, such as Ethibond, is easier to work with and has better knot stability. Although Ethibond is more expensive than nylon, its characteristics and added patient comfort suggest that it may be preferable. Absorbable suture materials, such as polyglycolide and polylactide polymers (Dexon, Vicryl), have been used strictly for subcutaneous and mucosal closures. Their highly reactive nature allows them to be broken down and absorbed over weeks. Chromic catgut, another absorbable material, has been shown to be safe and effective for the closure of scalp wounds in children.[44]

Needles

Surgical needles are available in a variety of sizes and shapes with a myriad of other characteristics. Cutting needles may be reverse cutting, conventional cutting, taper cut, or precision point. Most emergency wounds may be closed using a conventional cutting needle. In addition to its sharp point, it has two opposing cutting edges, with a third on the inside curve. Precision point needles are similarly shaped but are honed 24 extra times and maintain their added sharpness longer. These needles are used for delicate plastic or cosmetic surgery. Noncutting needles are reserved for organ repair and subcutaneous suturing. Cutting needles also may be used to repair subcutaneous tissue. Needle nomenclature is confusing and varies with the manufacturer.

Tape

Tape closure may be superior to sutures and staples if applied in the appropriate circumstances. Generally, the laceration should be linear and subjected to weak static and dynamic forces. Tape is not considered for wounds requiring meticulous tissue approximation. Compared with other closure materials, application of tape is associated with lower risk of infection, less expense, and less physician time. In addition, a painful injection of local anesthetic is not needed.

The ideal wound closure tape must allow water and gas exchange and possess elasticity, strength, and optimal adhesiveness. To maximize adhesive properties, tincture of benzoin should be painted on the skin adjacent to the wound. Care must be taken to avoid introducing benzoin compound in the wound itself. A nonwoven, microporous tape, which is not reinforced, has been found to fulfill these properties best.[45,46]

Staples

Staples offer several advantages over sutures. Monofilament stainless steel staples offer less risk of infection than even the least reactive suture.[47] The time necessary to accomplish closure may be significantly lessened. Acceptable wounds must be linear and subjected to weak skin forces. Wounds requiring accurate approximation of tissue are not candidates for staple closure. Staples also are uncomfortable while in situ and on removal. Stapled wounds gain tensile strength sooner, and the staples can be removed 1 to 3 days

earlier than sutures. After removal, the staples should be replaced with wound closure tape for continued reinforcement.

Various stapling devices are available. The device must allow good visual access and flexible positioning for difficult angles. A precocking mechanism is necessary to allow the physician to hold the staple securely during its placement. The angle of staple delivery is important. One brand releases the staple perpendicular to the wound with its crossbar flush with the skin; this can result in cross-hatching on the skin or tissue strangulation if placed too deeply. The device needs an ejector spring for smooth staple release and must handle without producing fatigue.

Tissue Adhesives

European and Canadian physicians have used tissue adhesives (butyl 2-cyanoacrylates) for many years. In August 1998, octyl-2-cyanoacrylates were approved for use in the United States. Tissue adhesives offer many advantages over traditional sutures. The emergency physician can apply the adhesive quickly and easily with a minimum of patient discomfort. In addition, suture removal in 7 to 10 days is unnecessary because the adhesive sloughs off the skin in about that time. Evidence indicates that adhesives not only provide their own dressing, but also have antibacterial properties and may decrease the rate of wound infections.[48,49] Considering time and materials, closing wounds with adhesives is less expensive than traditional suturing and carries no risk of needle-stick injuries.[50]

Tissue adhesives achieved cosmetic results similar to traditional sutures in randomized trials.[50,51] Tissue adhesive may be applied in high-tension areas, but only if used in conjunction with subcutaneous or subcuticular sutures. If used alone, tissue adhesives are not recommended for areas of higher tension or frequent repetitive movements, such as joints or hands.

Other disadvantages of tissue adhesives include the inability to use antibacterial or other petroleum-based products on the wound, the recommendation not to swim, and the greater risk of dehiscence. The tensile strength of tissue adhesives is significantly less than that of sutures. Despite these disadvantages, tissue adhesives represent a tremendous advance in the management of routine uncomplicated lacerations in nontension areas. Patients routinely prefer tissue adhesives over traditional sutures.[49]

Application of tissue adhesive begins with routine skin and wound preparation. The area must be dried and adequate hemostasis achieved before application of the adhesive. The wound margins should be approximated as meticulously as possible, and care should be taken to prevent adhesive from getting between the wound margins. Adhesive between the wound margins delays healing and increases the likelihood of wound dehiscence. The adhesive should be applied to the entire length of the wound sufficient to cover 5 to 10 mm of skin adjacent to the margins. Three layers of adhesive are to be applied. The physician should allow 30 to 45 seconds for the first layer to polymerize, then apply the subsequent two layers allowing about 10 seconds between applications. Special care must be taken to ensure that the adhesive does not run off and disturb adjacent tissues. This is especially true of wounds near the eye. Newer, high-viscosity formulations are now available and help to limit this risk. Wounds may get wet but should not be immersed in water and should be blotted dry and not vigorously rubbed. An additional dressing may be desired by the patient but is not necessary.[52]

Antibiotic Prophylaxis

Routine antibiotic prophylaxis for simple wounds has no scientific basis. A meta-analysis compared the rates of infection in patients with simple, nonbite wounds receiving antibiotics with control groups. Of 1734 patients enrolled in the seven studies, patients treated with antibiotics had a slightly greater incidence of infection. The authors concluded that prophylactic antibiotics had no role in simple, nonbite lacerations.[53] Routine antibiotic use also has complications; allergic reactions are common and may result in significant morbidity and unnecessary cost.

Although irrigation and debridement are the most important means of preventing wound infections, antibiotic prophylaxis is recommended in some circumstances. Prophylaxis must be tailored to each patient. Some recommendations are supported by scientific data, whereas others have few data to support their use and are based on custom.

Contamination, Crush, and Host Factors

Antibiotic prophylaxis is often provided for patients with wounds with gross contamination, patients with severe crush injuries, and immunocompromised patients. Some authors recommend not closing these wounds and instead using delayed primary closure. If circumstances require wound closure despite the infection risk, many emergency physicians recommend prophylaxis despite scarce data.[54]

Some authors believe that a patient with significant crush injury requires antibiotics. Crush injuries are high-risk wounds because they produce more devitalized tissue.[55] A definitive answer may not be forthcoming because it would be difficult to complete a well-controlled prospective, blind study.

Patients with certain risk factors have increased wound infection rates. A prospective study of more than 23,000 surgical wounds showed an increased rate of wound infection in patients with diabetes, obesity, malnutrition, chronic renal failure, advanced age, and chronic steroid use.[56] Because of higher rates of infection, some authors suggest the use of antibiotics in these patients, again based on individual circumstances.[57] No controlled studies of antibiotic prophylaxis in these patients exist, however. Finally, some authors advocate prophylaxis for other host factors, such as prosthetic joints or risk for endocarditis.[58,59] Little evidence exists to support either recommendation.

Bites and Puncture Wounds

Antibiotics are indicated for through-and-through intraoral lacerations, cat bites, some dog bites, some human bites, some puncture injuries to the foot, open fractures, and wounds involving exposed tendons or joints.

Cat Bites

Prophylaxis is required for patients with cat bites. These bites tend to be deep puncture wounds that are difficult to irrigate adequately. These wounds also tend to become infected at a much higher rate than other types of bites. Cat bites have been reported to cause infections in 10% to 40% of all wounds. In one study, 12.9% of patients had signs of infection when they presented to the emergency department, and 15.9% eventually developed infection. Other authors report that 80% of these bites become infected. Antibiotics seem to decrease the incidence of infection.[60]

The organisms found in cat bites include *Staphylococcus* species, *Streptococcus* species, and, most often, *Pasteurella multocida*. *P. multocida* is usually found in infected cat bite wounds and is present in the normal oral flora of 70% of all cats. *P. multocida* is sensitive to penicillin, but the infection is often polymicrobial. *P. multocida* is resistant to dicloxacillin, cephalexin, and clindamycin, and there are many erythromycin-resistant strains. Amoxicillin with clavulanate is the current recommendation for antibiotic prophylaxis for cat bites.[54]

Dog Bites

Antibiotic prophylaxis for dog bites is more controversial. The infection rate has been reported as 6% to 16% for patients not receiving antibiotics. Dog bites tend to be more crush injuries with tearing and avulsions rather than puncture wounds. As such, dog bites usually are more amenable to irrigation and debridement. Seven of eight randomized trials of dog bite wounds showed no benefit with antibiotics. Pooled data for meta-analysis did show, however, a small but statistically significant benefit from antibiotics.[54,61] It may be logical to limit use of antibiotics to high-risk wounds, such as hand injuries.

Hand Bites

In addition to the previous bite wound recommendations, antibiotic prophylaxis of injuries to the metacarpophalangeal joints is advised. These wounds are assumed to be human bites until proved otherwise. Also known as "fight bites," these wounds have a high incidence of infection. Patients without signs of infection may be managed as outpatients. Patients with early signs of infection must be admitted for intravenous antibiotics and aggressive debridement and irrigation. The choice of antibiotics reflects the predominant organisms of hand bite infections. *Streptococcus* and *Staphylococcus* species are common, but *Eikenella corrodens* and *Bacteroides* species also are typical pathogens. Because *Eikenella* is often resistant to clindamycin, first-generation cephalosporins, and erythromycin, patients with early infection should receive amoxicillin with clavulanate. Patients with later infection should receive intravenous extended-spectrum antibiotics (e.g., ampicillin with sulbactam).

Intraoral Lacerations

Lacerations of the oral mucosa involve bacteria-rich oral secretions and may become infected slightly more often (6% to 12%) than other wounds. Although few data suggest a clear indication for prophylactic antibiotics, one study showed that patients benefit from antibiotics if they are compliant with their regimen. Rates of infection for complex through-and-through lacerations may be twice the rates for simple mucosal lacerations. It may be reasonable to limit antibiotic use to complex lacerations. Penicillin is an appropriate choice of antibiotic.

Puncture Wounds of Foot

Puncture wounds of the foot are seen frequently in the emergency department. These wounds often are caused by common nails, although other objects (e.g., glass, metal, wood) must be considered. Despite their simple appearance, these wounds may produce significant morbidity. The infection rate for puncture wounds has been reported to be 15%.[61,62] Most wounds occur on the plantar surface, from the neck of the metatarsal to the toes. Simple cellulitis accounts for half of these infections. More significant infections include septic arthritis, abscesses, and osteomyelitis. *Pseudomonas* organisms cause 90% of osteomyelitis cases from puncture wounds. No data suggest a benefit from prophylactic antibiotics, but given the high risk of infection and serious complications, their use should be strongly considered in select puncture wounds. Consideration of *Pseudomonas* organisms when the puncture went through a rubber-soled shoe is essential. Patients with puncture wounds to the foot require early follow-up.

Drains, Dressings, and Immobilization

Drains

Drains probably have no role in emergency department wound care. In general, drains are placed when a collection of fluid exists or may develop. The presence of a drain reduces the wound's resistance to infection, regardless of the materials used in its construction, and the use of drains should be avoided.[63,64] In wounds likely to collect fluid (e.g., around the elbow or knee), it is preferable to place the extremity at rest with a plaster splint or perform delayed primary closure.

Dressings

Various dressing materials are available. The microenvironment created by a dressing affects the biology of healing. The optimal wound climate must not interfere with the activity of fibroblasts and macrophages. The production of granulation tissue and migration of epithelial cells across the wound must be optimized.

Several factors should be considered when choosing the appropriate dressing. Dressings that prevent evaporation of water and keep tissues moist are helpful. A drying wound produces a thick, hardened scab that impedes the process of epithelialization. Excess fluid can lead to maceration of tissue and may be a potential culture medium for bacterial proliferation. Gaseous permeability is essential because epithelialization is accelerated greatly in the presence of oxygen. The wound-covering product should be impermeable to bacteria and other particulate matter that can contaminate the wound. It is important not to traumatize newly established tissue during dressing changes. The optimal dressing should have a nonadherent surface, be permeable to gases, and have a capacity to absorb some fluid but not allow desiccation. The outer barrier of the product should be impermeable to bacteria but permeable to water vapor.

Partial-thickness wounds (e.g., abrasions, burns, "road rash," ulcers) have improved healing with much less patient discomfort when vapor-permeable membranes are used.[65-67] Wounds treated with vapor-permeable membranes fill with granulation tissue before re-epithelialization of the defect. This response seems to be unique to moist wound healing. The fluid that collects under the membrane apparently has a factor that stimulates fibroblasts to multiply at an accelerated rate.[67] Studies are ongoing to identify and isolate these factors. Currently, plastic surgeons and dermatologists use these dressings extensively. These products have a role in the emergency department because of their well-documented advantages over traditional dressings.

Using vapor-permeable dressings on lacerations is unnecessary and impractical. These wounds should be covered with an antibiotic ointment or aloe vera to aid healing and prevent desiccation.[68,69] A microporous polypropylene dressing can be used to cover the area and prevent further contamination. The wound seals itself within 24 hours and no longer requires a dressing.[70]

Immobilization

Wounds in proximity to joints must be immobilized as part of routine care. Splinting the injured body part places the injury at rest and hastens healing. Failure to splint appropriately exposes the healing tissue to the dynamic forces of muscular contractions, ultimately slowing the healing process and increasing scar size. In addition, immobilization decreases lymphatic flow and minimizes spread of microflora from the wound.

DISPOSITION

Wound Care Instructions

It is difficult for patients to identify and recognize the signs of infection (Box 56-2).[71] Discharge instructions must be clear, understandable, and reasonably comprehensive. Instructions should include daily care,

BOX 56-2. Wound Care Instructions

A. Elevate the injured extremity above the level of the heart. Wear a sling when appropriate
B. Cleanse daily in a gentle fashion to remove debris and crusting that develops. Use dilute hydrogen peroxide
C. Immobilization should be maintained at least until suture removal
D. Signs of infection
  1. Redness
  2. Increasing pain
  3. Swelling
  4. Fever
  5. Red streaks progressing up an extremity
E. Wound check
  1. As needed to check signs of infection
  2. Routine at 48 hours for high-risk wounds
F. Suture removal (*Note*: Suture may be removed earlier if Steri Strips reinforce the wound.)
  1. Face: 3-5 days (always replace with Steri Strips)
  2. Scalp: 7-10 days
  3. Trunk: 7-10 days
  4. Arms and legs: 10-14 days
  5. Joints: 14 days

BOX 56-3. Summary of Wound Care

A. Stabilize patient
B. History (include tetanus immunization and allergies)
C. Physical examination
  1. Neurovascular examination
  2. Anesthesia: bupivacaine 0.5% without epinephrine, regional or local
  3. Bloodless field: tourniquet or sphygmomanometer for extremities
  4. Sterile examination of anatomic structures, skin, nerves, tendons, blood vessels, bones, muscles, fascia, other (ducts, cartilage)
  5. Consult if indicated
D. X-ray films to detect injury to bone or presence of foreign bodies (xeroradiograph or ultrasound)
E. Wound preparation
  1. Cut—do not shave—surrounding hair
  2. Prepare surrounding skin with povidone-iodine (Betadine) solution
  3. Sharp debridement of foreign matter and devitalized tissue
  4. High-pressure irrigation with saline, 1% Betadine, an antibiotic solution, or a nonionic solution
F. Wound closure
  1. Tape, staples, or suture
  2. Do not use subcutaneous sutures unless the wound is under high tension
G. Antibiotics
  1. Apply topical antibiotics
  2. No systemic antibiotics unless wound is very high risk
H. Dress and immobilize: consider a transparent gas-permeable dressing
I. Wound care instructions (see Box 56-2)
  1. Signs of infection
  2. Elevation
  3. Wound check if necessary
  4. Suture removal as soon as possible

observation for signs of infection, suture removal dates, and a follow-up source. During the first 24 to 48 post-traumatic hours, the injured extremity should be elevated. Elevation lessens edema, hastens healing, and mollifies pain. The wound should be protected as described previously or should be cleaned daily to remove crust formations. It is safe to bathe and get the wound wet 24 hours after injury.[70,72] Daily swabbing with half-strength hydrogen peroxide rids the wound of debris and any blood clot that forms between the sutured edges. Hydrogen peroxide should not be used after separation of the scab because it is toxic to the epithelium and may produce bullae.

Wound infection is difficult for the untrained observer to distinguish from the inflammatory response of injury and subsequent healing. Patient education in this regard should be cautious and straightforward (e.g., return or follow-up for redness, swelling, increased pain, fever, pus, or red lines progressing up an extremity). An injury classified as high risk must be reexamined 48 hours after the trauma, regardless of its appearance.

Suture removal times vary, but generally are about 4 days for the face and 7 to 14 days for other body parts (see Box 56-2). Considerations include cosmetics, dynamic forces in proximity to the injury, static skin tension, blood supply, and anticipated healing rates.

Tetanus Immunization

The reported incidence of tetanus in the United States in 1998 was 0.014 per 100,000 population.[73] Most tetanus patients are older than 50 years old. Immunization status needs to be considered in all patients with wounds, regardless of severity. Forty percent of all cases of tetanus occur in individuals who have either minor wounds or no recollection of injury. These numbers raise serious questions regarding the validity of separating immunization recommendations according to clean and tetanus-prone wounds. Studies show that many people are inadequately immunized, especially elderly women.[74] Also, patient immunization histories are often unreliable. Given the inability to predict which wounds are high risk, all wounds should be approached with suspicion.

The usual incubation period for tetanus is 7 to 21 days (range 3 to 56 days). Immunization should be given as soon as possible but can be given days or weeks after the injury. The dose of tetanus toxoid (T) or diphtheria and tetanus toxoids (dT) is 0.5 mL intramuscularly, regardless of the patient's age. The tetanus immune globulin (TIG) dose is 250 U in patients 10 years old or older, 125 U in children 5 to 10 years old, and 75 U in children younger than 5 years old (Table 56-3). A single injection of TIG provides protective levels of passive antibodies for at least 4 weeks. The immune globulin and toxoid may be given during the same visit but should be administered with a different syringe at separate sites.

Because studies suggest that 10% to 40% of the U.S. population is inadequately immunized against diph-

Table 56-3. Tetanus Prophylaxis for All Patients with All Wounds*

Immunization History	dT (0.5 mL)	TIG (250 IU)
Fully immunized <10 yr since booster	No	No
Fully immunized >10 yr since booster	Yes	No
Incomplete series (<3 injections)	Yes[†]	Yes

*Consider more frequent immunization for elderly patients.
†Refer these patients to complete their series; dT in 6 weeks and 6 months.
dT, Diphtheria and tetanus toxoids; TIG, tetanus immune globulin. All injections are intramuscular.

theria, diphtheria vaccination should be given along with tetanus toxoid (dT).[75] The combined-injection dT is slightly more painful but does not present additional concerns. All three injections (T, TIG, dT) are safe and effective in pregnancy.[76]

SUMMARY

Box 56-3 summarizes the principles of wound care management.

KEY CONCEPTS

- Risk factors for wound infection include prolonged time since injury; crush mechanism; deep penetrating wounds; high-velocity missiles; and contamination with saliva, feces, soil, or other foreign matter.

- The most effective intervention to decrease infection is thorough cleansing, using saline irrigation at about 8 psi. Attaching a 19-gauge needle to a 35-mL syringe creates an irrigant force of 7 to 8 lb psi, which decreases bacterial counts.

- Soaking wounds in povidone-iodine (Betadine) is more toxic than beneficial to healthy tissue.

- Antibiotics are indicated for through-and-through intraoral lacerations, cat bites, some dog bites, some human bites, puncture injuries to the foot, open fractures, and wounds involving exposed tendons or joints.

- High-risk wounds should not be sutured primarily but may be repaired in 4 to 5 days (i.e., delayed primary closure).

- Tetanus immunization should be given soon after injury, but can be given days or weeks later. The usual incubation period for tetanus is 7 to 21 days (range 3 to 56 days).

REFERENCES

1. Trott AT: *Wounds and Lacerations: Emergency Care and Closure,* 2nd ed. St Louis, Mosby, 1997.
2. Jackson DS, Rovee DT: Current concepts in wound healing: Research and theory. *J Enterostom Ther* 15:133, 1988.
3. Hunt TK: The physiology of wound healing. *Ann Emerg Med* 17:1265, 1988.
4. Edlich RF, et al: Principles of emergency wound management. *Ann Emerg Med* 17:1284, 1988.
5. Tobin GR: Closure of contaminated wounds. *Surg Clin North Am* 64:639, 1984.
6. Perelman VS, et al: Sterile versus nonsterile gloves for repair of uncomplicated lacerations in the emergency department: A randomized controlled trial. *Ann Emerg Med* 43:362, 2004.
7. Avner JR: Lacerations involving glass: The role of routine roentgenograms. *Am J Dis Child* 146:600, 1992.
8. Hill R, et al: Ultrasound for the detection of foreign bodies in human tissue. *Ann Emerg Med* 29:353, 1997.
9. Manthey D, et al: Ultrasound versus radiograph in foreign body detection. *Ann Emerg Med* 28:7, 1996.
10. Fariss BL: Anesthetic properties and toxicity of bupivacaine and lidocaine for infiltration anesthesia. *J Emerg Med* 5:375, 1987.
11. Barker W, et al: Damage to tissue defenses by a topical anesthetic agent. *Ann Emerg Med* 11:307, 1982.
12. Maguire WM: Epinephrine induced vasospasm reversed by phentolamine digital block. *Am J Emerg Med* 8:46, 1990.
13. Marcaine package insert. New York, Winthrop Pharmaceuticals, 1998.
14. Parham SM, Pasieka JL: Effect of pH modification by bicarbonate on pain after subcutaneous lidocaine injection. *Can J Surg* 39:31, 1996.
15. Coventry DM: Alkalinization of bupivacaine for sciatic nerve blockade. *Anaesthesia* 44:467, 1989.
16. Brogan GX, et al: Comparison of plain, warmed, and buffered lidocaine for anesthesia of traumatic wounds. *Ann Emerg Med* 26:121, 1995.
17. Heggenbarth MA, et al: Comparison of topical tetracaine, adrenalin, and cocaine anesthesia with lidocaine infiltration for repair of lacerations in children. *Ann Emerg Med* 19:63, 1990.
18. Bonadio WA, et al: Half-strength TAC topical anesthesia for selected dermal lacerations. *Clin Pediatr* 27:495, 1988.
19. Blackburn PA, et al: Comparison of tetracaine-adrenaline-cocaine (TAC) with topical lidocaine-epinephrine (TLE): Efficacy and cost. *Am J Emerg Med* 13:315, 1995.
20. Terndrup TE: Plasma cocaine and tetracaine levels following application of topical anesthesia in children. *Ann Emerg Med* 21:162, 1992.
21. Dailey RH: Fatality secondary to misuse of TAC solution. *Ann Emerg Med* 17:159, 1988.
22. Ernst AA, et al: LAT (lidocaine-adrenaline-tetracaine) versus TAC (tetracaine-adrenaline-cocaine) for topical anesthesia in face and scalp lacerations. *Am J Emerg Med* 13:151, 1995.
23. Zempsky WT, Karasic RB: EMLA versus TAC for topical anesthesia of extremity wounds in children. *Ann Emerg Med* 30:163, 1997.
24. Incaudo G, et al: Administration of local anesthetics to patients with a history of prior adverse reaction. *J Allergy Clin Immunol* 61:339, 1978.
25. Swanson JG: Assessment of allergy to local anesthetic. *Ann Emerg Med* 12:316, 1983.
26. Pollack CV, Swindle GM: Use of diphenhydramine for local anesthesia in "caine"-sensitive patients. *J Emerg Med* 7:611, 1989.
27. Viljanto J: Disinfection of surgical wounds without inhibition of normal wound healing. *Arch Surg* 115:253, 1980.
28. Alexander JW, et al: The influence of hair-removal methods on wound infections. *Arch Surg* 118:347, 1983.
29. Dimick AR: Delayed wound closure: Indications and techniques. *Ann Emerg Med* 17:1303, 1988.
30. Angeras MH, et al: Comparison between sterile saline and tap water for the cleaning of acute traumatic soft tissue wounds. *Eur J Surg* 158:347, 1992.
31. Valente JH, et al: Wound irrigation in children: Saline solution or tap water? *Ann Emerg Med* 41:609, 2003.
32. Fernandez R, Griffiths R, Ussia C: Water for wound cleansing. *Cochrane Database Syst Rev* 4:CD003861, 2002.
33. Oberg MS: Povidone-iodine solutions in traumatic wound preparation. *Am J Emerg Med* 5:553, 1987.

34. Welsh AP: A comparison of wound irrigation solutions used in the emergency department. *Ann Emerg Med* 19:704, 1990.

35. Brown LL, et al: Evaluation of wound irrigation by pulsatile jet and conventional methods. *Ann Surg* 187:170, 1978.

36. Rogness H: High-pressure wound irrigation. *J Enterostom Ther* 12:27, 1985.

37. Hollander JE, et al: Irrigation in facial and scalp lacerations: Does it alter outcome? *Ann Emerg Med* 31:73, 1998.

38. Tobin GR: An improved method of delayed primary closure: An aggressive management approach to unfavorable wounds. *Surg Clin North Am* 64:659, 1984.

39. Berk WA, Osbourne DD, Taylor DD: Evaluation of the "golden period" for wound repair: 204 cases from a third world emergency department. *Ann Emerg Med* 17:496, 1988.

40. Shepard GH: Wounds treated by the healing of delayed primary closure: A clinical study. *Milit Med* 146:473, 1981.

41. Quinn J: Suturing versus conservative management of lacerations of the hand: Randomized controlled trial. *BMJ* 325:299, 2002.

42. McLean NR, et al: Comparison of skin closure using continuous and interrupted nylon sutures. *Br J Surg* 67:633, 1980.

43. Swanson NA, Tromovitch TA: Suture materials, 1980s: Properties, uses and abuses. Int J Dermatol 21:373, 1982.

44. Sharp WV, et al: Suture resistance to infection. *Surgery* 91:61, 1982.

45. Chusak RB, Dibbell DG: Clinical experience with polydioxanone monofilament absorbable sutures in plastic surgery. *Plast Reconstr Surg* 72:217, 1983.

46. Start NJ: The use of chromic catgut in the primary closure of scalp wounds in children. *Arch Emerg Med* 6:216, 1989.

47. Rodeheaver GT, Halverson MJ, Edlich RF: Mechanical performance of wound closure tapes. *Ann Emerg Med* 12:203, 1983.

48. Rodeheaver GT: Performance of new wound closure tapes. *J Emerg Med* 5:451, 1987.

49. Ritchie AJ, et al: Staples versus sutures in the closure of scalp wounds: A prospective double-blind randomized trial. *Injury* 20:217, 1989.

50. Quinn JV, et al: N-2-butylcyanoacrylate: Risk of bacterial contamination with an appraisal of its antimicrobial effects. *J Emerg Med* 13:581, 1995.

51. Osmond MH, et al: Economic comparison of a tissue adhesive and suturing in the repair of pediatric facial lacerations. *J Pediatr* 126:892, 1995.

52. Quinn JV, et al: A randomized trial comparing octylcyanoacrylate tissue adhesive and sutures in the management of lacerations. *JAMA* 277:1527, 1997.

53. Simon HK, et al: Long-term appearance of lacerations repaired using a tissue adhesive. *Pediatrics* 99:193, 1997.

54. Singer JA, Thode HC: A review of the literature on octylcyanoacrylate tissue adhesive. *Am J Surg* 187:2, 2004.

55. Cummings P, Del Beccaro MA: Antibiotics to prevent infection of simple wounds: A meta-analysis of randomized studies. *Am J Emerg Med* 13:396, 1995.

56. Hollander JE, Singer AJ: Laceration management. *Ann Emerg Med* 34:356, 1999.

57. Cardany CR, et al: The crush injury: A high risk wound. *J Am Coll Emerg Physicians* 5:965, 1976.

58. Cruse PJ, Foord R: A five-year prospective study of 23,649 surgical wounds. *Arch Surg* 107:206, 1973.

59. Singer AJ, Hollander JE, Quinn JV: Evaluation and management of traumatic lacerations. *N Engl J Med* 337:1142, 1997.

60. Edlich RF, et al: Antimicrobial treatment of minor soft tissue lacerations: A critical review. *Emerg Med Clin North Am* 4:561, 1986.

61. Kaplan EL: Prevention of bacterial endocarditis. *Circulation* 56:139A, 1977.

62. Elenbaas RM, McNabney WK, Robinson WA: Evaluation of prophylactic oxacillin in cat bite wounds. *Ann Emerg Med* 13:155, 1984.

63. Resnick CD, Fallat LM: Puncture wounds: Therapeutic considerations and a new classification. *J Foot Surg* 29:147, 1990.

64. Inaba AS, et al: An update of the evaluation and management of plantar puncture wounds and *Pseudomonas* osteomyelitis. *Pediatr Emerg Care* 8:38, 1992.

65. MaGee C, et al: Potentiation of wound infection by surgical drains. *Am J Surg* 131:547, 1976.

66. Edlich RF, et al: Technical factors in wound management. In Hunt TK (ed): *Fundamentals of Wound Management.* New York, Appleton-Century-Crofts, 1979.

67. Hutchinson JJ, et al: Wound infection under occlusive dressings. *J Hosp Infect* 17:83, 1991.

68. Madden MR: Comparison of an occlusive and a semi-occlusive dressing and the effect of the wound exudate upon keratinocyte proliferation. *J Trauma* 29:924, 1989.

69. Alper JC, Vittimberga G: How and when to apply membrane dressings. *Consultant* 28:142, 1988.

70. Leyden JJ, Sulzberger MB: Topical antibiotics and minor skin trauma. *Am Fam Physician* 23:121, 1981.

71. Davis RH, et al: Oral and topical activity of aloe vera. *J Am Podiatr Med Assoc* 79:559, 1989.

72. Chrintz H, et al: Need for surgical wound dressing. *Br J Surg* 76:204, 1989.

73. Seaman M, Lammers R: Inability of patients to self-diagnose wound infections. *J Emerg Med* 9:215, 1991.

74. Noe JM: Can stitches get wet? *Plast Reconstr Surg* 81:82, 1988.

75. Summary of notifiable diseases in the United States, 1998. *MMWR Morb Mortal Wkly Rep* 47:1-93, 1999.

76. Stair TO: Tetanus immunity in emergency department patients. *Am J Emerg Med* 7:563, 1989.

77. Edwards KM: Diphtheria, tetanus, and pertussis immunizations in adults. *Infect Dis Clin North Am* 4:85, 1990.

78. Briggs GG, Freeman RK, Yaffe SJ: *Drugs in Pregnancy and Lactation.* Baltimore, Williams & Wilkins, 1986.

57 Foreign Bodies

Stephen H. Thomas and David F. M. Brown

PERSPECTIVE

History

When people ingest or insert foreign bodies, a brief history might be sufficient to guide management and predict the process required for definitive resolution. The technical intervention required for foreign body removal may be more complex, sometimes requiring substantial expertise. Cases involving a toddler who coughs persistently after eating peanuts or a psychiatric patient with abdominal pain and a history of ingesting foreign objects should be diagnosed easily and rapidly. Sometimes the presence of a foreign body might require a meticulous history and insightful care, however. Some people are at higher risk to have a foreign body present, such as neurologically impaired patients, edentulous individuals, patients with certain psychiatric diagnoses, incarcerated individuals, and individuals at the extremes of age. In this same group, definitive history is not obtained easily.[1] Sometimes the clinician must use situational clues: A toddler left alone with an infant may have inserted a foreign body, or a prisoner with abdominal cramps may have ingested a foreign body for secondary gain. Even when patients are fully cooperative, the diagnosis of foreign body ingestion or insertion can be difficult. The presentation may be for a seemingly unrelated problem, and sequelae from foreign bodies may be delayed by months, years, or even decades.[2]

Physical Examination

Depending on the location of the foreign body, the physical examination can provide direct or indirect evidence of foreign bodies or their complications. Specifics are described in the following sections, but a recurring theme is that meticulous examination frequently aids in providing a diagnosis.

Diagnostic Imaging

Plain radiography, classically the primary technique used for foreign body detection, is often the test of first choice. In appropriate circumstances, plain films can aid determination of the location, size, and number of foreign objects present. Even when the foreign body is not visualized, radiographs may show secondary changes (e.g., pulmonary air trapping) providing clues to foreign body presence. To assist in the localization of the object, two views—anteroposterior and lateral—are usually necessary. Objects such as metal or gravel, which are denser than the tissue in which they are embedded, usually are easy to visualize on plain radiographs. Organic material, which has a density similar to that of human tissue, may not be seen on plain films.

PRINCIPLES OF DISEASE

When the foreign body is localized, it usually is removed, either in the emergency department or in specialized areas, such as interventional radiology, endoscopy, or operating suites. Although foreign body removal is not always feasible or desirable, extraction is indicated in most cases. Removal frequently is vexing for the physician and the patient, so an initial discussion outlining the need for the procedure is recommended.

When the foreign body represents an immediate threat to the patient, as is the case with an airway foreign body, the need for urgent extraction is obvious. Trauma-related foreign bodies, such as knives and bullets, pose important management issues (see other trauma chapters). Even in cases in which no immediate life threat exists, some foreign bodies should be removed because of the threat of injury from the nature or constituents of the foreign body. Cocaine can kill a body packer,[3] an impacted button battery can cause fatal electrochemical tissue damage,[4] and an insect can damage otic structures.[5]

In the absence of immediate life threat or constituent-related foreign body danger, additional complications can occur. In luminal obstruction, the foreign body may become lodged and may exert pressure on the adjacent tissue, risking necrosis and perforation. The object also may serve as a nidus for infection that is recurrent or refractory to treatment until removal of the foreign body. These patients often seek medical attention for secondary symptoms. Specific recommendations for foreign body removal are presented in the following sections outlining foreign body management by anatomic location.

EYE

Clinical Features

Although wooden and metallic fragments are found most frequently, ophthalmic foreign objects vary from dust particles to lost contact lenses to missiles associated with penetrating trauma.[6] The diagnosis usually is

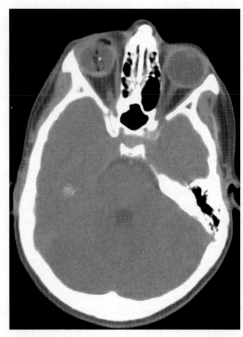

Figure 57-1. Computed tomography scan shows right intraocular foreign body (BB pellet) in intoxicated patient without known trauma history.

self-evident. Extraocular and intraocular foreign bodies may be subtle in presentation, however, with mild symptoms and uncharacteristic histories involving seemingly trivial trauma, such as brushing against a bush or falling. In some cases, foreign bodies are identified in intoxicated patients who present with an abnormal ocular examination and no known history of trauma (Figure 57-1). Emergency department presentation can be delayed by days or even years after the initial incident.[6,7] Early diagnosis and appropriate care and follow-up minimize the risks of delayed sequelae, such as endophthalmitis, which may occur 48 hours after foreign body introduction, or sight-threatening siderosis bulbi.[8,9] Controversy about foreign body removal (and its timing) has not diminished the importance of making the initial diagnosis.

History

Most patients complain of a foreign body sensation (often on blinking) and cannot see the foreign body. If the object is corneal, the patient may be able to see something in the visual field or may see the foreign body when looking in the mirror. The patient also may complain of tearing and conjunctival reddening. Foreign bodies that create corneal injury and are no longer present may account for symptoms identical to those noted in the presence of a foreign body. Additionally, patients may present with symptoms in the absence of any history of known foreign body. In these cases, the occupational and social history, including pets and hobbies, may shed light on the diagnosis. Another important component of the history is whether radial keratotomy has been performed. This procedure is associated with potential for foreign body entrap-

ment in the corneal incisions, which can gape 6 years postprocedure.[10]

Physical Examination

The initial survey should include standard elements of emergency department eye examination. Early visual acuity is an important predictor of final visual outcome in cases of intraocular foreign body.[11] During slit-lamp examination, the emergency physician may detect a corneal foreign body by the shadow it casts on the iris. The slit lamp also can facilitate identification of rust rings, and fluorescein can aid in detecting abraded corneal epithelium. The inner aspects of both lids must be examined. The upper lid should be everted by instructing the patient to look downward while upward traction on the eyelashes is applied and an applicator stick is placed, to act as a fulcrum, on the proximal edge of the tarsal plate. Multiple small foreign bodies can be overlooked. After locating and removing one foreign body, the examiner should continue with a complete examination.

Diagnostic Strategies

The foreign body may have penetrated the anterior eye structures and entered the globe (see Figure 57-1). If the history and mechanism of injury are compatible with ocular penetration, or if a small wound of the globe is noted, anteroposterior and lateral radiographs of the orbit are a reasonable initial step when the foreign body is thought to be radiopaque.[12] Computed tomography (CT) is a preferred first choice when intraocular penetration is strongly suspected because of the multiple advantages of spiral CT.[8,13] Scanning time is faster, less radiation is delivered to the lens, and multiplanar reconstruction minimizes streak artifacts and affords better localization of intraorbital objects. Fluorescein staining ordinarily is avoided when penetration of the globe is clear because it may make further evaluation or surgery more difficult. In cases when penetration has not been suspected, however, the identification of rivulets of fluorescein tracking from the puncture are helpful in identifying the fact that intraocular penetration has occurred.

Two ultrasound techniques can be useful in searching for foreign bodies. Standard B-scan ultrasound has been shown to detect foreign bodies missed on ophthalmologic examination and missed or not fully characterized on other imaging studies.[7,9] The newer technique of ultrasound biomicroscopy has been shown to be extremely helpful in foreign body imaging. The sensitivity of this modality is sufficiently high that it detects foreign bodies not visible by direct or indirect ophthalmologic examination, traditional B-scan ultrasound, or CT.[12] Owing to a lack of reported case series and justifiable concerns about eye damage from mobilization of ferromagnetic foreign objects,[14] use of magnetic resonance imaging (MRI) for ophthalmologic foreign body imaging is controversial.[8,15]

In some cases, orbital trauma is associated with central nervous system injury. When the workup indicates a potential for injury or foreign body involving

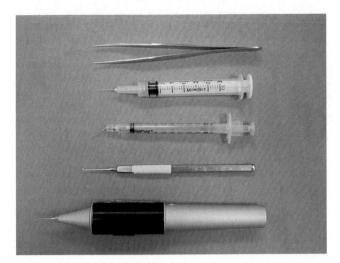

Figure 57-2. Instruments for removal of an ocular foreign object: forceps, needle (straight or bent) mounted on a syringe "handle," angled eye spud, and rotating straight-tip eye spud.

the brain, imaging of the intracranial compartment should be obtained.[16]

Management

In nearly all cases, therapy is removal of the foreign body. If the object is located on the bulbar or palpebral conjunctiva (*not* the cornea), it often can be removed easily by sweeping the site with a moist cotton-tipped applicator. Usually, other instruments are required (Figure 57-2). Occasionally, if the foreign body is large, it may be extracted with forceps. For small corneal foreign bodies, after applying topical anesthesia, it is often necessary to use an eye spud or small-gauge needle to move gently underneath one end of the object and pick it out, preferably under magnification. If this is unsuccessful or if the foreign body is deeply embedded, the patient should be referred for object removal. This is particularly true with metallic foreign bodies, where early removal decreases the size of the rust ring. Too-vigorous attempts at removal may cause anterior chamber perforation. It also is prudent to avoid significant corneal procedures in patients who have had a laser-assisted in situ keratomileusis (LASIK) procedure for nearsightedness, given the increased risks.

After the removal of a corneal foreign body that leaves no rust ring, treatment is essentially the same as for corneal abrasion. In cases in which foreign bodies may have elicited an allergic response, topical steroids have been employed. Therapy of patients with a rust ring is controversial, but it is prudent to recommend evaluation within 24 to 48 hours by an ophthalmologist to consider removal.

EAR

Clinical Features

Foreign bodies of the ear are more likely to prove problematic for the emergency physician than foreign bodies in other locations. This is not caused by diag-nostic difficulty, but by problems associated with removal of objects from a sensitive anatomic area in an often uncooperative patient population.[17] In terms of specific objects found in ears, different series list varying culprits. Most reports prominently feature insects, beans, plastic toys, and small spherical objects such as pearls, pebbles, or beads.[17,18]

History

Patients usually state something is in the ear. If the foreign body is an insect, the patient may feel motion or hear buzzing, although less specific complaints may include itching, discharge, or otalgia. Similar secondary symptoms may be present when noninsect foreign bodies are lodged in the ear canal. This type of presentation is especially common in children, who may fear telling of foreign object insertion into the ear; the problem is ignored until secondary problems prompt an emergency department visit.

In patients with ear complaints and travel or camping history or poor living conditions, specific information may suggest insects inhabiting the external ear canal. Infestation with Korean mites, Malaysian ticks, and Omani beetles has been associated with varying degrees of morbidity in patients spending time in those regions.[5,19] In most U.S. cases, the cockroach is the culprit.[17-19]

Patients with ear foreign bodies may present with secondary symptoms related to pathology in structures adjacent to otic structures. Malocclusion may be the chief complaint if the foreign body erodes to the temporomandibular joint.[20] Similar erosion has caused otic foreign bodies to manifest as eustachian tube dysfunction, parapharyngeal abscess, or mastoiditis with progression to fatal brain abscess and meningitis.[21,22] Such events are rare. The emergency physician should ask patients about prior attempts at foreign body removal. These efforts may have injured the ear canal; caused tympanic membrane perforation; pushed the foreign body deeper into the canal; or caused enlargement of the foreign object, especially if it is vegetable matter.

Physical Examination

The external auditory canal is cylindrical with an elliptic cross section (Figure 57-3). A thin layer of sensitive epithelium covers an outermost cartilaginous portion and an inner bony segment. There are two anatomic points of narrowing (and foreign object lodging) within the canal: (1) near the inner end of the cartilaginous portion of the canal and (2) at the point of bony narrowing called the *isthmus.*

The first factor crucial to successful examination is adequate lighting that can be directed by the emergency physician. This may be a strong light source and a head mirror, a headlamp, an operating otoscope, or an operating microscope. A large-size speculum is essential to obtain an adequate field of view and to enable four-quadrant injection of local ear canal anesthesia when necessary for foreign body removal. As with any examination involving the external auditory canal, the emergency physician should grasp the pinna of the ear and

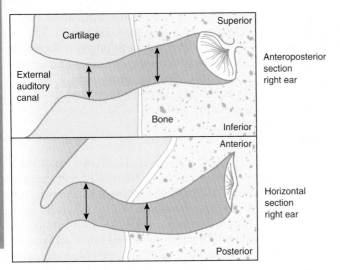

Figure 57-3. Horizontal and vertical cross sections of external ear canal showing points of anatomic narrowing.

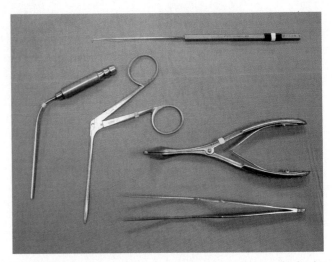

Figure 57-4. Instruments that may be useful for removal of a foreign body from ear canal or nares: right-angle probe, suction catheter, alligator forceps, nasal speculum, and bayonet forceps.

retract it in a posterosuperior direction to straighten the canal and afford a more complete view of the canal and tympanic membrane.

Inspection of the tympanic membrane is important because it may have been ruptured by the foreign object or by prior removal attempts.[5,23] If so, medical documentation should indicate that this was present before attempts at foreign object removal. If one foreign object is identified in the ear canal or in the nose, the emergency physician must search for additional objects in the ears or nose, given the risk of multiple objects.[23,24]

Diagnostic Strategies

Diagnostic imaging rarely plays a role in the emergency department workup of suspected otic foreign bodies. The primary indication is to identify complications from foreign body presence. CT or MRI may be performed to characterize infectious or erosive sequelae of ear canal foreign objects.

Management

The emergency physician should inform the patient about the extreme sensitivity of the auditory passage and the likely discomfort and potential for minor bleeding. Sedation may be important to minimize patient discomfort and reduce risks of iatrogenic trauma. Less often, foreign body removal requires local anesthesia of the external ear canal. This procedure, which may cause patient discomfort and iatrogenic injury, is performed by injecting all four quadrants of the canal with lidocaine using a tuberculin syringe inserted through the otic speculum. In most cases of a refractory foreign body and an uncooperative patient, definitive management should be performed in the operating room under general anesthesia.

When the ear canal is inhabited by an insect, it is important to kill or immobilize the insect to facilitate its removal. Immobilization reduces the chance of patient discomfort or ear damage caused by an insect attempting to evade forceps introduced into the ear

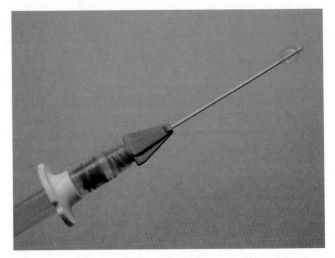

Figure 57-5. Balloon-tipped catheter that can be used for removal of otic or nasal foreign bodies.

canal. Different immobilizing agents have different reported success rates. Efficacious formulations include lidocaine as a 10% spray or less concentrated liquid, 2% lidocaine gel, mineral oil with 2% or 4% lidocaine, and alcohol.[5]

Several extrication methods may prove effective, and various instruments may be useful (Figure 57-4). Small objects often can be removed by the application of suction with a small plastic catheter. With soft or irregularly shaped objects, it is often possible to grasp the foreign body with forceps (alligator forceps may be best) and remove it either in one piece or in fragments. If the object cannot be grasped, it may be possible to remove it by passing a blunt-tipped right-angle hook beyond the foreign body and gently coaxing it out. Alternatively a balloon-tipped catheter can be passed distal to the object, with subsequent attempts to withdraw the (inflated) balloon and extract the object (Figure 57-5).

Indirect methods for foreign body removal also have been used with some success. The irrigation technique takes advantage of the elliptic shape of the external ear canal. A stream of warm water should be directed at the foreign body's periphery, with the hope that the jet of water will be directed past the object, against the tympanic membrane, and finally against the posterior aspect of the foreign body, driving it out of the canal. One report of an electric ear syringe found that it outperformed other techniques in removal of foreign bodies from the ear canal.[25] There were no significant complications using the technique, and it was well tolerated by children and adults. The emergency physician should use a room-temperature irrigant and consider complications of foreign body enlargement if the object can expand when wet (e.g., beans, seeds). This modality should not be used if there is a known history of or clinically suspected tympanic membrane perforation.

Removal of objects from the middle ear with cyano-acrylate adhesive–tipped swabs has been recommended in the past. This technique carries the risk, however, of contaminating the ear canal with a substance that is difficult to remove and has been associated with tympanic membrane rupture.[26,27] Insufficient evidence exists to condone or condemn this technique.

If these methods are unsuccessful or if the patient, especially a child, is uncooperative or in too much distress, the emergency physician should cease removal efforts and refer the patient to an otolaryngologist. Primary operative intervention frequently is indicated in very young children and in patients in whom the emergency physician and the ear-nose-throat (ENT) physician believe nonsurgical attempts are unlikely to be successful. In one series, nearly one third of pediatric patients with foreign bodies had the objects removed at surgery.[18]

Inappropriately prolonged efforts at foreign object removal can result in wasted time, unnecessary patient discomfort, and high potential for complications. Prolonged or inexpert attempts at foreign body removal incur several potential risks. Increasing patient apprehension, distal foreign body displacement, ear canal or tympanic membrane damage, and induction of localized tissue edema may necessitate surgical intervention when otherwise unnecessary.[17,28]

Otic foreign bodies are associated with many sequelae, but these are usually not serious. The most common effects in one series, all occurring in approximately 1 in 10 pediatric patients, were ear canal laceration, otitis externa, and cervical adenitis. Noniatrogenic tympanic membrane perforation was rare.[17]

After removal of the foreign body, canal examination should be repeated to ensure the lack of retained material and to evaluate otic anatomy. In cases in which the tympanic membrane is ruptured and the middle ear is at risk for infection, appropriate oral antibiotics are recommended. Topical antimicrobial therapy decreases the risk of external otitis; one method packs the meatus with ribbon gauze impregnated with a broad-spectrum antibiotic.[5] Follow-up evaluation should occur within 2 to 3 days.

NOSE

Clinical Features

The nose is perhaps the most common site for the insertion of foreign bodies by children.[29] The foreign bodies most often found include beans, sponge pieces, pebbles, plastic toy fragments, and other small round objects.[30] Perhaps because most people are right-handed, more than two thirds of nasal foreign bodies were right-sided in one series.[24] Compared with patients with ear canal foreign bodies, children with nasal foreign bodies tend to be younger (most commonly <5 years old).[23,24]

Nasal foreign bodies are less problematic than foreign bodies in other locations. Serious sequelae are rare. The infrequent intranasal alkaline button battery, which may cause electrical or chemical burns with liquefaction necrosis, is an exception to this rule.[23,30-32]

History

Although most patients seek medical attention within 24 hours, patients with nasal (versus ear canal) foreign bodies are more likely to present with secondary symptoms and delays of 1 week.[23] Nasal foreign bodies may be asymptomatic, sometimes identified as incidental findings on radiographs.

Patients seen in the emergency department with nasal foreign bodies usually have one of two histories. With the first type of presentation, the patient admits to, or is seen, placing an intranasal object. This is the most common history. Other patients present with a constellation of signs and symptoms: purulent, unilateral, malodorous nasal discharge or even persistent epistaxis. These patients often are misdiagnosed and treated with antibiotics for supposed sinusitis. Unresolving sinusitis despite appropriate antibiotic therapy should alert the emergency physician to the possibility of nasal foreign body.[23,24]

Foreign objects placed intranasally may purposefully or inadvertently end up in the sinuses. These foreign bodies require more invasive intervention, and psychiatric evaluation of the patient may be indicated when self-injury is suspected. When the history suggests a foreign body, but none is identified on nares examination, the emergency physician should consider imaging the sinuses.

Physical Examination

As with foreign bodies of the ear canal, it is important to prepare the patient (and the parents) for examination and subsequent removal attempts. Because of risks of iatrogenic movement of the foreign body further posteriorly or into the airway, children may need to be restrained to permit the examination. Physical examination sometimes can be delayed until after insufflation of the nares is attempted. The nasal mucosa is normally quite sensitive, and this sensitivity is increased by any infection or irritation. Examination is facilitated by provision of topical anesthesia and vasoconstriction to the nasal mucosa. Examination should include both nares, with adequate lighting and visualization with a nasal speculum. The emergency physician should note the presence of the foreign body and any secondary tissue damage. Necrosis of the nasal mucosa and septum may accompany button battery impaction.[32] During the examination, the emergency physician should take care not to dislodge or drive the foreign body posteriorly into the nasopharynx and risk aspiration. In some circumstances, it may be prudent to place patients in the lateral decubitus position, perhaps with additional Trendelenburg angulation, to help prevent aspiration of objects that are pushed into the posterior pharynx.

Diagnostic Strategies

Diagnostic imaging does not play a major role. When intrasinus foreign bodies are suspected, CT can be helpful. Rarely, CT or MRI may be indicated to visualize suspected foreign bodies or their complications.

Management

The emergency physician can remove most nasal foreign bodies effectively. Although the avoidance of iatrogenic injury is paramount, the structures local to an intranasal foreign body are not as sensitive or easily damaged as structures in other body cavities (e.g., the ear canal) that may harbor foreign objects. As a result, the need for subspecialty consultation and operating room removal is relatively rare.[23,24,30]

In some cases, positive pressure applied to the patient's mouth achieves rapid foreign body dislodgment while obviating the need for restraint, sedation, and other requirements attendant to more invasive removal techniques. This technique is a quick and safe primary intervention. The underlying principle is that a short burst of air blown into the mouth of a child, with finger occlusion of the nonobstructed naris, may force the foreign object out of the nose. Pretreatment with vasoconstrictive spray may improve chances of success.[33] The insufflation is preferably applied as a "kiss" from a parent, but also can be provided by a manual ventilation bag. The insufflation technique is quite useful, particularly in preschoolers who are likely to be uncooperative with other removal modalities. Many children can be instructed to take a deep breath and blow hard through their nose, as a parent closes the unaffected naris. An otherwise troublesome removal usually can be accomplished quickly and easily.[29,33,34]

When positive-pressure insufflation is not warranted or is unsuccessful, instruments and removal techniques may be required (see Figures 57-4 and 57-5).[30] Regardless of the method, the patient (usually a child) may benefit from some combination of restraint, sedation, and pretreatment with vasoconstrictive (e.g., nebulized racemic epinephrine) and anesthetic (e.g., benzocaine spray).[33] Adequate illumination is essential. Necessary instruments include a blunt-tipped right-angle probe, suction catheter, and alligator forceps. The forceps are used when the foreign body is to be directly grasped,

and the right-angle probe is used in an attempt to reach proximal to the foreign object and displace it forward. Other useful instruments include Fogarty vascular and Foley catheters; "specialized" balloon-tipped catheters also are available in many emergency departments (see Figure 57-5).[24,30] Suction is primarily necessary for removing purulent secretions and any blood that may obscure the field. In some cases, suction can be used to withdraw foreign bodies directly. Suction may be useful with hard-to-grasp objects or small soft objects not tightly lodged in place.

AIRWAY

Clinical Features

Although improved diagnostic and therapeutic techniques have reduced substantially fatality rates from foreign body inhalation, airway tract foreign objects still cause significant mortality and anoxic brain damage.[35,36] Approximately 3000 patients annually die from asphyxia related to foreign object aspiration.[37]

Alternatively, airway foreign objects can present less dramatically than acute respiratory distress and can go undiagnosed for years.[38,39] Delay is common. Only half of patients in one pediatric series of lower respiratory tract foreign body presented within 1 day of aspiration; an additional 20% presented during the first week, and another 20% presented after a delay of more than 1 week.[35] Patients with uncharacteristic presentations may have unusual foreign body introduction mechanisms, such as ingestion or penetrating trauma.[40] Patients with altered mental status from a variety of etiologies are at risk for occult aspiration, which may be difficult to diagnose (Figure 57-6).

Airway foreign bodies include pins, needles, jewelry, thermometers, pencils, and metal and plastic toys. The primary reason to characterize the type of air-

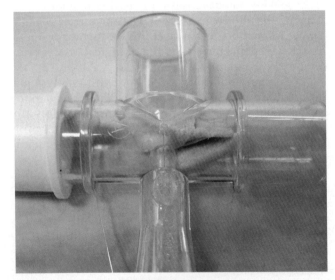

Figure 57-6. Chewing gum found on introduction of suction catheter placed through an endotracheal tube, in a patient found unresponsive after opioid overdose.

way foreign object is to determine the likelihood of radiopacity. Most airway foreign bodies are not visible with plain films.[40] In one 8-year pediatric series of foreign body aspiration, the most commonly identified objects were nuts (59%) or other vegetable material (23%) not likely to be visualized on plain films.[41] In another classic paper describing childhood asphyxiation with foreign bodies, nearly half of fatal choking cases were due to food aspiration, with hot dogs (17%), candy (10%), nuts (9%), and grapes (8%) most prominent.[42] In another report, more than 90% of pediatric aspiration cases were of organic (usually nut) classification.[43]

Airway foreign bodies are seen more commonly in pediatric patients. In one case series covering 2 decades, 75% of patients were younger than 9 years old.[43] Peak incidence of aspiration is in the second year of life, with a brisk decline after age 3.[43,44] Mastication difficulty secondary to premature molar teeth contributes to pediatric food aspiration.[35] Also, the fact that children explore their environment with their hands and mouth translates into aspiration of nonfood objects. In adults, the peak aspiration incidence is in the 60s.[43] Adults are more likely than children to have nonfood items aspirated into the airway.[44]

Children and adults also differ with respect to anatomic location of aspirated foreign bodies. This is crucial because foreign body location plays a major role in determining associated morbidity or mortality risk. In adults, 75% of foreign bodies lodge in the proximal airways (larynx, trachea, main bronchi). In children, less than half of foreign objects are located proximally, with bronchial tree locations the most common.[43]

Foreign bodies can be located as proximally as the oropharynx, with retained intraoral bodies having been found in the medial pterygoid space.[45] The foreign object can be slightly distal, causing airway obstruction at the laryngeal or subglottic level. Foreign body impaction at this level often is caused by inappropriately executed attempts to finger sweep an oropharyngeal foreign body.[44] Subglottic foreign bodies are difficult to identify and may be associated with diagnostic delay in most cases.[46] The emergency physician must be able to glean historical clues to differentiate epiglottitis, asthma, and laryngotracheobronchitis from subglottic foreign body.

Airway foreign bodies usually pass beyond the laryngeal inlet[44] and may cause drastic obstruction. Tracheal foreign bodies have a surprisingly high incidence of lack of symptoms or worrisome clinical findings, however.[41] Foreign bodies passing beyond the trachea are less likely to cause acute hypoxic crisis, but can cause substantial respiratory embarrassment and can be difficult to remove. In adults, bronchial foreign bodies are found more often in the right bronchial tree. In one large series, 69% of bronchial foreign bodies were right sided.[43] Because the main bronchi branch from the trachea at more equal angles in children, the left-right distribution of lower airway foreign bodies is approximately equal.[35,41] Foreign objects can be bilateral, with 3.6% of patients in one series having foreign bodies in right and left main bronchi.[43]

History

Clinical presentation can range from chronic nonspecific respiratory complaints to acute airway obstruction.[35] In most aspiration cases, foreign body presence is suspected after a thorough history. In the most dramatic cases, patients have a history of what is commonly termed the "cafe coronary." The patient attempts to swallow a food (usually meat) bolus larger than the esophagus can accept. The bolus lodges in the hypopharynx or trachea. Often there is confusion over whether the patient is having a myocardial infarction or has an obstructing foreign body, but the conscious cardiac patient is able to speak. Patients with airway foreign bodies may have noisy breathing, inspiratory stridor, vomiting, and possibly slight hemoptysis.[44]

Some patients may give a history similar to cafe coronary, with resolution of major symptoms. These symptoms, known as the *penetration syndrome,* occur in half of patients aspirating and include a choking sensation accompanied by respiratory distress with coughing, wheezing, and dyspnea.[43] Symptom resolution may result from the patient spontaneously clearing the foreign body by coughing. In some cases, coughing does not eject the foreign body completely, but rather impacts it in the subglottic region.[44] The emergency physician should maintain concern for retained airway foreign object in cases in which the patient history is one of perceived foreign body followed by cough with incomplete (or even complete) posttussive symptom resolution.

In a 20-year series of adult and pediatric patients with suspected foreign body aspiration, sudden onset of choking and intractable cough were present in half, with eventual foreign body identification.[43] In addition to coughing and choking, stridor is a frequent component of an acute aspiration episode in patients of all ages.[44] Symptom distribution is similar in adult and pediatric patients,[43] but choking and wheezing appear more prominently in the pediatric literature. In one series of 87 pediatric patients with suspected foreign body, 96% had a history of a choking crisis.[41] Wheezing has been reported in 75% of patients age 8 to 66 months with airway foreign bodies.[35]

Most patients aspirating objects have persistent symptoms (e.g., cough, wheezing, dyspnea) after manifesting penetration syndrome, but 20% have no ongoing symptoms.[43] Many patients have a history of alarming symptoms followed by few ongoing complaints; the emergency physician should not dismiss aspirated foreign body from consideration in such patients. With sudden onset of dyspnea and odynophagia, an impacted subglottic object may be present. If the object is known to be sharp and thin, the emergency physician should suspect embedding between the vocal cords or in the subglottic region, with resultant partial obstruction.[44]

Other components of the history may provide clues to airway foreign body presence and location. Even when the history cannot be obtained directly or does not suggest aspirated foreign object, the emergency physician can infer foreign body presence in certain patients. Trauma patients who present to the emergency department with injured and loose teeth may aspirate teeth during emergency laryngoscopy and oral intubation.[43] Besides the intubated or obtunded patient with only indirect historical evidence of aspiration (see Figure 57-6), conscious and alert patients may not give a direct history of aspiration owing to lack of dramatic airway symptoms or remoteness of the aspiration event and secondary problems (e.g., pneumonia). In some cases, such as penetrating trauma or blast injuries, the patient may be unaware of the potential for aspiration and not attribute symptoms to this entity.[40] Patients aspirating needles may have minimal or no symptoms, with chronic hemoptysis or odynophagia the only manifestation of these or similar foreign bodies.[43,44]

There is conflicting evidence regarding the role of neurologic disease in aspiration. Patients with deficits may be unaware or unable to report problems such as denture displacement; this inability has been associated with disastrous results in the case of airway obstruction from dental hardware.[47] Neurologic impairment may result in atypical or absent histories in cases of foreign body aspiration.[40] Reports of adult[43] and pediatric[41] series have identified little role, however, for neurologic impairment in foreign body aspiration. An atypical history is a concern in neurologically impaired patients, but the problem of foreign body aspiration with atypical history is uncommon in this patient population.

The child with respiratory difficulty after eating can represent a diagnostic dilemma. Children with stridor or other respiratory symptoms may have esophageal bolus impaction. The pediatric trachea is soft, especially posteriorly, and may be compressed by a large esophageal body pressing anteriorly on the trachea. In addition, the trachea itself may be displaced anteriorly and kinked, causing a partial obstruction.

Other components of the history can help diagnose and characterize foreign bodies in patients with aspiration of nonfood objects. These items may be aspirated by children who are exploring their environment, by psychiatric patients, or by individuals who normally "store" small items in their mouths. The latter group includes repairmen, construction workers, seamstresses, and others who keep nails, pins, and other paraphernalia in their mouths for quick access.

Regardless of the nature of the foreign body, patients with a retained airway foreign object may present only with infectious complications. A foreign object may cause retropharyngeal abscess. More distally in the airway tract, a patient with atypical or recurrent pneumonia may have pulmonary infection secondary to persistence of a foreign object serving as a nidus of infection. In some cases, the respiratory infection associated with retained pulmonary foreign body is silent, but seeds distant organs with organisms, raising suspicion of an airway foreign body. In patients with *Eikenella corrodens* brain abscess, clinically occult respiratory foreign bodies have been found.[48]

Patients may present to the emergency department with diagnoses of diseases thought to be infectious but actually have foreign bodies in the airway. A careful history should be obtained in the setting of suspected croup or epiglottitis because a foreign body in the trachea or larynx may have a clinical presentation similar to these infectious entities.

Physical Examination

Physical findings depend on degree of airway obstruction and duration of the object's presence in the respiratory system. Small objects causing no obstruction may produce no findings or may manifest as infectious complications. In many cases, however, the physical assessment is helpful in diagnosis and characterization of airway foreign bodies.

Cyanosis is present in 10% of patients, and coughing, audible wheezing, or overt respiratory distress occurs in 25% to 37% of patients with aspirated objects.[43] Patients may be stridorous or hoarse with upper airway foreign objects, and sternal retractions may be noted in patients with intratracheal foreign bodies.[49,50] More than half of children in one series had initial oxygen saturation values of 95% or less.[43] Patients with secondary infection may have fever.

Oropharyngeal examination may reveal a foreign body posteriorly or "donor sites" of fractured teeth. The examination should include a search for fractured or missing dental prostheses, which sometimes can be lodged in pharyngeal areas for days and can account for sudden deterioration in status when the airway becomes occluded, as can occur after coughing.[47] Oropharyngeal examination frequently can be augmented by indirect or direct laryngoscopy or nasopharyngoscopy. These procedures should be performed only with ready availability of definitive airway management necessities and should be postponed or omitted when the emergency physician believes that the stress of the procedure could risk airway compromise. The advantage of these modalities is that they allow excellent visualization of the proximal airway, which is important diagnostically and therapeutically. Indirect laryngoscopy can prove useful in detection of radiolucent structures.

Assessment of the neck may reveal accessory muscle use. Tracheal palpation may reveal a thud, indicating movement of a mobile foreign body against the tracheal wall. Abnormal inspiratory sounds may be heard on tracheal auscultation.[44] Coughing may result from local irritation caused by bronchial foreign bodies. Localized or apparently generalized wheezing was noted on auscultation in half of patients with lower respiratory tract foreign bodies in one pediatric series.[35] The emergency physician should keep in mind the dictum that "all that wheezes is not asthma." If a main stem bronchus is completely obstructed, breath sounds are absent on the involved side. Occasionally a foreign body acts as a one-way valve, allowing air into the lung during inspiration, but permitting none to exit during expiration. The involved lung becomes hyperexpanded, which may be detected as hyperresonance to percussion.

Diagnostic Imaging

In the stable patient, plain radiography of the neck and chest remains the mainstay of airway foreign body imaging.[40] Air trapping may be shown when inspiratory and expiratory films are compared. Other imaging techniques of potential utility are fluoroscopy, CT, and MRI, although bronchoscopy and microlaryngoscopy remain the ultimate diagnostic maneuvers.[49]

A normal radiograph cannot rule out an aspirated foreign body in a patient with a suggestive history. Plain films have been reported to provide 10% false-negative and 10% false-positive rates.[41,43] In another series of 87 patients with suspected aspiration, 70 of whom had objects confirmed on bronchoscopy, overall sensitivity and specificity of plain radiography were 70.3% and 62.5%. X-ray findings were indirect in most cases; radiopaque foreign bodies were found in only a few cases. This series included foreign bodies in the upper airway (at the level of the trachea); plain radiographs in these patients were frequently negative.[41] If doubt exists as to the radiopacity of the suspected foreign body, and if the patient has brought a piece of the object, it may be tested for radiodensity by placing it over the shoulder during taking of the radiographs. Specific findings on plain radiography are categorized as direct (i.e., identification of the foreign body itself) or indirect (e.g., hyperinflation). Direct foreign body identification is relatively uncommon.[44] When subglottic foreign body impaction is suspected, plain soft tissue radiographs of the neck are the best initial step, provided that they are performed under the close supervision of a physician trained in provision of airway management. In some of these patients, plain radiography may definitively show an intratracheal foreign body and can provide a rapid diagnosis.[44]

Indirect or secondary signs, such as narrowing of the subglottic space from an embedded foreign object, are an important aid in foreign body radiography.[44] Air trapping and atelectasis are the most common early clues to airway foreign body presence, with bronchiectasis and bronchial stenosis developing later.[40] In air trapping, a comparison of inspiratory and expiratory films shows a flat, fixed diaphragm on the involved side, and the heart and mediastinum shift to the uninvolved side during expiration (Figure 57-7). In one pediatric series, air trapping was found in 90% of patients with lower airway foreign bodies.[35] The small caliber of the airways may explain the relatively higher frequency of air trapping in children compared with adult patients.[43] If obstruction becomes complete, the involved lung becomes atelectatic; patients with persistent atelectasis should have foreign objects considered as the explanation. An additional indirect radiographic sign of more proximal foreign bodies is prevertebral swelling or soft tissue emphysema seen on neck films.[40]

When a foreign body is seen on the chest radiograph, but its exact location (airway or esophagus) is in doubt, the anteroposterior orientation of the object may help (Figure 57-8). Esophageal foreign bodies usually are oriented in the coronal plane (Figure 57-9), with airway objects oriented in the sagittal plane (Figure 57-10). X-rays also can provide useful information by showing whether the object is within, or outside of, the tracheal air column (Figure 57-11; see Figures 57-9 and 57-10).

Fluoroscopy was used historically, but has been largely supplanted by advances in bronchoscopy. Fluoroscopy has identified air trapping, but one case series reported a relatively low 77% sensitivity for foreign body presence using this finding.[35,40] CT, especially

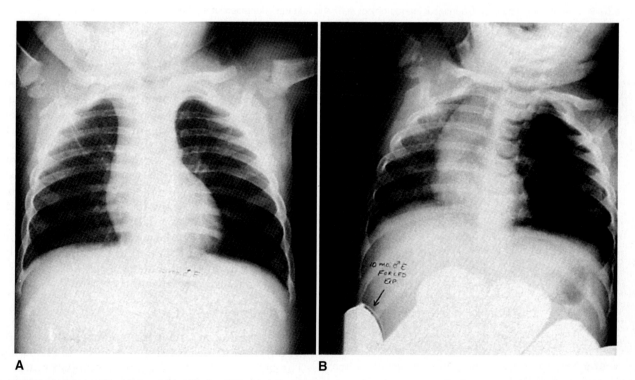

A   **B**

Figure 57-7. A, "Normal" inspiratory chest film in child with left main stem bronchus foreign body. **B,** Forced expiratory view shows expanded lung on the left with shift of mediastinum to uninvolved right side.

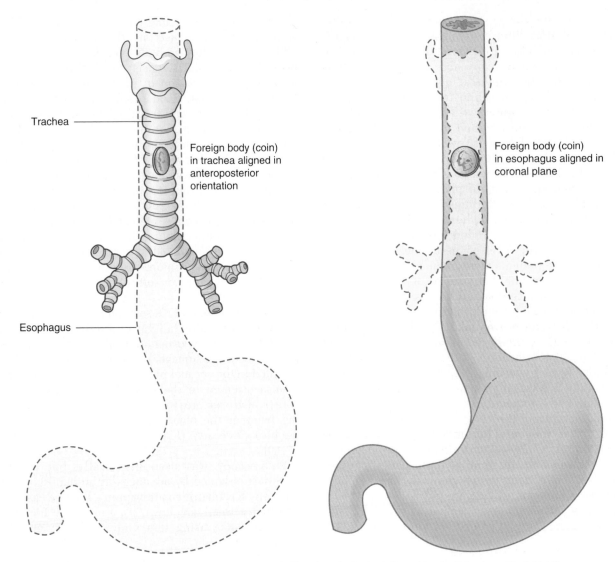

Trachea

Foreign body (coin)
in trachea aligned in
anteroposterior
orientation

Esophagus

Foreign body (coin)
in esophagus aligned in
coronal plane

Figure 57-8. Coronal orientation of esophageal foreign object *(left)* and sagittal orientation of tracheal foreign object *(right).*

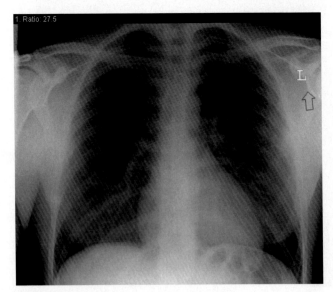

Figure 57-9. Esophageal foreign body (pull tab from beer can), oriented in the coronal plane.

helical, is useful in evaluating patients with suspected airway foreign bodies when plain films are negative. Even when an aspirated object is radiolucent, and often when the object cannot be identified by standard thoracic CT, helical CT has visualized the foreign body when it is of greater density than surrounding tissues. Helical CT can obviate the need for diagnostic flexible bronchoscopy, allowing direct progression to therapeutic rigid bronchoscopy for foreign object identification. CT also can be useful in delineating specific anatomic changes caused by foreign bodies. MRI may be useful in cases of aspiration of nuts, especially in children. The high fat content of the nut translates to its relatively easy visualization on MRI.[40]

Management

Management of an airway tract foreign body is removal, which generally leads to rapid recovery of the patient.[43] The emergency physician can accomplish removal in some patients. When the foreign object is distal to the oropharynx, however, subspecialty consultation is the

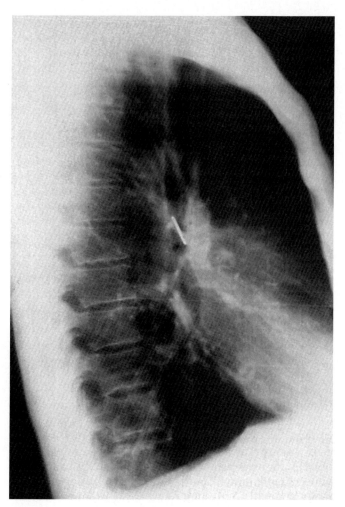

Figure 57-10. Lateral x-ray study of chest shows aspirated coin in tracheal air column.

safest and most expeditious means for foreign body removal. As a general rule, early bronchoscopy in any patient with a suspected foreign body is key to reducing morbidity and mortality.[35]

The emergency physician may need to act definitively in a patient with critical airway obstruction and impending or actual respiratory arrest. The emergency physician has three options: (1) attempt to force the foreign body out with maneuvers, (2) perform laryngoscopy with attempts at removal under direct visualization, or (3) control the patient's airway.

Some maneuvers to remove foreign bodies acutely are accomplished without direct visualization. These attempts may be directed at the proximal or distal respiratory tract. Proximal foreign body removal without direct visualization is attempted using the finger sweep, but this technique is losing favor in pediatric and adult patients. In infants, the larynx is higher, at the level of the fourth cervical vertebra; by age 4 years, it is at the C5-6 level. Blind finger sweeping has resulted in conversion of partial to complete airway obstruction when objects are displaced into the subglottic space. Finger sweeping also is less preferable in adults; abdominal thrusts and back blows are safer and at least as efficacious.[44] These procedures produce increased intraluminal pressure in the trachea and force objects out into the pharynx, from which they are easily removed.[51]

The optimal management of a choking infant is controversial as to whether back blows, chest thrusts, or abdominal thrusts should be the initial intervention. Data are limited, but the American Heart Association, National Academy of Science, American Academy of Pediatrics, and American Thoracic Society recommend

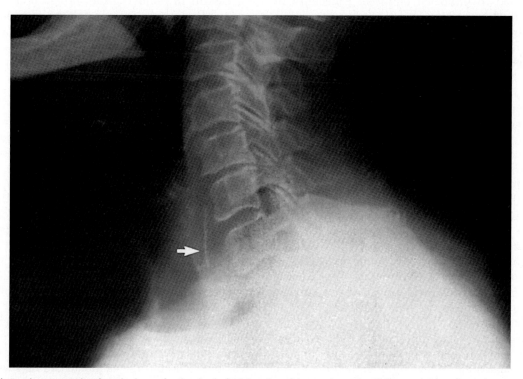

Figure 57-11. Lateral x-ray study of neck shows foreign body (chicken bone) in esophageal soft tissue shadow *(arrow)*.

four back blows with the patient in a head-down position, followed by chest thrusts. Intubation or needle cricothyroidotomy may be performed if consistent with the setting.[52]

If indirect efforts fail to remove foreign bodies from patients in extremis, direct laryngoscopic visualization during intubation may reveal a proximal foreign object that can be removed with Magill forceps. If a foreign body is not visualized on laryngoscopy, the emergency physician may choose to intubate the patient. Intubation may force the foreign body distally, especially if the endotracheal tube tip is passed beyond the carina. Placement of the endotracheal tube into the right main stem bronchus may displace the foreign body into the right bronchus, allowing oxygenation and ventilation through the left-sided pulmonary tree when the endotracheal tube is withdrawn back to normal position proximal to the carina. In cases in which intubation fails because of positioning of the foreign object, surgical cricothyrotomy (needle cricothyrotomy in young children) is indicated. Cricothyrotomy may bypass proximal obstruction and provide sufficient oxygenation to bridge the time gap to definitive care by surgical subspecialists.

Patients who do not require immediate intubation or cricothyrotomy for complete airway obstruction may require airway management for other indications. These patients may have poor oxygenation or may require assisted ventilations during transport to surgery. In either case, if airway obstruction is not too proximal or too complete, the emergency physician should consider placement of a laryngeal mask airway. The laryngeal mask airway offers easy airway access, excellent visualization, and safe respiratory management during bronchoscopic procedures. The laryngeal mask airway allows use of larger bronchoscopes than those employed in intubated children. Especially in pediatric patients requiring bronchoscopy, the laryngeal mask airway may be an appropriate airway.[43]

In noncritical situations, the only airway foreign objects generally amenable to emergency physician removal are those in the oropharynx, which are best removed by forceps under direct laryngoscopic visualization performed after topical anesthesia. Care should be taken when foreign objects appear to be impaled in the oropharynx because postremoval hemorrhage can occur. Also, special care should be taken to prevent posterior displacement of oropharyngeal foreign objects or dropping of incompletely grasped foreign bodies into the airway. These complications are risked in patients who are uncooperative; in these patients, consultation for removal in the operating room is the best course. Removal of a laryngeal foreign object, even with general anesthesia, can be dangerous. Risks include hemorrhage, laryngeal trauma, and airway obstruction from the mobilized foreign object; subspecialty consultation also is indicated for laryngeal foreign body removal.[44]

The management decisions of other subspecialists depend on the clinical presentation but involve fiberoptic (diagnostic) versus rigid bronchoscopy. In patients with lesser overall clinical suspicion, fiberop-

tic bronchoscopy may be indicated, but rigid bronchoscopy is the optimal first step when clinical suspicion is high.[35] Foreign body removal usually is achieved with rigid bronchoscopy under general anesthesia, but in unusual circumstances, flexible bronchoscopy under local anesthesia may suffice for foreign body location and removal.[43]

Even after foreign body removal, sequelae may occur. Airway fish bones, even after removal, can cause deep tissue infection, such as cervical spondylodiskitis.[50] A patient with an airway foreign body should be observed for development of sequelae. In pediatric patients, education should focus on preventive efforts to reduce the likelihood of a repeat aspiration episode.

GASTROINTESTINAL TRACT

Foreign bodies in the gastrointestinal tract can be seen in all age groups. There is no requirement for predisposing anatomic or pathologic conditions.[53] Series have noted, however, that ingested foreign bodies are relatively more common in pediatric, edentulous, incarcerated, and psychiatric patients.[1,54-56]

Complications associated with foreign body ingestion account for an estimated 1500 deaths annually in the United States.[57] Perforation occurs in approximately 3% of cases and most frequently involves the esophagus or the ileocecal region.[58] Because ingested objects are expected to pass spontaneously in 80% to 90% of patients with normal anatomy, initial management is usually expectant, with radiographic and stool follow-up to confirm passage.[1,58] Direct foreign body removal using surgical intervention is usually unnecessary. In one pediatric series, endoscopy—including esophagoscopy, laryngoscopy, and anoscopy—was successful in removing the foreign body in 98.8% of cases.[56] Early endoscopy should be considered in cases of potential toxicity (e.g., button battery ingestion), altered anatomy (e.g., prior abdominal surgery), or sharp foreign bodies.[1]

Pharynx and Esophagus

Foreign bodies lodged in the pharynx and esophagus are usually a sharp object (e.g., fishbone) that is impaled in the wall of the pharynx, hypopharynx, or esophagus or a large bolus, usually food, that cannot pass beyond the anatomic points of esophageal constriction. The constriction locations are the (1) proximal esophagus at the level of the cricopharyngeal muscle and thoracic inlet, or radiographically the clavicular level; (2) midesophagus at the level of the aortic arch and carina; and (3) distal esophagus just proximal to the esophagogastric junction, or radiographically a level two to four vertebral bodies cephalad to the gastric bubble. Foreign bodies may lodge at any level of the esophagus (or remainder of the gastrointestinal tract) with abnormal anatomy.[59] The complication rate for esophageal foreign body ingestion is estimated at less than 2%, but the sequelae can be severe. Complications become more likely with increasing impaction time and include esophageal erosion or perforation, tracheal compression, mediastinitis, esophagus-to-airway or esophagus-to-vascular fistulae, extraluminal migration, and formation of strictures or false esophageal diverticula.[59-61]

History

A useful history is usually available from the patient or caregivers.[59] Because natural curiosity leads them to ingest a myriad of nonfood items, children are particularly likely to present with esophageal foreign bodies. The object most often encountered is a coin, constituting more than half of ingested foreign bodies in some series.[4,56] Other common objects are foods, toys, bones, batteries, wood, and glass.[59,60] In one series of 104 consecutive cases, one third were sharp objects.[57]

The button (disk) battery can cause esophageal rupture.[4] These batteries cause pathologic changes through pressure, electrical current, corrosives leakage, or heavy metal poisoning.[62] Batteries containing potassium can produce liquefaction necrosis, and batteries containing mercury can cause mercury poisoning.[63] The identification of button batteries has therapeutic and prognostic ramifications.

An ingested object in place for longer than 24 hours is more likely to cause mucosal erosion, and management plans for ingested bodies are different when the objects have been in the gastrointestinal tract for a long duration.[59] Children usually present to the emergency department within 6 hours of foreign object ingestion. The most frequent presenting symptoms are dysphagia, drooling, retching, and vomiting. Pain, usually odynophagia, may be the major complaint. Anorexia, wheezing, or chest or neck pain also may be present. Patients may complain that they can feel the object in the throat or chest and are unable to pass it any farther. The victim often is able to localize the foreign body accurately, particularly in the upper esophagus, and should be asked to indicate the level of obstruction.[64] Drooling is consistent with high-grade obstruction. Patients rarely have complaints of shortness of breath or air hunger resulting from a large foreign body in the esophagus impinging anteriorly and compressing the trachea. Infants and children may experience coughing, choking, and significant respiratory compromise from foreign bodies lodged in the upper esophagus.[59]

Patients may present with late sequelae. Foreign bodies serving as a nidus for infection result in complaints (e.g., fever) consistent with the infectious process.[59] Signs of mediastinitis indicate esophageal perforation. Perforation of the esophagus with erosion into the vasculature or pulmonary tree can result in presentations ranging from hemoptysis to pulmonary abscess to life-threatening hemorrhage.[61,65]

The history should include any known esophageal anatomic abnormality or prior instrumentation. A patient with a history of esophageal stenting should be considered to have stent migration when the history is dysphagia. Migration typically occurs within the first week of placement, but has been reported up to 1 year after initial placement.[66]

Physical Examination

Examination begins with a careful search of the pharynx and hypopharynx. This search may reveal the foreign body or identify an oropharyngeal mucosal scratch that can cause foreign body symptoms even in the absence of an impacted object. Oropharyngeal examination also may provide indirect clues; for example, a missing dental plate on examination should lead the emergency physician to suspect this item as a possible gastrointestinal tract foreign object.[67] The base of the tongue, vallecula, supraglottic area, epiglottis, and piriform sinus should be examined. Topical anesthesia facilitates the examination. If adequate visualization is not obtained with the indirect laryngoscopy mirror, fiberoptic nasopharyngoscopy or direct laryngoscopy should be performed.

Subcutaneous emphysema found by neck palpation indicates probable esophageal perforation. Drooling and inability to handle secretions are secondary indicators of esophageal impaction. Esophageal object detection generally requires esophagoscopy, however, because these foreign bodies are not otherwise amenable to detection by physical examination.[68]

Diagnostic Imaging

Because the clinical presentation and examination are infrequently sufficient to diagnose or exclude a foreign body, radiography is routine.[60] The initial step is generally a chest radiograph and lateral cervical spine x-ray study using soft tissue technique (see Figures 57-9 and 57-11). The primary utility of plain radiography lies in detection of radiopaque objects. Overall the sensitivity of plain radiography for detection of esophageal foreign bodies is relatively poor.[68-71] Plain radiography has identified metal foreign objects missed on direct (including endoscopic) examination, however.[72] In patients who are transferred to the emergency department from an outlying hospital, repeat radiography may be useful to assess whether the foreign object has passed into the stomach in the interval since prior films.[59]

Esophageal foreign objects usually align themselves in the coronal plane and are posterior to the tracheal air column on lateral view. Coins in the esophagus lie in the coronal position in virtually all cases because the opening into the esophagus is much wider in this orientation.[59] Certain common foreign bodies are not radiopaque; for example, fish and chicken bones are frequently ingested, are difficult to visualize directly or radiographically, and often scratch the esophageal mucosa. Plain films of the neck and chest have sensitivity of 25% for impacted fish bones.[69] Although some studies suggest that technique variation improves fish bone detection, plain films remain insufficiently sensitive.[73,74] Studies have found that plain films are false-negative in 30% to 55% of cases and false-positive in 24% of cases.[69-71]

When plain films fail to visualize foreign bodies and suspicion remains high, one option is contrast esophagography, which can be useful with radiopaque and sometimes with radiolucent foreign bodies.[40,59] If perforation is not a concern, barium may be used as the contrast medium because it provides higher quality images. If an esophageal leak is suspected, water-soluble contrast solution should be used; a barium follow-up study may be considered if the initial contrast study is equivocal or suspicion remains high. When initial contrast films are not definitive, patients may be asked to swallow a contrast-soaked cotton ball, which may localize the foreign body by lodging proximal to the object. Contrast studies, even performed with barium, have limitations when the suspected object is an impacted bone.[68] In one series using barium-soaked cotton balls, false-positive and false-negative rates were 26.9% and 40%.[71] Barium swallow yields better results, but risks aspiration and coats the object and esophagus, reducing effectiveness of subsequent endoscopy.[68,75]

CT scans with coronal and sagittal reconstructions are useful in identifying foreign bodies or characterizing further objects seen on plain films.[56,72] CT has been recommended as the primary diagnostic modality because it can give information about foreign body size, type, location, and orientation with respect to other anatomic structures.[54] In one study, non–contrast-enhanced CT interpreted by resident physicians detected all impacted bony foreign bodies found by esophagoscopy; the one false-positive result was caused by esophageal calcification, and no false-negative results occurred. Overall, CT use reduced the incidence of negative esophagoscopies. This study portends a potentially important role for CT in imaging of impacted bony foreign objects.[68] CT also can assist with identification of complications. CT identified a fistulous (later fatal) esophagoaortic tract in a patient who had swallowed a bone splinter 1 week earlier.[65] Also, CT may be used in patients with positive plain films and negative esophagoscopy to search for objects that have migrated from the intraluminal to extraluminal space.[54]

A relatively inexpensive and noninvasive modality reported to be useful in detection and characterization of metal foreign bodies is the hand-held metal detector. Use of a commercial hand-held metal detector (Super Scanner; Garrett Security Systems, Garland, Tex) has been studied in 176 pediatric patients with suspected esophageal metallic foreign bodies, with positive and negative predictive values of approximately 90% and 100%.[76] The hand-held metal detector easily detects aluminum foreign bodies missed by radiography. The hand-held metal detector avoids time, radiation, and costs associated with radiography and may obviate the need for radiography when patients with suspected coin ingestion have no foreign body detected or have an object detected below the diaphragm.[60,76]

Management

Pharyngeal foreign bodies visualized by direct or indirect laryngoscopy usually can be removed with a forceps or clamp. The emergency physician should guard against the possibility of inducing trauma during extraction attempts.[72]

Management of esophageal foreign bodies depends on many factors. With esophageal food bolus or coin, the emergency physician may provide management. With sharp objects, displaced esophageal stents, or impacted button batteries, more invasive management is necessary.[59,77] Management strategy depends on the nature of the foreign body, the length of time the object has been lodged, and the expertise and experience of the clinicians managing the case.[59] In addition, the patient's age and prior medical and surgical history may be relevant.[56] The overall success rate for nonsurgical removal of objects from the esophagus is greater than 95%.[71]

The first basic strategy for esophageal foreign body management is applicable only if the object is known to be an impacted food bolus. In these cases, pharmacologic maneuvers may be tried to move the bolus into the stomach. Glucagon (0.5 to 2 mg) given intravenously has been used to relieve distal food obstructions. The drug acts by lowering the smooth muscle tone at the lower esophageal sphincter without inhibiting normal esophageal peristalsis. A concern is that glucagon, if given too rapidly, may cause vomiting and risk rupture of an obstructed esophagus. Other pharmacologic agents have been employed with mixed success. Gas-forming agents have been used, and some investigators suggest that this be the procedure attempted first or in combination with glucagon. After confirmation of distal food obstruction using contrast radiography, a solution of tartaric acid followed by sodium bicarbonate is administered. This mixture produces carbon dioxide, and the resulting pressure may push the bolus into the stomach. Patients who complain of chest pain at presentation should not be given gas-forming agents because they may have esophageal perforation. Two other agents used for distal food bolus impaction are nitroglycerine and nifedipine. Both of these agents have a relaxing action on the lower esophageal sphincter, and are safe (if only marginally effective) maneuvers for therapy of impacted food bolus. A last approach, enzymatic degradation of an impacted meat bolus using the proteolytic enzyme papain, has fallen into disfavor because of risks of esophageal perforation.

The preferred strategy for esophageal foreign body removal is endoscopy. Flexible endoscopy does not require general anesthesia, can be performed in a sedated (nonintubated) patient, and may be diagnostic and therapeutic in the case of foreign bodies such as coins.[56] The high overall success of endoscopy has prompted some experts to recommend that patients with symptoms starting within 48 hours of emergency department presentation be taken directly to endoscopy if no suspected complication is evident.[68]

Another removal strategy, best suited for smooth, nonimpacted and blunt objects, employs a contrast-filled balloon catheter and fluoroscopy. A Foley catheter is introduced into the esophagus, and the balloon is passed beyond the foreign body, inflated with radiographic contrast material, and withdrawn under fluoroscopic monitoring; the object is extracted with the catheter. To minimize risk of foreign body aspiration, this procedure should be performed with the patient in a steep, head-down position and is contraindicated in patients with airway compromise, complete esophageal obstruction, or an inability to cooperate.

The final strategy for active foreign body removal, bougienage, involves pushing the foreign object into the stomach. Strict criteria determine eligibility for this procedure, which generally is not performed by the emergency physician. Bougienage has been found in one study to be equally safe, more efficient, and much less expensive than endoscopy.[78] Although many patients were ineligible because of delayed presentation, bougienage was successful in more than 80% of attempts, with no complications.

The fifth approach, expectant management hoping for spontaneous foreign object passage into the stomach, may be the method used most often. This approach is best suited for patients presenting within 24 hours of ingestion and who have a radiographically identified "safe" (e.g., coin) object in the distal esophagus.[59] The button battery is associated with specific expectant management issues. If a disk battery has been ingested, its location must be ascertained, with immediate removal if it has lodged in the esophagus. If the button battery has passed distal to the esophagus, the patient can be observed, with follow-up radiography to confirm spontaneous passage through the gastrointestinal tract.[62]

After the removal of an esophageal foreign body, regardless of the method used, a follow-up esophagogram is frequently necessary to evaluate esophageal anatomy and patency. Referral for evaluation of dysphagia and obstruction should be made.

Stomach and Bowel

Foreign bodies that reach the stomach rarely cause major difficulties. Observation and expectant management are usually appropriate[62] because ingested foreign bodies reaching the stomach usually are propelled by peristalsis through the length of the gastrointestinal tract, with expulsion in a few days. Objects may pass beyond the esophagus and still become impacted, however, most often at the gastric outlet or the ileocecal valve, although complications can arise at any point throughout the intestinal portion of the gastrointestinal tract.[55] If the foreign body is a *bezoar,* a mass of undigestible food or nonfood material, there may be a palpable mass on abdominal examination. Otherwise, the physical examination is relatively unhelpful, only rarely revealing indirect evidence of foreign body presence or complications.

History

Signs and symptoms of intraluminal objects range from none, to vague abdominal pain, to obstruction or perforation-associated peritonitis. Most patients have a specific history of ingested items, however, or the circumstances indicate the likelihood and character of an intestinal foreign object. Occasionally, emergency physicians encounter patients with psychiatric or secondary-gain reasons for foreign body ingestion. Prisoners may view foreign body ingestion as a way out of jail (Figure 57-12).

Hiding of illicit drugs is an important motivation for foreign body ingestion. Rupture of these drug-containing packages, especially when cocaine is involved, can result in rapid and lethal consequences.[3] Less often, packages can cause bowel obstruction. Even when obstruction is not present, vomiting may be reported. *Body packing,* which entails systematic gastrointestinal tract placement of previously prepared drug packages, should be clinically differentiated from *body stuffing,* which denotes hurried ingestion of hastily prepared packages in the face of imminent police presence.[79] Body stuffers are more likely to experience toxicity because of the poor packaging of drugs and are less likely to have positive plain radiography findings.[80] Drugs most often seen with body packing or body stuffing are cocaine and heroin, with amphetamines and cannabinoids seen less frequently.

Another important component of the history is medical implants in the gastrointestinal tract. Dental implants can migrate and cause complications in the distal gastrointestinal tract.[67] Expandable esophageal stents migrate in 25% of patients; the migrated stent usually is located in the stomach, but small bowel obstruction also can occur.

Patients with gastrointestinal tract foreign bodies should be asked about history possibly related to bezoar presence. A habit of chewing hairs can result in trichobezoars, which infrequently extend from the stomach into the small intestine as a "tail" (Rapunzel syndrome). Phytobezoars (composed of vegetable matter) and lactobezoars (from milk curds) also have caused complications, usually in the stomach.[81] Infants with lactobezoars from undigested formula may have a history of prematurity and often are receiving formulas that have a high casein-to-whey ratio. Other bezoars may be composed of infectious (e.g., fungal bezoars) or inorganic (e.g., lithobezoar) material.[82]

Other specific intestinal foreign bodies, previously mentioned in the discussion of esophageal impaction, are important in the distal gastrointestinal tract. Button batteries can rupture in the intestines, and fish bones have penetrated through the gastric mucosa.

Diagnostic Imaging

The initial imaging modality is plain radiography, which is often diagnostic (Figure 57-13). Two-view plain radiography has proved useful for situations ranging from body stuffing to coin ingestion. Plain radiography is positive in approximately 90% of body packers, but is nearly always negative in body stuffers and is usually negative in patients ingesting crack vials.[79,80,83,84] Plain radiography usually identifies drug packets, but false-negative results do occur, and follow-up contrast radiography or CT is recommended.[85]

Contrast-enhanced upper gastrointestinal radiography has intermediate success in patients with suspected body stuffing or body packing. Contrast administration also has proved useful in outlining

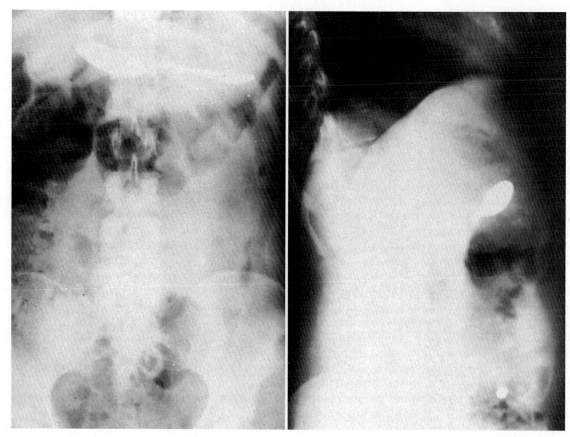

Figure 57-12. Radiographs of a prisoner who swallowed a spoon.

bezoars. CT can identify foreign bodies in the stomach and intestines and can help diagnose package ingestions in body stuffers. In these patients, contrast-enhanced CT outlines the bag containing the illicit drug; contrast administration also can help by identifying air trapped in the package. CT has had false-negative results, however, in detection of drug packages.[79,81] CT also has proved useful in determining whether complications of foreign body perforation are present.[73]

Ultrasound is useful for pediatric patients and for characterization of bezoars. Ultrasound also may help identify complications. Overall, ultrasound is of marginal utility, however, in foreign body evaluation, with disappointing efficacy for detection of items such as drug-containing packages.[79]

Management

The general rule for the management of gastric or intestinal foreign bodies is observation. Blunt objects can be expected to pass easily through the bowel, with expulsion verifiable by stool examination. If there is particular concern, serial radiographs may be obtained. Sharp objects may be recovered using fiberoptic gastroscopy, although they traverse the gastrointestinal tract without incident in 90% of cases.[56] Early removal generally is required for objects wider than 2 cm because they do not pass the pylorus or longer than 6 cm because they do not clear the duodenal sweep. Surgery is required in less than 1% of intestinal foreign body cases.[1] When chosen, observation should be continued until (1) the object is found in the patient's stool; (2) the object causes bowel obstruction or perforation, requiring immediate surgical intervention; or (3) the object shows no evidence of progression through the gastrointestinal tract on two radiographic examinations performed 24 hours apart, indicating impaction and mandating active removal. In some cases, the identity of the foreign body dictates management. In a body packer or body stuffer, regardless of external (i.e., law enforcement) pressures, the emergency physician should perform only interventions justified medically as reasonable steps to prevent injury from the ingested object or substance. If urgent drug package retrieval is unnecessary, the patient should be admitted for close observation for package passage or signs of toxicity. Monitoring of drug levels can be helpful. Usually the package passes through the gastrointestinal tract spontaneously. This passage can be facilitated with polyethylene glycol solution or laxatives or both. If cocaine-containing packets have been ingested, alkalinization of gastric contents (to enhance hydrolysis of cocaine to its inactive metabolite benzoylecgonine) may be of therapeutic assistance.

Immediate removal of drug-containing packages should be considered if the patient develops intestinal obstruction or drug intoxication. Most experts, citing

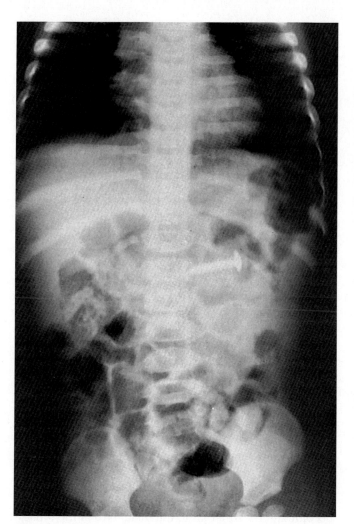

Figure 57-13. Radiograph of a child after ingestion of a screw (which ultimately passed after observation).

bezoars, specific therapy exists. Infants with lactobezoars should be changed to elemental diets and observed because most cases resolve without surgery.

Rectum

Anorectal foreign bodies seem to be increasing in frequency. Most result from retrograde introduction, typically as a result of sexual practices that patients might be reluctant to discuss. Prompt diagnosis is crucial because delay in definitive treatment is strongly associated with complications.

History

Patients with anorectal foreign bodies are often hesitant to give accurate histories. Studies have found that 33% of patients with self-introduced anorectal foreign bodies do not initially admit to insertion, but rather present with vague complaints of anal pain or constipation. Other complaints include rectal pain, bleeding, or inability to void when large objects impinge on the urethra. History also may be lacking in body packers, who may present with toxicity symptoms; fatal cardiovascular collapse can occur with ruptured cocaine packages.

It is possible for ingested food or objects to lodge in the rectum after passing through the proximal gastrointestinal tract. Rectal foreign masses of fish bones have been noted in many patients, all of whom strenuously denied transanal insertion. If patients do admit to transanal foreign body placement, the emergency physician might gain more accurate information about size, shape, and physical characteristics to plan imaging and extraction. The duration that the object has been in the anorectum has implications for mucosal failure and rupture.

Physical Examination

Patients with anorectal perforation may have findings of peritonitis or abdominal tenderness. On digital rectal examination, the foreign body might be directly palpated; this is the method of diagnosis in half of patients. In the absence of direct foreign body palpation, digital rectal examination may reveal findings (e.g., bloody discharge, loose sphincter tone) that raise suspicion for anorectal foreign body.

When the digital rectal examination is negative or when better visualization is required, anoscopy is the next step. Although the anoscope's diameter limits the size of foreign bodies that may be extracted through the instrument, anoscopy affords an improved view of the nature and positioning of the object. Similarly, rigid sigmoidoscopy may be performed, with special care taken to minimize pressure on possibly ischemic anorectal mucosa. In many patients, especially patients in whom multiple examinations or removal attempts have been made, sedation and analgesia may be required to enable invasive examination techniques. When there is any doubt about the integrity of the anorectal mucosa, invasive examination is best done in the operating room under general anesthesia.

risks of package rupture and drug toxicity, contend that endoscopic removal of cocaine-containing packages is never indicated. Endoscopic removal has been reported to be safe and effective, however, in an asymptomatic patient who ingested a single package.[86]

Button batteries represent another foreign body type with specific management implications. Intact batteries ingested into the stomach can be observed without the immediate removal necessary in cases of esophageal impaction. Repeat radiographs should be taken the next day to ensure movement of the battery into the intestinal tract, with films every 3 to 4 days thereafter to confirm continued distal movement. As with illicit drug-containing packages, administration of polyethylene glycol solution may speed distal movement. If the foreign body has not been passed after the first few clear-liquid stools, repeat radiography may identify the battery in the rectum, where it may be digitally evacuated.[62] Surgery is indicated for failure of the battery to progress, for radiographic signs of battery rupture, or for development of symptoms such as abdominal pain.[59]

Management of bezoars depends on type and location. Dietary therapy, endoscopic removal, and enzymatic dissolution frequently are used. For some

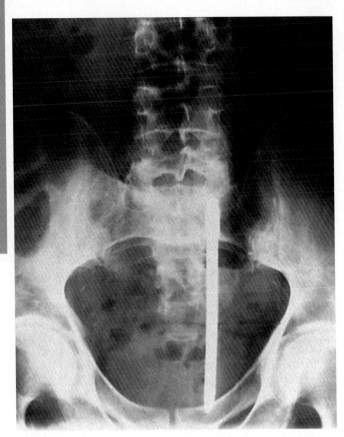

Figure 57-14. Radiograph of a patient who inserted a screwdriver into the rectum. The screwdriver was removed during proctoscopy.

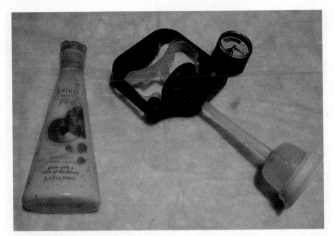

Figure 57-15. Vacuum device used to remove a difficult-to-grasp rectal foreign body.

Diagnostic Imaging

The foreign body may be detected on a plain abdominal radiograph (Figure 57-14). Plain films were diagnostic in nearly half of patients in one series and are recommended as the initial imaging technique. An important secondary finding is free intra-abdominal air secondary to anorectal perforation. If the object is not visualized on plain films, a contrast study can be performed, taking care to minimize hydrostatic pressures on potentially compromised mucosa. Water-soluble contrast should be used if perforation is suspected. Specialized imaging, such as CT, is not usually part of the imaging workup, but may be indicated if complications are suspected.

Management

Using patience and judicious sedation and analgesia, the emergency physician often can remove rectal foreign bodies. Surgical intervention may be necessary on occasion, depending on the nature of the foreign body and the presence of damage or perforation of the rectal wall. In one series, transanal removal under sedation was successful in 40% of patients, with the remainder undergoing general anesthesia with transanal removal (43%) or laparotomy (10%).[87]

Initial efforts at foreign body removal in the emergency department should begin with the examiner's digit. Small rectal objects occasionally can be hooked by the finger and withdrawn; this is the initial technique in patients who do not have signs of peritoneal irritation from bowel wall perforation. The digits should be lubricated with lidocaine jelly, and abdominal pressure may be applied in an attempt to mobilize foreign objects distally.

When digital extraction fails, the emergency physician should attempt to use an anoscope or small vaginal speculum to visualize the foreign body. Ring forceps are placed through the visualizing apparatus to grasp and remove the object. Sometimes the mucosa may become tightly adherent to the distal end of the foreign body, creating a vacuum that prevents object withdrawal. Passage of a Foley catheter beyond the foreign object with proximal air inflation usually breaks the vacuum and permits retrieval. Passage of the catheter, followed by air inflation and balloon filling, may allow object removal with gentle catheter traction.

When the emergency physician possesses the appropriate expertise and equipment, or if consultants are available, the next step may be removal with a vacuum device (Figure 57-15) or forceps; sigmoidoscopy may be a necessary adjunct to such an approach. As with other removal means, the physician should be careful to minimize risk of anorectal perforation. Removal of occult anorectal foreign objects after administration of an enema for symptomatic relief of anal pain was successful in 10% of patients in one series. Experts caution against possible perforation, however, when enemas or cathartics are administered to patients with known rectal foreign bodies, especially foreign bodies with sharp edges.

After removal of the foreign object, rectal trauma should be considered. When foreign body retrieval has been simple and the patient does not show increased pain, tenderness, or rectal bleeding, further evaluation for rectal trauma is likely unnecessary. If any of these is present, postremoval sigmoidoscopy may identify small abrasions requiring close follow-up, but generally hospitalization is necessary only if a rectal laceration or perforation is found. Appropriate antibiotics are indicated in all cases of suspected bowel wall perforation and peritonitis. Long-term follow-up has identified few or no sequelae in patients with rectal foreign bodies. In one study tracking patients for more than 5 years, investigators found no problems with fecal incontinence or recurrence of rectal foreign objects.[87]

GENITOURINARY TRACT

The literature describes a wide variety of genitourinary tract foreign objects, ranging from easily extracted tampons and condoms to penile rings removed only with great difficulty.[88]

History

An accurate history may not be readily obtained because most foreign bodies are placed by the patients themselves. Reports have validated the value of a history, however, as a means to diagnose genitourinary objects.[89] In children who fear parental disapproval of foreign object placement, secondary signs are the usual presentation. They are brought to medical attention when parents note foul-smelling, purulent discharge or bleeding from the urethra or vagina or both. Another common infant presentation is penile constriction caused by inadvertent wrapping of hairs around the shaft, usually just proximal to the corona.[90]

In older children, rubber bands or string may be placed around the genitalia. In adolescents and adults, metal objects are placed for autoerotic stimulation. Constricting bands may be placed proximal to the scrotum or more often on the penile shaft. These patients frequently have presentations delayed by 12 hours or more. The swelling that renders these constricting bands so difficult to remove also hinders the physical examination, emphasizing the need for an accurate history.[90]

Occasionally an object (e.g., tampon) is forgotten until it causes purulent discharge. Secondary symptoms also can bring foreign bodies to physicians' attention in rare cases of genitourinary tract perforation by foreign bodies from the genitourinary tract or elsewhere. Migration of an intrauterine device into the bladder has occurred, with associated cystolithiasis. In another unusual case, a sewing pin caused perforation through the appendix and into the bladder.

Genitourinary tract foreign bodies may be infectious. The term *bezoar,* traditionally considered to delineate indigestible material in the gastrointestinal tract, also has been used to describe foreign collections in the bladder. One common urinary tract bezoar is the *Candida* bezoar, seen in immunodepressed patients or in patients with diabetes mellitus, neurogenic bladder, antibiotic use, or an indwelling urinary catheter.[91]

Physical Examination

Patients of all ages require a careful gentle examination because they are often anxious about the anatomic region being examined. In a pediatric patient, a nasal speculum may be used to help visualize a vaginal foreign body. Thorough vaginal examination is indicated in patients with symptoms of vaginitis, with the search directed for infectious agents and foreign bodies. A vaginal foreign body may be palpated during digital rectal examination.

In children and adults, the presence of blood or discharge at the urethral meatus or vagina should be noted. Patients with intraurethral foreign objects also may have perineal induration and a high incidence of associated infection, which may progress to sepsis syndrome.[88] In males with penile shaft swelling, the emergency physician must perform careful inspection for constricting objects. In an infant with penile swelling, a coronal constricting hair should be sought.[90]

In patients with penile rings, especially most who present after some hours' delay, examination may reveal a swollen penis with mottling, duskiness, and excoriation. The interruption of venous and lymphatic outflow results in increasing penile enlargement with risks of tissue damage. Damage is especially likely if the patient previously has tried removal of the constriction.[90] Urethrocutaneous fistulae, relatively common in infants and children, should be sought in any patient with a constricting band.

Examination may reveal only indirect evidence of other genitourinary objects as well. Multiple abscesses in an enlarged scrotum have been reported in a patient presenting with acute infection from embedded metallic objects placed (by the patient) decades before emergency department presentation.[89] Any genitourinary examination abnormalities should prompt the emergency physician to question the patient about possible foreign bodies.

Diagnostic Imaging

Often, no imaging is necessary, but plain films may be used to seek urethral or bladder radiopaque foreign bodies. Plain radiography also has proved useful in unusual cases of embedded metallic objects not palpable because of pain.[89] Urethrocystography may be useful in identifying and locating genitourinary tract foreign objects and has been an aid to surgical planning for these patients.[88] Intravenous urography may reveal a filling defect in the case of a bladder foreign body, or it can reveal delayed renal excretion as a general finding suggesting foreign object–related renal function impairment. Ultrasound is useful to investigate for hydronephrosis. Acoustic shadowing may not be seen depending on the foreign body nature; *Candida* bezoars lack acoustic shadowing. These bezoars and other genitourinary tract objects are generally identifiable on CT.[91]

Management

Vaginal foreign bodies usually are removed easily. If the object has been present for some time and there is associated vaginitis, it should be treated. In males or females, foreign bodies located just inside the urethral meatus usually can be grasped with a clamp and removed. The overriding goal is to avoid causing further damage to the already traumatized urethra. After failure of one or two attempts at removal by the emergency physician, the best course is early consultation. Objects located in the proximal urethra or bladder usually require cystoscopy for extrication. One exception is the *Candida* bezoar, which generally is treated with antifungal agents.[91]

Constricting penile foreign bodies must be removed as early as possible because progressive swelling makes removal more difficult. Sedation and analgesia may be necessary. Also, care must be taken when removing constricting objects with instruments such as ring cutters; penile shaft lacerations may result from the tautness of the thin underlying skin. Hair and string foreign bodies are removed relatively easily with forceps and scissors or scalpel. Wrapping the penis with string and mobilizing the ring distally (as is done for digital foreign bodies) have been successful.[90] Other approaches have been used to remove penile constricting bands. A cast saw, the vibrating blade of which reduces risk of skin damage, may be useful for removal of some objects, such as acrylic rings. After penile ring removal and confirmation of ability to void, patients usually can be discharged with close follow-up.[90] Consultation should be obtained for patients with penile trauma.

SOFT TISSUES

Soft tissue foreign bodies present unique diagnostic and management dilemmas. Foreign bodies not only may be present in patients with known wounds, but also in patients with secondary symptoms who are unaware or uncertain of foreign body entry.

History

All patients with wounds should be considered for soft tissue foreign body contamination, and evaluation of soft tissue injury should include foreign objects. In straightforward cases, patients present with symptoms such as pain or foreign body sensation and may report specifically a foreign body. In more difficult cases, patients present with symptoms related to complications. Soft tissue infections, especially recurrent, should suggest a foreign body serving as a nidus. Careful history in patients with soft tissue complaints should include a search for antecedent trauma, no matter how remote, which may have resulted in foreign body entry.

Physical Examination

The diagnosis is frequently obvious on visual inspection or standard wound evaluation. Besides location of the foreign body, the examination should address injuries collateral to the object's presence. Distal neurovascular function should be tested.

Diagnostic Imaging

Anteroposterior and lateral radiographs of the involved area of the body are valuable. Plain radiography has been shown to be greater than 98% sensitive when the foreign body is metal or other radiopaque material, such as gravel.[92,93] If silver nitrate sticks were used to achieve hemostasis before imaging, the deposited metal can be expected to appear on plain radiography.[94]

One common foreign body is glass, which has shown radiopacity.[92,93] In one cadaver study, nonleaded glass was visualized with 90% sensitivity and a false-positive rate of 10%; glass color and location were unimportant, but a volume of less than 15 mm^3 was associated with risk of failed visualization.[95] Other items are not easily seen on plain radiographs, which are insensitive for detection of vegetable (e.g., wooden) material or plastic objects.[92,93] Xeroradiography, recommended in the past, has fallen out of favor. This technique has no advantage over plain films and has been discarded in favor of other modalities (e.g., CT) when plain films are negative and suspicion remains.[93,96]

Fluoroscopy has received attention as a diagnostic and therapeutic tool. In an ex vivo beef model, emergency physician–operated fluoroscopy had 100% sensitivity for gravel, metal, and glass; sensitivity was 90% for graphite and 0% for plastic and wood.[97] Another evaluation of C-arm imaging in a chicken leg model also found 100% of gravel, metal, and glass objects, although sensitivities for wood and plastic were low.[98] One advantage of fluoroscopy is that it can guide removal and later confirm absence of foreign objects.

When plain radiographs are negative and foreign body suspicion remains, ultrasound or CT is the next step.[96,99] Ultrasound is readily available in many emergency departments and has been the subject of intensive but disappointing study. Even radiologists, interpreting scans done in an animal model, have low detection rates for gravel (40%), metal (45%), glass (50%), cactus spine (30%), wood (50%), and plastic (40%); overall, false-negative and false-positive rates were 50% and 30%.[92] In another study, using a cadaver hand model, ultrasound proved 93% sensitive for wood and 73% sensitive for plastic foreign bodies, but specificity was only 59%.[100] A third study, using credentialed sonographers and radiologist interpretations in a chicken breast model, found some utility for ultrasound in the emergency department. The investigators concluded that a 7.5-MHz probe was better at shallow depths and that a 5-MHz probe should be used for deeper searching.[101] The study found that wood had the best acoustic shadow, followed by plastic; other materials investigated (paper clip, glass, needle) had lesser shadowing and were more difficult to detect. In another artificial setting, ultrasound was the only modality among plain radiography, CT, and xeroradiography that clearly identified wood and plastic foreign bodies.[102] Overall, given the availability of ultrasound in the emergency department, it is reasonable to employ this technique with the understanding that a positive test is much more useful than a negative one, after which CT is still necessary to rule out a foreign object.

In addition to characterizing objects seen on plain films, CT is useful for items (e.g., plastic, wood) missed on plain radiographs.[93,103] CT also is valuable in localizing small or deep objects and delineating anatomic positioning.[96,99] Newer generation image viewers increase utility of CT, with console-read imaging manifesting higher detection rates for wood and plastic than hard-copy CT film.[103] CT also is useful for identifying foreign body sequelae (e.g., abscess).

MRI can assist in identifying foreign body complications.[99] Soft tissue objects can induce a chronic inflammatory reaction and lytic or blastic osseous changes that allow MRI to locate foreign bodies.[104] In other cases, MRI is less optimal. Gravel, found easily on most modalities, causes MRI streaking because of ferromagnetic material. MRI also has identified foreign objects of wood and plastic; however, CT is usually adequate for detection of these types of foreign bodies.[93]

Management

The most important determinant of successful foreign body removal is knowledge of the object's precise location. Standard radiopaque markers can aid in wound localization. For small objects, needles placed in the soft tissues can help pinpoint the location of foreign objects seen on radiographs. Fluoroscopy may allow simultaneous visualization and removal. When objects are not radiopaque, judicious probing of wounds with fine-gauge needles or forceps may allow tactile detection of the foreign body.

To remove a foreign body, it may be necessary to extend the original wound or, if it is located away from the entrance site, to make a separate incision. The emergency physician can perform limited wound extension or make separate incisions in regions where adequate analgesia and a bloodless field can be achieved. When objects are deeply embedded, it may be better to leave them in place rather than create large surgical wounds to effect removal.

After foreign body removal, the emergency physician should consider tetanus prophylaxis and antibiotic coverage when warranted by clinical circumstances. Patients with contaminated hand wounds and wooden splinters may be candidates for prophylaxis. Patients with suspected vascular or neurologic injuries require early evaluation, possibly but not always in the emergency department, by appropriate subspecialists. Some soft tissue foreign bodies are not suspected or detected and can lead to infectious sequelae. Careful discharge instructions and timely follow-up are crucial in these patients.

KEY CONCEPTS

- If the history and mechanism of injury are compatible with ocular penetration or if a small puncture wound of the globe is noted, anteroposterior and lateral radiographs of the orbit are an appropriate initial step when the foreign body is thought to be radiopaque. CT and ultrasound are complementary diagnostic studies.

- Inappropriately prolonged emergency department efforts at removal of otic foreign bodies can result in wasted time, unnecessary patient discomfort, and potential for complications, including tympanic membrane damage.

- Unresolving sinusitis despite appropriate antibiotic therapy should alert the emergency physician to the possibility of nasal foreign body.

- Most airway foreign bodies are seen in pediatric patients and may not be visible on plain films. A normal radiograph does not rule out an aspirated foreign body.

- Esophageal foreign bodies (e.g., coins) usually are oriented in the coronal plane, and airway objects usually are oriented in the sagittal plane, parallel to the tracheal rings.

- The patient with critical airway obstruction and impending or actual respiratory arrest requires one of three options: (1) forced expulsion of the foreign body; (2) direct laryngoscopy with attempted manual removal; or (3) cricothyroidotomy, other transtracheal ventilation, or intubation, while pushing the foreign body distally.

- Esophageal foreign bodies typically are found at one of the three constriction locations: (1) proximal esophagus at the level of the cricopharyngeal muscle and thoracic inlet—radiographically, the clavicular level; (2) midesophagus at the level of the aortic arch and carina; and (3) distal esophagus just proximal to the esophageal-gastric junction—radiographically, a level two to four vertebral bodies cephalad to the gastric bubble.

- In cases involving body packers or body stuffers, regardless of external (i.e., law enforcement) pressures, the emergency physician should perform only interventions justified medically as reasonable steps to prevent injury resulting from the ingested object or substance.

ACKNOWLEDGMENT

The authors recognize the contributions of Peter T. Pons, MD, who prepared this chapter in previous editions.

REFERENCES

1. Mirhej MA, Koch J, Stansell J: A novel approach to ring-type foreign body removal. *Gastrointest Endosc* 49:243, 1999.
2. Langer D, et al: Relapsing pneumonia due to a migrating intrathoracic foreign body in a World War II veteran shot 53 years ago. *J Intern Med* 245:405, 1999.
3. Heinemann A, et al: Body-packing as cause of unexpected sudden death. *Forensic Sci Int* 92:1, 1998.
4. Samad L, Ali M, Ramzi H: Button battery ingestion: Hazards of esophageal impaction. *J Pediatr Surg* 34:1527, 1999.
5. Bhargava D, Victor R: Carabid beetle invasion of the ear in Oman. *Wild Environ Med* 10:157, 1999.
6. Bullock JD, et al: Unusual orbital foreign bodies. *Ophthalmic Plast Reconstr Surg* 15:44, 1999.

7. Khoury JM, O'Day DM: Retained intraocular metallic foreign body masquerading as a ciliary body melanoma with extrascleral extension. *Arch Ophthalmol* 117:410, 1999.

8. Coday MP, Colby K: Nailing down the diagnosis. *Arch Ophthalmol* 117:548, 1999.

9. O'Duffy D, Salmon JF: Siderosis bulbi resulting from an intralenticular foreign body. *Am J Ophthalmol* 127:218, 1999.

10. Soong K: Foreign body entrapment in radial keratotomy incisions. *Arch Ophthalmol* 117:836, 1999.

11. Chiquet C, et al: Intraocular foreign bodies: Factors influencing visual outcome. *Acta Ophthalmol Scand* 77:321, 1999.

12. Deramo VA, et al: Ultrasound biomicroscopy as a tool for detecting and localizing occult foreign bodies after ocular trauma. *Ophthalmology* 106:301, 1999.

13. Laktis A, et al: Evaluation of intraocular foreign bodies by spiral computed tomography and multiplanar reconstruction. *Ophthalmology* 105:307, 1998.

14. Kelly WM, et al: Ferromagnetism of intraocular foreign body causes unilateral blindness after MR study. *AJNR Am J Neuroradiol* 7:243, 1986.

15. Lakits A, Prokesch R, Bankier A: MRI for metallic foreign bodies? [letter]. *Ophthalmology* 106:1233, 1999.

16. Arunkumar MJ, Selvapandian S, Rajshekhar V: Penetrating intracranial wooden object: Case report and review of CT morphology, complications, and management. *Surg Neurol* 51:617, 1999.

17. Dubois M, Francois M, Hamrioui R: Foreign bodies in the ear: Report of 40 cases. *Arch Pediatr* 5:970, 1998.

18. Ainsley JF, Cunningham MJ: Treatment of aural foreign bodies in children. *Pediatrics* 101:638, 1998.

19. Indudharan R, et al: Human otoacariasis. *Ann Trop Med Parasitol* 93:163, 1999.

20. Tang C, Levine R, Shankar L: The mysterious case of persistent malocclusion. *Ann Plast Surg* 41:420, 1998.

21. Jones RL, Chavda SV, Pahor AL: Parapharyngeal abscess secondary to an external auditory meatus foreign body. *J Laryngol Otol* 111:1086, 1997.

22. Goldman SA, et al: Fatal meningitis and brain abscess resulting from foreign body-induced otomastoiditis. *Otolaryngol Head Neck Surg* 118:6, 1998.

23. Balbani APS, et al: Ear and nose foreign body removal in children. *Int J Pediatr Otorhinolaryngol* 46:37, 1998.

24. Francois M, Hamrioui R, Narcy P: Nasal foreign bodies in children. *Eur Arch Otorhinolaryngol* 255:132, 1998.

25. Jones I, Moulton C: Use of an electric ear syringe in the emergency department. *J Accid Emerg Med* 15:327, 1998.

26. Pollock HD: Glue ear: Cyanoacrylic. *Arch Otolaryngol Head Neck Surg* 114:1188, 1988.

27. Abadir WF, Nakhla V, Chong P: Removal of superglue from the external ear using acetone: Case report and literature review. *J Laryngol Otol* 109:1219, 1995.

28. Engelsma RJ, Lee WC: Impacted aural foreign body requiring endaural incision and canal widening for removal. *Int J Pediatr Otorhinolaryngol* 44:169, 1998.

29. Finkelstein JA: Oral Ambu-bag insufflation to remove unilateral nasal foreign bodies. *Am J Emerg Med* 14:57, 1996.

30. Kadish HA, Corneli HM: Removal of nasal foreign bodies in the pediatric population. *Am J Emerg Med* 15:54, 1997.

31. Alvi A, Bereliani A, Zahtz GD: Miniature disc battery in the nose: A dangerous foreign body. *Clin Pediatr* 36:427, 1997.

32. Kim KK, Kim JR, Kim JY: Button battery impaction in nasal cavity. *J Korean Med Sci* 14:210, 1999.

33. Douglas AR: Use of nebulized adrenaline to aid expulsion of intra-nasal foreign bodies in children. *J Laryngol Otol* 110:559, 1996.

34. Manca D: Up your nose: Quick and somewhat dirty method of removing foreign bodies from children's noses. *Can Fam Physician* 43:223, 1997.

35. Bodart E, et al: Foreign body aspiration in childhood: Management algorithm. *Eur J Emerg Med* 6:21, 1999.

36. Reilly JS, et al: Prevention and management of aerodigestive foreign body injuries in children. *Pediatr Clin North Am* 43:1403, 1996.

37. National Safety Council: *Accident Facts.* Itasca, Ill, The Council, 1995.

38. Massachusetts General Hospital: Weekly clinicopathological exercises: Case 33-1997—a 75-year-old man with chest pain, hemoptysis, and a pulmonary lesion. *N Engl J Med* 337:1220, 1997.

39. al-Majed SA, et al: Overlooked inhaled foreign bodies: Late sequelae and the likelihood of recovery. *Respir Med* 91:293, 1997.

40. Kavanaugh PV, Mason AC, Muller NL: Thoracic foreign bodies in adults. *Clin Radiol* 54:353, 1999.

41. Metrangolo S, et al: Eight years' experience with foreign body aspiration in children: What is really important for a timely diagnosis? *J Pediatr Surg* 34:1229, 1999.

42. Harris CS, et al: Childhood asphyxiation by food: A national analysis and overview. *JAMA* 251:2231, 1984.

43. Baharloo F, et al: Tracheobronchial foreign bodies. *Chest* 115:1357, 1999.

44. Sharma HS, Sharma S: Management of laryngeal foreign bodies in children. *J Accid Emerg Med* 16:150, 1999.

45. Ferretti C, Kruger L, Tsakiris P: Foreign body in the medial pterygoid space. *S Afr J Surg* 37:53, 1999.

46. Halvorson D, et al: Management of subglottic foreign bodies. *Ann Otol Rhinol Laryngol* 105:541, 1996.

47. Baigel GD: An unfortunate cause of death [letter]. *Anesthesia* 54:917, 1999.

48. Sane SM, Faerber EN, Belani KK: Respiratory foreign bodies and *Eikenella corrodens* brain abscess in two children. *Pediatr Radiol* 29:327, 1999.

49. Walner DL, et al: Utility of radiographs in the evaluation of pediatric upper airway obstruction. *Ann Otol Rhinol Laryngol* 108:378, 1999.

50. Ooij AV, et al: Cervical spondylodiscitis after removal of a fishbone. *Spine* 24:574, 1999.

51. Heimlich HJ: A life saving maneuver to prevent food choking. *JAMA* 234:298, 1975.

52. Abman SH, Fan LL, Cotton EK: Emergency treatment of foreign-body obstruction of the upper airway in children. *J Emerg Med* 2:7, 1984.

53. Brown DC, Doughty JC, George WD: Surgical treatment of oesophageal obstruction after ingestion of a granular laxative. *Postgrad Med J* 75:106, 1999.

54. Chee LWJ, Sethi DS: Diagnostic and therapeutic approach to migrating foreign bodies. *Ann Otol Rhinol Laryngol* 108:177, 1999.

55. Tander B, et al: An unusual foreign body in the bowel lumen causing obstruction in a neonate. *J Pediatr Surg* 34:1289, 1999.

56. Kim JK, et al: Management of foreign bodies in the gastrointestinal tract: An analysis of 104 cases in children. *Endoscopy* 31:302, 1999.

57. Schwartz GF, Polsky HS: Ingested foreign bodies of the gastrointestinal tract. *Am Surg* 42:236, 1976.

58. Goodfellow PB, Nockolds CL, Johnson AG: Foreign body perforation of lymphoma. *J R Soc Med* 91:545, 1998.

59. McGahren ED: Esophageal foreign bodies. *Pediatr Rev* 20:129, 1999.

60. Seikel K, et al: Handheld metal detector localization of ingested metallic foreign bodies. *Arch Pediatr Adolesc Med* 153:853, 1999.

61. Dahiya M, Denton JS: Esophagoaortic perforation by foreign body (coin) causing sudden death in a 3-year-old child. *Am J Forensic Med Pathol* 20:184, 1999.

62. Namasivayam S: Button battery ingestion: A solution to a management dilemma. *Pediatr Surg Int* 15:383, 1999.

63. Kulig K, et al: Disk battery ingestion. *JAMA* 249:2502, 1983.

64. Connolly AAP, et al: Ingested foreign bodies: Patient guided localization is a useful clinical tool. *Clin Otolaryngol* 17:520, 1992.

65. Pons J, et al: A fatal aorto-esophageal fistula due to a foreign body: A foreseeable accident? *Presse Med* 28:781, 1999.

66. May A, et al: Extrication of migrated self-expanding esophageal metal stents. *Gastrointest Endosc* 49:524, 1999.

67. Ghori A, Dorricott NJ, Sanders DS: A lethal ectopic denture: An unusual case of sigmoid perforation due to unnoticed swallowed dental plate. *J R Coll Surg Edinb* 44:203, 1999.

68. Eliashar R, et al: Computed tomography diagnosis of esophageal bone impaction: A prospective study. *Ann Otol Rhinol Laryngol* 108:708, 1999.

69. Evans RM, et al: The lateral neck radiograph in suspected impacted fish bones: Does it have a role? *Clin Radiol* 46:121, 1992.

70. Sundgren PC, Burnett A, Maly PV: Value of radiography in the management of possible fishbone ingestion. *Ann Otol Rhinol Laryngol* 103:628, 1994.

71. Derowe A, Ophir D: Negative findings of esophagoscopy for suspected foreign bodies. *Am J Otolaryngol* 15:41, 1994.

72. Lowinger DSG, et al: Retrieval of an extraluminal swallowed sharp foreign body. *Aust N Z J Surg* 69:399, 1999.

73. Horii K, et al: Successful treatment of a hepatic abscess that formed secondary to fish bone penetration by percutaneous transhepatic removal of the foreign body: Report of a case. *Surg Today* 29:922, 1999.

74. Abdullah BJJ, Kaur H, Ng KH: An in vitro study comparing two different film-screen combinations in the detection of impacted fish bones. *Br J Radiol* 71:930, 1998.

75. Ginsberg GG: Management of ingested foreign objects and food bolus impaction. *Gastrointest Endosc* 41:33, 1995.

76. Doraismwamy NV, Baig H, Hallam L: Metal detector and swallowed metal foreign bodies in children. *J Accid Emerg Med* 16:123, 1999.

77. Dunlap L, Oregon E: Removal of an esophageal foreign body using a Foley catheter. *Ann Emerg Med* 10:101, 1981.

78. Calkins CM, Christians KK, Sell LL: Cost analysis in the management of esophageal coins: Endoscopy versus bougienage. *J Pediatr Surg* 34:412, 1999.

79. Eng JGH, et al: False-negative abdominal CT scan in a cocaine body-stuffer. *Am J Emerg Med* 17:702, 1999.

80. Keys N, et al: Cocaine body stuffers: C case series. *J Toxicol Clin Toxicol* 33:517, 1995.

81. Gayer G, et al: Bezoars in the stomach and small bowel: CT appearance. *Clin Radiol* 54:228, 1999.

82. Rathi P, Rathi V: Colonic lithobezoar. *Indian J Gastroenterol* 18:89, 1999.

83. Sporer KA, Firestone J: Clinical course of crack cocaine body stuffers. *Ann Emerg Med* 29:596, 1997.

84. Hoffman RS, et al: Prospective evaluation of crack vial ingestions. *Vet Hum Toxicol* 32:164, 1990.

85. Gherardi R, et al: A cocaine body packer with normal abdominal plain radiograms. *Am J Forensic Med Pathol* 11:154, 1990.

86. Choudary AM, et al: Endoscopic removal of a cocaine packet from the stomach. *J Clin Gastroenterol* 27:155, 1998.

87. Kouraklis G, et al: Management of foreign bodies in the rectum: Report of 21 cases. *J R Coll Surg Edinb* 42:246, 1997.

88. Johnin K, et al: Percutaneous transvesical retrieval of foreign bodies penetrating the urethra. *J Urol* 161:915, 1999.

89. Rammos L, et al: Multiple recurrent scrotal abscesses and metallic foreign bodies. *Prog Urol* 9:541, 1999.

90. Schuster G, Stockmal P: Genital incarceration with metal rings: Their safe removal. *Tech Urol* 5:116, 1999.

91. el Fakir Y, et al: Imaging of urinary *Candida* bezoars. *Prog Urol* 9:513, 1999.

92. Russell RC, et al: Detection of foreign bodies in the hand. *J Hand Surg* 16:2, 1991.

93. Madan SI, Heilpern KL: Silver nitrate as a radiopaque foreign body. J Emerg Med 17:1045, 1999.

94. Arbona N, et al: Is glass visible on plain radiographs? A cadaver study. *J Foot Ankle Surg* 38:264, 1999.

95. Flom LL, Ellis GL: Radiologic evaluation of foreign bodies. *Emerg Med Clin North Am* 10:163, 1992.

96. Wyn T, et al: Bedside fluoroscopy for the detection of foreign bodies. *Acad Emerg Med* 2:979, 1995.

97. Cohen DM, et al: Miniature C-arm imaging: An in vitro study of detecting foreign bodies in the emergency department. *Pediatr Emerg Care* 13:247, 1997.

98. Donaldson JS: Radiographic imaging of foreign bodies in the hand. *Hand Clin* 7:125, 1991.

99. Hill R, et al: Ultrasound for the detection of foreign bodies in human tissue. *Ann Emerg Med* 29:353, 1997.

100. Turner J, et al: Ultrasound-guided retrieval of small foreign objects in subcutaneous tissue. *Ann Emerg Med* 29:731, 1997.

101. Ginsburg MJ, Ellis GL, Flom LL: Detection of soft-tissue foreign bodies by plain radiography, xerography, computed tomography, and ultrasonography. *Ann Emerg Med* 19:701, 1990.

102. Reiner B, et al: Evaluation of soft-tissue foreign bodies: Comparing conventional plain film radiography, computed radiography printed on film, and computed radiography displayed on a computer workstation. *AJR Am J Roentgenol* 167:141, 1996.

103. Laor T, Barnewolt CE: Nonradiopaque penetrating foreign body: "A sticky situation." *Pediatr Radiol* 29:702, 1999.

104. Uzumcu J: Medical application of the Dremel Multipro rotary tool [letter]. *Acad Emerg Med* 7:308, 2000.

ANIMAL BITES

PERSPECTIVE

Epidemiology

The true incidence of bites will always be difficult to determine because so many are not reported. In 1994, it is estimated that 4.7 million persons in the United States had been victims of dog bites but only about 800,000 (17%) sought medical attention.[1] Approximately 368,000 person were treated in U.S. emergency departments for dog-bite related injuries in 2001.[2]

The range in reported incidence is wide; interviews with families in Hermosillio, Mexico, in 1988 revealed an annual incidence of 2497 dog bites per 100,000 population.[3] Data from a surveillance network in Switzerland suggest there are 190 dog bites and 80 cat bites per 100,000 persons annually in that country.[4]

Dog bites represent approximately 0.4% of all emergency department visits and account for 60% to 90% of bite injuries treated in emergency departments.[5] Cat bites represent 1% to 15% of treated bites, rodents up to 7%, and other species (monkeys, ferrets, raccoons, foxes, livestock, bats, minks, kinkajous, other wild animals) less than 2% of bites.[6,7]

Children and young adults are the most frequent victims of animal bites, and males are bitten more often than females.[2,3,7,8] Most cat bites occur in or near the home of the victim. In the United States, more than half of dog bites occur at home and about one third in a public place.[5] Approximately 80% of dog bites inflicted on individuals younger than 18 years old are from the family or neighbor's dog.[2] This is not the case elsewhere in the world. In Bangkok, for instance, dog bites are more likely to be inflicted by stray or "community" dogs and to occur in public places.[8]

About 200 fatal attacks by dogs occur each decade in the United States.[9] The majority of the victims are children younger than 10 years of age. The breeds most frequently responsible are pit bulls, Rottweilers, and German shepherds. In at least half the cases, the attack involved an unrestrained dog on the owner's property. For most of the fatalities in children younger than 1 year of age, the attack involved a pet dog and a child who was sleeping or in a crib.[9]

Animal bites can usually be treated on an outpatient basis. Hospitalization is most often required for plastic surgery or repair of deep structures in fresh wounds, or for subsequent infection. Approximately 2% of victims who seek care for dog bites are hospitalized.[2] Patients with dog bites are usually hospitalized at the time of the injury for operative repair, whereas most hospitalizations for cat bites are a result of infection that occurs several days after the initial bite.[10]

PRINCIPLES OF DISEASE

Bites are traumatic injuries that can cause damage to skin, muscle, nerves, blood vessels, tendons, joints, and bones. Wounds can be lacerations, contusions, scratches, tears, or deep punctures. Contamination with oral flora from the biting animal makes local wound infection the principal treatment concern, along with rabies and tetanus.

Dogs

Injury

The jaws of adult dogs can exert approximately 200 pounds per square inch of pressure, enough to perforate sheet metal, but the teeth generally are not sharp. Most dog bites are large, relatively superficial crush injuries that damage skin and muscle but rarely reach tendon, bone, joint, or nerve. The wounds may be contusions with ecchymosis and hematoma, without any break in the skin, or large gaping wounds. Punctures occur less often. The large wound and emotional trauma of a dog bite typically precipitate an early visit for medical attention.[11]

The lower extremities are most frequently injured in dog bites, but face, neck, and scalp wounds are common sites for dog bites in young children.[2,4,5,11,12] In children up to 2 years old, dog bites can perforate the cranium, resulting in depressed skull fractures, brain laceration, intracranial abscess, and meningitis[13-15]; fractures of facial bones can also occur. In adults, dog bites rarely result in fracture, vascular injury, or tendon and nerve damage. However, bites from police dogs that are trained to hold their grasp until given the command to release pose a significant risk of complications, in particular vascular injury. Infection, fracture, and nerve or tendon injury are also more common in cases of bites from police dogs than those from civilian dogs.[16]

The overall incidence of infections from dog bites is 5% to 10%, only slightly higher than the 3% to 7% infection rate for nonbite lacerations that have been sutured. However, dog bites on the hand have a higher risk of infection, 12% to 30%. Dog bites to the face have a lower risk of infection (1-5%) than bites elsewhere.[4,11,17-23]

Bacteriology

More than 100 different organisms have been isolated from infected dog bites. Most infected wounds are polymicrobial.[10,18,24,25] No one organism is responsible for more than 30% of infections.[18,25] The organisms found in infected wounds are common mouth flora from the biting animal. *Staphylococcus aureus*, α-hemolytic and β-hemolytic streptococci, *Capnocytophaga canimorsus*, *Klebsiella*, *Bacillus subtilis*, *Pseudomonas*, and Enterobacteriaceae are among the more frequently isolated aerobic organisms.[24,26] NO-1, a gram-negative rod sensitive to β-lactams, quinolones, aminoglycosides, tetracycline, and sulfonamides, has recently been identified as a rare source of localized infection from dog and cat bites.[27] Anaerobic organisms isolated from infections include *Bacteroides*, *Fusobacterium*, *Peptostreptococcus*, and *Actinomyces* species; these bacteria rarely produce β-lactamase. Anaerobic organisms are almost always recovered with aerobic species in cultures of infected wounds.[24-26,28]

Although much attention is focused on *Pasteurella multocida*, its role in causing infections in dog bites may be overestimated.[18,29] *P. multocida* is found in the mouths of 77% of cats but only 13% of dogs.[30] *Pasteurella* species are isolated in 25% to 50% of infected dog bite wounds in some studies, but one study of infected dog bites found no *Pasteurella*.[10,24,25] The *Pasteurella* species that have usually been isolated from dogs, such as *P. stomatis*, *P. canis*, and *P. dagmatis*, are less virulent varieties.[24,30] When *P. multocida* is isolated from infected dog bites, it is frequently found in mixed culture with other organisms; when isolated from infected cat bites, *P. multocida* is often the sole pathogen.[10]

Capnocytophaga canimorsus

Capnocytophaga canimorsus, formerly known as dysgonic fermenter 2, is a fastidious gram-negative rod that causes overwhelming sepsis. It is part of the normal oral flora of both dogs and cats. More than 100 cases have been documented since the organism's discovery in 1976.[31-33] About 90% of cases are attributed to contact with a dog, primarily bites or scratches, but in approximately one quarter of cases, only dog contact (without a bite) was documented. Six infections have resulted from contact with cats. About 10% of cases are unrelated to any animal exposure. The disease tends to strike patients with alcoholic liver disease, functional or surgical asplenia, or lung disease or those taking corticosteroids. However, in 40% of victims, no underlying illness is identified.[31-37]

The illness begins within 2 to 3 days of exposure and is characterized by hypotension, disseminated intravascular coagulation, and renal failure. Purpura, particularly on the face, and petechiae are frequent findings and may progress to symmetric peripheral gangrene.[38] Cutaneous gangrene at the site of the bite strongly suggests *C. canimorsus*.[39] Waterhouse-Friderichsen syndrome (adrenal hemorrhage with cutaneous ecchymoses) occurs, as well as metastatic infection, resulting in endocarditis, meningitis, peritonitis, and pneumonitis. The mortality rate is 30%, with 70% of deaths in immunocompromised patients.[39]

Capnocytophaga canimorsus grows slowly and requires special media and growth conditions. The laboratory should be notified when this organism is suspected to prevent cultures from being misidentified or discarded prematurely. Although cultures can take up to 14 days, the organism can sometimes be identified in the patient's blood smear at the time of presentation, or in blood culture media before macroscopic growth.[36,39,40]

Cats

Injury

The typical cat bite is a puncture wound. Abrasions, lacerations, and avulsions can also result.[41] Cats have long, slender, pointed teeth that can penetrate tendons, joints, and bone, inoculating bacteria deep into these tissues. The majority of these bites occur on the hand.[4,41]

Wound Infection

The reported incidence of infection in cat bites is 30% to 50%, although this may be an overestimate, since many patients present for treatment of cat bites only after an infection develops.[4,6,7,41] In a prospective emergency department study of patients with cat bites, the overall infection rate was 16%, and most infections were present when the patient first sought care.[41] Nevertheless, 24% of the infections required admission to the hospital. Cat bites have a substantially higher risk of infection than dog bites. The puncture wound itself is difficult to explore, irrigate, or debride. Location on the hand increases the risk of infection.

Pasteurella multocida

Another important factor is the presence of *Pasteurella multocida*, a highly virulent, gram-negative, facultatively anaerobic rod found in the oral cavity or nasopharynx of 70% to 90% of healthy cats.[30] Wound infections and abscesses caused by *P. multocida* have occurred after cat scratches as well as bites and less often from dog bites or from open wounds that had been licked by dogs.[29] *P. multocida* infections have also been reported after the bite of an opossum, rat, lion, rabbit, pig, wolf, monkey, and cougar.[42-44]

Pasteurella multocida wound infections appear to have a distinctly earlier onset, causing a rapidly progressive cellulitis that may be apparent within 6 hours and is easily identifiable within 24 hours, whereas infections from other pathogens are usually not evident for 2 to 3 days. Presenting features include erythema, warmth, swelling, and tenderness. Purulent drainage, lymphangitis, and adenopathy may occur. In addition to cellulitis, *P. multocida* can cause abscess, tenosynovitis, joint infections, and osteomyelitis at the site of a bite and can seed arthritic joints and prosthetic valves, causing septic arthritis, endocarditis, and osteomyelitis at sites distant to the bite.[44-46] Meningitis and pericarditis due to *P. multocida* after a bite have also been reported.[45,47,48] Underlying liver disease and malignancy appear to be risk factors for bacteremia from *P. multocida,* and an association with human immunodeficiency virus (HIV) has also been described.[46]

In vitro, *P. multocida* is sensitive to penicillin, ampicillin, tetracycline, fluoroquinolones, amoxicillin-clavulanate, second- and third-generation cephalosporins, and trimethoprim-sulfamethoxazole.[49,50] The organism is resistant to vancomycin and clindamycin and shows borderline susceptibility to aminoglycosides. Oral first-generation cephalosporins may not be effective.[51] Semisynthetic penicillins such as oxacillin and dicloxacillin have been reported to have only minimal activity against *P. multocida* in vitro.[51] Erythromycin is a relatively poor agent against *P. multocida,* but the extended-spectrum macrolide azithromycin shows good in vitro activity against this organism.[49,50,52] The relevance of these in vitro data to wound care is unclear. Culture-proven *P. multocida* infections have resolved after treatment with erythromycin, and oral cephalothin has been used to successfully treat a *P. multocida* infection that failed to respond to erythromycin. Oxacillin was effective in a study of prophylactic antibiotics for cat bite wounds.[53]

Rodents

Rodent bites result in small puncture wounds with a low risk of local wound infection. These bites are frequently seen in laboratory workers, in children in lower socioeconomic areas who are bitten while sleeping, and occasionally in pet owners.[54] A number of diseases can be transmitted by rodent bites or scratches, including rat-bite fever, leptospirosis, tularemia, sporotrichosis, murine typhus, and plague, although nonbite contacts are the more common routes of transmission of systemic disease to humans. Rat-bite fever, caused by *Streptobacillus moniliformis* or *Spirillum minus* is rare but can result from any rodent bite. It usually manifests 1 to 3 days after the bite with abrupt onset of fever, chills, myalgias, and headache followed by a rash. Abscesses form in many organs including brain, myocardium, and soft tissues. Involvement of joints occurs in 50% of cases, resulting in an asymmetric migrating polyarthritis.[55]

Primates

Monkey and other primate bites are said to have a high wound infection rate. The infecting organisms have not been well described, with the exception of one case of wound infection due to *Eikenella corrodens* and a case of osteomyelitis due to *P. multocida.*[44,56] Old World macaque monkeys (rhesus macaques, cynomolgus, and other Asiatic macaque monkeys) may harbor *Cercopithecine herpesvirus 1,* also called *Herpesvirus simiae* or more simply, B virus, which is fatal to humans if not treated early. Most victims of B virus in the United States were laboratory workers who were bitten or scratched by monkeys or who sustained scratches from cages; many of the exposures were considered trivial at the time.[57,58] This virus has been found to be highly prevalent in adult macaque monkeys, making them unsuitable pets.[59]

The disease in monkeys resembles that of human herpesviruses; monkeys can shed virus without symptoms but are more likely to shed when ill, under stress, immunocompromised, or breeding. Virus can be found in the conjunctiva, buccal mucosa, and genital areas, but most infected monkeys do not display any lesions.[57] B virus can enter host cells within 5 minutes, making immediate wound care at the scene the most important step in prevention of transmission. Deep puncture wounds that are difficult to clean, inadequately cleansed wounds, and wounds of the face, neck, or thorax pose greater risks of infection.

The incubation period is 2 days to 5 weeks, with most cases presenting within 5 to 21 days. The illness usually, but not always, is heralded by the appearance of vesicles at the site of the injury, sometimes associated with tingling, pain, or numbness. In some cases, the illness starts with peripheral or central nervous system symptoms, or it can begin as a flulike illness. Eventually, paresthesias at the site ascend along the infected extremity, and the victim develops headache, confusion, cranial nerve palsies, hemiparesis, and ultimately coma and death. The case-fatality rate is approximately 70%.[57] Treatment is most successful if begun when vesicles first appear.[58] With aggressive treatment, however, survival is possible even after central nervous system symptoms develop.[57]

Ferrets

The European ferret (*Mustela putorius furo*) is now the third most popular pet in the United States, with an estimated 5 to 7 million pet ferrets in 4 to 5 million households. The ferret is descended from the polecat, a member of the weasel, mink, and wolverine family. In the past, hunters bred ferrets to hunt rats and rabbits; they are extremely ferocious and tenacious with their prey. Although domesticated for more than 2000 years, the ferret appears to retain its instinctive propensity for attacking suckling animals and an attraction to the neck of its victim. Ferrets are known to attack infants and young children suddenly and without provocation, even in the presence of an adult. They usually attack around the face and neck, and often have to be pried off the victim. Extensive cosmetic repair after such attacks has been required.[60,61] Locking ferrets in a cage may not be an adequate safeguard; ferrets have been known to escape and hide for several days.

Little is known about the bacteriology of ferret bites. Rabies, although uncommon, has been contracted by ferrets, but there has not been a documented case of transmission to humans.[62] In experimentally induced rabies, ferrets develop clinical signs (ataxia, paresis, anorexia, fever, hyperactivity) within 16 to 96 days after inoculation and secrete rabies in their saliva from 2 days before to 6 days after the onset of overt illness, which is similar to the way the illness behaves in other animals.[63] The Centers for Disease Control and Prevention (CDC) guidelines for managing ferret bites are similar to those for other domestic animal bites with regard to rabies, allowing a 10-day observation period after the bite, rather than immediate sacrifice and testing.[64] A rabies vaccine for ferrets is available.[65] Ferrets should be vaccinated at 3 months and yearly thereafter.

Pigs

Pig bites are often deep but can be deceptively small on the surface.[66] They require careful exploration and debridement. Pathogens include *Pasteurella aerogenes, P. multocida, Escherichia coli, Bacteroides, Proteus,* and α-hemolytic and β-hemolytic streptococci.[42,66] Despite antibiotics and appropriate wound care, pig bites have a high risk of infection.

Domestic Herbivores

The bites of horses result in severe soft tissue contusions, but virtually all heal uneventfully. Cattle do not have upper incisors, so they virtually never bite. Camels are well known for biting their handlers, particularly in the winter, reportedly in sudden vengeance for offenses committed previously. Unlike most other herbivores, the camel has canine teeth and can cause deep wounds, fractures, and amputations, most involving the handler's upper limbs. These wounds are reported to have a very high rate of infection.[67,68] Most domestic herbivores carry *P. multocida.* Because antibiotics are added to the feed of most domestic herbivores, bacterial isolates from these animals are frequently resistant to common antibiotics.

Wild Animals

Human encounters with large wild animals, such as wolves, coyotes, large cats, elephants, or bears, usually result in massive trauma and often death from some combination of biting, swiping, throwing, goring, and trampling. Attacks by animals may result in major blunt or penetrating trauma, with severe arterial blood loss, airway damage, intracranial and subarachnoid penetration, broken ribs and vertebrae, pneumothoraces, and intraperitoneal bleeding.[15,69] Hyenas are known for their tremendously strong jaws and their frequency of attacks on humans in Africa. Hyenas target the face and can literally rip off a face or a head with one clean massive bite. Bites of bears usually result in a series of punctures, with crushing and tearing of soft tissues, and underlying fractures, particularly of facial bones and those of the upper extremity. Big cats tend to go for the nape of the neck; their teeth may enter the pharynx, esophagus, and intervertebral space.[69] A common killing mechanism is to shake the victim by the neck, which results in hyperextension injuries. The wounds grow *P. multocida,* staphylococci, and streptococci.

Systemic Infection

Approximately 150 systemic diseases of mammals can be transmitted by some route and in some form to humans. Leptospirosis, rat-bite fever, cat-scratch disease (*Bartonella henselae*), tularemia, *Erysipelo-*

Table 58-1. Risk Factors in Bite Wound Infections

Factor	High Risk	Low Risk
Species	Cat	Dog
	Human	Rodent
	Probably primate	
	Pig	
Location of wound	Hand	Face
	Below knee	Scalp
	Through-and-through oral	Mucosa
	Over joint	
Wound type	Puncture	Large
	Extensive crush	Superficial
	Contaminated	Clean
	Old	Recent
Patient	Elderly	
	Diabetic	
	Prosthetic valve	
	Peripheral vascular disease	
	Asplenic	
	Alcoholic	
	Steroids, cytotoxic drugs	

thrix, hepatitis B, bubonic plague, rabies, tetanus, and sporotrichosis have been transmitted through bites or scratches, but with the exceptions of rabies and tetanus, this mode of transmission is rare.[70] Patients with these systemic illnesses present weeks or months after the exposure, so a history of animal contact must be elicited.

Infection Risk Factors

Location of Wound

In studies of nonbite lacerations, wounds on the hand and those below the knee have a greater propensity for infection and a higher risk of morbidity compared with wounds on other areas of the body (Table 58-1).[71-73] The hand contains many poorly vascularized structures that do not resist infection well. The fascial spaces and tendon sheaths communicate, so an infection quickly spreads throughout the entire hand. For dog bites, the infection rate of hand wounds is as high as 30%, regardless of suturing, whereas the infection rate of dog bites elsewhere averages 9%.[20,21] In a series of cat bites, hand wounds had an infection rate of 19%, lower extremity wounds 20%, and arm, neck, or trunk wounds 5% or less.[41] Nonbite lacerations of the head and neck have a lower risk of infection than wounds elsewhere on the body.[71,72] Similarly, dog bites of the face and neck (including punctures) have an infection rate of only 0% to 5% even when sutured.[17,18,23] Severe facial wounds that warrant hospital admission and operative repair have a substantially higher infection rate.

Delay in Care

The age of the wound may be one of the most important factors contributing to the risk of infection. In studies of nonbite wounds, delay in seeking care is associated with a higher risk of infection and complications.[71,73] Dog bites in patients who delay care by

BOX 58-1. Basic Wound Care For Bites

Arrival at Emergency Department
Elevate
Ice
Evaluate
  Airway-breathing-circulation
  History
    Circumstances of bite, biting animal, captivity status
    Diabetes, alcohol, spleen, peripheral vascular disease,
      steroids, tetanus
  Neurovascular examination distal to wound
  Radiographs as indicated

Wound Preparation
Clean skin; do not shave
If rabies is a concern, scrub wound with soap and water and
  rinse
Anesthetize
Irrigate, explore, debride

Wound Closure Factors
Species
Type of wound
Location of wound

Aftercare
Dressing
Splint extremities
Tetanus prophylaxis
Prophylactic antibiotics in selected cases
Rabies prophylaxis as indicated

10 to 24 hours have a substantially increased risk of becoming infected.[17,19] Time to presentation, presence of infection at presentation, and subsequent morbidity are strongly correlated in human bites of the hand.[74,75]

Host

Patients with underlying illnesses (e.g., diabetes, peripheral vascular disease) and those taking steroids are at increased risk for infection and poor healing.[72,73] Immunocompromised patients are probably at a higher risk for infection. Elderly patients in general have a higher risk of infection than other age groups for nonbite lacerations and dog bites.[11,72,76]

MANAGEMENT

First Aid and Wound Preparation

Animal bites should be treated as contusions, with immediate ice and elevation (Box 58-1). Direct pressure with a clean cloth or gauze for 10 minutes will stop most bleeding. Washing the wound with soap and water, ideally with a fine-pore sponge to minimize additional tissue trauma, substantially decreases the risk of rabies infection if done within 3 hours,[64] so should be carried out before hospital arrival if possible.

History

Practitioners should elicit the circumstances of the bite, the biting animal, and whether the animal is in cap-

tivity and has been immunized against rabies. Specific inquiry should be made about risks for poor wound healing (e.g., diabetes, peripheral vascular disease, smoking) and risks for increased susceptibility to *C. canimorsus*, specifically immune status, lung disease, steroid use, splenectomy, or alcoholism. Tetanus immunization status, allergies to medications, and availability and reliability of follow-up care should also be assessed.

Evaluation and Repair

Radiographs of the injured area may be indicated to detect possible fracture, foreign body, or joint penetration, although they are rarely necessary in dog bites in adults and older children. Infants and small children (up to 2 years old) who sustain substantial bite wounds to the scalp should have skull films or preferably a computed tomography scan.[15] Evidence of skull perforation should prompt neurosurgical consultation and admission to the hospital.

Following a careful neurovascular examination of the injured area, the wound should be anesthetized and explored, looking for foreign body and injuries to nerves, tendons, and arteries. After cleaning with soap and water, wound irrigation followed by debridement is recommended. There is no compelling evidence that extension of the wound to promote irrigation diminishes the chance of infection.

Much controversy and few data surround the question of suturing animal bites. Sound practice dictates that when a wound is at high risk for infection, it should not be sutured unless there is strong experimental evidence of the safety of the practice. To date, only dog bites have undergone controlled studies.[19] The infection rate in 169 wounds was the same for sutured bites as for those left to heal by secondary intention (7.7%). This was true even for dog bites on the hand, which had a higher infection rate (12%), but with no significant difference between sutured and unsutured wounds. Observational studies demonstrate an equivalent infection rate for sutured dog bites and unsutured wounds.[11,17,18,77] Sutured dog bites of the face have a very low infection rate, even when punctures are sutured and no prophylactic antibiotics are used.[23] Sutured cat bites primarily on the face developed no infections in one study, whereas another study of selectively sutured cat bites found an infection rate of 4.4%. In both studies, patients received antibiotic prophylaxis.[41,77]

The following guidelines are suggested, even though data are limited (Table 58-2). Thorough wound cleansing and irrigation are presumed. Bite wounds of the face and scalp from any species can be sutured. It is probably safe to suture most uncomplicated dog bites. Lower extremity and hand wounds are at higher risk for infection and should be handled with extra caution (i.e., rarely sutured). Cat bites and primate bites on the face or scalp can be considered for suture repair, but sutures should be avoided in other locations. Puncture wounds from any species should not be closed. Contaminated wounds, wounds more than 12 hours old, or wounds infected at presentation should not be sutured. Patients at risk for infection or poor wound healing should be treated conservatively, with sutures avoided in higher risk wounds. Proper alternatives include delayed primary closure or allowing healing by secondary intention. Patients and physicians can be reassured when small wounds are left open; a study comparing suturing versus conservative treatment of uncomplicated, full-thickness hand wounds less than 2 cm demonstrated no difference in functional or cosmetic outcome.[78] No current evidence shows that use of topical adhesive results in a lower infection rate than sutures.

A simple, sterile dry dressing is sufficient to protect the wound. Delayed primary closure requires that the wound be kept moist, usually with a wet saline dressing. Abrasions should be covered with a topical antibiotic and dry sterile dressing. Bites of the hands or over joints should be immobilized with a bulky soft dressing or a splint. Bite wounds are considered tetanus prone (see Table 58-5).[79] It is prudent to encourage patients to have wound checks within 1 to 3 days after the bite. Early follow-up is particularly important when the risk of a *Pasteurella* infection is high.

Prophylactic Antibiotics

Dog Bites

Prophylactic antibiotics are not indicated for most routine dog bite wounds, except of the hand.[18,20,21,80] Additionally, other high-risk wounds (e.g., deep structure injury) and high-risk patients have traditionally been excluded from studies on prophylactic antibiotics and would probably benefit.[21] Therefore, a reasonable approach is to give prophylactic antibiotics to victims of high-risk dog bite wounds but not to those with low-risk wounds (see Table 58-2).

For prophylaxis, 5 days of an antibiotic that covers *Staphylococcus aureus* and streptococcus is likely sufficient (Table 58-3).

On the other hand, for treatment of established dog bite infection, coverage of *P. multocida* should be included. Second- and third-generation cephalosporins and amoxicillin-clavulanate are all excellent first-line agents. For the adult allergic to penicillin, a combination of clindamycin plus a fluoroquinolone can be used. For penicillin-allergic children, clindamycin plus trimethoprim-sulfamethoxazole (TMP-SMX) is acceptable.

Capnocytophaga canimorsus

There are no studies on prevention of *C. canimorsus* infection, but it is prudent to give patients with known risks prophylactic antibiotics after a dog or cat bite.[32,35-37,39] It would be logical to include in this population other immunocompromised patients, in-

Table 58-2. Recommendations for Wound Closure and Antibiotics in Bite Cases

Species	Suturing	Prophylactic Antibiotics
Dog	All (+/− hands and feet)	High risk only*
Cat	Face only	All
Rodent	Yes (rarely needed)	No
Monkey	No	Yes
Human		
Hand bites	No	Yes
Other locations	Yes	Not necessary unless other high-risk concerns are present*
Self-inflicted		
Mucosa	Yes	No
Through-and-through	Yes	Yes

*Hand wounds; deep punctures; heavy contamination; significant tissue destruction; >12 hours old; joint, tendon, or bone involvement; patients with diabetes, peripheral vascular disease, or corticosteroid use.

Table 58-3. Suggested Regimens for Prophylactic Antibiotics in Bite Wounds

Species	Nonallergic Patient	Penicillin-Allergic Patient
Dog, most other animals	Dicloxacillin Cephalexin	Erythromycin TMP-SMX[†]
Cat	Cefuroxime Amoxicillin-clavulanate Dicloxacillin + penicillin	Extended spectrum quinolone* Azithromycin TMP-SMX[†]
Dog, cat; patient without spleen, alcoholic, or lung disease (*C. canimorsus*)	Penicillin Amoxicillin-clavulanate	Clindamycin Erythromycin Azithromycin or clarithromycin
Human (CFIs),[‡] monkey	Cefuroxime Cefaclor Amoxicillin-clavulanate Ampicillin + first-generation cephalosporin Ampicillin + dicloxacillin	Extended spectrum quinolone* TMP-SMX[†]
Human: not CFI	Dicloxacillin or cephalexin	Erythromycin
Human: through-and-through	Penicillin	Clindamycin

*Includes levofloxacin, moxifloxacin, sparfloxacin. Quinolones not approved for children and pregnant women.
[†]Sulfonamides should not be given to pregnant women.
[‡]Anaerobic coverage not necessary unless established infection; 50% of human mouth anaerobes resistant to penicillin.
CFI, closed-fist injury; TMP-SMX, trimethoprim-sulfamethoxazole.

cluding those with diabetes. In vitro, *C. canimorsus* is susceptible to penicillin G, ampicillin, carbenicillin, cephalothin, ceftizoxime, clindamycin, erythromycin, tetracycline, fluoroquinolones, vancomycin, and chloramphenicol, although one clinical case of resistance to penicillin, erythromycin, and clindamycin has occurred.[35,36] *C. canimorsus* displays variable susceptibility to TMP-SMX, and it appears to be resistant to all aminoglycosides. For prophylaxis, consider amoxicillin-clavulanate or penicillin. For treatment of established infection, an intravenous second- or third-generation cephalosporin, amoxicillin-sulbactam, or clindamycin plus a fluoroquinolone (in adults) is acceptable (see Table 58-3).

Cat Bites

Only one small randomized controlled study on the use of prophylactic antibiotics in cat bites has been published, demonstrating reduced infection with prophylaxis.[53] Cat bites have a high likelihood of infection, and patients with infected cat bites often require hospitalization.[7] Therefore, it is prudent to prescribe prophylactic antibiotics for cat bites.

Pasteurella multocida should be specifically covered, as should *S. aureus* and *Streptococcus* species. *P. multocida* is resistant to dicloxacillin, cephalexin, and clindamycin, and many strains are resistant to erythromycin. Excellent coverage and convenience are afforded by a second-generation cephalosporin such as cefuroxime, which needs to be taken only twice a day. Amoxicillin-clavulanate is also a good choice, although it requires more frequent dosing and has substantial side effects. A less expensive but more complicated regimen is the combination of dicloxacillin and penicillin. For the penicillin-allergic patient, options include the extended-spectrum macrolides, fluoroquinolones, or TMP-SMX. In vitro testing suggests that azithromycin is slightly more effective than clarithromycin against *P. multocida,* but no clinical data are available.[50,52]

Extended-spectrum fluoroquinolones cover *P. multocida* and have good staphylococcal and streptococcal coverage.[49] Given the many other alternatives for prophylaxis, however, the use of fluoroquinolones as first-line agents is not recommended because of cost, lack of clinical experience, and concerns that overuse will result in resistance. Additionally, these drugs are not approved for children or pregnant women.

TMP-SMX offers reasonable coverage against *P. multocida* as well as staphylococci and streptococci and is a low-cost, although not ideal, alternative (see Table 58-3). Tetracycline is not advisable for *P. multocida* coverage because it achieves low tissue levels at a very slow rate and is not very effective against common bite pathogens, including streptococci, staphylococci, diphtheroids, *Bacteroides,* and anaerobic gram-positive cocci.[49,51,81] When used together, however, tetracycline and erythromycin have a synergistic effect against *Pasteurella.*[82]

For very high-risk bites, such as cat bites on the hands, patients should receive an antibiotic in the

emergency department. Intravenous treatment is preferable because it achieves detectable levels in the wound much sooner than the oral or intramuscular route. However, even an oral dose of antibiotic at the time of treatment is preferable to giving patients a prescription that may not be filled for 24 hours. The usual course for prophylaxis is 5 days.

Other Animal Bites

Patients who sustain pig bites or camel bites, especially on the hand, should receive antibiotic prophylaxis. Rodent bites and bites from most other species have a lower risk of wound infection, so prophylaxis generally is not indicated.

Monkey Bites

Although there are no data on the use of prophylactic antibiotics, monkey bites are considered to have a high risk for bacterial infection.[56] Antibiotics are advisable for full-thickness bites, particularly those on the hand. Management of these wounds and selection of antibiotics should follow recommendations for human bites (see Tables 54-2 and 54-3).

Prevention of B virus requires *immediate* local wound care (Box 58-2). This should be performed at the scene of the exposure before medical evaluation is sought.[57] The wound should be washed with povidone-iodine, chlorhexidine, or a detergent soap solution for at least 15 minutes; eyes and mucous membranes should be irrigated with sterile saline or running water for at least 15 minutes. It is recommended that workers with potential exposures be referred by their occupational health care provider to a person knowledgeable about B virus, as treatment decisions are complex; however, most laboratories will provide workers with written information and appropriate kits for specimen collection if they are referred to an emergency department.

Clinicians examining patients with fresh monkey bites from macaque monkeys, in particular rhesus and cynomolgus, should determine the risk of exposure by evaluating the time, source, location, and type of exposure, and timeliness and adequacy of cleansing and examining the wound (see Box 58-2). Cleansing should be repeated. The health status of the monkey should be determined, and, if it can be done safely, the facility should examine the monkey for active lesions. Cultures of bite or scratch wounds or splashes should never be done prior to cleansing but are often negative after cleansing. However, a positive culture for B virus would prompt prophylaxis if not previously given. Prophylaxis with antiviral therapy is recommended only where the risk of transmission is high (Table 58-4) because human cases of infection are extremely rare, despite thousands of potential exposures each year, and treatment may interfere with seroconversion, confounding diagnostic testing. The recommended therapy is valacyclovir, 1 g PO q8h for 14 days (or alternatively, acyclovir, 800 mg PO five times daily for 14 days). Prophylaxis, when indicated, can be given up to 5 days after the exposure.[57] Patients should be counseled

BOX 58-2. Initial Management of Monkey Bites with Potential Exposure to *Herpesvirus simiae**

First Aid (within 5 min of exposure)

Wounds: wash wound thoroughly with a solution containing detergent soap (e.g., povidone-iodine or chlorhexidine) for at least 15 minutes. Rinse well.

Consider washing skin with 0.25% hypochloride† (Dakin's solution), followed by detergent solution, for 10-15 min. (Note: causes rapid deactivation of herpesviruses but is more toxic). Do not use for mucous membranes or eyes.

Eyes, nose, mucous membranes: irrigate immediately with sterile saline or running water for at least 15 min.

Assessment
Human Victim

Assess adequacy of cleansing. Repeat cleansing regardless.

Determine date, time, location, description of injury, type of fluid or tissue contacted.

Evaluate victim's health, medications and tetanus status.

Examine wound, perform full physical examination including neurologic examination.

Consider obtaining serum samples for serologic analysis.

Consider culture of wound or exposed mucosa (after cleansing).

Determine need for postexposure prophylaxis (rabies, B virus, bacteria, other).

Nonhuman Primate

Identify the monkey, species, and responsible veterinarian.

Assess monkey's health and involvement in research studies and known serologic status.

Note: monkey should be assumed to be seropositive for B virus.

If safe, monkey should be examined for mucosal lesions, conjunctivitis.

Consider culturing lesions if present, as well as conjunctiva and buccal mucosa.

Consider serologic testing if status is unknown.

Counseling and Prophylaxis
Prophylaxis

If indicated: valacyclovir 1 g PO q8 hours × 14 days (or acyclovir 800 mg PO five times daily × 14 days)

Counseling

Educate patient and family regarding significance of the injury and symptoms of B virus.

Advise patient to avoid activities involving exchange of body fluids.

Ensure that occupational health care provider and supervisor have been notified.

Provide a card patient can carry with information on B virus and number to call in emergency.

Ensure follow-up appointment.

---

*Bites or scratches from monkeys; contaminated needlestick injuries; open wounds in contact with contaminated object in Old World macaques.
†Balance risk of infection with toxicity to tissues. Prepare with household bleach 1:20 in water.
Modified from Cohen JI, et al: Recommendations for prevention of and therapy for exposure to B virus (*cercopithecine herpesvirus 1*). *Clin Infect Dis* 35:1191, 2002.

Table 58-4. Recommendations for Postexposure Prophylaxis for Persons Exposed to B Virus (Herpesvirus simiae)

Prophylaxis Recommended
Skin exposure (with loss of skin integrity) or mucosal exposure to a high-risk source: macaque that is ill, immunocompromised, known to be shedding virus, or has visible lesions compatible with B virus
Inadequately cleaned skin or mucosal exposure
Laceration of head, neck, or torso
Deep puncture bite
Needlestick associated with tissue or fluid from the nervous system, lesions suspicious for B virus, eyelids, or mucosa
Puncture or laceration after exposure to objects (a) contaminated with fluid from monkey oral or genital lesions or with nervous system tissues or (b) known to contain B virus.
Postcleaning culture-positive B virus

Prophylaxis Considered
Mucosal splash that has been adequately cleaned
Laceration (with loss of skin integrity) that has been adequately cleaned
Needlestick involving blood from an ill or immunocompromised macaque
Puncture or laceration occurring after exposure either to objects contaminated with body fluid (other than from a lesion) or potentially infected cell culture

Prophylaxis Not Recommended
Skin exposure in which the skin remains intact
Exposure associated with nonmacaque species of nonhuman primates.

Modified from Cohen JI, et al: Recommendations for prevention of and therapy for exposure to B virus (*cercopithecine herpesvirus 1*). *Clin Infect Dis* 35:1191, 2002.

about the signs and symptoms of B virus infection and told to immediately seek care if any occur. Patients with high-risk exposures should be told to avoid activities that involve exchange of bodily fluids, including saliva. Close follow-up for the next 4 weeks is essential.

DISPOSITION

Patients with life-threatening or limb-threatening injuries or with severe cosmetic defects requiring operative repair, particularly children, should be admitted to the hospital. Most other patients can be discharged with close follow-up. Many U.S. cities and counties have animal bite reporting laws. These require the emergency department to obtain details on the biting incident, the animals involved, and names of owners and submit a report shortly after the victim is treated. Public health officials may be able to locate escaped animals or those that are potentially ill based on these reports, as well as provide consultation regarding the need for rabies prophylaxis and animal management.

Treatment of Infected Bites

Patients who present or return with infected bites should be assessed for complications such as retained foreign body, tenosynovitis, joint infection, or fracture.

Abscesses should be drained. Patients with wound infection and fever, systemic symptoms, lymphangitis, or deep structure involvement should be hospitalized for intravenous antibiotics and possible surgical intervention. In addition, high-risk patients (e.g., diabetic, immunosuppressed, elderly) with localized infections, those with peripheral vascular disease, and those likely to be noncompliant with therapy require hospitalization, although intravenous antibiotic treatment in a short-stay unit or at home with a visiting nurse may be a suitable alternative. Empiric, broad-spectrum antibiotic coverage should be started and the affected area elevated and immobilized. Anaerobic coverage, not usually necessary for prophylaxis, should be included for infected bite wounds. Wound or blood cultures are usually not necessary unless the patient fails to respond to the first line of therapy.[83,84] Healthy patients with localized infections can be managed on oral antibiotics at home with close follow-up. The infected area should be immobilized with a splint; the patient should be instructed in strict elevation of the infected area and assessed daily until the infection has resolved.

HUMAN BITES

PERSPECTIVE

Epidemiology

Human bites of the hand, especially the clenched-fist or closed-fist injury (CFI), or fight bite, are associated with a high incidence of infectious complications. These include septic arthritis, tenosynovitis, and osteomyelitis, as well as surgical amputation necessitated by infection.[74,75] Most simple human bites elsewhere on the body are probably no more significant than ordinary lacerations. The reported rate of infectious complications in human bites of the hand is 25% to 50%.[85] The majority of infections already exist when the patient first presents for care.[74,75] The high infection rate results from a combination of factors: the location on the hand, the position of the hand at the time of injury, the mechanism of entry, associated injuries, the bacteriology of the human mouth, and a delay in seeking care.

PRINCIPLES OF DISEASE

Fight Bites

The CFI is a ragged laceration most often found over the metacarpal joints of the middle finger and ring finger. It results when an individual strikes another person's mouth with a closed fist. Associated traumatic injuries include the "boxer's fracture" (distal fourth or fifth metacarpal), amputations, foreign bodies, and extensor tendon lacerations. Penetration of the joint occurs in up to 62% of wounds; up to 58% involve

injury to the bone.[86] The presence of an extensor tendon laceration is highly predictive of joint penetration. Patients who have deep structure involvement have significantly more morbidity than those who do not. Another type of fight bite is an actual bite, usually on the finger, which may penetrate the proximal or distal interphalangeal joint; this can result in a traumatic amputation.

Bacteriology

Information on the bacteriology of human bites comes almost exclusively from hand bites, with the vast majority of these being CFIs. Infected wounds are polymicrobial, with an average of five organisms per wound.[87] Streptococci and S. aureus are the most common aerobic pathogens. Gram-negative rods and anaerobes are more frequently isolated from infected human bites than other types of hand infections, including those from animal bites. The presence of anaerobes in mixed infection may be associated with a worse outcome.

Eikenella corrodens, a facultatively anaerobic gram-negative rod harbored in human dental plaque, is found in 25% to 29% of CFI infections.[28] It acts synergistically with aerobic organisms, most frequently streptococci, and is thought to account for greater morbidity in these wounds.[87] E. corrodens is susceptible to penicillin, ampicillin, second- and third-generation cephalosporins, carbenicillin, tetracycline, and the fluoroquinolones.[49,81] Resistance to penicillin has been reported.[50] E. corrodens is resistant to penicillinase-resistant penicillins, methicillin, nafcillin, aminoglycosides, clindamycin, vancomycin, and metronidazole.[51] Susceptibility to first-generation cephalosporins and erythromycin is suboptimal.[50,81]

Other Human Bites

Human bites in locations other than the hand have about the same rate of infection as ordinary lacerations, if proper local wound care is administered. Human bites of the face have about a 2.5% infection rate.

In children, approximately 70% of human bites are abrasions, which generally do not become infected. The reported infection rate of human bites in children is 9% to 12%. Most of these infections are already established at the time of the initial visit, usually in patients who have delayed care for more than 12 to 18 hours.[88,89]

Wounds from the victim's own teeth, usually a result from a fall or a seizure, can be considered bites. Wounds that only involve the mucosa or tongue have a low infection rate, from 0% to 12%. Mucocutaneous (through-and-through) lacerations have an infection rate of 30%. Organisms cultured from these infected wounds include Streptococcus, S. aureus and epidermidis, Bacteroides, Corynebacterium, Neisseria, and Haemophilus haemolyticus.[90]

Transmission of Disease

Human bites have resulted in the transmission of actinomycosis, syphilis, tuberculosis, herpes, hepatitis C, and hepatitis B.[91,92] Herpetic whitlow, infection of the distal phalanx from herpes simplex virus, is a well-known occupational hazard of nurses, physicians, dentists, and oral hygienists. Although HIV is secreted at some time in the saliva of up to 44% of infected patients, the CDC does not consider human bites to carry a risk of transmission unless there is exposure to blood in the process.[93,94] HIV is not often present in the saliva of most infected patients, and when it is, the titer of virus is very low.[92] Cases in which HIV has convincingly been transmitted through a bite involved significant amounts of blood mixed with the saliva.[95,96] Nevertheless, when a significant bite has occurred, and particularly if the biter is known to be HIV positive, it is reasonable to consult with infection control experts locally or at the CDC. The potential risk of HIV transmission to the person inflicting the bite should also be considered.

MANAGEMENT

The approach to the human bite depends on the location and the mechanism of injury. Any laceration or puncture in the vicinity of the metacarpophalangeal joint should be considered a CFI unless proved otherwise. Full-thickness bites on the hand should be considered high risk. Hand radiographs should be obtained, looking for fractures, dislocations, retained teeth, or air in the joint.[74,75] A skyline view, but not standard finger views, will demonstrate vertical articular fractures of the metacarpals.[97]

The wound should be assessed for established infection and a careful neurovascular examination performed, with particular attention to the extensor function. The wound should then be anesthetized and explored in a bloodless field to look for foreign bodies, tendon laceration, or joint penetration. It is essential that the wound be examined through the full range of motion, including the position at the moment of injury. The wound should be irrigated and debrided. Wounds that demonstrate tendon lacerations should be presumed to have joint involvement as well, and this finding should prompt consultation with a hand surgeon.

Although there are no controlled studies on suturing human bites, the high rate of infection and complications of human bites on the hand mandate that they be left open. The wound should be covered with a dry sterile dressing and the hand splinted in a position of function either with a plaster splint or by packing the palm with bulky gauze and wrapping the hand in a mitten-type dressing. Human bites are tetanus-prone wounds (Table 58-5).[79,98] Human bite injuries elsewhere on the body should generally be treated as typical lacerations. Treatment includes irrigation, aggressive debridement, and suturing if anatomy permits and cosmetic considerations are important.[99]

Antiviral Agents

Victims of bites from persons potentially infected with HIV or hepatitis should receive exceptionally rapid,

Table 58-5. Guidelines for Tetanus Prophylaxis

History of Adsorbed Tetanus Toxoid (Doses)	Clean, Minor Wounds		All Other Wounds*	
	Td[†]	TIG	Td[†]	TIG
Unknown or <3	Yes	No	Yes	Yes
≥3[‡]	No[§]	No	No[¶]	No

*Such as, but not limited to, wounds contaminated with dirt, feces, soil, and saliva; puncture wounds; avulsions; and wounds resulting from missiles, crushing, burns, and frostbite.
†For children < 7 years old, DTP (DT, if pertussis vaccine is contraindicated) is preferred to tetanus toxoid alone. For persons ≥ 7 years of age, Td is preferred to tetanus toxoid alone.
‡If only three doses of *fluid* toxoid have been received, a fourth dose of toxoid, preferably an adsorbed toxoid, should be given.
§Yes, if >10 years since last dose.
¶Yes, if >5 years since last dose. (More frequent boosters are not needed and can accentuate side effects.)
DTP, diphtheria, tetanus, and pertussis antigen; Td, tetanus, diphtheria antigen; TIG, tetanus immune globulin.
From the Centers for Disease Control: Diphtheria, tetanus, and pertussis: Recommendations for vaccine use and other preventive measures—recommendations of the Immunization Practices Advisory Committee (ACIP). *MMWR Morb Mortal Wkly Rep* 40:1, 1991.

vigorous, and thorough wound cleansing with soap and water, to remove saliva, and irrigation with virucidal agents such as 1% povidone-iodine. A baseline HIV blood test and hepatitis antibodies at the time of injury should be obtained or arranged, along with a follow-up test in 6 months. If the bite involved blood, hepatitis B and HIV prophylaxis may be warranted. Consultation with the CDC's postexposure prophylaxis hotline regarding possible blood-borne exposures is available 24 hours a day (1-888-448-4911; http://www.ucsf.edu/hivcntr/).

Prophylactic Antibiotics

Antibiotic prophylaxis is recommended for all human bites of the hand (see Tables 58-2 and 58-3). One randomized, placebo-controlled study of hospitalized patients with uninfected human bites on the hand found no infections in patients who received antibiotics, whereas those who received placebo had a 47% infection rate.[85] However, good results have been achieved without prophylactic antibiotics when patients present early and appropriate wound cleansing is administered.[74,75] Antibiotics are indicated for high-risk human bite wounds elsewhere on the body, including deep punctures, severe crush injuries, contaminated wounds, older wounds, and wounds in patients with underlying illnesses. The antibiotic selected should offer coverage for gram-positive organisms and *E. corrodens,* such as a second-generation cephalosporin or amoxicillin-clavulanate, and should be given for 5 days.

Mucosal lacerations from a person's own teeth, including those of the tongue, should be irrigated well. Suturing is advisable only for deeper and larger wounds. Although such wounds may have a higher risk of infection, prophylactic antibiotics do not necessarily reduce the incidence.[90] Through-and-through lacerations, from a tooth puncture through the skin of the

BOX 58-3. Indications for Hospital Admission for Human Bites of the Hand

Wound >24 hours old
Established infection
Penetration of joint or tendon sheath
Bone involvement
Foreign body
Unreliable patient or poor home situation
Diabetic or suppressed immune status

lower lip, may require a layered closure and are at high risk of infection. Prophylactic antibiotics probably reduce the risk of infection.[90] Penicillin for 5 days remains the regimen of choice.

Infected Wounds

Infected human bites of the hand require both aerobic and anaerobic cultures, and the patient should be treated with intravenous antibiotics that cover gram-positive organisms, *E. corrodens,* and anaerobes. Up to 50% of anaerobes isolated from human bite wounds produce β-lactamase and are resistant to penicillin.[51] Treatment options include amoxicillin-sulbactam, cefoxitin, and ticarcillin-clavulanate. Penicillin-allergic patients can receive clindamycin plus TMP-SMX or clindamycin plus a fluoroquinolone, although data for these regimens are limited.

DISPOSITION

Patients with Infection

All patients with infected human bites of the hand should be hospitalized (Box 58-3). Localized infections of human bites not on the hand can usually be treated without hospitalization if the patient has no lymphangitis or systemic symptoms and can be followed closely.

Patients without Infection

Reliable, otherwise healthy patients who present within 24 hours without infection and have no tendon, joint, or bone damage can be treated at home with close follow-up, preferably within 1 to 2 days.[74,75] Discharge instructions should include immobilization, elevation, and sterile dressing changes every 6 hours.

High-risk patients, such as those with delayed presentation or deep structure involvement, require prophylactic parenteral antibiotics and close evaluation. Hospitalization is generally recommended. Although many human bites are a consequence of mutual aggression, the physician must keep in mind that the patient may be the victim—or perpetrator—of child, spousal, or elder abuse.[100] All states require reporting of suspected child abuse; laws vary for spousal or elder abuse. In all cases, details of the incident should be documented and the wound carefully described in the record. Counseling or referral should be offered when appropriate.

KEY CONCEPTS

■ Prophylactic antibiotics are not indicated for routine dog bite wounds but are recommended for dog bites of the hand and in high-risk patients.

■ Patients at risk for *C. canimorsus* should receive prophylactic antibiotics for this organism after a dog bite.

■ Cat bites have a high rate of infection and all warrant prophylactic antibiotics.

■ In general, when a wound is at high risk for infection, it should not be sutured.

■ Prophylactic antibiotics are recommended for all human bites of the hand as well as for high-risk wounds, including deep punctures, severe crush injuries, contaminated wounds, older wounds, and wounds in patients with underlying illnesses. Ordinary bites, such as those exchanged among children, are not high risk for infections or complications and do not require prophylaxis.

■ All bites are considered tetanus-prone wounds.

REFERENCES

1. Sacks JJ, Kresnow M, Houston B: Dog bites: How big a problem? *Inj Prev* 2:52, 1996.
2. Nonfatal dog bite-related injuries treated in hospital emergency departments—United States, 2001. *MMWR Morb Mortal Wkly Rep* 52:605, 2003.
3. Eng T, et al: Urban epizootic of rabies in Mexico: Epidemiology and impact of animal bite injuries. *Bull World Health Organ* 71:615, 1993.
4. Matter HC, Sentinella A: The epidemiology of bite and scratch injuries by vertebrate animals in Switzerland. *Eur J Epidemiol* 14:483, 1998.
5. Weiss HB, Friedman DI, Cohen JH: Incidence of dog bite injuries treated in emergency departments. *JAMA* 279:51, 1998.
6. Aghababian R, Conte J: Mammalian bite wounds. *Ann Emerg Med* 9:79, 1980.
7. Kizer K: Epidemiologic and clinical aspects of animal bite injuries. *JACEP* 8:134, 1979.
8. Bhanganada K, et al: Dog-bite injuries at a Bangkok teaching hospital. *Acta Trop* 55:249, 1993.
9. Dog-bite-related fatalities—United States, 1995-1996. *MMWR Morb Mortal Wkly Rep* 46:463, 1997.
10. Feder H, Shanley J, Baerbera J: Review of 59 patients hospitalized with animal bites. *Pediatr Infect Dis J* 6:24, 1987.
11. Dire D, Hogan D, Riggs M: A prospective evaluation of risk factors for infections from dog-bite wounds. *Acad Emerg Med* 1:258, 1994.
12. Overall KL, Love M: Dog bites to humans: Demography, epidemiology, injury, and risk. *J Am Vet Med Assoc* 218:1923, 2001.
13. Kenevan R, Gottlieb V, Rich J: A dog bite injury with involvement of cranial content: Case report. *Mil Med* 150:502, 1985.
14. Pinckney L, Kennedy L: Fractures of the infant skull caused by animal bites. *Am J Radiol* 135:179, 1980.
15. Steinbok P, Flodmark O, Scheifele D: Animal bites causing central nervous system injury to children. *Pediatr Neurosci* 12:96, 1986.
16. Hutson HR, et al: Law enforcement K-9 dog bites: Injuries, complications, and trends. *Ann Emerg Med* 29:637, 1997.
17. Callaham M: Treatment of common dog bites: Infection risk factors. *JACEP* 7:83, 1978.
18. Callaham M: Prophylactic antibiotics in common dog bite wounds: A controlled study. *Ann Emerg Med* 9:410, 1980.

19. Maimaris C, Quinton D: Dog-bite lacerations: A controlled trial of primary wound closure. *Arch Emerg Med* 15:156, 1988.

20. Cummings P: Antibiotics to prevent infections in patients with dog bite wounds: A meta-analysis of randomized trials. *Ann Emerg Med* 23:535, 1994.

21. Callaham M: Prophylactic antibiotics in dog bite wounds: Nipping at the heels of progress. *Ann Emerg Med* 23:577, 1994.

22. Hollander JE, et al: Wound registry: Development and validation. *Ann Emerg Med* 25:675, 1995 (erratum, 26:532, 1995).

23. Guy R, Zook E: Successful treatment of acute head and neck dog bite wounds without antibiotics. *Ann Plast Surg* 17:45, 1987.

24. Talan DA, et al: Bacteriologic analysis of infected dog and cat bites, Emergency Medicine Animal Bite Infection Study Group. *N Engl J Med* 340:85, 1999.

25. Ordog G: The bacteriology of dog bite wounds on initial presentation. *Ann Emerg Med* 15:1324, 1986.

26. Goldstein EJ: Bite wounds and infection. *Clin Infect Dis* 14:633, 1992.

27. Kaiser RM, et al: Clinical significance and epidemiology of NO-1, an unusual bacterium associated with dog and cat bites. *Emerg Infect Dis* 8:171, 2002.

28. Goldstein E, Citron D, Wield B: Bacteriology of human and animal bite wounds. *J Clin Microbiol* 8:667, 1978.

29. Holst E, et al: Characterization and distribution of *Pasteurella* species recovered from infected humans. *J Clin Microbiol* 30:2984, 1992.

30. Ganiere JP, et al: Characterization of *Pasteurella* from gingival scrapings of dogs and cats. *Comp Immunol Microbiol Infect Dis* 16:77, 1993.

31. Butler T, et al: Unidentified gram-negative rod infection: A new disease of man. *Ann Intern Med* 86:1, 1977.

32. Lion C, Escande F, Burdin JC: *Capnocytophaga canimorsus* infections in human: Review of the literature and case report. *Eur J Epidemiol* 12:521, 1996.

33. Valtonen M, et al: *Capnocytophaga canimorsus* septicemia: Fifth report of a cat-associated infection and five other cases. *Eur J Clin Microbiol Infect Dis* 14:520, 1995.

34. Chadha V, Warady BA: *Capnocytophaga canimorsus* peritonitis in a pediatric peritoneal dialysis patient. *Pediatr Nephrol* 13:646, 1999.

35. Carpenter P, Heppner B, Gnann J: DF-2 bacteremia following cat bites. *Am J Med* 82:621, 1987.

36. Job L, et al: Dysgonic fermenter-2: A clinico-epidemiologic review. *J Emerg Med* 7:185, 1989.

37. Howell J, Woodward G: Precipitous hypotension in the emergency department caused by *Capnocytophaga canimorsus*. *J Emerg Med* 8:312, 1990.

38. Findling J, Pohlmann G, Rose H: Fulminant gram-negative bacillemia (DF-2) following a dog bite in an asplenic woman. *Am J Med* 68:154, 1980.

39. Kullberg BJ, et al: Purpura fulminans and symmetrical peripheral gangrene caused by *Capnocytophaga canimorsus* (formerly DF-2) septicemia: A complication of dog bite. *Medicine (Baltimore)* 70:287, 1991.

40. Depres-Brummer P, et al: *Capnocytophaga canimorsus* sepsis presenting as an acute abdomen in an asplenic patient. *Neth J Med* 59:213, 2001.

41. Dire DJ: Cat bite wounds: Risk factors for infection. *Ann Emerg Med* 20:973, 1991.

42. Ejlertsen T, et al: *Pasteurella aerogenes* isolated from ulcers or wounds in humans with occupational exposure to pigs: A report of 7 Danish cases. *Scand J Infect Dis* 28:567, 1996.

43. Kizer KW: *Pasteurella multocida* infection from a cougar bite: A review of cougar attacks. *West J Med* 150:87, 1989.

44. Tan C, Ti T, Lee E: *Pasteurella multocida* osteomyelitis of the cervical spine in a patient on chronic hemodialysis. *Singapore Med J* 31:400, 1990.

45. Layton CT: *Pasteurella multocida* meningitis and septic arthritis secondary to a cat bite. *J Emerg Med* 17:445, 1999.

46. Morris JT, McAllister CK: Bacteremia due to *Pasteurella multocida*. *South Med J* 85:442, 1992.

47. Kumar A, Devlin HR, Vellend H: *Pasteurella multocida* meningitis in an adult: Case report and review. *Rev Infect Dis* 12:440, 1990.

48. Al-Allaf AK, Harvey TC, Cunnington AR: Pericardial tamponade caused by *Pasteurella multocida* infection after a cat bite. *Postgrad Med J* 77:199, 2001.

49. Goldstein EJ, et al: In vitro activity of Bay 12-8039, a new 8-methoxyquinolone, compared to the activities of 11 other oral antimicrobial agents against 390 aerobic and anaerobic bacteria isolated from human and animal bite wound skin and soft tissue infections in humans. *Antimicrob Agents Chemother* 41:1552, 1997.

50. Goldstein E, Nesbit C, Citron D: Comparative in vitro activities of azithromycin, Bay 3118, levofloxacin, sparfloxacin, and 11 other oral antimicrobial agents against 194 aerobic and anaerobic bite wound isolates. *Antimicrob Agents Chemother* 39:1097, 1995.

51. Goldstein E, Citron D, Vagvolgyi A: Susceptibility of bite wound bacteria to seven oral antimicrobial agents, including RU-985, a new erythromycin: Considerations in choosing empiric therapy. *Antimicrob Agents Chemother* 29:556, 1986.

52. Fass R: Erythromycin, clarithromycin, and azithromycin: Use of frequency distribution curves, scattergrams, and regression analyses to compare in vitro activities and describe cross-resistance. *Antimicrob Agents Chemother* 37:2080, 1993.

53. Elenbaas R, McNabney W, Robinson W: Evaluation of prophylactic oxacillin in cat bite wounds. *Ann Emerg Med* 13:155, 1984.

54. Hudsmith L, et al: Clinical picture: Rat bite fever. *Lancet Infect Dis* 1:91, 2001.

55. Stehle P, et al: Rat bite fever without fever. *Ann Rheum Dis* 62:894, 2003.

56. Janda DH, et al: Nonhuman primate bites. *J Orthop Res* 8:146, 1990.

57. Cohen JI, et al: Recommendations for prevention of and therapy for exposure to B virus (*cercopithecine herpesvirus 1*). *Clin Infect Dis* 35:1191, 2002.

58. Holmes GP, et al: B virus (*Herpesvirus simiae*) infection in humans: Epidemiologic investigation of a cluster. *Ann Intern Med* 112:833, 1990.

59. Ostrowski SR, et al: B-virus from pet macaque monkeys: An emerging threat in the United States? *Emerg Infect Dis* 4:117, 1998.

60. Applegate JA, Walhout MF: Childhood risks from the ferret. *J Emerg Med* 16:425, 1998.

61. Paisley J, Lauer B: Severe facial injuries to infants due to unprovoked attacks by pet ferrets. *JAMA* 259:2005, 1988.

62. Rupprecht CE, et al: Current issues in rabies prevention in the United States: Health dilemmas, public coffers, private interests. *Public Health Rep* 111:400, 1996.

63. Niezgoda M, et al: Pathogenesis of experimentally induced rabies in domestic ferrets. *Am J Vet Res* 58:1327, 1997.

64. Human rabies prevention—United States, 1999: Recommendations of the Advisory Committee on Immunization Practices (ACIP). *MMWR Recomm Rep* 48(RR-1):1, 1999.

65. Compendium of Animal Rabies Control, 1999. National Association of State Public Health Veterinarians, Inc. *MMWR Recomm Rep* 48(RR-3):1, 1999.

66. Van Demark RES, Van Demark REJ: Swine bites of the hand. *J Hand Surg Am* 16:136, 1991.

67. al Boukai A, et al: Camel bites: Report of severe osteolysis as late bone complications. *Postgrad Med J* 65:900, 1989.

68. Ogunbodede EO, Arotiba JT: Camel bite injuries of the orofacial region: Report of a case. *J Oral Maxillofac Surg* 55:1174, 1997.

69. Wiens M, Harrison P: Big cat attack: A case study. *J Trauma* 40:829, 1996.

70. Tan JS: Human zoonotic infections transmitted by dogs and cats. *Arch Intern Med* 157:1933, 1997.

71. Baker MD, Lanuti M: The management and outcome of lacerations in urban children. *Ann Emerg Med* 19:1001, 1990.

72. Singer AJ, Hollander JE, Quinn JV: Evaluation and management of traumatic lacerations. *N Engl J Med* 337:1142, 1997.

73. Glass K: Factors related to the resolution of treated hand infections. *J Hand Surg* 7:388, 1982.

74. Dreyfuss U, Singer M: Human bites of the hand: A study of one hundred six patients. *J Hand Surg* 10:884, 1985.

75. Perron AD, Miller MD, Brady WJ: Orthopedic pitfalls in the ED: Fight bite. *Am J Emerg Med* 20:114, 2002.

76. Dire D, Hogan D, Riggs M: A prospective evaluation of risk factors for dog bite wound infections. *Ann Emerg Med* 19:961, 1990.

77. Chen E, et al: Primary closure of mammalian bites. *Acad Emerg Med* 7:157, 2000.

78. Quinn J, et al: Suturing versus conservative management of lacerations of the hand: Randomised controlled trial. *BMJ* 325:299, 2002.

79. Centers for Disease Control: Diphtheria, tetanus and pertussis—recommendations for vaccine use and other preventive measures: Recommendations of the Immunization Practices Advisory Committee (ACIP). *MMWR Morb Mortal Wkly Rep* 40:1, 1991.

80. Dire DJ, Hogan DE, Walker JS: Prophylactic oral antibiotics for low-risk dog bite wounds. *Pediatr Emerg Care* 8:194, 1992.

81. Goldstein EJ, et al: Activities of HMR 3004 (RU 64004) and HMR 3647 (RU 66647) compared to those of erythromycin, azithromycin, clarithromycin, roxithromycin, and eight other antimicrobial agents against unusual aerobic and anaerobic human and animal bite pathogens isolated from skin and soft tissue infections in humans. *Antimicrob Agents Chemother* 42:11272, 1998.

82. Burrows GE, Ewing P: In vitro assessment of the efficacy of erythromycin in combination with oxytetracycline or spectinomycin against *Pasteurella haemolytica*. *J Vet Diagn Invest* 1:299, 1989.

83. Newell P: Value of needle aspiration in bacteriologic diagnosis of cellulitis in adults. *J Clin Microbiol* 26:401, 1988.

84. Perl B, et al: Cost-effectiveness of blood cultures for adult patients with cellulitis. *Clin Infect Dis* 29:1483, 1999.

85. Zubowicz VN, Gravier M: Management of early human bites of the hand: A prospective randomized study. *Plast Reconstr Surg* 88:111, 1991.

86. Dellinger EP, et al: Hand infections: Bacteriology and treatment—a prospective study. *Arch Surg* 123:745, 1988.

87. Phair IC, Quinton DN: Clenched fist human bite injuries. *J Hand Surg (Br)* 14:86, 1989.

88. Baker MD, Moore SE: Human bites in children: A six-year experience. *Am J Dis Child* 141:1285, 1987.

89. Schweich P, Fleisher G: Human bites in children. *Ped Emerg Care* 1:51, 1985.

90. Steele M, et al: Prophylactic penicillin for intraoral wounds. *Ann Emerg Med* 18:847, 1989.

91. Morgan MG, Mardel SN: Clenched fist actinomycosis in a penicillin-allergic female [Letter]. *J Infect* 26:222, 1993.

92. Richman KM, Rickman LS: The potential for transmission of human immunodeficiency virus through human bites. *J Acquir Immune Defic Syndr* 6:402, 1993.

93. Updated U.S. Public Health Service Guidelines for the Management of Occupational Exposures to HBV, HCV, and HIV and Recommendations for Postexposure Prophylaxis. *MMWR Recomm Rep* 50(RR-11):1, 2001.

94. Groopman J, Salahuddin S, Sarngadharan M: HTLV-III in saliva of people with AIDS-related complex and healthy homosexual men at risk for AIDS. *Science* 226:447, 1984.

95. Pretty IA, Anderson GS, Sweet DJ: Human bites and the risk of human immunodeficiency virus transmission. *Am J Forensic Med Pathol* 20:232, 1999.

96. Vidmar L, et al: Transmission of HIV-1 by human bite. (Letter). *Lancet* 347:1762, 1996.

97. Eyres KS, Allen TR: Skyline view of the metacarpal head in the assessment of human fight-bite injuries. *J Hand Surg Br* 18:43, 1993.

98. Agrawal K, et al: Tetanus caused by human bite of the finger. *Ann Plast Surg* 34:201, 1995.

99. Donkor P, Bankas DO: A study of primary closure of human bite injuries to the face. *J Oral Maxillofac Surg* 55:479, 1997.

100. Fischer H, Hammel PW, Dragovic LJ: Images in clinical medicine: Human bites versus dog bites. *N Engl J Med* 2003;349:e11.

CHAPTER

59 Venomous Animal Injuries

Edward J. Otten

Young primates appear to be born with only three inborn fears—of falling, snakes and the dark.[1]

PERSPECTIVE

Epidemiology

Venomous animals account for considerable morbidity and mortality worldwide. Snakes alone are estimated to inflict 2.5 million venomous bites annually, with approximately 125,000 deaths. The actual numbers may be much larger. Southeast Asia, India, Brazil, and parts of Africa lead the world in snakebite mortality.[2] It is impossible to estimate the worldwide morbidity and mortality resulting from other venomous animals such as bees, wasps, ants, and spiders.

Approximately 45,000 snakebites occur annually in the United States; 7000 to 8000 are inflicted by venomous snakes, and 5 to 10 result in death. Table 59-1 categorizes fatalities caused by venomous animals in the United States for the 20-year period from 1950 to

Table 59-1. Venomous Animal Fatalities in the United States, 1950-1969

Animal	Fatalities
Hymenoptera	
Bees	175
Wasps	127
Yellow jackets	33
Hornets	12
Ants	5
Ticks	3
Spiders	92
Unidentified insects	53
Coelenterata	2
Stingray	1
Snakes	
Rattlesnakes	159
Water moccasins	9
Copperheads	2
Coral	3
Cobra	3
Unidentified	67
Animal, not coded	44
Total	**790**

Table 59-2. Venomous Animal Injuries and Deaths, 1983-2002

Animal	Envenomations	Deaths
Coelenterates	11,021	0
Fish	21,145	0
Ants	38,704	0
Bees/wasps/hornets	294,719	19
Caterpillars/centipedes	34,318	0
Other arthropods	193,520	1
Copperheads	7,506	1
Rattlesnakes	12,860	16
Water moccasins	1,303	0
Coral snakes	800	0
Exotic snakes	1,423	2
Nonvenomous snakes	29,983	0
Unknown snakes	29,877	2
Black widow spiders	43,263	0
Brown recluse spiders	30,816	6
Other/unknown spiders	202,549	0
Scorpions	164,973	3

Data compiled from Litovitz TL, et al: American Association of Poison Control Centers data published in the *American Journal of Emergency Medicine*, vol 2-21, 1984-2003.

1969.[3-6] Insects were responsible for 52% of the fatalities; snakes, 30%; and spiders, 13%. More specifically, bees were responsible for the most fatalities, followed by rattlesnakes, wasps, and spiders. Historically, most of the recorded spider deaths were caused by the black widow, although the brown recluse spider had been implicated in an increasing number of deaths.

The American Association of Poison Control Centers began collecting data in 1983 on deaths caused by venomous animals. Their 20-year experience shows a significant number of exposures by bite or sting but relatively few deaths (Table 59-2).[7] Although these data include most of the United States, there is no requirement that hospitals, emergency departments, coroners, or public health agencies report deaths or exposure to Regional Drug and Poison Information Centers. This decline may be caused by an actual decrease in mortality or may be due to inadequate reporting. Meaningful morbidity data, such as the number of amputations, hospitalizations, and disabilities, do not exist. The number of exposures and deaths from exotic snakes seems to be increasing, possibly because of interest in collecting so-called hot or venomous varieties such as cobras, mambas, and vipers. The morbidity from marine animal injuries is increasing in proportion to the number of people exposed to the ocean and the number of private collectors, but the number of deaths has not increased dramatically. An increase in outdoor recreational activities such as camping, scuba diving, and wilderness trekking puts more people in proximity to venomous animals and increases the risk of envenomation. Most exposures occur from April to October, when animals are most active and potential victims are outdoors and involved in activities that might increase their risk for envenomation. Of course, many spider bites and exotic animal envenomations that occur indoors can take place at any time. Most deaths seem to occur in very young, elderly, and inappropriately treated patients.

Venom Delivery

Animals that have developed specific venom glands and venom delivery systems can be found in every class, including most recently birds.[8] The toxin and toxic apparatus vary from class to class. For example, the rattlesnake has modified salivary glands and maxillary teeth and uses this system primarily to obtain food. The bee has a modified ovipositor that is used mainly for defense. Poisonous and venomous animals are not the same and should be differentiated. Animals can be considered *poisonous* because of various toxins distributed in their tissues. For example, certain shellfish, toads, and barracuda have been known to cause death after ingestion. However, only animals with specific glands for producing venom connected to an apparatus for delivering that venom to another animal can be considered *venomous*.

Most venomous animal injuries seen in the emergency department are minor problems, but some injuries must be given priority. Venomous snakebites, black widow spider bites, certain marine animal envenomations, and anaphylactic reactions to insect stings are life-threatening emergencies requiring immediate attention.

VENOMOUS REPTILES

Snakes

Snakes first appeared in the late Cretaceous period, and venomous snakes evolved about 50 million years later in the Miocene epoch. Of the 3000 species of snakes, about 10% to 15% are venomous. Of the 14 families of snakes, 5 contain venomous species. Snakes are distributed throughout most of the earth's surface, including fresh and salt water. The major exceptions are the Arctic and Antarctic zones, New Zealand, Malagasy, and many small islands. Most snakebites occur in tropical and subtropical climates, especially in agricultural settings where the inhabitants go barefoot. Sea snakes are found only in the Pacific and Indian oceans. Snakes are *poikilotherms*, which accounts for their distribution and activity. Their inability to raise their body temperature above ambient levels restricts their activity to a fairly narrow temperature range, about 25° C to 35° C. All snakes are carnivorous, and their venom apparatus evolved for the purpose of obtaining food.

Epidemiology

The incidence of reported venomous snakebites is greatest in the southern United States, which has the largest number of venomous snakes. States having the highest death rates were North Carolina, Arkansas, Texas, and Georgia. The anatomic distribution of snakebites is not surprising. Of all snakebites, 97% occur on the extremities, with two thirds on the upper extremities and one third on the lower extremities. This is a reversal of the previous trend and may reflect bites being provoked rather than accidental. Bites that occur accidentally are considered "legitimate," whereas bites that occur when attempting to handle or disturb a snake are considered "illegitimate." Men are bitten nine times more frequently than women.[9]

Imported venomous snakes have recently been an increasing problem throughout the United States. In the past, only zoos, research centers, and herpetologists have kept exotic venomous snakes. Today, however, hundreds of people are raising deadly venomous snakes without the necessary precautions, such as specialized cages, safe handling techniques, and rapid access to specific antivenin. They place not only themselves in danger but also their families and the general public.

Classification and Characteristics

The five venomous families of snakes are the Colubridae, Hydrophiidae, Elapidae, Viperidae, and Crotalidae. The Colubridae, though representing 70% of all species of snakes, have very few venomous members dangerous to humans; these include the boomslang and bird snake. The Hydrophiidae are sea snakes. The Elapidae are more common and include the cobras, kraits, mambas, and coral snakes. The Viperidae, or true vipers, are represented by Russell's viper, the puff adder, the Gaboon viper, the saw-scaled viper, and the European viper. The Crotalidae, or pit vipers, are sometimes considered a separate family or a subfamily of the Viperidae. Among the pit vipers are the most common American venomous snakes, such as rattlesnakes, water moccasins, copperheads, the bushmaster, and the fer-de-lance. Several species of Asian pit vipers are responsible for bites in Okinawa and bites by imported snakes in the United States.[10-12]

Pit vipers, the most prevalent venomous snakes in the United States, are native to every state except Maine, Alaska, and Hawaii. They are classified into three main groups: true rattlesnakes (genus *Crotalus*), copperheads and water moccasins (genus *Agkistrodon*), and pygmy and Massasauga rattlesnakes (genus *Sistrurus*). Pit vipers account for 98% of all venomous snakebites in the United States.[13,14]

The Colubridae and Hydrophiidae families have few venomous members and are responsible for even fewer injuries. Some colubrid species found in the United States that were previously thought to be harmless may indeed be venomous. Examples are the Lyre snake and the wandering garter snake. No deaths have been reported, but the problem has generated much interest among herpetologists and toxicologists.[15] The yellow-bellied sea snake (family Hydrophiidae) has been found off the coast of southern California and western Mexico, but bites by this snake are rare. The yellow-bellied sea snake *(Pelamis platurus)* has a bright yellow underside.

The other major group of venomous snakes in the United States is the *coral* snakes. The eastern coral snake *(Micrurus fulvius)* is found in North Carolina, South Carolina, Florida, Louisiana, Mississippi, Georgia, and Texas. The western or Sonoran *(Micruroides euryxanthus)* coral snake is native to Arizona and New Mexico. Although both species are generally quite shy unless handled, the eastern coral snake is considered deadly. There are no records of fatalities caused by the western species.

Coral snakes can be readily identified by their color pattern. At first glance, they resemble one of several varieties of king snake found in the southern United States. The coral snake can be differentiated from the king snake by two characteristics: the nose of the coral snake is black, and the red and yellow bands are adjacent on the coral snake but separated by a black band on the king snake. The popular rhyme is as follows:

Red next to yellow, kill a fellow.

Red next to black, venom lack.

This rhyme can be used only in the United States; Brazilian coral snakes have red next to black bands, and some coral snakes have no red bands.

Identification

In the identification of venomous snakes, two principles should be kept in mind: only experts should handle live snakes, and even dead snakes can envenom careless handlers.[16] It is not difficult to differentiate between pit vipers and harmless snakes (Figure 59-1). Pit vipers, as their name implies, have a characteristic pit midway between the eye and the nostril on both sides of the head. This pit is a heat-sensitive organ that enables the snake to locate warm-blooded prey. Pit vipers can be identified through other methods, but this characteristic is 100% consistent. The triangular shape of the head, the presence of an elliptic pupil, the arrangement of subcaudal plates, the tail structure, and the presence of fangs are useful characteristics but may be inconsistent. An individual specimen may not fit the classic description, depending on the age of the snake, the time of the year, and the condition of the tail and

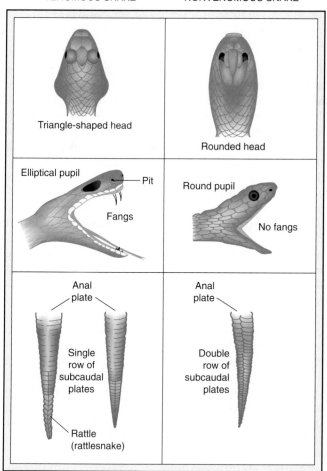

Triangle-shaped head

Rounded head

Elliptical pupil — Pit

Fangs

Round pupil

No fangs

Anal plate

Anal plate

Single row of subcaudal plates

Double row of subcaudal plates

Rattle (rattlesnake)

Figure 59-1. Identification of venomous and nonvenomous snakes.

mouthparts. A person should never attempt to identify pit vipers by color or skin patterns.[13,14]

Size is not an important factor in identifying various snakes and lizards. Venomous snakes range in length from several inches to several feet. Although a 6-ft eastern diamondback rattlesnake is much more dangerous than a 10-inch copperhead, all venomous snakes are able to envenom from birth and should be treated as though they are dangerous.

Exotic snakes that are *not* pit vipers are not as easily identified. If possible, they should be safely transported to an expert for positive identification. Local zoos, herpetology groups, and colleges often have individuals who can identify unknown snakes. Usually, however, a person bitten by an exotic snake knows the type of snake or at least the common name of the snake.

Other Reptiles

Only two venomous lizards are found in the world, both in the southwestern United States and Mexico. They are the Gila monster *(Heloderma suspectum)* and the Mexican beaded lizard *(Heloderma horridum)*. Fortunately, both these lizards are nonaggressive and rarely encountered. Bites usually result from handling the animals in captivity.[17] The Gila monster and the Mexican beaded lizard are easily identifiable. Both

Table 59-3. Compounds Identified in Snake Venoms

Components	Examples
Nonprotein Compounds (5-10%)	
Metals	Copper, zinc, sodium, magnesium
Free amino acids	Glycine, valine, isoleucine
Peptides	Pyroglutamylpeptide
Nucleosides	Adenosine, guanosine, inosine
Carbohydrates	Neutral sugars, sialic acid
Lipids	Phospholipids, cholesterol
Biogenic amines	Spermine, histamine, serotonin
Protein Components (90-95%)	
Enzymes	Proteolytic enzymes, collagenases, phospholipase A, nucleotidase, hyaluronidase, acetylcholinesterase, amino acid oxidase
Polypeptides	Crotoxin, cardiotoxin, crotamine

have thick bodies, beaded scales, and either white and black or pink and black coloration.

Principles of Disease

Toxins

The two main factors influencing the pathophysiology of any venomous animal injury are the toxic properties of the venom and the victim's response to these toxins. In the past, snake venoms were classified as either neurotoxic or hematotoxic, depending on the observed response of the victim to the various venoms. Modern toxicologic investigation has shown that this classification is inadequate because most snake venoms studied contain compounds that have other toxic properties. It is true, however, that the venom of a particular species of snake may show a clinical response, predominantly neurotoxic or hematotoxic.[18]

The toxic components of snake venom can be classified into four broad categories: enzymes, polypeptides, glycoproteins, and low-molecular-weight compounds. They can also be classified as protein and nonprotein compounds (Table 59-3). *Proteins*, which account for most of the toxic manifestations, make up 90% to 95% of venom. Symptoms can generally be classified as local or systemic. Local effects are usually caused by enzymatic action on the various cellular and noncellular structures in the victim's tissues. These enzymes can cause coagulation, anticoagulation, cell lysis, hemorrhage, hemolysis, and the destruction of nucleic acid, mitochondria, and other organelles.

Polypeptides are structurally smaller and more rapidly absorbed than proteins and account for the venom's systemic effects on the heart, lungs, kidneys, presynaptic and postsynaptic membranes, and other organ systems.

Phospholipase A can inhibit electron transfer at the level of cytochrome *c* and render mitochondrial-bound enzymes soluble. It can hydrolyze phospholipids in nerve axons, break down acetylcholine vesicles at the myoneural junction, cause myonecrosis, and induce lysis of red cell membranes. This single enzyme has been identified in all venoms of Hydrophiidae, Elapidae, Viperidae, and Crotalidae thus far investigated.[19,20]

Elapidae and Hydrophiidae venoms have predominantly systemic effects, whereas Colubridae, Viperidae, and Crotalidae venoms have mainly local effects. There are many exceptions to this general division. For example, the venom of the Mojave rattlesnake (*Crotalus scutulatus*) may show minimal local effects and deadly systemic effects, whereas the venom of the cobra (*Naja naja*) may cause extensive local tissue destruction.[19,21]

Venom Delivery

The mechanism for delivering venom is fairly standard among snakes. It consists of two venom glands, hollow or grooved fangs, and ducts connecting the glands to the fangs. The glands, which evolved from salivary glands, are located on each side of the head above the maxillae and behind the eyes. Each gland has an individual muscle and a separate nerve supply that allow the snake to vary the amount of venom injected. The venom duct leads from the anterior portion of the gland along the maxilla to the fangs. Pit vipers have fangs that are large anterior maxillary teeth. These teeth are hollow and rotate outward from a resting position to a striking position. The coral snake has fixed, hollow maxillary teeth that are much smaller than those of pit vipers. The fangs in most snakes are shed and replaced regularly, and it is not unusual to see a snake with double fangs on one or both sides of its mouth.[5,21,22]

The snake can control the amount of venom injected. In biting a human, a prey much too large to swallow, the snake may become confused or disoriented, especially if injured or surprised. However, the snake may inject more than 90% of the contents of the gland for the same reasons.

Clinical Features

The signs and symptoms of a venomous snakebite vary considerably and depend on many factors. From 30% to 50% of venomous snakebites result in little or no envenomation. A person with impaired cardiovascular, renal, or pulmonary function is less able to cope with even moderately severe envenomation. Because of these multiple variables, the individual clinical response is the only way to judge the severity of a venomous snakebite.[11] Factors that influence the effects of a snakebite are the age, health, and size of the snake; the relative toxicity of the venom; the condition of the fangs; whether the snake has recently fed or is injured; the size, age, and medical problems of the victim; and the anatomic location of the bite.

Local envenomation, if left untreated, can cause serious systemic problems (e.g., disseminated intravascular coagulation, pulmonary edema, shock) as the toxic products are absorbed. The victim's autopharmacologic response to the envenomation must also be taken into account. An IgE-mediated anaphylactic-type reaction may develop in victims of a previous snakebite when re-exposed to the venom. Many venoms contain enzymes that trigger the release of bradykinin, histamine, and serotonin from the patient's cells, which may cause fatal anaphylactic reactions. A wave of effects ranging from minimal pain to multisystem failure and death can occur over a period of several days.

Pit Vipers

The most consistent symptom associated with pit viper bites is immediate burning pain in the area of the bite, whereas pain may be minimal with bites of Elapidae and other exotic snakes. With pit vipers, the severity of pain is probably related to the amount of venom injected or the degree of swelling. Edema surrounding the bite that gradually spreads proximally is a common finding. This edema is usually subcutaneous, begins early, and may involve the entire extremity. Compartment syndrome has been described; however, it is unusual even with severe edema. It has been reported more frequently in models involving intracompartmental venom injection.[23] Most fangs do not penetrate into the fascial compartments, although muscle destruction may result from direct toxicity. Mortality is less frequent with distal bites to the toe and finger and is greatly increased with intravenous bites. In fact, an intravenous bite from any venomous snake is likely to be fatal. Petechiae, ecchymosis, and serous or hemorrhagic bullae are other local signs. Necrosis of skin and subcutaneous tissue is noted later and may result from inadequate doses of antivenin. Many systemic symptoms, such as weakness, nausea, fever, vomiting, sweating, numbness and tingling around the mouth, metallic taste in the mouth, muscle fasciculations, and hypotension, often occur after pit viper envenomation.

Death from pit viper bites is associated with disruption of the coagulation mechanism and increased capillary membrane permeability. Ultimately, these two processes lead to massive pulmonary edema, shock, and death. Heart and kidney damage occurs secondary to these mechanisms. Specific toxins in certain species may act directly on specific organs, such as the heart or skeletal muscle. An allergic type of reaction may add to this process through release of histamine and bradykinin.[24,25]

Coral Snakes

Signs and symptoms can vary considerably with bites of coral snakes, Mojave rattlesnakes, and many exotic snakes, especially cobras and Australian elapids. Little pain and swelling may occur. Many of these species' venoms contain compounds that block neuromuscular transmission at acetylcholine receptor sites and have direct inhibitory effects on cardiac and skeletal muscle. Ptosis is common and often the first outward sign of envenomation. Other signs and symptoms include vertigo, paresthesias, fasciculations, slurred speech, drowsiness, dysphagia, restlessness, increased salivation, nausea, and proximal muscle weakness. The usual cause of death is respiratory failure.[14]

Gila Monster

Gila monster bites are generally associated with pain, edema, and weakness. Hypotension is common with severe bites. Envenomation involves secretion of the venom from glands along the lower jaws. The venom is introduced into the victim through grooved teeth and a chewing mechanism. Gila monster bites are seldom fatal.[17]

Infection

Although snakebite envenomation has been stressed here, any bite or puncture wound carries a risk for bacterial contamination. Gram-negative organisms predominate when snake venom and mouthparts are cultured. Even though several studies have shown that prophylactic antibiotics are not indicated for snakebite, tetanus, osteomyelitis, cellulitis, or gas gangrene may occur in cases of snakebite with or without envenomation. This is especially true when a large amount of local tissue destruction has occurred, treatment has been delayed, or inappropriate first aid was attempted.[26]

Management

Prehospital Care

All snakebites should be considered an emergency, and any victim should be medically evaluated. The initial 6 to 8 hours after a snakebite is critical. During this time, medical therapy can help prevent the morbidity associated with severe envenomation. Effective prehospital care can be important.[27]

Prehospital care is relatively simple if guided by four basic concepts. First, the estimated time until arrival at a medical facility, as well as the skill of the on-scene assistants, must be considered when instituting first aid. The victim should be separated from the snake if possible to prevent further bites. A stick, pole, or other object longer than the snake can be used to move the snake away from the victim or, if necessary, to kill the snake by striking it behind the head. Rapid transportation to a medical facility is the best first aid for a snakebite.

Second, spread of the venom should be slowed if possible; several methods are known. The patient's excitement and physical activity, movement of the bitten area, alcohol consumption, and greater depth of the bite increase the spread of venom. Except for the last factor, these issues can be addressed by calming the victim, immobilizing the bitten area, and not giving anything by mouth. A new method of first aid for venomous snakebites has been developed in Australia. The *immobilization and compression technique*, also called the Commonwealth Serum Laboratory technique, slows uptake of Elapidae venom and mock venom in humans. The bitten extremity is either wrapped in an elastic bandage or placed in an air splint. In another technique from Australia called the *Monash method*, a thick pad and bandage are placed over the bite wound and extremity. Both these methods have similar postulated mechanisms of action: the lymphatic vessels and superficial veins are collapsed, and the proximal spread of venom is slowed. Although this method is successful

as first-aid therapy for Elapidae bites, its use for pit vipers has not been demonstrated.[29-31] If less than 30 minutes has elapsed since the bite, a constricting band applied tightly enough to impede superficial venous and lymph flow, but not arterial blood flow, may be used. The band should be loose enough to admit a finger between the band and the skin after application. It should be used with caution to prevent the development of a tourniquet effect under swollen tissue, which may cause more destruction than the snakebite.[28] Incision of bite wounds should be avoided because of lack of proven efficacy and potential danger to underlying structures. The use of ice is not helpful in slowing the spread of venom, but an ice bag wrapped in a towel and applied to the bite area helps relieve pain. Ice water immersion and packing of the extremity in ice are dangerous and only contribute to tissue destruction. The use of suction devices has not been shown to be beneficial.[32,33]

Third, when feasible, the snake should be identified or brought to the treating facility with the victim. This should be done safely; usually, only experts should handle live snakes. Dead snakes can be placed in a hard container such as a bucket or ice chest. Care should be taken to not touch the head of the snake because envenomation can occur even after death. Live snakes should not be pursued to capture them. It is more important to get the victim to definitive medical care. Fourth, additional medical interventions should be initiated, if available. Cardiac monitoring, intravenous fluids, analgesics, and blood samples may be helpful, especially with signs of envenomation.

Emergency Department Care

Many snakes do not envenom their victims when they bite, which has provided false support for the historical use of whiskey, clam juice, or split chickens. The only proven therapy is antivenin. Emergency department care of a snakebite must focus on supportive care and rapid treatment with antivenin. Rapid decision making is required to determine the optimal type, amount, and route of administration of the antivenin. By the time that the emergency physician examines a snakebite victim, the venom may have already caused much damage both locally and systemically. In this case the emergency physician must be prepared to support the victim's cardiovascular and respiratory systems.

The snake should be identified if possible, but this may not be easy. The presence of pits is the most consistent factor in identifying pit vipers, and the color pattern can help identify a coral snake. Most large cities have either zoos or herpetologic societies whose members can help identify exotic or unknown snakes. Fortunately, most victims of exotic snakebite are collectors and can positively identify the snake.

Patient History

Specific historical information should include time elapsed since the bite, circumstances surrounding the bite, the number of bites, whether first aid was administered and what type, location of the bite, and any symptoms (e.g., pain, numbness, nausea, tingling around the mouth, metallic taste in the mouth, muscle cramps, dyspnea, dizziness). A brief medical history should include the last tetanus immunization, medications, and cardiovascular, hematologic, renal, and respiratory problems. An allergy history with emphasis on symptoms after exposure to horse or sheep products, previous injection of horse or sheep serum, and a history of asthma, hay fever, or urticaria should be obtained if considering antivenin treatment.

Patient Examination

The bite area should be examined for signs of fang marks or scratches and local envenomation (e.g., edema, petechiae, ecchymosis, bullae). The area distal to the bite should be checked for pulses. A general physical examination should be performed with emphasis on the cardiorespiratory system. A thorough neurologic examination should be performed and recorded, especially if a Mojave rattlesnake, coral snake, or exotic snake is suspected. If the bite involves an extremity, the circumference of the extremity at the site of the bite and approximately 5 inches proximal to the bite should be measured and recorded. These data aid in objectively estimating both spread of the venom and the effect of antivenin.

Initial Medical Care

If the bite occurred less than 30 minutes before arrival in the emergency department, first-aid measures can be instituted, including a constricting band until antivenin can be obtained. Snakebite victims with clinical evidence of envenomation should have a large-bore intravenous line with normal saline placed in an unaffected extremity. An electrocardiogram, complete blood count, urinalysis, coagulation studies, and levels of fibrinogen, fibrin split products, electrolytes, blood urea nitrogen, and creatinine should be obtained. The patient's blood should be typed and crossmatched for 4 U of packed red blood cells.

The patient's vital signs must be monitored closely. Snakebite victims are often hypotensive because of third-space losses and hemorrhage. In an edematous extremity, the distal pulse may have to be examined with a Doppler instrument. If a compartment syndrome is suspected, a pressure monitor should be inserted and surgical consultation obtained. Pressure greater than 30 mm Hg may require fasciotomy.

At this point the emergency physician should determine the severity of the bite and decide whether to administer antivenin. The more distal the bite on the extremity, the less toxicity associated with the bite.[34] Intravenous bites may be rapidly fatal.[25] Bites occurring on the trunk, neck, and face have increased risk because of rapid transit of the venom.

Antivenin

The emergency physician should determine the type of antivenin to administer, how much, and over what period.[14] If the bite is from a pit viper, the problem is

Table 59-4. Antivenin Dosage for Pit Viper Envenomation*

Envenomation	FabAV[†]	Wyeth AV
Moderate	4-6 vials	4-6 vials
Severe	8-12 vials	5-10 vials
Very severe	12-18 vials	10-20+ vials

*Dosage based on initial findings and clinical response to antivenin.
†If this dose elicits a clinical response, an additional two vials at 6, 12, and 18 hours is recommended.

not too difficult. Wyeth, the former manufacturer of a polyvalent pit viper antivenin in the United States, supplies complete instructions on the grading of bites, the method of horse serum testing, and the protocol for administration with each vial. These instructions classify envenomation into five levels, starting with grade 0 (no sign of envenomation) to grade IV (very severe envenomation). The amount of antivenin to be given is correlated with the grade of envenomation (Table 59-4). Bites by copperheads usually cause a moderate amount of edema but generally do not require antivenin. Others have advocated slightly different grading systems and higher doses of antivenin. Grades 0 and I correspond to *minimal* envenomation, grade II represents *moderate* envenomation, and grades III and IV correspond to *severe* envenomation.[35]

Grading Envenomation

- *Grade 0 (minimal).* There is no evidence of envenomation, but snakebite is suspected. A fang wound may be present. Pain is minimal, with less than 1 inch of surrounding edema and erythema. No systemic manifestations are present during the first 12 hours after the bite. No laboratory changes occur.
- *Grade I (minimal).* There is minimal envenomation, and snakebite is suspected. A fang wound is usually present. Pain is moderate or throbbing and localized to the fang wound, surrounded by 1 to 5 inches of edema and erythema. No evidence of systemic involvement is present after 12 hours of observation. No laboratory changes occur.
- *Grade II (moderate).* There is moderate envenomation, more severe and widely distributed pain, edema spreading toward the trunk, and petechiae and ecchymoses limited to the area of edema. Nausea, vomiting, giddiness, and a mild elevation in temperature are usually present.
- *Grade III (severe).* The envenomation is severe. The case may initially resemble a grade I or II envenomation, but the course is rapidly progressive. Within 12 hours, edema spreads up the extremity and may involve part of the trunk. Petechiae and ecchymoses may be generalized. Systemic manifestations may include tachycardia, hypotension, and a subnormal temperature. Laboratory abnormalities may include an elevated white blood cell count, creatine phosphokinase, prothrombin time, and partial thromboplastin time, as well as elevated fibrin degradation products and D-dimer. Decreased platelets and fibrinogen are common. Hematuria, myoglobinuria,

increased bleeding time, and renal or hepatic abnormalities may also occur.

- *Grade IV (severe).* The envenomation is very severe and is seen most frequently after the bite of a large rattlesnake. It is characterized by sudden pain, rapidly progressive swelling that may reach and involve the trunk within a few hours, ecchymoses, bleb formation, and necrosis. Systemic manifestations, often commencing within 15 minutes of the bite, usually include weakness, nausea, vomiting, vertigo, and numbness or tingling of the lips or face. Muscle fasciculations, painful muscular cramping, pallor, sweating, cold and clammy skin, rapid and weak pulse, incontinence, convulsions, and coma may also be observed. Intravenous bites may result in cardiopulmonary arrest soon after the bite. The course of coral snakebites may be delayed and manifested as a variety of neurologic symptoms, including weakness, ptosis, stupor, bulbar paralysis, and other cranial nerve dysfunction, as well as nausea, abdominal pain, and headache.

Administration of Antivenin. Any victim of a venomous snakebite with moderate or severe envenomation is a candidate for antivenin. The choice of antivenin depends on the species of snake, and the antivenin may be horse serum– or sheep-derived Fab fragments. Wyeth laboratories, producer of the polyvalent antivenin for Western Hemisphere pit vipers, no longer manufactures that antivenin. Many zoos and hospitals still maintain vials of this antivenin until it can be replaced with the ovine-derived Fab antivenin (FabAV). This antivenin is derived from four species of U.S. pit vipers and has not been studied with regard to bites from Mexican, Central American, or South American pit vipers. The Wyeth antivenin was derived from two U.S. species, one Mexican and Central American species, and one South American species and was efficacious against most of the world's pit vipers. Most antivenin for exotic snakes is derived from horse serum, and the eastern coral snake antivenin is also horse serum derived. Skin testing was commonly performed before administering horse serum–derived antivenin, but it is not medically indicated because of the inaccuracy of the test. Moreover, testing with normal horse serum may itself precipitate an allergic reaction, and even a positive test may not preclude treatment if a patient has sustained severe envenomation.

Dosage and Precautions

1. Because anaphylaxis may occur whenever horse serum is administered, appropriate therapeutic agents (e.g., oxygen supply, airway support, epinephrine, other injectable pressors) must be ready for immediate use. Any patient requiring antivenin should have two intravenous lines inserted. If an allergic reaction occurs, the line with the antivenin can be clamped and the other line used for resuscitation. Administering 0.3 mg of 1:1000 epinephrine subcutaneously before administration of antivenin may prevent allergic reactions from horse serum–derived antivenin and, if not contraindicated, should be used.

2. The initial dosage of antivenin is prepared (see Table 59-4). The smaller the body of the patient, the larger the relative initial dose that may be required. A bitten child usually receives more venom in proportion to body weight and thus requires more antivenin to neutralize it. Because children seem to have less resistance and less body fluid with which to dilute the venom, they may require twice the adult dosage of antivenin. The total fluid requirements of children are less, however, so the antivenin should be given in a more concentrated solution. All antivenin should be administered intravenously.

3. Pregnancy is not a contraindication to antivenin therapy.

4. Administration of antivenin at or around the site of the bite is not recommended.

5. The need for subsequent doses is based on the patient's clinical response. The patient is monitored closely after the initial dose, and local and systemic symptoms, as well as laboratory findings, are determinants of the need for further antivenin. Additional injections of one to five vials of antivenin are administered every 1 to 2 hours if symptoms progress.

6. Even with a history or signs of allergy, patients with severe envenomation should be treated with a diluted form of antivenin and epinephrine.

Current treatment of pit viper envenomation in the United States is to use an FabAV polyvalent antivenin rather than the horse serum product. This is designed to limit the allergic reactions associated with horse serum antivenin by using antigen-binding fragments (Fabs) of sheep (ovine) immunized against four species of venomous snake found in the United States. CroFab has been shown to be as effective as the Wyeth antivenin, with fewer allergic reactions. Because of more rapid clearance of smaller Fab fragments by the kidney, however, a repeat dose regimen must be used to prevent the recurrence of coagulopathy. The duration of action of the venom may be longer than the therapeutic effect of the antivenin. Initial studies have shown promise for a new affinity-purified, mixed monospecific ovine Fab antivenin. This product has been tested with favorable results in humans after minimal to moderate crotalid envenomation.[36-39] Its efficacy in pit vipers from South America or Asia has not been proved, nor has its usefulness for copperhead bites. The use of enzyme-linked immunosorbent assay in the diagnosis of Viperidae and Elapidae bites, especially in Australia, Asia, and Africa, has led to more certain criteria for identifying the responsible snake in a patient with suspected envenomation. Active immunization against specific snakes, similar to that for certain jellyfish and hymenopterans, is being attempted in the Amami Islands. Purification of antivenin by separation of active fractions may lead to safer administration of horse serum–derived antivenin. In the next 10 years, snakebite management will probably change radically throughout the world. Phytotherapy (botanical therapy) and other nonantivenin drug therapies for snakebite have been shown to be efficacious in experimental animals, and some centers have successfully treated snakebite with medical support only.[40-47]

Coral and Exotic Snakes. All victims of bites by the *eastern coral snake (Micrurus fulvius)* should be given antivenin (also manufactured by Wyeth) even before any symptoms develop. The toxicity of this venom has a rapid onset, and once symptoms develop, it may be too late to reverse the effects with antivenin. The recommended dose is three to five vials in 300 to 500 mL of normal saline.[42] No antivenin exists for the venom of the *Arizona (Sonoran) coral snake*, which fortunately is less dangerous. Treatment of this type of snakebite is supportive.

The problems with bites of exotic snakes are threefold: positive identification of the specimen is sometimes difficult, even for experts; specific antivenin is not always readily available; and even if the antivenin is available, the instructions for reconstitution and dosage may not be written in English. Many zoos maintain a supply of antivenin for their venomous snakes, and this may be the best source of antivenin for an exotic species. Some collectors keep appropriate antivenin on hand for the species that they collect. The Antivenin Index at the Arizona Poison Center (602-626-6016) can assist in identifying sources of exotic antivenin. As with coral snakes, many patients do not show any early signs after envenomation by exotic snakes. The antivenin should be administered before neurologic changes develop.[35]

Wound Care

The wound should be cleansed and immobilized. Elevation at or above heart level may relieve some of the pain. If the snake is a pit viper and the wound is on an extremity, a constricting band that does not occlude arterial blood flow should be applied proximal to any swelling caused by the bite. A constricting band should not be applied, however, if more than 30 minutes has elapsed since the bite occurred. Some authors have previously advised excision of the bitten area, but such management is no longer recommended. Patients should be immunized against tetanus. The use of broad-spectrum antibiotics has not been shown to be useful in uncomplicated snakebites. If there has been a long delay in treatment or if signs of secondary infection develop, ampicillin-clavulanate can be administered. Analgesics should be given as needed to relieve severe pain.[11] The wound should be examined for remains of embedded fangs or teeth and these removed.

Patients admitted to the hospital should have the laboratory tests mentioned previously performed, then serial determinations of platelets, prothrombin time, and urinalysis every 4 hours to check for myoglobin and hemoglobin. Blood products should be administered, including packed red blood cells, fresh frozen plasma, and other coagulation factors as needed. Usually, it is best to wait until antivenin therapy has been started or the use of the blood products may be futile. Daily comprehensive laboratory tests should be performed. Awake patients who have no nausea or abdominal pain can be given oral fluids. Strict measurements of intake and output should be recorded. Local wound care should involve daily cleansing with soap and water and the application of a sterile dress-

ing. Surgical consultation should be obtained for debridement or skin grafting. Fasciotomy is not usually indicated unless compartment pressures are elevated above 300 mm Hg. Debridement should probably not be performed earlier than 3 days after the bite, until the coagulopathy has resolved. Surgical exploration of the bite wound is not necessary and may be harmful. Skin grafts are occasionally necessary after bites by pit vipers that produce large necrotic areas. Physical therapy is often needed and should begin soon after the acute phase of the envenomation is over.[6,10,11,31]

Serum Sickness

In most patients who receive more than 10 vials of horse serum–derived antivenin and in about 15% of those who receive FabAV, serum sickness develops up to a week later. The administration of diphenhydramine plus cimetidine, and in severe cases a tapering dose of steroids, can be used to treat this problem. Serum sickness is the only indication for the use of steroids with snakebite.[43-45]

Other Envenomation

Gila monster and *Mexican beaded lizard* bites are treated similar to pit viper bites in regard to first aid. No definitive medical treatment exists. Antivenin is not commercially available at this time. Local wound care, tetanus prophylaxis, the use of antibiotics and analgesics, and supportive care are the extent of emergency department treatment available for this type of envenomation.[17]

Envenomation by the yellow-bellied sea snake causes severe muscle necrosis with the release of large amounts of myoglobin. Although a polyvalent antivenin is available from Australia, maintenance of adequate urine output, alkalinization of urine, and general supportive care are usually sufficient.[10,35]

Disposition

If no envenomation is evident after clinical examination and the snake was either nonvenomous or a pit viper, the victim can be observed for 6 to 8 hours. With some snakebites, however, toxicity is delayed by up to 8 hours. If no sign of envenomation is seen after 8 hours, the patient may be discharged. These patients should be given tetanus immunization and wound care instructions and referred for follow-up within 24 to 48 hours. They should be told to return to the emergency department immediately if any symptoms of envenomation develop.

If only local pain and minimal edema have occurred and the snake is thought to be nonvenomous or a pit viper, the patient should be closely watched for 12 hours in the emergency department. Then, if the pain and swelling have decreased and no systemic symptoms have developed, the patient may be treated with the same precautions as a patient with no signs of envenomation. Any patient with moderate or severe envenomation should be admitted to an intensive care unit for constant monitoring during antivenin therapy. Depending on the severity of the bite, blood products, vasopressors, and invasive monitoring may be necessary.

Any patient bitten by a coral snake, a Mojave rattlesnake, or an exotic snake is at risk for severe neurologic sequelae that may not become manifested for many hours. As a result, they should be admitted to the hospital, preferably to an intensive care unit, where blood tests can be performed periodically and the patient can be monitored closely. Arrangements should be made to have a respirator, Swan-Ganz catheter, and dialysis equipment available if necessary. Appropriate antivenin should be obtained and treatment initiated at the earliest onset of symptoms.

VENOMOUS ARTHROPODS

Arthropods are animals with segmented bodies and jointed appendages. This phylum (Arthropoda) contains approximately 80% of all known animals. Arthropods first appeared in the Cambrian period of the Paleozoic era 600 million years ago. The living members of this phylum are categorized into 12 classes. Two classes, the Insecta and the Arachnida, are of particular interest in that numerous venomous species have evolved that are harmful to humans. Many species have developed venom glands and an apparatus for delivering the venom to obtain food. Others have developed venom delivery systems used solely for defense, most of which are found in the order Hymenoptera.[18]

Arthropods account for a higher percentage of deaths from envenomation than snakes do. They are found inside dwellings, as well as in deserts, forests, and lakes. Although most arthropods are more active in April through October, many are active throughout the colder months. Arthropods are also active 24 hours a day, and many can fly, thus increasing their range. This high level of contact results in millions of cases of envenomation annually. Most fatalities result from an autopharmacologic response by the victim rather than the toxicity of the venom. An individual stung by a bee may have a small amount of pain and local swelling or, in severe cases, an anaphylactic reaction and death.

Arthropods use three main methods of delivering venom: stinging, biting, and secreting venom through pores or hairs. Some arthropods combine two systems, one for offense and the other for defense. Generally, venom systems found on the oral pole of an animal are used for offensive purposes or food acquisition, whereas systems found on the caudal pole are used for defense. Humans are not considered prey for any venomous animal, and therefore bites from venomous animals are defensive, accidental, reflexive, or a mistake. Many venomous arthropods are omitted from this discussion because of their infrequent contact with humans or the relative impotence of their venom.[21,48,49]

Hymenoptera

Hymenoptera is a familiar order of arthropods that is composed of the families of bees, wasps, hornets, yellow jackets, and ants. Many of these species are social insects, and their defense response is related to protection of the group rather than the individual organism. Although most members of this order are stinging insects, several species of ant can bite and sting simultaneously.

Bees and wasps have similar mechanisms of delivering venom. Female insects of this type have modified ovipositors that protrude from the abdomen and act as hypodermic needles to administer the venom. The barbed stinging apparatus of the bee is quite prominent. The stinging action pulls the stinger from the bee, thereby eviscerating the insect. This action also kills the bee.[50]

The wasp, which has an unbarbed stinger, may inflict many stings without damaging itself or its stinging apparatus. The venom is produced in one or two tubular glands that empty into a venom reservoir. The venom reservoir has a duct that connects to the stinger. The venom itself is composed of several classes of substances varying in composition among different species. Proteins, as in snake venom, make up most of the venom by dry weight. Peptides, amino acids, carbohydrates, lipids, and other low-molecular-weight substances are also found. The most common enzymes are phospholipase A and hyaluronidase. Peptides are common in some species and compose up to 50% of the dry weight. Most of the toxicity of the venom results from substances of low molecular weight (e.g., bradykinin, acetylcholine, dopamine, histamine, serotonin). Many other antigenic substances have been identified in bee and wasp venom, and they account for the induction of hypersensitivity and anaphylaxis in humans.[21,51-53]

Clinical Features

The signs and symptoms of bee and wasp stings vary, depending on the degree, type, and location of envenomation, as well as the characteristics of the victim. Bee and wasp venom can cause serious injury other than allergic types of reactions, depending on the number of stings, the species of insect, the size and previous health of the victim, and the anatomic area stung. For example, a sting in the tongue or throat may quickly compromise the airway. Honeybee venom causes a much greater release of histamine per gram than other hymenoptera venom does and thus is more dangerous. Certain species of honeybee release a pheromone, isoamylacetate, when the ovipositor is pulled from the abdomen after stinging a victim. This pheromone attracts other bees to the victim and thus incites multiple stings.

There is little antigenic overlap between species, which may explain the variability in reaction to stings reported by victims. Victims who are allergic to honeybees and who mistakenly identify a yellow jacket as a honeybee may not have a systemic reaction and thus may think that they are no longer allergic to honeybees.[54-56]

The most consistent finding is immediate pain at the site of the sting, followed by local swelling, redness, and itching. A sensitive victim may experience swelling, urticaria, coughing, wheezing, coma, and respiratory arrest. Some large and especially venomous hornets have been known to cause muscle necrosis and renal damage. Most serious reactions to bee stings occur in the first 30 minutes; however, the local effects of a sting may persist for 2 to 3 days. Delayed hypersensitivity may occur 7 to 10 days after the sting.

"Killer Bees"

Health officials have been concerned about a particularly aggressive species of bee imported from Africa into Brazil in 1956 that has been known to attack humans and cattle with fatal results. This bee has managed to compete with native species and is gradually replacing some of these species while still retaining its aggressive behavior. Envenomation from these aggressive arthropods is most dangerous to very young or elderly patients and those with concomitant medical conditions.[57] Killer bees have colonized northern Mexico and have now moved into the southern United States, including California, Arizona, and Texas, where the mean high temperature is at least 60° F.[58,59] This type of bee is not more toxic, only more aggressive.

Fire Ants

Another unwelcome import to the United States is the fire ant. This insect is a member of the family Formicidae and is another of the Hymenoptera that is harmful to humans. Several species of fire ant are known, some native to North America and some imported. The species responsible for 95% of clinical cases, *Solenopsis invicta*, was imported from Brazil to Alabama in the 1930s. This ant is now found in nine southern states and is replacing many native species and inhabiting new niches. The only limiting factor keeping the fire ant from progressive migration seems to be cold winters. This ant is small and light reddish brown to dark brown. Its venom is unique to the animal kingdom in that it is 99% alkaloid. The other 1% is quite immunogenic and can sensitize an individual to the venom. Properties of this venom include hemolysis, depolarization of membranes, activation of the alternative complement pathway, and general tissue destruction. The sting is produced when the ant bites the victim with its jaws and, while holding tight, pivots around and stings the victim with its ovipositor. The sting usually produces a sterile pustule within 24 hours. Other symptoms include local burning, redness, and itching. With multiple stings and in sensitive individuals, urticaria, angioedema, dyspnea, nausea, vomiting, wheezing, dizziness, and respiratory arrest may occur. Approximately 10% of victims have some degree of hypersensitivity reaction.[60-62]

Management

Home Care

First aid for Hymenoptera envenomation depends on the degree of reaction to the sting. With simple stings, an ice bag wrapped in a towel and applied to the sting area usually relieves the pain and swelling. In the event of an anaphylactic reaction, basic life support should

be administered until further medical help can be obtained. Many people allergic to Hymenoptera envenomation carry an emergency insect sting kit containing a tourniquet, epinephrine in a 1:1000 dilution, and an antihistamine. These kits are readily available, and both the patient and the patient's family should be instructed in the treatment of a severe allergic reaction.

Emergency Department Care

No specific antivenin exists for Hymenoptera stings. Treatment consists of local wound care and general supportive measures. A history of any previous allergic reactions to bee stings, hay fever, asthma, or drug reactions should be obtained. The circumstances surrounding the sting and the number and location of stings should be noted. A patient with a single sting and only a local reaction should have the sting area inspected for evidence of a venom apparatus, which is removed by scraping the edge of a scalpel blade parallel to the skin and lifting the apparatus away from the skin without squeezing the venom sac. An ice bag wrapped in a towel may then be applied and the patient given an oral antihistamine (e.g., 50 mg of diphenhydramine). The patient should be monitored and, if no further reaction is observed, may be discharged with instructions to return to the emergency department if wheezing, dyspnea, hives, or burning occurs.

Adults in whom a severe urticarial reaction or hypotension develops should be given 0.3 mL of epinephrine in a 1 : 1000 dilution subcutaneously, 50 mg of diphenhydramine intravenously, and cimetidine, 300 mg intravenously. Patients with severe hypertension, cerebrovascular disease, or heart disease should be given epinephrine cautiously because of the potential for adverse reactions. Children should be given 0.01 mL/kg of body weight of a 1 : 1000 dilution of epinephrine subcutaneously and 1 mg/kg of diphenhydramine intravenously. These patients must be watched closely for signs of respiratory problems and treated accordingly. After 1 hour these individuals should be totally free of symptoms (except for some itching around the sting site). Symptom-free patients should be discharged and given antihistamines every 6 hours for the next 24 hours. They should be given the same instructions as patients with a minor reaction. Patients with allergic reactions to a single sting should be given an emergency insect sting kit and instructed in its use. They may be referred to an allergist for desensitization.

Wheezing should be treated with a β$_2$-agonist given by hand-held nebulizer and repeated as necessary. A second large-bore intravenous line with normal saline should be established. These patients should be monitored closely and given an intravenous steroid (e.g., 125 mg of methylprednisolone) plus 50 mg of diphenhydramine and 150 mg of cimetidine intravenously. Admission is warranted for any anaphylactic reaction. Patients who have life-threatening reactions may be given 0.1 mg of epinephrine in at least a 1 : 10,000 dilution, very slowly intravenously. The subcutaneous route should be used for all but the most extreme reactions.

Treatment of allergic reactions to fire ant stings is the same. The skin lesions should be kept clean with soap and water. Ice bags may be applied initially to relieve burning and pain. Prophylactic antibiotics are not needed.

Of patients who have a systemic reaction to an insect sting, 60% can have a future allergic reaction if they have a positive skin test. These patients should be desensitized to any specific venom to which they are allergic. Purified insect venom is currently available for most Hymenoptera, including fire ants.[63] Patients seen in the emergency department with systemic reactions to stings should be referred for skin testing and desensitization. These patients should be given emergency insect sting kits with instructions for use and should avoid activities that place them in proximity to Hymenoptera species.[54-56,64]

Spiders and Scorpions

The class Arachnida contains the largest number of venomous species known, with approximately 34,000 species of venomous spiders and 1400 species of venomous scorpions. Virtually all known species are venomous, but most are not harmful to humans. Only about 50 species of arachnids in the United States cause human illness because most species do not have fangs or stingers sufficiently long to penetrate human skin. Humans fear spiders and scorpions, which is well founded in certain cases. Ticks, which also belong to this class, are less feared but probably cause more morbidity because of transmission of infectious diseases such as Rocky Mountain spotted fever and Lyme disease. Some spider bites are never diagnosed because of lack of significant symptoms and the fact that they occur while the victim is sleeping. Many non–spider bites are incorrectly diagnosed as spider bites, and unfortunately, there is no "gold standard" for making the diagnosis.

Black Widow Spider

The black widow spider, *Latrodectus mactans*, may be the best known venomous spider in the world. Several other closely related species of *Latrodectus* or widow spiders are found throughout the United States, including *Latrodectus hesperus*, which is common in Arizona and other western states. The diagnosis and treatment of the bites of all species are the same.

The black widow is found throughout the United States (except Alaska) and in southern Canada. The female is about twice as large as the male, and although both are venomous, only the female is able to envenom humans. The black widow is glossy black, occasionally with red stripes, and has a bright red marking on the abdomen. This marking may have an hourglass shape or may appear only as two spots. Abdominal markings may vary, and related *Latrodectus* species may be similar in appearance and toxicity. The combined length of the black widow's head and abdomen is about 0.5 inch, and the spider is about 1½ inches long, including the legs. It is found in protected places such as under rocks, in woodpiles, and in outhouses and stables. The female is not aggressive except when guarding her eggs.

The venom apparatus of the black widow is a modified first appendage of the head known as the chelicera. The spider is able to control the amount of venom injected into its prey. The venom of the black widow is complex and contains both protein and nonprotein compounds.

Spiders normally use the venom to paralyze their prey and also to liquefy the tissues of the prey for digestion. The venom probably evolved from digestive glands analogous to the salivary glands in snakes. The ingredient most toxic to humans is thought to be a neurotoxin. This toxin destabilizes neuronal membranes by opening ionic channels, causing depletion of acetylcholine from presynaptic nerve terminals, and increasing the frequency of spontaneous miniature end plate potentials at neuromuscular junctions.[21,65]

Clinical Features

The classic symptomatology of the black widow bite is initially a pinprick sensation that may be followed by minimal local swelling and redness. If the area is examined closely, two small fang marks may be noticed. Sometimes the bite is not felt, especially if the victim is working when the bite occurs. From 15 minutes to an hour later, dull crampy pain develops in the area of the bite and gradually spreads to include the entire body. Usually, the pain is concentrated in the chest after upper extremity bites or in the abdomen after lower extremity bites. The abdomen may become boardlike, and the patient may complain of severe crampy pain. The abdominal manifestation may mimic pancreatitis, a peptic ulcer, or acute appendicitis, except that abdominal tenderness is usually minimal. Pregnant women may go into premature labor and precipitous delivery. Associated symptoms include dizziness, restlessness, ptosis, nausea, vomiting, headache, pruritus, dyspnea, conjunctivitis, facial swelling, sweating, weakness, difficulty speaking, anxiety, and cramping pain in all muscle groups. The patient is usually hypertensive, and cerebrospinal fluid pressure is sometimes elevated. There may be electrocardiographic changes similar to those produced by digitalis.[18,21,66]

In adults, the signs and symptoms begin to abate after several hours and usually disappear in 2 to 3 days. A small child bitten by a black widow spider, however, may not survive.[67] As with snake envenomation, the volume of distribution of black widow venom is much smaller in children than in adults. A dose that may cause only a few hours of pain in an adult may lead to complete cardiac decompensation and respiratory arrest in a child. Adult patients with preexisting hypertension, cerebrovascular disease, or cardiovascular disease are also at greater risk for complications. Symptoms usually persist for 8 to 12 hours and then subside, although in severe cases muscle cramps may continue for several days.

Management

First aid for a black widow spider bite consists of applying an ice pack to the bite area for relief of pain and transporting the victim to a hospital where supportive, symptomatic, and definitive treatment can be administered. The rescuer should obtain the specimen if at all possible because many dangerous spiders resemble harmless species, and vice versa. The patient should be monitored closely en route to the hospital and basic life support initiated if necessary. Bites in the neck or mouth area may cause airway compromise through muscle spasm. Emergency department care consists of obtaining a history of the circumstances surrounding the bite, a description of the appearance of the spider, any significant past medical history, present medications, and allergies to insect bites, horses, or horse serum.

The wound site should be inspected for fang marks and cleansed with soap and water. Tetanus immunization should be instituted. The patient should be observed for about 6 hours. If symptoms do not develop and the spider was not positively identified as a black widow, the patient may be discharged with instructions to return to the emergency department if any symptoms develop.

All patients with symptoms of moderate envenomation, pregnant women, children, and those with preexisting cardiovascular disease or hypertension should be admitted to the hospital, have intravenous lines inserted, and have a complete blood count, electrolytes, blood urea nitrogen, creatinine, coagulation studies, urinalysis, and an electrocardiogram performed. Acute hypertensive problems should be treated with nitroprusside if diastolic pressure rises above 120 mm Hg.

Symptomatic treatment usually involves controlling the muscle cramps responsible for most of the discomfort associated with the bite. Diazepam or other benzodiazepines given intravenously are useful for relieving muscle spasms. Dantrolene sodium has been used both orally and intravenously to provide muscle relaxation for *Latrodectus* envenomation.[68] Parenteral analgesics may be necessary to control pain. These drugs may affect an already-compromised respiratory condition, and thus their use must be closely monitored. Patients with moderate symptoms should be admitted to the hospital and monitored until symptoms subside; usually 1 day is sufficient. Pregnant women should undergo fetal monitoring, and those with severe symptoms should be admitted to an intensive care unit with cardiovascular monitoring.

Latrodectus Antivenin

In general, pediatric patients, pregnant women, and the elderly may need to be given *Latrodectus* antivenin (Lyovac), which is derived from horse serum. Clinical judgment must be used to adjust the age and category of patients needing antivenin. Antivenin should be administered to patients with severe envenomation manifested as seizures, respiratory failure, or uncontrolled hypertension; to pregnant women; and to patients not able to stand the stress of the envenomation. The dose of the antivenin is one vial diluted in 50 mL of normal saline and administered intravenously over a period of 15 minutes. Precautions for allergic reactions should be taken before administering anti-

venin. A dose of subcutaneous 1:1000 epinephrine may prevent allergic reactions when given before horse serum antivenin. This antivenin is also useful with other species of the *Latrodectus* genus.[66]

Brown Recluse Spider

Several deaths were attributed to the brown recluse spider, *Loxosceles reclusa*, in the 1950s, primarily in the south-central United States, thus drawing the attention of toxicologists. Many species of *Loxosceles* are venomous to humans, and at least five are found in the United States. These spiders are about 1 inch long, including leg span, and range in color from tan to dark brown. The most distinguishing mark is a violin-shaped darker area found on the cephalothorax. Close examination may reveal that the brown recluse has three pairs of eyes rather than the usual four.[18,69]

These spiders, as their name implies, are not aggressive and are usually found under rocks, in woodpiles, and occasionally in attics and closets. Their range is concentrated in the south-central United States, especially Missouri, Kansas, Arkansas, Louisiana, eastern Texas, and Oklahoma. However, they have been reported in several large cities outside this range.

The venom apparatus is similar to that of most spiders, including the black widow. The composition of brown recluse venom has not been totally determined, but sphingomyelinase D is a primary component. The local tissue destructive effects are thought to be primarily caused by hemolytic enzymes and a levarterenol-like substance that induces severe vasoconstriction. The systemic symptoms seem to be an allergic phenomenon and vary according to the individual's immune response to the venom.[70,71]

Clinical Features

The symptoms of a brown recluse spider bite are both local and systemic. Initially, they are similar to those caused by bites of many other spiders and other conditions, including pyoderma gangrenosum, furuncles, viral and fungal infections, and foreign body reactions. The victim may notice some burning pain in the area of the bite. Some victims do not notice the initial bite at all. Pain usually develops within 3 to 4 hours, and a white area of vasoconstriction begins to surround the bite. A bleb then forms in the center of this area, and an erythematous ring arises on the periphery. The lesion at this stage resembles a bull's-eye. The bleb darkens, necroses over the next several hours to days, and continues to spread slowly and gravitationally, with involvement of skin and subcutaneous fat.

Systemic symptoms include fever, chills, rash, petechiae, nausea, vomiting, malaise, and weakness. Hemolysis, thrombocytopenia, shock, jaundice, renal failure, hemorrhage, and pulmonary edema are the usual signs of severe envenomation. Fatalities are more common in children, most often the result of severe intravascular hemolysis.[71,72]

Management

First aid for a brown recluse spider bite is simple. The specimen is secured if possible and the victim transported to a medical facility. Emergency department treatment is as complicated as the first aid is simple. Because the lesion develops over a period of days, there may not be any local treatment of the lesion that is effective. The physician should try to determine whether any systemic toxicity is present. A history of the circumstances surrounding the bite, the time elapsed since the bite, and any past history of allergic reactions, medications, or medical problems should be obtained. If a specimen is available, an attempt should be made to identify it. The assistance of a local entomologist should be obtained if necessary. If signs of systemic toxicity develop, an intravenous line should be placed in an unaffected extremity, and a complete blood count, electrolyte levels, blood urea nitrogen level, and creatinine level should be determined and coagulation studies and urinalysis performed. The wound should be washed with soap and water and tetanus prophylaxis given. Vital signs and urine output should be monitored closely. Excision of the lesion has not been shown to aid healing and may be detrimental.[73] Lesions have been known to cause extensive scarring, infection, and necrosis. Bites that are in fatty areas, such as the thigh or buttocks, may cause more extensive necrosis. All patients should be observed in the emergency department if envenomation is suspected but no signs are present and the elapsed time is less than 6 hours. If no sign of envenomation is present after 6 hours, the patient may be discharged with instructions to return to the emergency department if any signs or symptoms develop.

Dapsone, 50 to 200 mg/day, has been shown to be helpful in preventing local effects of the venom.[74] If used within 48 hours, it may limit the size of the lesion that develops. However, dapsone may cause methemoglobinemia and hemolysis in patients with glucose-6-phosphate dehydrogenase deficiency. Hyperbaric oxygen has been shown to decrease lesion size in animals.[75-77] Analgesics and antibiotics should be used as indicated during the course of the disease, although infection is not common. All patients with signs of systemic envenomation should be admitted to the hospital and monitored closely with daily blood counts, urinalysis, and urine output. Dialysis may be necessary if acute renal failure develops, and surgical consultation should be obtained for evaluation of the wound.

The Instituto Butantan in Sao Paulo, Brazil, produces an antivenin for *Loxosceles* bites, but it is not available in the United States. Research is currently being conducted to produce a rabbit serum antivenin against *Loxosceles*, but it is not yet commercially available.[78]

Other Spiders

Several other spiders can cause envenomation but are uncommon in the United States. Some of these spiders are large and can be quite aggressive. Most are imported either intentionally or as stowaways on cargo ships. Tarantulas, wandering spiders, funnel-web spiders, pallid spiders, and crab spiders are a few of the imported venomous spiders. Many of these species can cause envenomation similar to that of the brown recluse spider, and some produce neurotoxins.

Antivenin is produced for some of these groups (e.g., Brazilian *Phoneutria* spp., Australian *Atrax* spp.) but is usually available only in the country where the species is generally found.[79] Emergency care therefore involves symptomatic and supportive treatment. An outbreak of bites by a species of *Tegenaria*, known as the hobo or aggressive house spider, has been reported. This species was imported from Europe to the Pacific Northwest. This spider is a small brown spider with a herringbone pattern on its abdomen. The lesions are similar to those caused by the brown recluse spider, but systemic symptoms include headache and weakness. Treatment is largely supportive.[69]

Tarantulas are popular pets in the United States, and most native species are relatively nontoxic. Tarantulas are unusual in that the abdominal hairs can be thrown by the spider and embedded in human skin and the eye. These hairs can cause allergic reactions and severe conjunctivitis and must be removed under a slit lamp or by an ophthalmologist. A recent import from Thailand, the cobalt blue tarantula, *Haplopelma lividum*, is a very aggressive spider with toxic venom.

Scorpions

Scorpions are arachnids that resemble crustaceans and are among the oldest terrestrial animals. Scorpions are found throughout the world, and several species are located in the southwestern United States. Only one species, *Centruroides exilicauda*, which is found in Arizona, is particularly dangerous. Scorpions are nocturnal predatory animals that usually spend the day under rocks, logs, or floors and in crevices. *C. exilicauda*, or the "bark scorpion," is found on or near trees.

The scorpion has a tail-like structure that is actually the last six segments of its abdomen. The last segment, or the telson, contains the two venom glands and stinger. The toxicity of scorpion venom varies greatly from species to species. Generally, the less dangerous species produce more local reactions, and the more dangerous species cause more systemic reactions. Several proteins have been identified in their venom; some cause hemolysis, local tissue destruction, and hemorrhage. The venom of *C. exilicauda* is predominantly a neurotoxin that causes or enhances repetitive firing of axons by activation of sodium channels.[18]

Clinical Features

Envenomation causes severe and immediate pain at the sting site. Local edema and erythema may or may not be present, depending on the species. After envenomation by *C. exilicauda*, the victim may have heightened sensitivity to touch in the area of the sting along with local numbness and weakness. The diagnosis is often made by tapping on the site of the sting and causing an increase in pain at the site. Systemic symptoms may then develop, including anxiety, restlessness, muscle spasms, nausea, vomiting, excessive salivation, sweating, itching of the nose and throat, hyperthermia, blurred vision, myoclonus, hypertension, hemiplegia, syncope, cardiac dysrhythmias, and respiratory arrest. Various systemic complications may occur, depending on the species of scorpion. *Tityus trinitatus* scorpion stings cause pancreatitis to develop in 80% of its victims. A wave of symptoms sometimes occurs over a 24-hour period, or respiratory failure may develop in the first 30 minutes. As with most envenomation, children are at a greater risk for severe reactions. A grading system has been developed to guide management of bark scorpion stings.

Management

First aid for a scorpion sting consists of applying an ice bag to the area of the sting and transporting the victim to the hospital. A history of the circumstances surrounding the bite, any previous medical problems, and a description of the scorpion if no specimen is present should be obtained. It is relatively difficult for a layperson to differentiate the various scorpions. For *C. exilicauda* envenomations that occur in Arizona, a goat-derived antivenin is available from the Antivenom Production Laboratory of Arizona State University.[80] Expert advice should be obtained before the use of this antivenin. Narcotic analgesics and barbiturates have been reported to increase the toxic effects of the venom and should be avoided.

Antivenin should be given in all cases of severe envenomation. All victims should be observed for 24 hours, and children should be admitted to the hospital and monitored closely. Intravenous diazepam or another benzodiazepine may be used for myoclonus and muscle spasms. Phenobarbital, previously used in large doses in children, may be more dangerous than efficacious. Atropine may be administered to control hypersalivation and bradycardia. Nitroprusside and prazosin have been used to control hypertension. Ventilatory assistance may be necessary, especially in children.[81]

Other Arthropods

Ticks have been known as vectors of human disease for some time. Certain female ticks also secrete a toxin that causes a progressive ascending paralysis in humans and animals. The precise mechanism and structure of the toxin are unknown. The two species responsible in the United States are *Dermacentor andersoni* (wood tick) and *Dermacentor variabilis* (dog tick). The bite of the tick is usually painless, but the victim later has difficulty walking, weakness, flaccid paralysis, slurred speech, and visual disturbances. The victim is usually a child, often with a history of recent outdoor activity. Treatment is removal of the offending tick before the paralysis has progressed too far. Any patient seen with ascending paralysis should be closely examined for the presence of a tick, especially on the head and back.

Several species of *beetles* and *caterpillars* secrete irritating substances that cause severe burning pain, numbness, pustular contact dermatitis, edema, nausea, vomiting, and headache. Oropharyngeal exposure can cause mucosal edema and irritation.[82] No deaths have

been reported. Treatment consists of washing the area thoroughly with soap and water and removing any spines present. Spines can be removed with adhesive tape or by applying white glue or facial peel. Locally applied ice bags and baking soda and water paste may be of benefit. Analgesics should be used as needed, and supportive therapy may be necessary for severe envenomation.

Centipedes can inflict bites causing erythema and edema. Treatment is usually local soaks and the use of analgesics. *Conenose bugs*, or "kissing bugs," may cause severe local and systemic allergic reactions. Treatment with antihistamines and supportive care, depending on the degree of reaction, are all that is necessary. Many other arthropods can cause local skin reactions and severe allergic reactions, depending on the individual's sensitivity. These patients should be treated symptomatically with local steroid creams, antihistamines, and other symptomatic supportive measures.[83]

VENOMOUS MARINE ANIMALS

Epidemiology

Almost 2000 species of animals found in the ocean are either venomous or poisonous to humans, and many can produce severe illness or fatalities. An estimated 40,000 to 50,000 marine envenomations occur annually. In recent years, the number of injuries caused by these animals has been increasing dramatically because of the greater number of scuba divers, snorkelers, surfers, and others engaging in water sports. These animals are not usually aggressive, and many are completely immobile. Most of the venomous marine animals injure humans with defense or food-procuring devices. Most venomous marine animals in the United States are found along the California, Gulf of Mexico, and southern Atlantic coasts. These animals range in complexity from sponges to bony fishes and contain some of the most complex and toxic venoms known.[20]

Venom Delivery

In general, venomous marine animals may be divided into three main classes according to the mechanism of venom delivery: bites, nematocysts, and stings.

Bites

Biting animals include several species of cephalopods, most often octopi. Although popular media portray a giant deadly creature that squeezes its victims to death, the most dangerous octopi are seldom larger than 20 cm. Several fatalities have been reported after a bite by the blue-ringed octopus, *Hapalochlaena maculosus*. Most victims are bitten on the upper extremity as they disturb this normally nonaggressive creature. The octopus has a pair of modified salivary glands that secrete venom into the wound produced by the animal's beak.[21] The venom contains a potent vasodilator and an inhibitor of neuromuscular transmission similar to tetrodotoxin.[84,85] No known antivenin exists, and treatment is largely supportive, with respiratory support the most important lifesaving intervention.[86-88]

Nematocysts

The second type of venom mechanism is the nematocyst found in coelenterates (Cnidaria). This group of animals includes the Portuguese man-of-war, true jellyfish, fire corals, stinging hydroids, sea wasps, sea nettle, and anemones. Most of these organisms are sessile, but some are free floating. Because of their large numbers, this group accounts for the greatest number of envenomations by marine animals.[18]

Many different types of nematocysts are known, but the basic mechanism is a "spring-loaded" venom gland that can, on mechanical or chemical stimulation, suddenly evert and discharge a structure that penetrates the prey and delivers the venom through a connecting tube. These nematocysts, found on the animal's tentacles, can number in the hundreds of thousands. Tentacles can be up to 100 ft long in some giant species. Nematocysts can still function even if the animal is dead or if the tentacles are separated from the animal's body. These stinging cells can remain active for weeks after an animal becomes beached. Often, not all nematocysts fire on initial contact but may discharge later during attempted rescue and treatment. Certain marine species have evolved methods of using ingested nematocysts for their own defense.

Toxicity

Nematocyst venom contains various peptides, phospholipase A, proteolytic enzymes, hemolytic enzymes, quaternary ammonium compounds, serotonin, and other toxic compounds. The venom of the coelenterates is antigenic, and allergic reactions are often seen. The severity of the envenomation is related to several factors. First, the severity of the injury is directly proportional to the number of nematocysts discharged. Second, the toxicity varies from species to species. It is unlikely that the victim or the treating physician is able to identify the species from the appearance of the wound. Symptoms may range from simple isolated stinging to respiratory paralysis, cardiovascular collapse, and death. Therefore, the diagnosis must be made according to the clinical findings. Third, the victim's autopharmacologic response to the venom may turn a relatively minor envenomation into a fatal anaphylactic reaction. Any clinician who regularly treats this type of injury should become acquainted with the common species in the particular area.[89]

Although lethal and potentially lethal jellyfish occur worldwide, the extremely toxic specimens are found off the coast of Australia and in other Indo-Pacific waters. Probably the most notable and most toxic coelenterate is the box jellyfish (*Chironex fleckeri*), also known as the "sea wasp." More dangerous than the famed great white shark, this small animal causes several deaths along the Australian coast annually.[90]

Cardiac arrest may occur within minutes, and early aggressive resuscitation offers the best chance of recovery. Intravenous verapamil and box jellyfish antivenin are advocated for use in treatment.[91,92]

Another north Australian jellyfish, *Carukia barnesi*, also produces a devastating envenomation known as *Irukandji syndrome*. Although no reported deaths from this small box jellyfish have been reported, its envenomation produces severe toxic heart failure requiring intensive care and treatment.[93]

The Portuguese man-of-war *(Physalia physalis)* is found along the southern U.S. coastline. This organism is not a true jellyfish but a hydroid colony and is most often included in the jellyfish literature. Envenomation is usually limited to local pain and paresthesias, but it may progress systemically to nausea, headache, chills, and even cardiopulmonary collapse. This organism has also been responsible for several deaths.[94,95]

Most other envenomations are minimal, and the danger is either drowning after being stung or an allergic reaction to the venom. The symptoms resulting from coelenterate envenomation usually consist of a severe burning sensation accompanied by raised erythematous lesions where nematocysts have discharged into the skin. The symptoms may progress, depending on the species and the number of nematocysts, to include nausea, vomiting, chest pain, muscle cramps, dyspnea, diarrhea, cough, convulsions, angioedema, and respiratory arrest. The initial pain and redness may last from a few hours to 2 or 3 days, depending on the therapy.

A related type of envenomation is caused by various species of coral, particularly fire coral *(Millepora)*. These injuries combine nematocyst envenomation with wound contamination. Animal protein and calcareous material left behind in these wounds cause infection and chronic inflammation.

Stings

Some marine animals cause a "sting" that is produced by a specialized apparatus that punctures the victim's skin and then introduces venom. Common examples of this type of animal are sea urchins, cone shells, bristle worms, sea snakes, crown-of-thorns starfish, stingrays, scorpion fish, weever fish, catfish, stonefish, rabbit fish, and zebra fish. Sea urchins, cone shells *(Conus californicus)*, catfish, scorpion fish, and stingrays account for most of the venomous marine animal injuries in the United States.[96]

Sea Urchins

Sea urchins belong to the Echinoderm family along with starfish and sea cucumbers. These animals produce injury and envenomation mostly through toxin-coated spines. These spines often break off and introduce calcareous material and debris into the wound, thereby potentiating severe infection. Symptoms most often include severe local burning, pain, and discoloration, but they may progress systemically in some patients. The degree of symptoms is usually related to the number of spines involved and the species of animal encountered.

Cone Shells

Cone shells are much more toxic than sea urchins, and some species have been responsible for fatalities in the Indo-Pacific region. The venom apparatus is a tubular gland that connects to several teeth at the end of a retractable proboscis. All envenomations reported have occurred in persons handling the shells. The venom contains several proteins, protein-carbohydrate complexes, and 3-indolyl derivatives that act mainly on skeletal muscle and cause variably spastic and flaccid paralysis.[97] Symptoms may or may not include pain, depending on the species. Severe envenomation may cause diplopia, slurred speech, numbness, weakness, paralysis, and respiratory arrest. Onset and regression of symptoms may vary from minutes to days. Currently, no antivenin is available for cone shell envenomation.

Stingray

The stingray is a member of the shark family. It is a broad, flat fish with a long, whiplike tail that may have one or more stingers with barbed ends. They vary in size from a few inches to several feet, and the stingers are proportional to the size of the fish. The stinger is encased in an integumentary sheath and contains venom glands. Stingrays bury themselves in the sand of shallow water, where they can be easily stepped on inadvertently. The sheath and stinger are often broken or left in the wound. The victim experiences an immediate, intense pain in the area of the wound, which may spread to the entire extremity. Systemic symp-toms include salivation, nausea, vomiting, diarrhea, syncope, muscle cramps, fasciculations, dyspnea, cardiac dysrhythmias, and convulsions. The exact composition of the venom is unknown. Enzymes, proteins, serotonin, and a cholinergic substance have been identified, but the exact toxin responsible for most of the severe symptoms is yet to be isolated. The presence of foreign material may also impair healing and cause infection.

Bony Fishes

Bony fishes inflict their wounds through spines located on their fins. The spines and venom glands are encased in a sheath, and grooves along the spines act as channels for the venom. These fish injuries are typically encountered when the fish are stepped on in shallow water or handled by fishermen. The venom is made up of several classes of proteins, most of which are heat labile. The family Scorpaenidae includes three groups of species categorized by venom apparatus: zebra fish, scorpion fish, and stonefish. Zebra fish include the popular aquarium resident the lionfish. Scorpion fish produce intense pain that can spread to the entire affected extremity within minutes.[98] Stonefish envenomation may cause serious and even life-threatening systemic illness, but manifestations such as cardiac and respiratory symptoms can be prevented by early administration of the appropriate antivenin.[21,99] Saltwater catfish produce envenomation through contact with dorsal and pectoral spines.[100]

Management

Much of the venom can be neutralized at the scene, and most fatalities can be prevented. The most important step is to remove the victim from the water. Drownings after minimal envenomation may account for more fatalities than the end effects of severe envenomation. The patient should be questioned about the circumstances of the bite, allergies, and systemic symptoms. If a severe allergic reaction has occurred, the victim should be treated for this emergency before attending to the wound. The type of wound care largely varies according to the type of venom apparatus involved. As with all wounds encountered in the emergency department, appropriate cleansing, debridement, and tetanus prophylaxis are paramount. Prophylactic antibiotics should be used when indicated and when residual foreign body is suspected. Specific antivenins are available for some species, such as the box jellyfish and stonefish.

Bite injuries should be treated with basic life support measures and general wound care consisting of cleansing, debridement, and irrigation. Systemic signs and symptoms are treated accordingly, with aggressive attention paid to the cardiac and respiratory systems.

Nematocysts

Nematocyst injuries are treated by first removing the nematocysts without allowing them to discharge. Tentacles should be removed with a gloved hand or forceps. The remaining nematocysts should be fixed by pouring vinegar (dilute acetic acid) over the wound area. Baking soda and alcohol have also been shown to be effective, and deactivation of nematocysts may be species specific. Fresh water should not be used because it may stimulate continued nematocyst discharge.[101] Other methods include scraping off residual material with the use of a shaving cream or baking soda slurry. The affected area should then be debrided and judiciously washed. Most lifeguard stations in areas where coelenterate stings are common have the necessary materials for this regimen. Supportive pharmacologic therapy (e.g., analgesics, antihistamines, steroid creams) is indicated for all but the most trivial envenomation. Delayed cutaneous reactions may persist despite optimal therapy.[102,103]

Bony Fishes

Puncture injuries are treated by removing the spine or sting if possible. An x-ray film should be taken of the involved area because many spines and sheaths are radiopaque. Sea urchin spines usually break off in the wound; they are so fragile that removing them is difficult without the proper instruments. The stinger of the stingray should be removed with forceps, although these stingers with their sheaths have been known to penetrate body cavities and require surgery for removal. Though not usually present in the wound itself, the fish spines of bony fish should be removed with forceps. In all cases the wound should be copiously irrigated. Most venoms injected through puncture wounds are heat labile. Significant analgesia can be achieved by submersion of the wound in water as hot as the person can tolerate for 30 to 90 minutes.[98]

Patients envenomed by unknown or unfamiliar organisms should be observed for systemic signs and symptoms. Careful discharge instructions should warn the patient to return for increasing pain, numbness, difficulty breathing, and signs of infection.

 KEY CONCEPTS

- Snake venom exhibits neurotoxicity and hematotoxicity, but one usually predominates, depending on the type of snake.
- The amount of crotalid antivenin given depends on the grade of envenomation, from 0 (minimal or no sign of envenomation) to IV (severe envenomation).
- Pit vipers have a characteristic pit found midway between the eye and the nostril on both sides of the head.
- Arthropods account for more deaths from envenomation than snakes do.
- Nematocyst (jellyfish) stings should be immediately neutralized with vinegar.
- Spider bites may be difficult to diagnose without identification of the offending spider.

REFERENCES

1. Sagan C: *The Dragons of Eden.* New York, Random House, 1977.
2. White J: Bites and stings from venomous animals: A global overview. *Ther Drug Monit* 22:65, 2000.
3. Parrish HM: Analysis of 460 fatalities from venomous animals in the United States. *Am J Med Sci* 245:129, 1963.
4. Parrish HM: *Poisonous Snakebites in the United States.* New York, Vantage, 1980.
5. Russell FE: Snake venom poisoning in the United States. *Annu Rev Med* 31:247, 1980.
6. Ennik F: Deaths from bites and stings of venomous animals. *West J Med* 133:463, 1980.
7. Litovitz TL, et al: 1998 annual report of the American Association of Poison Control Centers Toxic Exposure Surveillance System. *Am J Emerg Med* 17:435, 1999.
8. Dumbacher JP, et al: Homobatrachotoxin in the genus *Pitohui*: Chemical defense in birds? *Science* 258:799, 1992.
9. Morandi N, Williams J: Snakebite injuries: Contributing factors and intentionality of exposure. *Wilderness Environ Med* 8:152, 1997.
10. Kunkel DB: Bites of venomous reptiles. *Emerg Med Clin North Am* 2:563, 1984.
11. Kunkel DB, et al: Reptile envenomations. *J Toxicol Clin Toxicol* 21:503, 1983.
12. Gold BS, Barish RA: Venomous snakebites: Current concepts in diagnosis, treatment, and management. *Emerg Med Clin North Am* 10:249, 1992.
13. Davidson TM, Schafer SF, Jones J: North American pit vipers. *J Wilderness Med* 3:397, 1992.
14. Gold BS, Wingert WA: Snake venom poisoning in the United States: A review of therapeutic practice. *South Med J* 87:579, 1994.
15. Gomez HF, et al: Human envenomation from a wandering garter snake. *Ann Emerg Med* 23:1119, 1994.
16. Suchard JR, LoVecchio F: Envenomations by rattlesnakes thought to be dead [letter]. *N Engl J Med* 340:1930, 1999.
17. Strimple PD, et al: Report on envenomation by a Gila monster *(Heloderma suspectum)* with a discussion of venom apparatus, clinical findings, and treatment. *Wilderness Environ Med* 8:111, 1997.
18. Auerbach PS (ed): *Wilderness Medicine,* 4th ed. St Louis, CV Mosby, 2001.
19. Tu AT: *Reptile Venoms and Toxins: The Handbook of Natural Toxins.* New York, Marcel Dekker, 1991.
20. Tu AT: *Venoms: Chemistry and Molecular Biology.* New York, John Wiley & Sons, 1977.
21. Minton SA: *Venom Diseases.* Springfield, Ill, Charles C Thomas, 1974.
22. Russell FE: Snake venom poisoning. *Vet Hum Toxicol* 33:584, 1991.
23. Garfin SR, et al: Rattlesnake bites and surgical decompression: Results using a laboratory model. *Toxicon* 22:177, 1984.
24. Burgess JL, Dart RC: Snake venom coagulopathy: Use and abuse of blood products in the treatment of pit viper envenomation. *Ann Emerg Med* 20:795, 1991.
25. Curry SC, Kunkel DB: Toxicology rounds: Death from a rattlesnake bite. *Am J Emerg Med* 3:227, 1985.
26. Goldstein EJ, et al: Bacteriology of rattlesnake venom and implications for therapy. *J Infect Dis* 140:818, 1979.
27. Norris RL: Snakebite scenario [letter]. *Wilderness Environ Med* 10:55, 1999.
28. Burgess JL, et al: Effects of constriction bands on rattlesnake venom absorption: A pharmacokinetic study. *Ann Emerg Med* 21:1086, 1992.
29. Anker RL, et al: Retarding the uptake of "mock venom" in humans: Comparison of three first-aid treatments. *Med J Aust* 1:212, 1982.
30. Anker RL, et al: Snakebite: Comparison of three methods designed to delay uptake of "mock venom." *Aust Fam Physician* 12:365, 1983.
31. Blackman JR, Dillon S: Venomous snakebite: Past, present, and future treatment options. *J Am Board Fam Pract* 5:399, 1992.
32. Gold BS: Snake venom extractors: A valuable first aid tool [letter]. *Vet Hum Toxicol* 35:255, 1993.
33. Forgey WW: More on snake-venom and insect-venom extractors [letter]. *N Engl J Med* 328:516, 1993.
34. Moss ST, et al: Association of rattlesnake bite location with severity of clinical manifestations. *Ann Emerg Med* 30:58, 1997.
35. Otten EJ: Antivenin therapy in the emergency department. *Am J Emerg Med* 1:83, 1983.
36. Dart RC, et al: Affinity-purified, mixed monospecific crotalid antivenom ovine Fab for the treatment of crotalid venom poisoning. *Ann Emerg Med* 30:33, 1997.
37. Consroe P, et al: Comparison of a new ovine antigen binding fragment (Fab) antivenin for United States Crotalidae with the commercial antivenin for protection against venom-induced lethality in mice. *Am J Trop Med Hyg* 53:507, 1995.
38. Seifert SA, et al: Relationship of venom effects to venom antigen and antivenom serum concentrations in a patient with *Crotalus atrox* envenomation treated with a Fab antivenom. *Ann Emerg Med* 30:49, 1997.
39. Clark RF, et al: Successful treatment of crotalid-induced neurotoxicity with a new polyspecific crotalid Fab antivenom. *Ann Emerg Med* 30:54, 1997.
40. Otten EJ, McKimm D: Venomous snakebite in a patient allergic to horse serum. *Ann Emerg Med* 12:624, 1983.
41. Buntain WL: Successful venomous snakebite neutralization with massive antivenin infusion in a child. *J Trauma* 23:1012, 1983.
42. Kitchens CS, Van Mierop LH: Envenomation by the Eastern coral snake *(Micrurus fulvius fulvius)*: A study of 39 victims. *JAMA* 258:1615, 1987.
43. Lawrence WT, Giannopoulos A, Hansen A: Pit viper bites: Rational management in locales in which copperheads

and cottonmouths predominate. *Ann Plast Surg* 36:276, 1996.

44. Sutherland SK: Antivenom use in Australia: Premedication, adverse reactions and the use of venom detection kits. *Med J Aust* 157:734, 1992.

45. Heard K, O'Malley GF, Dart RC: Antivenom therapy in the Americas. *Drugs* 58:5, 1999.

46. Chippaux JP, Goyffon M: Venoms, antivenoms and immunotherapy. *Toxicon* 36:823, 1998.

47. Selvanayagam ZE, et al: ELISA for the detection of venoms from four medically important snakes of India. *Toxicon* 37:757, 1999.

48. Kunkel DB: Arthropod envenomations. *Emerg Med Clin North Am* 2:579, 1984.

49. Binder LS: Acute arthropod envenomation: Incidence, clinical features and management. *Med Toxicol Adverse Drug Exp* 4:163, 1989.

50. Normann SA: Venomous insects and reptiles. *J Fla Med Assoc* 83:183, 1996.

51. Reisman RE: Insect stings. *N Engl J Med* 331:523, 1994.

52. Incorvaia C, Pucci S, Pastorello EA: Clinical aspects of Hymenoptera venom allergy. *Allergy* 54(Suppl 58):50, 1999.

53. Cohen SG, Bianchine PJ: Hymenoptera, hypersensitivity, and history: A prologue to current day concepts and practices in the diagnosis, treatment, and prevention of insect sting allergy. *Ann Allergy Asthma Immunol* 74:198, 1995.

54. Valentine MD: Allergy to stinging insects. *Ann Allergy* 70:427, 1993 (erratum, 71:96, 1993).

55. Valentine MD: Insect-sting anaphylaxis [editorial]. *Ann Intern Med* 118:225, 1993.

56. Valentine MD: Insect venom allergy: Diagnosis and treatment. *J Allergy Clin Immunol* 73:299, 1984.

57. Ariue BK: Multiple Africanized bee stings in a child. *Pediatrics* 94:115, 1994.

58. Sherman RA: What physicians should know about Africanized honeybees. *West J Med* 163:541, 1995.

59. Winston ML: The Africanized "killer" bee: Biology and public health. *Q J Med* 87:263, 1994.

60. Freeman TM: Hymenoptera hypersensitivity in an imported fire ant endemic area. *Ann Allergy Asthma Immunol* 78:369, 1997.

61. Freeman TM: Insect and fire ant hypersensitivity: What the primary care physician needs to know. *Compr Ther* 23:38, 1997.

62. Freeman TM: Imported fire ants: The ants from hell! *Allergy Proc* 15:11, 1994.

63. Stafford CT: Hypersensitivity to fire ant venom. *Ann Allergy Asthma Immunol* 77:87, 1996.

64. Hamilton RG, et al: Selection of Hymenoptera venoms for immunotherapy on the basis of patient's IgE antibody cross-reactivity. *J Allergy Clin Immunol* 92:651, 1993.

65. Rauber A: Black widow spider bites. *J Toxicol Clin Toxicol* 21:473, 1983.

66. Clark RF, et al: Clinical presentation and treatment of black widow spider envenomation: A review of 163 cases. *Ann Emerg Med* 21:782, 1992.

67. Woestman R, Perkin R, Van Stralen D: The black widow: Is she deadly to children? *Pediatr Emerg Care* 12:360, 1996.

68. Ryan PJ: Preliminary report: Experience with the use of dantrolene sodium in the treatment of bites by the black widow spider *Latrodectus hesperus*. *J Toxicol Clin Toxicol* 21:487, 1983.

69. Blackman JR: Spider bites. *J Am Board Fam Pract* 8:288, 1995.

70. Anderson PC: Spider bites in the United States. *Dermatol Clin* 15:307, 1997.

71. Salm RJ, et al: Brown recluse spider bite: Two case reports and review. *J Am Podiatr Med Assoc* 88:37, 1998.

72. Wright SW, et al: Clinical presentation and outcome of brown recluse spider bite. *Ann Emerg Med* 30:28, 1997.

73. Futrell JM: Loxoscelism. *Am J Med Sci* 304:261, 1992.

74. King LE Jr, Rees RS: Dapsone treatment of a brown recluse bite. *JAMA* 250:648, 1983.

75. Hobbs GD: Brown recluse spider envenomation: Is hyperbaric oxygen the answer [editorial]? *Acad Emerg Med* 4:165, 1997.

76. Hobbs GD, et al: Comparison of hyperbaric oxygen and dapsone therapy for *Loxosceles* envenomation. *Acad Emerg Med* 3:758, 1996.

77. Maynor ML, et al: Brown recluse spider envenomation: A prospective trial of hyperbaric oxygen therapy. *Acad Emerg Med* 4:184, 1997.

78. Gomez HF, et al: Intradermal anti-*Loxosceles* Fab fragments attenuate dermonecrotic arachnidism. *Acad Emerg Med* 6:1195, 1999.

79. Miller MK, et al: Clinical features and management of *Hadronyche* envenomation in man. *Toxicon* 38:409, 2000.

80. Bond GR: Antivenin administration for *Centruroides* scorpion sting: Risks and benefits. *Ann Emerg Med* 21:788, 1992.

81. Gateau T, Bloom M, Clark R: Response to specific *Centruroides sculpturatus* antivenom in 151 cases of scorpion stings. *J Toxicol Clin Toxicol* 32:165, 1994.

82. Lee D, Pitetti RD, Casselbrant ML: Oropharyngeal manifestations of lepidopterism. *Arch Otolaryngol Head Neck Surg* 125:50, 1999.

83. Lynch PJ, Pinnas JL: "Kissing bug" bites: *Triatoma* species as an important cause of insect bites in the Southwest. *Cutis* 22:585, 1978.

84. Sutherland SK, Lane WR: Toxins and mode of envenomation of the common ringed or blue-banded octopus. *Med J Aust* 1:893, 1969.

85. Flachsenberger WA: Respiratory failure and lethal hypotension due to blue-ringed octopus and tetrodotoxin envenomation observed and counteracted in animal models. *J Toxicol Clin Toxicol* 24:485, 1986.

86. Edmonds C: A non-fatal case of blue-ringed octopus bite. *Med J Aust* 2:601, 1969.

87. Williamson JA: The blue-ringed octopus [letter]. *Med J Aust* 140:308, 1984.

88. Williamson JA: The blue-ringed octopus bite and envenomation syndrome. *Clin Dermatol* 5:127, 1987.

89. Auerbach PS: Marine envenomations. *N Engl J Med* 325:486, 1991.

90. Fenner PJ, Williamson JA: Worldwide deaths and severe envenomation from jellyfish stings. *Med J Aust* 165:658, 1996.

91. Lumley J, et al: Fatal envenomation by *Chironex fleckeri*, the north Australian box jellyfish: The continuing search for lethal mechanisms. *Med J Aust* 148:527, 1988.

92. Burnett JW, Calton GJ: Response of the box-jellyfish (*Chironex fleckeri*) cardiotoxin to intravenous administration of verapamil. *Med J Aust* 2:192, 1983.

93. Fenner P, Carney I: The Irukandji syndrome: A devastating syndrome caused by a north Australian jellyfish. *Aust Fam Physician* 28:1131, 1999.

94. Kaufman MB: Portuguese man-of-war envenomation. *Pediatr Emerg Care* 8:27, 1992.

95. Stein MR, et al: Fatal Portuguese man-o'-war (*Physalia physalis*) envenomation. *Ann Emerg Med* 18:312, 1989.

96. Cain D: Weever fish sting: An unusual problem. *Br Med J (Clin Res Ed)* 287:406, 1983.

97. Gray WR, Olivera BM, Cruz LJ: Peptide toxins from venomous *Conus* snails. *Annu Rev Biochem* 57:665, 1988.

98. Kizer KW, McKinney HE, Auerbach PS: Scorpaenidae envenomation: A five-year poison center experience. *JAMA* 253:807, 1985.

99. Lehmann DF, Hardy JC: Stonefish envenomation [letter]. *N Engl J Med* 329:510, 1993.

100. Blomkalns AL, Otten EJ: Catfish spine envenomation: A case report and literature review. *Wilderness Environ Med* 10:242, 1999.
101. Burnett JW, Rubinstein H, Calton GJ: First aid for jellyfish envenomation. *South Med J* 76:870, 1983.
102. Reed KM, Bronstein BR, Baden HP: Delayed and persistent cutaneous reactions to coelenterates. *J Am Acad Dermatol* 10:462, 1984.
103. Auerbach PS, Hays JT: Erythema nodosum following a jellyfish sting. *J Emerg Med* 5:487, 1987.

CHAPTER

60 Thermal Burns

Richard F. Edlich, Marcus L. Martin, and William B. Long III

PERSPECTIVE

Epidemiology

Compared with other natural disasters, burns exert a catastrophic influence on people in terms of human life, suffering, disability, and financial loss. Approximately 1.4 million persons in the United States sustain burns each year; an estimated 54,000 to 180,000 are hospitalized.[1] Work-related burns account for 20% to 25% of all serious burns.[2]

Burn wounds can be classified into six groups on the basis of the mechanism of injury: scalds, contact burns, fire, chemical (see Chapter 61), electrical (see Chapter 140), and radiation (see Chapter 144). This chapter addresses the first three types of burns. Scald burn injuries can be caused by liquids, grease, or steam. Liquid scalds can be further divided into spill and immersion scalds. Fire burn injuries can be subdivided into flash and flame burns. The mechanism of burn injury can be used as a predictor of outcome. For example, patients with flame burns and electrical burn injuries often require hospitalization (Figure 60-1). In contrast, most patients with burns caused by either contact with hot surfaces or sun exposure are managed as outpatients.

The highest incidence of burn injury occurs during the first few years of life and between 20 and 29 years of age. Serious burn injuries occur most often in males (67%). The highest incidence of serious burn injury occurs in young adults (ages 20 to 29), followed by children younger than 9 years. Individuals older than 50 sustain the fewest serious burn injuries (2.3%). The major causes of severe burn injury are flame burns (37%) and liquid scalds (24%). For children younger than 2 years, liquid scalds and hot surface burns account for nearly all serious burn injuries. After 2 years of age, flame burn is the most common cause of serious burn injury, accounting for nearly one third of all cases. In persons 80 years of age and older, hot surface exposure is a major cause (22%) of serious burns.

Five percent of hospitalized burn patients die as a result of their burn injuries; most are caused by flame burns. Liquid scald burns account for the second largest number of deaths. In structural fires, approximately one half of all burn victims, many with only moderate-sized burns of less than 40% of the body surface area, die of asphyxiation or carbon monoxide (CO) poisoning before reaching the hospital.

Flame burn injuries are associated with recurring scenarios regarding the most likely burn victims, the circumstances surrounding the burn, the burned victim's response to the situation, and the role of garments in the burn injury. The white population is most often involved (67%), and the highest incidence occurs in the 15- to 29-year-old age group. A flammable liquid is involved in most cases (66%), and gasoline is the most common liquid (63%). The high incidence of gasoline burns during the summer months reflects the increased use in the northern and midwestern United States of gasoline products in farming or for recreational purposes (e.g., bonfires, burning leaves, boating, yard work).[3] The most common contributing factor in flame burn injuries is the consumption of alcohol (26%).

The patient's or bystander's response to burn incidents has considerable influence on the magnitude of burn injury. When the response is timely and effective, the magnitude of burn injury is reduced (except when flammable liquids are involved). When flammable accelerants are present, the burning process persists even when the victim is rolling on the ground. In this setting, removal of the burning garments or smothering the flames is more likely to be an effective measure.

During the past two decades, deaths from burn injuries have decreased. This decline has been attributed to improved firefighting techniques and improved emergency medical services. The use of smoke detectors has significantly reduced the severity of burn injuries, with an estimated 80% reduction in mortality and 74% decline in injuries from residential fires. Educational programs reminding homeowners to lower the thermostat on water heating units as well as teaching children to extinguish flaming cloth by stopping, dropping, and rolling have had a significant impact. Consequently, all medical leaders agree that the best treatment of burn injuries is prevention.

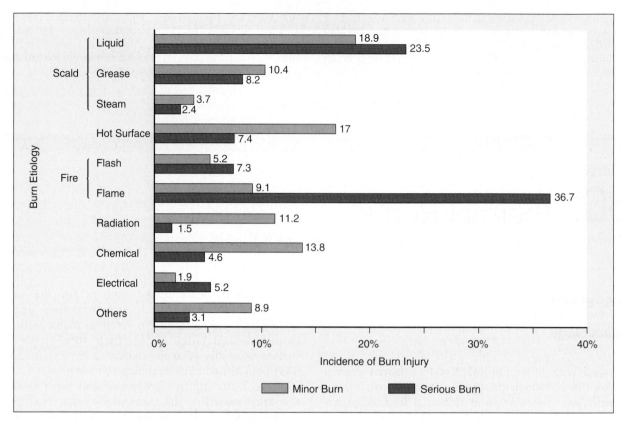

Figure 60-1. Burn incidence and severity according to etiology.

Burn injuries are extremely complex and elicit physiologic and metabolic interactions involving all major organ systems. These pathophysiologic changes occur in a time-dependent manner. One of the major goals of this chapter is to describe a system of care of burn injuries and to review current modes of surgical therapy with discussions of wound care and modern burn dressings.

PRINCIPLES OF DISEASE

Anatomy

Skin is the largest organ of the body. It has three major tissue layers. The outermost layer, the epidermis, is composed of stratified epithelium. The epidermis has two components, an outer layer of anucleate cornified cells (stratum corneum) covering inner layers of viable cells (malpighian layers), from which the cornified surface cells arise by differentiation. The stratum corneum acts as a barrier to impede the entrance of microorganisms and toxic substances while allowing the body to retain water and electrolytes. The malpighian layers provide a continuous production of cornified cells. The malpighian layers can be further subdivided into the germinal basal cell layer, the stratum spinosum, and the stratum granulosum. Beneath the epidermis is the dermis, which is composed of a dense fibroelastic connective tissue stroma, containing collagen and elastic fibers, and an extracellular gel called the *ground substance*. This amorphous gel is composed of an acid mucopolysaccharide protein combined with salts, water, and glycoproteins; it is believed to contribute to salt and water balance, to serve as a support for other components of the dermis and subcutaneous tissue, and to participate in collagen synthesis. The dermal layer contains an extensive vascular and nerve network and special glands and appendages that communicate with the overlying epidermis.

The dermis can be divided into two parts. The most superficial portion, the papillary dermis, is molded against the epidermis and contains superficial elements of the microcirculation of the skin. It consists of a relatively cellular, loose connective tissue with collagen and elastic fibers that are smaller in diameter and fewer in number than the underlying reticular dermis. Within the papillary dermis, dermal elevations indent the inner surface of the epidermis. Between the dermal papillae are peglike downward projections of the epidermis called rete pegs. In the reticular portion of the dermis, the collagen and elastic fibers are thicker and greater in number. Fewer cells and less ground substance are found in the reticular dermis than in the papillary dermis. The thickness of the dermis varies from 1 to 4 mm in different anatomic regions and is thickest in the back, followed by the thigh, abdomen, forehead, wrist, scalp, palm, and eyelid. Its thickness varies with the individual's age. The dermis is thinnest in very old people, in whom it is often atrophic, and in very young children, in whom it is not fully developed.

The third layer of skin is the subcutaneous tissue, which is composed primarily of areolar and fatty connective tissue. This layer shows great regional variations in thickness and adipose content. It contains skin appendages, glands, and hair follicles. The hair follicles extend in deep narrow pits or pockets that traverse the dermis to varying depths and usually extend into the subcutaneous tissue. Each hair follicle consists of a shaft that projects above the surface and a root that is embedded within the skin. There are two types of sweat glands in skin: apocrine and eccrine. The *apocrine glands* are called peridermal because they have a duct that opens into a hair follicle. The eccrine glands are simple, coiled, tubular glands usually extending into the papillary dermis. The *eccrine glands* are classified as etricheal because their duct opens onto the skin surface independently of a hair follicle. The eccrine glands are found over the entire body surface, except the margins of the lips, eardrum, inner surface of the prepuce, and glans penis. The apocrine glands are largely confined to the axillary and perineal region and do not become functional until just after puberty. The *sebaceous glands* are connected with the hair follicles. They are simple or branched alveolar glands. Sebaceous glands unconnected with hair follicles occur along the margin of the lips, in the nipples, in the glans and prepuce of the penis, and in the labia minora. Depending on the depth of burn injury, epithelial repair can be accomplished from local epithelial elements and skin appendages.

When skin is burned, the damaged stratum corneum allows the invasion of microorganisms, and the Langerhans cells, which mediate local immune responses, are also damaged. Burn patients with severe injuries have a diminished systemic immune response, making them susceptible to serious infections.

Pathophysiology

Thermodynamics of Burn Injury

The severity of burn injury is related to the rate at which heat is transferred from the heating agent to the skin. The rate of heat transfer depends on the (1) heat capacity of the agent, (2) temperature of the agent, (3) duration of contact with the agent, (4) transfer coefficient, and (5) specific heat and conductivity of the local tissues.

Heat Capacity

The capacity of a material to hold heat energy is determined by both the specific heat and the heat capacity of the material. The *specific heat* of a material is defined as the ratio of the amount of heat required to raise an equal mass of a reference substance, usually water, one degree in temperature. *Heat capacity* refers to the quantity of heat a material contains when it comes in contact with skin. The quantity of heat stored depends on the specific heat of the material and the amount and temperature of the material.

The importance of heat capacity as a determinant of the severity of burn injury is best illustrated by comparing the amount of heat stored in 10 g of two differ-

ent materials (copper and water) heated to the same temperature (100° C). The specific heat of water is 4.2178 W-sec/g-K (watts times seconds of heat per gram of mass times degrees in kelvin), and the specific heat of copper is 0.3831 W-sec/g-K. If these two materials come in contact with skin, they give up their heat by cooling, and the skin accepts the heat by increasing its temperature. If the temperature of each material decreases by 60° C (140° F), the water gives up 2530 W-sec of heat, whereas copper transfers only 230 W-sec of heat. Even if the initial temperatures of the two materials are identical, the heat available from water is much more likely to produce a severe injury. The specific heat of water (the most common cause of scald burns) is the highest of all the gases, metals, and solids so far tested, with the exception of ammonia and ether.

Temperature

The initial temperature of a material at the instant of contact is also an important determinant of burn severity. Many materials (e.g., water) cannot be heated beyond a certain temperature without changing state. Water can be heated only to 100° C (212° F) at atmospheric pressure before it ceases to be a liquid and vaporizes. When other liquids reach a specific temperature, they ignite or oxidize, combining with oxygen. The temperature at which the vapors of a volatile liquid mixed with air spontaneously ignite is designated as the *flash point* of the liquid. A *flammable* liquid is defined as any liquid having a flash point less than 37.8° C. Liquids with a flash point above this temperature are considered *combustible* liquids (Table 60-1). In addition to their high temperatures, burning liquids may ignite the victim's clothing, exacerbating the injury.

Duration of Contact

Human skin can tolerate temperatures up to 40° C (104° F) for a relatively long time before irreversible injury occurs (Figure 60-2).[4] Higher temperatures cause an almost logarithmic increase in tissue destruction. The duration of contact between a liquid and the skin depends on both the viscosity of the liquid and the manner in which it is applied to the victim's skin. When a hot liquid is splashed on a person (*spill scalds*), it usually flows down the body, having a rate of descent that depends on the fluid's viscosity. Although water streams to the ground unless impeded by clothing,

Table 60-1. Flash Points of Combustible Liquids

Liquid	Flash Points	
	°C	°F
Corn oil	249	480
Lard	215	419
Cottonseed oil	306	581
Olive oil	276	527
Peanut oil	282	540
Oleomargarine	232	450

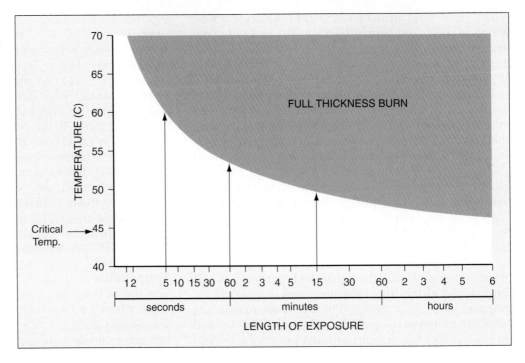

Figure 60-2. Relationship between temperature and duration of exposure in the development of full-thickness burn injury.

viscous oils and greases usually cling to a victim's skin, prolonging the duration of exposure and the extent of injury.

In *immersion scalds* the duration of contact between the hot liquid and the skin is considerably longer than with spill scalds, increasing the severity of injury. Certain populations are at high risk for immersion scald burns, including children younger than 5 years, elderly persons (65 and older), and disabled people.[5] These individuals tend to have a slower reaction time and a physical inability to escape from hot water. Immersion burns usually cover a very large percentage of total body surface area (TBSA), almost twice that of other scald burns, which contributes to their high rate of morbidity and mortality.[6,7]

Child abuse accounts for a large proportion of immersion scald burns. Immersion burns caused by child abuse can be distinguished from accidental burns by the pattern and site of the burn, the histories given by the caregiver and patient, and a medical history or scars representing previous abuse. Nonaccidental burns often have clear-cut edges, as found in "stocking" scalds, in which a child's foot has been held in scalding water. Spill scald burns, on the other hand, more often have uneven fuzzy edges as a result of the victim's attempts to escape the hot liquid. Burns from abuse tend to occur on the back of hands and feet, the buttocks and perineum, and the legs. Accidental burns, such as those caused by a child spilling a cup of coffee, more often occur on the head, trunk, and palmar surface of hands and feet. Physical evidence of previous injuries (e.g., crater-like cigarette burn scars, bruises) also suggests abuse.

Heat Transfer

Even when a substance possesses sufficient heat to cause a burn injury, it does not do so unless its heat can be transferred to the skin. The ability to transfer heat between two different materials is regulated by the *heat transfer coefficient*, which is defined as the amount of heat that passes through a unit area of contact between two materials when the temperature difference between these materials is one degree.

Three different methods of heat transfer exist: conduction, convection, and radiation. The simplest method of heat transfer is *conduction*, which occurs when a hot solid object comes in direct contact with the skin. *Convection* is the transfer of heat by a material that involves the physical movement of the material itself and is determined not only by heat conduction but also by energy storage and mixing motion. Convection is most important as the mechanism of energy transfer between skin and a heated liquid or gas. Hot water spilling on skin transfers heat by convection between the water droplets and the skin surface. Steam or very hot air also transfers heat to the skin by convection.

In each of these three methods of heat transfer, the amount of energy transferred is determined by the heat transfer coefficient associated with the two materials involved. Because the convective heat transfer coefficient of steam is 30 times greater than that of water, it transfers 30 times more heat to the skin than water (Table 60-2). As a result, steam causes a more severe thermal injury than heated water when the length of exposure is identical.

Tissue Conductivity

The conductivity of the specific tissue involved significantly affects the extent of burn injury. Heat transfer within skin is influenced by the thermal conductivity of the heated material, the area through which heat is transferred, and the temperature gradient within the material. Water content, natural oils or secretions

Table 60-2. Heat Transfer Coefficients for Various Agents

Agent	Convective Heat Transfer Coefficient (watts/m^2 × °C)
Air	5-15
Water	150-3000
Steam	5500-100,000

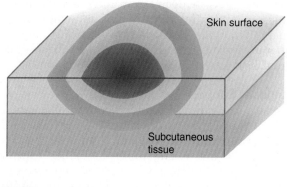

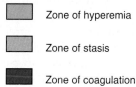

Zone of hyperemia

Zone of stasis

Zone of coagulation

Figure 60-3. Three concentric zones of burn injury.

of the skin, and the presence of insulating material (e.g., cornified keratin layer of skin) influence tissue conductivity. In addition, alterations in local tissue blood flow profoundly affect heat transfer and distribution. The inability to conduct heat away from a contact point efficiently results in varying degrees of tissue injury.

Because skin is a relatively poor conductor of heat, it provides an extensive barrier to heat injury. The degree to which it resists injury depends on its anatomic configuration. Its uppermost layer, the epidermis, is relatively uniform in thickness in all body regions (75 to 100 μm), except for the soles and palms, where it is thicker (0.4 to 0.6 mm). The rarity of full-thickness injury to the palms and soles of the feet can be attributed to their thick epithelial cover.

The ultimate outcome of a burn injury is also influenced by the depth of epidermal appendages in the burned tissue, which varies according to the age of the patient. Very young and old individuals have superficial appendages, which makes both groups more susceptible to full-thickness burn injury. By contrast, the epidermal appendages of the human scalp and male beard are very deep, making these sites more refractory to severe burn injury.

Burn Wound Injury

The first day after burn injury, three concentric zones of tissue injury characterize a full-thickness burn: the zones of coagulation, stasis, and hyperemia (Figure 60-3).[8]

The central zone of *coagulation* has the most intimate contact with the heat source. It consists of dead or dying cells as a result of coagulation necrosis and absent blood flow. It usually appears white or charred.

The intermediate zone of *stasis* is usually red and may blanch on pressure, giving the impression that it has an intact circulation. After 24 hours, however, the circulation through its superficial vessels has often ceased. Petechial hemorrhages may be present. By the third day the intermediate zone of stasis becomes white because its superficial dermis is avascular and necrotic.

The outer zone of *hyperemia* is a red zone that blanches on pressure, indicating that it has intact circulation. By the fourth day, this zone has a deeper red color. Healing is present by the seventh day.

Transformation of the zone of stasis to coagulation occurs and has been related to many factors, including progressive dermal ischemia. Experimental studies have implicated prostaglandins, histamine, and bradykinin as the chemical mediators of this progressive vascular occlusion.[9] They can produce edema by altering endothelial cell and basement membrane function to enhance permeability. When this ischemia persists, the zone of stasis eventually becomes a full-thickness burn injury.

When Robson and colleagues[9] discovered various prostaglandin derivatives in burn wounds, they suggested that an imbalance in the vasoconstrictive and vasodilatory prostanoids produces a progressive tissue loss in the zone of stasis. In acute burn wounds, an increased level of oxygen free radicals, such as xanthine oxidase, appeared to be involved in the formation of burn edema. This edema formation can be attenuated by pretreatment with xanthine oxidase inhibitors.[10]

Systemic Inflammatory Response

In patients whose burns exceed 30% of TBSA, cytokines and other mediators are released into the systemic circulation, causing a systemic inflammatory response. Because vessels in burned tissue exhibit increased vascular permeability, an extravasation of fluids into the burned tissues occurs. Hypovolemia is the immediate consequence of this fluid loss, which accounts for decreased perfusion and oxygen delivery. In patients with serious burns, release of catecholamines, vasopressin, and angiotensin causes peripheral and splanchnic bed vasoconstriction that can compromise in-organ perfusion. Myocardial contractility may also be reduced by release of the inflammatory cytokine tumor necrosis factor α. In deep third-degree burns, hemolysis may be encountered, necessitating blood transfusions to restore blood loss. A decrease in pulmonary function can occur in severely burned patients without evidence of inhalation injury from the bronchoconstriction caused by humoral factors, such as histamine, serotonin, and thromboxane A_2. A decrease in lung and tissue compliance is a manifestation of this reduction in pulmonary function. Burned skin exhibits increased evaporative water loss associated with obligatory concurrent heat loss, which can cause hypothermia.

Nutritional Support

Because burn injury causes a hypermetabolic state that is characterized by a dramatic increase in resting energy expenditure, nutritional support is essential, especially by the enteral route, to reduce intestinal villous atrophy. Deitch and colleagues[11] reported a syndrome of decreased bowel mucosal integrity, capillary leak, and decreased mesenteric blood flow, which allowed bacterial translocation into the portal circulation. These translocated bacteria significantly alter hepatocyte function and spread systemically to cause systemic sepsis. Adequate resuscitation that ensures mesenteric blood flow can prevent the potential development of multisystem organ failure. Enteral nutrition with glutamine has a tropic effect on the enterocytes that preserve mucosal integrity.

Infection

In patients with major burn injuries, infection remains the major cause of death. Immune consequences of this injury have been identified and are specific deficits in neutrophil chemotaxis, phagocytosis, and intracellular bacterial killing. Cell-mediated immunity, as measured by skin testing, is also compromised, which has been related to both decreased lymphocyte activation and suppressive mediators present in the serum of burn patients. A reduction in immunoglobulin synthesis has also been encountered in these seriously ill patients.

Burn Shock

Severe burn injury causes a coagulation necrosis of tissue that initiates a physiologic response in every organ system that is directly proportional to the size of the burn. Tissue destruction results in increased capillary permeability with profound egress of fluid from the intravascular space to the tissues adjacent to the burn wound. Inordinate amounts of fluid are lost by evaporation from the damaged surface, which is no longer able to retain water. This increase in capillary permeability, coupled with evaporative water loss, causes hypovolemic shock.

Other Physiologic Changes

Cardiac. Other physiologic changes seen with thermal injury are, to a large extent, a response to diminished circulating blood volume. The immediate cardiovascular response to thermal injury is a reduction in cardiac output accompanied by an elevation in peripheral vascular resistance. In the absence of heart disease, ventricular ejection fraction and velocity of myocardial fiber shortening are actually increased during thermal injury.[12] With replacement of plasma volume, cardiac output increases to levels that are above normal. This hyperdynamic state is a reflection of the hypermetabolic flow phase of thermal injury.

Pulmonary. Alterations in pulmonary function after burn injury are similar to those seen with other forms of traumatic injury. Minute ventilation usually increases immediately. After resuscitation, respiratory rate and tidal volume progressively increase, resulting in minute ventilation that may be twice normal. Pulmonary vascular resistance also increases after burn injury, which may be a manifestation of the release of vasoactive amines and other mediators.[13] This increase in pulmonary vascular resistance may provide a protective effect during fluid resuscitation by reducing pulmonary capillary hydrostatic pressure and lowering susceptibility to pulmonary edema. In the absence of inhalation injury, no significant change occurs in pulmonary capillary permeability after cutaneous thermal injury.[14]

Renal. In the immediate postburn period, glomerular filtration rate and renal blood flow are reduced in proportion to the reduction in intravascular volume. Gastrointestinal dysfunction also appears to be proportional to the magnitude of thermal injury. In patients with burned areas in excess of 25% of TBSA, gastroparesis is commonly noted until the third to fifth postburn day.

Hematologic. Burn shock may be complicated by an acute erythrocyte hemolysis caused by both direct heat damage and a decreased half-life of damaged red blood cells (RBCs). In major burns, the RBC mass may be reduced 3% to 15%. RBCs also exhibit a decreased half-life because of a microangiopathic hemolytic anemia that may persist for up to 2 weeks.

Depth of Burn Injury

The depth of burn injury is often classified according to degrees. In *first-degree burns*, minor epithelial damage of the epidermis exists. Redness, tenderness, and pain are the hallmarks of the injury. Blistering does not occur, and two-point discrimination remains intact. Healing takes place over several days without scarring. The most common causes of first-degree burns are flash burns and sunburns.

The two types of *second-degree burns* are superficial partial-thickness and deep partial-thickness burns. In these burn injuries, some portion of the skin appendages remains viable, allowing epithelial repair of the burn wound without skin grafting. The *superficial partial-thickness burn* involves the epidermis and superficial (papillary) dermis, often resulting in thin-walled, fluid-filled blisters (Figure 60-4A). These burns appear pink, moist, and soft and are exquisitely tender when touched by a gloved hand. They heal in approximately 2 to 3 weeks, usually without scarring, by outgrowth of epithelial buds from the viable pilosebaceous units and sweat glands residing in the papillary and reticular dermis. The *deep partial-thickness burn* extends into the reticular dermis (Figure 60-4B). The skin color is usually a mixture of red and blanched white. Blisters are thick walled and are often ruptured.

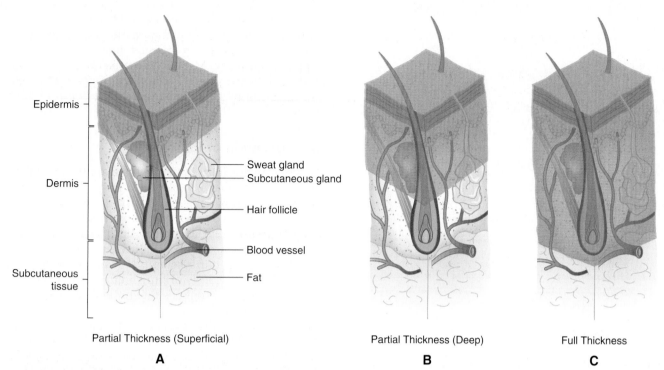

Figure 60-4. First-, second-, and third-degree burns. Stippled areas indicate depth of burn injury. **A,** Superficial partial-thickness burn. **B,** Deep partial-thickness burn. **C,** Full-thickness burn injury.

Two-point discrimination may be diminished, but pressure applied to the burned skin can be felt. This injury may undergo spontaneous epithelialization from the few viable epithelial appendages at this deepest layer of dermis and may heal in 3 to 6 weeks (if no infection arises). Because these burns have less capacity for reepithelializing, a greater potential for hypertrophic scar formation exists. Contraction across joints, with resulting limitation in range of motion, is a common sequela. Splash scalds often cause second-degree burns.

Third-degree burns are full-thickness burns that destroy both epidermis and dermis (Figure 60-4C). The capillary network of the dermis is completely destroyed. The burned skin has a white or leathery appearance with underlying clotted vessels and is anesthetic (numb). Unless a third-degree burn is small enough to heal by contraction (<1.0 cm in diameter), skin grafting is always necessary to resurface the injured area. Third-degree burns are caused by immersion scalds, flame burns, and chemical and high-voltage electrical injuries.

Fourth-degree burns involve full-thickness destruction of the skin and subcutaneous tissue, with involvement of the underlying fascia, muscle, bone, or other structures. These injuries require extensive debridement and complex reconstruction of specialized tissues and invariably result in prolonged disability. Fourth-degree burns result from prolonged exposure to the usual causes of third-degree burns.

Metabolic Response to Therapy

The degree of metabolic alteration experienced by burn patients is directly related to the extent of injury. The *ebb phase* is the initial decrease in cardiac output and metabolic rate. After fluid resuscitation, the cardiac output becomes normal and then increases to above normal levels, with a simultaneous increase in resting energy expenditure (*flow phase*). A severe burn can double the metabolic central rate, which can be blunted by 40% to 60% using occlusive dressings and increased room temperature. The central temperature is reset to 38.5° C at 5 to 15 days after the burn injury. In burns over 60% or more of TBSA, the central temperature can remain elevated for up to 2 months because of direct stimulation of the hypothalamus by inflammatory mediators and cytokines.

Burn injury causes the release of massive amounts of amino acids from muscle. This response is caused by increases in cortisol and decreases in growth hormone and insulin, with resultant increased proteolysis of muscle protein and release of amino acids. Anabolic growth hormone treatment has been shown to increase protein synthesis in muscle, increase muscle mass, and accelerate wound healing after burn injury. Potential anabolic hormones (e.g., insulin-like growth factor, insulin, dehydroepiandrosterone, oxandrolone) are being evaluated for their effects on wound healing.

CLINICAL FEATURES

Burn Wound Assessment

The *rule of nines* is a practical technique for estimating the extent of TBSA involved in a burn injury. This approach divides the major anatomic areas of the body into percentages of TBSA (Figure 60-5A). For the adult,

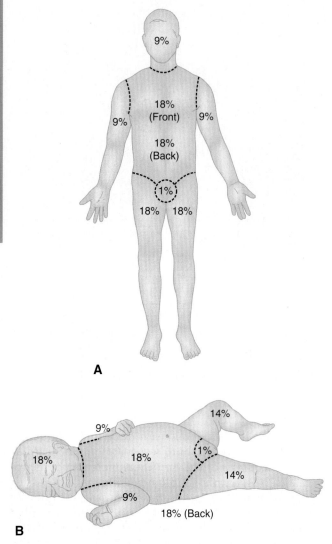

Figure 60-5. Rule of nines: percentages of total body area. **A,** Adult. **B,** Infant.

it allots 9% of the TBSA to the head and neck and to each upper extremity, 18% each to the anterior and posterior portions of the trunk, 18% to each lower extremity, and 1% to the perineum and genitalia. The area of a patient's palm represents approximately 1% of the TBSA and can be helpful in calculating scattered areas of involvement. In estimating the extent of burn injury, the extent of involvement of each anatomic area (e.g., an arm or leg) must be calculated separately and the total derived from the simple addition of the burned anatomic sites. The primary difference between the TBSA of the adult and infant reflects the size of the infant's head (18%), which is proportionally larger than that of the adult (Figure 60-5B), and the lower extremities (14%), which are proportionately smaller than those of the adult.

When possible, an attempt should be made to subdivide the TBSA further into partial-thickness and full-thickness percentages to facilitate categorization and subsequent management of patients. The depth of burn injury can be evaluated by numerous techniques, including burn wound biopsy, vital dyes, ultrasound studies, fluorescein fluorometry, thermography, light reflectance, magnetic resonance imaging, and laser Doppler flowmetry. Most of these techniques are not used in standard practice, but laser Doppler and light reflectance show promise of measuring depth of burn injury.

Categorization of Patients

The severity of a burn injury depends on the (1) extent, depth, and location of the burn injury; (2) age of the patient; (3) etiologic agents involved; (4) presence of inhalation injury; and (5) coexisting injuries or preexisting illnesses. The American Burn Association has used these parameters to establish guidelines for the classification of burn severity.[15] This classification creates three categories of burn injury (major, moderate, and minor) and defines the optimal setting for the management of each.

Major burn injury includes (1) partial-thickness burns involving more than 25% of TBSA in adults or 20% of TBSA in children younger than 10 and adults older than 50; (2) full-thickness burns involving more than 10% of TBSA; (3) burns involving the face, eyes, ears, hands, feet, or perineum that may result in functional or cosmetic impairment; (4) burns caused by caustic chemical agents; (5) high-voltage electrical injury; (6) burns complicated by inhalation injury or major trauma; and (7) burns sustained by high-risk patients (e.g., those with underlying debilitating diseases). These injuries are best managed in a specialized burn center staffed by a team of professionals with expertise in the care of burn patients, including both acute care and rehabilitation.

Moderate burn injury includes (1) partial-thickness burns of 15% to 25% of TBSA in adults or 10% to 20% of TBSA in children and older adults and (2) full-thickness burns involving 2% to 10% of TBSA that do not present a serious threat of functional or cosmetic impairment of the eyes, ears, face, hands, feet, or perineum. The moderate category *excludes* high-voltage electrical injury, all burns complicated by inhalation injury or other trauma, and burns sustained by high-risk patients. Patients with moderate burn injuries should be hospitalized for their initial care but not necessarily at a burn center.

Minor burn injury includes (1) partial-thickness burns involving less than 15% of TBSA in adults or 10% of TBSA in children and older adults and (2) full-thickness burns involving less than 2% of TBSA that do not present a serious threat of functional or cosmetic risk to eyes, ears, face, hands, feet, or perineum. These burns can usually be managed safely in the outpatient setting.

MANAGEMENT

Optimal management of burn victims is provided by an echelon system of burn care that is developed on a regional basis. Organization of burn care should begin at the site of injury and continue through prehospital care and transportation to the closest burn center, or to the closest emergency department with advanced life support capability, followed by transfer to a burn center when appropriate.

Prehospital Care

Fires usually emit smoke, which victims may inhale, especially in closed spaces. Smoke inhalation can cause both pulmonary parenchymal damage and CO and other toxic poisoning, which may have life-threatening consequences. The prehospital care provider should look for signs of inhalation injury (e.g., dyspnea, burns of mouth and nose, singed nasal hairs, sooty sputum, brassy cough). If one or more of these signs are present, humidified oxygen should be administered with a nonrebreathing reservoir mask at a rate of 10 to 12 L/min. The patient who has airway involvement should be intubated early in the course because edema can develop and make intubation increasingly difficult.

Treatment of burn shock in the prehospital setting should consist of elevating the patient's legs 12 inches off the ground and administering humidified oxygen. If rescue personnel have advanced life support capability and transport time is expected to be prolonged, these treatments are complemented by intravenous (IV) fluid administration. Fluid resuscitation need not be initiated if transportation to a hospital can be accomplished in less than 30 minutes. When the transport time is longer than 30 minutes, the indications for fluid resuscitation are thermal injuries involving greater than 20% of TBSA or evidence of burn shock. Fluid resuscitation is not recommended for children at the scene of the accident because of the difficulties encountered in cannulating small veins. When fluid resuscitation is indicated in an adult, lactated Ringer's (LR) solution or normal saline (NS) without glucose should be administered through a large-bore percutaneous catheter, preferably inserted through unburned skin. The arm is the preferred site for cannulation. The IV flow rates should be determined by the patient's clinical status.

When ventilatory and circulatory competence is restored, a secondary survey should be performed. All burned clothing and skin should be washed with cool water. The burn wound should be immersed in cold water (1° C to 5° C) for approximately 30 minutes if transport cannot be undertaken immediately. This cooling must be initiated as soon as possible because cooling has no therapeutic benefit if delayed more than 30 minutes after burn injury. Local cooling of less than 9% of TBSA can be continued longer than this 30-minute interval to relieve pain; however, the prolonged cooling of a larger percentage of TBSA can cause severe hypothermia, which may result in cardiac arrest. Ice should not be applied directly to the burn wound because it may result in increased tissue injury through frostbite.

The beneficial effects of immediate cold water treatment of burned skin appear to result from several factors. First, cold inhibits lactate production and acidosis, thereby promoting catecholamine function and cardiovascular homeostasis. Cold also inhibits burn wound histamine release, which in turn blocks local and remote histamine-mediated increases in vascular permeability. This minimizes edema formation and intravascular volume losses.[16] Finally, cold suppresses the production of thromboxane, which has been implicated as the mediator of vascular occlusion and progressive dermal ischemia after burn injury.[17]

Burn victims often complain of feeling chilled as a result of the loss of water and heat through the burned skin. Placing a clean sheet under the patient first, then covering the patient with another clean sheet followed by clean blankets, can minimize heat loss. The inside of the transport vehicle should be heated enough to make the patient comfortable. If a vehicle with advanced life support capability can transport the burn patient to a specialized burn treatment facility within 30 minutes, the patient should be transferred directly to this facility, bypassing other hospitals. If the transport time to the specialized burn treatment facility is longer than 30 minutes, the patient should be transported to the nearest emergency department with advanced life support capability.

Emergency Department Treatment

When the patient arrives in the emergency department, the emergency department personnel perform a rapid initial assessment of respiratory and cardiovascular status, establish the extent of burn injury, and determine the need for special procedures. Emergency department treatment focuses on airway and respiratory care and fluid resuscitation.

Airway and Respiratory Care

The natural history of upper airway burn injury is the development of edema that narrows the airway 12 to 24 hours after injury. The tongue and oral mucosa become edematous much more quickly, within minutes to hours. Consequently, intubation rather than observation is recommended in patients with signs of upper airway injury, such as stridor, inspiratory grunting, wheezing, or tachypnea.

Fiberoptic bronchoscopy is a simple, safe, and accurate method of diagnosing acute inhalation injury.[18] It reveals the anatomic level and severity of large airway injury; identification of supraglottic and infraglottic involvement is helpful in predicting pulmonary complications. Fiberoptic bronchoscopy can also aid in intubating patients with inhalation injury.[19] Because fiberoptic bronchoscopy has been associated with the development of severe hypoxemia, especially in elderly burn patients, supplementary oxygen should be administered through the bronchoscope.[20]

When the airway is secured and the patient is oxygenated, further treatment includes maintenance of pulmonary toilet, relief of mechanical restriction of chest wall motion, and prevention of respiratory failure. When collagen is burned, it loses its elasticity, its fibers are shortened, and it becomes rigid. This can occur very quickly with fourth-degree and severe third-degree burns. When combined with accumulation of burn edema in interstitial spaces, this may result in respiratory insufficiency or ischemia of an extremity. The compressive effect of a full-thickness burn of the neck may contribute to airway compromise. Without tracheostomy, the tight neck eschar accentuates pharyngeal edema and draws the neck into flexion, compressing the pharyngeal airway. A vertical incision through the eschar extending from the sternal notch to the chin helps maintain a patent airway. If the respiratory insufficiency is caused by a constricting eschar of the anterior thorax that limits respiratory excursion, escharotomy is imperative. Lateral incisions are made in the anterior axillary lines that extend 2 cm below the clavicle to the 9th or 10th rib. The top and bottom of the incisions are then joined so that a square across the anterior chest is formed.

If respiratory failure ensues, mechanical ventilation is necessary. Airway resistance is often increased after inhalation injury by edema, debris within the airway, or bronchospasm. The goal of mechanical ventilation should be to accept a slightly acidic environment (pH > 7.32) to minimize the mean airway pressure required for ventilation. To keep airway pressures to a minimum, ventilator settings may need to be adjusted to slightly higher respiratory rates (16 to 20 breaths/min) and smaller tidal volumes (7 to 8 mL/kg).

Experimental evidence from baboons with moderate smoke inhalation has demonstrated that the barotrauma index (rate times pressure product) is significantly increased during regular ventilation compared with high-frequency flow interruption ventilation.[21] Histologic damage of pulmonary parenchyma is also greater in the group treated with conventional ventilation. The usefulness of high-frequency flow interruption ventilation appears to be due to its ability to recruit damaged, collapsed alveoli and keep them open in expiratory ventilation. Maintaining alveolar recruitment at low mean alveolar pressures helps minimize barotrauma and allows improved distribution of ventilation. Two retrospective studies demonstrated a decreased incidence of pneumonia and mortality in patients with inhalation injury when high-frequency percussive ventilation was used compared with conventional "volume-limited" ventilation.[22,23] The oscillating ventilator, which superimposes high-frequency ventilation into conventional tidal volume breaths, may be an even better method of ventilation after smoke injury. This method reduces barotrauma and aids in the removal of airway casts by causing vibratory air movements. Airway casts and plug formation can be decreased by nebulized heparin treatment (5000 units in 10 mL of NS every 4 hours), which inhibits fibrin clot formation in the airway.

CO is present in smoke, and its affinity for hemoglobin is 280 times that of oxygen. A CO level is obtained for all patients with suspected inhalation injury. Patients should receive 100% oxygen until their carboxyhemoglobin (COHb) level is less than 10% because the elimination half-life of COHb depends on oxygen tension. In room air, the half-life of CO-bound hemoglobin is 4 hours. Under 100% oxygen, the half-life of CO-bound hemoglobin decreases to 45 minutes. Administration of 100% oxygen increases the gradient for oxygen binding to hemoglobin, and unbound CO is exhaled through the lungs.

Patients who have elevated COHb levels associated with a pH of less than 7.4 should be treated with hyperbaric oxygenation. Because serum COHb levels do not reflect tissue levels, clinical symptoms should be evaluated when considering hyperbaric oxygen therapy. These include a history of unconsciousness, the presence of neuropsychiatric abnormalities, and the presence of cardiac instability or cardiac ischemia.

Specific therapy for cyanide poisoning in patients with inhalation injury is another consideration. Cyanide causes tissue hypoxia by uncoupling oxidative phosphorylation by binding to mitochondrial cytochrome aa_3.[33] Empirical treatment for cyanide toxicity should be considered for patients with unexplained severe metabolic acidosis associated with elevated central venous oxygen content, normal arterial oxygen content, and a low COHb level.

Patients with moderate burns should have at least one large-bore IV line placed through unburned skin, and those with severe burns should have at least two lines initiated. When a burn patient requires considerable fluid resuscitation or has evidence of cardiopulmonary disease, a central venous line is indicated. Patients with massive burns or respiratory injury and elderly patients with severe burns or cardiac disease should be monitored with a Swan-Ganz catheter to avoid fluid overload or inadequate replacement of volume.

The microvascular injury caused by a burn produces increased vascular permeability with edema formation that results in ongoing plasma volume loss. Maximal edema formation occurs 8 to 12 hours after injury for small burns and 24 hours after injury for large burns. The purpose of fluid resuscitation is to restore effective plasma volume, avoid microvascular ischemia, and maintain vital organ function. The amount of fluid required varies with the patient's age, body weight, and extent of TBSA burned. Careful mapping of the burned areas over the entire body, including the back, should be performed to estimate the fluid requirements during the first 48 hours after injury. Typically, burns greater than 20% of TBSA require IV fluid resuscitation because the accompanying gastrointestinal ileus precludes sufficient oral intake.

Although different formulas for fluid resuscitation have been recommended, all regimens emphasize that adequate resuscitation is evidenced by a normal urine output (1 mL/kg/hr in children younger than 2 years, 0.5 mL/kg/hr in older children, and at least 30 to 40 mL/hr in adults), a normal sensorium, and stable vital signs. The *Parkland formula* for fluid resuscitation of burn patients is used as follows: LR solution (4 mL/kg/% TBSA burned) is administered intravenously in the first 24 hours, with one half given in the first 8 hours and the other half over the next 16 hours. The percent TBSA used for the formula includes only second- and third-degree burn injuries. The fluid loss must be calculated from the time of injury, and fluid replacement must take into account the fluid administered by prehospital personnel. To avoid overhydration, patients with inhalation injuries should be resuscitated with substantially less than formula predictions, with acceptance of a urinary output in the range of 0.3 to 0.5 mL/kg/hr.

After a burn injury, there are significant losses of intravascular protein through endothelial leaks in the burned vessels. When endothelial integrity is restored 24 hours after the injury, some clinicians favor the administration of 5% albumin at 0.5 mL/kg/% TBSA to maintain dynamic forces between the extracellular spaces and the intravascular system. In addition, a low-dose dopamine infusion (3 to 5 μg/kg/min) is beneficial in restoring renal and splanchnic blood flow in patients with major burn injury.

Resuscitation with hypertonic saline solutions reduces the required fluid volume.[24] The volume of fluid administered using hypertonic fluid solutions is notably less, yet fluid requirements and percent weight gain have not decreased with hypertonic saline compared with Ringer's solution. The anticipated benefits of fewer escharotomies and limited ileus have not been uniformly encountered. On the contrary, hypertonic saline resuscitation has been associated with an increased occurrence of acute tubular necrosis and hyperchloremic metabolic acidosis, which can exacerbate the metabolic acidosis of hypovolemic shock. Therefore, hypertonic saline is not currently recommended for resuscitation of burn patients.[25-30]

When the patient's survival is extremely unlikely after burn injury, the clinician must be encouraged not to begin fluid resuscitation. Elderly patients with large burns (>80% of TBSA) do not survive. This decision must be made after thoughtful communication with family members. When resuscitation is not undertaken, patients should be made pain free, kept warm, and allowed to remain in a room with family members.

Pediatric Considerations

Most of the burn care in children is similar to that in adults, yet some relevant physiologic differences need to be considered in the care of burned children. The Parkland formula is effective in estimating fluid loss in adults, yet it underestimates the evaporative fluid loss and maintenance needs in children. Compared with adults, children have a larger TBSA relative to weight than adults and generally have somewhat greater fluid needs during resuscitation. The *Galveston formula* for fluid resuscitation in children should be used as follows: 5% dextrose in LR (5000 mL/m² of TBSA burned plus 2000 mL/m²) is administered IV in the first 24 hours. One half is given in the first 8 hours, and the other half is given over the next 16 hours. Dextrose should be added to the resuscitation fluid in children

to prevent hypoglycemia because children have smaller glycogen stores than adults.

In infants younger than 6 months, temperature is regulated by *nonshivering thermogenesis*, a metabolic process by which stores of brown fat are catabolized under the influence of norepinephrine, which requires large amounts of oxygen. Consequently, prolonged hypothermia in burned infants may result in excessive lactate production and acidosis. After 6 months, infants and children are able to shiver. Because they have greater evaporative water loss relative to weight than adults, infants and children are especially susceptible to hypothermia; therefore, the ambient temperature should be kept high to decrease radiant and evaporative heat loss from burned infants and children to the environment.

Renal Function Differences

Differences in renal function between infants and adults may have important therapeutic implications in treating burned children. The glomerular filtration rate in infants does not reach adult levels until 9 to 12 months because of an imbalance in maturation of tubular and glomerular functions. During this interval, infants have approximately half the osmolar concentrating capacity of adults, and a water load is handled inefficiently. The rate of water excretion is time dependent and decreases as water loading continues. During the first several weeks of life, infants are likely to retain a larger portion of a water load administered as part of burn resuscitation. The hyposmolarity of LR solution, when used in accordance with the Parkland formula, already accounts for the free water needs of infants during the first 24 hours after the burn injury. Additional water often results in fluid overloading.

Catheterization of the Patient

A Foley catheter is placed into the bladder to monitor the effectiveness of IV fluid replacement. Burns of the perineum are also best cared for with an indwelling Foley catheter to decrease urinary soilage of the wound. In patients with major burn injuries who require IV fluid resuscitation, a nasogastric (NG) tube is passed for initial evacuation of fluid and air from the stomach and feeding access. Removal of the gastric contents prevents vomiting and aspiration, sequelae of the ileus that commonly occur soon after burn injuries involving more than 20% of TBSA. Early feeding through the NG tube within 6 to 8 hours of the burn injury diminishes the hypermetabolic response and maintains intestinal integrity.

Transportation of Patients

After stabilization of the burned patient in the emergency department, patients with severe burn injury should be transferred to burn centers. The American Burn Association has established criteria for optimal treatment of burn patients, including both indications for admission to a hospital and criteria for transfer to a burn center.

Ground, helicopter, or fixed-wing aircraft may transport burn patients. In addition to the condition of the patient, the mode of transportation (ambulance versus helicopter) depends on such factors as distance, terrain, and prevailing weather. The safety and costs of using helicopters in the transport of burn patients have been questioned. Helicopters transport patients more rapidly than ambulances and, because a nurse or physician usually staffs them, provide a higher level of medical expertise during transport. For burn patients, a helicopter offers little advantage over a ground ambulance if the distance is less than 30 miles. Helicopter transfers may be efficacious if the distance is 30 to 150 miles or if the transfer time is greater than 30 minutes. Over 150 miles, fixed-winged aircraft are best to transport patients.

When a burn patient is being transferred from an emergency department to a burn center, early physician-to-physician contact with the burn center is essential. A standard check sheet facilitates assessment of the patient's physiologic status by both the referring and receiving physician. Airway patency, IV access, and other injuries are evaluated prior to transfer. Burn wounds should be covered with dry dressings but use of antimicrobial creams should be postponed until admission to the burn center. The burn wound is considered a dirty wound and tetanus prophylaxis instituted accordingly. Prophylactic antibiotics are not indicated.

Burn Center Treatment

Treatment of the patient in the burn center involves three important considerations: supportive care, burn wound management, and nutritional support.

Specific Management

Pain

The requirement for pain medication is inversely proportional to the depth of burn injury. Full-thickness burns, which appear white, brown, or leathery with clotted vessels, are painless because their intrinsic sensory nerves are damaged. In contrast, partial-thickness burns, in which the skin is red with blisters, have intact nerves and are extremely painful. For more than 160 years, morphine has been advocated for the management of pain in burn patients. Its analgesic effect can be easily titrated with incremental IV doses. Morphine has two pharmacologic advantages for use in burn patients: a low amount of protein binding (30%) and a major active metabolite that is conjugated in the liver and removed by glomerular filtration. This rapid elimination may require that doses as high as 50 mg/hr be used in severely burned adults. Any respiratory depression caused by morphine can be rapidly reversed by small doses of naloxone.

Gastrointestinal Issues

A Foley catheter and nasogastric tube should be placed.

Acute upper gastrointestinal erosions and ulcers may occur in patients with severe burn injuries. These lesions are often called stress ulcers or erosions (Curling's ulcer). The most common clinical finding in such patients is painless gastrointestinal hemorrhage. In high-risk patients the occurrence of stress ulcerations can be reduced by the use of antacids to neutralize gastric contents, supplemented by H_2 receptor antagonists to inhibit gastric acid secretion. This prophylaxis is best initiated immediately after admission to the burn center.

Carboxyhemoglobin and Cyanide

A CO level should be obtained in all patients with a suspected inhalation injury. Such patients should receive 100% oxygen until their COHb level is shown to be less than 10% because the elimination half-life for COHb depends on oxygen tension. Patients who have elevated COHb levels associated with a pH of less than 7.4 should be treated with hyperbaric oxygenation.[31] Because serum COHb levels do not reflect tissue levels, clinical symptoms should be evaluated when considering hyperbaric oxygen therapy. These include a history of unconsciousness, the presence of neuropsychiatric abnormalities, and cardiac instability or cardiac ischemia.[32]

Empirical therapy for possible cyanide poisoning may be necessary.

Burn Wound Care

All wound management is undertaken using powder-free gloves because of the demonstrated toxicity of glove powders to tissue.

Major Burns

Escharotomy

A full-thickness circumferential burn of an extremity can result in vascular compromise. Loss of Doppler ultrasound signals in the radial and ulnar arteries and digital vessels is an indication for escharotomies of the upper extremity.[34] Loss of signal in the dorsalis pedis or posterior tibialis artery indicates the need for escharotomy of the lower extremity. Interstitial tissue pressure is usually slightly negative, and the normal arterial capillary perfusion pressure is approximately 5 to 7 mm Hg. After burn injury, rises in interstitial tissue pressure occlude arterial capillary inflow and venous outflow; escharotomies of the full-thickness burn prevent this ischemic injury. A period of 3 to 8 hours is required for edema to develop sufficiently to increase tissue pressure. When tissue compartment pressures are greater than 40 mm Hg, escharotomies of the full-thickness burn prevent ischemic injury. It is important to note that the most common cause of absent pulses in an extremity is hypovolemia with peripheral vasoconstriction, not increased interstitial pressure.

Escharotomies are performed on the medial and lateral aspects of the extremity and extend the length of the constricting eschar. Incisions are made using either a scalpel or a high-frequency electrical current, with release of the edematous tissues ensuring ade-

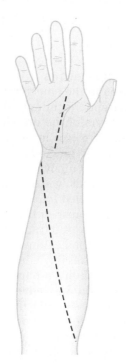

Figure 60-6. Skin incisions for digital escharotomy and palm decompression.

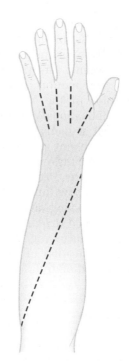

Figure 60-7. Decompression of interossei muscles by skin incisions.

quate depth. After prolonged vascular compromise, escharotomy may cause reperfusion injury to the extremity, with reactive hyperemia and edema of the compartment muscles. In this case, a fasciotomy is required to restore perfusion to the extremity.

For full-thickness circumferential burns of the upper extremity, the fingers are first decompressed by a digital escharotomy along each side of the burned finger, cutting down to fat. The palm is decompressed by an incision along the palmar crease (Figure 60-6). At the wrist, the incision continues ulnarward to avoid injury to the palmar cutaneous branch of the median nerve.

When intrinsic muscle involvement is suspected, decompression of the interossei muscles is accomplished through short longitudinal skin incisions made in the intermetacarpal spaces and carried down to the dorsal interossei muscles (Figure 60-7). Decompression of the leg is accomplished by midmedial and midlateral incisions. Each toe is decompressed in a manner similar to that used for the fingers.

Dressings

If transfer to a burn center is imminent, wound care should consist of simply wrapping the patient in a clean dry sheet. If disposition is delayed, however, treatment is begun by (1) gentle cleansing with either sterile saline or commercial products containing poloxamer 188 (e.g., Shur-Clens); (2) debridement of blisters, except those on the palms and soles; and (3) application of a topical antibacterial agent, according to the burn center's preference.[35] Topical antimicrobial agents are used to limit bacterial and fungal colonization of burn wounds until complete reepithelialization occurs. Silver sulfadiazine (Silvadene), mafenide acetate (Sul-

famylon), and 0.5% silver nitrate solution are the most frequently used topical antibacterial agents. Agents such as bacitracin and polymyxin B are less bactericidal but also less toxic to reepithelialization of the burn wound. Topical nystatin can be added to the antibacterial agents to prevent fungal growth. The water-soluble carrier poloxamer 188 can be used with these antimicrobial agents.[36] This gel can be easily washed from the wound surface after dressing changes. Sterile gauze followed by sterile sheets can then be used to cover the wounds and body.

Minor Burn Treatment in the Emergency Department

Blisters and Tetanus

All minor burns should first be cleansed with sterile saline or poloxamer 188. Treatment of burn blisters remains controversial. Exposing an unbroken blister can lead to local wound infection, but studies have demonstrated that burn blister fluid confined by necrotic skin can result in closed-space infection.[37,38] Most authors recommend that blisters on the palms or soles be left intact. Other blisters, particularly when large enough to preclude the application of an adequate dressing, should either be aspirated sterilely or be opened with a No. 15 knife blade and the surface of the blister removed.

Tetanus prophylaxis should be provided if indicated. As required under the National Childhood Injury Act, all health care providers in the United States who administer any vaccine shall, prior to administration of the vaccine, provide a copy of the Vaccine Information Statement (VIS) produced by the Centers for Disease

Control to the parent or legal representative of any child to whom the provider intends to administer such vaccine or to any adult to whom the provider intends to administer such vaccine. The VIS must be supplemented with visual presentation or oral explanations, as appropriate. Copies of the VIS are available at http://cdc.gov/nip/publications/VIS. Copies are available in English as well as many other languages. Prophylactic antibiotics are not recommended. Topical antimicrobial agents have little value in the outpatient management of minor burns. Because these agents lose their antibacterial activity within 6 to 24 hours after application, frequent dressing changes are necessary. Unfortunately, removal and reapplication of the cream are painful and time consuming. As a result, many patients resort to reapplication of the cream without initial removal, an invitation to infection.

Ointment and Dressings

Burn wounds can be treated by either open or closed technique. Open therapy of minor burn injuries is usually reserved for burns of the face. These burns are covered by bacitracin ointment, which is reapplied every 6 hours after gently washing the skin.

An enormous variety of synthetic dressings have been developed. First-generation film dressings (e.g., thin films, hydrocolloidal hydrogel foams, alginate) are based on the concept that epidermal regeneration occurs best in a moist environment.[39] Second-generation microenvironmental wound dressings combine the fluid-retaining properties of the film dressings with the absorptive properties of the hydrocolloid. In theory, wound fluid is absorbed by the central membrane through the porous inner layer. The external layer allows moisture vapor to escape but is impermeable to exterior fluids and bacteria. Although second-generation dressings have many desirable features, they are relatively expensive.

A simple, less costly alternative to these synthetic dressings can be reliably used in minor burns.[40] After cleansing and debridement, strips of sterile fine-mesh gauze (type 1) soaked in 0.9% sodium chloride are placed over the entire wound. This layer of gauze is then covered by multiple layers of fluffed 4 × 4-inch coarse-mesh gauze (type 6), which are secured by an inelastic roller-gauze dressing. The gauze dressing is attached to unburned skin using a microporous tape.

When possible, the site of injury should be elevated above the patient's heart. Elevation of the injured site limits accumulation of fluid in the interstitial spaces of the wound. The healing burn extremity with little edema resumes normal function more rapidly than the extremely edematous extremity. Early mobilization of the injured area within 24 hours after injury limits the development of joint stiffness, a particularly challenging problem in both elderly persons and workers who do heavy labor.

Oral analgesics should be routinely prescribed for patients with painful burns, and wound care instructions should be given to the patient before departure.

A follow-up appointment should be scheduled in 2 to 3 days.

Follow-up and Complications

If the patient returns to the emergency department for a follow-up visit, aseptic technique should be used to remove the outer layers of the dressing gently so that the bottom, fine-mesh gauze layer can be visualized. If the gauze is adherent to a relatively dry and pink burn wound, it should be covered again by layers of 4 × 4-inch coarse-mesh gauze and secured. The patient should be instructed to return in 5 to 7 days for reevaluation. Because most superficial partial-thickness burns heal in 10 to 14 days, spontaneous separation of the gauze from the healing burn wound should be evident at the next dressing change.

If the burn wound exhibits a purulent discharge, the fine-mesh gauze should be removed and the burn wound cleansed. Silver sulfadiazine cream should be applied twice daily to the burn wound and the area dressed with a sterile roller-gauze dressing. The patient should be instructed to wash the burn wound gently in clean water to remove this cream before applying additional cream.

The potential complications of minor burn injury should be reviewed with each patient. The patient must be aware that burn wound infection is a continual threat that can convert a partial-thickness burn to a full-thickness burn. The risk of hypertrophic scar formation, as well as pigmentary skin changes, should also be discussed. The patient should be reminded to use a sun-blocking agent over the healed wounds for at least 6 months after injury to prevent the development of permanent pigmentary changes caused by sun exposure.

Hot Tar Burns

Burns from hot tar present a challenging clinical problem. When tar that is heated to a liquid form inadvertently comes into contact with a worker's skin, it transfers sufficient heat to cause a burn injury. As it cools on the skin surface, the tar solidifies, making removal difficult.

The term *hot tar* refers to two distinct groups of materials: coal tar pitches and petroleum-derived asphalts. These two groups are often mistakenly considered synonymous because of similar industrial applications. They are both used for paving and roofing purposes and are used directly in the construction of roofing membranes. However, coal tar and petroleum asphalts are dissimilar in origin and chemical composition. Asphalt cements and roofing asphalts are high-molecular-weight naphthenic and paraffinic hydrocarbons that are produced from crude petroleum by a process that does not involve thermal conversion or cracking. In contrast, coal-derived tars are composed primarily of highly condensed-ring aromatic and heterocyclic hydrocarbons that are obtained by the high-temperature carbonization of bituminous coal.

Both products are heated to maintain a liquid form. Substantially lower temperatures (275° F to 300° F) are

BOX 60-1. Admission Guidelines for Patients with Moderate Burns

Any partial-thickness* burn injury involving 10%-20% of BSA in adults (>10 or <50 years of age)

Any partial-thickness* burn involving 5%-10% of BSA in patients less than 10 years of age

---

*These partial-thickness burns must not involve the eyes, ears, face, hands, feet, or perineum.

BSA, body surface area.

BOX 60-2. Transfer Guidelines for Patients with Severe Burns

Any burn >10% of total BSA in patients <10 and >50 years old

Burns involving >20% of total BSA in any patient

Full-thickness burns involving >5% of total BSA

Significant burns of hands, face, feet, genitalia, perineum, or major joints

Significant electrical injury

Significant chemical injury

Significant inhalation injury, concomitant mechanical trauma, preexisting medical disorders

Patients with special psychosocial or rehabilitative care needs

---

BSA, body surface area.

needed to achieve desirable application viscosities for paving roads than are necessary for roofing purposes (450° F to 500° F). The higher temperatures account for the deeper burn injuries associated with burns from roofing asphalt or pitch.

After coming in contact with the skin, the tar rapidly cools, solidifies, and becomes enmeshed in the hair. This cooling process should be expedited by the addition of cold water to the tar at the scene of the accident. Cooling the tar with cold water limits tissue damage and prevents further spread of the tar. Washing the tar with water should be continued until the tar has hardened and is cool. After the tar is cooled, the wet skin should be dried with towels to prevent the development of systemic hypothermia. Adherent tar should not be removed at the scene of the accident.

Definitive care of the tar burn injury in the emergency department includes early removal of the tar because it may serve as an occlusive barrier over the injured skin that encourages bacterial growth, with subsequent conversion of a partial-thickness burn to a full-thickness injury. The adherence of tar to skin is not a direct bond between the epidermis and the tar but rather a consequence of the tar becoming enmeshed in the hair.

Numerous organic solvents have been proposed to remove tar. Aromatic (naphthalene) and aliphatic (hexane) hydrocarbon solvents are useful for asphalts, whereas coal tars are susceptible only to aromatic hydrocarbons. Unfortunately, many of these aromatic and short-chain hydrocarbons are systemically absorbed and have potential side effects. Long-chain aliphatic hydrocarbons and waxes have been used for tar removal without evidence of local or systemic toxicity. These substances are oleaginous colloidal suspensions of solid microcrystalline waxes in petroleum oil (e.g., polymyxin-neomycin-bacitracin [Neosporin] ointment). Antibiotic ointments with a broad spectrum of activity, including bacitracin (400 units/g), polymyxin B (5000 units/g), and neomycin (5 mg/g), complement the action of the solvent by lowering the incidence of infection. These agents need to be removed and reapplied hourly until all the tar is removed. This approach has been used successfully to remove even tar layered over conjunctiva.

Unfortunately, the cost of using antibiotic ointments to treat tar burns covering a large percentage of TBSA can be substantial. Besides the cost of the antibiotic

preparations, multiple applications are necessary to remove the tar. The use of readily available topical agents may offer a rapid, cost-effective means of tar removal. Sunflower oil has been shown to remove both asphalt and coal-based tar. This inexpensive, nonirritating agent removes adherent tar in 30 minutes.[41] Likewise, butter can emulsify tar in 20 to 30 minutes.[42] Reapplication may be required when large areas are involved, but butter provides another nontoxic alternative for tar removal. Baby oil has been shown to provide similar results in 1 to 1½ hours.[43] Commercial surface-active agents such as polyoxyethylene sorbitan (Tween 80) and polysorbate (De-Solv-It), alone or in combination with a petrolatum ointment, are relatively inexpensive, safe, and effective means of tar removal. Their water solubility is believed to be an additional advantage over petrolatum ointment, which is not as easily removed from skin with water as are these surface-active agents.

DISPOSITION

As mentioned, the American Burn Association has established criteria for optimal treatment of burn patients, including the indications for admission to a hospital (Box 60-1) and the criteria for transfer to a burn center (Box 60-2).[44] The safety and costs of using helicopters in the transport of burn patients have been questioned.[6,45,46]

When a burn patient is being transferred from an emergency department to a burn center, early physician-to-physician contact with the burn center is essential. The use of a standard check sheet facilitates assessment of the patient's physiologic status by both the referring physician and the receiving physician. Prophylactic antibiotics are not indicated. The use of antimicrobial creams on the burn wound should be postponed until admission to the burn center. The burn wound should be considered a dirty wound, and tetanus prophylaxis should be instituted accordingly.

KEY CONCEPTS

- *Thermal burns:* Compared with other natural disasters, burns exert a catastrophic influence on people in terms of human life, suffering, disability, and financial loss. More than an estimated 2 million people in the United States suffer burn injuries, most of which are minor and cared for primarily in the emergency department.

- Thermal burns are commonly classified as scald burns, contact burns, and fire burns.

- The severity of burn injury is related to the rate at which heat is transferred from the heating agent to the skin. The rate of heat transfer depends on the (1) heat capacity of the agent, (2) temperature of the agent, (3) duration of contact with the agent, (4) transfer coefficient, and (5) specific heat and conductivity of the local tissues.

- The depth of burn injury is often classified according to degrees: first-degree burns, second-degree burns (superficial partial-thickness and deep partial-thickness), third-degree burns, and fourth-degree burns.

- The first day after burn injury, three concentric zones of tissue injury characterize a full-thickness burn: the zones of coagulation, stasis, and hyperemia.

- The *rule of nines* is a practical technique for estimating the extent of total body surface area involved in a burn injury.

- The severity of a burn injury depends on the (1) extent, depth, and location of the burn injury; (2) age of the patient; (3) etiologic agents involved; (4) presence of inhalation injury; and (5) coexisting injuries or preexisting illnesses.

- Optimal management of burn victims is provided by an echelon system of burn care that is developed on a regional basis. Organization of burn care should begin at the site of injury and continue through prehospital care and transportation to the closest burn center, or to the closest emergency department with advanced life support capability, followed by transfer to a burn center when appropriate.

- When the patient arrives in the emergency department, the department staff perform a rapid initial assessment of respiratory and cardiovascular status, establish the extent of burn injury, and determine the need for special procedures. Emergency department treatment focuses on airway and respiratory care and fluid resuscitation, along with determination of the need to transfer to a burn center.

- After stabilization of the burned patient in the emergency department, patients with severe burn injury are transferred to burn centers. The American Burn Association has established criteria for optimal treatment of burn patients, including both indications for admission to a hospital and criteria for transfer to a burn center.

- Treatment of the patient in the burn center involves three important considerations: supportive care, burn wound management, and nutritional support.

- Definitive care of the tar burn injury in the emergency department includes early removal of the tar because it may serve as an occlusive barrier over the injured skin that encourages bacterial growth, with subsequent conversion of a partial-thickness burn to a full-thickness injury. The adherence of tar to skin is not a direct bond between the epidermis and the tar but rather a consequence of the tar becoming enmeshed in the hair.

- Intubation rather than observation is recommended in burn patients with signs of upper airway injury.

- Aggressive fluid resuscitation is required for patients with burns over 20% of TBSA in order to restore effective plasma volume, avoid microvascular ischemia, and maintain vital organ function.

- The most common error is overhydration. Adequate resuscitation is evidenced by a normal urine output, normal sensorium, and stable vital signs.

- Dextrose is added to the resuscitation fluid in children to prevent hypoglycemia because children have smaller glycogen stores than adults.

- Because morphine is rapidly eliminated, doses as high as 50 mg/hr may be required for analgesia in severely burned adult patients.

REFERENCES

1. Centers for Disease Control/National Highway Traffic Safety Administration: Position papers from the Third National Injury control conference: Setting the national agenda for injury control in the 1990s. Atlanta, U.S. Department of Health and Human Services, Public Health Service, CDC, 1992, p 285.

2. Inansci WI, Guidotti TL: Occupation related burns: 5-year experience of an urban burn center. *J Occup Med* 29:730, 1987.

3. Williams JB, Ahrenholtz DH, Solem LD, Warren W: Gasoline burns: The preventable cause of thermal injury. *J Burn Care Rehabil* 11:446, 1990.

4. Moritz AR, Henrique FC Jr: Studies of thermal injury: The relative importance of time and surface temperature in the causation of cutaneous burns. *Am J Pathol* 23:695, 1947.

5. Weaver AM, Himel HN, Edlich RF: Immersion scald burns: Strategies for prevention. *J Emerg Med* 11:397, 1993.

6. Walker AR: Fatal tap water scald burns in the USA. *Burns* 16:49, 1990.

7. Feldman KW, Schaller RT, Feldman JA, McMillon M: Tap water burns in handicapped children. *Pediatrics* 62:1, 1978.

8. Jackson DM: The diagnosis of the depth of burning. *Br J Surg* 40:588, 1953.

9. Robson MC, Del Beccaro EJ, Heggers JP: The effect of prostaglandins in the dermal microcirculation after burning and the inhibition of the effect by specific pharmacological agents. *Plast Reconstr Surg* 63:781, 1979.

10. Friedel HP, Till GO, Trentz O: Roles of histamine, complement and xanthine oxidase in thermal injury of skin. *Am J Pathol* 135:203, 1989.

11. Deitch EA, Rutan R, Waymack JP: Trauma, shock, and gut translocation. *New Horiz* 4:289, 1996.

12. Aulick LH, Wilmore DW, Mason AD Jr, Pruitt BA Jr: Influence of the burn wound on peripheral circulation in thermally injured patients. *Am J Physiol* 223:520, 1977.

13. Demling RH, et al: Early lung dysfunction after major burns: Role of edema and vasoactive mediators. *J Trauma* 26:959, 1985.

14. Harms BA, Bodai BI, Kramer GC, Demling RH: Microvascular fluid and protein flux in pulmonary and systemic circulations after thermal injury. *Microvasc Res* 23:77, 1982.

15. American Burn Association: Guidelines for service standards and severity classifications in the treatment of burn injury. *Am Coll Surg Bull* 69:24, 1984.

16. Boykin JV Jr, Eriksson E, Sholley MM, Pittman RN: Histamine-mediated delayed permeability response after scald burn inhibited by cimetidine or cold-water treatment. *Science* 209:815, 1980.

17. Heggers JP, Loy GL, Robson MC, Del Beccaro EJ: Cooling and the prostaglandin effect in the thermal injury. *J Burn Care Rehabil* 3:350, 1980.
18. Becker DG, Himel HN, Nicholson WD, Edlich RF: Salvage of a patient with burn inhalation injury and pancreatitis. *Burns* 19:444, 1993.
19. Pruitt BA Jr, Goodwin CW: Burn injury. In Moore E (ed): *Early Care of the Injured Patient*, 4th ed. New York, Decker, 1990, pp 297-298.
20. Hunt JL, Agee RN, Pruitt BA Jr: Fiberoptic bronchoscopy in acute inhalation injury. *J Trauma* 15:641, 1975.
21. Cioffi WG, et al: Decreased pulmonary damage in primates with inhalation injury treated with high-frequency ventilation. *Am Surg* 218:328, 1993.
22. Rue LW 3rd, et al: Improved survival of burned patients with inhalation injury. *Arch Surg* 128:772, 1993.
23. Cioffi WG Jr, et al: Prophylactic use of high-frequency percussive ventilation in patients with inhalation injury. *Am Surg* 213:575, 1991.
24. Kien ND: Small-volume resuscitation using hypertonic saline improves organ perfusion in burned rats. *Anesth Analg* 83:782, 1996.
25. Tokyay R, et al: Effects of hypertonic saline dextran resuscitation on oxygen delivery, oxygen consumption, and lipid peroxidation after burn injury. *J Trauma* 32:704, 1992.
26. Horton JW, White J, Hunt JL: Delayed hypertonic saline dextran administration after burn injury. *J Trauma* 38:281, 1995.
27. Onarheim H, Missavage AE, Kramer GC, Gunther RA: Effectiveness of hypertonic saline-dextran 70 for initial fluid resuscitation of major burns. *J Trauma* 30:597, 1990.
28. Demling RH: Improved survival after massive burns. *J Trauma* 23:179, 1983.
29. Griswold JA, Anglin BL, Love RT Jr, Scott-Conner C: Hypertonic saline resuscitation: Efficacy in a community-based burn unit. *South Med J* 84:692, 1991.
30. Gunn ML, et al: Prospective, randomized trial of hypertonic sodium lactate versus lactated Ringer's solution for burn shock resuscitation. *J Trauma* 29:1261, 1989.
31. Strohl KP, Feldman NT, Saunders NA, O'Conner N: Carbon monoxide poisoning fire victims, a reappraisal of prognosis. *J Trauma* 20:78, 1980.
32. Grim PS, Gottlieb LJ, Boddie A, Batson E: Hyperbaric oxygen therapy. *JAMA* 263:2216, 1990.
33. Fitzpatrick JC, Cioffi WG: Inhalation injury. *Trauma Q* 11:114, 1994.
34. Edlich RF, et al: Technical considerations for fasciotomies in high voltage electrical injuries. *J Burn Care Rehabil* 1:22, 1980.
35. Bryant CA, et al: Search for a nontoxic scrub solution for periorbital lacerations. *Ann Emerg Med* 13:317, 1984.
36. Rockwell WB, Ehrlich HP: Should burn blister fluid be evacuated? *J Burn Care Rehabil* 11:93, 1990.
37. Garner WL, et al: The effects of burn blister fluid on keratinocyte replication and differentiation. *J Burn Care Rehabil* 14:127, 1993.
38. Gear AJ, et al: A new sliver sulfadiazine water soluble gel. *Burns* 23:387, 1997.
39. Nangia A, Hung CT: Preclinical evaluation of skin substitutes. *Burns* 16:358, 1990.
40. Haynes BW Jr: Outpatient burns. *Clin Plast Surg* 1:645, 1974.
41. Turegun M, Ozturk S, Selmanpakoglu N: Sunflower oil in the treatment of hot tar burns. *Burns* 23:442, 1997.
42. Tiernan E, Harris A: Butter in the initial treatment of hot tar burns. *Burns* 19:437, 1993.
43. Juma A: Bitumen burns and the use of baby oil. *Burns* 20:363, 1994.
44. American Burn Association: Hospital and prehospital resources for optimal care of patients with burn injury: Guidelines for development and operation of burn centers. *J Burn Care Rehabil* 11:97, 1990.
45. Dimick AR, Dietz PA: An unexpected burden: The safety of air ambulances [letter]. *JAMA* 259:3405, 1988.
46. Fromm RE Jr, Varon J: Air medical transport. *J Fam Pract* 36:313, 1993.

CHAPTER

61 Chemical Injuries

Richard F. Edlich, Marcus L. Martin, and William B. Long III

PERSPECTIVE

Chemical injuries are commonly encountered following exposure to acids, alkalis, and highly reactive substances. Injury to the skin, eyes, lung, and other organ systems can be disabling or life threatening. Injury can result from commonly used chemicals, including hydrofluoric acid, formic acid, hydrous ammonia, cement, and phenol. Other specific chemical agents that cause burns include white phosphorus, elemental metals, nitrates, hydrocarbons, and tar.

Since World War II, the number of chemicals that have been developed, produced, and used worldwide has increased dramatically. More than 65,000 chemicals are available on the market, and an estimated 60,000 new chemicals are produced each year. Unfortunately, the effects on human health of many of these chemicals are unknown.

Toxic chemical releases, whether from manufacturing plants, during transport, or while in use, are prevented through federal and state regulation along with sound industry practices. The federal Superfund Amendments and Reauthorization Act contains extensive provisions for emergency planning and the rights of communities to know about toxic chemical releases. In addition to state health departments, there are five national sources of information in the United States on death and injuries caused by chemical releases: the National Response Center (NRC), Department of Transportation (DOT), Hazardous Materials Information System (HMIS), Acute Hazardous Events (AHE) database, and American Association of Poison Control Centers (AAPCC).[1,2] These resources are valuable for accidental exposures to chemical agents, but they must be greatly expanded to address chemical terrorism.

Health departments from five states (Colorado, Iowa, Michigan, New Hampshire, and Wisconsin) evaluated 3125 emergency chemical-release events involving 4034 hazardous substances that occurred from 1990 to 1992. Of these events, 77% involved stationary facilities and 23% were transportation related. In 88% of the events, a single chemical was released. The most commonly released hazardous substances were volatile organic compounds (18%), herbicides (15%), acids (14%), and ammonia (11%). These events resulted in 1446 injuries and 11 deaths. Respiratory irritation (37%) and eye irritation (23%) were the most commonly reported symptoms. Chemical exposures can also occur at home or as the result of an attack.

Many common products once believed to be innocuous (e.g., cement, gasoline) are now regarded as potentially hazardous and the cause of serious injury and illness. Exposure to these agents can be reduced significantly through educational programs, cautionary labeling of toxic products, and appropriate use of protective clothing.

When poison control centers identify new products that are toxic to skin, information systems must include these products to ensure that injured patients are given the benefit of new data.[3] Concomitantly, this information is shared with the manufacturer and Consumer Products Safety Commission (CPSC) to recognize and address the problem nationally. For example, numerous cases of serious, permanent injury and occasionally death caused by exposure to sulfuric acid drain cleaners have been recorded by the CPSC. As a result, the CPSC currently proposes banning the retail sale of this agent.

PATHOPHYSIOLOGY

Most chemical agents damage the skin by producing a chemical reaction rather than a hyperthermic injury.[4] Although some chemicals produce considerable heat as the result of an exothermic reaction when they come into contact with water, their ability to produce direct chemical changes in the skin accounts for the most significant injury. The specific chemical changes depend on the agents, including acids, alkalis, corrosives, oxidizing and reducing agents, desiccants and vesicants, and protoplasmic poisons. The degree of skin destruction is determined mainly by the concentration of the toxic agent and the duration of its contact. When the skin is exposed to toxic chemicals, its keratinous covering is destroyed, and its underlying dermal tissues are exposed to continued necrotizing action.

Both inorganic and organic acids denature the proteins of the skin, resulting in a coagulum, the color of which depends on the acid involved. Nitric acid burns result in a yellow eschar, whereas sulfuric acid eschar is black or brown. Burns caused by hydrochloric acid or phenol tend to range from white to grayish-brown. After the initial exposure, cellular dehydration and further protein denaturation or coagulation occur. This dehydrative effect results in the characteristic dry surface of acid burns that depends on the nature of the acid.

Alkali burns are those caused by lime (cement), ammonia, and caustics (sodium hydroxide, potassium hydroxide). Alkali dissolves protein and collagen, resulting in alkaline complexes of these molecules. Cellular dehydration (as in acid burns) and saponification of fatty tissue also occur. Acid burns are characterized by "dry" edema and extensive fluid loss. Neutralization of alkali exposure is accomplished by first irrigating the burned site with a large amount of water to dilute any unreacted alkali remaining on the wound surface. This protects the wound from further damage caused by heat released during the neutralization reaction.

After skin contact, the absorption of some agents may cause systemic toxicity. For example, dichromate poisoning produces liver failure, acute tubular necrosis, and death. Oxalic acid and hydrofluoric acid injuries may result in hypocalcemia. Tannic acid or phosphorus may cause nephrotoxicity. Absorption of phenol may be associated with central nervous system (CNS) depression and hypotension. Inhalation injury may result from exposure to toxic fumes, particularly when the exposure occurs within a closed space.

COMMUNITY PREPAREDNESS AND HAZMAT RESPONSE

Hazardous materials (HAZMATs) are substances that can cause physical injury and damage the environment if improperly handled. These substances can be encountered in the home, in urban (industrial) areas, in rural (agricultural) areas, or in any location involved in their release. HAZMAT accidents are particularly dangerous for responding personnel, who are in danger of exposure from the time of arrival on the scene until containment of the accident.[5] The population of the surrounding community is also usually endangered. The Superfund Amendments and Reauthorization Act of 1986 mandated community preparedness for dealing with HAZMAT accidents. Before a community develops its plans for responding to HAZMAT accidents, it needs to determine what types of materials are likely to be involved.[6-8]

For those exposed to potentially dangerous chemicals at home, it is best to remove the chemical from the anatomic site by irrigation with copious amounts of water. A friend or a relative then must telephone the regional poison control center certified by the AAPCC. If the chemical is judged to be dangerous, arrangements should be made to transfer the victim to the nearest emergency department for definitive care. The emergency department should be notified as soon as possible after the incident to allow the staff to prepare for receiving the patient.

Identify and Assess Hazardous Environment

The paramedics and members of the HAZMAT response team (usually firefighters) must work together to identify toxic chemicals and assess hazardous environments. Placards, shipping papers, United Nations chemical identification numbers, and markings on shipping containers help identify the offending agent. In some cases, chemical analysis may be required to identify the agent. The presence of carbon monoxide, cyanide, hydrogen sulfide, oxygen, and combustible gases can be detected using different instruments. Colorimetric detector tubes can approximate the concentrations of chemicals in the air. Alpha, beta, and gamma radiation detectors can record radioactive contamination. The 24-hour hotline of Chemtrec (Chemical Transportation Emergency Center in Arlington, Virginia; 800-424-9300) can provide helpful information regarding the identification and management of HAZMATs. At the scene of the incident, members of the HAZMAT team should wear self-contained breathing apparatus (SCBA) and protective apparel.

For more than 30 years, Chemtrec (Chemical Transportation Emergency Center) has been providing the crucial information needed to assist emergency response personnel in handling HAZMAT incidents in the safest possible manner. It is a mission that Chemtrec personnel perform extremely well.

On average, Chemtrec (www.chemtrec.org) handles 22,000 HAZMAT incidents annually. The organization receives 150 calls a day, all of them handled by a skilled team of emergency specialists with access to a database of 2.8 million material safety data sheets (MSDSs).

Chemtrec capabilities were significantly enhanced over the past year. The Chemtrec call center in Arlington was completely renovated to accommodate additional on-duty emergency services specialists and technology upgrades to support the call center operations. Seven specialists now work in the call center, with three to four per shift.

The 800 number (800-424-9300) has caused some confusion. Chemtrec officials stress that the number is just for emergencies. It is not a customer service phone number. When the Chemtrec phone number is listed on paperwork (such as MSDSs, invoices, and labels), it is important to state clearly that this is an emergency number. Placement of a customer service phone number near the company name can help solve the problem.

The HAZMAT emergency clearinghouse also manages the chemical industry's mutual aid emergency response network. Chemtrec was established to provide chemical shippers with timely emergency response and technical assistance at the scene of chemical transportation incidents. The network is composed of emergency response teams from participating chemical companies and teams provided by for-hire contractors.

When calls for help come in, Chemtrec's specialists provide immediate assistance and can link emergency responders in the field with shipper or product manufacturers. The specialists provide technical information to responders, along with important medical support information.

Contingency Plan

The contingency plan for HAZMAT management can be divided into two parts: initiation of the site plan and the evacuation. Initiation of the site plan begins after identifying the HAZMAT and assessing the surrounding environment. When the substance is identified, the health risks to the environment are determined. A command post away from the exposure site is essential for a widespread HAZMAT incident because it allows coordination of the activities of paramedics, HAZMAT team, firefighters, police, and representatives from the state and local government and the manufacturer and shipper.

Coping with HAZMAT Incidents

In dealing with HAZMAT incidents, two distinct goals must be achieved: (1) the material must be contained, fire and explosions must be extinguished, and the site must eventually be cleaned and (2) exposed persons must be treated. Decontamination is initiated by removing and isolating the victim's clothes in plastic bags. Liquid chemicals are washed off the victim's body with water, whereas dry chemicals are first brushed off, followed by copious irrigation with water delivered under low pressures. The priority of decontamination should progress from cleansing of contaminated wounds to eyes, mucous membranes, skin, and hair. While decontamination is being performed, primary and secondary surveys of the patient are conducted to detect life-threatening injuries, and appropriate steps are taken to stabilize the patient's condition (e.g., administration of oxygen to dyspneic patients). Ideally, the patient should be thoroughly decontaminated before arrival in the emergency department.

Hospital personnel involved in decontamination should wear chemical-resistant clothing, with built-in hood and boots, at least two layers of gloves, protective eyewear, and some form of respiratory protection. The minimum level of respiratory protection for hospital personnel during decontamination has not been established.

MANAGEMENT

Acid and Alkali

Skin Injury

Chemical burns continue to destroy tissue until the causative agent is inactivated or removed.[6] For example, when hydrotherapy is initiated within 1 minute after skin contact with either an acid or alkali, the skin injury is much less severe than when treatment is delayed for 3 minutes. Early treatment is followed by a return of the pH of skin to normal. When the contact time exceeds 1 hour, the pH of a sodium hydroxide (NaOH) burn cannot be reversed. Similarly, a brief washing of a hydrochloric acid (HCl) burn more than

15 minutes after exposure does not significantly alter the acidity of the damaged skin.

Hydrotherapy

Because contact time is a critical determinant of the severity of injury, hydrotherapy of skin exposed to a toxic liquid chemical should be initiated immediately by the victim or witness to the injury. When a worker's clothes are soaked with such agents, valuable time is lost if clothing is removed before copious washing is begun. Gentle irrigation with a large volume of water under low pressure for a long time dilutes the toxic agent and washes it out of the skin. During hydrotherapy, the patient's clothes should be removed by the rescuer, wearing powder-free rubber gloves to prevent hand contact with the chemical.

After exposure to strong alkalis, prolonged hydrotherapy is especially important to limit the severity of the injury. In experimental animals, the pH of chemically burned skin does not approach a normal concentration unless more than 1 hour of continuous irrigation has been maintained, and pH often does not return to normal for 12 hours despite hydrotherapy. In contrast, with HCl skin burns the pH usually returns to normal within 2 hours after initiation of hydrotherapy. The mechanism by which NaOH maintains an alkaline pH despite treatment is related to the byproducts of its chemical reaction to skin. Alkalis combine with proteins or fats in tissue to form soluble protein complexes or soaps. These complexes permit passage of hydroxyl ions deep into the tissue, limiting their contact with the water diluent on the skin surface. Acids, on the other hand, do not form complexes, and their free hydrogen ions are easily neutralized.

Regardless of the causative agent, hydrotherapy should be continued when the patient arrives in the emergency department. If the chemical is localized in the patient's hand, the injured part can be immersed in a sink under flowing tap water. For other anatomic sites the patient should be placed supine in a hydrotherapy tank in which the temperature of the water can be regulated. Hydrotherapy treatment should be continued for 2 to 3 hours in the case of acid burns and for at least 12 hours in the case of strong alkali burns.

When it comes in contact with a solid chemical (e.g., lye), clothing must be removed before instituting hydrotherapy. All visible solid particles must be removed from the patient's skin during copious irrigation with water. The water should be delivered to the wound at the lowest possible pressure because high-pressure irrigation (e.g., shower) may disperse the liquid or solid chemical into the patient's or rescuer's eyes.

Water is the agent of choice for decontaminating acid and alkali burns of the skin. The deleterious effects of attempting to neutralize acid and alkali burns were first noted in experimental animals in 1927.[9] In every instance, animals with alkali or acid burns that were washed with water survived longer than animals treated with chemical neutralizers. The striking difference between the results of these two treatment methods is attributed to the additional trauma of the heat generated by the neutralization reaction superimposed on the existing burn. Although the same effect may occur when certain chemicals come in contact with water, large volumes of water tend to limit this exothermic reaction.

Scientists are beginning to question the belief that neutralization of an alkaline burn of the skin with acid does, indeed, increase tissue damage because of the exothermic nature of acid-based reactions.[10] In experimental studies in animals, surgeons demonstrated that topical treatment of alkaline burns with a weak acid such as 5% acetic acid (i.e., household vinegar) resulted in rapid tissue neutralization and reduction of tissue injury in comparison with water irrigation alone. The observed benefits of treating alkaline burns with 5% acetic acid in the rat model are significant and require clinical testing.

Ocular Injury

Acid and alkali injuries involving the eye are among the most disastrous of chemical burns.[4] Alkali substances are the most toxic chemicals, and *anhydrous ammonia* appears to be the worst offender. Even alkali burns that seem to be mild can result in devastating injury because alkalis tend to react with the lipid in the corneal epithelial cells to form a soluble soap that penetrates the corneal stroma. The alkali moves rapidly through the stroma and the endothelial cells to enter the anterior chamber. Anhydrous ammonia can penetrate into the anterior chamber in less than 1 minute.

Alkali usually kills each tissue layer of the anterior segment of the eye that it touches. The result is occlusive vasculitis about the corneoscleral limbus, which makes repair of these tissues difficult. As the tissues of the anterior segment of the eye degenerate, perforation follows, with the development of endophthalmitis and loss of the eye. If perforation can be prevented, recovery of sight may be possible through eventual corneal transplantation. Experimental studies conclude that the destruction of corneal stroma can be minimized by drug therapy (e.g., *N*-acetylcysteine, steroids).[4] However, drug therapy has limited therapeutic usefulness because of the need for frequent applications, the significant number of clinical failures, and the potential side effects.

The eye tolerates acid burns better than alkali burns because, as with other living tissue, this organ has a significant acid-buffering capacity. Acid is rapidly neutralized by the tear film, the proteins present in tears, and the conjunctival epithelial cells. Consequently, acid typically causes epithelial and basement membrane damage but rarely damages deep endothelial cells. Acid burns that injure the periphery of the cornea and conjunctiva often heal uneventfully, leaving a clear corneal epithelium. In contrast, acid burns of the central part of the cornea may lead to corneal ulcer formation with neovascularization and scarring, requiring later reconstruction.

Irrigation

Regardless of the nature of the chemical involved, immediate institution of copious irrigation is most important. At the scene of injury the victim should submerge the eyes in tap water and continuously open and close them. In the emergency department, hydrotherapy is most easily accomplished by using a low-flow stream of 0.9% sodium chloride from intravenous (IV) tubing. Topical anesthetic agents help improve patients' cooperation. Irrigation should then continue until the pH of the conjunctival sac returns to its physiologic level (pH 7.4). The initial slit-lamp examination of alkali burns often reveals corneal erosion, swelling of the corneal epithelium, and clouding of the anterior chamber. All eyes that demonstrate a corneal abrasion should be treated with an emollient broad-spectrum antibiotic ointment instilled in the conjunctival sac (e.g., chloramphenicol, gentamicin).

Ophthalmologic consultation and close follow-up are warranted in all significant exposures, and hospitalization for continuous irrigation may occasionally be required. Measurement of intraocular pressure should be performed serially to detect any pressure increases. The injured eye should be treated with a long-acting cycloplegic, a mydriatic, and occasionally a carbonic anhydrase inhibitor for 2 weeks or until the pain disappears. This treatment decreases the potential for pupillary constriction, increased intraocular pressure, and early glaucoma. The mobility of the globe should be encouraged to avoid the development of conjunctival adhesions (symblepharon).

Amniotic membrane patching has been demonstrated to be useful for achieving a desirable outcome for acute ocular chemical burns.[11,12] The human placenta was obtained shortly after elective cesarean delivery from a donor mother. Human immunodeficiency virus, hepatitis virus type B, hepatitis virus type C, and syphilis were serologically excluded. Temporary amniotic membrane patching with modifications in suture placement was performed in patients with acute chemical injury. Clinical results suggest that immediate amniotic membrane patching is quite useful for managing moderately severe acute ocular chemical injury by facilitating rapid epithelialization and pain relief and by securing ocular surface integrity.

Hydrofluoric Acid

During 1985 and 1986, the AAPCC Data Collection System received 2367 reports of human exposures to hydrofluoric acid (HF). Four fatalities occurred, three from ingestion and one as a result of dermal exposure. Significant local and systemic toxicity can result from exposure of eye, skin, or lung to HF.

Inhalation Injury

Inhalation of HF vapor is rare and usually involves explosions that produce fumes or high concentrations of liquid HF (>50%) that has soaked the clothing of the upper body.[13] Patients' outcomes vary considerably depending on the concentration and duration of exposure to HF. Inhalation and skin exposure to 70% HF have caused pulmonary edema and death within 2 hours.[10] Pulmonary injuries that are not evident until several days after exposure can also occur. Although the patient has no respiratory symptoms and a normal chest radiograph initially, massive purulent tracheobronchitis that is refractory to treatment may develop. Respiratory symptoms may persist for months after inhalation of HF fumes. Sustained irritation of the larynx and pharynx with fibrinous, granulating deposits on thickened vocal cords may cause a persistent cough and hoarseness.

After the patient is removed from the source, the clothes and skin should be decontaminated. If respiratory symptoms are present, the patient should be monitored with pulse oximetry, receive humidified oxygen using a nonrebreathing reservoir bag-mask system, and be evaluated for laryngeal edema, pneumonitis, pulmonary edema, pulmonary hemorrhage, and systemic toxicity. The treatment of HF inhalation injury is primarily symptomatic. Administration of 2.5% to 3% calcium gluconate solution by nebulizer as a therapy for inhalation of HF has been suggested but not tested.[14] Asymptomatic patients with possible HF inhalation should be admitted for observation.

Ocular Injury

Exposure of the eye to HF vapors produces more extensive damage than that of other acids at a similar concentration. The extent of damage by HF depends on its concentration. Exposure of rabbits to 0.5% HF caused mild initial conjunctival ischemia that resolved in 10 days.[15] Exposure to 8% HF caused severe initial ischemia that was still noted after 65 days. Corneal opacification and necrosis followed exposure to 20% HF.

Immediate and copious irrigation of the exposed eyes should be initiated at the scene of exposure and continued for at least 30 minutes during transport to the emergency department, where an ophthalmologic examination can be performed promptly.[16] Local ophthalmic anesthetic drops enhance patients' comfort and cooperation during irrigation and evaluation.

In experimental animals, single irrigations with 1 L of water, isotonic saline, or magnesium chloride are the only treatments that have been found to be therapeutically beneficial without causing toxicity.[15] Benefits include decreased epithelial loss and reduced corneal inflammation. Repeated irrigations over time have no therapeutic merit and are associated with an increased occurrence of corneal ulceration. Patients with significant ocular exposure to HF should be seen immediately by an ophthalmologist.

Skin Injury

A large number of personnel in industry and research handle concentrated solutions of HF. Relatively dilute solutions of HF (0.6% to 12%) are available to the public in the form of rust removal and aluminum cleaning products. During handling of containers containing

HF, contamination of inadequately protected fingers and hands often results in a chemical burn injury.

HF skin burns have distinct characteristics. The exposure causes progressive tissue destruction; intense pain can be delayed for hours but can persist for days if untreated. The skin at the site of contact develops a tough, coagulated appearance. Untreated sites progress to indurated, whitish, and blistered vesicles that contain caseous, necrotic tissue. In exposure of the digits, HF has a predilection for subungual tissue. Severe untreated burns may progress to full-thickness burns and may even result in the loss of digits.

Initial Care

The initial treatment of HF skin exposure is immediate irrigation with copious amounts of water for at least 15 to 30 minutes. Most exposures to dilute solutions of HF respond favorably to immediate irrigation. Severe pain or any pain that persists after irrigation denotes a more severe burn that requires detoxification of the fluoride ion. Detoxification is accomplished by promoting the formation of an insoluble calcium salt.

All blisters should be removed because necrotic tissue may harbor fluoride ions. The fluoride ion can then be detoxified through topical treatment, local infiltrative therapy, or intra-arterial infusion of calcium. Calcium gluconate (2.5%) gel is the preferred topical agent.[17] Because skin is impermeable to calcium, topical treatment is effective only for mild, superficial burns. Because this gel is not stocked in most hospital pharmacies, it must be formulated by mixing 3.5 g of calcium gluconate powder in 150 mL of a water-soluble lubricant (e.g., glycerin–hydroxyethyl cellulose [K-Y] jelly). The gel should be secured by an occlusive cover (e.g., powder-free latex glove).

Infiltration Therapy

Subcutaneous. Infiltrative therapy is necessary to treat deep and painful HF burns. Calcium gluconate is the agent of choice and can be administered by either direct infiltration or intra-arterial injection. A common technique involves injecting 10% calcium gluconate subcutaneously through a 30-gauge needle at a maximum dose of 0.5 mL/cm^2 of skin.[18] Using 5% calcium gluconate, by diluting the solution with an equal amount of isotonic saline, has been shown to reduce irritation of tissues and decrease subsequent scarring.[17] Patients treated in this manner should be hospitalized for observation and toxicologic consultation.

Despite its wide acceptance, notable disadvantages are present with the infiltration technique, especially when treating digits. A regional nerve block is recommended because the injections may be very painful. Removal of the nail to expose the nail bed is required if subungual tissue is involved. Vascular compromise can occur if excessive fluid is injected into the skin exposure sites, and unbound calcium ions have a direct toxic effect on tissue. Because of these disadvantages with subcutaneous infiltration, intra-arterial infusion of calcium is being used more often.

Intra-arterial. An intra-arterial catheter is placed in the appropriate vascular supply close to the site of HF exposure (e.g., radial, ulnar, or brachial artery). Various dilute solutions of calcium salts have been infused over 4 hours, including (1) a 10-mL solution of 10% calcium gluconate or calcium chloride mixed in 40 to 50 mL of 5% dextrose in water (D5W), repeated if pain returns within 4 hours; (2) a 10-mL solution of 20% calcium gluconate in 40 mL of normal saline for radial or ulnar artery infusion; and (3) 20 mL of 20% calcium gluconate in 80 mL of normal saline for brachial artery infusion, repeated at 12-hour intervals if needed.[19,20] If more than 6 hours have elapsed since the time of HF exposure, tissue necrosis cannot be prevented, even though pain relief can occur up to 24 hours after exposure.

The intra-arterial infusion technique also has potential disadvantages. Arterial spasm or thrombosis may result in significant skin loss. The intra-arterial procedure is more costly because it requires hospitalization for use of the infusion pump and monitoring of serum calcium if repeated infusions are used.

Systemic Toxicity

HF binds calcium and magnesium with strong affinity. Systemic fluoride toxicity, including dysrhythmias and hypocalcemia, can result from ingestion, inhalation, or dermal exposure to HF.[21] Consequently, patients with significant HF exposure should be hospitalized and monitored for cardiac dysrhythmias for 24 to 48 hours.

Hypocalcemia can occur after significant exposures to HF and should be corrected with 10% calcium gluconate administered IV. If left untreated, a burn caused by 7 mL of 99% HF can theoretically bind all available calcium in a 70-kg person. A prolonged QT interval on the electrocardiogram (ECG) is a reliable indicator of hypocalcemia.

Formic Acid

Formic acid is a caustic organic acid used in industry and agriculture.[22] It causes cutaneous injury by coagulation necrosis. Systemic toxicity occurs after absorption and is manifest by acidosis, hemolysis, and hemoglobinuria. Hemolysis is the result of the direct effect of formic acid on the red blood cells.

Copious wound lavage should be instituted immediately. Acidosis should be treated by sodium bicarbonate. Mannitol may be used to expand plasma volume and promote osmotic diuresis in patients with hemolysis. Exchange transfusions and hemodialysis may be needed in patients with severe formic acid poisoning.

Anhydrous Ammonia

Ammonia is used in the manufacture of explosives, petroleum, cyanide, plastic, and synthetic fibers.[23,24] It is also widely used as a cleaning agent and as a coolant in refrigerator units. As an agricultural fertilizer, ammonia is ideal because of its high nitrogen content (82%).

The sudden release of liquid ammonia can cause injury through two different mechanisms. It has an extremely low temperature (–33° C) and freezes any tissue it touches. Ammonia vapors readily dissolve in the moisture in skin, eyes, oropharynx, and lungs to form hydroxyl ions, which cause chemical burns through liquefaction necrosis. The severity of injury is directly related to the concentration of and duration of exposure to ammonia.

Treatment consists of prompt irrigation of the eyes and skin with water and management of inhalation injury. If necessary, the airway should be secured by nasal or oral intubation. A large-diameter tube should be used to prevent distal airway obstruction from sloughing of mucosa. After intubation, lower airway injury should be managed with positive end-expiratory pressure ventilation.

Cement

Cement burns are alkali burns.[25] When dry cement is combined with water, hydrolysis occurs. The resulting mixture is essentially a solution of slated lime saturated in water and initially has a pH of 10 to 12. As hydrolysis continues, the pH may continue to rise to 12 or 14, which is comparable to that of sodium or potassium hydroxide or lye. In addition, a contact dermatitis from chromate (a trace element) has been reported.

The best treatment of cement burns is immediate copious irrigation until the substance is completely gone, a practice performed by the experienced worker who habitually washes off the cement throughout the day. Prominent warning labels on packages containing cement products direct the user to wear protective gloves when using the product in either its wet or dry state.

Cement burns of the lower extremities respond well to immediate copious irrigation followed by coverage with a medicated bandage (e.g., Gelcast Unna's boot) that allows the patient to ambulate.

Phenol and Derivatives

Phenols are used industrially as starting materials for many organic polymers and plastics. They are used widely in the agricultural, cosmetic, and medical fields. Because of their antiseptic properties (first appreciated by Lister), they are used in many commercial germicidal solutions. A number of phenol derivatives (e.g., hexylresorcinol, resorcinol) are more bactericidal than phenol itself.

Phenol is an aromatic acidic alcohol. This compound and its derivatives are highly reactive, corrosive contact poisons that damage cells by denaturing and precipitating cellular proteins. Their characteristic odor usually signals their presence. After penetrating the dermis, phenol produces necrosis of the papillary dermis. This necrotic tissue may temporarily delay its absorption. Therefore, when skin comes in contact with phenol, treatment must be instituted immediately. The exposed area should be irrigated with large volumes of water delivered under low pressure. Because dilute solutions of phenol are more rapidly absorbed through skin than concentrated solutions, gentle swabbing of the skin surface with sponges soaked in water should be avoided. Because phenol may become trapped in the victim's hair or beard, any hair that has come into

contact with the chemical agent should be removed as soon as possible.

In animal studies, exposure to as little as 0.625 mg/kg of phenol causes death.[6] In humans, absorbed phenol causes profound CNS depression, resulting in coma and death from respiratory failure. Marked hypotension may occur as a result of central vasomotor depression in addition to a direct effect on the myocardium and small blood vessels. Phenol is also a powerful antipyretic that decreases body temperature. Metabolic acidosis may result from shock as well as from the direct effect of the acidic phenol.

A number of substituted phenols (e.g., resorcinol, picric acid) have systemic actions distinct from those of phenol. CNS stimulation often occurs after absorption of resorcinol. Picric acid hemolyzes red blood cells and causes acute hemorrhagic glomerulonephritis and liver injury.

Dilute solutions of phenol are used by plastic surgeons for chemical face peels.[26] Phenol (which is usually mixed with water, soap, and croton oil for this application) can produce a partial-thickness burn of predictable depth in a controlled manner. It has been the standard for many years for new technologies in skin resurfacing to remove both coarse and fine wrinkles, irregular pigmentation, and actinic keratoses.

The concentration of phenol is kept sufficiently low to reduce the occurrence of systemic complications. Interestingly, higher concentrations of phenol result in a shallower burn depth. A higher concentration of phenol results in increased coagulation of the keratin in the skin, thus forming a barrier to further penetration. Histologic studies have demonstrated that 100% concentrations of phenol produce 35% to 50% less penetration than a 50% phenol solution.

The physician performing phenol chemical peels should be concerned about the possibility of rapid phenol absorption. When phenol was applied to more than 50% of the facial surface in less than 30 minutes, a high incidence of cardiac arrhythmias was reported. When the application time over the same area was increased to 60 minutes, arrhythmias were avoided. Because of the complication of cardiac arrhythmias, all patients undergoing phenol peeling should be monitored electrocardiographically and have an IV line in place.

After application of the phenol solution, the skin is covered with an occlusive dressing consisting of either multiple layers of waterproof tape or petroleum jelly to prevent evaporation of the phenol, allowing increased penetration and burn depth. The peeled skin is maintained by daily cleansing and consequent reapplication of ointment, which keeps the surface moist and prevents desiccation. If this protocol is followed, healing is completed within 5 to 7 days.

Polyethylene Glycol Therapy

Experimental studies indicate that water alone is effective in reducing the severity of burns and preventing death in animals with skin exposed to phenol and its derivatives. However, the most effective treatment is undiluted polyethylene glycol (PEG) of molecular weight 200 to 400 or isopropanol (isopropyl alcohol). PEG should be stocked in hospitals located near areas of phenol use and can often be found in the chemical section of hospital pharmacies. A quick wipe of the skin with PEG solutions reduces mortality and burn severity in experimental animals. These solutions can be used in phenol burns of the face because they are not irritating to the eyes. Decontamination with water should be performed until a PEG solution is obtained. Large amounts of water must be used because small amounts of water are detrimental, enhancing dermal absorption of phenol. Removal of the phenol should be undertaken in a well-ventilated room so that hospital personnel are not exposed to high concentrations of phenol fumes.

Systemic Toxicity

The treatment of systemic symptoms is purely symptomatic. Respiratory depression may require ventilatory support. Hypotension should be treated with isotonic crystalloid fluid and pressor agents as needed. Metabolic acidosis may require treatment with sodium bicarbonate. Alkalinization also prevents precipitation of hemoglobin in the urine that occurs with hemolysis. Hemochromogen excretion in the urine can be enhanced by administering IV mannitol, which causes an osmotic diuresis. Anticonvulsants may be required to treat seizures resulting from CNS stimulation.

White Phosphorus

White phosphorus is a yellow, waxy translucent solid element that burns in the air unless preserved in oil.[6] When it ignites spontaneously in air, it is oxidized to phosphorus pentoside, which forms metaphosphoric and orthophosphoric acids with the addition of water. The capability of phosphorus to ignite spontaneously in air at temperatures greater than 34° C (93.2° F) has encouraged its use as an incendiary agent in military weapons and fireworks. After the explosion of a phosphorous munition, flaming droplets may become embedded beneath the skin, where they oxidize adjacent tissue unless removed. In nonmilitary industry, white phosphorus is used in the manufacture of insecticides, rodent poisons, and fertilizers.

Tissue injury from white phosphorus appears to be caused primarily by heat production rather than by liberation of inorganic acids or cellular dehydration from the hygroscopic phosphorus pentoside. The ultimate result of this thermal injury is often a painful partial-thickness or full-thickness burn.

Metabolic derangements have been identified after white phosphorus burns. Serum electrolyte changes consist of decreased serum calcium and increased serum phosphorus. ECG abnormalities include prolonged QT interval, bradycardia, and ST segment–T wave changes. These ECG changes may explain the sudden early death occasionally seen in patients with apparently inconsequential white phosphorus burns.

Prehospital care includes immediate removal of contaminated clothing followed by submersion of the injured skin in cool water. Warm water should be avoided because white phosphorus becomes a liquid at 44° C (111.2° F). Phosphorus particles should be removed from the victim's skin and submerged in water. The burned skin should be covered with towels soaked in cool water during transport to the emergency department.

After the patient's arrival in the emergency department, the burned skin should be washed with a suspension of 5% sodium bicarbonate and 3% copper sulfate in 1% hydroxyethyl cellulose. (This must be made by hospital pharmacies.) Phosphorus particles become coated with black cupric phosphide, allowing their easy identification. Copper sulfate also decreases the rate of oxidation of the phosphorus particles, limiting their damage to the underlying tissue. However, blackened particles can still elicit tissue injury and should be removed.

If absorbed systemically, copper sulfate is toxic. Absorption of copper sulfate can be minimized by the surface-active agent in the suspension as well as by sodium lauryl sulfate. Before the advent of these agents, prolonged treatment of phosphorus burns with copper sulfate solutions led to systemic copper poisoning, which is manifested by vomiting, diarrhea, hemolysis, oliguria, hematuria, hepatic necrosis, and cardiopulmonary collapse. After the burned skin is subjected to a suspension of copper sulfate for 30 minutes, the antidote must be thoroughly washed from the skin. This washing limits the development of systemic copper toxicity. An alternative approach is to use a Wood's lamp to identify the phosphorus particles because they fluoresce under ultraviolet light.

After hydrotherapy and treatment with the appropriate antidote, definitive management of the skin burns in the hospital intensive care unit setting is accomplished as with any other burn wound.

Nitrates

Toxic *methemoglobinemia* is a well-recognized hazard of ingestion of nitrates and nitrites.[27] Occasionally, severe methemoglobinemia has been reported in patients sustaining burn injury from molten sodium and potassium nitrates. In these cases, methemoglobinemia is caused by absorption of nitrates through burned skin. The diagnosis of methemoglobinemia should be sought in a cyanotic patient who is unresponsive to oxygen therapy and whose blood appears chocolate brown in color. Methemoglobin levels less than 20% to 30% are usually asymptomatic and require no treatment. Patients with levels greater than 30%, with or without symptoms, should be treated by high-flow oxygen and IV methylene blue administered slowly at a dose of 1 to 2 mg/kg body weight. Exchange transfusions may also benefit severe cases by rapidly decreasing circulating methemoglobin concentration.[28]

Hydrocarbons

Cutaneous injury from immersion in gasoline and other hydrocarbons may occur in individuals involved in motor vehicle accidents. The solvent properties of hydrocarbons cause cell membrane injury and dissolution of lipids, resulting in skin necrosis. Although full-thickness injuries can occur, most injuries are partial thickness.[29] Once the gasoline damages the protective skin barrier, the hydrocarbons are absorbed. The absorption of hydrocarbons produces systemic toxicity that causes neurologic, pulmonary, cardiovascular, gastrointestinal, and hepatic injuries.[30]

Treatment of individuals exposed to gasoline includes immediate removal from the site of exposure, removal of all clothing, copious irrigation, and transfer to the emergency department while continuing copious irrigation. Management in the emergency department consists of wound care of burn injuries and a search for evidence of systemic toxicity.

Tar

Burns from hot tar are a challenging clinical problem. Hot liquefied tar that comes in contact with skin transfers heat to cause burn injury. Tar then cools and solidifies on the skin surface, making removal difficult. Hot tar includes two distinct groups of materials: coal tar pitches and petroleum-derived asphalts. Both products are heated to maintain liquid form. Paving roads requires tar temperatures from 275° F to 300° F, and roofing demands higher tar temperatures of 450° F to 500° F. Deeper burn injuries are associated with burns from roofing asphalt. Mechanisms of injury include cauldron explosion, falling from buildings, trucks rolling over, pipe explosion, spillage from buckets, and industrial accidents.

When hot tar touches skin, it rapidly cools, solidifies, and becomes enmeshed in the hair. It is important to facilitate this cooling process by adding cold water to the tar at the scene of the accident. Cooling tar with cold water limits the amount of tissue damage and prevents the spread of tar. Tar should be continually washed with water until it has cooled and hardened. After cooling, the skin should be dried with towels to prevent systemic hypothermia.

Adherent tar should not be removed at the scene of the accident. In the emergency department, definitive care of tar burn injury involves early removal of tar because it occludes injured skin and encourages bacterial growth. This can convert a partial-thickness burn to a full-thickness burn. Tar adheres to skin because it is enmeshed in the hair, not because of a direct bond between epidermis and tar.

Solvents used to remove tar ideally should have a close structural affinity to tar. Asphalts are susceptible to both aromatic (e.g., naphthalene) and aliphatic (e.g., hexade) hydrocarbon solvents; coal tars are susceptible only to aromatic hydrocarbons. The cleansing capacity of these solvents is enhanced by prolonged contact with tar. Broad-spectrum antibiotic ointments such as bacitracin (400 U/g), polymyxin B (5000 U/g), and neomycin (5 mg/g) may be added to lower the incidence of infection. Antimicrobial petrolatum ointments should be removed and reapplied every hour until all tar is removed. The process of tar removal usually takes

12 to 48 hours. Antibiotic ointment has been used successfully to remove even tar layered over corneas and conjunctivas.

An alternative to petrolatum ointments is surface-active agents, such as polyoxyethylene sorbitan (Tween 80) and polysorbate (De-Solv-It). These are more water soluble and more easily removed from skin with water than petrolatum ointments. These surface-active agents are an effective, safe, and inexpensive means of removing tar from skin. NISA baby oil, sunflower oil, mayonnaise, and butter have also been used to remove adherent tar from skin, taking from 30 to 90 minutes for complete removal. Sunflower oil has proved effective and safe in removing tar without further skin damage.

Elemental Metals

The elemental metals *sodium* and *potassium* are harmless unless activated by water, which causes an exothermic reaction with the release of heat and the generation of hydrogen gas and hydroxide.[31] The evolved heat is sufficient to ignite the hydrogen gas, which results in greater heat and additional thermal burns. The formation of the hydroxide compound may also result in significant chemical injury to tissue. The reaction occurs more rapidly with elemental potassium than with sodium. These deleterious effects of potassium have been attributed to trace amounts of potassium superoxide released on exposure to room air. Water lavage is therefore dangerous in these circumstances.

In the prehospital setting, only a class D fire extinguisher (containing sodium chloride, sodium carbonate, or graphite base) or sand should be used to suppress the flames. When the fire is extinguished, the metal is covered by oil (e.g., mineral, cooking), which isolates the metal from water. The patient should be transported to the emergency department for wound debridement and cleansing. Small pieces of metal should be removed from the skin. Sodium fragments should be placed in isopropyl alcohol, containing no more than 2% water, whereas potassium particles should be inserted into terbutyl alcohol for safe deposit.

CHEMICAL TERRORISM

The reality of chemical agents as terrorist weapons is a part of news, public policy, and medical preparedness. The sarin gas attack in the Tokyo subway in March 1995 resulted in 12 deaths and more than 5000 casualties.[32] It was subsequently learned that the responsible cult, Aum Shinrikyo, had stored enough of the potent nerve gas, VX, to kill up to 4 million people. In addition, these agents continue to be used in modern warfare, despite being banned by the 1925 Geneva Convention. The Iraqi army used sulfur mustard and nerve gases extensively and caused mass casualties in their 6-year war with Iran.[33] As terrorist organizations begin to use nonconventional weapons such as chemical and biologic agents, the civilian medical community needs to better understand their characteristics and pathophysiology.

Response

The U.S. federal government recognizes the emerging threat of terrorism and the potential of these organizations to use nonconventional weapons. In 1997 the U.S. Congress enacted the Defense Against Weapons of Mass Destruction Act, with a $52.6 million appropriation.[34] Subtitle A of this document established the Domestic Preparedness Program to enhance the government's capability to respond to terrorist attacks with these weapons. The act also focuses on improving local and state agencies to address these threats and to train communities.

The government's direct response was delineated in Presidential Decision Directive 39 (PDD-39), signed by President Clinton in 1995.[35] For all cases of domestic terrorism, the Federal Bureau of Investigation (FBI) is assigned to oversee crisis management and to investigate the case for eventual prosecution. The Federal Emergency Management Agency (FEMA) is to coordinate assistance to state and local governments, provide emergency relief, and protect public health and safety. The sophisticated operations necessary to deal with a large-scale chemical attack could overwhelm local HAZMAT teams, and thus other agencies have been designated to provide operational support, including the U.S. Departments of Defense, Energy, and Transportation and the Environmental Protection Agency.

Appropriate casualty triage remains a critical component when dealing with nonconventional weapons. Overall death rates increase when triage systems are poorly coordinated.[36] Triage should be performed by specially trained emergency medical personnel who are familiar with these agents and with the use of personal protective equipment (PPE). The emergency department could be quickly overwhelmed with masses of noncritically injured survivors. Ideally, triage would be conducted both at the scene of the attack and again at a second point before emergency department arrival.

Emergency Department Preparedness

Once in the emergency department, noncritical victims should be rapidly removed from the acute setting. Steps should be taken to ensure that other patients and staff are not secondarily exposed. For those directly handling the casualties, PPE such as full-face respiratory masks, SCBAs, and impermeable suits should be available.[37] The use and location of decontamination showers should be well known, and negative flow isolation rooms should be available. A surveillance system should be established to identify groups at high risk and to evaluate medical interventions. Many of these agents can cause long-term adverse health outcomes, and registries should be established to facilitate appropriate follow-up.

Table 61-1. Classification of Chemical Warfare Agents

Class	Example	Treatment
Blistering agents	Sulfur mustard	Hydrotherapy Puncture and drain blisters Moist dressings 100% O$_2$ if inhaled Hydrotherapy followed by antibiotic-based steroid ointment for ocular injury
Nerve agents	Sarin Tabun VX	Atropine Pralidoxime (Protopam)
Choking gases	Phosgene	Supportive care
Cyanide agents	Hydrogen cyanide	Amyl nitrite Sodium nitrite 100% O$_2$

Chemical Agents

Chemical agents can be classified as (1) blistering agents, (2) nerve agents, (3) choking gases, or (4) cyanide agents (Table 61-1). *Blistering agents*, such as sulfur mustard, have been regarded as the chemical weapon of choice in modern warfare. First used in World War I, sulfur mustard is often referred to as the "king of war gases" because of its ability to incapacitate opponents.[38] *Nerve agents*, such as sarin gas, have been receiving increasing public attention. The first nerve gas synthesized was tabun, and although it was developed in Germany before World War II, it was not documented for military purposes until the Iraqis used the agent in the 1980s.[33] *Choking gases*, such as phosgene, were first developed during World War I. Phosgene is also used extensively in the industrial setting for the preparation of polyurethanes.[39] *Cyanide agents*, such as hydrogen cyanide, were first discovered in the 18th century by the Swedish chemist Carl Wilhelm Scheele.[40] Although Scheele gave no indication of its lethal characteristics, hydrogen cyanide has become one of the most toxic chemicals known, with potential deadly consequences if used by a terrorist organization.

Blistering Agents

Sulfur mustard is a vesicant and alkylating agent known by various names, including mustard gas, Yperite, and HD.[41] It is a bifunctional alkylating agent that can form covalent bonds, resulting in direct damage to DNA. It causes severe vesication of the skin, and at high doses it exerts systemic cytotoxic effects on the hematologic system and intestinal mucosa. Sulfur mustard is stored as an oil-based liquid and is readily aerosolized when attached to a bomb or shell. Because it is slowly vaporized, it poses a particular risk in closed-space or cool environments. Several minutes of exposure result in skin or eye injury, and exposure for longer than 30 minutes can lead to respiratory injury and death.

No specific antidote exists for mustard gas. The most effective therapy is rapid decontamination with water and supportive care. All blisters should be opened and covered with moist dressings. Eyes should be irrigated with water for at least 5 minutes. A mydriatic agent should be applied and topical antibiotic therapy instituted. Tetanus prophylaxis is mandatory. Inhalation injury requires the use of 100% oxygen and additional supportive measures.

Nerve Agents

The nerve agents, such as sarin and tabun, are members of the class of agents known as *organophosphates*.[41] These are among the most potent synthetic toxic agents known, and submilligram doses are lethal in mice. These agents tend to be odorless and are irreversible cholinesterase inhibitors. Metabolism of acetylcholine at the nerve endings is blocked, leading to a toxic buildup of this neurotransmitter and eventually paralysis. Complications include seizures, respiratory failure, pulmonary edema, and hypotension. Nerve agents are rapidly absorbed through the skin and pulmonary membranes, with a rapid onset of action. Symptomatic relief can be provided with atropine. Because it is an irreversible inhibitor of acetylcholine, pralidoxime is given and serves to reactivate the enzyme cholinesterase. Atropine must be given repeatedly until the agent has been completely metabolized (several hours to days).

Choking Agents

Phosgene is the most common type of choking agent and has been used in warfare.[42] Phosgene has a characteristic odor of freshly mown grass or moldy hay, which may assist in the diagnosis. This class causes pronounced irritation of the upper and lower respiratory tracts. Coughing, tearing, shortness of breath, and chest pain are common symptoms. Pulmonary edema can result, with onset often several hours after exposure. Most patients, however, recover without long-term effects, although secondary bacterial pneumonia has been reported. Treatment for exposure to these agents remains supportive, with oxygen supplementation as required.

Cyanide

Cyanide, or hydrocyanic acid, interferes with aerobic metabolism, and death may occur within minutes of exposure.[42] When cyanide is absorbed, it reacts with the trivalent iron of cytochrome oxidase in mitochondria. Because the utilization of oxygen is blocked, venous blood is highly oxygenated and may appear as red as arterial blood. Initially, hyperpnea and headache occur, but ultimately, hypoxic convulsions and respiratory arrest result in death. Thus, rapid diagnosis and treatment are essential. A characteristic odor of bitter almonds is noted.

To treat cyanide poisoning, amyl nitrite is given in the inhaled form, and sodium nitrite is administered IV (10 mL of a 3% solution). These substances oxidize hemoglobin to methemoglobin, which competes favorably with cytochrome oxidase for the cyanide ion,

allowing reactivation of normal cellular respiration. Hyperbaric oxygen therapy potentiates the effects of nitrites and is clinically useful.[38]

🔑 KEY CONCEPTS

- *Chemical injury*: The degree of skin destruction is determined mainly by the concentration of the toxic agent and the duration of its contact.

- Chemical injuries are commonly encountered after exposure to acids and alkalis, including hydrofluoric acid, formic acid, anhydrous ammonia, cement, and phenol. Other specific chemical agents that cause chemical burns include white phosphorus, elemental metals, nitrates, hydrocarbons, and tar.

- More than 65,000 chemicals are available on the market, and an estimated 60,000 new chemicals are produced each year.

- Hazardous materials (HAZMATs) are substances that can cause physical injury and damage the environment if improperly handled.

- *Hazardous materials*: In dealing with HAZMAT incidents, two distinct goals must be achieved: (1) the HAZMAT must be contained, fire and explosions must be extinguished, and the site must eventually be cleaned and (2) those exposed to the HAZMAT must be treated.

- For more than 30 years, Chemtrec (Chemical Transportation Emergency Center) has been providing the crucial information needed to assist emergency response personnel in handling HAZMAT incidents in the safest possible manner.

- When calls for help come in, Chemtrec's specialists provide immediate assistance and can link emergency responders in the field with shippers or product manufacturers.

- The management of chemical injuries must be individualized for the specific chemical and continue from the time of injury to rehabilitation.

- *Terrorism*: Nonconventional chemical weapons may be placed into four major classifications: blistering agents, nerve agents, choking gases, and cyanide agents.

REFERENCES

1. Hall HI, Dhara VR, Price-Green PA, Kaye WE: Surveillance for emergency events involving hazardous substances—United States, 1990-1992. *MMWR CDC Surveill Summ* 43(SS-2):1, 1994.
2. Litovitz TL, Normann S, Veltri JC: 1985 annual report of the American Association of Poison Control Centers National Data Collection System. *Am J Emerg Med* 5:405, 1986.
3. Litovitz TL, Martin TG, Schmitz B: 1986 annual report of the American Association of Poison Control Centers National Data Collection System. *Am J Emerg Med* 5:405, 1987.
4. Rodeheaver GT, Hiebert JM, Edlich RF: Initial treatment for chemical skin burns and eye burns. *Comp Ther* 8:37, 1982.
5. Binder S: Deaths, injuries, and evacuations from acute hazardous materials release. *Am J Public Health* 79:1042, 1989.
6. Kirk MA, Cisek J, Rose SR: Emergency department response to hazardous vehicle incidents. *Emerg Med Clin North Am* 12:461, 1994.
7. DeAtley C: Hazardous materials exposure mandates integrated patient care. *Occup Health Saf* 60:40, 1991.

8. Plante DM, Walker JS: EMS response at a hazardous material incident: Some basic guidelines. *J Emerg Med* 7:55, 1989.
9. Davidson EC: The treatment of acid and alkali burns. *Ann Surg* 35:481, 1927.
10. Andrews K, Mowlavi A, Milner M: The treatment of alkaline burns of the skin by neutralization. *Plast Reconstr Surg* 6:1918, 2003.
11. Sridhar MS, Bansal AK, Sangwan VS, Rao GN: Amniotic membrane transplantation in acute chemical and thermal injury. *Am J Ophthalmol* 130:134, 2000.
12. Kobayashi A, et al: Temporary amniotic membrane patching for acute chemical burns. *Eye* 17:149, 2003.
13. Mayer L, Guelich J: Hydrogen fluoride inhalation and burns. *Arch Environ Health* 7:445, 1963.
14. Trevino MA, Herrmann GH, Sprout WL: Treatment of severe hydrofluoric acid exposures. *J Occup Med* 25:861, 1983.
15. McCulley JP, et al: Hydrofluoric acid burns of the eye. *J Occup Med* 25:447, 1983.
16. Caravati EM: Acute hydrofluoric acid exposure. *Am J Emerg Med* 5:143, 1988.
17. Mackinnon MA: Treatment of hydrofluoric acid burns. *J Occup Med* 28:804, 1986.
18. Dibbell DG, et al: Hydrofluoric acid burns of the hand. *J Bone Joint Surg Am* 52:931, 1970.
19. Vance MV, et al: Digital hydrofluoric acid burn treatment with intra-arterial calcium infusion. *Ann Emerg Med* 15:890, 1988.
20. Kohnlein HE, Merkle P, Springorium HW: Hydrogen fluoride burns: Experiments and treatment. *Surg Forum* 24:50, 1973.
21. Reynolds KE, Whitford GM, Pashley DH: Acute fluoride toxicity: The influence of acid-base status. *Toxicol Appl Pharmacol* 45:415, 1978.
22. Sigurdsson J, Bjornsson A, Gudmundsson ST: Formic acid burns: Local and systemic effects. *Burns* 9:358, 1983.
23. Birken GA, Fabri PJ, Carey LC: Acute ammonia intoxication complicating multiple trauma. *J Trauma* 21:820, 1981.
24. Arwood R, Hammond J, Ward GG: Ammonia inhalation. *J Trauma* 25:444, 1983.
25. Pike J, Patterson A Jr, Arons MS: Chemistry of cement burns: Pathogenesis and treatment. *J Burn Care Rehabil* 9:258, 1988.
26. Stuzin JM: Phenol peeling and the history of phenol peeling. *Clin Plast Surg* 25:1, 1998.
27. Harris JC, Rumack BH, Peterson RG, McGuire BM: Methemoglobinemia resulting from absorption of nitrates. *JAMA* 242:2869, 1979.
28. Kirby NG: Sodium nitrate poisoning treated by exchange transfusions. *Lancet* 1:594, 1955.
29. Hansbrough JF, et al: Hydrocarbon contact injuries. *J Trauma* 24:250, 1985.
30. Simpson LA, Cruse CW: Gasoline immersion injury. *Plast Reconstr Surg* 67:54, 1981.
31. Clare RA, Krenzelok EP: Chemical burns secondary to elemental metal exposure: Two case reports. *Am J Emerg Med* 6:355, 1988.
32. Lillibridge SR, Sidell FR: *A Report on the Casualties from the Tokyo Subway Incident by the US Medical Team.* Atlanta, Centers for Disease Control and Prevention, 1995.
33. United Nations Security Council: Report of the Specialists Appointed by the Secretary General to Investigate Allegations by the Islamic Republic of Iran Concerning the Use of Chemical Weapons (UN Report No. S/16433). New York, United Nations, 1986.
34. Department of Defense: Report to Congress: Domestic Preparedness Program in the Defense against Weapons of Mass Destruction. Washington, DC, Department of Defense, 1997.
35. Federal Emergency Management Agency: Federal Response Plan. FEMA 229(11), 1997.
36. Brismar B, Bergenwald L: The terrorist bomb explosion in Bologna, Italy, 1980: An analysis of the effects and injuries sustained. *J Trauma* 22:216, 1982.
37. Brennan RJ, Waeckerle JF, Sharp TW, Lillibridge SR: Chemical warfare agents: Emergency medical and emergency public health issue. *Ann Emerg Med* 34:191, 1999.
38. Borak J, Sidell FR: Agents of chemical warfare: Sulfur mustard. *Ann Emerg Med* 21:303, 1992.
39. Wyatt JP, Allister CA: Occupational phosgene poisoning: A case report and review. *J Accid Emerg Med* 12:212, 1995.
40. Turrina S, Neri C, De Leo D: Effect of combined exposure to carbon monoxide and cyanides in selected forensic cases. *J Clin Forensic Med* 11:262, 2004.
41. Kavidar H, Adams SC: Treatment of chemical and biological warfare injuries: Insights derived from the 1984 Iraqi attack on Majnoon Island. *Mil Med* 4:171, 1991.
42. Slater MS, Trunkey DD: Terrorism in America: An evolving threat. *Arch Surg* 132:159, 1997.

Section V **VIOLENCE AND ABUSE**

CHAPTER

62 Injury Prevention and Control

Stephen W. Hargarten and Jeffrey W. Runge

PERSPECTIVE

The science of injury control is based on the model of injury, or trauma, as a disease rather than the consequence of fate or random occurrences. The principles of disease control are applied to injury as they have been applied successfully to infectious diseases. Although this model has achieved wide acceptance in the public health community, it depends on acceptance by the medical community for success.[1,2] Control of a disease this widespread can be achieved only through broad interdisciplinary effort, including that of medicine, public health, policy makers, law enforcement, and an educated citizenry (Box 62-1).

Emergency medicine plays a pivotal role in the care of injured patients and in injury control. One third of all emergency department visits are for the care of

BOX 62-1. Scientific Approach to Injury Control: Prevention, Acute Care, and Rehabilitation

Prevention
- Epidemiology—understanding the patterns of disease
- Biomechanics—understanding how the agent interacts with the host
- Public and patient education
- Public policy and law enforcement
- Engineering enhancements to the vector and the environment
- Outcome studies of prevention interventions
- Emergency preparedness

Acute Care
- Trauma system development, including surge capacity for disasters
- Emergency medical services medical direction
- Triage protocols—matching the injuries to the source of care
- Emergency care
- Definitive in-hospital care
- Outcome studies of trauma care

Rehabilitation
- Short-term
- Long-term
- Long-term outcome studies

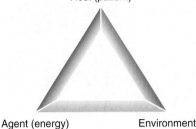

INJURY TRIANGLE

Host (patient)

Agent (energy)   Environment

Figure 62-1. An injury occurs by the interaction of the host and agent with an environment conducive to injury. Alteration of any of these interactions prevents the injury.

injuries.[3,4] Injury is the leading cause of death for many age groups (Table 62-1). Each year, one in four Americans is injured severely enough to seek medical attention.[5,6] An estimated 23 to 28 million people are annually treated in emergency departments for injuries, of which 90% are not admitted to the hospital.[3,7] The emergency physician may be the patient's only interface with the health care system. In addition to providing state-of-the-art acute care, this is also an opportunity for emergency medicine to take a leadership role, with state-of-the-art clinical preventive services for these injured patients,[8,9] working with surgeons, pediatricians, and colleagues in other specialties to decrease injuries through clinical and policy-relevant research and education.[10]

PRINCIPLES OF THE DISEASE OF INJURY

Injury is a harmful event caused by the acute transfer of energy to a patient that results in tissue and organ damage.[11] Acute injuries also include the absence of energy and hypothermia and hyperthermia. The major injury events include falls, car crashes, gunshots, drowning, and poisonings. The energy may be in various forms (kinetic, chemical, thermal, radiation, and electrical) and usually involves a vehicle of transmission, such as a car or a gun. Injury is similar to other diseases in which the interaction between the agent and the host in an environment conducive to exposure results in the disease (Figure 62-1). In this model, energy is the agent that is delivered to the host (victim) by a vehicle of transmission in an environment with increased risk. Likewise, injury control is similar to other forms of disease control, with the goal of preventing or attenuating the transfer of energy to the host by several methods: separating the host from the agent through modification of the environment, equipping the host with protection against the agent, or eliminating or modifying the vector that transmits the energy.[12-17]

The first step in the control of injuries is the recognition that injury is a disease. Common public perception is that injuries are accidents or random and unexpected events, similar to the way infectious disease was regarded before the discovery of bacteria. Using the disease model of injury is a prerequisite to a scientific approach to addressing the problem. Kinetic energy accounts for the overwhelming number of injuries, encountered through interactions with motorized vehicles, firearms, piercing or blunt instruments, and falls. Similar to other diseases, characteristics of the host affect prevention strategies, acute care, and rehabilitation outcomes. These include physical characteristics, such as age, gender, size, and motor skills, and mental and behavioral characteristics, such as intelligence, fatigue, alcohol use and abuse, emotional lability, social norms, and lifestyle. Risk for injury and death vary by age (see Table 62-1), and interventions for decreasing injury should be age-specific. To decrease the likelihood of an injury, changes in some of these predisposing factors can be made in the host (e.g., through improvement in driving skills).

Energy is transmitted to the host through a *vehicle,* such as motorized and nonmotorized vehicles (i.e., bicycles, skateboards), firearms, piercing instruments, explosives, and cigarettes. Modifying the vehicle by elimination or modification of design and separating the vector from the host are important methods of injury reduction and control. Understanding the biomechanical forces released during an injury event is crucial to understanding vehicle modification.[18-20]

For an injury to occur, host-agent interaction and energy transmission take place in an *environment.* Environmental modifications are effective means of injury control. If the environment does not permit energy transmission, the risk for injury, including intentional injuries to the host (victim), is reduced.[21] In contrast to altering host risk factors, environmental

Table 62-1. Injuries, Including Motor Vehicle Crashes as a Leading Cause of Death in the United States, 2001

Rank	Infants 1	Toddlers 1-3	Young Children 4-7	Children 8-15	Youth 16-20	Young Adults 21-24	Other Adults 25-34	35-44	45-64	Elderly ≥65	All Ages	Years of Life Lost
1	Perinatal period 13,734	Congenital anomalies, 496	MV traffic crashes, 533	MV traffic crashes, 1546	MV traffic crashes, 5979	MV traffic crashes, 4136	MV traffic crashes, 6759	Malignant neoplasms, 16,569	Malignant neoplasms, 139,785	Heart disease, 582,730	Heart disease, 700,142	Malignant neoplasms, 23% (8,614,131)
2	Congenital anomalies, 5513	MV traffic crashes, 421	Malignant neoplasms, 400	Malignant neoplasms, 829	Homicide, 2414	Homicide, 2738	Homicide, 5204	Heart disease, 13,326	Heart disease, 98,885	Malignant neoplasms, 390,214	Malignant neoplasms, 553,768	Heart disease, 22% (8,110,571)
3	Heart disease, 479	Accidental drowning, 393	Exposure to smoke/fire, 178	Suicide, 447	Suicide, 1879	Suicide, 1924	Suicide, 5070	MV traffic crashes, 6891	Stroke, 15,518	Stroke, 144,486	Stroke, 163,538	MV traffic crashes, 5% (1,700,952)
4	Homicide, 332	Homicide, 362	Congenital anomalies, 168	Homicide, 391	Malignant neoplasms, 814	Accidental poisoning, 771	Malignant neoplasms, 3994	Suicide, 6635	Diabetes, 14,913	Chronic lower resp. dis., 106,904	Chronic lower resp. dis., 123,013	Stroke, 5% (1,687,683)
5	Septicemia, 312	Malignant neoplasms, 321	Accidental drowning, 164	Congenital anomalies, 324	Accidental poisoning, 566	Malignant neoplasms, 768	Heart disease, 3160	HIV, 5867	Chronic lower resp. dis., 14,490	Influenza/pneumonia, 55,518	Diabetes, 71,372	Chronic, lower resp. dis., 4% (1,444,745)
6	Influenza/pneumonia, 299	Heart disease, 200	Homicide, 133	Accidental drowning, 293	Heart disease, 398	Heart disease, 543	Accidental poisoning, 2507	Accidental poisoning, 5036	Chronic liver disease, 13,009	Diabetes, 53,707	Influenza/pneumonia, 62,034	Suicide, 3% (1,079,822)
7	MV traffic crashes, 139	Exposure to smoke/fire, 170	Heart disease, 82	Heart disease, 273	Accidental drowning, 326	Accidental drowning, 211	HIV, 2101	Homicide, 4268	Suicide, 9259	Alzheimer's, 53,245	Alzheimer's, 53,852	Perinatal period, 3% (1,070,154)
8	Nephritis/nephrosis, 133	Septicemia, 96	MV nontraffic crashes, 51	Exposure to smoke/fire, 140	Congenital anomalies, 244	Congenital anomalies, 206	Stroke, 601	Chronic liver disease, 3336	MV traffic crashes, 8750	Nephritis/nephrosis, 33,121	MV traffic crashes, 42,443	Diabetes, 3% (1,014,201)
9	Stroke, 108	Influenza/pneumonia, 92	Benign neoplasms, 46	MV nontraffic crashes, 125	Accidental falls, 114	HIV, 167	Diabetes, 595	Stroke, 2491	HIV, 5437	Septicemia, 25,418	Nephritis/nephrosis, 39,480	Homicide, 3% (924,263)
10	Meningitis, 78	Perinatal period, 63	Septicemia, 33	Chronic lower resp. dis., 102	Acc. dischg. of firearms, 114	Accidental falls, 134	Congenital anomalies, 458	Diabetes, 1958	Nephritis/nephrosis, 5106	Hypertension renal dis., 16,397	Septicemia, 32,238	Chronic liver disease, 2% (623,998)
All	27,568	4288	2703	6672	15,851	14,940	41,683	91,674	412,204	1,798,420	2,416,425	All causes, 100% (36,866,317)

MV, motor vehicle.
From National Center for Statistics and Analysis, Subramanian R: Motor Vehicle Crashes as a Leading Cause of Death in the United States, 2001 (DOT HS 809 695). Washington, DC, National Highway Traffic Safety Administration, 2003.

Table 62-2. Haddon's Strategies for Preventing the Transfer of Energy to the Host

Technique	Car Crash	Falls
1. Prevent the initial marshalling of energy	Manual task/Breathalyzer ignition interlocks Use of alternative transportation	Remove floor obstacles Prevent unnecessary climbing
2. Reduce the amount of energy marshaled	Speed reduction Vehicle mass restrictions	Climbing height restrictions
3. Prevent the release of energy	Breakaway light poles, roadway obstacle removal	Ambulation aids for elderly Worker safety harnesses
4. Modify the rate of spatial distribution of the release of energy from its source	Autobody crumple zones Safety belts, air bags Water barrel barriers	Land with a "roll" Use of safety nets
5. Separate the energy from the host in space or time	Reduce traffic density Homogeneous traffic flow Increase following distance Sidewalks for pedestrians	Safety zones at edge of raised work areas
6. Separate the energy from the host by barrier	Guardrails, concrete median barriers	Guardrails for scaffolds, raised work areas
7. Modify the surface or structure of impact	Collapsible steering columns, padded pillars and bolsters, safety glass	Padded flooring Helmets and hard hats
8. Strengthen the host receiving the energy	Detect and treat premorbid medical conditions	Prevent/treat osteoporosis and strengthen hip flexion in elderly patients
9. Rapidly detect and evaluate damage and counter its continuation and extension	911 and EMS availability Trauma systems planning and implementations, and provision of state-of-the-art emergency care	911 and EMS availability Trauma systems planning and implementation, and provision of state-of-the-art emergency care
10. Reparative and rehabilitative measures	Provision of state-of-the-art trauma care, rehabilitation, and aftercare	Provision of state-of-the-art trauma care, rehabilitation, and aftercare

modifications require no cooperation or action on the part of the host and are more effective when implemented. Examples are safer road design and lighting, removal of throw rugs and raised thresholds from the homes of elderly persons, and separating bicycle paths and sidewalks from the roadway.[16,22]

William Haddon,[23] the first physician administrator for the National Highway Traffic Safety Commission, described this approach in a landmark article on injury control in 1970. Any type or cluster of injuries can be prevented or reduced in severity using this matrix when the environment, vector, and population most at risk are identified. Examples for reducing car crash injuries are given in Table 62-2. The key to energy transfer reduction or prevention is understanding that injuries are predictable, following age, gender, and other related patterns, and that relying solely on human factors for prevention has significant limits. A fragile item sent through the mail arrives at its destination intact only if it is properly packaged to reduce the energy we anticipate being delivered to the package. Likewise, injuries to people can be prevented by using the cells of Haddon's method to mitigate the energy transfer of predictable events. A simple analysis of the injury event using Haddon's method for any injured patient seen in the emergency department provides an example for generating individual and population-based prevention strategies.[24]

Injury and Public Health

Since 1900, there have been an estimated 2 million injury deaths and hundreds of millions of injuries in the United States.[25] The avoidance of personal injury is a goal of modern public health, but until the 1940s and

1950s, unintentional injuries were attributed primarily to human error, and prevention was based on educating people to act safely.[13] Unsafe roads were built. Motorized vehicles and other consumer products were manufactured with safety design flaws.[26] Using the disease model, this would be similar to supplying contaminated tap water in homes and relying on the education of people to purify their own drinking water.[14]

In the 1920s, attributing vehicle crashes to poor driver performance led to mandatory licensing of drivers. In the 1930s, when it was realized that vehicle crashes were due to human error and mechanical factors, President Roosevelt called for automobiles to be made more crashworthy.[15] In 1942, DeHaven, a former World War I pilot turned physiologist, pondering over his own survival in an airplane crash when another occupant had been killed, suggested structural provisions be made to vehicles that would distribute the forces of energy over the human body to attenuate injury in crashes. He advocated a focus on defining the physical factors that influence survival rather than the human error that caused the crash.[15] Physical factors became a focus of interest as the United States embarked on its space program. Air Force researchers, led by Stapp and Gell,[27] showed that people could withstand splashdown with a sled that decelerates from 30 to 0 mph over a stopping distance of 2 feet. This demonstration was considered to be a significant advance in understanding of the biomechanics of sudden deceleration.

The recognition that injuries could be addressed similar to diseases began in the 1940s, when Gordon, an epidemiologist, suggested that injuries have epidemic patterns, seasonal variation, long-term trends, and demographic distribution and can be examined

Table 62-3. Typical Haddon Matrix (Constructed for Motor Vehicle Injury)

	Host	Agent/Vector	Environment
Pre-event	Alcohol use Fatigue Experience and judgment Vision Amount of travel Stature Medications Motor skills Cognitive function	Brake condition Tire quality Center of gravity Jackknife tendency Ease of control Load weight Speed capacity Ergonomic controls Mirrors Visual obstructions	Visibility of hazards Road curvature and gradient Shoulder height Surface coefficient of friction Divided highways, one-way streets Intersections, access control Weather Signalization Speed limits
Event	Safety belt use Age Gender Bone density Stature	Speed at impact Direction of impact Vehicle size Automatic restraints Air bag Character of contact surfaces Load containment Deformation zones Fuel system integrity	Impaired driving laws Speed limits of traffic Recovery areas Guard rails Characteristics of fixed objects Median barriers Roadside embankments
Postevent	Age Physical condition Medications Preexisting medical conditions Social situation		911 access EMS response Triage and transfer protocols EMS training Quality of emergency care Location of appropriate emergency department Access to definitive care Access to rehabilitation services

Adapted from Baker S, et al: *The Injury Fact Book*, 2nd ed. New York, Oxford University Press, 1992.

with methodologies applied to infectious diseases. Gordon also believed that, similar to infectious diseases, injury results from the interaction of the agent, the host, and the environment.[15] In the 1960s, Haddon developed a two-dimensional approach to injury analysis by dividing the factors of agent, host, and environment into three phases: preinjury, injury, and postinjury. This phase-factor matrix has become a mainstay of injury control and prevention development. Any injury event can be broken down into the component factors, allowing specific interventions to target specific factors (Table 62-3).[16,24]

In 1985, the publication *Injury in America: A Continuing Public Health Problem* by the National Research Council and the Institute of Medicine called on the public health and health care community to address the injury epidemic.[17] In the 1990s, the Secretary of Health and Department of Human Services developed a national plan for injury control.[2] The permanent establishment of the National Center for Injury Prevention and Control in the Centers for Disease Control and Prevention was an acknowledgment by the U.S. government that the control of injuries belongs in the disease control community, including health care providers such as emergency physicians.

Methods of Prevention

The evolution of injury control and prevention began as soon as the first injury occurred. The pain of injury is still a powerful stimulus for avoidance behaviors. Early prevention technology is seen in the instruments and garb of the earliest armies, shielding people from the delivery of harmful kinetic energy by instruments of early warfare. Such technology included helmets, shields, and suits of armor. As the human ability to deliver kinetic energy became more sophisticated, prevention technology did not keep pace.[19,20] The invention of firearms and the automobile represented new plateaus in people's ability to harness kinetic energy for use.[28,29] The cultural belief was that individuals could avoid vehicular injury by safe driving, and if not, an "accident" occurred. It took more than 50 years after the invention of the automobile for policy makers to acknowledge that behavior modification alone is insufficient to mitigate high-energy transmission to persons in a hazardous environment. Cars were not uniformly equipped with seat belts until the 1960s.[29] It took another 2 decades before air bags became standard safety features in cars, despite rapid advancements in understanding energy delivery and dissipation in motor vehicle crashes in the 1950s.[19,20,30]

Implementation of effective injury control and prevention strategies depends on collaborative efforts with health care providers (e.g., emergency physicians, surgeons, and pediatricians), epidemiologists, biomechanical engineers, public policy makers, law enforcement officers, and members of the legal profession.[22,30,31] A major challenge is the wide diversity of disciplines and interests involved in safety and injury control, many of which are isolated from one another.[13] In the 1990s, important strides were made in community-based injury prevention and control programs that rely on coalitions of existing resources with the support of the National Highway Traffic Safety Administration (NHTSA), the Centers for Disease Control and Prevention, and the State and Territorial Injury Prevention Directors Association. These community coalitions were created to garner existing resources and implement injury countermeasures using the triad of public education, enforcement of laws, and engineering modification of hazardous devices and environmental conditions.[22]

INJURY CONTROL IN MEDICAL PRACTICE

Physicians traditionally have focused on treating the patient after the disease has occurred. As the causes of many diseases have become increasingly understood, education about risk assessment and clinically based prevention have been integrated into medical practice, particularly in areas such as infectious (immunizations) and cardiovascular (smoking cessation) disease. Emergency physicians are incorporating risk assessment, counseling, and referral of patients in high-risk groups for injury, such as with domestic violence patients.[8] The Joint Commission for Hospital Accreditation has been instrumental in addressing injury prevention through emergency department requirements for domestic violence patients.

Emergency physicians and nurses are pivotal in the recording and accumulation of data about the injury event, which become useful for epidemiologic analysis of the disease in the community, region, and state. Injury control techniques can be incorporated easily into emergency medicine practice as well.[32-35] A rational approach to improve trauma care in a community (Box 62-2) requires that emergency physicians, surgeons, pediatricians, and physiatrists, as the physicians primarily responsible for patients with injuries, assume specific roles and activities in promoting injury control. Documentation of injury information in the medical record, assessing risk factors in individual patients, counseling and referral, provision of systematized acute trauma care, and public heath advocacy all are important in the practice of injury control.[36-38]

Injury Epidemiology and Documentation

Gathering accurate data is essential to the science of injury control. To understand the characteristics of a disease—its endemic populations, cyclical variations, geographic characteristics, and effectiveness of interventions—consistent and comprehensive data must be gathered across the population of injured patients. Data may be used for research,[39,40] implying an in-depth examination of a particular question or for surveillance, which is the ongoing monitoring of disease patterns and characteristics.[35,41] The goal of injury data collection is to discover who is being injured, what is injuring them, and the circumstances surrounding the injury.[42,43]

Until more recently, good data on the disease of injury have been lacking, and gaps still exist.[44] Before

1980, the only large civilian databases on injury available for study were mortality data collected by coroners and medical examiners. The Fatal Analysis Reporting System, a comprehensive dataset on all car crash deaths in the United States, was established by the National Highway Safety Administration in 1975.[45] It has been a useful tool for examining the epidemiology of car crashes and has been used by injury control researchers for examining important questions.[39]

Because death results in only 1 in 1000 people who receive medical care for an injury, many conclusions based solely on mortality data are limited.[3,25] The advent of trauma registries in the 1980s increased the sample from the 0.1% of patients who die to a larger proportion of patients admitted for injury (i.e., patients admitted to trauma centers). Mortality data and patients receiving care in trauma centers are skewed toward the most severe injuries, however, and epidemiologic conclusions based on those data are important but have limitations.[46]

Approximately 90% of injured patients seeking medical care for injury are treated and discharged from the emergency department, many of whom experience significant morbidity resulting in long-term disability and significant cost to society.[3,25,35,41] In recognition of the importance to the national health care agenda, the Centers for Disease Control and Prevention has developed Data Elements for Emergency Department Systems to define the minimum data essential to the understanding of the disease for physicians and information systems developers.[47,48] The most crucial data element for the understanding of injury is the *E code*. The E-code is a system for identifying the cause of injury in a patient's medical record, according to a classification published in the *International Classification of Diseases (ICD-9-CM).*[22] The "E" stands for external cause of injury, such as car crash, fall, or bicycle crash. The causes of injury in a population cannot be extracted from diagnosis codes in medical records. These are "N" codes—the nature of the injury, such as skull fracture, laceration, or contusion. Because injury prevention depends on identifying the etiologic agent/vehicle causing injuries and not the end result, the only way to accomplish this systematically is by E-coding patient visits. Some states now have E-coded all emergency department discharges, and these statewide data are useful for injury control and prevention program development and evaluation.[35,41]

The notion that E-coding is expensive has been dispelled, and visits should be able to be coded easily in the emergency department.[42,43] The greatest barrier to the collection of E codes in the emergency department is the lack of adequate physician documentation to assign an accurate E code retrospectively from the medical record.[3,49,50] The first step in data gathering is to document completely and legibly the cause of injury on patient records. With cause of injury recorded, injuries in a given population can be examined by emergency physicians and others. Because injury problems in a community differ greatly from region to region, community-specific injury control efforts can be generated, implemented, and evaluated.[22,40]

E-coded hospital records can provide the *who, what,* and *when* of injury. The question of *where* can be either place of occurrence or place of residence, both of which are important and have implications for planned countermeasures. Hospital records are helpful in determining place of residence of injured patients, which is useful for community education in high-risk neighborhoods. Location-of-injury data are available only from other sources, such as emergency medical services (EMS), police, or traffic engineering. These data are more likely to be useful for environmental modification through engineering enhancements, police enforcement, or hazard removal. Linkage of these records to patient visits, either manually for specific research studies or electronically for surveillance, is the next step in gaining a comprehensive understanding of the epidemiology of injury.[51,52] Statewide injury data linkages exist in some states and are available for surveillance information[53] and research and for unintentional and intentional injuries.[7,33,40]

Interest and opportunity to apply injury control principles are growing for medical injuries. Medical injuries account for an estimated 50,000 to 98,000 deaths each year in the United States, with hundreds of thousands of nonfatal events occurring in emergency departments, intensive care units, and operating rooms.[44] Emergency physicians have begun to assume leadership roles in addressing this important area of injuries.[54,55] Application of injury control principles for the identification of injury patterns and for the development and evaluation of injury prevention strategies has great potential but has received limited attention.[56,57] Emergency physicians can play an important role in using injury control principles and science for reducing medical injuries.

Risk Factor Assessment

Biomechanical Risk Factors

Biomechanical factors responsible for the injury event are challenging to understand fully, occurring in car crashes in less than a tenth of a second. Emergency physicians are not trained in engineering principles and have had limited exposure to this "pathophysiology" during medical school or residency training. Ascertaining the forces released to the patient during a blunt (car crash, fall) or penetrating (gunshot, stabbing) injury event leads to a directed approach to injury management. Contrast this scientific evidence-based approach with the practice of obtaining cervical spine radiographs for any patient with a head strike of any severity.[58-61] Extensive research has been done using crash dummies, mathematical models, and computer models to understand the mechanical forces applied in injury events and human impact tolerance.[19,20] Although used extensively by the engineering community for design of products, such knowledge also is valuable to the trauma physician in guiding evaluation and treatment based on energy transfer, tissue tolerance, and risk of occult injury.[11]

Injury occurs when energy is delivered to the host in levels that exceed tissue and organ tolerance. This energy can be expressed in G forces. The G force that results from a motor vehicle crash, for instance, can be expressed using the following formula:

$$G = \frac{\Delta V^2}{\text{Stopping distance} \times k}$$

In this equation, ΔV is the change in velocity, *stopping distance* is the distance over which the change in velocity occurs, and k is a constant. G force is inversely related to stopping distance. To minimize energy transfer to the body during a car crash, one must maximize the stopping distance during the event. The formula shows that doubling the stopping distance reduces the G force by half, but doubling the speed quadruples the force. Less G force is applied as velocity is reduced over increasing distance, which allows the restrained occupant to "ride down" with the vehicle as it slows during preimpact braking or as it deforms during a crash. The same principle underlies engineering features, such as interior padding and collapsible steering columns, water barrel barriers at bridge abutments, and flexible guardrails, all designed to increase stopping distance. This principle is a major underpinning of automobile and highway safety engineering.[19,20,62]

The addition of the air bag in the mid-1980s was a significant improvement in safety engineering by increasing occupant stopping distance during a crash. The NHTSA estimates that 10,271 lives have been saved by air bags 2002.[63] Although these benefits have been largely confined to frontal crashes, increasing stopping distance and reducing head deceleration in side impacts through the use of side curtain air bags are expected to save hundreds of lives per year when fully deployed in the fleet.

As with many newly developed safety countermeasures, there were unintended consequences of air bags in the 1990s. First-generation air bags deployed with tremendous force to protect unbelted occupants. These early air bags deployed aggressively at speed of 140 to 200 mph over about 50 msec.[64] Such forces can be lethal to children seated in the front passenger seat, especially when unrestrained by safety belts, or infants seated in rear-facing infant seats exposed to the front seat air bag.[65,66] The NHTSA has documented 149 children killed as a result of air-bag deployment as of 2003.[63] A new generation of advanced, less aggressive air bags has been used in the vehicle fleet since the late 1990s, which is expected to reduce injuries associated with air-bag deployment. For an emergency physician to estimate risk when assessing a patient from a motor vehicle crash, it is essential to understand the differences in risk posed by seating position, restraint type and use, and vehicle type. This information also must be understood to counsel patients properly on safety belt and child restraint use.[39,67]

Understanding mechanisms of injury leads to more effective patient counseling to protect patients and their families against injury. Children less than 55 inches tall should ride in only the rear seats of vehicles. Infant seats should never be positioned in the front seat within range of the air bag. Infants 12 months old and younger and weighing 20 lb or less should always ride in a rear-facing infant seat, and children older than 12 months and weighing more than 20 lb should ride forward facing in a convertible or toddler seat. A booster seat should be used for children weighing 40 to 80 lb, allowing for better seat belt positioning and discouraging the child from sitting out of position to see out the windows. If circumstances dictate that a smaller child must ride in the front passenger seat, that seat should be positioned as far to the rear as possible and a seat belt should always be worn.[67] Federal rules from the U.S. Department of Transportation allow for air bags to be disabled if there are circumstances necessitating that small children ride in the front seat and for certain medical conditions.[68] Physicians caring for short-stature individuals should counsel these patients about the risk of air-bag injuries and recommend they sit with at least 10 inches between the sternum and the steering wheel equipped with an air bag. This distance should be measured objectively because people tend not to estimate this distance correctly.[69]

Other safety features have been associated with specific injuries. Automatic "passive" shoulder belts that require manual fastening of the lap portion may result in "submarining" of the torso toward the floorboard when the lap portion is not fastened, while the shoulder belt squeezes the lower rib cage. Such a mechanism explains the association of these devices with liver, spleen, and lung injuries.[70]

Knowing the contact surface in fall injuries may guide diagnostic and therapeutic interventions because soft, forgiving surfaces increase stopping distance compared with concrete or packed earth.[19,20] Understanding the biomechanical risks of other injuries, such as tissue forces from the ballistics of bullet wounds, can guide treatment decisions.[18,71]

Behavioral and Comorbid Risk Factors

Recognition of patients at high risk of injury affords opportunity for intervention. Counseling a patient about specific ways to avoid injury in the "teachable moment" after injury is more likely to have an effect than diffuse public education.[72] Family or friends can be recruited to enforce the message to patients or to assist patients in modifying their behavior or environment. Other patient encounters may be used as an opportunity to counsel high-risk patients, such as children at developmental stages that put them at risk for auto-pedestrian injuries, climbing injuries, or poisoning. It is particularly important to explore the circumstances surrounding injuries to children. A brief review of the injury incident would help physicians and parents identify risks for future injury and opportunities for intervention.[73] Children who come to the emergency department for an injury are likely to be injured again, commonly during falls and motor vehicle crashes.[74] When injury admissions in preschool-age children were examined for previous emergency department visits, children admitted to the hospital for trauma were twice as likely as community controls to have been treated previously in the emergency department for injury and more likely to have been in the emergency department more than once.[75]

Risk factors for intentional injury are complex and involve behavioral, social, and environmental factors. Risk factors vary by type of trauma, but risks for all types are higher for people in the following categories: male, low income, illicit drug involvement, previous arrest, and young age.[75-77] In studies using psychosocial inventories, recidivists are more likely to have a low sense of autonomy, to have low levels of spirituality, and to have been a victim of crime in the past.[75] As a practical matter in the emergency department, the most obvious risk factor for future violent injury is having had prior violent injury. A history of prior significant trauma is a strong predictor of trauma recidivism, with 10 times the risk of patients with no prior trauma.[77,78] Emergency departments should have protocols in place for the detection and referral of patients likely to be victims of trauma in the future, including victims of domestic violence,[8] and for children younger than 18 years injured intentionally, regardless of the age of the perpetrator. In many states in the United States, there are mandatory reporting laws for gunshot wounds, stabbing, and other violent acts. Physicians should be familiar with local laws regarding reporting to law enforcement.[79,80]

In the case of motor vehicle injury, the three behavioral risk factors most likely to result in future crash are speeding, seat belt nonuse, and driving after drinking alcohol. Giving patients the necessary data for them to make an accurate self-assessment about their risks is the essence of patient behavioral intervention.[81] These messages can be delivered during, and should be part of, every injury patient encounter, when it is feasible. Particularly important in this context is the screening and referral for alcohol use disorders (AUDs). Alcohol-related crash injury is a national epidemic in the

United States, claiming more than 17,000 lives annually and injuring an estimated 870,000 persons.[82] The reductions in alcohol-related deaths seen in the 1980s and 1990s have been due to more stringent laws to curb impaired driving, more vigilant public education, and a societal shift toward the condemnation of driving while impaired as socially undesirable. These changes have not had significant effects on people with AUD, however. Of patients seen in the emergency department after a motor vehicle crash, 17% to 20% meet criteria for AUD.[83,84] Patients with AUD have higher rates of illness and motor vehicle crash injury than the rest of the population, and patients with AUD are more likely to drive after drinking.[79]

Emergency physicians have a unique role to play in the identification of high-risk patients. In particular, patients with AUD should be detected and referred for formal evaluation and treatment. A structured approach to these patients is necessary to detect and treat the disease and must be brief and effective if it is to be used in a busy emergency department. Screening techniques validated in the emergency department and methods of brief intervention are described thoroughly.[79]

Successfully treating AUD leads to reductions in alcohol consumption and consequently fewer impaired driving episodes, which leads to a reduction in alcohol-related crash injuries. Evidence suggests that being treated for injury in the emergency department may be an important motivational opportunity to reduce drinking and presents a "teachable moment."[79,84-86]

Motor vehicle crashes are the leading cause of death for children older than 24 months in the United States (Table 62-4; see also Table 62-1). The risk of death in a motor vehicle crash can be reduced by half with the use of an age-appropriate child restraint. Emergency physicians should understand the various restraint types and recommendations for their use based on age, weight, and height. Every pediatric visit to the emergency department involves transportation to and from the emergency department. Every pediatric visit is an opportunity to counsel parents on the safe transport of their children.

The current recommendation by the NHTSA is that infants should be transported in a rear-facing infant seat in the back seat until they are 12 months old and weigh 20 lb. After reaching this milestone, children may be transported in forward-facing child restraints until they reach the weight limitation for the particular child restraint, usually about 40 lb and 4 years of age. Some child restraints may be designed to remain rear facing for longer periods, as is the practice in much of Europe. At 40 lb, children should be placed in a belt-positioning booster seat until the height of 57 inches or the auto manufacturer's recommendation for appropriate height for belt fit.

Acute Care

The acute care component of injury control involves trauma system planning, direction of out-of-hospital medical care, and provision of systematized resuscitative care after the injury event, whether it occurs close to or far from a trauma center.[87] A crucial part of injury assessment for the trauma physician is identification of local resources for management of the trauma patient. Algorithms and transfer agreements for referral of the patient to definitive care should be established, in the absence of a trauma system with defined triage and transfer protocols, to avoid the secondary injury that may occur from delays in transfer or inappropriate care.[88] Likewise, an environment with ready availability of trauma physician specialists should have clear protocols in place for use of those resources.[89] Cost-effective mobilization of trauma care resources dictates that in-hospital triage criteria be developed for the care of the injured patient to avoid the unneeded overuse of trauma surgery teams.[38,91]

In the early 1990s, less than 25% of the United States was served by an organized trauma system.[90] Trauma systems can be created that recognize and complement the exigencies of budgetary, geographic, and political constraints that are specific to states or regions. Such flexibility is often impossible when a trauma system is based only on the locations of hospitals that seek trauma center verification or designation.[91]

An *inclusive* trauma care system is one that comprises all acute care and rehabilitation facilities that treat injured patients and deals with the issues of community access, EMS dispatch and response, triage, transport and transfer protocols, training, communications, availability of definitive care and rehabilitation, and a data collection system. In an inclusive trauma care system, every injured patient, not only patients who live near trauma centers, is cared for by a part of the system. Every hospital has a part in an inclusive trauma system according to the services it is capable of offering, whether it is the expeditious transfer of patients, the treatment of patients without neuro-trauma, or the definitive care provided at a trauma center. The system should be designed to monitor patient outcomes and system performance.[92]

Out-of-hospital care is an integral part of injury control.[37] EMS response, triage, and treatment are the first critical steps in damage control after an injury event has occurred. Triage protocols must be well established to avoid unnecessary delays in definitive care.[88] EMS providers have a unique vantage point to help the trauma physician assess a patient's risk factors for immediate injuries and the risk of injury recurrence. EMS providers can observe the environment for information about mechanism of injury. Accurately reporting vehicle damage and other environmental circumstances associated with the injury event elucidates important biomechanical risk factors.[93] EMS providers also have become more involved in primary injury prevention, through injury risk identification, documentation of injury data, and safety education programs.[37]

Emergency Medicine Leadership: Advocacy of Public Policy

Passing and enforcing laws are more effective than education in effecting individual behavior change for

Table 62-4. Ten Leading Causes of Injury Deaths by Age Group, 2000

Rank	<1	1-4	5-9	10-14	15-24	25-34	35-44	45-54	55-64	≥65	All Ages
1	Unintentional suffocation, 526	Unintentional MV traffic, 563	Unintentional MV traffic, 731	Unintentional MV traffic, 916	Unintentional MV traffic, 10,323	Unintentional MV traffic, 6716	Unintentional MV traffic, 6757	Unintentional MV traffic, 5210	Unintentional MV traffic, 3372	Unintentional fall, 10,273	Unintentional MV traffic, 41,994
2	Unintentional MV traffic, 162	Unintentional drowning, 493	Unintentional drowning, 201	Unintentional drowning, 174	Homicide firearm, 3963	Homicide firearm, 3074	Unintentional poisoning, 4663	Unintentional poisoning, 3061	Suicide firearm, 1833	Unintentional MV traffic, 7218	Suicide firearm, 16,586
3	Homicide other spec., classifiable, 129	Unintentional fire/burn, 297	Unintentional fire/burn, 183	Suicide suffocation, 168	Suicide firearm, 2267	Suicide firearm, 2453	Suicide firearm, 3191	Suicide firearm, 2858	Unintentional fall, 949	Unintentional unspecified, 5364	Unintentional fall, 13,322
4	Homicide unspecified, 125	Unintentional suffocation, 151	Homicide firearm, 50	Homicide firearm, 137	Unintentional poisoning, 1160	Unintentional poisoning, 2380	Homicide firearm, 1906	Suicide poisoning, 1303	Unintentional poisoning, 688	Suicide firearm, 3869	Unintentional poisoning, 12,757
5	Unintentional drowning, 75	Homicide unspecified, 126	Unintentional suffocation, 45	Suicide firearm, 110	Suicide suffocation, 1134	Suicide suffocation, 1252	Suicide poisoning, 1465	Homicide firearm, 959	Suicide poisoning, 531	Unintentional suffocation, 3353	Homicide firearm, 10,801
6	Unintentional fire/burn, 39	Unintentional pedestrian, other, 97	Unintentional other land transport, 43	Unintentional fire/burn, 84	Unintentional drowning, 646	Suicide poisoning, 746	Suicide suffocation, 1381	Unintentional fall, 871	Unintentional suffocation, 412	Adverse effects, 2050	Unintentional unspecified, 6673
7	Undetermined suffocation, 36	Homicide other spec., classifiable, 74	Unintentional pedestrian, other, 33	Unintentional other land transport, 80	Homicide cut/pierce, 409	Undetermined poisoning, 475	Undetermined poisoning, 1048	Suicide suffocation, 843	Unintentional fire/burn, 380	Unintentional fire/burn, 1205	Suicide suffocation, 5688
8	Homicide suffocation, 26	Homicide other spec., NEC, 48	Unintentional natural/environment, 20	Unintentional suffocation, 72	Suicide poisoning, 304	Homicide cut/pierce, 420	Unintentional fall, 608	Undetermined poisoning, 637	Adverse effects, 376	Unintentional natural/environment, 764	Unintentional suffocation, 5648
9	Unintentional unspecified, 24	Unintentional fall, 36	Homicide other spec., NEC, 19	Unintentional firearm, 49	Unintentional other land transport, 279	Unintentional drowning, 419	Unintentional drowning, 480	Unintentional fire/burn, 446	Homicide firearm, 367	Unintentional poisoning, 707	Suicide poisoning, 4859
10	Homicide other spec., NEC 20	Unintentional natural/environment, 33	Unintentional struck by or against, 19	Unintentional pedestrian, other, 36	Unintentional fall, 237	Unintentional fall, 303	Homicide cut/pierce, 466	Unintentional suffocation, 396	Suicide suffocation, 343	Suicide suffocation, 560	Unintentional fire/burn, 3187

MV, motor vehicle; NEC, not elsewhere classified.
Source: National Center for Health Statistics (NCHS), Vital Statistics System.
Produced by Office of Statistics and Programming, National Center for Injury Prevention and Control, CDC.

increasing safety actions such as seat belt and helmet usage.[15,30] Emergency physicians and other trauma physicians, such as pediatricians, surgeons, and orthopedists, are well positioned to provide lawmakers with factual information coupled with the perspective of first-hand experience of the effects of injury. Effective prevention interventions and policies with documented cost savings are more likely to occur when sound, scientific studies are made available to policy makers.[94] Most public health regulations and traffic safety laws are under the jurisdiction of state legislatures and city and county governments. These policy makers are generally much more accessible to physicians and are in need of local expertise than policy makers at the federal level. Emergency physician leadership needs to accept its important advocacy role for reducing injuries and incorporate injury control as a professional activity.[10,95,96]

Community education aimed at people not yet injured may be effective when coming from an emergency physician. Emergency physicians are in a leadership role to deliver the message to school systems, the local housing authority, law enforcement, community service organizations, and policy makers.[33,34] Trauma physicians can be effective spokespersons for injury prevention through the news media, especially after a newsworthy injury event, and can reframe the event from one of personal blame and behavior failure to a broader biosocial issue that requires environmental and policy interventions.[97]

Public policy also determines where resources are used in a community. Environmental modifications and elimination of hazards are effective, but often expensive. In contrast to education and law enforcement, environmental modifications are *passive countermeasures,* in that they do not require any action by persons after they are in place. Such modifications might be lengthening a "walk" signal at a busy intersection to reduce auto-pedestrian injuries, especially in the elderly,[98] increasing lighting in areas where personal assaults occur,[21] or changing a playground surface from hard-packed earth to wood mulch.[99] The need for such modifications may be known only if the physician is alert to the circumstances by asking "How did this happen?" and documenting the location and circumstances of injuries seen in daily practice.

🔑 KEY CONCEPTS

- Injury is the second most costly disease to society and the most serious disease of young people.

- Through interdisciplinary research, a better understanding of the epidemiology and biomechanics of injury will lead to new prevention strategies. These strategies would complement advances in acute care and trauma systems, which improve care to the patient after the injury occurs.

- Emergency physicians can incorporate injury control techniques into daily practice.

- Emergency physicians are increasingly leaders in addressing and preventing injuries and complex biosocial problems.

REFERENCES

1. Teutsch SM: A framework for assessing the effectiveness of disease and injury prevention. *MMWR Morb Mortal Wkly Rep* 41:1, 1992.
2. Centers for Disease Control: *The National Agenda for Injury Control, 1992.* Atlanta, CDC, 1992.
3. Rice DP, et al: *Cost of Injury in the United States: A Report to Congress.* San Francisco, Institute for Health & Aging, University of California, and Injury Prevention Center, The Johns Hopkins University, 1989.
4. McCaig LF, Burt CW: National Hospital Ambulatory Medical Care Survey: 2001 Emergency Department Summary: Advance data from Vital and Health Statistics (No. 335). Hyattsville, Md, National Center for Health Statistics, 2003.
5. Baker SP, et al: *The Injury Fact Book.* New York, Oxford University Press, 1992.
6. Consumer Product Safety Commission National Electronic Injury Surveillance System (NEISS). Available at: http://www.cpsc.gov/cpscpub/pubs/3002.html.
7. Muelleman RL, et al: Missouri's emergency department E-code data reporting: A new level of data resource for injury prevention and control. *J Public Health Manage Pract* 3:8, 1997.
8. Krasnoff M, Moscati R: Domestic violence screening and referral can be effective. *Ann Emerg Med* 40:485, 2002.
9. Cortes L, Hargarten SW: Preventive care in the emergency department: A systematic literature review on emergency department-based interventions that address smoke detectors in the home. *Acad Emerg Med* 8:925, 2001.
10. Gruen RL, et al: Physician-citizens—public roles and professional obligations. *JAMA* 1:94, 2004.
11. Martinez R: Injury control: A primer for physicians. *Ann Emerg Med* 19:72, 1990.
12. Rosenberg M, Fenley MA: *Violence in America: A Public Health Approach.* New York, Oxford University Press, 1991.
13. National Committee for Injury Prevention and Control: *Injury Prevention: Meeting the Challenge.* Oxford, Oxford University Press, 1989.
14. Mohan D: *Injury Control and Safety Promotion: Ethics, Science and Practice.* New York, Taylor & Francis, 2000.
15. Robertson L: The problem, history and concepts. In: *Injury Epidemiology.* New York, Oxford University Press, 1992.
16. Haddon W: A logical framework for categorizing highway safety phenomenon and activity. *J Trauma* 12:193, 1972.
17. Committee on Trauma Research, Commission on Life Sciences, National Research Council, Institute of Medicine: *Injury in America: A Continuing Public Health Problem.* Washington, D.C., National Academy Press, 1985.
18. Yoganandan N, et al: Dynamic analysis of penetrating trauma. *J Trauma* 42:266, 1997.
19. Whiting WC, Zernicke RF: *Biomechanics of Musculoskeletal Injury.* Champaign, Ill, Human Kinetics, 1998.
20. Nahum AM, Melvin J (eds): *Accidental Injury: Biomechanics and Prevention,* 2nd ed. New York, Springer-Velag, 2001.
21. Mair JS, Mair M: Violence prevention and control through environmental modifications. *Annu Rev Public Health* 24:209, 2003.
22. Christoffel T, Gallagher S: *Injury Prevention and Public Health.* Gaithersburg, Md, Aspen, 1999.
23. Haddon W: On the escape of tigers: An ecologic note (strategy options in reducing losses in energy-damaged people and property). *MIT Technol Rev* 72:44, 1970.
24. Lambrecht CJ, Hargarten SW: Hunting-related injuries and deaths in Montana: The scope of the problem and a framework for prevention. *J Wilderness Med* 4:175, 1993.

25. Committee on Trauma Research, Commission on Life Science, National Research Council, Institute of Medicine: *Injury in America: A Continuing Public Health Problem.* Washington, D.C., National Academy Press, 1985.

26. Freed LH, Vernick JS, Hargarten SW: Prevention of firearms-related injuries and deaths among youth—a product orientated approach. *Pediatr Clin North Am* 45:427, 1998.

27. Stapp JP, Gell CF: Human exposure to linear declarative force in the backward and forward facing seated positions. *Milit Surg* 109:106, 1951.

28. Karlson T, Hargarten SW: *Reducing Injury and Death: A Public Health Sourcebook on Guns.* New Brunswick, NJ, Rutgers University Press, 1997.

29. Nader R: *Unsafe at Any Speed: The Designed-In Dangers of the American Automobile.* New York, Grossman, 1965.

30. Chistoffel T, Teret SP: *Protecting the Public: Legal Issues in Injury Prevention.* New York, Oxford University Press, 1993.

31. Rivara F, et al: *Injury Control: A Guide to Research and Program Evaluation.* Cambridge, Cambridge University Press, 2001.

32. Anglin D, Hutson HR, Kyriacou DN: Emergency medicine residents' perspectives on injury prevention. *Ann Emerg Med* 28:31, 1996.

33. Hargarten SW, Karlson T: Injury control: A crucial aspect of emergency medicine. *Emerg Med Clin North Am* 11:255, 1993.

34. Bernstein E, et al: The emergency physician's role in injury prevention. *Pediatr Emerg Care* 4:207, 1988.

35. Ribbeck BM, et al: Injury surveillance: A method for recording E codes for injured emergency department patients. *Ann Emerg Med* 21:37, 1992.

36. Rivara F, Thompson DC, Patterson MQ: Prevention of bicycle-related injuries: Helmets, education, and legislation. *Annu Rev Public Health* 19:293, 1998.

37. Garrison HG, et al: The role of emergency medical services in primary injury prevention. Consensus workshop, Arlington, Virginia, August 25-26, 1995. *Ann Emerg Med* 30:84, 1997.

38. Mann N, et al: Research recommendations and proposed action items to facilitate trauma system implementation and evaluation. *J Trauma* 47(Suppl):S75-S78, 1999.

39. Cummings P, Rivara F: Car occupant death according to the restraint use of other occupants: A matched cohort study. *JAMA* 291:343, 2004.

40. Runge J: Linking data for injury control research. *Ann Emerg Med* 35:613, 2000.

41. Wadman MC: The pyramid of injury—Using E-codes to accurately describe the burden of injury. *Ann Emerg Med* 42:468, 2003.

42. Sniezek JE, Finklea JF, Graitcer PL: Injury coding and hospital discharge data. *JAMA* 262:2270, 1989.

43. Muelleman RL, Hansen K, Sears W: Decoding the E-code. *Nebr Med J* 78:184, 1993.

44. Institute of Medicine: *To Err is Human: Building a Safer Health System.* Washington DC, National Academy Press, 1999.

45. National Highway Traffic Safety Administration, Office of Statistics and Analysis: *Fatal Accident Reporting System, 1975 Annual Report.* Washington, D.C., U.S. Department of Transportation, 1976.

46. Waller J: *Injury Control: A Guide to the Causes and Prevention of Trauma.* Lanham, Md, Lexington Books, DC Heath, 1995.

47. Centers for Disease Control and Prevention: *Data Elements for Emergency Department Systems (DEEDS).* Washington, D.C., U.S. Department of Health & Human Services, 1996.

48. Hirshon, JM, for the SAEM Public Health Task Force Preventive Care Project. The rationale for developing public health surveillance system based on emergency department data. *Acad Emerg Med* 7:1428, 2000.

49. Schwartz RJ, Nightingale BS, Jacobs LM: Accuracy of E-codes assigned to emergency department records. *Acad Emerg Med* 2:615, 1995.

50. Sheane K, Wright A, Bierlein LA: *A Comprehensive Statewide Injury Surveillance System: What Are the Issues?* Tempe, Ariz, Morrison Institute for Public Policy, 1995.

51. Johnson SW, Walker J: *The Crash Outcome Evaluation System (CODES)* (DOT HS 808 338). Washington, D.C., Department of Transportation, National Highway Traffic Safety Administration, 1996.

52. Hargarten SW, et al: Characteristics of firearms involved in fatalities. *JAMA* 275:42, 1996.

53. National Violent Injury Statistics System Work Group: *Violent Death Reporting System Training Manual.* Milwaukee, Wis, FIC & NVISS, 2002.

54. Adams JG, Bohan JS: System contributions to error. *Acad Emerg Med* 7:1189, 2000.

55. Kyriacou DN, Cohen JH: Errors in emergency medicine: Research strategies. *Acad Emerg Med* 7:1201, 2000.

56. Brasel KJ, et al: Evaluation of error in medicine: Application of a public health model. *Acad Emerg Med* 7:1298, 2000.

57. Layde PM, et al: Patient safety efforts should focus on medical injuries. *JAMA* 287:1993, 2002.

58. Norcross ED, et al: Application of American College of Surgeons' field triage guidelines by pre-hospital personnel. *J Am Coll Surg* 181:539, 1995.

59. Ryan GA, et al: Neck strain in car occupants: Injury status after 6 months and crash-related factors. *Injury* 25:533, 1994.

60. Velmahos GC, et al: Radiographic cervical spine evaluation in the alert asymptomatic blunt trauma victim: Much ado about nothing? *J Trauma* 40:768, 1996.

61. Ono K, Kanno M: Influences of the physical parameters on the risk to neck injuries in low impact speed rear-end collisions. *Accid Anal Prev* 28:493, 1996.

62. Peterson TD, et al: Motor vehicle safety: Current concepts and challenges for emergency physicians. *Ann Emerg Med* 34:384, 1999.

63. National Center for Statistics and Analysis: *Special Crash Investigations: Counts of Airbag Related Fatalities and Seriously Injured Persons.* Washington, D.C., National Highway Traffic Safety Administration, 2004.

64. National Highway Traffic Safety Administration: Update: Air bag-related fatalities to children—United States, 1993-1996. *MMWR Morb Mortal Wkly Rep* 49:1073, 1996.

65. Arbogast KB, Durbin DR, Kallan MJ, Winston FK: Effect of vehicle type on the performance of second generation air bags for child occupants. *Ann Proc Assoc Adv Auto Med* 47:85, 2003.

66. Moran SG, et al: Relationship between age and lower extremity fractures in frontal motor vehicle collisions. *J Trauma* 65:261, 2003.

67. Durbin DR, et al: Belt-positioning booster seats and reduction in risk of injury among children in vehicle crashes. *JAMA* 289:2835, 2003.

68. Jolly BT: Air bags—the changing landscape. *Ann Emerg Med* 31:783, 1998.

69. Segui-Gomez M, Levy J, Graham JD: Airbag safety and the distance of the driver from the steering wheel. *N Engl J Med* 339:132, 1998.

70. Augenstein JS, et al: Chest and abdominal injuries suffered by restraint occupants (950657). Detroit, Society of Automotive Engineers, 1995.

71. Pryor JP, et al: Nonoperative management of abdominal gunshot wounds. *Ann Emerg Med* 43:344, 2004

72. Hazinski MF, et al: Pediatric injury prevention. *Ann Emerg Med* 22:456, 1993.

73. Mace SE, et al: Injury prevention and control in children. *Ann Emerg Med* 38:405, 2001.

74. McCaig LF, Burt CW: Poisoning-related visits to emergency departments in the United States, 1993-1996. *J Toxicol Clin Toxicol* 37:817, 1999.

75. Redeker N, et al: Risk factors of adolescent and young adult trauma victims. *Am J Crit Care* 4:370, 1995.

76. Cooper C, et al: Repeat victims of violence: Report of a large concurrent case-control study. *Arch Surg* 135:837, 2000.

77. Kaufmann CR, Branas CC, Brawley M: A population-based study of trauma recidivism. *J Trauma* 45:325, 1998.

78. Sayfan J, Berlin Y: Previous trauma as a risk factor for recurrent trauma in rural northern Israel. *J Trauma* 43:123, 1997.

79. National Highway Traffic Safety Administration: Identification and referral of impaired drivers through emergency department protocols (DOT HS 809 412). Washington, D.C., U.S. Department of Transportation, 2002.

80. Hargarten SW: Docs and cops: A collaborating or colliding partnership? *Ann Emerg Med* 38:438, 2001.

81. Miller WR, Rollnick S: Motivational Interviewing: Preparing People to Change Addictive Behavior. New York, Guilford Press, 1991.

82. Maio RF, et al: Alcohol abuse/dependence in motor vehicle crash victims presenting to the emergency department. *Acad Emerg Med* 4:256, 1997.

83. Cherpitel CJ: Alcohol consumption among emergency room patients: Comparison of county/community hospitals and an HMO. *J Stud Alcohol* 54:432, 1993.

84. Becker BM, et al: Alcohol use among sub-critically injured emergency department patients and injury as a motivator to reduce drinking. *Acad Emerg Med* 2:784, 1995.

85. CDC: Alcohol problems among emergency department patients, proceedings of a research conference on identification and intervention. CDC, National Center for Injury Prevention and Control. Available at: www.cdc.gov/ncipc.

86. Hungerford DW, Pollock DA: Emergency department services for patients with alcohol problems: research directions. *Acad Emerg Med* 10:79, 2003.

87. Mullins RJ, et al: Population-based research assessing the effectiveness of trauma systems. *J Trauma* 47(Suppl):S59, 1999.

88. Mullins RJ, et al: Survival of seriously injured patients first treated in rural hospitals. *J Trauma* 52:1019, 2002.

89. Shatney CH, Sensaki K: Trauma team activation for 'mechanism of injury' blunt trauma victims: Time for a change? *J Trauma* 37:275, 1994.

90. Eastman AB: Blood in our streets: The status and evolution of trauma care systems. *Arch Surg* 127:677, 1992.

91. MacKenzie EJ, et al: National inventory of hospital trauma centers. *JAMA* 289:1515, 2003.

92. Trunkey DD: Trauma centers and trauma systems. *JAMA* 289:1566, 2003.

93. Augenstein JS, et al: Occult abdominal injuries to airbag-protected crash victims: A challenge to trauma systems. *J Trauma* 38:502, 1995.

94. Thacker SB, et al: Assessing prevention effectiveness using data to drive program decisions. *Public Health Rep* 109:187, 1994.

95. Physician's charter and the new professionalism. *Lancet* 359, 2002, p 520.

96. Medical professionalism in the new millennium: A physician charter. *Ann Intern Med* 136:243, 2002.

97. Woodruff K: Physicians as advocates: Promoting healthy public policy via the media. *California Physician* 11:48, 1994.

98. Retting RA, Ferguson SA, McCartt AT: A review of evidence-based traffic engineering measures designed to reduce pedestrian-motor vehicle crashes. *Am J Public Health* 93:1456, 2003.

99. Lewis LM, et al: Quantitation of impact attenuation of different playground surfaces under various environmental conditions using a tri-axial accelerometer. *J Trauma* 35:932, 1993.

CHAPTER

63 Forensic Emergency Medicine

William S. Smock

PERSPECTIVE

Clinical forensic medicine is the application of postmortem forensic medical knowledge and techniques to live patients in a clinical setting. European and British physicians, known as police surgeons, forensic physicians, forensic medical examiners, or forensic medical officers,[1] have performed clinical forensic examinations for more than 200 years.[2] The Metropolitan Police Force in London employs 20 full-time medical officers who perform forensic evaluations on prisoners and victims of physical and sexual assault.[3] Clinical forensic medicine programs are also well established in Asia, Latin America, and Australia.[4]

All patients who are victims of assault, abuse, trauma, or a terrorist event have forensic needs. When emergency physicians treat injuries without considering the forensic issues, they may misinterpret wounds, miss victims of abuse or domestic violence, and inadequately document the nature of injuries. During the provision of patient care, evidence that can be of critical significance to criminal or civil proceedings can be lost, discarded, or inadvertently washed away.[5-14] Wound evaluation and evidence collection take on additional significance when the patients are victims of a terrorist incident. Their wounds may contain radioactive materials, trace evidence, or bomb fragments that will be an important component of the criminal investigation.[15]

In 1991 the University of Louisville School of Medicine and the Kentucky Medical Examiner's Office established a clinical forensic medicine training and consultative program in the United States.[7,8,13,14] A forensically trained emergency physician or a forensic pathologist and a forensic nurse respond to the emergency department or other inpatient facility on a 24-hour basis. Consultations are initiated by a treating physician or a local, state, or federal law enforcement agency.

Forensic examinations are conducted with the consent of the patient, legal guardian, or court or by implied consent. The evaluation includes a history and physical examination, photographs, and anatomic diagrams.[15,16] Evidentiary material, including clothing, hair, blood, saliva, bullets, and bomb fragments, is collected when indicated or when ordered by the court. If a patient has been admitted from the emergency department to surgery, an evaluation is done in the operating suite in concert with the trauma surgeons.

Evaluations of gunshot and stab wounds, physical or sexual abuse, domestic violence, explosion-related injuries, and motor vehicle–related trauma should be adequately documented and include photographs as well as a narrative and diagram for possible use in future legal actions.[5-9,12,13,15,16] However, in one trauma center, 70% of cases had improper or inadequate documentation, and 38% had potential evidence improperly secured, incorrectly documented, or inadvertently discarded.[6] Surgeon General Dr. Richard Carmona and Prince reported that trauma physicians "usually have little or no training in the forensic aspects of trauma care and therefore necessary evidence may often be overlooked, lost, inadvertently discarded or its admissibility denied because of improper handling or documentation."[6]

It is easy to overlook or destroy both gross and trace evidence. Misinterpretation of physical injuries and evidence may be recorded in the medical record and complicate future legal proceedings.[2,4-14,16-20]

FORENSIC ASPECTS OF GUNSHOT WOUNDS

Firearm-related deaths, 29,737 in 2002, are the second leading cause of injury-related deaths in the United States after motor vehicle trauma.[21] Emergency physicians treat more than 115,000 victims of gunshot wounds each year, principally from handguns.[22] The direct and indirect costs associated with gunshot wounds have been estimated at $14 billion annually.[23,24]

Errors of Interpretation and Terminology

The emergency physician is in the ideal position to evaluate and document the state of a gunshot wound before it is disturbed, distorted, or destroyed by surgical intervention. Such evaluation requires a basic understanding of ammunition, ballistics, and relevant forensic terminology.[4-9,13,16,17,20] Documentation of gunshot wounds should include the anatomic location, size, shape, and characteristics of the wound. Wounds should be described according to the standard anatomic position with the arms to the side and palms up.

Clinicians should not describe wounds as "entrance" or "exit," but should document a detailed description of the appearance and location of a wound with the use of appropriate forensic terminology without speculating on an interpretation or the caliber of the bullet.[13,25,26] Despite common belief, exit wounds are *not* always larger than the entrance wound, and wound size does not correspond to bullet caliber.[13,16,17,25-28]

The size of any wound (entrance or exit) is determined by five factors: the size, shape, configuration, and velocity of the projectile at the instant of its impact with tissue and the physical characteristics of the impacted tissue itself. If the projectile is slow and its shape unchanged on exiting the skin, the exit wound may be equal to or smaller than its corresponding entrance wound.[13,25,29] If the projectile increases its surface area by fragmenting or changing its configuration while maintaining substantial velocity, the exit wound may be significantly larger than the entrance wound.[13,25,29-33] If the bullet strikes bone, fragments may extrude from the exit wound and contribute to the size and shape of the wound. Tissue elasticity also affects the wound size, so entrance or exit wound size may be smaller, equal to, or larger than the projectile that caused it.[13,31-33] Palm or sole wounds may appear only as slits and are easily mistaken for stab wounds.[25,32,33]

Inappropriate terminology should not be used to describe wounds.[6,33,34] Soot rather than the obsolete term *powder burns* should describe the carbonaceous material associated with close-range wounds.[25,27,32,33] Powder burns are literally the burns associated with the coincidental ignition of clothing by the flaming black powder used in muzzle loaders, antique weapons, and blank cartridges. Such burns do not occur with the smokeless powder used in modern commercial ammunition. *Powder burns*, therefore, is an obsolete and potentially misleading expression.

It is unnecessary to write in the medical record the manner of a gunshot victim's death. Whether a death is accidental, suicidal, or homicidal is the responsibility of the coroner or medical examiner and should be determined only after a detailed investigation of the scene and circumstances of the incident. The patient's position at the time of injury can be established only after an examination of the scene and collection of all forensic evidence.

An emergency physician, nurse, or paramedic may be required to render "factual" or "expert" testimony in a criminal case. Such testimony, without an appropriate forensic examination or adequate forensic training, may deny the criminal justice system, a suspect, or the patient access to short-lived evidence. This evidence could assist in the identification of entrance versus exit or the range of fire and affect the determination of a suspected assailant's innocence or guilt.[13,15,16,19,20,25,32] The speculation over the number and type of wounds in the assassination of President Kennedy is one example of the legal implications of the forensic evaluation.[19,20,35]

Forensic Aspects of Handguns

The Weapon

Four categories of handguns exist: single-shot weapon (usually a target pistol); derringer (a small, concealable weapon, usually with two barrels); revolver (a weapon with a rotating cylinder that advances with the pull of the trigger); and autoloading or semiautomatic pistol (which fires with each pull of the trigger), most popular because the magazine, or clip, can hold up to 17 cartridges versus the 5 or 6 cartridges of revolvers.

An automatic submachine gun fires pistol ammunition as long as the trigger is held until its ammunition is exhausted. A submachine gun's magazine may hold up to 60 cartridges. Weapons such as the Israeli UZI and the Heckler & Koch MP-5 use 9-mm or .40-caliber ammunition and are commonly used by police special weapons and tactics (SWAT) teams. Semiautomatic versions of the submachine gun are available to the general public, and kits to make these weapons fully automatic, though illegal, are sold through gun magazines.

Handgun Ammunition

This discussion is limited to handgun and submachine gun ammunition. The cartridge, or round, is composed of a primer, cartridge case, powder, and bullet (Figure 63-1). The bullet is the missile or projectile that is propelled out of the end of the muzzle.

The primer is a small explosive charge located in the base of the cartridge that ignites the gunpowder. The primer is a chemical compound that may contain lead, barium, or antimony. These compounds may be deposited on the hands of the shooter, on the victim of a close-range assault, and on objects within a room in which the weapon is discharged.

The cartridge case is typically made of brass, although other materials may be used. The function of the cartridge case is to expand slightly and seal the chamber against the escaping gases.[32] On detonation, a cartridge case is imprinted with unique microscopic marks that are valuable evidence and should be preserved for law enforcement.

The gunpowder found in all commercial cartridges, except blanks, is smokeless powder made with a single base (nitrocellulose) or a double base (nitrocellulose and nitroglycerin). Gunpowder comes in different shapes and sizes, including ball powder, flattened ball powder, flake powder, cylindrical powder, and in some cartridges, a combination of powders.[32]

When a weapon is discharged, not all the gunpowder is consumed in the combustion process. A percentage of the unburned gunpowder will travel out of the end of the muzzle for a distance, depending on the physical characteristics of the powder.

Blank cartridges, muzzleloaders, and other antiques or replicas may use black powder. Black powder (a combination of potassium nitrate, charcoal, and sulfur) does not burn as efficiently as smokeless powder and results in a large flame and white smoke.

The bullet is forced from the muzzle of a handgun at velocities ranging from 700 ft/sec to 1600 ft/sec (in magnum loads). The term *magnum* indicates that additional gunpowder has been added to the cartridge case to increase the velocity of the projectile. The most common bullet types include the round nose, full metal jacket, hollow point, wadcutter, and semiwadcutter. Bullets generally have a solid core of lead or steel and have a jacket if the bullet core is covered with a metal, usually copper or aluminum. If the jacket covers the entire projectile, it is called a full metal jacket, and if the jacket leaves some portion of the core exposed, it is semijacketed.

The term *hollow point* denotes a hole in the tip of the bullet that causes expansion on contact with tissue. Recent additions to the armamentarium include bullets such as the Winchester Black Talon and the Federal Hydra-Shok, which supposedly increase tissue damage.

Bullet caliber is described in 100ths of an inch or in millimeters. Handgun bullets range from .22 caliber, or 5.56 mm, to .45 caliber, or 11.3 mm. A bullet's weight is measured in grains, with 7000 grains/lb.

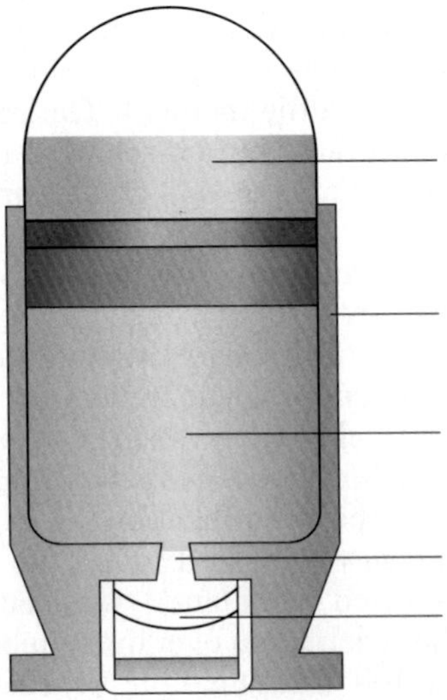

Handgun Wound Ballistics

Wound ballistics is the study of the effects of penetrating projectiles on the body.[30,36,37] Many misconceptions surround the science of wound ballistics.[30,37-41]

Injury results from the transference of a bullet's kinetic energy to the relatively stationary tissue. Wound severity is directly related to the amount of kinetic energy transferred to the tissue and direct tissue damage, not to the total amount of kinetic energy possessed by the bullet itself.[30,32,36] Bullets fired from rifles generally have a higher velocity than those fired from handguns, 1500 to 4000 ft/sec versus 700 to 1600 ft/sec in handguns. Therefore, rifled bullets have more kinetic energy and a *theoretically* higher wounding potential, but wound severity is the result of many variables such as bullet velocity, weight, deformation, and fragmentation on impact with tissue and the characteristics and location of the impacted tissue itself.[29,34,36,37]

Figure 63-1. A cartridge consists of several distinct components: bullet, cartridge case, gunpowder, flash hole, and primer.

- Bullet
- Cartridge case
- Powder
- Flash hole
- Primer

The principal mechanism of tissue damage is crushing. A bullet traveling through tissue generates two cavities, one permanent and the other temporary. The temporary cavity, a result of tissue stretching, lasts 5 to 10 msec from its generation until its collapse and leaves behind the permanently crushed tissue, the permanent cavity.[30,32,36] The size of the permanent cavity varies with the size, shape, and configuration of the bullet. A hollow-point bullet that mushrooms can increase its diameter 2.5 times on impact and will increase the area of tissue crushing 6.25 times over that of a non-deformed bullet.[32]

Forensic Evaluation of Handgun Wounds

Entrance Wounds

Range of fire is the distance from the muzzle to the victim and can be divided into four general categories: contact, near contact or close range, intermediate or medium range, and indeterminate or distant range. The size of the entrance wound does not correlate with the caliber of the bullet[13,31,32] because entrance wounds over elastic tissue will contract around the tissue defect and have a diameter much less than the caliber of the bullet.[25,32]

Contact Wounds

In contact wounds, the barrel or muzzle is in actual contact with the skin or clothing. Contact wounds can be subdivided into tight contact, in which the muzzle is pushed hard against the skin, and loose contact, in which the muzzle is incompletely or loosely held against the skin or clothing.

In a tight-contact wound, all material—the bullet, gases, soot, incompletely burned pieces of gunpowder, and metal fragments—is driven into the wound. These wounds can vary from a small hole with seared blackened edges from the discharge of hot gases and an actual flame to a gaping stellate wound (Figure 63-2). Large wounds occur when the wound is inflicted over thin or bony tissue and the injected hot gases cause the skin to expand to such an extent that the skin stretches and tears. These tears will have a triangular shape, with the base of the triangle overlying the entrance wound. Tears are generally associated with .32 caliber or greater, or magnum loads. Large stellate contact wounds are easily misinterpreted as exit wounds if based solely on their size.[13,25,32] Stellate tears are not pathognomonic for contact wounds, however. Tangential wounds, ricochet or tumbling bullets, and some exit wounds may also be stellate in appearance but lack

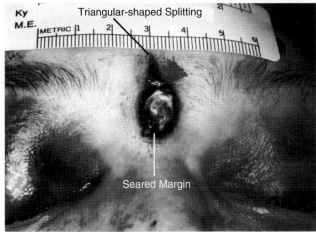

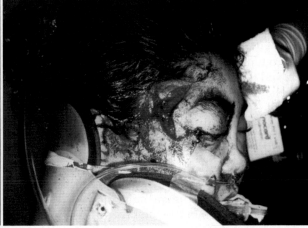

A

B

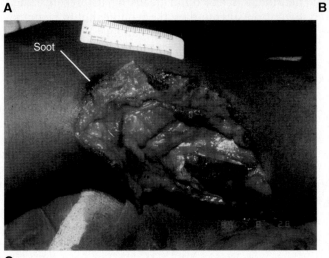

C

Figure 63-2. A, Tight-contact entrance wound from a .38-caliber revolver. The wound margins are seared from the discharge of hot gases and an actual flame from the end of the barrel. The triangular-shaped tear is the result of tissue expansion from the discharge of gases into the tissue. **B,** Tight-contact entrance wound with large stellate tears from a .380 semiautomatic pistol. The large triangular-shaped tears are the result of rapid expansion of gases under the skin. **C,** Tangential-contact wound from a 9-mm pistol on the medial aspect of the left calf. The presence of soot at the superior aspect indicates a close range of fire. The patient initially reported that he was shot from a distance of 3 to 4 ft and later admitted that he accidentally shot himself while withdrawing his pistol from his boot. Large wounds as seen in **B** and **C** may be misinterpreted as exit wounds because of their size.

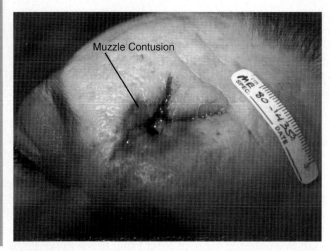

Figure 63-3. A "muzzle contusion" is a contusion caused by skin expansion against the barrel of the weapon. Muzzle contusions are associated with contact wounds.

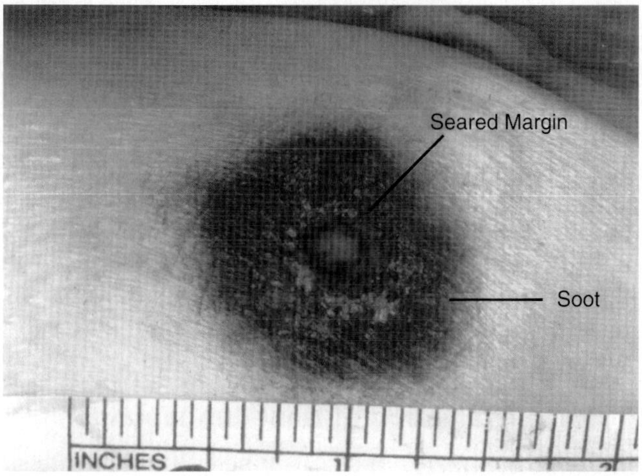

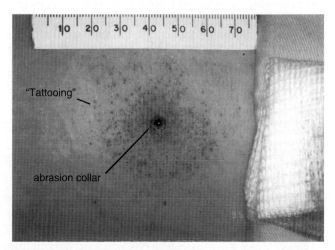

Figure 63-4. Close-range wound with soot deposition. Soot is associated with a range of fire of 6 inches or less.

soot and powder within the wound and seared wound margins.[13,25,32]

In some tight-contact wounds, expanding skin is forced back against the muzzle of the gun, and a characteristic pattern called a muzzle contusion is formed (Figure 63-3).[13,25,32] Patterns like these should be documented before wound debridement or surgery because they are helpful in determining the type of weapon (revolver or semiautomatic).[13,16]

When a gun's muzzle or barrel is not in complete (or with loose) contact or is angled relative to the skin, the soot and gunpowder residue are present both within and surrounding the wound. The angle between the muzzle and the skin determines the soot pattern. A perpendicular loose- or near-contact wound results in searing of skin and deposition of soot around the wound. A tangential-, loose-, or near-contact wound produces elongated searing and a soot deposit around the wound.

Close-Range Wounds

Close range is the maximum range at which soot is deposited on the wound or clothing, usually with a muzzle-to-target distance of less than 6 inches. Beyond 6 inches the soot usually falls away and does not reach the target. On rare occasion, soot has been noted on victims as far away as 12 inches.[31-33] The concentration of the soot varies inversely with the muzzle-to-target distance and is influenced by the type of gunpowder, ammunition, barrel length, caliber, and type of weapon (Figure 63-4).

At close range, the partially and unburned pieces of gunpowder have dispersed inadequately to cause powder tattooing. A precise range of fire, for example, 1 cm versus 10 cm, cannot be determined from an examination of the wound. A forensic crime laboratory can attempt to reproduce the patient's soot pattern on a target by test-firing the offending weapon at different ranges with ammunition similar to that causing the wound. The accuracy of this test depends principally on an exact and detailed description of the patient's

Figure 63-5. "Tattooing" results from contact with pieces of unburned gunpowder. These punctate abrasions are associated with an intermediate range of fire, generally less than 36 inches. The density of these abrasions depends on the length of the gun's barrel, the distance from the muzzle to the skin, the type of gunpowder used, and the presence of any intervening objects.

soot pattern. Because soot can be removed with debridement or wound cleansing, its presence and configuration surrounding the wound should be noted and photographed unless the patient's clinical condition precludes such attention to detail.[13,16]

Intermediate-Range Wounds

"Tattooing," or "stippling," is pathognomonic for an intermediate-range gunshot wound. It appears as punctate abrasions and is caused by contact with partially burned and wholly unburned pieces of gunpowder (Figure 63-5). Tattooing, or stippling, cannot be wiped away. Tattooing rarely occurs on the palms of the hands or the soles of the feet because of the thickness of the epithelium.[32]

Tattooing occurs as close as 1 cm and as far away as 1 m but is generally found at distances of 60 cm or less.[31-33,42] The density of the tattooing and the associated pattern depend on the length of the barrel, the

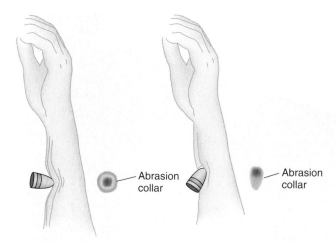

Figure 63-6. An "abrasion collar" is the abraded area surrounding the entrance wound created by the bullet when it indents and passes through the epithelium. The collar or rim is the result of friction between the bullet and the epithelium. The width of the abrasion collar will vary with the angle of impact.

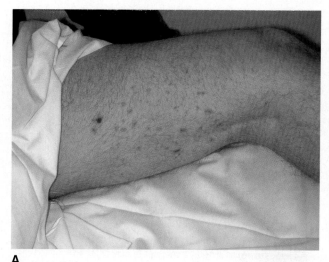

A

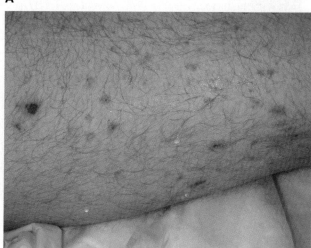

B

Figure 63-7. **A** and **B**, "Pseudotattooing," or punctate abrasions from glass fragments, not unburned gunpowder, on the medial aspect of the thigh associated with a gunshot wound. The leg was showered with glass fragments after the round penetrated the windowpane.

caliber, the type of ammunition/gunpowder, the muzzle-to-skin distance, and the presence of intermediate objects. Clothing, hair, or other intermediate barriers may prevent tattooing from occurring. Ball powder, because of its shape, travels farther and has greater penetration than flattened ball powder does.[32] Flattened ball powder travels farther than flake powder.[32] The presence of partially or entirely unburned pieces of gunpowder and gunpowder residue on clothing or skin is a clue that can aid in determination of the range of fire. If gunpowder penetrates even thin clothing, it will generally lack the energy to penetrate skin.

Long-Range Wounds

A long-range wound is inflicted from a distance far enough away that only the bullet makes contact with the skin. There is no tattooing or deposition of soot with distant entrance wounds. As the bullet penetrates the skin, the skin is indented, which results in the creation of an "abrasion collar," or interchangeably, an abrasion margin, abrasion rim, or abrasion ring (Figure 63-6). This collar is an abraded area of tissue that surrounds an entry wound, the result of friction between the bullet and the epithelium. The width of the abrasion collar varies with the angle of impact. Most entrance wounds will have an abrasion collar. Entrance wounds on the palms and soles are exceptions in that they usually appear slitlike.[32]

The abrasion collar is not the result of thermal changes associated with a hot projectile. The edges of a contact or close-range wound may be seared by the release of hot gases and flame. This clinical finding may overlap or obscure the abrasion collar. When an abrasion collar is the only superficial clinical finding present, the physician may also use the term *indeterminate range* to describe the range of fire. A wound inflicted from a distance of 10 ft will appear the same as a wound inflicted from 50 or 100 ft. An exact range of fire cannot be determined with a distant wound.

Determining the range of fire may be complicated by clothing that prevents the deposition of soot and powder on the skin. When such a wound is examined without the overlying clothing or without information regarding the crime scene, the wound may appear to be from a distant range of fire. In reality, the range may have been close or intermediate. Conversely, a projectile discharged from a distant range of fire may mimic an intermediate range if it strikes an object such as glass, which fragments. As with unburned gunpowder, when the glass fragments strike the skin, they may also cause punctate abrasions resulting in pseudotattooing (Figure 63-7).[32,43]

Atypical Entrance Wounds

Some atypical entrance wounds are indicative of a bullet having encountered an intermediate object, such as a window, wall, or door, before striking the victim. The intermediate object may change the bullet's size, shape, or path. Such changes can result in entrance wounds with large stellate configurations that mimic

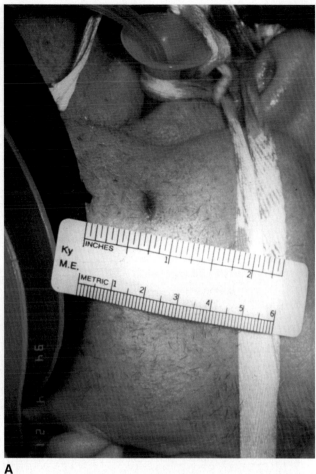

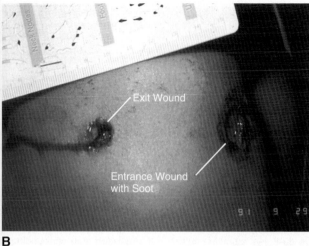

A

B

Figure 63-8. A, Slitlike exit wound from a .22-caliber bullet. **B,** Perforating gunshot wound to the left deltoid area with soot deposition around the larger entrance wound. No soot is present around the smaller exit wound. Exit wounds are *not* consistently larger than their corresponding entrance wounds.

close-range or contact wounds.[44,45] Ricochet bullets may also produce atypical entrance wounds.

Graze wounds occur as a result of tangential contact with a passing bullet. The directionality of the bullet can be determined from close examination of the wound.[32,46,47] The bullet produces a trough with the formation of skin tags on the lateral wound margins. The bases of these skin tags point toward the weapon and away from the direction of bullet travel.[46]

Exit Wounds

Exit wounds are the result of a bullet pushing and stretching the skin from inside out. The skin edges are generally everted with sharp, but irregular margins. Abrasion collars, soot, and tattooing are never seen at an exit wound.

Exit wounds have a variety of shapes and configurations and are *not* consistently larger than their corresponding entrance wounds (Figure 63-8). The exit wound's size is determined primarily by the amount of energy possessed by the bullet as it exits the skin and by the bullet's size and configuration. On entering the skin, a bullet's configuration will change from its usual nose-first attitude to tumbling and yawing. A bullet with sufficient energy to exit the skin sideways, or one that has increased its surface area by mushrooming, will produce an exit wound larger than its entrance wound.[13,25,32]

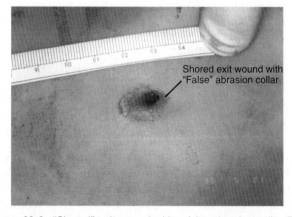

Figure 63-9. "Shored" exit wound with a false abrasion collar. This type of wound occurs when the skin in the region of the exiting bullet is in contact with a supporting structure (e.g., a wall, floor, or mattress). The skin is slapped against the supporting structure, which results in a false abrasion collar.

Atypical Exit Wounds

A "shored-exit" wound is a wound that has an associated false abrasion collar. If the skin is pressed against or supported by a firm object or surface at the moment that the bullet exits, the skin can be compressed between the exiting bullet and the supporting surface (Figure 63-9).[33,48] Examples of supporting structures include belts, floors, walls, doors, chairs, and mattresses.

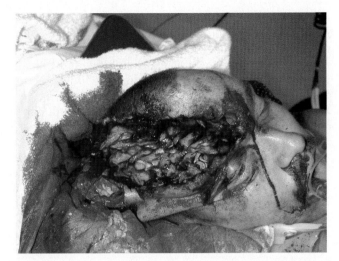

Figure 63-10. This patient sustained a high-velocity gunshot wound to the forehead. High-velocity rifle rounds, because of their kinetic energy, can cause massive damage when the energy is transferred to underlying tissue.

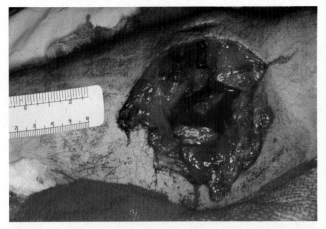

Figure 63-11. Exit wound from a high-velocity rifle round. Exit wounds from high-velocity rounds are generally larger than their corresponding entrance wounds. The large size is due to energy transfer from the projectile to underlying tissue with the expulsion of tissue, principally bone.

On rare occasion, soot may also be present at an atypical exit wound site.[49] If a contact entrance wound is located close to its associated exit wound, soot can be propelled through the short wound track and appear faintly on the exit wound surface.

Forensic Evaluation of Centerfire Rifle Wounds

Projectiles discharged from centerfire rifles have the potential to inflict massive tissue damage (Figure 63-10). A bullet's wounding potential is based on the kinetic energy that it possesses. The calibers of centerfire bullets, .223 to .308, are similar in diameter to handgun ammunition, but their wounding potential is greatly enhanced by the velocity of the round.[32] The higher the velocity of a projectile, the greater the potential to inflict tissue damage based on the formula kinetic energy = mass × velocity^2/g. Injuries result from the transference of energy from the projectile to organs and bony structures. With high-velocity rounds greater than 2000 ft/sec, a temporary cavity is formed along the wound tract. The temporary cavity may approach 11 to 12 times the diameter of the bullet and can result in tissue damage away from the physical tract taken by the projectile itself.[36] Temporary cavitation, in combination with direct tissue disruption and energy transfer from a fragmenting or yawing (turning sideways) projectile, is what determines the size of the internal injury and that of the exit wound. Because of the amount of energy possessed and transferred to underlying tissue, exit wounds associated with centerfire rifles, in contrast to those associated with handguns, are generally larger than their corresponding entrance wounds (Figure 63-11).[32]

Entrance wounds associated with high-velocity, centerfire projectiles do not significantly differ from those of handguns. Entrance wounds will generally exhibit abrasion collars or microtears on the skin surface (Figure 63-12). Wounds will also have associated soot

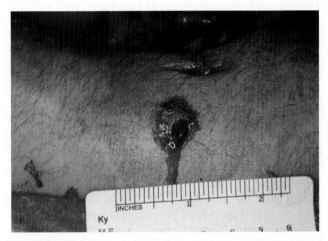

Figure 63-12. Entrance wound from a high-velocity rifle round. Entrance wounds of high-velocity projectiles will also display an abrasion collar.

deposition and tattooing, but because of a number of variables, such as muzzle length, amount of power in a given cartridge, muzzle configuration, and type of gunpowder (ball versus cylindrical), the range of fire in rifle wounds is not as clearly defined as in handgun wounds. Determination of an exact range of fire for rifles and shotguns is best established through controlled testing performed by a firearms examiner at a crime laboratory.

High-velocity lead core and jacketed bullets generally break up into hundreds of fragments, called a "lead snowstorm," on entering tissues and create significant tissue damage (Figure 63-13).[32] If the tissue is deep, the bullet fragments may fail to exit and remain embedded. Thus, it is possible to sustain an injury with a high-velocity round and not exhibit an exit wound. High-velocity rounds with steel cores will almost uniformly exit intact and continue down range. Both of these facts can confound a forensic investigator's efforts to find an adequate projectile sample to submit to the firearms examiner as evidence for ballistic analysis.

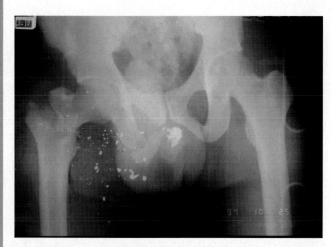

Figure 63-13. "Lead snowstorm" from a high-velocity rifle round. High-velocity projectiles have a tendency to fragment into hundreds of tiny particles on contact with bone. This fragmentation contributes to the massive tissue damage associated with these projectiles.

Microscopic Examination of Wounds

The debrided epithelial margins of wounds should be submitted to the pathology department for histologic examination to help determine the projectile's entrance, exit, and range of fire.[49-52]

Evidence

A victim's clothing may yield information about a bullet's range of fire and help distinguish entrance from exit wounds.[5,11,13,31-33,53,54] Clothing fibers deform in the direction of the passing projectile.[53,54] Gunpowder residue and soot will be deposited on clothing as they are on skin. Residue may be invisible to the naked eye but can be visualized with standard forensic staining techniques for nitrates and vaporized lead. Some bullets, as they make initial contact with clothing, leave a lead or lubricant residue that is termed *bullet wipe*. Articles of clothing removed from a wounded patient need to be placed in separate paper bags to avoid cross-contamination of evidence.

A gunshot residue (GSR) test may determine whether a victim or suspect has fired a weapon.[33,55-63] The GSR test checks for the presence of invisible residue from the primer: barium nitrate, antimony sulfide, and lead peroxide. There are two methods of checking for residue: the palms and the dorsum of the hands can be swabbed with a 5% nitric acid solution and analyzed by atomic absorption spectrophotometry, or tape or an adhesive disk can be placed on the hands and removed for examination under a scanning electron microscope.

The specificity and sensitivity of the GSR test are unclear.[33,58,62,63] Residue will be deposited on the hands of the individual who fired a weapon in only 50% of cases.[33] Residue may spread about a crime scene, and secondary contact with the weapon or furniture on which residue was deposited will result in a false-positive test. The possibility of transferring residue from police officers to suspects has also been reported.[63] The sensitivity of the test decreases with time, and law enforcement agents may not have access to a patient

during the "golden hour."[33] Factors that decrease the test's sensitivity include washing the skin with alcohol or povidone-iodine (Betadine), placing tape on the skin, rubbing the hands against clothing, and placing plastic bags over the patient's hands, which precipitates moisture on the skin. If a GSR test is to be performed or if soot is noted on the patient's hand, paper bags should be placed over the hands early during treatment of the patient.

The bullet, the bullet jacket, and the cartridge case are invaluable when identifying or excluding a weapon.[13,31,32] When a weapon is discharged, it imprints multiple unique microscopic marks on the side of the bullet and on the bottom or side of the cartridge case.[13,31,32] The bullet's markings result from its contact with the tool marks, or "rifling," in the gun's barrel. The marks on the cartridge case result from contact with the firing pin, the breechblock, the magazine of semiautomatic weapons, and the extractor and ejector mechanisms. The emergency physician must work diligently to preserve these microscopic fingerprints and not obliterate the markings by removing a bullet with hemostats or pickups.[13,33] Bullets should be handled with gloves and surgical instruments covered with gauze to ensure the preservation of these microscopic "fingerprint" marks. It is not necessary to place initials or other markings on the bullet if adequate notes are made in the patient's medical record regarding the chain of custody.

Radiographs also help locate retained projectiles and may be of evidentiary value when determining the number of projectiles and the direction of fire.[31-33,42,53]

FORENSIC ASPECTS OF PHYSICAL ASSAULT

Identifying Assault Victims

Studies estimate that 22% to 33% of the patients in an urban emergency department are victims of domestic violence, yet only a small percentage of these patients are recognized as such.[18,64-77] In one study of emergency department visits, 43% of abused patients were treated for acute trauma 6 or more times before they were identified as victims of abuse; nearly half of these patients were seen at least 12 times.[78]

Every weapon leaves a mark, design, or pattern stamped or imprinted on or just below the epithelium. The epithelial imprints of these weapons, called *pattern injuries*, are consistently reproducible.[13,79] These injuries fall into three major categories according to their source: blunt force, sharp force, and thermal.

Knowledge of pattern injuries and accurate documentation regarding the anatomic location of the injuries make determining what implement, tool, or weapon was responsible for producing each wound much easier.

Blunt Force Pattern Injuries

The most common blunt force injury is a contusion, along with abrasions and lacerations. A weapon with a

BOX 63-1. Commonly Inflicted Pattern Injuries

- Slap marks with digits delineated
- Looped or flat contusions from belts or cords
- Circular contusions from fingertip pressure
- Parallel contusions with central clearing from linear objects
- Contusions from shoe heels and soles
- Semicircular contusions and abrasions from bite marks

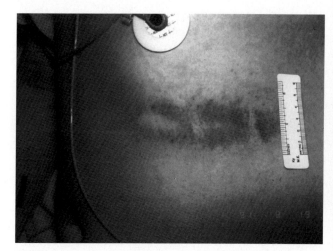

Figure 63-15. Pattern contusion with parallel lines and central clearing from contact with a baseball bat.

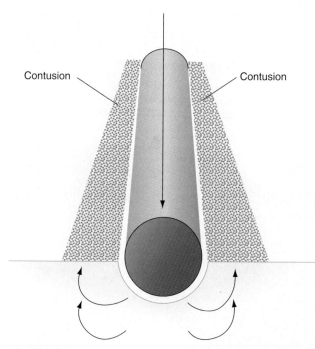

Contusion   Contusion

Figure 63-14. A direct blow from a linear object results in a pattern contusion with central clearing surrounded by parallel linear contusions. The blood directly beneath the impacting object is displaced laterally and accounts for the distinctive contusion.

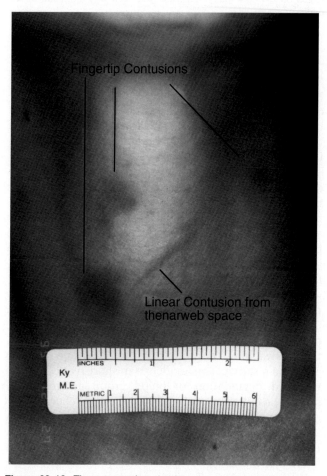

Fingertip Contusions

Linear Contusion from thenarweb space

Figure 63-16. Three somewhat circular contusions and a linear contusion on the anterior aspect of the neck. These injuries resulted from hand and fingertip pressure applied during an attempted strangulation.

unique shape or configuration may stamp a mirror image of itself on the skin (Box 63-1).[79]

Pattern Contusions

A pattern contusion is a common injury that helps identify the causative weapon. A blow from a linear object leaves a contusion that is characterized by a set of parallel lines separated by an area of central clearing (Figure 63-14).[13,79] The blood underlying the striking object is forcibly displaced to the sides, which accounts for the pattern's appearance (Figure 63-15).

Circular or linear contusions should suggest abuse or battery. Circular contusions 1.0 to 1.5 cm in diameter are consistent with fingertip pressure and grab marks (Figure 63-16). One commonly overlooked anatomic location where fingertip pressure contusions are often present is the medial aspect of the upper part of the arm.[79] Contact with the sole of a shoe from a kick or stomp may also leave a pattern contusion that can assist in identifying the patient's assailant.

The emergency physician may be requested to evaluate injuries that allegedly occurred as a result of police brutality. Specific pattern contusions can include parallel contusions from contact with a flashlight or nightstick. Handcuff or shackle marks are seen as narrow parallel contusions or abrasions on the wrists or ankles. Handcuff and shackle marks are generally more prominent on the lateral aspects of the extremity.[33]

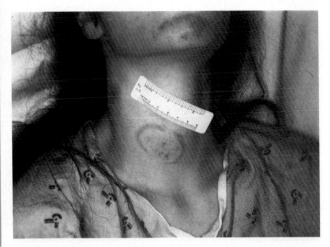

Figure 63-17. Bite mark with two semicircular arched contusions over the anterior lateral aspect of the patient's neck. A bite mark can be used to identify the assailant if the injury is correctly documented by a forensic photographer or forensic odontologist. A circular contusion on the right lateral aspect of the neck was the result of fingertip pressure.

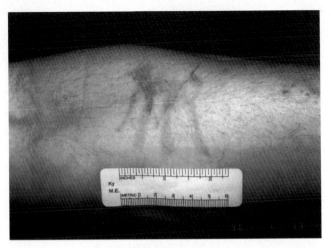

Figure 63-18. Four fingernail scratch marks on the medial aspect of a forearm.

The emergency physician should record a history and document the injuries with diagrams and photographs when possible. The investigation of all the circumstances surrounding the incident is best reviewed by an internal affairs or professional standards unit of the investigating law enforcement agency and not by the emergency physician.

A bite mark may appear as a pattern contusion, an abrasion, or a combination of both (Figure 63-17). Bite marks vary greatly in the quality of their identifiable features, depending on the anatomic location of the bite and the motion of the teeth relative to the skin. Some bite marks may not be readily identifiable as a bite and appear as a nonspecific contusion, abrasion, or contused abrasion.

When an acute bite mark is identified, the emergency physician should not wash away potential evidence. The skin surface should be swabbed with a sterile cotton-tipped applicator moistened with sterile saline. Such swabbing may detect the presence of the assailant's saliva. This evidence is short lived because of rapid degradation of blood group antigens and should be collected and sent to the crime laboratory as quickly as possible. Eighty percent of the population secretes an ABO blood group protein antigen in saliva. DNA from buccal cells may also be deposited over an acute bite mark.[13]

When available, a forensic odontologist can evaluate a bite wound with accuracy. The use of alternative light sources, such as ultraviolet or infrared, may reveal a pattern contusion within or under the epithelium that is not visible to the naked eye.[33] These light sources are routinely used by forensic odontologists on faint, old, or difficult bite marks. Assailants have been identified from bite marks up to 6 months after injury.

The emergency physician may be asked to render an opinion regarding the age of a contusion. The development of a contusion is based on a number of variables: the amount of blunt force applied to the skin, the vas-

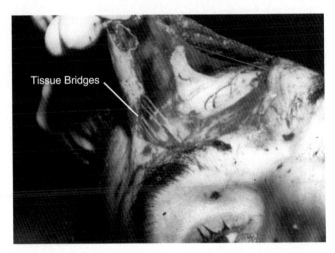

Figure 63-19. A laceration is the result of blunt trauma and characteristically displays tissue bridges and crushed wound margins.

cularity of the tissue, the fragility of the blood vessels, the density of the tissue, and the amount of blood that escapes into the surrounding tissue.[80,81] As a result, no reproducible standard for dating a contusion based on its color is possible.[81]

Pattern Abrasions

A *pattern abrasion* is a rubbing or scraping away of the superficial layers of the epidermis (Figure 63-18). The presence of such pattern injuries, though not important from the standpoint of treatment, may be invaluable from a forensic and injury reconstruction perspective.[79]

Pattern Lacerations

A *pattern laceration* is defined as a tear produced by blunt trauma and should not be confused with an incised wound produced when a sharp-edged implement (knife or scalpel) is drawn across the skin.[13] A pattern laceration has characteristically abraded or crushed skin edges and unique "tissue bridges" (Figure 63-19).

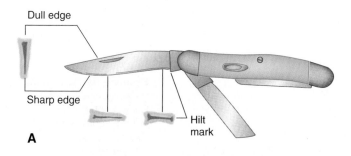

A

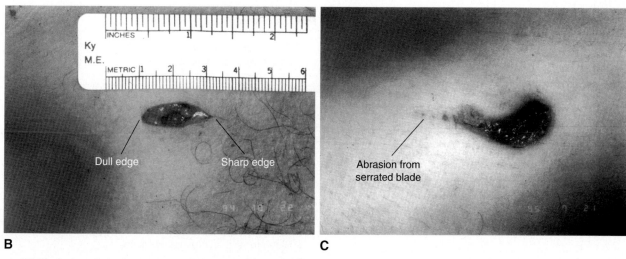

B   **C**

Figure 63-20. A, A stab wound with a single-edged knife blade will cause a wound to be formed with a sharp edge and a dull edge. If the blade penetrates to its hilt, a "hilt mark" may be seen overlying the sharp edge. **B**, Single-edged stab wound. **C**, Single-edged stab wound made by a serrated blade. Abrasions from the blade's serrated edges are seen on the left margin of the wound.

Sharp Force Pattern Injuries

Two types of sharp force injuries may be encountered. An *incised wound* is longer than it is deep, and a *stab wound* is defined as a puncture wound that is deeper than it is wide. The wound margins of sharp force injuries are clean and lack the abraded edges of injuries resulting from blunt force.

Forensic information can be gathered during the examination of a stab wound. Some of the characteristics of a knife blade, single edged or double edged, can be determined from visual inspection (Figure 63-20A and B).[13,79] Additional characteristics, such as serrated versus sharp, can be determined if the blade was drawn across the skin during insertion or withdrawal (Figure 63-20C). Serrated blades do not always leave these characteristic marks.[13,79]

Thermal Pattern Injuries

A thermal pattern injury is a common form of abuse or battery. The detailed history of the incident should include the position of the patient relative to the thermal source. When this information is available and reliable, it will help determine whether the injury was intentional or accidental.[79]

Immersion or dipping burns are characterized by a sharp or clear line of demarcation between burned and unburned tissue. In contrast, splash burns are characterized by an irregular or undulating line or by isolated areas of thermal injury, usually round or oval, caused by droplets of hot liquid.

The severity of a thermal or scald injury depends on the length of time of contact and the temperature. Water causes full-thickness burns in 1 second at 158° F (70° C) and 600 seconds at 120° F (48.9° C) (Figure 63-21).[82] Law enforcement agents routinely measure the household's or institution's water temperature in any investigation involving a scald injury.

FORENSIC ASPECTS OF MOTOR VEHICLE TRAUMA

Law enforcement officials investigating an incident involving serious injuries from a motor vehicle crash or pedestrian collision benefit from information regarding injury patterns and collection of trace evidence from the victim. This information can help determine whether an occupant was the driver or a passenger. It may also help identify a suspect vehicle involved in a hit-and-run pedestrian collision. A pedestrian's position (standing or lying) when struck in the roadway may be determined. The treating physicians may be involved in subsequent legal proceedings that arise in both civil and criminal court.

Determination of a vehicle occupant's role may be simple, if the driver is pinned behind the steering wheel, or complex, if the vehicle's occupants are

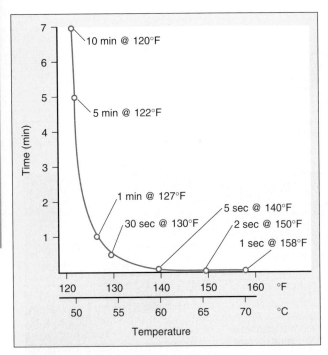

Figure 63-21. Relationship between water temperature and the duration of contact required to produce a full-thickness thermal injury (From Katcher ML: Scald burns from hot tap water. *JAMA* 246:1219, 1981.)

ejected. Many impaired drivers claim to be passengers. Short-lived evidence or pattern injuries that might be destroyed or altered in the delivery of patient care should optimally be preserved.[83,84]

The emergency physician should avoid rendering an opinion on an occupant's position because it is difficult to determine based solely on statements and physical findings in the emergency department.[83,84] Such an opinion is better based on an examination of the scene, the vehicle, other occupants, and information regarding trace evidence. Expert opinions are best rendered only after forensic examinations, including postmortem examinations, are performed on all the vehicle's occupants and all forensic evidence has been evaluated (Box 63-2).[33,83-85]

Pattern Injuries

Matching pattern injuries with components within a vehicle often reveals an occupant's position during a portion of the vehicle's collision sequence.[83-85] Common pattern contusions, abrasions, and lacerations occur as a result of contact with steering wheels, air bags, air bag module covers, window cranks, radio knobs, door latches, dashboard components, and front and side window glass.[83-86] An occupant's movement and subsequent contact with a vehicle's components are dictated by the force applied to the vehicle through its interaction with the environment. Vehicle occupants, restrained or unrestrained, will initially move toward the primary area of impact.[83,84] This movement within the vehicle, called occupant kinematics, is described as a motion parallel to and opposite the direction of the force developed by the impacting

BOX 63-2. Evidence Collection—Driver versus Passenger

Victim
Examine for Pattern Injuries
Steering wheel contusion
Radio knob contusion
Window crank contusion
Striated incised facial wounds
"Dicing" wounds

***Examine Clothing for Transferred Material*[*†]**
Glass (front and side windows)
Fibers
Pedal imprint on shoe
Dashboard components

Collect Biologic Standards[†]
Hair
Blood

Collect Clothing Standards[†]
Damage

Vehicle
Examine for Pattern Damage
Steering wheel
Radio/knobs/dashboard
Window crank/side door
Windshield (laminated glass)
Side/rear window (tempered glass)

Collect Standards
Glass
Carpets and seats
Gas and brake pedals
Broken dashboard components

Examine for Transferred Material of Pedestrian
Hair on windshield/components
Blood on windshield/components

Examine for Transferred Material on Car Occupants
Fabric fibers
Imprinted fabric pattern

---
*Each article of clothing should be collected in a separate paper bag. This avoids cross-contamination, and wet material will dry. Do not collect evidence in plastic bags because moisture will condense within the bag and may degrade biologic material.
†Each article should be marked with the patient's name, item collected, date and time collected, location of collection, name of the collector, and name of law enforcement official to whom the evidence was given. This information will preserve the "chain of custody."

object.[83,84] Applying the principles of occupant kinematics will predict in what direction a particular occupant will move and therefore what component will be struck.

A deploying air bag may induce a pattern abrasion on the face, cornea, forearms, or other exposed tissue. Pattern lacerations, specific fracture patterns, and amputations are seen when the deploying air bag module cover impacts the hand or forearm (Figure 63-22).[86,87] Correlation of these injuries to the driver or passenger air bag system is helpful in assessing an occupant's role.[86,87]

Both laminated glass (windshield) and tempered glass (side and rear windows) produce pattern injuries.

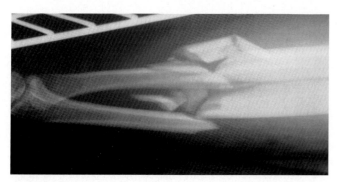

Figure 63-22. Comminuted, bending-type fracture of the radius and ulna from impact with a deploying air bag module cover.

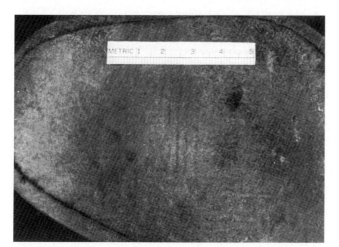

Figure 63-23. Imprint of a brake pedal on a leather-soled shoe. This information will assist in determining the occupant's role and in determining whether the patient's foot was on the brake or accelerator pedal at the moment of impact.

The windshield is composed of two layers of glass laminated together with a thin layer of clear plastic sandwiched between. Laminated glass breaks into shards on impact. Tempered, or "safety," glass is a single layer of glass that breaks into small cubes when fractured. Shattered tempered glass from side and rear windows imparts a "dicing" pattern to the skin, whereas shattered laminated windshield glass causes linear incised wounds.

Trace Evidence

Clothing, shoes, and biologic standards (hair and blood) may determine an occupant's role.[83,86,87] Examination of the soles of leather shoes may reveal an imprint of the gas or brake pedal (Figure 63-23). Preservation of clothing permits a comparison of clothing fibers with fibers transferred to vehicle components during the crash.[83,86-88] Imprints of fabric may also be transferred to components within the vehicle, including the steering wheel. Contact with the windshield often transfers hair and tissue to the glass. Glass collected from within a patient's wound can be matched with a particular window within the vehicle. Airbags are also a tremendous source of trace evidence, including skin, blood, makeup, and hair.[87]

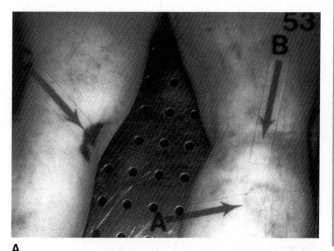

A

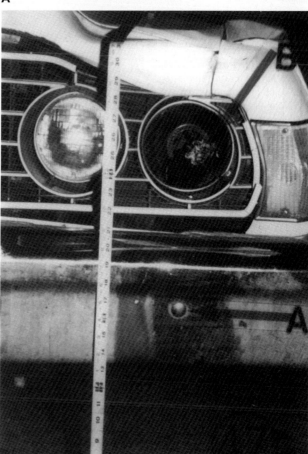

B

Figure 63-24. A, A circular pattern contusion on the posterior aspect of a pedestrian's left calf was the result of contact with the head of a bolt. The location of the contusion provides information about the configuration of the patient at the moment that the car struck him. The patient was struck from the rear. **B,** A puncture wound on the posterior aspect of the left thigh resulted from contact with the head-light filament.

Evaluation of Pedestrian Collisions
Pattern Injuries

Approximately 75,000 persons are killed or seriously injured annually in pedestrian collisions[89]; 82% are struck by a vehicle's front bumper/grill area. A standing adult struck by the front of a vehicle will sustain

BOX 63-3. Evidence Collection—Pedestrian Collisions

Victim

Examine for Pattern Injuries
Height of bumper injuries
    Contusion
    Fracture
Head/neck injuries
Crush injuries

Examine Clothing for Transferred Material[*†]
Paint
Glass (windshield, headlight)
Oil or grease

Collect Biologic Standards[†]
Hair
Blood or tissue

Collect Clothing Standards[†]
Damage or tears

Vehicle

Examine for Pattern Damage
Bumper height and damage
Specific components
Windshield damage
Wheels and undercarriage

Collect Standards
Paint
Glass
Oil or grease

Examine for Transferred Material
Hair
Blood or tissue

Examine for Transferred Material
Fabric fibers
Imprinted fabric pattern

---

[*]Each article of clothing should be collected in a separate paper bag. This avoids cross-contamination, and wet material will dry. Do not collect evidence in plastic bags because moisture will condense within the bag and may degrade biologic material.
[†]Each article should be market with the patient's name, item collected, date and time collected, location of collection, name of the collector, and name of law enforcement official to whom the evidence was given. This information will preserve the "chain of custody."

"bumper injuries," which include open and closed fractures of the tibia and fibula, soft tissue damage, and pattern injuries from vehicle components and hardware.[33]

The height of bumper injuries, measured from the heel and including the height of the patient's shoe, can be correlated with the height of the vehicle's bumper to determine whether the vehicle was braking at the moment of impact. Application of the brake results in dipping of a vehicle's front end. The presence or absence of braking may help determine the driver's intent. The presence of bumper injuries at one height on one leg and at another height on the other may indicate that the pedestrian was walking or running at the moment of impact, with one leg elevated. Examination of the soles may show lateral striations when a patient has been dragged.

A victim who is struck from behind may have pattern contusions on the calf or thigh (Figure 63-24), whereas

pattern contusions from a grill on the anterior aspect of the thigh indicate that the pedestrian was standing and facing the vehicle. Victims who are run over may display a tire tread pattern. Tire marks and the absence of bumper injuries may indicate that the patient was supine or prone in the roadway (Box 63-3).

KEY CONCEPTS

- Knowledge of wound mechanics and production, as well as wound appearance, can provide practicing emergency physicians with important clues to the forensic interpretation of injuries.
- Diagram and photograph wounds and injuries.
- The medical record should accurately document objective findings but should not speculate on the cause or mechanism.

REFERENCES

1. McLay WDS: _Clinical Forensic Medicine._ London, Pinter, 1990.
2. Eckert W: The development of forensic medicine in the United Kingdom from the 18th century. _Am J Forensic Med Pathol_ 13:124, 1992.
3. Payne-James JJ, Dean PJ: Assault and injury in clinical forensic medical practice. _Med Sci Law_ 34:202, 1994.
4. Goldsmith MF: US forensic pathologists on a new case: Examination of living patients. _JAMA_ 256:1685, 1986.
5. Smialek JE: Forensic medicine in the emergency department. _Emerg Med Clin North Am_ 1:1685, 1983.
6. Carmona R, Prince K: Trauma and forensic medicine. _J Trauma_ 29:1222, 1989.
7. Smock WS, Nichols GR, Fuller PM: Development and implementation of the first clinical forensic medicine training program. _J Forensic Sci_ 38:835, 1993.
8. Smock WS: Development of a clinical forensic medicine curriculum for emergency physicians in the USA. _J Clin Forensic Med_ 1:27, 1994.
9. Smock WS, Ross CS, Hamilton FN: Clinical forensic medicine: How ED physicians can help with the sleuthing. _Emerg Legal Briefings_ 5:1, 1994.
10. Eckert WG, et al: Clinical forensic medicine. _Am J Forensic Med Pathol_ 7:182, 1986.
11. Mittleman RE, Goldberg HS, Waksman DM: Preserving evidence in the emergency department. _Am J Nurs_ 83:1652, 1983.
12. Godley DR, Smith TK: Some medicolegal aspects of gunshot wounds. _J Trauma_ 17:866, 1977.
13. Smock WS: Forensic emergency medicine. In Olhaker JS, Jackson MC, Smock WS (eds): _Forensic Emergency Medicine._ Philadelphia, Lippincott, Williams & Wilkins, 2001.
14. Busuttil A, Smock WS: Training in clinical forensic medicine in Kentucky. _Police Surgeon_ 14:26, 1990.
15. Wade C (ed): _FBI Forensic Sciences Handbook. An FBI Laboratory Publication._ Quantico, Va, Federal Bureau of Investigation, 2003.
16. Smock WS: Forensic photography. In Stack LB, Storrow AB, Morris A, Patton DR (eds): _Handbook of Medical Photography._ Philadelphia, Hanley & Belfus, 2001, pp 397-408.
17. Collins KA, Lantz PE: Interpretation of fatal, multiple, and exiting gunshot wounds by trauma specialists. _J Forensic Sci_ 39:94, 1994.
18. McLeer SV, et al: Education is not enough: A systems failure in protecting battered women. _Ann Emerg Med_ 18:651, 1989.

19. Breo DL: JFK's death: The plain truth from the MDs who did the autopsy. *JAMA* 267:2794, 1992.

20. Randall T: Clinicians' forensic interpretations of fatal gunshot wounds often miss the mark. *JAMA* 269:2058, 1993.

21. Centers for Disease Control and Prevention: Death, preliminary data for 2002. *Natl Vital Stat Rep* 52:13, 2004.

22. Surveillance for fatal and nonfatal firearm-related injuries—United States, 1993-1998. *Mor Mortal Wkly Rep CDC Surveill Summ* 13:1, 2001.

23. Voelker R: Taking aim at handgun violence. *JAMA* 273:1739, 1995.

24. Annest JL, et al: National estimates of nonfatal firearm-related injuries. *JAMA* 273:1749, 1995.

25. Dana SE, DiMaio VJM: Gunshot trauma. In Payne-James J, Busuttil A, Smock W (eds): *Forensic Medicine: Clinical and Pathological Aspects.* London, Greenwich Medical Media, 2003, pp 149-168.

26. Fackler ML, Riddick L: Clinicians' inadequate descriptions of gunshot wounds obstruct justice: Clinical journals refuse to expose the problem. In *Proceedings of the American Academy of Forensic Sciences,* vol 2. Colorado Springs, Colo, McCormick-Armstrong, 1996, p 150.

27. Smock WS: Forensic medicine, pattern injuries of domestic violence, assault and abuse. In Knoop KH, Stack LB, Storrow AB (eds): *Atlas of Emergency Medicine,* 2nd ed. New York, McGraw-Hill, 2002, pp 565-576.

28. Marlowe AL, Smock WS: The forensic evaluation of gunshot wounds by prehospital personnel. In *Proceedings of the American Academy of Forensic Sciences,* vol 2. Colorado Springs, Colo, McCormick-Armstrong, 1996, p 149.

29. DiMaio VJM, Spitz WU: Variations in wounding due to unusual firearms and recently available ammunition. *J Forensic Sci* 17:377, 1972.

30. Fackler ML: Wound ballistics: A review of common misconceptions. *JAMA* 259:2730, 1988.

31. Fatteh A: *Medicolegal Investigation of Gunshot Wounds.* Philadelphia, JB Lippincott, 1976.

32. DiMaio VJM: *Gunshot Wounds,* 2nd ed. Boca Raton, Fla, CRC Press, 1999.

33. Spitz WU: *Medicolegal Investigation of Death,* 3rd ed. Springfield, Ill, Charles C Thomas, 1993.

34. Rich NM: Missile injuries. *Am J Surg* 139:414, 1980.

35. Breo DL: JFK's death, part II—Dallas MDs recall their memories. *JAMA* 267:2791, 1992.

36. Sellier KG, Kneubuehl BP: *Wound Ballistics and the Scientific Background.* Amsterdam, Elsevier, 1994.

37. Le Garde LA: *Gunshot injuries,* 2nd ed, revised. Mt. Ida, Ark, Lancer Militaria, 1991.

38. Lindsey D: The idolatry of velocity, or lies, damn lies, and ballistics. *J Trauma* 20:1068, 1980.

39. Lindsey D: Review of management of gunshot wounds by Ordog. *Am J Emerg Med* 7:117, 1989.

40. Fackler ML: Review of management of gunshot wounds by Ordog. *Ann Emerg Med* 17:1004, 1988.

41. Barach EM, Tomlanovich MC: Letter to editor. *J Trauma* 28:1610, 1988.

42. Mason JK: *The Pathology of Trauma,* 2nd ed. London, Hodder & Stoughton, 1993.

43. Dixon DS: Tempered plate glass as an intermediate target and its effects on gunshot wound characteristics. *J Forensic Sci* 27:205, 1982.

44. Stahl CJ, et al: The effect of glass as an intermediate target on bullets: Experimental studies and report of a case. *J Forensic Sci* 24:6, 1979.

45. Donoghue ER, et al: Atypical gunshot wounds of entrance: An empirical study. *J Forensic Sci* 29:379, 1984.

46. Dixon DS: Determination of direction of fire from graze gunshot wounds. *J Forensic Sci* 25:272, 1980.

47. Dixon DS: Determination of direction of fire from graze gunshot wounds of internal organs. *J Forensic Sci* 29:331, 1984.

48. Dixon DS: Characteristics of shored exit wounds. *J Forensic Sci* 26:691, 1981.

49. Adelson L: A microscopic study of dermal gunshot wounds. *Am J Clin Pathol* 35:393, 1961.

50. Murphy GK: The study of gunshot wounds in surgical pathology. *Am J Forensic Med Pathol* 1:123, 1980.

51. Finck PA: Ballistic and forensic pathologic aspects of missile wounds: Conversion between Anglo-American and metric-system units. *Mil Med* 130:545, 1965.

52. Torre C, Varetto L, Ricchiardi P: New observations on cutaneous firearm wounds. *Am J Forensic Med Pathol* 7:186, 1986.

53. Dixon DS: Gunshot wounds: Forensic implications in a surgical practice. In Ordog GJ (ed): *Management of Gunshot Wounds.* New York, Elsevier, 1988.

54. Lee HC, Palmbach T, Miller MT: *Henry Lee's Crime Scene Handbook.* San Diego, Calif, Academic Press, 2001.

55. Wolten GM, et al: Particle analysis for the detection of gunshot residue—I: Scanning electron microscopy/energy dispersive x-ray characterization of hand deposits from firing. *J Forensic Sci* 24:409, 1979.

56. Andrasko K, Maehly AC: Detection of gunshot residues on hands by scanning electron microscopy. *J Forensic Sci* 22:279, 1977.

57. Matricardi VR, Kilty JW: Detection of gunshot particles from the hands of a shooter by SEM. *J Forensic Sci* 22:725, 1977.

58. Wolten GM, et al: Particle analysis for the detection of gunshot residue—II: Occupational and environmental particles. *J Forensic Sci* 24:423, 1979.

59. Wolten GM, et al: Particle analysis for the detection of gunshot residue—III: The case record. *J Forensic Sci* 24:864, 1979.

60. Tillman J: Automated gunshot residue particle search and characterization. *J Forensic Sci* 32:62, 1987.

61. Kee TG, Beck C: Casework assessment of an automated scanning electron microscope/microanalysis system for the detection of firearms discharge particles. *J Forensic Sci Soc* 27:321, 1987.

62. Zeichner A, Levin N: Casework experience of GSR detection in Israel, on samples from hands, hair, and clothing using an autosearch SEM/EDX system. *J Forensic Sci* 40:1082, 1995.

63. Gialamas DM, et al: Officers, their weapons and their hands: An empirical study of GSR on the hands of non-shooting police officers. *J Forensic Sci* 40:1086, 1995.

64. Goldberg WG, Tomlanovich MC: Domestic violence victims in the emergency department. *JAMA* 251:3259, 1984.

65. Tilden VP: Response of the health care delivery system to battered women. *Issues Ment Health Nurs* 10:309, 1989.

66. Randall T: Domestic violence intervention calls for more than treating injuries. *JAMA* 254:939, 1990.

67. McLeer SV, Anwar RA: The role of the emergency physician in the prevention of domestic violence. *Ann Emerg Med* 16:1155, 1987.

68. Morrison LJ: The battering syndrome: A poor record of detection in the emergency department. *J Emerg Med* 6:521, 1988.

69. Tilden VP, Shepherd P: Increasing the rate of identification of battered women in an emergency department: Use of a nursing protocol. *Res Nurs Health* 10:209, 1987.

70. Goldberg W, Carey AL: Domestic violence victims in the emergency setting. *Top Emerg Med* 3:65, 1982.

71. Delahunta EA: Hidden trauma: The most missed diagnosis of domestic violence. *Am J Emerg Med* 13:74, 1995.

72. Grunfeld AF, et al: Detecting domestic violence against women in the emergency department: A nursing triage model. *J Emerg Nurs* 20:271, 1994.

73. Isaac NE, Sanches RL: Emergency department response to battered women in Massachusetts. *Ann Emerg Med* 23:85, 1994.

74. Abbott J, et al: Domestic violence against women: Incidence and prevalence in an emergency department population. *JAMA* 273:1763, 1995.

75. Gremillion DH, Evins G: Why don't doctors identify and refer victims of domestic violence? *N C Med J* 55:428, 1994.

76. Education about adult domestic violence in U.S. and Canadian medical schools, 1987-88. *MMWR Morb Mortal Wkly Rep* 38(2):17, 1989.

77. Chambliss LR, Bay RC, Jones RF: Domestic violence: An educational imperative? *Am J Obstet Gynecol* 172:1035, 1995.

78. Stark E, Flitcraft A, Frazier W: Medicine and patriarchal violence: The social construction of a "private" event. *Int J Health Serv* 9:461, 1979.

79. Smock WS: Recognition of pattern injuries in domestic violence victims. In Siegel JA, Saukko PJ, Knupfer GC (eds): *Encyclopedia of Forensic Sciences.* San Diego, Calif, Academic Press, 2000, pp 384-390.

80. Adelson L: *The Pathology of Homicide.* Springfield, Ill, Charles C Thomas, 1974.

81. Wilson EF: Estimation of the age of cutaneous contusions in child abuse. *Pediatrics* 60:750, 1977.

82. Katcher ML: Scald burns from hot tap water. *JAMA* 246:1219, 1981.

83. Smock WS, et al: The forensic pathologist and the determination of driver versus passenger in motor vehicle collisions. *Am J Forensic Med Pathol* 10:105, 1989.

84. Smock WS: Driver versus passenger in motor vehicle collisions. In Siegel JA, Saukko PJ, Knupfer GC (eds): *Encyclopedia of Forensic Sciences.* San Diego, Calif, Academic Press, 2000, pp 24-32.

85. Blackbourne BD: Injury-vehicle correlations in the investigation of motor vehicle accidents. In Wecht CH (ed): *Legal Medicine Annual 1980.* New York, Appleton-Century-Crofts, 1980.

86. Smock WS, Nichols GR: Air bag module cover injuries. *J Trauma Injury Infect Crit Care* 38:489, 1995.

87. Smock WS: Airbag related injuries and deaths. In Siegel JA, Saukko PJ, Knupfer GC (eds): *Encyclopedia of Forensic Sciences.* San Diego, Calif, Academic Press, 2000, pp 1-8.

88. Laing DK, et al: A fiber data collection for forensic scientists: Collection and examination methods. *J Forensic Sci* 32:364, 1987.

89. National Highway Traffic Safety Administration: *Traffic Safety Facts 2002.* Washington, DC, Department of Transportation, 2003.

CHAPTER

64 Child Maltreatment

Carol D. Berkowitz

PERSPECTIVE

Background

Child maltreatment is an all-encompassing term that includes all forms of child abuse: physical abuse, sexual abuse, emotional abuse, child neglect (physical, emotional, educational), and factitious disease by proxy (also known as *Munchausen syndrome by proxy*).[1] Although the recognition of these conditions by the medical community has occurred at different times, the pivotal report describing child physical abuse occurred in 1962 with the publication of the article "The Battered Child Syndrome" by Kempe and colleagues.[2] The article noted the presence of a complex of physical findings, including fractures, cutaneous bruises, and internal injuries. Since that time, multiple articles and books have described the spectrum of the disorders. During the 1980s, much of the literature focused on child sexual abuse, including the refinement of understanding of normal anogenital anatomy of prepubescent children.[3] *Child sexual abuse* is defined as the involvement of children and adolescents in sexual activity to which they cannot give consent, based on their developmental level, involving an age disparity between the victim and the perpetrator and for the sexual gratifica-

tion of the older individual. Child sexual abuse may involve physical contact between the child and the adult or the involvement of the child in other activities, such as photography or the production of pornographic material.

The role of the physician in caring for an abused child is multifold. Most importantly, the physician must recognize which presenting complaints are attributable to child abuse and initiate medical management of diagnosed medical conditions, some of which may be life-threatening. Differentiating between inflicted injuries, noninflicted injuries, and other medical conditions is paramount to the correct diagnosis and the proper management of the case. In addition, the clinician has the primary responsibility for reporting the suspicion of child abuse to the appropriate authorities which usually include child protective services and law enforcement.

Epidemiology

There are nearly 1 million cases of suspected child abuse and an equal number of child neglect cases noted annually in the United States. Table 64-1 summarizes the data by category of abuse or neglect as noted by the 1996 National Incidence Surveillance report.[4] This process asks individuals who have contact with chil-

Table 64-1. Overview of Incidence of Child Abuse

Type	No. of cases
Physical abuse	381,700
Sexual abuse	217,700
Emotional abuse	204,500
Total abuse	*803,900*
Physical neglect	338,901
Emotional neglect	212,800
Educational neglect	397,300
Total neglect	*949,001*

Data from National Incidence Surveillance Data, 1996.

dren (e.g., teachers) to record cases in which they suspect a child has been abused or neglected. Although child abuse occurs across the spectrum of race, ethnicity, and socioeconomic class, certain factors are associated with an increased prevalence of abuse,[5] including poverty, social isolation, parental alcohol and substance abuse, parental mental illness, and domestic violence.

PRINCIPLES OF DISEASE

Child Physical Abuse

Child physical abuse refers to the infliction of injury on any part of a child's body. Injuries may be manifest in the form of cutaneous bruises, burns, skeletal fractures, internal hemorrhage, organ perforation, and brain injury.

Bruises may appear as petechiae or ecchymoses. They occur at the point of impact between the striking object, such as the hand, and the child's body. Often they mirror the form of the inflicting object and may appear as a hand print, belt outline, or other object (Figure 64-1). These bruises are referred to as *patterned injuries*. When the blow occurs at high velocity, the bruising may resemble the outline of the object as the soft tissue in the center of the impacted field moves laterally (negative image). When the thrust of the strike is slower, the central portion of the skin also may be discolored (positive image). The extent of an injury is influenced by many factors, including the force of blow and the area struck. Frequently the struck area initially may be only erythematous, swollen, or tender, and 24 hours may lapse before bleeding into the skin and subsequent discoloration is noted. The degree of discoloration and the rapidity of resolution of the discoloration are influenced by the location of the injury; large muscle masses, such as the buttocks, can hold larger volumes of blood, and resolution takes longer. In general, extravasated blood goes through a predictable color change pattern as it resolves, progressing from purple to green to yellow and eventually to brown. In general, a minimum of 18 hours needs to elapse before a bruise achieves a yellow color.[6-8] Accidentally incurred bruises tend to occur over bony prominences, such as the shin and forehead. In addition, nonambulatory children (<1 year old) do not readily sustain acci-

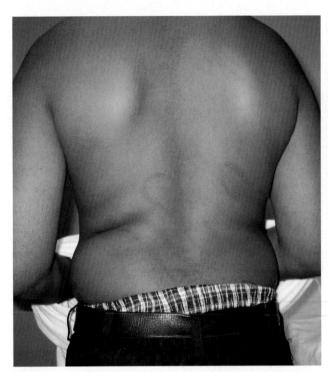

Figure 64-1. Electrical cord bruising on a child's back. (Courtesy of Dr. Marianne Gausche-Hill.)

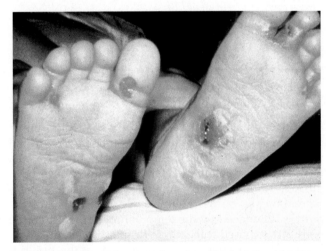

Figure 64-2. Cigarette burns on the soles of the feet of a child. (Courtesy of the EMSC Slide Set, National EMSC Resource Alliance.)

dental cutaneous injuries ("those who don't cruise, don't bruise").[9] Bites also produce a patterned injury. The distance between the maxillary canine teeth helps establish whether the perpetrator was a child (<2.5 cm), which is often alleged, or an adult (>3 cm).

Burns may be inflicted through contact with a dry hot object or through immersion in hot water. Commonly inflicted burns are secondary to contact with a cigarette. Such burns are usually circular, measuring 8 to 10 mm (Figure 64-2). Initially they have a blistered appearance, but then become ulcerated and crust over. Burn injuries also may assume a patterned appearance resembling the configuration of the hot object, such as a heating grid or an iron. Immersion burns occur when

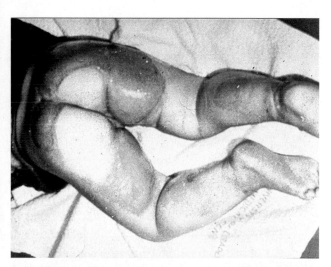

Figure 64-3. Immersion burn. (Courtesy of the EMSC Slide Set, National EMSC Resource Alliance.)

Table 64-2. Time to Cause First-Degree or Second-Degree Burn with Various Water Temperatures

Water Temperature °F(°C)	Exposure (seconds)
125.6 (52)	70
129.2 (54)	30
132.8 (56)	14
136.4 (58)	6
140 (60)	3
143.6 (62)	1.6
147.2 (64)	1

Table 64-3. Suspicious Fractures

Spiral fractures (long bones, preambulatory)
Metaphyseal fractures
Rib fractures
Scapula fractures
Spinous process fractures
Skull
   Multiple
   Complex
   Depressed
   Wide (>3 cm)
   Growing
   Involving >1 cranial bone
   Nonparietal

a child or infant is placed in hot water. Such burns often involve the anogenital area and may represent punishment for toilet training accidents or the hands or feet (glove-stocking distribution), which have been dunked in hot water. Immersion burns are usually second-degree burns (Figure 64-3). The extent of the burn is influenced by the temperature of the water, the body site exposed (the skin is thinner in certain areas, such as the anogenital region), the age of the individual (younger children and elderly adults have thinner skin), and the duration of the contact (Table 64-2).[10] Accidental burns can occur in children and usually involve scald injuries, which happen when children spill hot liquids such as coffee down their shirts. Spill burns have a characteristic drip appearance with more extensive and severe injury proximal to the point of contact and less extensive and milder injury more distally. Disposable diapers are very absorbent of heat as well as of liquids. Scald burns in the anogenital area that are attributed to hot beverages falling into a child's diaper should be scrutinized carefully.[11]

Skeletal injuries may involve any of the bones in the body. Although approximately 42% of boys and 27% of girls have sustained a fracture before the age of 16 years, certain fractures are highly suspicious of an inflicted injury (Table 64-3).[12] In particular, spiral fractures, metaphyseal fractures, rib fractures, and certain types of skull fractures should raise concern about inflicted trauma. Spiral fractures require a twisting motion, in which a rotational force is exerted on the bone. Sometimes they can occur accidentally when there is entrapment of an extremity. Generally a substantial amount of force must be applied for a long bone, such as the femur, to fracture, even in a child. The force required to fracture a femur is equivalent to being struck by a car. Metaphyseal fractures occur because of a yanking or pulling on an extremity. On x-ray, they may appear as chips or what is referred to as a *bucket-handle injury* of the long bone. They usually are noted in children younger than 2 years old. Rib fractures, particularly posterior rib fractures in a small infant, are virtually pathognomonic for inflicted injury.[13] The rib cage, because of its archlike structure, must be subjected to a good deal of force to cause disruption. Rib fractures do not result as a consequence of cardiopulmonary resuscitation.[14] Although children may sustain simple linear skull fractures, most often in the parietal area, after a fall to a solid surface, more complex skull fractures, such as fractures that cross suture lines, are depressed, or are comminuted, are unlikely except when associated with a major traumatic event, such as a motor sehicle crash (MVC).

Head injuries, including those associated with shaken baby syndrome, account for most child abuse–related fatalities. The syndrome includes evidence of head trauma in association with retinal hemorrhages and skeletal injuries and occurs generally in infants younger than 1 year of age, but may be seen in children 3 years old. Most often, there is no evidence of an impact injury to the head, such as a scalp hematoma or skull fracture. The impact may be against a soft or compressible surface, such as the mattress of the crib. Such an impact results in a rapid deceleration of the head, and the brain experiences a coup-contrecoup injury by moving back and forth within the confines of the skull.[15] Shaking of an infant or young child subjects the brain to rotational acceleration, which is capable of generating greater force and speed than linear acceleration, the type of acceleration that occurs with a fall. Rotational acceleration occurs when a discus thrower spins around before releasing the discus. It has been postulated that severe repeated shaking of an infant or young child can lead to disruption of the neuronal cells, with or without the presence of either subarachnoid or subdural hemorrhage. Hemorrhage is a marker for the event, but may be of limited clinical significance, and death, when it occurs, may not be related to bleeding, brain compression, or brain displacement. Injury to the brain cells is referred to as *traumatic axonal injury*.[16] This injury results in disruption of the cell membrane and subsequent cerebral edema. Cerebral edema impedes the cerebral circulation with resultant brain death. At autopsy, special staining techniques allow for the recognition of axonal injury, which may be diffuse (diffuse axonal injury).[17]

Retinal hemorrhages are another common associated finding and are reported to be present in about 75% of cases of shaken baby syndrome.[18] The pathophysiology of retinal hemorrhages is uncertain. It is unclear whether bleeding is a result of increased intracranial pressure that is transmitted to the eye or occurs directly within the eye itself, perhaps through increased pressure along the retinal vein with subsequent disruption of the vessel. Retinal hemorrhages may involve the area in front of the retina (preretinal hemorrhages), the vitreous, and the subretina in addition to the retina. Hemorrhages may be described as "dot and blot" hemorrhages or flame or splinter hemorrhages. Clinically, the hemorrhages may be localized or extend to the ora serrata (the retinal edge).

Abdominal trauma accounts for about 10% of injuries in abused children and represents the second most common type of fatal injury, implicated in 40% to 50% of abuse-related deaths.[19] Trauma is often blunt and includes blows and kicks to the abdomen. Frequently, there is no external evidence of the injury because the force has been transmitted to the intra-abdominal structures. Injuries can include lacerations to the liver (more commonly) or the spleen. In addition, children may develop duodenal hematomas, an injury that leads to symptoms of upper intestinal obstruction. Perforations of the intestine or other hollow viscera can follow a blow to the abdomen with subsequent progression to secondary peritonitis. Pancreatitis is also a sequela of inflicted abdominal trauma, and the latter is said to be the most common mechanism of non–medication-associated pancreatitis in children.

Child Sexual Abuse

Physical findings present when a child or adolescent has been sexually abused depend on the nature of the abuse, the time since the abuse, and whether the abuse was repetitive or isolated. Acute injuries include disruptions (tears) of the hymen, petechiae, hematomas, or rarely vaginal tears. The prepubescent hymen is significantly more fragile and more easily traumatized than the postpubertal hymen, which thickens and becomes redundant under the influence of estrogen. Evidence of recent trauma also may be visible in the anal area. Acutely, there may be lacerations that appear as perianal fissures, which are characteristically wider distal to the anus. There may be posttraumatic dilation, or alternatively anal spasm may occur in response to submucosal injury. In abused boys, the penis rarely has a noticeable injury. More recent studies have evaluated genital healing that occurs after traumatic injury.[20] Physical changes in the anogenital area also may be noted when there has been prior or recurrent sexual abuse. Changes include loss of hymenal tissue and the appearance of u-shaped disruptions in the hymenal contour. Anal findings include the presence of scars and changes in anal tone and the anal contour.[21]

CLINICAL FEATURES

Signs and Symptoms

Child Physical Abuse

Children who have been physically abused may have complaints related to the abuse, or injuries may be noted during the course of an evaluation for an unrelated medical condition. Infants with head injuries may present with nonspecific symptoms that go unrecognized as being related to inflicted head trauma. Jenny and coworkers[22] reported that 31% of infants ultimately diagnosed with inflicted head injury had been evaluated previously in an emergency department and diagnosed with another condition. Infants with head injury may present with apnea, an apparent life-threatening event, vomiting, or a seizure. Clinicians must remain alert that these symptoms may be related to intracranial bleeding or elevated intracranial pressure. A careful physical examination should include an attempt to visualize the eye grounds to determine if there is any evidence of retinal hemorrhages. Bruises on a young infant's face are suspicious of head injury.

Refusal to use an extremity or to weight bear may be an indication of fracture. Similarly, swelling of an extremity may be a sign of a skeletal injury.

Children with abdominal injuries may present with abdominal pain, vomiting, abdominal distention, or shock. In cases of inflicted trauma, the history may be unrevealing or be inconsistent with the medical findings. It is common for a parent to state that he or she is uncertain how a child sustained the injury, or that the child was well at bedtime and awoke in the morning refusing to walk or with severe abdominal pain. Caregivers always should be queried about how they think the injury was sustained. In cases of inflicted head trauma, the scenario often includes a young infant left in the care of a male friend or partner of the mother who has gone to work or to run errands. The male companion asserts that the infant was fine, sleeping in the crib when the companion went to take a shower or make some coffee, and when he returned to check on the infant, the infant was not breathing or was seizing. Often the mother is called before calling 911, or the infant is scooped up by the individual and carried to a hospital. The part of the history that is omitted is that the infant was crying, and the companion shook the infant and thrust the infant back into the crib. The infant sustained acute traumatic axonal injury and stopped crying. The infant is then left unattended, seemingly asleep. As bleeding and cerebral edema develop, other symptoms intervene. Sometimes a family member fallaciously relates a history of a fall, usually from a bed (about 18 to 24 inches above the ground) to a floor that is often carpeted. Or the family member may relate that a young sibling, for instance an 18-month-old, hit or jumped on the infant. Such events are not consistent with severe intracranial injuries.

Histories of falls also are related in children presenting with severe inflicted abdominal trauma. Although falls may lead to bruises of the abdominal wall and rarely splenic injuries, they are unlikely to cause duodenal hematomas, intestinal perforation, or liver lacerations.[23] In addition to obtaining a history of the current event, past medical, developmental, and social histories are important. In children presenting with acute injuries consistent with physical abuse, there is always the possibility that the findings or their severity may be related to an underlying medical condition. A careful medical history may help exclude such conditions or bring these disorders into consideration. A history of epistaxis and bleeding gums in a child who presents with bruises suggests an underlying coagulopathy. A family history of fractures raises the possibility of a bone disorder, such as osteogenesis imperfecta. Documenting a developmental history is important when attempting to assess the likelihood that children's injuries were related to their own activity. It is crucial to be suspicious of injuries in young infants who have limited motor skills. A caregiver may allege that a 3-week-old infant sustained a head injury when he or she fell after having been placed in the center of the bed, but a 3-week-old infant is developmentally unable to scoot or roll from the center to the edge of the bed. The developmental history should document major milestones, such as age of rolling over, sitting unsupported, crawling, and walking.

A social history also is important. It may be helpful for a social worker to assist with a comprehensive social interview, but the clinician can obtain basic information, such as family financial resources (e.g., are the parents working?), where the family lives, what the family's support system is (is there extended family around?), whether there has been domestic violence within the family unit, whether there is substance abuse, and whether the family has ever been reported to protective children's services.

A comprehensive physical examination should be conducted. Growth parameters should be obtained and plotted to determine if there is evidence of growth impairment or failure to thrive. The child should always be completely undressed to allow for visualization of the entire cutaneous surface and an assessment of the child's overall nutritional status and hygiene. It is helpful to have a diagram or outline of the body to allow for precise documentation of the size and location of bruises. Often such diagrams are incorporated into state-generated forms used for the formal reporting of suspected abuse. In addition to the routine examination, there should be a thorough inspection of the infant to detect areas of swelling or tenderness as might occur with fractures. The abdomen should be palpated carefully for tenderness or masses. A careful ophthalmologic examination should be carried out. It is fre-

quently difficult to visualize the fundi of young infants without the benefit of pupil dilation and an indirect ophthalmoscope. Specialized retinal cameras allow for documentation of the findings.

Child Sexual Abuse

Children who have been sexually abused may present with complaints related to an abusive event (e.g., "My Uncle Joey touched me"), anogenital injuries, or other related anogenital physical findings, such as a vaginal discharge. Some children present with stress-related symptoms, such as recurrent headaches or abdominal pain. Concerns about sexual abuse may be raised by divorcing parents when child custody is in dispute. Other patients, particularly older children and adolescents, may be brought to the emergency department by investigative agencies for a physical examination because of a disclosure about recent or prior abuse, even in the absence of any physical or medical complaints.

The medical evaluation should include a history of the events surrounding the alleged molestation. If the child is verbal and willing to disclose to the clinician, this information should be obtained and recorded in the medical record using the patient's own words as much as possible. The report with the disclosure is admissible as evidence. In other cases, the history may be related by other individuals, such as parents, social workers, or law enforcement officers, who are accompanying the patient. The history should include who did what, when, where, and how often. To facilitate communication and understand what the child is discussing, inquiring about the terms the child uses for different parts of the body and the use of anatomically detailed dolls are helpful.

Past medical history also should be noted, including previous anogenital injuries, surgeries, or symptoms such as the presence of vaginal discharges or recurrent urinary tract infections. Stool patterns should be noted and, if constipation is reported, whether any anal medications (suppositories or enemas) are used. In postpubertal girls, a menstrual history, including age of menarche and type of sanitary protection, should be recorded.

The physical examination should include a full head-to-toe assessment to determine if there are acute nongenital injuries (e.g., grip marks or oral injuries) or dermatologic conditions, such as lichen planus, which may explain changes in the anogenital area. The anogenital examination should note the level of pubertal development, recording if the child is prepubertal or at a more advanced stage of sexual maturity.[24] Prepubertal children should be examined using a multimethod approach.[25] Initially, children should be evaluated in the supine position. The labia majora and surrounding tissues should be assessed for evidence of injuries or other abnormalities. Separation or traction should be applied the labia to visualize the structures covered by the labia majora.[26] In prepubertal children, the labia majora are large and full and cover the underlying area. The labia minora are small and delicate and do not fully encircle the vaginal orifice. The clitoris and urethra should be examined. The hymen should be inspected visually for evidence of disruptions and irregularities. The hymen should be precisely described—the phrase "hymen intact" is not sufficiently descriptive for the purposes of a forensic medical assessment. An appropriate description would be: "hymen pink, annular, with smooth thin edge and no disruptions." Some examiners include the size of the hymenal orifice (e.g., "hymenal orifice 3 mm in supine position using traction"). Although the hymenal diameter is said to measure about 1 mm per year of age, an enlarged hymenal orifice without other changes in the hymen is not thought to have forensic significance. Prepubertal girls also should be examined in the prone knee-chest position. The hymen often relaxes more fully in this position, allowing for a more thorough assessment. Speculum examinations are neither indicated nor appropriate for a prepubertal child. If intravaginal trauma is suspected on the basis of vaginal hemorrhage, examination of the child in the operating room under anesthesia is mandatory. Postpubertal adolescents should be examined using a traditional pelvic examination table with stirrups. Findings of forensic significance in an adolescent with a history of prior sexual abuse relate to the appearance of the hymen and the surrounding tissues. In cases of acute sexual assault, a full evidentiary assessment, including speculum examination for the purpose of evaluation and collection of forensic material, is indicated.

DIAGNOSTIC STRATEGIES

Child Physical Abuse

Diagnostic studies should be done to determine the extent of the injuries, detect occult injuries, and exclude medical conditions that may account for the findings. If there is evidence of hemorrhage, such as cutaneous bruises or intramuscular hematomas, coagulation studies are indicated. As a baseline, these studies would include a platelet count, prothrombin time, and partial thromboplastin time. It would be appropriate also to obtain a complete blood count to rule out a blood dyscrasia, such as leukemia in a child who presents with multiple ecchymoses. Occasionally, rarer coagulation deficiencies may present with bruising; the detection of such disorders requires more specific diagnostic studies. In a child with suspected burn injuries, skin cultures are appropriate to rule out infections with *Staphylococcus aureus,* such as occur with bullous impetigo.

In general, children younger than age 2 to 3 years with suspected inflicted injuries should be evaluated with a skeletal series, sometimes referred to as a *trauma X* or *trauma series.* A trauma series includes x-rays of the skull, long bones, ribs, and vertebrae. The presence of multiple fractures, particularly ones in different stages of healing, is the hallmark of the battered child syndrome. Acutely, some fractures, such as rib injuries, may not be readily visible. Repeat studies in 1 to 2

weeks show evidence of callus formation and make the fracture more readily appreciated. Alternatively a radionucleotide bone scan can detect subtle injuries and should be obtained if there is a skeletal injury but a negative skeletal survey.

Urinalysis, liver function studies, and serum amylase and lipase should be considered in children with symptoms of abdominal injury, such as vomiting, abdominal pain, or guarding. Elevated aspartate aminotransferase greater than 450 IU/dL and alanine aminotransferase greater than 250 IU/dL are sensitive signs of liver injury.[27] Plain x-rays are rarely helpful, but should be considered if clinical findings suggest perforation or obstruction. Computed tomography (CT) scan of the abdomen is a more precise way of delineating any abdominal injury. CT scan of the head is indicated when symptoms are consistent with head trauma or in an infant with facial bruising. CT scans may reveal extra-axial hemorrhage or findings consistent with cerebral edema. If the child is sufficiently stable, magnetic resonance imaging is helpful in determining the age of the hemorrhages and in assessing whether there has been prior intracranial hemorrhage.

In recent years, certain metabolic disorders have been described that also may be associated with intracranial hemorrhage. In particular, glutaric aciduria type I may be mistaken for inflicted head trauma.[28] Urinalysis for organic and amino acids would detect this condition.

A careful ophthalmologic examination is crucial. The examination is best done by a pediatric ophthalmologist. Photographic recording of the retinal findings is an important part of the diagnostic workup. Photographing cutaneous injuries is also important and frequently can be carried out by a police criminalist, whose equipment includes color bars for accurate documentation of the coloration of the bruising.

Child Sexual Abuse

Child sexual abuse assessments are sometimes best done with equipment that allows for magnification of the genital tissue. An otoscope or hand-held magnifier is usually available in an emergency department. Centers that evaluate sexually abused children often use colposcopes with photographic or video capability or both to allow for recording of the physical findings. Magnification allows for the detection of microtrauma or small changes in the hymen that may not be readily apparent to the naked eye. Toluidine blue is a stain that is used to increase the ease with which minor injuries are detected. The dye is selectively taken up by exposed endothelial cells. The collection of forensic specimens for the detection of sperm or for the retrieval of DNA of the alleged perpetrator is indicated in cases of acute sexual assault.

Evaluating a child or adolescent for the presence of a sexually transmitted disease depends on many factors, including disease prevalence in the community, patient symptoms, and the nature of the abuse. In cases of acute assault, the recommendation is often to treat the patient prophylactically against sexually

Table 64-4. Sexually Transmitted Disease Prophylaxis or Treatment After Sexual Abuse/Assault

Disease	Treatment
	Child, or Weight <45 kg
Gonorrhea	Ceftriaxone 125 mg IM (1 dose)
	Spectinomycin 40 mg/kg IM (1 dose)
Chlamydia	Erythromycin base 50 mg/kg/dose QID × 10-14 days
Gardnerella	Metronidazole 5 mg/kg/dose PO TID × 7 days
	or Clindamycin 10 mg/kg/dose PO TID × 7 days
	or Amoxicillin/clavulanic acid 20 mg/kg/dose PO BID × 7 days
Trichomonas	Metronidazole 10 mg/kg/dose PO TID × 7 days
Syphilis	Ceftriaxone 50 mg/kg/dose IM (1 dose)
HSV (first clinical episode)	Acyclovir 80 mg/kg divided TID × 7-10 days
Hepatitis B*	HBIG 0.06 mg/kg IM + vaccine series
HIV	Contact local infectious disease specialist before starting zidovudine, 160 mg/m² PO q 6 hr × 28 days, and lamivudine, 4 mg/kg PO BID × 28 days, and nelfinavir, 20–30 mg/kg PO TID × 28 days
	Adolescent, or Weight >45 kg
Gonorrhea	Ceftriaxone 250 mg IM
Chlamydia	Azithromycin 1 g PO, or doxycycline, 100 mg PO BID × 7 days
Gardnerella	Metronidazole 2 g PO (or 500 mg PO BID × 7 days)
Trichomonas	Metronidazole 2 g PO (or 500 mg PO BID × 7 days)
Syphilis	Ceftriaxone 250 mg IM (incubating)
HSV (first clinical episode)	Acyclovir 400 mg PO TID (× episode) 7-10 days, or valacyclovir, 1 g PO BID × 7-10 days
Hepatitis B*	HBIG 0.06 mg/kg IM + vaccine series
HIV	Contact local infectious disease specialist before starting Combivir (ziduvidine/lamivudine), 1 tablet PO BID × 28 days, and indinavir, 800 mg PO q 8 hr × 28 days

*Unimmunized child and perpetrator with acute hepatitis B infection.
HBIG, hepatitis B immunoglobulin; HIV, human immunodeficiency virus; HSV, herpes simplex virus.
Adapted from *APLS: The Pediatric Emergency Medicine Resource,* 4th ed. Gausche-Hill M, Fuchs S, Yamamoto L (eds): Sudbury, Mass, Jones & Bartlett Publishers, 2004.

transmitted diseases such as gonorrhea and chlamydia. The decision to offer prophylaxis against human immunodeficiency virus is often based on disease prevalence and other risk factors (Table 64-4).

Part of the assessment of a sexually abused child may include a detailed interview. Forensic interviews are carried out by an individual with expertise in interviewing children, such as a social worker or clinical psychologist. Although the preliminary interview may be carried out in an emergency department, a more in-depth interview often takes place in a diagnostic center where it may be videotaped or observed (through a one-way mirror) by other individuals, such as law enforcement officers or criminal prosecutors, to minimize the number of times a child or adolescent needs to be questioned about the alleged abusive events.

DIFFERENTIAL CONSIDERATIONS

Child Physical Abuse

The major differential diagnosis when considering child abuse is unintentional injury. Differentiating between inflicted and noninflicted injuries requires the consideration of multiple factors, including the developmental stage of the child, the extent of the injuries, whether the injuries appear to have occurred over a period of time, whether there were witnesses to the alleged event, whether medical care was sought in a timely manner, and whether the injuries could have

been sustained in the stated manner. It is important for the evaluating clinician to have an understanding of normal child development, particularly the acquisition of motor skills. Children who are ambulatory, particularly toddlers and young school-age children, are prone to bruises over bony prominences, such as the shins and forehead. Noninflicted bruises are usually unilateral, occurring on the side where a fall or collision with a solid object has occurred.

Mongolian spots are bluish discolorations that are seen normally over the buttocks and lower spine in children with darker complexions (Figure 64-4). Mongolian spots can appear on other parts of the body, such as the face and upper arm. They are usually present from birth but may not appear until the infant is several weeks old. When seen in a typical location, they are readily recognized as Mongolian spots. When located elsewhere on the body, they may be mistaken for bruises. Bruises resolve over time, Mongolian spots remain unchanged (do not go through purple-green-yellow-brown transformation) because they are undistributed melanocytes.

Phytophotodermatitis also may be mistaken for bruises. This is a condition that develops on sun-exposed areas of the body that have been in contact with certain fruits or juices, such as lime or lemon juice. The lesion appears as a brown discoloration, which may take the shape of the dripped juice or the object with which the juice came in contact. For instance, if a mother is making lemonade, has the

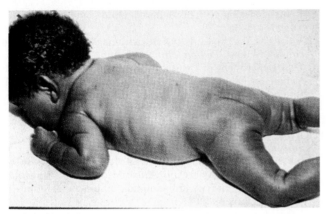

Figure 64-4. Mongolian spots in an infant. (Courtesy of the EMSC Slide Set, National EMSC Resource Alliance.)

lemon juice on her hand, and holds her child, a brown discoloration in the form of a handprint may appear if the child is in the sun. These lesions fade over time, and with a careful history and physician familiarity with the condition, the correct diagnosis can be made.

Burns also may occur unintentionally. Unintentional burns are usually secondary to spills and may take the form of drip marks down a child's chest. Bullous impetigo can be mistaken for second-degree burns because of its blister-like appearance. Culturing the lesion reveals the presence of *S. aureus* in the case of bullous impetigo. Certain dermatologic conditions, such as epidermolysis bullosa, also may cause bullous lesions that may resemble second-degree burns. The history and generalized appearance of these lesions help establish the correct diagnosis.

Fractures may occur unintentionally. In young infants, fractures may be a result of birth-related injuries. The most common fractures sustained during birth are clavicular and humeral fractures. These fractures may not be appreciated immediately after birth, but become apparent when callus formation is noted. Ambulatory children may sustain fractures related to falls. A toddler's fracture, also referred to as a *CAST fracture* (*c*hildhood *a*ccidental *s*piral *t*ibial fracture), occurs when there is a twisting injury to the tibia as the child falls on it.[29] In general, the fracture is a nondisplaced distal fracture of the tibia that is detected when a child presents with a limp. Sometimes the fracture may not be apparent on the initial x-ray, and a bone scan shows the presence of increased bony uptake.

Fractures occur with increased frequency and with lower amounts of force in certain conditions. Premature infants may experience osteopenia of prematurity (sometimes referred to as *rickets of prematurity*), which can be mistaken for metaphyseal fracture.[30] In addition, osteopenic bones may fracture more easily. Osteopenia can be noted on a plain film of the bones. Osteogenesis imperfecta is a condition in which the bone is more brittle and easily disrupted.[31] There are four types of osteogenesis imperfecta, each with a different gene frequency. The overall incidence of osteogenesis imperfecta is 1 in 20,000. Generally, osteogenesis imperfecta is associated with other clinical findings, such as blue sclerae and brown discoloration of the teeth (dentogenesis imperfecta). Rarely, bone fragility may be present in isolation. Scurvy, congenital syphilis, and congenital rubella are associated with bony changes that may be misinterpreted as evidence of prior bony injury.

Cerebral edema may occur with infection, such as encephalitis and meningitis, or after a hypoxic event. The history and the presence of associated medical findings help with the differentiation of these conditions.

Child Sexual Abuse

Numerous medical conditions may be misdiagnosed as child sexual abuse. Accidental trauma, most commonly straddle injuries, may occur after a fall onto the perineum. Such falls occur with climbing on monkey bars, riding on boys' bicycles, or exiting from a swimming pool. Straddle injuries usually involve the labia minora, labia majora, or periurethral area. The hymen remains uninjured. Lichen sclerosis et atrophicus is a dermatologic condition of unclear etiology affecting prepubertal girls and boys and postmenopausal women. The hymen is unaffected, but the adjacent skin becomes atrophic and may sustain blood blisters or petechiae. Characteristically the skin in the perianal and perihymenal areas becomes hypopigmented and surrounds these orifices with a pale figure-of-eight configuration.

Urethral prolapse characteristically affects African-American girls between the ages of 5 and 8 years. The mucosal lining of the urethra slides forward and protrudes from the urethral orifice, appearing as an erythematous, edematous mass. Symptoms include pain and bleeding. Management may involve sitz baths, antibiotic ointment, or referral to an urologist for ligation. Vaginal discharge may occur secondary to conditions other than sexually transmitted diseases. *Shigella,* group A beta-hemolytic streptococcus, *Candida,* and pinworm infestation can cause a vaginal discharge.

Penile swelling may occur with priapism (often secondary to sickle cell disease), paraphimosis, or an infestation with chiggers. Fissures and tags in the perianal area may result from trauma, but also may be associated with constipation and inflammatory bowel disease. Group A beta-hemolytic streptococcus can cause painful inflammation with erythema in the perianal area. Affected children may be febrile and experience pain with defecation. Hemorrhoids are rare in children and are associated with conditions that lead to an elevation of intra-abdominal venous pressure as occurs with cirrhosis of the liver.

MANAGEMENT

The focus of management is to attend to serious or life-threatening injuries, such as significant head or abdominal trauma, and stabilize the patient. Physical problems requiring medical intervention, such as fractures, lacerations, burns, or sexually transmitted diseases, should be managed appropriately. Key to the ultimate management of the abused child is the precise recording of the pertinent history, particularly any disclosure made by the child, and the physical findings. Most states require the completion of a specific child abuse reporting form as a means of notifying the authorities about the suspected case of child abuse. In addition, many jurisdictions require immediate telephonic notification to initiate an investigation of the circumstances surrounding the abuse.

Disposition

Admission to the hospital may be warranted because of the patient's injuries, to complete the medical evaluation, and to protect the child while the evaluation is occurring. Many hospitals have *SCAN* (*S*uspected *C*hild *A*buse and *N*eglect) teams. These teams can offer expert consultation either in the emergency department or after the child has been admitted. *SCAN* teams usually have unique expertise in assessing the genital findings in prepubertal girls.

The outcome for an abused child varies with the nature, extent, and duration of the abuse. Some children die as a result of their inflicted injuries. Others have irreversible brain damage and may spend the remainder of their lives confined to wheelchairs or be blind or otherwise disabled. For other children, intervention and therapy for themselves and their offending parents may help reverse the adverse psychological effects of the abuse. The emergency physician has a key role in the early detection of the problem. The entire medical team along with social services, law enforcement, and the judicial system is responsible for implementing a treatment plan that prevents against recidivism.

 KEY CONCEPTS

- The emergency physician is mandated to report suspicion of child physical or sexual abuse.
- In infants and young children presenting with any injury, the emergency physician must consider child physical abuse as a diagnosis and especially with certain injuries, such as facial bruising; skull, rib, or midshaft humerus fractures; and patterned burns.
- Children who have been sexually abused may present with vague complaints, such as poor sleep pattern or abdominal pain, or may present with vaginal bleeding or discharge.
- Numerous conditions mimic child abuse and must be considered in the differential diagnosis, such as Mongolian spots, lichen sclerosis, impetigo, or urethral prolapse.

REFERENCES

1. Department of Health and Human Services Releases 2000 Child Abuse Report Data. AHA Legislative Activities, American Humane Association. Available at: http://www.americanhumane.org/actnoww/2000_abuse_data.htm.

2. Kempe CH, et al: The battered child syndrome. *JAMA* 181:17, 1962.

3. Woodling BA, Kossoris PD: Sexual misuse: Rape, molestation and incest. *Pediatr Clin North Am* 28:481, 1981.

4. U.S. Department of Health and Human Services National Center on Child Abuse and Neglect: The Third National Incidence Study of Child Abuse and Neglect (NIS-3). Washington, DC, U.S. Government Printing Office, 1996.

5. Sinal S, Petree AN, Herman-Giddens M: Is race or ethnicity a predictive factor in shaken baby syndrome? *Child Abuse Negl* 24:1241, 2000.

6. Jenny C: Cutaneous manifestations of child abuse. In Reece RM, Ludwig S (eds): *Child Abuse Medical Diagnosis and Management,* 2nd ed. Philadelphia, Lippincott Williams & Wilkins, 2001, pp 23-45.

7. Labbe J, Caouette G: Recent skin injuries in normal children. *Pediatrics* 108:271, 2001.

8. Schwartz AJ, Ricci LR: How accurately can bruises be aged in abused children? Literature review and synthesis. *Pediatrics* 97:254, 1996.

9. Sugar NF, Taylor JA, Feldman KW: Bruises in infants and toddlers: Those who don't cruise don't bruise. *Arch Pediatr Adolesc Med* 153:399, 1999.

10. Peck MD, Priolo-Kapel D: Child abuse by burning: A review of the literature and an algorithm for medical investigation. *J Trauma* 53:1013, 2003.

11. Johnson CF, Oral R, Gullberg L: Diaper burn: Accident, abuse or neglect? *Pediatr Emerg Care* 16:173, 2000.

12. Thompson S: Fractures, sprains, and dislocations. In Osborn LM, DeWitt TG, First LR, Zenel JA (eds): *Pediatrics.* Philadelphia, Elsevier Mosby, 2005.

13. Bullock B, et al: Cause and clinical characteristics of rib fractures in infants. *Pediatrics* 105:e48, 2000.

14. Feldman KW, Brewer DK: Child abuse, cardiopulmonary resuscitation, and rib fractures. *Pediatrics* 73:339, 1984.

15. Saternus K-S, Kernbach-Wighton G, Oehmichen M: The shaking trauma in infants—kinetic chains. *Forensic Sci Int* 109:203, 2000.

16. Geddes JF, Whitwell HL, Graham DI: Traumatic axonal injury: Practical issues for diagnosis in medicolegal cases. *Neuropathol Appl Neurobiol* 26:105, 2000.

17. Paterakis K, et al: Outcome of patients with diffuse axonal injury: The significance and prognostic value of MRI in the acute phase. *J Trauma* 49:1071, 2000.

18. Levin A: Retinal hemorrhages and child abuse. *Rec Adv Paediatr* 18:151, 2000.

19. Holmes JF, Sokolove PE, Land C, Kuppermann N: Identification of intra-abdominal injuries in children hospitalized following blunt torso trauma. *Acad Emerg Med* 6:799, 1999.

20. Heppenstall-Heger A, et al: Healing patterns in anogenital injuries: A longitudinal study of injuries associated with sexual abuse, accidental injuries, or genital surgery in the preadolescent child. *Pediatrics* 112:829, 2003.

21. McCann J, Voris J: Perianal injuries resulting from sexual abuse: A longitudinal study. *Pediatrics* 91:390, 1993.

22. Jenny C, et al: Analysis of missed cases of abusive head trauma. *JAMA* 281:621, 1999.

23. Joffe M, Ludwig S: Stairway injuries in children. *Pediatrics* 82:457, 1988.

24. Herman-Giddens ME, Bourdony CJ: *Assessment of Sexual Maturity in Girls.* Elk Grove Village, Ill, American Academy of Pediatrics, 1995.

25. McCann J, Voris J, Simon M, Wells R: Comparison of genital examination techniques in prepubertal girls. *Pediatrics* 85:182, 1990.

26. Heger AH, et al: Appearance of the genitalia in girls selected for nonabuse: Review of hymenal morphology and nonspecific findings. *J Pediatr Adolesc Gynecol* 15:27, 2002.

27. Hennes HN, et al: Elevated liver transaminase levels in children with blunt abdominal trauma: A predictor of injury. *Pediatrics* 86:87, 1990.

28. Hartley LM, Khwaja OS, Verity CM: Glutaric aciduria type 1 and nonaccidental head injury. *Pediatrics* 107:174, 2001.
29. Mellinek LB, Milker L, Egsieker E: Childhood accidental spiral tibial (CAST) fractures. *Pediatr Emerg Care* 15:10, 1999.
30. Miller ME: The bone disease of preterm birth: A biomechanical perspective. *Pediatr Res* 53:10, 2003.
31. Lachman RS, Krakow D, Kleinman PK: Differential diagnosis. II. Osteogenesis imperfecta. In Kleinman PK (ed): *Diagnostic Imaging of Child Abuse,* 2nd ed. St Louis, Mosby, 1998, pp 197-213.

CHAPTER

65 Sexual Assault

Laura Slaughter

PERSPECTIVE

Background

Several major advances in the evaluation and management of sexual assault victims (SAVs) have occurred. The formation of community-based multidisciplinary teams, which first took hold in California, is probably the most important. The development of the sexual assault response team (SART), comprising members of the district attorney's office, law enforcement, medical personnel including physicians and nurses, social service agencies, and victim advocates, brought together all of the major players to solve the logistical, medical, psychological, legal, and social problems incurred by SAVs. The commitment and mutual cooperation of the SART led to the development of standardized protocols for the care and treatment of SAVs. Many of these protocols have been adopted by jurisdictions throughout the United States; this has facilitated greatly the documentation for medical and legal purposes. The necessity of having trained forensic examiners is now well recognized, and SART programs and their forensic organizations have generated training on local, regional, and national levels. Clinical forensic examiners have taken the examination to a different level by employing new technologies, including colposcopy, special staining techniques, and alternative light sources. Much information about the characteristics, physical examination findings, and correlates of injury in SAVs is now available. This information makes the job of the forensic examiner more interesting, facilitates the management of the SAV, and ultimately assists in the identification of the perpetrator.

Epidemiology

An emergency department study has shown that the lifetime prevalence rate of female sexual assault is 39% significantly higher than in other studies. Although it is true that most SAVs do not seek medical care, of those who did, most (78%) were treated, and 61% had an evidentiary examination performed.[1] Sexual assault does not seem to be declining at the rate of other violent crimes; nearly every category of crime was significantly lower in 2001-2002 than in the preceding 2 years except for sexual assault.[2]

Women remain the predominant victims (94%) of sexual assault. Historically, sexual assault has been a largely unreported crime, with only about one third of SAVs coming forward. The major reasons given for not reporting include that the matter was personal, fear of reprisal, or fear of police bias. The closer the relationship between the victim and offender, the less likely the SAV has been to report the crime. The underreporting trend may be changing, however. Of SAVs who report the crime, most do so within 24 hours. A substantial proportion of SAVs report at or after 72 hours, and they are typically adolescents. There is a high positive correlation between reporting to the police and receiving medical treatment.[3]

Sexual assault is an extremely common crime, with estimates of one in three females and one in seven males being assaulted during a lifetime.[4] The mean age of the SAV is approximately 20 years old. She is most often single. Adolescents account for less than half of all victims seen, yet the incidence of sexual assault peaks in the 16- to 19-year age group.[5] For nearly 40% of SAVs, sexual assault is the first sexual experience.[6] A person known to the victim commonly perpetrates the assault. The younger the victim, the more likely the perpetrator is to be a relative. The location of the sexual assault varies with the victim and the type of perpetrator. In general, adults are assaulted in their own home, whereas adolescents are more likely to be assaulted in the assailant's residence.[7] Stranger assaults are less common; they are more likely to involve adults, occur outdoors, and include the use of a weapon.[8] Alcohol and drug use are common accompaniments to sexual assault.[9,10]

Most assaults involve penile-vaginal penetration,[4,7] and penile penetration is significantly associated with genital injury.[11] Typically, digital-vaginal penetration is the second most common sexual act reported. Oral genital contact occurs in less than 30%, and anal assault is slightly less common.[4,6,12,13] The use of a foreign object is unusual (≤10%).[4,7] Anal assault is associated with increased violence,[6,8,11] offender preference for anal sex,[14] and offender problems with sexual dysfunction.[15] Atypical types of assault seem to be increasing over time.[16]

The detection of genital injury is multifactorial and may depend in part on the forensic training of the examiner[6,17] and the technology[18,19] used to perform the examination. Regardless of the methods employed, injury is not an inevitable consequence of sexual assault.[18-20] Adolescent SAVs have been shown to sustain more anogenital injuries than their adult counterparts.[7,11]

Nongenital trauma occurs in 40% to 81% of SAVs,[4,11,18,21-23] and its presence is associated with genital injury.[6,11] The extremities are most commonly injured, followed by the head and neck. Serious injury involving hospitalization occurs in about 5%,[3] and death associated with sexual assault is estimated at 1% or less, although this latter figure is probably a gross underestimate. Psychological distress and interpersonal difficulties are the major sequelae after a sexual assault. These problems are exacerbated in SAVs with known attackers who delay reporting.[24]

MANAGEMENT

Emergency Department Preparation: Multidisciplinary Teams

A standardized approach to the management of the SAV is important. This approach should include the development of a multidisciplinary team that works together under a protocol. The protocol must address every detail, from the handling of the SAV's first call to dispatch to the referral for psychological support. The SAV must be taken out of the medical triage system that typifies the emergency department not only to provide privacy and security for the SAV, but also to prevent the deterioration of evidence. This approach ensures a consistent process of evaluation, treatment, and collection of evidence. The medical team must receive forensic training on interviewing and examination techniques; collecting, preserving, and storing evidence; and chain of custody issues. The team must be trained to use the examination form (in some states this form is 8 pages long) and be thoroughly familiar with the sexual assault kit (rape kit) provided by the state or local crime laboratory. Advocates, whether provided through law enforcement or by a separate entity, need to receive training from the SART about examination procedures and staff roles so that they can best advise and counsel the SAV. A SART program cannot be successful unless advocates believe that the SAV will be treated with respect and receive the best treatment available. Because the SART examiner is the first person on the medical team to greet the victim, a kind, calm, knowledgeable, and professional demeanor is of the utmost importance.

The emergency department also must be prepared for the unusual SAV with significant or life-threatening

BOX 65-1. Consent Issues in Sexual Assault Cases

Consents should specify that the sexual assault victim signature acknowledges:

- That hospitals and health care professionals are mandated reporters
- Receipt of information about victim compensation funds
- Specific understanding of the examination and evidence collection procedures
- Specific understanding of the use of photography in documenting physical and genital injuries
- That information collected will be sent to law enforcement and is obtainable by defense counsel
- That data without patient identity can be collected for valid educational and scientific interest
- That consent may be withdrawn at any time

injuries. In this instance, the emergency physician needs to delegate the forensic responsibility to another forensically trained staff member whose sole purpose is to collect the evidence and, if required, follow the SAV to surgery. In cases in which there is substantial injury, following the patient from intake allows the examiner to understand better and document the nature and extent of the trauma and continue the forensic process with little further distress to the patient.

Obtaining the History and Consent

Numerous consents must be obtained from the SAV, depending on state and local laws (Box 65-1). The forensic examiner must be knowledgeable about all statutes governing consent, including whether minors need parental consent. In some states, even if parental consent is not required, the forensic examiner still may be required to contact the parents and document the success or failure of this attempt. Although not part of the official consent process, most SAVs are concerned about access to the SART record and photographs, particularly, when the SART examination facility is within the hospital setting. Keeping these records separate from the primary hospital chart system has a precedent in the similar handling of psychiatric records. Surveys of SAVs have identified that they desire information about sexually transmitted diseases (STDs), pregnancy, emergency contraception, follow-up care, and physical and psychological health effects of sexual assault.[25] Providing written information on these topics with signature confirmation is warranted.

With the exception of the medical history, group history taking makes the most sense because everyone gathers the same information, and this saves time and avoids contradictions. Before getting started with the history, the SAV's immediate privacy and personal needs need to be addressed. Box 65-2 outlines some of the issues that may make the interview more comfortable for the patient and ensure reliable historical information from the patient. The group taking the history should include a law enforcement officer, patient advocate, medical assistant, and forensic examiner.

A detailed history is important. California was the first state to mandate a uniform examination protocol and specific training for examiners. The protocol subsequently has undergone revision (Figure 65-1).[26]

History of Type of Sexual Assault

Questions about sexual acts need to be explicit and phrased in terms understandable to the SAV. Language used by the SAV to describe sexual acts should be defined clearly for the examiner. The forensic examiner needs to be familiar and comfortable with the array of terms used to describe these details. Importantly, the forensic examiner must ascertain if the SAV voiced her lack of consent and whether that terminated the behavior. The SAV's own words should be used as often as possible and recorded in quotation marks to preserve the integrity of the interview. The experienced forensic examiner also gathers information about the sequence and type of sexual acts that occurred during an assault, including not only kissing, fondling, use of foreign objects, and digital manipulation, but also fetishism, voyeurism, or exhibitionism on the part of the suspect. Table 65-1 lists additional information, which may be useful for the investigation, but which may not be found routinely on sexual assault forms.

BOX 65-2. Preliminary Issues and Strategies in Preparing for Taking the History from a Sexual Assault Victim

- Provide quiet, confidential, safe environment
- Briefly review the interview and examination process in private with the sexual assault victim
- Explain sensitive/personal/embarrassing nature of questions and right to be interviewed without family or friends
- Show concern for immediate comfort (e.g., if thirsty take oral swabs first so the victim may drink)
- Provide advocacy
- Always conduct interview the same way
- Leave difficult questions until the end
- Explain why you are asking the question and the possible responses
- Explain that all questions must be asked

Drug and Alcohol Use

Inquiry about drug and alcohol use is crucial.[9,27-29] Similar to driving under the influence, a sexual assault may be the first indicator that the SAV has a drug or alcohol problem.[30] Data indicate that drug and alcohol abuse by the SAV leads to a concurrent increased risk of an additional assault in the next 2 years; assaulted drug users are at risk for an escalation of drug abuse after the assault.[31] These SAVs need prompt referral for counseling and drug rehabilitation programs. The use of drugs and alcohol is relevant to issues of consent, credibility, and corroboration.[32,33] Except for one,[34] studies have not found a correlation between substance use by the SAV and trauma.[6,7,35-37] The forensic examiner should order drug screening if the victim reports loss of consciousness or forced ingestion, appears confused, is amnesic or has other changes in physical or vital signs that are suspicious of drug use. National drug screening data from SAVs shows that the prevalence of drug use is higher among SAVs than the general population.[38,39] Drugs frequently are used in combination. The two most popular combinations are alcohol and marijuana, followed by alcohol and benzodiazepines.[10]

History of Child Abuse

A history of childhood abuse increases the risk of repeat victimization, with SAVs experiencing multiple episodes of child abuse at greatest risk. Researchers now believe that identification of this vulnerable group is a prerequisite for prevention.[40] The sexual assault examination may be the one time during which the question of prior abuse is raised. A positive answer provides sound justification for emergent referral for psychological services.

Mental Illness

About a quarter of SAVs presenting for evaluation have mental health problems. Many of these women are not forthcoming with this information. A history of mental illness has been shown, however, to increase the severity of the sexual and physical attack. The sexual assault often results in an exacerbation of the mental illness and higher rate of posttraumatic stress disorder.[41]

Table 65-1. Useful Information Not Routinely Found on Sexual Assault Forms

Useful Information	Reason
Positions used during the assault	Affects the location of injury
Positions used during the examination	Helps to orient pictures
Sexual dysfunction in the suspect	Associated with increased violence and anal attack
Repeated thrusting by suspect	May explain loss of seminal product
Victim assistance with insertion of penis	May explain lack of genital injury
Did penis remain in vagina after ejaculation?	May explain loss of seminal product
How do you know ejaculation occurred?	Helps determine where semen may be found
Prior sexual experience	Lack of sexual experience associated with increased hymenal trauma
Gravity and parity	May be a factor in genital injury
History of prior victimization	At increased risk for PTSD; need triage for counseling
Mental health problems	Increased severity of attack and worsening mental health problems
Past medical history	May explain physical or laboratory findings

PTSD, posttraumatic stress disorder.

FORENSIC MEDICAL REPORT: ACUTE (<72 HOURS)
ADULT/ADOLESCENT SEXUAL ASSAULT EXAMINATION

STATE OF CALIFORNIA
OFFICE OF CRIMINAL JUSTICE PLANNING

OCJP 923
Confidential Document

Patient Identification

A. GENERAL INFORMATION (print or type)   Name of Medical Facility:

1. Name of patient

Patient ID number

2. Address   City   County   State   Telephone (W)
                                                                       (H)

3. Age | DOB | Gender | Ethnicity   Date/time of arrival   Date/time of discharge

B. REPORTING AND AUTHORIZATION   Jurisdiction (□ city □ county □ other):

1. Telephone report made to law enforcement agency
Name of Officer   Agency   ID Number   Telephone   Reported by: Name/date/time

2. Responding Officer   Agency   ID Number   Telephone

3. I request a forensic medical examination for suspected sexual assault at public expense.

Telephone Authorization
Agency: Law enforcement officer   ID number   Agency
Authorizing party:
ID number: Telephone   Date   Time   Case Number
Date/time:

C. PATIENT INFORMATION

- I understand that hospitals and health care professionals are required by Penal Code Sections 11160–11161 to report to law enforcement authorities cases in which medical care is sought when injuries have been inflicted upon any person in violation of any state penal law. The report must state the name of the injured person, current whereabouts, and the type and extent of injuries.   (Initial)

- I have been informed that victims of crime are eligible to submit crime victim compensation claims to the State Victims of Crime (VOC) Restitution Fund for out-of-pocket medical expenses, psychological counseling, loss of wages, and job retraining and rehabilitation.   (Initial)

D. PATIENT CONSENT

Minors: Family Code Section 6927 permits minors (12 to 17 years of age) to consent to medical examination, treatment, and evidence collection for sexual assault without parental consent. See instructions for parental notification requirements for minors.

- I understand that a forensic medical examination for evidence of sexual assault at public expense can, with my consent, be conducted by a health care professional to discover and preserve evidence of the assault. If conducted, the report of the examination and any evidence obtained will be released to law enforcement authorities. I understand that the examination may include the collection of reference specimens at the time of the examination or at a later date. I understand that I may withdraw consent at any time for any portion of the examination.   (Initial)

- I understand that collection of evidence may include photographing injuries and that these photographs may include the genital area.   (Initial)

- I hereby consent to a forensic medical examination for evidence of sexual assault.   (Initial)

- I understand that data without patient identity may be collected from this report for health and forensic purposes And provided to health authorities and other qualified persons with a valid educational or scientific interest for demographic and/or epidemiological studies.   (Initial)

Signature   □ Patient   □ Parent   □ Guardian

DISTRIBUTION OF OCJP 923

□ Original - Law Enforcement   □ Copy within evidence kit - Crime Lab   □ Copy - Crime Lab   □ Copy - Child Protective Services (if patient is a minor)   □ Copy - Medical Facility Records

OCJP 923   1   07/01/01

E. PATIENT HISTORY

1. Name of person providing history: Relationship to patient:

2. Pertinent medical history:
- Last menstrual period

- Any recent (60 days) anal-genital injuries, surgeries, diagnostic procedures, or medical treatment that may affect the interpretation of current physical findings? □ No □ Yes   If yes, describe:

- Any other pertinent medical condition(s) that may affect the interpretation of current physical findings? □ No □ Yes

- Any pre-existing physical injuries? □ No □ Yes   If yes, describe:

3. Pertinent pre- and post-assault related history:
                                                    No Yes Unsure
- Other intercourse within past 5 days?   □   □   □
  If yes,
  anal (within past 5 days)?   When ___
  vaginal (within past 5 days)? When ___
  oral (within past 24 hours)?   When ___
- If yes, did ejaculation occur?   □   □   □*
  If yes, where?
- If yes, was a condom used?   □   □   □*
- Any voluntary alcohol use within 12 hours prior to assault?   □   □
- Any voluntary drug or alcohol use within 96 hours prior assault?   □   □   □*
- Any voluntary drug or alcohol use between the time of the assault and the forensic exam? □   □   □*

*If yes, collection of toxicology samples is recommended according to local policy. □ Blood □ Urine

4. Post-assault hygiene/activity: □ Not applicable if over 72 hours
                                       No Yes
- Urinated   □   □
- Defecated   □   □
- Genital or body wipes   □   □
  If yes, describe:
- Douched   □   □
  If yes, with what:
- Removed/inserted □ tampon □ diaphragm □
- Oral gargle/rinse   □   □
- Bath/shower/wash   □   □
- Brushed teeth   □   □
- Ate or drank   □   □
- Changed clothing   □   □
  If yes, describe:

5. Assault-related history:
                                       No Yes
- Loss of memory? If yes, describe: □   □*

- Lapse of consciousness? If yes, describe: □   □*

- *If yes, collection of toxicology samples is recommended according to local policy. □ Blood □ Urine
  Vomited? If yes, describe: □   □

- Non-genital injury, pain and/or bleeding?   □   □
  If yes, describe:

- Anal-genital injury, pain, and/or bleeding?   □   □
  If yes, describe:

OCJP 923   2   07/01/01

F. ASSAULT HISTORY

Patient Identification

1. Date of assault(s):   Time of assault(s):

2. Pertinent physical surroundings of assault(s):

3. Alleged assailant(s)   Age Gender Ethnicity Relationship to patient
                                                            Known Unknown
name(s)
#1.   M F
#2.   M F
#3.   M F
#4.   M F

4. Methods employed by assailant(s):
                              No Yes If yes, describe:
Weapons   □   □
  Threatened?   □   □
  Injuries inflicted?   □   □
  Types?
Physical blows   □   □

Grabbing/holding/pinching   □   □

Physical restraints   □   □

Choking/strangulation   □   □

Burns   □   □
(thermal and/or chemical)

Threat(s) of harm   □   □

Target(s) of threat(s)   □   □

Other methods   □   □

Involuntary ingestion of alcohol/drugs   □ No □ Yes □ Unsure
  If yes, □ Alcohol □ Drugs
  If yes, □ Forced □ Coerced □ Suspected
If yes, toxicology samples collected: □ Blood □ Urine □ None

5. Injuries inflicted upon the assailant(s) during assault? □ No □ Yes
If yes, describe injuries, possible locations on the body, and how they were inflicted.

Figure 65-1. Data collection form from State of California Forensic Medical Report for adults and adolescents, OCJP 923. (From Forensic Medical Report: Acute [<72 hours] Adult/Adolescent Sexual Assault Examination. State of California, Governor's Office of Criminal Justice Planning. www.ocjp.ca.gov)

G. ACTS DESCRIBED BY PATIENT

- Any penetration of the genital or anal opening, however slight, constitutes the act.
- Oral copulation requires only contact
- If more than one assailant, identify by number.

Patient Identification

1. **Penetration of vagina by:**

	No	Yes	Attempted	Unsure
Penis	☐	☐	☐	☐
Finger	☐	☐	☐	☐
Object	☐	☐	☐	☐

Describe the object: _____

Describe: _____

2. **Penetration of anus by:**

	No	Yes	Attempted	Unsure
Penis	☐	☐	☐	☐
Finger	☐	☐	☐	☐
Object	☐	☐	☐	☐

Describe the object: _____

Describe: _____

3. **Oral copulation of genitals:**

	No	Yes	Attempted	Unsure
Of patient by assailant	☐	☐	☐	☐
Of assailant by patient	☐	☐	☐	☐

Describe: _____

4. **Oral copulation of anus:**

	No	Yes	Attempted	Unsure
Of patient by assailant	☐	☐	☐	☐
Of assailant by patient	☐	☐	☐	☐

Describe: _____

5. **Non-genital act(s):**

	No	Yes	Attempted	Unsure
Licking	☐	☐	☐	☐
Kissing	☐	☐	☐	☐
Suction injury	☐	☐	☐	☐
Biting	☐	☐	☐	☐

Describe: _____

6. **Other act(s):**

No	Yes	Attempted	Unsure
☐	☐	☐	☐

Describe: _____

7. **Did ejaculation occur?**

No	Yes	Unsure
☐	☐	☐

If yes, note location(s):
☐ Mouth
☐ Vagina
☐ Anus/Rectum
☐ Body surface
☐ On clothing
☐ On bedding
☐ Other

Describe: _____

8. **Contraceptive or lubricant products:**

	No	Yes	Unsure
Foam used?	☐	☐	☐
Jelly used?	☐	☐	☐
Lubricant used?	☐	☐	☐
Condom used?	☐	☐	☐

Describe type/brand, if known: _____

OCJP 923   07/01/01

3

H. GENERAL PHYSICAL EXAMINATION

Record all findings using diagrams, legend, and a consecutive numbering system.

1. Blood Pressure	Pulse	Resp	Temp	2. Date/time examination
				Started
				Completed

3. Describe general physical appearance   4. Describe general demeanor

Patient Identification

5. Describe condition of clothing upon arrival. _____

6. Collect outer and underclothing if indicated. ☐ Findings   ☐ Not indicated
7. Conduct a physical examination. ☐ Findings ☐ No Findings
8. Collect dried and moist secretions, stains, and foreign materials from the body. Scan the entire body with a Wood's Lamp.
   ☐ Findings ☐ No Findings
9. Collect fingernail scrapings or cuttings according to local policy.

Diagram A   Diagram B

LEGEND: Types of Findings

AB Abrasion	DF Deformity	FB Foreign Body	MS Moist Secretion	PE Petechiae	TB Toludine Blue®
BI Bite	DS Dry Secretion	IN Induration	OF Other Foreign	PS Potential Saliva	TE Tenderness
BU Burn	EC Ecchymosis (bruise)	IW Incised Wound	Materials (describe)	SHX Sample Per History	V/S Vegetation/Soil
CS Control Swab	ER Erythema (redness)	LA Laceration	OI Other Injury	SI Suction Injury	WL Wood's Lamp®
DE Debris	F/H Fiber/Hair		(describe)	SW Swelling	

Locator #	Type	Description	Locator #	Type	Description

RECORD ALL CLOTHING AND SPECIMENS COLLECTED ON PAGE 8

OCJP 923   07/01/01

4

Figure 65-1, cont'd.

I. HEAD, NECK, AND ORAL EXAMINATION

Record all findings using diagrams, legend, and a consecutive numbering system.

1. Examine the face, head, hair, scalp, and neck for injury and foreign materials. ☐ Findings ☐ No Findings

5. Collect dried and moist secretions, stains, and foreign materials from the face, head, hair, scalp, and neck.
☐ Findings ☐ No Findings

5. Examine the oral cavity for injury and foreign materials (if indicated by assault history). Collect foreign materials.
Exam done: ☐ Not applicable ☐ Yes ☐ Findings ☐ No Findings

4. Collect 2 swabs from the oral cavity up to 12 hours post assault and prepare one dry mount slide from one of the swabs.

5. Collect head hair reference samples according to local policy.

Diagram C

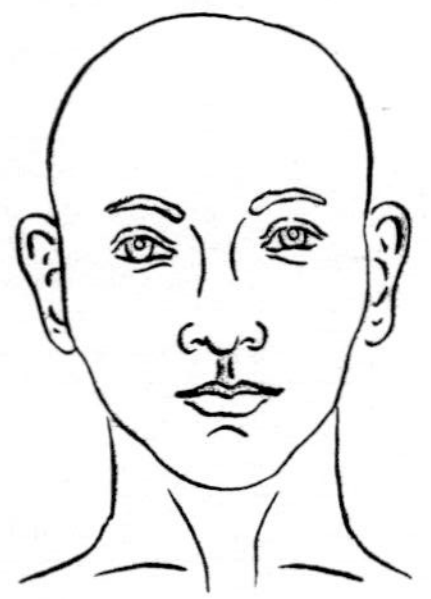

Diagram D

Patient Identification

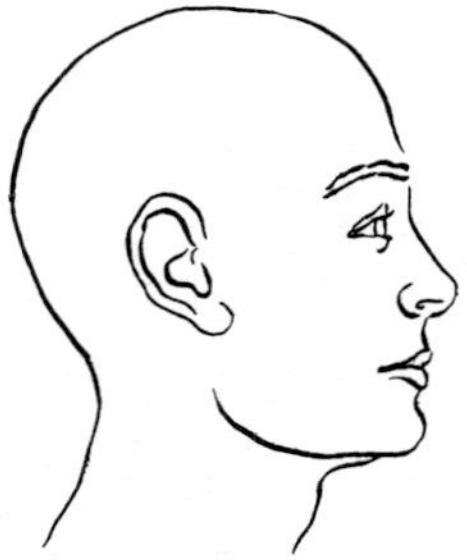

Diagram E

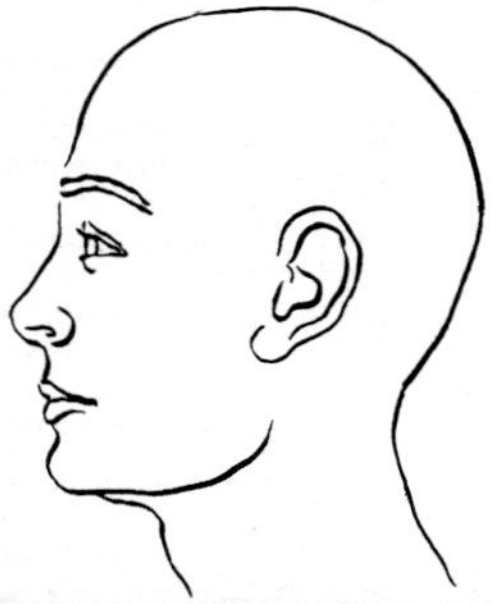

Diagram F

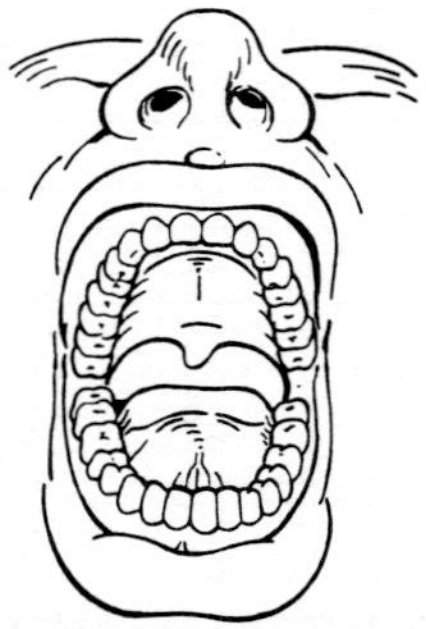

LEGEND: Types of Findings

AB	Abrasion	DF	Deformity	FB	Foreign Body	MS	Moist Secretion
BI	Bite	DS	Dry Secretion	IN	Induration	OF	Other Foreign
BU	Burn	EC	Ecchymosis (bruise)	IW	Incised Wound		Materials (describe)
CS	Control Swab	ER	Erythema (redness)	LA	Laceration	OI	Other Injury
DE	Debris	F/H	Fiber/Hair				(describe)

PE	Petechiae		TB	Toluidine Blue⊕
PS	Potential Saliva		TE	Tenderness
SHX	Sample Per History		V/S	Vegetation/Soil
SI	Suction Injury		WL	Wood's Lamp⊕
SW	Swelling			

Locator #	Type	Description

RECORD ALL SPECIMENS COLLECTED ON PAGE 8

OCJP 923   5   07/01/01

J. GENITAL EXAMINATION - FEMALES

Record all findings using diagrams, legend, and a consecutive numbering system.

1. Examine the inner thighs, external genitalia, and perineal area. Check the box(es) if there are assault related findings:
☐ No Findings
☐ Inner thighs ☐ Periurethral tissue/urethral meatus
☐ Perineum ☐ Perihymenal tissue (vestibule)
☐ Labia majora ☐ Hymen
☐ Labia minora ☐ Fossa navicularis
☐ Clitoris/surrounding area ☐ Posterior fourchette

2. Collect dried and moist secretions, stains, and foreign materials. Scan the area with a Wood's Lamp. ☐ Findings ☐ No Findings

3. Collect pubic hair combing or brushing.

4. Collect pubic hair reference samples according to local policy.

5. Examine the vagina and cervix. Check the box(es) if there are assault related findings.
☐ Vagina ☐ Cervix ☐ No Findings

6. Collect 4 swabs from the vaginal pool. Prepare one wet mount slide and one dry mount slide.

7. Collect 2 cervical swabs (if over 48 hours post assault).

8. Examine the buttocks, anus, and rectum (if indicated by history).
Exam done: ☐ Yes ☐ Not applicable
Check the box(es) if there are assault related findings:
☐ No Findings
☐ Buttocks ☐ Anal verge/folds/rugae
☐ Perianal skin ☐ Rectum

9. Collect dried and moist secretions, stains, and foreign materials.
☐ Findings ☐ No Findings

10. Collect 2 anal and/or rectal swabs and prepare one dry mount slide.

11. Conduct an anoscopic exam if rectal injury is suspected or if there is any sign of rectal bleeding. ☐ No ☐ Not applicable ☐ Yes
Rectal bleeding ☐ No ☐ Yes
If yes, describe:

12. Exam position used:
☐ Supine ☐ Other Describe:

Diagram G

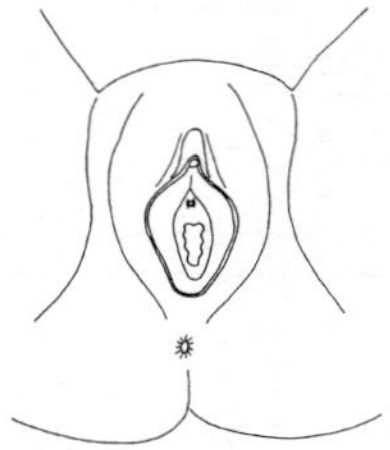

Diagram H

Patient Identification

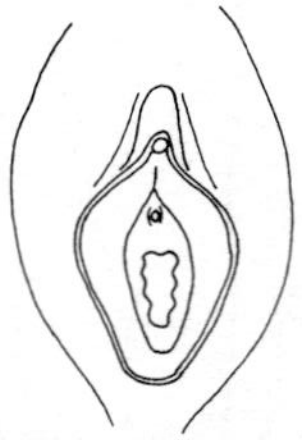

Diagram I

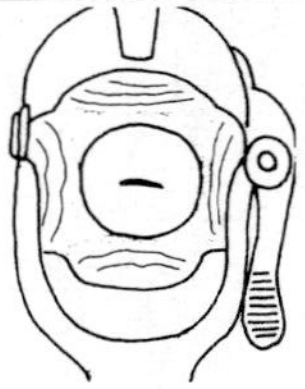

Diagram J

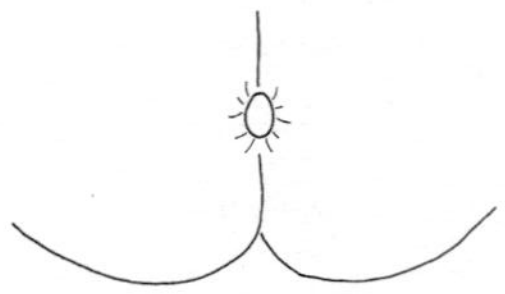

LEGEND: Types of Findings

AB	Abrasion	EC	Ecchymosis (bruise)	MS	Moist Secretion	SI	Suction Injury
BI	Bite	ER	Erythema (redness)	OF	Other Foreign	SW	Swelling
BU	Burn	F/H	Fiber/Hair		Materials (describe)	TB	Toluidine Blue⊕
CS	Control Swab	FB	Foreign Body	OI	Other Injury (describe)	TE	Tenderness
DE	Debris	IN	Induration	PE	Petechiae	V/S	Vegetation/Soil
DF	Deformity	IW	Incised Wound	PS	Potential Saliva	WL	Wood's Lamp⊕
DS	Dry Secretion	LA	Laceration	SHX	Sample Per History		

Locator #	Type	Description

RECORD ALL SPECIMENS COLLECTED ON PAGE 8

OCJP 923   6   07/01/01

Figure 65-1, cont'd.

BOX 65-4. Documentation of Findings During Sexual Assault Examination

Findings/evidence to be documented include:
- Preexisting injuries
- Acute injuries
- Tenderness or induration
- Foreign material
- Wood's lamp/alternate light source positive areas
- Secretions and stains
- Potential saliva/semen (per history)
- Swab collection sites (evidence and controls)
- Indicate any site where moist swab collection occurred

BOX 65-5. Information to Document on Standard Evidentiary Label

On each item in the rape kit:
- Full name of patient
- Medical record or case ID number
- Date of collection
- Time of collection
- Brief description of item with sampling site
- Initials of the examiner

BOX 65-6. Chain of Custody

Record of signatures, dates and times that:
   Document handling, transfer, and storage of evidence from the time of collection
   Provide sequential accountability of everyone who handled the evidence
   Document the location of the evidence at all times
   Ensures there has been no tampering, alteration, or loss of evidence before trial

For all transfers of evidence, documentation must include:
   Signature of person transferring custody
   Signature of person receiving custody
   Date of transfer
   Time of transfer

Documentation is written on sealed and packaged kit

BOX 65-7. Wood's Lamp and Alternate Light Source

Wood's Lamp
Screening tool for detection of stains, secretions, and injuries
Long-wave UV light (310-400 nm)
Dried semen usually fluoresces bright green/yellow or white
Moist semen fluoresces poorly or not at all
Other body fluids and substances may be seen
Room must be dark to use

Alternate Light Source
High-intensity, tunable light source
Uses 4 narrow bands: 450 nm, 485 nm, 525 nm, 570 nm
2 wide bands: white light, all wavelengths <530 nm
Colored goggles used to block the reflected light and pass only the fluorescent light
Because of absorptive differences between normal and damaged tissues, can detect injuries not seen with the naked eye
More accurate for certain body fluids and substances than Wood's lamp

second-guess what the laboratory may or may not recover based on rigid time frames. A report documents the retrieval of salivary DNA from a bite mark on a body that was submerged in water for more than 5 hours.[50] If there is a history of loss of consciousness or significant memory impairment, then all specimens should be collected. This opportunity for collection occurs only once.

Examination of the Skin

The forensic examiner needs to describe the SAV's demeanor and general appearance. The examiner should be especially careful to use specific terms and note responsiveness and ability to cooperate and give a history. All clothing worn during the assault should be inspected, collected, and photographed. A Wood's lamp or alternate light source should be used to detect dried secretions and to document the findings (Box 65-7).

The SAV should undress on the large square of paper from the rape kit after removing shoes. Another sheet of paper should be placed underneath this square to prevent contamination from the floor. The square paper is used to catch trace evidence and must be folded carefully and placed into evidence.

When the SAV is undressed, the forensic examiner uses the Wood's lamp or alternate light source over the body and documents positive fluorescence. Dried secretions should be removed with a cotton swab moistened with sterile, distilled water. If one side of the swab is flattened, and only that side is used to collect the specimen, the material is effectively concentrated. Conversely, wet secretions should be taken in the same manner using a dry swab. Swabs should be collected from areas of contact indicated by the SAV, even if there is no fluorescence or crusting seen. A double-swab technique is used to collect saliva from skin (Box 65-8).[51] Bite marks need special attention (Box 65-9).[52] Control swabs should be taken in areas next to the

containers (no plastic), labeled (Box 65-5), and sealed. Each container must be sealed securely with tape, and the examiner should initial or sign across the tape and onto the container/bag.

To preserve the integrity of the evidence, the SAV must not be left alone in the room with it, and the forensic examiner must wear powder-free gloves to prevent contamination of the evidence. If the evidence must be stored, a locked unit must be available. Preserving the chain of custody, a fundamental principle in the criminal justice system must be understood by all personnel (Box 65-6). A complete examination and historically relevant evidence collection should be performed regardless of the time between the assault and the examination. The forensic examiner must not

BOX 65-8. Double-Swab Technique for Recovery of Saliva from Human Skin

First swab—completely wet with sterile distilled water
  Roll over the surface of the skin using moderate pressure
    and circular motions
  Rotate swab on long axis to ensure maximal contact
  Air dry completely (≥30 min)
Second swab—used dry
  Apply with the same action as above to pick up all the
    moisture left behind
  Allow to dry completely (≥30 min)
Label each and submit *both swabs* with other evidence

BOX 65-9. Collection of Bite-mark Evidence

Take an orienting photograph before swabbing
  Be certain to take close-up photographs, and use a scale
  If the bite mark is on a rounded surface, more than one
    photograph is needed to avoid distortion
Notify law enforcement immediately so that they can contact
  a forensic odontologist, who may take additional pho-
  tographs and collect impressions
Serial photographs are recommended at 24-h intervals for
  5 days
Use the double-swab technique to obtain saliva sample (see
  Box 65-8)

material removed and labeled as such. All swabs must be dried in a stream of cool air at least 60 minutes before packaging. Swab-drying machines are available with locks to facilitate this process. To prevent contamination, only one person's evidence should be in the dryer at a time, and the drying chamber must be cleaned after each use with 10% bleach solution. The location of all foreign material should be documented on body diagrams and packaged in the standard fashion. Fingernail clippings or scrapings should be collected according to local custom and only if there is historical relevancy. All preexisting injuries and acute trauma needs to be documented in the report.

Diagrams of the body should be large enough to allow documentation to remain clear. If need be, copies of the state/local diagrams should be available in full-page format to accomplish this. The documentation process in some states is artistic, which means the forensic examiner draws the injury on the diagram. California has switched to a purely descriptive approach for uniformity and clarity (see Figure 65-1). Although the descriptive approach requires some adjustment, it is a superior method.

Head, Neck, and Oral Cavity

In examining the head, neck, and oral cavity, special attention should be given to the integrity of the frenulum, buccal surfaces, gums, and soft palate. The SAV should not be allowed to eat or drink before this examination. If the SAV gives a history of oral copulation with ejaculation, the upper and lower lips should be wiped using two moistened swabs. Next the examiner should swab from the gum to the tonsillar fossae, the upper first and second molars, behind the incisors, and the fold of the cheek. Lastly, using a 16-inch piece of unwaxed floss, with two knots tied about 2 to 3 inches apart in the center of the floss, the SAV should floss her teeth using only the section between the knots. While flossing, the patient should lean over a clean 8 × 10 piece of paper to catch any debris. The paper and floss are dried and placed in a bindled together. If the SAV is unable to use the floss, the examiner, wearing gloves and goggles, can perform this procedure.[53] Hair matted with secretions or debris should be cut out and packaged. Signs of manual or ligature strangulation may include neck injuries with petechiae of the skin and conjunctiva. Reference samples for head hair and saliva should be taken according to local custom, including buccal swabs made for DNA analysis. Reference standards are used to determine whether the evidence specimens are of SAV origin or are foreign. Additionally, they may help identify or eliminate potential suspects.

Anogenital Examination

The anogenital examination should begin with gross visualization of the inner thighs, external genitalia, perineal area, and anus, followed by Wood's lamp or alternate light source visualization. All trauma, secretions, and foreign material should be noted and appropriately handled. Gross visualization yields positive findings in 20% to 30% of cases (range 5% to 65%).[4,18,23,42,46,54] Genital trauma associated with sexual assault is considered to be a mounting injury because it occurs at the point of first contact of penis to vagina. This area, the posterior fourchette (soft tissue) or the perineal body (the juncture of the tendons of the superficial transverse perineal and the bulbocavernosus muscles), is inherently weak, and continued pressure results in tearing. The position of restraint, male straddling female, also effectively prevents the SAV from accommodating the erect penis. The angle of the erect penis is not the same as the angle the vagina makes with the vestibule (approximately 45 degrees). The vagina is considered a potential space. The lateral walls are more rigid than the anterior and posterior walls so that in its normal state the anterior wall is collapsed onto the posterior wall—hence the use of the speculum to lift the anterior wall during the gynecologic examination.[55] During voluntary intercourse, the changes that occur with sexual stimulation, the human sexual response, remove these normal anatomic barriers, and the female voluntarily tilts her pelvis.[56]

Typically, genital injury involves more than one site, is external, and is located posteriorly between 3, 6, and 9 o'clock (Figure 65-2). The posterior fourchette is the most common site of injury, as reported in several studies.[4,6,11,42] Injuries are usually the result of blunt force trauma, which produces tears, ecchymosis, abrasions, redness, and swelling. The latter two may be difficult to recognize without a follow-up examination,

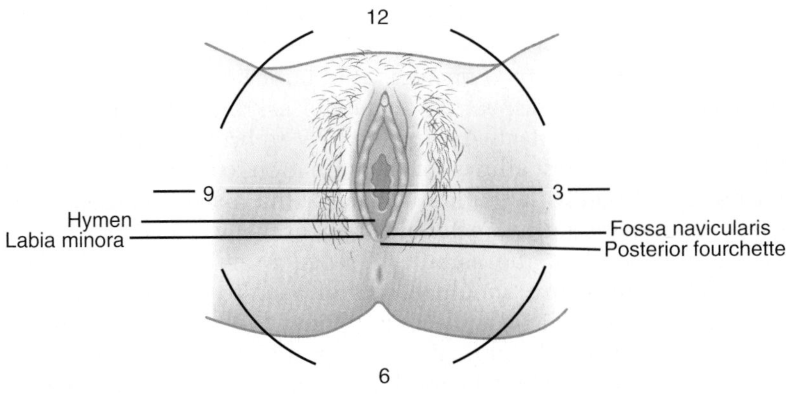

Figure 65-2. Typical genital injury between 3, 6, and 9 o'clock.

12

Hymen

Labia minora

9 — 3

Fossa navicularis

Posterior fourchette

6

BOX 65-10. Correlates of Genital Injury Found at the Time of Sexual Assault Examinations

Time to examination*
Nongenital injury associated with genital trauma
Penile penetration
Sexual inexperience and hymenal tearing
Postmenopausal
History of anal contact
History of stranger assault
History of nonconsensual intercourse
History of mental illness

*Increase in time since injury decreases likelihood of findings; other factors listed increase the likelihood of physical findings at the time of sexual assault examinations.

Table 65-2. Environmental Factors Associated with Intravaginal Epithelial Changes Seen with Visual Inspection, Colposcopy, or Acetic Acid Application

Factor	Findings*
Smoking	Edema, erythema, petechiae, abrasion
Tampon use at the time of examination	Erythema, petechiae, abrasion
Speculum manipulation	Laceration
Consenting intercourse	Erythema, petechiae, abrasion, ecchymosis
Herpetic infection	Microulcerations

*Findings on 56/314 inspections; considered to be minor; 80% of findings could be seen only with colposcope, and 26% of petechiae were seen only after acetic acid application.[61]

---

and some authors have suggested not reporting redness or swelling if a second examination is not performed.[6] Hymenal trauma is not the first site of injury, as myth would have it. Hymenal trauma is more common in adolescents and women without sexual experience.[6,11,42] Genital injury shows consistent topologic features, varying with the site and nature of the tissue. Tears are most commonly seen in the posterior fourchette and fossa navicularis. Abrasions typically occur on the labia minora. The hymen usually sustains damage in the form of ecchymoses or tears.[7,11] Many factors affect the prevalence of genital injury, and the forensic examiner should be familiar with them (Box 65-10).

Even though genital injury is statistically significantly associated with a history of nonconsent, genital trauma is not inevitable.[11,57,58] Whether this is true for adolescent SAVs has been questioned; in this study, the prevalence of injury between consenting and nonconsenting adolescents was not statistically different, but the localized pattern and severity of anogenital injuries between these two groups were.[59] Next, colposcopic magnification should be employed to document these areas photographically and to identify better the type of trauma seen. Colposcopy is the standard of care and is the best method for determining genital injury in the literature.[19,60] Certain environmental factors have been identified with colposcopically recognized genital changes; this is particularly true with intravaginal find-

ings (Table 65-2).[61] Frequently, trace evidence is seen only with the colposcope. We use adhesive notepaper (Post-it) to capture such tiny particles while visualized under the scope. The Post-it is folded and inserted into an envelope. Examiners must check with their local crime laboratories to see if this methodology is acceptable. Pubic hair brushings are collected by placing a sheet of paper under the patient's buttocks and brushing the pubic hair downward. The paper and brush should be bindled together and packaged. A pubic hair standard should be obtained according to local custom.

A warm speculum moistened with water should be inserted into the vagina. Inspection of the vagina and cervix should be performed first grossly, then with colposcopic photography. If the SAV reported bleeding, the source needs to be determined. Bleeding commonly is associated with hymenal, vaginal, or combined tears. Swabs from the vagina and cervix should be obtained according to local protocol, air-dried, and packaged. To check for motile sperm, the forensic examiner should inspect a wet mount slide. This method is useful because it gives a time frame for the assault and sufficient numbers of sperm (60 to 100) allow for identification of a suspect.[26] Semen is found about 50% of the time.[54] The forensic examiner should communicate this information to the investigator as soon as possible. The wet mount slide is dried and prepared for deposit into the rape kit. Aside from time and site of deposition (Table 65-3),[62-72] female and male factors influence the ability to find semen (Table 65-4). In the physiologic changes that accompany the human sexual response, the vagina lengthens and the cervix elevates, deforming the posterior wall into a seminal reservoir; swelling in the anterior vaginal wall prevents the egress of semen. Without these changes, the vagina is a short straight tube.[56] Typically a bimanual examination is not performed.

Table 65-3. Maximal Reported Time Intervals for Sperm Recovery

Body Cavity	Motile Sperm	Nonmotile Sperm
Vagina	6-28 hr	14 hr-10 days
Cervix	3-7 days	7.5-19 days
Mouth	—	2-31 hr
Rectum	—	4-113 hr
Anus	—	2-44 hr

Table 65-4. Factors Influencing Loss of Sperm and Seminal Fluid

Female Factors	Male Factors
Prior trauma to birth canal	Condom use
Lost on withdrawal of penis	Vasectomy
Vaginal hygiene (e.g., douching, wiping)	Azospermia
Repeated penile thrusting	Drug and alcohol abuse
Penis remains in the vagina after coitus	Sexual dysfunction
Change of posture	Failure to ejaculate

A rectal examination is performed as related by the history. Because SAVs are reluctant to report this type of activity, however, the forensic examiner should always inspect the anus and ask the SAV again about anal contact. Asking the SAV to bring her knees up to her chest allows this examination to be done easily and quickly. If trauma is seen or the history suggests anal penetration, rectal bleeding, or that a foreign object was used in the assault, a rectal examination, including anoscopy, should be performed. To avoid contamination with vaginal secretions, the perianal region is swabbed thoroughly with a moistened swab or 2 × 2 gauze, which is dried, labeled, and included in the rape kit. This procedure must be done after all vaginal samples, external secretions, and foreign material have been collected. A warm water–moistened anoscope is used to perform the procedure. The examiner observes grossly and colposcopically and photographs; swabs are collected under direct visualization beyond the tip of the scope. The source of any bleeding needs to be determined.

Special Staining Techniques

The use of special staining and lubrication techniques should be reserved until all photography and specimens are collected. On areas that are painful, 2% lidocaine gel can be used to obtain better visualization and pictures. Toluidine blue dye is a nuclear stain that has been shown to enhance gross visualization of external genital (vulvar) injuries (Figure 65-3). Toluidine blue dye has some spermicidal activity[57] and was shown in one small study not to influence DNA analysis.[73] Stain results depend on the presence or absence of a nucleated cell population at the exposed surface. Positive stain results can be seen with trauma, cancer, and areas of inflammation with a nucleated cellular infiltrate.

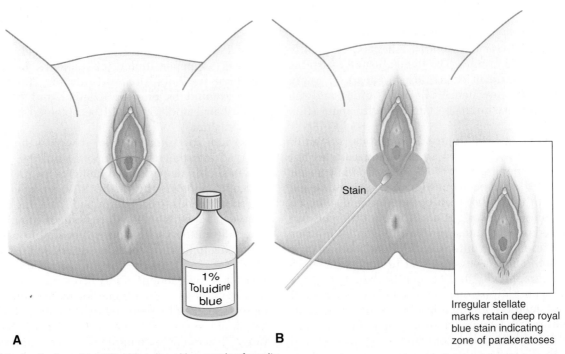

1%
Toluidine
blue

Stain

Irregular stellate marks retain deep royal blue stain indicating zone of parakeratoses

A

B

Figure 65-3. Application of toluidine blue dye with example of results.

Acutely, with tissue swelling and transudation, the dye may lift off quickly. Twenty-three categories of benign disease, including columnar epithelium, and mucus take up this stain.[74] Toluidine blue dye is nonspecific and should be used to enhance trauma seen with the colposcope or as an adjunct for gross visualization. It should not be used to date injuries. Diffuse staining or patchy uptake should not be reported.[58] Uptake should not be reported when no findings are seen with colposcopy.[19]

Photographic Documentation

Photographic documentation of the sexual assault examination has become increasingly important. Photographic documentation eliminates the problem of hyperbole in the forensic examiner's description and allows the court to see directly what the findings are. The entire examination should be photographically documented, not just the positive findings. All photographs must be labeled correctly to show patient identification, date, time, and examiner. Frequently this information can be combined with a color guide and ruler. Jurors usually want to know how pictures are identified. The forensic examiner must develop a standard photographic technique, making certain that the plane of the film is parallel with the injury to minimize distortion. Photos of skin are enhanced if the background is blue or green because the automatic lens adjusts according to the lightest part of the picture. The examiner should take pictures of lesions *first* without magnification, then take closer views as needed. The full extent of the injury needs to be captured. Using magnification usually requires more than one shot. The examiner should take lots of pictures because he or she has this opportunity only once (Box 65-11 outlines tips in performing photographic documentation in sexual assault cases). Pictures also are a concern for SAVs. Most SAVs worry about where the pictures are kept and whether their name will appear on the pictures. Keeping the SART record separate from the medical record is reassuring. Some groups go a step further and separate the pictures from the written reports.

Sexually Transmitted Diseases and Pregnancy

The risk of acquiring an STD after a sexual assault is small but varies by region and number of assailants (Table 65-5).[75] The gold standard for testing for STD has been culture, and this method is still recommended by the Centers for Disease Control and Prevention. Cultures are expensive; require a reassessment of the patient, which is often difficult; and have no forensic value. Many protocols no longer require or pay for this type of assessment. Additionally, many SAVs have pre-existing STDs. Most providers prefer preventive therapy (Box 65-12)[76,77]; this offers the SAV the psychological benefit of immediate protection from infection. For updated information and alternative therapies for patients who are pregnant or have specific allergies, the physician can consult www.cdc.gov and enter "std treatment." The efficacy of these regimens in preventing gonorrhea, trichomoniasis, bacterial vaginosis, and *Chlamydia trachomatis* genitourinary infections after sexual assault has not been evaluated. The forensic examiner should counsel patients about the possible toxicity of any regimen; gastrointestinal problems are

---

BOX 65-11. Tips in Photodocumentation of Sexual Assault Findings

Lens: best all around for bodily injury macro lens with focal length 100-105
Documentation
  Do not photograph more than one victim per roll
  Begin each roll with facial shot and ID number
Technique
  Background
    Avoid clutter
    Avoid reflective or bright light
    Use blue or green surgical towels for extremity shots
  Positioning
    The plane of the film should be parallel to the plane of the finding
    Textured finding (e.g., swelling, indentation)—take additional shots at a variety of tangential or oblique angles
  Anatomic context and scale
    Every finding should appear in at least 3 pictures—regional shots that orient the viewer to the finding's general location
    Close-ups that zoom in on the finding with the camera orientation the same as for the regional shot
    At least one close-up shot that includes a scale/color with victim's ID number on it
Review photos to make certain pictures of all findings and all areas of the anogenital anatomy were taken.

Table 65-5. Risk of Sexually Transmitted Disease After Sexual Assault

Disease	Risk
Gonorrhea	6-18%
Chlamydia	4-17%
Syphilis	0.5-3%
HIV	<1%

HIV, human immunodeficiency virus.

BOX 65-12. Centers for Disease Control Prophylaxis for Sexually Transmitted Disease* in Adult Sexual Assault Victims

Ceftriaxone 125 mg IM in a single dose
plus
Metronidazole 2 g orally in a single dose
plus
Azithromycin 1 g orally in a single dose
or
Doxycycline 100 mg orally twice a day for 7 days

Chlamydia, gonorrhea, *Trichomonas*, and bacterial vaginosis.

BOX 65-13. Hepatitis B Infection Prophylaxis for Sexual Assault Victims

Serologic testing not required
Give vaccination if sexual assault victim is unimmunized or uncertain
Follow-up doses at 1-2 mo and 4-6 mo (total of 3 doses)

BOX 65-14. Factors Influencing Probability of Human Immunodeficiency Virus Transmission

Sexual Assault Victim Factors: Susceptibility
Type of sexual contact   ↑ anal than vaginal
Presence of STDs   ↑
Presence of genital/anal trauma   ↑
Exposure to ejaculate   ↑
Cervical ectopy   ↑
Contraceptive method
  Barrier   ↓
  IUD   ?
  Nonoxynol 9   ↑
  Pills   ↑↓
Menstruation   ↓
Currently pregnant   ?

Assailant Factors: Infectiousness
Presence of foreskin   ↑
Late stage of infection   ↑
Primary HIV infection   ↑
Viral load in the genital tract   ↑
Presence of STDs or genital lesions   ↑
Antiretroviral therapy   ↓

↑ increased probability.
↓ decreased probability.
↑↓ evidence to support increased and decreased probability.
? Unknown effect.
STDs, sexually transmitted diseases; HIV, human immunodeficiency virus.

especially common, and the forensic examiner should consider antiemetic medication, particularly if emergency contraception also is prescribed. All patients should be advised to abstain from alcohol for 24 hours after metronidazole use and from sexual intercourse until the treatment is completed.

Hepatitis B

Hepatitis B vaccination (Box 65-13) is recommended for SAVs who are not immunized without the use of hepatitis B immune globulin. Although the hepatitis B virus is found in highest concentrations in the blood of persons infected, it is efficiently transmitted by percutaneous or mucous membrane exposure to infectious body fluids. Sexual transmission among adults accounts for most hepatitis B virus infections in the United States. In the 1990s, heterosexual transmission accounted for about 40% of these infections. Risk factors for hepatitis B virus include multiple sexual partners (more than one sex partner in a 6-month period) or a recent history of an STD. Currently, testing to determine antibody levels in immunocompetent persons is not necessary because most fully vaccinated persons have long-lasting protection, and relatively high rates of protection are achieved after each vaccine dose. Typically, protective antibody response develops in 50%, 70%, and 90% over the three-dose regimen.[77] The forensic examiner should give the vaccination even if the completion of the series is not assured. Some protocols may not cover this cost.

Human Immunodeficiency Virus

Although human immunodeficiency virus (HIV) exposure is of great concern to SAVs, the risk of seroconversion is likely low. The forensic examiner needs to be familiar with the local epidemiology of HIV and acquired immunodeficiency syndrome; the nature of the assault; and any HIV risk behaviors exhibited by the assailant, such as high-risk sexual practices, injection drug use, or crack cocaine use. Specific circumstances affecting the SAV and assailant, if known, can increase the probability of transmission (Box 65-14). The rate of HIV transmission in sexual assault is likely to be higher than in consenting intercourse because of the possible presence of genital trauma; based on this assumption, some authors recommend offering prophylaxis to all SAVs within 72 hours. Findings relative to the biologic plausibility of effective postexposure prophylaxis are based solely on treatment of health care workers who have occupational exposure. Whether these data can be extrapolated to sexual assault is unknown. Because the

seminal fluid of all HIV-infected men contains IgG antibodies to HIV in fairly high titers, a test for these antibodies in the cervicovaginal washing in a seronegative SAV would provide a rapid rationale for treatment. No studies are available that explore these issues. The Centers for Disease Control and Prevention recommends that therapy be considered in cases in which the risk for HIV is likely high and that all such cases be referred for consultation with an HIV specialist. Costs may not be covered by local protocols, and postexposure prophylaxis needs to be provided in the context of a comprehensive counseling, treatment, and follow-up program. To maximize the likelihood of success, therapy should be initiated as soon as possible, no later than 72 hours after the assault so that expeditious referral is prudent.[77]

Follow-up Testing

For SAVs who do not want postexposure prophylaxis, repeat HIV testing is recommended at 6 weeks, 3 months, and 6 months. If a suspect is apprehended, HIV testing can be done with his consent or a blood sample held and tested at a later date after a court order has been obtained on the SAV's behalf. Some states permit testing of the suspect at the SAV's request in cases of sexual assault. Although gonorrhea and *Chlamydia* prophylaxis generally eliminates incubating syphilis, the Centers for Disease Control and Prevention still recommends follow-up serologic testing for it at 6 weeks after the assault.[77] Many protocols do not require serologic testing and do not cover this cost.

Table 65-6. Types of Emergency Contraception for Sexual Assault Victims

Class	Dose	Brands	Comments
Combined oral	100 μ of ethinyl estradiol + 0.5 mg levonogestrel twice 12 hr apart	Preven Ovral*	Decreases risk to 2% 50% nausea 20% emesis Requires antiemetic
Progestin only	1.5 mg levonorgestrel once or 0.75 mg twice 12 hr apart	Plan B	Decreases risk to 1% 22% nausea 8% emesis
Copper T IUD Antiprogestins	10 mg of mifepristone	ParaGard T 380A Not yet available	

*Other hormonal contraceptives that are useful can be found at www.not-2-late.com.

Pregnancy Prophylaxis

There is a 2% to 4% risk of pregnancy from random unprotected intercourse; this figure reaches nearly 50% in women 19 to 26 years old, who are at their most fertile period, when combined with midcycle exposure. Before any medication is given to a SAV, pregnancy testing must be done. This includes SAVs already taking oral contraceptives, SAVs with an intrauterine device, and SAVs post–tubal ligation. If the pregnancy test is positive, and the SAV desires to continue the pregnancy, she should be considered to be pregnant and treated as such with appropriate antibiotic choices for STD prophylaxis and follow-up for repeat pregnancy testing in 10 days. The immediate use of an emergency contraceptive can reduce the risk of pregnancy to 1% to 2%. Its effectiveness depends on the regimen used and the time interval between exposure and treatment (Table 65-6). Data show that an emergency contraceptive should be offered 5 days after unprotected sex. There are no absolute contraindications to the use of hormonal emergency contraception, even for women who have contraindications to the long-term use of combination hormonal contraception. In women who have active migraine headaches with neurologic symptoms or a history of stroke, pulmonary embolus, or deep vein thrombophlebitis, a progestin-only emergency contraceptive or the insertion of an intrauterine device should be considered first. Evidence suggests that there is not an increase in ectopic pregnancy with emergency contraceptive use. Although there are no studies large enough to quantify the teratogenicity of hormonal emergency contraception, no increase in birth defects has been detected among infants exposed to daily oral contraceptive use.[78]

Debriefing

Regardless of any physical injury, psychological distress is always present after a sexual assault, and the forensic examiner needs to acknowledge that from the beginning of the examination. Establishing a quiet and calm place for the examination and explaining the need for questions, examination, and evidence collection techniques reassure the SAV and give back to her a sense of control and safety. At the termination of

BOX 65-15. Rape Trauma Syndrome

Acute Phase
Expressed
    Crying
    Anger
Restlessness
    Controlled
    Calm, quiet
    Emotionless
Somatic and emotional reactions are prominent
    Increased muscle tension
    Headaches
    Genitourinary disturbances
    Fear/guilt
    Fatigue
    Gastrointestinal disturbances
    Anger/self-blame

Outward Adjustment Phase
Alteration of daily routines
Change of residence
Change phone numbers
Seeking family support (often without giving reason)
Fears and phobic reactions
Daytime anxiety
Nightmares

Integration Phase
Survivor accepts the rape as part of her life
Survivor begins to integrate the crisis into her life experiences

the examination, the forensic examiner should spend time reviewing the physical and genital injuries and address modes of therapy as appropriate. The examiner should discuss any pending laboratory data and how results will be communicated (phone, written, or both) with the SAV. The method of communication must be acceptable to the SAV. The examiner should review all medications and vaccinations (e.g., tetanus), discuss side effects, and provide contact phone numbers in case of problems or questions. The examiner should review the common psychological problems (Box 65-15) and reinforce the need for counseling. The advocate who has been present during the examination can be a personal contact already established with the SAV. Nonetheless, contact numbers for rape crisis, local crisis intervention, social services, drug and alcohol services, and emergency psychiatric services should be reviewed in detail, and all referrals should be discussed before departure. Compensation for victims of crime should be discussed and appropriate referrals made.

A follow-up examination of all SAVs should be scheduled.[77,79-81] This examination is particularly important for SAVs with genital injury. It documents the healing of injury and differentiates those findings that may be confused with trauma, such as hypervascularity, telangiectasis, and cherry red spots.[11] Its utility extends to nonspecific injuries, such as swelling or redness, which are difficult to detect and create frequent interobserver disagreements.[6] This examination also gives the forensic examiner an opportunity to review any problems and encourage counseling, if it has not already begun. All of these plans should be in written format because most SAVs do not remember what is said during a time of crisis.

Male Victims

Male sexual assault is vastly underreported. Most victims seen come from institutional settings with few from the nonincarcerated population. Factors considered to be barriers to reporting this crime include societal beliefs that a man can defend himself and fear that his sexual orientation is suspect. The need to maintain emotional control makes disclosure stressful. Men need to be accorded the same sensitivity and support as their female counterparts.[82]

Except for their anatomic differences, the procedures for the history, physical examination, evidence collection, and medical treatment are the same. Some notable differences in the assault characteristics from the characteristics seen in female SAVs include a predilection for anal and oral sexual contact with subsequent injury seen in 50% to 67%, more common use of the prone position during the assault, a higher incidence of nongenital trauma (80% in one study), use of a weapon, assault by a stranger or multiple assailants, and a history of abduction. Injuries to the penis and scrotum area occur less often and may be the result of a non–sexually related injury (e.g., kicks).[83] In one study, the use of colposcopy, in addition to anoscopy, increased physical examination findings in men. As with female SAVs, colposcopy is recommended because of its additional utility for photographic documentation and collection of trace evidence.[84]

Male Suspect Examination

The importance of the male suspect examination must not be overlooked. The SAV and suspect are the two pieces of the forensic puzzle in a sexual assault. If they are evaluated and treated in the same location, it is crucial that they not come in contact with each other. Expectations about this examination must be tempered by the forensic examiner's knowledge of the suspect's rights and the time elapsed between the assault and the examination. Presumed innocent, the suspect must be handled with the same courtesy and respect as any other patient.

If the forensic examiner is the same for the SAV and suspect, the examination is facilitated by the examiner's knowledge of the SAV's history. If a different examiner is used, he or she must know the history as given by the victim, and this usually can be obtained from law enforcement. The history obtained from the officer is *not* the history that is recorded on the suspect evaluation form. The history on the examination form must come from the suspect, but he has the right to remain silent on the events surrounding the assault. If after understanding his rights, he chooses to give information about the events under inquiry, the examiner should have him sign the consent and record his statements on the suspect form. Most suspects voluntarily give this information. For suspects in custody, the consent is not necessary because state law provides for the collection of perishable evidence. The forensic examiner should be knowledgeable about local laws, and a protocol should be developed to handle suspects who resist the collection of evidence. The interview and examination, for security reasons, is performed with law enforcement present at all times. The forensic examiner needs to record suspect statements verbatim, using quotation marks just as is done with the SAV. Medical information about preexisting conditions and hygiene is focused on factors that could influence interpretation of current findings. If there is a history indicating the possible transfer of biologic material between the SAV and suspect, appropriate specimens should be collected regardless of hygiene or timing.

The physical examination follows the same format as the SAV examination. Injury to the suspect occurs less often than to the SAV, however. Swabs of the penis, including the glans, shaft, and base (but excluding the urethral meatus), scrotum, and sulcus of the foreskin, if present, are taken. In contrast to the SAV examination, identifying features, such as tattoos and scars, should be noted and documented photographically. Reference samples, including blood, saliva, and hair, should be taken in accordance with local protocol. Typically, STD cultures and serology are performed, although they may not be required or paid for in current state protocol, and advice, information about pending results, and treatment are given as indicated.

KEY CONCEPTS

- The role of the emergency physician as forensic examiner is to provide a thorough examination as the basis for a report.
- Findings must be accurately, reliably, and clearly documented.
- Ultimately the forensic examiner must be able to analyze and explain findings and medical information in an understandable format for the court.
- SAVs require information and treatment for STDs, hepatitis, HIV, and pregnancy prevention.

REFERENCES

1. Feldhaus K, Houry D, Kaminsky B: Lifetime sexual assault prevalence rates and reporting practices in an emergency department population. *Ann Emerg Med* 36:23, 2000.
2. Rennison C, Rand M: Criminal victimization, 2002. In: Bureau of Justice Statistics National Crime Victimization Survey. Washington DC, U.S. Department of Justice, Office of Justice Programs, 2003.
3. Rennison C: Rape and sexual assault: Reporting to police and medical attention, 1992-2000. In: Bureau of Justice Statistics Selected Findings. Washington DC, U.S. Department of Justice, Office of Justice Programs, 2002.
4. Riggs N, Hourym D, Long G: Analysis of 1,076 cases of sexual assault. *Ann Emerg Med* 34:358, 2000.
5. Poirier M: Care of the female adolescent rape victim. *Pediatr Emerg Care* 18:53, 2002.
6. Adams J, Girardin B, Faugno D: Adolescent sexual assault: Documentation of acute injuries using photo-colposcopy. *J Pediatr Adolesc Gynecol* 14:175, 2001.
7. Jones J, et al: Comparative analysis of adult versus adolescent sexual assault: Epidemiology and patterns of anogenital injury. *Acad Emerg Med* 10:872, 2003.
8. Stermac L, Du Mont J, Kalemba V: Comparison of sexual assaults by strangers and known assailants in an urban population of women. *Can Med Assoc J* 153:1089, 1995.
9. Muehlenhard CL, Linton MA: Date rape and sexual aggression in dating situations: Incidence and risk factors. *J Counsel Psychol* 34:186, 1987.
10. Slaughter L: Involvement of drugs in sexual assault. *J Reprod Med* 45:425, 2000.
11. Slaughter L, et al: Patterns of genital injury in victims of sexual assault. *Am J Obstet Gynecol* 176:609, 1997.
12. Grossin C, et al: Analysis of 418 cases of sexual assault. *Forensic Sci Int* 131:125, 2003.
13. Sugar N, Fine D, Eckert L: Physical injury after sexual assault: Findings of a large case series. *Am J Obstet Gynecol* 190:71, 2004.
14. Hazelwood R, Warren J: The criminal behavior of the serial rapist. *FBI Law Enforcement Bull* 59:11, 1990.
15. Hazelwood R: The behavior-oriented interview of rape victims: The key to profiling. *FBI Law Enforcement Bull* 52:8, 1983.
16. Magid D, et al: Changes in sexual assault over time: a prospective comparison of 1974-1991. *Ann Emerg Med* 21:608, 1992.
17. Eckert LO, Sugar N, Fine D: Factors impacting injury documentation after sexual assault: Role of the examiner experience and gender. *Am J Obstet Gynecol* 190:1739, 2004.
18. Lenahan L, Ernst A, Johnson B: Colposcopy in evaluation of the adult sexual assault victim. *Am J Emerg Med* 16:183, 1998.
19. Slaughter L, Brown C: Colposcopy to establish physical findings in rape victims. *Am J Obstet Gynecol* 166:83, 1992.
20. Rossman L, Wynn B, Jones J: The sexual assault exam: A comparison of physical findings between an emergency department and a free-standing nurse examiner clinic. *Ann Emerg Med* 34:156, 1999.
21. Cartwright P: Factors that correlate with injury sustained by survivors of sexual assault. *Obstet Gynecol* 70:44, 1987.
22. Satin A, et al: The prevalence of sexual assault: A survey of 2404 puerperal women. *Obstet Gynecol* 167:973, 1992.
23. Bowyer L, Dalton M: Female victims of rape and their genital injuries. *Br J Obstet Gynaecol* 104:617, 1997.
24. Millar G, Stermac L, Addison M: Immediate and delayed treatment seeking among adult sexual assault victims. *Women Health* 35:53, 2002.
25. Campbell R, Bybee D: Emergency medical services for rape victims: Detecting the cracks in service delivery. *Womens Health* 3:75, 1997.
26. Office of Criminal Justice Planning: *California Medical Protocol for the Examination of Sexual Assault and Child Abuse Victims.* Sacramento, Office of Criminal Justice Planning, 2002.
27. Koss MP, Dinero TE, Seibel CA: Stranger and acquaintance rape: Are there differences in the victim's experience? *Psychol Women Q* 12:1, 1988.
28. Koss MP: Discriminant analysis of risk factors for sexual victimization among a national sample of college women. *J Consult Clin Psychol* 57:242, 1989.
29. Harrington MT, Leitenberg H: Relationship between alcohol consumption and victim behaviors immediately preceding sexual aggression by an acquaintance. *Violence Victims* 9:315, 1994.
30. O'Connor PG, Schottenfeld RS: Patients with alcohol problems. *N Engl J Med* 338:592, 1998.
31. Kilpatrick DG, et al: A 2-year longitudinal analysis of the relationships between violent assault and substance use in women. *J Consult Clin Psychol* 65:834, 1997.
32. Hammock GS, Richardson DR: Perceptions of rape: The influence of closeness of relationship, intoxication and sex of participant. *Violence Victims* 12:237, 1997.
33. Scully D, Marolla J: Convicted rapists' vocabulary of motive: Excuses and justifications. *Social Problems* 31:530, 1984.
34. Sugar NF, Fine DN, Eckert LO: Physical injury after sexual assault: Findings of a large case series. *Am J Obstet Gynecol* 190:71, 2004.
35. Ullman S, Brecklin L: Alcohol and adult sexual assault in a national sample of women. *J Substance Abuse* 11:405, 2000.
36. Seifert S: Substance use and sexual assault. *Substance Use Misuse* 34:935, 1999.
37. Sachs C, Chu L: Predictors of genitorectal injury in female vicims of sexual assault. *Acad Emerg Med* 9:1146, 2002.
38. Johnston LD, O'Malley PM, Bachman JG: National survey results on drug use: College students and young adults from the Monitoring the Future study, 1975-92. Washington DC, National Institute on Drug Abuse, 1993.
39. Johnston L: Contributions of drug epidemiology to the field of drug abuse prevention. *Substance Use Misuse* 32:1637, 1997.
40. Coid J, et al: Relation between childhood sexual and physical abuse and the risk of revictimisation in women: A cross-sectional survey. *Lancet* 358:450, 2001.
41. Eckert LO, Sugar N, Fine D: Characteristics of sexual assault in women with a major psychiatric diagnosis. *Am J Obstet Gynecol* 186:1284, 2002.
42. Biggs M, Stermac L, Dicinsky M: Genital injuries following sexual assault of women with and without prior sexual intercourse experience. *Can Med Assoc J* 159:33, 1998.
43. Wilbur L, et al: Survey results of women who have been strangled while in an abusive relationship. *J Emerg Med* 21:297, 2001.
44. Funk M, Schuppel J: Strangulation injuries. *Wisconsin Med J* 102:41, 2003.
45. Reznic M, Nachman R, Hiss J: Penile lesions—reinforcing the case against suspects of sexual assault. *J Clin Forensic Med* 11:78, 2004.
46. McGregor M, et al: Examination for sexual assault: Is the documentation of physical injury associated with the laying of charges? A retrospective cohort study. *Can Med Assoc J* 160:1565, 1999.
47. Gray-Eurom K, Seaberg D, Wears R: The prosecution of sexual assault cases: Correlation with forensic evidence. *Ann Emerg Med* 39:39, 2002.
48. Rambow B, Adkinson C, Frost T: Female sexual assault: Medical and legal implications. *Ann Emerg Med* 21:727, 1992.
49. Penttila A, Karhuman P: Medicolegal findings among rape victims. *Med Law* 9:725, 1990.

50. Sweet D, Shutler G: Analysis of salivary DNA evidence from a bite mark on a body submerged in water. *J Forensic Sci* 44:1069, 1999.

51. Sweet D, et al: An improved method to recover saliva from human skin: The double swab technique. *J Forensic Sci* 42:320, 1997.

52. Crowley S: *Sexual Assault: The Medical Legal Examination.* Stamford, Conn, Appleton & Lange, 1999.

53. Henry T: Lip swabs, floss, effective for collecting DNA evidence. *On the Edge* 9:7, 2003.

54. Ramin S, et al: Sexual assault in postmenopausal women. *Obstet Gynecol* 80:860, 1992.

55. Kaufman R, Faro S: *Benign Diseases of the Vulva and Vagina.* Chicago, Year Book Medical Publishers, 1994.

56. Masters W, Johnson V: *Human Sexual Response.* Boston, Little, Brown, 1966.

57. Lauber A, Souma M: Use of toluidine blue for documentation of traumatic intercourse. *Obstet Gynecol* 60:644, 1982.

58. McCauley J, et al: Toluidine blue in the corroboration of rape in the adult victim. *Am J Emerg Med* 5:105, 1987.

59. Jones J, et al: Anogenital injuries in adolescents after consensual sexual intercourse. *Acad Emerg Med* 10:1378, 2003.

60. Mancino P, et al: Introducing colposcopy and vulvovaginoscopy as routine examinations for victims of sexual assault. *Clin Exp Obstet Gynecol* 30:40, 2003.

61. Fraser I, et al: Variations in vaginal epithelial surface appearance determined by colposcopic inspection in healthy, sexually active women. *Hum Reprod* 14:1974, 1999.

62. Allard J: The collection of data from findings in cases of sexual assault and the significance of spermatozoa on vaginal, anal, and oral swabs. *Science and Justice* 37:99, 1997.

63. Keatings S, Allard J: What's in a name? Medical samples and scientific evidence in sexual assaults. *Med Sci Law* 43:187, 1994.

64. Collins K, et al: Identification of sperm and non-sperm male cells in cervicovaginal smears using fluorescence in situ hybridization: Applications in alleged sexual assault cases. *J Forensic Sci* 39:1347, 1994.

65. Collins KA, Bennett AT: Persistence of spermatozoa and prostatic acid phosphatase in specimens from deceased individuals during varied postmortem intervals. *Am J Forensic Med Pathol* 22:228, 2001.

66. Dahlke M, et al: Identification of semen in 500 patients seen because of rape. *Am J Clin Pathol* 68:740, 1977.

67. Rao P, et al: Identification of male epithelial cells in routine postcoital cervicovaginal smears using fluorescence in situ hybridization. *Am J Clin Pathol* 104:32, 1995.

68. Morrison A: Persistence of spermatozoa in the vagina and cervix. *Br J Venereal Dis* 48:141, 1972.

69. Davies A, Elizabeth W: The persistence of seminal constituents in the human vagina. *Forensic Sci* 3:45, 1974.

70. Davies A, Wilson E, Silverman A: the persistence of seminal constituents in the human vagina. *J Forensic Sci* 3:45, 1974.

71. Davies A: Spermatozoa in the anal canal and rectum and in the oral cavity of female rape victims [letter]. *J Forensic Sci* 24:541, 1979.

72. Enos W, Beyers J: Spermatozoa in the anal canal and rectum and in the oral cavity of female rape victims. *J Forensic Sci* 23:231, 1979.

73. Hochmeister M, et al: Effects of toluidine blue and destaining reagents used in sexual assault examinations on the ability to obtain DNA profiles from postcoital vaginal swabs. *J Forensic Sci* 42:316, 1997.

74. Collins C, Hansen L, Theriot E: A clinical stain for use in selection biopsy in patients with vulvar disease. *Obstet Gynecol* 28:158, 1966.

75. Jenny C, et al: Sexually transmitted diseases in victims of rape. *N Engl J Med* 322:13, 1990.

76. Magid D, et al: The epidemiology of female rape victims who seek immediate medical care. *J Interpersonal Violence* 19:3, 2004.

77. CDC: Sexually transmitted diseases treatment guidelines 2002. *MMWR Morbid Mortal Wkly Rep* 51(RR-6):69, 2004.

78. Westhoff C: Emergency contraception. *N Engl J Med* 348:1830, 2003.

79. Holmes M, Resnick H, Frampton D: Follow-up of sexual assault victims. *Am J Obstet Gynecol* 179:336, 1998.

80. AMA Council on Scientific Affairs: Violence against women: Relevance for medical practitioners. *JAMA* 268:3184, 1992.

81. American College of Obstetricians and Gynecologists: *Sexual Assault.* Technical Bulletin No. 242. Washington, D.C., ACOG, 1997.

82. Groth N, Burgess A: Male rape: Offender and victims. *Am J Psychiatry* 137:806, 1980.

83. Lipscomb G, et al: Male victims of sexual assault. *JAMA* 267:3064, 1992.

84. Ernst A, et al: The utility of anoscopy and colposcopy in the evaluation of male sexual assault victims. *Ann Emerg Med* 36:432, 2000.

CHAPTER

66 Intimate Partner Violence and Abuse

Patricia R. Salber

PERSPECTIVE

Background

Intimate partner violence and abuse (IPVA) poses a threat to the health and safety of millions of people around the world. In the United States, approximately 1 million people experience abuse by their intimate partners each year.[1] Affected individuals come from all economic, educational, social, racial, ethnic, and geographic groups.[1-4] National Institute of Justice statistics reveal that most victims of IPVA are women; however, male victimization also occurs in heterosexual and homosexual relationships.[1-3,5-7] Increasingly, it is recognized that children reared in violent homes are adversely affected by IPVA even if they only witness

Table 66-1. Tactics Used by Batterers to Gain Power and Control Over Their Partners

Category	Example
Verbal abuse	"You're stupid. It's a good thing I am here to take care of you."
Emotional abuse	A victim may be coerced into doing humiliating things (e.g., waiting in the car while her partner visits his mistress), or she may be forced to do things against her religious or moral principles (e.g., telling lies or stealing).
Using children	The partner threatens or actually takes the children away to force the victim to do what he wants.
Isolation	The victim is cut off from friends and family. There is no one she can talk to about the abuse.
Use of "male privilege"	"It's the man's right to choose where we live and how we live."
Economic abuse	All of the family's finances are controlled by the batterer. She has no independent access to any money.
Threats of or actual physical abuse of children or pets or destruction of property	"If you leave me, I will harm the children."
Sexual abuse	Sexual abuse (partner rape) occurs in many violent relationships.
Threats of physical abuse	"I will kill you if you leave me."
Physical abuse	Pushing, punching, slapping, throwing, choking, stabbing, shooting

From Salber P, Taliaferro E: *The Physician's Guide to Domestic Violence.* Volcano, Calif, Volcano Press, 1995.

violence in their homes.[8-11] In many families in which there is IPVA, the children themselves are physically and emotionally abused.[12-14] Although intergenerational transmission of family violence is not inevitable, some studies indicate that boys reared in violent homes are at increased risk of becoming abusers, and girls who witness or experience family violence are at increased risk of becoming victims when they become adults.[15,16] There is also evidence that child abuse or neglect is a risk factor for nonfamilial violence.[13,17] A series of articles, the Adverse Childhood Exposure studies, has documented that exposure to adverse childhood events, including growing up in a violent household, increases the risk for adverse health behaviors and outcomes years after the exposure.[18-21]

Definition

It is now common to use the terms *intimate partner violence* (IPV) and *intimate partner abuse* instead of older terms, such as "domestic violence," "spousal abuse," and "wife battering." This change in terminology is because violence and abuse occur in all types of relationships, whether adult or adolescent; current or former; dating, married, separated, or cohabiting; or heterosexual or homosexual. *IPVA* is a pattern of assaultive and coercive behaviors, including physical, sexual, and psychological attacks and economic coercion, that adults or adolescents use against their intimate partners.[22] A variety of tactics are used by perpetrators (Table 66-1), all of which are directed at gaining compliance from or control over the victim. These tactics and behaviors are carried out in frequent, sometimes daily, episodes.

Epidemiology

According to the Bureau of Justice Statistics (BJS), the number of victims of IPV has been declining. Using estimates from the 2001 National Crime Victimization Survey, the BJS reported 588,490 women and 103,220 men experienced rape, sexual assault, robbery, aggra-

vated assault, and simple assault at the hands of an intimate. These figures represent a 49% and 42% reduction in victimization rates compared with 1993.[3] Young women (age 16 to 34) experience the highest per capita rates of IPV, but significant rates of victimization also have been reported in girls 12 years old and in older women.[1] The rate of victimization of women remains substantially greater than that of men (5 per 1000 versus 0.9 per 1000).[3]

Two thirds of IPV against women and about half of IPV against men occur in the victim's home, and in 60% of cases the violence occurs between 6 PM and 6 AM. Children younger than age 12 were living in 43% of the households where IPV occurred. For men and women, divorced or separated persons experienced the highest rates of intimate partner victimization followed by never-married persons.[1]

Two thirds of female and male victims of IPV report being physically attacked, with the remaining third reporting threats or attempted physical violence. There is, however, a significant difference in outcomes of the attacks, with 50% of female victims reporting being injured compared with only 32% of male victims. The percentages of serious injuries, predominantly gunshot wounds, are similar in male and female victims. The percentage of female victims reporting minor injuries (42%) is significantly greater than the percentage of male victims (27%). Most injuries did not receive professional medical care. Only about half of all victims of IPV reported the violence to law enforcement authorities.[1]

The BJS reported that in 2000, slightly more than 1687 murders were attributable to intimates. In 74% of these cases, the victim was female. There has been a 22% decline in the number of women murdered by intimates since 1976.[3] The percentage of all female murder victims killed by intimates is 33% compared with 4% for male murder victims.[23] More than two thirds of spouse and ex-spouse victims were killed by guns[2]; however, boyfriend victims are more likely to be killed by knives compared with other IPV victims.[22]

The presence of a firearm in the home is a homicide risk factor for women in particular.[24,25] Most women who are killed with a gun are killed by their intimate partner.[26,27]

Research on intimate murders suggests that men and women have different reasons for killing their partner. Men apparently kill after an escalating pattern of abuse, frequently in response to the woman's attempt to leave the abusive relationship.[28] Women apparently kill their male partners in self-defense or in retribution for prior acts of violence.[23]

PRINCIPLES

Risk Factors for Injury Related to Intimate Partner Violence

Female patients are at risk for injuries if they have a current or former male partner with one or more of the following characteristics: alcohol or substance abuse, recent unemployment or intermittent employment, arrest in the past, less than a high school education, and having experienced abuse as a child.[29,30]

Effect of Intimate Partner Violence and Abuse on the Emergency Department

The number of nonfatally injured victims who present for treatment in the emergency department and other health care settings is enormous. In 1994, the National Electronic Injury Surveillance System documented 243,000 emergency department visits related to IPV. Extrapolating this number to the United States as a whole suggests that at least 5.6 million emergency department visits were made for IPV that year.[23] This number is significantly greater than the 1.4 million estimate generated by the Study of Injured Victims of Violence, a 1994 BJS study based on hospital record extractions and the 1.3 million estimate generated by the National Violence Against Women Study.[31,32] The latter two studies included all victims of interpersonal violence, not just victims of IPV.

Injuries account for only a portion of IPVA-related visits to the emergency department.[33-35] Victims of IPV also present with myriad noninjury complaints, including anxiety and depression, complications of pregnancy, and chronic pain syndromes. In addition, perpetrators of IPVA may withhold needed medications or prevent physician office visits; victims in these types of situations may present to emergency departments with exacerbations of chronic illness or other manifestations related to "noncompliance" with their medical regimen.

Research suggests that 4% to 15% of women who are seen in emergency departments are there because of symptoms related to IPVA.[32,36-38] Approximately 2% to 4% of all women seen in emergency departments are there for acute trauma related to IPV.[32,35,39] Of women seen in an urban emergency department, 54% had been assaulted, threatened, or made to feel afraid by partners at some time in their lives.[32] The 40% to 50% cumula-

tive prevalence of abuse of women by intimates has been documented in a variety of health care settings and is not limited to hospitals that care for indigent patients.[38] Women who have been battered seek care in emergency departments for a variety of medical, psychiatric, and trauma-related complaints more frequently than the average woman of the same age.[40] Ten percent of mothers of patients seen in a pediatric emergency department had been in abusive relationships within the last year, with 67% of the perpetrators being described as intimate partners.[41] Another study reported that 13% of men in an urban emergency department had experienced violence committed by a female intimate partner within the previous year.[6] No attempt was made to determine whether the violence was inflicted as a result of self-defense, mutual battering, or unilateral aggression.

Victims of IPV have been reported to have multiple visits to the emergency department for injuries and IPVA-related, noninjury chief complaints.[42] One study documented that 8% of women with current partners seen at an urban emergency department had sustained IPV-related injuries five or more times.[32] Several reports document that female victims of IPVA are more likely to present on the night shift compared with other categories of female patients.[33,41] This fact is important because in-hospital referral resources, such as social workers, may be less available at night.

Financial Effect of Intimate Partner Violence

Although it is difficult to know the true dollar costs for providing direct medical care to victims of IPV, it has been estimated to be approximately $1.8 billion annually.[43] One study reported that abused women had a 1.6-fold increased health care utilization and estimated costs compared with nonabused women.[44] Another study reported that compared with a random sample of general female enrollees, victims of IPV cost one health plan 92% more.[45] When other factors are added (e.g., days of work missed; decreased productivity in the workplace because of emotional, psychiatric, and medical sequelae of abuse; and loss of young individuals from the workforce because of early death or disability), the financial toll becomes immense.

CLINICAL FEATURES

Emergency Physician's Role in Intimate Partner Violence

Emergency physicians and other members of the emergency department team can play an important role in the lives of victims of IPV by doing the following[46,47]:
- Identify the abuse
- Validate the person's experience
- Assess immediate risk
- Document current and past events
- Refer victims to IPV experts

Identification

Presenting Signs and Symptoms

The most frequently recognized presentations of IPV are physical injuries. Victims of IPVA often have non-trauma presentations, however. Emergency physicians must understand that although certain types of injuries or other presentations may be more frequent in victims of IPVA, no injury or noninjury presentation has proved to be a definitive marker for this type of abuse.[34,41,48] Most IPVA prevention experts recommend routine screening as the best way to identify IPVA.[34,41,45,46,49]

Injury Presentations

The most common sites of injury are the head, face, neck, and areas that usually are covered by clothing, such as the chest, breast, and abdomen.[50-52] Maxillo-facial trauma is common and includes eye and ear trauma; hearing loss; soft tissue injuries; and fractures of the mandible, nasal bones, orbits, and zygomatico-maxillary complex.[53,54] Injuries suggesting a defensive posture (e.g., forearm fractures or bruising) also occur in IPVA. Strangulation by abusive intimate partners is common and may cause delayed stroke in young women secondary to carotid artery dissection.[55,56]

The possibility of IPV should be suspected when the stated mechanism of injury does not explain adequately the injuries sustained. For example, it is extremely unlikely that an isolated periorbital ecchymosis would be caused by falling off a chair and landing on the floor. Multiple injuries, especially if they are in various stages of healing, should raise the question of physical abuse, similar to what is seen in child abuse. Victims of IPV may be prevented from leaving the house to obtain medical care for injuries. They may present at a later time with injuries that appear old, such as fading bruises or partially healed lacerations. Patients who describe themselves as "accident-prone," who are recognized by emergency department staff as frequent visitors, or who have hospital records showing recurrent emergency department or clinic visits should be asked directly if any of their injuries were caused by violence in the home. Injuries from a variety of "accidents" may be caused by IPV. Some motor vehicle crashes are caused by batterers' deliberate actions, and falls down stairs may be from pushes.

Medical Presentations

Victims of IPV may have a wide variety of medical complaints. These complaints may be the result of the stress of the living situation or may be used as an opportunity to seek a temporary safe haven in a medical setting. Pain is a common presenting symptom and may manifest as a chronic pain syndrome, such as chronic abdominal pain, pelvic pain, headaches, or neck pain.[57-60] Patients with functional gastrointestinal disorders self-report high rates of sexual and physical abuse; it has been postulated that the abuse may lower the gastrointestinal symptom threshold, increase

intestinal motility, or modify the appraisal of bodily symptoms owing to altered cognition (e.g., feeling ineffective and unable to control the symptoms) and affecting treatment-seeking behaviors.[61]

Women who are victims of IPVA also may have exacerbations or poor control of chronic medical conditions, such as diabetes, hypertension, or heart disease. These women may be prevented from obtaining or taking their medications or from seeking medical care. This is especially likely to be true for women with physical limitations.

Women who are victims of IPVA may be seen in the emergency department with physical symptoms related to stress, anxiety, or depression; sleep and appetite disturbances; decreased energy or fatigue; difficulty concentrating; palpitations; dizziness; paresthesias; dyspnea; and chest pain.[62] Patients with vague or diffuse complaints can be particularly difficult and often frustrating to assess; however, these symptoms also may be manifestations of IPV and need to be taken seriously and assessed compassionately.

Obstetric and Gynecologic Manifestations

When sexual coercion occurs in the context of an abusive relationship, the victim may be unable to use protection against unwanted pregnancy or sexually transmitted diseases.[63,64] Women may present with vaginal infections, pelvic inflammatory disease, chronic pelvic pain, or urinary tract infections. Some women who are positive for human immunodeficiency virus may have contracted the virus from coerced sexual activity in the context of a violent relationship.[65,66] In addition, sexual assault (marital rape) occurs commonly in the most violent relationships. Sexual violence is not limited to heterosexual relationships. Lesbian victims of IPVA report high levels of sexual violence, and a study documented that homosexual and bisexual men experience patterns, forms, and frequencies of physical, emotional, and sexual abuse similar to what has been documented in heterosexual and lesbian IPVA.[7,67]

Studies examining violence during pregnancy report a prevalence of 4% to 8%.[68] Violence during pregnancy threatens the health of the mother and the fetus. Women may present to the emergency department with complications of pregnancy directly or indirectly related to IPVA. Examples include placental abruption, premature labor and delivery, and injuries to the mother or fetus. In addition, there is an increase in behaviors associated with poor pregnancy outcome, such as smoking, alcohol and drug use, low maternal weight gain, and presentation in labor without prenatal care.[69]

The relationship between violence and pregnancy in teens is notable. One study reported that half of births to the youngest teenagers resulted from second-degree statutory rape.[70] The prevalence of IPV during teen pregnancy has been reported to be 22%.[71]

Mental Health Presentations

Women who are victims of IPVA may have anxiety, hyperventilation, panic disorders, posttraumatic stress disorder, dissociation, and phobias.[51,72,73] In one study, 42% of women seen in a psychiatric emergency department had experienced one or more physical assaults within an adult relationship.[74] Women who attempt or commit suicide often have a history of IPVA.[75] During a 16-year study period, 22 of 117 female victims of IPV seen for emergency care had made 82 suicide attempts.[76]

Substance Abuse

The use of alcohol and drugs seems to increase after physical abuse begins. Substance abuse is generally believed to be a consequence of the physical abuse, rather than a cause.[51] Physicians may play an unwitting role in the overuse or abuse of psychoactive or sedating prescription medications by victims of IPV as they diagnose and attempt to treat the psychiatric and somatic manifestations of abuse, such as anxiety, panic symptoms, or chronic pain syndromes. Substance abuse, particularly of alcohol and cocaine, by *perpetrators* has been identified as a risk factor for physical aggression and injuries related to IPV.[29] The combination of alcohol abuse and availability of firearms is particularly deadly.[24]

Barriers to Diagnosis

Despite the frequency with which victims of IPV are seen in emergency departments, IPV often remains unrecognized by emergency department personnel.[33,77] There are a variety of reasons for the failure to diagnose. A survey of emergency department medical directors and nurse managers in California found that patient factors (e.g., the patient's fear of repercussions, denial, failure to volunteer information, and use of drugs and alcohol) were perceived to be the greatest barriers to the identification of IPV.[78]

Victims of IPVA may be reluctant to disclose because of fear of retribution or fear that they could lose their children, because of denial of the abuse, because of embarrassment, because of fear of police involvement, because of lack of trust in the health care provider, or because they were not yet ready to leave the relationship.[79,80] One study found that only 2.6% of female IPV victims seen in the emergency department volunteered information about the abuse.[33] A subset of women describe the abuse, however, if asked directly in a manner that shows compassion and establishes trust that the information will remain confidential.[79,80] There is also evidence that, in general, patients believe health care providers should inquire about IPVA.[79-81]

Physicians do not ask about IPVA for a variety of reasons. Almost 40% of physicians in one study cited close identification with their patients as a barrier that prevented them from considering the possibility of IPV. This simply was not a problem they could conceive of occurring in their patient population. More than half the physicians stated that they were reluctant to ask about IPV because they were afraid such inquiries would offend their patients.[82] Other reasons include frustration that the victim will return to the abusive partner, concerns about misdiagnosis,

lack of time, personal discomfort, reluctance to intrude into familial privacy, and lack of 24-hour social service support.[77]

DIAGNOSTIC STRATEGIES

Routine Screening for Intimate Partner Violence and Abuse

Because of a paucity of peer-reviewed studies, the U.S. Preventive Services Task Force recommendation statement on screening for IPV is that there is insufficient evidence to recommend for or against routine screening of women for IPV.[83] Many IPV prevention experts recommend universal screening, however, for IPVA of all adolescent girls and women who present for medical care.[36,41,48,77,84-87] Some experts also recommend screening men for IPVA.[36] The rationale for universal screening is based on the prevalence of IPVA in society, the high association of IPV with an array of health problems, the lack of definitive markers to identify IPVA, and the low level of suspicion and inquiry on the part of physicians.

Women seen in the emergency department without IPV injuries often return to the emergency department later with such injuries.[88] Of domestic homicide victims, 44% had been seen in an emergency department within 2 years of the homicide.[89] These findings reinforce that routine screening may offer emergency physicians an opportunity to intervene to prevent future morbidity and mortality associated with IPV.

Women who are victims of IPVA have a general unwillingness to volunteer information when not asked, but have a high level of acceptance and response when asked in a constructive and supportive manner about the presence of IPVA in their lives. Screening increases identification rates, involves minimal to modest cost, and poses little risk to patients when implemented in a manner that ensures confidentiality and safety.[90-92] There is anecdotal information that screening in and of itself helps victims of IPV by enabling them to define what is happening, by offering them an opportunity to discuss the abuse, and by showing that health providers care about the issue and can serve as a resource for them.

National clinical guidelines on routine screening have been published (Box 66-1).[48] Screening should be performed in a nonjudgmental and supportive manner in a setting where the patient feels safe. To do this requires finding time to talk with the patient, apart from anyone who many have accompanied her or him to the emergency department, in a private setting where the questions and answers cannot be overheard. Some emergency departments have found it useful to use a written screening instrument administered in a private setting (Figures 66-1 and 66-2). Some emergency departments have had nurses screen at triage (acceptable only if done in a private place that others cannot see or hear) or during the process of obtaining vital signs and initial nursing history. Some emergency physicians prefer to inquire directly about IPVA during the course of their evaluation.

BOX 66-1. Screening Guidelines for Emergency Departments and Urgent Care

Who Should Be Screened for Intimate Partner Violence (IPV)?

All adolescent and adult patients regardless of cultural background. Parents or caregivers of children in pediatric care.

Note: The majority of IPV perpetrators are male, so screening all patients increases the likelihood of screening perpetrators for victimization. We recommend routinely screening men only if additional precautions can be taken to protect victims whose batterers claim to be abused. Training providers on perpetrator dynamics and the responses to lesbian, gay, transgender, bisexual, and heterosexual victims is critical, regardless of policies to screen all patients or women only.

Who Should Screen for Intimate Partner Violence?

Screening and initial response should be conducted by a health care provider who:

- Has been educated about the dynamics of IPV, the safety and autonomy of abused patients, and elements of culturally competent care
- Has been trained how to ask about abuse, to provide information about IPV and local community resources, and to intervene with identified victims
- Is authorized to record in the patient's medical record
- Has a clearly defined role in an emergency or urgent care setting

Who Should Provide Further Assessment and Intervention for IPV?

Responses to intimate partner victims are most efficient and effective when coordinated in a multi-disciplinary manner and in collaboration with domestic violence advocates so that no single provider is responsible for the entire intervention. All providers in emergency or urgent care settings should be trained and achieve basic competence regarding how to identify and respond to IPV. Site-specific policies should be developed that clarify each provider's role in implementing specific elements of the protocol.

What Should Patients Screen For?

Screen patients for current and lifetime exposure to IPV victimization, including direct questions about physical, emotional, and sexual abuse.

Note: Because of the long-term impact of abuse on a patient's health, we recommend integrating screening for current and lifetime exposure into routine care. However, we acknowledge there will be times (particularly in emergency/urgent care) when screening for lifetime exposure to abuse will not always be possible due to time constraints.

How Should Screening for Present and Past IPV Victimization Occur?

Screening should be:

- Conducted routinely, regardless of the presence or absence of indicators of abuse
- Conducted orally as part of a face-to-face health care encounter
- Included in written or computer-based health questionnaires
- Direct and nonjudgmental, using language that is culturally/linguistically appropriate
- Conducted in private: friends, relatives (except children under 3), or caregivers should not be present
- Confidential: prior to screening patients should be informed of any reporting requirements or other limits to provider/patient confidentiality
- Assisted, if needed, by interpreters who have been trained to ask about abuse and who do not know the patient or the patient's partner, caregiver, friends, or family socially

When Should Screening Not Occur?

- When provider cannot secure a private space in which to conduct screening
- When there are concerns that screening the patient is unsafe for either patient or provider
- When the provider is unable to secure an appropriate interpreter

If Screening Does Not Occur:

- Note in chart that screening was not completed and schedule a follow-up appointment, (or if in an emergency or urgent care setting, refer patient to a primary care provider)
- Have posters, safety cards, and patient education materials about IPV available in examination or waiting rooms, bathrooms, or on discharge instructions

From James L, Lee D, Marjavi A, et al: National Consensus Guidelines on Identifying and Responding to Domestic Violence Victimization in Health Care Settings. The Family Violence Prevention Fund, San Francisco, 2002, pp 11-13. Copies available through the Fund (1-888-RxAbuse).

All questioning about IPV should use direct, specific language (e.g., "Has your partner ever punched or kicked you?") as opposed to asking if a person is battered or a victim of IPV. This is because some women may not understand that what has happened to them is battering or IPV (Box 66-2).

MANAGEMENT

Validation of the Patient's Experience

It is important that emergency physicians verbally acknowledge that hitting, punching, or other violent acts are not part of a normal and healthy relationship and are a form of abuse. Failure to do so may be interpreted by patients as confirming a perpetrator's common assertions that he or she will get away with it and no one cares that the battering occurs. *Validation* involves telling the victim that violent behavior is wrong and that nothing he or she has done or has failed to do makes the violence acceptable. Finally, patients should be given a clear message that help is available. The patient should know that emergency department personnel can assist her or him to contact IPV experts (trained social workers or advocates) affiliated with the hospital or in the community. These experts can help the person work through the logistics of leaving or assist with other safety strategies if the person chooses to stay in the relationship.

Validation has been documented to serve as a turning point for women in abusive relationships.[79,80] Knowing this may be helpful for physicians who are frustrated by their inability to "fix" the problem of IPV at the time

Over the past several years, domestic violence has come to be recognized as an important, often overlooked, health issue in our society. The Mercy Hospital of Pittsburgh's mission is to care for our patients who are in need. **We would like to help you identify whether you are a victim of abuse or neglect. To receive help is** *your* **decision — let us know if you have questions or would like to discuss your situation further.** Following are some questions to help you and us evaluate if you are in an abusive situation. Please respond to them openly.

This information is part of your healthcare record. Your responses will not be released to anyone without your written consent, except as otherwise provided by law. If you do not feel comfortable talking today, you can call us at (extension).

1. Do you feel safe at home? ☐ Yes ☐ No
   If no, why do you feel this way?
   _____
   _____
   _____

2. We all have disagreements – when ☐ Yes ☐ No
   you and your partner or a family
   member argue, have you ever been
   physically hurt or threatened?

3. Do you feel your partner or a ☐ Yes ☐ No
   family member controls (or tries to
   control) your behavior too much?

4. Does he/she threaten you? ☐ Yes ☐ No

5. Has your partner (or other family ☐ Yes ☐ No
   member) ever hit, pushed, shoved,
   punched or kicked you?

6. Have you ever felt forced to engage ☐ Yes ☐ No
   in unwanted sexual acts/contact
   with your partner or other family
   member?

If there are problems, we would like to help — please let us know.

1. Would you like to discuss your ☐ Yes ☐ No
   situation?

2. Would you like additional ☐ Yes ☐ No
   information on domestic violence?

3. Declined referral. ☐ Yes

Figure 66-1. Example of a domestic violence screening questionnaire. (Courtesy of Mercy Hospital of Pittsburgh.)

of the emergency department visit.[86] Leaving an abusive relationship is a process that requires advance planning to accomplish safely and successfully.

Assess Immediate Risk

Safety assessment is a crucial part of the evaluation of victims of IPV. To perform this assessment appropriately, the emergency physician must understand the correlates of lethality in IPV. An escalating pattern of violence can signal an increased risk of a fatal outcome.[93] Threats to kill the victim, the children, or self must be taken seriously because more than half of murder-suicides occur in the setting of spousal or consortial relationships, often with a prior history of IPV.[94]

Other risk factors for serious injury or death include substance abuse, especially with drugs associated with an increase in violence, such as crack cocaine or amphetamines; stalking or other behaviors suggestive of obsession with the victim; the presence of a firearm in the home; and evidence of violent behavior outside the home.[24,93]

The most dangerous period for battered women is when they attempt to leave the relationship. Of domestic assaults reported to law enforcement agencies, 75% are inflicted after separation of the couple.[95] Women are most likely to be murdered when attempting to report abuse or to leave an abusive relationship.[93] During the early separation period, batterers often retaliate by abducting the children; more than half of the 350,000 children kidnapped by parents each year occur in the context of IPVA.[96] In some instances, the heightened period of danger can last for several years. Box 66-3 lists questions that can be used to assess a battered woman's immediate safety. In addition, two published tools can be helpful when assessing danger: the *Danger Assessment* instrument (Box 66-4) and the *Lethality Checklist* (Box 66-5). These instruments are recommended as helpful adjuncts but should never be used as a substitute for clinical judgment.

Every effort should be made to ensure that patients at high risk see or speak with an IPV specialist before discharge from the emergency department. IPV specialists, such as social workers or community-based advocates, can help the victim assess the situation; discuss options; develop a detailed safety plan; and arrange a safe haven, including shelter, if appropriate. If the patient is willing, arrangements should be made to speak with an IPV specialist before discharge. All patients should be advised of the option of calling law enforcement. Mandatory reporting laws are discussed in the section entitled "Legal Considerations."

Documentation

Detailed and accurate documentation is important in cases of IPV for many reasons. The medical record may be the only evidence that the abuse has taken place. This documentation can provide pivotal information when criminal or civil legal remedies, such as divorce or child custody, are sought. Good documentation also is useful for physicians who are concerned about being unavailable for clinical practice because of court appearances. A legible, detailed, and accurate medical record may substitute for a personal appearance by a physician. Finally, emergency department records are an important source of injury surveillance data. Basic surveillance data, such as the identity and relationship to the victim of the assailant, the object or force used, the site of assault, information on referral, and documentation of police involvement, are often missing from emergency department charts.[97]

The medical record should include the chief complaint and a description of the event in the patient's own words. The patient should be asked specifically when and how the abuse was inflicted and the name and relationship of the perpetrator. It is preferable to

How often does your partner:	Never (1)	Rarely (2)	Sometimes (3)	Fairly often (4)	Frequently (5)
Physically hurt you?					
Insult you or talk down to you?					
Threaten you with harm?					
Scream or curse at you?					

To score:

1. Give the following points for each answer:

Never   = 1
Rarely   = 2
Sometimes = 3
Fairly often = 4
Frequently = 5

2. Add up the points   **Total Score:**

If you scored 10 or more, you have a troubled or distressed relationship that could result in harm for you or your children. Please get help by calling **1-800-799-SAFE**. If you are in danger, call 911 now.

In addition, ask yourself these three questions:

• Has your partner ever threatened suicide?
• Has your partner ever attacked you or physically hurt you in public?
• Has your partner ever strangled or choked you?

If the answer to any of these questions is yes, the probability of potential harm to you and/or your children is great. Please seek help as soon as you can safely do so. (REF: Violence Intervention Prevention (VIP) Center of Parkland Health and Hospital Systems, Dallas, TX. Contact 214-590-0403 for more information.)

Call **1-800-799-SAFE (7233)** or make an appointment at the VIP Center at **214-590-2926** or your nearest shelter or domestic violence agency as soon as possible. If you are in danger now, call 911.

Figure 66-2. Domestic violence screening instrument.

record "the patient states her husband, John Jones, punched her in the left eye yesterday evening about 11 PM," instead of writing "hit in face by fist" or "the patient alleges her husband hit her," as the term *alleges* insinuates that it may not have occurred.

Prior episodes of abuse should be described in detail regardless of whether that abuse required medical care. Any history of abuse of the children or other dependents also should be recorded. Changes in the pattern of abuse should be noted. It is particularly important to determine and document whether the abuse pattern is escalating and whether the perpetrator is abusing alcohol or other substances and whether he or she has access to a firearm. A complete physical examination should be performed, paying close attention to areas of the body in which physical signs of abuse could be hidden, such as the scalp and areas usually concealed by clothing. If sexual abuse is suspected, a sexual assault examination should be performed.

Areas of tenderness and injuries that are not visible should be noted on a preprinted or hand-drawn outline of a human body. This includes injuries to the scalp concealed by hair and soft tissue injuries that are not yet discolored. After obtaining the patient's consent, all visible injuries should be photographed. Until recently, the use of instant photography (e.g., Polaroid camera)

was recommended. In many areas of the United States, digital photography is replacing the use of 35-mm and instant photography, despite initial concerns that digital photographs could be inadmissible because they could be altered.[98] The advantages of digital photographs include better visualization of difficult to photograph injuries, such as strangulation marks or bruising on dark-skinned individuals. The ability to check the adequacy of the photographs before the patient leaves the emergency department is equal to instant photography, and digital photographs can be transmitted easily and rapidly to law enforcement, if indicated. At least two views of each injury and at least one photograph that includes the patient's face should be obtained. A ruler or other measuring device should be included in the photograph whenever possible. The name of the patient; identifying data such as medical record number, date, and names of the photographer; and the names of any witnesses should be written on the back of each photograph before attaching it to the medical record. If a standard camera is used, the film should be removed from the camera and, after appropriate labeling, placed in a locked drawer for safekeeping until it can be developed and added to the patient's record. Consideration should be given to having the patient return in 1 or 2 days to obtain pho-

BOX 66-2. Screening Questions for Possible Victims of Domestic Violence

Framing Questions

Sometimes it feels awkward to introduce the subject of abuse suddenly, particularly if there are no obvious indications a woman is being abused. The following are examples of ways providers can introduce the issue:

- "We now know domestic violence is a very common problem. About 25% of women in this country are abused by their partners. Has that ever happened to you?"
- "Because violence is common in women's lives, I now ask every woman in my practice about domestic violence."
- "I don't know if this is a problem for you, but many of the women I see as patients are dealing with abusive relationships. Some are too afraid or uncomfortable to bring it up themselves, so I've started asking about it routinely."
- "Some women think they deserve abuse because they have not lived up to their partners' expectations, but no matter what someone has or hasn't done, no one deserves to be beaten. Have you ever been hit or threatened because of something you did or didn't do?"
- "Because so many women I see in my practice are involved with someone who hits them, threatens them, continually puts them down, or tries to control them, I now ask all my patients about abuse."
- "Many of the lesbians and gay men we see here are hurt by their partners. Does your partner ever try to hurt you?"

Direct Questions

However one initially raises the issue of domestic violence, it is important to include direct and specific questions:

- "Did someone hit you? Who was it? Was it your partner or husband?"
- "Has your partner or ex-partner ever hit you or physically hurt you? Has he ever threatened to hurt you or someone close to you?"
- "I'm concerned that your symptoms may have been caused by someone hurting you. Has someone been hurting you?"
- "Does your partner ever try to control you by threatening to hurt you or your family?"

- "Has your partner ever forced you to have sex when you didn't want to? Has he ever refused to practice safe sex?"
- "Has your freedom been restricted or are you kept from doing things that are important to you (like going to school, working, seeing your friends or family)?"
- "Does your partner frequently belittle you, insult you, and blame you?"
- "Do you feel controlled or isolated by your partner?"
- "Do you ever feel afraid of your partner? Do you feel you are in danger? Is it safe for you to go home?"
- "Is your partner jealous? Does he frequently accuse you of infidelity?"

Indirect Questions

In some clinical settings, it may be appropriate to start the inquiry with an indirect question before proceeding to more direct questions. The following are examples of this approach:

- "Have you been under any stress lately? Are you having any problems with your partner? Do you ever argue or fight? Do the fights ever become physical? Are you ever afraid? Have you ever gotten hurt?"
- "You seem to be concerned about your partner. Can you tell me more about that? Does he ever act in ways that frighten you?"
- "You mentioned that your partner loses his temper with the children. Can you tell me more about that? Has he ever hit or threatened to physically harm you or the children?"
- "How are things going in your relationship or marriage? All couples argue sometimes. Are you having fights? Do you fight physically?"
- "You mentioned that your partner uses alcohol. How does he act when he is intoxicated? Does his behavior ever frighten you? Does he ever become violent?"
- "Like all other couples, gay couples have various ways of resolving their conflicts. How do you and your partner deal with conflicts? What happens when you disagree? What happens when your partner doesn't get his (her) way?"

From Salber P, Taliaferro E: *The Physician's Guide to Domestic Violence*. Volcano, Calif, Volcano Press, 1995.

BOX 66-3. Questions to Ask to Assess the Patient's Immediate Safety

1. What is the pattern of the physical abuse?

Has the amount of physical violence increased in frequency and severity over the past year?

How often does the batterer attack, hit, or threaten you?

Has he ever beaten you when you were pregnant?

Have you ever been hospitalized as a result of the abuse?

Is he violent toward your children?

Is he violent outside of your home?

2. Has your partner threatened or tried to kill you?

Has the batterer ever threatened to kill you with a weapon? Has he ever used a weapon? Is there a gun in the house?

Has the batterer ever tried to choke you?

Has he ever threatened to kill you?

Have you ever been afraid you might die while the batterer was attacking you?

3. Are drugs or alcohol involved?

Does he get drunk every day or almost every day?

Does he use "upper drugs," such as amphetamines (speed), angel dust (PCP), cocaine, or crack cocaine?

4. How much control does he have over you?

Does he control your daily activities, such as where you can go, who you can be with, or how much money you can have?

Is he violent and constantly jealous of you? Has he ever said that if he cannot have you, no one else can?

Has he ever used threats or tried to commit suicide to get you to do what he wants?

5. Are you thinking of suicide or homicide?

Have you ever thought of or attempted to commit suicide because of problems in the relationship? Do you have a plan? A weapon?

Have you ever thought of or attempted to kill your batterer? Are you considering this now? Do you have a plan? A weapon?

Adapted from Salber P, Taliaferro E: *The Physician's Guide to Domestic Violence*. Volcano, Calif, Volcano Press, 1995.

BOX 66-4. Danger Assessment

Several risk factors have been associated with homicide (murder) of batterers and battered women in research conducted after the killings have taken place. We cannot predict what will happen in your case, but we would like you to be aware of the danger of homicide in situations of severe battering and for you to see how many of the risk factors apply to your situation. (The *he* in the questions refers to your husband, partner, ex-husband, or whoever currently is physically hurting you.)

A. On a calendar, please mark the approximate dates during the past year when your partner beat you. Write on that date how long each incident lasted in approximate hours and rate the incident according to the following scale:

1. Slapping, pushing; no injuries and/or lasting pain
2. Punching, kicking; bruises, cuts, and/or continuing pain
3. "Beating up"; severe contusions, burns, broken bones
4. Threat to use weapon; head injury, internal injury, permanent injury
5. Use of weapon; wounds from weapon

(If any of these descriptions for the higher number apply, use the higher number.)

B. Answer these questions yes or no.

_____ 1. Has the physical violence increased in frequency during the past year?

_____ 2. Has the physical violence increased in severity during the past year and/or has a weapon or threat with weapon been used?

_____ 3. Does he ever try to choke you?

_____ 4. Is there a gun in the house?

_____ 5. Has he ever forced you into sex when you did not wish to have sex?

_____ 6. Does he use drugs? ("uppers" or amphetamines, speed, angel dust, cocaine, crack, street drugs, heroin, or mixtures)

_____ 7. Does he threaten to kill you and/or do you believe he is capable of killing you?

_____ 8. Is he drunk every day or almost every day (in terms of quantity or alcohol)?

_____ 9. Does he control most or all of your daily activities? (For instance, does he tell you whom you can be friends with, how much money you can take with you shopping, or when you can take the car?) If he tries but you do not let him, check here _____

_____ 10. Have you ever been beaten by him while you were pregnant? If you have never been pregnant by him, check here _____

_____ 11. Is he violently and constantly jealous of you? For instance, does he say, "If I can't have you, no one can."

_____ 12. Have you ever threatened or tried to commit suicide?

_____ 13. Has he ever threatened or tried to commit suicide?

_____ 14. Is he violent toward your children?

_____ 15. is he violent outside the home?

_____ TOTAL YES ANSWERS

Thank you. Please talk with your physician, advocate, or counselor about what the danger assessment means in terms of your situation.

From Campbell J: *Assessing Dangerousness: Violence by Sexual Offenders, Batterers, and Child Abusers*. Thousand Oaks, Calif, Sage Publications, 1995.

BOX 66-5. Lethality Checklist

This checklist consists of 19 items. The higher the number of items checked, the greater the danger.

1. Perpetrator objectifies partner (e.g., calls her names, body parts, animals).
2. Perpetrator blames victim for perceived injuries to herself.
3. Perpetrator is unwilling to turn victim loose.
4. Perpetrator is obsessed with victim.
5. Perpetrator is hostile, angry, or furious.
6. Perpetrator appears distraught.
7. The relationship is extremely tense, volatile.
8. Perpetrator is extremely jealous, blaming the victim for all types of promiscuous behavior.
9. Perpetrator has been involved in previous incidents of significant violence.
10. Perpetrator has killed pets.
11. Perpetrator has made threats.
12. Perpetrator has made previous suicide attempts.
13. Perpetrator is threatening suicide.
14. Perpetrator has access to victim.
15. Perpetrator has access to guns.
16. Perpetrator uses alcohol.
17. Perpetrator uses amphetamines, speed, cocaine, crack, or other drugs.
18. Perpetrator has thoughts or desires of hurting partner.
19. Perpetrator has no desire to stop violence or control behavior.

From Salber P, Taliaferro E: *The Physician's Guide to Domestic Violence*. Volcano, Calif, Volcano Press, 1995.

tographs of soft tissue injuries after discoloration has developed.

The chart should include specific information on whether a social worker, IPV advocate, or law enforcement officer was contacted; whether or not the patient was seen by any of these individuals before discharge; and the results of these contacts. If an IPV specialist or law enforcement officer did not see the patient before discharge, the chart should include the details of the assessment of the patient's immediate risk of injury. If the patient is not at risk for immediate harm and if he or she prefers, up-to-date referral information should be given so that the patient can arrange follow-up independently; this also should be recorded in the chart. Similar to any other high-risk diagnosis, physicians must be sure specialist referral was made and that there

BOX 66-6. Considerations When Planning Disposition: Safety Planning

1. Does she think it is safe to go home?
Where is her batterer now? Was he arrested? Was he arrested and released?
Does he have access to a firearm or other weapon?
Has he been threatening to kill her? Does she believe him?
Has he been harassing her or stalking her? Are his abusive behaviors escalating?

2. Does she have friends or family with whom she can stay?
Would she feel safe at their homes, or is she afraid her batterer would come after her there?
Is she confident they would not inadvertently collude with the batterer by having him come get her, mistakenly thinking that they are helping to preserve the family or relationship?

3. Where are her children or other dependents?
Does she think they are safe?
Is she afraid they would be harmed if she did not go home?

4. Does she want immediate access to a shelter or other temporary living situation?
If she does not want to go to a shelter now, be sure to give her the telephone numbers in case she wants or needs to go at a later time.

If she wants to go to a shelter, but there are no beds available, what are her options? Motel vouchers? Overnight in the emergency department? Admission to the hospital?

5. Does she need immediate medical or psychiatric intervention?
Does she require admission or urgent follow-up for her medical condition(s)?
Is she suicidal? Homicidal?
Does she need urgent crisis counseling to help her deal with the stress of the abuse? If so, arrange for appropriate appointments or referrals.
If none of the above apply, be sure to give her telephone numbers to the domestic violence or crisis hotline in your community. Be sure to let her know how she can get in touch with you or an appropriate person in your department if she needs to.

6. If she wants to go home.
Be sure a definite follow-up appointment is scheduled—either with you or with an appropriate referral primary care provider. Also be sure she has information about community referrals.

7. She should be advised to have a safety plan (see Box 66-7).

From Salber P, Taliaferro E: *The Physician's Guide to Domestic Violence.* Volcano, Calif, Volcano Press, 1995.

---

is a high likelihood that the patient will follow up, or the physician should arrange for the specialist to see the patient before discharge.

Referral

Appropriate referral mechanisms must be established for every emergency department based on the resources of the hospital, health system, managed care organization, and community. For larger departments, 24-hour coverage by a medical social worker or an on-site IPV specialist (i.e., advocate) may be warranted. For smaller departments, appropriate referral may consist of a list of hospital or community resources. Such lists should be revised at least annually to ensure that the telephone numbers are correct and the services are still available. If 24-hour on-site services are not available, it can be helpful to work with local IPV advocates to set up referral patterns that are appropriate for the particular circumstances of the hospital and available IPV community resources.

DISPOSITION

Some victims of IPV require hospitalization for treatment of serious injuries or other health effects of IPV. Most patients are discharged from the emergency department, however. For some women, discharge to a domestic violence shelter or safe house may be necessary. For other women, safety can be ensured more easily through friends or relatives with whom they can stay. In some communities, motel vouchers or other alternatives to shelter may be available. Occasionally, the only alternative to ensure immediate safety may be

an overnight stay in the emergency department or admission to the hospital (under an assumed name).

Considerations when arranging disposition and planning for the safety of a victim of IPVA are outlined in Box 66-6. Although the emergency physician may be tempted to make the decision for a battered woman, the patient is in the best position ultimately to determine whether and where it is safest for her to go. She knows the batterer; she may be afraid for the safety of her loved ones, such as her children, parents, or siblings; and she may know, from prior attempts to leave, that the criminal justice system cannot ensure her safety from this individual. One of the most important questions to ask the victim is whether she thinks it is safe for her to go home. The decision to go home or not to go home ultimately must be made by the patient and respected by her physician. All victims of IPV should be given a personalized safety plan (Box 66-7) before discharge, regardless of whether they return to the violent relationship. On-call or on-site IPV specialists can help the patient fill out the plan.

Legal Considerations

Many states have laws that require health care providers to report known or suspected cases of IPV to the police. The indications for initiating a report (serious injuries, injuries with a weapon, or any injury), the persons or institutions who are required to report, and the agency to which the abuse must be reported vary by state. In some jurisdictions, the criminal justice response to victims of IPV may place the victim at increased, not decreased, risk of harm. A report that triggers a police home visit and not arrest or an arrest with only a few hours in jail may enrage the perpetra-

BOX 66-7. Elements of a Safety Plan

1. Safety during a violent incident that occurs in the home

Try to avoid arguments in small rooms, rooms with access to weapons (e.g., the kitchen), or rooms without access to an outside door.

Be aware that alcohol and other drugs can decrease your ability to act quickly to protect yourself and your children.

Know which doors, windows, or fire escapes you and your children would use if you have to escape quickly to safety. Know where you would go once you have left the house. If possible, practice taking this route.

If you can, tell a friend or neighbor to call the police if they hear suspicious noises coming from your home.

Arrange to use a code word with your children or friends so that they know when they should call for help.

Teach your children how to use the telephone to contact the police and fire department.

The following items should be hidden in a place you can access quickly in case of an emergency:

Identification for self and children (e.g., driver's license, passports, green cards, birth certificates, social security cards)

Important documents (e.g., school and health records, welfare identification, insurance records, automobile titles, lease or rental agreement, mortgage papers, marriage license, and address book)

Copies of any protective orders, divorce or custody papers, or other court documents

Money, checkbook, bankbook, and credit card (in your own name if possible)

A small supply of any prescription medicines or a list of the drugs and their dosages

Clothing, toys, and other comfort items for self and children

Items of special sentimental value and small sellable objects

Extra set of car, house, office, and safety deposit box keys

Telephone numbers and addresses of family, friends, and community agencies

2. Safety if you no longer live with the batterer

Change the locks on the doors and windows as soon as possible.

Be sure the doors are secure (e.g., steel/metal instead of wood).

Install extra locks, window bars, outdoor lights that detect the approach of a person, and an electronic security system.

Install smoke detectors, purchase fire extinguishers, and have rope ladders for upper floor windows.

3. Safety on the job and in public

Is there someone at work who can be informed of the situation? A coworker? Supervisor? Employment assistance person?

Can you use voice mail, the receptionist, or a coworker to help screen calls or visitors at work?

Have a plan for arriving and leaving work and other public places safely. Vary the time of arrival and departure; vary the route.

Adapted from *Personalized safety plan*, Office of the City Attorney, City of San Diego, April, 1990. Copies of a "fill in the blank" personalized safety plan can be obtained from The Family Violence Prevention Fund, 383 Rhode Island Street, Suite 304, San Francisco, 94103-5133, telephone 415-252-8900, fax 415-252-8991.

---

tor and lead to retaliation and more serious injury or death.[99] Victims of IPV must be apprised of the duty to report and its ramifications. Emergency physicians also have a duty to warn the person at risk if they become aware of a patient's intent to harm a third party. If commitment to a psychiatric facility is planned, the third party is temporarily protected, and the psychiatric facility then determines the need to warn.[51]

Victims of IPVA often need legal help as they seek to protect themselves and their children. Civil protection orders are available to battered women in every state and the District of Columbia. Help with obtaining protection orders and information on other legal services for victims of IPV often can be obtained through community domestic violence shelters or agencies. Community legal resources should be included in any written referral material given to victims of IPV.

IMPROVING EMERGENCY DEPARTMENT RESPONSE TO VICTIMS OF INTIMATE PARTNER VIOLENCE AND ABUSE

Every emergency department should have a plan for the continuing education of all staff about the dynamics, identification, and appropriate interventions for IPV. Research has documented that to be effective at changing provider behavior, traditional continuing medical education needs to be combined with enabling processes.[100] Examples of enablers for IPVA include chart stamps[34] or examination room posters that remind providers to discuss IPV.[101] Educational materials and background information on IPV can be obtained by calling or e-mailing one of the following organizations:

- The Family Violence Prevention Fund's Health Technical Assistance Center (1-888-Rx-Abuse)
- National Domestic Violence Hotline (1-800-799-SAFE); identify yourself as a provider and state your question

Many state and local medical societies, the American Medical Association, the American College of Emergency Physicians, and other specialty societies also provide materials on the medical response to IPV.

Some victims of IPV may have had previous medical encounters in which the violence was ignored or not responded to. IPV victims have stated that brochures and IPV posters help them talk about their abuse.[102] Palm cards, brochures, and posters placed in strategic locations in the hospital (e.g., examining rooms, women's restrooms) and lapel buttons with messages of concern about IPV may be helpful in establishing the emergency department and emergency physicians as a resource for victims of IPV.[103]

An effective approach to IPVA requires consistent responses from a variety of hospital-based resources. To ensure coordination of these responses, it may be helpful for the hospital to form an IPVA committee composed of physician and nurse representatives from each of the medical specialties and a representative from administration, social services, substance abuse services, and the clergy. It is useful for representatives from the community referral resources (e.g., battered women's advocates, legal services, law enforcement, and the district attorney's office) to attend committee meetings on a regular basis. Such committees have been helpful in developing a coordinated response to meet the complex needs of victims of IPV.

 KEY CONCEPTS

- Although most victims of IPV are women, male victimization also occurs. IPV is found in heterosexual and homosexual relationships.

- IPVA is a pattern of assaultive and coercive behaviors, including physical, sexual, and psychological attacks and economic coercion, that adults or adolescents use against their intimate partners.

- Female patients are at risk for injuries if they have a current or former male partner with one or more of the following characteristics: alcohol or substance abuse, recent unemployment or intermittent employment, arrest in the past, less than a high school education, having experienced abuse as a child.

- No injury or noninjury presentation has proved to be a definitive marker for IPVA. Most experts recommend routine screening as the best way to identify IPVA.

- Abused women may be unwilling to volunteer information, but have a high level of acceptance and response when asked directly about the presence of IPVA in their lives.

- Screening for IPVA increases identification rates, involves minimal to modest cost, and causes little risk to patients when implemented in a manner that ensures confidentiality and safety. Screening should be performed in a non-judgmental and supportive manner in a setting in which the patient feels safe.

- Safety assessment is a crucial part of the evaluation of victims of IPV. The most dangerous period for battered women is when they attempt to leave the relationship.

- Many states have laws that require health care providers to report known or suspected cases of IPV to the police. The indications for initiating a report (serious injuries, injuries with a weapon, or any injury), the persons or institutions who are required to report, and the agency to which the abuse must be reported vary by state.

- Every emergency department should have a plan for the continuing education of all staff about the dynamics and identification of and the appropriate interventions for IPV.

REFERENCES

1. Rennison M, Welchans S: *Intimate partner violence.* Washington, DC, U.S. Department of Justice, May 2000 (revised January 31, 2002), NCJ 178247.
2. Matson C, Klaus P: *Criminal victimization in the United States, 2001 statistical tables.* National Crime Victimization Survey, Washington, DC, U.S. Department of Justice, January 2003, NCJ 197064.
3. Rennison CM: *Intimate partner violence, 1993-2001.* Washington, DC, U.S. Department of Justice, February 2003, NCJ 197838.
4. Watts C, Zimmerman C: Violence against women, global scope and magnitude. *Lancet* 359:1232, 2002.
5. Waldner-Haugard L, Gratch L, Magruder B: Victimization and perpetration rates of violence in gay and lesbian relationships: Gender issues explored. *Violence Vict* 12:173, 1997.
6. Mechem CC, et al: History of domestic violence among male patients presenting to an urban emergency department. *Acad Emerg Med* 6:786, 1999.
7. Merrill GS, Wolfe VA: Battered gay men: An exploration of abuse, help seeking, and why they stay. *J Homosex* 39:1, 2000.
8. McFarlane JM, Groff JY, O'Brien JA, Watson K: Behaviors of children who are exposed and not exposed to intimate partner violence: An analysis of 330 black, white, and hispanic children. *Pediatrics* 112:e202, 2003.
9. Campbell JC, Lewandowski LA: Mental and physical health effects of intimate partner violence on women and children. *Psychiatr Clin North Am* 20:353, 1997.
10. Knapp JF: The impact of children witnessing violence. *Pediatr Clin North Am* 45:355, 1998.
11. Kernic MA, et al: Behavioral problems among children whose mothers are abused by an intimate partner. *Child Abuse Negl* 27:1231, 2003.
12. Christian CW, et al: Pediatric injury resulting from family violence. *Pediatrics* 99:E8, 1997.
13. Bowen K: Child abuse and domestic violence in families of children seen for suspected sexual abuse. *Clin Pediatr* 39:33, 2000.
14. Wright RJ, Wright PO, Isaac NE: Response to battered mothers in the pediatric emergency department: A call for an interdisciplinary approach to family violence. *Pediatrics* 99:186, 1997.
15. Hanson RK, et al: Correlates of battering among 997 men: Family history, adjustment, and attitudinal differences. *Violence Vict* 12:191, 1997.
16. Silverman JG, Williamson GM: Social ecology and entitlements involved in battering by heterosexual college males: Contributions of family and peers. *Violence Vict* 12:147, 1997.
17. Maxfield MG, Widom CS: The cycle of violence: Revisited 6 years later. *Arch Pediatr Adolesc Med* 150:390, 1996.
18. Felitti VJ, et al: Relationship of childhood abuse and household dysfunction to many of the leading causes of death in adults: The adverse childhood experience (ACE) study. *Am J Prev Med* 14:245, 1998.
19. Dube SR, et al: The impact of adverse childhood experiences on health problems: Evidence from four birth cohorts dating back to 1900. *Prev Med* 37:268, 2003.
20. Dube SR, et al: Adverse childhood experiences and personal alcohol abuse as an adult. *Addict Behav* 27:713, 2002.
21. Dube SR, et al: Childhood abuse, household dysfunctions and the risk of attempted suicide throughout the lifespan: Findings from the adverse childhood experiences study. *JAMA* 286:3089, 2001.
22. Ganley AL: Understanding domestic violence. In Lee D, Durborow N, Salber PR (eds): *Improving the Health Care Response to Domestic Violence: A Resource Manual for Health Care Providers.* San Francisco, The Family Violence Prevention Fund, 1998, pp 15-45.
23. *Homicide trends in the US: Intimate homicide.* U.S. Department of Justice Statistics, Office of Justice Programs, Bureau of Justice Statistics. Available at www.ojp.usdoj.gov/bjs/homicide/intimates.htm (page updated November 21, 2002).
24. Kellerman A, Heron S: Firearms and family violence. *Emerg Med Clin North Am* 17:699, 1999.
25. Wiebe D: Homicide and suicide risks associated with firearms in the home: A national case-control study. *Ann Emerg Med* 41:771, 2003.

26. Bailey JE, et al: Risk factors for violence death of women in the home. *Arch Intern Med* 157:777, 1997.

27. Morocco KE, Runyan CW, Butts JD: Female intimate partner homicide: A population-based study. *J Am Med Womens Assoc* 58:20, 2003.

28. Block CR, Christakos A: Intimate partner homicide in Chicago over 29 years. *Crime Delinquency* 4:496, 1995.

29. Kyriacou DN, et al: Risk factors for injury to women from domestic violence. *N Engl J Med* 341:1892, 1999.

30. Fahs-Steward W, Golden J, Schumacher JA: Intimate partner violence and substance use: A longitudinal day-to-day examination. *Addict Behav* 28:1555, 2003.

31. Rand M: *Violence-related injuries treated in hospital emergency departments, special report.* Washington, DC, U.S. Department of Justice, Bureau of Justice Statistics, 1997, NCJ 156921.

32. Tjaden P, Thoennes N: *Prevalence, incidence, and consequences of violence against women: Findings from the national violence against women survey.* NIJCDC, November 1-15, 1998, NCJ 172837.

33. Abbott J, et al: Domestic violence against women: Incidence and prevalence in an emergency department population. *JAMA* 273:1763, 1995.

34. Olson L, et al: Increasing emergency physician recognition of domestic violence. *Ann Emerg Med* 27:741, 1996.

35. Muelleman RL, Lenaghan PA, Pakieser RA: Nonbattering presentation to the ED of women in physically abusive relationships. *Am J Emerg Med* 6:128, 1998.

36. Abbott J: Injuries and illnesses of domestic violence. *Ann Emerg Med* 29:781, 1997.

37. Ernst A, et al: Domestic violence in an inner-city ED. *Ann Emerg Med* 30:190,1997.

38. Morrison LF, Allan R, Grunfeld A: Improving the detection rate of victims of domestic violence using direct questions in the ED [abstract]. *Acad Emerg Med* 3:505, 1996.

39. Dearwater SR, et al: Prevalence of intimate partner abuse in women treated at community hospital emergency departments. *JAMA* 280:433, 1998.

40. Bergman B, Brismar B: A 5-year follow-up study of 117 battered women. *Am J Public Health* 81:1486, 1991.

41. Duffy SJ, et al: Mothers with histories of domestic violence in a pediatric emergency department. *Pediatrics* 103:1007, 1999.

42. Fanslow JL, Norton RN, Spinola CG: Indicators of assault-related injuries among women presenting to the emergency department. *Ann Emerg Med* 132:341, 1998.

43. Miller TR, Cohen MA, Wiersma B: *Crime in the United States: Victim Costs and Consequences (Final Report to the National Institutes of Justice).* Washington, DC, Urban Institutes and National Public Services Research Institute, 1995.

44. Ulrich YC, et al: Medical care utilization patterns in women with diagnosed domestic violence. *Am J Prev Med* 24:9, 2003.

45. Wisner CL, et al: Intimate partner violence against women: Do victims cost health plans more? *J Fam Pract* 48:439,1999.

46. Gerbert B, et al: Simplifying the physician's response to domestic violence. *West J Med* 175:329, 2000.

47. Gerbert B, et al: Physicians' response to victims of domestic violence: Toward a model of care. *Women Health* 35:1, 2002.

48. Lee D, James L, Sawires P: *Preventing Domestic Violence: Clinical Guidelines on Routine Screening.* San Francisco, The Family Violence Prevention Fund, 1999.

49. Haywood Y, Haile-Mariam T: Violence against women. *Emerg Med Clin North Am* 17:603, 1999.

50. Muelleman RL, Lenaghan PA, Pakeiser RA: Battered women: Injury locations and types. *Ann Emerg Med* 28:486, 1996.

51. Warshaw C: Identification, assessment and intervention with victims of domestic violence. In Lee D, Durborow N, Salber P (eds): *Improving the Health Care Response to Domestic Violence: A Resource Manual for Health Care Providers.* San Francisco, The Family Violence Prevention Fund, 1998, pp 49-86.

52. Perricante VJ, Ochs HA, Dodson TB: Head, neck and facial injuries as markers of domestic violence in women. *J Oral Maxillofac Surg* 57:760, 1999.

53. Zacharides N, Komoura F, Konsolaki-Agouridaki E: Facial trauma in women resulting from violence by men. *J Oral Maxillofac Surg* 48:1250, 1990.

54. Le B, et al: Maxillofacial injuries associated with domestic violence. *J Oral Maxillofac Surg* 59:1277, 2001.

55. Wilbur L, et al: Survey results of women who have been strangled while in an abusive relationship. *J Emerg Med* 21:297, 2001.

56. Malek AM, et al: Patient presentation, angiographic features and treatment of strangulation-induced bilateral dissection of the cervical internal carotid artery: Report of three cases. *J Neurosurg* 92:481, 2000.

57. Fillingim RB, Wilkinson CS, Powell T: Self-reported abuse history and pain complaint among young adults. *Clin J Pain* 15:75, 1999.

58. Alexander RW, et al: Sexual and physical abuse in women with fibromyalgia: Association with outpatient health care utilization and pain medication usages. *Arthritis Care Res* 11:102, 1998.

59. Green CR, et al: Do physical and sexual abuse differentially affect chronic pain states in women? *J Pain Symptom Manage* 18:420, 1999.

60. Elliott BA, Johnson MM: Domestic violence in a primary care setting: Patterns and prevalence. *Arch Fam Med* 4:113, 1995.

61. Drossman DA, et al: Psychosocial aspects of the functional gastrointestinal disorders. *Gut* 45(Suppl 2):II-25, 1999.

62. Salber PR: Introduction. In Lee D, Durborow N, Salber P (eds): *Improving the Health Care Response to Domestic Violence: A Resource Manual for Health Care Providers.* San Francisco, The Family Violence Prevention Fund, 1998, pp 1-11.

63. Kalichman SC, et al: Sexual coercion, domestic violence, and negotiating condom use among low-income African American women. *J Womens Health* 7:371, 1998.

64. Davila YR, Brackley MH: Mexican and Mexican American women in a battered women's shelter: Barriers to condom negotiation for HIV/AIDS prevention. *Issues Mental Health Nurs* 20:333, 1998.

65. He H, et al: Violence and HIV sexual risk behaviors among female sex partners of male drug users. *Womens Health* 27:161, 1998.

66. El-Bassel N, et al: Partner violence and sexual HIV-risk behaviors among women in an inner-city emergency department. *Violence Vict* 13:377, 1998.

67. Renzetti C: *Violent Betrayal: Partner Abuse in Lesbian Relationships.* Newbury Park, Calif, Sage Publications, 1992.

68. Gazmarian JA, et al: Prevalence of violence against pregnant women. *JAMA* 275:1915, 1996.

69. Peterson R, et al: Violence and adverse pregnancy outcomes: A review of the literature and directions for future research. *Am J Prev Med* 13:366, 1997.

70. Gessner BD, Perham-Hester KA: Experience of violence among teenage mothers in Alaska. *J Adolesc Health* 22:383, 1998.

71. Parker B, et al: Physical and emotional abuse in pregnancy: A comparison of adult and teenage women. *Nurs Res* 42:173, 1993.

72. Roberts GL, et al: How does domestic violence affect women's mental health? *Womens Health* 28:117, 1998.

73. Gleason WJ: Mental disorders in battered women: An empirical study. *Violence Vict* 8:53, 1993.

74. Briere J, et al: Lifetime victimization history, demographics, and clinical status in female psychiatric emergency room patients. *Nerv Ment Dis* 185:95, 1997.

75. Kaplan ML, et al: Suicidal behavior and abuse in psychiatric outpatients. *Compr Psychiatry* 36:229, 1995.

76. Bergman B, Brismar B: Suicide attempts by battered wives. *Acta Psychiatr Scand* 83:380, 1991.

77. McGrath ME, et al: Violence against women: Provider barriers to intervention in emergency departments. *Acad Emerg Med* 4:297, 1997.

78. Lee D, et al: *California hospital emergency department's response to domestic violence-survey report.* San Francisco, The Family Violence Prevention Fund, August 1993.

79. Rodriguez MA, Quiroga SS, Bauer HM: Breaking the silence: Battered women's perspectives on medical care. *Arch Fam Med* 5:153, 1996.

80. Gerbert B, et al: How health care providers help battered women: The survivors perspective. *Womens Health* 29:115, 1999.

81. Caralis PV, Musialowski R: Women's experiences with domestic violence and their attitudes and expectations regarding medical care of abuse victims. *South Med J* 90:1075, 1997.

82. Sugg NK, Innui T: Primary care physicians' response to domestic violence: Opening Pandora's box. *JAMA* 267:65, 1992.

83. U.S. Preventive Services Task Force: Screening for family and intimate partner violence: Recommendation statement. *Ann Intern Med* 140:382, 2004.

84. Chescheir N: Violence against women: Response from clinicians. *Ann Emerg Med* 26:766, 1966.

85. Gerbert B, et al: A qualitative analysis of how physicians with expertise in domestic violence approach the identification of victims. *Ann Intern Med* 131:578, 1999.

86. Gerbert B, et al: Interventions that help victims of domestic violence: A qualitative analysis. *J Fam Pract* 49:889, 2000.

87. Lachs M: Screening for family violence: What's an evidence-based doctor to do? [editorial]. *Ann Intern Med* 140:399, 2004.

88. Muelleman RL, Liewer JD: How often do women in the emergency department without violence injuries return with such injuries? *Acad Emerg Med* 5:982, 1998.

89. Wadman MC, Muelleman RL: Domestic violence homicides: ED use before victimization. *Am J Emerg Med* 17:689, 1999.

90. Krasnoff M, Muscati R: Domestic violence screening and referral can be effective. *Ann Emerg Med* 40:485, 2002.

91. Rhodes KV, et al: "Between me and the computer": Increased detection of intimate partner violence using a computer questionnaire. *Ann Emerg Med* 40:476, 2002.

92. Ernst AA, Weiss SJ: Intimate partner violence from the emergency medicine perspective. *Womens Health* 35:71, 2002.

93. Campbell J (ed): *Assessing Dangerousness: Potential for Further Violence of Sexual Offenders, Batterers, and Child Abusers.* Newbury Park, Calif, Sage Publications, 1995.

94. Marzuk PM, Tardiff K, Hirsch CS: The epidemiology of murder-suicide. *JAMA* 267:3170, 1992.

95. Jones RF: Domestic violence: Let our voices be heard. *Obstet Gynecol* 81:1, 1993.

96. Grief G, Hegar R: *When Parents Kidnap.* New York, Free Press, 1992.

97. Houry D, Feldhaus K, Nyquist S: Emergency department documentation in cases of intentional assault. *Ann Emerg Med* 34:715, 1999.

98. Halperin K: *Black-and-blue in ones and zeros: Digital photography is revolutionizing the prosecution of domestic violence cases.* Available at www.salon.com/tech/feature/2002/07/10/digital_violence/print.html (accessed February 28, 2004).

99. Hyman A, et al: Laws mandating reporting of domestic violence: Do they promote patient well-being? *JAMA* 273:1781, 1995.

100. Davis D: Does CME work? An analysis of the effect of educational activities on physician performance or health care outcomes. *Int J Psychiatry Med* 28:21, 1998.

101. Salber P, McCaw B: Barriers to screening for intimate partner violence: Time to reframe the question. *Am J Prev Med* 19:276, 2000.

102. McCauley J, et al: Inside "Pandora's box": Abused women's experience with clinicians and health services. *J Gen Intern Med* 13:549, 1998.

103. Lee D, Durborow N, Salber PR (eds): *Improving the Health Care Response to Domestic Violence: A Resource Manual for Health Care Providers.* San Francisco, The Family Violence Prevention Fund, 1998.

CHAPTER

67 Elder Abuse and Neglect

Deirdre Anglin and Diana C. Schneider

PERSPECTIVE

Background

Currently, 12.4% of the population in the United States is estimated to be 65 years of age or older.[1] The elderly segment of the population is expected to increase to 16.3% of the population by 2020[2] and 20.7% of the population by 2050.[2] Further, the "oldest" old (85 years of age and older) will make up an increasing proportion of the population.[2] With advanced age, vulnerabilities increase, such as significant physical and cognitive decline, expended financial resources, and uncertain medical insurance. As the U.S. population ages, maltreatment of elders is increasingly identified. Further, the World Health Organization has recognized that abuse and neglect of elders is a global health problem.[3]

The first reports of "granny battering" appeared in the medical literature in 1975.[4,5] In 1978 the U.S. House of Representatives Select Committee on Aging held hearings on elder abuse. This committee concluded that elder abuse was a nationwide problem that suffered from severe underreporting. The committee recommended that the federal government assist states to develop agencies responsible for collecting reports and identifying and managing cases of elder abuse.[6] In 1985 the Elder Abuse Prevention, Identification and Treatment Act was introduced into Congress to standardize definitions of elder abuse. In 1990, the House Select Committee met to determine what progress had been made in the problems related to elder abuse. They concluded that elder abuse was increasing and that it continued to remain woefully underreported, even though 80% of states had statutes mandating reporting of elder abuse. Further, the committee noted that the federal government had not passed legislation to provide assistance to the states to deal effectively with the national problem of elder abuse.[7] In 1991, the National Institute on Elder Abuse was established to focus increased attention on the issue of elder abuse. An amendment to the Older Americans Act in 1992 established a national elder abuse policy and provided some funding. In the same year, the Joint Commission on Accreditation of Healthcare Organizations (JCAHO) set standards for emergency departments that included having criteria for the detection and management of elder abuse among patients.[8]

Elderly individuals may be isolated from society as a result of physical illness, disability, mental illness (e.g., dementia), and age. Visits to physicians by elderly persons may provide their only contact outside the family. Elderly persons frequently present to the emergency department for medical care. Therefore, emergency physicians have the opportunity to diagnose suspected elder abuse and initiate further evaluation by elder abuse teams and Adult Protective Services.[9] However, a survey suggests that emergency physicians may lack awareness and adequate training about elder abuse. In this survey, 79% of emergency physicians reported they had treated a case of elder abuse in the previous year, but only 50% said they had reported the abuse. Of respondents, 28% believe elder abuse is rare and 84% rarely ask their patients directly about elder abuse. Only 31% of emergency physicians responded that they are aware of a written protocol for elder abuse in the emergency departments where they practice, and just 38% said they are familiar with their state laws pertaining to elder abuse. In addition, only 40% responded that they are aware of types of community services available for victims of elder abuse, and only 25% could recall education during their residencies about elder abuse.[10]

Epidemiology

It has been estimated that 2 million elders are abused annually.[7] According to the National Elder Abuse Incidence Study, the median age of victims of elder abuse is 77.9 years, and two thirds of victims are women. Of the identified elder abuse victims, 66% are white, 19% black, and 10% Hispanic. More than two thirds of perpetrators of elder abuse are family members, primarily spouses and grown children, and the overwhelming majority of victims live with the perpetrators. A total of 77% of victims are unable or only somewhat able to care for themselves; 60% of victims are either very confused or occasionally confused. In addition, 37% of elder abuse victims are moderately depressed and 6% are severely depressed.[11] Surveys of noninstitutionalized elderly people in the community have revealed that between 3% and 5% had experienced elder abuse or neglect, and the rates of psychological abuse were even higher.[12] Numerous studies have shown that as few as 1 in 14 cases of elder abuse is actually reported.[12]

DEFINITIONS AND TYPES OF ELDER ABUSE

Some of the difficulty in establishing the true incidence and prevalence of elder abuse stems from the lack of uniformity of definitions of elder abuse, both among researchers and in legislation. Definitions vary from state to state and often lack objective criteria for reliably establishing a medical diagnosis. Elder abuse is a form of family violence, along with child abuse and intimate partner violence. There are three main categories of elder abuse: domestic elder abuse, institutional elder abuse, and self-neglect or self-abuse. *Domestic elder abuse* includes any form of elder abuse that occurs in the elder's home or the caregiver's home, by a family member or the caregiver. *Institutional abuse* includes any form of elder abuse that occurs in a residential facility for elderly persons, usually by individuals who are hired to provide care. *Self-neglect* or *self-abuse* is the result of the behavior of an elderly person and threatens the well-being of that individual. Self-neglect usually involves the refusal or failure of elderly individuals to provide themselves with basic necessities, such as food, water, shelter, medications if indicated, and appropriate personal hygiene. In 45% of cases of self-neglect, elders 80 years of age or older are involved.[13] Self-neglect does not include mentally competent elderly individuals who understand the consequences of their decisions.

In addition to the three main categories of elder abuse, 33 forms of elder abuse have been described.[14] These forms of elder abuse can be grouped into six types: physical abuse, sexual abuse, emotional or psychological abuse, neglect, abandonment, and financial or material exploitation.[13] In a study of reported cases of elder abuse, 55% involved neglect, 15% physical abuse, 12% exploitation, 8% emotional abuse, and 0.3% sexual abuse.[13] Victims of elder abuse are often subjected to multiple types of elder abuse.

Physical abuse is defined as the intentional use of physical force that may result in bodily injury, physical pain, or impairment.[13] Physical abuse is the most readily detected type of elder abuse. It includes slapping, hitting, kicking, pushing, pulling hair, and burning. Physical abuse may include overmedication or undermedication, the use of physical restraints, or force-feeding. It may also involve the use of household objects as weapons, as well as the use of firearms and knives.

Sexual abuse is defined as any type of sexual contact with an elderly person that is nonconsensual.[13] It may include sexual assault, sexual coercion, verbal and physical sexual advances, and indecent exposure. Sexual abuse also occurs if an elderly individual is incapacitated and therefore incapable of giving informed consent.

Emotional or *psychological abuse* is defined as intentional infliction of suffering, pain, and distress through verbal or nonverbal means.[13] Emotional abuse may include such acts as insulting or demeaning comments, name calling, threats of deprivation, isolation, and humiliation. Emotional abuse may accompany physical abuse or other forms of abuse.

Neglect is defined as the failure or refusal of caregivers to fulfill any of their duties or obligations to an elderly individual, which has resulted or is likely to result in serious harm to the elderly individual.[13] Neglect is the most common type of elder abuse.[15] Neglect may be either unintentional or intentional. However, intent is often very difficult to prove. Unintentional neglect may result from the inability of the caregiver to carry out responsibilities because of physical or mental inability or a lack of knowledge of how to care properly for the elderly individual. Neglect may consist of withholding of food, water, clothing, shelter, medications, medical equipment (e.g., walker, cane, glasses, hearing aids, dentures), or medical appointments.

Abandonment is defined as the desertion of an elderly person by the caregiver, custodian, or an individual who is responsible for providing care.[13] As many emergency physicians are aware, elderly patients may be abandoned in the emergency department. One survey reported that a median of 24 elderly patients were abandoned annually per emergency department, with 46% living alone and no longer being able to look after themselves and 41% being left in the emergency department by family members or a caregiver.[16] Abandonment may be considered a form of neglect.

Financial or *material exploitation* is defined as the illegal or improper use of an elderly person's money, property, or assets.[13] Financial exploitation includes denying an elderly person his or her home; stealing money or belongings; and coercing an elderly individual into signing contracts, changing a will, or assigning durable power of attorney to someone against his or her wishes.

ETIOLOGY AND RISK FACTORS FOR ELDER ABUSE

There are several theories of the etiology of elder abuse.[17] More recent focus has been directed toward the abusing relative or caregiver. The social learning or transgenerational violence theory proposes that chil-

BOX 67-1. Potential Risk Factors for Elder Abuse[17,19]

Caregiver Risk Factors
Alcohol or drug abuse
Mental illness
Financial stress
Stress resulting from caring for the elder (e.g., a lack of resources)
Outside factors resulting in stress (e.g., unemployment)
Financial dependence on the elder
Unrealistic expectations regarding caregiver responsibilities
Lack of caregiving skills
Long duration of time as a caregiver

Elder Risk Factors
Physical/functional impairment
Financial dependence on the caregiver
Cognitive impairment/dementia
Social isolation
History of family violence
Aggressive behavior
Female
Advanced age
Incontinence
Frequent falls

Environmental/Family Factors
Shared living situation
Overcrowded living conditions
Lack of family/community support
Socially isolated

Risk Factors for Institutional Abuse
Poor working conditions
Inadequate training, experience, and supervision of caregivers
Low wages
Low staff-to-patient ratio

dren who grow up in an abusive household may go on to be abusive against their own children and perhaps parents. Another theory, the stressed caregiver theory, proposes that as a caregiver becomes increasingly stressed (from caregiving or other causes) elder abuse is more likely to occur. Some researchers theorize that it is the psychopathology of the abuser that leads to elder abuse. Proponents of the isolation theory contend that as elderly individuals become more socially isolated as a result of illness, disability, and age, they are at increased risk for abuse. Those who adhere to the dependency theory believe that increasing frailty is the underlying etiology for elder abuse, whereas others contend that frailty only prevents many elders from protecting or defending themselves and the true etiology lies with the abuser.[18] It is now recognized that no single theory can account for all situations of abuse or neglect. An integrated theoretical model may describe all potential factors involved, and each circumstance may involve some components to a greater degree than others.[18]

Although numerous risk factors for elder abuse have been proposed, research is lacking and the list is far from definitive (Box 67-1). Therefore, emergency physicians should be alert to the possibility of abuse among all elderly patients. Risk factors for elder abuse may be divided into four main categories: caregiver risk factors for abusing, elder risk factors for being abused, environmental risk factors, and institutional abuse risk factors.

CLINICAL FEATURES

In addition to the risk factors stated previously, other findings suggestive of elder abuse are abandonment of the patient in the emergency department by the caregiver, frequent visits to the emergency department, lack of compliance with medical appointments and medications, and the use of numerous physicians and emergency departments for care rather than one primary care physician ("doctor hopping").

Elderly patients are four times more likely to present to the emergency department by ambulance than nonelderly patients.[20] When elders present to the emergency department by ambulance, the emergency medical technicians or paramedics may be invaluable in identifying at-risk elders on the basis of their assessment of the home situation and the family dynamics at the home.[21] Prehospital care providers should be questioned about the cleanliness and upkeep of the home; the availability of electricity, heat, water, and sanitation; infestation by rodents or vermin; and the safety of the interior of the home for the older patient.

The American Medical Association (AMA) has recommended that all health care providers routinely ask their older patients about abuse, even in the absence of signs of abuse.[22] Patients should always be questioned in as private a situation as possible, after the family or caregiver has left the room. If the patient suffers from dementia or is unable to answer questions for other reasons, individuals who have knowledge about the patient, other than the caregiver, should be questioned, such as other family members, visiting home nurses and assistants, therapists, primary care physician, or neighbors. If a translator is needed, someone other than a family member or the caregiver should be utilized. To broach the subject of elder abuse, the emergency physician should begin by asking about the patient's care in general and then focus on abuse and specific types of abuse (Box 67-2). Factors that have been shown to have a significant association with suspected elder abuse include a brittle support system, feeling lonely, expressing conflict with family or friends, alcohol abuse, short-term memory problems, and psychiatric illness.[24] One study has determined that emergency department nurses can be trained to screen older patients for neglect and appropriately refer them for care.[25] However, no validated screens for elder abuse have yet been adequately tested in the emergency department. If elder abuse or neglect is identified, the patient should be questioned further about the duration and frequency of the abuse, the nature of the abuse, and whether there has been intervention or assistance in the past because of the abuse.

There is increasing evidence that elder abuse is associated with adverse health outcomes including

---

BOX 67-2. Questions for Use in Screening Patients for Elder Abuse[19,23]

General
Do you feel safe where you live?
Are you afraid of anyone where you live?
Who assists you if you need help?
Who makes your meals?
Who helps you take your medications?
Who manages your checkbook?
Do you have frequent arguments with your family/caregiver?
What happens when you argue?

Physical Abuse
Have you been hit, slapped, or kicked?
Have you ever been locked in a room?
Have you ever been tied down?
Have you ever been forced to eat?

Sexual Abuse
Has anyone ever touched you sexually without your consent?

Psychological or Emotional Abuse
Do you feel alone?
Are you yelled at where you live?
Has your family/caregiver ever threatened to punish you or have you put in an institution?

Neglect
Are you left alone often at home?
Do you need to use hearing aids, glasses, and dentures, a walker, or a cane? Are they readily accessible to you?
Does your family/caregiver ever fail to help you when you need help?

Financial or Material Abuse
Has anyone ever taken anything from you without asking?
Have you been forced to sign a will, power of attorney, or any documents that you did not understand?
Does your family/caregiver rely on you for housing or financial support?

---

increased dementia, depression, and premature death.[26,27] Therefore, a thorough, well-documented medical history and physical examination should be performed.[22] When the medical history of an elderly patient is taken, it should be elicited from the patient and caregiver separately and alone. Potential historical indicators of abuse are listed in Box 67-3. As part of the medical history, the patient and caregiver should be asked about routine medications. The discovery of caregivers who are unfamiliar with daily medications and other necessary medical care of the elderly patient (e.g., dressing changes) should raise the suspicion of elder abuse. If injuries are noted, the patient should be questioned about how the injuries occurred. Patients should be asked directly whether anyone has hit, punched, or kicked them. If the injuries occurred as a result of interpersonal violence, the relationship between the patient and abuser should be ascertained. Providers should inform their patients if they are mandated to report abuse when it is disclosed by a patient. However, most states mandate reporting elder abuse even if it is only reasonably suspected. Because elders

BOX 67-3. Indicators from the Medical History of Possible Ongoing Elder Abuse

Implausible history of injury mechanism
Inconsistent history of injury mechanism between the patient and caregiver
Delay between onset of medical illness or injury and seeking medical attention
Unexplained injuries
Elderly patient referred to as "accident prone"
Past history of frequent injuries
Noncompliance with medications, appointments, or physician directions
Caregiver not able to give details of the patient's medical history or routine medications
Caregiver answers the questions regarding the patient
Patient or caregiver reluctant to answer questions
Strained patient-caregiver interaction

BOX 67-4. Signs of Physical Abuse, Sexual Abuse, and Neglect That May Be Noticed on the Physical Examination

Physical Abuse
Contusion
Contusions on bilateral upper arms (grab marks)
Abrasions
Burns (e.g., from cigarettes, irons, immersion)
Sprains
Patterned injuries (e.g., marks consistent with the shape of a belt, fingers, electrical cord)
Traumatic alopecia
Bite marks
Restraint marks (e.g., involving wrists, ankles, and torso)
Fractures
Multiple injuries in various stages of healing
Blunt head trauma
Intra-abdominal injuries (e.g., liver, spleen)
Gag marks
Ocular injuries (e.g., hyphema, retinal detachment)

Physical Signs of Sexual Abuse
Evidence of genital, rectal, or oral trauma (e.g., contusions, lacerations, erythema)
Evidence of sexually transmitted disease

Physical Signs of Neglect
Dehydration
Evidence that the patient has been lying in urine and stool
Malnutrition
Clothing inappropriate for the climate; dirty or severely worn
Poor body hygiene
Untreated injuries and medical problems
Poor oral hygiene
Skin breakdown (e.g., decubitus, pressure sores)

may be afraid to disclose abuse, it is important that providers reassure their patients that the goal is to provide a safer living environment for the elderly patient, not primarily to punish the caregiver. When a patient expresses fear about a report, the physician should give this information to Adult Protective Services in the report so that risk to the patient can be minimized.

When performing a physical examination of an elderly patient, the emergency physician should look for signs of physical abuse, sexual abuse, and neglect (Box 67-4). The emergency physician must use clinical skill and judgment to decide whether physical findings are suspicious for elder abuse or represent pathology. Illnesses that may resemble elder abuse occur frequently in older patients (e.g., easy bruising, fractures resulting from osteoporosis or osteopenia, dehydration). Elder abuse is included in the differential diagnosis of numerous conditions that occur frequently in the geriatric population. Elderly patients with multiple clinical findings consistent with elder abuse have a higher likelihood of being victims than patients with isolated findings. In addition, injuries and medical conditions for which no underlying etiology can be determined are more likely to be a result of abuse.

During the physical examination, the general appearance (e.g., cleanliness, hygiene, and dress) and behavior (e.g., agitated, fearful, withdrawn) of the patient should be noted. The skin should be examined for unexplained bruises, particularly of the head, face, torso, back, buttocks, or bilateral upper arms. Attention should be paid to the state of care of decubitus, if present. Head and facial injuries, including broken teeth, lacerations, or the absence of hair, may reflect abuse. If the genitourinary examination reveals evidence of trauma or vaginal bleeding and sexual abuse is suspected, a complete sexual assault examination, including collection of evidence, should be carried out as for other cases of sexual assault. The extremities should be examined for evidence of contractures that may indicate confinement for long periods, burns in a glove-stocking distribution related to immersion, and

wrist and ankle lesions from restraints. The patient's gait should be observed. If there has been a recent change in the patient's ability to ambulate, further imaging studies should be performed to rule out an occult fracture (e.g., hip fracture). A thorough neurologic examination should be performed with careful attention to an alteration in the patient's mental status, focal neurologic findings, and dementia. The recent development of focal neurologic deficits may be a result of blunt head trauma. Long-standing focal neurologic deficits, such as hemiparesis from a cerebrovascular accident, suggest increased needs for care of the elder. The elderly patient's mental status should be assessed. Subtle changes in the elder's mental status may be the only signs of ongoing abuse. Dehydration and malnutrition are the most frequent physical findings of neglect.

An elderly patient who is being emotionally or psychologically abused may display deterioration in mental health and show signs of posttraumatic stress disorder. The patient may demonstrate fear, anxiety, or infantile behavior in the presence of the caregiver and may also exhibit poor self-esteem. On questioning, the elderly patient may admit to ambivalent feelings toward the family member who is the caregiver as well as express feelings of mistrust related to the caregiver. The caregiver may also be emotionally abusive in the presence of the emergency physician. Elderly patients who are being physically abused, sexually abused, or neglected also demonstrate findings similar to those of emotionally abused elderly patients.

DIAGNOSTIC STRATEGIES

When elder abuse is suspected, laboratory investigations and imaging studies should be obtained as indicated by the history and physical examination. The emergency physician should have a lower threshold for ordering imaging studies for elderly patients secondary to difficulty in obtaining a history in some cases, the increased frequency of osteopenia and osteoporosis, and the tendency of some elders to minimize pain. Metabolic laboratory tests may be helpful in determining electrolyte, nutritional, or endocrine abnormalities. Toxicologic studies may be helpful to document compliance with medications, overmedicating or undermedicating by the caregiver, and, in severe cases of elder abuse, evidence of poisoning.

DOCUMENTATION

Accurate and thorough documentation of the history and physical examination in cases of suspected elder abuse is essential.[19,23] The history of any suspected types of abuse, as well as the mechanism of injury, should be documented in the patient's own words, if possible. Documentation should include details of the pertinent social history (e.g., caregiver's identity, living arrangements, functional status). A description of any injuries should include types of injuries (e.g., fractures, lacerations, contusions), number, size, location, color, and stage of healing or approximate ages of the injuries. When possible, photographs of the injuries should be taken before rendering treatment. In addition to photographs, the locations and types of injuries should be documented on a body map or diagram. In California, a statewide form has been developed for the purpose of documenting a forensic examination in cases of elder abuse.[28] At this time, its use is not mandated. The explanation given by the patient for the mechanism of each injury should be included in the history, as well as whether the explanation seems appropriate. If the explanations for the injuries seem reasonable, a statement reflecting that the physical examination is compatible with the history may be included in the medical record. The results of laboratory investigations and imaging studies should also be recorded. Follow-up plans, referrals, and interventions should be documented in the medical record. If a report is made to Adult Protective Services, the name of the individual contacted or the case number should be recorded. In addition, if law enforcement is contacted, the name and badge number of the officer taking the report should be documented. In cases of suspected elder abuse that result in legal action, thorough documentation may be critical in determining the outcome and ultimate care of the patient.

CAREGIVER INTERVIEW

Part of the assessment of a suspected victim of elder abuse involves interviewing the caregiver or suspected abuser. The needs of both the caregiver and the elder should be addressed. To obtain beneficial information and not create a confrontational situation with the caregiver or suspected abuser, questioning should proceed in a nonthreatening and nonjudgmental manner. The goal is not to punish the caregiver but rather to stop the abuse. Accusations are likely only to curtail the amount of information the caregiver provides to the emergency physician. The caregiver or suspected abuser should be interviewed separately from the patient. Conducting separate interviews may reveal discrepant histories between the caregiver and the patient. Initially, questioning should be directed at the reason for presenting to the emergency department. Subsequently, questions should be directed at the patient's medical conditions and the daily care requirements, including routine medications and assistance with activities of daily living. Caring for an individual with chronic illness who frequently requires assistance with basic activities of daily living is a difficult and tiring task.[29] Therefore, verbal expressions of sympathy, explicit recognition of the challenges, and demonstrations of support can be beneficial for the caregiver and also promote information sharing. Statements such as "Caring for your mother must be a difficult task. Do you ever feel anger or resentment toward her?" may actually allow the family member or caregiver to express valid frustrations. Questions should also explore whether any recent stresses have occurred in the household, whether the caregiver feels that the patient is a financial burden, and whether any respite services or other home help has been made available.

INTERVENTIONS AND REFERRALS

When elder abuse is suspected or identified, provision for immediate care needs, situational assessment, long-term care planning, and steps to prevent future abuse are all required. Emergency department interventions in elder abuse differ from those in child abuse primarily because the physician should respect the wishes of the mentally competent elderly adult. The older adult should be able to live in the least restrictive environment possible, and institutionalization should not automatically be regarded as a solution to ending the abuse. For many elders, the prospect of being institutionalized is worse than continuing to live in an abusive situation. In addition, providing home care assistance, respite care, and other in-home resources to the caregiver and elderly patient is more cost effective than institutionalization.[23] Therefore, one of the goals of management of elder abuse is to keep the family unit together, when possible, rather than have the elder removed from the home.

If there is immediate danger, the patient should be removed from the home. Hospitalization may be required for injuries and ongoing medical problems.

However, in the absence of an acute medical illness, medical insurance companies and third-party payers may not cover the cost of hospitalization, and a safe-house placement may be required.[30] Physicians should be aware of the diagnostic codes for adult maltreatment syndrome (unspecified) (ICD-9: 995.8; ICD-10: suspected T76.91, confirmed T74.91) and the additional codes for specific types of abuse.[31,32]

If the patient refuses intervention, the emergency physician must determine whether the patient is competent to make his or her own decisions. In some instances a psychiatric consultation for the determination of competence may be required. If the elderly patient is found not to be competent to make his or her own decisions, Adult Protective Services should be notified to arrange court-ordered guardianship. The wishes of a competent elderly patient must be respected even if the patient desires to return to an abusive situation.

In suspected cases of elder abuse that pose a less imminent threat, interventions should be individualized.[22] If the patient wants to return home and may be safely discharged from the emergency department, a follow-up plan should be established. This is best accomplished by a multidisciplinary team consisting of the patient's primary care physician, nurses, social workers, and occupational therapists or a geriatrics assessment team. Another approach includes Adult Protective Services caseworkers as members of the geriatric team.[33] The follow-up assessment should consist of an evaluation of the patient's functional, cognitive, medical, and emotional status. Social and financial resources should also be determined. The frequency, severity, and intent of the abuse should be assessed. At least one home visit should be included as part of the assessment.

The needs of the caregiver should also be assessed. Support services such as in-home services, respite care, psychological counseling, employment referrals, and alcohol and drug abuse rehabilitation program referrals should be provided, as needed. For the short term, the emergency physician may assist the caregiver by obtaining increased involvement from other family members or friends, close follow-up with the patient's primary care physician, a social services consultation, home nursing assistance, and the involvement of Adult Protective Services. Other referrals that may be beneficial for both the elderly patient and the caregiver include senior centers, medical transport services, Medicare referral, Meals-on-Wheels, senior's housing, Social Security benefits, religious communities, home health, adult day care, hospice care, and victim assistance. Ultimately, if the caregiver has severe personal problems that cannot be resolved, the only solution may be separation of the elder from the caregiver. If the elderly patient is competent and does not wish to accept interventions, he or she should nonetheless be educated about elder abuse and given referral materials. Some cases of elder abuse are actually intimate partner violence, committed by the elder's spouse.[12] In these cases intimate partner violence advocacy services should be notified.

Elderly victims should be educated about elder abuse and the likelihood that it will increase in frequency and severity over time. All emergency departments should have protocols for the management of suspected cases of elder abuse to facilitate management and ensure appropriate care for these elderly patients.[34] This recommendation has been made by the AMA, the American College of Emergency Physicians, and other professional medical organizations.[22,34] Some emergency departments also have access to in-house elder abuse response teams that can be mobilized to assist the emergency physician with the management of these complex cases.[35]

REPORTING REQUIREMENTS

In all 50 states and the District of Columbia laws have now been enacted that pertain to the reporting and investigation of elder abuse. However, the definitions of elder abuse and requirements of the laws vary from state to state.[36] In 44 of the states, physicians are mandated to file a report if they know or reasonably suspect that elder abuse has occurred, and in an additional 2 states physicians are mandated to report only if the suspected victim resides in a nursing home.[37] Many of the states with mandatory reporting requirements also grant immunity to physicians who report suspected elder abuse. Most state laws also have a penalty for failure to report.[38] These penalties usually consist of a fine or a jail sentence, or both. At this time, there are no known cases of health care providers being convicted for failure to report elder abuse. In most states, Adult Protective Services are designated as the agency responsible for receiving and investigating all reports of suspected elder abuse. The laws vary widely concerning the age at which "elder" is defined, with most states defining it as 60 years or older. In addition, the laws vary in their definitions of the circumstances of the abuse, types of abuse, the reporting and investigation of the abuse, and specifics regarding domestic and institutional abuse. Additional criminal laws regarding assault and battery, theft, fraud, rape, and murder may also pertain to elder abuse. Laws concerning guardianship and conservatorship, durable powers of attorney, intimate partner violence, and family violence may also be related to elder abuse. Emergency physicians should become familiar with state laws pertaining to elder abuse and their duty to report in the state in which they practice.

There are several issues regarding the mandatory reporting laws for elder abuse. Some physicians are concerned that reporting elder abuse constitutes a breach of confidentiality with their patients. Others are concerned that mandatory reporting may deter elders from seeking medical care. The AMA has stated that physicians should inform their patients of their legal obligation to report elder abuse and the medical necessity to intervene in cases of elder abuse. The AMA also emphasizes that the goal is to end the abuse by facilitating access to resources for the patient and the family.[22] There is a great need for standardization of legislation and increased funding to provide adequate service delivery to elder abuse victims and their families.[36]

Elder abuse is often underrecognized or underreported by emergency physicians. Reasons include[17,23] a lack of awareness of the prevalence of elder abuse, ageism (discrimination against the elderly), lack of knowledge of the appropriate management of suspected elder abuse, lack of an emergency department protocol for suspected elder abuse, lack of time to conduct a time-consuming evaluation of the suspected abuse, the emergency physician's concern about litigation, the emergency physician's concern about having to take time away from the practice to testify in court, and the ethical issue of not wanting to breach physician-patient confidentiality. One study reported that only 2% of reports of elder abuse were made by physicians.[39] Physicians were most likely to report physical abuse and least likely to report exploitation.[39]

Elderly patients may also contribute to the difficulty in identifying elder abuse, willingly or unwillingly, because of isolation resulting from illness or age; inability to report abuse; reluctance to disclose the elder abuse owing to embarrassment or guilt; fear of retaliation by the abuser; wanting to protect the abuser, who is often a spouse or a child; fear of the consequences of the discovery of the abuse; fear of institutionalization; cultural or ethnic beliefs and backgrounds; and feeling that they are a burden to their families.

INSTITUTIONAL ABUSE

Approximately 5% of all elderly individuals reside in institutions such as nursing homes, board and care homes, and other assisted-living facilities.[40] With the growing elderly population, this percentage is estimated to increase significantly in the future. In 1976, the Older Americans Act established the Long-Term Care Ombudsman Program to monitor nursing homes and board and care facilities and to investigate cases of suspected elder abuse. This program is present in all 50 states. In 1987, the Nursing Home Reform Act included the right to be free from physical, sexual, and emotional abuse as well as isolation. Elderly residents of institutions may be subjected to abuse by other patients, visitors, and staff. A random survey of staff in long-term care institutions in one state revealed that 10% of nurses' aides reported committing at least one act of physical violence in the previous year and 40% at least one act of psychological abuse.[41] Risk factors for institutional abuse are shown in Box 67-1. A study examining ombudsman data from six states found that a higher percentage of complaints lodged on behalf of minorities were verified, yet a lower percentage were fully resolved.[42] When patients from long-term care facilities present to the emergency department for medical care, emergency physicians should be alert to signs of possible abuse. These cases should be reported to the state long-term care ombudsman for further investigation.

ABUSE OF PERSONS WITH DISABILITIES

In most states, the laws protecting elders from abuse also protect persons with disabilities, often referred to as "dependent adults," "vulnerable adults," or "disabled adults." Included are persons aged 18 or older who have developmental, mental, or physical disabilities. Little is known about abuse and neglect of persons with disabilities; however, adults with disabilities are reported to be at higher risk for abuse than persons without disabilities.[43] In particular, persons with developmental disability are at high risk for abuse. The best conservative estimate is that people with developmental disability are 4 to 10 times more likely to be victims of crime (or abuse) than people without disabilities[44]; the most pronounced are robbery (12.7 times higher) and sexual assault (10.7 times higher).[45] One study found that 83% of women with developmental disabilities had been sexually assaulted and that, of those, nearly 50% had been sexually assaulted 10 or more times.[46] Emergency physicians should have a heightened awareness of the greater likelihood of abuse when managing patients with disabilities and understand the mandated reporting laws and resources available to disabled victims in their state.

FUTURE DIRECTIONS

Residency training should include education in identifying and managing elder abuse and the reporting requirements for elder abuse. Emergency physicians should also educate their patients and the community about the problem of elder abuse and the resources available in the community to assist elders and their caregivers. They should advocate for increased availability and funding of in-home services for elders. Further, they should engage in research on elder abuse to increase the understanding of risk factors for elder abuse, develop validated screens for the detection of elder abuse, determine effective management protocols, and evaluate effective preventive interventions.

 KEY CONCEPTS

- Emergency physicians should routinely ask all elderly patients about abuse, even in the absence of signs and symptoms of abuse. Emergency physicians should be alert to the possibility of elder abuse.
- The needs of the caregiver should be assessed and support offered.
- An elderly patient who is in immediate danger should be hospitalized or otherwise removed from the home. If the patient is not in imminent danger, assistance may be provided to the caregiver. The family unit should be preserved whenever possible.
- The wishes of a competent elderly patient must be respected, even if the patient is not willing to accept interventions.
- In 44 states emergency physicians are mandated to report cases of known or suspected elder abuse to Adult Protective Services.

REFERENCES

1. Table ST-EST 2003-01res. Annual estimates of the resident population by selected age groups for the U.S. and states, Population Estimates Program. Washington, DC, Population Division, U.S. Census Bureau, 2004. Available at: http://eire.census.gov.popest/data/states/tables/ST-EST2003-01res.pdf. Accessed March 17, 2004.

2. Table 2a. Projection population of the United States, by age and sex: 2000 to 2050. Washington, DC, U.S. Census Bureau, 2004. Available at: http://www.census.gov/ipc/www/usinterimproj. Internet release date March 18, 2004; accessed March 18, 2004.

3. Krug EG, et al (eds): World Report on Violence and Health. Geneva, World Health Organization, 2002. Available at: www.who.int/violence_injury-prevention

4. Baker AA: Granny battering. Mod Geriatr 5:20, 1975.

5. Burston GR: Granny-battering. Br Med J 3:592, 1975.

6. U.S. House of Representatives Select Committee on Aging: Elder abuse: An examination of a hidden problem, 97th Congress (Comm. Publication No. 97-277), Washington, DC, 1981, US Government Printing Office.

7. U.S. House of Representatives Select Committee on Aging: Elder Abuse: A Decade of Shame and Inaction, 101st Congress (Comm. Publication No. 101-752). Washington, DC, Government Printing Office, 1990.

8. Joint Commission on Accreditation of Healthcare Organizations: Accreditation Manual for Hospitals. Oakbrook Terrace, Ill, Emergency Services, 1992.

9. Lachs MS, et al: ED use by older victims of family violence. Ann Emerg Med 30:448, 1997.

10. Jones JS, et al: Elder mistreatment: National survey of emergency physicians. Ann Emerg Med 30:473, 1997.

11. National Center on Elder Abuse: National Elder Abuse Incidence Study: Final Report. Washington, DC, U.S. Department of Health and Human Services, 1998. Available at: www.aoa.gov/abuse/report/default.htm

12. Pillemer K, Finkelhor D: The prevalence of elder abuse: A random sample survey. Gerontologist 28:51, 1998.

13. Tatara T, Kuzmeskus LM: Types of Elder Abuse in Domestic Settings. Elder Abuse Information Series, No. 1. Washington, DC, National Center on Elder Abuse (NCEA), 1999. Available at: www.gwjapan.com/NCEA

14. Jones JS: Elder abuse and neglect: Responding to a national problem. Ann Emerg Med 23:845, 1994.

15. Tatara T, Kuzmeskus LM: Trends in Elder Abuse in Domestic Settings. Elder Abuse Information Series, No. 2. Washington, DC, National Center on Elder Abuse (NCEA), 1997. Available at: www.gwjapan.com/NCEA

16. American College of Emergency Physicians Survey: Elderly abandonment survey: The abandonment of the elderly in the emergency department. Frontlines, Fall 1992.

17. Jones JS, Holstege C, Holstege H: Elder abuse and neglect: Understanding the causes and potential risk factors. Am J Emerg Med 15:579, 1997.

18. Gordon RM, Brill D: The abuse and neglect of the elderly. Int J Law Psychiatry 24:183, 2001.

19. Levine JM: Elder neglect and abuse: A primer for primary care physicians. Geriatrics 58:37, 2003.

20. Strange GR, Chen EH, Sanders AB: Use of emergency departments by elderly patients: Projections from a multicenter data base. Ann Emerg Med 21:819, 1992.

21. Gerson LW, Schelble DT, Wilson JE: Using paramedics to identify at-risk elderly. Ann Emerg Med 21:688, 1992.

22. American Medical Association: Diagnostic and Treatment Guidelines on Elder Abuse and Neglect. Chicago, AMA, 1992.

23. Kleinschmidt KC: Elder abuse: A review. Ann Emerg Med 30:463, 1997.

24. Shugarman LR, et al: Identifying older people at risk of abuse during routine screening practices. J Am Geriatr Soc 51:24, 2003.

25. Fulmer T, et al: Elder neglect assessment in the emergency department. J Emerg Nurs 26:436, 2000.

26. Lachs MS, et al: The mortality of elder mistreatment. JAMA 280:428, 1998.

27. Dyer CB, et al: The high prevalence of depression and dementia in elder abuse or neglect. J Am Geriatr Soc 48:205, 2000.

28. Governor's Office of Emergency Services, State of California: Forensic Medical Report: Elder and Dependent Adult Abuse and Neglect Examination—OES 602. OES, Sacramento, Calif, 2004. Available at: www.oes.ca.gov (accessed 2/10/05).

29. Levine C: The loneliness of the long-term care giver. N Engl J Med 340:1587, 1999.

30. Lachs MS, et al: Older adults: An 11-year longitudinal study of adult protective service use. Arch Intern Med 156:449, 1996.

31. Rudman WJ: Coding and Documentation of Domestic Violence. San Francisco, Family Violence Prevention Fund, 2000.

32. National Center for Health Statistics, Centers for Disease Control and Prevention: Draft International Classification of Diseases, 10th revision, Clinical Modification, 2003. Available at: www.cdc.gov/nchs/about/otheract/icd9/icd10cm.htm

33. Dyer CB, et al: Treating elder neglect: Collaboration between a geriatrics assessment team and adult protective services. South Med J 92:242, 1999.

34. American College of Emergency Physicians: Management of elder abuse and neglect. Ann Emerg Med 31:149, 1998.

35. National Research Council: Elder Mistreatment: Abuse, Neglect, and Exploitation in an Aging America. Washington, DC, National Academies Press, 2003.

36. Jogerst GJ, et al: Domestic elder abuse and the law. Am J Public Health 93:2131,2003.

37. National Center for Elder Abuse: State elder abuse laws. Available at: www.elderabusecenter.org/default.cfm?p=statelaws.cfm; accessed March 15, 2004.

38. Mallon WK, Kassinove A: Mandatory reporting laws and the emergency department. Top Emerg Med 21:63,1999.

39. Rosenblatt DE, Cho K, Durance PW: Reporting mistreatment of older adults: The role of physicians. J Am Geriatr Soc 44:65, 1996.

40. Stiegel LA: Recommended guidelines for state courts handling cases involving elder abuse. American Bar Association, 1995.

41. Pillemer K, Moore DW: Abuse of patients in nursing homes: Findings from a survey of staff. Gerontologist 29:314, 1989.

42. Huber R, et al: Data from long-term care ombudsman programs in six states: The implications of collecting resident demographics. Gerontologist 41:61, 2001.

43. Baladerian NJ: Recognizing abuse and neglect in people with severe cognitive and/or communication impairments. J Elder Abuse Neglect 9:93, 1997.

44. Sobsey D, Lucardie R, Mansell S: Violence and Disability: An Annotated Bibliography. Baltimore, Brookes Publishing, 1995.

45. Wilson C, Brewer N: The incidence of criminal victimization of individuals with an intellectual disability. Aust Psychol 27:114, 1992.

46. Sobsey D, Doe T: Patterns of sexual abuse and assault. J Sex Disabil 9:243, 1991.

CHAPTER

68 Youth, Gangs, and Violence

H. Range Hutson

PERSPECTIVE

There are 78 million youths in the United States younger than age 20 years, and there are expected to be around 81 million by 2010 with increasingly more ethnic minorities and older adolescents. The adolescent period is filled with many anatomic, physiologic, and psychological adjustments. Adolescents are particularly vulnerable to violence and injury because of developmental issues, including independence and autonomy, curiosity leading to experimentation (e.g., alcohol, drugs, sex), peer group pressure, immaturity, impulsivity, the feeling of invincibility, narcissism, and problems with self-identity.[1] Other factors that increase the vulnerability of adolescents to violence include the breakdown of family and community structure, media violence, and easy accessibility to lethal weapons (e.g., firearms).[2]

Violence is learned and is predictable and preventable.[3] A child's initial exposure to violence usually occurs in the home (e.g., intimate partner violence, child abuse, elder abuse, corporal punishment) and increases an adolescent's predisposition to violence. The degree to which adolescents are exposed to violence in the home, community, school, media, sports, and peer groups and the extent to which they are victims of violence are associated with their own use of violence.[4,5] Adolescent boys perpetrate more violence than girls, and, with the exception of rape, are exposed to more violent acts than girls. Adolescents who live in the inner city have greater exposure to violence than other youth.[5,6]

Injuries have been mistakenly called "accidents" because they have been viewed as unpredictable and uncontrollable. Epidemiologic research now shows that injuries, similar to other diseases, occur in highly predictable patterns and are controllable and preventable. Every year in the United States, approximately 16 million children and adolescents are treated in the emergency department for injuries, 600,000 are hospitalized, and 30,000 sustain permanent physical and neurologic sequelae from their injuries.

Injury is the leading cause of death during the child and adolescent period, causing more deaths than all other diseases combined.[7] Assaultive violence is a leading cause of injury, particularly in adolescence, and adolescents are more likely to be victims of violent crime than any other age group.[8] Physical fighting is one of the most important risk factors for homicides that occur among adolescents, particularly with boys.[9,10] Homicide is the second leading cause of death

between 15 and 19 years and the leading cause among African-American boys, who are six times more likely to die from homicide than white boys in this age group.[7] Homicide rates for children and adolescents are peaking at progressively earlier ages.[1,7] Adolescents are disproportionately represented as perpetrators and victims of violent acts,[5] with one third of individuals arrested for violent crimes (e.g., assault, rape, and homicide) in this age group.

VIOLENCE IN SCHOOLS

Many adolescents report that their greatest fear is school violence.[11] In a more recent national school survey, 35.7% of high school students reported having been in a physical fight, and 6.9% have carried a weapon to school (e.g., a gun, knife, or club). Boys are more likely than girls to carry a weapon, and 5.2% of students missed school because they felt unsafe at school or traveling to or from school.[12] The survey also revealed that 7.7% of students have been threatened or injured with a weapon while on school property.[12] Although the rates of physical fighting and weapon carrying have decreased since 1995,[13] the availability of firearms to urban adolescents is pervasive and not limited to groups at high risk for violence (e.g., gang members).[5,14]

Assaultive violence leading to homicides at school accounts for less than 1% of all homicides that occur among school-age children. Half of all school-associated violent deaths occur during transition periods during the school day (beginning of school, lunch period, end of school day). Most firearms used in school-related deaths are obtained from the perpetrator's home.[15]

Although school violence is decreasing, one form of school violence that is now being increasingly recognized is bullying. Bullying behavior is designed to intimidate or harm an individual or group of individuals. Verbal intimidation is the most common form; however, at times it may lead to physical violence. Bullying commonly starts in elementary school and continues throughout junior high and high school. Although bullying occurs among girls and boys, it is a much larger male phenomenon, especially when it is associated with physical violence.[16-19]

In the National Crime Victimization Survey, 15% of students report that street gangs are present in their school, and that in school or on their way to and from school students are twice as likely to fear being assaulted.[20] Gang members are seven times more likely to own a firearm than children and adolescents not in gangs.[21] For these reasons, many children and adolescents are fearful about going to school, resulting in more weapons being brought to school for personal safety.[22]

MEDIA VIOLENCE AND ITS EFFECT ON CHILDREN AND ADOLESCENTS

By age 18, children, on average, see 200,000 violent acts portrayed on television and spend more hours watching television than attending school.[23] When today's children and adolescents reach age 70, they will have spent 10 years watching television.[24] Despite public concern over media violence, Saturday morning children's programming still contains 20 to 25 violent acts per hour. Before age 8, children cannot consistently discriminate between real life and fantasy in entertainment. Through television and other forms of media violence, children and adolescents learn and imitate violent behavior, particularly if the aggressor is the hero or the heroine.[24,25] The more realistic the violence portrayed, the greater the probability the violence will be imitated by children and adolescents. Of young men incarcerated for violent crimes (e.g., homicide, rape, and assault), 22% to 34% consciously imitated crimes learned from television. In the media, violence is a quick, effective ending for arguments and disagreements and does not show the importance of patience, negotiation, and compromise in resolving conflicts and disagreements.[26] Media violence does not portray the true physical and psychological consequences of violent acts. This may lead children and adolescents passively to accept violence as a way of life, desensitizing them to future acts of violence and making them less likely to intervene when violent acts occur.[26]

ADOLESCENTS, DRUG ABUSE, AND VIOLENCE

In the United States, 3 million adolescents have alcoholism, and another 400,000 adolescents require treatment for drug abuse. Illicit drugs cost $75 billion per year for law enforcement, incarceration, legal costs, medical treatment/hospitalization, and drug prevention programs, in addition to $70 billion per year spent for the purchase of illicit drugs. Illicit drugs account for almost half of the 1 million individuals incarcerated, requiring an enormous amount of time for law enforcement and almost 50% of judiciary work time.[27]

From ages 10 to 13 years, children begin experimenting with a wide range of new behaviors. Cigarettes, alcohol, and other types of drugs are a normal part of the "coming of age" for many children, regardless of race, culture, socioeconomic status, or geographic location. Substance use follows a predictable pattern beginning with experimentation with cigarettes and alcohol, followed by marijuana, then cocaine. Other drugs, including opioids and hallucinogens, typically occur later in the sequence, following the use of cocaine. This does not mean that an adolescent necessarily progresses beyond a particular stage. Initially, with cigarettes and alcohol, the adolescent associates drugs with euphoria and pleasure. With regular use, tolerance and the need for particular drugs develop. At this stage, the adolescent is drug dependent and now uses the drug to prevent withdrawal symptoms, which may be physiologic or psychological in nature. For adolescents, any use of a drug is commonly perceived as drug abuse. Adolescents at greatest risk for a lifelong pattern of substance abuse typically begin using drugs before age 15. Adolescents who are the most seriously affected by substance abuse are usually those who are least involved in school or other meaningful activities.[28]

Substance use and abuse is associated with violent behavior. The precise relationship has not been completely elucidated, but drugs and violent behavior are related to drug use (pharmacologic violence), to drug procurement (economic violence), and to the illicit sale of drugs.[29,30] Alcohol is the most commonly used drug associated with violence. The pharmacologic effects of alcohol contribute significantly to the prevalence of adolescent fighting, suicide, homicide, unintentional injury and death, rape, and physical assaults.[31] Cocaine, barbiturates, phencyclidine (PCP), amphetamines, and anabolic steroids also play a role in such violence.[29,30] Economic violence can lead to intentional injury and death during the process of obtaining money to finance drug use. The illicit sale of drugs leads to several types of violence between buyers and sellers: robbery for money or drugs, arguments over quality or quantity of the drug, competition for territory or markets for the sale of drugs, and violence as a management strategy to discipline drug-selling subordinates.

FIREARMS

In the United States, eight children and adolescents are killed every day by firearms.[32] For every child killed with a firearm, four children sustain a firearm-related injury.[33] Sixty percent of firearm assaults are fatal, compared with 4% of knife assaults and fewer than 1% of assaults with blunt objects.[34] There are approximately 200 million privately owned firearms, of which 60 million are handguns.[35] Handguns are involved in most firearm injuries and deaths, although they make up less than one third of all firearms. About half of all households in the United States contain a firearm.[35] Most privately owned firearms are purchased with the idea that firearms increase personal safety and home security, but the risks of firearms kept in the home are often unrecognized.[36] A firearm in the home is 43 times more likely to kill a family member or friend than an intruder.[37] When a gun is fired in the home by an adolescent, the victim most often is the adolescent (35%), a friend (34%), a sibling (25%), or a parent or relative (6%).[1] Many firearms in the home are stored unlocked and loaded.[38,39] In one survey, approximately 75% of first-grade and second-grade students reported that their families had a firearm in the home, and the students knew exactly where it was located.[40] Before 8 years of age, few children can distinguish between a toy gun and a real gun.[41]

The United States has one of the highest firearm homicide rates in the industrialized world.[5] The availability of firearms increases the lethality of violent behavior,[2,42] and easy accessibility plays a major role in the morbidity and mortality of children and adolescents. In 2001, firearms were involved in 2937 child and adolescent deaths in the United States, most of which occurred in the 15- to 19-year-old age group.[43] In the last 20 years, there has been a 75% increase in child and adolescent deaths caused by firearms.[34] The firearm homicide rate for boys is three to four times that for girls.[7] Firearms are the second leading cause of death in all children 10 to 19 years old,[7] and the firearm death rate among U.S. children age 14 and younger is approximately 12 times greater than the firearm death rate among children in 25 other industrialized nations combined.[44] Firearm homicide rates are highest among African-American adolescent boys in urban areas in the United States.[45] For African-American male adolescents, firearm injury is the leading cause of death. Among adolescents, homicides occur most often in urban areas, and suicides occur most often outside urban areas.[46] A handgun is the weapon used in 82% of adolescent homicides[47]; most adolescent homicides are not premeditated but are impulsive, unplanned, and, in most cases, instantly regretted.[34]

NONPOWDER FIREARMS

Modern technology has transformed the BB gun from a toy to a potentially lethal weapon with a muzzle velocity in the range of small-caliber, low-velocity powder firearms. Other nonpowder firearms include pellet guns and air pistols that use spring-loaded, manual pump compression or pressurized carbon dioxide instead of gunpowder and can cause severe injury or death at close range.[35]

Nonpowder firearms are used predominantly by children and adolescents, with 80% of all injuries by nonpowder firearms in these age groups.[48] These injuries account for 21,000 emergency department visits and approximately 3 deaths per year.[49] Victims of nonpowder firearm injuries are overwhelmingly male.[50] Injuries to the extremities are the most common, with 25% of injuries to the eyes, head, face, or neck.[50] The most serious injuries are intracranial penetration in the region of the orbit or thin regions of the skull. Nonpowder firearm injuries are a common cause of blindness in adolescent boys; other complications include embolization and lead poisoning. Penetration of the heart and aorta occasionally results in death.[51] Overall, nonpowder firearm injuries are more numerous and less severe than powder firearm injuries, but head, chest, and abdominal wounds from these weapons may be erroneously regarded as trivial, with catastrophic results.

PREVENTION STRATEGIES FOR YOUTH VIOLENCE

Children and adolescents lack judgment and experience and cannot be expected to avoid violence and injury by their own accord.[52] To decrease youth violence, physicians and other health care providers should urge the media to do the following: (1) decrease the violence, use of weapons, and pain and suffering depicted in the media; (2) accurately portray the true consequences of violent acts; and (3) decrease the amount of violent lyrics and violent scenes in music videos and video games. Physicians should advise parents to monitor and limit their children's viewing of television, video games, music videos, movies, and the Internet.[53]

Health care providers can encourage schools to address youth violence.[5,54-56] Schools should be encouraged to teach conflict resolution and anger management skills, which represent an empowering step toward avoiding violence. They can make the learning environment physically safe by decreasing weapons among students. Students should be advised of the risk and legal consequences of carrying weapons to school. Depending on the school and local community, metal detectors and school safety police may be necessary. Schools must work jointly with local communities to decrease violence that occurs on the way to and from school and the overall level of violence in the community. Emergency physicians and other health care providers should encourage school-based counseling of children and adolescents concerning violence and injury prevention.[57] This may be a cost-effective method of preventing childhood and adolescent violence leading to injury.[58-60]

Physicians should educate children, adolescents, and their parents about drug use leading to abuse and dependency and the association between drugs and violence. Physicians also should advocate for increasing funding for alcohol and drug treatment centers for substance-dependent adolescents.

Physicians should educate parents about the risk of firearms kept in the home and, if a firearm is present, the proper storage procedures, as follows: unloaded, separated from ammunition, and in a locked box or cabinet. Parents should ask about firearms when their children visit other homes. Parents should know about the number of injuries from nonpowder firearms and allow their children to use nonpowder firearms only with goggles, chest protection, and adult supervision. Other strategies proposed to prevent firearm injuries in children and adolescents include legislation and regulation of the availability and manufacturing of firearms (e.g., safety devices) and the institution of a Firearm Fatality Reporting System.[35,58-62]

The medical record of victims of violence should include the circumstances of the violent event leading to the injury. The emergency physician also should document the victim's relationship to the perpetrator of the violent event, the use of alcohol or drugs by the victim, and whether the victim has a previous history of injuries caused by violence. Most important, the emergency physician should determine whether the victim plans to seek revenge and provide immediate counseling emphasizing a cooling off period to prevent further acts of violence. The risk of reinjury or death to the patient and others and the risk of criminal prosecution should be discussed. Emergency physicians and other health care providers may be legally bound to report to law enforcement officers if the patient threatens a specific individual.[63,64] All individuals at risk for reinjury caused by violence should be counseled by either health care providers or social services while in the emergency department.

VIOLENCE BY STREET GANGS

Street gangs are composed mainly of inner-city adolescents from the same socioeconomic background. Adolescents join street gangs for a sense of belonging, protection, status, adventure, and illegal monetary gain. Most inner-city adolescents do not join street gangs, however.

In the 1950s, street gang violence typically involved fistfights, blunt objects, knives, and occasionally firearms. Modern-day street gangs are larger, more numerous, more widespread, more violent, and no longer confined to the inner city. More gang members and innocent bystanders are injured or killed since firearms have become the weapons of choice.[65] Violent street gangs view themselves as the ultimate defenders of their neighborhood or turf. Gang members are willing to die, kill rival gang members, risk imprisonment, and unintentionally injure or kill innocent bystanders in defending their turf or retaliating for intrusions by rival street gangs. If a rival street gang insults, challenges, injures, or kills a member of another street gang, it is highly probable that an episode of violence will occur. Being injured, imprisoned, or killed defending the gang or turf often enhances a gang member's reputation and standing in the gang. The more violent the street gang, the greater the reputation of the gang members. Gang members commonly do not testify in court against rival gang members, but prefer to enforce their own brand of justice, violently, against rival street gangs. Common reasons for street gang violence include retaliation for previous shootings, rivalry, turf fights, arguments, and, at times, control over an illegal criminal enterprise. Injuries and homicides by violent street gangs occur in many ways, including walk-up shootings, drive-by shootings, stabbings, use of blunt force weapons, and arson. In most instances, street gang violence is intraracial (e.g., African American versus African American, Hispanic versus Hispanic).

Violent street gangs are active in 94% of U.S. cities with more than 100,000 people,[66] but also are present in many small cities and towns. It is estimated that there are 26,000 gangs and 840,500 gang members nationwide.[67,68] Modern street gangs nationwide have patterned themselves after the street gang subculture in the Los Angeles area (African-American street gangs [e.g., Crips, Bloods] and Hispanic street gangs). The street gang subculture has created its own style of dress,

form of verbal and nonverbal communication, music, camaraderie, and funeral rituals, which has made it possible for adolescents of any ethnic group or background to identify with the gang lifestyle.[69,70] There are African-American, Hispanic, Asian, and white gangs. Some white gangs differ from other ethnic gangs in that they are consistently involved in acts of hate violence.[68]

Life in the gang typically begins around age 13 as a "wannabe," with most adolescents joining ("jumping in") the gang at or around age 15. The peak years for violent street gang activity are between 15 and 21 years of age,[71] after which, gang members begin to migrate out. Some members stay active in the gang into their early 30s.[72]

Why the Increase in Street Gang Violence?

The underlying factors for the increase in intensity of street gang violence are unknown. Drug dealing and the use of automatic weapons are not major causative factors for the increase in gang violence.[65,73,74] The most likely reasons include the following: the growth in the number of gang members, the appeal of the bravado and violent image of gang members, greater levels of intergang violence, an increase in the sophistication of firearm weaponry in gang violence, an increasingly violent society, increased economic despair in urban communities, a breakdown in sociocultural institutions, and an increase in marginalization of urban children and adolescents.[75-77]

Drive-By Shootings

One of the most common violent acts committed by street gangs is the *drive-by shooting,* defined as gang members shooting at suspected rival gang members from a vehicle. Violent street gangs perpetrate more than 90% of all drive-by shootings. The primary purpose of a drive-by shooting is to create fear, terror, and intimidation among the members of rival street gangs. The secondary intent is to kill.[78] Drive-by shootings mainly occur at night in the inner city and generally last 5 to 15 seconds (although some may last 1 minute).[72] Most frequently, drive-by shootings occur on public streets, with gang members shooting into cars of suspected rival gang members that are being driven, are stopped at traffic lights, or are parked. Drive-by shootings also occur with gang members shooting into the homes of suspected rival gang members, in parks, and around public schools.[79] In many drive-by shootings, gang members flash their gang hand sign (a form of nonverbal gang communication) and yell their gang name. This makes it known to all rival gang members which gang actually was shooting at them. Most drive-by shooters are not apprehended by law enforcement.

Drive-by shootings are not random events.[79] No longer confined to the inner city, drive-by shootings are now a national phenomenon and in some regions of the United States have become endemic.[80] Drive-by shootings are a major public health problem because many individuals can be injured or killed in one incident.[81] In one study, 63% of children and adolescents who were shot at sustained a firearm injury, and 5.3% died from their injuries. There are 13 people injured for each individual killed in a drive-by shooting.[79] For adolescents and young adults, the lower extremity is the most frequently injured body region, followed by the upper extremity. The most frequent fatal injuries are to the chest and head.[79] Small children who are victims of drive-by shootings frequently sustain fatal firearm injuries to the head, neck, and chest. Most small children injured or killed in drive-by shootings are unintentionally caught in the crossfire of gang shootings.[82]

The weapon of choice in a drive-by shooting is a 9-mm semiautomatic handgun. Some semiautomatic handguns may fire 15 or more bullets before reloading. The high-capacity, rapid-fire mechanism of a semiautomatic firearm helps to explain why many individuals may be injured or killed in a single drive-by shooting.[72]

Firearms and Violent Street Gangs

For many gang members, firearms fulfill the need for power, status, protection, and progression from adolescence into adulthood that is no longer being met by traditional sociocultural institutions. Firearms are used in 95% of gang homicides[65] compared with 70% of all homicides.[83] Handguns—in particular, semiautomatic handguns—are the most commonly used weapon in gang shootings, followed by shotguns, which are used in 8% of all gang homicides.[65] Rifles are involved in 5% and assault weapons in 3% of gang homicides.[65]

Psychological Effects of Street Gang Violence on Children and Adolescents

Children and adolescents in some communities have higher exposure to street gang violence than in others.[5,84] Approximately 10% to 20% of inner-city children in Los Angeles have witnessed a homicide.[85] Among another group of inner-city adolescents, nearly 85% had witnessed at least one violent act, and 43.4% had witnessed a murder.[86] Children and adolescents living in the inner city are exposed to chronic, pervasive violence rather than isolated episodes of violence. The reactions of these children to this pervasive violence are consistent with those of children and adolescents living in war zones.[87]

On exposure to repetitive or extreme acts of violence, children and adolescents may show signs of sleep disturbance, difficulty concentrating in school, flashbacks, hypervigilance, increased risk-taking behavior, and a nihilistic, fatalistic orientation to the future.[88] Many of these children also may have a posttraumatic stress disorder. The severity of a child or adolescent's reaction to a gang shooting is related to the proximity to the shooting, the threat to the child or adolescent's own life, his or her relationship to others who may have been injured or killed in the shooting, and whether or not gang violence is endemic in the community.[88]

Children and adolescents exposed to large numbers of violent street gangs receive little or no counseling for the physical and psychological sequelae resulting from the violence. The net psychological effect of exposure to gang violence on children and adolescents is unknown but potentially desensitizes children and adolescents to violence and may lead to carrying a weapon out of fear for their own personal safety.

Preventing Gang Violence in the Emergency Department

With the increase in gang violence across the United States, emergency physicians and other health care providers have become vulnerable to injury and death resulting from gang incidents in the hospital environment. The development of guidelines for the prevention of gang violence is recommended to safeguard emergency physicians, other health care providers, patients, and visitors.[89]

In the past, recognition of local street gangs was determined by tattoos, "colors" (e.g., blue for Crips, red for Bloods), typical clothing (e.g., baggy pants, athletic team jackets), and accessories (e.g., sneakers, caps, belt buckles, bandannas), in addition to hand signs. This style of clothing and tattoos has now become popular in all segments of society, however. Information about local gangs may be obtained from community activists involved in gang prevention programs or local law enforcement agencies. All health care providers should be educated about the root causes of violent street gang formation, the effects of gang violence on the community, and the prevention of street gang violence.

Emergency Department Guidelines

1. On the arrival of paramedics with injured, known or suspected gang members, hospital security should be immediately involved, should be stationed in the emergency department and waiting area, and should secure the hospital perimeter.
2. Consistent with the primary survey examination, the patient should be undressed and searched for concealed weapons.
3. The evidence of previous major trauma (e.g., exploratory laparotomy, thoracotomy, thoracostomy scars) may be indicative of previous gang injuries.[90,91]
4. In a nonjudgmental fashion, emergency department health care providers should ask the patient whether he or she is a gang member.
5. Emergency department health care providers should not challenge or insult known or suspected gang members. In the street gang subculture, perceived disrespect often leads to a violent confrontation.
6. While the patient is in the emergency department, visitation should be limited, preferably to the patient's parents. Other visitors (e.g., friends and relatives) should be kept informed by periodic updates from the emergency department staff.
7. If admission is required, gang members should be admitted under "John or Jane Doe" status. Keeping their hospital location confidential may protect their identity and prevent them from incurring further injury by rival gang members while hospitalized and may prevent an outbreak of gang violence in the hospital.
8. Hospital security must be available 24 hours a day and must maintain high visibility and vigilance

when injured gang members are present in the emergency department.

9. When large numbers of gang members (in particular, rival gang members) are present in the emergency department or waiting area, hospital security should be present and local law enforcement should be advised.

10. Although concerned for their personal safety, emergency department personnel should not arm themselves with firearms or other weapons while on duty. Health care providers with weapons potentially could escalate the level of violence in the emergency department. Gang members might view health care providers as adversaries.

11. Community leaders who are experienced with local street gangs may act as mediators between the emergency department staff and members of violent street gangs. These mediators should be summoned to help decompress any hostile situations that may arise.

12. Hospitals should have evacuation plans for emergency department personnel and visitors in the event that extreme violence erupts within the emergency department.

13. The emergency department staff should be educated in the recognition and de-escalation of pre-violent aggressive behavior.

14. The emergency department should keep a log of all violent incidents that occur within the emergency department. This strategy helps to quantify the severity and weapon use in violent incidents and could help determine the necessity for other security measures (e.g., video cameras, metal detectors, bulletproof glass, armed safety police).

15. An external review of emergency department security by an appropriately credentialed security firm may identify security problems and solutions pertinent to their facility.

As long as gang violence exists in the community, spillover of the violence into the emergency department is inevitable. Although concerned about their own safety, emergency department personnel should deliver compassionate care to all members of violent street gangs, while minimizing their own risk of injury.

Prevention of Street Gang Violence

Law enforcement and the criminal justice system alone cannot solve the violence perpetrated by members of street gangs. The United States must develop a national policy on the issue of violent street gangs, with an emphasis on alleviating the root causes of violent street gang formation, including poverty, stressed families, lack of education, unemployment, underemployment, racism, marginalization, and a breakdown of sociocultural institutions. Although incarceration is a part of the solution, primary prevention through alleviating the root causes of violent street gang formation would be more effective. For truces among violent street gangs to be effective, they should be supported by concerted efforts to alleviate the root causes of violent street gang formation.[65]

Populations at greatest risk of perpetrating and being injured or killed in gang violence are adolescents and young adults, and intervention strategies should focus on these two age groups. Prevention measures should target children approaching these age groups. Preventive measures should include violence prevention programs in schools and the community, the teaching of nonviolent conflict resolution-mediation skills, the building of self-esteem, and the use of positive male and female role models. These strategies should be community controlled, integrated (with properly funded violent street gang prevention programs), age specific, and culturally appropriate to encourage adolescents to progress to adulthood nonviolently.[92]

Some gang members are receptive to leaving the gang after being injured or after a fellow gang member has been injured or killed in violent street gang activity.[93] Accordingly, preventive measures to break the cycle of gang membership should occur when injured gang members come to the emergency department. Hospital-based interventions should begin in the emergency department and continue throughout their hospitalization. When discharged from the hospital, counseling should continue to intervene further in breaking the cycle of violent street gang involvement. Because many individuals in the community, particularly children and adolescents, may experience the physical and psychological effects of violence, counseling should be made readily available.

Because firearms are the most frequently used weapons in gang violence, the United States must make a concerted effort to limit access to firearms by gang members through legislation, regulation, and community education.[35,61,62] Legislation and regulation should focus on limiting access to illegally obtained firearms because these are the weapons most commonly used in violent crimes.[94]

The solution to street gang violence must involve a multifaceted approach. Any prevention strategy with a unilateral focus would be unsuccessful in decreasing violent street gang activity and breaking the bonds of gang membership.

🔑 KEY CONCEPTS

- Adolescents are particularly vulnerable to violence and injury because of numerous developmental issues inherent in the adolescent age group.
- Contrary to popular belief, violence in schools is decreasing.
- Although the number of children and adolescents killed by firearms has decreased, emergency physicians should remain vigilant of the dangers of inappropriate use of firearms by children and adolescents.
- Emergency physicians should have an understanding of adolescent violent street gang involvement and how to minimize gang violence in the emergency department.
- Emergency physicians should understand and become proactive in preventing the multifaceted forms of adolescent violence (e.g., school, media, drug and alcohol related, firearm, and street gang).

REFERENCES

1. Committee on Adolescence: Firearms and adolescents. *Pediatrics* 89:784, 1992.

2. Webster DW, Wilson MEH: Gun violence among youth and the pediatrician's role in primary prevention. *Pediatrics* 94S:617, 1994.

3. Heath I: Treating violence as a public health problem. *BMJ* 325:726, 2002.

4. Durant RH, Pendergrast RA, Cadenhead C: Exposure to violence and victimization and fighting behavior by urban black adolescents. *J Adolesc Health* 15:311, 1994.

5. Dahlberg LL: Youth violence in the United States: Major trends, risk factors, and prevention approaches. *Am J Prev Med* 14:259, 1998.

6. Gladstein J, Rusonis EJ, Heald FP: Comparison of inner city and upper middle class youth exposure to violence. *J Adolesc Health* 13:275, 1992.

7. Murphy SL: Final data for 1998, National Vital Statistics Reports: 48(11). Hyattsville, Md, National Center for Health Statistics, 2000.

8. U.S. Department of Justice, Bureau of Justice Statistics: National Crime Victimization Survey (NCJ176353). Washington, DC, 1998.

9. Orpinas PK, et al: The co-morbidity of violence-related behaviors with health-risk behaviors in a population of high school students. *J Adolesc Health* 16:216, 1995.

10. Lowry R, et al: Weapon-carrying, physical fighting, and fight-related injury among U.S. adolescents. *Am J Prev Med* 14:122, 1998.

11. Wilson-Brewer R, Spivak H: Violence prevention in schools and other community settings: The pediatrician as initiator, educator, collaborator, and advocate. *Pediatrics* 94S:623, 1994.

12. Centers for Disease Control and Prevention: Youth risk behavior surveillance: United States, 1999. *MMWR Morb Mortal Wkly Rep* 49(SS-05):1, 2000.

13. Brener ND, et al: Recent trends in violence-related behaviors among high school students in the United States. *JAMA* 282:440, 1999.

14. Callahan CM, Rivara FP: Urban high school youth and handguns: A school-based survey. *JAMA* 267:3038, 1992.

15. Anderson M, et al: School-associated violent deaths in the United States, 1994-1999. *JAMA* 286:2695, 2001.

16. Nansel TR, et al: Bullying behaviors among US youth. *JAMA* 285:2094, 2001.

17. Nansel TR, et al: Relationships between bullying and violence among US youth. *Arch Pediatr Adolesc Med* 157:388, 2003.

18. Spivak H, Prothrow-Smith D: The need to address bullying—An important component of violence prevention. *JAMA* 285:2131, 2001.

19. Green S: Systemic vs. individualistic approaches to bullying [letter to the editor]. *JAMA* 286:787, 2001.

20. Chandler KA, et al: Students' Reports of School Crime: 1989 and 1995 (NCES 98-241/NCJ-169607). Washington, DC, U.S. Departments of Education and Justice, 1998.

21. Callahan CM, Rivara FP, Farrow JA: Youth in detention and handguns. *J Adolesc Health* 14:350, 1993.

22. Sheley JF, McGee ZT, Wright JD: Gun-related violence in and around inner-city schools. *Am J Dis Child* 146:677, 1992.

23. Charren P, Gelber A, Arnold M: Media, children, and violence: A public policy perspective. *Pediatrics* 94S:631, 1994.

24. American Academy of Pediatrics Committee on Public Education: Children, adolescents, and television. *Pediatrics* 107:423, 2001.

25. Kostinsky S, Bixler EO, Kettl PA: Threats of school violence in Pennsylvania after media coverage of the Columbine High School massacre. *Arch Pediatr Adolesc Med* 155:994, 2001.

26. Sege R, Dietz W: Television viewing and violence in children: The pediatrician as agent for change. *Pediatrics* 94S:600, 1994.

27. Buckley WF Jr, et al: The war on drugs is lost. *National Review* 158:34, 1996.

28. Ellickson PL, McGuigan KA: Early predictors of adolescent violence. *Am J Public Health* 90:566, 2000.

29. Fagan J: Interactions among drugs, alcohol, and violence. *Health Aff* 12:65, 1993.

30. National Research Council: Alcohol, other psychoactive drugs, and violence. In Reiss AJ, Roth JA (eds): *Understanding and Preventing Violence*. Washington, DC, National Academy Press, 1993.

31. Hingson R, Heeren T, Zakocs R: Age of drinking onset and involvement in physical fights after drinking. *Pediatrics* 108:872, 2001.

32. Centers for Disease Control: *National Vital Statistics Report*, vol 50 no 16, September 16, 2002.

33. Annest JL, Mercy JA, Gibson DR, Ryan GW: National estimates of non-fatal firearm related injuries. *JAMA* 273:1749, 1995.

34. Violence Prevention Task Force for the Eastern Association for the Surgery of Trauma: Violence in America: A public health crisis—the role of firearms. *J Trauma* 38:163, 1995.

35. Christoffel KK: Toward reducing pediatric injuries from firearms: Charting a legislative and regulatory course. *Pediatrics* 88:294, 1991.

36. Kellermann AL, et al: Gun ownership as a risk factor for homicide in the home. *N Engl J Med* 329:1084, 1993.

37. Kellermann AL, Reay DT: Protection or peril? An analysis of firearm-related deaths in the home. *N Engl J Med* 314:1557, 1986.

38. Stennies G, et al: Firearm storage practices and children in the home, United States, 1994. *Arch Pediatr Adolesc Med* 153:586, 1999.

39. Farah MM, Simon HK, Kellermann AL: Firearms in the home: Parental perceptions. *Pediatrics* 104:1059, 1999.

40. Telljohann SK, Price JH: A preliminary investigation of inner-city primary grade students' perceptions of guns. *J Health Educ* 25:41, 1994.

41. Kellerman AL: Gun ownership as a risk factor for homicide in the home. *N Engl J Med* 329:1084, 1993.

42. Cohall AT, Cohall RM: "Number one with a bullet": Epidemiology and prevention of homicide among adolescents and young adults. *Adolesc Med State Art Rev* 6:183, 1995.

43. Centers for Disease Control and Prevention, National Center for Injury Prevention and Control: Ten leading causes of death, National Center for Health Statistics, United States 2001. Available at www.cdc_gov/ncipc/osp/charts.htm (accessed 3/11/2005).

44. Centers for Disease Control and Prevention: Rates of homicide, suicide and firearm-related death among children—26 industrialized countries. *MMWR Morb Mortal Wkly Rep* 46:101, 1997.

45. Larkin GL: Screening for adolescent firearms carrying: One more way to save a life. *Ann Emerg Med* 42:808, 2003.

46. Fingerhut LA, Jones C, Makuc DM: Firearm and motor vehicle injury mortality: Variations by state, race, and ethnicity—United States, 1990-91. In: *Advance Data from Vital and Health Statistics* (No. 242). Hyattsville, Md, National Center for Health Statistics, 1994, pp 41-46.

47. Page RM, Hammermeister J: Weapon-carrying and youth violence. *Adolescence* 32:505, 1997.

48. McNeill AM, Annest JL: The ongoing hazard of BB and gun-related injuries in the United States. *Ann Emerg Med* 26:187, 1995.

49. U.S. Consumer Product Safety Commission–National Injury Information Clearing House: Gas air spring operated guns, calendar year 1/80-2/01.

50. Christoffel KK, et al: Childhood injuries caused by non-powder firearms. *Am J Dis Child* 138:557, 1984.

51. Mejia A, et al: Air gun injuries to the abdominal aorta: Report of two cases and review of the literature. *J Trauma Inj Infect Crit Care* 54:1235, 2003.

52. Wilson MH, et al: *Saving Children: A Guide to Injury Prevention.* New York, Oxford University Press, 1991.

53. American Academy of Pediatrics Task Force on Violence: The role of the pediatrician in youth violence prevention in clinical practice and at the community level. *Pediatrics* 103:173, 1999.

54. Greene MB: Youth violence in the city: The role of educational interventions. *Health Educ Behav* 25:175, 1998.

55. Garcia JM: African American youth: Essential prevention strategies for every pediatrician. *Pediatrics* 96:132, 1995.

56. Miller TR, Galbraith M: Injury prevention counseling by pediatricians: A benefit-cost comparison. *Pediatrics* 96:1005, 1995.

57. Pittel EM: How to take a weapons history: Interviewing children at risk for violence at school. *J Am Acad Child Adolesc Psychiatry* 37:1100, 1998.

58. Singer MI, Flannery DJ: The relationship between children's threats of violence and violent behaviors. *Arch Pediatr Adolesc Med* 154:785, 2000.

59. Cole TB: Taking aim at gun violence. *JAMA* 290:583, 2003.

60. Hayes DN, Sege R: Fights: A preliminary screening tool for adolescent firearms-carrying. *Ann Emerg Med* 42:798, 2003.

61. Wintemute GJ: The future of firearm violence prevention: Building on success. *JAMA* 282:475, 1999.

62. Kellermann AL, et al: The epidemiologic basis for the prevention of firearm injuries. *Ann Rev Public Health* 12:17, 1991.

63. Oppenheimer K, Swanson G: Duty to warn: When should confidentiality be breached? *J Fam Pract* 30:179, 1990.

64. Bloom JD, Rogers JL: The duty to protect others from your patients: Tarasoff spreads to the Northwest. *West J Med* 148:231, 1988.

65. Hutson HR, et al: The epidemic of gang-related homicides in Los Angeles County from 1979 through 1994. *JAMA* 274:1031, 1995.

66. Klein MW: *The American Street Gang: Its Nature, Prevalence, and Control.* New York, Oxford University Press, 1995.

67. Egley A Jr: Highlights of the 1999 National Youth Gang Survey (Fact Sheet #2000-20). Washington, DC, U.S. Department of Justice, Office of Juvenile Justice and Delinquency Prevention, 2003.

68. Huff CR (ed): *Gangs in America.* Thousand Oaks, Calif, Sage Publications, 2002.

69. Jackson RK, McBride WD: *Understanding Street Gangs.* Placerville, Calif, Custom Publishing, 1991.

70. Martinez FB: The impact of gangs and drugs in the community. In Cervantes RC (ed): *Substance Abuse and Gang Violence.* Newbury Park, Calif, Sage Publications, 1992.

71. Vigil JD: *Barrio Gangs: Street Life and Identity in Southern California.* Austin, Tex, University of Texas Press, 1988.

72. Hutson HR, Anglin D, Spears K: The perspectives of violent street gang injuries. *Neurosurg Clin N Am* 6:621, 1995.

73. Klein MW, Maxson CL, Cunningham LC: "Crack," street gangs, and violence. *Criminology* 29:701, 1991.

74. Meehan PJ, O'Carroll PW: Gangs, drugs, and homicide in Los Angeles. *Am J Dis Child* 146:683, 1992.

75. McGonigal MD, et al: Urban firearm deaths: A five-year perspective. *J Trauma* 35:532, 1993.

76. Greenberg M, Schneider D: Violence in American cities: Young black males is the answer, but what was the question? *Soc Sci Med* 39:179, 1994.

77. Kyriacou DN, et al: Socioeconomic risk factors from gang-related homicides in the City of Los Angeles. *J Trauma* 46:334, 1999.

78. Hutson HR, Anglin D, Mallon W: Injuries and deaths from gang violence: They are preventable. *Ann Emerg Med* 21:1234, 1992.

79. Hutson HR, Anglin D, Pratts MJ: Adolescents and children injured or killed in drive-by shootings in Los Angeles. *N Engl J Med* 330:324, 1994.

80. Hutson HR, Anglin D, Eckstein M: Drive-by shootings by violent street gangs in Los Angeles: A five year review from 1989-1993. *Acad Emerg Med* 3:300, 1996.

81. Eckstein M, Hutson HR, Anglin D: Drive-by shootings. *Ann Emerg Med* 25:107, 1995.

82. Hutson HR, et al: Caught in the crossfire of gang violence: Small children as innocent victims of drive-by shootings. *J Emerg Med* 12:385, 1994.

83. Federal Bureau of Investigation: *Crime in the United States—1993: Uniform Crime Reports.* Washington, DC, Federal Bureau of Investigation, U.S. Department of Justice, 1994.

84. Schubiner H, Scott R, Tzelepis A: Exposure to violence among inner city youth. *J Adolesc Health* 14:214, 1993.

85. Groves BM, et al: Silent victims: Children who witness violence. *JAMA* 269:262, 1993.

86. Fitzpatrick KM, Boldizar JP: The prevalence and consequences of exposure to violence among African-American youth. *J Am Acad Child Adolesc Psychiatry* 32:424, 1993.

87. Schwab-Stone ME, et al: No safe haven: A study of violence exposure in an urban community. *J Am Acad Child Adolesc Psychiatry* 34:1343, 1995.

88. Pynoos RS, et al: Life threat and posttraumatic stress in school-age children. *Arch Gen Psychiatry* 44:1057, 1987.

89. Hutson HR, Anglin D, Mallon W: Minimizing gang violence in the emergency department. *Ann Emerg Med* 21:1291, 1992.

90. Morrissey TB, Byrd R, Deitch EA: The incidence of recurrent penetrating trauma in an urban trauma center. *J Trauma* 31:1536, 1991.

91. Weisbeski Sims D, et al: Urban trauma: A chronic recurrent disease. *J Trauma* 29:940, 1989.

92. Neighbors HW, Braithwaite RL, Thompson E: Health promotion and African-Americans: From personal empowerment to community action. *Am J Health Promotion* 9:281, 1995.

93. Decker SH, Lauritsen JL: Breaking the bonds of membership: leaving the gang. In Huff CR (ed): *Gangs in America,* 2nd ed. Thousand Oaks, Calif, Sage Publications, 1996, pp 63-68.

94. Wright JD: Ten essential observations on guns in America. *Society* March/April:63, 1995.

Index

Note: Page numbers followed by b, f, and t refer to boxes, figures, and tables, respectively.

A priori probability, 3055-3056
"A" wave, jugular venous, in tricuspid stenosis
    and regurgitation, 1307
Abandonment of elderly, 1010
Abciximab, in myocardial infarction, 1186
Abdomen
  acute, in spinal cord injury, 2907
  anterior, 490
  contusions of, 494
  infection in, antibiotics for, 217
Abdominal aortic aneurysm, 1330-1340
  back pain in, 265t
  clinical features of, 1332-1333
  diagnostic strategies in, 1334-1336, 1334f-
    1336f, 1337-1338
  differential diagnosis in, 1336, 1336b
  disposition in, 1340
  epidemiology of, 1330, 1331t
  false, 1330, 1340
  management of, 1336-1339
  pathophysiology and natural history of, 1330-
    1331
  repair of
    endovascular, 1338-1339, 1339f
    late complications of, 1339-1340
    survival rate for, 1339
    traditional, 1338, 1339f
  ruptured, 1331
    abdominal pain in, 214t
    clinical features of, 1332-1333
    management of, 1336-1338
  types of, 1330, 1331f
Abdominal cramps
  in *Aeromonas hydrophila* gastroenteritis, 1467
  in *Bacillus cereus* food poisoning, 1471
  in *Clostridium difficile* enterocolitis, 1475
  in *Clostridium perfringens* food poisoning,
    1471
  in coccidian gastroenteritis, 1478
  in *Escherichia coli* food poisoning, 1474
  in hemorrhagic *Escherichia coli* serotype
    O157:H7 gastroenteritis, 1466
  in intestinal amebiasis, 1480
  in Meckel's diverticulum, 2613
  in *Plesiomonas shigelloides* gastroenteritis,
    1468
  in scombroid fish poisoning, 1472
  in staphylococcal food poisoning, 1470
  in *Vibrio* fish poisoning, 1472
  in *Vibrio parahaemolyticus* gastroenteritis, 1466
  in viral gastroenteritis, 1476
Abdominal distention
  in acute mesenteric ischemia, 1447
  in colonic volvulus, 1498
  in gastric volvulus, 1394
  in *Giardia* gastroenteritis, 1479
  in large bowel obstruction, 1496
  in malrotation with midgut volvulus, 2606
Abdominal examination
  in abdominal pain, 213, 215
  in abdominal trauma, 493-494
  in chest pain, 187t
  in constipation, 239
  in diarrhea, 233
  in fever, 135
  in multiple trauma, 309-310, 310f
  in nausea and vomiting, 202t
  in pelvic pain, 249, 250t
  in vaginal bleeding, 256t
Abdominal mass
  in abdominal aortic aneurysm rupture, 1333
  in abdominal trauma, 494
  in children, 2646

Abdominal migraine, 2679
Abdominal pain, 209-218. *See also* Pelvic pain.
  ancillary studies in, 215-216, 216t
  differential considerations in, 212-214, 212f,
    214t-215t, 216-217, 216t
  disposition in, 217-218
  empiric management of, 217, 218f-219f
  epidemiology of, 209
  extraabdominopelvic causes of, 211b
  history in, 213, 213b
  in abdominal trauma, 493
  in acute mesenteric ischemia, 1447
  in acute pancreatitis, 1429
  in adrenal insufficiency, 1997
  in appendicitis, 1452
  in *Bacillus anthracis* gastroenteritis, 1469
  in *Campylobacter* gastroenteritis, 1460
  in cholangitis, 1421
  in cholecystitis, 1420
  in cholelithiasis, 1418
  in chronic pancreatitis, 1435
  in ciguatera fish poisoning, 1473
  in coccidian gastroenteritis, 1477, 1478
  in colonic ischemia, 1504
  in colonic volvulus, 1498
  in diabetic ketoacidosis, 1963
  in diverticular disease, 1493
  in ectopic pregnancy, 2743
  in elderly person, 2828-2829, 2828t
  in esophageal perforation, 1385
  in gastric volvulus, 1394
  in gastritis, 1391
  in *Giardia* gastroenteritis, 1479
  in hemorrhagic *Escherichia coli* serotype
    O157:H7 gastroenteritis, 1466
  in inflammatory bowel disease, 1501
  in intussusception, 1442
  in irritable bowel syndrome, 1491
  in large bowel intussusception, 1500
  in large bowel obstruction, 1496
  in pancreatic carcinoma, 1437
  in parasitic infection, 2113
  in pelvic inflammatory disease, 1570
  in peptic ulcer disease, 1392
  in peritoneal dialysis patient, 1553
  in pregnancy, 2733, 2752-2756, 2753t
  in radiation proctocolitis, 1505
  in salmonellosis, 1463
  in shigellosis, 1464
  in small bowel obstruction, 1442
  in spontaneous bacterial peritonitis, 1412
  in staphylococcal food poisoning, 1470
  in systemic lupus erythematosus, 1811
  in uterine inversion, 2820
  in women, 1453, 1453t
  in *Yersinia enterocolitica* gastroenteritis, 1465
  locations of, 212f
  nonspecific, 211t
  observation in, 3063-3064, 3064b
  opioids for, 2925-2926
  pathophysiology of, 209-212, 210t-211t, 211b
  pediatric
    differential considerations in, 2611, 2612t
    in appendicitis, 2619
    in hemolytic uremic syndrome, 2654
    in Henoch-Schönlein purpura, 2615, 2653
    in inflammatory bowel disease, 2616
    in intussusception, 2610
    in osteogenesis imperfecta, 2700
    in renal stones, 2646
  physical examination in, 213, 215
  rapid assessment and stabilization in, 213
  white blood cell count in, 1889

Abdominal radiography. *See* Radiography,
  abdominal.
Abdominal surgery, small bowel obstruction
  after, 1441
Abdominal tenderness
  in abdominal trauma, 494
  in genitourinary trauma, 515
Abdominal trauma, 489-512
  anatomy and physiology in, 490
  cardiac tamponade in, 473
  clinical features in, 492-495
  diagnostic peritoneal lavage in, 499-501, 500t
  differential considerations in, 501-502
  epidemiology of, 489-490
  history in, 492-493
  iatrogenic, 492
  in elderly person, 346
  laboratory tests in, 495
  laparoscopy in, 501, 508
  local wound exploration in, 501
  management of, 502-510
  observation in, 3067-3068
  pancreatitis following, 1428
  pathophysiology of, 490-492
  pediatric, 340-342
    blunt, 492, 510
    epidemiology of, 489-490
    history in, 493
  physical examination in, 493-495
  prehospital care in, 502
  radiologic imaging in, 495-499, 496f-499f
Abdominal viscera, in pregnancy, 317
Abducens nerve, 1665t
Abductor digiti minimi, 580-581, 581f
Abductor digiti quinti nerve, compression of,
  heel pain in, 836-837
Abductor pollicis brevis, 580, 581f
Abductor pollicis longus, 581, 582f, 583f
Abrasion
  corneal, 289, 289f, 292, 294t, 933, 1047, 1047f
  facial, 390
  pattern
    in motor vehicle crashes, 964
    in physical assault, 962, 962f
  scalp, 372
Abrasion collar, in long-range handgun wounds,
  957, 957f
Abruptio placentae, 319-320, 2747-2748, 2809-
  2810
Abrus precatorius, 2471-2472, 2472f
Abscess, 2202-2207
  amebic, 1415-1416, 2106-2107
  anorectal, 1513-1515, 1513t, 1514f
  Bartholin, 1560, 2205, 2205f
  Bezold, 1072
  brain
    after head trauma, 370-371
    ancillary studies in, 1720
    cerebrospinal fluid analysis in, 1716-1719,
      1717t, 1718t, 1719f
    complications of, 1716
    diagnosis of, 1716-1720
    differential considerations in, 1720, 1721b
    disposition in, 1723
    epidemiology of, 1711
    etiology of, 1712
    headache in, 174t, 1641, 2678
    in cancer patient, 1920
    in otitis media, 1068
    lumbar puncture in, 1716, 1716b
    management of, 1722, 1723
    neuroimaging studies in, 1719-1720
    pathophysiology of, 1713, 1713f

Abscess *(Continued)*
   risk factors for, 171b
   signs and symptoms of, 1714-1715
  Brodie's, 2184
  collar-button, 617, 617f
  cutaneous, 2202-2204, 2203t
  epidural
   in vertebral osteomyelitis, 2184-2185
   spinal, 1684
  epiglottitic, 1115
  extradural, in otitis media, 1068
  hepatic, 1414-1417, 1415f, 1416f, 2113
  horseshoe, 1515
  in carbuncle, 2204
  in diverticular disease, 1494-1495
  in furuncle, 2204
  in hidradenitis suppurativa, 2204-2205
  intersphincteric, 1513t, 1514, 2206
  intra-abdominal, in appendicitis, 1453, 1458
  ischiorectal, 1513t, 1514, 2206
  necrotizing, 1515
  parapharyngeal, 1121-1123, 1122f
  paraspinal cold, in tuberculosis, 2159
  pelvirectal, 2206
  perianal, 2206
  periapical, 1028, 1030f, 1031, 1032
  periodontal, 1031, 1033
  perirectal, 1513t, 1514, 2205-2206, 2206f
  peritonsillar, 1117-1118, 1118f
  pilonidal, 2206-2207
  postanal, 1513t, 1514-1515
  pulmonary, 1033, 1134, 1134f
  pyogenic, 1414-1415, 1415f
  retrobulbar, 288, 295t
  retropharyngeal, 1120-1121, 1120f, 1121f,
   2522-2523, 2523f
  spinal, 1684, 1712, 1715, 1716
  subperiosteal
   in mastoiditis, 1072
   in osteomyelitis, 2175
  supralevator, 1513t, 1514
  tubo-ovarian, 248, 251t
Absence seizure, 1621
Absinthe, 2412
Abuse
  child, 968-976
   abdominal trauma in, 490
   bruises consistent with, 969-971, 969f, 970f,
    970t, 2502b
   diagnostic strategies in, 973-974
   differential considerations in, 974-975, 975f,
    2699-2701
   disposition in, 976
   epidemiology of, 968-969, 969t
   facial trauma in, 383
   head trauma in, 349, 367
   historical indicators of, 2501b
   history of, in sexual assault cases, 979
   immersion scalds in, 916
   in Munchausen's syndrome by proxy, 1761,
    1763, 1763t, 1765
   management of, 975-976
   physical abuse in, 969-971, 969f, 970f, 970t,
    972, 973, 974-975
   radiography in, 2699
   reporting of, 976
   sexual abuse in, 969, 971, 972-973, 974, 975
   sexually transmitted disease and, 973-974,
    974t
   signs and symptoms of, 971-973
   skeletal aspects of, 2698-2701
  elder, 1008-1015
   caregiver interview in, 1013
   clinical features of, 1011-1013, 1011b, 1012b
   definitions and types of, 1009-1010
   diagnostic strategies in, 1013
   documentation of, 1013
   epidemiology of, 1009
   etiology and risk factors for, 1010-1011,
    1010b
   future directions in, 1015
   institutional, 1009, 1015
   interventions and referrals in, 1013-1014
   reporting requirements in, 1014-1015
   screening for, 1011, 1011b
  intimate partner, 994-1006
   barriers to diagnosis of, 998
   clinical features of, 996-998
   definitions of, 995, 995t

Abuse *(Continued)*
   disposition in, 1004-1005, 1005b
   documentation of, 1000-1001, 1003-1004
   during pregnancy, 997, 2734-2735, 2734t
   epidemiology of, 995-996
   improving emergency department response
    to victims of, 1005-1006
   legal considerations in, 1004-1005
   referral in, 1004
   risk assessment in, 1000, 1002b, 1003b
   risk factors for injury related to, 996
   screening for, 998-999, 999b, 1000f, 1001f,
    1002b
   use of emergency department in, 996
   validation of patient's experience in, 999-
    1000
  of persons with disabilities, 1015
  sexual. *See* Sexual abuse; Sexual assault.
Acalculous cholecystitis, 1421, 2620, 2621
Acanthamoeba infection
  neurologic disorders in, 2107
  visual disturbances in, 2110
Acanthosis nigricans
  in diabetes mellitus, 1972
  internal malignancy associated with, 1862-
   1863
Acarbose, during pregnancy and lactation, 2790
Acceleration-deceleration injury, 352
Accessory muscles of respiration
  in asthma, 1084, 2534, 2535f
  in chronic obstructive pulmonary disease, 1100
Accessory ossicles of foot, 821-822, 822f
Accessory pathway, 1203
  atrial flutter with, 1229
  in Lown-Ganong-Levine syndrome, 1237
  in Wolff-Parkinson-White syndrome, 1235-
   1237, 1236f, 1237f
Accident prevention. *See* Injury prevention and
  control.
Accidental hypothermia, 2236-2252
  advanced life support in, 2245-2246
  cardiovascular agents for, 2246
  clinical features of, 2241-2242, 2242b
  diagnostic strategies in, 2242-2244
  disposition in, 2251
  dysrhythmia in, 2237-2238, 2246
  laboratory evaluation of, 2242-2244, 2243f
  management of, 2244-2251
  outcome of, 2251
  pathophysiology of, 2237-2239, 2238f, 2239t
  predisposing factors in, 2239-2241, 2240b
  rewarming techniques in, 2247-2251, 2247b,
   2250b
  septicemia following, 2247
  volume resuscitation in, 2245
Acclimatization
  to heat stress, 2255-2256
  to high altitude, 2297-2298, 2297b, 2298f
Acebutolol, 1209, 1321t
  overdose of, 2373t, 2374
Acetabular fracture, 728-729, 728b, 731, 731f,
  732f, 757
Acetaminophen, 2927
  alcohol interactions with, 2875-2876
  during pregnancy and lactation, 2781
  for migraine, 1633, 1633t, 2680
  for osteoarthritis, 1787
  for pediatric fever, 2511, 2514, 2515
  hepatotoxicity of, 1413
  in children, 2935
  in elderly person, 2826
  metabolism of, 2331-2332, 2332f
  overdose of, 2331-2337, 2332f
   antidotes to, 2329t
   chronic exposure in, 2334b, 2335
   clinical features of, 2332-2333
   diagnosis of, 2333-2335, 2333b, 2334b
   disposition in, 2337
   in children, 2335
   management of, 2333b, 2334b, 2335-2337
   risk assessment using treatment nomogram
    in, 2333-2335, 2334f
Acetazolamide
  for acute mountain sickness, 2301-2302
  for central retinal artery occlusion, 1057
  for closed-angle glaucoma, 1056
  for hyperuricemia, 1914
  for increased intraocular pressure, 292
Acetic acid, for neutralization of alkali burn, 932

Acetone
  isopropyl alcohol metabolism to, 2402, 2403f
  on breath, in diabetic ketoacidosis, 1964
Acetylcholine
  in delirium, 1646-1647
  in dementia, 1657
Acetylcholinesterase inhibitors, 2457-2462,
  2458b
  for myasthenia gravis, 1706
N-Acetylcysteine
  for acetaminophen overdose, 2331-2332, 2332f,
   2333b, 2334b, 2336-2337
  for contrast agent-induced renal failure, 1537
  in pregnancy, 2336-2337
  intravenous, 2336
Achalasia, 1397, 1398
Achilles tendon
  injury to, 1799-1800
  rupture of, 818, 1800
Acid, weak, for neutralization of alkali burn, 932
Acid burn, 931-933
  esophageal perforation from, 483
  ocular, 1046
  oral, 2381, 2383
  pathophysiology of, 930
Acid-base disorders, 1922-1932. *See also*
  Acidosis; Alkalosis; Ketoacidosis.
  diagnosis of, 1924
  in hypothermia, 2242-2243, 2243f
  in salicylate overdose, 2340
  mixed, 1931, 1931b
  physiologic buffers and, 1923
  pulmonary compensation in, 1923
  renal compensation in, 1923-1924
Acid-fast bacillus smear, in tuberculosis, 2147,
  2154, 2154f
Acidosis. *See also* Ketoacidosis.
  anion gap, 1927-1929, 1927b
   delirium in, 1651
   in cyanide poisoning, 2437
   in ethylene glycol poisoning, 2399, 2400-2401
   in methanol poisoning, 2396, 2397
   seizure in, 1622
  double-gap
   differential diagnosis in, 2397
   in ethylene glycol poisoning, 2400
   in methanol poisoning, 2397
  hypokalemia in, 1938
  lactic, 1928-1929
   in crush injury, 3007
   in sepsis, 2216
   in shock, 42-43, 43f
  metabolic, 1926-1930, 1927f, 1931b
   dialysis for, 1549
   etiology of, 1927-1929, 1927b
   in abdominal trauma, 495
   in acute renal failure, 1539, 2650
   in cyanide poisoning, 2437
   in diarrhea, 2624
   in salicylate overdose, 2340
   management of, 1929-1930
   physiologic compensation in, 1929
   renal compensation in, 1923-1924
   with high anion gap, 1927-1929, 1927b
   with normal anion gap, 1927b, 1929
  paradoxical central nervous system, from
   sodium bicarbonate, 1930
  respiratory, 1924-1926, 1925b, 1925f, 1931b
   causes of, 1925b
   clinical features of, 1924-1925
   in chronic obstructive pulmonary disease,
    1100
   management of, 1925-1926
   physiologic compensation in, 1925
Acoustic neuroma, 147t, 1668-1669
Acquired immunodeficiency syndrome. *See*
  HIV/AIDS.
Acrocyanosis, 1347, 1357
Acrodermatitis chronica atrophicans, in Lyme
  disease, 2124-2125
Acromial process fracture, 679, 680
Acromioclavicular joint
  anatomy of, 670-671, 671f
  dislocation at, 685-687, 686f, 687f
  osteoarthritis in, 687
Acromioclavicular ligaments, 670, 671f
ACTH (adrenocorticotropic hormone)
  for gouty arthritis, 1786
  for infantile spasms, 2666

Action potential of myocardial cells, 1200, 1201f, 1202f

Activated charcoal
  in acetaminophen overdose, 2336
  in amphetamine abuse, 2896
  in anticholinergic poisoning, 2349-2350
  in barbiturate overdose, 2483
  in beta blocker overdose, 2374
  in bipyridyl compound poisoning, 2466
  in NSAID overdose, 2343
  in opioid overdose, 2455
  in overdosed/poisoned patient, 2330
  in PCP intoxication, 2893
  in salicylate overdose, 2341

Activated protein C
  for sepsis, 2221-2222
  for septic shock, 53

Active compression-decompression–cardiopulmonary resuscitation, 89, 98

Active external rewarming, 2248

Acute abdomen, in spinal cord injury, 2907

Acute chest syndrome, in sickle cell disease, 1880

Acute confusional state, 2679. See also Confusion.

Acute coronary syndromes, 1154-1195. See also Angina; Myocardial infarction.
  atypical presentations in, 1158-1159, 1159t
  chest pain centers and, 1181-1182
  chest pain in, 183, 186, 186b, 188, 189f, 190t-191t
  chest radiography in, 1174, 1175f
  clinical features of, 1157-1161, 1158t, 1159t
  cocaine-related, 2391
  creatine kinase MB isoenzyme in, 1175f, 1176t, 1177-1178
  diagnostic strategies in, 1161-1181
  echocardiography in, 1179
  electrocardiography in, 1161-1174
    abnormalities in, 1161-1163, 1162f-1164f, 1162t
    additional lead, 1171-1173, 1172f, 1173f
    adjuncts in, 1171-1174
    anatomic location of infarct on, 1164-1166, 1164t, 1165f-1167f
    body surface mapping and, 1174
    limitations of, 1174
    noninfarct ST segment elevation and, 1166-1170, 1167f-1172f
    NSTEMI and, 1170-1171
    QT dispersion and, 1174
    serial, 1173-1174, 1173f
  epidemiology of, 1155
  graded exercise testing in, 1180-1181
  historical perspective of, 1154-1155
  in pregnancy, 2763t, 2766-2767
  management algorithm for, 189f
  management of, 1182-1195
    angiotensin-converting enzyme inhibitors in, 1185
    antiplatelet therapy in, 1185-1187
    antithrombotic therapy in, 1187-1188
    aspirin in, 1185
    beta blockers in, 1184-1185
    calcium channel blockers in, 1185
    clinical pathways for, 3039f-3041f
    direct thrombin inhibitors in, 1188
    glycoprotein IIb/IIIa receptor inhibitors in, 1186, 1194
    heparins in, 1187-1188
    morphine in, 1184
    nitroglycerin in, 1184
    pharmacologic, 1184-1188, 1195
    reperfusion in, 1189-1195
    thienopyridines in, 1186-1187
    time to treatment and, 1182-1184, 1183f, 1184f
  missed diagnosis of, 1160
  pathophysiology of, 1156-1157
  physical examination in, 1159, 1159t
  prehospital care in, 1157
  radionucleotide scanning in, 1179-1180
  risk factors for, 186b
  serum markers in, 1174-1179, 1175f, 1176t
  spectrum of disease in, 1155-1156
  transfer of patient with, 1195
  troponins in, 1175-1177, 1175f, 1176t

Acute lung injury. See Pulmonary edema, noncardiogenic.

Acute mountain sickness (AMS), 2300-2303, 2301b. See also Altitude; High-altitude illness.

Acute mountain sickness (AMS) (Continued)
  clinical presentation in, 2301
  epidemiology of, 2296
  management of, 2301-2302
  pathophysiology of, 2299-2300, 2299f
  prevention of, 2302-2303

Acute necrotic ulcerative gingivitis (ANUG), 1033, 1033f

Acute radiation syndrome, 2317t, 2321-2322, 2321f

Acute renal failure. See Renal failure, acute.

Acute respiratory distress syndrome (ARDS), 1141, 1141b
  in ethylene glycol poisoning, 2399
  in pancreatitis, 1429
  in sepsis, 2214, 2214b
  mechanical ventilation in, 32
  pulmonary contusion vs., 461

Acute seroconversion syndrome, in HIV infection, 2075

Acute stress disorder, 1746b

Acute tubular necrosis, 1534b, 1535-1537, 1536b
  in rhabdomyolysis, 1977, 1977f
  urinary findings in, 1527t

Acyclovir
  during pregnancy and lactation, 2785
  for bacterial meningitis, 2665
  for Bell's palsy, 1667
  for febrile, neutropenic cancer patient, 2838t
  for genital herpes, 1557t, 1559, 1858
  for herpes simplex esophagitis, 1387
  for herpes simplex meningoencephalitis, 1722
  for herpes simplex virus infection, 2042
  for herpes zoster, 2043
  for varicella, 1859, 2043
  in HIV/AIDS, side effects of, 2079t
  indications for, 2038
  prophylactic, in monkey bites, 888, 889t

Adaptive immune response, 2832-2834

Addison's disease, 1994, 1996, 1997

Adductor pollicis, 580, 581f

Adenocarcinoma, pancreatic, 1437-1438

Adenopathy. See Lymphadenopathy.

Adenosine
  during pregnancy and lactation, 2788
  for dysrhythmia, 1212-1213, 2586b
  for junctional tachycardia, 1234
  for pediatric resuscitation, 101t, 104
  for supraventricular tachycardia, 2588, 2589f
  for wide-complex tachycardia, 1240
  side effects of, 1212

Adenosine deaminase test, in tuberculosis, 2155

Adenosine triphosphate depletion
  in cerebral ischemia, 65
  in rhabdomyolysis, 1977

Adenovirus infection, 1289, 2034t, 2045

Adhesive capsulitis, 682, 698-699, 699t, 1797

Adhesive strips for ankle immobilization, 571, 572f

Adhesive-tipped swab for foreign body removal from ear, 863

Adie's tonic pupil, 1061

Adipocytes, glucose metabolism in, 1956

Adjustment disorder
  depression vs., 1740
  with anxiety, 1749

Admission. See Hospitalization.

Adnexal mass
  in ectopic pregnancy, 2743
  pelvic pain in, 250t

Adolescent
  abdominal pain in, 2611, 2612t
  alcohol consumption in, 2877
  antituberculous agents for, 2166, 2167b
  consent to treatment on behalf of, 3167-3168
  depression in, 1737
  developmental milestones in, 2496t, 2497
  gastrointestinal bleeding in, 2613-2614, 2614t
  refusal of medical care for, 3171
  substance abuse in, 2883, 2884
  suicide by, 1769
  violence and, 1017-1022
  vomiting in, 203, 208t, 2606t

Adrenal hemorrhage, 1995, 1995b

Adrenal insufficiency, 1994-1998
  acute, 1994-1996, 1995b
  autoimmune, 1996
  chronic, 1996
  clinical features of, 1996-1997, 1996t

Adrenal insufficiency (Continued)
  diagnosis of, 1997-1998
  in sepsis, 2214
  management of, 1998

Adrenergic medications
  for asthma, 1086-1088, 1087t, 2538, 2539t, 2540-2541
  for chronic obstructive pulmonary disease, 1105

Adrenocorticotropic hormone
  for gouty arthritis, 1786
  for infantile spasms, 2666

Adrenocorticotropic hormone stimulation test, in adrenal insufficiency, 1997-1998

Adult infectious botulism, 2013, 2015

Adult Protective Services, 1014

Adult resuscitation. See Resuscitation.

Advance directives, 3132, 3133, 3142
  honoring, 3144-3145, 3152
  initiating, 3153
  nonstandard, 3133

Advanced life support
  in hypothermia, 2245-2246
  in ICD patient, 1256-1257
  in pacemaker patient, 1255
  in pediatric resuscitation, 99, 99f
  prehospital, 78

Advanced life support (ALS) systems, 2986

Adynamic ileus, 1440, 1441b, 1443

Aeroesophageal foreign body, 2529-2530

Aeromonas hydrophila
  dysenteric colitis in, 229t
  gastroenteritis in, 1461t, 1462t, 1467-1468

Aerophobia, in rabies, 2065

Aerosol exposure, ocular trauma from, 1046

Affect, flattened, in schizophrenia, 1728

Affective disorders. See Mood disorders.

Affective processes, in clinical decision making, 130, 131t

Afterdepolarization
  dysrhythmias from, 1205
  early vs. delayed, 1201, 1202f

Afterload, in heart failure, 1260-1261, 1260f, 1261f

Age. See also Adolescent; Child; Elderly person; Infant; Neonate.
  fertility rate and, 2722
  fibrinolytic therapy eligibility and, 1190
  gestational. See Gestational age.
  high-altitude illness and, 2296
  risk for injury and death by, 942t, 949t

Agent Orange, 2463, 2463b

Aggression, 1768. See also Abuse; Combative patient; Violence.

Aging. See Elderly person.

Agitation
  in amphetamine abuse, 2896
  in anticholinergic poisoning, 2349
  in delirium, 1653-1654
  in depression, 1737
  in PCP intoxication, 2891, 2892
  in substance abuse, 2886
  in thought disorders, 1730
  violent behavior and. See Combative patient.

Agonal respiration, 97

Agoraphobia, 1746b, 1749

Agranulocytosis, antipsychotic-induced, 2448

AIDS. See HIV/AIDS.

Air
  compressed, esophageal perforation from, 483
  contaminated, in scuba diving–related disorders, 2283

Air bags, 946-947
  in pregnancy, 2735-2736
  injury from, 964, 965f

Air casts, for ankle immobilization, 571, 573f, 817

Air contrast enema, in intussusception, 2611

Air hunger, in chronic obstructive pulmonary disease, 1100

Air leak, persistent, 466

Air medical transport, 2994-2999
  administrative structure in, 2995
  aviation physiology and, 2994-2995, 2995t
  clinical concepts and patient care in, 2998-2999
  criteria for, 2998b
  efficacy and cost effectiveness of, 2999
  flight crew in, 2996
  future of, 2999

Air medical transport *(Continued)*
    medical direction in, 2996
    safety issues in, 2997, 2997b, 2997f, 2998b
    types of missions in, 2995
Air pollution, in COPD exacerbation, 1099
Air trapping, in airway foreign body aspiration, 866
Aircraft for medical transport, 2995-2996, 2996f
Airway. *See also* Airway management; Intubation; Mechanical ventilation; Ventilatory Support.
    adult vs. child, 2519, 2520f
    angioedema of, 1835
    cellulitis of, in epiglottitis, 1115
    contamination of, in urban search and rescue, 3008
    decision to intubate, 2-3
    difficult
        approach to, 8-9, 9f
        cricothyrotomy for, 22-23, 23f
        esophagotracheal combitube for, 20, 20f
        fiberoptic intubation of, 20-21, 22f
        identification of, 3-4, 3b, 4b, 5f
        in children, 2502, 2502b
        intubating laryngeal mask airway for, 19, 19f
        lighted stylet for, 19-20, 20f
        retrograde intubation of, 20
        special airway devices for, 18-23, 19f-23f
    failed, 8, 9, 10f
        special airway devices for, 18-23, 19f-23f
    failure to maintain or protect, as indication for intubation, 2
    foreign body in, 864-870, 867f-869f, 2529-2530, 2550-2551, 2551f
    inflammation of
        in asthma, 1080-1081, 1080f, 1083, 2532-2533
        in chronic obstructive pulmonary disease, 1097-1098
    reflex closure of, in physically disabled patient, 2907-2908
    remodeling of, in asthma, 1081, 1083
    rewarming of, 2248-2249, 2249t
    surgical, 22
        in multiple trauma, 306
        in neck trauma, 445
Airway management. *See also* Airway; Intubation; Mechanical ventilation; Ventilatory support.
    crash airway algorithm for, 7, 8f
    in anaphylaxis, 1830
    in cardiac arrest, 87
    in central nervous system infection, 1721
    in comatose patient, 158
    in dental infection, 1032
    in elderly trauma patient, 348
    in facial trauma, 389
    in foreign body aspiration, 868-870
    in heatstroke, 2264
    in hemoptysis, 280
    in laryngotracheal trauma, 447-448
    in multiple trauma, 306
    in myasthenia gravis, 1706
    in neck trauma, 444-445
    in neonatal resuscitation, 122
    in organophosphate poisoning, 2460
    in pregnant trauma patient, 322
    in seizure, 166, 1626
    in sepsis, 2218-2219
    in severe head trauma, 358-359
    in smoke inhalation, 921-922
    in spinal injuries, 436
    in subarachnoid hemorrhage, 1637
    in thermal burns, 921-923
    pediatric
        in anaphylaxis, 2549
        in cardiac arrest, 97-98, 105-109, 106f, 107b, 107t
        in epiglottitis, 2523-2524
        in neck trauma, 445
        in status epilepticus, 2672
        in trauma, 329, 332t
        in upper airway obstruction, 2521, 2521f
    prehospital, 2990, 2991
Airway muscles, weakness of, 138-139
Airway obstruction
    difficult airway and, 4
    in adult epiglottitis, 1115
    in asthma, 1081
    in chronic obstructive pulmonary disease, 1097, 1098

Airway obstruction *(Continued)*
    in foreign body impaction, 864-870, 867f-869f, 2529-2530, 2550-2551, 2551f.
    in pharyngitis, 276-277
    measurement of, 1084-1085
    pediatric, 2502, 2502b, 2519-2530, 2532-2552
        evaluation of, 2498, 2498f, 2521, 2521f
        in aeroesophageal foreign body, 2529-2530
        in anaphylaxis, 2546-2550
        in asthma, 2532-2544
        in bronchiolitis, 2544-2546
        in congenital lesions, 2522, 2524-2525, 2524f, 2527-2528, 2528f
        in croup, 2525-2527, 2526f, 2527b
        in epiglottitis, 2523-2524, 2524f
        in foreign body aspiration, 2550-2551, 2551f
        in laryngeal disease, 2524-2525, 2524f
        in retropharyngeal abscess, 2522-2523, 2523f
        in subglottic tracheal disease, 2525-2527
        in supraglottic disease, 2522-2524
        in tracheal disease, 2527-2529, 2529t
        pathophysiology of, 2519, 2520f
        stridor in, 2519-2520, 2521t
Airway pressure release ventilation, 33
Airway tuberculosis, 2151
Akathisia, antipsychotic-induced, 1732, 2446-2447
Akinesia, antipsychotic-induced, 1732
Alanine aminotransferase
    in acute pancreatitis, 1431, 1431t
    in alcoholic hepatitis, 1409
    in amebic abscess, 1416
    in viral hepatitis, 1404
Alarm systems, in emergency department, 2966
Albendazole, for *Enterobius vermicularis* gastroenteritis, 1482
Albumin
    administration of, after burn injury, 923
    as cardiac marker, 1178
    glycosylated, in diabetes mellitus, 1959
Albuterol
    for acute renal failure, 2650
    for asthma, 1086-1087, 1087t, 1088, 2538, 2539t, 2543t
    for chronic obstructive pulmonary disease, 1105
    for hyperkalemia
        in acute renal failure, 1539
        in chronic renal failure, 1545, 1545t
Alcohol. *See also* Ethanol.
    drug interactions with, 2875-2877, 2876t
    for wound cleansing, 848t
    metabolism of, 2859
    occupational testing for, 3080-3081
Alcohol consumption
    cardiovascular effects of, 2866
    deaths related to, 300
    during pregnancy, 2791-2792, 2791b, 2877-2878
    endocrine effects of, 2871
    gastrointestinal and hepatic effects of, 2867-2869
    hematologic effects of, 2873-2874, 2873t
    hypothermia and, 2240, 2874-2875
    in adolescents, 2877
    in ciguatera fish poisoning, 1473
    in elderly person, 2877
    metabolic effects of, 2871-2872, 2872t
    neurologic effects of, 2869-2870
    oncologic effects of, 2874
    physiologic effects of, blood alcohol levels and, 2859, 2859t
    psychiatric effects of, 2875
    pulmonary effects of, 2866-2867
    rhabdomyolysis from, 1979
    risks and benefits of, 2867b
    submersion injuries and, 2312, 2314
    trauma and, 2878
Alcohol intoxication, 2327t, 2328
    as diagnosis of exclusion, 2859-2860
    as injury risk factor, 948-949
    consent and, 3168-3169
    disposition in, 2879
    management of, 2860
    opioid/sedative/ethanol syndrome and, 2327t, 2328
    violence and, 1018

Alcohol withdrawal syndrome, 2860-2863
    clinical features of, 2860-2861
    differential considerations in, 2860
    disposition in, 2879
    hypertension in, 1314
    management of, 2861-2863
    pathophysiology of, 2860
    seizure in, 1623, 2863
Alcoholic cardiomyopathy, 2866
Alcoholic cirrhosis, 2868
Alcoholic fatty liver, 2868
Alcoholic hepatitis, 2868
Alcoholic ketoacidosis, 1927-1928, 1964-1965, 2872-2873
Alcoholic liver disorders, 1407, 1409, 2867-2868
    cirrhosis in, 1410
    hepatitis in, 1405, 1409
Alcoholic pancreatitis, 2868
    acute, 1426, 1427-1428
    chronic, 1434-1435
Alcohol-in-combination, emergency department visits related to, 2884f
Alcoholism, 2858-2880, 2859-2860
    definition and natural history of, 2858
    dementia in, 1658
    differential considerations in, 2859-2860
    hypertension in, 1314
    hypomagnesemia in, 1947
    hypophosphatemia in, 1951
    immune defects in, 2841-2842
    infection in, 2842, 2870-2871
    neuropathy in, 1692, 2869
    psychiatric and social problems in, 2879-2880
    screening test for, 2858
    sideroblastic anemia in, 1873
    suicide and, 1769
Alcohol-related seizure, 1623, 2863-2866, 2863b, 2879
Aldosterone, 527
    in heart failure, 1262
    in hypertension, 1311, 1312f
    in sodium homeostasis, 1933
Aldosterone receptor blockers, 1321t
Alexia, in ischemic stroke, 1609
Alexithymia, in somatoform disorders, 1753
Alfentanil, 2922t, 2923
Alice in Wonderland syndrome, 2679
Aliphatic petroleum distillates, toxicity of, 2428, 2429t
Alkalemia, in pregnancy, 1926
Alkali burn, 931-933
    esophageal perforation from, 483
    ocular, 1046, 1046f, 2384
    oral, 2381, 2381f, 2382-2383, 2382f
    pathophysiology of, 930
Alkaline batteries
    impaction of, 1384
    ingestion of, 2384-2385
Alkaline phosphatase
    in acute pancreatitis, 1431, 1431t
    in amebic abscess, 1416
    in hepatitis, 1404
    in peritoneal lavage, 501
    in pregnancy, 2726
    in pyogenic abscess, 1415
Alkalinization, urinary. *See* Sodium bicarbonate.
Alkalosis
    metabolic, 1930-1931, 1931b
        causes of, 1930, 1930b
        from vomiting, 201
        renal compensation in, 1924
        saline-resistant, 1931
        saline-responsive, 1930-1931
    respiratory, 1926, 1931b
        causes of, 1926, 1926b
        during acclimatization to high altitude, 2297-2298
        hypophosphatemia in, 1951
        in chronic obstructive pulmonary disease, 1100
        in salicylate overdose, 2340
Allen's test, 586, 588f, 1346
Allergens, sensitization to, 1819
Allergic airway inflammation, in asthma, 1080-1081, 1080f, 1083
Allergic conjunctivitis, 296t
Allergic contact dermatitis, 1851-1852, 1851f, 1852f
Allergic granulomatosis and angiitis, 1816

Allergic rhinitis, exercise-induced asthma and, 1082
Allergic sinusitis, 1123
Allergy. *See also* Anaphylaxis; Hypersensitivity reactions.
  classification of reactions in, 1821-1822
  immune system and, 1820-1822, 1820f
  immunopathology of, 1819
  incidence of, 1819
  pathophysiology of, 1822-1824, 1822f
  to antibiotics, 1826
  to aspirin/NSAIDs, 1828
  to bupivacaine, 846-847
  to contrast media, 1828
  to foods, 1826, 1848, 2547, 2548
  to herbal medicines, 2477, 2477t
  to hymenoptera stings, 1827, 2547
  to insulin, 1972
  to latex, 1826-1827, 2543
  to local anesthesia, 846-847, 1827, 2931
  to miscellaneous medications, 1827
  to opioid analgesics, 1828
  to pyrethrins and pyrethroids, 2467
  to sulfites, 1827
  to whole blood and immunoglobulins, 1827
Allis technique for hip reduction, 758-759, 759f
Alloantibodies, extrinsic, in hemolytic anemia, 1882
Allopurinol
  for gouty arthritis, 1786
  for hyperuricemia, 1914
All-terrain vehicle accidents, facial trauma from, 382
Almitrine, for chronic obstructive pulmonary disease, 1106
Aloe vera, for frostbite, 2232
Alogia, in schizophrenia, 1728
Alpha (α) error, 3051t, 3052
Alpha particles, 2319, 2320f
Alpha-adrenergic agonists
  central, 1321t
  for alcohol withdrawal syndrome, 2862
Alpha-adrenergic blocking agents, 1321t
  for hypertensive emergencies, 1319
Alphavirus, 2047-2048
Alprazolam, 2484, 2484t
ALTE (apparent life-threatening event), 2714, 2718-2720, 2718b, 2719b.
Alteplase. *See* Tissue plasminogen activator (t-PA).
Alternating current, electrical injury and, 2268
Alternative hypothesis, 3051, 3051t
Alternative medicine, cultural competent approach to, 3113-3114
Alternobaric vertigo, in scuba diving–related disorders, 2286, 2287t
Altitude. *See also* Acute mountain sickness (AMS); High-altitude illness.
  and underlying medical conditions, 2307-2309
  barometric pressure and, 2297
  definitions of, 2296
  dehydration and, 2995
  oxygenation and, 2307, 2307f, 2994, 2995t
  oxyhemoglobin dissociation curve and, 2296, 2297f, 2298
Aluminum antacids
  for hyperphosphatemia, 1953
  for upper gastrointestinal disorders, 1398
Alum-precipitated toxoid test, in vasa previa, 2810
Alveolar bone fracture, 1040
Alveolar gas equation, 2297, 2297b
Alveolar infiltration, in pulmonary contusion, 460, 460f
Alveolar osteitis, acute, 1034
Alzheimer's disease
  anxiety in, 1748
  clinical features of, 1658-1659
  diagnosis of, 1661
  epidemiology of, 1655
  palliative care in, 3154
  pathophysiology of, 1655
  treatment of, 1661-1662
Amanita muscaria mushroom, 2412-2413, 2412f
Amanita phylloides, 2479
Amantadine
  for influenza, 1139, 2035, 2037
  for neuroleptic malignant syndrome, 2449
Amblyomma americanum tick, 2121f

Ambulances
  air, 2995-2996, 2996f
  ground, 2988, 2988f
Amebiasis
  abscess in, 1415, 2106-2107
  drug therapy for, 2100t
  dysenteric colitis in, 229t
  dysentery in, 235, 1477t, 1480-1481
  hepatic abscess in, 1415-1416, 2113
  in HIV/AIDS, 1482-1483
  intestinal symptoms in, 1477t, 1480-1481
  pulmonary symptoms in, 2110
American College of Cardiology, clinical practice guidelines of, 3035, 3036f
American College of Emergency Physicians, clinical practice guidelines of, 3035
American Heart Association
  clinical practice guidelines of, 3035, 3036f
  dietary guidelines of, 3177, 3177b
American Medical Association
  clinical practice guidelines published by, 3037
  medical literature guidance of, 3046
American Sign Language, 2905
Amikacin
  for febrile, neutropenic cancer patient, 2838t
  for tuberculosis, 2163t
Amiloride hydrochloride, 1321t
Aminoglycosides
  acute tubular necrosis from, 1536
  during pregnancy and lactation, 2784
  for febrile, neutropenic cancer patient, 2838t
Aminophylline
  for anaphylaxis, 1831b, 1832-1833
  for asthma, 1090, 1090t
  for chronic obstructive pulmonary disease, 1105
Aminosalicylic acid
  for inflammatory bowel disease, 1502
  for tuberculosis, 2163t, 2164-2165
Aminosidine, for intestinal amebiasis, 1481
Amiodarone, 1209
  during pregnancy and lactation, 2788
  for atrial fibrillation, 1232b, 1233
  for cardiac arrest, 92
  for dysrhythmia, 2586b
  for hypertrophic cardiomyopathy, 1295-1296
  for pediatric resuscitation, 101t, 104-105
  for ventricular fibrillation and pulseless ventricular tachycardia, 112-113
  for ventricular tachycardia, 1242
  hepatotoxicity of, 1414
  hypothyroidism from, 1990
  prehospital use of, 2990-2991
  side effects of, 1209, 1210b
  thyrotoxicosis from, 1986
Amitriptyline
  for neuropathic pain, 1692
  metabolism of, 2352
  prophylactic, for migraine, 2680-2681
Amlodipine, 1321t
  for postpartum cardiomyopathy, 2821
  overdose of, 2377t
Ammonia, anhydrous, injury from, 934-935
Ammunition, handgun, 954, 954f
Amnesia
  alcohol-induced, 2869
  in delirium, 1649
  in dementia, 1658-1659
  in head trauma, 363
Amniorrhexis, 2807-2808, 2808t
Amniotic fluid, meconium in, 120, 120f
Amniotic fluid embolism, 2751-2752, 2821
Amniotic membrane, premature rupture of, 2807-2808, 2808t
Amniotic membrane patching, in acute ocular chemical injury, 933
Amoxapine
  metabolism of, 2352
  overdose of, 2354
Amoxicillin
  for Lyme disease, 1789, 2127t, 2128
  for otitis media, 1068, 1069, 1070t
  for pneumonia, 2557, 2558t, 2563
  for sinusitis, 1125
  prophylactic, for pediatric bacteremia, 2506
Amoxicillin-clavulanate
  for otitis media, 1068, 1069, 1070t
  prophylactic, in cat bites, 888
Amperage, electrical injury and, 2269, 2269t

Amphetamines
  abuse of, 2893-2896, 2894t, 2895b
  designer, 2408-2409, 2410-2411
  during pregnancy, 2793
  overdose of, 2392
Amphotericin
  hepatotoxicity of, 1414
  in HIV/AIDS, side effects of, 2079t
Amphotericin B
  for cryptococcal meningitis, 2081
  for febrile, neutropenic cancer patient, 2838-2839, 2838t
  for fungal meningitis, 1722
Ampicillin
  during pregnancy and lactation, 2784
  for meningococcal disease, 2023
  for pediatric fever, 2513-2514
AMPLE history, 330b
Amplification, of bodily functions, 1756
Ampulla, Vater's, carcinoma of, 1423
Amputation
  fingertip, 610, 610f
  foot, 838
  in frostbite, 2234
  in hand trauma, 612-613, 613b
  in peripheral vascular injury, 543
  penile, 532-533
Amrinone
  for acute pulmonary edema in hypotensive patient, 1270t, 1274
  for cardiogenic shock, 54
  for heart failure, in infants and children, 2583t, 2584
Amsel criteria, in bacterial vaginosis, 1568
Amyl nitrite, for cyanide poisoning, 939, 2438
Amylase
  in abdominal trauma, 495
  in acute pancreatitis, 1430
  in peritoneal lavage, 501
Amyloid angiopathy, intracerebral hemorrhage from, 1609
Amyloidosis
  cardiac, 1297
  pericarditis in, 1287
Amyotrophic lateral sclerosis, 1704
  clinical characteristics of, 1680t
  motor neuron disease in, 1700
Anabolic steroids, hepatotoxicity of, 1414
Anaerobic cellulitis, 2199, 2208
Anaerobic organisms, lower respiratory infection due to, 1130
Anal fissures, 1508, 1512-1513, 1512f, 1513t
Anal pruritus, 1509, 1517-1518, 1517b
  causes of, 1517, 1517b
  in *Enterobius vermicularis* gastroenteritis, 1481
  in parasitic infection, 2113-2114
Anal reflexes, in head trauma, 357
Analgesia, 2913-2935
  acute vs. chronic pain and, 2913-2914, 2914b
  definition of terms related to, 2914b
  during pregnancy and lactation, 2781, 2784
  during rewarming of frostbite, 2232
  evaluation and documentation of pain and, 2916-2917, 2917b, 2917t
  for abdominal pain, 217
  for acute pancreatitis, 1433
  for appendicitis, 1456
  for back pain, 264, 267, 710
  for chest pain, 184
  for chronic pancreatitis, 1436
  for dental caries pain, 1031
  for epididymitis, 2639
  for femoral and hip fractures, 749
  for knee trauma, 776
  for migraine, 1633-1634, 1633t
  for pleural effusion, 1151
  for procedures, 2938-2954, 2940t-2941t. *See also* Procedural sedation and analgesia.
  for red and painful eye, 291
  for reduction of glenohumeral joint dislocation, 689
  for renal stones, 2646
  for rib fracture, 455-456
  for sickle cell disease, 1880
  for thermal burns, 924
  for urolithiasis, 1591-1592
  in child, 2935-2936, 2946-2947, 2952-2954
  in elderly person, 2826-2827, 2936
  in ventilated patient, 31

Analgesia *(Cotinued)*
  intravenous regional anesthesia for, 2934
  local anesthesia for, 2930-2933, 2931t, 2932b, 2932t
  nitrous oxide–oxygen mixtures for, 2929-2930
  nonopioid/NSAID, 2926-2928, 2927b, 2927f
  nonpharmacologic interventions for, 2934
  of face, Dejeune onion skin pattern of, 420
  oligoanalgesia and, 2917-2918
  opioid, 2918-2926
    adjuvant agents with, 2921
    agonist-antagonist group of, 2924-2925, 2924b
    common therapeutic mistakes in, 2918-2921, 2919b
    for abdominal pain, 2925-2926
    intramuscular, disadvantages of, 2919-2920, 2919b
    mechanism of action of, 2918, 2918t
    oral, 2925
    parenteral, 2921-2924
    pathophysiology of pain and, 2914-2916, 2915f, 2915t, 2916f, 2916t
    patient-controlled, 2920
    prehospital, 2936
    priorities of pain management and, 2918
    sites and mechanisms of, 2916, 2916t
  skeletal muscle relaxants for, 2928-2929
  topical anesthesia for, 2933-2934
Analysis of variance, one-way, 3052-3053, 3052t
Anaphylactic shock
  causes of, 47
  treatment of, 52b, 54
Anaphylactoid purpura, 2615, 2615f
Anaphylactoid reaction, 1819
Anaphylaxis, 1818-1834. *See also* Allergy; Hypersensitivity reactions.
  biphasic, 1828
  classification of reactions in, 1821-1822
  clinical features of, 1825t, 1828-1829, 2547-2548
  complications of, 2548
  diagnosis of, 1829, 2548
  differential considerations in, 1829-1830, 2548-2549
  disposition in, 1833-1834, 2549-2550
  dyspnea in, 179t
  epidemiology of, 2547
  etiology of, 1819, 1824-1828, 1824b
  idiopathic, 1828
  immune complex–mediated agents in, 1827
  immune system and, 1820-1822, 1820f, 1821f
  immunoglobulin E–mediated
    agents associated with, 1826-1827
    signal transduction system in, 1822-1823, 1822f
  immunopathology of, 1819
  in children, 2546-2550
  incidence of, 1819
  management of, 1830-1833, 1831b, 2549
  mediators of, 1823, 1823b
  nonimmunologic activators of, 1828
  pathophysiology of, 1822-1824, 1822f, 2547
  physically induced, 1828
  physiologic effects of, 1824, 1825t
  prevention of, 1833-1834, 1834b
  risk factors for, 1819-1820
  to horse serum–derived antivenin, 901
  to snake venom, 898
  transfusion-related, 60
Anastomotic aneurysm, after abdominal aortic aneurysm repair, 1340
Anatomic abnormalities, neonatal resuscitation in, 121
Anatomic differences, in children vs. adults, 329, 329b, 329t, 335b
Anatomic snuffbox, 581, 583f, 625
Ancef, for catheter-related infections, 1363
Ancillary services, in medical screening examination, 3160-3161
Anembryonic gestation, 2740
Anemia, 1867-1884
  after head trauma, 353
  aplastic, 1875-1876, 1875t
  decreased red blood cell production in, 1870-1876, 1870b, 1871t
  definition of, 1867
  differential diagnosis in, 1869-1884, 1870b, 1871t
  emergent, 1868-1869, 1869b

Anemia *(Cotinued)*
  heart failure in, 1268
  hemolytic, 1868t, 1876-1884
    abnormal sequestration in, 1884
    ancillary evaluation of, 1877, 1877b
    aplastic crisis in, 2046, 2046f
    clinical features of, 1876-1877
    differential diagnosis in, 1878-1884, 1879b
    drug-induced, 1883, 1883b
    environmental causes of, 1883-1884
    extrinsic alloantibodies in, 1882
    extrinsic autoantibodies in, 1882-1883, 1883b
    extrinsic mechanical causes of, 1883
    in alcoholism, 2874
    intrinsic enzyme defects in, 1878-1879, 1879b
    intrinsic hemoglobin abnormality in, 1879-1882. *See also* Sickle cell disease.
    intrinsic membrane abnormality in, 1879
    jaundice in, 246
    laboratory studies in, 1877-1878, 1877b, 1877f, 1878f
    microangiopathic, 1883
  in acute renal failure, 1540
  in alcoholism, 2873-2874
  in chronic renal failure, 1543
  in lead poisoning, 2421
  in pregnancy, 2724, 2763t, 2767-2768
  in systemic lupus erythematosus, 1808
  in thalassemia, 1872-1873, 1872f
  in trichuriasis, 2107
  increased red blood cell destruction in, 1868t, 1876-1884
  iron deficiency, 1871-1872, 1871f, 1872t
    in alcoholism, 2873-2874
    in pregnancy, 2763t, 2767-2768
  macrocytic and megaloblastic, 1873-1875, 1874f, 1874t, 1875t, 2768, 2873
  microcytic, 1871-1873
  myelophthisic, 1876, 1876f
  nonemergent, 1869, 1870b
  normochromic and normocytic, 1875-1876, 1875t, 1876f
  of chronic disease, 1873, 1876
  pathophysiology of, 1867-1868, 1868b, 1868f
  pernicious, optic neuropathy from, 1060
  sickle cell, 1879-1882
    altitude and, 2308
    clinical features of, 1880-1881, 1881f, 1881t
    in pregnancy, 2763t, 2768
    management of, 1881-1882
    pathophysiology of, 1879-1880
    urinary tract infection in, 1578
  sideroblastic, 1873, 2874
Anemone, 909
Anesthesia, 2914b
  dissociative, in syringomyelia, 1683
  general, for critically ill asthmatic patient, 1093
  in Colles' fracture, 633, 634f
  in frostbite, 2230
  in red and painful eye, 291
  in wound care, 845-847
  intravenous regional, 2934
  isoflurane, for status epilepticus, 1627-1628, 1627t
  local, 2914b, 2930-2933, 2931t, 2932b, 2932t
    allergy to, 846-847, 1827, 2931
    buffering in, 846, 2932-2933, 2932b
    in calcific tendinitis, 698
    in wound care, 846
    ophthalmic, 1063b, 1064
    profiles of agents used for, 2930-2931, 2931t, 2932t
    toxicity of, 2931-2932
  topical, 2933-2934
Aneurysm
  aortic. *See* Aortic aneurysm.
  atherosclerotic, infection in, 1356, 1357t
  carotid artery, parapharyngeal abscess and, 1123
  cerebral, and subarachnoid hemorrhage, Hunt and Hess scale for, 1636, 1636t, 1637
  coronary artery, in Kawasaki disease, 2025, 2026, 2594
  false. *See* Pseudoaneurysm.
  left ventricular, ST segment elevation in, 1167, 1168f

Aneurysm *(Continued)*
  pathophysiology of, 1343
  peripheral arterial
    infected, 1356-1357, 1357t
    lower extremity, 1354
    traumatic, 1357
    upper extremity, 1354-1355
    visceral, 1355-1356
  renal artery, urolithiasis vs., 1591
  traumatic, 1357
Angiitis, allergic, 1816
Angina. *See also* Acute coronary syndromes; Chest pain.
  atypical, 1158-1159, 1159t
  classic, 1158, 1158t
  clinical features of, 1157-1161, 1158t, 1159t
  differential diagnosis in, 1159, 1159t
  history in, 1157-1159
  hypertension and, 1306
  in aortic stenosis, 1306
  in hemodialysis patient, 1551
  increasing or progressive, 1156
  Ludwig's, 1028, 1032, 1118-1119
  new-onset, 1156
  pathophysiology of, 1156-1157
  prehospital care in, 1157
  rest, 1156
  septicemia after, 1123
  stable, 1155-1156
  unstable
    definition of, 1156
    in differential diagnosis of chest pain, 190t-191t
    management of
      antiplatelet therapy in, 1185-1187
      beta blockers in, 1184-1185
      heparins in, 1187-1188
      morphine in, 1184
    missed diagnosis of, 1160
    ST segment depression in, 1163f
  variant (Prinzmetal), 1156
  Vincent's, 1033, 1111-1112, 1113
Anginal equivalent symptoms, 1158
Angioedema, 1834-1835
  hereditary, 1835
  in anaphylaxis, 1825t, 2547
Angiography
  computed tomography
    in anthrax exposure, 3025, 3025f
    in cervical vascular injury, 449
    in peripheral arteriovascular disease, 1348
    in pulmonary embolism, 1375-1377, 1377b
  coronary, in aortic rupture, 480-481
  digital subtraction
    in peripheral vascular injury, 543
    intravenous, in aortic rupture, 480-481
  in abdominal trauma, 499
  in acute mesenteric ischemia, 1448, 1448f
  in colonic ischemia, 1504
  in frostbite, 2231
  in gastrointestinal bleeding, 224
  in ischemic stroke, 1613
  in pelvic fracture, 732-734, 733f
  in pregnant trauma patient, 321t
  in proximity wounds, 543
  in severe head trauma, 362, 362t
  magnetic resonance
    in ischemic stroke, 1613
    in peripheral arteriovascular disease, 1348
Angioma, spider, in hepatitis, 1404
Angioplasty, coronary, percutaneous transluminal. *See* Percutaneous coronary intervention.
Angiostrongylus costaricensis, 2113
Angiotensin, 527
  in heart failure, 1262
  in hypertension, 1311, 1312f
  in sodium homeostasis, 1933
Angiotensin II receptor blockade, 1322t
  during pregnancy and lactation, 2788
  for chronic heart failure, 1276
Angiotensin-converting enzyme inhibitors, 1322t
  angioedema from, 1835
  during pregnancy and lactation, 2788
  for acute coronary syndromes, 1185
  for chronic heart failure, 1270t, 1275-1276
  for dilated cardiomyopathy, 1294
  for hypertension, 1320
  for postpartum cardiomyopathy, 2821
Anhedonia, in depression, 1736

Anhydrous ammonia, injury from, 934-935
Animal bite, 882-892
  antibiotic prophylaxis in, 887-889, 887t
  cats in, 883-884, 888
  disposition in, 889-890
  dogs in, 882-883, 887-888
  domestic herbivores in, 885
  epidemiology of, 882
  ferrets in, 884-885
  infected, treatment of, 889-890
  infection risks in, 885-886, 885t
  management of, 886-889, 886b, 887t, 889b, 889t
  osteomyelitis after, 2176
  pigs in, 885
  primates in, 884, 888-889, 889b, 889t
  reporting requirements for, 3172-3173
  rodents in, 884
  systemic infection in, 885
  wild animals in, 885
Anion gap
  calculation of, 1924
  in mixed acid-base disorders, 1931
  in rhabdomyolysis, 1981
Anion gap acidosis, 1927-1929, 1927b
  delirium in, 1651
  in cyanide poisoning, 2437
  in ethylene glycol poisoning, 2399, 2400-2401
  in methanol poisoning, 2396, 2397
  seizure in, 1622
Anisakiasis, 2100t, 2113
Anisocoria, 1061-1062
Ankle
  edema of, heat-induced, 2258-2259
  immobilization of, 571, 572f, 573f
  tendinopathy of, 1799-1800
Ankle trauma, 808-820
  anatomy and physiology in, 808, 809f, 810f
  clinical features of, 808, 810
  diagnostic strategies in, 810-811, 810f, 811f
  dislocation without fracture in, 820
  fracture in, 811-815, 812b, 812f-815f
  ligament injuries in, 815-818, 817b, 817f
  pathophysiology of, 808, 810f
  physical examination, 810
  soft tissue injuries in, 815-820
  tendon injuries in, 818-820, 819f
Ankle-brachial index, 541-542
Ankylosing spondylitis, 1789
Annular ligament, 647, 648f
Annulus fibrosus, 702, 702f
Anogenital examination
  in genitourinary trauma, 515
  in sexual assault victim, 986-988, 987f, 987t, 988t
Anogenital warts, 1563-1564, 1564f
Anorectal disorders, 1507-1522. See also
    Anorectal pain.
  abscesses and fistulas in, 1513-1515, 1513t, 1514f
  anal fissures in, 1508, 1512-1513, 1512f, 1513t
  anatomy and physiology in, 1507-1508, 1508f
  clinical features of, 1508-1509, 1508b
  fecal incontinence in, 1516-1517, 1516b
  foreign bodies and, 875-877, 876f, 1521-1522, 1522f
  hemorrhoids in, 1509-1512, 1510t, 1511b, 1511t, 1512f
  hidradenitis suppurativa in, 1515-1516
  history in, 1508-1509, 1508b
  in HIV/AIDS, 1520, 1520b, 2084
  levator ani syndrome in, 1516
  management of, 1509-1522
  pain and itching in, 1509
  physical examination in, 1509
  pilonidal disease in, 1515
  procidentia in, 1521, 1521f
  proctalgia fugax in, 1509, 1516
  pruritus ani in, 1509, 1517-1518, 1517b
  rectal bleeding in, 1508
  sexually transmitted disease and, 1518-1520, 1518t
  swelling and masses in, 1508-1509
Anorectal pain, 1509.
  in anal fissures, 1512-1513
  in appendicitis, 1452
  in hemorrhoids, 1510
  in levator ani syndrome, 1516
Anorexia
  in appendicitis, 2619
  in chronic renal failure, 1542
  palliative care for, 3154

Anoscopy, 1509
  in gastrointestinal bleeding, 224
  in sexual assault victim, 988
ANOVA, 3052-3053, 3052t
Anserine bursitis, 795-796, 1803-1804
Antacids
  during pregnancy and lactation, 2790
  for gastroesophageal reflux, 1389
  for peptic ulcer disease, 1392
  for upper gastrointestinal disorders, 1398
Antalgic gait
  in femoral neck stress fracture, 755-756
  pediatric, 764-765
Anterior chamber, nonpenetrating trauma to, 1048-1049, 1048f, 1049f
Anterior chamber angle recession, 1049
Anterior cord syndrome, 419f, 420, 1678, 1678f
Anterior cruciate ligament injury, 790-791, 792
  intercondylar eminence fracture and, 779
  meniscal tears and, 792, 793
  Segond fracture and, 777, 777f
  stability testing in, 773, 774
  tibial femoral knee dislocation and, 788
  tibial plateau fracture and, 778
Anterior drawer test
  of ankle, 816-817
  of knee, 773
Anterior elbow dislocation, 664f, 665-666
Anterior fat pad in elbow, 651, 651f
Anterior humeral line, 651, 651f
Anterior interosseous nerve, 586-589, 589f
Anterior superior iliac spine, avulsion of, 750, 750f
Anterior talofibular ligament, injury to, 816-817
Anterior tibial artery, 797
  anatomy of, 771
  injury to, 547
Anterior uveitis, 287, 287f, 289, 295t
Anteroposterior radiographs, in spinal injuries, 424, 426, 426f, 427f
Anthrax
  as biological weapon, 3021, 3024-3026, 3025f, 3026b, 3026f
  cutaneous, 1860, 1861f, 3025, 3026f
  gastrointestinal, 1461t, 1462t, 1468-1469, 3026
  inhalational, 3024-3025, 3025f
  oropharyngeal, 1469, 3026
  vaccine for, 3026
Antiallergy agents, ophthalmic, 1063b
Antiasthmatic agents, during pregnancy and lactation, 2789-2790
Antibiotics
  after miscarriage, 2742
  allergy to, 1826
  anaphylaxis to, 2547
  Clostridium difficile enterocolitis from, 1470t, 1474-1475
  diarrhea from, 233
  during pregnancy and lactation, 2758, 2784
  for abdominal infections, 217
  for acute necrotic ulcerative gingivitis, 1033
  for acute pancreatitis, 1434
  for acute septic arthritis, 2706, 2706t
  for adult epiglottitis, 1115
  for Aeromonas hydrophila gastroenteritis, 1461t, 1468
  for AIDS-related diarrhea, 1484, 1485t
  for anorectal sexually transmitted disease, 1519
  for anthrax exposure, 3026, 3026b
  for appendicitis, 1457
  for Bacillus anthracis gastroenteritis, 1461t, 1469
  for bacterial endocarditis, 2591
  for bacterial meningitis, 1721-1722, 1721t, 2663-2664, 2664t
  for bursitis, 1803
  for catheter-related infections, 1363
  for cellulitis, 2197, 2197t
  for central nervous system abscess, 1722
  for central nervous system infections in cancer patient, 1920
  for cholangitis, 1422
  for chronic obstructive pulmonary disease, 1106
  for Clostridium difficile enterocolitis, 1475
  for cystic fibrosis, 2564-2565
  for diphtheria, 2004
  for diverticular disease, 1494-1495, 1494b, 1495b

Antibiotics (Continued)
  for Escherichia coli food poisoning, 1474
  for esophageal perforation, 1386
  for febrile cancer patient, 1908b, 1909
  for fever, 137
  for impetigo, 1842-1843, 2202
  for infected aneurysm, 1356
  for infectious diarrhea, 229t-230t, 235
  for infective endocarditis, 1302
  for inflammatory bowel disease, 1502
  for intussusception, 2612
  for isosporiasis, 1478
  for Ludwig's angina, 1032, 1119
  for Lyme disease, 1292, 1789, 2127-2128, 2127t
  for malrotation with midgut volvulus, 2608
  for mastoiditis, 1072
  for meningococcal disease, 2023
  for neck masses, 1076
  for necrotizing enterocolitis, 2609
  for necrotizing otitis externa, 1071
  for neutropenia, 2516
  for neutropenic cancer patient, 2837-2839, 2838t
  for open fracture, 558
  for orofacial infections, 1032
  for osteomyelitis, 2187, 2189t
  for otitis externa, 1071
  for otitis media, 1068-1069, 1069t, 1070t
  for pacemaker-induced infection, 1250
  for peritonitis in dialysis patient, 1552-1553, 1553t
  for peritonsillitis, 1118
  for pertussis, 2006
  for plague, 3027-3028
  for Plesiomonas shigelloides gastroenteritis, 1461t, 1468
  for pneumococcal disease, 2018-2019
  for pneumonia, 1136-1139, 1138t, 1139t, 2557, 2558t, 2562-2563
  for prostatitis, 1586
  for purulent pericarditis, 1286
  for retropharyngeal abscess, 1121
  for Rocky Mountain spotted fever, 2136, 2136t
  for salmonellosis, 1461t, 1463
  for sepsis, 2221, 2221t
  for septic arthritis, 1785, 2178t, 2192
  for septic shock, 53
  for shigellosis, 1461t, 1464
  for sinusitis, 1125
  for small bowel obstruction, 1444
  for spinal epidural abscess, 1684
  for spinal infection, 712
  for spontaneous bacterial peritonitis, 1413
  for streptococcal pharyngitis, 1112-1113
  for tar removal, 927
  for tetanus, 2011
  for toxic shock syndrome, 2030, 2201
  for traveler's diarrhea, 1486-1487
  for urinary tract infections, 2643-2644
  for Vibrio fish poisoning, 1472
  for Yersinia enterocolitica gastroenteritis, 1465
  in asthma, 1090
  in comatose patient, 163
  injections of, medicolegal issues in, 3159
  ophthalmic, 1063b, 1064
  preoperative, in arterial injury, 544
  prophylactic
    for anthrax exposure, 3026
    for bacteremia, 2506
    for infective endocarditis, 1302, 1303b, 1303t
    for meningococcal disease, 2024
    for red and painful eye, 292
    for rheumatic fever, 2597
    for traveler's diarrhea, 1486-1487
    in abdominal trauma, 502
    in animal bite, 887-889, 887t
    in frostbite, 2232
    in hand amputation and ring avulsion injuries, 613
    in HIV/AIDS, 2089
    in human bites, 891-892
    in hypothermia, 2247
    in open ankle fractures, 814
    in open tibial shaft fracture, 800-801
    in severe head trauma, 361
    in wound management, 854-855
  resistance to, plasmids and, 1575
  topical, for burn injury, 925

Antibodies
  B cell, 2832
  diversity of, 1821
  Lyme disease, 2125
  meningococcal, 2021
Antibody-antigen specificity, 1821
Anticholinergic agents
  for anaphylaxis, 1832
  for asthma, 1089, 2539t, 2541
  for chronic obstructive pulmonary disease, 1105
  for dysphagia, 1398
  for nausea and vomiting, 206
  for vertigo, 146
  overdose of, 2345-2350, 2346b, 2346t, 2347f
    alcohol withdrawal syndrome vs., 2860
    antidotes to, 2329t
    clinical presentation in, 2347-2348, 2347t
    diagnosis of, 2349
    differential diagnosis in, 2348, 2348b
    disposition in, 2350
    management of, 2349-2350
    types of, 2345, 2346b, 2346t
Anticholinergic toxidrome, 2327, 2327t, 2347-2348
Anticoagulation
  during pregnancy and lactation, 2757, 2785-2786
  for acute mesenteric ischemia, 1449
  for cerebral venous thrombosis, 1671
  for dilated cardiomyopathy, 1294
  for ischemic stroke, 1615-1616
  in deep venous thrombosis, 1370
  in peripheral arteriovascular disease, 1349
  in pulmonary embolism, 1377
  postresuscitation, 86
Anticonvulsant therapy
  for alcohol withdrawal syndrome, 2862
  for neuropathic pain, 1692
  for seizure, 166-167, 166t
    during pregnancy and lactation, 2763t, 2769, 2786-2787
    immediate, 1626-1628, 1627t
    in children, prophylactic, 2674-2676, 2675t
    in intracerebral hemorrhage, 1616
    long-term, 1628-1629, 1629t
  for status epilepticus, 1627-1628, 1627t, 2672-2673, 2672t
  for trigeminal neuralgia, 1664, 1666
  in developmentally disabled patient, 2898-2899
  prophylactic, in head trauma, 361, 361b, 370
  side effects of, 1628t, 2674-2675
  withdrawal of, 2676
Antidepressants
  discontinuation syndrome with, 2365-2366
  FDA-approved, 2353t
  for depression, 1741
  for somatoform disorders, 1758
  overdose of, 2352-2366, 2354t
    bupropion in, 2361, 2361t
    cyclic antidepressants in, 2352-2357, 2353b, 2353f, 2354b, 2355f, 2357t
    mirtazapine in, 2362-2363
    monoamine oxidase inhibitors in, 2363-2365, 2363b-2365b, 2364t
    neurologic complications of, 2354t, 2356
    selective serotonin reuptake inhibitors in, 2357-2360, 2358b, 2358t, 2359b, 2360t
    trazodone in, 2361-2362
    venlafaxine in, 2362, 2362t
  suicide and, 1768
Antidiuretic hormone
  for cardiac arrest, 92
  for gastrointestinal bleeding, 225
  for heart failure, 1262-1263
  for pediatric resuscitation, 100, 103t
  for sepsis, 2213, 2219t, 2220
  in sodium homeostasis, 1933
Antidote, 2329t
  antivenin as
    Latrodectus, 906
    scorpion, 908
    snake, 900-902, 900t
  cyanide, 2329t, 2437-2438, 2440
  in benzodiazepine poisoning, 2326, 2329t, 2485-2486, 2485b
  in opioid overdose, 2948-2949
Antidromic tachycardia, in Wolff-Parkinson-White syndrome, 1235, 1237

"Antidumping" law, 3156
Antidysrhythmic devices. See Implantable cardioverter-defibrillator; Pacemaker(s).
Antidysrhythmic drugs
  adenosine as, 1212-1213
  class IA, 1206
  class IB, 1206-1207
  class IC, 1207-1208
  class II, 1208-1209, 1208t
  class III, 1209-1210
  class IV, 1210-1211
  classification of, 1204-1213, 1205b
  digitalis as, 1211-1212, 1211t
  during pregnancy and lactation, 2787-2788
  for adult resuscitation, 92-93
  for chronic heart failure, 1277
  for pediatric resuscitation, 109-113, 110f-113f, 110t
  heart failure from, 1269
  magnesium as, 1212
  prodysrhythmic effects of, 1205-1206
Antiemetic agents
  during pregnancy and lactation, 2790
  for nausea and vomiting, 203, 206, 208b, 208t
Antiepileptic agents. See Anticonvulsant therapy.
Antifibrillatory agents, 1209-1210
Antifreeze
  bittering agents in, 2402
  ingestion of, 2398-2402, 2401t
Antifungals, during pregnancy and lactation, 2785
Antigen detection, in central nervous system infection, 1718-1719
Antigen detection kits, cerebrospinal fluid, in bacterial meningitis, 2662
Antihelmintics, 2098t
Antihemophilic factor antibodies, in hemophilia A, 1901
Antihistamines
  during pregnancy and lactation, 2789-2790
  for anaphylaxis, 1831b, 1832
  for nausea and vomiting, 206
  for scombroid fish poisoning, 1472
  for upper airway angioedema, 1835
  for urticaria, 1848
Antihypertensive drug therapy
  agents used in, 1321t-1322t
  ambulatory, 1320, 1320t
  during pregnancy and lactation, 2762, 2763t, 2765t, 2788-2789
  for aortic dissection, 1328-1329
  for eclampsia, 2751
  for hypertensive emergencies, 1317-1319, 1317t
  for hypertensive urgency, 1320
  for intracerebral hemorrhage, 1616
  for ischemic stroke, 1614, 1614t
  in children, 2652-2653, 2653t
Antiinflammatory drugs
  after cerebral ischemia, 72
  in frostbite, 2233
  nonsteroidal. See Nonsteroidal antiinflammatory drugs.
Antilymphocyte monoclonal antibody preparations, for organ transplant patient, 2850-2851
Antimalarial drugs, 2098t
  for systemic lupus erythematosus, 1809
Antimotility agents
  for AIDS-related diarrhea, 1484
  for diarrhea, 235, 236t
Antimuscarinic agents, overdose of, 2345-2349. See also Anticholinergic agents, overdose of.
Antimyosin scanning, in myocarditis, 1290
Antinuclear antibodies, in systemic lupus erythematosus, 1808
Antioxidant therapy, after cerebral ischemia, 71
Antiparasitic agents, 2098-2099, 2098t, 2100t-2103t
Antiparkinsonian drugs
  anticholinergic toxicity of, 2345, 2346, 2346b, 2347t
  for prevention of antipsychotic-induced extrapyramidal symptoms, 1731
Antiphospholipid antibody syndrome, 1809-1810t
Antiplatelet therapy
  for acute coronary syndromes, 1185-1187
  for acute mesenteric ischemia, 1449
  for ischemic stroke, 1615
  postresuscitation, 86

Antiprotozoals, 2098t
Antipsychotic agents, 2446t
  agranulocytosis from, 2448
  atypical
    for agitation in delirious patient, 1654
    for rapid tranquilization, 2962
  complications of, 1732-1733
  extrapyramidal symptoms from, 2445, 2446-2447, 2449
  for agitation in delirious patient, 1654
  for mood disorders, 1741
  for rapid tranquilization, 2961-2962
  for thought disorders, 1730-1731, 1731b
  neuroleptic malignant syndrome from, 2445, 2447, 2447t, 2448, 2448t, 2449, 2961-2962
  overdose of, 2446, 2448-2449
  QT prolongation and torsades de pointes from, 2447, 2449
  seizures from, 2448, 2962
  side effects of, 2961-2962
  tardive dyskinesia from, 2445, 2447
  toxicity of, 2445-2450, 2446t
Antipyretics, 137
Antiretroviral therapy, 2039, 2087-2089, 2087t
  during delivery, 2810
  for HIV postexposure prophylaxis, 2091-2092, 3085t, 3086-3087
  in pregnancy, 2088-2089, 2764t, 2774
  rifamycins and, drug interactions between, 2166
Antiseptics, for wound cleansing, 847-848, 848t
Antisocial personality disorder, 2979b
  in alcoholism, 2875
  malingering and, 1763
Antistreptococcal antibody titers, in rheumatic fever, 1304
Antithrombotic therapy
  in acute coronary syndromes, 1187-1188
  in frostbite, 2232-2233
Antitoxin. See also Immunization; Vaccine.
  botulism, 1707-1708, 2016
  diphtheria, 1113, 2004
  equine, allergy to, 1827
Antituberculous agents
  during pregnancy and lactation, 2168, 2785
  first-line, 2162, 2163t, 2164
  fixed-dose combinations if, 2164
  for drug-resistant tuberculosis, 2166-2167, 2167b, 2167t
  for extrapulmonary tuberculosis, 2168
  for initial therapy, 2165-2166, 2165t
  for latent infection, 2168-2169, 2168t
  in children and adolescents, 2166, 2167b
  in HIV/AIDS, 2166
  noncompliance with, risk factors for, 2162
  second-line, 2163t-2164t, 2164-2165
  susceptibility testing for, 2154-2155
Antivenin
  Latrodectus, 906
  scorpion, 908
  snake, 900-902, 900t
Antiviral agents
  during pregnancy and lactation, 2785
  for myocarditis, 1290
  for pneumonia, 1139
  ophthalmic, 1063b, 1064
  prophylactic, in monkey bites, 888-889, 889t
Antiviral chemotherapy, 2035-2039, 2036t-2037t
Anton's syndrome, 1060
Anxiety
  endogenous, 1745
  exogenous, 1745, 1746b
  in cardiovascular disease, 1746-1747
  in drug intoxication and withdrawal states, 1748
  in endocrine disease, 1747
  in neurologic disorders, 1747-1748
  in primary psychiatric disorders, 1748-1749
  in pulmonary disease, 1747
  medical illness manifesting as, 1745-1746, 1746b
  somatoform disorders vs., 1757
Anxiety disorders, 1744-1752
  clinical features of, 1745, 1745b
  definitions of, 1746b
  differential considerations in, 1745-1749, 1746b
  disposition in, 1751-1752
  epidemiology of, 1744

Anxiety disorders (Continued)
  generalized, 1746b
  management of, 1749-1751
    pharmacological, 1750-1751, 1750t
    psychological, 1751
  not otherwise specified, 1746b
  pathophysiology of, 1744-1745
  substance-induced, 1746b
Anxiolytics, 1750-1751, 1751t
Aorta
  coarctation of, 1312, 2578-2579
  penetrating atherosclerotic ulcers of, 1325
Aortic aneurysm
  abdominal, 1330-1340
    back pain in, 265t
    clinical features of, 1332-1333
    diagnostic strategies in, 1334-1336, 1334f-
      1336f, 1337-1338
    differential diagnosis in, 1336, 1336b
    disposition in, 1340
    epidemiology of, 1330, 1331t
    false, 1330, 1340
    management of, 1336-1339
    pathophysiology and natural history of,
      1330-1331
    repair of
      endovascular, 1338-1339, 1339f
      late complications of, 1339-1340
      survival rate for, 1339
      traditional, 1338, 1339f
    ruptured, 1331
      abdominal pain in, 214t
      clinical features of, 1332-1333
      management of, 1336-1338
    types of, 1330, 1331f
  thoracic
    chronic, 482
    superior vena cava syndrome in, 1909
Aortic arch
  congenital anomalies of, dysphagia in, 1383
  right-sided, 2574
Aortic clamping
  in abdominal aortic aneurysm rupture, 1337
  in abdominal trauma, 502
  in aortic rupture, 481
Aortic compression, for postpartum hemorrhage,
  2819
Aortic dissection, 1324-1329
  abdominal aortic aneurysm vs., 1330
  anatomy and physiology in, 1324
  arterial embolism vs., 1352
  back pain in, 261, 265t
  chest pain in, 183, 186b, 190t-191t
  clinical features of, 1325-1326
  diagnostic strategies in, 1326-1328, 1326t,
    1327f, 1327t
  differential diagnosis in, 1328
  disposition in, 1329
  epidemiology of, 1324
  hypertension in, 1317
  management of, 1328-1329
  pathophysiology of, 1324-1325
  risk factors for, 186b
  Stanford classification of, 1325, 1325f
Aortic media, degeneration of, in aortic
  dissection, 1324-1325
Aortic regurgitation, 1307
  heart failure in, 1265
  in aortic dissection, 1326
  in pregnancy, 2763t, 2767
Aortic rupture, 476-482, 477f-479f, 481b, 510,
  511f
Aortic stenosis, 1306-1307
  heart failure in, 1265
  in pregnancy, 2763t, 2767
Aortic wall, intramural hemorrhage within, 1325
Aortoenteric fistula
  after abdominal aortic aneurysm repair, 1340
  in abdominal aortic aneurysm rupture, 1333
Aortography
  in aortic dissection, 1327
  in aortic rupture, 480-481
Aortoiliac occlusive disease, 1345, 1350
Aortovenous fistula, in abdominal aortic
  aneurysm rupture, 1333
APACHE-II system in acute pancreatitis, 1432
Apgar score, 122, 122t
Aphasia, in ischemic stroke, 1609
Aphthous stomatitis, 1036

Aphthous ulcers
  in Behçet's disease, 1814
  in HIV/AIDS, 2083
Aplastic anemia, 1875-1876, 1875t
Aplastic crisis
  in hemolytic anemia, 2046, 2046f
  in sickle cell disease, 1880
Apley's test, in meniscal tears, 774
Apnea
  definition of, 2714
  from etomidate, 2947
  in neonates, 119
  in pneumonia, 2562
  respiratory depression with, in GHB
    intoxication, 2489
  sleep, hypertension in, 1313
Apocrine glands, 915, 2255
  abscess of, in hidradenitis suppurativa, 2204-
    2205
Apolipoprotein E gene, in dementia, 1657
Apophyseal injuries/disorders, 2709-2711, 2711f
Apophysitis, 2709-2710
  of elbow, 2710-2711
  of hip, 2711
Apoptosis, after cerebral ischemia, 66
Apparent life-threatening event, 2714, 2718-2720,
  2718b, 2719b
Appearance
  in chest pain, 187t
  in dyspnea, 178t
  in headache, 172t
  in nausea and vomiting, 202t
  in pediatric assessment triangle, 2497-2498,
    2498t
  in vaginal bleeding, 256t
  toxic, as indication for lumbar puncture, 2659
Appendectomy, laparoscopic, 1457-1458
Appendicitis, 1451-1458
  abdominal pain in, 210t
  complications of, 1453-1454
  diagnosis of, 1454-1455
  differential diagnosis in, 1455, 1456t
  disposition in, 1458
  epidemiology of, 1451
  historical perspective in, 1451
  imaging studies in, 1454-1455, 1455f, 1456
  in children, 1452-1453, 2509b, 2618-2620,
    2620f
  in elderly person, 1453
  in pregnancy, 1453, 2752-2754, 2754f
  in women, 1453, 1453t
  management of, 1456-1458, 1457f
  nausea and vomiting in, 205t
  observation in, 1455, 3063, 3064
  pathophysiology of, 1451-1452
  pelvic pain in, 251t
  perforation in, 1452, 1453, 1458
Appendicolith, 2619, 2620f
Appendix, perforation of, 1452, 1453, 1458
Appendix testis
  in children, 2641
  torsion of, 1597
Appetite disturbance, in depression, 1737
Apprehension sign
  in anterior subluxation of glenohumeral joint,
    690, 691f
  in patellar dislocation, 786
Aqueous humor, 1055
Arachidonic acid, metabolism of, 1081f
Arbovirus
  group A, 2047-2048
  group B, 2049-2050
Arcanobacterium haemolyticum, in pharyngitis,
  1111, 1113, 1114
Arenavirus, 2034t, 2055-2056
Argentine hemorrhagic fever, 2055-2056
Aripiprazole, 2446t
  for thought disorders, 1731
Arm. See also Forearm entries.
  decompression of, in burn injury, 925
  delivery of, in shoulder dystocia, 2815
Aromatic petroleum distillates, toxicity of, 2428,
  2429t
Arousal
  disorders of, in sudden infant death syndrome,
    2716
  physiology of, 156
Arrhythmia. See Dysrhythmia.
Arsenic poisoning, 2329t, 2423-2424, 2424b

Arterial anatomy, 1342
Arterial aneurysm, peripheral
  infected, 1356-1357, 1357t
  lower extremity, 1354
  traumatic, 1357
  upper extremity, 1354-1355
  visceral, 1355-1356
Arterial blood gases
  during cardiopulmonary resuscitation, 80-81
  in asthma, 1085, 2537
  in chronic obstructive pulmonary disease, 1100
  in comatose patient, 162
  in cyanosis, 271
  in electrical and lightning injuries, 2276
  in hypothermia, 2242, 2243f
  in infants and children, 2572-2573
  in pulmonary contusion, 461
  monitoring of, 36-39
    capnography/capnometry in, 37-39, 38f
    pulse oximetry in, 36-37
    transcutaneous and conjunctival, 36
Arterial disease, in hypertension, 1312-1313
Arterial embolism, 1352-1353
  differential diagnosis in, 1352
  management of, 1352-1353
  pathophysiology of, 1343-1344
  physical examination in, 1346, 1347t
  vs. thrombosis in situ, 1347t
Arterial gas embolism
  in scuba diving-related disorders, 2285-2286
  recompression therapy for, 2288-2292, 2288b,
    2289f-2291f
  vs. pulmonary decompression sickness, 2288,
    2288t
Arterial injury
  in hip trauma, 761
  peripheral, 536-547. See also Arteriovascular
    disease, peripheral.
    clinical features of, 539-541, 540f
    diagnostic strategies in, 541-543
    disposition in, 547
    epidemiology of, 536-537
    of lower extremity, 546-547
    of upper extremity, 544-546
    pathophysiology of, 537-539, 538f
    treatment of, 543-544
Arterial insufficiency, 539, 1345-1346, 1350-1352
Arterial occlusion, acute, 1345, 1345f, 1352-1354,
  1353f
Arterial pressure index, in peripheral vascular
  injury, 541-542
Arterial spasm, reversible, posttraumatic, 538
Arterial supply
  to distal humerus and elbow, 648, 648f
  to femur and hip, 737, 737t, 738f
  to foot, 821
  to forearm, 640t
  to hand, 585-586, 587f, 588f
  to knee, 771
  to lower leg, 797
  to lower limb, 540f
  to nose, 1073, 1073f
  to pelvis, 717-718
  to upper limb, 540f
  to wrist, 622, 625f
Arterial thrombosis, 1344, 1347, 1347t, 1353-
  1354
Arteriography
  in cervical vascular injury, 449
  in knee trauma, 774
  in pelvic fracture, 732-734, 733f
  in peripheral arteriovascular disease, 1348
  in peripheral vascular injury, 542-543
  in popliteal artery injury, 546-547
  in subclavian artery injury, 545
  in thoracic outlet syndrome, 1360
  in tibial femoral knee dislocation, 788
Arteriosclerosis, hypertension in, 1312
Arteriovascular disease, peripheral, 1342-1366
  acute arterial occlusion in, 1345, 1345f, 1352-
    1354, 1353f
  arterial anatomy and, 1342
  arterial embolism in, 1343-1344, 1346, 1347t,
    1352-1353
  arterial thrombosis in, 1344, 1347, 1347t, 1353-
    1354
  arteriosclerosis obliterans in, 1350-1351
  arteriovenous fistula in, 538-539, 541, 1344,
    1347, 1360

Arteriovascular disease, peripheral (Continued)
  atheroembolism in, 1343-1344, 1353, 1353f
  Buerger's disease in, 1351-1352
  chronic arterial insufficiency in, 1345-1346,
    1350-1352
  clinical features of, 1344-1347
  diagnosis of, 1348
  drug abuse–related, 1360-1361
  history in, 1344-1346, 1345f
  inflammatory, 1344, 1347
  management of, 1348-1350
  pathophysiology of, 1342-1344
  physical examination in, 1346-1347, 1347t
  thoracic outlet syndrome in, 1358-1360, 1358f,
    1359f
  trauma in, 1344
  vasospastic disorders in, 1344
Arteriovenous anastomoses rewarming, 2248
Arteriovenous bridge fistula, prosthetic, 1365-
    1366
Arteriovenous fistula, 538-539, 541, 1344, 1347,
    1360
Arteriovenous malformations
  hemorrhage in, 1609
  seizure in, 1624
Arteriovenous rewarming, continuous, 2250t,
    2251
Arteritis
  giant cell (temporal)
    headache in, 1638
    ischemic stroke vs., 1611
    pericarditis in, 1284
  pathophysiology of, 1344
  Takayasu's, 1813
Arthralgia, in Henoch-Schönlein purpura, 2615,
    2653
Arthritis, 1776-1792. See also Osteoarthritis;
    Rheumatic disease.
  anatomy and physiology in, 1777, 1777f
  arthrocentesis in, 1780-1781
  clinical findings in, 1778-1779, 1779f, 1779t
  diagnosis of, 1779-1782, 1780t
  differential considerations in, 1782, 1782b
  disposition in, 1792
  electrocardiography in, 1782
  gonococcal, 1787-1788, 2190-2191
  gouty, 1785-1786
  historical perspective of, 1776-1777
  in chronic renal failure, 1543
  in hepatitis B, 1788
  in Lyme disease, 1788-1789, 2124, 2126
  in seronegative spondyloarthropathies, 1789-
    1790
  management of, 1782-1792, 1783f, 1784f
  monarticular, 1782-1787, 1783f
  pathophysiology of, 1777, 1777f
  polyarticular, 1303-1304, 1784f, 1787-1792,
    1790b, 2596
  pseudogout and, 1786-1787
  radiological findings in, 1779-1780, 1780t
  reactive, 1789-1790, 1791, 2192
  rheumatoid, 1791-1792
    in pregnancy, 2776
    myocarditis in, 1297
    pericarditis in, 1284
    skin lesions in, 1862t
  rubella, 1788
  septic, 1782-1785, 2174
    clinical features of, 1784-1785, 2188-2191
    complications of, 2190
    differential considerations in, 2191-2192
    disposition in, 2193
    etiology and microbiology of, 2177-2179,
      2178t
    gonococcal, 2190-2191
    history and physical examination in, 2188
    in atypical joints, 2191
    in disseminated gonococcal infection,
      1566
    in hand, 618
    in knee, 796
    in tuberculosis, 2159
    joint aspiration and joint fluid analysis in,
      2188-2190, 2189f
    management of, 1785, 2178t, 2192-2193
    pathophysiology and epidemiology of, 1782-
      1784, 2177
    pediatric, 2190, 2509b, 2704-2706, 2705t,
      2706t

Arthritis (Continued)
    pediatric limp from, 764
    with existing joint disease, 2191
  synovial fluid analysis in, 1781-1782, 1781t
  viral, 1788
Arthritis-dermatitis syndrome, 1566, 1788, 1843-
    1844, 1843f
Arthrocentesis
  in arthritis, 1780-1781
  in knee trauma, 774
Arthrography, in knee trauma, 774-775
Arthrometer, in anterior cruciate ligament injury,
    774
Arthropathy
  back pain in, 703, 705-706
  psoriatic, 1790
Arthroplasty, hip
  partial, 751, 752b
  total, 749-750, 750f
Arthropod envenomation, 903-908
Arthroscopy
  in ankle trauma, 811
  in intercondylar eminence fracture, 780
  in knee trauma, 774
  in meniscal tears, 793
  in septic arthritis, 2189
Arthrotomy, for infected hip, 2192
Articular cartilage destruction, in septic arthritis,
    2177
Articular humeral fractures, 661-664, 661f-663f
Articular surface, fracture extension into, 553
Artificial tears, 1063b, 1064
Ascariasis, 2100t, 2113
Ascending aortic rupture, 476, 477
Ascending reticular activating system, 156
Ascending sensory tracts, 1676, 1676f, 2915,
    2915f, 2916f
Ascites
  in chronic schistosomiasis, 2112, 2113f
  in cirrhosis, 1410, 1411
  in pancreatitis, 1427
  in spontaneous bacterial peritonitis, 1412
Ashman phenomenon, 1203, 1223, 1230, 1232f
Aspartate aminotransferase
  in acetaminophen overdose, 2335
  in acute pancreatitis, 1431, 1431t
  in alcoholic hepatitis, 1409
  in amebic abscess, 1416
  in viral hepatitis, 1404
Aspergilloma, in tuberculosis, 2151, 2151f
Aspergillus
  in febrile, neutropenic cancer patient, 2836
  in infective endocarditis, 1301
  in osteomyelitis, 2178-2179
Asphalt burns, petroleum-derived, 926-927, 937
Asphyxia, traumatic, in chest wall trauma, 459
Asphyxiants, simple, inhalation of, 2432-2433
Asphyxic asthma, sudden, 1084
Aspiration
  after vomiting, 202
  cavernosal, in priapism, 2636
  foreign body, 864-870, 867f-869f, 2529-2530,
    2550-2551, 2551f
  in hydrocarbon poisoning, 2428, 2431
  in physically disabled patient, 2907-2908
  in submersion injuries, 2312-2313
  meconium, resuscitation in, 120, 120f, 122
  of tooth, 395, 866
  pneumonia and, 1136
Aspiration pneumonia, in children, 2560
Aspiration techniques
  for confirmation of endotracheal tube
    placement, 6
  in bursitis, 1802
  in gonococcal arthritis, 2191
  in knee trauma, 776
  in osteomyelitis, 2182
  in peritonsillar abscess, 1118
  in pneumothorax, 1147
  in radial head and neck fracture, 664
  in septic arthritis, 2188-2190, 2189f, 2192
  in septic olecranon bursitis, 667
Aspirin
  allergy to, 1828
  during pregnancy and lactation, 2776, 2781
  for acute coronary syndromes, 1185
  for chest pain, 184
  for ischemic stroke, 1615
  for Kawasaki disease, 2027, 2596

Aspirin (Continued)
  for migraine, 2680
  for polycythemia, 1885
  for systemic lupus erythematosus, 1808
  gastritis from, 1390
  metabolism of, 2339-2340, 2340f
  overdose of, 2339-2342, 2340f
    chronic exposure in, 2340
    clinical features of, 2341, 2341b
    diagnosis of, 2341
    disposition in, 2342
    management of, 2341-2342, 2341b
  thrombocytopathy from, 1898-1899
Aspirin-exacerbated respiratory disease, 1082
Asplenia, immune defects in, 2842-2843
Assault
  by combative patient, 2963
  sexual. See Sexual assault.
Assisted-living facilities, institutional abuse in,
    1009, 1015
Asterixis, in hepatic encephalopathy, 1411
Asthma, 1078-1094. See also Status asthmaticus.
  acute severe, near fatal, and fatal, 1091-1093
  adrenergic medications for, 1086-1088, 1087t,
    2538, 2539t, 2540-2541
  altitude and, 2307
  anticholinergic agents for, 1089, 2539t, 2541
  anxiety in, 1747
  clinical features of, 1083-1084
  corticosteroid-resistant, 1089
  corticosteroids for, 1087t, 1088-1089, 2539t,
    2541-2543, 2543t
  critically ill patient with
    intubation and ventilator strategies for, 1092-
      1093
    noninvasive strategies for, 1091-1092
    refractoriness to treatment in, 1093
  definition of, 1078
  diagnosis of, 1083, 1084-1085, 1086t
  differential diagnosis in, 1086b
  disposition in, 1093-1094, 1094b
  dyspnea in, 179t
  epidemiology of, 1078-1079, 1079f
  exercise-induced, 1082
  genetic findings in, 1082-1083
  historic components in, 1084
  in aspirin-exacerbated respiratory disease, 1082
  in pregnancy, 1091, 2761-2762, 2763t, 2765t
  intubation in, 2542
  leukotriene modifiers for, 1090, 2542, 2543t
  magnesium sulfate for, 1087t, 1089-1090
  management of, 1086-1093, 1087t
    guidelines for, 1083
    home strategies for, 1086
    inpatient vs. observation or clinical decision
      unit, 1093
    planning discharge in, 1094, 1094b
    severity of attack and, 1086, 1087t
  menstruation-associated, 1082
  methylxanthines for, 1090, 1090t
  monitoring strategies in, 1085
  mortality in, 1078
    risk factors for, 1084b
  observation in, 3069-3070, 3070b
  oxygen therapy for, 1086, 1091-1092, 2538
  pathology of, 1083
  pathophysiology of, 1080-1083, 1080f, 1081f
  pediatric, 2532-2544
    clinical features of, 2534-2536
    complications of, 2535-2536, 2536b
    diagnosis of, 2536-2537, 2536f, 2537f
    differential diagnosis in, 2537, 2538b
    disposition in, 2542-2544
    epidemiology of, 2532
    factors associated with, 2533-2534, 2534b
    history in, 2534, 2534b
    management of, 2537-2542, 2539t, 2540f,
      2543t
    pathophysiology of, 2532-2533
    physical examination in, 2534-2535, 2535t
    prehospital care in, 2537
    severity assessment score for, 2503t
  physical examination in, 1084, 1086t
  prediction of relapse in, 1093
  psychological factors in, 1082
  pulmonary barotrauma and, 2285
  rapid sequence intubation in, 16
  reflux-induced, 1388-1389
  severity of, classification of, 2534t

Asthma *(Continued)*
 sudden asphyxic, 1084
 symptoms of, 1083-1084
Astrovirus, 2034t, 2057-2058
Asystole
 in hypothermia, 2238
 pediatric, 111-112, 112f, 2586t, 2590
 treatment of, 84-85
Ataxia
 cerebellar
  in high-altitude cerebral edema, 2306
  pediatric, 2681, 2682
 in multiple sclerosis, 1673
 pediatric, 2681-2682, 2681b
Ataxia telangiectasia, 2682
Atelectasis, in asthma, 2537, 2537f
Atenolol, 1321t
 during pregnancy and lactation, 2788
 for alcohol withdrawal syndrome, 2862
 overdose of, 2373t
Atheroembolism, 1343-1344, 1353, 1353f
Atherosclerosis
 coronary artery disease and, 1157
 in diabetes mellitus, 1970
 infected aneurysm in, 1356, 1357t
 pathophysiology of, 1342-1343
Athetoid cerebral palsy, 2904
Athletes
 injuries in. *See* Sports injuries.
 young, sudden death in, 2597-2599, 2597b
Atlantoaxial dislocation
 anterior, 399, 401, 402f
 rotary, 405-406, 408f
Atlantoaxial instability, in Down syndrome, 2901
Atlantoaxial separation, in retropharyngeal
  abscess, 1121
Atlanto-occipital dislocation, 399, 401, 402f
Atlas
 posterior neural arch fracture of, 410, 410f
 radiography of, 424, 424f-425f
Atmospheres absolute, 2280
Atmospheric cooling power, 2255
Atopic dermatitis, 1841-1842
Atopy
 in anaphylaxis, 1820, 2547
 in asthma, 2533
Atovaquone, in HIV/AIDS, side effects of, 2079t
Atracurium, in intubation, 14
Atrial clot, 1232
Atrial dysrhythmias, 1216
 in cocaine overdose, 2390
 in myocardial contusion, 469
Atrial fibrillation, 1230-1233, 1231f, 1232b, 1232f
 etiology of, 1230-1231, 1232b
 in hyperthyroidism, 1987
 in hypertrophic cardiomyopathy, 1296
 in hypothermia, 2238
 in infants and children, 2589
 in mitral stenosis, 1306
 ischemic stroke in, 1608
 observation in, 3070-3071, 3070b
 treatment of, 1231-1233, 1232b
Atrial fibrillation-flutter, 1231
Atrial flutter, 1229-1230, 1230f-1231f
 in infants and children, 2589
 with accessory pathway, 1229
Atrial parasystole, 1226
Atrial rupture, 470-472
Atrial septal defect, 2578
Atrial tachycardia, 1228-1229, 1228f, 1229f
 multifocal, 1228, 1229f
 nonparoxysmal, 1228
 paroxysmal, 1228
Atrioventricular block, 1218-1221
 antipsychotic-induced, 2447
 first-degree, 1218, 1219f
 in beta blocker overdose, 2374-2375
 in Lyme disease, 2123-2124, 2128
 second-degree
  Mobitz type I (Wenckebach), 1218-1219,
   1218t, 1219b, 1220f
  Mobitz type II, 1218, 1219-1220, 1220f
 third-degree (complete), 1220-1221, 1221f
Atrioventricular dissociation, isorhythmic, 1221
Atrioventricular node
 conduction and, 1202, 1202t, 1203, 1203f
 digitalis effects on, 2368
Atrium, penetrating injury to, 472
Atrophic vaginitis, 1569

Atropine
 for anaphylactic patient on beta blockers,
  1831b, 1833
 for asystole, 85
 for beta blocker overdose, 2375
 for bradycardia, 1215
 for calcium channel blocker–induced
  hypotension, 2377-2378
 for cardiac arrest, 93
 for complete atrioventricular block, 1221
 for digitalis toxicity, 2371
 for dysrhythmia, 2586b
 for nerve agent exposure, 3030-3031, 3031t
 for organophosphate poisoning, 2460
 for pediatric resuscitation, 99, 100, 101t-102t,
  103-104
 for pulseless electrical activity, 84
 for sinoatrial block, 1218
 for sinus node dysfunction, 1218
 in rapid sequence intubation, 11b
 mydriasis from, 1061
Attachment apparatus, 1027, 1027f
Attitudinal bias, 130
Attribution error, 130
Auditing systems for confidential medical
  records, 3103
Auditory symptoms, in vertigo, 144
Aura, migraine with, 2678, 2678b
Auscultation
 cardiac, in infants and children, 2571-2572,
  2572f
 for confirmation of endotracheal tube
  placement, 7
 of pregnant abdomen, 2728
Austin Flint murmur, in aortic regurgitation,
  1307
Authentication, in confidential medical records,
  3103
Authority gradients, as source of failures in
  emergency department, 3122
Authorization, in confidential medical records,
  3103
Autoimmune adrenal insufficiency, 1996
Autoimmune hemolytic anemia, 1882-1883,
  1883b
Autoimmune response, in systemic lupus
  erythematosus, 1806, 1808
Autoimmune thrombocytopenic purpura, 1897-
  1898
Automatic external defibrillators, in pediatric
  resuscitation, 113
Automaticity, altered, dysrhythmias from, 1204,
  1204f
Automobile cooling system, and body's heat
  dissipation mechanisms, 2256-2258, 2256f
Automotive products, bittering agents in, 2402
Autonomic arousal, 1745
Autonomic dysreflexia, in spinal cord injury,
  2906
Autonomic nervous system, 2459f
Autonomic neuropathy
 diabetic, 1971
 in alcohol withdrawal syndrome, 2861
 in tetanus, 2009
Autonomy, 3129, 3129b
Auto-pedestrian collisions. *See* Pedestrian
  collisions.
Autotransfusion, 59
 in hemothorax, 465
 in multiple trauma, 307-308
Avascular necrosis
 after fracture, 562
 after talar fracture, 824
 in knee trauma, 782
 in scuba diving–related disorders, 2286
 of femoral head, 739-741, 741b, 742f
  after femoral neck fracture, 740, 742f, 750-751
  pediatric, 767
 of proximal femoral epiphysis, 2706-2707,
  2707f
Aviation physiology, 2994-2995, 2995t
Aviator's fracture, 550t
Avolition, in schizophrenia, 1728
AVPU system, 330b
Avulsion, tooth, 389-390, 395, 1037-1040, 1038f,
  1039f
Avulsion fracture, 553, 554f
 femoral, 750, 750f
 fibular, 818

Avulsion fracture *(Continued)*
 of elbow, 2711, 2711f
 of greater tuberosity, in glenohumeral joint
  dislocation, 688
 of tibial tubercle, 798, 798f
 pelvic, 723-724, 724f
 sprains and, 566
Avulsion injuries
 nail bed, 611
 ring, in hand trauma, 612-613, 613b
 scalp, 372
Awake oral intubation, 12
Axillary artery, 540, 540f
 aneurysm of, 1354-1355
 injury to, 545
Axillary nerve
 anatomy of, 672
 injury to, after anterior glenohumeral joint
  dislocation, 687, 690
Axillary vein injury, 545
Axis, radiography of, 424, 424f-425f
Axonal injury
 in child abuse, 971
 in head trauma, 374
Axonotmesis, 559
Azathioprine, 2844
 for inflammatory bowel disease, 1502
 for myasthenia gravis, 1706
 for organ transplant patient, 2850
 in pregnancy, 2776
 toxicity of, 1417
Azidothymidine, in pregnancy, 2764t, 2774
Azithromycin
 during pregnancy and lactation, 2784
 for AIDS-related diarrhea, 1484
 for *Campylobacter* gastroenteritis, 1461, 1461t
 for chancroid, 1559t, 1563
 for *Chlamydia trachomatis* infection, 1559t,
  1565
 for chronic obstructive pulmonary disease,
  1106
 for granuloma inguinale, 1559t, 1563
 for Lyme disease, 1789, 2127t, 2128
 for *Mycobacterium avium* infection in
  HIV/AIDS, 2076
 for nongonococcal urethritis, 1565
 for pertussis, 2006
 for pharyngitis, 1113
 for pneumonia, 2558t
 for salmonellosis, 1463
 in HIV/AIDS, side effects of, 2079t
Azotemia. *See also* Uremia.
 evaluation of, 1533f, 1537
 prerenal, 1527t, 1532-1533, 1533b, 1538
Aztreonam, for febrile, neutropenic cancer
  patient, 2837, 2838t

B cell antibodies, 2832
B cells
 development of, 1820-1821, 1820f
 in asthma, 1080, 1080f
Babesiosis, 2104-2105, 2113, 2138-2140, 2139f
Babinski's sign
 in cerebral herniation, 355
 in head trauma, 357
Baby oil, for tar removal, 927
Bacille Calmette-Guérin (BCG) vaccine, 2170-
  2171, 2170b
Bacillus anthracis, 3024
Bacillus anthracis gastroenteritis, 1461t, 1462t,
  1468-1469
Bacillus cereus food poisoning, 1470t, 1471
Bacitracin ointment, for burn wounds, 926
Back, 490
 examination of, in back pain, 263
 gunshot wounds to, 506-507
 stab wounds to, 505
Back blows, for airway foreign body, 2530
Back pain, 260-267
 ancillary studies in, 264
 chronic, 713
 diagnostic approach to, 261-264, 261b, 262b,
  263f
 differential diagnosis in, 262t, 263f, 264, 265t-
  266t
 disposition in, 267
 empiric management of, 264, 266f, 267

Back pain (Continued)
  epidemiology of, 260-261
  functional, 703, 706
  history in, 261b, 262
  in diskitis, 1684
  in elderly person, 707
  in epidural abscess, 261, 265t, 703, 706, 712,
    1684
  in epidural hematoma, 1683
  in epidural spinal cord compression, 1919
  in pregnancy, 2733
  in spinal cord tumor, 1685
  in transverse myelitis, 1682
  low, 701-715
    anatomy and physiology in, 702, 702f
    clinical features of, 703-707, 704t, 705f
    differential considerations in, 709, 710b
    disposition in, 713
    epidemiology of, 701-702
    laboratory tests in, 707
    management of, 710-713, 711f
    pathophysiology of, 702-703
  pathophysiology of, 261
  pediatric, 703, 707, 713
  physical examination in, 261b, 262-264
  radiologic imaging in, 707-709, 708b, 708f-709f
  rapid assessment and stabilization in, 261-262,
    263f
  referred, 703, 706
  skeletal muscle relaxants for, 2928-2929
  uncomplicated, 703-704, 710-711
Baclofen
  for gastroesophageal reflux, 1390
  for spasticity in cerebral palsy, 2904
  for spasticity in multiple sclerosis, 1673
Bacteremia. See also Sepsis.
  definition of, 2212b
  gonococcal, 1566
  in AIDS-related diarrhea, 1483
  in infective endocarditis, 1301
  meningococcal, 2021, 2023
  pediatric fever and, 2505-2506, 2512, 2515
  pneumococcal, 2019
Bacterial infection
  hyperpyrexia in, 2506
  in bone or joint infections, 2177-2178, 2178t
  in botulism, 2012-2016
  in cancer patient with impaired cell-mediated
    immunity, 2839-2840
  in conjunctivitis, 296t
  in COPD exacerbation, 1099
  in croup, 2528-2529, 2529t
  in diarrhea, 228, 230b
  in diphtheria, 2001-2004, 2003b
  in endocarditis, prophylaxis for, 2590-2591,
    2591b
  in febrile cancer patient, 1908
  in Kawasaki disease, 2024-2027, 2025b
  in meningitis. See Meningitis, bacterial.
  in meningococcal disease, 2020-2024
  in organ transplant patient, 2848-2849, 2849f
  in otitis media, 1066-1067
  in peritonitis, 245-246, 1412-1413, 1441
  in peritonsillitis, 1117
  in pertussis, 2004-2007, 2005f, 2006b
  in pharyngitis, 274-275, 275t, 1109
  in pneumococcal disease, 2016-2020, 2020b
  in pneumonia, 1129, 1130-1131
    pediatric, 2555, 2556-2557, 2556f, 2557f,
      2558t, 2563f
  in prostatitis, 1586
  in sinusitis, 1123, 1124, 1125
  in tetanus, 2007-2012, 2008f, 2010b, 2012t,
    2013t
  in toxic shock syndrome, 2027-2031, 2028b,
    2029b, 2029t
  in tracheitis, 2528-2529, 2529t
  in vaginosis, 1567t, 1568-1569, 2758
  of hip and femur, pediatric limp from, 764
  serious, in children, signs of, 2658, 2659t
Bacterial pathogens
  in central nervous system infection, 1711t
  in contaminated blood products, 60-61
  in cutaneous abscess, 2203, 2203t
  in dental plaque, 1028
Bacteriology, in urinary tract infection, 1574-
  1575
Bacteriuria, 1573, 2757-2758
Bacteroides fragilis, in Ludwig's angina, 1032

Bad news, delivering, 3146-3147, 3146b
Bag/mask ventilation. See also Mask ventilation.
  difficult, evaluation of, 4, 4b
  in adult resuscitation, 87
  in neonatal resuscitation, 122
  in pediatric resuscitation, 108
Baker's cyst, 796, 797f
BAL (British anti-Lewisite), for mercury
  poisoning, 2426
Balanoposthitis, 2637-2638, 2638f
Balantidiasis, 2100t
Ballistic injury, nonpenetrating, in chest wall
  trauma, 458-459
Ballistics, handgun wound, 954-955
Balloon-tipped catheter for foreign body removal,
  862f, 863, 872-873
Ballottement, 2728
Bandage immobilization, 568-571
Bankart's fracture, in glenohumeral joint
  dislocation, 688
Barbiturates
  after cerebral ischemia, 71-72
  as induction agents, 15-16
  for GHB withdrawal, 2490
  for procedural sedation and analgesia, 2940t-
    2941t, 2945-2946
    in children, 2953
  for severe head trauma, 360-361
  overdose of, 2481-2483, 2482b, 2482f
  withdrawal from, 2482
Barium enema
  in appendicitis, 1454
  in colonic ischemia, 1504
  in colonic volvulus, 1498f
  in diverticular disease, 1493
  in intussusception, 2611, 2611f
Barlow provocative test, in developmental hip
  dysplasia, 2701, 2702b
Barodontalgia, in scuba diving–related disorders,
  2286
Barometric pressure, altitude and, 2297
Barosinusitis, in scuba diving–related disorders,
  2282
Barotitis, 2281-2282, 2282f, 2286-2287, 2287t,
  2292
Barotrauma, 2281
  external ear, 2282, 2292
  facial, 2282, 2293
  gastrointestinal, 2286
  inhalational, cocaine-induced, 2388
  inner ear, 2282, 2287-2288, 2287t, 2292
  middle ear, 2281-2282, 2282f, 2286-2287,
    2287t, 2292
  pulmonary, 2285-2286, 2293
Barrett's metaplasia, 1389
Bartholin abscess, 1560, 2205, 2205f
Bartholin cyst, 1559-1560
Barton bandage, for chronic temporomandibular
  joint dislocation, 1042
Bartonella, in infective endocarditis, 1301
Barton's fracture, 550t, 635-636, 636f
Bartter's syndrome, 1938
Basal ganglia lesions, in methanol poisoning,
  2396
Base deficit
  in abdominal trauma, 495
  in shock, 46, 47
Basic life support systems, 2985-2986
Basic life support techniques, in pediatric
  resuscitation, 97-99
Basilar artery migraine, 1632, 2679
  ataxia in, 2681
  vertigo in, 2683
Basilar impression, in osteogenesis imperfecta,
  2700-2701
Basilar skull fracture, 357, 358b, 373
  meningitis after, 370
Basophil(s), 2834
  activated, mediators of, 1823, 1823b
  normal values for, 1886t
Battered child syndrome, 973
Batteries
  impaction of, 1384
  ingestion of, 871, 873, 2384-2385
Battering. See Abuse.
Battery, 2967
Baumann's angle, 651-652, 651f, 2694, 2695f
Bayesian statistics, 3056
Bazin's disease, 1816

Beanbag shotgun shells, ballistic injury
  associated with, 458-459
Beau's lines, in Kawasaki disease, 2026
Bed rest
  for high-altitude pulmonary edema, 2304
  for myocarditis, 1290
Bee pollen, adverse effects of, 2476t
Bee stings. See Hymenoptera stings.
Behavior
  as symptom, 2976
  grossly disorganized, in schizophrenia,
    1728
  of difficult patient, classification of, 2978-2981,
    2978t. See also Difficult patient.
  violent. See Combative patient; Violence.
Behavioral disorders. See also Psychiatric
  disorders.
  in bacterial meningitis, 2658, 2659
  in hyperthyroidism, 1987
  in PCP intoxication, 2414, 2415-2416
  seizures vs., 2668
Behavioral risk factors, in injury prevention and
  control, 947-948
Behçet's disease, 1814-1815
Belladona alkaloids, anticholinergic toxicity of,
  2345, 2346, 2346b, 2347t
Bell's palsy, 1666-1667, 1668, 2123
Benazepril hydrochloride, 1322t
Bendroflumethiazide, during pregnancy and
  lactation, 2788
Bends, 2279, 2284
Beneficence, 3129, 3129b
Benign early repolarization, ST segment
  elevation in, 1166-1167, 1167f, 1168f
Benign paroxysmal positional vertigo, 147t,
  2683
Benign rolandic epilepsy, 2666
Bennett's fracture, 550t, 599-600, 599f
Benzalkonium chloride, for rabies postexposure
  prophylaxis, 2068
Benzathine penicillin
  for Lyme disease, 1789
  for rheumatic fever, 1791
  for scarlet fever, 1851
  for streptococcal pharyngitis, 1304
  for syphilis, 1856
Benznidazole, for Chagas' disease, 2112
Benzocaine, topical, 2933
Benzodiazepines
  as induction agents, 16
  during pregnancy and lactation, 2787
  for agitation, 1654, 2349
  for alcohol withdrawal syndrome, 2861-2862,
    2863
  for alcohol-related seizure, 2864, 2865
  for anxiety disorders, 1750-1751, 1751t
  for back pain, 267
  for bupropion-induced seizure, 2361
  for cocaine overdose, 2391
  for GHB withdrawal, 2490
  for PCP intoxication, 2416, 2892
  for procedural sedation and analgesia, 2940t-
    2941t, 2944-2945
    in children, 2953
  for psychedelic-induced intoxication, 2408
  for rapid tranquilization, 2962-2963
  for seizure, 166, 166t, 1626, 1627t
  for status epilepticus, 2672-2673, 2672t
  for tetanus, 2010-2011
  for thought disorders, 1731
  in heatstroke, 2265
  in ventilated patient, 30
  overdose of, 2483-2486, 2484t
    antidote to, 2326, 2329t, 2485-2486, 2485b
  prophylactic, in severe head trauma, 361
  reversal agents for, 2949
  withdrawal from, 2486, 2486b
Benztropine
  anticholinergic toxicity of, 2345
  for acute extrapyramidal symptoms, 2449
  for mood disorders, 1741
Bepridril, overdose of, 2376, 2377t
Bereavement, depression vs., 1740
Best interests, 3134
Beta₂ agonists
  during pregnancy and lactation, 2762, 2765t,
    2789
  for anaphylactic shock, 54
  for anaphylaxis, 1831b, 1832

Beta₂ agonists (Continued)
for asthma, 1086-1088, 1087t, 2538, 2539t, 2540-2541
for bronchiolitis, 2546
for chronic obstructive pulmonary disease, 1105
for hyperkalemia, 1941
for pneumonia, 2562
Beta blockers, 1208-1209, 1208t, 1321t
contraindications to, 1208
during pregnancy and lactation, 2788
for acute coronary syndromes, 1184-1185
for alcohol withdrawal syndrome, 2862
for anxiety disorders, 1751
for aortic dissection, 1328
for atrial fibrillation, 1232-1233
for atrial flutter, 1229
for atrial tachycardia, 1228
for chloral hydrate poisoning, 2487
for chronic heart failure, 1276-1277
for dilated cardiomyopathy, 1294
for glaucoma, 1063b
for hypertension, 1320
for hypertensive emergencies, 1318-1319
for hypertrophic cardiomyopathy, 1295
for junctional tachycardia, 1234
for migraine prophylaxis, 1634
for premature ventricular contractions, 1225
for tetanus, 2011
for thyroid storm, 1989
for torsades de pointes, 1244
for ventricular tachycardia, 1242-1243
for Wolff-Parkinson-White syndrome, 1237
heart failure from, 1269
overdose of, 2373-2376, 2373t, 2374b, 2375b
Beta (β) error, 3051t, 3052
Beta particles, 2319, 2320f
Betamethasone valerate, for phimosis, 2636
Beta-mimetics, for premature labor, 2806-2807, 2806b
Betaxolol, 1321t, 2373t
Betel nut
adverse effects of, 2476t
drug interactions with, 2478t
Bethanecol, for nausea and vomiting in children, 206
Beverages, MAOI toxicity and, 2364, 2364b
Bezoar
gastrointestinal, 873, 875
urinary tract, 877
Bezold abscess, in mastoiditis, 1072
Bias
attitudinal, 130
cognitive, 3122
confirmation, 132
definition of, 3059t
publication, 3050-3051, 3058
selection, 3049
visceral, 3122
Bicarbonate
in metabolic acidosis, 1929
in metabolic alkalosis, 1930
in respiratory acidosis, 1925
in respiratory alkalosis, 1926
inhalational, for irritant gas exposure, 2434-2435
sodium. See Sodium bicarbonate.
Bicarbonate–carbonic acid buffer system, 1923
Biceps muscle lesions, 697-698, 697f
Biceps tendon
long head of, 672, 673f, 697
rupture of, 668, 697-698
short head of, 697
subluxation and dislocation of, 698
Bicipital tendinopathy, 1797
Bicipital tenosynovitis, 697, 697f
Bier block, 2934
Bigemy, 1222, 1222f
Bile acid administration, for cholelithiasis, 1419
Bile duct(s)
common, obstruction of, in cholangitis, 1421, 1422f
extrahepatic, carcinoma of, 1423
Bilevel positive airway pressure, 28, 28f
in critically ill asthmatic patient, 1092
Biliary cirrhosis, 1410
Biliary colic, in cholelithiasis, 1418
Biliary pancreatitis, 1426, 1427, 1428, 1433, 1434
Biliary tract carcinoma, 1423

Biliary tract disorders, 1418-1423
abdominal pain in, 210t
in children, 2620-2621
nausea and vomiting in, 204t
obstructive, jaundice in, 243, 244f
Bilious vomiting, in malrotation with midgut volvulus, 2606
Bilirubin
in acute pancreatitis, 1431, 1431t
in hemolytic anemia, 1878
in hepatitis, 1404
in infants and children, 2601-2603, 2602t, 2603b, 2603t, 2604f-2605f
in pyogenic abscess, 1415
metabolism of, 243
Bimalleolar fractures, 813
Bioethics, 3127-3138
dilemmas in, 3130-3131, 3132-3137
emergency medicine guidelines and, 3044
in decision-making capacity and consent, 3133-3135, 3134b
in disasters and triage, 3136
in emergency medicine, 3131-3137, 3131b, 3131t
in HIV/AIDS, 2089-2090
in medical teaching/training, 3135-3136
in occupational medicine, 3077
in prehospital resuscitation, 3132-3133
in resuscitation research, 3136-3137
in withholding and withdrawing treatment, 3132
legal issues vs., 3128
professional etiquette vs., 3128
values and, 3128-3130, 3129b, 3130b
Bioethics committees
as surrogate decision-makers, 3135
role of, 3137-3138
Bioethics consultants, as surrogate decision-makers, 3135
Biofeedback, for anxiety disorders, 1751
Biologic weapon(s), 3023-3029, 3024b
anthrax as, 3021, 3024-3026, 3025f, 3026b, 3026f
botulinum toxin as, 2013
disaster preparedness for, 3018
infectious agents as, 3024, 3024b
plague as, 3027-3028, 3027f, 3028b
smallpox as, 3028-3029, 3028f, 3029f
warning signs of, 3024, 3024b
Biological factors, in suicide, 1767-1768
Biomechanical properties of skin, 843
Biomechanical risk factors, in injury prevention and control, 946-947
Biomechanics of head trauma, 352
Biophysical profile of fetus, 2802, 2802t
Bioprosthetic valve, complications of, 1308
Biopsy
endomyocardial
in dilated cardiomyopathy, 1294
in myocarditis, 1290, 1290f
rectal, in AIDS-related diarrhea, 1484
skin, in Rocky Mountain spotted fever, 2135
small bowel, in AIDS-related diarrhea, 1484
Bipolar disorder
clinical features of, 1738-1739
differential considerations in, 1740-1741
epidemiology of, 1735
hypomanic episode in, 1738
manic episode in, 1738-1739, 1738b
mixed, 1739
pathophysiology of, 1735-1736
stabilization in, 1741
treatment of, 1742
Bipyridyl compound poisoning, 2465-2466, 2465b
Bird's beak sign, in colonic volvulus, 1498f
Birth, transitional circulation at, 118-119, 119t, 2568
Birth defects
alcohol-related, 2791-2792, 2791b
drug-induced, 2779-2780, 2780b
Birth trauma, postpartum hemorrhage from, 2818
Bismuth
for diarrhea, 236t
for traveler's diarrhea, 1486
for upper gastrointestinal disorders, 1399
Bisoprolol fumarate, 1321t, 2373t
Bispectral Index monitoring, during procedural sedation and analgesia, 2942

Bisphosphonates
for hypercalcemia, 1946
for hypercalcemic cancer patient, 1916
Bite
animal, 882-892
antibiotic prophylaxis in, 887-889, 887t
cats in, 883-884, 888
disposition in, 889-890
dogs in, 882-883, 887-888
domestic herbivores in, 885
epidemiology of, 882
ferrets in, 884-885
infected, treatment of, 889-890
infection risks in, 885-886, 885t
management of, 886-889, 886b, 887t, 889b, 889t
pigs in, 885
primates in, 884, 888-889, 889b, 889t
reporting requirements for, 3172-3173
rodents in, 884
systemic infection in, 885
wild animals in, 885
antibiotic prophylaxis for, 854-855
human, 890-892, 891t, 892b
antibiotic prophylaxis in, 891-892
antiviral prophylaxis in, 891
in child abuse, 969
in clenched-fist injuries, 611
in extensor tendon injuries at metacarpophalangeal joint, 608
in sexual assault, 986b
infected, treatment of, 892, 892b
tetanus prophylaxis in, 891, 891t
to penis, 534
rabies transmission from, 2065
venomous, 894-911
arthropods in, 903-908
marine animals in, 908-909, 910
scorpions in, 907-908
snakes and other reptiles in, 895-903, 897f, 897t, 900t
spiders in, 905-907
venom delivery in, 895
Bite marks, in physical assault, 962, 962f
Bitolterol, for asthma, 2538, 2539t
Bittering agents, in automotive products, 2402
Bivalirudin, in myocardial infarction, 1188
BK virus, 2045-2046
Black widow spider bite, 905-906, 2329t
Bladder
anatomy of, 519
decompression of, for urinary retention, 1599
distention of, in spinal cord injury, 2906
dysfunction of, in multiple sclerosis, 1672
neurogenic, in spinal cord injury, 2908
physical examination of, 1572-1573
stones in, 1593
trauma to, 519-526, 521f-526f, 719
Bladder neck obstruction, 1538
Blanch sign of Steele, in slipped capital femoral epiphysis, 2708
Blastic crisis, in chronic myeloid leukemia, 1888
Blastomyces dermatitidis, in pneumonia, 1130
Bleach, ingestion of, 2380-2381
Blebs, in frostbite, 2231
Bleeding. See also Hemorrhage.
after hemodialysis, 1549
from arteriovenous fistula or graft, 1366
gastrointestinal, 220-227. See also Gastrointestinal bleeding.
in facial trauma, 389, 390
in hemothorax, 465
in neck trauma, 444
in peripheral vascular injury, 539
in radiation proctocolitis, 1505
nasal, 394
rectal, 1508
in Meckel's diverticulum, 2613
with defecation, 1508
vaginal, 254-259. See also Vaginal bleeding.
Bleeding diathesis
in alcoholism, 2874
in disseminated intravascular coagulation, 1903
in hyperviscosity syndrome, 1913
in pregnancy, 2753t
Bleeding disorders, 1892-1904
ancillary studies in, 1894-1895, 1894b
clinical features of, 1894-1895, 1894b

Bleeding disorders (Continued)
  differential diagnosis and management of,
    1895-1904
  disposition in, 1904
  in alcoholism, 2874
  in coagulopathies, 1899-1904
  in platelet disorders, 1896-1899, 1896b
  in vascular disorders, 1896, 1896b
  pathophysiology of, 1892-1894, 1893b, 1893f
Bleeding time, in bleeding disorders, 1895
Blepharitis, 293t, 1055
Blinding in clinical trials, 3049
Blindness. See also Visual loss.
  cortical, 1060
  legal, 2905
  postconcussive, 367
  river, 2109, 2109f
Blister
  burn, 925
  fracture, 563
  in frostbite, 2232, 2233f
  in mustard exposure, 3031
Blocking agents, for internal radioactive
    contamination, 2324
Blood
  leukodepleted, in hemorrhagic shock, 52
  occult, tests for, in gastrointestinal bleeding,
    222
  vomiting of, 221
Blood agents, as chemical weapons, 939, 3031-
    3032
Blood alcohol concentration (BAC), 2859
Blood alcohol tests, police-requested,
    medicolegal issues in, 3160
Blood banking, 57
Blood component therapy, 56-61
  clinical features in, 58
  decision making in, 58-59
  outcomes in, 59-61
  pathophysiologic principles in, 57-58, 58t
  therapeutic modalities in, 59
Blood culture
  in acute septic arthritis, 2705
  in AIDS-related diarrhea, 1483-1484
  in bacterial meningitis, 2662
  in central nervous system infection, 1720
  in gastrointestinal anthrax, 1469
  in infected aneurysm, 1356
  in infective endocarditis, 1301-1302
  in meningococcal disease, 2022
  in pediatric fever, 2510
  in pneumococcal disease, 2018
  in pneumonia, 1135, 2561
  in sepsis, 2216-2217
Blood dyscrasias, oral manifestations of, 1036
Blood flow. See also Circulation.
  cerebral, 350-352, 351f
    after brain resuscitation, 68
    autoregulation of, 351
      loss of, 354
    during cardiopulmonary resuscitation, 67
    during cerebral ischemia, 62, 63f-64f
    in hypothermia, 2238
    in stroke, 1606-1607
    restoration of, after cardiac arrest, 62-64
  during cardiopulmonary resuscitation, 76-77
  renal, in hypothermia, 2239
  to skin, in pediatric assessment triangle, 2498t,
    2499, 2499f
Blood gases, arterial. See Arterial blood gases.
Blood loss, anemia from, 1868
Blood pressure. See also Hypertension;
    Hypotension.
  in pregnancy, 316, 317t, 2725, 2727
  management of
    guidelines for, 3038
    in aortic rupture, 481
    in peripheral vascular injury, 543
  measurement of, 1310-1311
  monitoring of, 35-36
  normalization of, in sepsis, 2218
  pediatric, 2495, 2495t, 2571, 2571t, 2578, 2651t
Blood products, bacterial contamination of, 60-61
Blood protein buffers, 1923
Blood sample, in anemia, 1869
Blood smear
  in anemia, 1869
  in babesiosis, 2140
  in bleeding disorders, 1894

Blood smear (Continued)
  in hemolytic anemia, 1877, 1877f, 1878f
  in sickle cell disease, 1881, 1881f
Blood supply
  to face, 385, 385f
  to femur and hip, 737, 737t, 738f
  to foot, 821
  to forearm, 640t
  to hand, 585-586, 587f, 588f
  to knee, 771
  to lower leg, 797
  to nose, 1073, 1073f
  to pelvis, 717-718
  to shoulder, 672
  to wrist, 622, 625f
Blood tests
  in chronic obstructive pulmonary disease, 1101
  in gastrointestinal bleeding, 222
  in septic arthritis, 2189
Blood transfusion, 56-61
  adjuncts in, 58
  clinical features in, 58
  decision making in, 58-59
  hepatitis C infection risk in, 1403
  hypocalcemia after, 1943
  in autoimmune hemolytic anemia, 1883
  in gastrointestinal bleeding, 222
  in hemolytic uremic syndrome, 2655
  in kernicterus prophylaxis, 2603, 2604f
  in multiple trauma, 307-308
  in pelvic fracture, 723, 728, 731
  in peripheral vascular injury, 543
  in placenta previa or abruptio placentae, 2748
  in sickle cell disease, 1880
  in thalassemia, 1872-1873
  massive, 57-58
  outcomes in, 59-61
  pathophysiologic principles in, 57-58, 58t
  refusal of, 3171-3172
  therapeutic modalities in, 59
  thrombocytopenia after, 1897
  viral infection transmission and, 57t, 61
Blood typing, 57, 58
Blood urea nitrogen (BUN), 1527
  dialysis and, 1549
  in acute renal failure, 2649
  in hypothermia, 2243
  in nausea and vomiting, 203
Blood volume, in pregnancy, 316-317, 317t, 2724,
    2724f
Blood-borne pathogen exposure, 3081-3087,
    3084f, 3085t, 3086b
Bloodborne Pathogen Standard, 3082
Blood-brain barrier, 350
Bloody show, in labor and delivery, 2798-2799
Bloody stool, 221
  in hemolytic uremic syndrome, 2654
  in hemorrhagic Escherichia coli serotype
    O157:H7 gastroenteritis, 1466
  in inflammatory bowel disease, 2616
  in intussusception, 2610
  in Plesiomonas shigelloides gastroenteritis,
    1468
Blowout fracture, orbital wall, 393
"Blue bloater," 1099
Blue cohosh, adverse effects of, 2476t
Blue leg, painful, 1370
Blue toe syndrome
  in abdominal aortic aneurysm, 1332
  in arteriosclerosis obliterans, 1350
  in atheroembolism, 1343, 1353, 1353f
Blunt trauma
  abdominal
    diagnostic studies in, 507-508, 507t
    epidemiology of, 489
    history in, 493
    management of, 508-510, 508f, 509t, 510f,
      511f
    observation in, 3067
    pathophysiology of, 491-492
    physical examination in, 494-495
  chest
    aortic injury in, 476-482, 477f-479f, 481b
    cardiac injury in, 467-472
    esophageal injury in, 483-484
    flail chest and, 457
    observation in, 3068
  from lightning, 2271
  in physical assault, 960-962, 961f-962f

Blunt trauma (Continued)
  in pregnancy, 318, 2734
  in sternal fracture, 456
  ocular, 1044-1051
  peripheral vascular injury in, 536-547
    clinical features of, 539-541, 540f
    diagnostic strategies in, 541-543
    disposition in, 547
    epidemiology of, 536-537
    of lower extremity, 546-547
    of upper extremity, 544-546
    pathophysiology of, 537-539, 538f
    treatment of, 543-544
  renal, 527, 528-530, 530f
  to ear, 392
  to neck
    pathophysiology of, 442
    pharyngoesophageal injuries in, 446-447
    vascular injuries in, 448-450
  ureteral, 530
Bockhart, impetigo of, 2202
Body
  cooling of
    for comatose survivors of cardiac arrest, 69
    for heatstroke, 2263-2264, 2264b, 2265f
  rewarming of. See Rewarming.
  skin tension lines of, 844f
  viewing of, after death, 3148-3149
Body lice, 1853-1854, 1853f
Body packing/stuffing
  cocaine, 2391-2392
  management of, 874-875, 2886
  opioid, 2454
Body surface area assessment, in burn injury,
    919-920, 920f
Body surface mapping, in acute coronary
    syndromes, 1174
Body temperature
  abnormalities of. See Fever; Heat illness;
    Hyperthermia; Hypothermia.
  changes in, during air medical transport, 2995
  determination of, in children, 2508
  regulation of. See Thermoregulation.
Boehler's angle, 827, 827f
Boerhaave's syndrome, 201-202, 206t, 484
Bolivian hemorrhagic fever, 2056
Bone
  anatomy of, 2174-2175, 2175f
  as buffer, 1923
  fracture of. See Fracture.
  growing, 554, 556f, 2689
  infection of. See Osteomyelitis.
  needle aspiration of, in osteomyelitis, 2182
  of distal humerus and elbow, 647, 647f
  of foot, 820-821, 820f
  of forearm, 639
  of hand, 577-578, 579f-580f
  of hip and femur, 736-737, 737f
  of knee, 770, 771f
  of lower leg, 797
  of wrist, 622, 623f
  periosteal formation of, 2699
  plastic deformation of, 2690
Bone bruise, in knee, 781
Bone cancer, hypercalcemia in, 1914
Bone marrow transplantation
  for aplastic anemia, 1875-1876
  for sickle cell disease, 1881
Bone pain, in osteomyelitis, 2179
Bone scan
  in ankle trauma, 811
  in arthritis, 1780
  in foot trauma, 822
  in fracture, 558
  in frostbite, 2231
  in hip fracture, 746, 748f
  in knee trauma, 774
  in Legg-Calvé-Perthes disease, 2707
  in lower leg stress fractures, 804
  in osteomyelitis, 2180-2181, 2180f, 2181f
  in scaphoid fracture, 628
  in septic arthritis, 2189-2190
  in stress fracture of foot, 838
Bone tumor, osteomyelitis vs., 2186
Bonferonni correction for reducing risk of type I
    error, 3053-3054
Bonfils Intubating Fiberscope, 21, 22f
Bony fish injuries, 910-911
Borborygmi, in Giardia gastroenteritis, 1479

Borderline personality disorder, 2979b
  depression vs., 1740
  suicide and, 1769
Bordetella pertussis/parapertussis, 2004-2007,
  2005f, 2006b, 2559-2560
Borrelia burgdorferi, 2118. See also Lyme
  disease.
Borrelia spp., in relapsing fever, 2129
Bosworth fracture, 550t
Botanical poisoning. See Plant poisoning.
Botulinum toxin, 2013, 2014
  for anal fissures, 1513
Botulism, 1707-1708, 2012-2016
Bougienage, for foreign body removal, 873, 2617
Boutonniére deformity, 607, 607f
Bovine pustular stomatitis virus, 2040
Bowel. See Intestinal *entries;* Intestine(s); Large
  intestine; Small intestine.
Bowel sounds, in abdominal trauma, 494
Bowstring sign, in lumbar radiculopathy, 704
Boxer's fracture, 550t, 597, 597f
Boyle's law, 2280, 2281f, 2994
Brachial artery
  anatomy of, 540, 540f, 648, 648f
  injury to, 545, 665
Brachial plexus, 672, 1676
  compression of, thoracic outlet syndrome from,
    1358
  injury to, 1692-1693, 1693b
    axillary artery injury and, 545
    scapula fracture and, 680
    subclavian artery injury and, 545
  testing of, 674, 674t
Bracing, functional, for ankle immobilization,
  571
Bradycardia, 1215
  in beta blocker overdose, 2374-2375
  in hypothermia, 2237
  pediatric, 111, 111f, 2585, 2586t
  sinus, 1215-1216, 1216f
    from succinylcholine, 13
    in hypothyroidism, 1992
Bradycardia-tachycardia syndrome, 1231
Brain. See also Cerebral *entries.*
  anatomy and physiology of, 350-352, 351f
  cellular damage to, in head trauma, 352-353,
    353f
  contusion of, 374
  diffuse axonal injury in, 374
  inflammation of. See Encephalitis.
  membranes of, inflammation of. See
    Meningitis.
  pediatric, vulnerability of, 366
  swelling of. See Cerebral edema.
  traumatic injury to. See Head trauma;
    Traumatic brain injury.
Brain abscess
  after head trauma, 370-371
  ancillary studies in, 1720
  cerebrospinal fluid analysis in, 1716-1719,
    1717t, 1718t, 1719f
  complications of, 1716
  diagnosis of, 1716-1720
  differential considerations in, 1720, 1721b
  disposition in, 1723
  epidemiology of, 1711
  etiology of, 1712
  headache in, 174t, 1641, 2678
  in cancer patient, 1920
  in otitis media, 1068
  lumbar puncture in, 1716, 1716b
  management of, 1722, 1723
  neuroimaging studies in, 1719-1720
  pathophysiology of, 1713, 1713f
  risk factors for, 171b
  signs and symptoms of, 1714-1715
Brain damage
  seizure and, 2665
  violent behavior and, 2957
Brain death, 3141
Brain resuscitation, 62-73
  clinical outcomes in, 72-73
  experimental therapies in, 70-72
  pathophysiology of cerebral ischemia and, 62-
    67, 63f-64f
  standard strategies for, 67-70, 69t
Brain tumor
  ataxia in, 2681
  cerebral herniation in, 1918

Brain tumor *(Continued)*
  headache in, 1637-1638, 2678
  in pregnancy, 2732
Brainstem
  assessment of, in head trauma, 357
  in arousal, 156
Brainstem encephalitis, ataxia in, 2681
Brainstem reflex examination, in comatose
  patient, 159t, 160-161
Branham's sign, 1347
Brassaia, 2472
BRAT diet, for diarrhea, 235
Braxton-Hicks contractions, 2728, 2798
Breast
  cancer of
    hypercalcemia in, 1914
    superior vena cava syndrome in, 1909
  changes in, during pregnancy, 2724, 2728
Breast milk jaundice, 2601-2603, 2602t, 2603b,
  2603t, 2604f-2605f
Breast-feeding, in HIV/AIDS, 2774
Breath sounds
  in tension pneumothorax, 462
  in tuberculosis, 2150
Breath-holding spells
  definition of, 2714
  seizures vs., 2668
Breathing
  management of
    in cardiac arrest, 87
    in elderly trauma patient, 348
    in pediatric resuscitation, 98, 108-109
    in pediatric trauma, 329-330, 332t
  periodic, in acute mountain sickness, 2301,
    2302
  work of, in pediatric assessment triangle, 2498-
    2499, 2498f, 2498t, 2499f
Breathlessness. See Dyspnea.
Breech presentations, in labor and delivery,
  2811-2813, 2811b, 2812f, 2813b
Bretylium, 1209
"Bridegroom's palsy," 1695
Broca's aphasia, in ischemic stroke, 1609
Brodie's abscess, 2184
Bromocriptine, for neuroleptic malignant
  syndrome, 2449
Bronchial artery embolization, for hemoptysis, 282
Bronchial hyperresponsiveness, in asthma, 2533
Bronchiectasis
  hemoptysis in, 280
  in chronic obstructive pulmonary disease,
    1102-1103
Bronchiolitis, in children, 2509b, 2544-2546
Bronchitis
  chronic, 1097, 1100
  high-altitude, 2304
  laryngotracheal, 2525-2527, 2526f, 2527b
Broncholithiasis, hemoptysis in, 280
Bronchopleural fistula, 466
Bronchopulmonary dysplasia, 2565, 2565f
Bronchorrhea, in organophosphate poisoning,
  2459
Bronchoscopy
  in acute inhalation injury, 921
  in foreign body removal, 870, 2551
  in hemoptysis, 282
  in neck trauma, 445
  in tracheobronchial injury, 466
  in tuberculosis, 2154
Bronchospasm
  heroin-induced, 2452-2453
  in anaphylaxis, 1825t, 1829-1830
  in irritant gas exposure, 2434
Bronchostenosis, tuberculous, 2151
Bronchus, ruptured, subcutaneous emphysema
  and, 459
Broselow emergency tape, in pediatric
  resuscitation, 106, 114f-115f
Brow presentations, in labor and delivery, 2815-
  2816
Brown recluse spider bite, 906-907
Brown-Séquard syndrome, 418, 419f, 420, 1677-
  1678, 1678f
Brudzinski sign
  in bacterial meningitis, 2659
  in central nervous system infection, 1714
Brugada criteria, 1237, 1239f
Bruises, in child abuse, 969-971, 969f, 970f, 970t,
  2502b

Bruit, in arteriovenous fistula, 539, 541
Bruit de moulin, in myocardial rupture, 471
Brush ECG criteria, for risk stratification in acute
  coronary ischemia, 3065
B-type natriuretic peptide
  as cardiac marker, 1178
  in asthma, 1085
  in chronic obstructive pulmonary disease,
    1101, 1102
  in heart failure, 1269-1270
  in pulmonary embolism, predictive value of,
    1377, 1378t
Bubo, in tularemia, 2131
Bubonic plague, 3027, 3027f
Buccal space infection, 1028-1029
Bucket-handle fracture, 727, 729f
Bucket-handle tears, meniscal, 792
Buckle fracture, 800, 2690, 2690f
Buddy-taping
  of metacarpal or phalangeal fractures, 595, 595f
  of phalangeal fractures, 834
Budesonide
  for asthma, 1089
  for viral croup, 2526-2527
Buerger's disease, 1351-1352
Buerger's sign, 1346
Buffer systems, physiologic, 1923
Buffer therapy. See Sodium bicarbonate.
Buffering, in local anesthesia, 846, 2932-2933,
  2932b
Bufo toad, tryptamines obtained from, 2407
Bulk agents, for constipation, 241t, 242
Bullae, 1839t
  giant, pneumothorax vs., 1146
  in frostbite, 2231
  in pemphigus vulgaris, 1857, 1857f
  in varicella, 1858, 1859f
  subpleural, in pneumothorax, 1145
Bullet
  handgun, 954, 954f
  rubber, ballistic injury associated with, 458-459
Bullet resistant vests, ballistic injury associated
  with, 458-459
Bullosis diabeticorum, 1972
Bullous impetigo, 1842, 1843, 2202
Bullous myringitis, 1066-1067
Bullying behavior, 1017
Bumetanide, 1321t
  for acute renal failure, 2650
Bundle branch fascicles, 1202
Bunyavirus, 2034t, 2055
Bupivacaine, 2931, 2932t, 2933
  allergy to, 846-847
  for femoral and hip fractures, 749
  for local anesthesia, 846
  in knee trauma, 776
  in radial head and neck fracture, 664
Buprenorphine, 2924-2925, 2924b
Bupropion, overdose of, 2361, 2361t
Burkholderia cepacia, in cystic fibrosis, 2564-
  2565
Burn
  chemical, 929-939
    acid and alkali burns in, 931-933
    anhydrous ammonia in, 934-935
    caustics in, 2380-2385, 2381f, 2381t, 2382f
    cement burns in, 935
    chemical terrorism and, 937-939, 938t
    community preparedness and HAZMAT
      response in, 930-931
    elemental metals in, 937
    esophageal perforation from, 483
    formic acid in, 934
    hydrocarbon-related, 936-937
    hydrofluoric acid in, 933-934
    nitrates in, 936
    pathophysiology of, 930
    phenol and derivatives in, 935-936
    tar burns in, 937
    white phosphorus in, 936
  classification of, 913
  epidemiology of, 913-914, 914f
  feathering, 2273, 2273f
  in acute radiation syndrome, 2322
  in elderly person, 347
  in electrical and lightning injuries, 2267-2277
    clinical features of, 2271-2274, 2272f
    complications of, 2274
    differential considerations in, 2275

Burn *(Continued)*
disposition in, 2277
management of, 2275-2277, 2276b
mechanisms of, 2270-2271, 2270b
perioral, 391
physics of, 2267-2270, 2268t, 2269t
in mustard exposure, 3031
kissing, 2272, 2272f
management of, 920-927
pathophysiology of, 915-919
powder, 953
thermal, 913-928
airway management and respiratory care in, 921-923
anatomy of skin and, 914-915
burn shock and, 918
burn wound assessment in, 919-920, 920f
burn wound care in, 924-927, 925f
catheterization of patient in, 923
depth of burn injury in, 918-919, 919f
disposition in, 927, 927b
epidemiology of, 913-914, 914f
fluid resuscitation in, 921, 922-923
gastrointestinal disorders in, 924
in child abuse, 969-970, 970f, 970t
in lightning injury, 2273
in physical assault, 963, 964f
metabolic response to therapy in, 919
ocular, 1046
pain management in, 924
patient categorization in, 920
pediatric considerations in, 923
physiologic changes in, 917-918
prehospital care in, 921
thermodynamics of burn injury in, 915-917, 915t, 916f, 917t
transportation of patient in, 923-924
white phosphorus in, 936
zones of tissue injury in, 917, 917f
Burn center, patient transfer to, 927, 927b
Burn shock, 918
Burnout, in emergency physician, 3175-3176
Burow's solution, for tinea corporis, 1839-1840
Bursa
aspiration of, 1802
elbow, 649
radiohumeral, 649
radioulnar, flexor tendons and, 585, 586f
trochanteric, calcification of, 742, 744f
Bursitis, 568, 1801-1804
anserine, 1803-1804
calcific of femur and hip, 742, 744f
common sites for, 1796f
iliopsoas, 1803
ischiogluteal, 1803
knee, 795-796
olecranon and prepatellar, 1801-1803
septic, 1801-1803
subacromial, 693-696, 694t, 695f, 1803
subcalcaneal, 836
trochanteric, 1803
Burst fracture of vertical body, 411-412, 411f-413f, 426, 427f
Buspirone
for anxiety disorders, 1751, 1751t
for opioid withdrawal, 2456
overdose of, 2486
Butanediol, overdose of, 2488b, 2489
Butorphanol, 2924, 2924b
Butter, for tar removal, 927
Button (disk) batteries, ingestion of, 871, 873, 875, 2384-2385
Buttonhole deformity, 607, 607f
Butyrophenones
cardiotoxicity of, 2445
for alcohol withdrawal syndrome, 2862
for psychedelic-induced intoxication, 2408
for psychostimulant intoxication, 2410
Bypass, cardiopulmonary. *See* Cardiopulmonary bypass.
Bypass graft
coronary artery, previous, fibrinolytic therapy eligibility and, 1191
for peripheral arteriovascular disease, 1350

Cachexia, palliative care for, 3154
Café coronary, 865, 1383

Caffeine
for postdural puncture headache, 1641
sudden infant death syndrome and, 2719-2720
CAGE questions, for alcoholism, 2858
Caisson's disease, 2279, 2284
Calcaneofibular ligament injury, 816, 817
Calcaneus
fracture of, 826-827, 826f, 827f
stress fracture of, 836, 837
Calcification
in bursitis of femur and hip, 742, 744f
in hip trauma, 741-742, 743f-755f
in pancreatitis, 1435-1436, 1436f
in peritendinitis of femur and hip, 742
in tendinitis, 698
in tendinopathy, 568, 1797-1798
of gallstones, 1418, 1418f
Calcitonin
for hypercalcemia, 1915, 1946
in calcium homeostasis, 1941
Calcium
for beta blocker overdose, 2375
for hyperkalemia
in acute renal failure, 1539
in chronic renal failure, 1545, 1545t
for hypermagnesemia, 1950
for hypocalcemia, 1539, 1943-1944
for pediatric resuscitation, 101t, 104
imbalance of. *See* Hypercalcemia; Hypocalcemia.
in cerebral ischemia, 65
in phosphate homeostasis, 1950-1951
in resting membrane potential, 1199-1200, 1200f
in shock, 45
normal physiology of, 1941-1942
serum, measurement of, 1942
Calcium antacids, for upper gastrointestinal disorders, 1398
Calcium apatite crystals, in pseudogout, 1787
Calcium channel blockers, 1210-1211, 1321t
after cerebral ischemia, 71
antidotes to, 2329t
during pregnancy and lactation, 2788
for acute coronary syndromes, 1185
for atrial fibrillation, 1232-1233
for atrial flutter, 1229
for atrial tachycardia, 1228
for chronic heart failure, 1276
for dysphagia, 1398
for hypertrophic cardiomyopathy, 1295
for junctional tachycardia, 1234
for premature labor, 2807
for premature ventricular contractions, 1225
for ventricular tachycardia, 1243
for Wolff-Parkinson-White syndrome, 1235, 1237
heart failure from, 1269
overdose of, 2376-2379, 2377b, 2377t, 2378b
Calcium chelation, hypocalcemia from, 1943
Calcium chloride
for calcium channel blocker–induced hypotension, 2377-2378
for cardiac arrest, 93
for hyperkalemia, 1940-1941, 2650
for verapamil-induced hypotension, 1210
Calcium disodium edetate, for radioactive lead poisoning, 2324
Calcium disodium ethylenediaminetetraacetic acid, for lead poisoning, 2422
Calcium gluconate
for hydrofluoric acid burns, 933
for hyperkalemia, 1940-1941
Calcium hydroxide dust particles, in scuba diving–related disorders, 2283
Calcium hydroxide paste, for dentin fractures, 1037
Calcium hydroxyapatite crystals, in calcific tendinopathy, 1797
Calcium oxalate crystals, in ethylene glycol poisoning, 2398, 2399-2400
Calcium oxalate kidney stones, 1587
Calcium pumps, 1976, 1977f
Calcium pyrophosphate crystals
in pseudogout, 1786
in synovial fluid, 1782
"Calcium sign," in aortic dissection, 1326

Calculus
gallbladder, 1418-1419, 1418f, 1419f. *See also* Cholelithiasis.
renal, 1586-1593, 1586b, 1589f-1592f, 1593b. *See also* Urolithiasis.
vesical, 1593
Calf veins, 1368
isolated thrombosis of, 1370
Calicivirus, 2034t, 2057-2058
California encephalitis, 2055
Callus formation, in fracture healing, 564
Calpains
in cerebral necrosis, 66
inhibitors of, after cerebral ischemia, 72
Calyces, 527, 527f
Calymmatobacterium granulomatis, in granuloma inguinale, 1563
Cam walker, for ankle immobilization, 571
Campylobacter infection
in dysenteric colitis, 229t
in gastroenteritis, 1460-1461, 1461t, 1462t, 2625
Canalicular system, lacerations involving, 1051, 1051f
Cancer. *See also* site of cancer, e.g., Breast, cancer of.
acute tumor lysis syndrome in, 1911-1912, 1911b, 1912b
adrenal insufficiency in, 1996
alcoholism and, 2874
central nervous system infections in, 1920
cerebral herniation in, 1918
dyspnea in, 179t
encephalopathy in, 1920-1921
epidural spinal cord compression in, 1919-1920
fever in, 1907-1909, 1908b
HIV/AIDS and, 2079
hypercalcemia in, 1914-1916, 1915b, 1944-1945
hyperuricemia in, 1913-1914
hyperviscosity syndrome in, 1912-1913
hypophosphatemia in, 1951-1952
immune defects in, 2834-2841, 2836t, 2838t
neoplastic cardiac tamponade in, 1916-1918
neutropenia in, 2834-2839, 2836t, 2838t
oncologic emergencies in, 1907-1921
pediatric fever in, 2516
seizures in, 1919
skin lesions associated with, 1862-1864
superior vena cava syndrome in, 1909-1911, 1910f
Cancrum oris, 1033
Candesartan, 1322t
Candida albicans
in catheter-related infections, 1363
in diaper dermatitis, 1852
vaginitis in, in pregnancy, 2758
Candida bezoar, 877
Candida infection
in cancer patient with impaired cell-mediated immunity, 2840
in esophagitis, 1386, 1387
in febrile, neutropenic cancer patient, 2836
in HIV/AIDS, 2083-2084
in infective endocarditis, 1301
in osteomyelitis, 2178
in pericarditis, 1286
in pharyngitis, 275, 1112, 1113
skin lesions in, 1840-1841
Candidiasis
cutaneous, 1841
esophageal, 2083-2084
oral, 2083
vulvovaginal, 1567t, 1568
Canine search team, 3006
Canine space infection, 1028
Cannabis plants, 2411
"Can't intubate, can't oxygenate" situation, 8
Canthal tendon, lacerations involving, 1051
Capacity, decision-making, 3133-3134, 3134b
Capillary refill, delayed, in peripheral vascular injury, 539
Capitate
anatomy of, 622, 623f, 625
fracture of, 630
Capitellum
anatomy of, 647, 647f
fracture of, 661-662, 661f
in little leaguer's elbow, 663, 663f

Capitolunate angle, 626, 627f
Capnocytophaga canimorsus infection, in dog
  bites, 883, 887-888
Capnography/capnometry, 37-39, 38f
  during cardiopulmonary resuscitation, 81-82,
    81f
Capreomycin, for tuberculosis, 2163t
Capsaicin, toxicity of, 2472
Capsicum annum, 2472
Capsule
  hip, 736, 736f
  shoulder, 672, 673f
Capsulitis, adhesive, 682, 698-699, 699t, 1797
Captopril, 1322t
  during pregnancy and lactation, 2788
Caput medusae, in cirrhosis, 1410
Carbamate poisoning, 2329t, 2458b, 2461-2462
Carbamazepine
  during pregnancy and lactation, 2786
  for neuropathic pain, 1692
  for seizure, 2675, 2675t
  for tic douloureux, 1034
  for trigeminal neuralgia, 1664, 1666
  side effects of, 1628t
Carbon dioxide
  arterial pressure of
    end-tidal carbon dioxide and, 37-38
    in metabolic acidosis, 1929
    in metabolic alkalosis, 1930
    in pregnancy, 318
    in respiratory acidosis, 1925
    in respiratory alkalosis, 1926
    minute ventilation and, 1923
  end-tidal, 37-39, 38f
    during cardiopulmonary resuscitation, 81-82,
      81f
    for confirmation of endotracheal tube
      placement, 6, 6f
    in children, 2504
    monitoring of, during procedural sedation
      and analgesia, 2942-2943
  partial pressure of
    altitude and, 2297, 2297b
    cerebral blood flow and, 351, 351f
    transcutaneous, 36
  retention of, in chronic obstructive pulmonary
    disease, 1100
Carbon monoxide poisoning, 2438-2441
  cyanosis in, 271-272
  headache in, 174t
  in scuba diving–related disorders, 2283
  metabolic acidosis in, 1927
  nausea and vomiting in, 206t
  rhabdomyolysis in, 1979
  risk factors for, 171b
  with cyanide poisoning, 2440-2441
Carbon tetrachloride, toxicity of, 2887
Carbonated beverages, for esophageal obstruction,
  1384
Carbonic acid–bicarbonate buffer system, 1923
Carbonic anhydrase inhibitors
  for glaucoma, 1063b
  metabolic acidosis from, 1929
Carboxyhemoglobin toxicity
  cyanosis in, 271-272
  in burn injury, 922
Carbuncle, 1843, 2204
Carcinoma
  biliary tract, 1423
  hepatocellular, 1417
  pancreatic, 1437-1438
  scrotal, 2642
  testicular, 2642
Cardiac. *See also* Heart *entries.*
Cardiac agents. *See* Cardiovascular drugs.
Cardiac amyloidosis, 1297
Cardiac arrest, 75-94
  airway and breathing management in, 87
  algorithm for, 83f
  asystole and, 84-85
  cardiopulmonary resuscitation in, 88-90
  defibrillation in, 90-91
  epidemiology of, 76
  etiology of, 77-78, 78t
  factors preceding, 77
  history and physical examination in, 78-79, 79t
  in anaphylaxis, 1825t
  in critically ill asthmatic patient, 1093
  in electrical and lightning injuries, 2272, 2274

Cardiac arrest *(Continued)*
  in pulmonary embolism, 1379-1380
  monitoring in, 79-82, 80f-82f, 80t
  neurologic recovery after, 62-73
    clinical outcomes in, 72-73
    experimental therapies in, 70-72
    pathophysiology of cerebral ischemia and,
      62-67, 63f-64f
    standard strategies for, 67-70, 69t
  outcomes in, 93
  pacing in, 91
  pathophysiology of, 76-77
  pediatric, 97-116
    adenosine for, 101t, 104
    advanced life support techniques in, 99, 99f
    airway management in, 97-98, 105-109, 106f,
      107b, 107t
    amiodarone for, 101t, 104-105
    antidiuretic hormone for, 100, 103t
    atropine for, 99, 100, 101t-102t, 103-104
    basic life support techniques in, 97-99
    breathing management in, 98, 108-109
    calcium for, 101t, 104
    circulatory management in, 98-99, 109-113
    defibrillation and cardioversion in, 113
    epinephrine for, 111, 114
    etiology of, 109-113, 109t, 110f-112f, 110t
    family presence during, 114-116
    glucose for, 100, 101t, 103
    lidocaine for, 102t, 105
    magnesium for, 104
    pharmacologic therapy in, 100-105, 101t-
      103t, 109-113
    postresuscitation stabilization in, 113-114,
      113f
    procainamide for, 103t, 105
    rapid sequence intubation in, 107-108, 107b,
      107t
    sodium bicarbonate for, 100, 101t
    tape measurement system in, 114, 114f-115f
  pharmacologic therapy in, 91-93
  postresuscitation management of, 85-87, 86,
    88f
  pulseless electrical activity and, 84
  therapeutic modalities in, 87-93
  ventricular fibrillation and pulseless
    ventricular tachycardia and, 84
Cardiac auscultation, in infants and children,
  2571-2572, 2572b
Cardiac cellular electrophysiology, 1199-1201,
  1200f-1202f
Cardiac compression model of chest
  compression, 77, 98
Cardiac conduction, 1201-1203, 1202t, 1203f
Cardiac dysrhythmia. *See* Dysrhythmia.
Cardiac enzymes, in myocardial contusion, 469
Cardiac examination
  in chest pain, 187t
  in chronic obstructive pulmonary disease, 1100
  in dyspnea, 178t
  in spinal cord injury, 310
Cardiac glycosides, in oleander, 2474
Cardiac index, 1259
Cardiac markers
  in acute coronary syndromes, 1174-1179,
    1175f, 1176t
  in chest pain, 188
  in infants and children, 2575
  multiple use of, 1175-1179
Cardiac massage, open-chest, 89-90
Cardiac monitoring. *See also*
  Electrocardiography.
  during cardiopulmonary resuscitation, 79-82,
    80f-82f, 80t
  in hypothermia, 2245
  in myocardial infarction, 1173-1174, 1173f
Cardiac output
  during acclimatization to high altitude, 2298
  in heart failure, 1261
  in myocardial contusion, 468
  in pregnancy, 2725
Cardiac pacing. *See* Pacemaker(s); Pacing.
Cardiac sarcoidosis, 1297
Cardiac surgery
  in pregnancy, 2766
  pericarditis after, 1283
Cardiac tamponade, 1285-1286, 1286f
  acute, 473-476, 474f, 475f, 476t
  heart failure in, 1265

Cardiac tamponade *(Continued)*
  in children, 340
  in hemodialysis patient, 1550-1551
  in myocardial rupture, 471
  in uremic pericardial effusion, 1282
  neoplastic, 1916-1918
Cardiac trauma, 467-482
  acute pericardial tamponade in, 473-476, 474f,
    475f, 476t
  blunt, 467-472
  blunt aortic injury in, 476-482, 477f-479f, 481b
  chronic thoracic aneurysm and, 482
  in children, 340
  intracardiac injuries in, 472
  myocardial concussion in, 467
  myocardial contusion in, 467-470
  myocardial rupture in, 470-472
  penetrating, 472-476
  pericarditis after, 1283
Cardinal presentation(s)
  abdominal pain as
    diagnostic approach to, 212-216, 212f, 214t-
      216t
    differential considerations in, 212-214, 212f,
      214t-215t, 216-217, 216t
    disposition in, 217-218
    empiric management of, 217, 218f-219f
    pathophysiology of, 209-212, 210t-211t, 211b
  back pain as, 260-267
    diagnostic approach to, 261-264, 261b, 262b,
      263f
    differential diagnosis in, 262t, 263f, 264,
      265t-266t
    disposition in, 267
    empiric management of, 264, 266f, 267
  chest pain as, 183-188
    ancillary studies in, 185-186, 188t
    diagnostic table in, 188, 190t-191t
    differential considerations in, 183-184, 184t
    disposition in, 188, 192t
    epidemiology of, 183
    history in, 185, 186b, 186t
    management of, 188, 192f
    pathophysiology of, 183
    physical examination in, 185, 187t
    rapid assessment and stabilization in, 184-
      185, 184f
  coma and depressed level of consciousness as,
    156-164
    diagnostic approach to, 157-162, 158b, 159t,
      160f, 162f, 163f
    disposition in, 163
    empiric management of, 162-163
  confusion as, 150-155
    diagnostic approach to, 150-153, 151b, 152f,
      153f
    differential diagnosis in, 153, 154b, 154f
    disposition in, 154-155
    empiric management of, 154, 155f
  constipation as, 237-242
    diagnostic approach to, 238-239, 238b
    differential diagnosis in, 239, 240f
    disposition in, 242
    empiric management of, 239-242, 240f, 241t,
      242b
    pathophysiology of, 237
  cyanosis as, 268-273
    diagnostic approach to, 268-271, 270b, 270f
    differential diagnosis in, 270b, 271-273, 272f
    disposition in, 273
    empiric management of, 273
    pathophysiology of, 268, 269b, 269f
  diarrhea as, 227-236
    diagnostic approach to, 228-233, 230b, 231b
    differential diagnosis in, 228, 230b-231b, 234
    disposition in, 235-236
    empiric management of, 234-235, 234f, 236t
    pathophysiology of, 228, 229t-230t
  dizziness and vertigo as, 142-149
    diagnostic approach to, 143-146, 143b, 143t,
      145b, 145t, 148f
    differential diagnosis in, 143, 143b, 143t,
      146, 147t-148t
    disposition in, 146, 149
    management of, 146, 149f
    pathophysiology of, 142-143
  dyspnea as, 175-181
    diagnostic approach to, 176-177, 176t, 178t-
      180t

Cardinal presentation(s) (Continued)
  differential considerations in, 177, 179t, 180
  disposition in, 181
  empiric management of, 180-181, 182f
  fever as, 134-137
    diagnostic approach to, 135-137, 135b, 135t
    differential considerations in, 135, 135b, 135t, 137
    disposition in, 137
    empirical management of, 137
  gastrointestinal bleeding as, 220-227
    diagnostic approach to, 220-223, 221b
    differential diagnosis in, 220, 221b, 223
    disposition in, 225-227, 225b, 226t
    management of, 223-225, 223f
  headache as, 169-175, 173t
  hemoptysis as, 279-283, 281b, 282f
  jaundice as, 243-246
    diagnostic approach to, 243-244, 244f, 245f
    differential diagnosis in, 245, 246t
    empiric management of, 245-246, 247f
  nausea and vomiting as, 200-207
    diagnostic approach to, 201-203, 202t
    differential considerations in, 201-202, 201t, 203, 204t-206t, 207f
    disposition in, 207, 209
    management of, 203, 206, 207f, 208b, 208t
    pathophysiology of, 200-201, 201f
    pediatric considerations in, 203, 208t
    physical examination in, 202t
    rapid assessment and stabilization in, 201t
  pelvic pain as, 248-253
    diagnostic approach to, 248-250, 250t
    differential diagnosis in, 249b, 250, 251t-252t
    empiric management of, 250, 252-253, 252f, 253f
  pharyngitis as, 274-279
    diagnosis of, 275-278, 276t, 277f, 277t
    differential diagnosis in, 278
    management of, 278-279, 278f
    pathophysiology of, 274-275, 275t
  red and painful eye as, 283-297
    diagnostic approach to, 283-288, 284b, 285b, 287f
    differential diagnosis in, 288-290, 288f-291f
    disposition in, 293t-297t, 297
    empiric management of, 290-292, 293t-297t
  seizure as, 164-168
    diagnosis of, 165-168, 165t
    differential considerations in, 165-166, 165t
    disposition in, 168
    empiric management of, 166-167, 166t, 168
  syncope as, 193-198
    diagnostic approach to, 193-196, 194b, 195b, 195t, 196t
    differential diagnosis in, 194b, 196, 196t, 197t, 198f
    disposition in, 198
    empiric management of, 196, 198, 199f
  vaginal bleeding as, 254-259
    diagnostic approach to, 254-257, 255t, 256t
    differential diagnosis in, 255t, 257, 257t-258t
    disposition in, 259
    empiric management of, 257, 259, 259f, 260f
  weakness as, 138-141
    diagnostic approach to, 138-139, 139f, 139t, 140b, 140t
    differential diagnosis in, 138, 139t, 140, 140b
    disposition in, 141
    empiric management of, 140-141, 141b
Cardioembolic ischemic stroke, 1608
Cardiogenic pulmonary edema, 32, 1261-1262
Cardiogenic shock
  causes of, 47
  definition of, 49, 49b
  in myocardial infarction, 1160, 1194
  reperfusion therapy in, 1194
  treatment of, 52b, 54, 113-114, 113f, 1273
Cardiomegaly, with pulmonary edema, 1174, 1175f
Cardiomyopathy, 1293-1297
  alcoholic, 2866
  amyloidosis and, 1297
  connective tissue disorders and, 1297-1298
  dilated, 1293-1294
    heart failure in, 1264
    peripartum cardiomyopathy and, 1297
  heart failure in, 1264
  hypertrophic, 1294-1296

Cardiomyopathy (Continued)
    heart failure in, 1264
    sudden death in, 1298, 2597-2598
  inflammatory. See Myocarditis.
  ischemic, 1264
  peripartum, 1297
  postpartum, 2821
  restrictive, 1296-1297
    constrictive pericarditis vs., 1288
    heart failure in, 1264
  sarcoidosis and, 1297
Cardiopulmonary arrest, 79
Cardiopulmonary bypass
  during cardiac arrest, 90
  for rewarming in accidental hypothermia, 2250-2251, 2250t
  in aortic rupture, 481
  in myocardial rupture, 471-472
Cardiopulmonary decompensation, in pulmonary embolism, 1378, 1379f
Cardiopulmonary resuscitation
  active compression-decompression, 89, 98
  before defibrillation, 90
  blood flow during, 76-77
  brain resuscitation and, 67-68
  capnography in, 39
  cough, 90
  for cardiac arrest, 88-90
  for submersion victim, 2313-2314
  in hypothermia, 2245-2246
  in pediatric resuscitation, 98-99
  interposed abdominal compression, 89, 98
  previous, fibrinolytic therapy eligibility and, 1191
  vestibule or circumferential, 89
  withdrawing or discontinuing, 3144, 3152
Cardiothoracic injury, pediatric, 338-340
Cardiothoracic ratio, in infants and children, 2573
Cardiovascular collapse
  from local anesthesia, 2932
  in anaphylaxis, 1824, 1825t, 2548
  in carbon monoxide poisoning, 2439
  in cyclic antidepressant poisoning, 2352
  in pneumococcal disease, 2018
Cardiovascular depression, in septic shock, 46
Cardiovascular disorders
  after head trauma, 371
  altitude and, 2308
  anxiety in, 1746-1747
  in chronic renal failure, 1542
  in developmentally disabled patient, 2902
  in diabetes mellitus, 1970
  in HIV/AIDS, 2086
  in hyperviscosity syndrome, 1913
  in Kawasaki disease, 2025, 2026
  in opioid overdose, 2453
  in parasitic infection, 2111-2112
  in pregnancy, 2766-2767
  in Rocky Mountain spotted fever, 2134
  in sepsis, 2213-2214
  in serotonin toxicity, 2357t, 2360
  in systemic lupus erythematosus, 1807
  in thermal burns, 918
  pediatric, 2567-2599
    chest radiography in, 2573-2574, 2573f, 2574f
    circulatory changes related to, 2568-2569
    compensatory responses associated with, 2569, 2569b
    history in, 2570-2571, 2570b
  syncope in, 2685
Cardiovascular drugs
  during pregnancy and lactation, 2787-2789
  for hypothermia, 2246
  in elderly person, 2826
  overdose of, 2368-2379
  prehospital use of, 2990-2991
  syncope from, 195b
Cardiovascular emergencies
  air medical transport in, 2998-2999
  prehospital care in, 2990-2991
Cardiovascular system
  aging and, 345
  in accidental hypothermia, 2237-2238, 2238f
  in acclimatization and endurance training, 2256
  in electrical and lightning injuries, 2272
  in pregnancy, 316-317, 317t, 2725
  in thyrotoxicosis, 1986-1987
  sepsis and, 2219-2220

Cardiovascular trauma, 467-482. See also Cardiac trauma.
Cardioversion
  for atrial fibrillation, 1231-1232
  for pulseless electrical activity, 84
  for supraventricular tachycardia, 2587-2588
  for torsades de pointes, 1244
  for ventricular tachycardia, 1242
  for wide-complex tachycardia, 1239
  for Wolff-Parkinson-White syndrome, 1235, 1237
  in pediatric resuscitation, 113
Carditis
  in acute rheumatic fever, 2596
  in Lyme disease, 2123-2124, 2128
Care paths, 3038, 3039f-3041f
Care under fire in tactical emergency medical support, 3002-3003
Caregiver interview, in elder abuse, 1013
Caries, 1028-1029, 1030-1032, 1030f, 1031f
Carnitine, for diphtheria, 1291
Carotid artery
  aneurysm of, parapharyngeal abscess and, 1123
  dissection of
    after head trauma, 357-358
    headache in, 1638-1639, 1639f
  injury to, 448
  stroke involving, 1607, 1609
Carotid duplex scanning, in ischemic stroke, 1613
Carotid pulse, during cardiopulmonary resuscitation, 79
Carotid sinus massage
  for dysrhythmias, 1214, 1215
  in digitalis toxicity, 2371
Carpal bones
  anatomy of, 577-578, 579f, 622, 623f
  radiography of, 625-626, 626f, 627f
Carpal injuries, 627-632
  capitate fracture in, 630
  hamate fracture in, 629
  lunate fracture in, 629
  pisiform fracture in, 629
  scaphoid fracture in, 627-629, 628f
  trapezium fracture in, 630
  trapezoid fracture in, 630
  triquetral fracture in, 629
Carpal instability, 630-632, 630f-633f
Carpal tunnel, 578
Carpal tunnel syndrome, 639, 639f, 1696-1697, 1697b, 1697f
  in hypothyroidism, 1992
  in pregnancy, 2733
  thoracic outlet syndrome vs., 1360
Carpal tunnel view of wrist, 627, 627t
Carpometacarpal joint
  dislocation of
    finger, 603, 603f
    thumb, 604
  motions of, 578f
Carrying angle of elbow, 649, 649f, 650f
  loss of, after supracondylar fracture, 657-658
Cartridge, handgun, 954, 954f
Carvedilol, 1321t, 2373t
Caspase inhibitors, after cerebral ischemia, 72
CAST fracture, 975
Cast immobilization
  in Achilles tendon rupture, 818
  in carpal bone fractures, 628, 628f, 629
  in gastrocnemius strain, 804
  in humeral shaft fracture, 654-655, 654f
  in intercondylar eminence fracture, 780
  in Lisfranc injuries, 830
  in medial malleolar fracture, 813
  in metatarsal head and neck fractures, 832
  in metatarsal shaft fractures, 831
  in metatarsophalangeal dislocation, 835
  in patellar fracture, 785
  in peroneal tendon dislocation or tear, 819
  in posterior malleolar fracture, 813
  in sesamoid fractures, 835
  in Smith's fracture, 634-635
  in tibial plateau fracture, 779
  in tibial tubercle fracture, 799
Castration anxiety, 1746b
Casts
  air, for ankle immobilization, 571, 573f, 817
  fatty
    in proteinuria, 1532
    in urinary sediment, 1526, 1526f

Casts *(Continued)*
 in glomerulonephritis, 1534
 in urinary sediment, 1525-1527, 1526f
 plaster, 571-573
Cat
 bites by, 854, 883-884, 888
 rabies in, 2064, 2064f
Cataracts
 in electrical injuries, 2272
 in substituted phenol poisoning, 2464
Catastrophic casualty management, 3013-3014
Catatonia, in schizophrenia, 1728
Catecholamines
 for acute pulmonary edema in hypotensive
  patient, 1273-1274
 for beta blocker overdose, 2375
 for calcium channel blocker overdose, 2378
 for digitalis toxicity, 2368
 in anxiety disorders, 1744
 in torsades de pointes, 1244
Caterpillar bites, 908
Catfish envenomation, 910
Cathartics, for botulism, 2016
Catheter
 balloon-tipped, in foreign body removal, 862f,
  863, 872-873
 Foley
  in burn injury, 923
  in foreign body removal, 2617
  in genitourinary trauma, 515, 517, 518f
  in peripheral vascular injury, 543
 Groshong, 1363-1364, 1365f
 Hickman-Broviac, problems related to, 1361-
  1363, 1362b, 1362f, 1365f
 laceration of, 1363
 occluded indwelling, differential diagnosis in,
  1362b
 Quinton-Mahurkar, 1362f, 1364-1365
 Word, for Bartholin abscess, 1560
Catheterization
 central venous
  in adult resuscitation, 91-92
  in pediatric resuscitation, 99
  postresuscitation, 87
 in thermal burn, 923
 pulmonary artery, in shock, 50
 urinary
  in children, 2643
  in genitourinary trauma, 515, 517, 518f
  in hypothermia, 2244-2245
  in urinary retention, 1599-1600
Catheter-related infection, 1363
 in peritoneal dialysis patient, 1553
 of urinary tract, 1578-1579
Cationic protein, in asthma, 1081
Cauda equina syndrome, 420, 1678f, 1679
 back pain in, 261, 265t, 703, 706, 712
 in pelvic fracture, 720
 pseudoclaudication in, 1350
Causalgia, 562
Causes of death, 942t
Causes of injury deaths, 949t
Caustic keratoconjunctivitis, 288, 288f, 293t
Caustics
 dermal exposure to, 2384
 esophagitis from, 1386, 1387-1388
 ocular exposure to, 2384
 oral exposure to, 2380-2385, 2381f, 2381t, 2382f
Cavernosal aspiration, for priapism, 2636
Cavitation
 in pneumonia, 1134, 1134f
 nontuberculous, 2157
 tuberculous, 2153, 2153f
CD4 (helper) cell, 2833
CD4 count, in case definition of AIDS, 2071, 2072b
CD8 (suppressor) cell, 2833
Cecal bascule, 1497
Cecal volvulus, 1497-1498, 1499, 1499f
Cefazolin, for peritonitis in dialysis patient,
 1552, 1553t
Cefdinir, for otitis media, 1069
Cefepime, for febrile, neutropenic cancer patient,
 2837, 2838t
Cefixime
 for gonococcal arthritis, 1788
 for gonorrhea, 1559t, 1566
Cefotaxime
 for gonococcal dermatitis, 1843
 for Lyme disease, 2127t, 2128

Cefotaxime *(Continued)*
 for meningococcal disease, 2023
 for pediatric fever, 2513-2514, 2515
 for pneumococcal disease, 2019
 for pneumonia, 2558t
Cefotetan, for pelvic inflammatory disease, 1571t
Ceftizoxime, for gonococcal dermatitis, 1843
Ceftriaxone
 for anorectal sexually transmitted disease, 1519
 for bacterial meningitis, 1721, 1722
 for chancroid, 1559t, 1563
 for epididymitis, 1597t, 2639
 for fever, 2513, 2514, 2515
 for gonococcal arthritis, 1788
 for gonococcal dermatitis, 1843
 for gonorrhea, 1559t, 1566
 for Lyme disease, 1789, 2127t, 2128
 for mastoiditis, 1072
 for meningococcal disease, 2023
 for meningococcal meningitis, 1723
 for otitis media, 1069, 1070t
 for pelvic inflammatory disease, 1571t
 for pneumococcal disease, 2019
 for pneumonia, 2558t
 for prostatitis, 1586
 prophylactic
  for bacteremia, 2506
  for meningococcal disease, 2024
Cefuroxime
 for bacterial meningitis, 1721, 1722
 for Lyme disease, 1789
 for mastoiditis, 1072
 for otitis media, 1068, 1070t
 for pneumococcal disease, 2019
 for pneumonia, 2558t
 prophylactic, in cat bites, 888
Celecoxib, 2928
Celiac trunk, 1445
Cell membrane, myocardial, electrophysiology of,
 1199-1201, 1200f-1202f
Cell stimulation therapy, for febrile, neutropenic
 cancer patient, 2839
Cell-mediated immunity, 2833
 defects in, 2833
  from corticosteroids, 2843
  in cancer patient, 2839-2840
  in renal failure, 2842
 immunosenescence of, 2826
 in tuberculosis, 2148
Cellophane tape test, in *Enterobius vermicularis*
 gastroenteritis, 1481
Cellular phone, pacemaker oversensing due to,
 1254
Cellularity, cerebrospinal fluid, in bacterial
 meningitis, 2661-2662, 2661t
Cellulitis, 2196-2199, 2196t, 2196f, 2197t
 clostridial (anaerobic), 2208
 gram-negative and anaerobic, 2199
 in erysipelas, 2198
 in head and neck spaces, 1027, 1028-1029,
  1030f, 1117
 influenzae, 2199
 nonclostridial crepitant, 2208
 orbital, 293t, 2197-2198
 periorbital (preseptal), 1055, 2197-2198
 peritonsillar, 1117-1118, 1118f
 retropharyngeal, 1120-1121, 1120f, 1121f
 staphylococcal, 2198-2199
 streptococcal, 2198
 submandibular, 1028, 1032, 1118-1119
 synergistic necrotizing, 2209
 upper airway, in epiglottitis, 1115
Cement burn, 935, 2381
Cementum, 1026, 1027f
Centerfire rifle wounds, forensic evaluation of,
 959, 959f, 960f
Centers for Disease Control and Prevention, 2016,
 3019
Centipede bites, 908
Centor criteria, in pharyngitis, 1112
Central cord syndrome, 417-418, 419f, 1677, 1678f
Central herniation
 after head trauma, 356
 in cancer patient, 1918
Central log of patients presenting to emergency
 department, 3162
Central nervous system. *See also* Brain; Spinal
 cord.
 aging and, 345

Central nervous system *(Continued)*
 cyclic antidepressant effects on, 2354b
 degenerative diseases of, seizure in, 1624
 in acute radiation syndrome, 2321-2322
 in decompression sickness, 2284
 in electrical and lightning injuries, 2273-2274
 in fetal alcohol syndrome, 2791b, 2792
 in heatstroke, 2262
 in hypothermia, 2238
 in lead poisoning, 2421
 in submersion victim, 2313
 in systemic lupus erythematosus, 1807
 in thermoregulation, 2255
 in tuberculosis, 2160-2161, 2161f
 lymphoma of, in HIV/AIDS, 2082
 oxygen toxicity in, in scuba diving–related
  disorders, 2283
 tumor of, seizure in, 1624
 vasculitis of, seizure in, 1624
Central nervous system abscess
 ancillary studies in, 1720
 cerebrospinal fluid analysis in, 1716-1719,
  1717t, 1718t, 1719f
 complications of, 1716
 diagnosis of, 1716-1720
 differential considerations in, 1720, 1721b
 disposition in, 1723
 epidemiology of, 1711
 etiology of, 1712
 locations of, 1710-1711
 lumbar puncture in, 1716, 1716b
 management of, 1722, 1723
 neuroimaging studies in, 1719-1720
 pathophysiology of, 1713, 1713f
 signs and symptoms of, 1714-1715
Central nervous system acidosis, from sodium
 bicarbonate, 1930
Central nervous system depression
 in barbiturate overdose, 2482
 in benzodiazepine poisoning, 2484
 in chloral hydrate poisoning, 2487
 in flunitrazepam overdose, 2486
 in hydrocarbon poisoning, 2429
 in opioid overdose, 2452
Central nervous system infection, 1710-1723
 acute and subacute
  ancillary studies in, 1720
  cerebrospinal fluid analysis in, 1716-1719,
   1717t, 1718t, 1719f
  complications of, 1715-1716
  diagnosis of, 1716-1720
  differential considerations in, 1720, 1721b
  disposition in, 1723
  epidemiology of, 1711
  etiology of, 1711-1712, 1711b, 1712b
  lumbar puncture in, 1716, 1716b
  management of, 1721-1723, 1721t
  neuroimaging studies in, 1719-1720
  pathophysiology of, 1713, 1713b
  signs and symptoms of, 1714-1715
 after head trauma, 370-371
 definitions in, 1710-1711
 in cancer patient, 1920
 in HIV/AIDS, 2079-2082, 2080f
 slow virus, 2058
  dementia in, 1657-1658, 1659
Central pontine myelinolysis, in hyponatremia,
 1935
Central retinal artery occlusion, 283, 284f, 1057,
 1057f
Central retinal vein occlusion, 1057, 1057f
Central venous catheterization
 in adult resuscitation, 91-92
 in pediatric resuscitation, 99
 postresuscitation, 87
Central venous oxygen saturation, during
 cardiopulmonary resuscitation, 82, 82f
Central venous pressure
 in cardiac tamponade, 473
 in multiple trauma, 304, 307
 in shock, 51
 postresuscitation, 87
Central venous pressure lines, in sepsis, 2217
Cephalexin, for impetigo, 1843
Cephalosporins
 allergy to, 1826
 during pregnancy and lactation, 2784
 for febrile, neutropenic cancer patient, 2838t
 for orofacial infections, 1032

Cephalosporins (Continued)
for peritonitis in dialysis patient, 1552, 1553t
for pharyngitis, 1113
Cerebellar artery syndrome, posteroinferior, 420
Cerebellar ataxia
in high-altitude cerebral edema, 2306
pediatric, 2681, 2682
Cerebellar degeneration, alcoholic, 2870
Cerebellar disturbances
in hypothyroidism, 1992
in multiple sclerosis, 1672
in vertigo, 145
Cerebellar hemorrhage, 147t, 378
Cerebellotonsillar herniation, after head trauma, 356
Cerebral. See also Brain.
Cerebral anatomy, mood disorders and, 1735
Cerebral aneurysm, and subarachnoid
hemorrhage, Hunt and Hess scale for, 1636, 1636t, 1637
Cerebral artery
embolism to, in scuba diving–related disorders, 2285
stroke involving, 1607, 1609
Cerebral atrophy, in dementia, 1656-1657
Cerebral blood flow, 350-352, 351f
after brain resuscitation, 68
autoregulation of, 351
loss of, 354
during cardiopulmonary resuscitation, 67
during cerebral ischemia, 62, 63f-64f
in hypothermia, 2238
in stroke, 1606-1607
restoration of, after cardiac arrest, 62-64
Cerebral demyelination, in hyponatremia, 1935
Cerebral edema
after head trauma, 354
during cerebral ischemia, 64-65
high-altitude, 2296, 2299-2300, 2299f, 2305-2306, 2305b
in diabetic ketoacidosis, 1967
in salicylate overdose, 2340
in spinal cord injury, 2906
Cerebral hemodynamics, 350-352, 351f
Cerebral hemorrhage. See Intracerebral hemorrhage.
Cerebral herniation
after head trauma, 354-356, 355f
in cancer patient, 1918
Cerebral hypoperfusion
after brain resuscitation, 68
syncope and, 193, 194b
Cerebral hypoxia, during air medical transport, 2994-2995
Cerebral ischemia
neurologic recovery after, 62-73
clinical outcomes in, 72-73
experimental therapies in, 70-72
standard strategies for, 67-70, 69t
pathophysiology of, 62-67, 63f-64f
Cerebral malaria, 2104f, 2105
Cerebral palsy, 2903-2904
failure to thrive in, 2900
musculoskeletal disorders in, 2901-2902
Cerebral perfusion pressure, 352
during cardiopulmonary resuscitation, 80, 80f
Cerebral resuscitation, 62-73
clinical outcomes in, 72-73
experimental therapies in, 70-72
in near-hanging and strangulation, 451
pathophysiology of cerebral ischemia and, 62-67, 63f-64f
standard strategies for, 67-70, 69t
Cerebral thrombovasculitis, in Rocky Mountain spotted fever, 2134
Cerebral vasospasm, in traumatic subarachnoid hemorrhage, 377
Cerebral venous catheterization, problems related to, 1361-1366, 1362b, 1362f, 1364f, 1365f
Cerebral venous thrombosis, 1670-1671
Cerebritis, lupus, 1807
Cerebrospinal fluid
analysis of
in bacterial meningitis, 2661-2662, 2661t
in central nervous system infection, 1716-1719, 1717t, 1718t, 1719f
in delirium, 1652
in Guillain-Barré syndrome, 1690-1691
in headache, 173t

Cerebrospinal fluid (Continued)
in HIV/AIDS, 2080
in multiple sclerosis, 1672-1673
in subarachnoid hemorrhage, 1636-1637
leakage of, in midface fracture, 394
physiology of, 350
Cerebrospinal fluid shunt, in developmentally disabled patient, 2899
Cervical disk herniation, thoracic outlet syndrome vs., 1360
Cervical lymphadenopathy
in African trypanosomiasis, 2106
in Kawasaki disease, 2026
in peritonsillitis, 1117
in pharyngitis, 1109, 1110f
Cervical motion tenderness
in pelvic inflammatory disease, 1570
pelvic pain in, 250t
Cervical os, 250t
Cervical rib syndrome, thoracic outlet syndrome in, 1358
Cervical spine
anatomy of, 400f
cartilage space assessment of, 424
neurologic examination of, 415-417
pediatric, anatomic differences in, 335b
pseudosubluxation of, 421
subluxation of, 401, 404, 404f-405f, 427, 428f
Cervical spine immobilization, 435, 436
in comatose survivors of cardiac arrest, 70
in multiple trauma, 308
in spinal injuries, 435-436
Cervical spine injury
airway management in, 436
computed tomography in, 427, 429-431, 429b, 429f-432f
extension, 410-411, 410f-411f
vertebral artery injury from, 420, 420f
facial trauma and, 386
flexion, 399, 401-404, 402f-405f
head trauma with, 358
in children, 336-338, 337f
in elderly person, 413, 415f
in intubation, 17-18
in multiple trauma, 308-309
in neck trauma, 445
magnetic resonance imaging in, 431-435, 433f-436f
radiographic evaluation of, 420-427, 422f-428f
anteroposterior view in, 424, 426, 426f, 427f
cross-table lateral view in, 421, 424, 425f, 426f
flexion-extension views in, 428
indications for, 420-421
oblique views in, 426-428, 426f, 427f, 428f
odontoid view in, 424, 424f-425f
standard trauma series in, 421, 422f-424f
rotational, 405-409, 408f-410f
shear, 405, 406f-407f
stabilization in, 435-436
vascular damage in, 413, 415f
vertical compression, 411-413, 411f-414f
Cervical vertebrae, 399, 400f
Cervicogenic headache, 1642
Cervix
examination of
during labor, 2799, 2799f
in sexual assault victim, 987
in pregnancy, 2723
Cesarean section
in abruptio placentae, 2809
in circumvallate placenta, 2810
in face, brow, and compound presentations, 2816
in HIV-infected patient, 2810
in multiple gestations, 2816
in placenta previa, 2809
in umbilical cord prolapse, 2817
in uterine rupture, 2820-2821
in vasa previa, 2810
perimortem, 325-326
vaginal birth after, 2820
Cesium ingestion, radiogardase for, 3023, 3023t
Cestode infection, 2099t
Cetirizine, during pregnancy and lactation, 2790
Chadwick's sign, 2723, 2728, 2798
Chagas' disease, 2103t
fever in, 2105
myocarditis in, 1291, 2111-2112

Chain of custody in sexual assault cases, 985b
Chalazion, 293t, 1054, 1055f
Chalcosis, 1052
Chamomile, adverse effects of, 2476t
Chance's fracture, 550t
Chancre, syphilitic, 1560-1561, 1560f, 1855, 1855f
Chancroid, 1518t, 1519, 1557t, 1559t, 1562-1563, 1562f
Changuinola virus, 2047
Chaparral, adverse effects of, 2476t
Charcoal, activated. See Activated charcoal.
Charcot's triad in cholangitis, 1421
Charles' law, 2280, 2994
Chauffeur's fracture, 550t
Cheek injury, 391
Chelating agents
for arsenic poisoning, 2424
for internal radioactive contamination, 2324
for iron overdose, 2420
for lead poisoning, 2422-2423
for mercury poisoning, 2426
for rhabdomyolysis, 1982
Chemical injuries, 929-939
acid and alkali burns in, 931-933
anhydrous ammonia in, 934-935
caustics in, 2380-2385, 2381f, 2381t, 2382f
cement burns in, 935
chemical terrorism and, 937-939, 938t. See also Chemical weapons.
community preparedness and HAZMAT response in, 930-931
elemental metals in, 937
formic acid in, 934
hydrocarbon-related, 936-937
hydrofluoric acid in, 933-934
in pesticide poisoning, 2452-2469
nitrates in, 936
ocular, 1046, 1046f
pathophysiology of, 930
phenol and derivatives in, 935-936
tar burns in, 937
white phosphorus in, 936
Chemical peels, 935
Chemical vaginitis, 1569
Chemical weapons, 937-939, 938t, 3029-3032, 3030b, 3031b
blood agents (cyanide) as, 939, 3031-3032
disaster preparedness for, 3018
nerve gases as, 939, 3030-3031, 3030b, 3031b
pulmonary agents (phosgene, chlorine) as, 939, 3032
vesicants (mustard) as, 938-939, 3031
Chemoreceptor trigger zone, in nausea and vomiting, 200
Chemotaxis, 2834
Chemotherapy, acute tumor lysis syndrome in, 1911
Chemtrec (Chemical Transportation Emergency Center), 931
Cherenkov radiation, 2317
Chernobyl nuclear reactor incident, 2317
Cherry-red spot, in central retinal artery occlusion, 283, 284f, 1057, 1057f
Chest
examination of, in dyspnea, 178t
flail, 457-458, 457f, 458b, 460
low, 490
gunshot wounds to, 506
stab wounds to, 505
Chest compressions
abdominal trauma after, 492
cardiac compression model of, 77, 98
closed, 89
for critically ill asthmatic patient, 1093
for submersion victim, 2314
in hypothermia, 2245
in neonatal resuscitation, 123
in pediatric resuscitation, 98-99, 109
in ventricular fibrillation and pulseless ventricular tachycardia, 84
open, 89-90
thoracic pump model of, 77, 98
Chest pain, 183-188. See also Angina.
ancillary studies in, 185-186, 188t
cocaine-related, 2390-2391, 2390b, 2392, 2392b
diagnostic table in, 188, 190t-191t
differential diagnosis in, 183-184, 184t, 1159, 1159t

Chest pain (Continued)
    disposition in, 188, 192f
    epidemiology of, 183
    history in, 185, 186b, 186t
    in aortic dissection, 1325
    in aortic rupture, 478
    in dilated cardiomyopathy, 1293
    in esophageal motility disorders, 1396-1397
    in esophageal perforation, 1385
    in esophagitis, 1387
    in gastroesophageal reflux, 1388
    in hemodialysis patient, 1551
    in hypertrophic cardiomyopathy, 1295
    in mitral valve prolapse, 1305
    in myocarditis, 1290
    in neoplastic cardiac tamponade, 1917
    in pericarditis, 1280-1281
    in pneumothorax, 1145
    in pregnancy, 2732-2733
    in pulmonary embolism, 1372, 1380
    in tuberculosis, 2149
    management of, 188, 192f
    nonmyocardial, guidelines for, 192f
    observation in, 3064-3065, 3065b
    pathophysiology of, 183
    pediatric, 2570-2571, 2592
    physical examination in, 185, 187t
    rapid assessment and stabilization in, 184-185,
        184f
Chest pain centers, 1181-1182, 3064-3065,
    3065b
Chest Pain Evaluation in the Emergency Room
    (CHEER), 1181-1182
Chest radiography. See Radiography, chest.
Chest thrusts, for airway foreign body, 2530
Chest trauma. See Thoracic trauma.
Chest tube
    abdominal trauma after, 492
    in children, 339
    in hemothorax, 465
    in pleural effusion, 1151-1152
    in pneumothorax, 463, 464, 464b, 1147-1148
Chest wall trauma, 454-459
    costochondral separation in, 457
    flail chest in, 457-458, 457f, 458b
    nonpenetrating ballistic injury in, 458-459
    observation in, 3068-3069
    pneumothorax and, 461
    rib fracture in, 454-456, 454b, 455f
    sternal fracture in, 456-457
    subcutaneous emphysema and, 459-460
    traumatic asphyxia in, 459
Chickenpox. See Varicella.
Chilblains, 2228, 2230
Child, 2494-2720. See also Adolescent; Infant;
    Neonate.
    abdominal pain in
        differential considerations in, 2611, 2612t
        in appendicitis, 2619
        in hemolytic uremic syndrome, 2654
        in Henoch-Schönlein purpura, 2615, 2653
        in inflammatory bowel disease, 2616
        in intussusception, 2610
        in osteogenesis imperfecta, 2700
        in renal stones, 2646
    abuse of. See Child abuse.
    acetaminophen poisoning in, 2335
    acute bacterial meningitis in, 2657-2665
        clinical features of, 2658-2659, 2658t
        diagnosis of, 2659-2663, 2660b, 2661f, 2661t
        differential considerations in, 2663, 2663b
        management of, 2663-2665, 2664t
        pathophysiology of, 2657-2658
    acute mountain sickness in, 2301, 2302
    acute renal failure in, 2649-2651, 2649b
    acute rheumatic fever in, 2596-2597, 2596f
    acute septic arthritis in, 2704-2706, 2705t,
        2706t
    air medical transport of, 2999
    airway obstruction in, 2502, 2502b, 2519-2530,
        2532-2552
    altered consciousness in, 2502-2503
    analgesia in, 2935-2936, 2946-2947, 2952-2954
    anaphylaxis/anaphylactoid reactions in, 2546-
        2550
    anatomic and physiologic differences in, 329,
        329b, 329t, 335b, 2494-2495
    appendicitis in, 1452-1453, 2509b, 2618-2620,
        2620f

Child (Continued)
    assessment of
        appearance in, 2497-2498, 2498t
        circulation to skin in, 2498t, 2499, 2499f
        clinical interview in, 2500-2501, 2501b
        hands-on, 2499-2500
        physical examination in, 2501
        special health care needs and, 2503-2504
        triage tools in, 2500, 2500t
        work of breathing in, 2498-2499, 2498f,
            2498t, 2499f
    asthma in, 2532-2544
        clinical features of, 2534-2536
        complications of, 2535-2536, 2536b
        diagnosis of, 2536-2537, 2536f, 2537f
        differential diagnosis in, 2537, 2538b
        disposition in, 2542-2544
        epidemiology of, 2532
        factors associated with, 2533-2534, 2534b
        history in, 2534, 2534b
        management of, 2537-2542, 2539f, 2540f,
            2543t
        pathophysiology of, 2532-2533
        physical examination in, 2534-2535, 2535t
        prehospital care in, 2537
        severity assessment score for, 2503t
    ataxia in, 2681-2682, 2681b
    athletic, sudden death of, 2597-2599, 2597b
    atrial septal defect in, 2578
    automobile restraint seats for, 947, 948
    back pain in, 703, 707, 713
    bacterial endocarditis in, 2590-2591, 2591b
    benzodiazepine poisoning in, 2484-2485
    beta blocker overdose in, 2375
    biliary tract disorders in, 2620-2621
    blood pressure in, 2495, 2495t, 2571, 2571t,
        2651t
    bronchiolitis in, 2509b, 2544-2546
    bronchopulmonary dysplasia in, 2565, 2565f
    burns in
        in child abuse, 969-970, 970f, 970t
        unintentional, 975
    calcium channel blocker overdose in, 2378-2379
    cardiac arrest in, 97-116
        adenosine for, 101t, 104
        advanced life support techniques in, 99, 99f
        airway management in, 97-98, 105-109, 106f,
            107b, 107t
        amiodarone for, 101t, 104-105
        antidiuretic hormone for, 100, 103t
        atropine for, 99, 100, 101t-102t, 103-104
        basic life support techniques in, 97-99
        breathing management in, 98, 108-109
        calcium for, 101t, 104
        circulatory management in, 98-99, 109-113
        defibrillation and cardioversion in, 113
        epinephrine for, 111, 114
        etiology of, 109-113, 109t, 110f-112f, 110t
        family presence during, 114-116
        glucose for, 100, 101t, 103
        lidocaine for, 102t, 105
        magnesium for, 104
        pharmacologic therapy in, 100-105, 101t-
            103t, 109-113
        postresuscitation stabilization in, 113-114,
            113f
        procainamide for, 103t, 105
        rapid sequence intubation in, 107-108, 107b,
            107t
        sodium bicarbonate for, 100, 101t
        tape measurement system in, 114, 114f-115f
    cardiovascular disorders in, 2567-2599
        chest radiography in, 2573-2574, 2573f,
            2574f
        circulatory changes related to, 2568-2569
        compensatory responses associated with,
            2569, 2569b
        history in, 2570-2571, 2570b
        physical examination in, 2571-2575, 2571t,
            2572b
    causes of death in, 942t, 949t
    chest pain in, 2570-2571, 2592
    cholecystitis in, 1421
    cholelithiasis in, 1419
    cigarette ingestion by, 2474
    coarctation of the aorta in, 2578-2579
    congenital heart disease in, 2575-2582
        acyanotic, 2577-2579, 2577f
        chest radiography in, 2573-2574, 2574f

Child (Continued)
    clinical features of, 2575-2576, 2575t
    cyanotic, 2579-2581, 2579f, 2581b
    diagnosis of, 2576, 2576b
    ductal-dependent, 2576-2577, 2576b, 2577b
    incidence of, 2575, 2575t
    management of, 2576-2577, 2576b, 2577b
    postoperative complications of, 2581
    respiratory syncytial virus infection and,
        2581-2582, 2582b
    consent to treatment on behalf of, 3167-3168
    constipation in, 2612-2613
    croup in, 2525-2527, 2526f, 2527b
    cyanosis in
        central, cardiac vs. pulmonary, 2569, 2569b,
            2572
        in tetralogy of Fallot, 2580
        pathophysiology of, 269t, 2569
    cystic fibrosis in, 2564-2565, 2565f
    death of
        in emergency department, 2717
        prehospital issues related to, 3145-3146
    depression in, 1737
    developmental differences in, 2495-2497, 2496t
    diarrhea in, 227, 2623-2634, 2628b, 2628t
    difficult airway in, 2502, 2502b
    digitalis poisoning in, 2372, 2372t
    dysrhythmias in, 2584-2590, 2584b, 2586b,
        2587f-2589f
    Eisenmenger syndrome in, 2578
    electrocardiography in, 2574-2575, 2574t
    emergency department visits by
        readiness for, 2504
        reasons for, 2494, 2495t
    epiglottitis in, 2523-2524, 2524f
    factitious disorder in, 1762
    fever in, 2505-2517
        ancillary tests in, 2508-2510
        bacteremia and, 2505-2506, 2512, 2515
        chest radiography in, 2510
        clinical features of, 2508-2510
        disposition in, 2517
        history in, 2508
        hyperpyrexia and, 2506
        in cancer patient, 2516
        in congenital heart disease, 2517
        in heat exhaustion and heatstroke, 2510
        in HIV/AIDS, 2516
        in Kawasaki disease, 2511, 2512b
        in septic shock, 2511
        in sickle cell anemia, 2516-2517
        in toxic ingestion, 2510-2511
        in toxic shock syndrome, 2511, 2511b
        in ventriculoperitoneal shunts, 2517
        lumbar puncture and, 2660
        management of, 2511-2516, 2513b
        of unknown origin, 2507, 2507b
        pathophysiology of, 2505
        petechiae and, 2507-2508
        physical examination in, 2508, 2509b
        prehospital care in, 2511
        seizure and, 2507, 2666-2667, 2674, 2674b
        temperature determination in, 2508
    foreign bodies in
        airway, 2529-2530, 2550-2551, 2551f
        gastrointestinal, 2616-2617, 2617f
    fracture in, 554-557
        apophyseal, 2709-2711, 2711f
        child abuse and, 970, 970t, 2698-2701
        clavicle, 2692-2693, 2693f
        condylar, 660
        diaphyseal, 2699
        distal radius, 637-639, 637f, 638f, 638t
        elbow avulsion, 2711, 2711f
        epicondylar, 662-663, 662f
        femoral, 763-764, 763f
        greenstick, 554, 556f
        hand, 600
        healing of, 781
        metaphyseal, 2699
        Monteggia, 2697
        multiple, in osteogenesis imperfecta, 2700-
            2701, 2700f, 2700t
        nose, 392
        patterns of, 554-557, 557t, 2689-2692, 2690f-
            2692f, 2691f
        radius, 644, 644f
        rib, 2699
        skull, 334-335, 2699

Child (Continued)
supracondylar, 655-659, 656f-658f
supracondylar humeral, 2693-2697, 2694f-2696f, 2694t
toddler's, 2698, 2698f
torus, 554, 556f
trochanteric, 767
ulnar, 644, 644f
unintentional, 975
gastroesophageal reflux in, 2609-2610
gastrointestinal bleeding in, differential considerations in, 220, 221b, 2613-2614, 2614t
gastrointestinal disorders in, 2601-2621
general approach to, 2494-2504
genitourinary disorders in, 2635-2655
headache in, 2676-2681
acute, 2677
chronic-nonprogressive, 2679
chronic-progressive, 2677-2678
clinical features of, 2676-2677, 2677b
cluster, 2679
diagnosis of, 2679, 2680b
differential considerations in, 2677b
management of, 2680-2681
migraine, 2678-2679, 2678b
pathophysiology of, 2676
heart failure in, 2582-2584, 2583t
hematuria in, 2644-2645, 2645b
hemolytic uremic syndrome in, 2654-2655
Henoch-Schönlein purpura in, 2615, 2615f, 2653-2654
hip dysplasia in, 2701-2702, 2702b, 2702f
hip pain in, 764-765, 2702-2709, 2703b
Hirschsprung's disease in, 2612-2613
human bites in, 890
hypertension in, 2651-2653, 2651b, 2651t, 2652b, 2653t
hypertrophic pyloric stenosis in, 2603-2606, 2605f, 2606t
infectious diarrhea in, 2623-2634
clinical features of, 2626
complications of, 2626
dehydration in, 2629, 2629t
diagnosis of, 2626-2627
differential diagnosis in, 2627, 2627t
disposition in, 2628-2629, 2628b
epidemiology of, 2623-2624
etiology of, 2624-2626, 2628t
fluid and electrolyte management for, 2629-2634, 2630t, 2632b-2634b
management of, 2628, 2628t
pathophysiology of, 2624
inflammatory bowel disease in, 2615-2616
intubation of, 18, 99, 106-107, 108-109, 2519
intussusception in, 2509b, 2610-2612, 2611f, 2612t
iron overdose in, 2418-2419
jaundice in, 2601-2603, 2602t, 2603b, 2603t, 2604f-2605f
Kawasaki disease in, 2593-2596, 2594b, 2595f
lead poisoning in, 2421
Legg-Calvé-Perthes disease in, 2706-2707, 2707f
lower airway obstruction in, 2532-2552
in anaphylaxis, 2546-2550
in asthma, 2532-2544
in bronchiolitis, 2544-2546
in foreign body aspiration, 2550-2551, 2551f
marijuana intoxication in, 2411
Meckel's diverticulum in, 2613-2615, 2614t
musculoskeletal disorders in, 2689-2711
anatomy and physiology in, 2689
apophyseal, 2709-2711, 2711f
child abuse and, 970, 970t, 2698-2701
physeal, 2690, 2691f, 2691t, 2692, 2692f
myocarditis in, 2591-2592
nephrotic syndrome in, 2648-2649
neurologic disorders in, 2657-2686
noninvasive monitoring in, 2504
nursemaid's elbow in, 666, 666f, 2697-2698, 2697f
Osgood-Schlatter syndrome in, 2710
osteogenesis imperfecta in, 2700-2701, 2700f, 2700t
osteomyelitis in, 2183-2184, 2184f
pancreatitis in, 1428, 2618, 2618t
penile disorders in, 2635-2638, 2637f-2638f
peptic ulcer disease in, 1392

Child (Continued)
pericarditis in, 2592-2593, 2593f
periosteal new bone formation in, 2699
pertussis in, 2559-2560
pharmacokinetics of drugs in, 2935, 2952
plant poisoning in, 2471
pneumonia in, 2554-2564
aspiration, 2560
bacterial, 2555, 2556-2557, 2556f, 2557f, 2558t, 2563t
chlamydial, 2559, 2559f, 2563t
complications of, 2562
diagnosis of, 2560-2561, 2561f
differential diagnosis in, 2561, 2562b
epidemiology of, 2555
in immunocompromised host, 2560
management of, 2558t, 2562-2564
mycoplasmal, 2558-2559, 2563t
pathophysiology of, 2555
physical examination in, 2556
signs and symptoms of, 2555-2556
viral, 2555, 2557-2560, 2563t
poststreptococcal glomerulonephritis in, 2647-2648
procedural sedation and analgesia in, 2946-2947, 2952-2954
proteinuria in, 2646-2647
red and painful eye in, 292
refusal of medical care for, 3171
renal disorders in, 2635-2655
renal stones in, 2645-2646
renal tumor in, 2646
respiration in, physiology of, 338
resuscitation of, 97-116
adenosine for, 101t, 104
advanced life support techniques in, 99, 99f
airway management in, 97-98, 105-109, 106f, 107b, 107t
amiodarone for, 101t, 104-105
antidiuretic hormone for, 100, 103t
atropine for, 99, 100, 101t-102t, 103-104
basic life support techniques in, 97-99
breathing management in, 98, 108-109
calcium for, 101t, 104
cardiac rhythm and etiology of arrest in, 109-113, 109t, 110f-112f, 110t
circulatory management in, 98-99, 109-113
defibrillation and cardioversion in, 113
epinephrine for, 111, 114
family presence during, 114-116
glucose for, 100, 101t, 103
lidocaine for, 102t, 105
magnesium for, 104
pharmacologic therapy in, 100-105, 101t-103t, 109-113
postresuscitation stabilization in, 113-114, 113f
procainamide for, 103t, 105
rapid sequence intubation in, 107-108, 107b, 107t
sodium bicarbonate for, 100, 101t
tape measurement system in, 114, 114f-115f
termination of, 116
retropharyngeal abscess in, 2522-2523, 2523f
scrotal masses and swelling in, 2638-2642, 2639f-2640f
seizure in, 367, 2665-2676
after head trauma, 334
anticonvulsant therapy for, 2674-2676, 2675t
clinical features of, 2665-2667, 2666b
diagnosis of, 2670-2671
disposition in, 2674-2676, 2674b, 2675t
etiology of, 2667-2670, 2668b-2670b
febrile, 2507, 2666-2667, 2674, 2674b
management of, 2671-2673, 2671b, 2672t
pathophysiology of, 2665
precipitators of, identification and treatment of, 2673
secondary survey in, 2502
status epilepticus and, 2667, 2668b, 2672-2673, 2672t
septic arthritis in, 2190
Sever's disease in, 2710
shock in, 2499, 2503
slipped capital femoral epiphysis in, 2707-2709, 2708f
small bowel obstruction in, 1441
stroke volume in, decreased, causes of, 2569, 2569b

Child (Continued)
submersion injuries in, 2311, 2314-2315
surrogate decision-making for, 3134
syncope in, 2685-2686
tetralogy of Fallot in, 2579-2581, 2579f, 2580f, 2581b
thermal burns in, 923, 969-970, 970f, 970t
transient synovitis in, 2703-2704
trauma in, 328-342
abdominal, 340-342
blunt, 492, 510
epidemiology of, 489-490
history in, 493
cardiothoracic, 338-340
cervical spine, 336-338, 337f
clinical features of, 329-330
disposition in, 342
epidemiology of, 328
facial, 382, 383
general management principles in, 331-333, 332b, 332t, 333t
head, 333-336, 334b, 335b, 366-368, 369b
hip, 763-767, 763f, 765f-767f
primary survey in, 329-330, 329t, 331t-333t
renal, 528
secondary survey in, 330, 330b, 333, 333b, 2501, 2501b, 2502b
surgical indications in, 332b
upper airway obstruction in, 2519-2530
evaluation of, 2521, 2521f
in congenital lesions, 2522, 2524-2525, 2524f, 2527-2528, 2528f
in croup, 2525-2527, 2526f, 2527b
in epiglottitis, 2523-2524, 2524f
in foreign body aspiration, 2529-2530
in laryngeal disease, 2524-2525, 2524f
in retropharyngeal abscess, 2522-2523, 2523f
in subglottic tracheal disease, 2525-2527
in supraglottic disease, 2522-2524
in tracheal disease, 2527-2529, 2529t
pathophysiology of, 2519, 2520f
stridor in, 2519-2520, 2521f
urinary tract infection in, 1573, 1583-1585, 2510, 2642-2644, 2643b, 2643t
clinical features of, 1583, 1583t
diagnosis of, 1583-1584, 1584f
treatment of, 1584-1585
ventricular septal defect in, 2577
vertigo in, 2682-2685, 2683b, 2684b, 2684f
violence and, 1017-1022
vital signs in, 2495, 2495t
vomiting in, 203, 206, 208t, 2605, 2606t, 2627t, 2628b
vulnerability of, to weapons of mass destruction, 3021
Child abuse, 968-976
abdominal trauma in, 490
bruises consistent with, 969-971, 969f, 970f, 970t, 2502b
diagnostic strategies in, 973-974
differential considerations in, 974-975, 975f, 2699-2701
disposition in, 976
epidemiology of, 968-969, 969t
facial trauma in, 383
head trauma in, 349, 367
historical indicators of, 2501b
history of, in sexual assault cases, 979
immersion scalds in, 916
in Munchausen's syndrome by proxy, 1761, 1763, 1763t, 1765
management of, 975-976
physical abuse in, 969-971, 969f, 970f, 970t, 972, 973, 974-975
radiography in, 2699
reporting of, 976
sexual abuse in, 969, 971, 972-973, 974, 975
sexually transmitted disease and, 973-974, 974t
signs and symptoms of, 971-973
skeletal aspects of, 2698-2701
Child maltreatment, 968
Child neglect, refusal of medical care and, 3171
Child restraint seats, 947, 948
Childbirth. See Labor and delivery.
Chili pepper, drug interactions with, 2478t
Chinese liver fluke, 2100t
Chi-squared test, 3052t, 3053
Chlamydia conjunctivitis, 297t

Chlamydia pneumoniae, 1130, 1132, 2559
  in myocarditis, 1292
  in pharyngitis, 1109, 1111, 1113
Chlamydia psittaci, in pneumonia, 1131
Chlamydia trachomatis
  dysuria in, 1579-1580, 1579t
  in epididymitis, 1595, 1596
  in pharyngitis, 1111, 1113
  in pneumonia, 2559
  in pregnancy, 2758
  in sexually transmitted disease, 1518t, 1519,
    1559t, 1562, 1564-1565
  in urinary tract infection, 1579-1580, 1579t
Chloral hydrate
  for procedural sedation and analgesia, in
    children, 2954
  overdose of, 2487
Chloramphenicol
  during pregnancy and lactation, 2784
  for meningococcal disease, 2023
  for pneumonia, 2558t
  for Q fever, 2137
  for Rocky Mountain spotted fever, 1850, 2136,
    2136t
Chlorazepate, 2484, 2484t
Chlordiazepoxide, 2484, 2484t
  for alcohol withdrawal syndrome, 2862-2863
Chlorhexidine
  for prickly heat, 2259
  for skin disinfection, 847
Chlorinated hydrocarbon poisoning, 2462-2463,
  2462b
Chlorine, as chemical weapon, 3032
Chlorophenoxy compound poisoning, 2464-2465,
  2465b
Chloroquine, for systemic lupus erythematosus,
  1809
Chlorothiazide, 1321t
Chlorpheniramine, for anaphylaxis, 1831b, 1832
Chlorpromazine, 2446t
  hepatotoxicity of, 1414
  in heatstroke, 2265
  seizures from, 2962
Chlorpropamide
  overdose of, hypoglycemia from, 1961
  rash from, 1972
Chlorprothixene, 2446t
Chlorthalidone, 1321t
  during pregnancy and lactation, 2788
Choanal atresia, 121, 2522
Choking, in airway foreign body aspiration, 865,
  866
Cholangiopancreaticoduodenography, endoscopic
  retrograde, in abdominal trauma, 499
Cholangiopancreatography, endoscopic retrograde
  in acute pancreatitis, 1433
  in chronic pancreatitis, 1436
  in gallstone pancreatitis, 1434
  in jaundice, 244
  pancreatitis after, 1428
Cholangiopathy, AIDS, 1423
Cholangioscopy, endoscopic, in cholangitis, 1422
Cholangitis, 1421-1422, 1422f
Cholecystitis, 1419-1421, 1419f
  acalculous, 1421, 2620, 2621
  emphysematous, 1421
  jaundice in, 246
Cholecystography, oral, in cholelithiasis, 1419
Choledocholithiasis, 246
Cholelithiasis, 1418-1419, 1418f, 1419f
  in children, 2620-2621
  in cholangitis, 1421, 1422f
  in cholecystitis, 1419f, 1420
  in pregnancy, 1419, 2754-2755
  pancreatitis in, 1426, 1427, 1428, 1433, 1434
Cholestasis
  in drug-induced liver disorders, 1414
  in pregnancy, 1416-1417, 2726
  jaundice in, 243, 244f, 246
Cholesteatoma, in otitis media, 1067
Cholesterol gallstones, 1418
Choline acetyltransferase, in dementia, 1657
Cholinergic syndrome
  in organophosphate poisoning, 2459, 2459b
  in overdosed/poisoned patient, 2327t, 2328
  mushrooms associated with, 2479
Cholinergic urticaria, 1848
Cholinesterase inhibitors, for myasthenia gravis,
  1706

Chondrocalcinosis, in hypothyroidism, 1992
Chondrolysis, in slipped capital femoral
  epiphysis, 2709
Chondromalacia patellae, 786
Chopart's joint
  anatomy of, 820, 820f
  injuries to, 827
Chorea
  in acute rheumatic fever, 2596
  in rheumatic fever, 1304
Choreoathetoid movement, in cocaine overdose,
  2388
Choreoathetosis, paroxysmal, 2668
Chorioamnionitis, 2759, 2808, 2808b
Chorionic membrane, premature rupture of,
  2807-2808, 2808t
Choroid, 1045f
Chromic gut suture, 852t
Chromosomal abnormalities, miscarriage and,
  2740
Chronic disease, reporting requirements for,
  3173
Chronic obstructive pulmonary disease, 1097-
  1107
  acute decompensation in, causes of, 1101-1103,
    1103t
  acute exacerbations of
    causes of, 1099, 1103t
    management of, 1103-1106, 1103t-1105t
  altitude and, 2307, 2308
  anxiety in, 1747
  clinical features of, 1099-1100
  definition of, 1097
  diagnosis of, 1100-1101
  differential diagnosis in, 1101-1103
  disposition in, 1106, 1106t
  dyspnea in, 179t
  epidemiology of, 1097
  mechanical ventilation in, 31-32
  natural history of, 1099, 1099f
  palliative care in, 3154
  pathophysiology of, 1097-1098
  pharmacologic therapy for, 1105-1106
  physical examination in, 1099-1100
  pneumonia in, 1132
  pneumothorax in, 1102, 1143-1144, 1145
  staging severity of, 1098-1099, 1098t
  symptoms of, 1099
  ventilation and oxygenation in, 1103-1105,
    1103t-1105t
Chronic pain syndromes, 2913-2914, 2914b
Chronic recurrent multifocal osteomyelitis
  (CRMO), 2184
Churg-Strauss syndrome, 1816
Chvostek's sign, in hypocalcemia, 1943
Cicuta maculata, 2472, 2472f
Cicutoxin, 2472
Cidofovir, 2038
Cigarette burn, in child abuse, 969, 969f
Ciguatera fish poisoning, 1470t, 1473-1474
Cilastatin, for febrile, neutropenic cancer patient,
  2838t
Ciliary flush, in traumatic iridocyclitis, 1049,
  1049f
Ciliary muscle, 1045f
Cimetidine, 1390t
  for anaphylactic shock, 54
  for anaphylaxis, 2549
  for hymenoptera stings, 904
  for scombroid fish poisoning, 1472
Cimino-Brescia fistula, 1365-1366
Ciprofloxacin
  for anthrax exposure, 3026, 3026b
  for *Campylobacter* gastroenteritis, 1461
  for *Escherichia coli* food poisoning, 1474
  for gonococcal arthritis, 1788
  for gonococcal dermatitis, 1843-1844
  for granuloma inguinale, 1559t, 1563
  for infectious diarrhea, 235
  for meningococcal meningitis, 1723
  for *Plesiomonas shigelloides* gastroenteritis,
    1468
  for prostatitis, 1586
  for salmonellosis, 1463
  for shigellosis, 1461t, 1464
  for traveler's diarrhea, 1487
  for urinary tract infection, 1582
  for *Vibrio* fish poisoning, 1472
  prophylactic, for meningococcal disease, 2024

Circadian rhythm disruption, from shift work,
  performance and, 3123, 3123b
Circuit, AC vs. DC, electrical injury and, 2268
Circulation. *See also* Blood flow.
  fetal, 2568, 2568f
  in beta blocker overdose, 2375
  in cardiac arrest, 88-90
  in elderly trauma patient, 348
  in pediatric resuscitation, 98-99, 109-113
  in pediatric trauma, 330, 332t
  in pregnant trauma patient, 322-323
  neonatal, 2568-2569
  persistent fetal, 119
  transitional, at birth, 118-119, 119t, 2568
Circumcision, complications of, 2638
Circumferential cardiopulmonary resuscitation,
  89
Circumflex fibular artery, 771
Circumflex humeral arteries, 672
Circumvallate placenta, 2810
Cirrhosis, 1410-1411
  alcoholic, 2868
  hepatocellular carcinoma and, 1417
  immune defects in, 2841-2842
  infections in, 2842
  pipe-stem, in chronic schistosomiasis, 2112,
    2113f
  prerenal azotemia in, 1532-1533
  with ascites, 1410, 1411, 1412
Cisapride, for nausea and vomiting, 206
Citalopram, metabolism of, 2357
Citrate, hypocalcemia from, 1943
Civil protection order, in intimate partner
  violence and abuse, 1005
Clarithromycin
  during pregnancy and lactation, 2784
  for Lyme disease, 2127t, 2128
  for *Mycobacterium avium* infection in
    HIV/AIDS, 2076
  for pertussis, 2006
  for pharyngitis, 1113
  for pneumonia, 2558t
  in HIV/AIDS, side effects of, 2079t
Clark v. Baton Rouge General Medical Center, 3157
Claudication
  exercise-induced, in arteriosclerosis obliterans,
    1350
  intermittent, in chronic arterial insufficiency,
    1345
Clavicle
  anatomy of, 670, 671f
  fracture of, 676-679, 676f-679f
    in children, 2692-2693, 2693f
    subclavian artery injury and, 545
Clavicular splint, 569, 677, 678f
Clawhand, 586, 588f
Clay shoveler's fracture, 401, 403f, 550t
Clearblue One Step pregnancy test, 2729
Clenched-fist injury, 611, 890
Clenched-fist view of wrist, 627, 627t
Clindamycin
  for babesiosis, 2140
  for bacterial vaginosis, 1567t, 1568
  for orofacial infections, 1032
  for otitis media, 1069
  for pelvic inflammatory disease, 1571t
  for pneumonia, 2558t
  for toxic shock syndrome, 2030, 2201
  in HIV/AIDS, side effects of, 2079t
Clinical decision making
  diagnostic approach and, 125-130, 127f, 128b,
    129f
  errors in, 130-133, 131t, 133b
Clinical decision rules in emergency medicine,
  3035-3036
Clinical decision support (CDS) systems, 3098
Clinical decision unit, 1093. *See also*
  Observation medicine.
Clinical documentation, in material safety data
  sheet, 3081, 3082b
Clinical interview, in pediatric assessment, 2500-
  2501, 2501b
Clinical pathways, 3038, 3039f-3041f
  decision making errors in using, 131t, 132
Clinical practice guidelines. *See* Guidelines for
  emergency medicine.
Clinical protocols, 3038
Clinical question, in evidence-based medicine,
  3058

Clinical reasoning, 126
Clinical studies, 3046-3047
Clinical trials, 3047-3051, 3048f
Clonazepam, 2484, 2484t
  during pregnancy and lactation, 2787
  for seizure, 2675t
  side effects of, 1628t
Clonidine, 1321t
  during pregnancy and lactation, 2789
  for alcohol withdrawal syndrome, 2862
  for opioid withdrawal, 2455-2456
  withdrawal of, hypertension from, 1313-1314
Clonorchis sinensis, 2100t
Clopidogrel
  for acute coronary syndromes, 1186-1187
  for chest pain, 184
  thrombocytopenia from, 1898
Closed-fist injury, 611, 890
Closed-loop obstruction of small bowel, 1440
Close-range handgun wounds, 956, 956f
Clostridial cellulitis, 2208
Clostridial myonecrosis, 2208-2209
Clostridium botulinum poisoning, 1707-1708, 2012-2016
Clostridium difficile infection
  in antibiotic-associated enterocolitis, 1470t, 1474-1475
  in dysenteric colitis, 230t
  in pseudomembranous colitis, 2625
Clostridium difficile toxin test, 233
Clostridium perfringens food poisoning, 1470-1471, 1470t, 2625-2626
Clostridium tetani, 2007, 2008-2009. See also Tetanus.
Clot solubility testing in bleeding disorders, 1895
Clotrimazole
  during pregnancy and lactation, 2785
  for candidal esophagitis, 1387
  in HIV/AIDS, side effects of, 2079t
Cloxacillin, for staphylococcal scalded skin syndrome, 1845
Clozapine
  for psychosis in demented patient, 1662
  for thought disorders, 1731
  toxicity of, 2446, 2446t, 2448
"Club drugs," 2883-2884
Clubbing, in cyanosis, 270-271, 270f
Cluster headache, 1634-1635, 2679
Coagulation
  disseminated intravascular, 1903-1904, 1904t
    after head trauma, 371
    in anaphylaxis, 1825t
    in meningococcal disease, 2022
    in pregnancy, placental abruption and, 319-320
    in rhabdomyolysis, 1981
    in sepsis, 2214
  for epistaxis, 1074
  hypothermic, 2243-2244
  in pregnancy, 2725
  in wound healing, 842
  regulation of, 1894
  zone of, in burn injury, 917, 917f
Coagulation factors, 1892, 1893b, 1893f, 1894
  assays of, in bleeding disorders, 1895
  replacement of, for disseminated intravascular coagulation, 1904
Coagulation pathway
  disorders of. See Coagulopathy.
  in hemostasis, 1892, 1893f, 1894
Coagulation studies, 1894-1895, 1894b
Coagulopathy, 1899-1904
  in disseminated intravascular coagulation, 1903-1904, 1904t
  in heatstroke, 2262, 2265
  in hemophilia A, 1899-1902, 1901t, 1902t
  in hemophilia B, 1903
  in pancreatitis, 1430
  in rhabdomyolysis, 1981, 1983
  in sepsis, 2214
  in submersion victim, 2313
  in von Willebrand's disease, 1902-1903
  oral hemorrhage and, 1042
Coal tar burns, 926-927, 937
Coarctation of the aorta, 1312, 2578-2579
Cobalt blue lamp test of corneal damage, 287-288
COBRA, 3156
Cocaethylene, 2876

Cocaine
  alcohol interactions with, 2876
  cardiac effects of, 1292-1293
  during pregnancy, 2792-2793
  formulations of, 2386, 2387t
  metabolism of, 2386
  mydriasis from, 1061
  overdose of, 2386-2392
    body packing/stuffing and, 2391-2392
    clinical features of, 2386-2388, 2387b
    diagnosis of, 2388-2389
    differential diagnosis in, 2389, 2389b
    disposition in, 2392, 2392t
    emergency department visits related to, 2884f
    management of, 2389-2391, 2389b, 2390b
    pathophysiology of, 2386, 2387f
    rhabdomyolysis from, 1979
    seizure from, 1623
    topical, 846, 2933
Cocaine test, in Horner's syndrome, 1061-1062
Coccidia, gastroenteritis from, 1476-1479, 1477t
Coccidioides immitis
  in cancer patient with impaired cell-mediated immunity, 2840
  in pneumonia, 1130
Coccyx, 400f
  fracture of, 725
Cochleovestibular apparatus damage, in middle ear barotrauma, 2282
Cochrane Library, clinical practice guidelines in, 3035, 3042
Codeine, 2920, 2921t, 2925
  during pregnancy and lactation, 2784
  for migraine, 2680
  respiratory effects of, 2453t
Coffee bean sign
  in colonic volvulus, 1499
  in small bowel obstruction, 1443
Cognitive dispositions as source of failures in emergency department, 3122
Cognitive distortions, difficult patient and, 2975, 2976
Cognitive impairment
  assessment of, 151, 152f, 153f
    in delirium, 1649-1650, 1650f
    in systemic lupus erythematosus, 1811
    in thought disorders, 1730
  in delirium, 1649
  in dementia, 1658-1659
  in depression, 1737
  in elderly person, 2827
  in multiple sclerosis, 1672
Cognitive processes, in clinical decision making, 130, 131t, 132
Cognitive-behavioral therapy, for anxiety disorders, 1751, 1751t
Coining, 3114
Coital headache, 1642
Colchicine
  for gouty arthritis, 1786
  for pseudogout, 1787
Cold agglutinins, in autoimmune hemolytic anemia, 1883
Cold diuresis, 2239
Cold intolerance, in hypothyroidism, 1991
"Cold sores," 2230
Cold stress. See also Frostbite; Hypothermia.
  injuries associated with
    central, 2236-2252
    peripheral, 2228-2235
  physiology of, 2228-2229, 2236-2237, 2237f
Cold urticaria, 1848
Cold water treatment, of burned skin, 921
Cold-water head dunking, for dysrhythmias, 1214-1215
Colic
  biliary, in cholelithiasis, 1418
  in lead poisoning, 2421
  nonsteroidal antiinflammatory drugs for, 2926
  renal, 1586-1593, 1586b, 1589f-1592f, 1593b. See also Urolithiasis.
Colitis
  antibiotic-associated, *Clostridium difficile*, 1470t, 1474-1475
  dysenteric, infectious causes of, 228, 229t-230t
  ulcerative, 1500-1503, 1502b, 1502f, 1503b
    in children, 2615-2616
    skin lesions in, 1862t

Collagen, in wound healing, 842-843
Collagen vascular disease, oral manifestations of, 1035, 1035f
Collar-button abscess, 617, 617f
Collateral geniculate artery injury, in tibial femoral knee dislocation, 788
Collateral ligament
  of ankle, 808, 809f
  of knee
    anatomy of, 770, 771f
    injury to, 791-792
    stress test of, 774
  radial, 647, 648f
    injury to, 604
  stress test of, 774
  ulnar, 647, 648f
    injury to, 604
Colles' fracture, 632-633, 634f, 635f
  reverse, 633-635, 635f
Colloid solutions
  for anaphylaxis, 1833
  for hemorrhagic shock, 52
  for septic shock, 53
Colon
  congenital aganglionosis of, 2612-2613
  distention of, in large bowel obstruction, 1496, 1496f
  diverticula of, 1492-1495, 1494b, 1495b
  ischemia of, 1503-1504
  pathologic dilation of, 1501, 1502f
  trauma to, 489, 490
  volvulus of, 1497-1499, 1498f, 1499b, 1499f
Colonic inertia, in elderly person, 237
Colonoscopy
  in colonic ischemia, 1504
  in large bowel obstruction, 1496-1497
Colorado tick fever, 2047, 2140-2141
Colorectal cancer, large bowel obstruction in, 1495
Colostrum, 2724, 2728
Colposcopy, in sexual assault examination, 987, 987b
Coma, 156-164
  alcohol-induced, 2869
  diagnostic approach to, 157-162, 158b, 159t, 160f, 162f, 163f
  disposition in, 163
  drug-induced, 1991
  empiric management of, 162-163
  epidemiology of, 156
  hypothyroid, 1991
  in anticholinergic poisoning, 2348
  in barbiturate overdose, 2482
  in carbon monoxide poisoning, 2439
  in cardiac arrest survivors
    acute coronary syndrome diagnosis and, 86
    resuscitative hypothermia for, 68-70, 69t, 85-86
  in cyclic antidepressant poisoning, 2354t, 2356
  in eclampsia, 2749
  in hepatic encephalopathy, 1411
  in high-altitude cerebral edema, 2306
  in hyperviscosity syndrome, 1913
  in intracerebral hemorrhage, 1610
  in rabies, 2066
  in Rocky Mountain spotted fever, 2134
  myxedema, 1990, 1990b, 1991, 1991b, 1993-1994
  hypothermia and, 2239
  pathophysiology of, 156
  scoring methods for, 157, 157t
Combat casualty evacuation care (CASEVAC), 3003, 3003f
Combative patient, 2956-2969
  assault by, 2963
  diagnostic studies in, 2964
  differential considerations in, 2964-2965, 2965b
  disposition of, 2969
  epidemiology of, 2956-2957
  functional vs. organic etiology of, 2963, 2964t
  history taking and physical examination of, 2963-2964, 2964t
  medical clearance of, 2965
  medicolegal issues of, 2967-2969
  pathophysiology of, 2957
  physical restraints for, 2958-2961, 2960f
  preparation of emergency department for, 2965-2967

Combative patient (Continued)
   rapid tranquilization of, 2961-2963
   risk assessment and, 2957-2958
   verbal management techniques for, 2958
Combustible liquids, flash points of, 915, 915t
Comfrey, adverse effects of, 2476t
Commercial emergency department information
   technology systems, 3102
Comminuted fracture, 552, 552f, 2690, 2691f
Commitment, involuntary, in suicide, 1773
Common bile duct obstruction, in cholangitis,
   1421, 1422f
Common cold
   coronavirus infection in, 2051
   pharyngitis in, 1110
Common femoral artery
   anatomy of, 540, 540f
   bifurcation of, arterial embolism at, 1343
Common peroneal mononeuropathy, 1698-1699,
   1698f
Common peroneal nerve, 771
Commotio cordis
   in children, 340
   sudden death in, 2599
Commotio retinae, 1050
Communicable diseases, reporting requirements
   for, 3172
Communication
   in disaster response, 3015
   in emergency medical services, 2988-2989
   information technology for, 3098
   with hearing impaired patient, 2905
   with visually impaired patient, 2905
Community, disaster response experience in,
   3016-3017
Community preparedness, in chemical injuries,
   930-931
Comparative justice, 3129, 3129b
Comparison radiographs, in fracture, 557-558
Compartment pressure, measurement of, 561-562,
   561f
Compartment syndrome, 559-562, 560b, 561b,
   561f
   crush injury and, 3007-3008
   in foot, 838-839
   in hand, 614, 614f
   in lower leg, 804
   in peripheral vascular injury, 539
   in rhabdomyolysis, 1977-1978, 1980, 1983,
     1983f
   in thigh, 749
   in tibial femoral knee dislocation, 789
Compartments
   of knee, 770, 771f
   of lower leg, 797
   of thigh, 737, 737t, 738f
Competence
   capacity vs., 3133-3134, 3134b
   determination of, in refusal of medical care,
     3169
   elder abuse and, 1014
   impaired, consent in, 3168
   of combative or violent patient, 2967
Complement
   activation of, in cerebral ischemia, 66
   deficiencies of, 2833
   in anaphylaxis/anaphylactoid reactions, 2547
Complement pathway, 2832-2833
Complementary medicine, cultural competent
   approach to, 3113-3114
Complete blood count
   in abdominal pain, 215, 216t
   in arthritis, 1779
   in bacterial meningitis, 2662
   in bleeding disorders, 1894
   in central nervous system infection, 1720
   in delirium, 1651
   in headache, 173t
   in nausea and vomiting, 203
Complete fracture, 2690, 2691f
Complex regional pain syndrome, 562-563
Compound presentations, in labor and delivery,
   2815-2816
Compressed air, esophageal perforation from, 483
Compression
   for epistaxis, 1074
   for snakebite management, 899
   rhabdomyolysis from, 1978
Compressive optic neuropathy, 1060

Computed tomography
   before lumbar puncture, 1716, 1716t
   in abdominal aortic aneurysm, 1335, 1336f,
     1338
   in abdominal trauma, 496-498, 497f, 498f
   in acute mesenteric ischemia, 1447-1448
   in acute pancreatitis, 1432-1433
   in airway foreign body aspiration, 866-867
   in ankle trauma, 811
   in aortic dissection, 1327, 1327f, 1327t
   in aortic rupture, 479-480, 479f
   in appendicitis, 1454-1455, 1455f, 1456, 2619-
     2620
   in arthritis, 1780
   in back pain, 708
   in bacterial meningitis, 2662-2663
   in brain abscess, 371
   in brain contusion, 374
   in central nervous system infection, 1719-1720
   in cerebral venous thrombosis, 1670
   in cervical vascular injury, 449
   in chronic pancreatitis, 1436
   in colonic ischemia, 1504
   in comatose patient, 162
   in delirium, 1651
   in dementia, 1661
   in depressed skull fracture, 373
   in diverticular disease, 1493
   in elderly trauma patient, 347
   in electrical and lightning injuries, 2275-2276
   in epidural hematoma, 375, 375f, 376f
   in esophageal foreign body, 872
   in esophageal obstruction, 1383
   in esophageal perforation, 1385
   in facial fracture, 388, 389, 394f
   in flail chest, 457
   in foot trauma, 822
   in fracture, 558
   in gastrointestinal foreign body, 874
   in headache, 172, 173t, 2679
   in head-injured child, 368
   in hemoptysis, 281
   in HIV/AIDS, 2079-2080
   in intracerebral hemorrhage, 1613
   in ischemic stroke, 1612, 1612f
   in jaundice, 244
   in knee trauma, 774
   in large bowel obstruction, 1496
   in laryngotracheal trauma, 447
   in minor head trauma, 364
   in moderate head trauma, 363
   in multiple trauma, 312, 313
   in ocular foreign body, 860, 860f
   in osteomyelitis, 2181
   in pediatric head trauma, 336
   in pelvic fracture, 721-722, 723
   in pelvic pain, 250
   in peripheral vascular injury, 542
   in pneumonia, 1133
   in pneumothorax, 463
   in pregnant trauma patient, 321, 321t
   in pulmonary contusion, 460-461
   in red and painful eye, 288
   in renal disorders, 1528, 1528f
   in renal trauma, 528, 529f
   in rib fracture, 455
   in seizure, 168, 1625, 2671
   in septic arthritis, 2190
   in severe head trauma, 362, 362t
   in sinusitis, 1124, 1125f
   in skull fracture, 372
   in small bowel obstruction, 1443
   in soft tissue foreign body, 879
   in spinal injuries, 427, 429-431, 429b, 429f-
     432f, 430-431, 431f
   in sternoclavicular joint dislocation, 684, 684f
   in subarachnoid hemorrhage, 1636, 1637f
   in subdural hematoma, 376, 376f
   in *Toxoplasma gondii* infection, 2081, 2082f
   in ureteral trauma, 531
   in urinary tract infection, 1578
   in urolithiasis, 1589, 1589f
   of parapharyngeal abscess, 1122, 1122f
   of pyogenic abscess, 1415, 1415f
   of retropharyngeal abscess, 1121, 1121f
Computed tomography angiography
   in anthrax exposure, 3025, 3025f
   in bacterial meningitis, 1716, 1716t
   in cervical vascular injury, 449

Computed tomography angiography (Continued)
   in peripheral arteriovascular disease, 1348
   in pulmonary embolism, 1375-1377, 1377b
Computed tomography urogram, in renal stones,
   2645-2646
Computed tomography venography, in
   pulmonary embolism, 1377
Computer-based protocols, for emergency
   medicine guidelines, 3042-3044, 3043f
Computerized physician order entry (CPOE)
   systems, 3043, 3043f, 3101, 3102f
Conception, estimated date of, 2727
Concussion
   in children, 335
   in head trauma, 365-366, 367
   myocardial, 467
Conduction system, 1201-1203, 1202t, 1203f
Conductive hearing loss, 1072
Conductive heat transfer, 2255
Condylar fracture
   distal, 776-777
   in adults, 660-661, 661f
   in children, 660
   tibial, 777-779, 777f-778f
Condylomata lata, in syphilis, 1561, 1561f
Condylomata acuminata, 1518t, 1519-1520,
   1559t, 1563-1564, 1564f, 2045
Cone shells, 910
Confidence intervals, 3053
Confidentiality
   as value, 3129, 3129b
   of patient information, 3102-3103
Confirmation bias, 132
Confounding variables, 3049, 3055
Confusion, 150-155, 156
   acute, 2679
   after moderate head trauma, 363
   diagnostic approach to, 150-153, 151b, 152f,
     153f
   differential diagnosis in, 153, 154b, 154f
   disposition in, 154-155
   empiric management of, 154, 155f
   epidemiology of, 150
   guidelines for evaluation of, 1645-1646
   in delirium, 1645-1655
   in dementia, 1655-1662
   in rabies, 2065-2066
   pathophysiology of, 150
Confusional Assessment Method, in delirium,
   1650, 1650f
Congenital heart disease, 2575-2582
   acyanotic, 2577-2579, 2577f
   chest radiography in, 2573-2574, 2574f
   clinical features of, 2575-2576, 2575t
   cyanotic, 2579-2581, 2579f, 2581b
   diagnosis of, 2576, 2576b
   ductal-dependent, 2576-2577, 2576b, 2577b
   incidence of, 2575, 2575t
   management of, 2576-2577, 2576b, 2577b
   pediatric fever in, 2517
   postoperative complications of, 2581
   respiratory syncytial virus infection and, 2581-
     2582, 2582b
Congestive heart failure. See Heart failure.
Congo-Crimean hemorrhagic fever, 2055
Conium maculatum, 2472, 2473f
Conjunctiva, 1045f
   foreign body in, 1048
   laceration of, 1051
   nonpenetrating trauma to, 1046-1048, 1047f,
     1048f
Conjunctival blood gas monitoring, 36
Conjunctivitis
   gonococcal, 1566
   in anaphylaxis, 1825t
   in Kawasaki disease, 2025-2026
   red and painful eye in, 296t-297t
Connective tissue disorders
   myocarditis in, 1297-1298
   pericardial disease in, 1284
Conn's syndrome, hypokalemia in, 1938
Conoid ligament, 670-671, 671f
Conscience anxiety, 1746b
Conscious sedation, 2914b
Consciousness
   altered, 156-164. See also Coma; Mental status,
     altered.
     after head trauma, 354, 363-364
     definitions of, 156-157

Consciousness (Continued)
  diagnostic approach to, 157-162, 158b, 159t, 160f, 162f, 163f
  disposition in, 163
  empiric management of, 162-163
  epidemiology of, 156
  host defense impairment in, 1129
  in beta blocker overdose, 2374
  in central nervous system infection, 1714
  in children, 2502-2503
  in cyclic antidepressant poisoning, 2352
  in high-altitude cerebral edema, 2306
  in neoplastic cardiac tamponade, 1917
  in scuba diving–related disorders, 2285
  pathophysiology of, 156
  clouding of, 156
Consent
  federal vs. state laws governing, 3166
  for procedural sedation and analgesia, 2940
  implied, 3134, 3167
  in alcohol intoxication, 3168-3169
  in delirious patient, 1654-1655
  in impaired competence, 3168
  in patient given pain medications, 3169
  in sexual assault cases, 978, 979b
  informed, 3134, 3166
    emergency research without, 3136-3137
    for procedures on newly dead, 3149
    physician's role in, 3166-3167
  minors and, 3167-3168
  of combative or violent patient, 2967
  prisoners and, 3168
  "reasonable person" vs. "professional disclosure" standard in, 3166
Constipation, 237-242
  acute vs. chronic, 238b
  complications of, 239
  definition of, 237, 237t
  diagnostic approach to, 238-239, 238b
  differential diagnosis in, 239, 240f
  disposition in, 242
  empiric management of, 239-242, 240f, 241t, 242b
  epidemiology of, 237
  in children, 2612-2613
  in colonic volvulus, 1497, 1498
  in spinal cord injury, 2907
  palliative care for, 3154
  pathophysiology of, 237
Constrictive pericarditis, 1288
  heart failure in, 1265
  neoplastic, 1917
  restrictive cardiomyopathy vs., 1296
Consultation
  in HIV postexposure prophylaxis, 3086b
  in observation unit, 3063
  in poisoning, 2331
  in spinal cord injury, 311
Consumption, galloping, 2151
Contact burn, 913-928. See also Thermal burn.
Contact dermatitis, skin lesions in, 1851-1852, 1851f, 1852f
Contact dermatoconjunctivitis, 296t
Contact handgun wounds, 955-956, 955f, 956f
Contact lens
  corneal complications of, 1054
  superficial punctate keratitis from, 1054
Contaminated air, in scuba diving–related disorders, 2283
Contamination. See also Decontamination.
  of airway, in urban search and rescue, 3008
  of blood products, 60-61
  of herbal medicines, 2476-2477
  radioactive
    external, 2320
    internal, 2320, 2324
    management of, 2322-2324, 2323f
  wound, 2321
Continence
  loss of, 1516-1517, 1516b
  physiology of, 1507
Contingency management
  for factitious disorder, 1764-1765
  in HAZMAT incidents, 931
Continuous positive airway pressure (CPAP), 27-28
  in acute pulmonary edema, 1271, 1271f
  in sleep apnea in chronic heart failure, 1277

Continuous positive airway pressure (CPAP) (Continued)
  in submersion victim, 2314
  mask, 28
Contraception, emergency, after sexual assault, 991, 991t
Contractility, in heart failure, 1260f, 1261
Contraction-relaxation cycle, 1259
Contrast agents
  acute tubular necrosis from, 1536-1537
    prevention of, 1539
  allergy to, 1828
  anaphylaxis to, 2547
Contrast studies
  in abdominal trauma, 499, 499f
  in bladder trauma, 521-525, 521f-526f
  in esophageal foreign body, 871-872
  in esophageal perforation, 485, 485f
  in gastrointestinal foreign body, 873-874
  in urethral trauma, 517-519, 518f-520f
Contrecoup contusion, 352, 374
Controlled mechanical ventilation (CMV), 27
Contusion
  eyelid, 1044
  foot, 838
  in facial trauma, 390, 391
  in head trauma, 335, 374
  pattern
    in pedestrian collisions, 966
    in physical assault, 961-962, 961f, 962f
  renal, 530, 530f
  testicular, 534
Conus medullaris syndrome, 1678f, 1679
Convective heat transfer, 916, 917t, 2255
Convenience sample, 3048
Conversion disorder, 1755, 1755b
Convulsion, in shigellosis, 1464
Convulsive status epilepticus, 2667
Cooling system, automobile, and body's heat dissipation mechanisms, 2256-2258, 2256f
Cooling techniques
  for comatose survivors of cardiac arrest, 69
  for heatstroke, 2263-2264, 2264b, 2265f
Coombs and Gell classification of hypersensitivity reactions, 1821-1822
Coombs test, in hemolytic anemia, 1878
Co-oximetry, in carbon monoxide poisoning, 2439
COPD. See Chronic obstructive pulmonary disease.
Copper, corneal foreign body containing, 1052
Copper reduction tests, in diabetes mellitus, 1959, 1959b
Copper sulfate, for white phosphorus burn, 936
Copperheads, 896
Coprine in mushrooms, ethanol and, 2479
Cor pulmonale, in chronic obstructive pulmonary disease, 1100
Coracoacromial arch, 671f, 672
Coracoclavicular ligaments, 670-671, 671f
Coracoid process
  anatomy of, 671f, 672
  fracture of, 679, 680
Coral snakes, 896, 898
Cornea, 1045f
  abrasions of, 289, 289f, 292, 294t, 933, 1047, 1047f
  clouding of
    in alkali burn, 1046, 1046f
    in closed-angle glaucoma, 1056, 1056f
  damage to, testing of, 287-288
  diseases of, 1053-1054, 1054f
  foreign body in, 289, 289f, 292, 294t, 297, 1047, 1047f, 1048f
  herpes simplex virus infection of, 289, 290f, 295t
  laceration of, 1051, 1051f
  nonpenetrating trauma to, 1046-1048, 1046f, 1047f, 1048f
  ulcers of, 289, 289f, 294t, 1052, 1052f, 1054
Corner stitch suture, 851

Coronary angiography, in aortic rupture, 480-481
Coronary angioplasty, percutaneous transluminal. See Percutaneous coronary intervention.
Coronary artery
  aneurysm of, in Kawasaki disease, 2025, 2026, 2594
  anomalous, sudden death in, 1298
  congenital anomalies of, sudden death in, 2597
  dilation of, in Kawasaki disease, 2594
  embolism to, in scuba diving–related disorders, 2285
  laceration of, 472
Coronary artery bypass graft, previous, fibrinolytic therapy eligibility and, 1191
Coronary artery disease
  alcohol consumption and, 2866
  altitude and, 2308
  atherosclerotic plaques in, 1157
  cardiac arrest in, 77
  echocardiography in, 1179
  epidemiology of, 1155
  graded exercise testing in, 1180-1181
  historical perspective of, 1155
  in systemic lupus erythematosus, 1807
Coronary stents, in myocardial infarction, 1195
Coronary vasospasm, in acute coronary syndromes, 1157
Coronavirus, 2034t, 2050-2051
Coronoid fossa, 647, 647f
Corpus cavernosa
  anatomy of, 532, 532f
  rupture of, 533-534, 534f
Corpus luteum cyst rupture
  ectopic pregnancy vs., 2745
  pelvic pain in, 251t
Corpus spongiosum, 532, 532f
Corrigan's pulse, in aortic regurgitation, 1307
Cortical blindness, 1060
Cortical dysfunction, in confusion, 150
Corticospinal tract, lateral, 1676, 1676f
Corticosteroids. See also specific agents, e.g., Prednisone.
  adrenal insufficiency from, 1994-1995
  allergy to, 1827
  during pregnancy and lactation, 2762, 2765t, 2776, 2789
  for adhesive capsulitis, 699, 699t
  for anaphylactic shock, 54
  for anaphylaxis, 1833, 2549
  for asthma, 1087t, 1088-1089, 2539t, 2541-2543, 2543t
  for atopic dermatitis, 1842
  for bacterial meningitis, 1722, 2664-2665
  for Behçet's disease, 1815
  for Bell's palsy, 1667
  for bronchiolitis, 2546
  for bursitis, 1803
  for calcific tendinitis, 698
  for caustic ingestion, 2383
  for chronic obstructive pulmonary disease, 1105-1106
  for epicondylitis, 667
  for granulomatous vasculitis, 1814
  for Henoch-Schönlein purpura, 2615
  for hypercalcemia, 1946
  for hypercalcemic cancer patient, 1916
  for hypothermia, 2246
  for inflammatory bowel disease, 1502, 2616
  for knee bursitis, 796
  for meningococcal disease, 2023-2024
  for microscopic polyangiitis, 1814
  for migraine, 1633t, 1634
  for multiple sclerosis, 1673
  for myasthenia gravis, 1706
  for myxedema coma, 1994
  for nephrotic syndrome, 2648
  for optic neuritis, 1059-1060
  for organ transplant patient, 2850, 2851f
  for pharyngitis, 1113
  for polyarteritis nodosa, 1814
  for PROM, 2808
  for Rocky Mountain spotted fever, 2136-2137
  for sciatica, 711
  for sepsis, 2222
  for septic shock, 54
  for severe head trauma, 361
  for spinal injuries, 438
  for subacromial syndromes, 696

Corticosteroids (Continued)
  for superior vena cava syndrome, 1911
  for systemic lupus erythematosus, 1808-1809
  for thyroid storm, 1989
  for tuberculosis, 2168
  for viral croup, 2526-2527
  immunosuppressive effects of, 2843-2844
  medical indications for, 1995, 1996b
  ophthalmic, 1063b, 1064
  toxicity of, 1417
Corticotropin. See Adrenocorticotropic hormone.
Cortisol, in glucose regulation, 1957
Cortisone acetate, for adrenal insufficiency, 1998
Corynebacterium diphtheriae, 1110-1111, 2001, 2002. See also Diphtheria.
Costochondral separation, 457
Costoclavicular ligaments, 670, 671f
Costoclavicular syndrome, 1359
Cotton fever, in intravenous drug abuse, 2454
Cotton's fracture, 550t
Cough
  as host defense, 1128-1129
  in airway foreign body aspiration, 865, 866
  in asthma, 1083
  in bacterial tracheitis, 2528
  in bronchiolitis, 2545
  in chronic obstructive pulmonary disease, 1099, 1100
  in high-altitude pulmonary edema, 2303
  in pertussis, 2005
  in pneumonia, 2556
  in tuberculosis, 2149
  in viral croup, 2525
  whooping, 2559-2560
Cough cardiopulmonary resuscitation, 90
Cough headache, 1642
Counter Narcotics and Terrorism Operational Medical Support Program, 3003
Counterimmunoelectrophoresis, in central nervous system infection, 1718
Coup contusion, 374
Couplet, 1222
Coupling interval, 1222
Courts, as surrogate decision-makers, 3135
Cowpox virus, 2040
Coxiella burnetii, 1131, 2137
Coxsackie A virus infection, exanthems in, 1849
Coxsackie B virus infection
  in myocarditis, 1289
  in pancreatitis, 1428
Coxsackievirus, 2057
Coyote, rabies in, 2062-2063, 2064
Cozen's test, in lateral epicondylitis, 1798
Crack cocaine, 2386, 2387t
"Crack dancing," 2388
Cramps
  abdominal. See Abdominal cramps.
  heat, 2258, 2258b
Cranial decompression, in severe head trauma, 361
Cranial nerve examination, in head trauma, 357
Cranial neuropathy, 1664-1670, 1665t
  diabetic, 1669-1670
  eye movement disorders in, 1062-1063
  in ethylene glycol poisoning, 2399
  in Lyme disease, 2123
  in tetanus, 2009
Cranial osteomyelitis, after head trauma, 371
Craniofacial abnormalities, in fetal alcohol syndrome, 2791b, 2792
Cranium, anatomy and physiology of, 350
C-reactive protein
  as cardiac marker, 1178
  in appendicitis, 1454
  in immune response, 2831
  in osteomyelitis, 2179
Creatine, in nausea and vomiting, 203
Creatine kinase
  in electrical and lightning injuries, 2276
  in rhabdomyolysis, 1980-1981, 1981f, 1983, 1983f
Creatine kinase MB isoenzyme
  in acute coronary syndromes, 1175f, 1176t, 1177-1178
  in chest pain, 188
  in cocaine-related chest pain, 2388

Creatinine
  dialysis and, 1549
  in acute renal failure, 2649
  serum, 1527
Cremasteric reflex, 1594
  loss of, in testicular torsion, 1595
Crescent sign, in Legg-Calvé-Perthes disease, 2707, 2707f
Creutzfeldt-Jakob disease, 1657-1658, 1659, 2058
Cricoid cartilage fracture, 447
Cricothyrotomy
  difficult, evaluation of, 4
  for failed airway, 9, 10f
  in airway foreign body removal, 870, 2530
  in multiple trauma, 306
  in neck trauma, 445
  percutaneous, 22-23, 23f
  surgical, 22
  with transtracheal jet ventilation, 22, 22f
Crisis intervention, for difficult patient, 2976-2977, 2977b
Critical care unit, computer order entry system for, 3043, 3043f
Critical diagnostic syndromes, observation of, 3063-3069
Critical incident stress debriefing, 3018, 3176-3177
Critically appraised topic, 3059t, 3060
Crohn's disease, 1500-1503, 1502b, 1503b, 2615-2616
Cromolyn
  during pregnancy and lactation, 2789
  for chronic asthma, 2542, 2543t
Crossed straight leg raise test, in lumbar radiculopathy, 704
Cross-sectional studies, 3046-3047
Crotamiton, for scabies, 1855
Croup, 2051
  bacterial (membranous), 2528-2529, 2529t
  screening for, 2509b
  spasmodic, 2527
  viral, 2525-2527, 2526f, 2527b, 2529t
Cruciate ligament injury, 790-791, 792
  intercondylar eminence fracture and, 779
  meniscal tears and, 792, 793
  Segond fracture and, 777, 777f
  tibial femoral knee dislocation and, 788
  tibial plateau fracture and, 778
Crush injuries, 3007-3008
  antibiotic prophylaxis in, 854
  in foot trauma, 838
Crutches
  for ankle sprain, 817
  for proximal fibula fracture, 802
Cruzan v. Director, Missouri Department of Health, 3169
Cryoglobulinemia
  hyperviscosity syndrome in, 1912
  mixed, 1815
Cryotherapy
  for condylomata acuminata, 1564
  for orthopedic injuries, 573-574
  for tendinopathy, 1801
  for trigeminal neuralgia, 1666
Cryptococcal meningitis, 2081
Cryptococcus neoformans
  in cancer patient with impaired cell-mediated immunity, 2840
  in HIV/AIDS, 2081
Cryptogenic cirrhosis, 1410
Cryptosporidium gastroenteritis, 1476-1478, 1477t
  in HIV/AIDS, 1478, 1482, 1484, 2084
Crystallization, extracellular, in frostbite, 2229, 2229b
Crystalloids
  for anaphylactic hypotension, 2549
  for bacterial meningitis, 2663
  for cardiac tamponade, 475
  for gastrointestinal bleeding, 221
  for hemorrhagic shock, 52
  for pediatric infectious diarrhea, 2631
  for pulmonary contusion, 461
  for septic shock, 53
Crystalluria, in ethylene glycol poisoning, 2398, 2399-2400
Cubitus valgus, 659

Cubitus varus, 657-658
Cuboid
  dislocation of, 828
  fracture of, 828
Culdocentesis
  in ectopic pregnancy, 2745
  in vaginal bleeding, 256t, 257
Cultural blindness, 3112
Cultural competence, 3107-3117. See also Racial/ethnic differences.
  as tool for enhancing emergency department care, 3111-3116
  continuum of, 3111-3112
  institutional policies promoting, 3117, 3117b
  rationale for, 3108-3111, 3108t, 3109t
  recommendations for, 3116
  standards for, 3112-3113
  to cross barrier of different beliefs, values, and life experiences, 3113-3114
  to cross language barrier, 3112-3113
Cultural considerations, in prehospital end-of-life care, 3145
Cultural destructiveness, 3111-3112
Cultural incapacity, 3112
Cultural precompetence, 3112
Culture
  blood
    in acute septic arthritis, 2705
    in AIDS-related diarrhea, 1483-1484
    in bacterial meningitis, 2662
    in central nervous system infection, 1720
    in gastrointestinal anthrax, 1469
    in infected aneurysm, 1356
    in infective endocarditis, 1301-1302
    in meningococcal disease, 2022
    in pediatric fever, 2510
    in pneumococcal disease, 2018
    in pneumonia, 1135, 2561
    in sepsis, 2216-2217
  in central nervous system infection, 1719
  in diphtheria, 2003
  in febrile, neutropenic cancer patient, 2837
  in genital herpes, 1558-1559
  in gonorrhea, 1566
  in osteomyelitis, 2182
  in pertussis, 2006
  joint fluid, in septic arthritis, 2189
  sputum
    in chronic obstructive pulmonary disease, 1101
    in pneumonia, 1134-1135
    in tuberculosis, 2154-2155
  stool
    in Aeromonas hydrophila gastroenteritis, 1468
    in AIDS-related diarrhea, 1483
    in Bacillus anthracis gastroenteritis, 1469
    in Campylobacter gastroenteritis, 1460
    in Clostridium difficile enterocolitis, 1475
    in coccidial gastroenteritis, 1478
    in diarrhea, 233
    in Giardia gastroenteritis, 1479
    in hemorrhagic Escherichia coli serotype O157:H7 gastroenteritis, 1467
    in infectious diarrhea, 2626-2627
    in intestinal amebiasis, 1480
    in pediatric fever, 2510
    in Plesiomonas shigelloides gastroenteritis, 1468
    in salmonellosis, 1463
    in shigellosis, 1464
    in Vibrio fish poisoning, 1472
    in Vibrio parahaemolyticus gastroenteritis, 1466
    in Yersinia enterocolitica gastroenteritis, 1465
  throat, in pharyngitis, 1111, 1112
  urine
    in epididymitis, 2639
    in pediatric fever, 2509-2510
    in urinary tract infection, 1576-1577, 1577b
Culture (human), definition of, 3111
Cuneiform
  dislocation of, 828
  fracture of, 828
Curling's ulcers, in burn injured patient, 924
Current, direct vs. alternating, electrical injury and, 2268

Cushing's reflex/phenomenon, after head trauma, 354
Cutaneous abscess, 2202-2204, 2203t
Cutaneous anthrax, 1860, 1861f, 3025, 3026f
Cutaneous candidiasis, 1841
Cutaneous larva migrans, 2100t, 2109
Cutaneous mastocytosis, 1835
Cutaneous presentations. See Skin lesions; Skin rash.
Cutis marmorata, 2284, 2499, 2499f
Cyanide antidote kit, 2329t, 2437-2438, 2440
Cyanide poisoning, 2436-2438, 2437f
    antidotes to, 2329t, 2437-2438, 2440
    as chemical weapon, 939, 3031-3032
    carbon monoxide poisoning vs., 2439
    carbon monoxide poisoning with, 2440-2441
    cyanosis in, 271
Cyano-acrylate adhesive-tipped swab, for foreign body removal from ear, 863
Cyanosis, 268-273
    ancillary studies in, 271
    central, 269, 270b, 2889-2890
    diagnostic approach to, 268-271, 270b, 270f
    differential diagnosis in, 270b, 271-273, 272f
    disposition in, 273
    empiric management of, 273
    history in, 268-269
    in airway foreign body aspiration, 866
    in high-altitude pulmonary edema, 2303
    in nitrite abuse, 2889-2890
    pathophysiology of, 268, 269b, 269f
    pediatric
        cardiac vs. pulmonary, 2569, 2569b, 2572
        in tetralogy of Fallot, 2580
        pathophysiology of, 269t, 2569
    peripheral, 269, 270b
    physical examination in, 269-271, 270f
    pseudocyanosis and, 268
Cyanotic congenital heart disease, 2579-2581, 2579f, 2581b
Cyclic antidepressants
    central nervous system effects of, 2354b
    overdose of, 2352-2357, 2353f, 2354b, 2355f, 2357f
    peripheral nervous system effects of, 2353b
    pharmacodynamic effects of, 2353b
Cyclobenzaprine, for back pain, 2928-2929
Cyclooxygenase inhibitors, 1082, 2342
Cyclooxygenase-2 inhibitors, 2927-2928, 2927b, 2927f
    in aspirin-exacerbated respiratory disease, 1082
Cyclophosphamide
    for Goodpasture syndrome, 1816
    for granulomatous vasculitis, 1814
    for mixed cryoglobulinemia, 1815
Cycloplegics, 1063b, 1064
    for red and painful eye, 292, 297t
Cycloserine, for tuberculosis, 2163t, 2164-2165
Cyclospora cayetanensis gastroenteritis, 1477t, 1478-1479
Cyclosporine, 2844
    drug interactions with, 2850, 2850t
    during pregnancy and lactation, 2776
    for inflammatory bowel disease, 1503
    for myasthenia gravis, 1706
    for organ transplant patient, 2849-2850, 2850t
    nephrotoxicity of, 2850
    toxicity of, 1417
Cyclothymic disorder, 1739
CYP450 enzymes, in acetaminophen metabolism, 2332, 2332f
Cyproheptadine, for serotonin toxicity, 2360
Cyst, 1839t
    Baker's, 796, 797f
    Bartholin, 1559-1560
    corpus luteum, ruptured
        ectopic pregnancy vs., 2745
        pelvic pain in, 251t
    hydatid, 2102t, 2105-2106, 2106f, 2111, 2113
    leptomeningeal, in head-injured child, 368
    ovarian, 251t
    popliteal, 796, 797f
Cystic duct obstruction, cholecystitis in, 1420
Cystic fibrosis
    in children, 2564-2565, 2565f
    pneumonia in, 1132
Cystic myelopathy, in spinal cord injury, 2909
Cysticercosis, 2102t, 2105
Cystine kidney stones, 1587

Cystitis, 1573
    dysuria in, 1580-1581
    guidelines for management of, 3042
    in children, 2642, 2643, 2644
    in men, 1585
    in urinary tract infection, 1575
    treatment of, 1581-1582, 1581t
Cystography, retrograde
    computed tomography, in bladder trauma, 521, 525, 526f
    conventional, in bladder trauma, 521, 521f-526f
Cystostomy, for urinary retention, 1600, 1600f
Cytoid body, in malignant hypertension, 1315
Cytokines
    as anaphylaxis mediators, 1823, 1823b
    during resuscitation from hemorrhagic shock, 46
    in asthma, 1080, 1080f, 1081
    in bacterial meningitis, 2662
    in cerebral ischemia, 66-67
    in sepsis, 2213
    in shock, 43, 44f, 45
Cytomegalovirus infection, 2043-2044
    drugs for, 2036t
    in cancer patient with impaired cell-mediated immunity, 2840
    in esophagitis, 1387
    in gastroenteritis, 1482, 1484
    in HIV/AIDS, 1482, 1484, 2076, 2086
    in organ transplant patient, 2847-2848
    in pneumonia, 1130
    in retinitis, 2086
Cytotoxic cerebral edema
    after head trauma, 354
    in high-altitude cerebral edema, 2300
Cytotoxic diarrhea, 228
Cytotoxic hypersensitivity reactions, 1821

D-400, drug interactions with, 2478t
Dacroadenitis, 293t
Dacryocystitis, 293t, 1055, 1055f
Dalton's law, 2280, 2994-2995, 2995t
Dance's sign, in intussusception, 2611
Danger Assessment instrument, 1000, 1003b
Danger space, 1117
Danis-Weber classification of ankle fractures, 814f
Dantrolene
    for neuroleptic malignant syndrome, 1733, 2449
    for phenelzine overdose, 2365
Dapsone, in HIV/AIDS, side effects of, 2079t
Darkfield microscopy, in syphilis, 1561, 1856
Dashboard fracture, 550f
Data, definition of, 3097
Data access, information technology for, 3097
Data analysis in evidence-based medicine, 3051-3058, 3051t, 3057f
    confidence intervals in, 3053
    data dredging or torturing in, 3056
    hypothesis testing in, 3051-3058, 3051t, 3057f
    intention-to-treat analysis in, 3056-3057, 3057f
    interim analyses of accumulating data in, 3054
    meta-analysis in, 3057-3058
    multiple comparisons in, 3053-3054
    multivariate models in, 3054-3055
    prior probabilities and, 3055-3056
    statistical tests in, 3052-3053, 3052t
    subgroups in, 3054
Data collection, 3050
Data dredging or torturing, 3056
Data management, 3050
Databases, electronic, 3059, 3099
Datura stramonium poisoning, 2345, 2346, 2473, 2473t
D-dimer analysis
    in cerebral venous thrombosis, 1671
    in deep venous thrombosis, 1369-1370
    in pulmonary embolism, 1374-1375
DDT (dichlorodiphenyltrichloroethane), 2462-2463, 2462b
De Quervain's tenosynovitis, 1799
Death. See also End of life.
    autopsy after, 3149
    brain, 3141
    cardiopulmonary, 3141

Death (Continued)
    causes of, 942t
    definitions of, 3141
    epidemiology of, 3140-3141, 3140f
    field pronouncement of, 3144
    "good," 3142
    grief response after, 3149-3151, 3150b
    in emergency department, 3146-3151, 3146b, 3148b
    injury, causes of, 949t
    new, consent for procedures after, 3149
    of child
        in emergency department, 2717
        prehospital issues related to, 3145-3146
    reporting requirements for, 3172
    sedation for survivors after, 3149
    triage marker of, 2251
    viewing body after, 3148-3149
Death notification
    by phone, 3148
    empathy in, 3147-3149, 3148b
    training in, bioethical dilemmas in, 3135
Debacterol, for aphthous stomatitis, 1036
Debridement
    in open tibial shaft fracture, 801
    in wound management, 847
    surgical, in osteomyelitis, 2187
Decelerations, in fetal heart rate, 2801, 2803f
Decerebrate posturing
    in cerebral herniation, 355, 356
    in head trauma, 357
Decision analysis, 132
Decision making
    diagnostic approach and, 125-130, 127f, 128b, 129f
    errors in, 130-133, 131t, 133b
Decision-makers, surrogate, 3134-3135
Decision-making capacity, 3133-3134, 3134b
Decision-making process, as stressor for emergency physician, 3175
Decompression
    in burn injury, 925, 925f
    in cardiopulmonary resuscitation, 89, 98
    in pneumothorax, 1147
    in severe head trauma, 361
    in small bowel obstruction, 1444
    in thoracic outlet syndrome, 1360
    in urinary retention, 1599
    surgical, in spinal stenosis, 712
Decompression sickness, 2283-2285
    flying and, 2293-2294, 2293f
    recompression therapy for, 2288-2292, 2288b, 2289f-2291f
    type I, 2279, 2284
    type II, 2284-2285
Decongestants
    for sinusitis, 1125
    ophthalmic, 1063b
Decontamination
    gastrointestinal, 2330. See also specific type, e.g., Activated charcoal.
        in anticholinergic poisoning, 2349
        in barbiturate overdose, 2483
        in bipyridyl compound poisoning, 2466
        in hydrocarbon poisoning, 2431
        in iron overdose, 2420
        in mercury poisoning, 2426
        in opioid overdose, 2455
    in bipyridyl compound poisoning, 2466
    in chlorinated hydrocarbon poisoning, 2463
    in HAZMAT incidents, 931
    in mustard exposure, 3031
    in nerve agent exposure, 3030
    in organophosphate poisoning, 2460
    in pyrethrin and pyrethroid exposure, 2467
    in radiation exposure, 2322-2323, 2323f, 3023
    in toxic disasters, 3017
Decorticate posturing, in head trauma, 357
Decubitus ulcer
    in developmentally disabled patient, 2903
    in physically disabled patient, 2907
    in spinal injuries, 438
Deep fascia
    anatomy of, 842
    cervical, 442-443, 1027
Deep fascial space infection in hand, 617-618, 617f
Deep partial-thickness burn, 918-919, 919f
Deep peroneal nerve, 797

Deep sedation, 2938, 2939b
Deep tendon reflexes
    examination of, in spinal injuries, 417, 417t
    in head trauma, 357
    pseudomyotonic, in hypothyroidism, 1992
Deep vein thrombosis. See Venous thrombosis.
DEET
    overdose of, 2468-2469
    prophylactic, for tick-borne illness, 2142
Defasciculation, in rapid sequence intubation,
    11b
Defecation
    bleeding with, 1508
    normal, 237
    physiology of, 1507-1508
Defense Against Weapons of Mass Destruction
    Act, 938
Deferoxamine
    for iron overdose, 2420
    for thalassemia, 1872-1873
Defibrillation
    in cardiac arrest, 90-91
    in hypothermia, 2246
    in infants and children, 2586b
    in pacemaker patient, 1255
    in pediatric resuscitation, 113
    in ventricular fibrillation and pulseless
        ventricular tachycardia, 84, 112
    prehospital, 2990
Degenerative joint disease. See Osteoarthritis.
Degloving injuries, penile, 532
Dehydration. See also Hypovolemia.
    clinical assessment of, 2627t
    during air medical transport, 2995
    heat illness and, 2256
    in AIDS-related diarrhea, 1483
    in diabetic ketoacidosis, 1962, 1964, 1966
    in hypercalcemia, 1945
    in hyperglycemic hyperosmolar nonketotic
        coma, 1968, 1969
    in pediatric infectious diarrhea, 2629,
        2629t
    in *Plesiomonas shigelloides* gastroenteritis,
        1468
    in pneumonia, 2562
    observation in, 3071-3072, 3072b
    types of, by serum sodium, 2629t
Delayed primary wound closure, 849
Delbet classification of pediatric femoral
    fractures, 763, 763f
Delirium, 156, 1645-1655
    clinical findings in, 1648-1651, 1650f
    confusion vs., 150
    dementia vs., 1645, 1653, 1660
    diagnosis and ancillary studies in, 1651-1652
    diagnostic criteria for, 1645, 1645b
    differential diagnosis in, 1652-1653, 1652t,
        2348, 2348b
    disposition in, 1655
    etiology of, 1647-1648, 1647t
    in anticholinergic poisoning, 2348
    in HIV/AIDS, 2086
    management of, 1653-1655
    pathophysiology of, 1645-1647
Delirium tremens, 1653, 2861
Delivery. See Labor and delivery.
Delta gap
    calculation of, 1924
    in mixed acid-base disorders, 1931
Delta wave, in Wolff-Parkinson-White syndrome,
    1235
Delusional disorder, 1729
Delusions
    in amphetamine abuse, 2894
    in depression, 1737
    in schizophrenia, 1727
Dementia, 1655-1662
    advanced, palliative care in, 3154
    AIDS, 2081
    Alzheimer's. See Alzheimer's disease.
    clinical features of, 1658-1660, 1659t, 1660t
    cortical vs. subcortical, 1659, 1659t
    delirium vs., 1645, 1653, 1660
    depression vs., 1740-1741
    diagnosis of, 1660-1661, 1661b
    diagnostic criteria for, 1654, 1654b
    differential diagnosis in, 1660
    etiology of, 1656, 1656b
    pathophysiology of, 1656-1658

Dementia (Continued)
    pseudodementia (depression) vs., 1656, 1659-
        1660, 1660t
    treatment and disposition in, 1661-1662
Demyelinating polyneuropathy, 1690-1691, 1690b
Demyelination
    in hyponatremia, 1935
    in multiple sclerosis, 1681-1682
    in transverse myelitis, 1682
Dengue, 2049-2050
Dental bacterial plaque, 1028
Dental caries, 1028-1029, 1030-1032, 1030f, 1031f
Dental disorders, in developmentally disabled
    patient, 2903
Dental emergencies. See also Oral medicine.
    nontraumatic, 1027-1029, 1030f
    traumatic, 1036-1042
Dental infection
    airway management in, 1032
    extension of, into head and neck, 1027, 1028-
        1029, 1030f, 1032
    Ludwig's angina and, 1032, 1118-1119
Dental pain. See Oral pain.
Dentin fracture, 1037
Dentition. See Tooth (teeth).
Department of Homeland Security, 3018
Department of Transportation drug testing
    guidelines, 3080
Department of Veterans Affairs, 3018-3019
Dependent patient, 2978, 2978t, 2980
Dependent personality disorder, 2979b
Depolarization, 1200
Depolarizing agents, in intubation, 13-14
Depressed skull fracture, 373
Depression
    asthma and, 1082
    clinical features of, 1736-1738, 1736b, 1737b
    criteria for, 1736, 1736b
    differential considerations in, 1740-1741
    dysthmic, 1738
    epidemiology of, 1735
    in alcoholism, 2875
    in children and adolescents, 1737
    in elderly person, 1737-1738, 2827
    in HIV/AIDS, 2086-2087
    in pseudodementia, 1656, 1659-1660, 1660t
    in seasonal affective disorder, 1738
    masked (hidden), 1737
    panic attack in, 1748-1749
    pathophysiology of, 1735-1736
    postpartum, 1738, 2821-2822
    psychosocial theories of, 1736
    somatoform disorders vs., 1756-1757
    stabilization in, 1741
    substance-induced, 1739-1740, 1740b
    suicide and, 1737, 1768, 1769
    treatment of, 1741-1742
Dermacentor andersoni tick, 908
Dermacentor variabilis tick, 908, 2118f, 2121f
Dermatitis
    atopic, 1841-1842
    contact, 1851-1852, 1851f, 1852f
    diaper, 1852
    erythematous, 1863f
    gonococcal, 1566, 1843-1844, 1843f, 2191
    in arthritis-dermatitis syndrome, 1566, 1788,
        1843-1844, 1843f
    infectious eczematoid, in otitis media, 1067-1068
    seborrheic, in HIV/AIDS, 2085
Dermatoconjunctivitis, 296t
Dermatographism, in urticaria, 1848, 1848f
Dermatologic presentations. See Skin lesions;
    Skin rash.
Dermatomes, sensory, 418f
Dermatomyositis, 1708
    internal malignancy associated with, 1863
    neuromuscular dysphagia in, 1396
    skin lesions in, 1862t, 1863f
Dermatophyte infections, 1838-1840, 1839f, 1840f
Dermis, 842, 914
Dermopathy, diabetic, 1861f, 1862t, 1863f, 1971-
    1972
Descending aortic rupture, 476-477
Desferrioxamine, for rhabdomyolysis, 1982
Designer amphetamines, 2408-2409, 2410-2411
Desmopressin
    for hemophilia A, 1902
    for von Willebrand's disease, 1903
Detergents, ocular trauma from, 1046

Detorsion, in colonic volvulus, 1499
Developmental milestones, 2495-2497, 2496t
Developmentally disabled patient, 2898-2904,
    2900t-2902t
    abuse of, 1015
    cardiovascular disorders in, 2902
    cerebral palsy in, 2903-2904
    cerebrospinal fluid shunts in, 2899
    dental disorders in, 2903
    failure to thrive in, 2900-2901
    fractures in, 2901
    gastrointestinal disorders in, 2903
    musculoskeletal disorders in, 2901-2902
    psychiatric disorders in, 2903
    pulmonary disorders in, 2903
    seizures in, 2898-2899
    skin disorders in, 2903
Devil's claw, drug interactions with, 2478t
Dexamethasone
    for acute mountain sickness, 2302
    for adrenal insufficiency, 1998
    for asthma, 2539t, 2541
    for bacterial meningitis, 1722, 2664-2665
    for cerebral herniation, 1918
    for epidural spinal cord compression, 1919
    for high-altitude cerebral edema, 2306
    for meningococcal disease, 2024
    for septic arthritis, 2193
    for thyroid storm, 1989
    for viral croup, 2526, 2527
Dexamethasone suppression test, in dementia,
    1661
Dexon suture, 852t
Dextran, low-molecular-weight, in frostbite,
    2233
Dextromethorphan
    respiratory effects of, 2453t
    toxicity of, 2413-2414, 2415, 2416
Dextrose
    for acute renal failure, 2650
    for alcohol intoxication, 2860
    for alcohol withdrawal syndrome, 2861
    for alcoholic ketoacidosis, 2873
    for burn injured children, 923
    for comatose patient, 157-158
    for hypoglycemia, 1961
    for neonatal resuscitation, 123t, 124
    for pediatric infectious diarrhea, 2631
    for Wernicke-Korsakoff syndrome, 2869
Dezocine, 2924, 2924b
Diabetes insipidus
    causes of, 1936b
    hypernatremia in, 1935, 1936
Diabetes mellitus, 1955-1974
    anxiety in, 1747
    carpal tunnel syndrome in, 1697
    classification of, 1957, 1957b
    clinical features of, 1958-1959
    cranial mononeuropathy in, 1669-1670
    delirium in, 1649
    diagnosis of, 1959-1960, 1959b
    epidemiology of, 1958
    etiology and pathophysiology of, 1958
    gestational, 1957, 2772
    hyperglycemic hyperosmolar nonketotic coma
        in, 1968-1970, 1968b, 1969b
    hypoglycemia in, 1960-1961, 1960b, 1961b
    hypomagnesemia in, 1948
    immune defects in, 2841
    in alcoholism, 2871
    in pancreatitis, 1435
    in pregnancy, 1972, 2764t, 2771-2772
    infectious complications in, 1971, 2841
    ketoalkalosis in, 1963
    late complications of, 1970-1972
    mononeuropathy multiplex in, 1699
    myocardial infarction in, atypical presentations
        associated with, 1159
    nephropathy in, 1970
        in pregnancy, 1972
    neuropathy in, 1691-1692, 1970-1971
        in pregnancy, 1972
        lower extremity ulcers in, 1351, 1971
    new trends in, 1973
    oral manifestations of, 1035
    retinopathy in, 1970
        in pregnancy, 1972
    skin lesions in, 1861f, 1862t, 1863f, 1971-1972
    urinary tract infection in, 1578

Diabetic foot, 1971
  osteomyelitis in, 2185-2186
Diabetic ketoacidosis, 1928, 1962-1967
  complications of, 1967
  diagnosis of, 1963-1964
  differential considerations in, 1964-1965
  disposition in, 1967
  etiology of, 1963
  hypophosphatemia in, 1951
  in pregnancy, 1972, 2771-2772
  laboratory tests in, 1964, 1964t
  management of, 1965-1967, 1965b
  nausea and vomiting in, 205t
  pathophysiology of, 1962-1963, 1962t, 1963f
Diagnostic approach, clinical decision making
  and, 125-130, 127f, 128b, 129f
Diagnostic-therapeutic trial, in clinical decision
  making, 128
Dialysate, bloody, causes of, 1553
Dialysis
  for acute renal failure, 2650
  for acute tumor lysis syndrome, 1912, 1912b
  for barbiturate overdose, 2483
  for beta blocker overdose, 2375
  for bipyridyl compound poisoning, 2466
  for chronic heart failure, 1277
  for chronic renal failure, 1547-1554
    complications of, 1549-1554, 1550b, 1552b,
      1553t
    emergency, indications for, 1548-1549, 1548b
  for hyperkalemia, 1941
  for isopropyl alcohol poisoning, 2404
  for lithium toxicity, 2444
  for pulmonary edema in chronic renal failure,
    1546, 1548
  for rewarming in accidental hypothermia,
    2249, 2250t, 2251
  for salicylate overdose, 2342
  for toxic alcohol poisoning, 2401-2402
  for uremic pericarditis, 1282
  vascular access for, problems related to, 1364-
    1366
Dialysis disequilibrium syndrome, 1622
Diaper dermatitis, 1852
Diaphoresis
  in asthma, 1084
  in ciguatera fish poisoning, 1473
Diaphragm
  in pregnancy, 317
  injury to, laparotomy and, 504
Diaphragmatic hernia
  neonatal resuscitation in, 121
  traumatic, in children, 340, 341
Diaphyseal fracture, 2699
Diaphysis, 2175, 2175f
Diarrhea, 227-236
  acute vs. chronic, 228
  ancillary studies in, 233
  diagnostic approach to, 228-233, 230b, 231b
  differential diagnosis in, 228, 230b-231b, 234
  disposition in, 235-236
  empiric management of, 234-235, 234f, 236t
  epidemiology of, 227-228
  from abnormal motility, 228
  history in, 232
  hypokalemia from, 1938
  in Aeromonas hydrophila gastroenteritis, 1467
  in Bacillus anthracis gastroenteritis, 1469
  in Bacillus cereus food poisoning, 1471
  in Campylobacter gastroenteritis, 1460
  in ciguatera fish poisoning, 1473
  in Clostridium difficile enterocolitis, 1475
  in Clostridium perfringens food poisoning,
    1471
  in coccidial gastroenteritis, 1477, 1478
  in Escherichia coli food poisoning, 1474
  in Giardia gastroenteritis, 1479
  in hemolytic uremic syndrome, 2654
  in hemorrhagic Escherichia coli serotype
    O157:H7 gastroenteritis, 1466
  in HIV/AIDS, 1482-1484, 1482t, 1483b, 1485t,
    2084
  in inflammatory bowel disease, 1501, 2616
  in intestinal amebiasis, 1480
  in intussusception, 2610
  in parasitic infection, 2112, 2112f, 2113f
  in Plesiomonas shigelloides gastroenteritis,
    1468
  in salmonellosis, 1463

Diarrhea (Continued)
  in scombroid fish poisoning, 1472
  in shigellosis, 1464
  in staphylococcal food poisoning, 1470
  in Vibrio fish poisoning, 1472
  in Vibrio parahaemolyticus gastroenteritis,
    1466
  in viral gastroenteritis, 1476
  in Yersinia enterocolitica gastroenteritis, 1465
  infectious, 228, 230b
    pediatric, 2623-2634
    treatment of, 229t-230t, 235
  inflammatory, 228, 229t-230t
  metabolic acidosis in, 2624
  noninfectious, 228, 231b
  osmotic, 228, 2624
  pathophysiology of, 228, 229t-230t
  pediatric, 227, 2623-2634, 2628b, 2628t. See
    also Children, infectious diarrhea in.
  physical examination in, 232-233
  rapid assessment and stabilization in, 228,
    232
  secretory, 228, 2624
  severe, with blood and mucus. See Dysentery.
  traveler's, 1484-1487, 1486t, 1487b
Diastolic dysfunction
  in heart failure, 1267
  in restrictive cardiomyopathy, 1296
Diathermic rewarming, 2250
Diazepam, 2484, 2484t
  for alcohol withdrawal syndrome, 2862, 2863
  for alcohol-related seizure, 2864, 2865
  for cocaine overdose, 2389
  for febrile seizure, 2667
  for nerve agent exposure, 3030
  for psychostimulant intoxication, 2410
  for seizure, 166, 166t, 1626, 1627t
    in cancer patient, 1919
    in children, 2675t
  for status epilepticus, 2672-2673, 2672t
  for tetanus, 2011
  for vertigo, 146
  in ventilated patient, 30
  prophylactic, in severe head trauma, 361
Dichloroacetic acid, for condylomata acuminata,
  1564
Dichlorophenoxyacetic acid, 2465b
Diclofenac, 2927
Dicloxacillin
  during pregnancy and lactation, 2784
  for folliculitis, 1843
  for impetigo, 1843
  for staphylococcal scalded skin syndrome, 1845
Didanosine, 2079t
Dieffenbachia, 2473, 2473f
Diet
  BRAT, for diarrhea, 235
  diabetic, 1973
  during pregnancy, 2736
  high-fiber, for diverticular disease, 1494
  in acute pancreatitis, 1433-1434
  in burn injury, 918
Dietary guidelines
  for traveler's diarrhea prophylaxis, 1486
  of American Heart Association, 3177, 3177b
Dietary supplements, 2475-2477, 2476t
Diethylcarbamazine, for loiasis, 2110
Diethylenetriamine pentaacetic acid, for
  plutonium exposure, 3023
Difficult airway
  approach to, 8-9, 9f
  cricothyrotomy for, 22-23, 23f
  esophagotracheal combitube for, 20, 20f
  fiberoptic intubation of, 20-21, 22f
  identification of, 3-4, 3b, 4b, 5f
  in children, 2502, 2502b
  intubating laryngeal mask airway for, 19, 19f
  lighted stylet for, 19-20, 20f
  retrograde intubation of, 20
  special airway devices for, 18-23, 19f-23f
Difficult patient, 2972-2982
  as stressor for emergency physician, 3175
  behavioral classification of, 2978-2981, 2978t
  combative patient as, 2956-2969. See also
    Combative patient.
  definition of, 2972-2973
  emergency department factors in, 2973
  impaired patient-physician relationship and,
    2973, 2974f

Difficult patient (Continued)
  management of, 2973-2981
    crisis intervention in, 2976-2977, 2977b
    dealing with negative reactions in, 2975-
      2976
    general strategies in, 2973-2975, 2973b
    personality disorder classification of, 2978,
      2979b
    physician factors in, 2973
Diffuse axonal injury
  in child abuse, 971
  in head trauma, 374
Digital radiography, in fracture, 557
Digital subtraction angiography
  in peripheral vascular injury, 543
  intravenous, in aortic rupture, 480-481
Digitalis lanata, 2476
Digoxin (digitalis)
  as antidysrhythmic drug, 1211-1212, 1211t
  during pregnancy and lactation, 2787
  for acute pulmonary edema in hypotensive
    patient, 1270t, 1274
  for atrial flutter, 1229
  for chronic heart failure, 1276
  for heart failure, 2583, 2583t
  for junctional tachycardia, 1234
  hyperkalemia from, 1940
  misconceptions about, 1212
  overdose of, 2368-2373
    acute vs. chronic, 2369, 2370t
    antidotes to, 2329t
    clinical features of, 2369, 2370b
    diagnosis of, 2369-2370
    differential diagnosis in, 2370
    disposition in, 2372-2373
    dysrhythmias associated with, 2369b
    in children, 2372, 2372t
    management of, 2370-2371, 2372b
    pathophysiology of, 2368-2369, 2369b
    risk of, factors associated with, 2369b
  side effects of, 1211-1212, 1212b
Dihydrocodeine, respiratory effects of, 2453t
Dihydroergotamine, for migraine, 1633t, 1634
Dihydropyridines, 1321t
Dilated cardiomyopathy, 1293-1294
  heart failure in, 1264
  inflammatory. See Myocarditis.
  peripartum cardiomyopathy and, 1297
Dilation and curettage, after miscarriage, 2742
Dilation and evacuation, in ectopic pregnancy,
  2745
Diloxanide, for intestinal amebiasis, 1481
Diltiazem, 1211, 1321t
  during pregnancy and lactation, 2788
  for atrial flutter, 1229
  for dysphagia, 1398
  overdose of, 2376, 2377t
Dilutional thrombocytopenia, 1898
Dimenhydrinate, for vertigo, 146
Dimercaprol
  for arsenic poisoning, 2424
  for lead poisoning, 2422
2,3-Dimercaptosuccinic acid
  for arsenic poisoning, 2424
  for lead poisoning, 2422
  for mercury poisoning, 2426
Dinitrocresol, 2463, 2463b
Dinitrophenol, 2463, 2463b, 2464
Diphenhydramine
  anticholinergic toxicity of, 2345
  for acute extrapyramidal symptoms, 2449
  for anaphylactic shock, 54
  for anaphylaxis, 1831b, 1832, 2549
  for drug eruptions, 1845
  for hymenoptera stings, 904
  for local anesthesia, 847, 2931
  for OTC sleep aid overdose, 2487-2488, 2488t
  for scombroid fish poisoning, 1472
  for upper airway angioedema, 1835
  for vertigo, 146
Diphenoxylate
  for diarrhea, 236t
  overdose of, 2456
  respiratory effects of, 2453t
Diphtheria, 2001-2004, 2003b
  myocarditis in, 1291
  pharyngitis in, 1110-1111, 1113
  vaccine for, 2002, 2004, 2012, 2012t
Diphyllobothrium latum, 2102t, 2107

Diplegia, spastic, in cerebral palsy, 2904
Dipstick tests, in diabetes mellitus, 1959, 1959b
Dipylidium caninum, 2102t
Dipyridamole, for Kawasaki disease, 2027
Diquat poisoning, 2465-2466, 2465b
Direct antiglobulin test, in hemolytic anemia, 1878
Direct current, electrical injury and, 2268
Direct patient admission, medicolegal issues in, 3159
Direct thrombin inhibitors, in acute coronary syndromes, 1188
"Dirty bomb," 2316
Disability. *See also* Developmentally disabled patient; Physically disabled patient.
    assessment of, in pediatric trauma, 330, 330b, 331t, 332t
    in elderly trauma patient, 348
    vs. impairment, 3078
    work-related, types of, 3078
Disaster
    bioethical dilemmas in, 3136
    internal vs. external, 3010-3011
    PICE nomenclature vs., 3011-3012, 3011t, 3012b, 3012t
    role of informatics in, 3105
    scene of, organization of, 3014-3015
Disaster preparedness, 3010-3019
    comprehensive emergency management in, 3015
    definitions in, 3010-3012
    disaster response organizations and, 3018-3019
    external disaster plan in, 3015
    for catastrophic disasters, 3016-3017
    for focal disasters, 3016
    for nuclear, biologic, and chemical terrorism, 3017-3018
    for radiation exposure, 2323
    for toxic disasters, 3017
    for weapons of mass destruction, 3017-3018
    future directions in, 3019
    hazards analysis in, 3012
    hospital response in, 3015-3016
    internal disaster plan in, 3015
    nature of disasters and, 3010-3012
    need for local response in, 3017
    planning in, 3015-3016
    prehospital response in, 3014-3015
    stress management and, 3018
    triage in, 3012-3014, 3013f
Disaster preparedness committee, 3015
Discharge instructions
    in procedural sedation and analgesia, 2943
    in wound management, 855-856, 856b
    preprinted, 3102
Discoid rash, in systemic lupus erythematosus, 1806
Discontinuation syndrome, with antidepressants, 2365-2366
Discrimination, and health outcomes, 3109-3110
Disease and injury prevention. *See* Injury prevention and control.
Disease transmission
    in HIV/AIDS, 990, 990b, 2073, 2810
    in tuberculosis, 2147, 2169-2171, 2170b
    via human bite, 891
Disequilibrium syndrome, in hemodialysis patient, 1551
Dishwashing detergents, ingestion of, 2380, 2381t
Disinfection, skin, in wound care, 847
Disk herniation
    lumbar, 702-703, 704-705, 711-712
    magnetic resonance imaging in, 432, 433f
    radicular pain in, 264
Diskectomy, surgical, 711
Diskitis, in children, vertebral osteomyelitis vs., 2185
Dislocation, 564-566, 565f. *See also* Fracture-dislocation; Instability.
    ankle, 820
    atlantoaxial or atlanto-occipital, 399, 401, 402f, 405-406, 408f
    biceps tendon, 698
    carpal, 630-631, 630f-632f
    distal radioulnar joint, 636-637, 642-643, 643f
    elbow, 664-666, 664f, 665f
    facet
        bilateral, 404, 405f
        unilateral, 406, 408f-409f, 409

Dislocation *(Continued)*
    foot
        cuneiform, cuboid, or navicular, 828
        interphalangeal, 835-836
        Lisfranc, 828-831, 829f, 830f
        metatarsophalangeal, 835
        subtalar, 825-826, 825f
        total talar, 826
    hand, 600-604, 601f-603f
    hip, 756-759, 757f-759f
        arterial injury in, 761
        avascular necrosis after, 740
        pediatric, 763
        prosthetic, 749, 750f, 760
    in electrical and lightning injuries, 2273
    in Monteggia's fracture, 642, 642f
    knee
        patellar, 785-786, 785b
        tibial femoral, 787-790, 789f
    lens, 1049
    peroneal tendon, 818-819, 819f
    proximal tibiofibular joint, 802-803
    shoulder, 683-693
        acromioclavicular, 685-687, 686f, 687f
        glenohumeral, 687-693, 688f-694f
        scapulothoracic, 693
        sternoclavicular, 683-685, 684f-685f
        temporomandibular joint, 396, 1041-1042, 1041f
    testicular, 534
    thumb
        carpometacarpal joint, 604
        interphalangeal joint, 564, 565f, 603
Disopyramide, 1206, 2787
Displacement
    in extension supracondylar fracture, 656-657
    in femoral neck fracture, 751, 752b
    in medial epicondylar fracture, 662-663
    in olecranon fracture, 663
    in proximal humerus fractures, 681, 681f, 682f
Disposition requirements, 3164-3165, 3165t
Disseminated intravascular coagulation, 1903-1904, 1904t
    after head trauma, 371
    in anaphylaxis, 1825t
    in meningococcal disease, 2022
    in pregnancy, placental abruption and, 319-320
    in rhabdomyolysis, 1981
    in sepsis, 2214
Dissociative agent intoxication, 2413-2426, 2414t, 2415t
Dissociative anesthesia, in syringomyelia, 1683
Dissociative sedation, 2914b, 2938, 2939b
Distal femur
    anatomy of, 770, 771f
    epiphyseal fracture of, 780-781
    fracture of, 776-777
Distal fibula, avulsion fracture of, 818
Distal humerus
    anatomy of, 647, 647f
    fracture of, 655-661
        condylar, 660-661, 661f
        intercondylar, 659-660, 659f
        lateral condyle, 660
        medial condyle, 660
        supracondylar, 655-659, 656f-658f
            in children, 2693-2697, 2694f-2696f, 2694t
        transcondylar, 659, 659f
Distal interphalangeal joint
    dislocation of, 564, 565f, 601, 601f
    extensor tendon injury at, 605-607, 606f, 607f
Distal phalanx
    extensor tendon injury at, 605-607, 606f, 607f
    fracture of, 593-594, 593f
Distal radioulnar joint, 622, 623f, 639-640
    dislocation of, 636-637
        in Galeazzi's fracture, 642-643, 643f
Distal radius
    injuries to, 632-639, 634f-638f
        Barton's fracture in, 635-636, 636f
        Colles' fracture in, 632-633, 634f, 635f
        Hutchinson's fracture in, 636, 636f
        pediatric, 637-639, 637f, 638f, 638t
        radioulnar joint disruption in, 636-637
        Smith's fracture in, 633-635, 635f
    ulnar slant of, 625, 626f
    volar tilt of, 626, 626f
Distal tibiofibular syndesmotic ligament injury, 816, 817

Distributive justice, 3129, 3129b
Disulfiram, alcohol interactions with, 2876-2877
Diuresis
    cold, 2239
    forced, in crush injury, 3007
Diuretics, 1321t
    during pregnancy and lactation, 2788
    for acute pulmonary edema, 1270t, 1272
    for chronic heart failure, 1276
    for hyperkalemia in chronic renal failure, 1546
    for hypernatremia, 1936
    for hyponatremia, 1935
    for intracerebral hemorrhage, 1616
    for superior vena cava syndrome, 1911
    hypercalcemia from, 1945
    hypokalemia from, 1937
    hypomagnesemia from, 1947
    hypophosphatemia from, 1951
    metabolic alkalosis from, 1930
Dive history, focused, 2286b
Divers Alert Network (DAN), 2288
Diversion management, computerized, 3105
Diversity education, 3116, 3116b. *See also* Cultural competence.
Diversity of practice elements, as stressor for emergency physician, 3175
Diverticular disease, 1492-1495, 1494b, 1495b, 2848
Diverticulitis, abdominal pain in, 210t
Diverticulum, Meckel's, in children, 2613-2615, 2614t
Diving reflex, 2312
Diving-related disorders. *See* Scuba diving–related disorders.
Dizziness, 142-149
    diagnostic approach to, 143-146, 143b, 143t, 145b, 145t, 148f
    differential diagnosis in, 143, 143b, 143t, 146, 147t-148t
    disposition in, 146, 149
    management of, 146, 149f
    pathophysiology of, 142-143
DMSA (2,3-Dimercaptosuccinic acid)
    for arsenic poisoning, 2424
    for lead poisoning, 2422
    for mercury poisoning, 2426
DNA synthesis, in megaloblastic anemia, 1873
DNA viruses, 2034t, 2039-2046
DNAR (do-not-attempt-resuscitate) order, 3132, 3133
    in advance directives, honoring, 3144-3145
    initiating, 3153
DNIR (do-not-initiate-resuscitate) order, 3132
DNR (do-not-resuscitate) order, 3132
Dobutamine
    for acute pulmonary edema in hypotensive patient, 1270t, 1273-1274
    for anaphylaxis, 1833
    for heart failure, 2583t, 2584
    for sepsis, 2219t, 2220
    in pediatric resuscitation, 114
Documentation
    in injury prevention and control, 945-946
    information technology for, 3098, 3101-3102
    of child abuse, 972-973
    of elder abuse, 1013
    of facial trauma, 388
    of gunshot wounds, 953
    of informed consent, 3167
    of intimate partner violence and abuse, 1000-1001, 1003-1004
    of medical screening examination, 3162-3163
    of physical restraint use, 2959, 2960f
    of refusal of medical care, 3169-3170
    of sexual assault, 985b, 989, 989b
    of suicide attempt, 1774
    of testing in emergency department, 3158
Dog
    bites by, 854, 882-883, 887-888
    rabies in, 2061, 2062-2063, 2063f, 2064
Dog-ear deformity repair, 851
Doll's eye reflex, 161, 357, 2503
Domestic elder abuse, 1009
Domestic herbivore bite, 885
Domestic violence. *See* Intimate partner violence and abuse.
Domperidone, for nausea and vomiting in children, 206
Donepezil, for dementia, 1661

Donovanosis, 1559t, 1563
Donq quai, drug interactions with, 2478t
Dopamine
    for acute pulmonary edema in hypotensive
        patient, 1270t, 1273
    for acute renal failure, 1538, 2650
    for anaphylaxis, 1833
    for burn injury, 923
    for calcium channel blocker overdose, 2378
    for cyclic antidepressant poisoning, 2356
    for heart failure, 2583-2584, 2583t
    for hypothermia, 2246
    for sepsis, 2219t, 2220
    for septic shock, 53
    in mood disorders, 1735
    in neonatal resuscitation, 123t, 124
    in pediatric resuscitation, 114
    suicide and, 1768
Dopamine antagonists, during pregnancy and
        lactation, 2790
Dopexamine, for sepsis, 2222
Doppler ultrasonography
    color flow, 542, 774
    in knee trauma, 774
    in peripheral arteriovascular disease, 1346,
        1348
    in peripheral vascular injury, 541
    in testicular torsion, 1595, 2640
    in testicular trauma, 534, 535f
Dorsal Barton's fracture, 550t
Dorsal compartment of forearm, 640, 640t
Dorsal extrinsic ligaments of wrist, 622, 624f
Dorsal horn, in pain transmission, 2914-2915,
    2915f
Dorsal intercalated segment instability (DISI),
    631-632, 633f
Dorsal rhizotomy, for spasticity in cerebral palsy,
    2904
Dorsal subaponeurotic space infection, 617, 618
Dorsal surface of hand, 576, 577f, 608
Dorsal vein of penis, 532, 532f, 534
Dorzolamide, for increased intraocular pressure,
    292
Double blinding, 3049
Double decidual sac sign, 2730
Double vision, in botulism, 2014
Double-break pelvic fracture, 727
Double-bubble sign
    conditions associated with, 2607
    in hypertrophic pyloric stenosis, 2604, 2605f
    in malrotation with midgut volvulus, 2607
Double-gap acidosis
    differential diagnosis in, 2397
    in ethylene glycol poisoning, 2400
    in methanol poisoning, 2397
Douching, during pregnancy, 2736
Down syndrome, 2900t, 2901
Doxapram, for chronic obstructive pulmonary
        disease, 1106
Doxazosin, 1321t
Doxepin, for upper airway angioedema, 1835
Doxorubicin, cardiotoxicity of, 1292
Doxycycline
    during pregnancy and lactation, 2785
    for anorectal sexually transmitted disease, 1519
    for anthrax exposure, 3026, 3026b
    for Campylobacter gastroenteritis, 1461
    for Chlamydia trachomatis infection, 1559t,
        1565
    for ehrlichiosis, 2138
    for epididymitis, 1597t, 2639
    for granuloma inguinale, 1559t, 1563
    for Lyme disease, 1789, 2127, 2127t, 2128
    for lymphogranuloma venereum, 1559t, 1562
    for malaria, 2104
    for nongonococcal urethritis, 1565
    for Q fever, 2137
    for Rocky Mountain spotted fever, 1850, 2136,
        2136t
    for syphilis, 1856
    for Vibrio fish poisoning, 1472
    prophylactic, for tularemia, 2131
Doxylamine, in OTC sleep aids, overdose of,
    2487-2488, 2488t
Dracunculus medinensis, skin disorders in,
    2100t, 2108-2109
Drain cleaner, ingestion of, 2380, 2381t
Drainage
    in paronychia, 615, 615f

Drainage (Continued)
    in pericoronitis, 1035
    in septic arthritis, 2192, 2706
    of Bartholin cyst abscess, 2205, 2205f
    of cutaneous abscess, 2204
    of felon, 615, 616f
    of periodontal abscess, 1031, 1033
    of peritonsillar abscess, 1118
    of retropharyngeal abscess, 1121
Drains, in wound management, 855
Dressings
    for burn wounds, 925, 926
    in wound management, 855
    Jones compression, 570-571
Dressler syndrome, 1283
Drive-by shootings, 1020-1021
Drooling
    in developmentally disabled patient, 2903
    in epiglottitis, 2523
Drop arm test
    in rotator cuff tear, 696
    in rotator cuff tendinopathy, 1797
Droperidol, 2446t
    conduction disturbances from, 2962
    for delirium, 1654
    for PCP intoxication, 2416
    for rapid tranquilization, 2961-2962
    for thought disorders, 1730
    side effects of, 2961-2962
Drotrecogin alfa, for septic shock, 53
Drowning
    definition of, 2311
    submersion injuries and, 2311-2315
Drug(s). See also Medications.
    abuse of. See Substance abuse.
    anxiety from, 1746b, 1748
    aplastic anemia from, 1875, 1875t
    ataxia from, 2681
    birth defects from, 2779-2780, 2780b
    chronic renal failure from, 1544
    coma from, 1991
    cyanosis from, 269t
    delirium from, 1647-1648
    dementia from, 1656, 1658
    diarrhea from, 231b
    gingival hyperplasia from, 1036
    heart failure from, 1269
    hemolytic anemia from, 1883, 1883b
    hepatic injury from, 1413-1414, 1414t
    hypomagnesemia from, 1948
    immune thrombocytopenia from, 1897
    interactions of
        substance abuse and, 2884
        with alcohol, 2875-2877, 2876t
        with herbal medicines, 2477, 2478t
        with labor and delivery, 2811t
        with MAOIs, 2364, 2364b
    lupus erythematosus from, 1809, 1809t
    mood disorders from, 1739-1740, 1740b,
        1740f
    myasthenia gravis exacerbation from, 1706,
        1706b
    overdose of. See Poisoning/overdose.
    pancreatitis from, 1428, 1429b
    pharmacokinetics of
        in children, 2935, 2952
        in elderly person, 2826
    psychosis from, 1727b, 1728-1729
    reactions to
        in elderly person, 2826-2827
        in HIV/AIDS, 2079t, 2087
    rhabdomyolysis from, 1979
    safety of, during pregnancy and lactation,
        2781-2790, 2782t-2783t
    seizures from, 1623, 2669-2670, 2670b
    syncope from, 195, 195b
    toxicity of
        cardiac arrest and, 77
        in chronic renal failure, 1544, 1544b
        in heart transplant patient, 2852
        in organ transplant patient, 2849-2851,
            2850t, 2851f
    transfer of
        across placenta, 2780-2781
        during lactation, 2781
    urinary retention from, 1599, 1599b
    with anticholinergic effects, 2345, 2346t
    withdrawal from. See Withdrawal.
Drug Alert Warning Network (DAWN), 2883

Drug eruptions, skin lesions in, 1844-1845,
    1844f, 1845f, 1846t-1847t
Drug testing, occupational, 3080-3081
Drusen, in macular degeneration, 1059, 1059f
Dry mouth, in botulism, 2014
Dry skin, in HIV/AIDS, 2084-2085
Dry socket, 1034
Duchenne dystrophy, 2900t
Duchenne's sign, 586, 588f
Ductus arteriosus, closure of, 2568
    cardiac lesions associated with, 2576-2577,
        2576b, 2577b
Duke criteria for infective endocarditis, 1302
Duodenal atresia, malrotation with midgut
        volvulus vs., 2607
Duodenal C-loop, in malrotation with midgut
        volvulus, 2607, 2607f, 2608f
Duodenal perforation, 496, 497f
Duodenal rupture, 485, 485f
Duodenal ulcers, 1391-1394
Duplex ultrasonography, 449, 542
Dupuytren's fracture, 550t
Durable power of attorney, 3133
Dural leak, bacterial meningitis associated with,
    1712
Dural penetration, as indication for lumbar
        puncture, 2660
Dural sinus, 350
Duroziez's murmur, in aortic regurgitation, 1307
Dust contamination, in urban search and rescue,
    3008
Duty to act, legal rights and, 3128
Duty to warn third parties, 2967-2968
Dying. See Death; End of life.
Dynamic splinting, of metacarpal or phalangeal
        fractures, 595, 595f
Dysarthria, in ischemic stroke, 1609
Dysbarisms, 2280-2281, 2281f. See also Scuba
        diving–related disorders.
Dysentery, 2624
    amebic, 235, 1477t, 1480-1481
    in shigellosis, 1464
    infectious causes of, 228, 229t-230t
Dysesthesia, in ciguatera fish poisoning, 1473
Dysmetria, 145
Dyspepsia
    in peptic ulcer disease, 1391, 1392
    nonulcer, 1393
Dysphagia, 1395-1398
    clinical features of, 1396-1397
    diagnosis of, 1397-1398
    esophageal, 1397
    in esophageal obstruction, 1383
    in esophagitis, 1387
    in gastroesophageal reflux, 1388
    in neck masses, 1076
    management of, 1398
    oropharyngeal, 1396-1397
    pathophysiology of, 1395-1396, 1396b
Dyspnea, 175-181
    acute, differential diagnosis in, 1101-1103
    ancillary studies in, 177, 180t
    at rest, in high-altitude pulmonary edema,
        2303
    chest pain associated with, 185, 186t
    diagnostic approach to, 176-177, 176t, 178t-
        180t
    differential considerations in, 176, 176t, 177,
        179t, 180
    disposition in, 181
    empiric management of, 180-181, 182f
    epidemiology of, 176
    exertional, 176, 1269
    history in, 176-177
    in abdominal trauma, 493
    in aortic stenosis, 1306
    in asthma, 1083, 2534, 2535t
    in chronic obstructive pulmonary disease, 1099
    in dilated cardiomyopathy, 1293
    in heart failure, 1269
    in hemodialysis patient, 1551
    in neoplastic cardiac tamponade, 1917
    in pleural effusion, 1150
    in pneumothorax, 1145
    in pregnancy, 2725, 2753t
    in pulmonary embolism, 1372
    palliative care for, 3154
    pathophysiology of, 176
    physical examination in, 177, 178t, 179t

Dyspnea *(Continued)*
    rapid assessment and stabilization in, 181f
    symptoms associated with, 177
    terminology related to, 175-176
Dysproteinemia, hyperviscosity syndrome in, 1912
Dysrhythmia, 1199-1244
    after head trauma, 371
    alcohol consumption and, 2866
    anxiety in, 1746-1747
    atrial, 1216
    bradycardia, sinoatrial and atrioventricular block as, 1215-1221
    cardiac cellular electrophysiology and, 1199-1201, 1200f-1202f
    cardiac conduction and, 1201-1203, 1202t, 1203f
    chaotic, causes of, 1227b
    classification of, 1213
    electrocardiography in, 1213-1214, 1214b, 1214f
    extrasystoles and parasystole as, 1221-1226
    from altered automaticity, 1204, 1204f
    from phenol chemical peel, 935
    from succinylcholine, 13
    heart failure in, 1268
    in amphetamine abuse, 2895
    in anaphylaxis, 1825t
    in asthma, 2536
    in chloral hydrate poisoning, 2487
    in cocaine overdose, 2388, 2390
    in crush injury, 3007
    in hydrofluoric acid poisoning, 934
    in hypercalcemia, 1945
    in hyperkalemia, 1940
    in hyperthyroidism, 1987
    in hypertrophic cardiomyopathy, 1295
    in hypomagnesemia, 1948-1949
    in hypothermia, 2237-2238, 2246
    in hypothyroidism, 1992
    in myocardial contusion, 468-469
    in submersion victim, 2313
    maneuvers for diagnosis and treatment of, 1214-1215
    mechanisms for formation of, 1204-1205, 1204f
    narrow-complex tachycardia as, 1226-1235
    pediatric, 2584-2590, 2584b, 2586b, 2587f-2589f
        in cardiac arrest, 109-113, 109t, 110f-113f, 110t
        unstable, 110, 110t
    pharmacologic treatment of, 1204-1213, 1205b.
        See also Antidysrhythmic drugs.
    preexcitation and accessory pathway syndromes as, 1235-1237
    pseudodysrhythmias and, 1215, 1215f
    reentry mechanisms for, 1204-1205, 1204f
    sinus, 1216, 1216f
    stable, initial assessment of, 1213-1215, 1214b, 1214f
    triggered, 1205
    unstable, signs and symptoms of, 1213
    wide-complex tachycardia as, 1237-1244
Dysthmic disorder, 1738
Dystonia, antipsychotic-induced, 1732, 2446
Dysuria
    differential diagnosis in, 1579-1581, 1579t, 1580f
    in children, 2643, 2643t

E code in injury prevention and control, 945-946
Ear
    anatomy of, 384
    blunt trauma to, 392
    discharge from
        in malignant otitis externa, 1071
        in otitis externa, 1070
        in otitis media, 1067
    examination of, in facial trauma, 388
    external
        barotrauma to, 2282, 2292
        infection in. *See* Otitis externa.
    foreign body in, 861-863, 862f
    in decompression sickness, 2284
    inner, barotrauma to, 2282, 2287-2288, 2287t, 2292
    laceration of, 392

Ear *(Continued)*
    middle
        barotrauma to, 2281-2282, 2282f, 2286-2287, 2287t, 2292
        infection in. *See* Otitis media.
        pain in. *See* Otalgia.
Ear squeeze, 2281-2282, 2282f, 2286-2287, 2287t, 2292
Early asthmatic response, 1081
Earthquakes, disaster preparedness for, 3016, 3017
Eastern Association for the Surgery of Trauma, clinical practice guidelines of, 3037
Ebb phase, in recovery from burn injury, 919
Ebola virus, 2054
Ecchymoses, in chronic renal failure, 1543
Eccrine glands, 915, 2255
Echinacea, adverse effects of, 2476t
Echinococcal infection, pulmonary disorders in, 2110-2111
Echinococcus granulosus, 2102t, 2105-2106, 2106f, 2111, 2113
Echinococcus multilocularis, 2102t
Echocardiography
    during cardiopulmonary resuscitation, 82
    in acute coronary syndromes, 1179
    in aortic dissection, 1327, 1327t
    in aortic rupture, 480, 480f
    in cardiac tamponade, 474, 1285
    in cyanosis, 271
    in high-altitude pulmonary edema, 2304
    in hypertrophic cardiomyopathy, 1295
    in infective endocarditis, 1302
    in ischemic stroke, 1613
    in multiple trauma, 313
    in myocardial contusion, 469
    in neoplastic cardiac tamponade, 1917
    in pericardial effusion, 1285, 1285f
    in pericarditis, 1282
    in pulmonary embolism, 1377, 1378t
    in restrictive cardiomyopathy, 1296
Echovirus, 2057
Eclampsia, 1627, 2749-2751, 2750b
Economic violence, 1018
Ecstasy. *See* MDMA (methylenedioxymethamphetamine).
Ecthyma, impetigo vs., 2202
Ectopic pregnancy, 2742-2746
    ancillary studies in, 2745
    clinical features of, 2743
    diagnosis of, 2743-2744
    differential considerations in, 2745
    hormonal assays in, 2744
    management of, 2745-2746, 2746f
    miscarriage vs., 2741
    risk factors for, 2743, 2743b
    ultrasonography of, 2730, 2744, 2744b
Eczematoid dermatitis, in otitis media, 1067-1068
Eczematous rash, drug-induced, 1844, 1847t
Edema
    anorectal, 1508-1509
    burn, 917
    cerebral. *See* Cerebral edema.
    heat, 2258-2259
    in aortic rupture, 478
    in *Bacillus anthracis* gastroenteritis, 1469
    in diphtheria, 2003
    in frostbite, 2229, 2231
    in hypothyroidism, 1992
    in nephrotic syndrome, 1531
    in spinal cord injury, 2906, 2907
    in superior vena cava syndrome, 1910
    laryngeal, in anaphylaxis, 1825t, 2548
    peripheral, in parasitic infection, 2107-2108
    pulmonary. *See* Pulmonary edema.
    renal causes of, 2648
    scrotal, in children, 2638-2642, 2639f-2640f, 2641
Edrophonium test, in myasthenia gravis, 1705
Education
    diversity, 3116, 3116b. *See also* Cultural competence.
    patient
        information technology for, 3098-3099
        on back pain, 710-711
        on wound management, 855-856, 856b
Educational materials, on emergency seclusion and restraint, 2961
Educational programs, in emergency medical services, 2989

Efavirenz, for HIV/AIDS, 2088
Effective refractory period, 1200, 1202f
Effervescent agents, for esophageal obstruction, 1384
Effusion
    otitis media with, 1066, 1069-1070
    pericardial, 1284-1285, 1285f
        in cardiac tamponade, 474, 474f
        in chronic renal failure, 1542
        in HIV/AIDS, 1287
        in hypothyroidism, 1993
        in myocardial contusion, 468
        in pregnancy, 1287
        malignant, 1283-1284
        transudative vs. exudative, 1285
        uremic, 1282
    pleural, 1134, 1148-1153
        clinical features of, 1150-1151, 1151f
        exudative vs. transudative, 1149-1150, 1152, 1152b
        in pneumonia, 2561, 2562
        in superior vena cava syndrome, 1911
        in systemic lupus erythematosus, 1808
        in tuberculosis, 2152, 2152f, 2158-2159
        loculated, 1148
        malignant, 1149, 1153
        management of, 1151-1153, 1152b
        parapneumonic, 1148, 1149, 1152, 1153
        pathophysiology of, 1148-1150, 1149b, 1149f
Egg embryo–grown vaccine, allergy to, 1827
Ehlers-Danlos syndrome, aortic dissection in, 1324-1325
Ehrlichiosis, 2137-2138
Eighty percent rule, in neck masses, 1075
Eikenella corrodens infection, in human bites, 890
Eisenmenger syndrome, 2578
Elastoplast, for ankle immobilization, 571
Elbow
    apophysitis of, 2710-2711
    avulsion fracture of, 2711, 2711f
    examination of, 649-650, 649f, 650f
        in arthritis, 1778
    immobilization of, 569
    little leaguer's, 663, 663f, 2710-2711
    nursemaid's, 666, 666f, 2697-2698, 2697f
    ossification centers in, 652, 652f, 653t, 2694, 2694f, 2694t
    pain in, in apophysitis, 2710
    tendinopathy of, 668, 1798-1799
    tennis, 667, 1798-1799, 2710-2711
Elbow trauma, 647-668
    anatomy in, 647-649, 647f, 648f
    biceps tendon rupture in, 668
    clinical features of, 649-650, 649f, 650f
    dislocation in, 664-666, 664f, 665f
    epicondylitis in, 667, 1798-1799, 2710-2711
    humeral fractures in, 652-664
        articular surface, 661-664, 661f-663f
        distal, 655-661, 656f-661f
        shaft, 652-655, 653f, 654f
    management of, 652
    olecranon bursitis in, 667, 1801-1803
    radial head subluxation in, 666, 666f, 2697-2698, 2697f
    radiography in, 641f, 650-652, 651f
Elderly person, 2824-2830
    abdominal injuries in, 346
    abdominal pain in, 2828-2829, 2828t
    abuse of, 1008-1015
        caregiver interview in, 1013
        clinical features of, 1011-1013, 1011b, 1012b
        definitions and types of, 1009-1010
        diagnostic strategies in, 1013
        documentation of, 1013
        epidemiology of, 1009
        etiology and risk factors for, 1010-1011, 1010b
        future directions in, 1015
        institutional, 1009, 1015
        interventions and referrals in, 1013-1014
        reporting requirements in, 1014-1015
        screening for, 1011, 1011b
    alcohol consumption in, 2877
    anxiety in, 1750
    appendicitis in, 1453
    as intractable patient, 2980
    auto-pedestrian collisions in, 345
    back pain in, 707

Elderly person (Continued)
    burns in, 347
    causes of death in, 942t, 949t
    central retinal artery occlusion in, 1057, 1057f
    chronic salicylate toxicity in, 2340
    constipation in, 237
    delirium in, 1649
    depression in, 1737-1738
    diagnostic strategies in, 2828
    extremity injuries in, 346-347
    falls in, 344, 2829-2830
    fever in, 134
    head trauma in, 346
    heat illness in, 2256
    high-altitude illness in, 2296
    history taking in, 2827
    hypothermia in, 2239-2240, 2241
    immunizations in, 2829
    infections in, 2828
    macular degeneration in, 1059, 1059f
    motor vehicle crashes in, 344-345
    myocardial infarction in, 2828
    pancreatitis in, 1428
    pharmacologic considerations in, 2826-2827
    physical examination of, 2827-2828
    physiologic changes in, 345, 2825-2826, 2825t
    pneumonia in, 1131, 2828
    psychosocial considerations in, 2827
    rib fracture in, 456
    seizure in, 1624
    soft tissue injuries in, 347
    spinal cord injury in, 346
    spinal injuries in, 413, 415f
    substance abuse in, 2883
    suicide in, 1767, 1769-1770
    transcondylar fracture in, 659, 659f
    trauma in, 344-348, 2829
        background of, 344
        clinical features of, 347
        diagnostic strategies in, 347
        disposition in, 348
        epidemiology of, 344-345
        management of, 348
        pathophysiology of, 345
        specific disorders and injuries related to,
            345-347
Electrical alternans
    in cardiac tamponade, 474, 474f, 1285, 1286f
    in neoplastic cardiac tamponade, 1917
Electrical arc, 2270-2271
Electrical field strength, 2270
Electrical injuries, 2267-2277
    cardiac arrest in, 78
    clinical features of, 2271-2274, 2272f
    complications of, 2274
    differential considerations in, 2275
    disposition in, 2277
    in pregnancy, 2277
    management of, 2275-2277, 2276b
    mechanisms of, 2270-2271, 2270b
    perioral, 391
    physics of, 2267-2270, 2268t, 2269t
    rhabdomyolysis from, 1978
Electrocardiography
    during cardiopulmonary resuscitation, 79
    during procedural sedation and analgesia, 2943
    electrophysiologic correlates of, 1202, 1203f
    in acute coronary syndromes, 1161-1174
        abnormalities in, 1161-1163, 1162f-1164f,
            1162t
        additional lead, 1171-1173, 1172f, 1173f
        adjuncts in, 1171-1174
        anatomic location of infarct on, 1164-1166,
            1164t, 1165f-1167f
        body surface mapping and, 1174
        limitations of, 1174
        noninfarct ST segment elevation and, 1166-
            1170, 1167f-1172f
        NSTEMI and, 1170-1171
        QT dispersion and, 1174
        serial, 1173-1174, 1173f
    in aortic dissection, 1326, 1326t
    in arthritis, 1782
    in asthma, 1085
    in atrial flutter, 1229, 1230f-1231f
    in cardiac tamponade, 474, 474f, 1285, 1286f
    in chest pain, 185-186, 188t
    in chronic obstructive pulmonary disease, 1101
    in cocaine overdose, 2388

Electrocardiography (Continued)
    in cyanosis, 271
    in cyclic antidepressant poisoning, 2354, 2355f
    in dilated cardiomyopathy, 1293
    in dysrhythmias, 1213-1214, 1214b, 1214f
    in electrical and lightning injuries, 2272, 2275,
        2276b
    in gastrointestinal bleeding, 223
    in headache, 173t
    in heart transplant patient, 2853, 2853f
    in high-altitude pulmonary edema, 2304
    in hypertrophic cardiomyopathy, 1295
    in hypothermia, 2237, 2238f
    in lithium toxicity, 2442
    in mitral regurgitation, 1306
    in mitral stenosis, 1305
    in mitral valve prolapse, 1305
    in myocardial contusion, 468-469
    in myocarditis, 1289
    in nausea and vomiting, 203
    in neoplastic cardiac tamponade, 1917
    in pacemaker patient, 1248-1250, 1249f, 1250f,
        1255
    in pericarditis, 1281-1282, 1281f, 2592-2593,
        2593f
    in pregnancy, 318, 2725
    in pulmonary embolism, 1373, 1373f, 1378,
        1379f
    in syncope, 195, 196t
    in ventricular tachycardia, 1238-1239, 1241f-
        1243f
    15-lead, 1171-1173, 1172f, 1173f
    pauses on
        compensatory, 1224f
        noncompensatory, 1222, 1223
    prehospital, 2990
Electroconvulsive therapy, for depression, 1742
Electroencephalogram
    in ataxia, 2682
    in seizure, 168, 2671
Electrolyte disturbances, 1933-1953. See also
        specific electrolyte disturbances, e.g.,
        Hyperkalemia.
    alcohol-induced, 2871-2872, 2872t
    in asthma, 1085
    in bacterial meningitis, 2662
    in chronic obstructive pulmonary disease,
        1102
    in comatose patient, 161-162
    in delirium, 1648, 1649
    in diabetic ketoacidosis, 1962
    in hyperglycemic hyperosmolar nonketotic
        coma, 1968, 1969
    in hypothermia, 2243
    in infants and children, 2573
    in nausea and vomiting, 203
    in pediatric gastroenteritis, 2630-2634, 2630t,
        2632b-2634b
    in rhabdomyolysis, 1979-1980, 1982
    in sepsis, 2216
Electromagnetic spectrum, 2318, 2318f
Electromechanical dissociation, 84, 112
Electromyography
    in botulism, 2015
    needle, 1689
Electronic databases, 3059
Electronic fetal monitoring, 2800
Electronic medical information systems, 3098
Electronic thermometer, 2508
Electrophysiological studies, 1689
Electroporation theory, 2267
Electrothermal burns, 2270
Electrothermal heating formulas, 2268b
Elemental metals, skin injuries from, 937
Elephantiasis, 2107-2108
Elevated arm stress test, in thoracic outlet
        syndrome, 1359
Ellis classification of tooth fracture, 1036, 1036f
Embolectomy
    for acute arterial embolism, 1352
    for pulmonary embolism, 1379
Embolism
    amniotic fluid, 2751-2752, 2821
    arterial, 1352-1353
        differential diagnosis in, 1352
        management of, 1352-1353
        pathophysiology of, 1343-1344
        physical examination in, 1346, 1347t
        vs. thrombosis in situ, 1347t

Embolism (Continued)
    arterial gas
        in scuba diving-related disorders, 2285-2286
        recompression therapy for, 2288-2292,
            2288b, 2289f-2291f
        vs. pulmonary decompression sickness,
            2288, 2288t
    atheroembolism and, 1343-1344, 1353, 1353f
    fat, 563
    pulmonary. See Pulmonary embolism.
    superior mesenteric artery, 1445-1446, 1446b
    thromboembolism and, 1308, 1343-1344
    venous air, in neck trauma, 444, 450
Embolization
    in acute coronary syndromes, 1157
    in pelvic fracture, 732-734, 733f
    of bronchial arteries, for hemoptysis, 282
Emergence phenomena, from ketamine, 2946-
    2947
Emergency department
    as factor in difficult patient-physician
        relationship, 2973
    death in, 2717, 3146-3151, 3146b, 3148b
    dedicated, regulatory definition of, 3158
    design of, 3120
    information management in, 3099-3102, 3100t,
        3102f
    minority populations' use of, 3115-3116, 3115b
    nonemergency functions of, 3158-3160
    occupational health issues in
        blood-borne pathogen exposure protocol and,
            3081-3087, 3084t, 3085t, 3086b
        material safety data sheet and, 3081, 3082b
    overcrowding in, 3120-3121
    pediatric-ready, 2504
    performance shaping factors in, 3120t, 3121-
        3123
    process improvement and patient safety in,
        3119-3126
        problem areas and, 3124-3126, 3125t
        sources of failure and, 3119-3123, 3120f,
            3120t
    promoting wellness in, 3176-3178, 3176b, 3177b
    violence in, 2956-2969. See also Combative
        patient.
        epidemiology of, 2956-2957
        gang, 1021-1022
        management of, 2957-2963
        medicolegal issues related to, 2967-2969
        prevention of, 2965-2967
Emergency medical condition, 3156-3157
Emergency medical dispatcher, 2988
Emergency medical services, 2984-3032, 2987-
    2988
    air medical transport in, 2994-2999. See also
        Air medical transport.
    bioethical dilemmas in, 3132-3133
    communications in, 2988-2989
    disaster preparedness in, 3010-3019. See also
        Disaster preparedness.
    educational programs in, 2989
    end of life issues in, 3144-3146
    future directions in, 2992
    history of, 2984
    interfacility and specialized transport in, 2991-
        2992, 2991b, 2992b
    material resources in, 2987-2988, 2988f
    medical direction of, 2989-2990
    prehospital care and management controversies
        in, 2990-2991
    provider levels and scope of practice in, 2986-
        2987, 2987t
    quality/performance improvement in, 2989
    resource and contact information for, 2992
    systems for
        air medical transport integration with, 2997
        design of, 2984-2986, 2985f
        protocols in, 3014
        status management of, 2988-2989
    tactical emergency medical support in, 3000-
        3005. See also Tactical emergency medical
        support.
    urban search and rescue in, 3005-3008, 3006b,
        3008f
    weapons of mass destruction and, 3021-3032
Emergency medical services medical director,
    2989-2990
Emergency medical technician-basic, 2986-2987,
    2987t

Emergency medical technician–intermediate, 2987, 2987t
Emergency medical technician–paramedic, 2987, 2987t
Emergency Medical Treatment and Active Labor Act (EMTALA), 2991, 3156
Emergency medicine
    bioethics in, 3131-3137, 3131b, 3131t. See also Bioethics.
    certification in, information technology for, 3099
    clinical decision rules in, 3035-3036
    clinical pathways in, 3038, 3039f-3041f
    cultural competence and, 3107-3117
        as tool for enhancing emergency department care, 3111-3116
        continuum of, 3111-3112
        institutional policies promoting, 3117, 3117b
        rationale for, 3108-3111, 3108t, 3109t
        recommendations for, 3116
        standards for, 3112-3113
        to cross barrier of different beliefs, values, and life experiences, 3113-3114
        to cross language barrier, 3112-3113
    disaster preparedness in, 3010-3019. See also Disaster preparedness.
    end of life issues in, 3143-3154. See also Death; End of life.
    evidence-based, 3046-3060
        data analysis in, 3051-3058, 3051t, 3057f
        hypothesis testing in, 3051-3058, 3051t, 3057f
        medical literature and, 3046
        practice guidelines in, 3036f, 3037t
        randomized clinical trials in, 3047-3051, 3048f
        steps in, 3058-3060
        terms in, 3058, 3059t
        types of clinical studies in, 3046-3047
    failures in, 3119-3126
        problem areas for, 3124-3126, 3125t
        sources of, 3119-3123, 3120f, 3120t
    forensic, 952-966
    guidelines for, 3034-3044
        computer-based protocols for, 3042-3044, 3043f
        development of, 3035, 3036f
        implementation and outcomes of, 3038, 3042
        legal and ethical considerations in, 3044
        sources and adoption of, 3036-3038, 3037t
    information gaps in, 3121
    information technology in, 3097-3106
        Internet and, 3104
        networks and, 3104
        security and confidentiality of patient information and, 3102-3103
        standards and, 3103-3104
        telemedicine and, 3105-3106
        terminology in, 3097
        uses of, 3097-3099, 3104-3106
    injury control in, 940-950, 945b. See also Injury prevention and control.
    medicolegal issues in, 3156-3173. See also Medicolegal issues.
    observation in, 3062-3073
        approach in, 3062-3063
        in abdominal pain, 3063-3064, 3064b
        in asthma, 3069-3070, 3070b
        in atrial fibrillation, 3070-3071, 3070b
        in chest pain, 3064-3065, 3065b
        in congestive heart failure, 3071, 3071b
        in deep vein thrombosis, 3065-3066
        in dehydration, 3071-3072, 3072b
        in head trauma, 3069
        in infection, 3072-3073, 3072b, 3073t
        in syncope, 3066-3067, 3066b
        in trauma, 3067-3069
        in upper gastrointestinal bleeding, 3066
        of critical diagnostic syndromes, 3063-3069
        of emergency conditions, 3069-3073
        principles of, 3062, 3063b
        staffing requirements for, 3062-3063
    occupational medicine and, 3076-3081
        drug and alcohol testing in, 3080-3081
        overview of, 3076-3077
        return-to-work issues in, 3078-3080
        workers' compensation and, 3077-3078
    restricted access to, bioethical dilemnas in, 3137

Emergency medicine (Continued)
    stressors in, 3174-3175
    teamwork in, failure of, 3121-3122
Emergency physician
    and primary care physician, differences between, 3131, 3131t
    as advocate for injury prevention and control, 948, 950
    as factor in difficult patient-physician relationship, 2973
    as surrogate decision-maker, 3135
    burnout in, 3175-3176
    delivery of bad news by, 3146-3147, 3146b
    diagnostic and management decisions made by, 125, 126b. See also Clinical decision making.
    grief response in, 3150-3151
    impaired, 3176
    major stresses for, 3174-3175
    negative reactions of, 2975-2976
    role of, in informed consent, 3166-3167
    wellness strategies for, 3176-3178, 3176b, 3177b
Emergency preparedness committee, 3015
Emergency seclusion and restraint, 2958-2961, 2960f
Emesis. See Vomiting.
EMLA (eutectic mixture of local anesthetics), 846, 2933
Emotional abuse, of elder, 1010
Emotional lability, in delirium, 1649
Emotional upset, heart failure from, 1268
Empathy, in death notification, 3147-3149, 3148b
Emphysema
    in chronic obstructive pulmonary disease, 1100
    in esophageal perforation, 1385
    orbital, 1044, 1045f
    subcutaneous
        chest wall trauma and, 459-460
        in esophageal perforation, 484
        in scuba diving–related disorders, 2286
        tracheobronchial injury and, 466, 466f
Emphysematous cholecystitis, 1421
Empty can test, in rotator cuff tendinopathy, 1797
Empyema
    in pleural effusion, 1152, 1153
    in pneumonia, 2562
    in tuberculosis, 2150-2151
    subdural, in otitis media, 1068
Enalapril, 1322t
    during pregnancy and lactation, 2788
    for hypertensive emergencies, 1319
Enamel, 1026, 1027f
    fractures involving, 1036-1037
Encainide, 1208, 2788
Encephalitis, 1710
    alcohol withdrawal syndrome vs., 2860
    arboviral, 2047-2048
    brainstem, ataxia in, 2681
    California, 2055
    headache in, 174t, 1641
    in cancer patient, 1920
    in rabies, 2065
    otic, 1068
    risk factors for, 171b
    St. Louis, 2049-2050
    viral
        ancillary studies in, 1720
        cerebrospinal fluid analysis in, 1716-1719, 1717t, 1718t, 1719f
        complications of, 1715
        diagnosis of, 1716-1720
        differential considerations in, 1720, 1721b
        disposition in, 1723
        epidemiology of, 1711
        etiology of, 1712
        lumbar puncture in, 1716, 1716b
        management of, 1722, 1723
        neuroimaging studies in, 1719-1720
        pathophysiology of, 1713
        signs and symptoms of, 1714
Encephalomyelitis, postinfectious demyelinating, ataxia in, 2681
Encephalopathy
    hepatic, 1411-1412, 1411t
        clinical stages of, 245t
        grades of, 1411t
        in cirrhosis, 1411
        jaundice in, 246

Encephalopathy (Continued)
    HIV, 2081
    hypertensive, 1314-1315
        headache in, 1641
        pediatric, 2650, 2652
        seizure in, 1622
    in cancer patient, 1920-1921
    in Lyme disease, 2124
    in pertussis, 2006
    lead, 2421, 2422
    progressive multifocal, 2045-2046
        dementia in, 1658, 1659
        in HIV/AIDS, 2082
    spongiform
        dementia in, 1657-1658, 1659
        from inhaled heroin, 2452
    uremic, 1542
End of life, 3139-3154. See also Death.
    death notification and, 3147-3149, 3148b
    emergency medicine and, 3143-3154
    epidemiology of death and dying and, 3140-3141, 3140f
    futility and, 3141-3142
    goals of medicine and, 3142-3143
    grief response in, 3149-3151, 3150b
    hospice medicine at, 3143
    initiating discussion about issues in, 3152-3153, 3152t
    palliative care at, 3143, 3151-3154, 3152t
    prehospital considerations in, 3144-3146
    quality of life and, 3142
    transplantation requests at, 3151
Endobronchial tuberculosis, 2151
Endocarditis, 1300-1302
    clinical features of, 1301
    diagnostic strategies in, 1301-1302, 1302b
    in prosthetic valve patient, 1308
    in Q fever, 2137
    in systemic lupus erythematosus, 1807
    management of, 1302, 1302b
    pathophysiology of, 1301
    prophylaxis for, 1302, 1303b, 1303t
    risk factors for, 1302, 1303b
Endocrine disorders
    anxiety in, 1747
    dementia from, 1656
    diarrhea in, 231b
    in chronic pancreatitis, 1435
    in sepsis, 2214
Endocrine system
    alcohol consumption and, 2871
    in mood disorders, 1735-1736
Endoleak, after abdominal aortic aneurysm repair, 1340
Endometriosis
    pelvic pain in, 251t
    postpartum, 2821
    thoracic, 1144
Endomyocardial biopsy
    in dilated cardiomyopathy, 1294
    in myocarditis, 1290, 1290f
Endophthalmitis
    posttraumatic, 1052, 1052f
    red and painful eye in, 290, 296t
Endorphin, 2451
Endoscopic cholangioscopy, in cholangitis, 1422
Endoscopic retrograde cholangiopancreaticoduodenography, in abdominal trauma, 499
Endoscopic retrograde cholangiopancreatography
    in acute pancreatitis, 1433
    in chronic pancreatitis, 1436
    in gallstone pancreatitis, 1434
    in jaundice, 244
    pancreatitis after, 1428
Endoscopy
    esophageal perforation from, 482
    in AIDS-related diarrhea, 1484
    in diverticular disease, 1494
    in esophageal foreign body removal, 872
    in esophageal obstruction, 1383-1384
    in esophageal perforation, 485
    in esophagitis, 1387
    in gastrointestinal bleeding, 224
Endothelial cells
    in hemostasis, 1892, 1893f
    injury to, in frostbite, 2229
Endothelin-1, in heart failure, 1263

Endotracheal intubation. *See also* Airway management; Mechanical ventilation.
approach to, 7-8, 7f-9f
assessment of access for, 4, 5f
capnography in, 38-39
confirmation of tube placement in, 6-7, 6f
elevated intracranial pressure and, 17, 18t
hemodynamic consequences of, 16-17
in acute pulmonary edema, 1271, 1271f
in adult epiglottitis, 1115
in adult resuscitation, 87, 91
in airway foreign body removal, 870
in anaphylaxis, 1830
in asthma, 1092
in botulism, 2016
in chronic obstructive pulmonary disease, 1103-1113, 1105t
in flail chest, 458, 458b
in hypothermia, 2244
in Ludwig's angina, 1119
in neonatal resuscitation, 122
in submersion victim, 2314
in tracheobronchial injury, 466
of difficult airway
approach to, 8-9, 9f
cricothyrotomy for, 22-23, 23f
esophagotracheal combitube for, 20, 20f
fiberoptic, 20-21, 22f
identification in, 3-4, 3b, 4b, 5f
intubating laryngeal mask airway for, 19, 19f
lighted stylet for, 19-20, 20f
retrograde, 20
special airway devices for, 18-23, 19f-23f
outcomes in, 23
pediatric, 99, 106-107, 108-109, 330, 2519
pharmacologic agents in, 13-16
potential cervical spine injury in, 17-18
prehospital, 2990, 2991
rapid sequence, 9-12, 10b
in asthma, 16
in elevated intracranial pressure, 17, 18t
in head trauma, 358-359
in neck trauma, 444
in shock, 51
indications for, 7-8
paralysis with induction phase in, 11
pediatric, 18, 107-108, 107b, 107t
post-intubation management in, 11-12
prehospital, 2990, 2991
preoxygenation in, 10, 10f
preparations for, 9-10
pretreatment agents for, 10, 11b
tube placement in, 11
vs. blind nasotracheal intubation, 12
with competitive neuromuscular blocking agent and etomidate, 14-15, 15t
status asthmaticus and, 16, 17t
Endotracheal suctioning
in meconium aspiration, 120, 120f, 122
in ventilated patient, 31
Endovascular cooling, for comatose survivors of cardiac arrest, 69
Endovascular surgery
for abdominal aortic aneurysm, 1337, 1338-1339, 1339f
for aortic rupture, 482
End-stage renal disease. *See* Renal failure.
Endurance training, cardiovascular system in, 2256
Enema
for constipation, 241t, 242
in appendicitis, 1454
in colonic ischemia, 1504
in colonic volvulus, 1498f
in diverticular disease, 1493, 1494
in intussusception, 2611, 2611f
in large bowel obstruction, 1496-1497
Enophthalmos, in red and painful eye, 286
Enoxaparin
for prostatis, 1586
with tenecteplase, in myocardial infarction, 1194-1195
Enriched Air Nitrox (EAN), 2279-2280
Entactogen intoxication, 2408-2411, 2409f
Entamoeba histolytica infection
amebic abscess in, 1415, 2106-2107
amebic dysentery in, 235, 1477t, 1480-1481
drug therapy for, 2100t
dysenteric colitis in, 229t

Entamoeba histolytica infection *(Continued)*
hepatic abscess in, 1415-1416, 2113
in HIV/AIDS, 1482-1483
intestinal symptoms in, 1477t, 1480-1481
pulmonary symptoms in, 2110
Enteritis. *See also* Gastroenteritis.
bacterial, 1469-1475, 1480t
acute, 2625-2626
invasive, 1460-1469, 1461t, 1462t
toxin-induced, 1469-1475, 1480t
in HIV/AIDS, 1482-1484, 1482t, 1483b, 1485t
protozoal, 1476-1482, 1477t
viral, acute, 1475-1476
Enteritis necroticans, 1471
Enterobius vermicularis infection, 1479-1482
drug therapy for, 2100t
gastroenteritis in, 1479-1482
pruritus ani in, 2113-2114
Enterocolitis
antibiotic-associated, *Clostridium difficile*, 1470t, 1474-1475
in infants and children, 2613
necrotizing, 2608-2609, 2609f
Enteromonas hominis gastroenteritis, 1477t
Enteropathy, HIV-induced, 1482
Enterovirus infection, 1289, 2057
Entitled patient, 2978t, 2980
Entrance wounds
centerfire rifle, 959, 959f
handgun, 955-958, 955f-957f
Envenomation grading, 900-901. *See also* Venomous animal injuries.
Environmental control for tuberculosis, 2169-2170
Environmental exposures
accidental hypothermia in, 2236-2252
electrical and lightning injuries in, 2267-2277
frostbite in, 2228-2235
heart failure from, 1268
heat illness in, 2254-2265
high altitude illness in, 2296-2309
radiation injuries in, 2316-2325
scuba diving and dysbarism in. *See* Scuba diving–related disorders.
submersion injuries in, 2311-2315
Environmental factors
in COPD exacerbation, 1099
in hemolytic anemia, 1883-1884
Environmental somatization syndrome, 1753
Enzyme analysis, in electrical and lightning injuries, 2276
Enzyme defects, in hemolytic anemia, 1878-1879, 1879b
Enzyme-linked immunosorbent assay
for HIV, 2073-2074
in Lyme disease, 2125
pregnancy test using, 2728-2730, 2729f
Eosinophil(s), 2834
in asthma, 1081, 1083
normal values for, 1886t
Eosinophilic peritonitis, 1552
Eosinophilic pneumonia, tropical, 2110
Ephedrine/ephedra
abuse of, 2893
overdose of, 2393
Epicondyles, 770, 771f
anatomy of, 647, 647f
fracture of, 662-663, 662f
Epicondylitis, 667
lateral, 1798
medial, 1798-1799, 2710-2711
Epidemiology, in injury prevention and control, 945-946
Epidermal appendages, depth of, burn injury and, 917
Epidermis, 842, 914
Epididymal appendage, torsion of, 1597
Epididymis
anatomy of, 1594, 1594f
physical examination of, 1573
Epididymitis, 1595-1597, 1597t, 2638-2639, 2639f
Epidural abscess
back pain in, 261, 265t, 703, 706, 712, 1684
in vertebral osteomyelitis, 2184-2185
magnetic resonance imaging in, 708, 709f
spinal, 1684
Epidural hematoma, 374-375, 375f, 376f
back pain in, 265t
in cancer patient, 1919-1920

Epidural hematoma *(Continued)*
in children, 335
spinal, 1683-1684
Epidural spinal cord compression, in cancer patient, 1919-1920
Epigastric pain
differential diagnosis in, 1393
in acute pancreatitis, 1429
in chronic pancreatitis, 1435
in pancreatitis, 2618
Epiglottic abscess, 1115
Epiglottis, adult vs. child, 2519, 2520f
Epiglottitis, 2529t
adult, 1114-1116, 1115f, 1116f
pediatric, 2523-2524, 2524f
screening for, 2509b
Epilepsia partialis continua, 1621
Epilepsy. *See also* Seizure.
benign rolandic, 2666
brain damage and, 2665
childhood and juvenile, 2666
classification of, 2665-2667, 2666b
electroencephalogram in, 2671
febrile seizures and, 2666-2667
gestational, 1624
ictal events in, clinical features of, 1620-1622
migraine and, 2679
psychomotor, 1621
risk of, after seizure, 2674
temporal lobe, vertigo in, 148t
Epileptic syndromes, 2665-2667, 2666b
Epileptiform discharges, 2671
Epinephrine
for anaphylactic shock, 54
for anaphylaxis, 1830, 1831b, 1832, 2549
for asthma, 1088, 2539t, 2541
for asystole, 85
for bradycardia, 2585
for bronchiolitis, 2546
for cardiac arrest, 92
for digital trauma, 2932
for dysrhythmia, 2586b
for heart failure, 1263, 2583t, 2584
for hymenoptera stings, 904
for neonatal resuscitation, 123-124, 123t
for pediatric resuscitation, 111, 114
for sepsis, 2219t, 2220
for viral croup, 2526
in glucose regulation, 1957
topical, 846
EpiPen, 1834, 2550
Epiphyseal injuries
classification of, 555-556, 557t
distal radius, 638-639, 638f
proximal humerus, 682-683, 683f
proximal tibial, 780-781
Epiphyseal-shaft angle of Southwick, in slipped capital femoral epiphysis, 2709
Epiphysis, 2175, 2175f
of hand
anatomy of, 578, 580f
fracture of, 600
proximal femoral, avascular necrosis of, 2706-2707, 2707f
slipped capital femoral, 765-767, 765f, 766f, 2707-2709, 2708f
Epipremnum aureum, 2473
Episcleritis, red and painful eye in, 289-290, 290f, 295t
Episioproctotomy, in shoulder dystocia, 2815
Episiotomy, 2804
in shoulder dystocia, 2815
in vaginal breech delivery, 2813
Epistaxis, 863, 1072-1075, 1073f, 1074t
Epithelialization, in wound healing, 843
Eplerenone, 1321t
Eponychium, 589
Eprosartan, 1322t
Epstein-Barr virus, 2044
in organ transplant patient, 2848
in pharyngitis, 1111
Epulis, in pregnancy, 2726
Equine antitoxins, allergy to, 1827
Ergonovine, after miscarriage, 2742
Errors in medical inquiry and clinical decision making, 130-133, 131t, 133b
Erysipelas, 2198

Erythema, 1839t, 1844
  in Kawasaki disease, 2026
  malar, in systemic lupus erythematosus, 1863f
  palmar, in pregnancy, 2724
Erythema induratum, 1816
Erythema infectiosum, 1850, 2046, 2046f
Erythema marginatum, in rheumatic fever, 1304
Erythema migrans, in Lyme disease, 2122, 2122f
Erythema multiforme
  drug-induced, 1846t
  internal malignancy associated with, 1863
  skin lesions in, 1852-1853, 1853f
Erythema nodosum, 1816-1817
  drug-induced, 1847t
  internal malignancy associated with, 1863-1864
  skin lesions in, 1856-1857, 1856f
Erythematous dermatitis, in dermatomyositis, 1863f
Erythrocyte. See Red blood cell entries.
Erythrocyte sedimentation rate
  in acute septic arthritis, 2705
  in arthritis, 1779
  in back pain, 707
  in headache, 173t
  in osteomyelitis, 2179
  in pediatric fever, 2509
  in pregnancy, 318
  in red and painful eye, 288
  in temporal arteritis, 1060
  in transient synovitis, 2703
Erythrocytosis, 273, 1884-1885, 1884f, 1885b
Erythroderma, internal malignancy associated with, 1864
Erythromelalgia, 1357
Erythromycin
  alcohol interactions with, 2875
  during pregnancy and lactation, 2784
  for Campylobacter gastroenteritis, 1461, 1461t
  for diphtheria, 2004
  for epididymitis, 2639
  for folliculitis, 1843
  for granuloma inguinale, 1559t, 1563
  for impetigo, 1842-1843
  for Lyme disease, 1292, 1789, 2127t, 2128
  for lymphogranuloma venereum, 1559t, 1562
  for orofacial infections, 1032
  for pertussis, 2006
  for pharyngitis, 1113
  for pneumonia, 2558t
  for relapsing fever, 2129-2130
  for scarlet fever, 1851
  for syphilis, 1856
  for toxic shock syndrome, 2030
  hepatotoxicity of, 1414
Erythropoietin, in anemia, 1868
Escape rhythms, idiojunctional, 1216, 1218
Escharotomy, in burn care, 921, 924-925, 925f
Escherichia coli
  enterohemorrhagic, dysenteric colitis in, 229t
  in food poisoning, 1470t, 1474
  in gastroenteritis, 2626
  in urinary tract infection, 1574
Escherichia coli serotype O157:H7 infection, in hemorrhagic gastroenteritis, 1461t, 1462t, 1466-1467
Escherichia coli serotype O157:H7 toxin test, 233
Escitalopram, 2357
Esmolol, 1209
  for aortic dissection, 1328
  for hypertensive emergencies, 1319, 2653
  in aortic rupture, 481
  overdose of, 2373t
Esomeprazole, 1390t
Esophageal dilation, perforation from, 482-483
Esophageal disorders
  alcohol consumption and, 2867
  gastroesophageal reflux in, 1388
  in HIV/AIDS, 2083-2084
  of motility, 1395-1396, 1397
Esophageal dysphagia, 1397
Esophageal intubation, detection of, 6-7, 6f
Esophageal obturator airway
  abdominal trauma after, 492
  esophageal perforation from, 483
Esophageal sphincter, lower, defective, in gastroesophageal reflux, 1388
Esophageal stricture, from caustic ingestion, 2383
Esophageal web, 1383

Esophagitis, 1386-1388
  causes of, 1386
  clinical features of, 1387
  diagnosis of, 1387
  in gastroesophageal reflux, 1388
  in HIV/AIDS, 2083
  management of, 1387-1388
Esophagotracheal combitube, for intubation of difficult airway, 20, 20f
Esophagus
  anatomy and physiology of, 1382
  cancer of, from caustic ingestion, 2383
  compression of, 1383
  diffuse spasm of, 1397
  foreign body in, 868f, 869f, 870-873, 1382-1384, 2617, 2617f
  nutcracker, 1397
  obstruction of, 1382-1385
  pain in, causes of, 1387
  perforation/rupture of, 482-485, 482b, 484b, 485f, 1385-1386
    anatomy and physiology in, 482
    chest pain in, 183, 187, 190t-191t
    conditions that mimic, 484b
    diagnosis of, 484-485, 485f
    epidemiology of, 482
    etiology of, 482-484, 482b
    management of, 485
    spontaneous, from vomiting, 201-202, 206t, 484
  trauma to, 446-447
    from caustic ingestion, 483, 2381, 2382f, 2383
    subcutaneous emphysema and, 459
Essex-Lopresti fracture, 550t
Estate of Doe v ABC Ambulance, 2967
Estrazolam, 2484t
Etanercept, 2844
Ethambutol
  for Mycobacterium avium infection in HIV/AIDS, 2076
  for tuberculosis, 2162-2163, 2163t, 2164t
Ethanol. See also Alcohol entries.
  butanediol with, 2489
  chloral hydrate with, 2487
  coprine-containing mushrooms with, 2479
  flunitrazepam with, 2486
  for toxic alcohol poisoning, 2401, 2401t
Ethibond suture, 852t
Ethical case analysis in emergency medicine, 3131-3132, 3131b
Ethical codes, 3129
Ethical issues in medicine and biology. See Bioethics.
Ethionamide, for tuberculosis, 2163t, 2164-2165
Ethmoid sinus, 1123
Ethmoid sinusitis, 1124
Ethmoidal arteries, 1073, 1073f
Ethnic differences. See Racial/ethnic differences.
Ethnicity, definition of, 3111
Ethosuximide
  during pregnancy and lactation, 2787
  for pediatric seizure, 2675t
  side effects of, 1628t
Ethyl chloride, 2933
Ethylene glycol poisoning, 2398-2402, 2401t
  antidotes to, 2329t
  metabolic acidosis in, 1928
  pharmacology and metabolism in, 2398, 2399f
Ethylene oxide, allergy to, 1827
Etidocaine, 2931t
Etidronate, for hypercalcemia, 1946
Etomidate
  as induction agent, 15
  for procedural sedation and analgesia, 2940t-2941t, 2947-2948, 2951t, 2952
  for rapid sequence intubation, 15, 15t, 359
Eucalyptus oil, 2473
Euphorbia pulcherrima, 2474
Eustachian tube dysfunction, in otitis media, 1066
Euvolemic hypernatremia, 1936
Euvolemic hyponatremia, 1934, 1935
Evaporation, heat transfer by, 2255
Evidence collection
  in child abuse, 972-973
  in gunshot wounds, 960
  in intimate partner violence and abuse, 1000-1001, 1003-1004

Evidence collection (Continued)
  in motor vehicle crashes, 965, 965f
  in pedestrian collisions, 966b
  in sexual assault cases, 984-989, 985b-987b, 987f, 987t, 988f, 988t
Evidence-based medicine, 3046-3060
  data analysis in, 3051-3058, 3051t, 3057f
  hypothesis testing in, 3051-3058, 3051t, 3057f
  medical literature and, 3046
  practice guidelines in, 3036f, 3037t
  randomized clinical trials in, 3047-3051, 3048f
  steps in, 3058-3060
  terms in, 3058, 3059t
  types of clinical studies in, 3046-3047
Evisceration, in abdominal stab wound, laparotomy and, 504
Exanthem, 1848-1851
  drug-induced, 1844, 1846t
  in Rocky Mountain spotted fever, 2133-2134, 2133f, 2134f
Exanthem subitum, 1850, 2044
Exchange resins, for hyperkalemia, 1941
Exchange transfusion
  for Goodpasture syndrome, 1816
  for hyperviscosity syndrome, 1913
  for kernicterus prophylaxis, 2603, 2604f
  for myasthenia gravis, 1707
  for thrombotic thrombocytopenic purpura, 1898
Exercise
  anaphylaxis from, 1828
  asthma from, 1082
  during pregnancy, 2736
  hematuria from, 1603-1604
  rhabdomyolysis from, 1978
Exercises, shoulder
  in clavicle fracture, 677, 679f
  in proximal humerus fractures, 682
Exertional dyspnea, 176
Exertional headache, 1642
Exertional heatstroke, 2256, 2262
Exertional rhabdomyolysis, 1978
Exit blot, pacemaker failure to capture due to, 1253
Exit wounds
  centerfire rifle, 959, 959f
  handgun, 958-959, 958f
Exophthalmos, in red and painful eye, 286
Exotoxin(s)
  in diphtheria, 2002
  in toxic shock syndrome, 2029
Expiratory volume, 30
Exposure, in pediatric trauma, 330, 333t
Extension injuries, of cervical spine, 410-411, 410f-411f
Extension supracondylar fracture, 655-659, 656f-658f
Extension teardrop fracture, 410-411
Extensor carpi radialis brevis, 581, 582f, 583f
Extensor carpi radialis longus, 581, 582f, 583f
Extensor carpi ulnaris, 582, 582f, 583f
Extensor digiti minimi, 582, 582f, 583f
Extensor hallucis longus tendon, 838
Extensor indicis proprius, 581-582, 582f, 583f
Extensor pollicis brevis, 581, 582f, 583f
Extensor pollicis longus, 581, 582f, 583f
Extensor retinaculum
  of ankle, 808, 809f
  of knee, 770, 771f
Extensor tendons
  of hand
    anatomy of, 581-582, 582f, 583f
    trauma to, 605-608, 605f-607f
  of knee
    anatomy of, 770, 771f
    trauma to, 782-784, 783f, 784f
External disaster plan, 3015
External ear
  barotrauma to, 2282, 2292
  infection of. See Otitis externa.
External radiation exposure, 2320
External radioactive contamination, 2320
External rewarming, 2247, 2248
External rotation stress test, of ankle, 817
External rotation technique, for reduction of anterior glenohumeral joint dislocation, 689, 689f
Extra-articular fracture, of thumb metacarpal, 599

Extracorporeal blood rewarming, 2250-2251, 2250t
Extracorporeal membrane oxygenation
  for sepsis, 2222
  in pediatric resuscitation, 98-99
Extracorporeal shock wave lithotripsy
  for cholelithiasis, 1419
  for urolithiasis, 1593
Extradural abscess, in otitis media, 1068
Extrahepatic bile duct carcinoma, 1423
Extraocular movement disorders, 1062-1063
Extraocular muscle function, in red and painful eye, 286
Extraperitoneal bladder rupture, 526
Extrapyramidal symptoms
  dementia with, 1657
  from antipsychotic agents, 2445, 2446-2447, 2449
  prevention of, 1731
Extrasystoles, 1221-1225
Extravascular hemolytic transfusion reaction, 60
Extreme altitude, 2296
Extremity(ies)
  examination of
    in chest pain, 187t
    in cyanosis, 270-271, 270f
    in dyspnea, 178t
    in peripheral vascular injury, 541
  lower
    aneurysm of, 1354
    escharotomy of, 924
    immobilization of, 569-571, 570f, 572f, 573f
    isolated mononeuropathy of, 1694b, 1697-1699
    ulcers of, 1350-1351, 1972
    vascular injury of, 546-547
    venous anatomy of, 1368-1369
  trauma to
    in elderly person, 346-347
    in electrical and lightning injuries, 2273, 2277
  upper
    aneurysm of, 1354-1355
    deep venous thrombosis of, 1370
    distal, neurologic examination of, 2694t
    escharotomy of, 924-925, 925f
    fracture of, in elderly person, 346
    immobilization of, 569, 569f
    isolated mononeuropathy of, 1693-1697, 1694b
    vascular injury of, 544-546
  vascular disease of. See Peripheral arteriovascular disease; Venous thrombosis.
Extrinsic ligaments of wrist, 622, 624f
Exudative pericardial effusion, 1285
Exudative pleural effusion, 1149-1150, 1152, 1152b
Exudative retinal detachment, 1058
Eye, 1044-1064
  acute visual loss and, 1056-1061, 1057f-1059f
  anatomy of, 283, 284f, 384, 1045f
  anisocoria and, 1061-1062
  conjunctivitis of
    gonococcal, 1566
    in anaphylaxis, 1825t
    in Kawasaki disease, 2025-2026
    red and painful eye in, 296t-297t
  corneal disease and, 1053-1054, 1054f
  epidemiology of, 1044
  examination of
    in altered consciousness, 2502-2503
    in facial trauma, 387-388
    in red and painful eye, 285-288, 285b
    extraocular movement disorders and, 1062-1063
    eyelid and ocular soft tissue disorders and, 1054-1055, 1055f
  foreign body in, 859-861, 860f, 861f
  glaucoma and, 1055-1056, 1056f
  HIV/AIDS and, 2085-2086
  hypertension and, 1055
  laceration of, 392
  Lyme disease and, 2124
  nystagmus and, 1062
  ophthalmic drugs for, 1063-1064, 1063b
  opioid overdose and, 2453
  optic disk abnormalities and, 1062
  pressure of. See Intraocular pressure.

Eye (Continued)
  red and painful
    ancillary studies in, 288
    diagnostic approach to, 283-288, 284b, 285b, 287f
    differential diagnosis in, 288-290, 288f-291f
    disposition in, 293t-297t, 297
    empiric management of, 290-292, 293t-297t
    epidemiology of, 283
    history in, 285
    in infants and children, 292
    physical examination in, 285-288, 285b
    traumatic, 283, 290, 292, 297
  trauma to, 1044-1052. See also Ocular trauma.
  vertigo and, 2685
Eye drops, 1063
Eye movements
  disorders of, 1062-1063
  examination of, in comatose patient, 159t, 160-161
Eyebrow laceration, 392
Eyelid
  contusion of, 1044
  disorders of, 1054-1055, 1055f
  laceration of, 392, 1051, 1051f
  super glue adhered to, 1046
  thermal burns of, 1046

Fab antivenin, in snakebite, 901
Fab fragments
  for digitalis toxicity, 2371, 2372b
  for oleander poisoning, 2474
Face
  analgesia of, Dejeune onion skin pattern of, 420
  anatomy of, 383-386, 383f-386f
  barotrauma to, in scuba diving–related disorders, 2282, 2293
  blood supply to, 385, 385f
  edema of, in superior vena cava syndrome, 1910
  nerve supply to, 383-384
  skin of, 384-385, 384f
  skin tension lines of, 843f
  trauma to, 382-396
    anatomy and physiology in, 383-386, 383f-386f
    clinical features of, 386-388
    disposition in, 396
    epidemiology of, 382-383
    fractures and dislocations in, 392-396, 394f, 395f
    history in, 386-387
    imaging of, 388-389
    management of, 389-390
    pathophysiology of, 386, 387f
    penetrating, 386, 387f
    physical examination in, 387-388
    prehospital care in, 389-390
    soft tissue injuries in, 390-392
Face presentations in labor and delivery, 2815-2816
Facet dislocation
  bilateral, 404, 405f
  unilateral, 406, 408f-409f, 409
Facial auditory nerve oxalosis, in ethylene glycol poisoning, 2399
Facial expression, lines of, 384, 384f
Facial flushing, in scombroid fish poisoning, 1472
Facial nerve, 1665t
  paralysis of, 1666-1668
    clinical features of, 1667-1668
    diagnosis of, 1668
    disposition in, 1668
    in otitis media, 1067
    pathophysiology of, 1666-1667
    tumor of, paralysis from, 1667
Facial pain
  in multiple sclerosis, 1673
  in trigeminal neuralgia, 1664
Facial rash
  in dermatomyositis, 1708
  in systemic lupus erythematosus, 1806
Facial skeleton, 383, 383f
Factitious disorder, 1761-1765
  by proxy, 1761, 1763, 1765
  clinical features of, 1761-1762

Factitious disorder (Continued)
  diagnosis of, 1764
  differential considerations in, 1764, 1764b
  disposition in, 1765
  management of, 1764-1765
  somatoform disorders vs., 1757
Factor VII deficiency, 1899
Factor VIII deficiency
  assay for, 1899-1900
  in hemophilia A, 1900-1902
  in von Willebrand's disease, 1902-1903
Factor VIII replacement
  for hemophilia A, 1900-1902, 1901t, 1902t
  for von Willebrand's disease, 1902-1903
Factor IX deficiency, 1902
Failure to thrive, in developmentally disabled patient, 2900-2901
Failures in emergency care, 3119-3126
  problem areas for, 3124-3126, 3125t
  sources of, 3119-3123, 3120f, 3120t
Fainting, 2685
Falls
  in elderly person, 344, 2829-2830
  in pregnancy, 318
  injury control in, 943t
  mechanism of injury of, 302, 303t
False imprisonment, 2967
False labor, 2798
False negative, 3052
False positive, 3052
Famciclovir
  for genital herpes, 1557t, 1559, 1858
  for herpes simplex esophagitis, 1387
  indications for, 2038
Familial periodic paralysis, 1709
Family
  as surrogate decision-maker, 3134
  during pediatric resuscitation, 114-116, 3149
  in pediatric trauma, 330
Family relationships, promotion of, as wellness strategy for emergency physicians, 3177
Famotidine, 1390t
  for anaphylaxis, 2549
Fascial anatomy, 842
Fascial planes of head and neck, 1027, 1030f, 1116
Fasciculations, from succinylcholine, 13-14
Fasciitis, 2196t, 2207-2208
Fasciola hepatica, 2101t, 2113
Fascioliasis, fever in, 2105
Fasciolopsis buski, 2101t
Fasciotomy, for compartment syndrome, 562, 1983
Fasting, preprocedural, 2939-2940
Fasting hypoglycemia, 1961-1962
Fat embolism, 563
Fat pads
  in elbow and humeral trauma, 651, 651f
  in supracondylar fracture, 2694-2695, 2695f
Fatigue
  in multiple sclerosis, 1673
  in myasthenia gravis, 1705
  performance and, 3122-3123, 3122f, 3123b
Fatty casts
  in proteinuria, 1532
  in urinary sediment, 1526, 1526f
Fatty liver
  alcoholic, 2868
  in pregnancy, 1417, 2755-2756
Feathering burn, 2273, 2273f
Febrile seizures, 2507, 2666-2667, 2674, 2674b
Febrile transfusion reaction, 60
Fecal impaction
  in developmentally disabled patient, 2903
  in spinal cord injury, 2907
  management of, 1497
Fecal incontinence, 1516-1517, 1516b
Fecal leukocytes, in diarrhea, 233, 2627
Federal Hazard Communication Standard, 3081
Feeding intolerance, in necrotizing enterocolitis, 2608
Felbamate, 1628t
Felodipine, 1321t
  overdose of, 2377t
Felon, 615-616, 616f
Female
  HIV/AIDS in, 2072
  myocardial infarction in, atypical presentations associated with, 1159
  urine collection methods in, 1575

Feminism, in alcoholism, 2871
Femoral aneurysm, 1354
Femoral artery and vein
    anatomy of, 737, 738f
    injury to, 546
Femoral condyles, 770, 771f
Femoral fracture
    arterial injury in, 761
    arthroplasty for, 749-750, 750f
    avulsion, 750, 750f
    distal, 776-777
    distal epiphyseal, 780-781
    occult, 746, 748f
    open fracture care in, 748-749, 749t
    pain management in, 749
    pediatric, 763-764, 763f
    proximal, 750-752, 750f-751f, 752b
    stress, 755-756
    traction and immobilization in, 746, 748
    with minimal or no trauma, 755
Femoral head
    anatomy of, 736, 737f
    arterial supply to, 737, 738f
    avascular necrosis of, 739-741, 741b, 742f
        after femoral neck fracture, 740, 742f, 750-
            751
        pediatric, 767
    development of, 763, 763f
    dislocation of, 756-759, 757f-759f
    fracture-dislocation of, 759-760, 760f
Femoral neck
    anatomy of, 736, 737f
    development of, 763, 763f
    fracture of, 750-752, 750f-751f, 752b
        avascular necrosis after, 740, 742f, 750-751
        displaced, 751, 752b
        radiologic evaluation in, 746, 747f, 751f
        stress type, 755-756
Femoral nerve, 737
Femoral nerve block, for femoral and hip
        fractures, 749
Femoral neuropathy, in hip trauma, 762
Femoral pulse, during cardiopulmonary
        resuscitation, 79
Femoral shaft fracture, 755
    pediatric, 763-764
    subtrochanteric, 753-755, 754f
Femoral trauma, 735-768
    anatomy in, 736-738, 736f-738f, 737t
    clinical features of, 742-744
    diagnostic strategies in, 746, 747f, 748f
    epidemiology of, 735-736
    femoral and hip fractures in, 746-756
        arthroplasty for, 749-750, 750f
        avulsion type, 750, 750f
        compartment syndrome in, 749
        femoral shaft, 755
        greater or lesser trochanteric, 753, 753f
        history in, 742-743
        intertrochanteric, 752-753, 752f
        open fracture care in, 748-749, 749t
        pain management in, 749
        pathophysiology of, 739
        physical examination in, 743-744
        proximal femoral, 750-752, 750f-751f, 752b
        stress type, 755-756
        subtrochanteric, 753-755, 754f
        traction and immobilization in, 746, 748
        with minimal or no trauma, 755
    femoral head fracture-dislocation in, 759-760,
        760f
    hip dislocation in, 756-759, 757f-759f
    hip prosthesis dislocation in, 749, 750f, 760
    management of, 746-750
    muscular injuries in, 761-762
    neurologic injuries in, 762-763
    pathophysiology of, 739-742, 739f-745f
    pediatric considerations in, 763-767, 763f,
        765f-767f
    radiologic evaluation in, 746, 747f, 751f
    soft tissue injuries in, 761-763
    vascular injuries in, 762
Femur
    anatomy of, 736-738, 736f-738f, 737t
    calcifying lesions of, 741-742, 743f-755f
    immobilization of, 569-570, 570f
    neoplastic disease in, 742, 745f
    osteoporosis of, 739, 739f-741f
Fenamate, overdose of, 2343

Fennel, adverse effects of, 2476t
Fenoldopam, for hypertensive emergencies, 1318
Fentanyl, 2922t, 2923
    for procedural sedation and analgesia, 2940t-
        2941t, 2944, 2952-2953
    in intubation of patient with elevated
        intracranial pressure, 17
    in rapid sequence intubation, 11b
    respiratory effects of, 2453t
    sympatholytic dose of, 17
    with midazolam, for procedural sedation and
        analgesia, 2950, 2951t
Ferret bite, 884-885
Ferritin, serum, in pregnancy, 2768
Ferrous sulfate, for iron deficiency anemia, 1871
Fertility rate, age-specific, 2722
Fertilization, hormonal role in, 2723
Fetal alcohol syndrome, 2791-2792, 2791b, 2877-
        2878, 2901t
Fetal anticonvulsant syndrome, 2769
Fetal heart rate monitoring, in pregnant trauma
        patient, 39, 319, 323-324, 324f
Fetal pole, ultrasonography of, 2730, 2731f
Fetal stations, in labor and delivery, 2799, 2799f
Fetomaternal hemorrhage, Kleihauer-Betke test
        for, 321
Fetopelvic disproportion, 2811
Fetor hepaticus, in hepatic encephalopathy, 1411
Fetus
    abruptio placentae and, 2747-2748
    antenatal assessment of, 2800-2802, 2803f
    ballottement or palpation of, 2728
    biophysical profile of, 2802, 2802t
    circulation in, 2568, 2568f
    death of
        first- or second-trimester, 2740
        sonographic criteria for, 2741, 2741b
    diabetes effects on, 2772
    evaluation of, in pregnant trauma patient, 323-
        324, 323f, 323t, 324f
    hyperthyroidism effects on, 2773
    maternal chronic medical illness effects on,
        2761-2776, 2763t-2764t
    maternal drug therapy and, 2779-2780, 2780b
    maternal substance abuse and, 2791, 2791b
    radiographic identification of, 2730
    skull of, bony landmarks of, 2800f
    trauma to, 319
    ultrasonography of, 2741, 2741b, 2741t
    umbilical cord entanglement with, 2817-2818
Fever, 134-137
    altered mental status and, 136, 2509b
    diagnostic approach to, 135-137, 135b, 135t
    differential considerations in, 135, 135b, 135t,
        137
    disposition in, 137
    empirical management of, 137
    epidemiology of, 134
    hyperthermia vs., 2258
    in Aeromonas hydrophila gastroenteritis, 1467
    in alcoholism, 2870-2871
    in amebic abscess, 1415
    in anticholinergic poisoning, 2348
    in arthritis, 1778
    in Bacillus anthracis gastroenteritis, 1469
    in Campylobacter gastroenteritis, 1460
    in central nervous system infection, 1714
    in cholangitis, 1421
    in Clostridium difficile enterocolitis, 1475
    in Colorado tick fever, 2141
    in diarrhea, 232
    in elderly person, 134, 2827-2828
    in hemorrhagic Escherichia coli serotype
        O157:H7 gastroenteritis, 1467
    in HIV/AIDS, 2076
    in hyperthyroidism, 1986
    in infective endocarditis, 1301
    in intestinal amebiasis, 1480
    in Kawasaki disease, 2025
    in meningococcal disease, 2021
    in neutropenic cancer patient, 2834-2839,
        2836t, 2838t
    in osteomyelitis, 2179
    in otitis media, 1067
    in pancreatitis, 1429
    in pertussis, 2006
    in Plesiomonas shigelloides gastroenteritis,
        1468
    in pneumococcal disease, 2018

Fever (Continued)
    in purulent pericarditis, 1286
    in pyogenic abscess, 1414
    in Q fever, 2137
    in rheumatic fever, 1304
    in Rocky Mountain spotted fever, 2133
    in salmonellosis, 1463
    in septic arthritis, 1785, 2188
    in shigellosis, 1464
    in sickle cell disease, 1880-1881
    in staphylococcal food poisoning, 1470
    in toxic shock syndrome, 2029
    in Vibrio parahaemolyticus gastroenteritis,
        1466
    in viral gastroenteritis, 1476
    in Yersinia enterocolitica gastroenteritis, 1465
    pathophysiology of, 134-135
    pediatric, 2505-2517
        ancillary tests in, 2508-2510
        bacteremia and, 2505-2506, 2512, 2515
        chest radiography in, 2510
        clinical features of, 2508-2511
        disposition in, 2517
        history in, 2508
        hyperpyrexia and, 2506
        in appendicitis, 2619
        in bacterial meningitis, 2658, 2659
        in bacterial tracheitis, 2528
        in cancer patient, 2516
        in congenital heart disease, 2517
        in epiglottitis, 2523
        in heat exhaustion and heatstroke, 2511
        in hemolytic uremic syndrome, 2654
        in HIV/AIDS, 2516
        in Kawasaki disease, 2511-2512, 2512b
        in pneumonia, 2556
        in septic shock, 2511
        in sickle cell anemia, 2516-2517
        in toxic ingestion, 2511
        in toxic shock syndrome, 2511, 2511b
        in ventriculoperitoneal shunts, 2517
        lumbar puncture and, 2660
        management of, 2511-2516, 2513b, 2515f
        of unknown origin, 2507, 2507b
        pathophysiology of, 2505
        petechiae and, 2507-2508
        physical examination in, 2508, 2509b
        prehospital care in, 2511
        seizure and, 2507, 2666-2667, 2674, 2674b
        temperature determination in, 2508
    plus petechiae, as indication for lumbar
        puncture, 2660
    relapsing, 2129-2130
Feverfew, adverse effects of, 2476t
Fiber, dietary, for constipation, 241t, 242
Fiberoptic bronchoscopy, in acute inhalation
        injury, 921
Fiberoptic intubation, 20-21, 22f
Fibrin clot formation, 1892, 1893f, 1894
Fibrin deposition, in thrombosis, 1368
Fibrinogen
    in bleeding disorders, 1895, 1903
    in disseminated intravascular coagulation,
        1903-1904
    in placenta previa, 2748
    in pregnancy, 318
Fibrinolysis, in anaphylaxis, 1825t
Fibrinolytic therapy
    for acute arterial occlusion, 1349
    for stroke, 1613t, 1615, 1615b
    in cocaine overdose, 2391
    in myocardial infarction, 1189-1192, 1192b
        contraindications to, 1192b
        eligibility criteria for, 1190-1192
        reduced-dose, in PCI candidates, 1195
        selection of agent for, 1189-1190
        with glycoprotein inhibitor, 1194
    in pulmonary embolism, 1377-1378, 1378t,
        1379
    prehospital use of, 2991
Fibroproductive lesions, in tuberculosis, 2153
Fibula
    anatomy of, 797
    fracture of
        avulsion, 818
        distal, 818
        proximal, 801-802, 802f, 814f
        stress, 804
Fibular compression test, 816

Field care, tactical, 3003
Field communications in emergency medical services, 2988-2989
Field death pronouncement, 3144
Fifth disease, 1850, 2046, 2046f
Fifth metatarsal base fracture, 832, 833f, 834
Fight bite, 611, 890
Figure-of-eight splint
　for clavicle fracture, 2693
　in clavicle fracture, 677, 678f
　in sternoclavicular joint dislocation, 684
Filariasis, 2100t, 2107-2108
File drawer problem, in clinical trials, 3051
Filovirus, 2034t, 2054
Financial exploitation, of elder, 1010
Finger
　amputations and ring avulsion injuries of, 612-613, 613b
　boutonnière deformity of, 607, 607f
　carpometacarpal joint dislocation of, 603, 603f
　decompression of, in burn injury, 925
　distal interphalangeal joint dislocation of, 601, 601f
　distal phalanx fracture of, 593-594, 593f
　examination of, in arthritis, 1779
　extensor tendon injuries in, 605-608, 605f-607f
　felon of, 615-616, 616f
　flexor tendon injuries in, 608-609
　herpetic whitlow of, 616
　metacarpal fractures of, 595-599, 597f-598f
　metacarpophalangeal joint dislocation of, 602-603, 602f, 603f
　motions of, 578f
　proximal and middle phalangeal fractures of, 594-595, 594f-596f
　proximal interphalangeal joint dislocation of, 601-602
　radiography of, 592f
　swan neck deformity of, 607, 607f
　trigger, 585, 618
　vascular injuries of, 613-614
Finger drop, in radial mononeuropathy, 1695
Finger sweeping, for airway foreign body removal, 869
Finger traps, in Colles' fracture, 633, 635f
Fingernail
　paronychia and, 614-615, 615f
　structural framework of, 589
Finger-snapping test, in lateral epicondylitis, 1798
Fingertip
　anatomy of, 589, 589f
　injuries to, 609-611, 610f
Finkelstein's test, in De Quervain's tenosynovitis, 1799
Fioricet, for migraine, 2680
Fiorinal, for migraine, 2680
Fire ant stings, 904, 905, 1827
Fire burn, 913-928. See also Thermal burn.
Fire corals, 909
Fire departments, EMS systems incorporated into, 2985
Fire victim, simultaneous carbon monoxide and cyanide poisoning in, 2440-2441
Firearm injuries. See also Gunshot wounds; Shotgun wounds.
　death from, 300
　epidemiology of, 489
　nonpowder, 1019
　street gangs and, 1021
　suicide and, 1768
　youth, 1018-1019
Firethorn, 2475
First responder, 2986, 2987t
First stage of labor, 2799-2800, 2799f-2802f
First-degree atrioventricular block, 1218, 1219f
First-degree burn, 918, 919f
First-trimester fetal death, 2740
First-trimester vaginal bleeding, 2740-2741, 2746f
Fish poisoning
　ciguatera, 1470t, 1473-1474
　scombroid, 1470t, 1472-1473
　Vibrio, 1470t, 1471-1472
Fisher's exact test, 3052t, 3053
Fissure, anal, 1508, 1512-1513, 1512f, 1513t
Fistula
　anorectal, 1513, 1515
　aortoenteric

Fistula (Continued)
　after abdominal aortic aneurysm repair, 1340
　in abdominal aortic aneurysm rupture, 1333
　aortovenous, in abdominal aortic aneurysm rupture, 1333
　arteriovenous, 538-539, 541, 1344, 1347, 1360
　arteriovenous bridge, prosthetic, 1365-1366
　bronchopleural, 466
　perilymphatic, vertigo in, 2685
Fitz-Hugh–Curtis syndrome, 1570
Fixation
　in humeral shaft fracture, 655
　in metacarpal or phalangeal fractures, 595
　in open tibial shaft fracture, 801
　in pelvic fracture, 731-732
Flail chest, 457-458, 457f, 458b, 460
Flammable liquids, 915
Flank, 490
　gunshot wounds to, 506-507
　stab wounds to, 505
Flank pain
　in renal stones, 2646
　in urolithiasis, 1588, 1590, 1593b
Flash burn, 2272
Flash points, of combustible liquids, 915, 915t
Flatulence, in intestinal amebiasis, 1480
Flavivirus, 2034t, 2049-2050
Flecainide, 1208, 2788
Flexion injuries of cervical spine, 399, 401-404, 402f-405f
Flexion supracondylar fracture, 657f, 658-659
Flexion teardrop fracture, of cervical spine, 401, 403f
Flexion-extension radiographs, in spinal injuries, 427
Flexor carpi radialis, 582, 584f
Flexor carpi ulnaris, 582, 584f
Flexor digiti minimi, 580-581, 581f
Flexor digitorum profundus, 582, 584-585, 584f, 585f, 609
Flexor digitorum superficialis, 582, 584, 584f, 585f, 609
Flexor hallucis longus tendinitis, 820
Flexor hallucis longus tendon, 838
Flexor pollicis brevis, 580, 581f
Flexor pollicis longus, 582, 584f
Flexor pulley system, 582, 584f
Flexor retinaculum, 808, 809f
Flexor tendons, of hand, 582, 584-585, 584f, 585, 585f, 586f
　relationship to radial and ulnar bursae, 585, 586f
　trauma to, 608-609
Flexor tenosynovitis, 616-617
Flight crew in air medical transport, 2996
Flip test, in lumbar radiculopathy, 704
Floaters, eye, 1040
Flori-Methane spray, 2933
Flow phase in recovery from burn injury, 919
Fluconazole
　during pregnancy and lactation, 2785
　for candidal esophagitis, 1387
　for cryptococcal meningitis, 2081
　for esophageal candidiasis, 2083-2084
　for tinea capitis, 1839
　for vulvovaginal candidiasis, 1567t, 1568
　in HIV/AIDS, side effects of, 2079t
Fludrocortisone acetate, for adrenal insufficiency, 1998
Fluid
　depletion of. See Dehydration; Hypovolemia.
　excess of. See Hypervolemia.
Fluid and electrolyte disturbances
　in delirium, 1648, 1649
　in diabetic ketoacidosis, 1962
　in hyperglycemic hyperosmolar nonketotic coma, 1968, 1969
　in pediatric gastroenteritis, 2630-2634, 2630t, 2632b-2634b
Fluid challenge, for acute pulmonary edema in hypotensive patient, 1273
Fluid intake, heat illness and, 2256
Fluid restriction, for hyponatremia, 1935
Fluid resuscitation
　for diabetic ketoacidosis, 1966
　for diarrhea, 235
　for hyperglycemic hyperosmolar nonketotic coma, 1969
　for hypermagnesemia, 1950

Fluid resuscitation (Continued)
　for hyperuricemia, 1914
　for hypovolemic hypotension, 360
　for rhabdomyolysis, 1982
　for salicylate overdose, 2341-2342
　for sickle cell disease, 1881
　in abdominal aortic aneurysm rupture, 1337
　in cardiac tamponade, 475
　in crush injury, 3007-3008
　in elderly trauma patient, 348
　in gastrointestinal bleeding, 221
　in heatstroke, 2264-2265
　in hemorrhagic shock, 52
　in hypothermia, 2245
　in lithium toxicity, 2443
　in multiple trauma, 307
　in neonatal resuscitation, 123t, 124
　in pulmonary contusion, 461
　in sepsis, 2218, 2219, 2219t
　in septic shock, 53
　in severe head trauma, 360
　in shock, 52
　in thermal burns, 921, 922-923
　in toxic shock syndrome, 2030
　pediatric
　　in cardiac arrest, 109
　　in hypertrophic pyloric stenosis, 2605-2606
　　in infectious diarrhea, 2629-2634, 2630t, 2632b-2634b
　　in necrotizing enterocolitis, 2609
　prehospital, 2991
Fluid retention, from high altitude exposure, 2298
Fluke infection, 2100t-2101t
Flu-like illness, in anthrax exposure, 3025
Flumazenil
　for benzodiazepine reversal, 2949
　in benzodiazepine overdose, 2326
　in children, 2953
　in comatose patient, 163
Flunitrazepam, overdose of, 2486
Fluoride poisoning. See Hydrofluoric acid.
Fluorine-18-deoxyglucose positron emission tomography, in osteomyelitis, 2181
Fluoroquinolones
　during pregnancy and lactation, 2785
　for Escherichia coli food poisoning, 1474
　for pneumonia, 1136
　for tuberculosis, 2164t, 2165
　for urinary tract infection, 1581t, 1582, 1583
　prophylactic, in cat bites, 888
Fluoroscopy, in esophageal foreign body removal, 872-873
Fluoxetine, 2357
Fluphenazine, 2446t
　injectable, for psychotic relapse, 1732
Flurazepam, 2484, 2484t
Flush syndromes, anaphylaxis vs., 1829
Flutter waves, 1229, 1230f-1231f
Flying, decompression sickness and, 2293-2294, 2293f
Focused assessment with sonography for trauma (FAST), 312-313, 723
Fogarty catheter embolectomy, for acute arterial embolism, 1352
Fogarty catheter thrombectomy
　for arterial thrombosis, 1354
　for peripheral arteriovascular disease, 1349
Folate/folic acid
　deficiency of
　　causes of, 1873b
　　megaloblastic anemia from, 1873-1875, 1874f, 1874t, 1875t
　supplementation of, in pregnancy, 2768
Foley catheter
　in burn injury, 923
　in foreign body removal, 2617
　in genitourinary trauma, 515, 517, 518f
　in peripheral vascular injury, 543
Folinic acid
　for toxic alcohol poisoning, 2402
　for Toxoplasma gondii infection, 2082
Folk/alternative medicine, cultural competent approach to, 3113-3114
Folliculitis, skin lesions in, 1843
Follow-up
　in clinical trials, 3050
　in disposition requirements, 3164-3165
Fomepizole, for toxic alcohol poisoning, 2401

Food allergy, 1826, 1848, 2547, 2548
Food bolus impaction, management of, 872
Food poisoning
    Bacillus cereus, 1470t, 1471
    bacterial, 1469-1475, 1480t
    ciguatera, 1470t, 1473-1474
    Clostridium botulinum, 2012-2016
    Clostridium perfringens, 1470-1471, 1470t
    Escherichia coli, 1470t, 1474
    in salmonellosis, 1461-1463, 1461t, 1462t
    reporting requirements for, 1463b
    scombroid, 1470t, 1472-1473
    staphylococcal, 1469-1470, 1480t
    Vibrio, 1470t, 1471-1472
Foods
    MAOI toxicity and, 2364, 2364b
    tyramine-containing, 1313, 1314b
Foot
    diabetic, 1971
    edema of, heat-induced, 2258-2259
    in Kawasaki disease, 2026
    pain in, 836-837
    puncture wounds to
        antibiotic prophylaxis for, 855
        osteomyelitis after, 2185
    trench, 2228, 2230-2231
Foot drop, in common peroneal
        mononeuropathy, 1699
Foot trauma, 820-839
    anatomy and physiology in, 820-821, 820f
    calcaneal fracture in, 826-827, 826f, 827f
    clinical features of, 821
    compartment syndrome in, 838-839
    contusions and sprains in, 838
    crush injuries, amputations, and major
        vascular injuries in, 838
    cuboid fracture in, 828
    cuneiform fracture in, 828
    diagnostic strategies in, 821-822, 822f
    dislocation of cuneiform, cuboid, or navicular
        bones in, 828
    interphalangeal dislocations in, 835-836
    Lisfranc injuries in, 828-831, 829f, 830f
    metatarsal base fractures in, 832-834, 833f
    metatarsal head and neck fractures in, 832
    metatarsal shaft fractures in, 831-832
    metatarsophalangeal dislocations in, 835
    midtarsal joint injuries in, 827
    navicular fracture in, 827-828
    osteochondral fracture of talar dome in, 824-
        825, 825f
    pain in, 836-837
    phalangeal fractures in, 834
    sesamoid fractures in, 834-835
    stress fractures in, 837-838
    subtalar dislocation in, 825-826, 825f
    talar fracture in, 822-824, 823f, 824f
    tendon injuries in, 838
    total talar dislocation in, 826
Foramen magnum, 350
Foramen ovale, closure of, 2568
Forced air warming systems, 2248
Forced expiratory volume in 1 second (FEV_1)
    in asthma, 1084, 1086f, 2535t, 2536
    in chronic obstructive pulmonary disease,
        1098, 1098t, 1101
Forced vital capacity
    in chronic obstructive pulmonary disease,
        1098, 1098t
    weakness and, 139
Forearm arterial injury, 545-546
Forearm splint, 569
Forearm trauma, 639-644
    anatomy in, 639-640, 640t
    clinical features of, 640
    Galeazzi's fracture in, 642-643, 643f
    Monteggia's fracture-dislocation in, 642, 642f
    plastic deformation in, 644, 645f
    radiography in, 640-641, 640f
    shaft fractures of radius and ulna in, 641
    ulnar shaft fracture in, 641-642
Forefoot
    anatomy of, 820, 820f
    interphalangeal dislocations of, 835-836
    metatarsal base fractures of, 832-834, 833f
    metatarsal head and neck fractures of, 832
    metatarsal shaft fractures of, 831-832
    metatarsophalangeal dislocations of, 835
    pain in, 837

Forefoot *(Continued)*
    phalangeal fractures of, 834
    sesamoid fractures of, 834-835
Foreign body, 859-879
    anorectal, 875-877, 876f, 1521-1522, 1522f
    assessment for, 845, 859
    gastrointestinal, 870-877, 2616-2617, 2617f
    genitourinary, 877-878
    in airway, 864-870, 2529-2530, 2550-2551,
        2551f
        clinical features of, 864-865
        history in, 865-866
        imaging of, 866-868, 867f-869f
        management of, 868-870
        physical examination in, 866
    in bowel, 873-875, 875f
    in children
        airway, 2529-2530, 2550-2551, 2551f
        esophageal, 2617, 2617f
        gastrointestinal, 2616-2617, 2617f
    in ear, 861-863, 862f
    in esophagus, 868f, 869f, 870-873, 1382-1384,
        2617, 2617f
    in hand, 618-619
    in lower leg, 805
    in nose, 863-864
    in pharynx, 870-873
    in stomach, 873-875, 875f, 1384-1385
    lead, 2423
    management of, 859
    ocular, 859-861, 860f, 861f, 1051-1052
        conjunctival, 1048
        corneal, 292, 297, 1047, 1047f, 1048f
        oropharyngeal, 1384
    soft tissue, 878-879
Forensic emergency medicine, 952-966
    in auto-pedestrian collisions, 965-966, 966b,
        966f
    in gunshot wounds, 953-960, 954f-960f
    in motor vehicle trauma, 963-966, 964b, 965f-
        966f, 966b
    in physical assault, 960-963, 961b, 961f-964f
    in sexual assault, 984-989, 985b-987b, 987f,
        987t, 988f, 988t
Forensic science, tactical emergency medical
        support and, 3004
Formaldehyde
    ingestion of, 2384
    methanol metabolism to, 2395, 2396f
Formic acid
    methanol metabolism to, 2395, 2396f
    poisoning from, 934
Formication, in amphetamine abuse, 2894
Formoterol, for asthma, 1088
Forward elevation maneuver, for reduction of
        anterior glenohumeral joint dislocation, 689
Foscarnet
    for AIDS-related diarrhea, 1484
    for cytomegalovirus esophagitis, 1387
    for herpes zoster, 2043
    in HIV/AIDS, side effects of, 2079t
    indications for, 2038
Fosinopril, 1322t
Fosphenytoin
    for alcohol-related status epilepticus, 2865
    for seizure, 166, 166t, 1627, 1627t
    for status epilepticus, 2672t, 2673
    prophylactic, in severe head trauma, 361
    side effects of, 1628t
Fournier's syndrome, 2208
Four-pillar anterior ring injuries, pelvic, 725, 726f
Fourth stage of labor, 2805
Fourth-degree burn, 919, 919f
Fourth-nerve palsy, eye movement disorders in,
        1062-1063
Fox, rabies in, 2062, 2062f, 2063f
Foxglove plant, 2368, 2369f
Fractional excretion of sodium (FENa), 1527-
        1528, 1527t, 1528b
Fracture, 552-564
    alignment of, 552-553
    alveolar bone, 1040
    angulation of, 553, 554f
    ankle, 811-815, 812b, 812f-815f
    avascular necrosis after, 562
    blisters associated with, 563
    clavicle, 676-679, 676f-679f
        in children, 2692-2693, 2693f
        subclavian artery injury and, 545

Fracture *(Continued)*
    closed, 552
    comminuted, 552, 552f, 2690, 2691f
    compartment syndrome in, 559-562, 560b,
        561b, 561f
    complete vs. incomplete, 553
    complex regional pain syndrome after, 562-563
    complications of, 558-564, 563b
    cricoid cartilage, 447
    diagnostic modalities in, 557-558
    displacement of, 552-553, 553f
    eponyms for, 550t-551t, 554
    facial, 392-396, 394f, 395f
        dental and alveolar, 395
        forehead, 393
        imaging of, 388-389, 394f
        mandible, 394-395, 395f
        midface, 393-394, 394f
        orbit, 393
        temporomandibular joint, 395-396
        zygoma, 394
    fat embolism syndrome after, 563
    foot
        calcaneal, 826-827, 826f, 827f
        cuboid, 828
        cuneiform, 828
        Lisfranc, 828-831, 829f, 830f
        metatarsal base, 832-834, 833f
        metatarsal head and neck, 832
        metatarsal shaft, 831-832
        navicular, 827-828
        phalangeal, 834
        sesamoid, 834-835
        stress, 837-838
        talar, 822-824, 823f, 824f
        talar dome, osteochondral, 824-825, 825f
    forearm, 641-644
    hand
        distal phalanx, 593-594, 593f
        mechanism of injury in, 592-593, 592f
        metacarpal, 595-600, 597f-599f
        pediatric, 600
        proximal and middle phalangeal, 594-595,
            594f-596f
        terminology in, 592-593, 592f
    healing of, 564, 781
    hemorrhage associated with, 559, 559t
    hip, 746-756
        arthroplasty for, 749-750, 750f
        avulsion type, 750, 750f
        compartment syndrome in, 749
        femoral shaft, 755
        greater or lesser trochanteric, 753, 753f
        history in, 742-743
        intertrochanteric, 752-753, 752f
        open fracture care in, 748-749, 749t
        pain management in, 749
        pathophysiology of, 739
        physical examination in, 743-744
        proximal femoral, 750-752, 750f-751f, 752f
        stress type, 755-756
        subtrochanteric, 753-755, 754f
        traction and immobilization in, 746, 748
        with minimal or no trauma, 755
    humeral, 652-664
        articular surface, 661-664, 661f-663f
        distal, 655-661, 656f-661f
        proximal, 680-682, 681f, 682f
        proximal epiphyseal, 682-683, 683f
        shaft, 652-655, 653f, 654f
        supracondylar, 2693-2697, 2694f-2696f,
            2694t
    immobilization after
        casts for, 571-573, 573f
        complications of, 563, 564b
        splinting and bandaging for, 568-571, 569f,
            570f
    in developmentally disabled patient, 2901
    in electrical and lightning injuries, 2273
    in spinal cord injury patient, 2909
    infection and, 558, 558b
    knee
        distal femur, 776-777
        patellar, 784-785, 785f
        proximal intra-articular tibial, 777-781
    laryngeal, in near-hanging and strangulation,
        451
    lower leg
        proximal extra-articular tibial, 797-799

Fracture (Continued)
    proximal fibula, 801-802, 802f
    stress, 803-804
    tibial shaft, 799-801, 801f
  mandibular, 394-395, 395f
  nasal, 391-392
  nasoethmoid, 393-394
  nerve injuries in, 559, 559t
  nomenclature in, 550t-551t, 552-554, 552b, 553f-555f
  oblique, 552, 552f
  odontoid
    type II, 405, 406f-407f
    type III, 432f
    with anterior dislocation, 399, 401, 402f
  open, 552, 558, 558b
  orbital, 393, 1044, 1045f
  osteomyelitis after, 2185
  pathologic, 553
  pediatric, 554-557
    apophyseal, 2709-2711, 2711f
    child abuse and, 970, 970t, 2698-2701
    clavicle, 2692-2693, 2693f
    condylar, 660
    diaphyseal, 2699
    distal radius, 637-639, 637f, 638f, 638t
    elbow avulsion, 2711, 2711f
    epicondylar, 662-663, 662f
    femoral, 763-764, 763f
    greenstick, 554, 556f
    hand, 600
    healing of, 781
    metaphyseal, 2699
    Monteggia, 2697
    multiple, in osteogenesis imperfecta, 2700-2701, 2700f, 2700t
    nose, 392
    patterns of, 554-557, 557t, 2689-2692, 2690f-2692f, 2691t
    radius, 644, 644f
    rib, 2699
    skull, 334-335, 2699
    supracondylar, 655-659, 656f-658f
    supracondylar humeral, 2693-2697, 2694f-2696f, 2694t
    toddler's, 2698, 2698f
    torus, 554, 556f
    trochanteric, 767
    ulnar, 644, 644f
    unintentional, 975
  pelvic, 717-734
    acetabular, 728-729, 728b, 731, 731f, 732f
    anatomy in, 717-718, 718f
    and blunt abdominal trauma, 509, 510f
    classification of, 723, 723b
    clinical features of, 718-720
    diagnostic peritoneal lavage in, 722-723, 722f
    epidemiology of, 717
    general management of, 722f, 723
    gynecologic injury in, 720
    hemorrhage in, 718
      evaluation of, 722-723, 722f
      management of, 731-734, 731b, 733f
    high-energy, 726-728, 727b, 733f
    in bladder trauma, 520-521
    in elderly person, 346
    low-energy, 723-726, 724f
    neurologic injury in, 719-720
    open, 719
    penetrating injuries in, 720
    posterior urethral trauma and, 516, 516f
    prehospital care in, 718
    radiologic imaging in, 720-722, 721f
    retrograde urethrogram and, 517-518
    thoracic aortic injury in, 720
    urologic injury in, 719
    visceral and soft tissue injuries in, 719
  penile, 533-534, 534f
  peripheral vascular injury in, 544, 559
  rib, 454-456, 454b, 455f
    anatomy in, 455f
    aortic rupture and, 479
    flail chest and, 457
    in children, 2699
    in chronic obstructive pulmonary disease, 1102
    pneumothorax and, 461-462
    pulmonary contusion and, 460

Fracture (Continued)
  shoulder, 676-683
    clavicle, 676-679, 676f-679f
    proximal humeral epiphysis, 682-683, 683f
    proximal humerus, 680-682, 681f, 682f
    scapula, 679-680, 680f
  skull, 372-374
    basilar, 373
    clinical assessment and significance of, 372
    depressed, 373
    frontal, 393
    in children, 334-335, 2699
    linear, 372-373
    open, 373-374
  spinal
    anatomy and physiology in, 399, 402f
    back pain in, 706
    computed tomography in, 429-430, 429f
    disposition in, 439
    extension, 410-411, 410f-411f
    flexion, 399, 401-404, 402f-405f
    minor, 439
    rotational, 405-409, 408f-410f
    vertical compression, 411-413, 411f-414f
    with cord impingement, back pain in, 265t
  spiral, 552, 552f
  sternal, 456-457
  stress, 553
  thermal therapy for, 573-574
  tibial
    epiphyseal, 780-781
    proximal
      extra-articular, 797-799
      intra-articular, 777-781
    shaft, 799-801, 801f
    stress, 803-804
    subcondylar, 797-798
    tibial plateau, 777-779, 777f-778f
    tibial spine, 779-780, 780f
    tibial tubercle, 798-799, 798f
  tooth, 395, 1036-1037, 1036f
  transverse, 552, 552f
  wrist, 627-630, 632-636, 637-639
Fracture-dislocation, 564
  Monteggia's, 551t, 642, 642f, 2697
  of femoral head, 759-760, 760f
  thoracic spine, 410f
Frailty, trajectory of dying in, 3140f, 3141
Francisella tularensis, 1131, 2130-2132
Free radical scavengers, after cerebral ischemia, 71
Free radicals, in necrosis after cerebral ischemia, 66
Free wall rupture, in myocardial infarction, 1160
Freeze-thaw phase of frostbite, 2229, 2229b
Freiberg's disease, 837
Frenzel maneuver for middle ear barotrauma, 2292
Freon gas abuse, frostbite from, 296f, 2887
Fresh frozen plasma, 59, 307
Friction rub
  pericardial, 1281, 2592
  pleural, 1150
Friedreich's ataxia, 2682
Frontal sinus, 1123
Frontal sinusitis, 1126
Frontal skull fracture, 393
Frontotemporal dementia, 1657
Frostbite, 2228-2235
  clinical features of, 2230-2231
  diagnostic strategies in, 2231
  disposition in, 2233-2234
  from freon gas abuse, 296f, 2887
  management of, 2231-2233, 2232b
  pathophysiology of, 2229, 2229b
  predisposing factors in, 2229-2230, 2230b
  sequelae of, 2234, 2234b
  temperature regulation physiology and, 2228
Frostnip, 2230
Frozen shoulder, 682, 698-699, 699t, 1797
Full-thickness burn, 919, 919f
Fulminant hepatitis, 1404
Fundic soufflé, 2728
Funduscopic examination, in red and painful eye, 287

Fundus, normal, 1045f
Fungal infection
  during pregnancy and lactation, 2785
  in cancer patient with impaired cell-mediated immunity, 2840
  in febrile cancer patient, 1908
  in HIV/AIDS, 2079
  in meningitis
    complications of, 1715-1716
    management of, 1722
    pathophysiology of, 1713
    signs and symptoms of, 1714
  in organ transplant patient, 2848
  in otitis externa, 1070-1071
  in pharyngitis, 275, 1112, 1113
  in pneumonia, 1130
  in sinusitis, 1123, 1124, 1126
  of bone or joint, 2178-2179
  skin lesions in, 1838-1840, 1839f, 1840f
Fungal pathogens, in central nervous system infection, 1711t
Fungus ball, in tuberculosis, 2151, 2151f
Funic reduction in umbilical cord prolapse, 2817
Funnel plots for assessment of publication bias, 3058
Furazolidone, for *Giardia* gastroenteritis, 1479-1480
Furosemide, 1321t
  for acute pulmonary edema, 1270t, 1272
  for acute renal failure, 2650
  for heart failure, 2583
  for high-altitude pulmonary edema, 2304
  for hypercalcemia, 1915, 1946
  for hypermagnesemia, 1950
  for hyponatremic hypovolemia, 2631-2632
  for nephrotic syndrome, 2648
Furuncle, 1843, 2204
Furunculosis, in otitis externa, 1071
Fusospirochetes, in necrotizing ulcerative oral diseases, 1033
Futility, end of life and, 3141-3142

GABA (γ-Amino butyric acid) agonists, after cerebral ischemia, 71-72
GABA (γ-Amino butyric acid) receptor complex, 2481, 2482
Gabapentin
  for neuropathic pain, 1692
  for pediatric seizure, 2675t
  side effects of, 1628t
Gadolinium-enhanced magnetic resonance imaging, in osteomyelitis, 2182, 2182f
Gait abnormalities
  antalgic, 764-765, 765f
  cerebellar, 145
  in developmental hip dysplasia, 2702
  in femoral neck stress fracture, 755-756
  in slipped capital femoral epiphysis, 2708
Galeal laceration, 372, 850
Galeazzi's fracture, 550t, 642-643, 643f
Galeazzi's sign, in developmental hip dysplasia, 2701, 2702f
Gallbladder
  carcinoma of, 1423
  enlarged, in pancreatic carcinoma, 1437
  hydrops of, in children, 2620
  in pregnancy, 2726
  inflammation of, 1419-1421, 1419f
  porcelain, 1423
Gallium-labeled bone scan, in osteomyelitis, 2181, 2181f
Galloping consumption, 2151
Gallstone ileus, small bowel obstruction in, 1441
Gallstones, 1418-1419, 1418f, 1419f. See also Cholelithiasis.
Galveston formula, for fluid resuscitation of pediatric burn patient, 923
Gamekeeper's thumb, 604
Gamma globulin. See Immunoglobulin preparations.
Gamma rays, 2319, 2320f
Gamma/neutron exposure, 2319-2320
Ganciclovir
  for AIDS-related diarrhea, 1484
  for cytomegalovirus esophagitis, 1387

Ganciclovir (Continued)
  in HIV/AIDS, side effects of, 2079t
  indications for, 2038
Gang violence, 1017-1018, 1020-1022
Ganglion, hand, 618
Ganglionopathy, 1700, 1700b
Gangrene
  gas, 2208-2209
  in frostbite, 2229
  local gas, 2208
  Meleney's synergistic, 2208
Ganser's syndrome, 1729
Garlic, drug interactions with, 2478t
Gartland classification for extension-type
    supracondylar fracture, 2694t
Gas(es), pulmonary irritant, inhalation of, 2433t,
    2434-2435, 2434f
Gas embolism
  in scuba diving–related disorders, 2285-2286
  recompression therapy for, 2288-2292, 2288b,
    2289f-2291f
  vs. pulmonary decompression sickness, 2288,
    2288t
Gas gangrene, 2208-2209
Gas laws, 2280-2281, 2281f, 2994-2995, 2995t
Gas-forming agents, for food bolus impaction
    management, 872
Gasoline, dermal exposure to, 936-937
Gastric acid secretion, inhibitors of, 1390t, 1398-
    1399
Gastric emptying
  in pregnancy, 2726
  prolonged, gastroesophageal reflux in, 1388
Gastric fluid aspiration, pneumonia vs., 1136
Gastric infarction, 1394
Gastric injury, from alkali ingestion, 2381, 2381f,
    2382f
Gastric lavage
  in anticholinergic poisoning, 2349
  in gastrointestinal bleeding, 224
  in mercury poisoning, 2426
  in overdosed/poisoned patient, 2330
Gastric mucosa damage, causes of, 1391, 1391b
Gastric outlet obstruction
  in hypertrophic pyloric stenosis, 2603
  in peptic ulcer disease, 1393
Gastric tonography, in shock, 50-51
Gastric tube, in gastrointestinal bleeding, 223-224
Gastric ulcers, 1391-1394
Gastric volvulus, 1394-1395
Gastritis, 1390-1391
  nausea and vomiting in, 204t
  peptic ulcer disease vs., 1393
Gastrocnemius strain, 804
Gastroenteritis
  abdominal pain in, 211t
  Aeromonas hydrophila, 1461t, 1462t, 1467-
    1468
  Bacillus anthracis, 1461t, 1462t, 1468-1469
  Bacillus cereus, 1470t, 1471
  bacterial, 1469-1475, 1480t
    acute, 2625-2626
    invasive, 1460-1469, 1461t, 1462t
    toxin-induced, 1469-1475, 1480t
  Campylobacter, 1460-1461, 1461t, 1462t, 2625
  ciguatera, 1470t, 1473-1474
  Clostridium perfringens, 1470-1471, 1470t
  Cryptosporidium, 1476-1478, 1477t
  Cyclospora cayetanensis, 1477t, 1478-1479
  diarrhea and, 234
  Entamoebaa histolytica, 1477t, 1480-1481
  Enterobius vermicularis, 1479-1482
  Escherichia coli, 1470t, 1474, 2626
  Giardia, 1477t, 1479-1480
  hemorrhagic Escherichia coli serotype
    O157:H7, 1461t, 1462t, 1466-1467
  hepatitis A, 2625
  in HIV/AIDS, 1482-1484, 1482t, 1483b, 1485t,
    2084
  in salmonellosis, 1461-1463, 1461t, 1462t, 2625
  in shigellosis, 1461t, 1462t, 1464-1465, 2625
  Isospora belli, 1476-1478, 1477t
  nausea and vomiting in, 204t
  pediatric, 2623-2634
    clinical features of, 2626
    complications of, 2626
    dehydration in, 2629, 2629t
    diagnosis of, 2626-2627
    differential diagnosis in, 2627, 2627t

Gastroenteritis (Continued)
    disposition in, 2628-2629, 2628b
    epidemiology of, 2623-2624
    etiology of, 2624-2626, 2628t
    fluid and electrolyte management in, 2629-
      2634, 2630t, 2632b-2634b
    management of, 2628, 2628t
    pathophysiology of, 2624
  Plesiomonas shigelloides, 1461t, 1462t, 1468
  protozoal, 1476-1482, 1477t
  rotavirus, 1475-1476, 2624-2625
  scombroid, 1470t, 1472-1473
  staphylococcal, 1469-1470, 1480t, 2626
  Vibrio, 1470t, 1471-1472, 2626
  Vibrio parahaemolyticus, 1461t, 1462t, 1465-
    1466
  viral, acute, 1475-1476, 2624-2625
  Yersinia enterocolitica, 1461t, 1462t, 1465,
    2625
Gastroesophageal reflux, 1388-1390
  causes of, 1388, 1388b
  clinical features of, 1388-1389
  complications of, 1389
  diagnosis of, 1389
  hypertrophic pyloric stenosis vs., 2605
  in apparent life-threatening event, 2718
  in asthma, 1083-1084
  in developmentally disabled patient, 2903
  in infants and children, 2609-2610
  in sudden infant death syndrome, 2715
  management of, 1389-1390, 1390t
Gastrointestinal anthrax, 3026
Gastrointestinal barotrauma, in scuba
    diving–related disorders, 2286
Gastrointestinal bleeding, 220-227
  alcohol consumption and, 2867
  ancillary studies in, 222-223
  diagnostic approach to, 220-223, 221b
  differential diagnosis in, 220, 221b, 223
  disposition in, 225-227, 225b, 226t
  epidemiology of, 229
  history in, 221
  in abdominal stab wound, 504
  in acute renal failure, 1540
  in Bacillus anthracis gastroenteritis, 1469
  in burn-injured patient, 924
  in cirrhosis, 1411
  in hemodialysis patient, 1550
  in iron overdose, 2419
  management of, 223-225, 223f
  observation in, 3066
  pediatric, differential considerations in, 220,
    221b, 2613-2614, 2614t
  physical examination in, 222
  rapid assessment and stabilization in,
    220-221
  risk stratification in, 225-226, 225b, 226t
Gastrointestinal disorders, 1382-1423. See also
    specific disorders, e.g., Appendicitis.
  alcohol consumption and, 2867
  diarrhea in, 231b
  hypomagnesemia in, 1948
  in acute mountain sickness, 2301
  in arsenic poisoning, 2423
  in chloral hydrate poisoning, 2487
  in chronic renal failure, 1542
  in developmentally disabled patient, 2903
  in HIV/AIDS, 2082-2084
  in hyperthyroidism, 1987
  in multiple sclerosis, 1672
  in opioid overdose, 2453
  in parasitic infection, 2112-2114
  in sepsis, 2214
  in spinal injuries, 438
  in systemic lupus erythematosus, 1808
  in thermal burns, 918
  in tuberculosis, 2161-2162
  pelvic pain in, 249b
  upper, pharmacological agents for, 1398-1399
Gastrointestinal foreign bodies, 870-877, 2616-
    2617, 2617f
Gastrointestinal system
  in acute radiation syndrome, 2322
  in pregnancy, 317, 2726
Gastrointestinal vasculitis, in systemic lupus
    erythematosus, 1808
Gastropathy, 1390-1391
Gastrostomy tube, in developmentally disabled
    patient, 2900-2901

Gatifloxacin
  for tuberculosis, 2164t, 2165
  for urinary tract infection, 1582
"Gay bowel syndrome," 1518
Gaze deviations, in comatose patient, 160-161
Gelatin sponge, for epistaxis, 1074
Gene activation, in cerebral ischemia, 66
General anesthesia, 1093, 2938, 2939b
Generalized anxiety disorders, asthma and, 1082
Genetic factors
  in asthma, 1082-1083
  in violent behavior, 2957
Genetic factors in mood disorders, 1736
Genital discharge, in sexually transmitted
    diseases, 1564-1571
Genital herpes, 1557-1559, 1557t, 1558f, 1559f,
    1858
Genital ulcers, 1557-1564
  in Bartholin cyst and abscess, 1559-1560
  in chancroid, 1557t, 1559t, 1562-1563, 1562f
  in condylomata acuminata, 1559t, 1563-1564,
    1564
  in granuloma inguinale, 1559t, 1563
  in herpes simplex virus infection, 1557-1559,
    1557t, 1558f, 1559t, 1858
  in lymphogranuloma venereum, 1557t, 1559t,
    1562
  in syphilis, 1557t, 1559-1562, 1559t, 1560f, 1561f
Genital warts, 1518t, 1519-1520, 1563-1564,
    1564f, 2045
Genitalia
  examination of
    in genitourinary trauma, 515
    in sexual assault, 986-988, 987f, 987t, 988t
  male, anatomy of, 516f
Genitourinary disorders, 1524-1604. See also
    specific disorders, e.g., Renal failure.
  foreign body and, 877-878
  in infants and children, 2635-2655
  in opioid overdose, 2453
  in spinal injuries, 438
  in tuberculosis, 2159
Genitourinary infection. See also Sexually
    transmitted disease.
  in pregnancy, 2757-2759
Genitourinary trauma, 514-535
  bladder injuries in, 519-526, 521f-526f
  clinical features of, 515
  Foley catheter placement in, 515, 517, 518f
  in sexual assault, 986-988, 987f, 987t, 988t
  penile injuries in, 532-534, 532f-534f
  renal injuries in, 526-530, 527f, 529f-530f
  staining techniques in, 988-989, 988f
  testicular injuries in, 534-535, 535f
  ureteral injuries in, 530-531, 531f-532f
  urethral injuries in, 515-519, 516f-520f
Gentamicin
  during pregnancy and lactation, 2784
  for catheter-related infections, 1363
  for febrile, neutropenic cancer patient, 2838t
  for pediatric fever, 2513
  for pneumonia, 2558t
  for tularemia, 2131
Geriatric patient. See Elderly person.
German measles. See Rubella.
Germander, adverse effects of, 2476t
Gerstmann-Strassler syndrome, 2058
Gestation(s)
  anembryonic, 2740
  multiple
    incidence of, 2722
    labor and delivery in, 2816
Gestational age, 2722-2723
  fetal viability and, 323, 323t
  fundal height and, 2800, 2802f
  uterine size and, 323, 323f
Gestational diabetes mellitus, 1957, 2772
Gestational epilepsy, 1624
Gestational hypertension, 2749-2751, 2750b
Gestational sac, ultrasonography of, 2730, 2730f,
    2731f
GHB (γ-Hydroxybutyrate)
  overdose of, 2488-2490, 2488b
  withdrawal from, 2490
Ghon focus, in tuberculosis, 2152, 2152f
Giant cell arteritis
  headache in, 1638
  ischemic stroke vs., 1611
  pericarditis in, 1284

Giardia antigen test, in diarrhea, 233
Giardia infection
  drug therapy for, 2101t
  in gastroenteritis, 1477t, 1479-1480
Gila monster, 896, 898-899, 902
Ginger, adverse effects of, 2476t
Gingiva, 1027, 1027f
  hyperplasia of, drug-induced, 1036
  laceration of, 1040
  lesions of, in leukemic states, 1036
  resorption of, 1032-1033
  spontaneous hemorrhage of, 1042
Gingival sulcus, 1027, 1027f
Gingivitis, 1032-1033, 1033f
Ginkgo
  adverse effects of, 2476t
  drug interactions with, 2478t
Ginseng
  adverse effects of, 2476t
  drug interactions with, 2478t
Glandular injuries, in neck trauma, 450
Glandular tularemia, 2131
Glans penis, 532, 532f
Glasgow Coma Scale
  for adults, 157, 157t
  for pediatric patient, 331t, 334
  in head trauma, 356-357, 357t
Glatiramer acetate, for multiple sclerosis, 1673
Glaucoma, 1055-1056
  acute, headache in, 1640
  acute angle closure
    headache in, 174t
    red and painful eye in, 288, 289f, 295t
    risk factors for, 171b
  closed-angle, 1056, 1056f
  low-tension, 1055
  open-angle, 1055-1056
  pharmacologic management of, 1063b, 1064
Glenohumeral joint
  anatomy of, 672, 673f
  anterior subluxation of, 690, 691f
  dislocation of, 687-693, 688f-694f
    anterior, 687-690, 688f-690f
    inferior, 692-693, 692f-694f
    posterior, 691-692, 691f, 692f
Glenohumeral ligaments, 672, 673f
Glenoid fossa
  anatomy of, 672, 673f
  fracture of, 680
Glenoid labrum, 672, 673f
Glenoid rim fracture, in glenohumeral joint
    dislocation, 688
GlideScope, 21f
Glipizide
  during pregnancy and lactation, 2790
  for new-onset hyperglycemia, 1973
Global massage, for central retinal artery
    occlusion, 1057
Globe. *See* Sclera.
Globin production, decreased, in thalassemia,
    1872
Globus symptom, in neck masses, 1076
Glomerular filtrate, composition of, 1524
Glomerular filtration rate, 1524, 2725-2726
Glomerular proteinuria, 1531
Glomerulonephritis
  acute renal failure in, 1534, 1534b
  hypertension in, 1312
  in Goodpasture syndrome, 1816
  poststreptococcal, 2647-2648
Glossopharyngeal nerve, 1665t
Glucagon
  for anaphylactic patient on beta blockers,
    1831b, 1833
  for beta blocker overdose, 2375
  for calcium channel blocker overdose, 2378
  for diabetic ketoacidosis, 1963
  for esophageal obstruction, 1384
  for food bolus impaction management, 872
  for hypoglycemia, 1961
  in glucose regulation, 1956-1957
Glucocorticoids. *See also* Corticosteroids.
  excess of, hypertension in, 1313
  replacement of, for adrenal insufficiency, 1998
Gluconeogenesis, 1956
Glucose
  administration of
    for alcohol intoxication, 2860
    for alcohol withdrawal syndrome, 2861

Glucose *(Continued)*
    for alcoholic ketoacidosis, 2873
    for hyperkalemia, 1941
    for Wernicke-Korsakoff syndrome, 2869
    in coma, 157-158
    in neonatal resuscitation, 123t, 124
    in pediatric resuscitation, 100, 101t, 103
  cerebrospinal fluid
    in bacterial meningitis, 2661
    in central nervous system infection, 1718
  dipstick blood, in diabetes mellitus, 1960
  disturbances of. *See* Hyperglycemia;
      Hypoglycemia.
  impaired fasting, 1957
  impaired tolerance, 1957
  in pregnancy, 2771
  metabolism of, in pregnancy, 2724
  normal physiology of, 1955-1957
  regulation of, 1956-1957
  serum
    in bacterial meningitis, 2662
    in comatose patient, 157, 161
    in diabetes mellitus, 1959
    in diabetic ketoacidosis, 1964, 1964t
  urine, in diabetes mellitus, 1959, 1959b
Glucose oxidase tests, in diabetes mellitus, 1959,
    1959b
Glucose transporter (GLUT) proteins, 1958
Glucose-6-phosphate dehydrogenase deficiency,
    in hemolytic anemia, 1878-1879, 1879b
α-Glucosidase inhibitors, 1973
Glue, ocular trauma from, 1046
Glue sniffer's rash, 2430
Glutamate, in cerebral ischemia, 65
Glutamate antagonists, after cerebral ischemia, 71
Glutamine, in hepatic encephalopathy, 1411
Gluteus muscle strain, 761
Glyburide
  during pregnancy and lactation, 2790
  for new-onset hyperglycemia, 1973
Glycemic control, 1973
Glycogenolysis, 1956
Glycoprotein IIb/IIIa receptor inhibitors
  in acute coronary syndromes, 1186
  in myocardial infarction
    with fibrinolytic therapy, 1194
    with percutaneous coronary intervention,
      1186, 1194
  thrombocytopenia from, 1897
Glycosuria, in pregnancy, 2725-2726
Glyphosate poisoning, 2467-2468
Goal-directed therapy
  for postresuscitation care, 87, 88f
  for shock, 50-52, 51f
Goiter, toxic
  diffuse, 1985-1986, 1987
  in pregnancy, 2764t, 2772-2773
  multinodular, 1986
  uninodular, 1986
Goldenseal, adverse effects of, 2476t
Goldman protocol, for risk stratification in acute
    coronary ischemia, 3065
Gonococcal arthritis, 1787-1788, 2190-2191
Gonococcal dermatitis, 1566, 1843-1844, 1843f,
    2191
Gonococcal pharyngitis, 1111, 1112, 1113
Gonorrhea, 1518t, 1519, 1559t, 1565-1567,
    1565f
  diagnosis of, 1566
  disseminated, 1566
  epididymitis in, 1595
  in pregnancy, 2758-2759
  septic arthritis in, 1784
  treatment of, 1559t, 1566-1567
"Goodness of fit" measurement, 3055
Goodpasture syndrome, 1816
Gouty arthritis, 1785-1786
Graded exercise testing, in acute coronary
    syndromes, 1180-1181
Graft infection, after abdominal aortic aneurysm
    repair, 1339-1340
Grafting, vascular, for peripheral arteriovascular
    disease, 1349-1350
Graft-versus-host-disease, transfusion-associated,
    60
Gram stain
  in bacterial meningitis, 1718, 1718t, 2662
  in cutaneous abscess, 2203-2204
  in gonorrhea, 1566

Gram stain *(Continued)*
    in meningococcal disease, 2022
    in pneumococcal disease, 2018
    in sepsis, 2217
    in septic arthritis, 2189
    in urinary tract infection, 1576
Gram-negative bacteria
  in cellulitis, 2199
  in febrile, neutropenic cancer patient, 2835
  in sepsis, 2212
Gram-positive bacteria
  in febrile, neutropenic cancer patient, 2835-
    2836
  in sepsis, 2212
Grandiosity, in mania, 1739
Granular casts, in urinary sediment, 1526, 1526f
Granules, in hemostasis, 1892, 1893f
Granulocyte, 1886, 2834
Granulocyte colony-stimulating factor,
    recombinant, for febrile, neutropenic cancer
    patient, 2839
Granulocyte count, radiation dose and, 2321
Granulocytopenia, in febrile cancer patient, 1907-
    1909, 1908b
Granuloma inguinale, 1559t, 1563
Granulomatosis, allergic, 1816
Granulomatous disease
  hypercalcemia in, 1945
  oral manifestations of, 1035
Granulomatous vasculitis, 1814
Graupel, lightning and, 2267
Graves disease, 1985-1986, 1987, 2764t, 2772-
    2773
Gravidity, 2722
Gray (Gy), 2321
Grease, in high-pressure injection injuries to
    hand, 612
Greater trochanter fracture
  intertrochanteric, 752-753, 752f
  isolated, 753, 753f
  pediatric, 767
  subtrochanteric, 753-755, 754f
Greater tuberosity fracture, in glenohumeral joint
    dislocation, 688
Green tobacco sickness, 2374
Greenstick fracture, 554, 556f, 2690
  distal radius, 637
  midclavicular, 677, 678f
  tibial shaft, 800
Grief response, 3149-3151, 3150b
  complicated, 3150, 3150b
  depression vs., 1740
  in staff, 3150-3151
Griseofulvin, for tinea capitis, 1839
Groin pull, in hip trauma, 761-762
Groshong catheter, 1363-1364, 1365f
Ground substance, 914
Group A beta-hemolytic streptococcus (GABHS)
    infection
  in pharyngitis, 1109, 1110, 1111, 1112-1113,
    1114
  in pneumonia, 2557
Growing skull fracture, in head-injured child,
    368
Growth disturbances, in proximal tibial
    epiphyseal injuries, 781
Growth factors, hematopoietic, for acute
    radiation syndrome, 2324
Growth hormone, in glucose regulation, 1957
Growth plates, in hip, 763, 763f
Grunting, in pediatric assessment, 2498
Guaiac test, 222
Guanabenz, 1321t
Guanfacine, 1321t
Guanidine hydrochloride, for botulism, 2016
Guar gum, drug interactions with, 2478t
Guidelines for emergency medicine, 3034-3044
  clinical decision rules and, 3035-3036
  clinical pathways and, 3038, 3039f-3041f
  computer-based protocols for, 3042-3044,
    3043f
  decision making errors in using, 131t, 132
  development of, 3035, 3036f
  implementation and outcomes of, 3038,
    3042
  legal and ethical considerations in, 3044
  medical screening examination and, 3161
  on emergency seclusion and restraint, 2961
  sources and adoption of, 3036-3038, 3037t

Guillain-Barré syndrome
    neuropathy in, 1690-1691
    sensory ataxia in, 2682
    weakness in, 138, 140, 141
Guilt, in grief response, 3150
Guinea worm skin disorders, 2100t, 2108-2109
Gums, in pregnancy, 2726
Gunshot residue test, 960
Gunshot wounds. *See also* Firearm injuries.
    abdominal
        diagnostic studies in, 505
        history in, 493
        management of, 505-507, 506f
        pathophysiology of, 490-491
        physical examination in, 494
    forensic aspects of, 953-960, 954f-960f
    mechanism of injury of, 302, 303t
    nonpenetrating ballistic injury from, 458-459
    observation in, 3068
    peripheral vascular, 537
    to head, 368-370
    to neck, 441
    transcervical, 446
Gunstock deformity, after supracondylar fracture,
    657-658
Gut suture, 852t
Gutter splint
    in epiphyseal hand fracture, 600
    in metacarpal or phalangeal fractures, 595,
        596f
    in metacarpal shaft fracture, 599
Guyon's canal, 586
Gynecologic injury
    in intimate partner violence and abuse, 997
    in pelvic fracture, 720
Gynecologic problems, in pregnancy, 2752, 2753t
Gyromitrin, in mushrooms, 2479

HACEK group, in infective endocarditis, 1301
Haddon's strategies, for injury prevention and
    control, 943, 943t, 944t
Haemophilus ducreyi, in chancroid, 1562, 1563
Haemophilus influenzae
    in bacteremia, 2506
    in bone or joint infections, 2177, 2178t
    in epiglottitis, 1115, 1116
    in meningitis, 1723
    in pneumonia, 1129, 1132, 2557
    vaccine for, 1723
Hair follicle, 915
Hair perm relaxers, caustic injuries from, 2381
Hair removal, in wound care, 847
Hairpin splint, in distal phalanx fracture, 593,
    593f
Hairy leukoplakia, in HIV/AIDS, 2083
Halazepam, 2484t
Hallucination
    from ketamine, 2946-2947
    in delirium, 1649
    in depression, 1737
    in schizophrenia, 1727
Hallucinogen intoxication, 2406-2416. *See also*
    specific drugs.
    dissociative agents in, 2413-2426, 2414t, 2415t
    entactogens in, 2408-2411, 2409f
    marijuana and miscellaneous plants and fungi
        in, 2411-2413, 2412f
    mushrooms in, 2478-2479
    serotonin-like agents in, 2406-2408, 2407f
Hallux
    fracture of, 834
    interphalangeal dislocation of, 836
    pain in, 837
Halogenated hydrocarbons, 2428, 2429t
Haloperidol, 2446t
    for agitation in delirious patient, 1654
    for agitation in demented patient, 1662
    for alcohol withdrawal syndrome, 2862, 2863
    for mood disorders, 1741
    for PCP intoxication, 2416, 2892
    for rapid tranquilization, 2961-2962
    for thought disorders, 1730
    hepatotoxicity of, 1414
    injectable, for psychotic relapse, 1732
    side effects of, 2961-2962
    with lorazepam, for rapid tranquilization, 2963
Halothane, hepatotoxicity of, 1414

Hamate
    anatomy of, 622, 623f
    fracture of, 629
Hamman crunch
    in esophageal perforation, 484
    in subcutaneous emphysema, 459
Hamman's sign
    in esophageal perforation, 1385
    in pneumopericardium, 1288
Hammer fracture, 814
Hamstring injury, 761
Hand, 576-619
    bites of
        antibiotic prophylaxis for, 854-855
        human, 611, 890-892, 891t, 892b
        infection risks in, 885
    examination of, 590, 590b
    foreign body in, 618-619
    ganglion in, 618
    motions of, 576, 577f-578
    nontraumatic injury to, 618
    stenosing tenosynovitis in, 618
    structural framework of, 576-589
        blood supply and, 585-586, 587f, 588f
        fingertip and, 589, 589f
        muscle and tendon function and, 578, 580-
            585, 581f-585f
        nail and, 589
        nerve supply and, 586, 587, 588f, 589f
        skeleton and, 577-578, 579f-580f
        skin cover and, 576-577
        synovial spaces and, 585, 586f
    surface anatomy of, 576, 577f
Hand symptoms
    in Kawasaki disease, 2026
    in pregnancy, 2733
Hand trauma, 592-618
    amputations and ring avulsion injuries in, 612-
        613, 613b
    clenched-fist injuries in, 611
    clinical features of, 589-590, 590b
    compartment syndrome in, 614, 614f
    diagnostic strategies in, 590-591, 591f, 592f
    dislocations and ligamentous injuries in, 600-
        604, 601f-603f
    epidemiology of, 576
    fingertip injuries in, 609-611, 610f
    fracture in
        distal phalanx, 593-594, 593f
        mechanism of injury in, 592-593, 592f
        metacarpal, 595-600, 597f-599f
        pediatric, 600
        proximal and middle phalangeal, 594-595,
            594f-596f
        terminology in, 592-593, 592f
    high-pressure injection injuries in, 611-612
    infection in, 614-618, 615f-617f
    mutilating injuries in, 609
    nerve injuries in, 614
    radiologic evaluation of, 590-591, 591f, 592f
    soft tissue injuries in, 600
    tendon injuries in, 604-609, 605f-607f
    vascular injuries in, 613-614
Handguns
    forensic aspects of, 954-955, 954f
    wounds inflicted by, forensic evaluation of,
        955-960, 955f-960f
    youth violence and, 1018-1019
Hand-held metal detector, in esophageal foreign
    body, 872
Hanging and near-hanging, 450-451
Hanging cast technique, in humeral shaft
    fracture, 654-655, 654f
Hanging weight method, for reduction of anterior
    glenohumeral joint dislocation, 689, 689f
Hangman's fracture, 410, 411f, 421, 550t
Hank's solution, 1038-1039, 1039f
Hantaviruses, 1131, 2055
Haptoglobin, in hemolytic anemia, 1877-1878
Hare traction splint, 569-570, 570f, 746, 748
Haversian canals, 2175, 2175f
Hawkin's sign, in rotator cuff tendinopathy,
    1797
Hazard Communication Standard (HazCom),
    3081
Hazardous materials
    disaster preparedness and, 3012, 3017
    tactical emergency medical support and, 3004
HAZMAT response, in chemical injuries, 930-931

Head and neck. *See also* Ophthalmologic
    conditions; Oral medicine; Otolaryngologic
    conditions.
    cancer of
        central nervous system infections in, 1920
        hypercalcemia in, 1914
    examination of
        in fever, 135
        in head trauma, 357-358, 358b
        in sexual assault victim, 986
        in vertigo, 144-145
    fascial planes of, 1027, 1030f, 1116
    in electrical and lightning injuries, 2272
    lymph nodes in, 1075, 1075f
    space infections of, 1027, 1028-1029, 1030f,
        1032, 1116-1117, 1116f
        parapharyngeal, 1121-1123, 1122f
        peritonsillar, 1117-1118, 1118f
        retropharyngeal, 1120-1121, 1120f, 1121f
        submandibular, 1028, 1032, 1118-1119
Head bobbing, 2498
Head compression, 352
Head position, in comatose survivors of cardiac
    arrest, 70
Head tilt–chin lift maneuver, in pediatric
    resuscitation, 97
Head trauma, 349-379. *See also* Traumatic brain
    injury.
    abdominal trauma and, 509-510, 511f
    alcohol consumption and, 2878
    anatomy and physiology in, 350-352
    ataxia in, 2681
    biomechanics of, 352
    brain cellular damage and death in, 352-353,
        353f
    central nervous system infections after, 370-
        371
    cerebral hemodynamics and, 350-352, 351f
    complications after, 370-371
    concussion in, 365-366
    contusion in, 374
    diffuse axonal injury in, 374
    epidemiology of, 349
    epidural hematoma and, 374-375, 375f, 376f
    facial nerve paralysis from, 1667
    facial trauma and, 386
    headache following, 1640
    hemophilia A and, 1902
    history in, 356
    in child abuse, 970-971
    in elderly person, 346
    inflicted, 349, 367
    intracerebral hematoma and, 378, 378f
    intracranial hematoma and, 371
    management of, 358-366
    medical complications in, 371
    minor, 363-365, 364b
    moderate, 362-363
    neurologic complications in, 370-371
    neurologic examination in, 356-357, 357t
    observation in, 3069
    pathophysiology of, 353-356, 355f
    pediatric, 333-336, 334b, 335b, 366-368, 368b
    penetrating, 368-370
    physical examination in, 356-358, 358b
    scalp wounds in, 371-372
    seizure in, 370, 373, 1623, 2669
        in children, 334, 367
        prophylaxis against, 361, 361b
    severe, 358-362, 359f
    skull fractures in, 372-374
    subdural hematoma and, 375-377, 376f
    subdural hygroma and, 377
    traumatic intracerebellar hematoma and, 378
    traumatic subarachnoid hemorrhage and, 377
    vertigo in, 144, 147t, 2684
Headache, 169-175, 1631-1643
    acute, 2677
    after moderate head trauma, 363
    ancillary studies in, 172, 173t
    cervicogenic, 1642
    chronic-progressive, 2677-2678
    classification of, 1631, 1632b
    cluster, 1634-1635, 2679
    coital, 1642
    cough, 1642
    differential considerations in, 170, 170t, 171b,
        173-175, 174t
    disposition in, 175

Headache (Continued)
epidemiology of, 169
exertional, 1642
history in, 170-172, 170t
hypertensive, 1641
in acute glaucoma, 1640
in acute mountain sickness, 2300, 2301
in bacterial meningitis, 2659
in brain tumor, 1637-1638, 2678
in carotid and vertebral artery dissection, 1638-
   1639, 1639f
in central nervous system infection, 1714
in cerebral venous thrombosis, 1670
in giant cell arteritis, 1638
in high-altitude illness, 1642
in idiopathic intracranial hypertension, 1639-
   1640
in intracerebral hemorrhage, 1610
in intracranial infection, 1641
in pneumonia, 2556
in polycythemia, 1884
in Q fever, 2137
in Rocky Mountain spotted fever, 2134
in scombroid fish poisoning, 1472
in spinal cord injury, 2906
in subarachnoid hemorrhage, 1635-1637, 1636t,
   1637f, 2677
in trigeminal neuralgia, 1642
in Vibrio parahaemolyticus gastroenteritis, 1466
isolated benign, guidelines for management of,
   3038
management of, 175
medication-induced, 1642
migraine. See Migraine.
orofacial pain in, 1034
pathophysiology of, 169
pediatric, 2676-2681
   clinical features of, 2676-2677, 2677b
   diagnosis of, 2679, 2680b
   differential considerations in, 2677b
   management of, 2680-2681
   pathophysiology of, 2676
physical examination in, 172, 172t
postdural puncture, 1641
postpartum, 2732
posttraumatic, 1640
primary, 1631-1635
rapid assessment and stabilization in, 170
secondary, 1635-1642
tension, 1635, 2679
Healing
fracture, 564, 781
wound, 842-843
Health beliefs/values, racial/ethnic differences in,
   culturally competent approach to, 3113-3114
Health care
culturally competent, 3111-3116. See also
   Cultural competence.
information in, uses of, 3097-3099
Internet in, 3104
racial/ethnic differences in access to, 3108-
   3111, 3109t
Health care workers
hepatitis B exposure protocol for, 1406, 1408f,
   3083-3084, 3084t
HIV exposure protocol for, 2091-2092, 3083,
   3084-3087, 3085t, 3086b
Health insurance status, medical screening
   examination and, 3162
Health Level 7, 3104
Health promotion
for emergency physician, 3176-3178, 3176b,
   3177b
in pregnancy, 2735-2737
Hearing impaired patient, 2904-2905
Hearing loss
acute, as indication for lumbar puncture, 2660
in otitis media, 1067
sensorineural, in acoustic neuroma, 1668
sudden, 1072, 1073b
vertigo and, 144, 2684b, 2684f
Heart. See Cardiac; Cardiovascular; Coronary.
Heart disease. See Cardiovascular disorders;
   Coronary artery disease; Valvular heart
   disease.
Heart failure, 1258-1278
acute, 1266
acute pulmonary edema in, 1261-1262, 1270-
   1274. See also Pulmonary edema, acute.

Heart failure (Continued)
alcohol consumption and, 2866
cellular mechanisms of, 1259-1261, 1260f,
   1261f
chronic, 1266, 1274-1277, 1275t
classification of, 1266-1267, 1267b
clinical evaluation of, 1267-1270, 1268b
compensatory mechanisms in, 1262-1263
constrictive pericarditis vs., 1288
definition of, 1258
diagnostic testing in, 1269-1270
drug-induced, 1269
epidemiology of, 1259
forward vs. backward, 1267
high-output vs. low-output, 1266
history in, 1269
in aortic regurgitation, 1307
in cardiomyopathy, 1264
in coronary artery disease, 1263-1264
in dilated cardiomyopathy, 1293
in Kawasaki disease, 2026
in myocarditis, 1264-1265, 1268
in pericardial disease, 1265
in pulmonary disease, 1265-1266
in valvular heart disease, 1265, 1268
myocardial hypertrophy in, 1262
myocardial pathophysiology in, 1263
neurohormonal alterations in, 1262-1263
observation in, 3071, 3071b
palliative care in, 3154
pediatric, 2582-2584, 2583t
physical examination in, 1269
pleural effusion in, 1149
precipitating causes of, 1267-1269, 1268b
prerenal azotemia in, 1532-1533
rapid-onset, 1270
right-sided vs. left-sided, 1266-1267
stroke volume in, 1260, 1260f, 1262
systemic vascular resistance in, 1262
systolic vs. diastolic dysfunction in, 1267
thyrocardiac, 1987
transfusion-related, 60
treatment of, 1270-1277, 1270t
vs. chronic obstructive pulmonary disease,
   1101, 1102
without pulmonary congestion, 1274
Heart murmur
in aortic regurgitation, 1307
in aortic rupture, 478
in aortic stenosis, 1306
in arteriovenous fistulas, 1347
in chronic obstructive pulmonary disease, 1100
in hypertrophic cardiomyopathy, 1295
in infective endocarditis, 1301
in mitral regurgitation, 1306
in mitral stenosis, 1305
in mitral valve prolapse, 1305
in myocardial rupture, 471
in tetralogy of Fallot, 2580
in tricuspid stenosis and regurgitation, 1307
innocent (functional), 2572
pediatric, 2571-2572, 2572b
Heart rate
fetal, antenatal assessment of, 2800-2802, 2803f
fever and, 135
in heart failure, 1261
in pregnancy, 2727
pediatric, 2495, 2495t, 2571, 2571t
Heart rhythm, disorders of. See Dysrhythmia.
Heart sounds
fetal, 2727-2728
in aortic regurgitation, 1307
in chronic obstructive pulmonary disease,
   1100
in hypertrophic cardiomyopathy, 1295
in mitral stenosis, 1305
in pacemaker malfunction, 1254
in pneumopericardium, 1288
pediatric, 2571
Heart transplant, 2851-2854, 2852f, 2853f
Heartburn
in gastroesophageal reflux, 1388
in pregnancy, 2726
Heat capacity of material, burn injury and, 915
Heat cramps, 2258, 2258b
Heat edema, 2258-2259
Heat exhaustion, 2259-2260, 2259t
heatstroke vs., 2261
pediatric fever in, 2510

Heat illness. See also Hyperthermia.
fever vs., 2258
minor, 2258-2259
pathophysiology of, 2256-2258
predisposing factors in, 2256-2258, 2256f
rhabdomyolysis in, 1978-1979
Heat intolerance, in hyperthyroidism, 1986
Heat loss
increased, hypothermia and, 2240, 2240b
mechanisms of, 2236, 2255
minimization of, in burn care, 921
Heat production
decreased, hypothermia and, 2239-2240, 2240b
increased, heat illness and, 2257
physiology of, 2254-2255
Heat rash, 2259
Heat regulation, 2255-2256
Heat stress
acclimatization to, 2255-2256
physiology of, 2254-2256
Heat syncope, 2259
Heat transfer
burn injury and, 916
mechanisms of, 916, 917t, 2254-2255
Heat transfer coefficient, 916, 917t
Heated irrigation, for rewarming, 2250
Heatstroke, 2260-2265
classic, 2261-2262
clinical features of, 2261-2263, 2261b, 2261t
diagnostic strategies in, 2263, 2263b
exertional, 2256, 2262
Heatstroke, hyperthyroidism vs., 1988
management of, 2263-2265, 2264b, 2265f
pediatric fever in, 2510
physiology of, 2260-2261
Heavy metal poisoning, 2418-2426
arsenic in, 2423-2424, 2424b
iron in, 2418-2421, 2419t, 2420f, 2420t
lead in, 2421-2423, 2422t
mercury in, 2424-2426, 2425b, 2425t
Heel pain
in Sever's disease, 2710
subcalcaneal, 836-837
HEENT (head, eyes, ears, nose, and throat
   findings)
in headache, 172t
in nausea and vomiting, 202t
Hegar's sign, 2728, 2728f
Heimlich device, 1147
Heimlich maneuver, for foreign body removal,
   2530
Helicobacter pylori infection
in gastritis, 1390, 1391
in peptic ulcer disease, 1392, 1394, 1394b
Helicopters for medical transport, 2995-2996,
   2996f
in severe head trauma, 358
in trauma, 2998
landing zone safety issues of, 2997, 2997b,
   2997f, 2998b
Heliox
for asthma, 2542
for chronic obstructive pulmonary disease,
   1106
for critically ill asthmatic patient, 1091-1092
Heliox diving, 2280
Helium intoxication, solvent abuse vs., 2888
HELLP syndrome, in pregnancy, 245, 2749
Helmet use, in pregnancy, 2735-2736
HELPER mnemonic for shoulder dystocia, 2816b
Hemangioma, subglottic, 2525
Hemarthrosis
in anterior cruciate ligament injury, 790-791
in distal femur fracture, 777
in intercondylar eminence fracture, 779
in patellar dislocation, 786
in tibial plateau fracture, 777-778
Hematemesis, 221
Hematochezia, 221
Hematocrit
in abdominal trauma, 495
in acute pancreatitis, 1431
in gastrointestinal bleeding, 222
in hypothermia, 2243
normal values for, 1868t
pediatric, 2573
Hematologic disorders, 1878-1904. See also
   specific disorders, e.g., Anemia.
alcohol-induced, 2873-2874, 2873t

Hematologic disorders (Continued)
  in HIV/AIDS, 2087
  in pregnancy, 2767-2768
  in sepsis, 2214
  in systemic lupus erythematosus, 1808
  in thermal burns, 918
Hematologic studies
  in abdominal trauma, 495
  in hypothermia, 2243
  in sepsis, 2216
Hematoma
  epidural, 374-375, 375f, 376f
    back pain in, 265t
    in cancer patient, 1919-1920
    in children, 335
    spinal, 1683-1684
  in fracture healing, 564
  in peripheral vascular injury, 539
  in tibial femoral knee dislocation, 788
  intracerebral, 378, 378f
  mediastinal, sternal fracture and, 456
  orbital, 393
  pelvic, 718
  penile, 534
  perirenal, 498f
  retrobulbar, red and painful eye in, 288, 295t
  retroperitoneal, pelvic fracture and, 500
  subdural, 375-377, 376f
    headache in, 2678
    in children, 335
  subungual
    nail bed laceration and, 594
    nail bed trauma and, 610-611
Hematoma block, in Colles' fracture, 633, 634f
Hematopoietic growth factors, for acute radiation
    syndrome, 2324
Hematopoietic response
  in acute radiation syndrome, 2322
  to high altitude, 2298
Hematopoietic system, development of, 1820f
Hematuria, 1528-1530, 1601-1604
  causes of, 1529, 1529b, 1529t, 1601, 1601b,
    1602b, 1603t
  clinical features of, 1530, 1601-1602,
    1602b
  differential considerations in, 1603-1604
  evaluation of, 1529-1530
  exercise-induced, 1603-1604
  imaging studies in, 1530, 1603
  in bladder trauma, 520
  in glomerulonephritis, 1534
  in pelvic fracture, 719
  in renal trauma, 528
  in spinal cord injury, 310
  in ureteral trauma, 530-531
  in urologic trauma, 515
  laboratory studies in, 1530, 1602-1603
  pediatric, 2644-2645, 2645b
    in Henoch-Schönlein purpura, 2615
    in proteinuria, 2647
    in renal stones, 2645
  pseudohematuria and, 1604
Heme pigment, in urine, 1525
Hemiarthroplasty, for displaced femoral neck
    fracture, 751, 752b
Hemiparesis, in cerebral herniation, 355
Hemiplegic migraine, 1632, 2678-2679
Hemlock
  poison, 2472, 2473f
  water, 2472, 2472f
Hemodialysis
  complications of, 1549-1552, 1550b, 1552b
  for acute renal failure, 2650
  for acute tumor lysis syndrome, 1912, 1912b
  for barbiturate overdose, 2483
  for beta blocker overdose, 2375
  for bipyridyl compound poisoning, 2466
  for chronic renal failure, 1547
  for isopropyl alcohol poisoning, 2404
  for rewarming in accidental hypothermia,
    2250t, 2251
  for salicylate overdose, 2342
  for toxic alcohol poisoning, 2401-2402
  vascular access for, problems related to, 1364-
    1366
Hemodynamics
  cerebral, 350-352, 351f
  during pregnancy, 316-317, 317t
  of intubation, 16-17

Hemoglobin
  as buffer, 1923
  glycosylated, in diabetes mellitus, 1959
  in carbon monoxide poisoning, 2438
  in gastrointestinal bleeding, 222
  in pregnancy, 2724, 2725f
  intrinsic abnormality of, in sickle cell disease,
    1879-1882
  normal values for, 1868t
  pediatric, 2573
Hemoglobinemia, march, 1883
Hemoglobinopathies, traumatic hyphema and,
    1049
Hemoglobin-oxygen dissociation curve
  altitude and, 2296, 2297f
  in cyanosis, 268, 269f
  shift of, during acclimatization to high altitude,
    2298
Hemoglobin-oxygen transport, impaired, anemia
    from, 1868
Hemoglobinuria, paroxysmal nocturnal, 1879
Hemolysis
  extravascular, 1877
  in burn injury, 917
  in hypophosphatemia, 1952
  in prosthetic valve patient, 1308
  intravascular, 1876-1877
Hemolytic anemia, 1868t, 1876-1884
  abnormal sequestration in, 1884
  ancillary evaluation of, 1877, 1877b
  aplastic crisis in, 2046, 2046f
  clinical features of, 1876-1877
  differential diagnosis in, 1878-1884, 1879b
  drug-induced, 1883, 1883b
  environmental causes of, 1883-1884
  extrinsic alloantibodies in, 1882
  extrinsic autoantibodies in, 1882-1883, 1883b
  extrinsic mechanical causes of, 1883
  in alcoholism, 2874
  intrinsic enzyme defects in, 1878-1879, 1879b
  intrinsic hemoglobin abnormality in, 1879-
    1882. See also Sickle cell disease.
  intrinsic membrane abnormality in, 1879
  jaundice in, 246
  laboratory studies in, 1877-1878, 1877b, 1877f,
    1878f
  microangiopathic, 1883
Hemolytic disorders
  in alcoholism, 2874
  jaundice in, 243, 244f
Hemolytic transfusion reaction
  extravascular, 60
  intravascular, 59-60
Hemolytic uremic syndrome
  in hemorrhagic Escherichia coli serotype
    O157:H7 gastroenteritis, 1467
  pediatric, 2654-2655
Hemoperfusion
  in barbiturate overdose, 2483
  in bipyridyl compound poisoning, 2466
Hemoperitoneum, 498, 498f, 499
  diagnosis of, 507
  iatrogenic, 492
Hemophilia A, 1900-1902, 1901t, 1902t
Hemophilia B, 1903
Hemopneumothorax, spontaneous, 1146
Hemoptysis, 279-283
  diagnostic approach to, 280-281
  differential diagnosis in, 281, 281t
  disposition in, 282-283
  epidemiology of, 279
  in tuberculosis, 2149, 2151, 2162
  management of, 282, 282f
  massive, definition of, 279
  pathophysiology of, 280
Hemorrhage. See also Bleeding.
  adrenal, 1995, 1995b
  cerebellar, vertigo in, 147t
  fetomaternal, Kleihauer-Betke test for, 321
  hypertensive, 1608-1609, 1608b
  in abdominal trauma, 502
  in aortic rupture, 479, 479f, 480, 480f
  in arteriovenous malformations, 1609
  in cardiac tamponade, 473
  in fracture, 559, 559t
  in hand trauma, 613-614
  in hemodialysis patient, 1550
  in multiple trauma, 308, 312, 313f
  in myocardial rupture, 471

Hemorrhage (Continued)
  in pediatric trauma, 330, 332t
  in pelvic fracture, 718
    evaluation of, 722-723, 722f
    management of, 731-734, 731b, 733f
  in penetrating cardiac trauma, 472
  in peptic ulcer disease, 1393
  in peripheral vascular injury, 539, 543
  intracerebral
    alcohol consumption and, 2869-2870
    anatomy and physiology in, 1607
    cerebral herniation in, 1918
    clinical features of, 1610-1611, 1610t,
      1611f
    diagnosis of, 1613
    differential diagnosis in, 1611-1612
    disposition in, 1617
    epidemiology of, 1608-1609, 1608b
    in pertussis, 2006
    management of, 1616
    pathophysiology of, 1607
    volume of, measurement of, 1611, 1611f
  intracranial
    dysrhythmia after, 371
    hypertension in, 1316
  oral, 1036, 1042
  orbital, 1046
  pelvic pain and, 250
  postpartum, 258t, 2818-2820
  pulmonary, in Goodpasture syndrome, 1816
  retinal, 1050
    high-altitude, 2306-2307, 2307f
    in child abuse, 971
  retrobulbar, 1046
  spinal cord, magnetic resonance imaging in,
    434, 434f
  subarachnoid, 1635-1637, 1636t, 1637f
    diagnosis of, 1636-1637, 1637f
    dysrhythmia after, 371
    headache in, 174t, 1637, 2677
    Hunt and Hess scale for, 1636, 1636t
    in pregnancy, 2732
    risk factors for, 171b
    spinal, 1682
    traumatic, 377
    treatment of, 1637
  subconjunctival, 285, 296t, 1048, 1048f
  vitreous, 1050, 1058-1059
Hemorrhagic fever viruses, 2055-2056
Hemorrhagic gastroenteritis, in Escherichia coli
    serotype O157:H7 infection, 1461t, 1462t,
    1466-1467
Hemorrhagic shock
  causes of, 44f, 45-46
  definition of, 49, 49b
  in subclavian artery injury, 545
  treatment of, 52-53, 52b
Hemorrhoidal arteries, 1507
Hemorrhoids, 1509-1512, 1510t, 1511b, 1511t,
    1512f, 2726
Hemosiderosis, transfusional, 61
Hemostasis
  disorders of. See Bleeding disorders.
  physiology of, 1892-1894, 1893b, 1893f
Hemothorax
  in children, 339
  traumatic, 464-465, 465b, 465f, 1152
Henderson-Hasselbalch equation, 1923
Hennebert fistula test, in middle ear barotrauma,
    2282
Henoch-Schönlein purpura, 1815, 2615, 2615f,
    2653-2654
Henry's law, 2280-2281
Heparin
  during pregnancy and lactation, 2757, 2766,
    2785, 2786
  for arterial thrombosis, 1354
  for cerebral venous thrombosis, 1671
  for cervical vascular injury, 449
  for deep venous thrombosis, 1370
  for disseminated intravascular coagulation,
    1904
  for ischemic stroke, 1615-1616
  for peripheral arteriovascular disease, 1349
  for pulmonary embolism, 1377
  in acute coronary syndromes, 1187
  low-molecular-weight
    advantages of, 1188
    during pregnancy and lactation, 2757, 2786

Heparin *(Continued)*
  for deep vein thrombosis, 3065-3066
  in acute coronary syndromes, 1187-1188
  thrombocytopenia from, 1897
Hepatic abscess, 1414-1417, 1415f, 1416f, 2113
  amebic, 1415-1416
  pyogenic, 1414-1415, 1415f
Hepatic artery aneurysm, 1355
Hepatic encephalopathy, 1411-1412
  clinical stages of, 245t
  grades of, 1411t
  in cirrhosis, 1411
  jaundice in, 246
Hepatitis
  alcoholic, 1405, 1409, 2868
  chronic, 1416
  fulminant, 1404
  halothane-induced, 1414
  in developmentally disabled patient, 2903
  in pregnancy, 2755, 2775
  serologic markers in, 1405t
  transmission of, in human bites, 891
  viral, 1402-1406
    clinical features of, 1404
    diagnosis of, 1404-1405, 1405t
    disposition in, 1405-1406
    epidemiology of, 1402-1404, 1403f, 1403t
    management of, 1405-1406
    pathophysiology of, 1404
    postexposure prophylaxis for, 1406, 1407t, 1408f
Hepatitis A, 1402, 1403f, 1405, 2035t, 2057, 2625
Hepatitis B, 1402-1403, 1403f, 1403t, 1405, 1406, 1407t
  arthritis in, 1788
  chronic, with hepatitis D infection, 1404
  drugs for, 2036t
  hepatocellular carcinoma and, 1417
  in organ transplant patient, 2848
  in pregnancy, 2775
  occupational exposure protocol for, 1406, 1408f, 3083-3084, 3084t
  prophylaxis against, after sexual assault, 990, 990b
  vaccine for, 1406, 2035t
Hepatitis B immune globulin, for postexposure prophylaxis, 1406, 3083-3084, 3084t
Hepatitis B surface antigen, 1402-1403, 1403f, 1403t
Hepatitis B surface antigen status, postexposure prophylaxis and, 3083-3084, 3084t
Hepatitis C, 1403, 1405, 1406, 1408f, 2050
  drugs for, 2036t
  in kidney transplant patient, 2855
  in organ transplant patient, 2848
  in pregnancy, 2775
  occupational exposure protocol for, 3083, 3084
Hepatitis D, 1404, 1405
Hepatitis E, 1403-1404, 2058
Hepatitis G, 1404
Hepatocellular carcinoma, 1417
Hepatomegaly, in hepatitis, 1404
Hepatorenal syndrome, in cirrhosis, 1411
Hepatosplenomegaly, in tricuspid stenosis and regurgitation, 1307
Herbal medicines, 2475-2477, 2476t
  allergic reactions to, 2477, 2477t
  contamination of, 2476-2477
  drug interactions with, 2477, 2478t
  misidentification of, 2475-2476
Hernia
  diaphragmatic
    neonatal resuscitation in, 121
    traumatic, in children, 340, 341
  hiatal, gastroesophageal reflux in, 1388
  inguinal, 1598, 2641-2642
  obturator, 1441
  small bowel obstruction related to, 1441
Herniation
  cerebral
    after head trauma, 354-356, 355f
    in cancer patient, 1918
  disk
    lumbar, 702-703, 704-705, 711-712
    magnetic resonance imaging in, 432, 433f
    radicular pain in, 264
  impending, in multiple trauma, 308
Herniation syndromes, in children, 335-336

Heroin
  during pregnancy, 2793-2794
  emergency department visits related to, 2884f
  pharmacology of, 2452
  respiratory effects of, 2452-2453, 2453t
  route of administration of, 2451-2452
  toxicity of, 2452-2453
  withdrawal from, 2452, 2455-2456
Herpes B virus, 2044-2045
Herpes simplex virus infection, 2040-2042
  Bell's palsy and, 1667
  corneal involvement in, 289, 290f, 295t, 1054, 1054f
  drugs for, 2036t
  genital, 1557-1559, 1557t, 1558f, 1559t, 1858
  in cancer patient with impaired cell-mediated immunity, 2840
  in encephalitis, 1712
  in esophagitis, 1387
  in HIV/AIDS, 2085
  in organ transplant patient, 2848
  in pharyngitis, 1110, 1112, 1114
  in pregnancy, 2758
  in sexually transmitted disease, 1518t, 1519
  skin lesions in, 1857-1858, 1858f
Herpes zoster, 2042-2043
  ophthalmic, 1054
  skin lesions in, 1859-1860, 1860f
Herpes zoster oticus, 1071, 1667
Herpesvirus, 2034t, 2040-2045. *See also specific type, e.g.,* Herpes simplex virus infection.
Herpesvirus simiae, 884, 888-889, 889b, 889t, 2044-2045
Herpetic whitlow, 616
Heterotopic ossification
  after tibial femoral knee dislocation, 790
  of femur and hip, 741-742, 743f-754f
Heterotopic pregnancy, 2743
Hexachlorophene, for wound cleansing, 848t
Hiatal hernia, gastroesophageal reflux in, 1388
Hickman-Broviac catheter, problems related to, 1361-1363, 1362b, 1362f, 1365f
Hidradenitis suppurativa, 1515-1516, 1843, 2204-2205
High altitude
  definition of, 2296
  oxygenation at, 2307, 2307f
High-altitude cerebral edema (HACE), 2305-2306, 2305b
  clinical presentation in, 2306, 2306f
  epidemiology of, 2296
  management of, 2306
  pathophysiology of, 2299-2300, 2299f
High-altitude illness, 2296-2309. *See also* Acute mountain sickness (AMS).
  acclimatization and, 2297-2298, 2297b, 2298f
  and underlying medical conditions, 2307-2309
  environmental considerations in, 2297
  epidemiology of, 2296
  headache in, 1642
  pathophysiology of, 2298-2300, 2299f, 2300f
High-altitude pulmonary edema (HAPE), 2303-2305, 2303b
  ancillary tests in, 2300f, 2303-2304
  clinical presentation in, 2303
  differential diagnosis in, 2304
  disposition in, 2305
  epidemiology of, 2296
  management of, 2304-2305, 2305f
  pathophysiology of, 2298-2299, 2299f, 2300f
  prevention of, 2305
  re-entry, 2303
High-altitude retinal hemorrhage, 2306-2307, 2307f
High-frequency flow interruption ventilation, in burn care, 922
High-frequency ventilation, 33
High-pressure injection injuries, to hand, 611-612
High-pressure irrigation, for wound cleansing, 848
High-velocity missiles
  abdominal injuries from, 491
  in youth violence, 1019
Hill-Sachs deformity, 688, 688f
  reverse, 691, 692f
Hilum, 527, 527f
Hindfoot
  anatomy of, 820, 820f
  calcaneal fracture of, 826-827, 826f, 827f

Hindfoot *(Continued)*
  pain in, 836-837
  subtalar dislocation of, 825-826, 825f
  talar dome of, osteochondral fracture of, 824-825, 825f
  talar fracture of, 822-824, 823f, 824f
  total talar dislocation of, 826
Hip
  anatomy of, 736-738, 736f-738f, 737t
  apophysitis of, 2711
  calcifying lesions of, 741-742, 743f-755f
  development of, 763, 763f
  developmental dysplasia of, 2701-2702, 2702b, 2702f
  examination of, in arthritis, 1779, 1779f
  immobilization of, 569-570, 570f
  neoplastic disease in, 742, 745f
  normal radiograph of, 746, 747f
  osteoarthritis of, 739, 739f-741f
Hip adductor strain, 761
Hip arthroplasty
  partial, 751, 752b
  total, 749-750, 750f
Hip dislocation, 756-759, 757f-759f
  arterial injury in, 761
  avascular necrosis after, 740
  pediatric, 763
  prosthetic, 749, 750f, 760
Hip pain
  atraumatic, differential diagnosis of, 756b
  pediatric, 2702-2709, 2703b
    in acute septic arthritis, 2704-2706, 2705t, 2706t
    in apophysitis of hip, 2711
    in Legg-Calvé-Perthes disease, 2706-2707, 2707f
    in slipped capital femoral epiphysis, 765-767, 765f, 766f, 2707-2709, 2708f
    in transient synovitis, 2703-2704
    limp from, 764-765
Hip prosthesis, dislocation of, 749, 750f, 760
Hip trauma, 735-768
  anatomy in, 736-738, 736f-738f, 737t
  clinical features of, 742-744
  diagnostic strategies in, 746, 747f, 748f
  epidemiology of, 735-736
  femoral and hip fractures in, 746-756
    arthroplasty for, 749-750, 750f
    avulsion type, 750, 750f
    compartment syndrome in, 749
    femoral shaft, 755
    greater or lesser trochanteric, 753, 753f
    history in, 742-743
    in elderly person, 347
    intertrochanteric, 752-753, 752f
    open fracture care in, 748-749, 749f
    pain management in, 749
    pathophysiology of, 739
    physical examination in, 743-744
    proximal femoral, 750-752, 750f-751f, 752b
    stress type, 755-756
    subtrochanteric, 753-755, 754f
    traction and immobilization in, 746, 748
    with minimal or no trauma, 755
  femoral head fracture-dislocation in, 759-760, 760f
  hip dislocation in, 756-759, 757f-759f
  hip prosthesis dislocation in, 749, 750f, 760
  management of, 746-750
  muscular injuries in, 761-762
  neurologic injuries in, 762-763
  pathophysiology of, 739-742, 739f-745f
  pediatric considerations in, 763-767, 763f, 765f-767f
  radiologic evaluation in, 746, 747f, 751f
  soft tissue injuries in, 761-763
  vascular injuries in, 762
HIPAA (Healthcare Insurance Portability and Accountability Act), 3103
Hirschsprung's disease, 2612-2613
Hirudin, in myocardial infarction, 1188
His bundle, 1202
Histamine
  in anaphylaxis/anaphylactoid reactions, 1823, 1823b, 2547, 2548
  in asthma, 1080f, 1081
Histamine receptor antagonists, for anaphylactic shock, 54

Histamine₁-receptor blockers
  anticholinergic toxicity of, 2346b
  for anaphylaxis, 2549
  overdose of, 2487-2488, 2488t
Histamine₂-receptor blockers
  for acute pancreatitis, 1434
  for anaphylaxis, 2549
  for gastroesophageal reflux, 1389, 1390t
  for upper gastrointestinal disorders, 1390t,
      1398-1399
Histoplasma capsulatum
  in cancer patient with impaired cell-mediated
      immunity, 2840
  in pneumonia, 1130
Histoplasma infection, of pericardium, 1286
Histrionic personality disorder, 1755, 2979b
HIV virion, 2073
HIV/AIDS, 2056, 2071-2093
  acalculous cholecystitis in, 1421
  anorectal disorders in, 1520, 1520b, 2084
  antibiotic prophylaxis in, 2089
  antiretroviral therapy for, 2039, 2087-2089, 2087t
  bone or joint infections in, 2179
  cardiovascular disease in, 2086
  case definition of, 2071, 2072b
  central nervous system lymphoma in, 2082
  cholangiopathy in, 1423
  classification and staging of, 2075
  complications of, 2076-2087, 2076t, 2078b,
      2079t
  Cryptococcus neoformans in, 2081
  dementia in, 1658, 1659
  diarrhea in, 1482-1484, 1482t, 1483b, 1485t,
      2084
  disposition in, 2089, 2090b
  drug reactions in, 2079t, 2087
  drugs for, 2036t-2037t, 2039
  encephalopathy in, 2081
  enteropathy in, 1482
  epidemiology of, 2071-2073, 2072b, 2072f
  esophageal disorders in, 2083-2084
  ethical issues in, 2089-2090
  gastrointestinal disorders in, 2082-2084
  headache in, 1641
  hematologic disorders in, 2087
  historical background of, 2071
  immunization in, 2089
  in pregnancy, 2764t, 2774, 2810
  initial evaluation in, 2075
  intussusception in, 1441-1442
  liver disorders in, 2084
  Mycobacterium tuberculosis in, 1136, 1140-
      1141, 2078-2079
  myelopathy in, 1683
  myocarditis in, 1292
  neurologic disorders in, 2079-2082, 2080f
  neuropathy in, 1692, 2082
  nonoccupational exposure protocol for, 2092
  occupational exposure protocol for, 2091-2092,
      3083, 3084-3087, 3085t, 3086b
  ophthalmologic conditions in, 2085-2086
  oropharyngeal disorders in, 2083
  pancreatitis in, 1428
  parasitic co-infections in, 2114
  pediatric fever in, 2516
  pericardial disease in, 1287
  pneumonia in, 1135-1136, 1136f, 1138-1139,
      1140-1141, 2077-2078
  point-of-care testing for, 2074-2075, 2810
  primary HIV infection in, 2075
  progression of, predictors of, 2076
  progressive multifocal leukoencephalopathy in,
      2082
  psychiatric considerations in, 2086-2087
  pulmonary disease in, 2076-2079, 2076t
  renal disorders in, 2086
  rhabdomyolysis in, 1979
  sexually transmitted disease in, 2087
  skin disorders in, 2084-2085
  skin lesions in, 1861f, 1862t
  suicide in, 1770
  systemic symptoms of, 2076, 2078b
  tests for, 990, 2073-2075, 2810, 3087
  Toxoplasma gondii infection in, 2081-2082,
      2082f
  transmission of, 2073
    during labor and delivery, 2810
    in human bites, 891
    in sexual assault, 990, 990b

HIV/AIDS *(Continued)*
  tuberculosis in, 1136, 1140-1141, 2078-2079,
      2149, 2153-2154, 2166
  tuberculosis meningitis in, 2082
  with hepatitis C infection, 1403
HIV-associated nephropathy (HIVAN), 2086
Hives, 1834, 1834f, 1835
  drug-induced, 1844-1845, 1844f, 1846t-1847t
  skin lesions in, 1847-1848, 1848f
  transfusion-related, 60
HMG CoA reductase inhibitors, rhabdomyolysis
      from, 1979
HMPAO scan, in osteomyelitis, 2181
Hoarseness
  in airway foreign body aspiration, 866
  in neck masses, 1076
  in viral croup, 2525
Hodgkin's lymphoma, radiation-induced
      pericarditis in, 1284
Hohl's classification of tibial plateau fractures,
      778f, 779
Holiday heart syndrome, 1230-1231
Holly plant, 2474
Homan's sign, in deep venous thrombosis, 1369
Home monitoring for apparent life-threatening
      event or SIDS, 2720
Homeland Security, 3018
Homicide
  intimate partner, 995-996
  youth, 1017, 1019
Honey, infant botulism from, 2013
Honeybee stings. *See* Hymenoptera stings.
Hookworm infection, 2101t, 2107
Hordeolum, 293t, 1054
Horizontal mattress suture, 850
  half-buried, 851
Horner's syndrome, 416, 420, 1061-1062
Hornet stings. *See* Hymenoptera stings.
Horse serum–derived antivenin, 901
Horseshoe abscess, 1515
Hospice care, 3143, 3145
Hospital property, screening requirements related
      to, 3157-3158
Hospitalization
  direct, medicolegal issues in, 3159
  for alcohol-related problems, 2879-2880
  for burn injury, 927, 927b
  for chronic obstructive pulmonary disease,
      1106t
  for croup, 2527, 2527b
  for hemophilia A, 1902
  for nonemergent anemia, 1870b
  for pelvic inflammatory disease, 1571
  for pneumonia, 1138, 1140
  for seizure, 2674
  for suicide attempt, 1773
  for systemic lupus erythematosus, 1811-1812
  for tuberculosis, 2169
  for urolithiasis, 1592-1593, 1593b
  in disposition requirements, 3164
  of febrile, neutropenic cancer patient, 2839
Hospitals
  critical operational substrates for, 3012b
  disaster response experience in, 3016-3017
  disaster response plan for, 3015-3016
  EMS programs based in, 2985
Host defenses, against pneumonia, 1128-1129
Hot tar burns, 926-927
Housemaid's knee, 795
Human bite, 890-892, 891t, 892b
  antibiotic prophylaxis in, 891-892
  antiviral prophylaxis in, 891
  in child abuse, 969
  in clenched-fist injuries, 611
  in extensor tendon injuries, at
      metacarpophalangeal joint, 608
  in sexual assault, 986b
  infected, treatment of, 892, 892b
  tetanus prophylaxis in, 891, 891t
  to penis, 534
Human chorionic gonadotropin assays
  in ectopic pregnancy, 2744, 2745
  in pregnancy, 2728-2730, 2729f, 2741, 2741t
  in vaginal bleeding, 256-257, 256t
Human granulocytic ehrlichiosis, 2137-2138
Human herpesvirus-3. *See* Herpes zoster;
      Varicella-zoster virus.
Human herpesvirus-4. *See* Epstein-Barr virus.
Human herpesvirus-5. *See* Cytomegalovirus.

Human herpesvirus-6, 2044
Human herpesvirus-7, 2044
Human herpesvirus-8. *See* Kaposi's sarcoma.
Human immunodeficiency virus infection. *See*
      HIV/AIDS.
Human monocytic ehrlichiosis, 2137-2138
Human papillomavirus infection, 2034t, 2045
  drugs for, 2037t
  genital warts from, 1518t, 1519-1520
  in condylomata acuminata, 1563-1564, 1564f
  in HIV/AIDS, 2085
Human T-cell leukemia virus type 1, 2056
Hume fracture, 550t
Humeral head
  anatomy of, 647
  compression fracture of, 688, 688f
  impaction fracture of, 691, 692f
  manipulation of, in reduction of glenohumeral
      joint dislocation, 689, 689f
Humeral trauma, 647-668
  anatomy in, 647-649, 647f, 648f, 672, 673f
  biceps tendon rupture in, 668
  clinical features of, 649-650, 649f, 650f
  elbow dislocation in, 664-666, 664f, 665f
  epicondylitis in, 667, 1798-1799, 2710-2711
  fractures in, 652-664
    articular surface, 661-664, 661f-663f
    distal, 655-661, 656f-661f
    proximal, 680-682, 681f, 682f
    proximal epiphyseal, 682-683, 683f
    shaft, 652-655, 653f, 654f
    supracondylar, 2693-2697, 2694f-2696f,
        2694t
  management of, 652
  olecranon bursitis in, 667, 1801-1803
  radial head subluxation in, 666, 666f, 2697-
      2698, 2697f
  radiography in, 641f, 650-652, 651f
  soft tissue injuries in, 667-668
Humerus, immobilization of, 569
Humidity, evaporative heat loss and, 2255
Humoral immunity, 2832
  defects in, in cancer patient, 2840-2841
Hunter serotonin toxicity criteria, 2359b
"Hunting response," 2228
Huntington's disease, 1747
Hutchinson's fracture, 636, 636f
Hutchinson's sign, in ophthalmic herpes zoster,
      1054
Hyaline casts, in urinary sediment, 1526, 1526f
Hydatid cyst, 2102t, 2105-2106, 2106f, 2111,
      2113
Hydatidiform mole, 2746-2747
Hydralazine, 1321t
  during pregnancy and lactation, 2765t, 2788-
      2789
  for hypertension of pregnancy, 1317
  for hypertensive emergencies, 1318, 2653,
      2765t
Hydrazine, overdose of, antidotes to, 2329t
Hydrocarbons
  abuse of, 2886-2889, 2887t, 2888f, 2889b
  chlorinated, poisoning from, 2462-2463, 2462b
  dermal exposure to, 936-937, 2430, 2431
  for tar removal, 927
  poisoning from, 2428-2432, 2429t, 2430f, 2431f
Hydrocele
  acute, 1598
  in children, 2641
Hydrochlorothiazide, 1321t
  during pregnancy and lactation, 2788
  for hypertension, 1320
Hydrocodone, 2453t, 2920, 2921t, 2925
Hydrocortisone
  for adrenal insufficiency, 1998
  for anaphylactic shock, 54
  for asthma, 1088
  for diaper dermatitis, 1852
  for hypercalcemia, 1946
  for myxedema coma, 1994
  for sepsis, 2222
  for septic shock, 54
  for thyroid storm, 1989
  in hypothermia, 2246
Hydrofluoric acid
  antidotes to, 2329t
  dermal exposure to, 933-934, 2384
  hypocalcemia from, 1943
  ingestion of, 934, 2380, 2381t, 2383

Hydrogen peroxide
   for acute necrotic ulcerative gingivitis, 1033
   for wound cleansing, 848t
   ingestion of, 2384
Hydrogen sulfide poisoning, antidotes to, 2329t
Hydroids, stinging, 909
Hydromorphone, 2453t, 2920, 2921t, 2923-2924
Hydronephrosis, in urolithiasis, 1589, 1589f,
   1590f
Hydrophobia, in rabies, 2065
Hydrotherapy
   in acid and alkali burns, 932, 933
   whirlpool, for frostbite, 2234
Hydroxyamphetamine, in Horner's syndrome,
   1062
Hydroxychloroquine, for systemic lupus
   erythematosus, 1809
Hydroxyurea, for sickle cell disease, 1881
Hydroxyzine, 2446t
   adjuvant, with opioids, 2921
   for urticaria, 1848
Hymenal trauma, in sexual assault, 987
Hymenolepsis nana, 2102t
Hymenoptera stings, 903-905
   allergy to, 1827, 2547
   rhabdomyolysis from, 1979
Hyoscyamine, anticholinergic toxicity of, 2345
Hyperabduction syndrome, thoracic outlet
   syndrome in, 1359
Hyperaldosteronism
   hypokalemia in, 1938
   in hypertension, 1311
   metabolic alkalosis in, 1930
Hyperammonemia, in hepatic encephalopathy,
   1411
Hyperamylasemia, in hypothermia, 2243
Hyperbaric oxygen therapy
   for carbon monoxide poisoning, 2439-2440
   for frostbite, 2233
   for high-altitude cerebral edema, 2306
   for high-altitude pulmonary edema, 2304,
      2305f
   for myonecrosis, 2209
   for nitrite abuse, 2891
   for peripheral arteriovascular disease, 1350
   for scuba diving–related disorders, 2288-2292,
      2288b, 2289f-2291f
   for simultaneous carbon monoxide and
      cyanide poisoning, 2440-2441
Hyperbilirubinemia
   in hepatitis, 1404
   in pyogenic abscess, 1415
   pediatric, 2601-2603, 2602t, 2603b, 2603t,
      2604f-2605f
Hypercalcemia, 1944-1947
   causes of, 1944-1945, 1944b
   clinical features of, 1945-1946, 1945b
   dialysis for, 1548
   in adrenal insufficiency, 1997
   in cancer patient, 1914-1916, 1915b
   in hyperthyroidism, 1988
   in hypothyroidism, 1993
   in rhabdomyolysis, 1981
   management of, 1946-1947, 1946b
   nonneoplastic, 1914, 1914b, 1915, 1915f
Hypercapnia, permissive
   for chronic obstructive pulmonary disease,
      1104
   for critically ill asthmatic patient, 1092
Hypercarbia, in scuba diving–related disorders,
   2283
Hyperchloremia, in respiratory alkalosis, 1926
Hyperemesis gravidarum, 204t, 206, 2756
Hyperemia zone, in burn injury, 917, 917f
Hyperglycemia
   after cerebral ischemia, 70
   in alcoholism, 2871
   in hyperthyroidism, 1988
   in hypothermia, 2243
   in pancreatitis, 1429-1430
   in peritoneal dialysis patient, 1554
   new-onset, 1973
   seizure in, 1622
Hyperglycemic hyperosmolar nonketotic coma,
   in diabetes mellitus, 1968-1970, 1968b,
      1969b
Hyperhidrosis, in frostbite, 2234
Hyperinfection syndrome, in organ transplant
   patient, 2849

Hyperkalemia, 1939-1941
   cardiac arrest in, 77
   causes of, 1939-1940, 1940b
   dialysis for, 1548
   from succinylcholine, 14, 14t
   in acute renal failure, 1539, 2650
   in acute tumor lysis syndrome, 1911
   in adrenal insufficiency, 1997
   in chronic renal failure, 1545-1546, 1545t
   in crush injury, 3007
   in digitalis toxicity, 2370
   in familial periodic paralysis, 1709
   in hemodialysis patient, 1551
   in hemolytic uremic syndrome, 2655
   in hypothermia, 2243
   in rhabdomyolysis, 1981
   management of, 1940-1941
Hyperlipidemia, in nephrotic syndrome, 1531,
   2648
Hypermagnesemia, 1949-1950, 1949b
   dialysis for, 1548-1549
   in acute renal failure, 1539
Hypernatremia, 1935-1937
   causes of, 1935-1936, 1936b
   clinical features of, 1936
   euvolemic, 1936
   hypervolemic, 1936
   hypovolemic, 1936, 2629t, 2632, 2634b
   management of, 1936-1937
   seizure in, 1622, 2669
Hyperoxia test of cardiac vs. pulmonary
   cyanosis, 2572
Hyperparathyroidism
   hypercalcemia in, 1915, 1944
   hypertension in, 1313
Hyperphosphatemia, 1952-1953, 1953b
   hypocalcemia in, 1943
   in acute renal failure, 1539
   in acute tumor lysis syndrome, 1911
   in hemolytic uremic syndrome, 2655
   in rhabdomyolysis, 1981
Hyperpigmentation, mucocutaneous, in
   Addison's disease, 1997
Hyperpnea, 176
   in tetralogy of Fallot, 2581
Hyperpyrexia, pediatric fever and, 2506
Hypersensitivity reactions. See also Anaphylaxis.
   at insulin injection sites, 1971
   cytotoxic, 1821
   delayed, 1821-1822
   immediate, 1821
   immune complex, 1821
   in tuberculosis, 2148
Hypersensitivity vasculitis, 1815-1817
   Churg-Strauss syndrome as, 1816
   erythema nodosum as, 1816-1817
   Goodpasture syndrome as, 1816
   Henoch-Schönlein purpura as, 1815, 2615,
      2615f
   mixed cryoglobulinemia as, 1815
   panniculitis as, 1817
   serum sickness as, 1815-1816
Hypersplenism, hemolytic anemia in, 1884
Hypertension, 1310-1322
   altitude and, 2308
   arterial disease in, 1312-1313
   chronic, in pregnancy, 2762, 2763t, 2765t
   definition of, 1310
   determination of, 1310-1311
   diastolic vs. systolic, 1310
   essential, 1311
   fibrinolytic therapy eligibility and, 1191
   gestational, 2749-2751, 2750b
   headache in, 1641
   heart failure in, 1267-1268
   in amphetamine abuse, 2895
   in aortic dissection, 1317
   in aortic rupture, 478
   in chronic renal failure, 1316-1317
   in glucocorticoid excess, 1313
   in intracranial hemorrhage, 1316
   in MAOI toxicity, 2365
   in myocardial ischemia, 1316
   in pheochromocytoma, 1313
   in pregnancy, 1317, 2727, 2765t
   in pulmonary edema, 1316
   in sleep apnea, 1313
   in spinal cord injury, 2906
   in stroke syndromes, 1315-1316

Hypertension (Continued)
   in systemic lupus erythematosus, 1807
   in thyroid and parathyroid disease, 1313
   intracranial
      after head trauma, 353-354, 367
      headache and, 174t, 2677-2678
      idiopathic, 1639-1640, 1640b
      in developmentally disabled patient, 2899
      in high-altitude cerebral edema, 2306
      in pediatric patient, 334, 334b
      intubation and, 17, 18t
      risk factors for, 171b
      treatment of, 360, 367
   lower extremity ulcers in, 1351
   malignant, 1315
      acute renal failure in, 1535
      dialysis for, 1548
   mild or transient, 1320, 1322
   ocular, 1055
   pathophysiology of, 1311-1314
   pediatric, 2651-2653, 2651b, 2651t, 2652b,
      2653t
   pulmonary
      altitude and, 2308
      from high altitude exposure, 2298-2299
      in pregnancy, 2762, 2766
   renal disease in, 1311-1312
   renin-angiotensin-aldosterone system in, 1311,
      1312f
   renovascular, 526-527, 1311
   venous
      from arteriovenous fistula or graft, 1366
      in superior vena cava syndrome, 1910
Hypertensive emergencies
   clinical presentation in, 1314-1317, 1314b
   in cocaine overdose, 2388, 2390
   in PCP intoxication, 2893
   in pregnancy, 2762, 2763t, 2765t
   management of, 1317-1319, 1317t
   pediatric, 2652, 2653, 2653t
Hypertensive encephalopathy, 1314-1315
   headache in, 1641
   pediatric, 2650, 2652
   seizure in, 1622
Hypertensive hemorrhage, 1608-1609, 1608b
Hypertensive urgency
   clinical presentation and management of, 1319-
      1322, 1320t, 1321t-1322t
   pediatric, 2651, 2652-2653
Hyperthermia. See also Heat illness.
   after brain resuscitation, 68
   delirium in, 1648
   fever vs., 2258
   in amphetamine abuse, 2894, 2896
   in anticholinergic poisoning, 2348, 2349
   in cocaine overdose, 2388, 2389-2390, 2390b
   in cyclic antidepressant poisoning, 2354t, 2356
   in PCP intoxication, 2414-2415, 2416, 2892
   in psychostimulant overdose, 2408, 2410-2411
   in substituted phenol poisoning, 2464
   malignant, 14, 2257
   succinylcholine-induced, 14
Hyperthyroidism, 1985-1989
   anxiety in, 1747
   apathetic, 1986, 1988, 1988t
   clinical features of, 1986-1987, 1987b
   diagnosis of, 1987-1988
   differential considerations in, 1988, 1988t
   etiology of, 1985-1986, 1986b
   factitious, 1986
   heart failure in, 1268
   hypertension in, 1313
   in pregnancy, 2764t, 2772-2773
   in thyrotoxic periodic paralysis, 1709
   management of, 1988, 1989, 1989t
   skin lesions in, 1862t
Hypertonic saline
   for elevated intracranial pressure, 360
   for multiple trauma patient, 307
   for seizure in acute renal failure, 2650
Hypertriglyceridemia
   in alcoholism, 2871
   in diabetic ketoacidosis, 1964
   in pancreatitis, 1428
Hypertrophic cardiomyopathy, 1294-1296
   heart failure in, 1264
   sudden death in, 1298, 2597-2598
Hypertrophic pyloric stenosis, in infants and
   children, 2603-2606, 2605f, 2606t

Hyperuricemia
in acute renal failure, 1539-1540
in acute tumor lysis syndrome, 1911, 1912
in alcoholism, 2871
in cancer patient, 1913-1914
in rhabdomyolysis, 1981
Hyperventilation, 176
for cerebral herniation, 1918
for elevated intracranial pressure, 360, 367
for intracerebral hemorrhage, 1616
for scuba diving–related disorders, 2292
functional vs. organic, 1749
hypophosphatemia from, 1951
in chronic obstructive pulmonary disease, 1100
in cyclic antidepressant poisoning, 2356
Hyperventilation syndrome, 2668
Hyperventilation tetany, heat cramps vs., 2258
Hyperviscosity
cyanosis in, 273
in cancer patient, 1912-1913
in polycythemia, 1884
Hypervitaminosis A, fracture in, 2701
Hypervolemia
dyspnea in, 179t
hypernatremic, 1936
hyponatremic, 1934, 1935
in acute renal failure, 1540
in polycythemia, 1884
Hyphema
red and painful eye in, 290, 296t
traumatic, 1048-1049, 1048f
Hypnosis
for anxiety disorders, 1751
for pain management, 2934
Hypnotic, 2914b. See also Sedative hypnotics.
Hypoalbuminemia
in nephrotic syndrome, 2648
in rhabdomyolysis, 1981
pediatric, 2646
Hypobaria, in acute mountain sickness, 2300
Hypobaric hypoxia, 2297, 2298-2299, 2299f
Hypocalcemia, 1942-1944
alcohol-induced, 2871, 2872t
causes of, 1942-1943, 1942b
clinical features of, 1943, 1943b
in acute renal failure, 1539
in acute tumor lysis syndrome, 1911
in ethylene glycol poisoning, 2400
in hydrofluoric acid poisoning, 934
in pancreatitis, 1430
in rhabdomyolysis, 1976-1977, 1977f, 1981
management of, 1943-1944
seizure in, 1622, 2669
Hypocapnia, neurologic effects of, 351, 351f
Hypocarbia, ventilation-induced, 351, 351f
Hypochondriasis, 1755-1756
Hypogammaglobulinemia, in cancer patient, 2840-2841
Hypoglossal nerve, 1665t
Hypoglycemia
alcohol-induced, 2860, 2871
clinical features of, 1960-1961
confusion and, 150
diagnosis of, 1961
fasting, 1961-1962
hyperthyroidism vs., 1988
hypothermia and, 2239
in adrenal insufficiency, 1997, 1998
in alcoholic hepatitis, 1409
in chronic pancreatitis, 1435
in diabetes mellitus, 1960-1961, 1960b, 1961b
in hypothermia, 2243
in hypothyroidism, 1993, 1994
in neonates, 119
in nondiabetic patient, 1961-1962, 1962b
in opioid overdose, 2454
in overdosed/poisoned patient, 2326
in pregnancy, 1972
management of, 1961, 1961b
postprandial, 1961
seizure in, 166, 1622, 2669
unawareness of, 1960
vertigo in, 148t
Hypoglycemic agents, oral, 1972-1973
alcohol interactions with, 2877
overdose of, hypoglycemia from, 1961
rash from, 1972

Hypogonadism, male, in alcoholism, 2871
Hypokalemia, 1937-1939
alcohol-induced, 2871, 2872t
causes of, 1937-1938, 1938b
clinical features of, 1938-1939
hypomagnesemia in, 1947
in digitalis toxicity, 2370
in familial periodic paralysis, 1709
in hypercalcemic cancer patient, 1915-1916
in hypothermia, 2243
in respiratory alkalosis, 1926
management of, 1939
metabolic alkalosis in, 1930
rhabdomyolysis in, 1979
vomiting-induced, 201
Hypomagnesemia, 1947-1949
alcohol-induced, 2871, 2872t
causes of, 1947-1948, 1948b
clinical features of, 1948-1949
in digitalis toxicity, 2371
management of, 1949
seizure in, 1622, 2669
Hypomanic episode, 1738
Hyponatremia, 1933-1935
alcohol-induced, 2871, 2872t
causes of, 1933-1934, 1934b
clinical features of, 1934
diagnosis of, 1934
euvolemic, 1934, 1935
hypervolemic, 1934, 1935
hypovolemic, 1933-1934, 1935, 2629t, 2631-2632, 2633b
in adrenal insufficiency, 1997
in hypothyroidism, 1993, 1994
in nephrotic syndrome, 2648
management of, 1935
MDMA-induced, 2408
rhabdomyolysis in, 1979-1980
seizure in, 1622, 2669
Hyponychium, 589
Hypoparathyroidism
anxiety in, 1747
hypocalcemia in, 1942
seizure in, 1622
Hypophosphatemia, 1951-1952, 1951b, 1952b
alcohol-induced, 2871-2872, 2872t
rhabdomyolysis in, 1979
Hypotension
acute pulmonary edema with, 1273-1274
after brain resuscitation, 68
after head trauma, 353
fibrinolytic therapy eligibility and, 1191
from propofol, 2947
gastritis in, 1391
hypovolemic, 360, 367
in abdominal aortic aneurysm rupture, 1333
in adrenal insufficiency, 1997
in barbiturate overdose, 2482
in beta blocker overdose, 2374-2375
in cardiac tamponade, 473
in cyclic antidepressant poisoning, 2352, 2354-2356
in head trauma, 359-360, 370
in heatstroke, 2264, 2265f
in hemodialysis patient, 1550-1551, 1550b
in hip trauma, 743-744
in hypothyroidism, 1994
in isopropyl alcohol poisoning, 2403
in MAOI toxicity, 2365
in opioid overdose, 2453
in pregnancy, 316, 2725
in pulmonary embolism, 1372
in shock, 45
neurogenic, secondary to spinal shock, 437
orthostatic
from antipsychotic agents, 1732
in spinal cord injury, 2906
Hypotensive resuscitation, in peripheral vascular injury, 543
Hypotensive shock, in anaphylaxis, 2548
Hypothalamic-pituitary-adrenal axis
in mood disorders, 1735-1736
in sepsis, 2214
suppression of, adrenal insufficiency from, 1994-1995
Hypothalamus, in temperature regulation, 134
Hypothenar hammer syndrome, 1355
Hypothenar mass or eminence, 576, 577f
Hypothenar muscles, 580-581, 581f

Hypothermia
accidental, 2236-2252
advanced life support in, 2245-2246
cardiovascular agents for, 2246
clinical features of, 2241-2242, 2242b
diagnostic strategies in, 2242-2244
disposition in, 2251
dysrhythmia in, 2237-2238, 2246
laboratory evaluation of, 2242-2244, 2243f
management of, 2244-2251
outcome of, 2251
pathophysiology of, 2237-2239, 2238f, 2239t
predisposing factors in, 2239-2241, 2240b
rewarming techniques in, 2247-2251, 2247b, 2250b
septicemia following, 2247
volume resuscitation in, 2245
alcohol consumption and, 2874-2875
cardiac arrest from, 78
definition of, 2236
delirium in, 1648
in barbiturate overdose, 2482
in hypothyroidism, 1992, 1994
in neonates, 119
in opioid overdose, 2454
in submersion injuries, 2312, 2314
in urban search and rescue, 3008
oxygenation considerations during, 2249, 2249t
physiology of cold exposure and, 2236-2237, 2237f
resuscitative, 85-86
mild, 68-70, 69t
profound and selective, 70
rhabdomyolysis in, 1979
zones of, 2239t
Hypothermic coagulation, 2243-2244
Hypothesis testing, 3051-3058, 3051t, 3057f
Hypothetico-deductive process, clinical decision making by, 127, 127f, 131t, 132
Hypothyroidism, 1990-1994
causes of, 1990, 1990b
clinical features of, 1990-1992, 1991b, 1991t
congenital, 2773
diagnosis of, 1992-1993
differential considerations in, 1993
heart failure in, 1268
hypertension in, 1313
in lithium toxicity, 2443
in pregnancy, 2773
management of, 1993-1994
seizure in, 1622
skin lesions in, 1862t, 1863f
Hypotonic diuresis, in hyperglycemic hyperosmolar nonketotic coma, 1968
Hypoventilation
controlled
for chronic obstructive pulmonary disease, 1104
for critically ill asthmatic patient, 1092
in hypothyroidism, 1994
in pediatric cervical spine injury, 338
Hypovolemia. See also Dehydration.
differential diagnosis in, 2629, 2629t
from vomiting, 201
gastritis in, 1391
hypernatremic, 1936, 2629t, 2632, 2634b
hyponatremic, 1933-1934, 1935, 2629t, 2631-2632, 2633b
in acute renal failure, 1540, 2650
in adrenal insufficiency, 1997, 1998
in burn injury, 917
in chronic renal failure, 1543
in crush injury, 3007
in ectopic pregnancy, 2745
in gastrointestinal bleeding, 222-223
in hypercalcemia, 1945
in hyperglycemic hyperosmolar nonketotic coma, 1968
in septic shock, 46-47
isonatremic, 2629t, 2631, 2632b
Hypovolemic hypotension, in head trauma, 360, 367
Hypovolemic shock
in cardiac tamponade, 473
in diabetic ketoacidosis, 1966
mechanical ventilation in, 32
Hypoxemia
acute, differential diagnosis in, 1101-1103
confusion and, 150

Hypoxemia *(Continued)*
  from high altitude exposure, 2298-2299, 2299f
  in chronic obstructive pulmonary disease,
    1100, 1104-1105
  in pulmonary embolism, 1372
Hypoxia
  after brain resuscitation, 68
  after head trauma, 353
  during air medical transport, 2994-2995
  hypobaric, 2297, 2298-2299, 2299f
  in cyanide poisoning, 2436
  in neonates, 119
  in simple asphyxiant inhalation, 2433
  neurologic effects of, 351-352
  rhabdomyolysis in, 1979
Hypoxic (tet) spells, in tetralogy of Fallot, 2580-
    2581, 2580f, 2581b
Hypoxic ventilatory response, during
    acclimatization to high altitude, 2297-2298
Hypsarrhythmia, infantile spasms with, 2665-
    2666
Hysterectomy, for postpartum hemorrhage, 2819
Hysterical conversion reactions, visual loss in,
    1060-1061
Hysterical neurosis, conversion type, 1755,
    1755b

Iatrogenic injury
  abdominal trauma as, 492
  esophageal perforation as, 482-483
  peripheral vascular, 536-537
Ibotenic acid, 2479
Ibuprofen, 2927
  for back pain, 710
  for migraine, 2680
  in frostbite, 2232
  in HIV/AIDS, side effects of, 2079t
  overdose of, 2343
Ibutilide, 1209-1210
  for atrial fibrillation, 1232b, 1233
Ice packs
  for dysrhythmias, 1214-1215
  for heatstroke, 2264
  for supraventricular tachycardia, 2588
Ice test, in myasthenia gravis, 1705-1706
Ice therapy. *See* Cryotherapy.
Ichthyosis, acquired, internal malignancy
    associated with, 1864
Icterus gravidarum, 2726
Idiojunctional escape rhythms, 1216, 1218
Ileocecitis, in *Yersinia enterocolitica*
    gastroenteritis, 1465
Ileocolic intussusception, 2611
Ileoileal intussusception, 2611
Ileus
  adynamic, 1440, 1441b, 1443
  gallstone, small bowel obstruction in, 1441
  segmental, 1440
Ilex, 2474
Iliac artery and vein injury, 546
Iliac wing fracture, 724
Iliopsoas bursitis, 1803
Iliopsoas strain, 761
Iliotibial band syndrome, 793-794
Ilium, 717, 718f
Imidazole, for tinea versicolor, 1840
Imipenem, for febrile, neutropenic cancer
    patient, 2838t
Imipramine
  for neuropathic pain, 1692
  metabolism of, 2352
Imiquimod, for condylomata acuminata, 1564
Immersion burn, 916
  in child abuse, 969-970, 970f, 970t
  in physical assault, 963, 964f
Immersion foot, 2228, 2230-2231
Immersion syndrome, 2311-2312
Immersion therapy
  for heatstroke, 2264
  for rewarming, 2232, 2248
Immobilization
  casts for, 571-573, 573f. *See also* Cast
    immobilization.
  complications of, 563, 564b
  in acromioclavicular joint dislocations, 686
  in ankle sprain, 817
  in anterior glenohumeral joint dislocation, 690

Immobilization *(Continued)*
  in biceps tendon rupture, 697
  in bicipital tenosynovitis, 697
  in clavicle fracture, 677, 678f
  in condylar fracture, 660-661
  in epiphyseal hand fracture, 600
  in extension supracondylar fracture, 655-656
  in femoral and hip fractures, 746, 748
  in flexion supracondylar fracture, 659
  in humeral shaft fracture, 654-655, 654f
  in knee extensor tendon injuries, 783
  in knee ligament injuries, 792
  in mallet finger, 606, 606f
  in metacarpal or phalangeal fracture, 595, 595f,
    596f
  in metatarsal base fracture, 833
  in olecranon fracture, 663
  in Osgood-Schlatter disease, 799
  in patellar dislocation, 786
  in posterior elbow dislocation, 665
  in proximal fibular fracture, 802
  in proximal humeral epiphyseal fracture, 683
  in proximal humeral fracture, 682
  in proximal tibial epiphyseal injuries, 781
  in proximal tibiofibular joint dislocation, 803
  in rotator cuff tear, 696
  in scapula fracture, 680
  in snakebite management, 899
  in sprain, 566
  in sternoclavicular joint dislocation, 684
  in tibial femoral knee dislocation, 789
  in tibial shaft fracture, 800
  in ulnar shaft fracture, 642
  in wound management, 855
  splinting and bandaging for, 568-571, 569f,
    570f, 572f, 573f. *See also* Splint
    immobilization.
Immune complex hypersensitivity reactions, 1821
Immune complexes
  in Henoch-Schönlein purpura, 1815
  in vasculitis, 1812-1813
Immune complex–mediated agents, in
    anaphylaxis, 1827
Immune response
  acute-phase, 2831-2832
  adaptive, 2832-2834
  in asthma, 1080-1081, 1080f
  in bone or joint infection, 2176
  in Kawasaki disease, 2025
  in systemic lupus erythematosus, 1806, 1808
  in tuberculosis, 2148
  non–microbe-specific, 2831-2832
  pneumonia and, 1129
  reticuloendothelial system in, 2832
Immune system
  characteristics of, 1821
  development of, 1820-1821, 1820f
  in elderly person, 2826
  in pregnancy, 2724-2725
  physical barriers in, 2831
    disruption of, in cancer patient, 2841
  suppression of. *See* Immunocompromised
    patient.
Immune thrombocytopenia, 1896-1897
Immune-mediated transfusion reactions, 59-60
Immunization. *See also* Vaccine.
  during pregnancy, 2736
  for viral infection, 2033-2034, 2035t
  in bronchopulmonary dysplasia, 2565
  in elderly person, 2829
  in HIV/AIDS, 2089
Immunocompromised patient, 2831-2844, 2832t
  adaptive immunity in, 2832-2834
  alcoholism and, 2841-2842
  antibiotic prophylaxis in, 854
  cancer and, 2834-2841, 2836t, 2838t
  delirium in, 1649
  diabetes mellitus and, 2841
  immunosuppressive therapy in, 2843-2844
  infection in, 2834-2843, 2835t
  non–microbe-specific immunity in, 2831-2832
  organ transplantation and. *See* Organ
    transplant patient.
  pneumonia in, 1132, 2560, 2841
  renal failure and, 2842
  respiratory tract infection in, 2841
  reticuloendothelial system in, 2832
  splenectomy and functional asplenia and,
    2842-2843

Immunoglobulin(s)
  anaphylactic-type reactions to, 1827
  classes of, 1821, 2832
  structure of, 1821, 1821f
Immunoglobulin A, 2832
Immunoglobulin E, 2832
  in anaphylactic shock, 47
  in anaphylaxis, 2547
  in asthma, 1080, 1080f
Immunoglobulin E antibodies, 1819
Immunoglobulin E–mediated anaphylaxis
  agents associated with, 1826-1827
  signal transduction system in, 1822-1823,
    1822f
Immunoglobulin G, 2832
Immunoglobulin M, 2832
Immunoglobulin preparations
  for hepatitis B postexposure prophylaxis, 1406,
    3083-3084, 3084t
  for Kawasaki disease, 2027, 2596
  for measles, 1849
  for myasthenia gravis, 1707
  for myocarditis, 1290
  for rabies, 2068, 2068b
  for tetanus, 856, 857t, 2011
  for toxic shock syndrome, 2030-2031, 2201
  for varicella, 1859
  Rh (anti-D), in pregnancy, 2742, 2752
Immunomodulatory therapy, for myasthenia
    gravis, 1707
Immunopathology, 1819, 1821-1822
Immunoprophylaxis, for hepatitis, 1406,
    1407t
Immunosenescence, 2826
Immunosuppressive therapy
  agents used in, 2843-2844
  for diabetes mellitus, 1973
  for myasthenia gravis, 1706
  for myocarditis, 1290
  for organ transplant patient, 2849-2851, 2850t
  for systemic lupus erythematosus, 1809
Impact seizure, 334
  in children, 367
  in head trauma, 2669
Impaction fracture, 553, 555f
Impairment, disability vs., 3078
Impalement, in facial trauma, 386, 387f
Impartiality Test, in ethical case analysis, 3131-
    3132
Impetigo, 1842-1843, 2201-2202
Impingement, nerve root, 702-703
Impingement syndrome of shoulder, 693-696,
    694t, 695f, 1796-1797
Impingement test, 694, 695f
Implantable cardiac devices, 1246-1257. *See also*
    Pacemaker(s).
Implantable cardioverter-defibrillator, 1255-1257
  advanced life support in patient with, 1256-
    1257
  complications of, 1256
  disposition in, 1257
  for chronic heart failure, 1277
  indications for, 1246-1247, 1247b
  malfunction of, 1256, 1256b, 1257b
  terminology and components in, 1255-1256
Implements in situ, in abdominal stab wound,
    504, 505
Implied consent, of combative or violent patient,
    2967, 3134
Impotence, pelvic fracture and, 719
Imprisonment, false, 2967
Impulses, grouped, causes of, 1219, 1219b
Inborn errors of metabolism, ataxia in, 2682
Incarceration, penile, 532, 533f
Incident command system, 3014
Incised wounds, in physical assault, 963
Incision and drainage
  in paronychia, 615, 615f
  in pericoronitis, 1035
  of Bartholin cyst abscess, 2205, 2205f
  of cutaneous abscess, 2204
  of felon, 615, 616f
  of periodontal abscess, 1031, 1033
  of retropharyngeal abscess, 1121
Incontinence, fecal, 1516-1517, 1516b
Incorporation, radioactive, 2320
Indapamide, 1321t
India ink staining of cerebrospinal fluid, in
    central nervous system infection, 1718, 1719f

Indinavir, in HIV/AIDS, side effects of, 2079t
Indirect immunofluorescence assay (IFA)
  in babesiosis, 2140
  in ehrlichiosis, 2138
  in Rocky Mountain spotted fever, 2135
Indium-labeled bone scan, in osteomyelitis, 2181
Indomethacin, 2927
  during pregnancy and lactation, 2784
  for gouty arthritis, 1786
  for premature labor, 2807
  for reactive arthritis, 1790
Induction agents, 15-16, 2914b
Induration, 1839t
Infant. See also Neonate.
  abdominal pain in, differential considerations
    in, 2611, 2612t
  acute bacterial meningitis in, 2657-2665
    clinical features of, 2658-2659, 2658t
    diagnosis of, 2659-2663, 2660b, 2661f, 2661t
    differential considerations in, 2663, 2663b
    management of, 2663-2665, 2664t
    pathophysiology of, 2657-2658
  acute septic arthritis in, 2704-2706, 2705t,
    2706t
  airway foreign body in, 869-870, 2530
  apnea in, 2714
  apparent life-threatening event in, 2718-2720,
    2718b, 2719b
  atrial septal defect in, 2578
  automobile restraint seats for, 947, 948
  bacterial endocarditis in, 2590-2591, 2591b
  botulism in, 1707, 2013, 2015-2016
  burn injury in, 923
  cardiovascular disorders in, 2567-2599
    chest radiography in, 2573-2574, 2573f,
      2574f
    circulatory changes related to, 2568-2569
    compensatory responses associated with,
      2569, 2569b
    history in, 2570-2571, 2570b
    physical examination in, 2571-2575, 2571t,
      2572b
  causes of death in, 942t, 949t
  chest pain in, 2570-2571
  choanal atresia in, 2522
  coarctation of the aorta in, 2578-2579
  congenital heart disease in, 2575-2582
    acyanotic, 2577-2579, 2577f
    chest radiography in, 2573-2574, 2574f
    clinical features of, 2575-2576, 2575t
    cyanotic, 2579-2581, 2579f, 2581b
    diagnosis of, 2576, 2576b
    ductal-dependent, 2576-2577, 2576b, 2577b
    incidence of, 2575, 2575t
    management of, 2576-2577, 2576b, 2577b
    postoperative complications of, 2581
    respiratory syncytial virus infection and,
      2581-2582, 2582b
  cyanosis in
    central, cardiac vs. pulmonary, 2569, 2569b,
      2572
    in tetralogy of Fallot, 2580
    pathophysiology of, 2569
  developmental milestones in, 2496-2497, 2496t
  diarrhea in, 2628b, 2628t
  dysrhythmias in, 2584-2590, 2584b, 2586b,
    2587f-2589f
  Eisenmenger syndrome in, 2578
  electrocardiography in, 2574-2575, 2574t
  fever in
    management of, 2512-2514, 2513b
    pathophysiology of, 2505
  gastroesophageal reflux in, 2609-2610
  gastrointestinal bleeding in, differential
    considerations in, 220, 221b, 2613-2614,
    2614t
  gastrointestinal disorders in, 2601-2621
  heart failure in, 2582-2584, 2583t
  hip dysplasia in, 2701-2702, 2702b, 2702f
  Hirschsprung's disease in, 2612-2613
  HIV/AIDS in, 2774
  hypertrophic pyloric stenosis in, 2603-2606,
    2605f, 2606t
  hypomagnesemia in, 1948
  increased intracranial pressure in, 334, 334b
  infectious diarrhea in, 2623-2634
    clinical features of, 2626
    complications of, 2626
    dehydration in, 2629, 2629t

Infant (Continued)
  diagnosis of, 2626-2627
  differential diagnosis in, 2627, 2627t
  disposition in, 2628-2629, 2628b
  epidemiology of, 2623-2624
  etiology of, 2624-2626, 2628t
  fluid and electrolyte management in, 2629-
    2634, 2630t, 2632b-2634b
  management of, 2628, 2628t
  pathophysiology of, 2624
  intussusception in, 2509b, 2610-2612, 2611f,
    2612t
  jaundice in, 2601-2603, 2602t, 2603b, 2603t,
    2604f-2605f
  Kawasaki disease in, 2593-2596, 2594b, 2595f
  malrotation with midgut volvulus in, 2606-
    2608, 2607f, 2608f
  myocarditis in, 2591-2592
  necrotizing enterocolitis in, 2608-2609, 2609f
  neurologic disorders in, 2657-2686
  peptic ulcer disease in, 1392
  pericarditis in, 2592-2593, 2593f
  periodic breathing in, 2495
  pneumonia in, 1131
  red and painful eye in, 292
  renal and genitourinary disorders in, 2635-
    2655
  renal function in, 923
  stroke volume in, decreased, causes of, 2569,
    2569b
  sudden death of. See Sudden infant death
    syndrome.
  temperature determination in, 2508
  tetralogy of Fallot in, 2579-2581, 2579f, 2580f,
    2581b
  upper airway obstruction in, 2519-2530
    evaluation of, 2521, 2521f
    in congenital lesions, 2522, 2524-2525,
      2524f, 2527-2528, 2528f
    in croup, 2525-2527, 2526f, 2527b
    in epiglottitis, 2523-2524, 2524f
    in foreign body aspiration, 2529-2530
    in laryngeal disease, 2524-2525, 2524f
    in retropharyngeal abscess, 2522-2523, 2523f
    in subglottic tracheal disease, 2525-2527
    in supraglottic disease, 2522-2524
    in tracheal disease, 2527-2529, 2529t
    pathophysiology of, 2519, 2520f
    stridor in, 2519-2520, 2521t
  urinary tract infection in, 1583, 1583t, 2510,
    2642-2644, 2643b, 2643t
  ventricular septal defect in, 2577
  vomiting in, 203, 208t, 2605, 2606t, 2627t,
    2628b
  wheezing in, 2532-2533
Infantile spasms, 2665-2666
Infarction
  gastric, 1394
  lung, pulmonary embolism with, 1373
  myocardial. See Myocardial infarction.
  renal, urolithiasis vs., 1591
  spinal cord, 1683
  splenic, in sickle cell disease, 2308
Infection. See also Bacterial infection; Fungal
    infection; Parasitic infection; Viral infection.
  catheter-related, 1363
    in peritoneal dialysis patient, 1553
    of urinary tract, 1578-1579
  cerebrospinal fluid shunt–related, in
    developmentally disabled patient, 2899
  facial nerve paralysis from, 1666-1667
  fever in, differential diagnosis in, 135, 135t
  fracture and, 558, 558b
  from pacemaker, 1250
  heart failure in, 1268
  hypothermia and, 2241
  in acute renal failure, 1540
  in alcoholism, 2870-2871
  in atherosclerotic aneurysm, 1356, 1357t
  in burn injury, 918
  in chronic renal failure, 1543, 1546-1547
  in diabetes mellitus, 1971
  in elderly person, 2828
  in febrile cancer patient, 1907-1909, 1908b
  in hand trauma, 614-618, 615f-617f
  in heart transplant patient, 2853-2854
  in kidney transplant patient, 2855
  in liver transplant patient, 2854-2855
  in lung transplant patient, 2856

Infection (Continued)
  in neutropenic cancer patient, 2834-2839,
    2836t, 2838t
  in organ transplant patient, 2847-2849, 2847b
  observation in, 3072-3073, 3072b, 3073t
  of arteriovenous fistula or graft, 1366
  of vascular access for hemodialysis, 1549-1550
  rhabdomyolysis in, 1979
  seizure in, 1623
  susceptibility to, in sickle cell disease, 1880-
    1881
  thrombocytopenia in, 1897
  wound
    prophylaxis against, 854-855
    risk factors for, 844-845, 844b
Infectious agents
  as biologic weapons, 3024, 3024b
  in organ transplant patient, 2847b
Infectious diarrhea, 228, 230b
  pediatric, 2623-2634
    clinical features of, 2626
    complications of, 2626
    dehydration in, 2629, 2629t
    diagnosis of, 2626-2627
    differential diagnosis in, 2627, 2627t
    disposition in, 2628-2629, 2628b
    epidemiology of, 2623-2624
    etiology of, 2624-2626, 2628t
    fluid and electrolyte management in, 2629-
      2634, 2630t, 2632b-2634b
    management of, 2628, 2628t
    pathophysiology of, 2624
    treatment of, 229t-230t, 235
Infectious diseases, 2001-2225. See also specific
    diseases, e.g., Tuberculosis.
Infectious eczematoid dermatitis, in otitis media,
    1067-1068
Infectious esophagitis, 1386, 1387
Infectious mononucleosis, 1110, 1112, 1114
  cytomegalovirus in, 2043
  Epstein-Barr virus in, 2044
Infectious parotitis, 1428, 2052
Infective endocarditis, 1300-1302
  clinical features of, 1301
  diagnostic strategies in, 1301-1302, 1302b
  in prosthetic valve patient, 1308
  management of, 1302, 1302b
  pathophysiology of, 1301
  prophylaxis for, 1302, 1303b, 1303t
  risk factors for, 1302, 1303b
Inferior mesenteric artery, 1445
Infiltration therapy, for hydrofluoric acid burns,
    933
Inflammation
  after cerebral ischemia, 66-67
  allergic, in asthma, 1080-1081, 1080f, 1083
  in septic shock, 47
  in shock, 43, 44f, 45
  macular disorders from, 1059
  of bursa. See Bursitis.
  of joint. See Arthritis.
  of tendon. See Tendinitis/tendinopathy.
  systemic, in burn injury, 917-918
Inflammatory bowel disease, 1500-1503, 1502b,
    1502f, 1503b
  Aeromonas hydrophila gastroenteritis and, 1467
  arthritis in, 1790
  in children, 2615-2616
  pericarditis in, 1287
Inflammatory diarrhea, 228, 229t-230t
Inflammatory disorders. See also specific
    disorders, e.g., Arthritis.
  allergy, anaphylaxis, and hypersensitivity in,
    1818-1835
  arthritis as, 1776-1792
  bursitis as, 1801-1804
  myopathy in, 1708
  tendinopathy as, 1794-1801
  vasculitis as, 1812-1817
Inflammatory mediators
  in anaphylaxis, 1823, 1823b, 2547
  in asthma, 1081
  in sepsis, 2213
Inflammatory pancreatitis, 1435
Inflammatory pseudotumor, 293t
Infliximab, 2844
  for inflammatory bowel disease, 1503
Influenza, 2054-2055
  drugs for, 2037t

Influenza (Continued)
  in pneumonia, 1130, 1139
  pharyngitis in, 1110
  rhabdomyolysis in, 1979
  vaccine for, 2035t, 2055
Influenzae cellulitis, 2199
Information management
  definition of, 3097
  in emergency department, 3099-3102, 3100t, 3102f
  prehospital, 3099, 3101, 3105
Information technology in emergency medicine, 3097-3106
  Internet and, 3104
  networks and, 3104
  security and confidentiality of patient information and, 3102-3103
  standards and, 3103-3104
  telemedicine and, 3105-3106
  terminology in, 3097
  uses of, 3097-3099, 3104-3106
Informed consent, 3134, 3166
  emergency research without, 3136-3137
  for procedures on newly dead, 3149
  physician's role in, 3166-3167
Informed refusal of medical care, 3169-3170
Infrapatellar bursitis, 795-796
Infraspinatus muscle, 672, 673f
Inguinal hernia, 1598, 2641-2642
Inguinal lymphadenopathy, in lymphogranuloma venereum, 1562
Inhalation
  of anhydrous ammonia, 935
  of carbon monoxide, 2438-2441
  of cocaine, 2388
  of cyanide, 2436-2438, 2437f
  of heroin, 2451, 2452
  of hydrocarbons, 2428-2432, 2430f
  of hydrofluoric acid, 933
  of hydrogen sulfide, 2436-2438, 2437f
  of pulmonary irritants, 2433t, 2434-2435, 2434f
  of pyrethrins and pyrethroids, 2467
  of simple asphyxiants, 2432-2433
  of tobacco. See Smoking.
  smoke, 2435-2436
    carbon monoxide with cyanide poisoning in, 2440-2441
Inhalational anthrax, 3024-3025, 3025f
Injection pain, reducing, 2932-2933, 2932b
Injection therapy
  in adhesive capsulitis, 699, 699t
  in knee bursitis, 796
Injections, antibiotic and narcotic, medicolegal issues in, 3159
Injury prevention and control, 940-950
  acute trauma care and, 948
  advocacy of public policy for, 948, 950
  epidemiology and documentation in, 945-946
  in elderly person, 2829-2830
  in gang violence in emergency department, 1021-1022
  in pregnancy, 2735-2737
  in youth violence, 1020
  methods of prevention in, 944-945
  prehospital care in, 948
  principles of, 940, 941f, 943-945, 943t, 944t
  public health and, 943-944, 944t
  risk factor assessment in, 946-948
  scientific approach to, 940, 941b
Injury severity score (ISS), 300, 302b
Inner ear
  barotrauma to, 2282, 2287-2288, 2287t, 2292
  in decompression sickness, 2284
Innominate bone, 717, 718f
Inotropic agents, for sepsis, 2219t, 2220-2221
Inpatient, definition of, 3159
Insect repellent
  overdose of, 2468-2469
  prophylactic, for tick-borne illness, 2142
Insect sting kit, allergy to, 1827
Insect stings. See Hymenoptera stings.
Insecticide poisoning. See Pesticide poisoning.
Insomnia
  in acute mountain sickness, 2301, 2302
  in depression, 1737
  seizures vs., 2668
Inspiratory muscles, weakness of, 139
Inspiratory stridor, in pediatric assessment, 2498

Instability. See also Dislocation; Fracture-dislocation.
  atlantoaxial, 2901
  carpal, 630-632, 630f-633f
  shoulder, 674
Instinctual anxiety, 1746b
Institutional abuse, 1009, 1015
Institutional review boards, 3136, 3137
Instrument testing, for anterior cruciate ligament injury, 774
Insufficiency fracture, of femoral neck, 750-752, 750f-751f, 752b
Insufflation technique, for nasal foreign body, 864
Insulin
  allergy to, 1972
  deficiency of, diabetic ketoacidosis from, 1962
  in glucose regulation, 1956
  release of, 1956
Insulin preparations, allergy to, 1827
Insulin pumps, 1973
Insulin resistance
  in diabetes mellitus, 1966
  in pregnancy, 2724
Insulin therapy
  during pregnancy and lactation, 2790
  for calcium channel blocker overdose, 2378
  for diabetic ketoacidosis, 1965-1966
  for hyperkalemia, 1941
  skin problems associated with, 1971-1972
Integrity, personal, 3129, 3129b
Intention-to-treat analysis, 3056-3057, 3057f
Interaction term, 3055
Interclavicular ligaments, 670, 671f
Intercondylar eminence fracture, 779-780, 780f
Intercondylar fracture, 659-660, 659f
Intercostal retractions, in pediatric assessment, 2498, 2498f
Interdental papillae, edematous, in acute necrotic ulcerative gingivitis, 1033
Interferon-α, recombinant, indications for, 2038-2039
Interferon-β, for multiple sclerosis, 1673
Interferon-γ, in tuberculosis, 2155
Interleukin-4, in asthma, 1080, 1080f
Interleukin-13, in asthma, 1080, 1080f
Interleukin(s), in sepsis, 2213
Intermediate-range handgun wounds, 956-957, 956f
Intermittent claudication, in chronic arterial insufficiency, 1345
Intermittent mechanical ventilation (IMV), 27
Internal cervical os, miscarriage and, 2740
Internal disaster plan, 3015
Internal elastic lamina, 1342
Internal iliac arteries, 717-718
Internal radioactive contamination, 2320, 2324
International Classification of Diseases, 3104
International normalized ratio
  in bleeding disorders, 1895
  in hepatitis, 1404
Internet, in health care, 3104
Interossei muscles, 580, 581f
  decompression of, in burn injury, 925, 925f
Interosseous membrane, 797
Interpersonal Justifiability Test, in ethical case analysis, 3132
Interphalangeal joint, 578, 579f
  dislocation of
    distal, 601, 601f
    in foot, 835-836
    in thumb, 564, 565f, 603
    proximal, 601-602
  extensor tendon injury at
    distal, 605-607, 606f, 607f
    proximal, 607-608, 607f
  motions of, 578f
  stability testing of, 601
Interposed abdominal compression–cardiopulmonary resuscitation, 89, 98
Interpreter services
  and effective medical care, 3110-3111
  as standard of cultural competence, 3112-3113
  requirements for, 3161
  sign language, 2905
Interscapular pain, in aortic rupture, 478
Intersphincteric abscess, 1513t, 1514, 2206
Interstitial nephritis, acute, 1534-1535, 1534b
Intertriginous infections, in HIV/AIDS, 2085
Intertrochanteric fracture, 752-753, 752f

Intervertebral disk, 702, 702f
  herniation of
    lumbar, 702-703, 704-705, 711-712
    magnetic resonance imaging in, 432, 433f
    radicular pain in, 264
Intestinal amebiasis, 1477t, 1480-1481
Intestinal fluke, 2101t
Intestinal transit time, in pregnancy, 2726
Intestine(s). See also Gastrointestinal entries;
    Large intestine; Small intestine.
  decompression of, for small bowel obstruction, 1444
  distention of, in small bowel obstruction, 1440
  foreign body in, 873-875, 875f
  inflammation of. See Enteritis; Gastroenteritis.
  ischemia of. See Mesenteric ischemia.
  obstruction of
    abdominal pain in, 214t
    in Hirschsprung's disease, 2612
    in hypertrophic pyloric stenosis, 2603-2606, 2605f, 2606t
    in intussusception, 2610
    in malrotation with midgut volvulus, 2606-2608, 2607f, 2608f
    large bowel, 1495-1497, 1496f
    nausea and vomiting in, 205t
    small bowel, 1440-1444, 1441b, 1443f
  perforation of, in seat belt injuries, 491
  whole-bowel irrigation of
    in beta blocker overdose, 2374
    in cocaine body packing/stuffing, 2391
    in iron overdose, 2420
    in lithium toxicity, 2444
    in opioid overdose, 2455
    in overdosed/poisoned patient, 2330
Intimal flap
  in aortic rupture, 479, 479f, 480, 480f
  in peripheral vascular injury, 538
Intimate partner violence and abuse, 994-1006
  barriers to diagnosis of, 998
  clinical features of, 996-998
  definitions of, 995, 995t
  disposition in, 1004-1005, 1005b
  documentation of, 1000-1001, 1003-1004
  during pregnancy, 997
  epidemiology of, 995-996
  facial trauma from, 382-383
  improving emergency department response to victims of, 1005-1006
  in pregnancy, 2734-2735, 2734t
  legal considerations in, 1004-1005
  referral in, 1004
  risk assessment in, 1000, 1002b, 1003b
  risk factors for injury related to, 996
  screening for, 998-999, 999b, 1000f, 1001f, 1002b
  use of emergency department in, 996
  validation of patient's experience in, 999-1000
Intoxication. See Poisoning/overdose.
Intra-abdominal abscess, in appendicitis, 1453, 1458
Intra-aortic balloon pump counterpulsation, for cardiogenic shock, 54
Intra-arterial drug abusers, vascular abnormalities in, 1360-1361
Intra-arterial pressure monitoring, in heart failure, 1269, 1270t, 2773
Intra-articular fracture, of thumb metacarpal, 599-600, 599f
Intracardiac injection, in adult resuscitation, 92
Intracardiac injuries, traumatic, 472
Intracerebral hematoma, 378, 378f
Intracerebral hemorrhage
  alcohol consumption and, 2869-2870
  anatomy and physiology in, 1607
  cerebral herniation in, 1918
  clinical features of, 1610-1611, 1610t, 1611f
  diagnosis of, 1613
  differential diagnosis in, 1611-1612
  disposition in, 1617
  epidemiology of, 1608-1609, 1608b
  in pertussis, 2006
  management of, 1616
  pathophysiology of, 1607
  volume of, measurement of, 1611, 1611f
Intracranial abscess. See Brain abscess.
Intracranial hemorrhage
  dysrhythmia after, 371
  hypertension in, 1316

Intracranial hypertension
  after head trauma, 353-354, 367
  headache and, 174t, 2677-2678
  idiopathic, 1639-1640, 1640b
  in developmentally disabled patient, 2899
  in high-altitude cerebral edema, 2306
  in pediatric patient, 334, 334b
  intubation and, 17, 18t
  risk factors for, 171b
  treatment of, 360, 367
Intracranial infection, headache in, 1641
Intracranial lesion
  delirium in, 1649
  dementia in, 1660
  in head-injured child, 367
Intracranial pressure
  cerebral perfusion pressure and, 352
  elevated. See Intracranial hypertension.
Intracranial trauma, repetitive, dementia from, 1656
Intractable patient, 2978t, 2980-2981
Intramuscular opioid analgesia, disadvantages of, 2919-2920, 2919b
Intraocular pressure
  in red and painful eye, 286-287
  increased
    from succinylcholine, 14
    in central retinal artery occlusion, 1057
    in glaucoma, 1055, 1056
    in retrobulbar hemorrhage, 1046
    in traumatic hyphema, 1048
    reversal of, 292
  normal, 1055
Intraosseous access
  in adult resuscitation, 92
  in pediatric resuscitation, 99
Intraperitoneal air, 496, 496f, 504
Intraperitoneal bladder rupture, 526
Intraperitoneal hemorrhage, 493, 498, 498f
  in multiple trauma, 312, 313f
  peritoneal lavage in, 499-501, 500t
Intraperitoneal injury
  penetrating renal trauma and, 528
  single vs. multiple, 502
  vs. necessary laparotomy, 502
Intrathoracic dislocation, 697, 698f
Intravascular hemolytic transfusion reaction, 59-60
Intravenous drug abuse
  cotton fever in, 2454
  infective endocarditis in, 1300-1301
  skin lesions associated with, 1864, 1865f
  vascular abnormalities in, 1360-1361
Intravenous fluid therapy, in pediatric infectious
    diarrhea, 2630-2634, 2632b-2634b
Intravenous immunoglobulin. See
    Immunoglobulin preparations.
Intravenous pyelography
  in renal trauma, 528
  in ureteral trauma, 531, 531f
Intravenous regional anesthesia, 2934
Intrinsic ligaments of wrist, 622, 624f
Intubation. See also Mechanical ventilation.
  approach to, 7-8, 7f-9f
  awake oral, 12
  confirmation of tube placement in, 6-7, 6f
  decision criteria for, 2-3
  elevated intracranial pressure and, 17, 18t
  esophageal, detection of, 6-7, 6f
  fiberoptic, 20-21, 22f
  hemodynamic consequences of, 16-17
  in abdominal trauma, 494
  in acute pulmonary edema, 1271, 1271f
  in adult epiglottitis, 1115
  in adult resuscitation, 87, 91
  in airway foreign body removal, 870
  in anaphylaxis, 1830
  in asthma, 1092
  in barbiturate overdose, 2483
  in botulism, 2016
  in caustic ingestion, 2383
  in chronic obstructive pulmonary disease,
      1103-1113, 1105t
  in facial trauma, 389, 390
  in flail chest, 458, 458b
  in hypothermia, 2244
  in Ludwig's angina, 1119
  in multiple trauma, 306
  in neonatal resuscitation, 122

Intubation (Continued)
  in orofacial infections, 1032
  in sepsis, 2219
  in submersion victim, 2314
  in tracheobronchial injury, 466
  in weakness and ventilatory insufficiency, 141,
      141b
  induction agents in, 15-16
  measurement of potential difficulty in, 4-5
  nasogastric
    esophageal perforation from, 483
    in abdominal trauma, 494
    in acute pancreatitis, 1433-1434
    in burn injury, 923
    in gastric volvulus, 1394
    in gastrointestinal bleeding, 223-224
    in hypothermia, 2244
    in neck trauma, 444
    in small bowel obstruction, 1444
  nasotracheal, 12
    esophageal perforation from, 483
    in multiple trauma, 306
    in neck trauma, 444
  neuromuscular blocking agents in, 13-15
  of difficult airway
    approach to, 8-9, 9f
    cricothyrotomy for, 22-23, 23f
    esophagotracheal combitube for, 20, 20f
    fiberoptic, 20-21, 22f
    identification in, 3-4, 3b, 4b, 5f
    intubating laryngeal mask airway for, 19, 19f
    lighted stylet for, 19-20, 20f
    retrograde, 20
    special airway devices for, 18-23, 19f-23f
  oral access for, assessment of, 4, 5f
  outcomes in, 23
  pediatric, 18
    in asthma, 2542
    in bacterial tracheitis, 2529
    in status epilepticus, 2672
  pharmacologic agents in, 13-16
  potential cervical spine injury in, 17-18
  prehospital, 2990, 2991
  rapid sequence, 9-12, 10b
    in asthma, 16
    in elevated intracranial pressure, 17, 18t
    in head trauma, 358-359
    in neck trauma, 444
    in shock, 51
    indications for, 7-8
    paralysis with induction phase in, 11
    pediatric, 18, 107-108, 107b, 107t
    post-intubation management in, 11-12
    prehospital, 2990, 2991
    preoxygenation in, 10, 10f
    preparations for, 9-10
    pretreatment agents for, 10, 11b
    tube placement in, 11
    vs. blind nasotracheal intubation, 12
    with competitive neuromuscular blocking
        agent and etomidate, 14-15, 15t
  retrograde, 20
  status asthmaticus and, 16, 17t
  with sedation alone, 12
  without pharmacologic agents, 12-13
Intussusception
  in Henoch-Schönlein purpura, 2615
  in infants and children, 2509b, 2610-2612,
      2611f, 2612f
  large bowel, 1499-1500
  small bowel, 1441-1442
Inverse ratio ventilation (IRV), 33
Inversion stress test, 817
Involucrum, in osteomyelitis, 2175
Iodine exposure, as weapon of mass destruction,
    3023, 3023t
Iodine therapy, for thyroid storm, 1989
Iodine tincture, ingestion of, 2384
Iodoquinol, for intestinal amebiasis, 1481
Ionizing radiation, 2318f, 2319
Iothalamate meglumine contrast medium, in
    retrograde cystography, 521, 525
Ipratropium
  during pregnancy and lactation, 2762, 2765t,
      2789
  for anaphylaxis, 1832
  for asthma, 1087t, 1089, 2539t, 2541
  for chronic obstructive pulmonary disease,
      1105

Irbesartan, 1322t
Iridocyclitis, traumatic, 1049, 1049f
Iridodialysis, traumatic, 1049
Iridodonesis, in lens dislocation, 1049
Iris, 1045f
  flat or plateau, closed-angle glaucoma from,
      1056
  nonpenetrating trauma to, 1048-1049, 1048f,
      1049f
Iron
  caustic effects of, 2419
  corneal foreign body containing, 1047, 1048f,
      1052
  metabolic acidosis from, 1928
  overdose of, 2418-2421, 2419t, 2420f, 2420t
    antidotes to, 2329t
  preparations of, 2419t
  requirements for, in pregnancy, 2724
Iron deficiency anemia, 1871-1872, 1871f, 1872t
  in alcoholism, 2873-2874
  in pregnancy, 2763t, 2767-2768
Irradiation
  definition of, 2319
  microwave, 2319
    for rewarming in accidental hypothermia,
        2250
    vs. contamination and incorporation, 2319-
        2320
  whole-body, acute radiation syndrome after,
      2317t, 2321-2322, 2321f
Irrigation
  for foreign body removal from ear, 863
  heated, for rewarming, 2250
  in acid and alkali burns, 933
  in anhydrous ammonia exposure, 935
  in cement burn, 935
  in hydrofluoric acid exposure, 933, 934
  in ocular burns, 1046
  in red and painful eye, 290-291
  of wound, 848
Irritability
  in bacterial meningitis, 2658
  in pediatric assessment, 2498
Irritable bowel syndrome, 1490-1492, 1491b,
    1492b
Irritant laxatives, for constipation, 241t, 242
Irritants, ocular trauma from, 1046
Ischemia
  cerebral
    neurologic recovery after, 62-73
    clinical outcomes in, 72-73
    experimental therapies in, 70-72
    standard strategies for, 67-70, 69t
    pathophysiology of, 62-67, 63f-64f
  colonic, 1503-1504
  in frostbite, 2229, 2229b
  limb-threatening
    in acute arterial occlusion, 1345
    management of, 1351
  mesenteric. See Mesenteric ischemia.
  myocardial. See Myocardial ischemia.
  of tissue, in compartment syndrome, 560-561,
      560b, 561b, 561f
  transient. See Transient ischemic attack (TIA).
  warm, in peripheral vascular injury, 537
Ischemic central retinal vein occlusion, 1057
Ischemic heart disease. See Acute coronary
    syndromes; Coronary artery disease;
    Myocardial infarction; Myocardial ischemia.
Ischemic optic neuropathy, 1060
Ischemic penumbra, 1607
Ischemic stroke
  acute drug therapy for, 1615-1616, 1615t
  anatomy and physiology in, 1607
  antihypertensive drug therapy for, 1614, 1614t
  cardioembolic, 1608
  clinical features of, 1609-1610, 1610t
  diagnosis of, 1612-1613, 1612f
  differential diagnosis in, 1611
  disposition in, 1616-1617
  epidemiology of, 1607-1608, 1607t
  fibrinolytic therapy for, 1615, 1615t
  in central retinal artery occlusion, 1057
  management of, 1613-1616, 1613t, 1614t,
      1615b
  pathophysiology of, 1606-1607
  thrombotic, 1607-1608
  time goals in, 1613t
Ischial tuberosity avulsion fracture, 724, 724f

Ischiogluteal bursitis, 1803
Ischiorectal abscess, 1513t, 1514, 2206
Ischium, 717, 718f
Isoenzyme analysis, in electrical and lightning
     injuries, 2276
Isoflurane anesthesia, for status epilepticus,
     1627-1628, 1627t
Isolation
     in plague, 3027-3028
     in pneumonia, 1136, 1140-1141
     in tuberculosis, 2147, 2169-2170
Isonatremic hypovolemia, 2629t, 2631, 2632b
Isoniazid
     during pregnancy and lactation, 2785
     for tuberculosis, 2162, 2163t
     hepatotoxicity of, 1413
     in HIV/AIDS, side effects of, 2079t
     metabolic acidosis from, 1928
     overdose of, antidotes to, 2329t
Isopropyl alcohol poisoning, 2402-2404, 2403f
Isoproterenol
     for anaphylactic patient on beta blockers,
          1831b, 1833
     for calcium channel blocker overdose, 2378
     for torsades de pointes, 1244
Isorhythmic atrioventricular dissociation, 1221
Isospora belli gastroenteritis, 1476-1478, 1477t,
     2084
Isradipine, 1321t, 2377t
Itraconazole
     for candidal esophagitis, 1387
     for tinea capitis, 1839
     in HIV/AIDS, side effects of, 2079t
Ivermectin
     for Onchocerca volvulus infection, 2109
     for pediculosis, 1854
Ivory soap, for rabies postexposure prophylaxis,
     2068
Ixodes tick, 2117, 2118, 2118f, 2121f, 2139

J wave, in hypothermia, 2237, 2238f
Jacksonian march, 1621
Japanese encephalitis virus, 1723
Jarisch-Herxheimer-type reaction
     in Lyme disease, 2128
     in relapsing fever, 2130
Jaundice, 243-246
     diagnostic approach to, 243-244, 244f, 245f
     differential diagnosis in, 245, 246t
     empiric management of, 245-246, 247f
     epidemiology of, 243
     in cholangitis, 1421
     in drug-induced liver disorders, 1414
     in hepatitis, 1404
     in hyperthyroidism, 1987
     in pancreatic carcinoma, 1437
     in pregnancy, 2726, 2753t
     in pyogenic abscess, 1414-1415
     neonatal, 2601-2603, 2602t, 2603b, 2603t,
          2604f-2605f
Jaw-thrust maneuver, in pediatric resuscitation,
     97
JC virus, 2045-2046
Jefferson fracture, 412-413, 414f, 421, 550t
Jehovah's Witnesses, refusal of medical care by,
     3171-3172
Jellyfish, 909
Jequirty pea, 2471-2472, 2472f
Jerk test, in knee trauma, 774
Jimson weed poisoning, 2345, 2346, 2473,
     2473f
Jobe's sign, in rotator cuff tendinopathy, 1797
Joint
     anatomy of, 2175
     arthrocentesis of, 1780-1781
     aspiration of
          in gonococcal arthritis, 2191
          in septic arthritis, 2188-2190, 2189f, 2192
     clinical anatomy of, 1777, 1777f
     contractures of, in cerebral palsy, 2901
     dislocation of. See Dislocation.
     examination of, 1778-1779, 1779f
     infection of. See Septic arthritis.
     inflammation of. See Arthritis.
     injury to, in electrical and lightning injuries,
          2273
     subluxation of. See Subluxation.

Joint fluid analysis, in septic arthritis, 2188-2190,
     2189f
Joint pain
     causes of, 1778, 1778t
     in gouty arthritis, 1785
     in hypothyroidism, 1992
     in osteoarthritis, 1787
     in septic arthritis, 1784-1785, 2188
Joint prosthesis, infection after, 2191
Jones compression dressing, 570-571
Jones criteria for rheumatic fever, 1303, 1304b,
     1790b, 2596, 2596f
Jones fracture, 550t, 832
Judgment, substituted, 3134
Jugular vein injury, 448
Jugular venous "A" wave, in tricuspid stenosis
     and regurgitation, 1307
Jugular venous distention
     in constrictive pericarditis, 1288
     in tension pneumothorax, 462
Jumper's knee, 794
Junctional parasystole, 1226
Junctional tachycardia, 1233-1235, 1233f, 1234f
     nonparoxysmal, 1234
     paroxysmal, 1233-1234, 1233f, 1234f, 1235
     reentrant, 1233
Junin virus, 2055-2056
Juniper, adverse effects of, 2476t
Justice, distributive, 3129, 3129b
Juvenile epilepsy, 2666

Kanamycin, for tuberculosis, 2163t
Kaopectate, for diarrhea, 236t
Kaposi's sarcoma, 1861f, 2044, 2079, 2083, 2085
Karlea, drug interactions with, 2478t
Kawasaki disease, 2024-2027, 2025b
     diagnostic criteria for, 2512b
     myocarditis in, 1293
     pediatric, 2593-2596, 2594b, 2595f
     pediatric fever in, 2511, 2512b
Kayexalate, for hyperkalemia, 1545-1546, 1545t,
     1941
Kelly clamp, for oropharyngeal foreign body
     removal, 1384
Kemerovo virus, 2047
Keratitis
     epithelial, corneal, 1054
     red and painful eye in, 289, 289f, 290f, 294t-
          295t
     superficial punctate, 294t, 1054
     ultraviolet, 1046-1047
Keratoconjunctivitis
     in herpes zoster, 1054
     red and painful eye in, 288, 288f, 293t, 295t
Keratotomy, radial, altitude and, 2309
Kerion, 1839
Kernicterus
     in hyperbilirubinemia, 2602
     prevention of, 2603, 2604f-2605f
Kernig sign
     in bacterial meningitis, 2659
     in central nervous system infection, 1714
Kernohan's notch syndrome, in cerebral
     herniation, 355
Ketamine
     abuse of, 2893
     as induction agent, 16
     for critically ill asthmatic patient, 1092
     for hypoxic (tet) spells, 2581
     for procedural sedation and analgesia, 2940t-
          2941t, 2946-2947, 2950, 2951t, 2953
     toxicity of, 2413, 2415
Ketoacidosis
     alcoholic, 1927-1928, 1964-1965, 2872-2873
     diabetic, 1928, 1962-1967
          complications of, 1967
          diagnosis of, 1963-1964
          differential considerations in, 1964-1965
          disposition in, 1967
          etiology of, 1963
          hypophosphatemia in, 1951
          in pregnancy, 1972, 2771-2772
          laboratory tests in, 1964, 1964t
          management of, 1965-1967, 1965b
          nausea and vomiting in, 205t
          pathophysiology of, 1962-1963, 1962t, 1963f

Ketoconazole
     during pregnancy and lactation, 2785
     for candidal esophagitis, 1387
     for esophageal candidiasis, 2083
     for tinea versicolor, 1840
     hepatotoxicity of, 1414
     in HIV/AIDS, side effects of, 2079t
Ketones, urine, in diabetes mellitus, 1959
Ketoprofen, for gouty arthritis, 1786
Ketorolac, 2927
     for abdominal pain, 217
     for migraine, 2680
     for urolithiasis, 1591-1592
Ketosis, in isopropyl alcohol poisoning, 2403
Khat, 2393, 2893
Kidney. See also Renal entries.
     anatomy of, 527, 527f
     blood supply to, 527, 527f
     gluconeogenesis in, 1956
     physical examination of, 1572, 1573f
     size of, in chronic renal failure, 1543, 1543b
     transplantation of, 2855
     ureter, and bladder films (KUB)
          in bladder trauma, 521, 522f, 523f, 524f
          in urethral trauma, 518
          in urolithiasis, 1590, 1592f
Kidney stones, 1586-1593, 1586b, 1589f-1592f,
     1593b. See also Urolithiasis.
Kienbock's disease, 629
Kiesselbach's area, 1073f
Killer bees, 904
Kindling, 1623
Kingella kingae, in bone or joint infections, 2177,
     2178t
Kinky-hair syndrome, fracture in, 2701
Kissing burn, 2272, 2272f
Klebsiella pneumoniae, 1130, 1132
Kleihauer-Betke test, for fetomaternal
     hemorrhage, 321
Klein's line, in slipped capital femoral epiphysis,
     2708
Knee
     bursitis of, 795-796
     dislocation of, popliteal artery injury and, 546
     immobilization of, 570-571
     osteoarthritis in, 796
     septic arthritis in, 796
     tendinitis of, 794, 795
     tendinopathy of, 1799
Knee pain
     differential diagnosis in, 771-772
     in bursitis of knee, 795
     in iliotibial band syndrome, 794
     in lateral patellar compression syndrome, 794
     in patellofemoral pain syndrome, 786-787
     in peripatellar tendinitis, 794
     in plica syndrome, 794-795
     in popliteus tendinitis, 795
     in tibial tubercle fracture, 798
Knee trauma, 770-796
     anatomy and physiology in, 770-771, 771f
     arthrocentesis in, 774
     arthroscopy in, 774
     bone bruise in, 781
     clinical features of, 771-774
     collateral ligament injuries in, 791-792
     cruciate ligament injuries in, 790-791
     distal femur fracture in, 776-777
     extensor tendon injuries in, 782-784, 783f, 784f
     meniscal tears in, 792-793
     osteochondritis dissecans in, 781-782
     osteonecrosis in, 782
     overuse injuries in, 793-796
     patellar dislocation in, 785-786, 785b
     patellar fracture in, 784-785, 785f
     patellofemoral pain syndrome in, 786-787
     physical examination in, 772-773, 772b, 772f
     proximal intra-articular tibial fractures in, 777-
          781
          epiphyseal, 780-781
          tibial plateau, 777-779, 777f-778f
          tibial spine, 779-780, 780f
     radiologic evaluation in, 774-775
     soft tissue injuries in, 790-792
     stability testing in, 773-774
     tibial femoral knee dislocation in, 787-790,
          789f
Koplik's spots, in measles, 1849, 2053, 2053f
Korsakoff's psychosis, 2869

Kruskal-Wallis test, 3052t, 3053
Kuru, 2058
Kussmaul's respiration
 in diabetic ketoacidosis, 1963
 in metabolic acidosis, 1929
Kussmaul's signs, in neoplastic cardiac
  tamponade, 1917
Kyphosis, in pregnancy, 2727
Labetalol, 1321t
 during pregnancy and lactation, 2765t, 2788
 for aortic dissection, 1328
 for hypertensive emergencies, 1318-1319, 2653,
  2765t
 for intracranial hemorrhage–related
  hypertension, 1316
 for tetanus, 2011
 overdose of, 2373t, 2374
Labor and delivery, 2797-2822
 abruptio placentae and, 2809-2810
 amniotic fluid embolism and, 2821
 bloody show in, 2798-2799
 breech presentations in, 2811-2813, 2811b,
  2812f, 2813b
 chorioamnionitis in, 2808, 2808b
 circumvallate placenta and, 2810
 complicated, 2810-2816
 delivery preparations and techniques in, 2802,
  2804
 drug interactions in, 2811t
 emergency, epidemiology of, 2797
 episiotomy in, 2804, 2813, 2815
 face, brow, and compound presentations in,
  2815-2816
 false vs. true labor in, 2798
 human immunodeficiency virus transmission
  during, 2810
 in multiple gestations, 2816
 in spinal cord injured patient, 2769
 limitations of emergency department for, 2797
 malpresentations in, 2811-2816, 2811b, 2811t,
  2812f, 2813b, 2814f, 2815f, 2816b
 maternal complications of, 2818-2822
 normal, 2798-2805
 nursery care after, 2798, 2798b
 patient transfer considerations in, 2797-2798
 placenta previa and, 2808-2809
 postpartum cardiomyopathy and, 2821
 postpartum depression and, 2821-2822
 postpartum endometriosis and, 2821
 postpartum hemorrhage and, 258t, 2818-2820
 premature, 2805-2807, 2806b, 2807b
 PROM in, 2807-2808, 2808t
 routine adjuncts to, risk-benefit analysis of,
  2805t
 shoulder dystocia in, 2811, 2813-2815, 2814f,
  2815f, 2816b
 stages of, 2799-2805, 2809f
  first, 2799-2800, 2799f-2802f
  second, 2800-2804, 2802b, 2802t, 2803f
  third, 2804-2805
  fourth, 2805
 substance abuse and, 2791, 2791b
 third-trimester complications associated with,
  2805-2810
 umbilical cord–related emergencies in, 2817-
  2818, 2817t
 uterine inversion and, 2820
 uterine rupture and, 2820
 vasa previa and, 2810
Laboratory studies
 as source of failures in emergency department,
  3125
 during cardiopulmonary resuscitation, 82
 for pregnancy detection, 2728-2730, 2729f
 in abdominal trauma, 495
 in accidental hypothermia, 2242-2244, 2243f
 in acute pancreatitis, 1430-1432, 1431t, 1432b
 in anemia, 1869
 in arthritis, 1779
 in back pain, 264, 707
 in comatose patient, 161-162
 in confusion, 152-153
 in cyanosis, 271
 in delirium, 1651-1652
 in dementia, 1660-1661, 1661b
 in diabetic ketoacidosis, 1964, 1964t
 in disseminated intravascular coagulation,
  1903, 1904t
 in elderly trauma patient, 347

Laboratory studies (Continued)
 in electrical and lightning injuries, 2276
 in fever, 137
 in gastrointestinal bleeding, 222-223
 in hematuria, 1530, 1602-1603
 in hemolytic anemia, 1877-1878, 1877b, 1877f,
  1878f
 in hemoptysis, 281
 in jaundice, 243-244, 244f
 in multiple trauma, 304
 in neuromuscular disorders, 1704-1705
 in osteomyelitis, 2179
 in pediatric fever, 2508-2510
 in pediatric pneumonia, 2560-2561
 in pediatric seizure, 2671
 in pediatric trauma, 332-333
 in pneumonia, 1134-1135
 in pregnancy, 318, 2728-2730, 2729f
 in pregnant trauma patient, 324
 in proteinuria, 1532
 in renal trauma, 528
 in seizure, 168
 in severe head trauma, 361
 in tuberculosis, 2151-2152
 in urinary tract infection, 1575-1577, 1577b
 in urolithiasis, 1588-1589
 in vertigo, 145
 in weakness, 139
 renal, 1524-1528, 1526f, 1527t, 1528b, 1528f
Labyrinthitis
 in otitis media, 1067
 vertigo in, 146, 147t, 2683
Laceration
 cheek, 391
 conjunctival, 1051
 corneal, 1051, 1051f
 coronary artery, 472
 ear, 392
 eye, 392
 eyelid, 1051, 1051f
 liver, 497f
 management of, 842-857. See also Wound
  management.
 mouth, 391
 of extensor mechanism over distal
  interphalangeal joint, 607, 607f
 pattern
  in motor vehicle crashes, 964, 965f
  in physical assault, 962, 962f
 penile, 532
 renal, 530, 530f
 scalp, 371-372, 850
 testicular, 534
Lachman's test, in anterior cruciate ligament
  injury, 773
Lacrimal glands, 385
Lacrimal sac, infection of, 1055, 1055f
Lactate
 in acute mesenteric ischemia, 1447
 in cyanide poisoning, 2437
 in shock, 47
 postresuscitation levels of, 87
Lactate clearance index, in shock, 50
Lactate dehydrogenase
 in acute tumor lysis syndrome, 1911
 in hemolytic anemia, 1878
 in hepatitis, 1404
Lactation
 asthma during, 1091
 drug therapy during, safety of, 2781-2790,
  2782t-2783t
 drug transfer during, 2781
Lactic acid, cerebrospinal fluid, in central
  nervous system infection, 1718
Lactic acidosis, 1928-1929
 in crush injury, 3007
 in sepsis, 2216
 in shock, 42-43, 43f
Lactobezoar, 873
Lactulose, for hepatic encephalopathy, 1412
Lacunar stroke, 1608
Ladd's bands, 2606
Laënnec's cirrhosis, 1410
Lambert-Eaton myasthenic syndrome, 1705
Laminar fracture, 426, 427f
Lamivudine, in HIV/AIDS, side effects of,
  2079t
Lamotrigine
 during pregnancy and lactation, 2787

Lamotrigine (Continued)
 for pediatric seizure, 2675t
 side effects of, 1628t
Landing zone safety issues for helicopters, 2997,
  2997b, 2997f, 2998b
Langer's lines, 384, 384f
Language, developmental milestones in, 2495-
  2497, 2496t
Language barriers
 and effective medical care, 3110-3111
 culturally competent approach to, 3112-3113
Lansoprazole, 1390t
Laparoscopy
 in abdominal trauma, 501, 508
 in appendicitis, 1455, 1457-1458
 in ectopic pregnancy, 2745
 in pelvic pain, 250
 in small bowel obstruction, 1444
Laparotomy
 in abdominal aortic aneurysm, 1338, 1339f
 in acute mesenteric ischemia, 1448
 in blunt abdominal trauma, 507-510, 507t,
  508f, 509f
 in children, 510
 in penetrating abdominal trauma
  from gunshot wounds, 505-507, 506f
  from stab wounds, 503-505, 503f, 503t
Large intestine. See also Anorectal disorders;
  Colon; Rectum.
 disorders of, 1490-1506
  diverticular disease of, 1492-1495, 1494b,
   1495b
  inflammatory bowel disease and, 1500-1503,
   1502b, 1502f, 1503b
  intussusception of, 1499-1500
  irritable bowel syndrome and, 1490-1492,
   1491b, 1492b
  obstruction of, 1495-1497, 1496f
   causes of, 1499b
   in volvulus, 1497-1499, 1498f, 1499b,
    1499f
  pseudo-obstruction and, 1495-1496, 1497
  radiation proctocolitis and, 1505-1506
Larkspur, adverse effects of, 2476t
Laryngeal disease, pediatric upper airway
  obstruction in, 2524-2525, 2524f
Laryngeal dystonia, antipsychotic-induced, 2446
Laryngeal edema, in anaphylaxis, 1825t, 2548
Laryngeal foreign body, 870
Laryngeal fracture, in near-hanging and
  strangulation, 451
Laryngeal injury, in smoke inhalation, 2435
Laryngeal mask airway, 18-19, 19f
 in airway foreign body removal, 870
 in neonatal resuscitation, 123
 intubating, 19, 19f
Laryngeal papilloma, 2045, 2525
Laryngeal tuberculosis, 2151
Laryngeal web, 2525, 2525f
Laryngitis, 1114
Laryngomalacia, 2524, 2524f
Laryngoscopy
 direct
  awake, 8
  evaluation of suitability for, 4, 5f
 failed, 8
 fiberoptic, in neck trauma, 445
 grades in, intubation difficulty and, 5
 in adult epiglottitis, 1115, 1115f
 in confirmation of endotracheal tube
  placement, 6-7
 reflex sympathetic response to, 16-17
 video and rigid fiberoptic, 21, 22f
Laryngotracheal stenosis, 2525
Laryngotracheal trauma, 447-448
Laryngotracheobronchitis, viral, 2525-2527,
  2526f, 2527b
Larynx, adult vs. child, 2519, 2520f
Lasègue's sign, in lumbar radiculopathy, 704
Lassa fever virus, 2037t, 2055
Late asthmatic response, 1081
Lateral collateral ligament
 anatomy of, 770, 771f, 808, 809f
 injury to, 791-792
 stress test of, 774
Lateral compression pelvic fracture, 727, 729f
Lateral condyle
 anatomy of, 647, 647f, 770, 771f
 fracture of, 660-661, 661f

Lateral corticospinal tract, 1676, 1676f
Lateral elbow dislocation, 665
Lateral epicondylitis, 1798
Lateral femoral cutaneous mononeuropathy, 1698
Lateral malleolus
    anatomy of, 808, 809f
    fracture of, 812-813, 813f
Lateral meniscus injury, 792-793
Lateral patellar compression syndrome, 794
Lateral pharyngeal space, 1027, 1117
Lateral radiographs of spinal injuries, 421, 424,
    425f, 426f
Lateral retinacula, 770, 771f
Lateral spinothalamic tract, 1676, 1676f
Lateral talocalcaneal ligament injury, 816
Lateral tibiofemoral compartment, 770, 771f
Latex agglutination, in central nervous system
    infection, 1718-1719
Latex allergy, 1826-1827, 2547
Law enforcement, tactical emergency medical
    support in, 3000-3005
Laxatives
    abuse of, 239
    for constipation, 241t, 242
Löffler's syndrome, 2110
Le Fort fracture, 387, 393, 551t
Le Fort-Wagstaffe fracture, 551t
Lead
    blood level of, as biomarker, 2422
    encephalopathy caused by, 2421, 2422
    foreign body containing, 2423
    poisoning from, 2421-2423, 2422t
        antidotes to, 2329t
        sideroblastic anemia in, 1873
Lead snowstorm, from centerfire rifle wound,
    959, 960f
Learned helplessness, 1736
Leaving against medical advice, 3170-3171
Leaving without being seen, 3170
Lebombo virus, 2047
Left bundle branch block
    myocardial infarction in, predictors of, 1167,
        1170f
    ST segment elevation in, 1167, 1169, 1169f,
        1170f
Left ventricular aneurysm, 1167, 1168f
Left ventricular free wall rupture, 1160
Left ventricular hypertrophy, 1169-1170, 1172f
Left ventriculoplasty, for chronic heart failure,
    1277
Left-sided heart failure, 1266-1267
Leg. See also Lower leg.
    blue, painful, 1370
    decompression of, in burn injury, 925
    position of, in hip trauma examination, 744
    swelling of, in spinal cord injury, 2907
Leg pain
    in disk herniation, 705
    lower, differential diagnosis of, 803
Legal case precedents, for combative or violent
    patient, 2967-2968
Legal issues, 3156-3173
    combative patient and, 2967-2969
    consent to medical care and, 3166-3169
    disposition requirements and, 3164-3165,
        3165f
    emergency medical condition and, 3156-3157
    Emergency Medical Treatment and Active
        Labor Act and, 3156
    in blood transfusion, 58
    in intimate partner violence and abuse, 1004-
        1005
    in patient transfer during labor and delivery,
        2797
    medical screening examination and, 3160-3163
    of combative patient, 2967-2969
    refusal of medical care and, 3169-3172
    reporting requirements and, 3172-3173
    screening requirements and, 3157-3158
    stabilization requirements and, 3163-3164
    testing requests and requirements and, 3158-
        3160
Legal rights, 3128
Legg-Calvé-Perthes disease, in children, 2706-
    2707, 2707f
Legionella infection
    in cancer patient with impaired cell-mediated
        immunity, 2839-2840
    in rhabdomyolysis, 1979

Legionella pneumoniae, 1130, 1132
Legionella pneumophila, myocarditis in, 1292
Leishmaniasis
    cutaneous, 2108, 2108f
    drug therapy for, 2101t
    fever in, 2105
Lemierre's syndrome, parapharyngeal abscess
    and, 1123
LEMON approach for evaluation of difficult
    airway, 3-4, 3b, 4b, 5f
Lennox-Gastaut syndrome, 2666
Lens, 1045f
    dislocation of, 1049
    subluxation of, 1049
Leopold's maneuvers, 2800, 2801f, 2813
Leptomeningeal cyst, in head-injured child, 368
Leriche's syndrome, 1345
Lesser trochanter fracture
    intertrochanteric, 752-753, 752f
    isolated, 753, 753f
    pediatric, 767, 767f
    subtrochanteric, 753-755, 754f
LET (lidocaine, epinephrine, and tetracaine),
    2933
Lethality Checklist in intimate partner violence
    and abuse, 1000, 1003b
Lethargy, in pediatric assessment, 2498
Leucovorin, for toxic alcohol poisoning, 2402
Leukemia
    acute tumor lysis syndrome in, 1911
    central nervous system infections in, 1920
    chronic myeloid, 1887-1888, 1887f
    fever and granulocytopenia in, 1908
    gingival lesions in, 1036
    hypercalcemia in, 1914
    hyperuricemia in, 1913
    hyperviscosity syndrome in, 1912
    hypogammaglobulinemia in, 2840-2841
    immune thrombocytopenia in, 1897
    lymphocytosis in, 1888
Leukemoid reaction, 1888
Leukocyte. See White blood cell entries.
Leukocyte esterase, urinary, in urinary tract
    infection, 1575-1576
Leukocytosis
    causes of, 1887b
    in amebic abscess, 1416
    in appendicitis, 1454
    in asthma, 1085
    in pertussis, 2006
    in pyogenic abscess, 1415
    lymphocytic, 1887b, 1888
    neutrophil, 1887-1888, 1887b, 1887f
Leukoencephalopathy
    progressive multifocal, 2045-2046
        dementia in, 1658, 1659
        in HIV/AIDS, 2082
    spongiform, from inhaled heroin, 2452
Leukopenia, 52, 1888-1889, 1889t
Leukopheresis, for hyperviscosity syndrome,
    1913
Leukoplakia, hairy, in HIV/AIDS, 2083
Leukotriene modifiers
    during pregnancy and lactation, 2789
    for aspirin-exacerbated respiratory disease, 1082
    for asthma, 1090, 2542, 2543t
Leukotrienes
    as anaphylaxis mediators, 1823, 1823b
    in aspirin-exacerbated respiratory disease,
        1082
    in asthma, 1080f, 1081, 1081f
Levalbuterol, for asthma, 1087, 1087t, 2538
Levator ani syndrome, 1516
Levator scapulae muscle, 672, 673f
Levator tendon lacerations, 1051
Levitaractam, for seizure, 2675t
Levofloxacin
    for tuberculosis, 2164t, 2165
    for urinary tract infection, 1582
Levorphanol, respiratory effects of, 2453t
Levothyroxine
    for hypothyroidism, 1993-1994
    in hypothermia, 2246-2247
Lewy body dementia, 1656, 1657
Libman-Sachs vegetations, in systemic lupus
    erythematosus, 1807
Lice, 1853-1854, 1853f
Lichen sclerosis et atrophicus, 975
Lichen tropicus, 2259

Lichenification, 1839t, 1842
Licorice
    adverse effects of, 2476t
    drug interactions with, 2478t
Lidocaine, 1206-1207, 2931, 2931t, 2932, 2932t
    allergy to, 846-847
    buffered, 2932-2933
    cardiac, 847
    central nervous system toxicity of, 2932
    during pregnancy and lactation, 2787-2788
    epinephrine, and tetracaine combination, 2933
    for anal fissures, 1513
    for cardiac arrest, 92-93
    for digitalis toxicity, 2371
    for dysrhythmia, 2586b
    for intubation of asthmatic patient, 16
    for knee bursitis, 796
    for local anesthesia, 846
    for pediatric resuscitation, 102t, 105
    for premature ventricular contractions, 1225
    for rapid sequence intubation, 11b, 359
    for reduction of glenohumeral joint dislocation,
        689
    for rotator cuff tear, 696
    for ventricular fibrillation and pulseless
        ventricular tachycardia, 113
    for ventricular tachycardia, 1242
    for wide-complex tachycardia, 1239-1240
    topical, 846, 2933
Life experiences, racial/ethnic differences in,
    culturally competent approach to, 3113-3114
Life or limb threats, in clinical decision making,
    128
Lifestyle modification, for gastroesophageal
    reflux, 1389
Life-threatening event, apparent, 2714, 2718-
    2720, 2718b, 2719b
Ligamentous injuries
    carpally, 630-632, 630f-633f
    in ankle trauma, 815-818, 817b, 817f
    in hand, 600-604, 601f-603f
    spinal, 434, 435f, 439
Ligaments
    of ankle, 808, 809f, 810f
    of distal humerus and elbow, 647-648, 648f
    of hip, 736, 736f
    of knee, 770-771, 771f
    of lumbosacral spine, 702, 702f
    of pelvis, 717, 718f
    of shoulder, 670-671, 671f, 672, 673f
    of wrist, 622, 624f
Ligamentum flavum, 702
Ligase chain reaction test, in tuberculosis, 2155
Ligature strangulation, 450
Lighted stylet, for intubation of difficult airway,
    19-20, 20f
Lightning injuries, 2267-2277
    and distribution of lightning, 2268f
    clinical features of, 2271-2274, 2273f
    complications of, 2274
    differential considerations in, 2275
    disposition in, 2277
    management of, 2275-2277, 2276b
    mechanisms of, 2271, 2271b
    physics of, 2269-2270
    rhabdomyolysis from, 1978
Light's criteria, in pleural fluid analysis, 1152,
    1152b
Likelihood ratio, 3059t
Limaprost, in frostbite, 2232
Limb ischemia, in tibial femoral knee
    dislocation, 788
Limb-threatening ischemia
    in acute arterial occlusion, 1345
    management of, 1351
Limp
    child with, 764-765, 765f
    in Legg-Calvé-Perthes disease, 2706
    in slipped capital femoral epiphysis, 2708
Lindane, for Phthirus pubis infestation, 1569
Linear burns, 2273
Linear regression models, 3055
Linear skull fracture, 372-373
Lingual tonsillitis, 1114, 1114f
Linton tube, for gastrointestinal bleeding, 225
Lip
    laceration of, 391, 1040
    skin of, 384-385
Lip reading, 2905

Lipase
    in acute pancreatitis, 1430-1431
    serum
        in abdominal trauma, 495
        in nausea and vomiting, 203
Lipid-lowering therapy, rhabdomyolysis from, 1979
Lipoatrophy, insulin, 1971
Lipohyalinosis, 1608
Lipohypertrophy, insulin, 1971
Lipovnik virus, 2047
Lisfranc's joint
    anatomy of, 820, 820f
    fractures and dislocations of, 551t, 828-831, 829f, 830f
    sprains of, 838
Lisinopril, 1322t
Listeria infection, in cancer patient with impaired cell-mediated immunity, 2839-2840
Lister's tubercle, 581, 583f, 625
Lithium
    drug interactions with, 2442, 2443t
    for bipolar disorder, 1742
    hypercalcemia from, 1945
    toxicity of, 2442-2444, 2443t
Lithotripsy, extracorporeal shock wave
    for cholelithiasis, 1419
    for urolithiasis, 1593
Little leaguer's elbow, 663, 663f, 2710-2711
Livedo reticularis, 1347, 1357
Liver. *See also* Hepatic *entries.*
    alcohol metabolism in, 2859
    cancer of, 1417
    enlarged, in hepatitis, 1404
    fatty
        alcoholic, 2868
        in pregnancy, 1417, 2755-2756
    gluconeogenesis in, 1956
    in immune response, 2831
    injury to
        acetaminophen-induced, 2332-2333, 2334-2335, 2336, 2337
        drug-induced, 1413-1414, 1414t
        in children, 342
        in heatstroke, 2262
    transplantation of, 1417-1418, 2337, 2854-2855, 2854f
    trauma to, 489, 490, 491, 497f
Liver disorders, 1402-1418
    alcoholic, 1407, 1409, 2867-2868
        cirrhosis in, 1410
        hepatitis in, 1405, 1409
    chronic, end stage, 1410-1411. *See also* Cirrhosis.
    drug-induced, 1413-1414, 1414t
    encephalopathy in, 1411-1412, 1411t
    in HIV/AIDS, 2084
    in pregnancy, 1416-1417, 2755-2756
    inflammatory. *See* Hepatitis.
    spontaneous bacterial peritonitis in, 1412-1413
Liver enzymes
    in acetaminophen overdose, 2335
    in acute pancreatitis, 1431, 1431t
    in alcoholic hepatitis, 1409
    in amebic abscess, 1416
    in viral hepatitis, 1404
Liver function tests
    in abdominal trauma, 495
    in nausea and vomiting, 203
Living will, 3133
Lizards, venomous, 896, 898-899, 902
LOAD mnemonic, in rapid sequence intubation, 10, 11b
Lobar atelectasis, in chronic obstructive pulmonary disease, 1102
Local anesthesia, 2914b, 2930-2933, 2931t, 2932b, 2932t
    allergy to, 846-847, 1827, 2931
    buffering in, 846, 2932-2933, 2932b
    in calcific tendinitis, 698
    in wound care, 846
    ophthalmic, 1063b, 1064
    profiles of agents used for, 2930-2931, 2931t, 2932t
    toxicity of, 2931-2932
Local area network (LAN), 3104
Local disaster preparedness, 3017
Local gas gangrene, 2208

Local wound exploration, in abdominal trauma, 501
Locus ceruleus
    in anxiety disorders, 1744
    in mood disorders, 1735
Logistic regression models, 3055
Loiasis
    drug therapy for, 2100t
    visual disturbances in, 2110
Loma Prieta earthquake, 3016, 3017
Longitudinal studies, types of, 3047
Long-range handgun wounds, 957, 957f
Loop diuretics, 1321t
    for acute pulmonary edema, 1270t, 1272
    for chronic heart failure, 1276
Loperamide
    for diarrhea, 236t
    for traveler's diarrhea, 1487
Loratadine, during pregnancy and lactation, 2790
Lorazepam, 2484, 2484t
    for agitation in delirious patient, 1654
    for alcohol withdrawal syndrome, 2862, 2863
    for alcohol-related seizure, 2864, 2865
    for anxiety disorders, 1750
    for neuroleptic malignant syndrome, 2449
    for psychedelic-induced intoxication, 2408
    for psychostimulant intoxication, 2410
    for rapid tranquilization, 2962-2963
    for seizure, 166, 166t, 1626, 1627t, 1919
    for status epilepticus, 2672-2673, 2672t
    for thought disorders, 1731
    prophylactic, in severe head trauma, 361
Lordosis, in pregnancy, 2727
Losartan, 1322t
Low-back pain. *See* Back pain.
Lower airway obstruction, pediatric, 2532-2552
    in anaphylaxis, 2546-2550
    in asthma, 2532-2544
    in bronchiolitis, 2544-2546
    in foreign body aspiration, 2550-2551, 2551f
Lower esophageal sphincter, defective, in gastroesophageal reflux, 1388
Lower extremity
    aneurysm of, 1354
    escharotomy of, 924
    immobilization of, 569-571, 570f, 572f, 573f
    isolated mononeuropathy of, 1694b, 1697-1699
    ulcers of, 1350-1351, 1971
    vascular injury of, 546-547
    venous anatomy of, 1368-1369
Lower gastrointestinal bleeding, 220-227
    diagnostic approach to, 220-223, 221b
    differential diagnosis in, 220, 221b, 223
    disposition in, 225-227, 225b, 226t
    management of, 223-225, 223f
Lower leg
    arteries of, 540f, 797
    trauma to, 796-805
        anatomy and physiology in, 797
        compartment syndrome and, 804
        foreign bodies and, 805
        Osgood-Schlatter disease in, 799
        proximal extra-articular tibial fracture in, 797-799
        proximal fibula fracture in, 801-802, 802f
        proximal tibiofibular joint dislocation in, 802-803
        soft tissue injuries in, 547, 804-805
        stress fracture in, 803-804
        tibial shaft fracture in, 799-801, 801f
Lower respiratory tract infection
    in bronchiolitis, 2544-2546
    in pertussis, 2004-2007, 2005f, 2006b, 2559-2560
    in pneumococcal disease, 2016-2020, 2020b
    in pneumonia, 1128-1141, 2554-2564. *See also* Pneumonia.
Lower sulcus examination, in red and painful eye, 286
Lower urinary tract trauma
    bladder injuries in, 519-526, 521f-526f
    urethral injuries in, 515-519, 516f-520f
Low-molecular-weight dextran, for frostbite, 2233
Low-molecular-weight heparin
    advantages of, 1188
    during pregnancy and lactation, 2757, 2786

Low-molecular-weight heparin *(Continued)*
    for acute coronary syndromes, 1187-1188
    for deep vein thrombosis, 3065-3066
Lown classification of premature ventricular contractions, 1225, 1225t
Lown-Ganong-Levine syndrome, 1237
Low-output states, arterial embolism vs., 1352
Loxapine, 2446t
LSD (lysergic acid diethylamide), 2406-2408, 2407f
Lubeluzole, after cerebral ischemia, 71
Lubricants, for constipation, 241t, 242
Ludington's test, in biceps tendon rupture, 697
Ludwig's angina, 1028, 1032, 1118-1119
Lugol's iodine solution, for thyroid storm, 1989
Lumbar disk herniation, 432, 433f, 702-703, 704-705, 711-712
Lumbar plexus, 718
Lumbar puncture
    headache after, 1641
    in alcohol-related seizure, 2864
    in central nervous system infection, 1716, 1716b
    in cerebral venous thrombosis, 1670-1671
    in delirium, 1652
    in headache, 172, 173t
    in subarachnoid hemorrhage, 1636
    pediatric
        contraindications to, 2660
        in bacterial meningitis, 2659-2662, 2660b, 2661t, 2661t
        in febrile seizure, 2507
        in headache, 2679
        in seizure, 2671
        procedure for, 2660-2661, 2661f
    traumatic, 1717-1718
Lumbar spine
    anatomy of, 400f, 702, 702f
    vertebral osteomyelitis in, 2184
Lumbar vertebrae, 399, 400f
Lumbosacral plexopathy, 1692-1693, 1693b
Lumbosacral plexus, 1676
Lumbosacral spine, 702, 702f
Lumbrical muscles, 580, 581f
Lunate
    anatomy of, 622, 623f, 625
    dislocation of, 630, 632f
    fracture of, 629
Lung. *See also* Cardiopulmonary; Pulmonary; Respiration; Respiratory.
    abscess in, 1033, 1134, 1134f
    cancer of
        hypercalcemia in, 1914
        superior vena cava syndrome in, 1909
    collapsed. *See* Pneumothorax.
    examination of
        in chest pain, 187t
        in dyspnea, 178t
        in fever, 135
    fetal, 119
    infarction of, pulmonary embolism with, 1373
    transplantation of, 2855-2856
    uremic, 1542
Lung disease. *See* Pulmonary disorders; *specific diseases, e.g.,* Pneumonia.
Lung infection. *See* Respiratory tract infection.
Lung injury. *See* Pulmonary trauma.
Lungfluke, 2101t, 2110-2111
Lunotriquetral ligament, 622, 624f
Lunula, 589
Lupus erythematosus
    drug-induced, 1809, 1809t
    systemic, 1805-1812
        clinical features of, 1806-1808, 1806b
        diagnosis of, 1808
        disposition in, 1811-1812
        epidemiology of, 1805
        immune thrombocytopenia in, 1896-1897
        in pregnancy, 1810, 2775-2776
        management of, 1808-1810
        myocarditis in, 1297
        oral manifestations of, 1035, 1035f
        panniculitis in, 1817
        pathophysiology of, 1806
        pericarditis in, 1284
        skin lesions in, 1862t, 1863f
Luxatio erecta, 692-693, 692f-694f
Lye, ingestion of, 2380, 2381, 2381t

Lying, pathologic, in Munchausen's syndrome, 1762
Lyme disease, 2118-2129
    acute disseminated infection in, 2123-2124, 2128
    arthritis in, 1788-1789, 2124, 2126
    carditis in, 2123-2124, 2128
    clinical features of, 2119, 2121f, 2122-2125
    diagnosis of, 2125
    differential considerations in, 2126
    early, 2122-2123, 2122f, 2123t, 2127-2128
    epidemiology of, 2119, 2120f
    facial paralysis in, 1667, 1668
    in pregnancy, 2128-2129
    late, 2124-2125, 2128
    management of, 2126-2128, 2127t
    mononeuropathy multiplex in, 1699-1700
    myocarditis in, 1291-1292
    neurologic disorders in, 2123, 2128
    ophthalmologic disorders in, 2124
    vaccine for, 2126-2127
    vertigo in, 2683
Lymph node(s)
    in head and neck, 1075, 1075f
    regional, in tularemia, 2131
Lymphadenitis, tuberculous, 2158
Lymphadenopathy
    cervical
        in African trypanosomiasis, 2106
        in Kawasaki disease, 2026
        in peritonsillitis, 1117
        in pharyngitis, 1109, 1110f
    in genital herpes, 1558
    in plague, 3027
    in rubella, 1850
    in tuberculosis, 2152, 2152f
    inguinal, in lymphogranuloma venereum, 1562
    mediastinal, differential diagnosis in, 2157
Lymphangitis, traumatic, of penis, 534
Lymphatic system, of hand, 586
Lymphocyte(s), function of, 1886
Lymphocyte count
    and hematopoietic involvement in radiation exposure, 2322
    normal values for, 1886t
    radiation dose and, 2317t, 2321
Lymphocytic choriomeningitis virus, 2055
Lymphocytic leukemia
    acute, 1888
    chronic, 1888
Lymphocytosis, 1887b, 1888
    in leukemia, 1888
    in pneumonia, 2561
Lymphogranuloma venereum, 1518t, 1519, 1557t, 1559f, 1562
Lymphohematogenous dissemination of tuberculosis, 2147-2148
Lymphoma
    acute tumor lysis syndrome in, 1911
    central nervous system, in HIV/AIDS, 2082
    central nervous system infections in, 1920
    Hodgkin's, radiation-induced pericarditis in, 1284
    hyperuricemia in, 1913
    immune thrombocytopenia in, 1897
    superior vena cava syndrome in, 1909
Lymphomatoid granulomatosis, 1814
Lymphoproliferative disorders, in HIV/AIDS, 2079
Lysergic acid diethylamide, 2406-2408, 2407f
Lyssavirus, rabies from, 2065
"Lytic" cocktail, for procedural sedation and analgesia, in children, 2954

Mach effect, 558
Machupo virus, 2056
Macrocytic anemia, 1873-1875, 1874f, 1874t, 1875t
Macrocytosis, in alcoholism, 2873
Macroglobulinemia, Waldenstrom's, hyperviscosity syndrome in, 1912
Macroglossia, 2522
Macrolides
    during pregnancy and lactation, 2784
    for otitis media, 1069
Macrophage, 2834
Macula, 1045f

Macular disorders, 1059, 1059f, 1970
Macular purpura, 1839t
Macules, 1839t, 1844-1848
MADFOCS mnemonic, 1729t
Magnesium
    as antidysrhythmic drug, 1212
    for alcohol withdrawal syndrome, 2863
    imbalance of. See Hypermagnesemia; Hypomagnesemia.
    normal physiology of, 1947
Magnesium antacids, for upper gastrointestinal disorders, 1398
Magnesium sulfate
    for asthma, 1087t, 1089-1090, 2542
    for atrial flutter, 1229
    for atrial tachycardia, 1228
    for cardiac arrest, 93
    for diabetic ketoacidosis, 1966
    for digitalis toxicity, 2371
    for dysrhythmia, 2586b
    for eclamptic seizure, 1627-1628, 1627t
    for hypomagnesemia, 1949
    for junctional tachycardia, 1234
    for pediatric resuscitation, 104
    for premature ventricular contractions, 1225
    for tetanus, 2011
    for torsades de pointes, 113, 1244
    for ventricular tachycardia, 1242
    in pregnancy
        for asthma, 2762
        for eclamptic seizure prophylaxis, 2750, 2751
        for myocardial infarction, 2766
        for premature labor, 2806, 2806b
Magnesium wasting, in alcoholic hepatitis, 1409
Magnet, for pacemaker malfunction, 1251-1252, 1251b, 1252f-1254f
Magnetic resonance angiography
    in ischemic stroke, 1613
    in peripheral arteriovascular disease, 1348
Magnetic resonance cholangiopancreatography, in pancreatitis, 1433
Magnetic resonance imaging
    in abdominal trauma, 499
    in airway foreign body aspiration, 867
    in ankle trauma, 811
    in aortic dissection, 1327t, 1328
    in appendicitis, 1455
    in arthritis, 1780
    in back pain, 708, 709f
    in central nervous system infection, 1719-1720
    in cerebral venous thrombosis, 1670
    in deep venous thrombosis, 1370
    in delirium, 1651
    in epidural abscess, 708, 709f
    in foot trauma, 822
    in fracture, 558
    in frostbite, 2231
    in headache, 2679
    in hip fracture, 746
    in ischemic stroke, 1613
    in knee extensor tendon injuries, 783
    in knee ligament injuries, 791
    in knee trauma, 774-775
    in Legg-Calvé-Perthes disease, 2707
    in meniscal tears, 793
    in minor head trauma, 365
    in multiple sclerosis, 1673, 2910
    in osteomyelitis, 2181-2182, 2182f
    in peripheral vascular injury, 542
    in pregnancy, 2730
    in pregnant trauma patient, 321
    in scaphoid fracture, 628
    in seizure, 2671
    in septic arthritis, 2190
    in severe head trauma, 362, 362t
    in soft tissue foreign body, 879
    in spinal carcinoma, 712-713
    in spinal cord disorders, 1680
    in spinal injuries, 431-435, 433f-436f
    in tendinopathy, 1780
    in vertebral osteomyelitis, 2182f, 2185
    in vertigo, 146
Magnetic resonance spectroscopy, in multiple sclerosis, 2910
Magnetic resonance venography, in cerebral venous thrombosis, 1670
Magnolia officinalis, 2476

Ma-huang
    abuse of, 2893
    adverse effects of, 2476t
    drug interactions with, 2478t
Maisonneuve fracture, 551t, 802, 802f, 814f
Major basic protein, in asthma, 1081
Major burn injury, 920
Major histocompatibility complex antigens, 2833
Malabsorption
    alcohol consumption and, 2868-2869
    in chronic pancreatitis, 1435
Malaise
    in infective endocarditis, 1301
    in pneumonia, 2556
Malar erythema, in systemic lupus erythematosus, 1863f
Malaria
    anemia in, 2107, 2107f
    cerebral, 2104f, 2105
    drug therapy for, 2101t-2102t
    fever in, 2099, 2103-2104, 2104f
    visual disturbances in, 2110
Malathion, for Phthirus pubis infestation, 1569
Male
    cystitis in, 1585
    genitalia of, anatomy of, 516f
    hypogonadism in, 2871
    pyelonephritis in, 1585
    sexual assault of, 992
    urinary tract infection in, 1573, 1574, 1585-1586
    urine collection methods in, 1575
Malgaigne fracture, 551t, 727
Malignant disease. See Cancer.
Malignant hypertension, 1315
    acute renal failure in, 1535
    dialysis for, 1548
Malignant hyperthermia, 14, 2257
Malignant otitis externa, 1071
Malingering, 1761-1765, 2980
    clinical features of, 1763
    diagnosis of, 1764, 1764b
    differential considerations in, 1764
    disposition in, 1765
    management of, 1765
    somatoform disorders vs., 1757
    visual loss and, 1061
Mallampati score, 4, 5f
Malleolar fractures, 812-813, 813f
Mallet finger, 605-607, 606f, 607f
Mallory-Weiss tears, from vomiting, 201
Malnutrition
    hypothermia and, 2239
    in AIDS-related diarrhea, 1483
Malpighian layers, 914
Malpresentations, in labor and delivery, 2811-2816, 2811b, 2811t, 2812f, 2813b, 2814f, 2815f, 2816b
Malrotation
    of metacarpal or phalangeal fracture, 594, 594f, 595f
    of phalangeal fractures, 595
    with midgut volvulus, 2606-2608, 2607f, 2608f
Malunion, 564
    in Colles' fracture, 633
    in phalangeal fracture, 595
Mammalian bite. See Animal bite; Human bite.
Managed care, medical screening examination and, 3161-3162
Management decision making, 127, 131t, 132
Mandible, 384
    anatomy of, 1026, 1027f
    dislocation of, 1041-1042, 1041f
    fracture of, 394-395, 395f
Mandibular division of trigeminal nerve, 384
Maneuvers for diagnosis and treatment of dysrhythmias, 1214-1215
Mania, 1738-1739, 1738b
    differential considerations in, 1741
    stabilization in, 1741
    substance-induced, 1740, 1740b
Mannitol
    for acute renal failure, 1538, 2650
    for cerebral herniation, 1918
    for ciguatera fish poisoning, 1473-1474
    for closed-angle glaucoma, 1056
    for elevated intracranial pressure, 360, 367
    for heatstroke, 2264
    for hyperuricemia, 1914

Mannitol (Continued)
  for rhabdomyolysis, 1982
  neuroprotective effects of, 360
  preoperative, in arterial injury, 544
Mann-Whitney test, 3053
Mantoux test, 2156-2157, 2157b, 2158t
Manual strangulation, 450
Maoexipril, 1322t
Maprotiline, overdose of, 2352, 2354
Marburg virus, 2054
March fracture, 551t
March hemoglobinemia, 1883
Marfan syndrome, 2901t
  aortic dissection in, 1324-1325
  sudden death in, 2597
Marijuana use, 2411-2412
  during pregnancy, 2792
  emergency department visits related to, 2884f
Marine animal envenomations, 908-911
Mask, for tuberculosis exposure prophylaxis, 2170
Mask continuous positive airway pressure, 28
Mask ventilation. See also Bag/mask ventilation.
  heated, 2249
  laryngeal. See Laryngeal mask airway.
  mechanical, 29
Masked depression, 1737
Mass
  abdominal
    in abdominal aortic aneurysm rupture, 1333
    in abdominal trauma, 494
    in children, 2646
  adnexal
    in ectopic pregnancy, 2743
    pelvic pain in, 250t
  anorectal, 1508-1509
  hypothenar, 576, 577f
  neck, 1075-1076, 1075f, 1076b
  red blood cell, in thermal burns, 918
  scrotal, 1593-1598
    anatomy and physiology in, 1594, 1594f
    differential considerations in, 1594-1598
    in children, 2638-2642, 2639f-2640f
Masseter spasm
  from succinylcholine, 14
  in tetanus, 2009
Mast cells
  activated, mediators of, 1823, 1823b
  in asthma, 1080-1081, 1080f
Mastication, muscles of, 1026, 1027f
Mastocytosis, 1835
Mastoiditis, 1071-1072
Material exploitation of elder, 1010
Material resources, in emergency medical services, 2987-2988, 2988f
Material safety data sheet, 3081, 3082b
Mauriceau maneuver, 2813
Maxillary division of trigeminal nerve, 384
Maxillary sinus, 1123
  teardrop sign in, from orbital wall fracture, 1044, 1045f
Maxillary sinusitis, 1034, 1124, 1124f, 1125f
McBurney's point, 1451, 1452
McGill forceps, for oropharyngeal foreign body removal, 1384
McMurray's test, in meniscal tears, 774
McRoberts' maneuver, in shoulder dystocia, 2815, 2815f
MDMA (methylenedioxymethamphetamine), 2408-2409, 2410-2411
  abuse of, 2894, 2895
  overdose of, 2392-2393
  rhabdomyolysis from, 1979
Mean corpuscular hemoglobin (MCH), 1871t
Mean corpuscular hemoglobin concentration (MCHC), 1871t
Mean corpuscular volume (MCV), 1871t
Measles, 2052-2053, 2053f
  Kawasaki disease vs., 2594
  screening for, 2509b
  skin lesions in, 1849
  vaccine for, 2035t, 2053
Mebendazole, for Enterobius vermicularis gastroenteritis, 1482
Mechanical obstruction of small bowel, 1440
Mechanical ventilation
  abdominal trauma after, 492
  basic approaches to, 26-27
  evolving therapies in, 33

Mechanical ventilation (Continued)
  in asthma, 1092-1093
  in burn care, 922
  in chronic obstructive pulmonary disease, 1103-1113, 1105t
  in flail chest, 458, 458b
  in sepsis, 2219
  in submersion victim, 2314
  in tetanus, 2011
  initial settings and ongoing monitoring in, 29-30, 29t
  intubation for. See Intubation.
  mask, 29
  outcomes in, 33
  patient management in, 30-31
  special clinical circumstances in, 31-32
  techniques in, 27-28
Meckel's diverticulum, 2613-2615, 2614t
Meckel's scan, 2613
Meclizine, for vertigo, 146
Meconium aspiration, resuscitation in, 120, 120f, 122
Media
  in disaster response, 3015
  violence and, 1018
Medial collateral ligament
  anatomy of, 770, 771f, 808, 809f
  injury to, 778, 791-792
  stress test of, 774
Medial condyle
  anatomy of, 647, 647f, 770, 771f
  fracture of, 660-661, 661f
Medial elbow dislocation, 665
Medial epicondyle
  avulsion of, in little leaguer's elbow, 663, 663f
  fracture of, 662-663, 662f
Medial epicondylitis, 1798-1799, 2710-2711
Medial malleolus
  anatomy of, 808, 809f
  fracture of, 813, 814f
Medial meniscus, injury to, 792-793
Medial orbital wall fracture, 393
Medial patellar retinaculum injury, patellar dislocation and, 785
Medial retinacula, 770, 771f
Medial tibiofemoral compartment, 770, 771f
Median nerve, 586-587, 588f, 589f, 622, 625f, 648, 648f
  compression of, in pregnancy, 2733
  injury to
    in Colles' fracture, 633
    in posterior elbow dislocation, 665
    palmaris longus laceration and, 609
    neuropathy of, 639, 639f, 1696-1697, 1697b, 1697f
    palsy of, 587, 588f
Mediastinal crunch, in pneumopericardium, 1288
Mediastinal hematoma, sternal fracture and, 456
Mediastinal irrigation, for rewarming in accidental hypothermia, 2250
Mediastinal widening
  abdominal trauma and, 510, 511f
  in aortic rupture, 478-479, 478f
Medical clearance, of combative patient, 2965
Medical decision making
  information technology for, 3098
  racism in, 3110
Medical director, EMS, 2989-2990
Medical disorders
  abdominal trauma vs., 501-502
  anxiety associated with, 1745-1746, 1746b
  depression associated with, 1739, 1739b
  in intimate partner violence and abuse, 997
  psychosis associated with, 1728-1729, 1728b, 1729t
  somatoform disorders vs., 1757, 1757b
Medical informatics, 3097
Medical information systems, electronic, 3098
Medical inquiry, in clinical decision making, 125-126, 127f, 130, 131t, 132
Medical liability
  in tactical emergency medical support, 3004-3005
  motive and, 3161
Medical literature
  electronic databases of, 3059
  evaluation of, 3046. See also Evidence-based medicine.
  publication bias in, 3050-3051, 3058

Medical procedures
  abdominal trauma from, 492
  esophageal perforation as, 482-483
Medical records
  electronic
    confidentiality and, 3103
    integration with, 3105
  of patient presenting to emergency department, 3162-3163
Medical review officer (MRO), 3080
Medical screening examination, 3160-3163
  documentation of, 3162-3163
  implementation of, 3160-3161
  patient withdrawal of request for, 3162
  registration and authorization in, 3161-3162
  requirements for, 3157-3158
  use of ancillary services in, 3160-3161
Medical specialty exceptions in disposition requirements, 3164
Medical students, in observation unit, 3063
Medical teaching/training, bioethical dilemmas in, 3135-3136
Medical threat assessment in tactical emergency medical support, 3004
Medication errors, 3125-3126, 3125t
Medications. See also Drug(s).
  abbreviations and notations to avoid for, 3125, 3125t
  caustic injuries from, 2381
  in prehospital care, 2987-2988, 2990-2991
Medicine, goals of, 3142-3143
Medicolegal issues, 3156-3173
  combative patient and, 2967-2969
  consent to medical care and, 3166-3169
  disposition requirements and, 3164-3165, 3165f
  emergency medical condition and, 3156-3157
  Emergency Medical Treatment and Active Labor Act and, 3156
  in blood transfusion, 58
  in intimate partner violence and abuse, 1004-1005
  in patient transfer during labor and delivery, 2797
  medical screening examination and, 3160-3163
  of combative patient, 2967-2969
  refusal of medical care and, 3169-3172
  reporting requirements and, 3172-3173
  screening requirements and, 3157-3158
  stabilization requirements and, 3163-3164
  testing requests and requirements and, 3158-3160
Meditation, for anxiety disorders, 1751
Medulla, vomiting center in, 200, 201f
Mefenamic acid, overdose of, 2343
Megacolon, toxic, 1501, 1502f, 2613, 2616
Megaloblastic anemia, 1873-1875, 1874f, 1874t, 1875t
  in alcoholism, 2873
  in pregnancy, 2768
Melasma gravidarum, 2728
Melena, 221
Meleney's synergistic gangrene, 2208
Membrane potential, 1199-1200, 1200f
Memory loss
  alcohol-induced, 2869
  in delirium, 1649
  in dementia, 1658-1659
  in head trauma, 363
Menarche, median age of, 2722, 2723f
Ménière's disease
  acoustic neuroma vs., 1669
  vertigo in, 146, 147t, 2683
Meningioma, acoustic neuroma vs., 1669
Meningismus
  in HIV/AIDS, 2079
  in Rocky Mountain spotted fever, 2134
Meningitis, 1710
  after basilar fracture, 370
  ancillary studies in, 1720
  bacterial
    ancillary studies in, 1720
    cerebrospinal fluid analysis in, 1716-1719, 1717t, 1718t, 1719f
    complications of, 1715
    diagnosis of, 1716-1720
    differential considerations in, 1720, 1721b
    disposition in, 1723
    epidemiology of, 1711

Meningitis *(Continued)*
etiology of, 1711-1712, 1711b, 1712b
lumbar puncture in, 1716, 1716b, 2659-2662, 2660b, 2661f, 2661t
management of, 1721-1723, 1721t
neuroimaging studies in, 1719-1720
pathophysiology of, 1713
pediatric, 2657-2665
clinical features of, 2658-2659, 2658t
diagnosis of, 2659-2663, 2660b, 2661f, 2661t
differential considerations in, 2663, 2663b
management of, 2663-2665, 2664t
pathophysiology of, 2657-2658
rash in, 2658, 2659
signs and symptoms of, 1714
cerebrospinal fluid analysis in, 1716-1719, 1717t, 1718t, 1719f
complications of, 1715-1716
cryptococcal, 2081
diagnosis of, 1716-1720
differential considerations in, 1720, 1721b
disposition in, 1723
epidemiology of, 1711
etiology of, 1711-1712, 1711b, 1712b
fungal
complications of, 1715-1716
management of, 1722
pathophysiology of, 1713
signs and symptoms of, 1714
headache in, 174t, 1641
host factors predisposing to, 1714t
in cancer patient, 1920
in Lyme disease, 2123
in meningococcal disease, 1711-1712, 1714, 1715, 1720, 1721t, 1722-1723, 2021-2022
in otitis media, 1068
in pneumococcal disease, 1711, 1714, 1715, 1720, 1721t, 1723, 2019
in tuberculosis, 2160-2161
complications of, 1715
in HIV/AIDS, 2082
management of, 2161
signs and symptoms of, 1714
spinal, 2161
lumbar puncture in, 1716, 1716b
management of, 1721-1723, 1721t
neuroimaging studies in, 1719-1720
noninfectious causes of, 1712b
pathophysiology of, 1713
risk factors for, 171b
seizure in, 1623, 2669
signs and symptoms of, 1714
viral, 2663, 2664
ancillary studies in, 1720
cerebrospinal fluid analysis in, 1716-1719, 1717t, 1718t, 1719f
complications of, 1715
diagnosis of, 1716-1720
differential considerations in, 1720, 1721b
disposition in, 1723
epidemiology of, 1711
etiology of, 1712, 1712b
lumbar puncture in, 1716, 1716b
management of, 1722, 1723
neuroimaging studies in, 1719-1720
pathophysiology of, 1713
signs and symptoms of, 1714
Meningococcal disease, 2020-2024
Henoch-Schönlein purpura vs., 2615
in children, 2506, 2507, 2509b
meningitis in, 1711-1712, 1714, 1715, 1720, 1721t, 1722-1723, 2021-2022
pediatric bacteremia in, 2506
Meningococcal vaccine, 1723, 2024
Meningoencephalitis
arboviral, 2049
in Lyme disease, 2123
seizure in, 1623
Meningomyelocele, neonatal resuscitation in, 121
Meniscal tears, 792-793
anterior cruciate ligament injury and, 790
stability testing in, 774
Menkes' kinky-hair syndrome, fracture in, 2701
Menstruation
asthma associated with, 1082
catamenial pneumothorax and, 1144
current, fibrinolytic therapy eligibility and, 1192
toxic shock syndrome and, 2028

Mental illness. *See* Psychiatric disorders.
Mental retardation, abuse of persons with, 1015
Mental space infection, 1029
Mental status, altered. *See also* Consciousness, altered.
alcohol-induced, 2869
categories of, 153, 154f
confusion as, 150
definitions of, 156-157
differential diagnosis in, 2397
fever and, 136, 2509b
headache and, 170
in adrenal insufficiency, 1997
in hemodialysis patient, 1551-1552, 1552b
in hyperglycemic hyperosmolar nonketotic coma, 1968
in ischemic stroke, 1609
in isopropyl alcohol poisoning, 2403
in methanol poisoning, 2396
in nonconvulsive status epilepticus, 2667
in PCP intoxication, 2891, 2892
in toxic shock syndrome, 2029
treatable causes of, mnemonic for, 157, 157t
Mental status examination, 151, 152f, 153f
in delirium, 1649-1650, 1650f
in systemic lupus erythematosus, 1811
in thought disorders, 1730
Meperidine, 2922t, 2923
during pregnancy and lactation, 2784
for acute pancreatitis, 1433
for migraine, 1633t, 1634
oral, 2920, 2925
pharmacology of, 2452
toxicity of, 2452, 2453t
vs. morphine, 2920-2921, 2920t
Mepivacaine, 2931t, 2932t
Meralgia paresthetica, 1698, 2733
6-Mercaptopurine, for inflammatory bowel disease, 1502
Mercury
antidotes to, 2329t
poisoning from, 2424-2426, 2425b, 2425t
sources of, 2425b
Meropenem, for febrile, neutropenic cancer patient, 2838t
Mersilene suture, 852t
Mesalamine, for inflammatory bowel disease, 1502
Mescaline, 2409, 2409f
Mesenteric adenitis, appendicitis vs., 2620
Mesenteric artery, superior, 1445
embolism of, 1445-1446, 1446b
thrombosis of, 1446
Mesenteric ischemia
abdominal pain in, 214t
acute, 1444-1449
clinical features of, 1446-1447
diagnosis of, 1447-1448, 1448f
differential diagnosis in, 1448
in mesenteric venous thrombosis, 1446, 1446b
in superior mesenteric artery emboli, 1445-1446, 1446b
in superior mesenteric artery thrombosis, 1446
management of, 1448
chronic, 1444-1445
nonocclusive, 1446, 1446b
Mesenteric tear, in seat belt injuries, 491
Mesenteric venous thrombosis, acute mesenteric ischemia in, 1446, 1446b
Mesoridazine, toxicity of, 2445, 2446t
Mesothelioma, pericardial, 1916
Meta-analysis, 3057-3058
Metabolic acidosis, 1926-1930, 1927f, 1931b. *See also* Ketoacidosis.
dialysis for, 1549
etiology of, 1927-1929, 1927b
high anion gap, 1927-1929, 1927b
delirium in, 1651
in cyanide poisoning, 2437
in ethylene glycol poisoning, 2399, 2400-2401
in methanol poisoning, 2396, 2397
seizure in, 1622
in abdominal trauma, 495
in acute renal failure, 1539, 2650
in diarrhea, 2624
in salicylate overdose, 2340

Metabolic acidosis *(Continued)*
management of, 1929-1930
physiologic compensation in, 1929
renal compensation in, 1923-1924
with normal anion gap, 1927b, 1929
Metabolic alkalosis, 1930-1931, 1931b
causes of, 1930, 1930b
from vomiting, 201
renal compensation in, 1924
saline-resistant, 1931
saline-responsive, 1930-1931
Metabolic changes, in pregnancy, 2724
Metabolic disorders
delirium in, 1648, 1649
in acute tumor lysis syndrome, 1912
in opioid overdose, 2454
in substituted phenol poisoning, 2464
myopathy in, 1708-1709, 1978
neuropathy in, 1692
seizure in, 1622
Metabolic encephalopathy, in cancer patient, 1920-1921
Metabolic optic neuropathy, 1060
Metacarpal arches, 578, 580f
Metacarpal base fracture, 599
Metacarpal bones, 577-578, 579f-580f
Metacarpal fracture, 595-600, 597f-599f
Metacarpal head fracture, 596-597, 597f
Metacarpal neck fracture, 597-598, 597f, 598f
Metacarpal shaft fracture, 598-599, 598f
Metacarpophalangeal joint, 578, 579f
dislocation of
finger, 602-603, 602f, 603f
thumb, 603-604
extensor tendon injuries at, 608
laceration of, with metacarpal head fracture, 596-597
stability testing of, 601
Metal, elemental, skin injuries from, 937
Metal detector
in esophageal foreign body, 872
in esophageal obstruction, 1383
Metal poisoning, 2418-2426
arsenic in, 2423-2424, 2424b
iron in, 2418-2421, 2419t, 2420f, 2420t
lead in, 2421-2423, 2422t
mercury in, 2424-2426, 2425b, 2425t
Metaphyseal fracture, 2699
Metaphyseal spurs, normal-variant, 2699
Metaphysis, 2175, 2175f
Metaplasia, Barrett's, 1389
Metaproterenol, for chronic obstructive pulmonary disease, 1105
Metaraminol, for junctional tachycardia, 1234
Metastatic cancer
epidural spinal cord compression in, 1919
hyperuricemia in, 1913
Metatarsal base fractures, 832-834, 833f
Metatarsal bones
fractures of, 831-836
stress fracture of, 837
Metatarsal head and neck fractures, 832
Metatarsal shaft fractures, 831-832
Metatarsalgia, 837
Metatarsophalangeal dislocations, 835
Metered-dose inhaler plus spacer/holding chamber
for asthma, 2538, 2539t, 2540
for chronic obstructive pulmonary disease, 1105
instructions for, 1094b
nebulizer vs., 1087-1088
Metformin, 1972-1973
alcohol interactions with, 2877
during pregnancy and lactation, 2790
lactic acidosis from, 1928-1929
Methadone, 2922t, 2925
for opioid withdrawal, 2455
respiratory effects of, 2453t
Methamphetamine, 2393, 2893-2896
Methanol poisoning, 2395-2398, 2887
antidotes to, 2329t
disposition in, 2402
management of, 2400-2402, 2401t
metabolic acidosis in, 1928
pharmacology and metabolism in, 2395, 2396f
vs. ethylene glycol poisoning, 2397-2398
Methantheline, anticholinergic toxicity of, 2345

Methazolamide, for increased intraocular pressure, 292
Methcathinone, 2393, 2893
Methemoglobinemia, 268, 269b, 269f, 273, 936, 2889, 2891. *See also* Cyanosis.
Methemoglobin-forming agents, antidotes to, 2329t
Methicillin-nafcillin, for pneumonia, 2558t
Methicillin-resistant *Staphylococcus aureus*, 1130
Methimazole
    for hyperthyroidism in pregnancy, 2773
    for thyroid storm, 1988
Methohexital
    as induction agent, 15
    for procedural sedation and analgesia, 2940t-2941t, 2945-2946, 2949-2950, 2951t, 2953
Methotrexate, 2844
    for ectopic pregnancy, 2746
    for rheumatoid arthritis, 1791
Methoxamine, for junctional tachycardia, 1234
Methyl mercury poisoning, 2425, 2426
Methyldopa, 1321t, 2789
Methylene blue
    for methemoglobinemia, 273
    for nitrite abuse, 2890
Methylene chloride, toxicity of, 2887
Methylergonovine, after miscarriage, 2742
Methylparaben, allergy to, 847
Methylprednisolone
    for anaphylactic shock, 54
    for anaphylaxis, 2549
    for asthma, 1088, 2539t, 2541, 2543t
    for chronic obstructive pulmonary disease, 1106
    for Goodpasture syndrome, 1816
    for hypothermia, 2246
    for multiple sclerosis, 1673
    for optic neuritis, 1059-1060
    for rheumatologic disease, 2776
    for spinal cord injury, 309
    for spinal injuries, 438
    for systemic lupus erythematosus, 1809
    for temporal arteritis, 1060
Methylxanthines
    for asthma, 1090, 1090t
    for chronic obstructive pulmonary disease, 1105
    for postdural puncture headache, 1641
Methysergide, for migraine prophylaxis, 1634
Metoclopramide
    alcohol interactions with, 2875
    for gastroesophageal reflux, 1390
    for migraine, 2680
    for nausea and vomiting, 206
Metolazone, 1321t
Metoprolol, 1209, 1321t
    during pregnancy and lactation, 2788
    overdose of, 2373t
Metronidazole
    during pregnancy and lactation, 2758, 2785
    for amebic abscess, 1416
    for amebic dysentery, 235
    for bacterial vaginosis, 1567t, 1568
    for *Clostridium difficile* enterocolitis, 1475
    for *Giardia* gastroenteritis, 1479-1480
    for tetanus, 2011
    for trichomoniasis, 1567-1568, 1567t
Metropolitan Medical Response Systems, 3019
Mexican beaded lizard, 896, 902
Mexiletine, 1207
Mezlocillin, for cholangitis, 1422
Miconazole, during pregnancy and lactation, 2785
Microangiopathic hemolytic anemia, 1883
Microbiology
    in sepsis, 2216-2217
    in tuberculosis, 2154-2157, 2154f, 2157b, 2158t
Microcytic anemia, 1871-1873
Micrognathia, 2522
Microhematuria
    in bladder rupture, 521
    in kidney trauma, 528
    in pelvic fracture, 719
    in ureteral trauma, 531
Microreentry, 1204
Microscopic polyangiitis, 1813-1814
Microscopy, direct, in tuberculosis, 2154, 2154f

Microsomal ethanol-oxidizing system (MEOS), 2859
Microwave irradiation, 2319
    for rewarming in accidental hypothermia, 2250
Midazolam, 2484, 2484t
    as induction agent, 16
    for anxiety disorders, 1750
    for procedural sedation and analgesia, 2940t-2941t, 2944-2945
        in children, 2953
        with fentanyl, 2950, 2951t
    for seizure, 166, 166t, 1626, 1627t
    for status epilepticus, 2672t, 2673
    for tetanus, 2011
    in ventilated patient, 30
Midcarpal joint
    anatomy of, 622, 623f
    collapse of, 631-632, 632f, 633f
Middle ear
    barotrauma to, 2281-2282, 2282f, 2286-2287, 2287t, 2292
    infection of. *See* Otitis media.
Middle phalanx
    extensor tendon injuries at, 607
    fracture of, 594-595, 594f-596f
Midface fracture, 393-394, 394f
Midfoot
    anatomy of, 820, 820f
    cuboid fracture of, 828
    cuneiform fracture of, 828
    dislocation of cuneiform, cuboid, or navicular bones of, 828
    Lisfranc injuries in, 828-831, 829f, 830f
    navicular fracture of, 827-828
    pain in, 837
Midgut volvulus, malrotation with, 2606-2608, 2607f, 2608f
Midline lethal granuloma, oral manifestations of, 1035
Midpalmar space infection, 617-618, 617f
Midrin, for migraine, 2680
Midtarsal joint
    anatomy of, 820, 820f
    injuries to, 827
Migraine, 1631-1634
    basilar artery, 1632
    clinical features of, 1631-1633
    diagnosis of, 1633
    differential diagnosis in, 1633
    hemiplegic, 1632
    ophthalmoplegic, 1632
    pathophysiology of, 1631
    pediatric, 2678-2679, 2678b
    prophylactic therapy for, 1634
    seizure in, 1624
    seizures vs., 2668
    status migrainosus and, 1632-1633
    treatment of, 1633-1634, 1633t
    types of, 2678-2679
    with aura, 1631, 1632, 1632b, 2678, 2678b
    without aura, 1631, 1632b, 2678, 2678b
Miliaria rubra, 2259
Miliary tuberculosis, 2152, 2159-2160, 2160f
Military Assistance to Safety and Traffic (MAST) program, 2995
Military forces, disaster response responsibility of, 3019
Milk thistle, adverse effects of, 2476t
Milk-alkali syndrome, hypercalcemia in, 1945
Milker's node virus, 2040
Milrinone
    for acute pulmonary edema in hypotensive patient, 1274
    for cardiogenic shock, 54
    for heart failure, 2583t, 2584
Mineralocorticoids
    excess of, metabolic alkalosis in, 1930
    replacement of, for adrenal insufficiency, 1998
Minimal sedation, 2938, 2939b
Minimally conscious state, 156
Mini-mental state examination, 151, 152f, 1650, 1650f
Minor. *See also* Adolescent; Child.
    consent to treatment on behalf of, 3167-3168
    emancipated, 3168
    mature, 3168
    refusal of medical care for, by parent or guardian, 3171
Minor burn injury, 920

Minoxidil, 1321t
Minute ventilation
    carbon dioxide arterial pressure and, 1923
    during acclimatization to high altitude, 2297-2298
    in metabolic acidosis, 1929
Miosis
    in nerve agent exposure, 3030
    in opioid overdose, 2453
    traumatic, 1049
Mirtazapine, overdose of, 2362-2363
Miscarriage, 2740-2742
    clinical features of, 2740-2741
    diagnosis of, 2741, 2741b, 2741t
    differential considerations in, 2741
    ectopic pregnancy vs., 2745
    management of, 2741-2742
    pathophysiology of, 2740
    terminology in, 2740
Misoprostol
    after miscarriage, 2742
    for upper gastrointestinal disorders, 1399
Mist therapy, for viral croup, 2526
Mites
    in HIV/AIDS, 2085
    skin lesions in, 1854-1855, 1854f
Mithramycin, for hypercalcemic cancer patient, 1916
Mitochondrial function, in shock, 42, 43f
Mitral insufficiency, heart failure in, 1265
Mitral regurgitation, 1306
    heart failure in, 1265
    in pregnancy, 2763t, 2767
Mitral stenosis, 1305-1306
    in pregnancy, 2763t, 2767
Mitral valve prolapse, 1304-1305, 1747
Mixed cryoglobulinemia, 1815
Mixed venous oxygen saturation, in shock, 50
MOANS mnemonic, for evaluation of difficult bag/mask ventilation, 4, 4b
Mobitz type I (Wenckebach) second-degree atrioventricular block, 1218-1219, 1218t, 1219b, 1220f
Mobitz type II second-degree atrioventricular block, 1218t, 1219-1220, 1220f
Moderate burn injury, 920
Moderate sedation, 2938, 2939b
Molar pregnancy, 2741, 2746-2747
Molindone, 2446t
Molluscum contagiosum, 1861f, 2040, 2085
Monash method for snakebite management, 899
Mongolian spots, 974, 975f
Monitoring, 35-40
    blood gas, 36-39
        capnography/capnometry in, 37-39, 38f
        pulse oximetry in, 36-37
        transcutaneous and conjunctival, 36
    blood pressure, 35-36
    cardiac. *See also* Electrocardiography.
        during cardiopulmonary resuscitation, 79-82, 80f-82f, 80t
        in hypothermia, 2245
        in myocardial infarction, 1173-1174, 1173f
    core temperature
        in heatstroke, 2263
        in hypothermia, 2244
    during procedural sedation and analgesia, 2942-2943
    during ventilatory support, 29-30, 29t
    fetal
        electronic, 2800
        in pregnant trauma patient, 39, 319, 323-324, 324f
    home, for apparent life-threatening event or SIDS, 2720
    in asthma, 1085
    in cardiac arrest, 79-82, 80f-82f, 80t
    in heart failure, 1269, 1270t, 2773
    in multiple trauma, 304, 305
    in shock, 50
Monkey hand, 587, 588f
Monkeypox virus, 2040
Monoamine oxidase inhibitors
    classification of, 2363b
    for anxiety disorders, 1751, 1751t
    hypertension in patient taking, 1313, 1314b
    meperidine interactions with, 2923
    overdose of, 2363-2365, 2363b-2365b, 2364t

Monocytes, 1886t
Monomethylhydrazine, overdose of, 2329t
Mononeuropathy
    common peroneal, 1698-1699, 1698f
    diabetic, 1669-1670, 1971
    isolated, 1693-1699, 1694b
    lateral femoral cutaneous, 1698
    median, 1696-1697, 1697b, 1697f
    radial, 1693-1695, 1694f
    sciatic, 1697-1698, 1698f
    ulnar, 1695-1696, 1695f, 1696f
Mononeuropathy multiplex, 1699-1700, 1699b,
    1971
Monosodium urate crystals, in synovial fluid,
    1781-1782
Monospot tests, in pharyngitis, 1111
Monteggia fracture-dislocation, 551t, 642, 642f,
    2697
Montelukast, for asthma, 1090
Mood disorders, 1734-1742. See also Bipolar
    disorder; Depression.
    caused by general medical condition, 1739,
        1739b
    cerebral anatomy and, 1735
    clinical features of, 1736-1740, 1736b, 1737b,
        1738b
    cyclothymic disorder and, 1739
    diagnosis of, 1740
    differential considerations in, 1740-1741
    epidemiology of, 1735
    genetics of, 1736
    hypothalamic-pituitary-adrenocortical system
        in, 1735-1736
    management of, 1741-1742, 1741b
    neurotransmitters in, 1735
    psychosocial theories of, 1736
    substance-induced, 1739-1740, 1740b
    suicide and, 1769
    with psychotic features, 1729
Mood stabilizers, for bipolar disorder, 1742
Moral rules, 3130, 3130b
Moraxella (Branhamella) catarrhalis, 1130
Morbilliform rash, drug-induced, 1844, 1844f
Moricizine hydrochloride, 1207
Morphine, 2921-2923, 2921t
    during pregnancy and lactation, 2784
    for acute coronary syndromes, 1184
    for acute pancreatitis, 1433
    for acute pulmonary edema, 1270t, 1271-1272
    for anxiety disorders, 1750
    for burn patient, 924
    for high-altitude pulmonary edema, 2304
    for hypoxic (tet) spells, 2580-2581
    for knee trauma, 776
    for pulmonary edema in chronic renal failure,
        1546
    for sickle cell disease, 1880
    meperidine vs., 2920-2921, 2920t
    oral, 2925
    respiratory effects of, 2453
Morrison's pouch, 498, 498f
Morton's neuroma, 837
Morulae, in ehrlichiosis, 2138
Motility disorders. See also Constipation;
        Diarrhea.
    esophageal, 1388, 1395-1396, 1397
    in opioid overdose, 2453
    small bowel, 1440, 1441b, 1443
Motive, medical liability and, 3161
Motor disturbances
    in cerebral palsy, 2904
    in ischemic stroke, 1609
    in multiple sclerosis, 1672
    in spinal cord disorders, 1678f, 1679
Motor examination
    in head trauma, 357
    in spinal injuries, 416, 417t
Motor function, developmental milestones in,
    2495-2497, 2496t
Motor innervation of hand, 586-587, 588f, 589f
Motor neuron disease
    clinical characteristics of, 1680t, 1703t, 1704
    in amyotrophic lateral sclerosis, 1700
    upper vs. lower, 1704t
Motor strength, grading score for, 1704b
Motor tracts, 1676, 1676f
Motor vehicle crashes. See also Pedestrian
        collisions.
    aortic injury from, 476, 477

Motor vehicle crashes (Continued)
    biomechanical risk factors in, 946-947
    cardiac trauma from, 467
    death from, 300
    facial trauma from, 382, 383
    forensic aspects of, 963-966, 964b, 965f-966f,
        966b
    hip dislocation from, 756
    in elderly person, 344-345
    in pregnancy, 318
    injury control in, 943, 943t, 944t, 946-947, 948
    mechanism of injury of, 303t
    myocardial contusion from, 467
    myocardial rupture from, 470
    spinal injuries from, 399
    sternal fracture from, 456
Motorcycle accidents
    death from, 300
    facial trauma from, 382
Mottling of skin, in pediatric assessment, 2499,
    2499f
Mountain sickness, acute, 2296, 2299, 2299f,
    2300-2303, 2301b
Mouth. See also Oral entries.
    anatomy of, 384
    laceration of, 391
Movement disorders
    alcohol-induced, 2870
    pediatric, ataxia as, 2681-2682, 2681b
    seizures vs., 2668
Moxifloxacin, for tuberculosis, 2164t, 2165
MPTP, parkinsonism caused by, 2452
Mucin clot test, in acute septic arthritis, 2705,
    2706t
Mucocutaneous hyperpigmentation, in Addison's
    disease, 1997
Mucocutaneous lymph node syndrome. See
    Kawasaki disease.
Mucokinetic medications, for chronic obstructive
    pulmonary disease, 1106
Mucormycosis, 1123, 1124, 1126
Mucous clearance strategies, for chronic
    obstructive pulmonary disease, 1106
Muerto Canyon virus, 2055
Multicollinearity, 3055
Multiculturalism, 3107-3117. See also Cultural
        competence.
Multifocal atrial tachycardia, 1228, 1229f
Multi-infarct dementia, 1657
Multiple comparisons, and risk of type I error,
    3053-3054
Multiple gestations
    incidence of, 2722
    labor and delivery in, 2816
Multiple myeloma
    hypercalcemia in, 1914
    hyperuricemia in, 1913
    hyperviscosity syndrome in, 1912
Multiple organ dysfunction syndrome (MODS)
    definition of, 2211
    in pancreatitis, 1427, 1429
    in sepsis, 2213-2214
    in solvent abuse, 2888
    trajectory of dying in, 3140-3141, 3140f
Multiple sclerosis, 1671-1674, 2909-2911
    anxiety in, 1747-1748
    ataxia in, 2682
    clinical features of, 1672
    diagnosis of, 1672-1673
    differential considerations in, 1673
    disposition in, 1674
    in pregnancy, 2763t, 2769-2770
    management of, 1673
    optic neuritis and, 1059
    pathophysiology of, 1671-1672
    seizure in, 1624
    spinal cord lesions in, 1681-1682
    vertigo in, 148t, 2684
Multiple trauma, 300-314
    clinical features in, 309-311, 310f
    diagnostic strategies in, 311-313, 313f
    disposition in, 311
    epidemiology of, 300
    etiology of, 302, 303t
    examination and reassessment in, 305
    in elderly person, 345
    management of, 302-309, 304b
    monitoring in, 305
    prehospital care in, 302-304

Multiple trauma (Continued)
    radiologic imaging in, 311-313, 313f
    stabilization in, 305-309
    team approach in, 304
    trauma system and, 300-302, 301f, 302b
Multiple victim incidents, prehospital end-of-life
    issues related to, 3145
Multisystem disease, in tuberculosis, 2159-2160,
    2160f
Multivariate models, 3054-3055
Mumps, 1428, 2052
Mumps vaccine, 2035t
Munchausen's syndrome, 1761-1765
    by proxy, 1761, 1763, 1763t, 1765
    clinical features of, 1763
    diagnosis of, 1764
    differential considerations in, 1764, 1764b
    disposition in, 1765
    management of, 1765
Mupirocin, for impetigo, 1842
Murmur
    in aortic regurgitation, 1307
    in aortic rupture, 478
    in aortic stenosis, 1306
    in arteriovenous fistulas, 1347
    in chronic obstructive pulmonary disease,
        1100
    in hypertrophic cardiomyopathy, 1295
    in infective endocarditis, 1301
    in mitral regurgitation, 1306
    in mitral stenosis, 1305
    in mitral valve prolapse, 1305
    in myocardial rupture, 471
    in tetralogy of Fallot, 2580
    in tricuspid stenosis and regurgitation, 1307
    innocent, 2572
    pediatric, 2571-2572, 2572b
Murphy's sign
    in cholecystitis, 1420
    in pancreatitis, 1429
Muscarinic acetylcholine receptors, 2345, 2346,
    2347f
Muscimol, 2479
Muscle
    of forearm, 640t
    of hand, 578, 580-585, 581f-585f
    of hip and thigh, 737, 737t, 738f
    of knee, 770, 771f
    of lower leg, 797
    of shoulder, 672, 673f
    of upper arm, 648
Muscle contraction headache, in pregnancy, 2732
Muscle cramps, heat-induced, 2258, 2258b
Muscle fasciculations, in nerve agent exposure,
    3030
Muscle relaxation, in reduction of glenohumeral
    joint dislocation, 688-689
Muscle spasm, in tetanus, 2009
Muscle weakness. See Weakness.
Muscles of mastication, 1026, 1027f
Muscular dystrophy, 2900t
Musculocutaneous nerve, 672
Musculoskeletal disorders
    in chronic renal failure, 1542-1543
    in developmentally disabled patient, 2901-
        2902
    pediatric, 2689-2711
        anatomy and physiology in, 2689
        apophyseal, 2709-2711, 2711f
        child abuse and, 2698-2701
        physeal, 2690, 2691f, 2691t, 2692, 2692f
        rhabdomyolysis as. See Rhabdomyolysis.
Musculoskeletal pain, during pregnancy, 2733
Musculoskeletal system
    aging and, 345
    examination of, in spinal cord injury, 310-311
    in pregnancy, 2727
Musculoskeletal trauma. See Orthopedic injuries.
Mushrooms
    anticholinergic, 2412-2413, 2412f
    cholinergic, 2413
    psilocybin, 2406-2408, 2407f
    toxicity of, 2477-2479, 2478t
Mustard exposure, 938-939, 3031
Mutilating injuries, to hand, 609
Muzzle contusion, 956, 956f
Myalgia
    during pregnancy, 2733
    in rhabdomyolysis, 1979

Myasthenia gravis, 1705-1707, 1706b
  diagnosis of, 1705-1706, 1706b
  exacerbation of, drug-induced, 1706, 1706b
  in pregnancy, 2764t, 2770-2771
  management of, 1706-1707
  oropharyngeal dysphagia in, 1397
  weakness in, 141
Mycobacterial infection
  fungal and nontuberculous, 2157
  in cancer patient with impaired cell-mediated
    immunity, 2840
  in organ transplant patient, 2849
Mycobacterium avium, 2076
Mycobacterium tuberculosis. See also
    Tuberculosis.
  in HIV/AIDS, 1136, 1140-1141, 2078-2079
  in pneumonia, 1130-1131
Mycobacterium tuberculosis direct test (MTDT),
    2155
Mycophenolate, 2844
  for organ transplant patient, 2850, 2851f
Mycoplasma pneumoniae, 1130, 1132
  in children, 2558-2559, 2563t
  in myocarditis, 1292
  in pharyngitis, 1109, 1111, 1112, 1113
Mycotic aneurysm, 1356, 1357t
Mydriasis
  in psychedelic intoxication, 2408
  pharmacologic, 1061
  traumatic, 1049
Mydriatics, 1063b, 1064
  for red and painful eye, 292, 297t
Myelitis, 1710
  transverse, 1682
Myeloid leukemia, chronic, neutrophilia in,
    1887-1888, 1887f
Myeloma
  hypogammaglobulinemia in, 2840-2841
  multiple
    hypercalcemia in, 1914
    hyperuricemia in, 1913
    hyperviscosity syndrome in, 1912
Myelopathy
  clinical characteristics of, 1680t, 1703t, 1704
  cystic, in spinal cord injury, 2909
  in HIV/AIDS, 1683
Myeloperoxidase, as cardiac marker, 1178
Myelophthisic anemia, 1876, 1876f
Mylohyoid muscle, 1027
Myocardial biopsy
  in dilated cardiomyopathy, 1294
  in myocarditis, 1290, 1290f
Myocardial cell action potential, 1200, 1201f,
    1202f
Myocardial cell membrane, electrophysiology of,
    1199-1201, 1200f-1202f
Myocardial concussion, 467
Myocardial contusions
  in children, 340
  observation in, 3068
Myocardial dysfunction, after resuscitation, 77
Myocardial fibrosis and scarring, heart failure
    from, 1263-1264
Myocardial hypertrophy, 1169-1170, 1172f. See
    also Hypertrophic cardiomyopathy.
Myocardial infarction. See also Acute coronary
    syndromes.
  anatomic location of, 1164-1166, 1164t, 1165f-
    1167f
  angina in, 1158, 1158t
  anterior, 1164, 1165f
  anxiety in, 1746
  atypical symptoms of, 1158-1159, 1159t
  cardiogenic shock in, 54, 1160
  chest pain centers and, 1181-1182
  chest pain in, 183, 186, 188, 189f, 190t-191t
  clinical features of, 1157-1161, 1158t, 1159t
  cocaine-related, 2391
  creatine kinase MB isoenzyme in, 1175f, 1176t,
    1177-1178
  definition of, 1156
  Dressler syndrome after, 1189-1190, 1283
  early complications of, 1160-1161
  echocardiography in, 1179
  electrocardiography in, 1161-1174
    abnormalities in, 1161-1163, 1162f-1164f,
      1162t
    additional lead, 1171-1173, 1172f, 1173f
    adjuncts in, 1171-1174

Myocardial infarction (Continued)
  anatomic location of infarct on, 1164-1166,
    1164t, 1165f-1167f
  body surface mapping and, 1174
  fibrinolytic therapy eligibility and, 1190
  limitations of, 1174
  noninfarct ST segment elevation and, 1166-
    1170, 1167f-1172f
  NSTEMI and, 1170-1171
  QT dispersion and, 1174
  serial, 1173-1174, 1173f
  epidemiology of, 1155
  free wall rupture in, 1160
  graded exercise testing in, 1180-1181
  heart failure in, 1268
  historical perspective of, 1155
  in aortic dissection, 1326
  in diabetes mellitus, 1970
  in elderly person, 2828
  in Kawasaki disease, 2025, 2026, 2595
  in left bundle branch block, 1167, 1170f
  in pregnancy, 2766-2767
  inferior, 1164, 1165f, 1166, 1167f
  ischemic stroke after, 1608
  lateral, 1164, 1165f
  management of
    angiotensin-converting enzyme inhibitors in,
      1185
    antiplatelet therapy in, 1185-1187
    antithrombotic therapy in, 1187-1188
    aspirin in, 1185
    beta blockers in, 1184-1185
    calcium channel blockers in, 1185
    chest pain centers and, 1181-1182
    delay in, reasons for, 1183
    direct thrombin inhibitors in, 1188
    fibrinolytic therapy in, 1189-1192, 1192b
    glycoprotein IIb/IIIa receptor inhibitors in,
      1186, 1194
    heparins in, 1187-1188
    morphine in, 1184
    nitroglycerin in, 1184
    percutaneous coronary intervention in, 1186,
      1192-1193, 1195
    physical examination in, 1159, 1159t
    prehospital care in, 1157
    reperfusion therapy in, 1189-1195
      choice of, 1193-1194
      combination, 1194-1195
      in cardiogenic shock, 1194
      process time points for, 1183, 1184f
      time to, 1182-1184, 1183f, 1184f
    thienopyridines in, 1186-1187
    time to treatment and, 1182-1184, 1183f, 1184f
    transfer of patient with, 1195
  missed diagnosis of, 1160
  myoglobin in, 1175f, 1176t, 1178
  nausea and vomiting in, 205t
  non-ST segment elevation, 1170-1171
  observation in, 3064, 3065
  outcome of, time to treatment and, 1182-1184,
    1183f, 1184f
  pathophysiology of, 1156-1157
  pericarditis in, 1160, 1282-1283
  pneumothorax vs., 1146
  posterior, 1166, 1166f
  previous, fibrinolytic therapy eligibility and,
    1191
  Q waves in, 1156, 1164
  radionucleotide scanning in, 1179-1180
  right ventricular, 1166, 1167f, 1172-1173
  ST segment abnormalities in
    monitoring in, 1173-1174, 1173f
    regional, 1164t
  ST segment depression in, 1162-1163, 1163f,
    1171
  ST segment elevation, 1161-1162, 1162t, 1163f
  stroke in, 1161
  T wave in
    hyperacute, 1161, 1162f
    inverted, 1163-1164, 1164f, 1171
  time from symptom onset in, fibrinolytic
    therapy eligibility and, 1190-1191
  transmural, 1156
  troponins in, 1175-1177, 1175f, 1176t
  without chest pain, outcomes in, 1159
Myocardial ischemia
  acute
    observation in, 3064, 3065

Myocardial ischemia (Continued)
  risk stratification in, 3065
  time insensitive predictive instrument for,
    3065
  chest pain in, 188t, 189f
  heart failure in, 1268
  hypertension in, 1316
  in hypomagnesemia, 1949
  in pathophysiology of acute coronary
    syndromes, 1156-1157
  orofacial pain in, 1034
Myocardial lavage, for rewarming in accidental
    hypothermia, 2250
Myocardial stunning, 77
Myocarditis, 1289-1293
  clinical features of, 1289
  cocaine-related, 1292-1293
  diagnostic strategies in, 1289-1290
  differential diagnosis in, 1290
  disposition in, 1290-1291
  doxorubicin-related, 1292
  epidemiology of, 1289
  etiology of, 1289
  heart failure in, 1264-1265, 1268
  in Chagas' disease, 1291
  in connective tissue disorders, 1297-1298
  in diphtheria, 1291
  in HIV/AIDS, 1292
  in infants and children, 2591-2592
  in Kawasaki disease, 1293, 2025, 2594
  in Lyme disease, 1291-1292
  in meningococcal disease, 2022
  in Rocky Mountain spotted fever, 2134
  in systemic lupus erythematosus, 1807
  in trichinosis, 1291
  management of, 1290
  pathophysiology of, 1289
  risk factors for, 186b
  sudden death in, 1298
Myoclonic seizure, 1621
Myoclonus
  alcoholic, 2870
  from etomidate, 2947-2948
Myofascial pain, temporomandibular, 1034-1035
Myofibrils, 1259
Myoglobin
  in myocardial infarction, 1175f, 1176t, 1178
  in renal pathology of rhabdomyolysis, 1977
  in sarcoplasm, 1976
  release of. See Rhabdomyolysis.
  urine, in rhabdomyolysis, 1980
Myoglobinuria
  in electrical and lightning injuries, 2276
  in heatstroke, 2264
Myonecrosis, 2196t, 2208-2209
Myonephropathic-metabolic syndrome, in arterial
    embolism, 1343
Myopathy
  alcohol-induced, 2870
  clinical characteristics of, 1680t, 1703t, 1704
  in hyperthyroidism, 1987
  inflammatory, 1708
  metabolic, 1708-1709, 1978
Myosin heavy chain, mutation of, in
    hypertrophic cardiomyopathy, 1294
Myositis, 2196t, 2208-2209
Myositis ossificans–heterotopic ossification, of
    femur and hip, 741-742, 743f-754f
Myringitis, bullous, 1066-1067
Myringotomy, for otitis media with effusion,
    1069-1070
Myxedema, in hypothyroidism, 1863f
Myxedema coma, 1990, 1990b, 1991, 1991b,
    1993-1994, 2239

NADH methemoglobin reductase deficiency,
    cyanosis in, 268
Nadolol, 1209, 1321t, 2373t, 2374
Naegleria infection, neurologic disorders in,
    2107
Nafcillin, for staphylococcal scalded skin
    syndrome, 1845
Nägele's rule, 2727
Nail
  ingrown, 837
  paronychia and, 614-615, 615f
  structural framework of, 589

Nail bed
  avulsion of, 611
  laceration of, 594, 611
  trauma to, 610-611
Nail matrix, 589
Nalbuphine, 2924, 2924b
Nalmefene, for opioid overdose, 2455
Naloxone
  for alcohol intoxication, 2860
  for alcohol withdrawal syndrome, 2861
  for opioid overdose, 2328, 2455
  for opioid reversal, 2948-2949
  for overdosed/poisoned patient, 2326
  for Wernicke-Korsakoff syndrome, 2869
  in neonatal resuscitation, 123t, 124
Naproxen, for migraine, 2680
Narcissistic personality disorder, 2979b
Narcotic, 2451. See also Opioid(s).
Narrow-complex tachycardia, 1226-1235
  atrial fibrillation as, 1230-1233, 1231f, 1232b,
    1232f
  atrial flutter as, 1229-1230, 1230f-1231f
  atrial tachycardia as, 1228-1229, 1228f, 1229f
  in infants and children, 2586-2587, 2588f
  junctional tachycardia as, 1233-1235, 1233f,
    1234f
  P wave in, 1234f
  sinus tachycardia as, 1227-1228, 1227f
Nasal capnography, in asthma, 1085
Nasal congestion, in bronchiolitis, 2545
Nasal flaring, in pediatric assessment, 2498-2499,
  2499f
Nasal pack, for epistaxis, 1074, 1075
Nasal polyp, 1082
Nasoethmoid complex fracture, 393-394
Nasogastric intubation
  esophageal perforation from, 483
  in abdominal trauma, 494
  in acute pancreatitis, 1433-1434
  in burn injury, 923
  in gastric volvulus, 1394
  in gastrointestinal bleeding, 223-224
  in hypothermia, 2244
  in neck trauma, 444
  in small bowel obstruction, 1444
Nasogastric suctioning, metabolic alkalosis from,
  1930
Nasotracheal intubation, 12
  esophageal perforation from, 483
  in multiple trauma, 306
  in neck trauma, 444
National Clinicians' Postexposure Prophylaxis
  Hotline, 3083
National Disaster Medical System, 3018
National Guideline Clearing House, 3037, 3037t
National Heart Attack Alert Program, 1181
National Institute on Drug Abuse, drug testing
  guidelines of, 3080
National Institute on Elder Abuse, 1009
National Institutes of Health Expert Panel Report
  2, on asthma diagnosis and management,
  1083
Natriuretic peptides, in heart failure, 1263, 1269-
  1270
Natural killer cells, 2833
Naturalistic process, clinical decision making by,
  127, 131t, 132
Nausea, 200-207
  ancillary studies in, 202-203
  chest pain associated with, 185, 186t
  definition of, 200
  differential considerations in, 201-202, 201t,
    203, 204t-206t, 207f
  disposition in, 207, 209
  epidemiology of, 200
  history in, 202
  in abdominal aortic aneurysm rupture, 1333
  in abdominal trauma, 493
  in Aeromonas hydrophila gastroenteritis, 1467
  in appendicitis, 2619
  in Bacillus anthracis gastroenteritis, 1469
  in cholecystitis, 1420
  in cholelithiasis, 1418
  in chronic renal failure, 1542
  in ciguatera fish poisoning, 1473
  in esophagitis, 1387
  in gastritis, 1391
  in hemorrhagic Escherichia coli serotype
    O157:H7 gastroenteritis, 1467

Nausea (Continued)
  in infants and children, 203, 208t
  in opioid overdose, 2453
  in pancreatitis, 1429
  in Plesiomonas shigelloides gastroenteritis,
    1468
  in pregnancy, 204t, 206, 2756
  in salmonellosis, 1463
  in Vibrio fish poisoning, 1472
  in Vibrio parahaemolyticus gastroenteritis,
    1466
  in viral gastroenteritis, 1476
  management of, 203, 206, 207f, 208b, 208t
  palliative care for, 3153-3154
  pathophysiology of, 200-201, 201f
  physical examination in, 202, 202t
  rapid assessment and stabilization in, 201t, 202
Navicular
  accessory, 822, 822f, 837
  dislocation of, 828
  fracture of, 827-828
  stress fracture of, 837-838
Nebulizer, for asthma, 1087-1088
Neck. See also Head and neck.
  examination of, in dyspnea, 178t
  mass in, 1075-1076, 1075f, 1076b
  mobility of, difficult airway and, 4
  nuchal rigidity and
    causes of, 2663
    in bacterial meningitis, 2658, 2659
    in central nervous system infection, 1714
  zones of, 442, 442f, 443b
Neck stiffness
  causes of, 2663
  in bacterial meningitis, 2658, 2659
  in central nervous system infection, 1714
Neck swelling
  in aortic rupture, 478
  in Bacillus anthracis gastroenteritis, 1469
  in diphtheria, 2003
  in spinal cord injury, 2906
  in superior vena cava syndrome, 1910
Neck trauma, 441-451
  airway management in, 444-445
  anatomy in, 442-443, 442f, 443b
  clinical features of, 443, 443b
  diagnostic strategies in, 443
  disposition in, 446
  laryngotracheal injuries in, 447-448
  management of, 443-446
  near-hanging and strangulation in, 450-451
  nerve injuries in, 450
  pathophysiology of, 441-442, 442t
  pharyngoesophageal injuries in, 446-447
  thoracic duct, glandular, and retropharyngeal
    injuries in, 450
  tracheobronchial injury in, 466, 466f
  transcervical gunshot wounds in, 446
  vascular injuries in, 448-450
  venous air embolism in, 444, 450
  vertigo in, 144, 147t
Neck vein distention
  in neoplastic cardiac tamponade, 1917
  in superior vena cava syndrome, 1910
Necrobiosis lipoidica diabeticorum, 1972
Necrotizing abscess, 1515
Necrotizing anorectal infection, 1515
Necrotizing cellulitis, synergistic, 2209
Necrotizing enterocolitis, 2608-2609, 2609f
Necrotizing fasciitis, 2196t, 2207-2208
Necrotizing otitis externa, 1071
Necrotizing ulcerative oral diseases, 1033, 1033f
Needle, suturing, 853
Needle aspiration
  in osteomyelitis, 2182
  in peritonsillar abscess, 1118
Needle cricothyroidotomy
  for airway foreign body, 2530
  in pediatric resuscitation, 108
Needle cricothyrotomy, with transtracheal jet
  ventilation, 22, 22f
Needle decompression, for pneumothorax, 1147
Needle electromyography, 1689
Neer classification
  of proximal humerus fractures, 680-681, 681f
  of subacromial syndromes, 694, 694t, 695f
Neer's test, in rotator cuff tendinopathy, 1797
Negative predictive value, 3059t
Negative pressure rewarming, 2248

Negative reactions of physicians, 2975-2976
Negative symptoms in schizophrenia, 1726,
  1728
Neglect
  child. See Child abuse.
  elder, 1010. See also Elderly person, abuse of.
Neisseria gonorrhoeae, 1518t, 1519, 1559t, 1565-
  1567, 1565f. See also Gonorrhea.
Neisseria meningitidis, 2021. See also
  Meningococcal disease.
Nematocysts, in marine animal envenomations,
  909, 910
Nematode infections, parasites in, 2099t
Neologisms, in schizophrenia, 1727-1728
Neomycin, for hepatic encephalopathy, 1412
Neonatal abstinence syndrome, 2794
Neonatal resuscitation, 118-124
  chest compressions in, 123
  discontinuation of, 120
  disposition in, 124
  in anatomic abnormalities, 121
  in late decelerations of fetal heart rate, 2801
  in meconium aspiration, 120, 120f
  indications for, 119-120
  medications in, 123-124, 123t
  oxygen therapy, ventilation, and intubation in,
    122-123
  positioning, suctioning, and stimulation in,
    121-122
  preparation for, 121, 121b
  transition from fetal to extrauterine life and,
    118-119, 119t
Neonate. See also Infant.
  acute bacterial meningitis in, 2657, 2658-2659
  air medical transport of, 2999
  Apgar score of, 122, 122t
  apnea in, 119
  assessment of, 2804
  circulation in, 2568-2569
  clavicle fracture in, 2693
  developmental milestones in, 2496, 2496t
  fever in, management of, 2512-2514, 2513b
  herpes simplex virus infection in, 1559
  hyperthyroidism in, 2773
  hypoglycemia in, 119
  hypomagnesemia in, 1948
  hypothermia in, 119, 2239
  hypoxia in, 119
  jaundice in, 2601-2603, 2602t, 2603b, 2603t,
    2604f-2605f
  lupus erythematosus in, 1810
  necrotizing enterocolitis in, 2608-2609, 2609f
  osteomyelitis in, 2183-2184
  otitis media in, 1067
  pulmonic flow murmur of, 2572
  red and painful eye and, 292
  seizure in, 2667
  urinary tract infection in, 1583, 1583t
  vital signs in, 119t
  vomiting in, 203, 208t
Neoplasm. See Tumor.
Neoplastic cardiac tamponade, 1916-1918
Neoplastic constrictive pericarditis, 1917
Neoplastic pericardial tamponade, 1916-1918
Neostigmine, for myasthenia gravis, 1706
Nephritis, lupus, 1806-1807
Nephropathy
  diabetic, in pregnancy, 1972
  heroin, 2453
  HIV-associated, 2086
  pigment, 1536, 1536b
Nephrotic syndrome
  in children, 2648-2649
  proteinuria in, 1531, 1531b
Nephrotomography, bolus infusion intravenous
  pyelography with, in renal trauma, 528
Nephrotoxicity
  of acetaminophen, 2333
  of cyclosporine, 2850
  of ethylene glycol, 2398, 2399
Nephrotoxins, acute tubular necrosis from, 1536-
  1537, 1536b, 1538, 1539
Nerium oleander, 2474, 2474f
Nerve block
  for trigeminal neuralgia, 1666
  intercostal, for multiple rib fractures, 456
Nerve conduction studies, 1689
Nerve gases, 939, 2458b, 2461, 3030-3031, 3030b,
  3031b

Nerve injury
  in electrical and lightning injuries, 2271
  in fracture, 559, 559t
  in hand trauma, 614
  in high-altitude cerebral edema, 2306
  in hip trauma, 762-763
  in neck trauma, 450
  in pelvic fracture, 719-720
  in supracondylar fracture, 2696-2697
Nerve supply
  to distal humerus and elbow, 648-649, 648f
  to face, 383-384
  to femur and hip, 737-738
  to foot, 821
  to forearm, 640t
  to hand, 586-587, 588f, 589f
  to knee, 771
  to lower leg, 797
  to shoulder, 672
  to wrist, 622, 625f
Nervous system. *See* Central nervous system;
    Neurologic *entries*; Peripheral nervous
    system.
Nesiritide, for acute pulmonary edema, 1270t,
    1272
Networks, in medical information systems, 3104
Neurapraxia, 559
Neurocysticercosis, seizure in, 1623
Neuroendocrine tumor, pancreatic, 1437
Neurofibrillary tangles, in dementia, 1657
Neurofibromatosis, vertigo in, 2683
Neurogenic bladder, in spinal cord injury, 2908
Neurogenic hypotension, secondary to spinal
    shock, 437
Neurogenic obstruction of small bowel, 1440
Neurogenic pulmonary edema
  after head trauma, 371
  after seizure, 1625
Neurohormonal alterations, in heart failure,
    1262-1263
Neuroimaging studies
  in central nervous system infection, 1719-1720
  in headache, 2679, 2680b
  in HIV/AIDS, 2079-2080, 2080f
  in minor head trauma, 364-365
  in severe head trauma, 361-362, 362t
Neuroleptic agents. *See* Antipsychotic agents.
Neuroleptic malignant syndrome, 2257-2258,
    2961-2962
  clinical features of, 2447, 2447t
  differential diagnosis in, 2448, 2448t
  from antipsychotic agents, 1732-1733
  management of, 2449
  serotonin syndrome vs., 2359
Neurologic abnormalities
  in acoustic neuroma, 1668-1669
  in acute renal failure, 1540
  in antidepressant overdose, 2354t, 2356
  in bacterial meningitis, 2658
  in carbon monoxide poisoning, 2439
  in central nervous system infection, 1714
  in cerebral venous thrombosis, 1670
  in cervical vascular injury, 449
  in chronic renal failure, 1542
  in ciguatera fish poisoning, 1473
  in electrical and lightning injuries, 2273-2274,
    2274
  in epidural abscess, 1684
  in epidural hematoma, 1683
  in ethylene glycol poisoning, 2399
  in head trauma, 370-371
  in headache, 172t
  in heatstroke, 2260-2261, 2262
  in hemodialysis patient, 1551-1552, 1552b
  in HIV/AIDS, 1683
  in hypothermia, 2241
  in idiopathic spastic paraparesis, 1683
  in intracerebral hemorrhage, 1611
  in ischemic stroke, 1609-1610
  in lithium toxicity, 2442
  in MAOI toxicity, 2365
  in mitral valve prolapse, 1305
  in multiple sclerosis, 1672, 1681
  in opioid overdose, 2452
  in organophosphate poisoning, 2460
  in osteogenesis imperfecta, 2700-2701
  in serotonin toxicity of, 2360
  in shigellosis, 1464
  in spinal subarachnoid hemorrhage, 1682

Neurologic abnormalities *(Continued)*
  in substituted phenol poisoning, 2464
  in syringomyelia, 1682-1683
  in systemic lupus erythematosus, 1807
  in transverse myelitis, 1682
  in vitamin B$_{12}$ deficiency, 1874
  mushrooms associated with, 2478-2479
Neurologic disorders, 1606-1723
  airway foreign body aspiration and, 866
  anxiety in, 1747-1748
  cranial nerve, 1664-1670, 1665t
  delirium in, 1645-1655
  dementia in, 1655-1662
  headache in, 1631-1643
  in botulism, 1707-1708, 2014
  in HIV/AIDS, 2079-2082, 2080f
  in Lyme disease, 2123, 2128
  in pregnancy, 2768-2771
  in Rocky Mountain spotted fever, 2134
  in spinal cord injury, 2909
  pediatric, 2657-2686
  peripheral, 1687-1701
  seizure in, 1619-1629
  spinal cord, 1675-1685
  stroke in, 1606-1617
Neurologic emergencies, in cancer patient, 1918-
    1921
Neurologic examination
  in back pain, 263
  in chest pain, 187t
  in comatose patient, 159-161, 159t
  in dyspnea, 178t
  in facial trauma, 388
  in head trauma, 356-357, 357t
  in multiple trauma, 309
  in nausea and vomiting, 202, 202t
  in seizure, 168
  in spinal injuries, 415-417
  in vertigo, 145
  of distal upper extremity, 2694t
Neuroma
  acoustic, 147t, 1668-1669
  Morton's, 837
Neuromuscular blocking agents
  competitive, for rapid sequence intubation,
    14-15, 15t
  for critically ill asthmatic patient, 1092-1093
  for intubation, 13-15
  for tetanus, 2011
  in intubated, mechanically ventilated patient,
    31
Neuromuscular disorders, 1702-1709
  clinical characteristics of, 1680t, 1703-1704,
    1703t
  diagnosis of, 1704-1705
  differential considerations in, 1703t, 1704
  history in, 1703
  in hyperkalemia, 1940
  laboratory studies in, 1704-1705
  oropharyngeal dysphagia in, 1396
  physical examination in, 1703-1704
  weakness and, 139, 139t, 140b, 1702-1709
Neuromuscular junction, 1703
Neuromuscular junction disease, 1705-1708
  clinical characteristics of, 1680t, 1703t, 1704
  in botulism, 1707-1708, 2014
  in myasthenia gravis, 1705-1707, 1706b
  in tick paralysis, 1708
Neuronal theory of headache, 2676
Neuronitis, vestibular, vertigo in, 147t
Neuronopathy
  in amyotrophic lateral sclerosis, 1700
  sensory, 1700, 1700b
Neuroophthalmologic visual loss, 1059-1061
Neuropathic pain, 1692
Neuropathy, 1687-1701. *See also*
    Mononeuropathy; Polyneuropathy.
  alcoholic, 1692, 2869
  anatomy in, 1688-1689, 1688f
  ancillary studies in, 1700-1701, 1701b
  asymmetric proximal and distal, 1692-1693,
    1693b
  autonomic
    diabetic, 1971
    in alcohol withdrawal syndrome, 2861
    in tetanus, 2009
  clinical features of, 1689-1700, 1703t, 1704
  cranial, 1664-1670, 1665t
    diabetic, 1669-1670

Neuropathy *(Continued)*
  eye movement disorders in, 1062-1063
  in ethylene glycol poisoning, 2399
  in Lyme disease, 2123
  in tetanus, 2009
  diabetic, 1669-1670, 1691-1692, 1970-1971
    in pregnancy, 1972
    lower extremity ulcers in, 1351, 1972
  epidemiology of, 1688
  in alcoholism, 1692
  in Guillain-Barré syndrome, 1690-1691
  in hip trauma, 762-763
  in HIV/AIDS, 1692, 2082
  in Lyme disease, 2124
  in plexopathies, 1692-1693, 1693b
  median nerve, 639, 639f
  metabolic, 1692
  optic
    compressive, 1060
    glaucoma as, 1055-1056, 1056f
    in ethylene glycol poisoning, 2399
    in methanol poisoning, 2395-2396
    ischemic, 1060
    toxic and metabolic, 1060
    traumatic, 1050-1051
  pathophysiology of, 1689
  patterns and prototypes of, 1690t
  peripheral vascular injury and, 539
  toxic, 1691b, 1692
Neuroprotective agents, for ischemic stroke,
    1616
Neuropsychiatric symptoms, in cocaine overdose,
    2388
Neurosis, hysterical, conversion type, 1755,
    1755b
Neurotmesis, 559
Neurotoxin
  botulinum, 2014
  tetanospasmin, 2009
Neurotransmitters
  in anxiety disorders, 1744-1745
  in delirium, 1646-1647
  in mood disorders, 1735
Neurovascular bundle, proximity wounds and,
    540, 540f
Neutron exposure, 2319-2320, 2320f
Neutropenia, 1888-1889, 1889t
  in cancer patient, 1907-1909, 1908b, 2834-
    2839, 2836t, 2838t
  in children, 2516
Neutrophil(s), 2834
  function of, 1886
  in arthritis, 1777
  in asthma, 1083
  in bacterial meningitis, 2662
  normal values for, 1886t
Neutrophilia, 1887-1888, 1887b, 1887f
Nevirapine, for HIV/AIDS, 2088
Newborn. *See* Neonate.
Nicardipine, 1321t
  for hypertensive emergencies, 1319
  for premature labor, 2807
  overdose of, 2377t
Nicotiana tabacum, 2474
Nicotine
  dermal exposure to, 2474
  ingestion of, 2474
  inhalation of. *See* Smoking.
Nicotinic acetylcholine receptors, 2345, 2347f
Nifedipine, 1321t
  during pregnancy and lactation, 2788
  for anal fissures, 1513
  for aortic dissection, 1329
  for chilblains, 2230
  for dysphagia, 1398
  for high-altitude pulmonary edema, 2304-2305
  for premature labor, 2807
  for thrombosed hemorrhoids, 1512
  overdose of, 2376, 2377t
Nifurtimox, for Chagas' disease, 2112
Night terrors, 2668
Nightstick fracture, 551t
Nikolsky's sign, in pemphigus vulgaris, 1857
Nimodipine
  for aneurysmal subarachnoid hemorrhage, 1637
  overdose of, 2377t
9-1-1 universal emergency access number, 2988
Nisoldipine, 1321t
  overdose of, 2377t

Nitrates
  abuse of, 936, 2889-2891, 2890b
  burn injury from, 936
  for chronic heart failure, 1276
  for urinary tract infection, 1575-1576
Nitric oxide
  in cerebral ischemia, 65-66
  in heart failure, 1263
  in sepsis, 2213
Nitrogen bubble formation, decompression
    sickness and, 2283-2284
Nitrogen narcosis, in scuba diving–related
    disorders, 2283, 2293
Nitroglycerin
  for acute coronary syndromes, 1184
  for acute pulmonary edema, 1270t, 1272
  for anal fissures, 1513
  for aortic dissection, 1329
  for chest pain, 184
  for hypertensive emergencies, 1318
  for pulmonary edema in chronic renal failure,
    1546
  for pulmonary edema–related hypertension,
    1316
Nitroprusside
  during pregnancy and lactation, 2765t, 2789
  for acute pulmonary edema, 1270t, 1272-1273
  for aortic dissection, 1328
  for heart failure, 2583t, 2584
  for hypertension
    in MAOI toxicity, 2365
    pulmonary edema–related, 1316
  for hypertensive emergencies, 1317-1318, 2653,
    2765t
  for hypertensive encephalopathy, 1315
  for intracerebral hemorrhage, 1616
  for pulmonary edema in chronic renal failure,
    1546
Nitrous oxide intoxication, solvent abuse vs.,
    2888
Nitrous oxide-oxygen mixtures, for procedural
    sedation and analgesia, 2929-2930, 2940t-
    2941t, 2948, 2950, 2951t
Nitrox I, 2279
Nits, in pediculosis, 1853, 1853f
Nizatidine, 1390t
NMDA receptor antagonists, after cerebral
    ischemia, 71
"No harm" contract, in suicide, 1773-1774
Nocardiosis
  in cancer patient with impaired cell-mediated
    immunity, 2840
  in organ transplant patient, 2848
Nociception, 2914-2916, 2915f, 2915t, 2916f,
    2916t
Nociceptor, 2914, 2914b
Nocturnal enuresis, 2668
Nodule, 1839t, 1856-1857
  in milker's node virus, 2040
  in molluscum contagiosum, 2040
  in tuberculosis, 2151
  subcutaneous, in rheumatic fever, 1304
Noise stress, during air medical transport, 2995
Noninvasive positive pressure ventilation
    (NPPV), 28-29, 28f
  evolving therapies in, 33
  in asthma, 1091-1092
  in chronic obstructive pulmonary disease,
    1104, 1104t
  initial settings and ongoing monitoring in, 29-
    30, 29t
  outcomes in, 32-33
  patient management in, 31
  patient selection for, 29
Nonmaleficence, 3129, 3129b
Nonnucleoside reverse transcriptase inhibitors,
    2087t, 2088
  rifamycins and, drug interactions between, 2166
Nonparametric statistical tests, 3053
Nonpenetrating ballistic injury, in chest wall
    trauma, 458-459
Nonshivering thermogenesis, in burned infant,
    923
Nonsteroidal antiinflammatory drugs, 2925-2926,
    2927b, 2927f
  alcohol interactions with, 2876
  allergy to, 1828
  aspirin-exacerbated respiratory disease from,
    1082

Nonsteroidal antiinflammatory drugs (Continued)
  during pregnancy and lactation, 2776, 2781,
    2784
  for back pain, 267
  for colic syndromes, 2926
  for dental caries pain, 1031
  for gouty arthritis, 1786
  for migraine, 1633, 1633t, 2680
  for pericarditis, 1282
  for pseudogout, 1787
  for reactive arthritis, 1790
  for rheumatoid arthritis, 1791-1792
  for sprain, 566
  for strain, 567
  for subacromial syndromes, 696
  for systemic lupus erythematosus, 1808
  for tendinopathy, 568
  gastritis from, 1390
  guidelines for, 2928
  heart failure from, 1269
  in elderly person, 2826
  mechanisms of action of, 2927f
  ophthalmic, 1063b, 1064
  overdose of, 2342-2344
  peptic ulcer disease from, 1392, 1394
  pharmacokinetics of, 2342-2343
  physiology of, 2342
  renal insufficiency from, 1533
  routes of administration of, 2927
  safety of, 2926
  side effects of, 2926-2927
Nonunion, 564
Noradrenergic system, in mood disorders, 1735
Norepinephrine
  for acute pulmonary edema in hypotensive
    patient, 1273
  for cyclic antidepressant poisoning, 2356
  for sepsis, 2219t, 2220
  in anxiety disorders, 1744-1745
  in glucose regulation, 1957
  in heart failure, 1263
  in mood disorders, 1735
Norfloxacin
  for Plesiomonas shigelloides gastroenteritis,
    1468
  for prostatitis, 1586
  for salmonellosis, 1463
  for shigellosis, 1461t, 1464
  for traveler's diarrhea, 1487
Normal-pressure hydrocephalus, dementia in,
    1658, 1660
Normeperidine, 2923
Normochromic and normocytic anemia, 1875-
    1876, 1875t, 1876f
Norovirus gastroenteritis, 1475-1476
Northern Command (NorthCom), 3019
Northridge earthquake, 3016, 3017
Norwegian scabies, 1854, 1855
Nose. See also Nasal entries.
  anatomy of, 384
  choanal atresia of, 2522
  examination of, in facial trauma, 388
  foreign body in, 863-864
  fracture of, 391-392
  medial wall of, arterial supply to, 1073,
    1073f
  soft tissue injuries to, 391
Nosebleed, 394, 863, 1072-1075, 1073f, 1074t
Notification
  death
    by phone, 3148
    empathy in, 3147-3149, 3148b
    training in, bioethical dilemnas in, 3135
  of foodborne diseases and conditions, 1463b
  to referring physician, computerized, 3102
Noxious stimulus, 2914b
Nuchal rigidity
  causes of, 2663
  in bacterial meningitis, 2658, 2659
  in central nervous system infection, 1714
Nuchal signs, as indication for lumbar puncture,
    2659
Nuclear explosion injury, 2316-2317, 2317t
Nuclear reactor incidents, 2317
Nuclear studies. See Radionucleotide scanning.
Nuclear weapons, disaster preparedness for,
    3017-3018, 3022
Nucleic acid amplification tests (NAATs)
  for chlamydia, 1565

Nucleic acid amplification tests
    (NAATs) (Continued)
  for gonorrhea, 1566
  for tuberculosis, 2154
Nucleoside analogue reverse transcriptase
    inhibitors, 1928, 2087-2088, 2087t
Nucleus pulposus
  anatomy of, 702, 702f
  herniation of, 702-703
Null hypothesis, 3051, 3051f
Number needed to treat, 3059t, 3060
Numbness, in frostbite, 2230
Nurse staffing, for observation, 3062
Nursemaid's elbow, 666, 666f, 2697-2698, 2697f
Nursery care, in emergency department, 2798,
    2798b
Nursing home, institutional abuse in, 1009, 1015
Nutcracker esophagus, 1397
Nutcracker fracture, 828
Nutmeg, 2409-2410
Nutrition. See also Diet.
  in acute pancreatitis, 1433-1434
  in burn injury, 918
Nutritional deficiency
  dementia from, 1656
  hypothermia and, 2239
  in AIDS-related diarrhea, 1483
Nylon suture, 852t
Nystagmus, 1062
  in PCP intoxication, 2891
  vertigo and, 142-143, 144-145, 145t
Nystatin
  during pregnancy and lactation, 2785
  for oral thrush, 1841

Obese patient
  pulmonary embolism in, 1380-1381
  slipped capital femoral epiphysis in, 2708
Obidoxime, for organophosphate poisoning,
    2461
Oblique fracture, 552, 552f
Oblique radiographs, of spinal injuries, 426-428,
    426f, 427f, 428f
Observation medicine, 3062-3073
  approach in, 3062-3063
  in abdominal pain, 3063-3064, 3064b
  in asthma, 3069-3070, 3070b
  in atrial fibrillation, 3070-3071, 3070b
  in chest pain, 3064-3065, 3065b
  in congestive heart failure, 3071, 3071b
  in critical diagnostic syndromes, 3063-3069
  in deep vein thrombosis, 3065-3066
  in dehydration, 3071-3072, 3072b
  in emergency conditions, 3069-3073
  in head trauma, 3069
  in infection, 3072-3073, 3072b, 3073t
  in peripheral vascular injury, 544
  in syncope, 3066-3067, 3066b
  in trauma, 3067-3069
  in upper gastrointestinal bleeding, 3066
  principles of, 3062, 3063b
  staffing requirements for, 3062-3063
Observation unit, structure of, 3063
Observational study, longitudinal, 3047
Obsessive-compulsive disorder, 1746b, 1749
Obstetric trauma, 318-326, 320-321, 2733
  blunt, 318
  diagnostic strategies in, 320-321, 320t, 321t
  disposition in, 326
  fetal evaluation in, 323-324, 323f, 323t, 324f
  fetal injury in, 319
  fetomaternal hemorrhage and, 321
  management of, 321-326, 322f
  maternal resuscitation in, 322-323
  penetrating, 318-319
  perimortem cesarean section in, 325-326
  placental injury in, 319-320
  prehospital end-of-life issues related to, 3145
  primary survey in, 322-323
  secondary survey in, 323
  uterine injury in, 320
Obstipation, in large bowel obstruction, 1496
Obstructive acute renal failure, 1533-1534,
    1533b, 1538
Obstructive biliary tract disorders, jaundice in,
    243, 244f
Obstructive pancreatitis, 1435

Obstructive pulmonary disorders, chronic, 1097-
1107. *See also* Chronic obstructive
pulmonary disease.
Obtundation, 156, 2865
Obturator dislocation, 756, 757f
Obturator hernia, 1441
Obturator sign, in appendicitis, 1452, 2619
Occlusive injury in peripheral vascular trauma,
537-538, 538f
Occult blood tests, in gastrointestinal bleeding,
222
Occupational health issues in emergency
department
blood-borne pathogen exposure protocol and,
3081-3087, 3084t, 3085t, 3086b
material safety data sheet and, 3081, 3082b
tuberculosis prevention and, 2170-2171,
2170b
Occupational medicine, 3076-3081
definition of, 3076
drug and alcohol testing in, 3080-3081
ethical issues in, 3077
overview of, 3076-3077
return-to-work issues in, 3078-3080
workers' compensation and, 3077-3078
Octreotide
for diarrhea, 236t
for gastrointestinal bleeding, 225
Ocular bobbing, 161
Ocular dipping, 161
Ocular foreign body, 859-861, 860f, 861f
Ocular hypertension, 1055
Ocular migraine, 2679
Ocular tonometry, in red and painful eye, 286-
287
Ocular trauma, 1044-1052
acid and alkali burns in, 1046, 1046f
blunt, 1044-1051
complications of, 1052, 1052f
in acid and alkali burns, 932
in anhydrous ammonia exposure, 935
in bipyridyl compound exposure, 2466
in child abuse, 971
in hydrofluoric acid exposure, 933
in methanol poisoning, 2395-2396
in mustard exposure, 3031
of anterior chamber and iris, 1048-1049, 1048f,
1049f
of cornea and conjunctiva, 1046-1048, 1047f-
1048f
of orbit and lid, 1044, 1045f, 1046, 1051-1052
of posterior segment, 1050-1051, 1050f
of sclera and lens, 1049-1050, 1050f
penetrating, 290, 1051-1052, 1051f
red and painful eye in, 283, 290, 292, 297
Oculocephalic testing
in comatose patient, 161
in head trauma, 357
Oculogyric crisis, antipsychotic-induced, 2446
Oculomotor nerve, 1665t
Oculovestibular testing
in comatose patient, 161, 162f
in head trauma, 357
Odds, 3059t
Odds ratio, 3059t
Odontalgia. *See also* Oral pain.
atypical, 1034
in scuba diving–related disorders, 2286
Odontoid fracture
type II, 405, 406f-407f
type III, 432f
with anterior dislocation, 399, 401, 402f
Odontoid radiographs, of spinal injuries, 424,
424f-425f
Odors, in poisoning, 2327, 2327t
Odynophagia
in achalasia, 1397
in esophagitis, 1387
in gastroesophageal reflux, 1388
in neck masses, 1076
Ofloxacin
for gonococcal dermatitis, 1843-1844
for pelvic inflammatory disease, 1571t
for prostatitis, 1586
Ogilvie's syndrome, 1495-1496
Ointment
for burn wounds, 926
ophthalmic, 1063
OKT3, for organ transplant patient, 2850-2851

Olanzapine
for agitation in delirious patient, 1654
for mood disorders, 1741
for rapid tranquilization, 2962
for thought disorders, 1730-1731
toxicity of, 2446, 2446t, 2448
Oleander, 2474, 2474f
Olecranon
anatomy of, 647, 647f
fracture of, 663
Olecranon bursa, 649
Olecranon bursitis, 667, 1801-1803
Olfactory nerve, 1665t
Oligoanalgesia, 2917-2918
Olmesartan, 1322t
Omeprazole, 1390t
Onchocerca volvulus, 2100t, 2109, 2109f
Oncologic emergencies, 1907-1921
acute tumor lysis syndrome in, 1911-1912,
1911b, 1912b
central nervous system infections in, 1920
cerebral herniation in, 1918
encephalopathy in, 1920-1921
epidural spinal cord compression in, 1919-
1920
fever in, 1907-1909, 1908b
hypercalcemia in, 1914-1916, 1915b
hyperuricemia in, 1913-1914
hyperviscosity syndrome in, 1912-1913
neoplastic cardiac tamponade in, 1916-1918
seizures in, 1919
superior vena cava syndrome in, 1909-1911,
1910f
Oncovirus, type C, 2056
Ondansetron
during pregnancy and lactation, 2790
for nausea and vomiting, 203
One-way analysis of variance (ANOVA), 3052-
3053, 3052t
Onychia, candidal, 1841
Open fracture, 552, 558, 558b
classification of, 749t
of ankle, 813-814
of hip, 748-749, 749t
of pelvis, 719
of skull, 373-374
of tibial shaft, 800-801
Open-book pelvic fracture, 727, 728f, 733f
Open-chest cardiac massage, 89-90
Ophthalmia, sympathetic, 1052
Ophthalmic division of trigeminal nerve, 383-384
Ophthalmic drugs, 1063-1064, 1063b
Ophthalmologic conditions, 1044-1064
acute visual loss and, 1056-1061, 1057f-1059f
anatomy in, 1045f
anisocoria and, 1061-1062
corneal disease and, 1053-1054, 1054f
epidemiology of, 1044
extraocular movement disorders and, 1062-
1063
eyelid and ocular soft tissue disorders and,
1054-1055, 1055f
glaucoma and, 1055-1056, 1056f
in Graves disease, 1987
in HIV/AIDS, 2085-2086, 2085f-2087f
in Lyme disease, 2124
in opioid overdose, 2453
nystagmus and, 1062
ocular trauma and, 1044-1052. *See also* Ocular
trauma.
ophthalmic drugs for, 1063-1064, 1063b
optic disk abnormalities and, 1062
Ophthalmologic system, in pregnancy, 2727
Ophthalmologists, disposition requirements
related to, 3164
Ophthalmoplegia, in diabetes mellitus, 1669-
1670
Ophthalmoplegic migraine, 1632, 2679
Opioid(s), 2918-2926
adjuvant analgesic agents with, 2921
agonist-antagonist group of, 2924-2925, 2924b
allergy to, 1828
classification of, 2921t-2922t
common therapeutic mistakes in, 2918-2921,
2919b
during pregnancy, 2784, 2793-2794
for abdominal pain, 217, 2925-2926
for acute pancreatitis, 1433
for appendicitis, 1456

Opioid(s) *(Continued)*
for back pain, 264, 267
for chronic pancreatitis, 1436
for dental caries pain, 1031
for migraine, 1633t, 1634
for procedural sedation and analgesia, 2940t-
2941t, 2944, 2952-2953
for sickle cell disease, 1880
for urolithiasis, 1592
in children, 2935, 2952-2953
in elderly person, 2826-2827
in HIV/AIDS, side effects of, 2079t
in rapid sequence intubation, 11b
in ventilated patient, 31
injection of
medicolegal issues in, 3159
skin lesions associated with, 1864-1865,
1865f, 2453-2454
intramuscular, disadvantages of, 2919-2920,
2919b
mechanism of action of, 2918, 2918t
oral, 2925
overdose of, 2327t, 2328, 2451-2456
antidotes to, 2329t
clinical features of, 2452-2454, 2453t
diagnosis of, 2454
differential diagnosis in, 2454
disposition in, 2455
management of, 2454-2455
pathophysiology and pharmacology of, 2451-
2452
parenteral, 2921-2924
patient given, informed consent in, 3169
receptors for, 2451
reversal agents for, 2948-2949
withdrawal from, 2451-2456
alcohol withdrawal syndrome vs., 2860
clinical features of, 2454
diagnosis of, 2454
differential diagnosis in, 2454
disposition in, 2455
management of, 2455-2456
pathophysiology and pharmacology of, 2452
Opioid receptors, 2918, 2918t
Opioid/sedative/ethanol syndrome, 2327t, 2328
Opisthorchis felineus, 2101t
Opium tincture, for diarrhea, 236t
Opponens digiti minimi, 580-581, 581f
Opponens pollicis, 580, 581f
Opportunistic infections
after liver transplantation, 1417
allograft rejection and, 2848-2849, 2849f
in cancer patient, that mimic neoplasms, 2841
respiratory, 1135-1136
Opsoclonus-myoclonus syndrome, ataxia in,
2681
Opsonin, 2834
Opsonization, 2833
Optic disk papilledema, 1062
Optic nerve, 1045f, 1665t
blunt injury to, 1050-1051
Optic neuritis, 1059-1060
in multiple sclerosis, 1672, 2910
Optic neuropathy
compressive, 1060
glaucoma as, 1055-1056, 1056f
in ethylene glycol poisoning, 2399
in methanol poisoning, 2395-2396
ischemic, 1060
toxic and metabolic, 1060
traumatic, 1050-1051
Oral cavity
examination of, 1029-1030, 1029f, 1030f
pyogenic granuloma in, 1035
Oral contraceptives, hepatotoxicity of, 1414
Oral flora, 1128
Oral hemorrhage, 1036, 1042
Oral hypoglycemic agents, 1972-1973
alcohol interactions with, 2877
overdose of, hypoglycemia from, 1961
rash from, 1972
Oral infection, extension of, into head and neck,
2229, 2230-2231, 2232f
Oral medicine
acute necrotic ulcerative gingivitis and, 1033,
1033f
alveolar bone fracture and, 1040
anatomy in, 1026-1027, 1027f-1030f
aphthous stomatitis and, 1036

Oral medicine (Continued)
  atypical odontalgia and, 1034
  blood dyscrasias and, 1036
  dental caries and, 1028-1029, 1030-1032,
    1030f, 1031f
  drug-induced gingival hyperplasia and, 1036
  examination of oral cavity in, 1029-1030, 1029f
  nontraumatic dental emergencies and, 1027-
    1029, 1030f
  oral hemorrhage and, 1042
  oral manifestations of systemic disease and,
    1035, 1035f
  oral pain and, 1033-1034
  paroxysmal pain of neuropathic origin and, 1034
  pathophysiology of, 1027-1029
  pericoronitis and, 1035
  periodontal disease and, 1032-1033
  postextraction pain and, 1034
  soft tissue injuries and, 1040
  subluxated and avulsed teeth and, 1037-1040,
    1038f, 1039f
  temporomandibular joint dislocation and,
    1041-1042, 1041f
  temporomandibular myofascial pain
    dysfunction syndrome and, 1034-1035
  tooth fracture and, 1036-1037, 1036f
Oral mucosa
  in Kawasaki disease, 2026
  laceration of, 391, 1040
    antibiotic prophylaxis for, 855
  ulcers of, 1036
Oral pain
  atypical, 1034
  dental caries and, 1030-1031
  in acute necrotic ulcerative gingivitis, 1033,
    1033f
  in cracked tooth and split root syndromes,
    1033-1034
  in maxillary sinusitis, 1034
  in pericoronitis, 1035
  in pulp exposure, 1037
  in sinusitis, 1124
  in temporomandibular myofascial pain
    dysfunction syndrome, 1034-1035
  paroxysmal, of neuropathic origin, 1034
  periapical abscess and, 1033
  postextraction, 1034
  root canal, 1033
Oral pharynx, visibility of, assessment of, 4, 5f
Oral rehydration therapy
  for diarrhea, 234-235
  for pediatric infectious diarrhea, 2629-2630,
    2630t
  for Vibrio fish poisoning, 1472
Oral thrush, 1840-1841
Oral ulcers, 1036
  in Behçet's disease, 1814
  in HIV/AIDS, 2083
OraQuick test, for HIV, 2074
Orbit
  contusion of, 1044
  examination of, in facial trauma, 387-388
  foreign body in, 1051-1052
  hemorrhage of, 1046
Orbital cellulitis, 293t, 2197-2198
Orbital emphysema, 393, 1044, 1045f
Orbital fracture, 393
Orbital hematoma, 393
Orbital septum, laceration through, 1051
Orbital tumor, red and painful eye in, 294t
Orbital wall fracture, traumatic, 1044, 1045f
Orbivirus, 2047
Orchitis, 1598
  in children, 2639
  in mumps, 2052
Order entry systems, computerized, 3043, 3043f,
  3101, 3102f
Orelline/orellanine, in mushrooms, 2479
Organ damage, in sickle cell disease, 1881, 1881t
Organ radiosensitivity, 2321, 2321f
Organ system dysfunction
  definition of, 2211
  in pancreatitis, 1427, 1429
  in sepsis, 2213-2214
  in solvent abuse, 2888
  trajectory of dying in, 3140-3141, 3140f
Organ transplant patient, 2846-2856
  complications in, 2847-2851, 2850t, 2851f
  disposition of, 2856

Organ transplant patient (Continued)
  drug toxicity in, 2849-2851, 2850t, 2851f
  heart, 2851-2854, 2852f, 2853f
  immune defects in, 2846-2847
  immunosuppressive therapy for, 2849-2851,
    2850t
  infectious complications in, 2847-2849, 2847b
  kidney, 2855
  liver, 2854-2855, 2854f
  lung, 2855-2856
  pancreas, 2856
  rejection in, 2848-2849, 2849f
Organic brain syndrome, 1645-1662. See also
  Delirium; Dementia.
Organoaxial volvulus, 1394
Organogenesis, drug exposure during, 2781
Organophosphate poisoning, 2457-2461, 2458b,
    2459b, 2459f
  antidotes to, 2329t
  as chemical weapon, 939, 3030-3031, 3030b,
    3031b
O'Riain wrinkle test, in nerve injuries, 559
Ornithodoros tick, 2117
Oropharyngeal anthrax, 3026
Oropharyngeal disorders, in HIV/AIDS, 2083
Oropharyngeal dysphagia, 1396-1397
Oropharynx
  examination of
    in airway foreign body aspiration, 866
    in facial trauma, 388
  foreign body in, 870, 1384
  inflammation or irritation of. See Pharyngitis.
Orphaned patient, as problem area in emergency
  care, 3124-3125
Orthodromic tachycardia, in Wolff-Parkinson-
  White syndrome, 1235, 1237
Orthomyxovirus, 2034t, 2054-2055
Orthopedic consultation, for ankle fractures, 812,
  812b
Orthopedic infections, 2174-2194. See also
  Osteomyelitis; Septic arthritis.
Orthopedic injuries. See also specific anatomic
  locations.
  ankle, 808-820
  dislocations in, 564-566, 565f. See also
    Dislocation.
  elbow and humerus, 647-668
  femur and hip, 735-768
  foot, 820-839
  forearm, 639-644
  fractures in, 552-564. See also Fracture.
  hand, 589-618
  in spinal cord–injured patient, 2909
  injury prevention and control in, 940-950
  knee, 770-796
  low back pain and, 701-715
  lower leg, 796-805
  management principles in, 549-552, 550t-551t
  pelvic, 717-734
  shoulder, 670-699
  soft tissue injuries in, 566-568. See also Soft
    tissue injuries.
  subluxation in, 564-566. See also Subluxation.
  treatment modalities for
    casts in, 571-573, 573f
    splinting and bandaging in, 568-571, 569f,
      570f
    thermal therapy in, 573-574
  wrist, 622-639
Orthopedic repair, vascular repair vs., 544
Orthopedic surgeons, disposition requirements
  related to, 3164
Orthopnea, 176, 177
  in heart failure, 1269
Orthoses, knee, in Osgood-Schlatter disease, 799
Orthostatic hypotension
  from antipsychotic agents, 1732
  in spinal cord injury, 2906
Orthostatic proteinuria, 1531, 2647
Orthotic supports, in sesamoid fractures, 835
Ortolani reduction maneuver in developmental
  hip dysplasia, 2701, 2702b
Orungo virus, 2047
Os acromiale, 680
Os peroneum, 822, 822f, 837
Os tibiale externum, 822, 822f, 837
Os trigonum, 822, 822f
Os trigonum syndrome, 836
Os vesalianum, 822, 822f

Osborn wave, in hypothermia, 2237, 2238f
Oseltamivir
  for influenza, 2055
  indications for, 2037-2038
Osgood-Schlatter disease, 798, 799, 2710
Osmol gap, elevated
  differential diagnosis in, 2397
  in ethylene glycol poisoning, 2400
  in isopropyl alcohol poisoning, 2403
  in methanol poisoning, 2397
Osmotic agents
  for constipation, 241t, 242
  for elevated intracranial pressure, in severe
    head trauma, 360
Osmotic diarrhea, 228, 2624
Osmotic equilibrium, 1933
Ossicles, accessory, of foot, 821-822, 822f
Ossification, heterotopic
  after tibial femoral knee dislocation, 790
  of femur and hip, 741-742, 743f-754f
Ossification centers
  in elbow, 652, 652f, 653t, 2694, 2694f, 2694t
  in hip, 763, 763f
Osteitis, alveolar, acute, 1034
Osteoarthritis, 1787
  of hip, 739, 739f-741f
  of knee, 796
Osteochondral fracture
  of talar dome, 824-825, 825f
  patellar dislocation and, 786
Osteochondritis dissecans, in knee trauma, 781-
  782
Osteochondroma, in femur, 742, 745f
Osteoclast inhibitors, for hypercalcemia, 1946
Osteocytes, 2175
Osteodystrophy, renal, 1542-1543
Osteogenesis imperfecta, 975, 2700-2701, 2700f,
  2700t, 2901t
Osteoid osteoma, in femur, 742, 745f
Osteomyelitis, 558, 2174-2187
  anatomy in, 2174-2175, 2175f
  chronic, 2186
  classification of, 2174
  clinical features of, 2179-2186
  complications of, 2186
  cranial, after head trauma, 371
  diagnostic imaging in, 2179-2182, 2179f-2183f
  differential considerations in, 2186
  disposition in, 2187
  epidemiology of, 2174
  etiology and microbiology of, 2177-2179, 2178t
  hematogenous, 2175-2176, 2183, 2184f
  history in, 2179
  imaging in, 2179f-2182f
  in children, 2183-2184, 2184f, 2516
  in diabetic foot, 2185-2186
  in hand, 618
  in sickle cell anemia, 2186
  in tuberculosis, 2159
  laboratory studies in, 2179
  management of, 2186-2187, 2189t
  pathophysiology of, 2175-2176
  pediatric limp and, 764-765
  physical examination in, 2179
  posttraumatic, 2185
  skull-base, 1071
  vertebral, 261, 265t, 2159, 2178, 2182, 2182f,
    2184-2185
Osteonecrosis
  after fracture, 562
  after talar fracture, 824
  in knee trauma, 782
  in scuba diving–related disorders, 2286
  of femoral head, 739-741, 741b, 742f
    after femoral neck fracture, 740, 742f, 750-
      751
    pediatric, 767
  of proximal femoral epiphysis, 2706-2707,
    2707f
Osteopenia of prematurity, 975
Osteoporosis, of femur, 739, 739f-741f
Ostiomeatal complex, 1123
Otalgia
  differential diagnosis in, 1068
  in mastoiditis, 1072
  in neck masses, 1076
  in otitis externa, 1070
  in otitis media, 1067
  referred, 1076

Otic encephalitis, in otitis media, 1068
Otitis externa, 1070-1071
    facial paralysis and, 1667
    necrotizing (malignant), 1071
Otitis media, 1066-1070
    acute, 1066, 1068-1069, 1069t, 1070t
    chronic suppurative, 1066, 1067
    facial paralysis and, 1667
    mastoiditis and, 1071
    recurrent, 1066
    screening for, 2509b
    with bronchiolitis, 2545
    with effusion, 1066, 1069-1070
Otolaryngologic conditions, 1066-1077
    epistaxis and, 1072-1075, 1073f, 1074t
    mastoiditis and, 1071-1072
    neck masses and, 1075-1076, 1075f, 1076b
    necrotizing otitis externa and, 1071
    otitis externa and, 1070-1071
    otitis media and, 1066-1070, 1069t, 1070t
    sialolithiasis and, 1075
    sudden hearing loss and, 1072, 1073b
Otolith, 142
Otomycosis, 1070-1071
Otorrhea
    in malignant otitis externa, 1071
    in otitis externa, 1070
    in otitis media, 1067
Ototoxic drugs, vertigo from, 2683
Ottawa Ankle Rules, 810-811, 3036, 3042
Ottawa Knee Rule, 774
Outcome data, collection of, 3050
Ovarian abscess, 248, 251t
Ovarian cyst, 251t
Ovarian torsion, 251t
Oven cleaner, ingestion of, 2381t
Overcrowding in emergency department, 3120-3121
Overdose. See Poisoning/overdose.
Overdose history, 2326, 2326b
Overflow proteinuria, 1531
Overuse injuries
    of foot, 836-838
    of knee, 793-796
    tendinopathy and bursitis in, 1794-1801
Overwhelming postsplenectomy infection (OPSI), 2018
Ovulation, cyclic, hormonal role in, 2723
Oxacillin, for pneumonia, 2558t
Oxalic acid, in ethylene glycol poisoning, 2398
Oxalosis, facial auditory nerve, in ethylene glycol poisoning, 2399
Oxazepam, 2484, 2484t
Oxidative stress, in chronic obstructive pulmonary disease, 1098
Oxime therapy, for organophosphate poisoning, 2461
Oxprenolol, overdose of, 2373t
Oxycodone, 2920, 2921t, 2925
    during pregnancy and lactation, 2784
    for migraine, 2680
    respiratory effects of, 2453t
Oxycontin, 2920
Oxygen
    desaturation of, in rapid sequence intubation, 10, 10f
    partial pressure of
        altitude and, 2297, 2307, 2307f
        cerebral blood flow and, 351-352, 351f
        conjunctival, 36
    saturation of
        during cardiopulmonary resuscitation, 82, 82f
        in asthma, 2537
        in shock, 50
    toxicity of, in scuba diving–related disorders, 2283
Oxygen therapy
    during procedural sedation and analgesia, 2942
    for acute mountain sickness, 2302-2303
    for acute pulmonary edema, 1271
    for asthma, 1086, 1091-1092, 2538
    for burns, 921
    for carbon monoxide poisoning, 2439-2440
    for cardiac arrest, 93
    for chronic obstructive pulmonary disease, 1103-1105, 1103t-1105t
    for cluster headache, 1635

Oxygen therapy (Continued)
    for cyanosis, 271, 273
    for high-altitude cerebral edema, 2306
    for high-altitude pulmonary edema, 2304
    for pulmonary edema, in chronic renal failure, 1546
    for scuba diving–related disorders, 2292
    for sepsis, 2218
    for sickle cell disease, 1880
    for toxic shock syndrome, 2030
    hyperbaric
        for carbon monoxide poisoning, 2439-2440
        for frostbite, 2233
        for high-altitude cerebral edema, 2306
        for high-altitude pulmonary edema, 2304, 2305f
        for myonecrosis, 2209
        for nitrite abuse, 2891
        for peripheral arteriovascular disease, 1350
        for scuba diving–related disorders, 2288-2292, 2288b, 2289f-2291f
        for simultaneous carbon monoxide and cyanide poisoning, 2440-2441
    in neonatal resuscitation, 122, 123, 123t
    in postresuscitation care, 86-87, 86f
Oxygenation
    altitude and, 2307, 2307f, 2994, 2995t
    before rapid sequence intubation, 10, 10f
    failure of, as indication for intubation, 2-3
    for sepsis, 2222
    in hypothermia, 2249, 2249t
    in pediatric resuscitation, 98-99
Oxygen-enriched air, 2279-2280
Oxygen-enriched Tri-Mix, 2280
Oxyhemoglobin dissociation curve
    altitude and, 2296, 2297f
    in cyanosis, 268, 269f
    shift of, during acclimatization to high altitude, 2298
Oxymetazoline, for sinusitis, 1125
Oxymorphone, respiratory effects of, 2453t
Oxytocin, during labor and delivery, 2805

P wave
    in complete atrioventricular block, 1221
    in multifocal atrial tachycardia, 1228, 1229f
    in narrow-complex tachycardia, 1234f
    in sinoatrial block, 1216
P′ wave
    in junctional tachycardia, 1233
    in premature atrial contractions, 1222-1223, 1222f, 1223f
    in premature junctional contractions, 1223
    in premature ventricular contractions, 1224
Pacemaker(s), 1246-1255
    components of, 1247-1248
    DDD, 1248t, 1249, 1249f, 1251, 1252f
    DDDR, 1248t
    defibrillation in patient with, 1255
    electrocardiography with, 1248-1250, 1249f, 1250f
    failure to capture by, 1252-1253, 1252f
    for atrial tachycardia, 1228
    for bradycardia, 1215
    for complete atrioventricular block, 1221
    for digitalis toxicity, 2371
    for Mobitz type II second-degree atrioventricular block, 1220
    for sinoatrial block, 1218
    for sinus node dysfunction, 1218
    for torsades de pointes, 1244
    inappropriate rate by, 1254
    inappropriate sensing by, 1253
    indications for, 1246-1247, 1247b
    infection from, 1250
    leads for, 1247-1248
        problems with, 1253
    malfunction of
        disposition in, 1255
        management of, 1254-1255
        types of, 1251-1254, 1251b, 1252f-1254f
    oversensing by, 1253-1254, 1254f
    terminology of, 1247, 1248t
    thrombophlebitis from, 1250
    undersensing by, 1253, 1253f
    ventricular, ICDs as, 1255

Pacemaker(s) (Continued)
    VVI, 1248t, 1249, 1249f, 1251
        with fusion beats, 1250, 1250f
    VVIR, 1248t
Pacemaker cells
    action potential of, 1200-1201, 1201f
    in atrioventricular node, 1203
    in sinoatrial node, 1201-1202
    infranodal, 1203
Pacemaker syndrome, 1250-1251
Pacing
    external noninvasive, in hypothermia, 2246
    for pediatric bradycardia, 111
    in adult resuscitation, 91
Packed red blood cells, 52, 58-59
Paget's disease of bone, hypercalcemia in, 1915, 1915f
Pain. See also specific anatomic locations, e.g., Abdominal pain.
    acute vs. chronic, 2913-2914, 2914b
    anginal. See Angina.
    definition of, 2914b
    evaluation and documentation of, 2916-2917, 2917b, 2917t
    in abdominal aortic aneurysm, 1332-1333
    in acute arterial occlusion, 1345
    in aortic dissection, 1325
    in arthritis, 1778, 1778t
    in cholangitis, 1421
    in cholecystitis, 1420
    in cholelithiasis, 1418
    in chronic arterial insufficiency, 1345, 1346
    in compartment syndrome, 561
    in dislocation, 564
    in diverticular disease, 1493
    in frostbite, 2230
    in Osgood-Schlatter syndrome, 2710
    in peptic ulcer disease, 1392
    in peptic ulcer perforation, 1393
    in sickle cell disease, 1880
    in snakebite, 898
    in sprain, 566
    in strain, 567
    in tendinopathy, 568
    in thoracic outlet syndrome, 1359
    in toxic shock syndrome, 2200
    ischemic rest, in chronic arterial insufficiency, 1346
    management of. See Analgesia.
    palliative care for, 3153
    pathophysiology of, 2914-2916, 2915f, 2915t, 2916f, 2916t
    undertreatment of, 2917-2918
Pain behavior, 2916-2917
Pain conduction pathways, 2914-2916, 2915f, 2915t, 2916f, 2916t
Pain disorder, 1755
Pain scales, 2916, 2917b, 2917t
Pain threshold, 2915-2916
Painful arc syndrome
    in calcific tendinitis, 698
    in rotator cuff tear, 696
    shoulder, 693-696, 694t, 695f
Paint, in high-pressure injection injuries to hand, 612
Paint sniffer, 2430, 2430f
Paint thinner, in high-pressure injection injuries to hand, 612
Palivizumab, for respiratory syncytial virus prophylaxis, 2582, 2582b
Palliative care, 3143, 3151-3154
    establishing goals of, 3151-3153, 3152t
    in advanced dementia, 3154
    in chronic obstructive pulmonary disease, 3154
    in heart failure, 3154
    in renal failure, 3154
    medical treatment options in, 3153-3154, 3153b
    prehospital care end-of-life issues related to, 3145
Pallor, in pediatric assessment, 2499
Palmar erythema, in pregnancy, 2724
Palmar lesions, in Kawasaki disease, 2594, 2595f
Palmar rash, in syphilis, 1561, 1561f
Palmar surface of hand, 576, 577f
Palmaris longus
    anatomy of, 582, 584f
    laceration of, 609

Palpation
in peripheral vascular injury, 541
of fetus, 2728
of knee, 772-773, 772f
of spine, 416
Palpitations
in mitral valve prolapse, 1305
in scombroid fish poisoning, 1472
Palsy. *See also* Paralysis.
Bell's, 1666-1667, 1668, 2123
bridegroom's, 1695
cerebral, 2903-2904
failure to thrive in, 2900
musculoskeletal disorders in, 2901-2902
fourth-nerve, eye movement disorders in, 1062-1063
median nerve, 587, 588f
radial nerve, 586, 588f
humeral shaft fracture and, 655
in radial mononeuropathy, 1695
Saturday night, 1694-1695
sixth-nerve, eye movement disorders in, 1063
third-nerve
anisocoria in, 1061
eye movement disorders in, 1062
ulnar nerve, 586, 588f
Pamidronate
for hypercalcemia, 1946
for hypercalcemic cancer patient, 1916
Pancarditis, in rheumatic fever, 1304
Pancreas
anatomy and physiology of, 1426, 1427f
carcinoma of, 1437-1438, 1817
transplantation of, 1973, 2856
tumor of, 1437
Pancreatic disorders, 1426-1438
Pancreatic enzymes, 1426
in abdominal trauma, 495
in acute pancreatitis, 1430-1431
replacement of, in chronic pancreatitis, 1436
Pancreatitis
acute, 1426-1434
abdominal pain in, 215t
clinical features of, 1429
complications of, 1429-1430, 1430f
diagnosis of, 1430-1433
differential diagnosis in, 1433, 1433b
imaging studies in, 1432-1433
laboratory tests in, 1430-1432, 1431t, 1432b
management of, 1433-1434
pathophysiology of, 1427
prognostic scoring systems for, 1431-1432, 1432b
alcoholic, 2868
chronic, 1434-1437
classification of, 1435
clinical features of, 1435
diagnosis of, 1435-1436, 1436f
management of, 1436-1437
drug-induced, 1428, 1429b
etiology of, 1427-1428, 1428b, 1429b
in child abuse, 971
in children, 2618, 2618t
nausea and vomiting in, 205t
panniculitis in, 1817
severe, definition of, 1432, 1432b
Pancuronium
for tetanus, 2011
in intubation, 14, 31
Panencephalitis, sclerosing, subacute, 2054
Panic attack, 1746b, 1748-1749, 2668
in primary psychiatric disorders, 1748-1749
management of, 1749-1751, 1750t
Panic buttons, in emergency department, 2966
Panic disorder
asthma and, 1082
primary, depression with, 1748-1749
suicide and, 1769
with agoraphobia, 1746b
Panic reactions
in marijuana intoxication, 2411
in psychedelic intoxication, 2408
in psychostimulant intoxication, 2410
Panniculitis, 1817
Panoramic radiography, 1030, 1030f
Panorex imaging of facial fracture, 388
Pantoprazole, 1390t
Papaverine, for acute mesenteric ischemia, 1449
Papaya, drug interactions with, 2478t

Papillae, interdental, edematous, in acute necrotic ulcerative gingivitis, 1033
Papillary dermis, 914
Papillary examination, in overdosed/poisoned patient, 2326
Papilledema
in cerebral venous thrombosis, 1670
of optic disk, 1062
Papilloma, laryngeal, 2045, 2525
Papillomavirus infection, 2034t, 2045
drugs for, 2037t
genital warts from, 1518t, 1519-1520
in condylomata acuminata, 1563-1564, 1564f
in HIV/AIDS, 2085
Papular purpura, 1839t
Papule
scaly, skin disorders with, 1841-1842
skin disorders with, 1839t, 1851-1856
Paracentesis, in ascites, 1410
Paradoxical central nervous system acidosis, from sodium bicarbonate, 1930
Paradoxical undressing, in hypothermia, 2241
Paragonimus westermani, 2101t, 2110-2111
Parainfluenza, 2051
in bronchiolitis, 2544
in pneumonia, 1130, 2555, 2557
Paraldehyde poisoning, metabolic acidosis in, 1928
Paralysis. *See also* Palsy.
facial nerve, 1666-1668
flaccid, in botulism, 2014
in acute arterial occlusion, 1345
in botulism, 1707
in rabies, 2065
induced, in intubated, mechanically ventilated patient, 11
periodic, 1708-1709
familial, 1709
hyperkalemia in, 1940
hypokalemia in, 1938
thyrotoxic, 1709, 1987
tick, 1708, 2141-2142
Todd's, 1625
vocal cord, 2524-2525
Paralysis with induction phase of rapid sequence intubation, 11
Paralytic PICE, 3012, 3012b
Paralytic poliomyelitis, 2056-2057
Paramedic, 2987, 2987t
Parametric statistical tests, 3053
Paramyxovirus, 2034t, 2051-2054
Paranoid personality disorder, 2979b
Parapharyngeal abscess, 1121-1123, 1122f
Parapharyngeal space, 1027, 1117
Paraphimosis, 2637, 2637f
Parapneumonic pleural effusion, 1148, 1149, 1152, 1153
Parapoxviruses, 2040
Paraquat poisoning, 2465-2466, 2465b
Parasitic infection, 2096-2104
abdominal pain in, 2113
anemia in, 2107
cardiovascular disease in, 2111-2112
challenges related to, 2096
diarrhea in, 228, 230b, 2112, 2112f, 2113f
drug therapy for, 2098-2099, 2098t, 2100t-2103t
fever in, 2099, 2103-2105
gastrointestinal disorders in, 2112-2114
in cancer patient with impaired cell-mediated immunity, 2840
in HIV/AIDS, 2114
neurologic disorders in, 2105-2107
peripheral edema in, 2107-2108
pruritus ani in, 2113-2114
pulmonary disorders in, 2110-2111
skin disorders in, 2108-2109
travel history and, 2097, 2099t
visual disturbances in, 2109-2110
Parasitic pathogens, in central nervous system infection, 1711t
Parasitosis, delusion of, in amphetamine abuse, 2894
Paraspinal cold abscess, in tuberculosis, 2159
Parasystole, 1225-1226, 1226b, 1226f
Parathyroid disease, hypertension in, 1313
Parathyroid hormone
in calcium homeostasis, 1941-1942
in phosphate homeostasis, 1950
Paravaccinia, 2040

Paregoric, respiratory effects of, 2453t
Parental advice
on simple febrile seizures, 2674b
on vomiting and diarrhea, 2628b
Parental consent, 3167-3168
Parental refusal of medical care, 3171
Paresthesia
in acute arterial occlusion, 1345
in ciguatera fish poisoning, 1473
in frostbite, 2234
in hypothyroidism, 1992
in thoracic outlet syndrome, 1359
Parity, 2722
Parkinsonian motor dysfunction
in antipsychotic overdose, 2447
in methanol poisoning, 2395
Parkinson's disease, anxiety in, 1747-1748
Parkland formula, for fluid resuscitation of burn patient, 922-923
Paromomycin, for AIDS-related diarrhea, 1484
Paronychia, 614-615, 615f, 1841
Parotid gland and duct, 385, 386f
Parotitis, infectious, 1428, 2052
Paroxysmal atrial tachycardia, 1228
Paroxysmal choreoathetosis, 2668
Paroxysmal nocturnal dyspnea, 176
Paroxysmal nocturnal hemoglobinuria, hemolytic anemia in, 1879
Paroxysmal pain of neuropathic origin, 1034
Paroxysmal supraventricular tachycardia, 1233-1235, 1233f, 1234f
Paroxysmal tachycardia, in Wolff-Parkinson-White syndrome, 1235
Paroxysmal vertigo, benign, 147t, 2683
Parsley, adverse effects of, 2476t
Partial thromboplastin time (PTT)
abnormal, differential diagnosis in, 1899-1900
in bleeding disorders, 1895
in pregnancy, 318
Partial-thickness burn, 918-919, 919f
Parvovirus B19 infection, 1850, 2046, 2046f
Pascal's law, 2280
Pasteurella multocida infection
in cat bites, 883-884, 888
in dog bites, 883
Patch, 1839t
Patchy skin disorders, 1838-1841
Patella
anatomy of, 770, 771f
dislocation of, 564, 565f, 785-786, 785b
fracture of, 784-785, 785f
lateral compression of, 794
Patella alta, 782, 783, 784f
Patella baja, 782
Patellar tendinitis, 794
Patellar tendinopathy, 1799
Patellar tendon
anatomy of, 770, 771f
injury to, 761, 782-784, 783f, 784f
Patellofemoral compartment, 770, 771f
Patellofemoral joint, 770, 771f
Patellofemoral pain syndrome, 786-787
Patent ductus arteriosus, 2568
Patent foramen ovale, decompression sickness and, 2284
Pathogen exposure, blood-borne, 3081-3087, 3084t, 3085t, 3086b
Pathologic apnea, 2714
Pathologic fracture, tibial shaft, 799-800
Pathologic lying, in Munchausen's syndrome, 1762
Patient
combative, 2956-2969
assault by, 2963
diagnostic studies in, 2964
differential considerations in, 2964-2965, 2965b
disposition of, 2969
epidemiology of, 2956-2957
functional vs. organic etiology of, 2963, 2964t
history taking and physical examination of, 2963-2964, 2964t
medical clearance of, 2965
medicolegal issues of, 2967-2969
pathophysiology of, 2957
physical restraints for, 2958-2961, 2960f
preparation of emergency department for, 2965-2967

Patient (Continued)
  rapid tranquilization of, 2961-2963
  risk assessment and, 2957-2958
  verbal management techniques for, 2958
difficult, 2972-2982
  as stressor for emergency physician, 3175
  behavioral classification of, 2978-2981, 2978t
  combative patient as, 2956-2969. See also
    Combative patient.
  definition of, 2972-2973
  emergency department factors in, 2973
  impaired patient-physician relationship and,
    2973, 2974f
  management of, 2973-2981
    crisis intervention in, 2976-2977, 2977b
    dealing with negative reactions in, 2975-
      2976
    general strategies in, 2973-2975, 2973b
    personality disorder classification of, 2978,
      2979b
  physician factors in, 2973
Patient education
  information technology for, 3098-3099
  on back pain, 710-711
  on wound management, 855-856, 856b
Patient information, security and confidentiality
  of, 3102-3103
Patient population in clinical trials
  definition of, 3048
  measurement of baseline characteristics of, 3049
  recruitment and enrollment of, 3048-3049
Patient rights, 2967
Patient safety in emergency department, 3119-
  3126
  problem areas and, 3124-3126, 3125t
  sources of failure and, 3119-3123, 3120f, 3120t
Patient Self-Determination Act, 3144
Patient transfer
  disposition requirements related to, 3165,
    3165b
  in acute coronary syndromes, 1195
  in labor and delivery, 2797-2798
  in myocardial infarction, 1195
  interfacility and specialized, 2991-2992, 2991b,
    2992b
  to burn center, 927, 927b
Patient transport
  by air, 2994-2999
    administrative structure in, 2995
    aviation physiology and, 2994-2995, 2995t
    clinical concepts and patient care in, 2998-
      2999
    criteria for, 2998b
    efficacy and cost effectiveness of, 2999
    flight crew in, 2996
    future of, 2999
    medical direction in, 2996
    safety issues in, 2997, 2997b, 2997f, 2998b
    types of missions in, 2995
  interfacility and specialized, 2991-2992, 2991b,
    2992b
Patient-controlled analgesia, 2920
Patient-physician relationship
  and racial/ethnic disparities in health
    outcomes, 3109-3110
  pathology of, difficult patient and, 2973, 2974f
Pattern injuries
  in child abuse, 969, 969f
  in intimate partner violence and abuse, 997
  in motor vehicle crashes, 964-966, 965f
  in pedestrian collisions, 965-966, 965f
  in physical assault, 960-963, 961b, 961f-964f
Pattern recognition process, clinical decision
  making by, 126, 131t, 132
Pavlik harness, for developmental hip dysplasia,
  2702
PCP (phencyclidine) intoxication, 2413, 2414-
  2415, 2414t, 2415t, 2416, 2882b, 2891-2893
  during pregnancy, 2792
  rhabdomyolysis in, 1979
Peak expiratory flow rate (PEFR)
  in asthma, 1084, 1086t, 2535t, 2536, 2536f
  in chronic obstructive pulmonary disease, 1101
Peak inspiratory pressure, 30
Pedestrian collisions
  death from, 300
  forensic aspects of, 965-966, 966b, 966f
  in elderly person, 345
  mechanism of injury of, 303t

Pediatric assessment triangle, 2497-2499
  appearance in, 2497-2498, 2498t
  circulation to skin in, 2498t, 2499, 2499f
  interpretation of, 2500t
  work of breathing in, 2498-2499, 2498f, 2498t,
    2499f
Pediculosis, skin lesions in, 1853-1854, 1853f
Pelvic examination
  in abdominal pain, 213, 215
  in fever, 135
  in genitourinary trauma, 515
  in pelvic fracture, 718-719
  in pelvic pain, 249, 250t
  in vaginal bleeding, 256t
Pelvic fracture, 717-734
  acetabular, 728-729, 728b, 731, 731f, 732f
  anatomy in, 717-718, 718f
  and blunt abdominal trauma, 509, 510f
  classification of, 723, 723b
  clinical features of, 718-720
  diagnostic peritoneal lavage in, 722-723,
    722f
  epidemiology of, 717
  general management of, 722f, 723
  gynecologic injury in, 720
  hemorrhage in, 718
    evaluation of, 722-723, 722f
    management of, 731-734, 731b, 733f
  high-energy, 726-728, 727b, 733f
  in bladder trauma, 520-521
  in elderly person, 346
  low-energy, 723-726, 724f
  neurologic injury in, 719-720
  open, 719
  penetrating injuries in, 720
  posterior urethral trauma and, 516, 516f
  prehospital care in, 718
  radiologic imaging in, 720-722, 721f
  retrograde urethrogram and, 517-518
  thoracic aortic injury in, 720
  urologic injury in, 719
  visceral and soft tissue injuries in, 719
Pelvic hematoma, 718
Pelvic inflammatory disease, 1569-1571
  appendicitis vs., 1453, 1453t
  clinical features of, 1570
  differential diagnosis in, 1570-1571
  ectopic pregnancy after, 2743
  in pregnancy, 2759
  pelvic pain in, 248, 251t
  treatment of, 1571, 1571t
Pelvic ligaments, 717, 718f
Pelvic pain, 248-253. See also Abdominal pain.
  diagnostic approach to, 248-250, 250t
  differential diagnosis in, 249b, 250, 251t-252t
  empiric management of, 250, 252-253, 252f,
    253f
  epidemiology of, 248
  pathophysiology of, 248
Pelvic vessel embolization, for postpartum
  hemorrhage, 2819
Pelvirectal abscess, 2206
Pelvis, anatomy of, 717-718, 718f
Pemphigus vulgaris, skin lesions in, 1857, 1857f
Penbutolol sulfate, 1321t
Pendular shoulder exercises, 679f
Penetrating trauma
  abdominal
    diagnosis and management of, 502-507
    epidemiology of, 489
    history in, 493
    in children, 342
    observation in, 3067-3068
    pathophysiology of, 490-491
    physical examination in, 494
  cardiac, 472-476
  chest
    observation in, 3068-3069
    pneumothorax and, 462
  esophageal, 483-484
  facial, 386, 387f
  head, 368-370
  in pelvic fracture, 720
  in pregnancy, 318-319
  neck
    in transcervical gunshot wounds, 446
    mandatory vs. selective exploration of, 445-
      446
    pathophysiology of, 441-442, 442t

Penetrating trauma (Continued)
  pharyngoesophageal injuries in, 446-447
  vascular injuries in, 448-450
  ocular, 1051-1052, 1051f
  peripheral vascular, 536, 537
  renal, 528, 530
  ureteral, 530
Penetration syndrome, in airway foreign body
  impaction, 865
Penicillamine
  for lead poisoning, 2422
  for mercury poisoning, 2426
  for radioactive lead poisoning, 2324
Penicillin
  allergy to, 1826
  during pregnancy and lactation, 2775, 2784
  for Bacillus anthracis gastroenteritis, 1469
  for diphtheria, 2004
  for diphtheria-related myocardial disease, 1291
  for febrile, neutropenic cancer patient, 2838t
  for Lyme disease, 1292, 1789
  for mastoiditis, 1072
  for orofacial infections, 1032
  for pharyngitis, 1113
  for pneumonia, 2558t
  for scarlet fever, 1851
  for streptococcal pharyngitis, 1304
  for syphilis, 1856
  for tetanus, 2011
  in frostbite, 2232
  prophylactic, in rheumatic fever, 2597
Penicillin G
  for Lyme disease, 1789, 2127t, 2128
  for meningococcal disease, 2023
  for pneumococcal disease, 2019
  for syphilis, 1559t, 1562
Penicillin V, for rheumatic fever, 1791
Penile disorders, in children, 2635-2638, 2637f-
  2638f
Penile entrapment and tourniquet injuries, 878,
  2638
Penis
  anatomy of, 532, 532f
  physical examination of, 1573
  trauma to, 532-534, 532f-534f
Pennyroyal, adverse effects of, 2476t
Pentachlorophenol, 2463, 2463b
Pentamidine
  for pneumonia, in HIV-infected patient, 1139
  in HIV/AIDS, side effects of, 2079t
Pentazocine, 2924, 2924b
Pentobarbital
  for GHB withdrawal, 2490
  for status epilepticus, 1627, 1627t, 2672t, 2673
Pentoxifylline, in frostbite, 2233
Penumbra, ischemic, 1607
Pepper sprays, capsaicin in, 2472
Peptic ulcer disease, 1391-1394
  abdominal pain in, 210t
  causes of, 1391-1392, 1391b
  clinical features of, 1392
  complications of, 1393
  diagnosis of, 1393
  in spinal cord injury, 2907
  management of, 1393-1394, 1394t
  nausea and vomiting in, 204t
PERC rule, 1372b, 1374
Perceptual disturbances, in delirium, 1649
Percutaneous coronary intervention, in
  myocardial infarction, 1192-1193
  after fibrinolytic therapy, 1193
  facilitated, 1195
  guidelines on, 1193-1194
  in cardiogenic shock, 1194
  with glycoprotein IIb/IIIa receptor inhibitors,
    1186, 1194
Percutaneous cricothyrotomy, 22-23, 23f
Percutaneous embolotherapy, for hemoptysis,
  282
Percutaneous transluminal angioplasty, for acute
  mesenteric ischemia, 1449
Percutaneous transluminal peripheral
  angioplasty, for peripheral arteriovascular
  disease, 1349
Percutaneous transtracheal jet insufflation, in
  neck trauma, 445
Percutaneous transtracheal ventilation, in
  multiple trauma, 306
Perforating wounds to head, 369

Performance shaping factors, as source of failures in emergency department, 3120t, 3121-3123
Perfumes, caustic injuries from, 2381
Perianal abscess, 2206
Perianal itching, 1509
Periapical abscess, 1028, 1030f, 1031, 1032
Pericardial disease, 1280-1298. See also Pericardial effusion; Pericarditis.
    acquired immunodeficiency syndrome and, 1287
    cardiac tamponade in, 1285-1286, 1286f
    connective tissue disorders and, 1284
    epidemiology of, 1280
    etiology of, 1280, 1281b
    heart failure in, 1265
    neoplastic, 1283-1284
    pneumopericardium in, 1287-1288
    pregnancy and, 1287
    uremic, 1282
Pericardial effusion, 1284-1285, 1285f
    in cardiac tamponade, 474, 474f
    in chronic renal failure, 1542
    in HIV/AIDS, 1287
    in hypothyroidism, 1993
    in myocardial contusion, 468
    in pregnancy, 1287
    malignant, 1283-1284
    transudative vs. exudative, 1285
    uremic, 1282
Pericardial friction rub, 1281, 2592
Pericardial knock, in constrictive pericarditis, 1288
Pericardial mesothelioma, 1916
Pericardial rupture, 471
Pericardial tamponade. See Cardiac tamponade.
Pericardial tumor, malignant, 1283-1284
Pericardiocentesis
    in cardiac tamponade, 475, 1286
    in hemodialysis patient, 1551
    in myocardial rupture, 471
    in neoplastic cardiac tamponade, 1917-1918
    in pericardial effusion, 1285
Pericardiotomy
    in myocardial rupture, 471
    pericarditis after, 2581
Pericarditis
    chest pain in, 183, 186b, 190t-191t
    constrictive, 1288
        heart failure in, 1265
        neoplastic, 1917
        restrictive cardiomyopathy vs., 1296
    epidemiology of, 1280
    etiology of, 1280, 1281b
    iatrogenic, 1287
    idiopathic, 1280-1282, 1281f
    in acute renal failure, 1540
    in amyloidosis, 1287
    in chronic renal failure, 1542
    in giant cell arteritis, 1284
    in hemodialysis patient, 1551
    in HIV/AIDS, 1287
    in infants and children, 2592-2593, 2593f
    in inflammatory bowel disease, 1287
    in pregnancy, 1287
    in rheumatoid arthritis, 1284
    in Sjögren's syndrome, 1284
    in systemic lupus erythematosus, 1284, 1807
    infarct, 1160
    miscellaneous infectious causes of, 1284
    neoplastic, 1916
    pathophysiology of, 1280
    post-myocardial infarction, 1282-1283
    post-pericardiotomy, 2581
    posttraumatic, 1283
    purulent, 1286-1287
    radiation-induced, 1284, 1916-1917
    risk factors for, 186b
    ST segment elevation in, 1167, 1167f, 1168f
    tuberculous, 1287, 2151
    uremic, 1282
Pericardium, anatomy and physiology of, 1280
Pericoronitis, 1035
Perihepatitis, 1570
Perilunate dislocation, 630, 631f
Perilymphatic fistula, vertigo in, 2685
Perindopril, 1322t
Perineal laceration, 719
Periodic breathing
    definition of, 2714

Periodic breathing (Continued)
    in acute mountain sickness, 2301, 2302
    in infants, 2495
Periodic paralysis, 1708-1709
    familial, 1709
    hyperkalemia in, 1940
    hypokalemia in, 1938
    thyrotoxic, 1709, 1987
Periodontal abscess, 1031, 1033
Periodontal disease, 1032-1033
    in diabetes mellitus, 1035
    in HIV/AIDS, 2083
Periodontal ligament, 1027, 1027f
Periodontal surgery, hemorrhage after, 1042
Periodontitis, 1032-1033
Periodontium, anatomy of, 1027, 1027f
Perionychium, 589
Perioral tremor, antipsychotic-induced, 2447
Periorbital cellulitis, 294t, 2197-2198
Periorbital edema
    in hypothyroidism, 1992
    in superior vena cava syndrome, 1910
Periosteum, in children, 2689
Periostitis, physiologic, 2699-2700
Peripatellar tendinitis, 794
Peripheral arterial aneurysm
    infected, 1356-1357, 1357t
    lower extremity, 1354
    traumatic, 1357
    upper extremity, 1354-1355
    visceral, 1355-1356
Peripheral arteriovascular disease, 1342-1366
    acute arterial occlusion in, 1345, 1345f, 1352-1354, 1353f
    arterial anatomy and, 1342
    arterial embolism in, 1343-1344, 1346, 1347t, 1352-1353
    arterial thrombosis in, 1344, 1347, 1347t, 1353-1354
    arteriosclerosis obliterans in, 1350-1351
    arteriovenous fistula in, 538-539, 541, 1344, 1347, 1360
    atheroembolism in, 1343-1344, 1353, 1353f
    Buerger's disease in, 1351-1352
    chronic arterial insufficiency in, 1345-1346, 1350-1352
    clinical features of, 1344-1347
    diagnosis of, 1348
    drug abuse–related, 1360-1361
    history in, 1344-1346, 1345f
    inflammatory, 1344, 1347
    management of, 1348-1350
    pathophysiology of, 1342-1344
    physical examination in, 1346-1347, 1347t
    thoracic outlet syndrome in, 1358-1360, 1358f, 1359f
    trauma in, 1344
    vasospastic disorders in, 1344
Peripheral nerve disorders. See Mononeuropathy; Neuropathy; Polyneuropathy.
Peripheral nerve fibers, in pain transmission, 2914, 2915t
Peripheral nervous system
    anatomy of, 1688-1689, 1688f
    cyclic antidepressant effects on, 2353b
Peripheral vascular injury, 536-547
    clinical features of, 539-541, 540f
    diagnostic strategies in, 541-543
    disposition in, 547
    epidemiology of, 536-537
    of lower extremity, 546-547
    of upper extremity, 544-546
    pathophysiology of, 537-539, 538f
    treatment of, 543-544
Peripheral venous access
    in adult resuscitation, 91
    in pediatric resuscitation, 99
Perirectal abscess, 1513t, 1514, 2205-2206, 2206f
Perirenal hematoma, 498f
Peristaltic activity, decreased, causes of, 1440, 1441b
Peritalar dislocation, 825-826, 825f
Peritendinitis, calcifying, of femur and hip, 742
Peritoneal dialysis
    chronic ambulatory, 1547
    complications of, 1552-1554, 1553t
    continuous cyclic, 1547
    for acute renal failure, 2650

Peritoneal dialysis (Continued)
    for chronic renal failure, 1547-1548
    for rewarming in accidental hypothermia, 2249
Peritoneal irritation, in ectopic pregnancy, 2743
Peritoneal lavage
    in abdominal trauma, 499-501, 500t
    in multiple trauma, 312
    in pregnant trauma patient, 321
Peritoneal signs
    in abdominal stab wound, 503
    in small bowel obstruction, 1442
Peritoneal violation, laparotomy and, 504, 506
Peritonitis
    bacterial
        in small bowel obstruction, 1441
        spontaneous, 245-246, 1412-1413
    eosinophilic, 1552
    from corticosteroids, 2844
    iatrogenic, 492
    in peritoneal dialysis patient, 1552-1553, 1553t
    in tuberculosis, 2161-2162
    pelvic pain in, 250t
Peritonsillar abscess, 1117-1118, 1118f
Peritonsillar space, 1117
Peritonsillitis, 1117-1118, 1118f
Permethrin
    for pediculosis, 1854
    for Phthirus pubis infestation, 1569
    for Sarcoptes scabiei infestation, 1569
    for scabies, 1855
    prophylactic, for tick-borne illness, 2142
Permissive hypercapnia
    for chronic obstructive pulmonary disease, 1104
    for critically ill asthmatic patient, 1092
Pernicious anemia, optic neuropathy from, 1060
Pernio, 2228, 2230
Peroneal arteries
    anatomy of, 797
    injury to, 547
Peroneal nerve, 797
    anatomy of, 771, 797
    injury to
        in proximal tibial epiphyseal fracture, 781
        in tibial femoral knee dislocation, 788
        in tibial plateau fracture, 778
        in tibial shaft fracture, 800
Peroneal retinaculum, 808, 809f
Peroneal tendon dislocation or tear, 818-819, 819f
Perphenazine, 2446t
Perseverations, speech, in schizophrenia, 1728
Persistent fetal circulation, 119
Personal integrity, 3129, 3129b
Personal protective equipment
    for tuberculosis, 2170
    in tactical emergency medical support, 3004
    in terrorism incidents, 3013
Personality changes, in central nervous system infection, 1714
Personality disorders
    classification of, 2978, 2979b
    with brief psychotic episodes, 1729
Perthes' disease, 767
Perthes-Bankart lesion, in anterior glenohumeral joint dislocation, 690
Pertussis, 2004-2007, 2005f, 2006b, 2559-2560
Pes anserinus, 770, 771f
Pesticide poisoning, 2452-2469
    bipyridyl compounds in, 2465-2466, 2465b
    carbamate insecticides in, 2458b, 2461-2462
    chlorinated hydrocarbon pesticides in, 2462-2463, 2462b
    chlorophenoxy compounds in, 2464-2465, 2465b
    DEET in, 2468-2469
    glyphosate in, 2467-2468
    hydrocarbons in, 2430
    organophosphate insecticides in, 2457-2461, 2458b, 2459b, 2459f
    pyrethrins and pyrethroids in, 2466-2467, 2467b
    substituted phenols in, 2463-2464, 2463b
Petechiae
    fever and, as indication for lumbar puncture, 2660
    in infective endocarditis, 1301

Petechiae (Continued)
in meningococcal disease, 2022
pediatric fever and, 2507-2508
Petroleum asphalt burns, 926-927, 937
Petroleum distillates, toxicity of, 2428, 2429t
Peyote, 2409, 2409f
Peyronie's disease, 534
pH
in metabolic acidosis, 1929
in metabolic alkalosis, 1930
in mixed acid-base disorders, 1931
in respiratory acidosis, 1925
in respiratory alkalosis, 1926
of blood
changes in, compensatory responses to, 1923-1924
normal values for, 1923
Phagocytes, 2834
Phagocytosis, 2834
Phalangeal bones, 577-578, 579f-580f
Phalanx
extensor tendon injury at
distal, 605-607, 606f, 607f
proximal, 608
fracture of, 834
distal, 593-594, 593f
proximal, 594-595, 594f-596f
Phalen's sign, in carpal tunnel syndrome, 639, 639f, 1697
Pharmacokinetics
in children, 2935, 2952
in elderly person, 2826
Pharyngeal pain, in pharyngitis, 1109
Pharyngitis, 274-279, 1109-1114
ancillary studies in, 277-278, 277t
clinical features of, 1109-1111, 1110f
diagnosis of, 275-278, 276t, 277f, 277t, 1111-1112
differential diagnosis in, 278, 1112
disposition in, 1113-1114
epidemiology of, 274
etiology of, 1109
high-altitude, 2304
history in, 275-276
in children, screening for, 2509b
in epiglottitis, 2523
in lingual tonsillitis, 1114
in parapharyngeal abscess, 1122
management of, 278-279, 278f, 1112-1113
pathophysiology of, 274-275, 275t
physical examination in, 276-277, 276t
streptococcal, 274-275, 1109, 1110, 1111, 1112-1113, 1114
adult epiglottitis vs., 1115
in rheumatic fever, 1303, 1304
Pharyngoesophageal trauma, 446-447
Pharyngomaxillary space, 1121-1123, 1122f
Pharynx, foreign body in, 870-873
Phencyclidine intoxication, 2413, 2414-2415, 2414t, 2415t, 2416, 2882b, 2891-2893
during pregnancy, 2792
rhabdomyolysis in, 1979
Phenelzine, overdose of, 2365
Phenobarbital
during pregnancy and lactation, 2787
for alcohol-related status epilepticus, 2865
for bupropion-induced seizure, 2361
for cyclic antidepressant poisoning, 2356
for seizure, 166t, 167, 1627, 1627t, 1628t
in children, 2675, 2675t
for status epilepticus, 2672t, 2673
overdose of, 2482, 2483
side effects of, 1628t
Phenol and derivatives
burn injury from, 935-936
for wound cleansing, 848t
ingestion of, 2384
poisoning from, 936, 2463-2464, 2463b
Phenothiazine
adjuvant, with opioids, 2921
anticholinergic toxicity of, 2346b
cardiotoxicity of, 2445
during pregnancy and lactation, 2790
for nausea and vomiting, 203, 208b, 208t
Phenoxybenzamine
for hypertensive emergencies, 1319
in frostbite, 2233
Phentolamine
for cocaine overdose, 2390, 2391
for hypertension, 1319, 2653

Phentolamine (Continued)
in cocaine overdose, 2390
in MAOI toxicity, 2365
Phenylbutazone, overdose of, 2343
Phenylephrine
for sepsis, 2219t, 2220
for sinusitis, 1125
mydriasis from, 1061
Phenylephrinemethoxamine, for junctional tachycardia, 1234
Phenylpropanolamine, during pregnancy and lactation, 2790
Phenytoin, 1207
alcohol withdrawal syndrome and, 2865-2866
drugs affecting levels of, 1207b
during pregnancy and lactation, 2786
for alcohol-related status epilepticus, 2865
for digitalis toxicity, 2371
for seizure, 166, 166t, 1626-1627, 1627t, 1628t
in cancer patient, 1919
in children, 2675, 2675t
for status epilepticus, 2672t, 2673
gingival hyperplasia in, 1036
hyperglycemic hyperosmolar nonketotic coma from, 1969
prophylactic, in head trauma, 361, 370
side effects of, 1628t
Pheochromocytoma
anxiety in, 1747
hypertension in, 1313
Phimosis, in children, 2636
Phlebotomy, for polycythemia, 1885
Phlegmasia cerulea dolens, 1352, 1370
Phlegmonous gastritis, 1390, 1391
Phobia, 1746b, 1749
Phosgene, as chemical weapon, 939, 3032
Phosphate
for hypophosphatemia, 1952
imbalance of. See Hyperphosphatemia; Hypophosphatemia.
in diabetic ketoacidosis, 1966
normal physiology of, 1950-1951
Phosphodiesterase inhibitors
for beta blocker overdose, 2375
for calcium channel blocker overdose, 2378
for chronic heart failure, 1276
Phosphorus. See Phosphate.
Photographic documentation
in intimate partner violence and abuse, 1001, 1003
in sexual assault cases, 989, 989b
Photosensitivity, drug-induced, 1845, 1847t
Phototherapy, for kernicterus prophylaxis, 2603, 2605f
Phrenic nerve injury, 450
Phthirus pubis infestation, 1569
Physeal injuries, 2690, 2691f, 2691t, 2692, 2692f
Physical abuse
in pregnancy, 318
of child, 969-971, 969f, 970f, 970t, 972, 973, 974-975
of elder, 1009-1010
of intimate partner, 995-996, 997. See also Intimate partner violence and abuse.
Physical assault
by combative patient, 2963
forensic aspects of, 960-963, 961b, 961f-964f
victim identification in, 960
Physical fitness, as wellness strategy for emergency physicians, 3177-3178, 3177b
Physically disabled patient, 2904-2911
abuse of, 1015
hearing impairment in, 2904-2905
multiple sclerosis in, 2909-2911
pulmonary disorders in, 2907-2908
spinal cord injury in, 2905-2909
visual impairment in, 2905
Physician, emergency. See Emergency physician.
Physician staffing, for observation, 3062-3063
Physician-patient relationship
and racial/ethnic disparities in health outcomes, 3109-3110
pathology of, difficult patient and, 2973, 2974f
Physiologic jaundice of the newborn, 2601-2603, 2602t, 2603b, 2603t, 2604f-2605f
Physostigmine, for anticholinergic poisoning, 2350
Phytobezoar, 873

Phytolacca americana, 2474-2475, 2474f
Phytophotodermatitis, 974-975
Pick's disease, dementia in, 1657, 1659
Picornavirus, 2034t, 2056-2057
Picric acid, 935
Picture Archiving and Communications Systems and Imaging Systems, 3101
Piece of pie sign, in lunate dislocation, 630
Piedmont fracture, 551t
Pierre Robin syndrome, neonatal resuscitation in, 121
Pigment nephropathy, 1536, 1536b
Pigmentation changes
in Addison's disease, 1997
in pregnancy, 2723-2724, 2728
Pigmented gallstones, 1418, 2620
Pigmenturia, differential diagnosis in, 1981-1982, 1981b
Pill esophagitis, 1386, 1387
Pilocarpine, for closed-angle glaucoma, 1056
Pilon fractures, 814-815, 815f
Pilonidal abscess, 2206-2207
Pilonidal disease, 1515
Pimozide, 2446t
Pinch-off syndrome, 1362, 1363
Pindolol, 1321t, 2373t, 2374
Ping-pong fracture, in head-injured child, 368
Pinguecula, 296t, 1053-1054
"Pink puffer," 1099
Pinworm, 1479-1482
drug therapy for, 2100t
gastroenteritis in, 1479-1482
pruritus ani in, 2113-2114
Pipe-stem cirrhosis, in chronic schistosomiasis, 2112, 2113f
Pirbuterol, for asthma, 2538, 2539t
Pisiform
anatomy of, 622, 623f, 625
fracture of, 629
Pit viper envenomation, 896-897, 897f, 898, 900t
Pittsburgh Knee Rule, 774
Pituitary gland, in pregnancy, 2726
Pityriasis rosea, 1841
Pivot shift test, in knee trauma, 774
Placenta
abruption of, 319-320, 2747-2748, 2809-2810
circumvallate, 2810
delivery of, 2804-2805
drug transfer across, 2780-2781
examination of, 2805
retained, postpartum hemorrhage from, 2819
surgical removal of, 2819
Placenta accreta, increta, and percreta, 257-258, 257t, 2819
Placenta previa, 257, 257t, 2748, 2808-2809
Plague, 1131, 3027-3028, 3027f, 3028b
Plant poisoning, 2471-2479
anticholinergic agents in, 2345, 2346t
botanical identification in, 2471-2475, 2472f-2475f
epidemiology of, 2471
herbal medicines and, 2475-2477, 2476t
mushrooms in, 2477-2479, 2478f
unintentional childhood exposure in, 2471
Plantar fascial rupture, 836
Plantar fasciitis, 836
Plantaris strain and rupture, 804
Plaque, 1839t
dental bacterial, 1028
skin disorders with, 1838-1841
Plasma exchange
for Goodpasture syndrome, 1816
for hyperviscosity syndrome, 1913
for myasthenia gravis, 1707
for thrombotic thrombocytopenic purpura, 1898
Plasmids, antibiotic resistance and, 1575
Plasmodium falciparum, 2104. See also Malaria.
Plaster cast, 571-573
Plaster splint, 569
Plastic deformation of forearm, 644, 645f
Platelet(s)
adhesion defects of, 1898
aggregation defects of, 1899
in hemostasis, 1892, 1893b, 1893f
release defects of, 1898-1899
Platelet count
in bleeding disorders, 1895

Platelet count *(Continued)*
  in gastrointestinal bleeding, 222
  in pregnancy, 2725
Platelet disorders. *See also specific disorders,*
      e.g., Thrombocytopenia.
  differential diagnosis in, 1896-1899, 1896b
  in alcoholism, 2874
  in polycythemia, 1884
Platelet transfusions, 59, 1899
  in acute radiation syndrome, 2324
  in disseminated intravascular coagulation,
      1904
  in multiple trauma, 307
Platelet-activating factor, as anaphylaxis
      mediator, 1823, 1823b
Platysma muscle, 443
Plesiomonas shigelloides
  dysenteric colitis in, 229t
  gastroenteritis in, 1461t, 1462t, 1468
Plethysmography, in deep venous thrombosis,
      1370
Pleural disease
  pleural effusion and, 1148-1153
  spontaneous pneumothorax and, 1143-1147
Pleural effusion, 1134, 1148-1153
  clinical features of, 1150-1151, 1151f
  exudative vs. transudative, 1149-1150, 1152,
      1152f
  in pneumonia, 2561, 2562
  in superior vena cava syndrome, 1911
  in systemic lupus erythematosus, 1808
  in tuberculosis, 2152, 2152f, 2158-2159
  loculated, 1148
  malignant, 1149, 1153
  management of, 1151-1153
  parapneumonic, 1148, 1149, 1152, 1153
  pathophysiology of, 1148-1150, 1149b, 1149f
Pleural fluid analysis, 1152-1153, 1152b
Pleural fluid cell count, 1152
Pleural friction rub, 1150
Pleural irritation, in pneumonia, 2556
Pleuritic chest pain
  in esophageal perforation, 484
  in pneumothorax, 1145
Pleuritis, 1148, 1150
  uremic, 1542
Plexopathy
  brachial, 1692-1693, 1693b
  in pelvic fracture, 720
  lumbosacral, 1692-1693, 1693b
Plica syndrome, 794-795
Plicamycin, for hypercalcemia, 1946
Plummer-Vinson syndrome, esophageal web in,
      1383
PMA (paramethylenedioxymethamphetamine),
      2409
Pneumatic antishock garment, 2991
Pneumatocele, 1134
Pneumatosis intestinalis, in necrotizing
      enterocolitis, 2609, 2609f
Pneumococcal disease, 2016-2020, 2020b
  after splenectomy, 2842-2843
  drug-resistant, 1137-1138, 2019
  in children, 2556, 2557, 2557f
  meningitis in, 1711, 1714, 1715, 1720, 1721t,
      1723, 2019
  pediatric bacteremia in, 2505
Pneumococcal vaccine, 1129, 1723, 2017, 2019-
      2020, 2020b
Pneumocystis pneumonia (PCP), 1130, 2110
  chest radiography in, 1136, 1136f
  in cancer patient with impaired cell-mediated
      immunity, 2840
  in HIV/AIDS, 1135-1136, 2077-2078, 1140
  in organ transplant patient, 2848, 2849f
  pneumothorax in, 1144
Pneumomediastinum
  in asthma, 2536
  in scuba diving–related disorders, 2286, 2293
  spontaneous, 1146
  subcutaneous emphysema and, 459
  tracheobronchial injury and, 466, 466f
Pneumonia, 1128-1141
  aspiration, 1136, 2560
  atypical, 1131-1132
  bacterial, 1129, 1130-1131
    in children, 2555, 2556-2557, 2556f, 2557f,
      2558f, 2563t
    tuberculosis vs., 2157

Pneumonia *(Continued)*
  chlamydial, 2559, 2559f, 2563t
  clinical features of, 1131-1132
  diagnostic strategies in, 1132-1135, 1133f,
      1134f
  differential diagnosis in, 1136
  disposition in, 1140-1141, 1140t
  dyspnea in, 179t
  epidemiology of, 1128
  etiologic agents in, 1129-1131
  high-altitude pulmonary edema vs., 2304
  host defenses and, 1128-1129
  in alcoholism, 2870
  in bronchopulmonary dysplasia, 2565, 2565f
  in chronic obstructive pulmonary disease,
      1102, 1106
  in elderly person, 2828
  in HIV-infected patient, 1135-1136, 1136f,
      1138-1139, 1140-1141
  in immunocompromised patient, 2560, 2841
  in pertussis, 2006
  in physically disabled patient, 2907
  in pulmonary contusion, 461
  isolation in, 1136, 1140-1141
  management of, 1136-1139, 1138t, 1139t
  mortality in, 1128, 1140, 1140t
  mycoplasmal, 2558-2559, 2563t
  observation in, 3072, 3072b, 3073t
  pediatric, 2554-2564
    complications of, 2562
    diagnosis in, 2560-2561, 2561f
    differential diagnosis in, 2561, 2562b
    epidemiology of, 2555
    management of, 2558t, 2562-2564
    pathophysiology of, 2555
    physical examination in, 2556
    screening for, 2509b
    signs and symptoms of, 2555-2556
  Pneumocystis, 1130, 2110
    chest radiography in, 1136, 1136f
    in cancer patient with impaired cell-
      mediated immunity, 2840
    in HIV/AIDS, 1135-1136, 2077-2078, 1140
    in organ transplant patient, 2848, 2849f
    pneumothorax in, 1144
  tropical eosinophilic, 2110
  viral, 1129, 1130, 1139, 2555, 2557-2560, 2563t
Pneumonia Severity Index, 3072, 3073t
Pneumonic plague, 3027
Pneumonitis, in systemic lupus erythematosus,
      1808
Pneumopericardium, 1287-1288
Pneumoperitoneum
  iatrogenic, 492
  peptic ulcer perforation and, 1393
Pneumothorax, 1134, 1143-1147
  catamenial, 1144
  chest pain in, 183, 184, 186b, 187, 190t-191t
  clinical features of, 1145-1146, 1145f, 1146f
  communicating, 462, 462f, 464
  dyspnea in, 179t
  etiology of, 1143-1144, 1144b
  in abdominal trauma, 497f
  in asthma, 2536
  in chronic obstructive pulmonary disease,
      1102, 1143-1144, 1145
  in scuba diving–related disorders, 2286, 2293
  in tuberculosis, 2150, 2150f
  management of, 1146-1148
  occult, 463
  open, 339
  outcome of, 1148
  pathophysiology of, 1144-1145, 1144f
  risk factors for, 186b
  simple, 461-462, 461f, 463-464, 464b
  subcutaneous emphysema and, 459
  tension, 339, 462, 462f, 463f, 464
  tracheobronchial injury and, 466
  traumatic, 338-339, 461-464, 461f-463f, 464b
Podofilox
  for condylomata acuminata, 1564
  for genital warts, 1520
Poikilocytosis, in myelophthisic anemia, 1876,
      1876f
Poinsettia, 2474
Poison hemlock, 2472, 2473f
Poisoning/overdose, 2418-2426. *See also*
      Substance abuse.
  acetaminophen, 2331-2337, 2332f

Poisoning/overdose *(Continued)*
  antidotes to, 2329t
  chronic exposure in, 2334b, 2335
  clinical features of, 2332-2333
  diagnosis of, 2333-2335, 2333b, 2334b
  disposition in, 2337
  in children, 2335
  management of, 2333b, 2334b, 2335-2337
  risk assessment using treatment nomogram
      in, 2333-2335, 2334f
  anticholinergic, 2345-2350, 2346b, 2346t,
      2347f
    antidotes to, 2329t
    clinical presentation in, 2347-2348, 2347t
    diagnosis of, 2349
    differential diagnosis in, 2348, 2348b
    disposition in, 2350
    management of, 2349-2350
  antidepressant, 2352-2366
    bupropion in, 2361, 2361t
    cyclic antidepressants in, 2352-2357, 2353b,
      2353f, 2354b, 2355f, 2357t
    mirtazapine in, 2362-2363
    monamine oxidase inhibitors in, 2363-2365,
      2363b-2365b, 2364t
    neurologic complications of, 2354t, 2356
    selective serotonin reuptake inhibitors in,
      2357-2360, 2358b, 2358t, 2359b, 2360t
    trazadone in, 2361-2362
    venlafaxine in, 2362, 2362t
    antidotes to, 2329t
  antipsychotic agent, 2445-2450, 2446t
  arsenic, 2423-2424, 2424b
  aspirin, 2339-2342, 2340f
    clinical features of, 2341, 2341b
    diagnosis of, 2341
    disposition in, 2342
    management of, 2341-2342, 2341b
  cardiovascular drug, 2368-2379
    beta blockers in, 2373-2376, 2373t, 2374b,
      2375b
    calcium channel blockers in, 2329t, 2376-
      2379, 2377b, 2377t, 2378b
    digitalis in, 2368-2373
  caustic, 2380-2385, 2381f, 2381t, 2382f
  cocaine, 2386-2392
    body packing/stuffing and, 2391-2392
    clinical features of, 2386-2388, 2387b
    diagnosis of, 2388-2389
    differential diagnosis in, 2389, 2389b
    disposition in, 2392, 2392t
    management of, 2389-2391, 2389b, 2390b
  dialysis for, 1549
  digitalis, 2368-2373
    acute vs. chronic, 2369, 2370t
    antidotes to, 2329t
    clinical features of, 2369, 2370b
    diagnosis of, 2369-2370
    differential diagnosis in, 2370
    disposition in, 2372-2373
    in children, 2372, 2372t
    management of, 2370-2371, 2372b
    pathophysiology of, 2368-2369, 2369b
  ethanol. *See* Alcohol intoxication; Alcoholism.
  general approach to, 2325-2331
    consultation in, 2331
    decontamination in, 2330
    disposition in, 2330-2331
    initial, 2326-2327
    overdose history in, 2326, 2326b
    physical examination in, 2326-2327, 2327t
    toxic syndromes in, 2327-2328, 2327t
  hallucinogen, 2406-2416
    dissociative agents in, 2413-2426, 2414t,
      2415t
    entactogens in, 2408-2411, 2409f
    marijuana and miscellaneous plants and
      fungi in, 2411-2413, 2412f
    serotonin-like agents in, 2406-2408, 2407f
  heavy metal, 2418-2426
    arsenic in, 2423-2424, 2424b
    iron in, 2418-2421, 2419f, 2420f, 2420t
    lead in, 2421-2423, 2422f
    mercury in, 2424-2426, 2425b, 2425t
  hydrocarbon, 2428-2432, 2429t, 2430f, 2431f
  inhaled toxin, 2436-2441, 2443t
    carbon monoxide in, 2438-2441
    cyanide and hydrogen sulfide in, 2436-2438,
      2437f

Poisoning/overdose *(Continued)*
    pulmonary irritants in, 2433t, 2434-2435, 2434f
    simple asphyxiants in, 2432-2433
    smoke in, 2435-2436
  lithium, 2442-2444, 2443t
  nonsteroidal antiinflammatory drug, 2342-2344
  odors in, 2327, 2327t
  opioid, 2327t, 2328, 2451-2456
    antidotes to, 2329t
    clinical features of, 2452-2454, 2453t
    diagnosis of, 2454
    differential diagnosis in, 2454
    disposition in, 2455
    management of, 2454-2455
    pathophysiology and pharmacology of, 2451-2452
  pesticide, 2452-2469
    bipyridyl compounds in, 2465-2466, 2465b
    carbamate insecticides in, 2458b, 2461-2462
    chlorinated hydrocarbon pesticides in, 2462-2463, 2462b
    chlorophenoxy compounds in, 2464-2465, 2465b
    DEET in, 2468-2469
    glyphosate in, 2467-2468
    hydrocarbons in, 2430
    organophosphate insecticides in, 2457-2461, 2458b, 2459b, 2459f
    pyrethrins and pyrethroids in, 2466-2467, 2467b
    substituted phenols in, 2463-2464, 2463b
  plant, 2471-2479
    anticholinergic agents in, 2345, 2346t
    botanical identification in, 2471-2475, 2472f-2475f
    epidemiology of, 2471
    herbal medicines and, 2475-2477, 2476t
    mushrooms in, 2477-2479, 2478t
    unintentional childhood exposure in, 2471
  sedative hypnotic, 2327t, 2328, 2481-2490
    barbiturates in, 2481-2483, 2482b, 2482f
    benzodiazepines in, 2483-2486, 2484t
    buspirone in, 2486
    chloral hydrate in, 2487
    flunitrazepam in, 2486
    γ-hydroxybutyrate in, 2488-2490, 2488b
    OTC sleep aids in, 2487-2488, 2488t
    zolpidem and zaleplon in, 2486-2487
  suicide by, 1768
  sympathomimetic, 2386-2393
  toxic alcohol, 2395-2404
    ethylene glycol in, 2398-2402, 2401t
    isopropyl alcohol in, 2402-2404
    methanol in, 2395-2398
Pokeweed, 2474-2475, 2474f
Police dogs, bites by, 882
Poliomyelitis, 1704
  paralytic, 2056-2057
Poliovirus, 2035t, 2056-2057
Polle syndrome, 1761, 1763, 1765
Poloxamer, for sickle cell disease, 1880
Polyarteritis nodosa, 1813-1814
Polyarthritis, 1303-1304, 1784f, 1787-1792, 1790b, 2596
Polycythemia, 273, 1884-1885, 1884f, 1885b
Polycythemia vera, 1885, 1885b
Polydioxanone suture, 852t
Polydipsia, psychogenic, 1934
Polyethylene glycol therapy, for phenol burn, 935-936
Polymerase chain reaction testing
  in bacterial meningitis, 2662
  in central nervous system infection, 1719
  in HIV, 2074
  in trichomoniasis, 1567
  in tuberculosis, 2155
Polymorphonuclear leukocytes. *See* Neutrophil(s).
Polymyalgia rheumatica, 1638
Polymyositis, 1396, 1708
Polyneuropathy
  demyelinating, 1690-1691, 1690b
  distal symmetrical sensorimotor, 1691-1692, 1691b
Polyomaviruses, 2034t, 2045-2046
Polyoxyethylene amine, in glyphosate poisoning, 2467-2468
Polyoxyethylene sorbitan, for tar removal, 927

Polyp, nasal, 1082
Polypropylene suture, 852t
Polysorbate, for tar removal, 927
Polytetrafluoroethylene (PTFE) vascular shunt, in arterial injury, 544
Polythiazide, 1321t
Pontine myelinolysis, central, in hyponatremia, 1935
Popliteal aneurysm, 1354
Popliteal artery, 540, 540f
  anatomy of, 771
  injury to, 546-547
    in proximal tibial epiphyseal fracture, 781
    in tibial femoral knee dislocation, 787, 788, 789
    in tibial plateau fracture, 778
Popliteal cyst, 796, 797f
Popliteal disease, pain in, 1345
Popliteal fossa, 771
Popliteofibular ligament, 770-771, 771f
Popliteus tendinitis, 795
Porcelain gallbladder, 1423
Porphyrin, defective synthesis of, in sideroblastic anemia, 1873
Portuguese man-of-war, 909
Positional testing, in vertigo, 145, 145f
Positional vertigo, benign, 147t, 2683
Positioning, in neonatal resuscitation, 122
Positive airway pressure
  bilevel, 28, 28f
    in critically ill asthmatic patient, 1092
  continuous, 27-28
    in acute pulmonary edema, 1271, 1271f
    in sleep apnea in chronic heart failure, 1277
    in submersion victim, 2314
Positive end-expiratory pressure (PEEP), 27-28
Positive predictive value, 3059t
Positive-pressure insufflation technique, for nasal foreign body, 864
Positive-pressure ventilation
  adverse effects of, 26b
  basic approaches to, 26-27
  modes of, 27-28
  noninvasive, 28-29, 28f
    evolving therapies in, 33
    in asthma, 1091-1092
    in chronic obstructive pulmonary disease, 1104, 1104t
    initial settings and ongoing monitoring in, 29-30, 29t
    outcomes in, 32-33
    patient management in, 31
    patient selection for, 29
Positive symptoms in schizophrenia, 1726, 1727-1728
Positron emission tomography
  in minor head trauma, 365
  in osteomyelitis, 2181
Postanal abscess, 1513t, 1514-1515
Postconcussive syndrome, 366
Postdural puncture headache, 1641
Posterior arch, 717, 718f
Posterior columns, 1676, 1676f
Posterior cruciate ligament injury, 790-791, 792
  stability testing in, 773-774
  tibial femoral knee dislocation and, 788
Posterior drawer test, in posterior cruciate ligament injury, 773-774
Posterior elbow dislocation, 664-665, 664f, 665f
Posterior fat pad, in elbow, 651, 651f
Posterior fossa, epidural hematoma in, 375, 376f
Posterior longitudinal ligament, 702
Posterior malleolus, fracture of, 813
Posterior neural arch fracture, of atlas, 410, 410f
Posterior sag sign, in posterior cruciate ligament injury, 774
Posterior segment, traumatic injury to, 1050-1051, 1050f
Posterior tibial artery
  anatomy of, 797
  injury to, 547
Posterior tibial nerve
  compression of, heel pain in, 836-837
  injury to
    in tibial femoral knee dislocation, 788
    tibial shaft fracture and, 800
Posteroinferior cerebellar artery syndrome, 420
Posterolateral corner, 770, 771f

Postexposure prophylaxis
  for hepatitis, 1406, 1407t, 1408f
  for hepatitis B, 1406, 3083-3084, 3084t
  for hepatitis C, 3083, 3084
  for HIV, 3083, 3084-3087, 3085t, 3086b
  for rabies, 2066-2069, 2067t, 2068b
Postexposure testing, for HIV, 3087
Postmortem teaching, bioethical dilemmas in, 3136
Postnecrotic cirrhosis, 1410
Postoperative pancreatitis, 1428
Postpartum cardiomyopathy, 2821
Postpartum depression, 2821-2822
Postpartum endometriosis, 2821
Postpartum hemorrhage, 258t, 2818-2820
Postprandial hypoglycemia, 1961
Postresuscitation syndrome, 77
Poststreptococcal glomerulonephritis, 2647-2648
Poststreptococcal reactive arthritis, 1791
Post-test odds, 3059t
Post-test probability, 3059t
Posttraumatic corneal ulcer, 1052, 1052f
Posttraumatic headache, 1640
Posttraumatic osteomyelitis, 2185
Posttraumatic pericarditis, 1283
Posttraumatic pseudoaneurysm, 789-790, 1356-1357, 1357f
Posttraumatic reversible arterial spasm, 538
Posttraumatic seizure, 370, 373, 1623
  prophylaxis against, 361, 361b
Posttraumatic stress disorder, 1746b
  panic attack in, 1749
  suicide and, 1769
Posttraumatic syrinx, 435, 436f, 2909
Postural strangulation, 450
Posturing, in head trauma, 357
Potassium
  administration of
    for diabetic ketoacidosis, 1966
    for digitalis toxicity, 2370
    for hypokalemia, 1939
    for metabolic alkalosis, 1931
  imbalance of. *See* Hyperkalemia; Hypokalemia.
  in resting membrane potential, 1200, 1200f
  normal physiology of, 1937
  serum, in diabetic ketoacidosis, 1964, 1964t
  serum pH and, 1924
  skin injury from, 937
Potassium channel antagonists, after cerebral ischemia, 71
Potassium chloride
  for alcoholic ketoacidosis, 2873
  ingestion of, gastric injury from, 2381, 2381f, 2382f
Potassium hydroxide, ingestion of, 2380, 2381t
Potassium hydroxide (KOH) examination, in dermatophyte infections, 1838
Potassium iodide
  for erythema nodosum, 1856-1857
  for internal radioactive contamination, 2324
  for radioactive iodine exposure, 3023, 3023t
  for thyroid storm, 1989
Potassium loss, in salicylate overdose, 2340
Potassium phosphate, for hypophosphatemia, 1952
Potassium-sparing diuretics, 1321t
Potential injury-creating event (PICE) nomenclature, 3011-3012, 3011t, 3012b, 3012t
Pott's disease, 261, 265t, 2159, 2178, 2182, 2182f, 2184-2185
Pott's fracture, 551t
Povidone-iodine
  for rabies postexposure prophylaxis, 2068
  for skin disinfection, 847
  for wound cleansing, 847-848, 848t
Powder burn, 953
Power of attorney, durable, 3133
Power of clinical trial, 3051t, 3052
Poxviruses, 2034t, 2039-2040, 2039f
PPD testing, 2156-2157, 2157b, 2158t
PR interval, 1202
  in first-degree atrioventricular block, 1218
  in infants and children, 2574, 2574t
  in Wolff-Parkinson-White syndrome, 1235
PR segment, in pericarditis, 1281, 1282
Practice guidelines. *See* Guidelines for emergency medicine.

Practice patterns, computer-based analysis of, 3099
Practolol, overdose of, 2373t
Pralidoxime
 for nerve agent exposure, 3030-3031, 3031t
 for organophosphate poisoning, 2461
Prazosin, 1321t
Prechiasmal visual loss, 1059
Precordial thump, 90
Prednisolone
 for asthma, 1088, 2539t, 2541, 2543t
 for caustic ingestion, 2383
Prednisone
 during pregnancy and lactation, 2776, 2789
 for anaphylaxis, 2549
 for asthma, 1088, 1089, 2539t, 2541, 2543t
 for autoimmune hemolytic anemia, 1883
 for Bell's palsy, 1667
 for chronic obstructive pulmonary disease, 1106
 for Churg-Strauss syndrome, 1816
 for contact dermatitis, 1852
 for erythema multiforme, 1853
 for giant cell arteritis, 1638
 for gouty arthritis, 1786
 for Henoch-Schönlein purpura, 1815
 for hypercalcemic cancer patient, 1916
 for inflammatory bowel disease, 2616
 for inflammatory myopathy, 1708
 for kerion, 1839
 for Lyme disease–related myocarditis, 1292
 for mixed cryoglobulinemia, 1815
 for nephrotic syndrome, 2648
 for pemphigus vulgaris, 1857
 for pericarditis, 1282
 for Pneumocystis pneumonia in HIV/AIDS, 2078
 for rheumatic fever, 1791
 for rheumatoid arthritis, 1791
 for systemic lupus erythematosus, 1809
 for Takayasu's arteritis, 1813
 for temporal, 1813
 immunosuppressive effects of, 2843-2844
 prophylactic, for cluster headache, 1635
Preeclampsia, 2749-2751, 2750b
Preexcitation, 1203, 1235-1237, 1236f, 1237f
Preexposure prophylaxis, for rabies, 2069, 2069t
Prefreeze phase of frostbite, 2229, 2229b
Pregnancy, 2722-2872
 abdominal pain in, 2733, 2752-2756, 2753t
 abruptio placentae in, 2747-2748, 2809-2810
 acetaminophen overdose in, 2336-2337
 acute complications of, 2739-2759
  early, 2740-2747
  late, 2747-2752
  medical and surgical problems associated with, 2752-2759, 2753t
 acute coronary syndromes in, 2763t, 2766-2767
 acute fatty liver of, 1417, 2755-2756
 air medical transport in, 2999
 alcohol consumption during, 2877-2878
 alkalemia in, 1926
 altitude and, 2308-2309
 amniotic fluid embolus in, 2751-2752
 anatomic changes in, 317-318
 anemia in, 2724, 2763t, 2767-2768
 antituberculous agents during, 2168
 appendicitis in, 1453, 2752-2754, 2754f
 asthma in, 1091, 2761-2762, 2763t, 2765t
 bacterial vaginosis in, 1568
 bleeding diathesis in, 2753t
 carbon monoxide poisoning in, 2440
 cardiomyopathy in, 1297
 carpal tunnel syndrome in, 1697
 chest pain in, 2732-2733
 cholelithiasis in, 1419, 2754-2755
 cholestasis in, 1416-1417
  intrahepatic, 2756
 chorioamnionitis in, 2759
 chronic medical illness during, 2761-2776, 2763t-2765t
 decompression sickness in, 2285
 definitions related to, 2722-2723
 depression following, 1738
 diabetes mellitus in, 1972, 2764t, 2771-2772
 differential considerations in, 2731-2733
 disease and injury prevention in, 2735-2737
 domestic violence in, 997, 2734-2735, 2734t

Pregnancy (Continued)
 drug therapy during, safety of, 2781-2790, 2782t-2783t
 dyspnea in, 2725, 2753t
 ectopic, 2742-2746
  ancillary studies in, 2745
  clinical features of, 2743
  diagnosis of, 2743-2744
  differential considerations in, 2745
  hormonal assays in, 2744
  management of, 2745-2746, 2746f
  miscarriage vs., 2741
  pelvic pain in, 251t
  risk factors for, 2743, 2743b
  ruptured, abdominal pain in, 214t
  ultrasonography of, 2730, 2744, 2744b
  vaginal bleeding in, 257, 257t
 electrical injuries in, 2277
 emergency equipment needs in, 2735
 epidemiology of, 2722, 2723f
 epilepsy in, 2763t, 2768-2769
 genitourinary infections in, 2757-2759
 gynecologic problems in, 2752, 2753t
 headache in, 2732
 heart failure in, 1268
 hemorrhoids in, 1510
 hepatitis in, 2775
 heterotopic, 2743
 history in, 2727
 HIV/AIDS in, 2764t, 2774, 2810
 hyperemesis gravidarum in, 2756
 hypertension in, 1317, 2727, 2765t
  chronic, 2762, 2763t, 2765t
  gestational, 2749-2751, 2750b
  pulmonary, 2762, 2766
 hypomagnesemia in, 1948
 jaundice in, 2726, 2753t
 laboratory studies in, 2728-2730, 2729f
 liver disorders in, 1416-1417, 2755-2756
 Lyme disease in, 2128-2129
 miscarriage in, 2740-2742, 2741b
  ectopic pregnancy vs., 2745
 molar, 257, 2741, 2746-2747
 multiple sclerosis in, 2763t, 2769-2770
 musculoskeletal pain in, 2733
 myasthenia gravis in, 2764t, 2770-2771
 nausea and vomiting in, 204t, 206, 2756
 pancreatitis in, 1428
 pelvic inflammatory disease in, 2759
 pelvic pain in, 248, 249b, 250, 252
 pericardial disease in, 1287
 physical examination in, 2727-2728
 physiologic changes in, 316-317, 317t, 2723-2727, 2724f-2726f, 2727t
 placenta previa in, 2748, 2808-2809
 prevention of, after sexual assault, 991, 991t
 pulmonary embolism in, 1380
 pyelonephritis in, 2754, 2757, 2758
 radiologic studies in, 2730-2731, 2730f, 2731f
 renal disorders in, 2771
 rheumatic diseases in, 2775-2776
 salicylate poisoning in, 2342
 seizure in, 1624, 2753t, 2763t, 2768-2769
 sexually transmitted diseases in, 2758-2759
 spinal cord injury in, 2770
 spurious, 2731-2732
 substance abuse in, 2736, 2790-2794, 2791b, 2883
 syphilis in, 1562, 2764t, 2775
 systemic lupus erythematosus in, 1810, 2775-2776
 thromboembolic disease in, 317, 2756-2757
 thyroid disorders in, 2764t, 2772-2773
 trauma in, 318-326, 2733
  blunt, 318
  diagnostic strategies in, 320-321, 320t, 321t
  disposition in, 326
  fetal evaluation in, 323-324, 323f, 323t, 324f
  fetal injury in, 319
  fetomaternal hemorrhage and, 321
  management of, 321-326, 322f
  maternal resuscitation in, 322-323
  penetrating, 318-319
  perimortem cesarean section in, 325-326
  placental injury in, 319-320
  prehospital end-of-life issues related to, 3145
  primary survey in, 322-323
  secondary survey in, 323
  uterine injury in, 320

Pregnancy (Continued)
 trichomoniasis in, 1568
 tuberculosis in, 2764t, 2773-2774
 ultrasonography in, third trimester, 2802, 2802b, 2802t
 urinary tract infection in, 1578, 2757-2758
 vaginal bleeding in, 2727
  differential diagnosis in, 2753t
  during second half, 2747-2748
  epidemiology of, 254
  first-trimester, 2740-2741, 2746f
  pathophysiology of, 254
  third-trimester, 2808-2810
  treatment of, 257, 259
 vaginitis in, 2758
 valvular heart disease in, 2763t, 2767
 vulvovaginal candidiasis in, 1568
Pregnancy test, 2728-2730, 2729f
 in abdominal pain, 216
 in appendicitis, 1454
 in pelvic pain, 249
Pregnancy tumor, 1035
Prehospital care
 airway management in, 2990
 controversies in, 2990-2991
 during air medical transport, 2998-2999
 end-of-life issues in, 3144-3146
 equipment in, 2988
 in abdominal trauma, 502
 in acute coronary syndromes, 1157
 in alcohol withdrawal syndrome, 2861
 in anaphylaxis, 1830
 in aortic rupture, 481
 in bleeding disorders, 1894
 in cardiac tamponade, 475
 in cardiovascular emergencies, 2990-2991
 in central nervous system infection, 1721
 in delirium, 1653
 in eclampsia, 2750
 in elder abuse, 1011
 in elderly trauma patient, 348
 in facial trauma, 389-390
 in injury prevention and control, 948
 in ischemic stroke, 1613-1614
 in PCP intoxication, 2415
 in pediatric asthma, 2537
 in pediatric fever, 2511
 in pelvic fracture, 718
 in respiratory emergencies, 2990
 in severe head trauma, 358
 in snakebite, 899
 in spinal injuries, 435
 in splinting and bandaging of fractures, 568, 569f
 in sudden infant death syndrome, 2717
 in suicide, 1771
 in thermal burns, 921
 in trauma emergencies, 2991
 medications in, 2987-2988, 2990-2991
 protocols for, 2989
Prehospital directives, 3132-3133
Prehospital information systems, 3099, 3101, 3105
Prehospital response, in disaster preparedness, 3014-3015
Prehospital resuscitation, bioethical dilemmas in, 3132-3133
Prehypertension, 1310
Preload
 in heart failure, 1259-1260, 1260f
 normalization of, in sepsis, 2218
Premature atrial contractions, 1222-1223, 1222f, 1223f
Premature infant
 sudden death in, 2714-2715
 symptomatic, definition of, 2714
Premature junctional contractions, 1223-1224
Premature labor, 2805-2807, 2806b, 2807b
Premature rupture of membranes, 2807-2808, 2808t
Premature ventricular contractions, 1223t, 1224-1225, 1224f
 causes of, 1224, 1224b
 Lown classification of, 1225, 1225t
 treatment of, 1225
Prematurity, apnea of, definition of, 2714
Preoxygenation, in rapid sequence intubation, 10, 10f
Prepatellar bursitis, 795-796, 1801-1803

Prerenal azotemia, 1527t, 1532-1533, 1533b, 1538
Preschool children
　developmental milestones in, 2496t, 2497
　fever in, management of, 2515
Prescriptions, medicolegal issues in, 3160
Preseptal cellulitis, 2197-2198
Pressure urticaria, 1848
Pressure-cycled ventilation, 27
Pressure-support ventilation (PSV), 27
Pressure-volume relationships
　and scuba diving–related disorders, 2281f
　in dysbarisms, 2280-2281, 2281f
Preterm labor, 2805-2807, 2806b, 2807b
Pretest odds, 3059t
Pretracheal layer, 442-443
Prevention and control of injury, 940-950
　acute trauma care and, 948
　advocacy of public policy for, 948, 950
　epidemiology and documentation in, 945-946
　in elderly person, 2829-2830
　in gang violence in emergency department,
　　1021-1022
　in pregnancy, 2735-2737
　in youth violence, 1020
　methods of prevention in, 944-945
　prehospital care in, 948
　principles of, 940, 941f, 943-945, 943t, 944t
　public health and, 943-944, 944t
　risk factor assessment in, 946-948
　scientific approach to, 940, 941b
Preventive services
　for elderly person, 2829-2830
　in tactical emergency medical support, 3004
　medicolegal issues in, 3159
Prevertebral space, 1027, 1117
Priapism
　in children, 2635-2636
　in sickle cell disease, 1880
Prickly heat, 2259
Primaquine, for malaria, 2104
Primary care physician, emergency physician
　　and, differences between, 3131, 3131t
Primary survey
　in obstetric trauma, 322-323
　in pediatric trauma, 329-330, 329t, 331t-333t
Primate bite, 884, 888-889, 889b, 889t
Primidone, during pregnancy and lactation, 2787
Prinzmetal angina, 1156
Prion disease, 1657-1658, 1659, 2058
Prisoners
　consent and, 3168
　foreign body ingestion by, 873, 874f
Private patient, screening requirements for, 3157
Probability, 3051t, 3052
　a priori, 3055-3056
　post-test, 3059t
　pretest, 3059t
Probenecid
　during pregnancy and lactation, 2784
　for gouty arthritis, 1786
Problem patient. See Combative patient; Difficult
　　patient.
Problem-solving, developmental milestones in,
　　2495-2497, 2496t
Procainamide, 1206
　during pregnancy and lactation, 2787
　for atrial fibrillation, 1232b, 1233
　for dysrhythmia, in infants and children,
　　2586b
　for pediatric resuscitation, 103t, 105
　for ventricular tachycardia, 1242
　for wide-complex tachycardia, 1240
　for Wolff-Parkinson-White syndrome, 1237
Procaine, 2931t
Procedural sedation and analgesia, 2938-2954
　agents for, 2940t-2941t
　barbiturates for, 2945-2946
　benzodiazepines for, 2944-2945
　consent prior to, 2940
　contraindications to, 2939
　discharge criteria and instructions after, 2943
　drug selection and administration in, 2949-
　　2952, 2950t, 2951b
　etomidate for, 2940t-2941t, 2947-2948
　fasting prior to, 2939-2940
　in children, 2952-2954
　ketamine for, 2940t-2941t, 2946-2947
　monitoring of, 2942-2943
　nitrous oxide for, 2940t-2941t, 2948

Procedural sedation and analgesia (Continued)
　opioids for, 2944
　personnel providing, 2941-2942
　preprocedure patient assessment in, 2938-2940
　propofol for, 2940t-2941t, 2947
　recovery from, 2943
　reversal agents in, 2948-2949
　route of administration for, 2943-2944
　sedation continuum and, 2938, 2939f
　supplies and equipment for, 2942
　terminology in, 2938, 2939b
Process improvement in emergency department,
　　3119-3126
　problem areas and, 3124-3126, 3125t
　sources of failure and, 3119-3123, 3120f, 3120t
Prochlorperazine, 2446t
　for migraine, 1633t, 1634, 2680
　for nausea and vomiting, 203, 208b, 208t
　for vertigo, 146
Procidentia, 1521, 1521f
Proctalgia fugax, 1509, 1516 See also Anorectal
　　pain
Proctitis
　Chlamydia trachomatis, 1519
　herpes, 1519
　radiation, 1520-1521
Proctocolitis, radiation, 1505-1506
Proctosigmoidoscopy, in gastrointestinal
　　bleeding, 224
"Professional disclosure" standard, 3166
Professional relationships, as stressor for
　　emergency physician, 3175
Professional values, 3129, 3129b
Progesterone, serum, in ectopic pregnancy, 2744
Progressive multifocal leukoencephalopathy,
　　2045-2046
　dementia in, 1658, 1659
　in HIV/AIDS, 2082
Prokinetic agents, for nausea and vomiting, 206,
　　208b
Prolactin, serum, in pregnancy, 2726
PROM (premature rupture of membranes), 2807-
　　2808, 2808t
Promethazine, 2446t
　for migraine, 2680
　for vertigo, 146
Pronation, of hand, 577f
Pronator quadratus line, 626, 628f
Prone sleeping, in sudden infant death
　　syndrome, 2715
Propafenone, 1208
Propantheline, anticholinergic toxicity of, 2345
Proparacaine, for red and painful eye, 291
Propofol
　for procedural sedation and analgesia, 2940t-
　　2941t, 2947, 2950-2952, 2954
　for status epilepticus, 1627, 1627t, 2672t, 2673
　for tetanus, 2011
　in cyclic antidepressant poisoning, 2356
Proportional assist ventilation, 33
Propoxyphene, 2452, 2453, 2453t, 2920
Propranolol, 1209, 1321t
　alcohol interactions with, 2875
　for alcohol withdrawal syndrome, 2862
　for chloral hydrate poisoning, 2487
　for hypoxic (tet) spells, 2581
　for migraine prophylaxis, 1634
　for tetanus, 2011
　for thyroid storm, 1989
　overdose of, 2373t, 2374
　prophylactic, for migraine, 2680
Propylthiouracil
　for hyperthyroidism in pregnancy, 2773
　for thyroid storm, 1988
Prospective observational study, 3047
Prostacyclin
　as anaphylaxis mediator, 1823, 1823b
　in heart failure, 1262
Prostaglandin
　as anaphylaxis mediator, 1823, 1823b
　for upper gastrointestinal disorders, 1399
　in asthma, 1080f, 1081, 1081f
　in burn edema, 917
　in frostbite, 2229
　in heart failure, 1262
　in sepsis, 2213
Prostaglandin E1, for ductal-dependent
　　congenital heart disease, 2576-2577, 2577b
Prostaglandin E2, in fever, 134

Prostaglandin synthetase inhibitors, for
　　premature labor, 2807
Prostate, physical examination of, 1573
Prostatitis, 1585-1586
Prosthesis, joint, infection after, 2191
Prosthetic graft, for peripheral arteriovascular
　　disease, 1350
Prosthetic valve
　complications of, 1307-1308
　endocarditis as complication of, 1300
Protease inhibitors
　for HIV/AIDS, 2087t, 2088
　rifamycins and, drug interactions between,
　　2166
Protease-antiprotease relationship, in chronic
　　obstructive pulmonary disease, 1098
Protective body armor, nonpenetrating ballistic
　　injury associated with, 458-459
Protective equipment
　for tuberculosis, 2170
　in tactical emergency medical support, 3004
　in terrorism incidents, 3013
Protein
　cerebrospinal fluid
　　in bacterial meningitis, 2661
　　in central nervous system infection, 1718
　urine, 1525
Protein buffers, 1923
Protein C, in sepsis, 2214
Protein kinases, in cerebral ischemia, 66
Proteinuria, 1530-1532
　clinical features of, 1531
　glomerular, 1531
　in children, 2646-2647
　in glomerulonephritis, 1534
　in nephrotic syndrome, 1531, 1531b
　in preeclampsia/eclampsia, 2749-2751, 2750b
　laboratory studies in, 1532
　orthostatic, 1531
　overflow, 1531
　tubular, 1531
Proteolytic enzymes, in sarcoplasm, 1976
Proteus infection, in urinary tract infection,
　　1583
Prothrombin time (PT)
　abnormal, 1899
　in bleeding disorders, 1895
　in factor VII deficiency, 1899
　in gastrointestinal bleeding, 222
　in hepatitis, 1404
　in pregnancy, 318
Protocols, decision making errors in using, 131t,
　　132
Proton pump inhibitors
　for gastroesophageal reflux, 1389-1390, 1390t
　for gastrointestinal bleeding, 224-225
　for upper gastrointestinal disorders, 1390t,
　　1399
Protozoal gastroenteritis, 1476-1482, 1477t
　Cryptosporidium, 1476-1478, 1477t
　Cyclospora cayetanensis, 1477t, 1478-1479
　Entamoeba histolytica, 1477t, 1480-1481
　Enterobius vermicularis, 1479-1482
　Giardia, 1477t, 1479-1480
　Isospora belli, 1476-1478, 1477t
Protozoal infections
　drug therapy for, 2098t
　parasites in, 2099t
Proximal femoral epiphysis, avascular necrosis
　　of, 2706-2707, 2707f
Proximal femoral fracture, 750-752, 750f-751f,
　　752b
Proximal fibula, fracture of, 801-802, 802f, 814f
Proximal humeral epiphysis, fracture of, 682-683,
　　683f
Proximal humerus
　anatomy of, 672, 673f
　fracture of, 680-682, 681f, 682f
Proximal interphalangeal joint, 578, 579f
　dislocation of, 601-602
　extensor tendon injuries at, 607-608, 607f
Proximal phalanx
　extensor tendon injuries at, 608
　fracture of, 594-595, 594f-596f
Proximal radioulnar joint, 639-640
Proximal radius, 647, 647f
Proximal tibia
　anatomy of, 770, 771f
　fracture of

Proximal tibia *(Continued)*
  extra-articular, 797-799
  intra-articular, 777-781
Proximal tibiofibular joint, dislocation of, 802-803
Proximity wounds, 540, 540f, 543
Pruritus
  in anaphylaxis, 1829, 2548
  in atopic dermatitis, 1842
  in ciguatera fish poisoning, 1473
  in decompression sickness, 2284
  in HIV/AIDS, 2084-2085
  in *Sarcoptes scabiei* infestation, 1569
  internal malignancy associated with, 1864
Pruritus ani, 1509, 1517-1518, 1517b
  causes of, 1517, 1517b
  in *Enterobius vermicularis* gastroenteritis, 1481
  in parasitic infection, 2113-2114
Pruritus gravidarum, 2726, 2756
Prussian blue, for cesium and thallium ingestion, 3023, 3023t
Pseudarthrosis, 564
Pseudoaneurysm, 538, 538f, 1348
  after abdominal aortic aneurysm repair, 1340
  infected, in drug abusers, 1361
  posttraumatic, 789-790, 1356-1357, 1357t
  repair of, 544
Pseudocholinesterase activity, conditions and drugs that reduce, 13, 13b
Pseudoclaudication, in spinal stenosis, 705
Pseudoclawing, 595
Pseudocoarctation syndrome, in aortic rupture, 478
Pseudocyanosis, 268
Pseudocyst, pancreatic, 1427, 1430, 1430f, 1435
Pseudodementia, 1656, 1659-1660, 1660t
Pseudodysrhythmias, 1215, 1215f
Pseudoephedrine
  during pregnancy and lactation, 2790
  prophylactic, for middle ear barotrauma, 2292
Pseudofracture, 558
Pseudogout, 1786-1787
Pseudohematuria, 1604
Pseudohyperkalemia, 1939
Pseudohyperphosphatemia, 1952
Pseudohyponatremia, 1933
Pseudohypoparathyroidism, hypocalcemia in, 1943
Pseudohypotension, in aortic dissection, 1326
Pseudologica fantastica, in Munchausen's syndrome, 1762
Pseudomembranous colitis, in *Clostridium difficile* infection, 2625
Pseudomonas aeruginosa
  in bone or joint infections, 2178, 2178t
  in cystic fibrosis, 2564
Pseudoneurologic symptoms, 1755, 1755b
Pseudoparkinsonism, from antipsychotic agents, 1732
Pseudoseizure, 1624-1625, 2668
Pseudosubluxation, cervical spine, 337, 337f, 421
Pseudotattooing, in long-range handgun wounds, 957, 957f
Pseudotumor cerebri
  headache in, 2678
  in pregnancy, 2732
Pseudotumor sign, in small bowel obstruction, 1443
Psilocybin, 2406-2408, 2407f, 2478-2479
Psittacosis, pneumonia in, 1131
Psoas sign, in appendicitis, 1452, 2619
Psoriatic arthropathy, 1790
Psychedelics, ingestion of, 2406-2408, 2407f
Psychiatric consultation, for somatoform disorders, 1758-1759
Psychiatric disorders
  anxiety disorders as, 1744-1752
  factitious disease and malingering as, 1761-1765
  in developmentally disabled patient, 2903
  in intimate partner violence and abuse, 997-998
  in substance abuse, 2885
  mood disorders as, 1734-1742
  panic attack in, 1748-1749
  seizures vs., 2668
  sexual assault and, 979
  somatoform disorders as, 1753-1759
  suicide and, 1768, 1769

Psychiatric disorders *(Continued)*
  thought disorders as, 1726-1733
  violent behavior and, 2957
Psychiatric interview, 1730
Psychiatric presentations, hypothermia-induced, 2242
Psychiatric short-procedure unit, 1733
Psychic pain, in grief response, 3149
Psychoactive substances
  ingestion of, 2406-2408, 2407f
  syncope from, 195b
Psychogenic casualties, in terrorism incidents, 3013
Psychogenic polydipsia, 1934
Psychological abuse of elder, 1010
Psychological issues
  after sexual assault, 991-992, 991b
  in alcoholism, 2879-2880
  in asthma, 1082
  in elderly person, 2827
  in HIV/AIDS, 2086-2087
Psychological symptoms, factitious disorder with, 1761-1762
Psychological techniques, in pain management, 2934
Psychomotor agitation. *See* Agitation.
Psychomotor epilepsy, 1621
Psychomotor processes, in clinical decision making, 130, 131t
Psychomotor retardation, in depression, 1737
Psychosis, 1726-1733
  clinical features of, 1726-1728
  delirium vs., 1652, 1652t
  depression with, 1737
  diagnosis of, 1728
  disposition in, 1733
  in anticholinergic poisoning, 2348
  in HIV/AIDS, 2087
  in psychostimulant intoxication, 2410
  in systemic lupus erythematosus, 1807
  Korsakoff's, 2869
  LSD-induced, 2408
  management of, 1730-1733, 1731b
  organic vs. functional, 1727b, 1728-1729, 1728b, 1729t, 1771t
  panic attack in, 1748
  psychiatric diagnoses associated with, 1729
  suicide and, 1769
Psychosocial considerations
  in elderly person, 2827
  in sudden infant death syndrome, 2717, 2717b
Psychosocial stress, somatoform disorders and, 1753
Psychosocial support, for bipolar disorder, 1742
Psychosocial theories of mood disorders, 1736
Psychostimulant intoxication, 2408-2409, 2410-2411
Psychotherapy
  for anxiety disorders, 1751
  for depression, 1741-1742
  for somatoform disorders, 1758-1759
Psychotic disorder, brief, 1729
Psychotropics, for dysphagia, 1398
Psyllium, drug interactions with, 2478t
PTCA (percutaneous transluminal coronary angioplasty). *See* Percutaneous coronary intervention.
Pterygium, 296t, 1053-1054
Ptosis, in coral snakebite, 898
Pubic dislocation, reduction of, 759
Pubic ramus, fracture of, 724-725
Pubis, 717, 718f
Public health, injury prevention and control and, 943-944, 944t
Public health reporting, syndromic surveillance and, 3105
Public utility model, for EMS programs, 2985
Publication bias, 3050-3051, 3058
Puffy hand syndrome, in intravenous drug abusers, 1361
Pulled elbow, 666, 666f, 2697-2698, 2697f
Pulled muscle. *See* Strain.
Pulmonary. *See also* Lung; Respiration; Respiratory.
Pulmonary abscess, 1033, 1134, 1134f
Pulmonary agents, as chemical weapons, 3032
Pulmonary angiography, in pulmonary embolism, 1375-1377, 1377b

Pulmonary artery, congenital absence of, high-altitude pulmonary edema and, 2303
Pulmonary artery catheterization, in shock, 50
Pulmonary artery occlusive pressure (PAOP), in heart failure, 1260, 1260f
Pulmonary barotrauma, in scuba diving–related disorders, 2285-2286, 2293
Pulmonary compensation, in acid-base disorders, 1923
Pulmonary contusion, 340, 460-461, 460f
Pulmonary decompression sickness, 2284-2285, 2288, 2288t
Pulmonary disorders. *See also specific diseases, e.g.,* Asthma.
  altitude and, 2307-2308, 2307f
  anxiety in, 1747
  aspirin-exacerbated, 1082
  chronic
    in children, 2565, 2565f
    nonobstructive, 1102-1103
    obstructive, 1097-1107. *See also* Chronic obstructive pulmonary disease.
  heart failure in, 1265-1266
  in airway foreign body aspiration, 866
  in chronic renal failure, 1542
  in Churg-Strauss syndrome, 1816
  in developmentally disabled patient, 2903
  in HIV/AIDS, 2076-2079, 2076t
  in hydrocarbon poisoning, 2428
  in hypothyroidism, 1992
  in intracerebral hemorrhage, 1610
  in opioid overdose, 2452-2453, 2453t
  in pancreatitis, 1429
  in parasitic infection, 2110-2111
  in physically disabled patient, 2907-2908
  in sepsis, 2214, 2214b
  in substance abuse, 2885
  in systemic lupus erythematosus, 1808
  in thermal burns, 918
  infectious. *See* Respiratory tract infection.
  pleural, 1143-1153
Pulmonary edema
  acute
    in mitral regurgitation, 1306
    pathophysiology of, 1261-1262
    treatment of, 1270-1274, 1271f
    with adequate perfusion, 1271-1273
    with hypotension, 1273-1274
  cardiogenic, 1261-1262
  cardiomegaly with, 1174, 1175f
  dialysis for, 1548
  high-altitude, 2296, 2298-2299, 2299f, 2300f, 2303-2305, 2303b
  hypertension in, 1316
  in chronic renal failure, 1542, 1546, 1546b, 1546f
  in cyclic antidepressant poisoning, 2354
  in near-hanging and strangulation, 450-451
  in peritoneal dialysis patient, 1554
  in salicylate overdose, 2340, 2341
  in scuba diving–related disorders, 2286
  in spinal injuries, 438
  neurogenic
    after head trauma, 371
    after seizure, 1625
  noncardiogenic, 1261
    in barbiturate overdose, 2482
    in irritant gas exposure, 2434, 2435
    in opioid overdose, 2453
    in overdosed/poisoned patient, 2330
    in sickle cell disease, 1880
    in smoke inhalation, 2435
    transfusion-related, 60
Pulmonary embolism, 1371-1381. *See also* Venous thrombosis.
  anticoagulation in, 1377
  chest pain in, 183, 186b, 190t-191t, 1372, 1380
  clinical course in, unpredictability of, 1378-1380, 1379f
  complications of, predictors of, 1377, 1378t
  diagnosis of, 1372-1377, 1373f, 1375f, 1376t, 1377b
  dyspnea in, 179t
  heart failure in, 1269
  high-altitude, 2304
  in chronic obstructive pulmonary disease, 1102
  in elderly person, 1368
  in mitral stenosis, 1306
  in obese patient, 1380-1381

Pulmonary embolism (Continued)
  in pregnancy, 1380, 2733, 2756-2757
  in spinal cord injury, 2906
  management of, 1377-1381
  massive, 1372f, 1378f
  pathophysiology of, 1371-1372, 1371t, 1372b,
    1372f
  pleural effusion in, 1150-1151
  pneumothorax vs., 1146
  risk factors for, 186b, 1371, 1371t
  rule-out criteria for, 1372b, 1374
  thrombolytic therapy in, 1377-1378, 1378t,
    1379
  with lung infarction, 1373
Pulmonary function tests
  in asthma, 1084-1085, 1086f, 2535t, 2536,
    2536f
  in chronic obstructive pulmonary disease, 1101
Pulmonary hemorrhage, in Goodpasture
  syndrome, 1816
Pulmonary hypersecretion, in organophosphate
  poisoning, 2459
Pulmonary hypertension
  altitude and, 2308
  from high altitude exposure, 2298-2299
  in pregnancy, 2762, 2766
Pulmonary irritants, inhalation of, 2433t, 2434-
  2435, 2434f
Pulmonary laceration, 461
Pulmonary oxygen toxicity, in scuba
  diving–related disorders, 2283
Pulmonary system
  aging and, 345
  alcohol consumption and, 2866-2867
  in hypothermia, 2239
  in pregnancy, 2725
  in transition from fetal to extrauterine life, 118-
    119, 119t, 2568
Pulmonary trauma, 459-466
  hemothorax in, 464-465, 465b, 465f
  in bipyridyl compound poisoning, 2466
  in electrical and lightning injuries, 2274
  in hydrocarbon poisoning, 2428
  in scuba diving–related disorders, 2285-2286,
    2293
  in smoke inhalation, 2435
  in submersion victim, 2312-2313
  pneumothorax in, 461-464, 461f-463f, 464b
  pulmonary contusion in, 460-461, 460f
  pulmonary laceration in, 461
  subcutaneous emphysema in, 459-460
  tracheobronchial injury in, 466, 466f
Pulmonary tularemia, 2131
Pulmonary vascular bed, destruction of, in
  chronic obstructive pulmonary disease,
  1097-1098
Pulmonary vascular occlusion, 1371-1372
Pulmonary vascular resistance, in thermal burns,
  918
Pulmonic flow murmur of neonates, 2572
Pulp, 1026, 1027f
  exposure of, fractures resulting in, 1037
Pulpitis, 1031
Pulpotomy, 1037
Pulse
  absent
    in electrical and lightning injuries, 2271
    in pulmonary embolism, 1380
    in tibial femoral knee dislocation, 788
  during cardiopulmonary resuscitation, 79
  in aortic regurgitation, 1307
  in peripheral arteriovascular disease, 1346
  in peripheral vascular injury, 539, 541
Pulse oximetry, 36-37
  during procedural sedation and analgesia, 2942
  in asthma, 1085, 2537
  in bronchiolitis, 2545
  in children, 2504
  in chronic obstructive pulmonary disease,
    1100
  in comatose patient, 162
  in confirmation of endotracheal tube
    placement, 7
  in cyanosis, 270
  in delirium, 1651
  in peripheral vascular injury, 541
  in pneumonia, 1134
  in pulmonary embolism, 1377, 1378t
Pulseless disease, 1813

Pulseless electrical activity
  capnography in, 82
  in infants and children, 112, 2586t, 2590
  treatment of, 84, 112
Pulseless ventricular tachycardia, treatment of,
  84, 112-113, 112f
Pulsus alternans, in neoplastic cardiac
  tamponade, 1917
Pulsus paradoxus
  in asthma, 1084, 2534, 2535t
  in cardiac tamponade, 473
Punctate burns, 2273
Puncture wounds, antibiotic prophylaxis for,
  855
Pupil
  Adie's tonic, 1061
  Horner's, 1061-1062
Pupillary abnormalities
  in intracerebral hemorrhage, 1610-1611
  in red and painful eye, 286
Pupillary block, in closed-angle glaucoma, 1056,
  1056f
Pupillary examination, in head trauma, 357
Purkinje fibers, 1202
  digitalis effects on, 2368
Purpura, 1839t
  anaphylactoid, 2615, 2615f
  causes of, 1864b
  drug-induced, 1844-1845, 1845f, 1847t, 1864b
  Henoch-Schönlein, 1815, 2615, 2615f, 2653-
    2654
  in meningococcal disease, 2022
  internal malignancy associated with, 1864
  thrombocytopenic
    autoimmune, 1897-1898
    oral manifestations of, 1036
    thrombotic, 1467, 1898
Purulent arthritis, gonococcal, 2191
Pustule, 1839t
Putaminal lesions, in methanol poisoning, 2396,
  2397
Pyarthrosis, pediatric limp and, 764-765, 765f
Pyelography
  intravenous
    in renal trauma, 528
    in ureteral trauma, 531, 531f
    in urinary tract infection, 1578
    in urolithiasis, 1589, 1592f
  retrograde, in ureteral trauma, 531, 531f-532f
Pyelonephritis
  acute, 1573
  hypertension in, 1312
  in children, 2642, 2643, 2644
  in kidney transplant patient, 2855
  in men, 1585
  in pregnancy, 2757, 2758
    appendicitis vs., 2754
  in urinary tract infection, 1575, 1581t, 1582-
    1583
  observation in, 3072-3073
  urolithiasis vs., 1590
Pyloric stenosis
  in infants and children, 2603-2606, 2605f,
    2606t
  malrotation with midgut volvulus vs., 2608
Pyogenic abscess, 1414-1415, 1415f
Pyogenic granuloma, 1035
Pyopneumopericardium, 1287-1288
Pyracantha, 2475
Pyrantel pamoate, for Enterobius vermicularis
  gastroenteritis, 1482
Pyrazinamide, for tuberculosis, 2162, 2163t,
  2164t
Pyrazolone, overdose of, 2343
Pyrethrin and pyrethroid poisoning, 2466-2467,
  2467b
Pyridostigmine, for myasthenia gravis, 1706
Pyridoxine
  deficiency of, seizure in, 2667
  for gyromitrin-containing mushroom
    poisoning, 2479
  for sideroblastic anemia, 1873
  for toxic alcohol poisoning, 2402
Pyrilamine, anticholinergic toxicity of, 2345
Pyrimethamine
  for isosporiasis, 1478
  for Toxoplasma gondii infection, 2082
  in HIV/AIDS, side effects of, 2079t
Pyrogens, 134, 2258

Pyruvate kinase deficiency, in hemolytic anemia,
  1878
Pyuria, in urinary tract infection, 1576

Q fever, 1131, 2137
Q waves, in myocardial infarction, 1156, 1164
QRS axis, in infants and children, 2574-2575,
  2574t
QRS complex, 1202-1203
  in atrial fibrillation, 1230, 1231f
  in complete atrioventricular block, 1221
  in infants and children, 2574, 2574t
  in premature atrial contractions, 1222
  in premature ventricular contractions, 1224
  in Wolff-Parkinson-White syndrome, 1235
QRS prolongation
  in cyclic antidepressant poisoning, 2352, 2354
  in OTC sleep aid overdose, 2488
QT dispersion, in acute coronary syndromes,
  1174
QT interval, 1203, 2574, 2574t
QT prolongation
  antipsychotic-induced, 2447, 2449
  classification and causes of, 1244b
  seizures vs., 2668
  submersion injuries and, 2312
  sudden death in, 2598-2599
Quadriceps, overuse of, popliteus tendinitis and,
  795
Quadriceps angle, in patellar dislocation, 785
Quadriceps tendon
  anatomy of, 770, 771f
  injury to, 761, 782-784, 783f, 784f
Quadriplegia
  in cerebral herniation, 356
  spastic, in cerebral palsy, 2904
Quality of life, end of life and, 3142
Quality/performance improvement, in emergency
  medical services, 2989
Quazepam, 2484t
Quetiapine
  for thought disorders, 1731
  toxicity of, 2446, 2446t
Quick Confusion Scale, 151, 153f
Quinapril hydrochloride, 1322t
Quincke's sign, in aortic regurgitation, 1307
Quinidine, 1206
  during pregnancy and lactation, 2787
  immune thrombocytopenia from, 1897
Quinine
  for babesiosis, 2140
  for malaria, 2104
  thrombocytopenia from, 1897, 1898
Quinsy, 1117-1118, 1118f
Quinton-Mahurkar catheter, 1362f, 1364-1365

Rabeprazole, 1390t
Rabies, 2061-2069
  clinical features of, 2065-2066
  epidemiology of, 2061-2065, 2062f-2064f
  pathophysiology of, 2065
  postexposure prophylaxis for, 2066-2069,
    2067t, 2068b
  preexposure prophylaxis for, 2069, 2069t
  vaccine for, 2035t, 2068, 2068b
Raccoon, rabies in, 2062, 2062f, 2063-2064,
  2063f
Race, definition of, 3111
Racial/ethnic differences. See also Cultural
  competence.
  demographics of, 3108, 3108t
  discrimination based on, health consequences
    of, 3110
  in atypical symptoms of myocardial infarction,
    1159
  in health beliefs, values, and life experiences,
    3113-3114
  in health care access and outcomes, 3108-3111,
    3109t
  in hepatitis A infection, 1402
  in HIV/AIDS, 2072
  in sudden infant death syndrome, 2713
  in use of emergency department, 3115-3116,
    3115b
Racism, 3110

Radial artery, 540f, 585-586, 587f, 588f, 622, 625f
　injury to, 545-546
Radial bursa, flexor tendons and, 585, 586f
Radial collateral ligament, injury to, 604
Radial deviation, of hand, 577f
Radial head, 647
　dislocation of, in Monteggia's fracture, 642, 642f
　fracture of, 663, 663f, 664
　subluxation of, 666, 666f, 2697-2698, 2697f
Radial keratotomy, altitude and, 2309
Radial length measurement, 625, 626f
Radial mononeuropathy, 1693-1695, 1694f
Radial neck, fracture of, 664
Radial nerve, 586, 588f, 589f, 622, 625f, 648, 648f
　palsy of, 586, 588f
　　humeral shaft fracture and, 655
　　in radial mononeuropathy, 1695
Radial styloid, 625
Radial surface, of hand, 576, 577f
Radiation
　external, 2320
　heat transfer by, 2255
　ionizing, 2318f, 2319
　nonionizing, 2318-2319, 2318f
　types of, and possible hazards, 2319-2320, 2320f
Radiation absorbed dose, 2321
Radiation accident protocol, 2322-2323
Radiation burns, ocular, 1046-1047
Radiation dose
　indicators of, 2317t, 2321, 2321f
　median lethal whole-body, 2322
Radiation Emergency Assistance Center/Training Site, 2324-2325
Radiation exposure, 2316-2325
　as weapon of mass destruction, 3022-3023, 3023t
　disaster preparedness for, 3017-3018
　disposition in, 2324
　epidemiology of, 2316-2318, 2317t
　intrauterine, 320, 320t, 2731, 2731t
　management of, 2322-2325, 2323f
　pathophysiology of, 2318-2320, 2318f
　prehospital care in, 2322-2323
　resources for, 2324-2325
　signs and symptoms of, 2321-2322, 2321f
　types of, 2320-2321
Radiation therapy
　acute tumor lysis syndrome from, 1911
　esophagitis from, 1386, 1388
　pericarditis after, 1284
　proctocolitis from, 1505-1506
Radicular artery of Adamkiewicz, 1676
Radicular pain
　in diskitis, 1684
　in epidural abscess, 1684
　in epidural hematoma, 1683
　in intervertebral disk herniation, 264
　in spinal cord tumor, 1685
　pathophysiology of, 261
Radiculopathy
　in Lyme disease, 2123
　lumbar, 704
Radiocarpal joint, 622, 623f
Radiogardase, for cesium and thallium ingestion, 3023, 3023t
Radiography
　abdominal
　　in abdominal aortic aneurysm, 1334, 1334f
　　in abdominal pain, 216, 216t
　　in abdominal trauma, 495-496, 496f, 497f
　　in constipation, 239
　　in iron overdose, 2420, 2420f
　　of calcified gallstones, 1418, 1418f
　chest
　　in airway foreign body aspiration, 867, 867f-869f, 2551, 2551f
　　in anthrax exposure, 3025, 3025f
　　in aortic dissection, 1326-1327, 1326t
　　in aortic rupture, 478-479, 478f
　　in asthma, 1085, 2537, 2537f
　　in bronchiolitis, 2545
　　in cardiac tamponade, 474, 475f, 1285
　　in chest pain, 186, 188, 188t
　　in chronic obstructive pulmonary disease, 1100-1101
　　in confirmation of endotracheal tube placement, 7

Radiography (Continued)
　in cyanosis, 271
　in cystic fibrosis, 2564, 2565f
　in esophageal obstruction, 1383
　in esophageal perforation, 484-485, 485f
　in fever, 137
　in flail chest, 457-458
　in heart failure, 1269
　in hemoptysis, 281
　in hemothorax, 465, 465f
　in high-altitude pulmonary edema, 2299, 2300f, 2303
　in HIV/AIDS, 2076t, 2077
　in hydrocarbon poisoning, 2430, 2431f
　in hypothyroidism, 1993
　in mitral regurgitation, 1306
　in mitral stenosis, 1305
　in multiple trauma, 312
　in neoplastic cardiac tamponade, 1917
　in osteomyelitis, 2179-2180, 2179f, 2180f
　in pacemaker malfunction, 1254-1255
　in pediatric cardiovascular disorders, 2573-2574, 2573f, 2574f
　in pediatric fever, 2510
　in pericardial effusion, 1285
　in pleural effusion, 1150, 1151f
　in *Pneumocystis carinii* pneumonia, 1136, 1136f
　in pneumonia, 1132-1134, 1133f, 1134f, 2561, 2561f
　in pneumothorax, 462f, 463, 1145, 1145f, 1146f
　in pulmonary embolism, 1373
　in rib fracture, 454, 454b, 455f
　in sepsis, 2217
　in tetralogy of Fallot, 2580
　in tuberculosis, 2152-2154, 2152f-2153f, 2159, 2159f
　computed (digital), in fracture, 557
　in acromioclavicular joint dislocation, 686, 687f
　in acute mesenteric ischemia, 1447
　in acute pancreatitis, 1432
　in acute renal failure, 1538
　in adult epiglottitis, 1115-1116, 1116f
　in airway foreign body aspiration, 866-867, 867f-869f
　in ankle trauma, 810-811, 810f, 811f
　in anterior glenohumeral joint dislocation, 688, 688f
　in appendicitis, 1454, 2619, 2620f
　in arthritis, 1779-1780, 1780f
　in back pain, 264, 707-708, 708b, 708f-709f
　in calcaneal fracture, 826-827, 826f, 827f
　in calcific tendinitis, 698
　in cervical vascular injury, 449
　in child abuse, 973, 2699
　in chronic pancreatitis, 1435-1436, 1436f
　in clavicle fracture, 2693, 2693f
　in colonic ischemia, 1504
　in diarrhea, 233
　in distal tibiofibular syndesmotic ligament injury, 816
　in diverticular disease, 1494
　in elbow and humeral trauma, 641f, 650-652, 651f
　in elderly trauma patient, 347
　in esophageal foreign body, 868f, 869f, 871
　in esophageal perforation, 1385
　in facial fracture, 389
　in fetal identification, 2730
　in foot trauma, 821-822, 822f
　in forearm trauma, 640-641, 640f
　in fracture, 557-558
　in frostbite, 2231
　in hematuria, 1530
　in hip dislocation, 757, 758f
　in hypothermia, 2244
　in inferior glenohumeral joint dislocation, 693, 694f
　in inflammatory bowel disease, 1502, 1502f
　in intercondylar eminence fracture, 780
　in intussusception, 2611, 2611f
　in knee extensor tendon injuries, 783, 784f
　in knee ligament injuries, 791
　in knee trauma, 774
　in Legg-Calvé-Perthes disease, 2707, 2707f
　in Lisfranc injuries, 829-830, 830f
　in lower leg stress fractures, 803-804

Radiography (Continued)
　in metatarsal base fractures, 832, 833f
　in multiple trauma, 308-309, 312
　in osteoarthritis of knee, 796
　in osteochondral fracture of talar dome, 825, 825f
　in patellar dislocation, 786
　in patellar fracture, 784-785, 785f
　in patellofemoral pain syndrome, 787
　in pediatric cervical spine injury, 337, 337f
　in pediatric pyarthrosis, 765, 765f
　in pediatric trauma, 333
　in pelvic fracture, 720-721, 721f
　in peripheral vascular injury, 541
　in posterior elbow dislocation, 665, 665f
　in posterior shoulder dislocation, 691, 692f
　in pregnant trauma patient, 320, 320t
　in proximal tibial epiphyseal injuries, 781
　in red and painful eye, 288
　in renal disorders, 1528
　in retropharyngeal abscess, 1120-1121, 1120f
　in scaphoid fracture, 628
　in septic arthritis, 2189
　in sesamoid fractures, 835
　in shoulder trauma, 674-676, 674f-676f
　in sinusitis, 1124, 1124f
　in slipped capital femoral epiphysis, 2708, 2708f
　in small bowel obstruction, 1443, 1443f
　in supracondylar fracture, 2694-2695, 2695f
　in talar fracture, 823, 824f
　in tendinopathy, 1800-1801
　in tibial femoral knee dislocation, 788, 789f
　in tibial plateau fracture, 778-779
　in tibial shaft fracture, 800, 801f
　in tibial tubercle fracture, 798
　in upper airway obstruction, 2521, 2521f
　in wrist trauma, 625-627, 626f-628f, 628t
　of normal hip, 746, 747f
　of teeth, 1030, 1030f
　skull
　　in head-injured child, 336, 368
　　in minor head trauma, 364-365
　　in severe head trauma, 362, 362t
　　in skull fracture, 372
Radiohumeral bursa, 649
Radiology, misinterpretation errors in, 3125
Radionucleotide scanning, 2319
　in acute coronary syndromes, 1179-1180
　in appendicitis, 1454
　in cholecystitis, 1420
　in frostbite, 2231
　in myocardial contusion, 469
　in testicular torsion, 2640
　in urinary tract infection, 1578
　of bone. See Bone scan.
Radiosensitivity, organ and tissue, 2321, 2321f
Radioulnar joint
　distal
　　anatomy of, 622, 623f, 639-640
　　dislocation of, 636-637, 642-643, 643f
　proximal, 639-640
Radius, 639
　distal. See Distal radius.
　fracture of
　　in Galeazzi's fracture, 642-643, 643f
　　pediatric, 644, 644f
　　plastic deformation of, 644, 645f
　　proximal, 647, 647f
　　shaft fracture of, with ulnar shaft fracture, 641
Radon exposure, 2317-2318, 2318f
RAFFT score, for substance abuse in adolescents, 2884
Rales
　in bronchiolitis, 2545
　in high-altitude pulmonary edema, 2303
　in tuberculosis, 2150
Ramipril, 1322t
Ramsay Hunt syndrome, 1071, 1667
Randomization, 3049
Range of motion
　of elbow, 650
　of foot, 821
　of knee, 773
　of shoulder, 674
Ranitidine, 1390t
　during pregnancy and lactation, 2790
　for anaphylaxis, 1831b, 1832, 2549

Ranke complex, in tuberculosis, 2152
Ranson's criteria for acute pancreatitis, 1431-1432, 1432b
Rape trauma syndrome, 991-992, 991b
Rapid diagnostic tests, for viral antigens, 1135
Rapid diagnostic treatment unit. *See* Observation medicine.
Rapid sequence intubation, 9-12, 10b
  in asthma, 16
  in elevated intracranial pressure, 17, 18t
  in head trauma, 358-359
  in neck trauma, 444
  in shock, 51
  indications for, 7-8
  paralysis with induction phase in, 11
  pediatric, 18, 107-108, 107b, 107t
  post-intubation management in, 11-12
  prehospital, 2990, 2991
  preoxygenation in, 10, 10f
  preparations for, 9-10
  pretreatment agents for, 10, 11b
  tube placement in, 11
  vs. blind nasotracheal intubation, 12
  with competitive neuromuscular blocking agent and etomidate, 14-15, 15t
Rapid streptococcal tests, 1111
Rapid tranquilization, 2914b
  for mood disorders, 1741
  for thought disorders, 1730-1731, 1731b
  of combative patient, 2961-2963
Rash. *See also* Skin lesions.
  drug-induced, 1844, 1847t
  glue sniffer's, 2430
  heat, 2259
  in bacterial meningitis, 2658, 2659
  in Colorado tick fever, 2141
  in dermatomyositis, 1708
  in disseminated gonococcal infection, 1566
  in ehrlichiosis, 2138
  in erythema infectiosum, 1850
  in gonococcal arthritis, 1788
  in halothane-induced hepatitis, 1414
  in Henoch-Schönlein purpura, 1815, 2615, 2615f, 2653
  in herpes zoster, 1859, 1860f
  in Kawasaki disease, 2026, 2594, 2595f
  in Lyme disease, 2122, 2122f
  in measles, 1849, 2053, 2053f
  in Rocky Mountain spotted fever, 1849, 2133-2134, 2133f, 2134f
  in roseola infantum, 1850
  in rubella, 1850
  in scarlet fever, 1851, 1851f
  in smallpox, 2039, 2039f, 3028-3029, 3028f, 3029f
  in syphilis, 1561, 1561f
  in systemic lupus erythematosus, 1806
  in toxic shock syndrome, 1847, 2029, 2200
  oral hypoglycemic agent–induced, 1972
Rat-bite fever, 884
Rattlesnake bite, 896, 2329t
Raynaud's disease, 1347, 1357
Raynaud's phenomenon, 273, 1357
Reactionary anxiety, 1746b
Reactive arthritis, 1789-1790, 1791, 2192
Reactive hypochondriasis, 1756
Reactive oxygen species, in cerebral necrosis, 66
Reanastomosis, end-to-end, in arterial injury, 544
"Reasonable person" standard, 3166
Reassurance, in somatoform disorders, 1757-1758
Rebleeding, in traumatic hyphema, 1048-1049
Rebreathers, in diving, 2280
Recommendations for emergency medicine. *See* Guidelines for emergency medicine.
Rectal biopsy, in AIDS-related diarrhea, 1484
Rectal bleeding, 1508
  in Meckel's diverticulum, 2613
  with defecation, 1508
Rectal examination, 1573
  in abdominal pain, 213, 215
  in abdominal trauma, 494
  in back pain, 263
  in constipation, 239
  in diarrhea, 233
  in gastrointestinal bleeding, 222
  in genitourinary trauma, 515
  in pelvic fracture, 719
  in sexual assault victim, 988

Rectal pain, 1509
  in anal fissures, 1512-1513
  in appendicitis, 1452
  in hemorrhoids, 1510
  in levator ani syndrome, 1516
Rectal sphincter tone, in head trauma, 357
Rectal tonography, in shock, 50-51
Rectum
  disorders of. *See* Anorectal disorders.
  foreign bodies in, 875-877, 876f, 1521-1522, 1522f
Recurrent laryngeal nerve, injury to, 450
Red and painful eye, 283-297
  ancillary studies in, 288
  diagnostic approach to, 283-288, 284b, 285b, 287f
  differential diagnosis in, 288-290, 288f-291f
  disposition in, 293t-297t, 297
  empiric management of, 290-292, 293t-297t
  epidemiology of, 283
  history in, 285
  in infants and children, 292
  physical examination in, 285-288, 285b
  traumatic, 283, 290, 292, 297
Red blood cell casts
  in glomerulonephritis, 1534
  in urinary sediment, 1526, 1526f
Red blood cell count
  decreased. *See* Anemia.
  in alcoholism, 2874
  in hypothermia, 2243
  in pregnancy, 318
  increased, 273, 1884-1885, 1884f, 1885b
  normal values for, 1868t
  peritoneal lavage, 500, 500t
Red blood cell indices, normal values for, 1871t
Red blood cell mass, in thermal burns, 918
Redistributive hyponatremia, 1933
Red-red tears, meniscal, 792
Reduction
  of dislocation, 565-566
    ankle, 820
    anterior elbow, 666
    carpometacarpal joint, 603
    distal interphalangeal joint, 601
    glenohumeral joint, 688-690, 689f, 690f
    hip, 757-759, 758f-759f
    hip prosthesis, 760
    inferior glenohumeral joint, 693, 694f
    metacarpophalangeal joint, 602-603, 602f
    metatarsophalangeal joint, 835
    patellar, 786
    posterior elbow, 665
    posterior glenohumeral joint, 691-692
    proximal interphalangeal joint, 602
    proximal tibiofibular joint, 803
    sternoclavicular, 684-685, 685f
    subtalar, 826
    temporomandibular joint, 1041-1042, 1041f
    tibial femoral knee, 788-789
  of femoral head fracture-dislocation, 759-760, 760f
  of fracture
    ankle, 812
    Colles', 633, 634f
    displaced supracondylar, 657, 658f
    distal femur, 776-777
    humeral shaft, 654, 654f
    intercondylar, 659-660, 659f
    intercondylar eminence, 780
    metacarpal neck, 597-598, 598f
    metatarsal shaft, 831
    phalangeal, 834
    proximal humeral epiphysis, 683
    supracondylar, 2695, 2696f
    talar, 824
  of radial head subluxation, 666, 666f, 2697-2698
Red-white tears, meniscal, 792
Reentry mechanisms, for dysrhythmias, 1204-1205, 1204f
Refeeding syndrome, hypophosphatemia in, 1951
Referral
  in elder abuse, 1013-1014
  in intimate partner violence and abuse, 1004
  in substance abuse, 2886
Referred pain
  abdominal, 212
  to back, 703, 706

Reflex(es)
  brainstem, in comatose patient, 159t, 160-161
  cremasteric, 1594
    loss of, in testicular torsion, 1595
  deep tendon
    in head trauma, 357
    in spinal injuries, 417, 417t
    pseudomyotonic, in hypothyroidism, 1992
  diving, 2312
  doll's eye, 161, 2503
  in hypothermia, 2241
  in spinal cord disorders, 1679-1680
Reflex airway closure in physically disabled patient, 2907-2908
Reflex sympathetic dystrophy, 562-563
Reflex sympathetic response to laryngoscopy, 16-17
Reflex syncope, 2685
Reflux
  gastroesophageal. *See* Gastroesophageal reflux.
  vesicoureteral, in urinary tract infection, 1574
Refractory periods of action potential, 1200, 1202f
Refusal of medical care
  by Jehovah's Witnesses, 3171-3172
  federal rules governing, 3170-3171
  for minors, by parent or guardian, 3171
  informed, 3169-3170
  medicolegal issues in, 3169-3172
Regional anesthesia
  in wound care, 845-846
  intravenous, 2934
Regional health information network (RHIN), 3104
Regression models, 3055
Regurgitation
  in achalasia, 1397
  in gastroesophageal reflux, 1388
Rehydralyte, for pediatric infectious diarrhea, 2630, 2630t
Reimplantation
  in hand trauma, 613, 613b
  of avulsed tooth, 1038f, 1040
  penile, 533
Reiter syndrome, arthritis in, 1789-1790
Rejection
  in heart transplant patient, 2852-2853, 2853f
  in kidney transplant patient, 2855
  in liver transplant patient, 2854
  in lung transplant patient, 2855-2856
  opportunistic infections associated with, 2848-2849, 2849f
  phases of, 2849
Relapsing fever, 2129-2130
Relative afferent pupillary defect (RAPD), in red and painful eye, 286
Relative refractory period, 1200, 1202f
Relative risk, 3059t
Relaxation, as wellness strategy for emergency physicians, 3178
Relevance of study, 3059, 3059t
Reliability, 3059, 3059t
Religious values, 3129-3130, 3130b
Remifentanil, 2922t, 2923
Renal artery
  aneurysm of, urolithiasis vs., 1591
  fibromuscular dysplasia of, hypertension in, 1311-1312
  stenosis of, hypertension in, 1312
  trauma to, 529, 530
Renal blood flow, in hypothermia, 2239
Renal cell carcinoma, urolithiasis vs., 1590
Renal colic, 1586-1593, 1589f-1592f, 1593b, 2645-2646. *See also* Urolithiasis.
Renal compensation
  in acid-base disorders, 1923-1924
  in metabolic acidosis, 1923-1924
  in metabolic alkalosis, 1924
Renal dialysis. *See* Dialysis.
Renal disorders
  diagnosis of, 1525-1528, 1527t, 1528b
  hypermagnesemia in, 1949
  hypomagnesemia in, 1947-1948
  in acetaminophen poisoning, 2333
  in acute tumor lysis syndrome, 1911
  in diabetes mellitus, 1970
  in ethylene glycol poisoning, 2398, 2399
  in heatstroke, 2262
  in HIV/AIDS, 2086

Renal disorders (Continued)
in hypertension, 1311-1312
in hyperuricemia, 1913
in infants and children, 2635-2655
in lithium toxicity, 2443
in pregnancy, 2771
in spinal cord injury, 2908
in submersion victim, 2313
in thermal burns, 918
in tuberculosis, 2159
Renal failure
acute, 1532-1540
clinical features of, 1532b, 1537
diagnosis of, 1537-1538
disposition in, 1540
in acute interstitial nephritis, 1534-1535,
1534b
in acute tubular necrosis, 1534b, 1535-1537,
1536b
in children, 2649-2651, 2649b
in glomerulonephritis, 1534, 1534b
in prerenal azotemia, 1532-1533, 1533b,
1538
in renal vascular disease, 1534b, 1535
in rhabdomyolysis, 1977, 1977f
intrinsic, 1534-1537, 1534b
management of, 1538-1540
organ system effects of, 1540
pigment-induced, 1536, 1536b
postrenal (obstructive), 1533-1534, 1533b,
1538
prevention of, 1538-1539
volume and metabolic complications of,
1539-1540
chronic, 1540-1554
causes of, 1541, 1541b, 1543, 1544b
clinical features of, 1542-1543, 1542f
definition of, 1541
diagnosis of, 1543-1544, 1543b, 1544b
dialysis for, 1547-1554
complications of, 1549-1554, 1550b,
1552b, 1553t
emergency, 1548-1549, 1548b
hyperkalemia in, 1545-1546, 1545t
hypertension in, 1316-1317
infection in, 1543, 1546-1547
kidney size in, normal or large, 1543, 1543b
management of, 1544-1554
pulmonary edema in, 1542, 1546, 1546b,
1546f
reversible factors and treatable causes of,
1543, 1544b
uremia in, 1541-1543, 1542f
hyperphosphatemia in, 1952
hypocalcemia in, 1943
immune defects in, 2842
in crush injury, 3007
in ethylene glycol poisoning, 2399, 2400
in HIV/AIDS, 2086
in hyperuricemia, 1913
in pregnancy, 2771
in salicylate overdose, 2340
in sepsis, 2214
in tetanus, 2009
infections in, 2842
metabolic acidosis in, 1929
palliative care in, 3154
pseudo-, in isopropyl alcohol poisoning, 2403-
2404
renal function evaluation in, 1524-1528, 1526f,
1527t, 1528b, 1528f
seizure in, 1622
Renal function tests, 1524-1528, 1526f, 1527t,
1528b, 1528f
Renal infarction, urolithiasis vs., 1591
Renal ischemia, in acute tubular necrosis, 1536
Renal osteodystrophy, 1542-1543
Renal pedicle injuries, 530
Renal pelvis, 527, 527f
Renal trauma, 342, 526-530, 527f, 529f-530f
Renal tuberculosis, urolithiasis vs., 1590-1591
Renal tubular acidosis, hypokalemia in, 1937
Renal tumor, 2646
Renal vascular disease, 1534b, 1535
Renal vein
thrombosis of, urolithiasis vs., 1591
trauma to, 529-530
Renewal, as wellness strategy for emergency
physicians, 3178

Renin-angiotensin-aldosterone system, 527
in heart failure, 1262
in hypertension, 1311, 1312f
in sodium homeostasis, 1933
Renovascular hypertension, 1311
in renal trauma, 526-527
Reovirus infection, 2034t, 2046-2047
Colorado tick fever in, 2140-2141
gastroenteritis, 1475-1476
Repaglinide, 1973
Reperfusion, cerebral, after cardiac arrest, 62-64
Reperfusion therapy
for acute mesenteric ischemia, 1449
in myocardial infarction, 1189-1195
choice of, 1193-1194
combination, 1194-1195
in cardiogenic shock, 1194
process time points for, 1183, 1184f
time to, 1182-1184, 1183f, 1184f
Repolarization, 1200
abnormalities of, in ventricular tachycardia,
1242
early, benign, ST segment elevation in, 1166-
1167, 1167f, 1168f
Reporting requirements, 3172-3173
in child abuse, 976
in elder abuse, 1014-1015
in hepatitis, 1406
in intimate partner violence and abuse, 1004-
1005
Reptile envenomation, 895-903, 897f, 897t,
900t
Rescue, search and, urban, 3005-3008, 3006b,
3008f
Rescue breathing, in pediatric resuscitation, 98
Research question, definition of, 3047-3048
Reserpine, 1321t
intra-arterial, for frostbite, 2233
Residents, in observation unit, 3063
Resistance, electrical injury and, 2268-2269,
2269b, 2269t
Resorcinol, 935
Resource limitations, as stressor for emergency
physician, 3175
Respiration
accessory muscles of
in asthma, 1084
in chronic obstructive pulmonary disease,
1100
agonal, 97
Kussmaul's
in diabetic ketoacidosis, 1963
in metabolic acidosis, 1929
Respiratory acidosis, 1924-1926, 1925b, 1925f,
1931b
causes of, 1925b
clinical features of, 1924-1925
in chronic obstructive pulmonary disease,
1100
management of, 1925-1926
physiologic compensation in, 1925
Respiratory alkalosis, 1926, 1931b
causes of, 1926, 1926b
during acclimatization to high altitude, 2297-
2298
hypophosphatemia in, 1951
in chronic obstructive pulmonary disease,
1100
in salicylate overdose, 2340
Respiratory arrest, 97
asthma-related, 2540
definition of, 79
in organophosphate poisoning, 2459
Respiratory depression
in barbiturate overdose, 2482
in benzodiazepine poisoning, 2484
with apnea, in GHB intoxication, 2489
Respiratory disease. See Pulmonary disorders.
Respiratory distress
acute, 1141, 1141b
in ethylene glycol poisoning, 2399
in pancreatitis, 1429
in sepsis, 2214, 2214b
mechanical ventilation in, 32
pulmonary contusion vs., 461
in anaphylaxis, 1829
in cystic fibrosis, 2564-2565, 2565f
in pediatric airway obstruction, 2519-2530,
2532-2552

Respiratory distress (Continued)
evaluation of, 2521, 2521f
in aeroesophageal foreign body, 2529-2530
in anaphylaxis, 2546-2550
in asthma, 2532-2544
in bronchiolitis, 2544-2546
in congenital lesions, 2522, 2524-2525,
2524f, 2527-2528, 2528f
in croup, 2525-2527, 2526f, 2527b
in epiglottitis, 2523-2524, 2524f
in foreign body aspiration, 2550-2551, 2551f
in laryngeal disease, 2524-2525, 2524f
in retropharyngeal abscess, 2522-2523, 2523f
in subglottic tracheal disease, 2525-2527
in supraglottic disease, 2522-2524
in tracheal disease, 2527-2529, 2529t
pathophysiology of, 2519, 2520f
stridor in, 2519-2520, 2521t
in pneumonia, 2554-2564
severe acute, 1130, 2034t, 2050-2051
Respiratory dyskinesia, antipsychotic-induced,
2447
Respiratory emergencies, prehospital care in,
2990
Respiratory failure
cardiac arrest in, 77
in acute respiratory distress syndrome, 1141
in botulism, 2015
in chronic obstructive pulmonary disease, 1100
in meningococcal disease, 2022
in myasthenia gravis, 1706
in pulmonary embolism, 1378-1379
in tetanus, 2009
Respiratory insufficiency
in botulism, 1707
in hypophosphatemia, 1952
Respiratory muscles
accessory
in asthma, 1084, 2534, 2535t
in chronic obstructive pulmonary disease,
1100
weakness of, 139
Respiratory rate
fever and, 135
in asthma, 1084
in infants and children, 2495, 2495t, 2571,
2571t
Respiratory stimulants, for chronic obstructive
pulmonary disease, 1106
Respiratory syncytial virus infection, 2051-2052
congenital heart disease and, 2581-2582, 2582b
drugs for, 2037t
in bronchiolitis, 2544-2545
in pneumonia, 1130, 2555, 2557
Respiratory tract infection
high-altitude pulmonary edema and, 2299
host defenses against, 1128-1129
in diphtheria, 2001-2004, 2003b
in HIV/AIDS, 2076-2079, 2076t
in immunocompromised patient, 2841
in meningococcal disease, 2020-2024
lower
in bronchiolitis, 2544-2546
in pertussis, 2004-2007, 2005f, 2006b, 2559-
2560
in pneumococcal disease, 2016-2020, 2020b
in pneumonia, 1128-1141, 2554-2564. See
also Pneumonia.
upper, 1109-1126
in adult epiglottitis, 1114-1116, 1115f, 1116f
in deep space infections of head and neck,
1116-1117, 1116f
in laryngitis, 1114
in lingual tonsillitis, 1114, 1114f
in Ludwig's angina, 1118-1119
in parapharyngeal abscess, 1121-1123, 1122f
in peritonsiillitis, 1117-1118, 1118f
in pharyngitis, 1109-1114, 1110f
in retropharyngeal abscess, 1120-1121, 1120f,
1121f
in sinusitis, 1123-1126, 1124f, 1125f
pediatric screening for, 2509b
Restaurant syndromes, anaphylaxis vs., 2548-
2549
Restless legs syndrome, in chronic renal failure,
1542
Restraint
in delirium, 1653-1654
in PCP intoxication, 2416

Restraint (Continued)
  in suicide, 1772
  physical
    for combative patient, 2958-2961, 2960f
    in alcohol withdrawal syndrome, 2861
    in PCP intoxication, 2892
    in thought disorders, 1730
Restrictions, return-to-work, 3079
Restrictive cardiomyopathy, 1296-1297
  constrictive pericarditis vs., 1288
  heart failure in, 1264
Resuscitation
  adult, 75-94
    airway and breathing management in, 87
    algorithm for, 83f
    cardiopulmonary resuscitation in, 88-90
    defibrillation in, 90-91
    epidemiology of cardiac arrest and, 76
    etiology of cardiac arrest and, 77-78, 78t
    history and physical examination in, 78-79, 79t
    in asystole, 84-85
    in pulseless electrical activity, 84
    in ventricular fibrillation and pulseless ventricular tachycardia, 84
    monitoring in, 79-82, 80f-82f, 80t
    outcomes in, 93
    pacing in, 91
    pathophysiology of cardiac arrest and, 76-77
    pharmacologic therapy in, 91-93
    postresuscitation management of cardiac arrest and, 85-87, 88f
    therapeutic modalities in, 87-93
  brain, 62-73
    clinical outcomes in, 72-73
    experimental therapies in, 70-72
    pathophysiology of cerebral ischemia and, 62-67, 63f-64f
    standard strategies for, 67-70, 69t
  family presence during, 3149
  fluid. See Fluid resuscitation.
  honoring advance directive wishes to withhold, 3144-3145, 3152
  hypotensive, in peripheral vascular injury, 543
  in electrical and lightning injuries, 2275
  in heatstroke, 2264-2265, 2265f
  in hemorrhagic shock, 46, 52-53
  myocardial dysfunction after, 77
  neonatal, 118-124
    chest compressions in, 123
    discontinuation of, 120
    disposition in, 124
    in anatomic abnormalities, 121
    in late decelerations of fetal heart rate, 2801
    in meconium aspiration, 120, 120f
    indications for, 119-120
    medications in, 123-124, 123t
    oxygen therapy, ventilation, and intubation in, 122-123
    positioning, suctioning, and stimulation in, 121-122
    preparation for, 121, 121b
    transition from fetal to extrauterine life and, 118-119, 119f
  of elderly trauma patient, 348
  of implantable cardioverter-defibrillator patient, 1256-1257
  of pregnant patient, 322-323
  pediatric, 97-116
    adenosine for, 101t, 104
    advanced life support techniques in, 99, 99f
    airway management in, 97-98, 105-109, 106f, 107b, 107t
    amiodarone for, 101t, 104-105
    antidiuretic hormone for, 100, 103t
    atropine for, 99, 100, 101t-102t, 103-104
    basic life support techniques in, 97-99
    breathing management in, 98, 108-109
    calcium for, 101t, 104
    cardiac rhythm and etiology of arrest in, 109-113, 109t, 110f-112f, 110t
    circulatory management in, 98-99, 109-113
    defibrillation and cardioversion in, 113
    epinephrine for, 111, 114
    family presence during, 114-116, 3149
    glucose for, 100, 101t, 103
    lidocaine for, 102t, 105
    magnesium for, 104

Resuscitation (Continued)
    pharmacologic therapy in, 100-105, 101t-103t, 109-113
    postresuscitation stabilization in, 113-114, 113f
    procainamide for, 103t, 105
    rapid sequence intubation in, 107-108, 107b, 107t
    sodium bicarbonate for, 100, 101t
    tape measurement system in, 114, 114f-115f
    termination of, 116
  research in, bioethical dilemmas in, 3136-3137
  training in, bioethical dilemmas in, 3135
Resuscitative hypothermia, for comatose survivors of cardiac arrest, 68-70, 69t
Retching, definition of, 200
Reticular activating system, 156
Reticulocyte count
  in normochromic and normocytic anemia, 1875
  in sickle cell disease, 1881
Reticulocytes, 1868, 1868f
Reticuloendothelial system, 2832
Retina, 1045f
  blunt injury to, 1050, 1050f
  detachment of, 1050, 1050f, 1057-1058
  tear of, 1050, 1057-1058
Retinal hemorrhage, 1050
  high-altitude, 2306-2307, 2307f
  in child abuse, 971
Retinitis, cytomegalovirus, in HIV/AIDS, 2086
Retinopathy
  diabetic, 1970, 1972
  fibrinolytic therapy eligibility and, 1191
Retrobulbar abscess, 288, 295t
Retrobulbar emphysema, 294t
Retrobulbar hematoma, 288, 295t
Retrobulbar hemorrhage, 1046
Retrograde cystography
  computed tomography, in bladder trauma, 521, 525, 526f
  conventional, in bladder trauma, 521, 521f-525f
Retrograde intubation, 20
Retrograde pyelography, 531, 531f-532f
Retrograde urethrogram, 517-519, 518f-520f
Retroperitoneal air, 497f
Retroperitoneal hematoma, pelvic fracture and, 500
Retropharyngeal abscess, 1120-1121, 1120f, 1121f
  in children, 2522-2523, 2523f
Retropharyngeal injuries, in neck trauma, 450
Retropharyngeal space, 1027
  soft tissues of, 424, 426f
Retrospective observational study, 3047
Retrosternal pain, in aortic rupture, 478
Retrovirus, 2034t, 2056
Return-to-work issues, in occupational medicine, 3078-3080
Reverse straight leg raise test, in lumbar radiculopathy, 704
Revised trauma score (RTS), 300
Rewarming
  active, 2247-2251, 2247b
    core, 2248-2251
    external, 2248
  airway, 2248-2249, 2249t
  arteriovenous, continuous, 2250t, 2251
  arteriovenous anastomoses, 2248
  diathermic, 2250
  external, 2247, 2248
  extracorporeal blood, 2250-2251, 2250t
  forced air, 2248
  heated irrigation for, 2250
  in accidental hypothermia, 2247-2251, 2247b, 2250b
  in frostbite, 2231-2232, 2232b
  negative pressure, 2248
  peritoneal lavage, 2249
  venovenous, 2250t, 2251
Reynolds' pentad in cholangitis, 1421
Rh (anti-D) immunoglobulin, in pregnancy, 2742, 2752
Rhabdomyolysis, 1975-1983
  acute tubular necrosis in, 1536
  anatomy and physiology in, 1976, 1977f
  clinical features of, 1980
  diagnosis of, 1980-1981, 1981f
  differential considerations in, 1981-1982, 1981b

Rhabdomyolysis (Continued)
  disposition in, 1983
  etiology of, 1978-1980, 1978b
  in amphetamine abuse, 2896
  in electrical and lightning injuries, 2276
  in hypokalemia, 1939
  in hypophosphatemia, 1952
  in hypothermia, 2243
  in overdosed/poisoned patient, 2330
  in PCP intoxication, 2892-2893
  management of, 1982-1983, 1983f
  pathophysiology of, 1976-1978, 1977b, 1977f
  pigmenturia in, 1981-1982, 1981b
  psychostimulant-induced, 2408
Rhabdovirus, 2034t, 2054
Rhegmatogenous retinal detachment, 1058
Rheumatic disease. See also specific diseases, e.g., Arthritis.
  historical perspective of, 1776-1777
  in hypothyroidism, 1992
  in pregnancy, 2775-2776
  in systemic lupus erythematosus, 1806
  orofacial pain in, 1034
  sites and types of, 1777f
  synovial fluid analysis in, 1781-1782, 1781t
Rheumatic fever, 1303-1304, 1304b
  acute, 1790-1791, 1790b, 2596-2597, 2596f
  after streptococcal pharyngitis, 1112, 1114
  mitral stenosis after, 1305
Rheumatic heart disease, infective endocarditis in, 1300
Rheumatoid arthritis, 1791-1792
  in pregnancy, 2776
  myocarditis in, 1297
  pericarditis in, 1284
  skin lesions in, 1862t
Rheumatoid factor, in rheumatoid arthritis, 1791
Rhinitis
  allergic, exercise-induced asthma and, 1082
  in anaphylaxis, 1825t
  in asthma, 1084
  vs. sinusitis, 1125
Rhinitis medicamentosa, 1125
Rhinovirus, 2057
Rhizotomy, dorsal, for spasticity in cerebral palsy, 2904
Rhododendron, 2475
Rhomboid muscle, 672, 673f
Rib fracture, 454-456, 454b, 455f
  anatomy in, 455f
  aortic rupture and, 479
  flail chest and, 457
  in children, 2699
  in chronic obstructive pulmonary disease, 1102
  pneumothorax and, 461-462
  pulmonary contusion and, 460
RICE therapy, for ankle sprain, 817
Rickets
  fracture in, 2701
  of prematurity, 975
Rickettsia rickettsii, 2132. See also Rocky Mountain spotted fever.
Rifabutin
  for tuberculosis, 2163t
  in HIV/AIDS, side effects of, 2079t
Rifamate, for tuberculosis, 2164
Rifampin
  during pregnancy and lactation, 2785
  for meningococcal meningitis, 1722-1723
  for pharyngitis, 1113
  for tuberculosis, 2162, 2163t
  prophylactic, for meningococcal disease, 2024
Rifamycins, antiretroviral therapy and, drug interactions between, 2166
Rifater, for tuberculosis, 2164
Rifle wounds, centerfire, forensic evaluation of, 959, 959f, 960f
Rift Valley fever virus, 2055
Right bundle branch block, in pulmonary embolism, 1378, 1379f
Right subclavian artery, anomalous, dysphagia in, 1383
Right to refuse medical care, 3169-3172
Right ventricular collapse, in cardiac tamponade, 474, 474f
Right ventricular myocardial infarction, 1166, 1167f, 1172-1173

Rights
 legal, 3128
 patient, 2967
Right-sided aortic arch, 2574
Right-sided heart failure, 1266-1267
Rigidity
 in appendicitis, 1452
 nuchal
  causes of, 2663
  in bacterial meningitis, 2658, 2659
  in central nervous system infection, 1714
Rigors, in pneumonia, 2556
Rimantadine, for influenza, 1139, 2035, 2037
Ring avulsion injuries, in hand trauma, 612-613, 613b
Risk assessment
 combative patient and, 2957-2958
 in acetaminophen overdose, 2333-2335, 2334f
 in anaphylaxis, 1819-1820
 in ectopic pregnancy, 2743, 2743b
 in elder abuse, 1010-1011, 1010b
 in endocarditis, 1302, 1303b
 in injury prevention and control, 946-948
 in intimate partner violence and abuse, 1000, 1002b, 1003b
 in pulmonary embolism, 186b, 1371, 1371t
 in sudden infant death syndrome, 2714-2716, 2715b
 in tuberculosis, 2149-2150, 2149b, 2150b
Risk management, 3156-3173
 consent to medical care and, 3166-3169
 disposition requirements and, 3164-3165, 3165t
 emergency medical condition and, 3156-3157
 Emergency Medical Treatment and Active Labor Act and, 3156
 medical screening examination and, 3160-3163
 refusal of medical care and, 3169-3172
 reporting requirements and, 3172-3173
 screening requirements and, 3157-3158
 stabilization requirements and, 3163-3164
 testing requests and requirements and, 3158-3160
Risk stratification
 in acute coronary ischemia, 3065
 in gastrointestinal bleeding, 225-226, 225b, 226t
 in minor head trauma, 363-364, 364b
 in suicide, 1772-1773
Risperidone
 for agitation, in delirious patient, 1654
 for mood disorders, 1741
 for thought disorders, 1730-1731
 toxicity of, 2446, 2446t
Ritgen maneuver, modified, 2804
Ritodrine, for premature labor, 2806-2807, 2806b
Ritonavir, in HIV/AIDS, side effects of, 2079t
River blindness, 2109, 2109f
RNA viruses, 2034t, 2046-2058
Roberts v. Galen, 3164
Rochester method, for hip reduction, 759
Rocky Mountain spotted fever, 2132-2137
 clinical features of, 2132-2134, 2133f, 2133t, 2134f
 diagnosis of, 2134-2135, 2135b
 differential considerations in, 2135
 management of, 2136-2137, 2136t
 skin lesions in, 1849-1850
Rocuronium
 for tetanus, 2011
 in rapid sequence intubation, 15, 15t, 16
Rodent bite, 884
Roentgen-equivalent-man (rem), 2321
Rofecoxib, 2927-2928
Rolandic epilepsy, benign, 2666
Rolando's fracture, 551t, 600
Rome II criteria for irritable bowel syndrome, 1491, 1491b
Root, 1026, 1027f
 split, 1033-1034
Root canal pain, 1033
Rosary pea, 2471-2472, 2472f
Roseola infantum, 1850, 2044
Rotational injuries, cervical spine, 405-409, 408f-410f
Rotator cuff, 672, 673f
 calcific tendinitis of, 698
 hemorrhage into, in scapula fracture, 680
 tears of, 696

Rotator cuff (Continued)
 in anterior glenohumeral joint dislocation, 690
 tendinitis of, 693-696, 694t, 695f
 tendinopathy of, 1796-1797
Rotavirus, 2047
Rotavirus gastroenteritis, 1475-1476, 2624-2625
Roundup, 2467-2468
Roundworm, 2100t, 2113
Rovsing's sign, in appendicitis, 1452, 2619
R-plasminogen activator (r-PA), in myocardial infarction, 1189-1190
Rubber bullet, ballistic injury associated with, 458-459
Rubella, 2048-2049, 2049f
 arthritis in, 1788
 skin lesions in, 1850
Rubella vaccine, 2035t, 2048-2049
Rubeola, 2052-2053, 2053f
 Kawasaki disease vs., 2594
 screening for, 2509b
 skin lesions in, 1849
Rubin syndrome, 1910
Rubin's maneuver, in shoulder dystocia, 2815, 2815f
Rue, adverse effects of, 2476t
Rule of 80, in neck masses, 1075
Rule of nines, in burn wound assessment, 919-920, 920f
Rule-using process, clinical decision making by, 126, 131t, 132
Rumination, definition of, 201
Rust remover, ingestion of, 2381t
Rust ring, in iron-containing corneal foreign body, 1047, 1048f

Saccharomyces boulardii, 1475
Sacral plexus, 718
Sacrum, 400f
 fracture of, 725-726
SAD PERSONS scale, 1770, 1770t, 1772
Safety concerns, as stressor for emergency physician, 3175
Safety issues
 in air medical transport, 2997, 2997b, 2997f, 2998b
 in emergency department, 3119-3126
 in intimate partner violence and abuse, 1004b
 in suicide, 1772
Sager splint, 570, 570f
Sail sign
 in infants and children, 2573, 2574f
 in supracondylar fracture, 2695, 2695f
St. John's wort
 adverse effects of, 2476t
 drug interactions with, 2478t
St. Louis encephalitis, 2049-2050
Salicylates
 during pregnancy and lactation, 2781
 for rheumatic fever, 1791
 for rheumatoid arthritis, 1791-1792
 lactic acidosis from, 1929
 metabolism of, 2339-2340, 2340f
 overdose of, 2339-2342, 2340f
  chronic exposure in, 2340
  clinical features of, 2341, 2341b
  diagnosis of, 2341
  disposition in, 2342
  management of, 2341-2342, 2341b
Salicylic acid, for prickly heat, 2259
Saline
 for diabetic ketoacidosis, 1966
 for diarrhea, 235
 for elevated intracranial pressure, 360
 for hypercalcemia, 1946
 for hyperglycemic hyperosmolar nonketotic coma, 1969
 for hypernatremia, 1936-1937
 for hyponatremia, 1935
 for hypovolemia, in adrenal insufficiency, 1998
 for metabolic alkalosis, 1930-1931
 for multiple trauma patient, 307
 for rhabdomyolysis, 1982
 for seizure in acute renal failure, 2650
 for wound cleansing, 848
Saliva
 microorganisms in, 1128

Saliva (Continued)
 recovery of, in sexual assault examination, 985, 986b
Salivary glands, 385-386, 386f
 stones of, 1075
Salmeterol
 for asthma, 1088
 for chronic asthma, 2542, 2543t
 for chronic obstructive pulmonary disease, 1105
Salmonella infection
 in cancer patient with impaired cell-mediated immunity, 2839-2840
 in dysenteric colitis, 229t
 in gastroenteritis, 1461-1463, 1461t, 1462t, 1482, 2625
Salpingitis, 248, 251t
Salt depletion heat exhaustion, 2259-2260
Salt solutions, for heat cramps, 2258
Salt tablets, heat illness and, 2256
Salter-Harris fracture classification system, 551t, 555-556, 557t, 2690, 2691f, 2691t, 2692, 2692f
Salvia, 2412
SAMPLE mnemonic, 2501, 2501b
Sample size, 3052
Sandifer's syndrome, 2610, 2668
Saphenous vein, thrombosis of, 1370
Saphenous vein graft, in arterial injury, 544
Saquinavir, in HIV/AIDS, side effects of, 2079t
Sarcoidosis
 cardiac, 1297
 hypercalcemia in, 1945
 in chronic obstructive pulmonary disease, 1103
Sarcolemma
 damage to, in rhabdomyolysis, 1976-1977, 1977f
 ionic pumps in, 1976, 1977f
Sarcomeres, 1259
Sarcoplasmic reticulum, 1259
Sarcoptes scabiei, 1569
Sarin exposure, 2461
 as chemical weapon, 939, 3030-3031, 3030b, 3031b
 in children, 3021
Saturday night palsy, 1694-1695
"Save-a-Tooth" system, 1038-1039, 1039f
Saw palmetto, adverse effects of, 2476t
Scabies
 in HIV/AIDS, 2085
 skin lesions in, 1854-1855, 1854f
Scald burn, 913-928. See also Thermal burn.
Scalded skin syndrome, staphylococcal, 1845, 2199
Scalenus anticus syndrome, thoracic outlet syndrome in, 1359
Scales, 1838-1841, 1839t
Scalp
 abrasion of, 372
 anatomy and physiology of, 350
 avulsion of, 372
 laceration of, 371-372, 850
Scalp injury complexes, in children, 334
Scaly papules, skin disorders with, 1841-1842
Scaphoid fracture, 627-629, 628f
Scaphoid tubercle, 622, 623f, 625
Scaphoid view of wrist, 627, 627t
Scapholunate angle, 626, 627f
Scapholunate dissociation, 630, 631f
Scapholunate joint, 625
Scapholunate ligament, 622, 624f
Scapula
 anatomy of, 672, 673f
 fracture of, 679-680, 680f
 manipulation of, in reduction of glenohumeral joint dislocation, 689-690, 690f
Scapular neck, fracture of, 680
Scapulothoracic dislocation, 693
Scarlet fever, 1110, 1851, 1851f
Schatzki's ring, 1383
Scheduling systems, computerized, 3104-3105
Schefflera, 2472
Schistosomiasis
 chronic, 2112, 2112f, 2113f
 drug therapy for, 2102t
 fever in, 2105
 neurologic disorders in, 2107
Schizoaffective disorder, 1729
Schizocytes, in hemolytic anemia, 1877, 1877f

Schizophrenia, 1726-1733
  alcohol withdrawal syndrome vs., 2860
  clinical features of, 1726-1728
  criteria for, 1727, 1727b
  diagnosis of, 1728
  differential considerations in, 1727b, 1728-
    1729, 1728b, 1729t
  disposition in, 1733
  in alcoholism, 2875
  management of, 1730-1733, 1731b
  panic attack in, 1748
  phases of, 1726-1727
  suicide and, 1769
Schizophreniform disorder, 1729
School-age children
  developmental milestones in, 2496t, 2497
  fever in, management of, 2515-2516
Schools, violence in, 1017-1018
Schwannoma, 147t, 1668-1669
Sciatic mononeuropathy, 1697-1698, 1698f
Sciatic nerve, 738
Sciatic neuropathy, in hip trauma, 762-763
Sciatica, 702-703, 704-705, 711-712
Scintigraphy. See Radionucleotide scanning.
Sclera, 1045f
  laceration of, 1051
  penetration of, red and painful eye in, 296t
  traumatic rupture of, 1049-1050, 1050f
  whitening of, in alkali burn, 1046, 1046f
Scleritis, 289-290, 290f, 295t
Scleroderma
  myocarditis in, 1297-1298
  oral manifestations of, 1035
Scleroderma renal crisis, 1535, 1543-1544
Sclerosing cholangitis, 1422
Sclerosing panencephalitis, subacute, 2054
Scoliosis, in cerebral palsy, 2901
Scombroid fish poisoning, 1470t, 1472-1473
Scopolamine
  anticholinergic toxicity of, 2345, 2346
  for nausea and vomiting, 206
  mydriasis from, 1061
Scorpion bites, 907-908
Scorpion fish envenomation, 910
Scratch, rabies transmission from, 2065
Screening
  for alcoholism, 2858
  for elder abuse, 1011, 1011b
  for gestational diabetes, 2772
  for HIV, 2074-2075
  for intimate partner violence and abuse, 998-
    999, 999b, 1000f, 1001f, 1002b
  for pediatric upper respiratory tract infection,
    2509b
  for substance abuse in adolescents, 2884
  for tuberculosis, 2169
  requirements for, 3157-3158. See also Medical
    screening examination.
  toxicologic. See Toxicologic screen.
Scrofula, 2158
Scrotal pain, in testicular torsion, 1595, 2640
Scrotal skin loss, 532
Scrotum
  anatomy of, 1594, 1594f
  carcinoma of, in children, 2642
  dog bites to, 534-535
  masses and swelling of, 1593-1598
    anatomy and physiology in, 1594, 1594f
    differential considerations in, 1594-1598
    in children, 2638-2642, 2639f-2640f
  physical examination of, 1573, 1594
Scuba diving–related disorders, 2279-2294
  alternobaric vertigo in, 2286, 2287t
  arterial gas embolism in, 2285-2286, 2288,
    2288t
  avascular osteonecrosis in, 2286
  barodontalgia in, 2286
  barosinusitis in, 2282
  clinical features of, 2281-2286
  contaminated air in, 2283
  decompression sickness in, 2283-2285
  diagnostic strategies in, 2286-2287, 2286b,
    2287f, 2287t
  differential considerations in, 2287-2288, 2288t
  disposition in, 2293-2294, 2293f
  external ear barotrauma in, 2282, 2292
  facial barotrauma in, 2282, 2293
  gastrointestinal barotrauma in, 2286

Scuba diving–related disorders (Continued)
  inner ear barotrauma in, 2282, 2287-2288,
    2287t, 2292
  management of, 2288-2293
  middle ear barotrauma in, 2281-2282, 2282f,
    2286-2287, 2287t, 2292
  nitrogen narcosis in, 2283, 2293
  not requiring recompression therapy, 2292-
    2293, 2292b
  oxygen toxicity in, 2283
  pathophysiology of, 2280-2281, 2281f
  pneumomediastinum in, 2286, 2293
  pneumothorax in, 2286, 2293
  pulmonary barotrauma in, 2285-2286, 2293
  pulmonary edema in, 2286
  recompression therapy for, 2288-2292, 2288b,
    2289f-2291f
  subcutaneous emphysema in, 2286
  temporomandibular joint dysfunction in,
    2283
Sea nettle, 909
Sea urchin, 909-910
Sea wasp, 909
Search and rescue, urban, 3005-3008, 3006b,
    3008f
Seasonal affective disorder, 1738
Seat belt
  injuries from, 341, 491-492, 947
  use during pregnancy, 2735-2736
"Seatbelt sign," 491-492
Seatworm, 1479-1482
Sebaceous glands, 915
Seborrheic dermatitis, in HIV/AIDS, 2085
Seclusion, emergency, 2958-2961, 2960f
Second impact syndrome, 365-366
Second stage of labor, 2800-2804, 2802b, 2802t,
    2803f
Secondary assessment of victim endpoint (SAVE)
    system, 3013
Secondary survey
  in obstetric trauma, 323
  in pediatric trauma, 330, 330b, 333, 333b
Second-degree burn, 918-919, 919f
SECONDS mnemonic, 1779-1780
Second-trimester fetal death, 2740
Secretory diarrhea, 228, 2624
Security
  in emergency department, 2965-2966
  of patient information, 3102-3103
Sedation, 2938-2954
  agents for, 2940t-2941t
  barbiturates for, 2945-2946
  benzodiazepines for, 2944-2945
  consent prior to, 2940
  continuum of, 2938, 2939f
  contraindications to, 2939
  definitions of, 2914b, 2938, 2939b
  discharge criteria and instructions after, 2943
  drug selection and administration in, 2949-
    2952, 2950t, 2951b
  etomidate for, 2940t-2941t, 2947-2948
  fasting prior to, 2939-2940
  for agitation in delirious patient, 1653-1654
  for PCP intoxication, 2892
  in children, 2952-2954
  in cocaine overdose, 2389
  in comatose survivors of cardiac arrest, 70
  in PCP intoxication, 2416
  in severe head trauma, 358
  in ventilated patient, 30-31
  ketamine for, 2940t-2941t, 2946-2947
  monitoring of, 2942-2943
  nitrous oxide for, 2940t-2941t, 2948
  opioids for, 2944
  personnel providing, 2941-2942
  preprocedure patient assessment in, 2938-2940
  propofol for, 2940t-2941t, 2947
  rapid, 2914b
    for mood disorders, 1741
    for thought disorders, 1730-1731, 1731b
    of combative patient, 2961-2963
  recovery from, 2943
  reversal agents in, 2948-2949
  route of administration for, 2943-2944
  supplies and equipment for, 2942
  terminology in, 2938, 2939b
Sedative hypnotics
  in elderly person, 2827
  overdose of, 2481-2490

Sedative hypnotics (Continued)
  barbiturates in, 2481-2483, 2482b, 2482f
  benzodiazepines in, 2483-2486, 2484t
  buspirone in, 2486
  chloral hydrate in, 2487
  flunitrazepam in, 2486
  γ-hydroxybutyrate in, 2488-2490, 2488b
  opioid/sedative/ethanol syndrome and,
    2327t, 2328
  OTC sleep aids in, 2487-2488, 2488t
  zolpidem and zaleplon in, 2486-2487
Segmental ileus, 1440
Segond fracture, 777, 777f
Seidel's test, in corneal laceration, 287-288, 1051,
    1051f
Seizure, 164-168, 1619-1629. See also Epilepsy.
  absence, 1621
  after cerebral ischemia, 70
  alcohol-related, 2863-2866, 2863b, 2879
  ataxia in, 2682
  brain damage and, 2665
  cerebrospinal fluid shunt–related, in
    developmentally disabled patient, 2899
  classification of, 164, 165t, 1619-1620, 2665,
    2666b
  clinical features of, 1620-1625
  confusion after, 154
  diagnosis of, 165-168, 165t, 1625-1626
  differential considerations in, 165-166, 165t,
    1626
  disposition in, 168
  drug-induced, 1623, 2669-2670, 2670b
  epidemiology of, 164
  episodic disorders that mimic, 2668b
  febrile, as indication for lumbar puncture,
    2660
  focal (partial), 164, 1620, 1621
  from antipsychotic agents, 2448
  generalized, 164, 1620, 1621
  history in, 167
  ictal events in, properties of, 167
  imaging studies in, 168
  in acute renal failure, 2650
  in amphetamine abuse, 2896
  in anticholinergic poisoning, 2349
  in apparent life-threatening event, 2719
  in arteriovenous malformations, 1624
  in asthma, 2536
  in beta blocker overdose, 2374
  in bupropion overdose, 2361
  in cancer patient, 1919
  in central nervous system degenerative
    diseases, 1624
  in central nervous system infection, 1721
  in central nervous system tumor or vasculitis,
    1624
  in cerebral venous thrombosis, 1670
  in chlorinated hydrocarbon poisoning, 2462,
    2463
  in cicutoxin poisoning, 2472
  in cyclic antidepressant poisoning, 2354t, 2356
  in developmentally disabled patient, 2898-
    2899
  in eclampsia, 1627, 2749-2750, 2751
  in HIV/AIDS, 2079
  in infectious diseases, 1623
  in mefenamic acid poisoning, 2343
  in metabolic disorders, 1622
  in migraine, 1624
  in organophosphate poisoning, 2459
  in pertussis, 2006
  in pregnancy, 1624, 2753t, 2763t, 2768-2769
  in severe head trauma, prophylaxis against,
    361, 361b
  in stroke, 1624
  in systemic lupus erythematosus, 1807
  laboratory tests in, 168
  management of
    immediate, 166-167, 166t, 168, 1626-1628,
      1627t, 1628t
    long-term, 1628-1629, 1629t
  myoclonic, 1621
  neonatal, 2667
  pathophysiology of, 164-165, 1620
  pediatric, 367, 2665-2676
    after head trauma, 334
    anticonvulsant therapy for, 2674-2676, 2675t
    clinical features of, 2665-2667, 2666b
    diagnosis of, 2670-2671

Seizure (Continued)
  disposition in, 2674-2676, 2674b, 2675t
  etiology of, 2667-2670, 2668b-2670b
  febrile, 2507, 2666-2667, 2674, 2674b
  management of, 2671-2673, 2671b, 2672t
  pathophysiology of, 2665
  precipitators of, identification and treatment of, 2673
  secondary survey in, 2502
  status epilepticus and, 2667, 2668b, 2672-2673, 2672t
  physical examination in, 167-168
  postictal states in, 1625
  posttraumatic, 370, 373, 1623
   prophylaxis against, 361, 361b
  primary. See Epilepsy.
  pseudoseizure and, 1624-1625, 2668
  rapid assessment and stabilization in, 166-167, 166t
  reactive, 1622-1624
  recurrent
   diagnosis of, 1625-1626
   risk of, 2674
  submersion injuries and, 2312
  syncope vs., 194
  temporal lobe, 1621
  terminology in, 1620
  tonic, 1621
  toxin-induced, 1623
Selection bias, 3049
Selective serotonin reuptake inhibitors, 2328
  for anxiety disorders, 1751, 1751t
  for depression, 1741
  for neuropathic pain, 1692
  metabolism of, 2357
  overdose of, 2357-2360, 2358b, 2358t, 2359b, 2360t
Selenium sulfide
  for tinea capitis, 1839
  for tinea versicolor, 1840
Self-destructive patient, 2978t, 2981
Self-neglect, by elder, 1009
Sellick's maneuver, in rapid sequence intubation, 11b
Semicircular canal, 142
Senescent forgetfulness, dementia vs., 1660
Sengstaken-Blakemore tube, in gastrointestinal bleeding, 225
Senile plaques, in dementia, 1657
Sensitivity analyses, 3058
Sensitization, to allergens, 1819
Sensorineural hearing loss, 1072
Sensorium, altered, in cholangitis, 1421
Sensory ataxia, 2682
Sensory dermatomes, 418f
Sensory disturbances
  in carpal tunnel syndrome, 1697
  in ischemic stroke, 1609
  in multiple sclerosis, 1672
  in spinal cord disorders, 1678f, 1679
  in syringomyelia, 1683
Sensory examination
  in lumbar radiculopathy, 704, 705f
  in spinal injuries, 417, 418f
Sensory nerves, to hand, 587, 589f
Sensory neuronopathy, 1700, 1700b
Sensory tracts, ascending, 1676, 1676f, 2915, 2915f, 2916f
Sentinel loop, 1440
Sentinel pile, in anal fissures, 1512
Separation anxiety, 1746b
Sepsis, 2211-2222. See also Bacteremia.
  as indication for lumbar puncture
   in immunocompromised child, 2660
   in young infant, 2659
  clinical features of, 2214-2216
  definitions in, 2211, 2212b
  diagnosis of, 2216-2217
  differential considerations in, 2217, 2218b
  disposition in, 2222
  epidemiology of, 2211-2212
  in asplenic patient, 2842-2843
  in cholangitis, 1421
  in febrile cancer patient, 1907-1909, 1908b
  in pneumococcal disease, 2017-2018
  inflammatory mediators in, 2213
  management of, 2217-2222, 2218f, 2219t, 2221t
  mortality in, 2216, 2216t
  pathophysiology of, 2212-2213

Sepsis (Continued)
  pelvic pain and, 250
  progression of disease in, 2211, 2212f
  severe
   definition of, 2211, 2212b
   treatment of, 51, 51f
Septal branch of superior labial artery, 1073, 1073f
Septal defects, traumatic, 472
Septal myomectomy, for hypertrophic cardiomyopathy, 1296
Septic arthritis, 1782-1785, 2174
  clinical features of, 1784-1785, 2188-2191
  complications of, 2190
  differential considerations in, 2191-2192
  disposition in, 2193
  etiology and microbiology of, 2177-2179, 2178t
  gonococcal, 2190-2191
  history and physical examination in, 2188
  in atypical joints, 2191
  in disseminated gonococcal infection, 1566
  in hand, 618
  in knee, 796
  in tuberculosis, 2159
  joint aspiration and joint fluid analysis in, 2188-2190, 2189f
  management of, 1785, 2178t, 2192-2193
  pathophysiology and epidemiology of, 1782-1784
  pathophysiology of, 2177
  pediatric, 2190, 2509b, 2704-2706, 2705t, 2706t
  pediatric limp from, 764
  with existing joint disease, 2191
Septic bursitis, 1801-1803
Septic olecranon bursitis, 667
Septic shock
  adrenal insufficiency in, 1995-1996
  causes of, 46-47
  clinical features of, 2215
  definition of, 49, 49b, 2211, 2212b
  differential considerations in, 2218b
  pediatric fever in, 2511
  treatment of, 51, 51f, 52b, 53-54
Septic thrombosis, 1123, 1363
Septicemia
  following hypothermia, 2247
  postanginal, parapharyngeal abscess and, 1123
Septicemic plague, 3027
Sequestra, in osteomyelitis, 2175
Sequestration
  abnormal, hemolytic anemia, 1884
  splenic, 1896
Serologic tests
  in babesiosis, 2140
  in Colorado tick fever, 2141
  in hepatitis, 1405t
  in Lyme disease, 2125
  in pneumonia, 1135
  in Q fever, 2137
  in Rocky Mountain spotted fever, 2135
  in syphilis, 1561-1562
  in tuberculosis, 2156
Serotonin
  in mood disorders, 1735
  suicide and, 1768
  violent behavior and, 2957
Serotonin reuptake inhibitors
  nonselective, 2328
  selective, 2328
   for anxiety disorders, 1751, 1751t
   for depression, 1741
   for neuropathic pain, 1692
   metabolism of, 2357
   overdose of, 2357-2360, 2358b, 2358t, 2359b, 2360t
Serotonin syndrome, 2328, 2358-2359
  antidotes to, 2329t
  clinical manifestations of, 2358b
  diagnostic criteria for, 2358-2359, 2359b
  differential diagnosis in, 2359
  drugs associated with, 2359b
  lithium-induced, 2442
  opioid-induced, 2452
Serotonin-like agents, psychoactive, ingestion of, 2406-2408, 2407f
Serratus anterior muscle, 672, 673f
Sertraline, metabolism of, 2357
Serum sickness, 901, 1815-1816
Sesamoid fractures, 834-835

Severe acute respiratory distress syndrome (SARS), 1130, 2034t, 2050-2051
Sever's disease, 2710
Sexual abuse
  of child, 969, 971, 972-973, 974, 975
  of elder, 1010
  of intimate partner, 997
Sexual assault, 977-992
  debriefing after, 991-992, 991b
  emergency department preparation for victim of, 978
  epidemiology of, 977-978
  examination protocol in, 980f-983f
  male victim of, examination of, 992
  medicolegal issues in, 3159-3160
  obtaining history and consent in, 978-979, 978b, 979b, 979t, 984
  of intimate partner, 997
  perpetrators of
   detection avoidance methods used by, 984
   sexual dysfunction in, 984, 984b
   suspected, examination of, 992
  physical examination and evidence collection in, 984-989, 985b-987b, 987f, 987t, 988f, 988t
  pregnancy prophylaxis and, 991, 991t
  sexually transmitted disease and, 989-990, 989b, 989t
Sexual dysfunction
  in depression, 1737
  in multiple sclerosis, 1672
  in perpetrators of sexual assault, 984, 984b
  pelvic fracture and, 719, 720
Sexual intercourse, during pregnancy, 2736
Sexually transmitted disease, 1556-1571
  after sexual assault, 989-990, 989b, 989t
  anorectal involvement in, 1518-1520, 1518t
  differential diagnosis in, 1557t
  epididymitis and, 1595, 1596-1597, 1597t
  in bacterial vaginosis, 1567t, 1568-1569
  in Bartholin cyst and abscess, 1559-1560
  in candidiasis, 1567t, 1568
  in chancroid, 1557t, 1559t, 1562-1563, 1562f
  in Chlamydia trachomatis, 1559t, 1564-1565
  in condylomata acuminata, 1559t, 1563-1564, 1564
  in granuloma inguinale, 1559t, 1563
  in herpes simplex virus infection, 1557-1559, 1557t, 1558f, 1559t
  in HIV/AIDS, 2087
  in lymphogranuloma venereum, 1557t, 1559t, 1562
  in nongonococcal urethritis, 1565
  in pelvic inflammatory disease, 1569-1571
  in pregnancy, 2758-2759
  in syphilis, 1557t, 1559-1562, 1559t, 1560f, 1561f
  in trichomoniasis, 1567-1568, 1567t
  prophylaxis against, after sexual assault, 973-974, 974t, 989-990, 989t
  treatment of, 1559t
  with genital discharge, 1564-1571
  with genital ulcers, 1557-1564, 1557t
Shaken-baby syndrome, 367, 970-971
Shear injuries, cervical spine, 405, 406f-407f
Sheep liver fluke, 2101t, 2113
Shenton's line, in hip dislocation, 757, 758f
Shepherd's purse, adverse effects of, 2476t
Shift work
  performance and, 3122-3123, 3122f, 3123b
  rational approaches to, 3123b
  strategies for, 3176, 3177b
Shigella infection
  in dysenteric colitis, 229t
  in gastroenteritis, 1461t, 1462t, 1464-1465, 2625
  in myocarditis, 1292
Shikani Optical Stylet, 21, 22f
Shin splints, 804-805
Shingles, 1054, 1859-1860, 1860f, 2042-2043
Shivering thermogenesis, 2236, 2247
Shock, 41-55
  acid-base calculations in, 1924
  anaphylaxis vs., 1830
  burn, 918
  cardiogenic
   causes of, 47
   definition of, 49, 49b
   in myocardial infarction, 1160, 1194

Shock (Continued)
  reperfusion therapy in, 1194
    treatment of, 52b, 54, 113-114, 113f, 1273
  classification of, 41-42, 42b
  clinical features of, 47-49, 47b, 48f, 49b
  compensated, in children, 2499
  epidemiology of, 42
  goal-directed therapy for, 50-52, 51f
  heart function in, 45
  hemorrhagic
    causes of, 44f, 45-46
    definition of, 49, 49b
    in subclavian artery injury, 545
    treatment of, 52-53, 52b
  hypovolemic
    in cardiac tamponade, 473
    in diabetic ketoacidosis, 1966
    mechanical ventilation in, 32
  in bacterial meningitis, 2663
  in children, 2499, 2503
  in meningococcal disease, 2022
  in multiple trauma, 307-308
  in pancreatitis, 1429
  management of, 50-54, 51f, 52b
  monitoring perfusion status in, 50
  pathophysiology of, 42-47, 43f, 44f
  septic. See also Sepsis.
    adrenal insufficiency in, 1995-1996
    causes of, 46-47
    clinical features of, 2215
    definition of, 49, 49b, 2211, 2212b
    differential considerations in, 2218b
    pediatric fever in, 2511
    treatment of, 51, 51f, 52b, 53-54
  spinal, 436-437, 1677
    complete spinal cord lesion vs., 417
    neurogenic hypotension secondary to, 437
  toxic. See Toxic shock syndrome.
  undifferentiated, classification of, 48f
  ventilation in, 51-52
  volume replacement in, 52
  vs. hemodynamic changes in pregnancy, 316-317, 317f
Shored-exit wound, 958-959, 958f
Shotgun wounds. See also Firearm injuries
  abdominal, 491, 507
  peripheral vascular, 537
Shoulder
  exercises for
    in clavicle fracture, 677, 679f
    in proximal humerus fractures, 682
  frozen, 682, 698-699, 699t, 1797
  immobilization of, 569, 677, 678f
  pain in
    in ectopic pregnancy, 2743
    sources of, 672, 674
  physical examination of, 674, 674t, 1778
  tendinopathy of, 1796-1798
Shoulder dystocia, 2811, 2813-2815, 2814f, 2815f, 2816b
Shoulder girdle, 670, 671f
Shoulder trauma, 670-699
  anatomy in, 670-672, 671f, 673f
  clinical features of, 672, 674, 674t
  dislocations in, 683-693
    acromioclavicular, 685-687, 686f, 687f
    glenohumeral, 687-693, 688f-694f
    scapulothoracic, 693
    sternoclavicular, 683-685, 684f-685f
  fractures in, 676-683
    clavicle, 676-679, 676f-679f
    proximal humeral epiphysis, 682-683, 683f
    proximal humerus, 680-682, 681f, 682f
    scapula, 679-680, 680f
  radiography in, 674-676, 674f-676f
  soft tissue injuries in, 693-699
    adhesive capsulitis, 698-699, 699t
    biceps muscle lesions, 697-698, 697f
    calcific tendinitis, 698
    rotator cuff tears, 696
    subacromial syndromes and impingement, 693-696, 694t, 695f
Shrug sign, in rotator cuff tendinopathy, 1797
Shudder attacks, 2668
Shunt
  cerebrospinal fluid, in developmentally disabled patient, 2899
  vascular, in arterial injury, 544
  ventriculoperitoneal, pediatric fever in, 2517

Sialolithiasis, 1075
Siberian ginseng
  adverse effects of, 2476t
  drug interactions with, 2478t
Sick sinus syndrome, 1218
Sickle cell disease, 1879-1882
  altitude and, 2308
  clinical features of, 1880-1881, 1881f, 1881t
  in pregnancy, 2763t, 2768
  management of, 1881-1882
  osteomyelitis in, 2186
  pathophysiology of, 1879-1880
  pediatric fever in, 2516-2517
  urinary tract infection in, 1578
Sickle cell trait, 1880
Sickle cell–ß-thalassemia, 1882
Sideroblastic anemia, 1873, 2874
Sigmoid volvulus, 1497, 1498, 1498f, 1499
Sign language, 2905
Signet ring sign, in scapholunate dissociation, 630, 631f
Sign-overs, 3124
Silent perilobular fibrosis, 1435
Silk suture, 852t
Silver nitrate, for epistaxis, 1074
Simon's foci, in tuberculosis, 2152
Simple asphyxiants, inhalation of, 2432-2433
Simple obstruction of small bowel, 1440
Simple triage and rapid treatment (START) technique, 3012-3013, 3013f
Simulator technology, 3099, 3099f
Sin Nombre virus, 2055
Sinding-Larsen-Johansson disease, 794
Singh score for hip osteoporosis, 739, 740f-741f
Sinoatrial block, 1216-1218, 1217f
Sinoatrial node, 1201-1202, 1203f
  digitalis effects on, 2368
Sinus, nasal, 384
Sinus bradycardia, 1215-1216, 1216f
  from succinylcholine, 13
  in hypothyroidism, 1992
Sinus dysrhythmias, 1216, 1216f
Sinus node dysfunction, 1218
Sinus tachycardia, 1227-1228, 1227f
  in hyperthyroidism, 1987
  in myocardial contusion, 468
  in pediatric cardiac arrest, 109-110, 109t
Sinus thrombosis, lateral venous, in otitis media, 1068
Sinusitis, 1123-1126, 1124f, 1125f
  allergic vs. infectious, 1123
  clinical features of, 1124
  complications of, 1125-1126
  diagnostic strategies in, 1124, 1124f, 1125f
  differential diagnosis in, 1125
  management of, 1125
  maxillary, oral pain in, 1034
Sirolimus, 2844
Sixth disease, 1850
Sixth-nerve palsy, eye movement disorders in, 1063
Sjögren's syndrome
  myocarditis in, 1297
  pericarditis in, 1284
Skeletal muscle
  hyperactivity of, in organophosphate poisoning, 2459-2460
  ionic pump function of, 1976, 1977f
Skeletal muscle relaxants, for analgesia, 2928-2929
Skeletal system. See also Bone; Musculoskeletal system; Orthopedic entries.
  aging and, 345
  in electrical and lightning injuries, 2273
Skeletal tuberculosis, 2159
Skew deviation, 160
Skier's thumb, 604
Skin
  anatomy of, 842, 914-915
  biomechanical properties of, 843
  biopsy of, in Rocky Mountain spotted fever, 2135
  changes in
    in acute radiation syndrome, 2322
    in pregnancy, 2723-2724, 2728
  disinfection of, in wound care, 847
  dry, in HIV/AIDS, 2084-2085
  examination of
    in dyspnea, 178t
    in sexual assault victim, 985-986, 985b, 986b

Skin (Continued)
  injury to. See also Chemical injuries; Thermal burn.
    in acid and alkali burns, 931-933
    in anhydrous ammonia exposure, 935
    in bipyridyl compound exposure, 2466
    in chlorinated hydrocarbon exposure, 2463
    in elderly person, 347
    in electrical and lightning injuries, 2272-2273, 2272f, 2273f
    in frostbite, 2229
    in hydrofluoric acid exposure, 933-934
    in organophosphate exposure, 2460
    in substituted phenol exposure, 2464
    in tobacco workers, 2474
  of hand, 576-577
  of scalp, 350
  resistance of, 2269b
Skin abscess, 2202-2204, 2203t
Skin disorders, 1838-1865
  carbuncle as, 1843
  in developmentally disabled patient, 2903
  in HIV/AIDS, 2084-2085
  in parasitic infections, 2108-2109
  in spinal injuries, 438
  in traumatic asphyxia, 459
  with erythema, 1839t, 1844
  with exanthems, 1848-1851
  with nodular lesions, 1856-1857
  with papular lesions, 1851-1856
  with pustules, 1842-1844
  with red macules, 1844-1848
  with scales, plaques, and patches, 1838-1841
  with scaly papules, 1841-1842
  with vesicular lesions, 1857-1860
Skin lesions. See also Skin rash.
  definitions of, 1839t
  from opioid injection, 1864-1865, 1865f, 2453-2454
  in anaphylaxis, 1829
  in atopic dermatitis, 1841-1842
  in Candida infection, 1840-1841
  in chronic renal failure, 1542, 1542f
  in Churg-Strauss syndrome, 1816
  in contact dermatitis, 1851-1852, 1851f, 1852f
  in cutaneous anthrax, 1860, 1861f, 3025, 3026f
  in decompression sickness, 2284
  in dermatomyositis, 1708, 1862t, 1863f
  in diabetes mellitus, 1861f, 1862t, 1863f, 1971-1972
  in diaper dermatitis, 1852
  in diphtheria, 2003, 2004
  in drug eruptions, 1844-1845, 1844f, 1845f, 1846t-1847t
  in erythema infectiosum, 1850
  in erythema multiforme, 1852-1853, 1853f
  in erythema nodosum, 1816, 1856-1857, 1856f
  in folliculitis, 1843
  in fungal infection, 1838-1840, 1839f, 1840f
  in gonococcal dermatitis, 1566, 1843-1844, 1843f
  in herpes simplex virus infection, 1857-1858, 1858f
  in herpes zoster, 1859-1860, 1860f
  in hidradenitis suppurativa, 1843
  in HIV/AIDS, 1861f, 1862t, 2085
  in hypersensitivity vasculitis, 1815
  in hyperthyroidism, 1862t, 1987
  in hypothyroidism, 1862t, 1863f
  in impetigo, 1842-1843, 2202
  in inflammatory vascular disease, 1347
  in Lyme disease, 2122, 2122f, 2124-2125
  in measles, 1849
  in meningococcal disease, 2022
  in mustard exposure, 3031
  in panniculitis, 1817
  in pediculosis, 1853-1854, 1853f
  in pemphigus vulgaris, 1857, 1857f
  in pityriasis rosea, 1841
  in rheumatoid arthritis, 1862t
  in Rocky Mountain spotted fever, 1849-1850, 2133-2134, 2133f, 2134f
  in roseola infantum, 1850
  in rubella, 1850
  in scabies, 1854-1855, 1854f
  in scarlet fever, 1851, 1851f
  in smallpox, 1860, 1860f, 1861f, 2039, 2039f
  in staphylococcal scalded skin syndrome, 1845, 2199

Skin lesions *(Continued)*
in syphilis, 1855-1856, 1855f
in systemic lupus erythematosus, 1806, 1862t, 1863f
in toxic epidermal necrolysis, 1845-1846, 1846f
in toxic shock syndrome, 1846-1847
in ulcerative colitis, 1862t
in urticaria, 1847-1848, 1848f
in varicella, 1858-1859, 1859f
malignant diseases associated with, 1862-1864
nodular, 1856-1857
papular, 1851-1856
systemic diseases associated with, 1860, 1861f, 1862t, 1863f
vesicular, 1857-1860
Skin rash. *See also* Skin lesions.
drug-induced, 1844, 1847t
glue sniffer's, 2430
heat, 2259
in bacterial meningitis, 2658, 2659
in Colorado tick fever, 2141
in dermatomyositis, 1708
in disseminated gonococcal infection, 1566
in ehrlichiosis, 2138
in erythema infectiosum, 1850
in gonococcal arthritis, 1788
in halothane-induced hepatitis, 1414
in Henoch-Schönlein purpura, 1815, 2615, 2615f, 2653
in herpes zoster, 1859, 1860f
in Kawasaki disease, 2026, 2594, 2595f
in Lyme disease, 2122, 2122f
in measles, 1849, 2053, 2053f
in Rocky Mountain spotted fever, 1849, 2133-2134, 2133f, 2134f
in roseola infantum, 1850
in rubella, 1850
in scarlet fever, 1851, 1851f
in smallpox, 2039, 2039f, 3028-3029, 3028f, 3029f
in syphilis, 1561, 1561f
in systemic lupus erythematosus, 1806
in toxic shock syndrome, 1847, 2029, 2200
oral hypoglycemic agent–induced, 1972
Skin tension lines, 843, 843f, 844f
Skinfold asymmetry, in developmental hip dysplasia, 2701
Skull
anatomy of, 350
fetal, 2800f
radiography of
in minor head trauma, 364-365
in pediatric head trauma, 336, 368
in severe head trauma, 362, 362t
in skull fracture, 372
Skull fracture, 372-374
basilar, 373
clinical assessment and significance of, 372
depressed, 373
frontal, 393
in children, 334-335, 2699
linear, 372-373
open, 373-374
Skull-base osteomyelitis, 1071
Skullcap, adverse effects of, 2476t
Skunk, rabies in, 2062, 2062f, 2063, 2063f, 2064
Sleep aids, OTC, overdose of, 2487-2488, 2488t
Sleep apnea, hypertension in, 1313
Sleep deprivation, from shift work, performance and, 3123, 3123b
Sleep disturbance
in acute mountain sickness, 2301, 2302
in depression, 1737
seizures vs., 2668
Sleep talking, 2668
Sleeping, prone, sudden infant death syndrome and, 2715
Sleep-wake disturbances, in delirium, 1649
Sleepwalking, 2668
Sling and swathe, 569, 677, 678f
Sling immobilization
in clavicle fracture, 677, 678f
in scapula fracture, 680
Slipped capital femoral epiphysis, 765-767, 765f, 766f, 2707-2709, 2708f
Slit ventricle syndrome, in developmentally disabled patient, 2899
Slit-lamp examination
in corneal trauma, 1047, 1047f, 1051, 1051f

Slit-lamp examination *(Continued)*
in red and painful eye, 287, 287f
in traumatic hyphema, 1048, 1048f
of ocular foreign body, 860
Slow virus infections, 1657-1658, 1659, 2058
SLUDGE mnemonic, 2328, 2459, 2459b
Small intestine
biopsy of, in AIDS-related diarrhea, 1484
disorders of, 1440-1449
ischemia of, 1444-1449. *See also* Mesenteric ischemia.
motility disorders of, 1440, 1441b, 1443
obstruction of, 1440-1444, 1441b, 1443f
adynamic ileus in, 1440, 1441b, 1443
causes of, 1441-1442, 1441b, 1500b
clinical features of, 1442
complications of, 1442
diagnosis of, 1442-1443, 1443f
differential diagnosis in, 1443-1444
in malrotation with midgut volvulus, 2607, 2607f, 2608f
management of, 1444
mechanical vs. neurogenic, 1440
pseudoobstruction and, 1440
trauma to, 489, 490
volvulus of, 1441
Smallpox, 2034f, 2039-2040, 2039f, 3028-3029, 3028f, 3029f
skin lesions in, 1860, 1860t, 1861f
vaccine for, 2035t, 3029
Smith's fracture, 551t, 633-635, 635f
Smoke inhalation, 2435-2436
airway management and respiratory care in, 921-922
carbon monoxide with cyanide poisoning in, 2440-2441
prehospital care in, 921
Smoking
Buerger's disease and, 1351, 1352
chronic obstructive pulmonary disease and, 1098
Snakebite, 895-903, 897f, 897t, 900t, 1979
Sniffing position, in pediatric resuscitation, 105, 106f
Snowbird technique for reduction of anterior glenohumeral joint dislocation, 689
Snowblower injuries, 609
Snowmobile injuries, 609
Soap, for rabies postexposure prophylaxis, 2068
Social phobia, 1746b, 1749
Social problems, in alcoholism, 2879-2880
Social relationships, promotion of, as wellness strategy for emergency physicians, 3177
Social/adaptive milestones, 2495-2497, 2496t
Societal factors, in suicide, 1767-1768
Societal values, 3129, 3129b
Soda lime dust particles, in scuba diving–related disorders, 2283
Sodium
dietary excess of, heart failure from, 1268
fractional excretion of, 1527-1528, 1527t, 1528b
imbalance of. *See* Hypernatremia; Hyponatremia.
normal physiology of, 1933
serum
in bacterial meningitis, 2662
in diabetic ketoacidosis, 1964, 1964t
skin injury from, 937
urine, 1527-1528, 1527t, 1528b, 1934
Sodium bicarbonate
for acute renal failure, 2650
for cardiac arrest, 93
for cyanide poisoning, 2437
for cyclic antidepressant poisoning, 2355, 2356
for diabetic ketoacidosis, 1966-1967
for hyperkalemia, 1941
in acute renal failure, 1539
in chronic renal failure, 1545, 1545t
for hyperuricemia, 1914
for metabolic acidosis, 1929-1930
for pediatric asystole, 111-112
for pediatric bradycardia, 111
for pediatric resuscitation, 100, 101t
for QRS prolongation in OTC sleep aid overdose, 2488
for rhabdomyolysis, 1982
for salicylate overdose, 2342
for sepsis, 2219t, 2220

Sodium bicarbonate *(Continued)*
for toxicant-induced metabolic acidosis, 2400-2401
for ventricular fibrillation and pulseless ventricular tachycardia, 84
for white phosphorus burn, 936
topical anesthetic with, 846
Sodium channel antagonists, after cerebral ischemia, 71
Sodium chloride
for hyponatremia, 1935
hypertonic, in cyclic antidepressant poisoning, 2356-2357
in hydrotherapy for acid and alkali burns, 933
Sodium hydroxide, ingestion of, 2380, 2381, 2381t
Sodium nitrite, for cyanide poisoning, 939, 2438
Sodium phosphate
for hypercalcemia, 1915
for hypophosphatemia, 1952
Sodium thiosulfate
for cyanide poisoning, 2438
for simultaneous carbon monoxide and cyanide poisoning, 2440
Sodium-calcium exchanger, 1199-1200, 1200f
Sodium-potassium pump, 1200, 1200f, 1976, 1977f
Soft tissue examination, in spinal cord injury, 311
Soft tissue infection, 2195-2209
clinical characteristics of, 2195-2196, 2196t
in abscess, 2202-2207. *See also* Abscess.
in cellulitis, 2196-2199, 2196t, 2197t
in impetigo, 2201-2202
in myonecrosis, 2196t, 2208-2209
in necrotizing fasciitis, 2196t, 2207-2208
in toxic shock syndrome, 2199-2201, 2200b, 2201b
superficial, antibiotics for, 2197, 2197t
Soft tissue injuries, 566-568. *See also specific types, e.g.,* Sprain.
foreign body in, 878-879
from dentoalveolar trauma, 1040
in ankle trauma, 815-820
in elbow and humeral trauma, 667-668
in elderly person, 347
in eye, 1054-1055, 1055f
in facial trauma, 390-392
in hand, 600
in hip trauma, 761-763
in lower leg trauma, 804-805
in pelvic fracture, 719
in shoulder, 693-699
in wrist trauma, 639, 639f
wound management in, 842-857
Solar urticaria, 1848
Solid-organ transplant patient. *See* Organ transplant patient.
Solvents, inhaled, 2428-2432, 2430f, 2886-2889, 2887t, 2888f, 2889b
Soman, 2461, 3030-3031, 3030b, 3031b
Somatic pain, 211-212
Somatization, 1753
Somatization disorder, 1754-1755, 1754b
Somatoform disorders, 1753-1759
clinical features of, 1753-1756, 1754b, 1755b
diagnosis of, 1756
differential considerations in, 1756-1757, 1757b
disposition in, 1759
management of, 1757-1759
panic attack in, 1748
undifferentiated, 1755
Somatoform pain disorder, 1755
Somatostatin analogues, for gastrointestinal bleeding, 225
Somogyi phenomenon, in hypoglycemia, 1960
Sore throat. *See* Pharyngitis.
Sotalol, 1210, 2373t
Space infections of head and neck, 1027, 1028-1029, 1030f, 1032, 1116-1117, 1116f
parapharyngeal, 1121-1123, 1122f
peritonsillar, 1117-1118, 1118f
retropharyngeal, 1120-1121, 1120f, 1121f
submandibular, 1028, 1032, 1118-1119
Space of Poirier, 622, 624f
Spasmodic croup, 2527
Spastic paraparesis, idiopathic, 1683

Spasticity
  in cerebral palsy, 2904
  in multiple sclerosis, 1673, 2910
Spathiphyllum, 2475
Specificity, 3059t
Spectinomycin, for gonococcal dermatitis, 1843
Specula, 2735
Speech
  disorganized, in schizophrenia, 1727-1728
  pressured, in mania, 1739
Speech disorders
  in botulism, 2014
  in neck masses, 1076
Speed's test, in bicipital tendinopathy, 1797
Sperm, recovery of, in sexual assault victim, 987-
    988, 988t
Spermatic cord, torsion of, in children, 2639-
    2640, 2640f
Sphenoid sinus, 1123
Sphenoid sinusitis, 1124, 1126
Sphenopalatine artery, 1073, 1073f
Spherocytosis, in hemolytic anemia, 1877, 1878f
Sphygmomanometer, in wound assessment, 845
Spider angioma, in hepatitis, 1404
Spider bites, 905-907, 2329t
Spider nevi, in pregnancy, 2724
Spill scalds, 915-916
Spilled teacup sign, in lunate dislocation, 630,
    632f
Spinal abscess, 1684, 1712, 1715, 1716
Spinal accessory nerve, 1665t
Spinal arteries, 1676
Spinal carcinoma
  back pain in, 261, 703, 706, 712-713
  magnetic resonance imaging in, 712-713
  radiography in, 708, 709f
Spinal column
  anatomy of, 399, 400f-401f
  injuries of. *See* Spinal injuries.
Spinal cord
  infarction of, 1683
  ligaments of, 401f
  membranes of, inflammation of. *See*
    Meningitis.
  pain transmission in, 2914-2915, 2915f,
    2916f
  tracts in, illustration of, 2916f
  tumor of, 1685
  vascular damage to, 413, 415f
Spinal cord compression, 1680-1681, 1681t,
    1683-1685
  epidural, in cancer patient, 1919-1920
  with superior vena cava syndrome, 1910
Spinal cord disorders, 1675-1685
  anatomy in, 1676, 1676f
  classification of, 1677-1679, 1678f
  clinical features of, 1679-1680
  demyelinating
    in multiple sclerosis, 1681-1682
    in transverse myelitis, 1682
  diagnosis of, 1680
  differential considerations in, 1680-1681,
    1681b
  in diskitis, 1684-1685
  in epidural abscess, 1684
  in epidural hematoma, 1683-1684
  in HIV/AIDS, 1683
  in idiopathic spastic paraparesis, 1683
  in subarachnoid hemorrhage, 1682
  in syringomyelia, 1682-1683
  management of, 1681
Spinal cord syndromes, 417-420, 419f, 420f,
    1677-1679, 1678f
  anterior, 419f, 420, 1678, 1678f
  Brown-Séquard, 418, 419f, 420, 1677-1678,
    1678f
  cauda equina, 1678f, 1679
  central, 417-418, 419f, 1677, 1678f
  conus medullaris, 1678f, 1679
  transverse, 417, 1677, 1678f
Spinal fracture
  anatomy and physiology in, 399, 402f
  back pain in, 706
  computed tomography in, 429-430, 429f
  disposition in, 439
  extension, 410-411, 410f-411f
  flexion, 399, 401-404, 402f-405f
  minor, 439
  rotational, 405-409, 408f-410f

Spinal fracture *(Continued)*
  vertical compression, 411-413, 411f-414f
  with cord impingement, back pain in, 265t
Spinal hemorrhage, magnetic resonance imaging
    in, 434, 434f
Spinal immobilization, 435, 436
Spinal infection, back pain in, 703, 706, 712
Spinal injuries, 398-439, 2905-2909
  airway management in, 436
  anatomy and physiology in, 399, 400f-402f
  autonomic dysreflexia in, 2906
  classification of, 399, 399t, 413
  clinical features of, 415-420
  complete (transverse), 417, 1677, 1678f
  computed tomography in, 427, 429-431, 429b,
    429f-432f
  definitive treatment and prognosis in, 438-439
  disposition in, 439
  epidemiology of, 399
  extension, 410-411, 410f-411f
  flexion, 399, 401-404, 402f-405f
  gastrointestinal disorders in, 438, 2907
  genitourinary disorders in, 438
  in children, 336-338, 337f
  in decompression sickness, 2284
  in elderly person, 346, 413, 415f
  in electrical and lightning injuries, 2273-2274
  in multiple trauma, 309
  in pregnancy, 2770
  incomplete, 417-420, 419f, 420f, 437-438, 1677-
    1679, 1678f
  ligamentous, 434, 435f, 439
  magnetic resonance imaging in, 431-435, 433f-
    436f
  management of, 435-439, 437f
  motor examination in, 416, 417t
  neurologic disorders in, 2909
  neurologic examination in, 415-417
  orthopedic disorders in, 2909
  orthostatic hypotension in, 2906
  pathophysiology of, 399, 401-413
  prehospital care in, 435
  primary, 413, 415f
  pulmonary edema in, 438
  radiographic evaluation of, 420-427, 422f-428f
    anteroposterior view in, 424, 426, 426f, 427f
    cross-table lateral view in, 421, 424, 425f,
      426f
    flexion-extension views in, 428
    indications for, 420-421
    oblique views in, 426-428, 426f, 427f, 428f
    odontoid view in, 424, 424f-425f
    standard trauma series in, 421, 422f-424f
  reflex examination in, 417, 417t
  rotational, 405-409, 408f-410f
  secondary, 413, 416f
  sensory examination in, 417, 417t, 418f
  shear, 405, 406f-407f
  skin disorders in, 438
  stabilization in, 435-436
  thromboembolic disease in, 2906-2907
  urinary tract disorders in, 2908-2909
  vascular damage in, 413, 415f
  vertical compression, 411-413, 411f-414f
  without radiographic abnormality, 420
Spinal nerve, 1688f, 1689
Spinal shock, 436-437, 1677
  complete spinal cord lesion vs., 417
  neurogenic hypotension secondary to, 437
Spinal stenosis, back pain in, 705, 712
Spinal trigeminal tract, damage to, Dejeune onion
    skin pattern from, 420
Spinal tuberculosis, 261, 265t, 2159, 2178, 2182,
    2182f, 2184-2185
Spinning sensation, 144
Spinoreticular tract, 2915, 2915f, 2916f
Spinothalamic tract, 2915, 2915f, 2916f
  lateral, 1676, 1676f
Spiral fracture, 2690, 2691f
Spirochetemia, in Lyme disease, 2119
Spironolactone, 1321t
  for chronic heart failure, 1276
Splash burns, 963, 2271
Spleen
  infarction of, in sickle cell disease, 2308
  trauma to, 341, 489, 490, 491
Splenectomy
  immune defects in, 2842-2843
    pneumococcal infection after, 2018

Splenic artery aneurysm, 1355
Splenic sequestration, 1880, 1896
Splenomegaly
  in hepatitis, 1404
  in tricuspid stenosis and regurgitation, 1307
Splint immobilization, 568-571, 569f, 570f
  in ankle sprain, 817
  in carpal tunnel syndrome, 639
  in clavicle fracture, 677, 678f, 2693
  in developmental hip dysplasia, 2702
  in distal femur fracture, 776-777
  in distal phalanx fracture, 593, 593f
  in humeral shaft fracture, 654, 654f
  in mallet finger, 606, 606f
  in medial epicondylar fracture, 662
  in metacarpal neck fracture, 597
  in metacarpal or phalangeal fractures, 595,
    595f, 596f
  in pelvic fracture, 723
  in sternoclavicular joint dislocation, 684
  in tibial shaft fracture, 800
Split root syndromes, 1033-1034
Spondylitis
  ankylosing, arthritis in, 1789
  back pain in, 703, 706, 712
  radiography in, 708, 709f
Spondyloarthropathies, seronegative, arthritis in,
    1789-1790
Spondylolisthesis, degenerative
  back pain in, 703, 705, 712
  radiography in, 708, 708f
Spongiform encephalopathy, dementia in, 1657-
    1658, 1659
Spongiform leukoencephalopathy, from inhaled
    heroin, 2452
Spontaneous bacterial peritonitis, 245-246, 1412-
    1413
Sports injuries
  concussion in, 365-366, 367
  in facial trauma, 382
  in foot trauma, 837-838
  in hip trauma, 761-762
Spousal abuse. *See* Intimate partner violence and
    abuse.
Sprain, 566-567
  ankle, 815-818, 817b, 817f
  foot, 838
Spurious pregnancy, 2731-2732
Sputum, mucopurulent, in pneumonia, 1132
Sputum studies
  in chronic obstructive pulmonary disease,
    1101
  in pneumonia, 1134-1135
  in tuberculosis, 2154-2155, 2154f
Squeeze test, 816
ST segment
  depression of
    differential diagnosis in, 1163, 1163f
    in myocardial infarction, 1162-1163, 1163f,
      1171
    reciprocal, 1162-1163, 1163f
  elevation of
    differential diagnosis in, 1161-1162, 1162t
    electrocardiographic differential diagnosis of,
      1166-1170, 1167f-1172f
    in benign early repolarization, 1166-1167,
      1167f, 1168f
    in left bundle branch block, 1167, 1169,
      1169f, 1170f
    in left ventricular aneurysm, 1167, 1168f
    in left ventricular hypertrophy, 1169-1170,
      1172f
    in pericarditis, 1167, 1167f, 1168f
    in ventricular paced rhythms, 1169, 1171f
    in myocardial infarction, 1164t, 1173-1174,
      1173f
  in pericarditis, 1281, 1282
ST segment elevation myocardial infarction
    (STEMI), 1161-1162, 1162t, 1163f
Stab wounds
  abdominal
    diagnostic studies in, 502
    history in, 493
    management of, 502-505, 503f, 503t
    pathophysiology of, 490
    physical examination in, 494
  acute cardiac tamponade from, 473
  in physical assault, 963, 963f
  observation in, 3068-3069

Stab wounds (Continued)
 peripheral vascular, 537
 to neck, 442
Stabilization
 in abdominal pain, 213
 in anaphylaxis, 1830
 in back pain, 261-262, 263f
 in central nervous system infection, 1721
 in cervical spine injuries, 435-436
 in chest pain, 184-185, 184f
 in coma, 157-158
 in confusion, 150-151
 in diarrhea, 228, 232
 in dyspnea, 181f
 in fever, 135
 in gastrointestinal bleeding, 220-221
 in hemoptysis, 280
 in mood disorders, 1741
 in multiple trauma, 305-309
 in nausea and vomiting, 201t, 202
 in pediatric trauma, 329
 in seizure, 166-167, 166t
 in syncope, 196, 198, 199f
 in vaginal bleeding, 254-255
 in weakness, 138-139
 mechanical. See Fixation.
 medicolegal requirements for, 3163-3164
 of avulsed tooth, 1038f, 1040
 postresuscitation
  adult, 85-87, 88f
  pediatric, 113-114, 113f
Staffing requirements for observation, 3062-3063
Staining techniques, in sexual assault
  examination, 988-989, 988f
Stainless steel wire suture, 852t
Stanford classification of aortic dissection, 1325,
  1325f
Staphylococcal infection
 in catheter-related infections, 1363
 in cellulitis, 2198-2199
 in dacryocystitis, 1055
 in food poisoning, 1469-1470, 1480t
 in gastroenteritis, 2626
 in impetigo, 1842, 2202
 in infective endocarditis, 1301
 scalded skin syndrome in, 1845, 2199
Staphylococcus aureus
 in bone or joint infections, 2177, 2178t
 in pneumonia, 1130, 2556-2557, 2556f
 in septic arthritis, 1784
 in toxic shock syndrome, 2027-2031, 2028b,
  2029b, 2029t, 2199-2200, 2200b
 methicillin-resistant, 1130
Staphylococcus lugdenesis, 1301
Staphylococcus saprophyticus, 1574
Staples
 for scalp laceration repair, 850
 for wound closure, 853
"Star of Life," 2988, 2988f
Stasis, zone of, in burn injury, 917, 917f
Statins, rhabdomyolysis from, 1979
Statistical analysis
 bayesian, 3056
 in clinical trials, 3050
Statistical tests, 3052-3053, 3052t
Status asthmaticus, 1083, 1091, 2535-2536
 intubation and, 16, 17t
 mechanical ventilation in, 32
Status epilepticus, 167, 1621, 1622b
 alcohol-related, 2865
 complications of, 2668b
 convulsive vs. nonconvulsive, 2667
 in children, 2667, 2668b, 2672-2673, 2672t
 in pregnancy, 2769
 treatment of, 1627-1628, 1627t
Status migrainosus, 1632-1633
Steakhouse syndrome, 1383
Steal phenomenon, in arteriovenous fistula or
  graft, 1366
Steatorrhea, in viral gastroenteritis, 1476
Steatosis, in alcoholic liver disorders, 1409
Stellate tear, in handgun contact wound, 955-
  956, 955f
"STEMI alert" system, 1193
Stener fracture, 551t
Stenosing tenosynovitis, in hand, 618
Stensen's duct, 385, 386f
Stephania tetrandra, 2476
Sternal fracture, 456-457

Sternbach's diagnostic criteria for serotonin
  syndrome, 2359b
Sternoclavicular arthritis, 2191
Sternoclavicular joint
 anatomy of, 670, 671f
 dislocation, 683-685, 684f-685f
Sternoclavicular ligaments, 670, 671f
Steroids. See Corticosteroids.
Stevens-Johnson syndrome, 1853, 1853f
Still's murmur, 2572
Stimson technique
 for anterior glenohumeral joint dislocation
  reduction, 689, 689f
 for hip reduction, 758, 758f
Stimulation, in neonatal resuscitation, 122
Stinging hydroids, 909
Stingray, 910
Stings
 hymenoptera, 903-905
  allergy to, 1827, 2547
  rhabdomyolysis from, 1979
 venomous, marine animals in, 909-910, 911
Stokes sign
 in neoplastic cardiac tamponade, 1917
 in superior vena cava syndrome, 1910
Stomach. See also Gastric entries.
 foreign body in, 873-875, 875f, 1384-1385
 inflammation of. See Gastroenteritis.
 perforation of, in peptic ulcer disease, 1393
 secretory cells of, 1391
Stomatitis
 aphthous, 1036
 vesicular, 2054
Stomatocytosis, in alcoholism, 2874
Stomatognathic system, anatomy of, 1026-1027,
  1027f-1030f
Stonefish envenomation, 910
Stool culture
 in Aeromonas hydrophila gastroenteritis, 1468
 in AIDS-related diarrhea, 1483
 in Bacillus anthracis gastroenteritis, 1469
 in Campylobacter gastroenteritis, 1460
 in Clostridium difficile enterocolitis, 1475
 in coccidial gastroenteritis, 1478
 in diarrhea, 233
 in Giardia gastroenteritis, 1479
 in hemorrhagic Escherichia coli serotype
  O157:H7 gastroenteritis, 1467
 in infectious diarrhea, 2626-2627
 in intestinal amebiasis, 1480
 in pediatric fever, 2510
 in Plesiomonas shigelloides gastroenteritis,
  1468
 in salmonellosis, 1463
 in shigellosis, 1464
 in Vibrio fish poisoning, 1472
 in Vibrio parahaemolyticus gastroenteritis,
  1466
 in Yersinia enterocolitica gastroenteritis,
  1465
Stool examination
 in diarrhea, 233
 in gastrointestinal bleeding, 222
Stool softener, for constipation, 241t, 242
Stools
 black tarry, 221
 bloody, 221
  in hemolytic uremic syndrome, 2654
  in hemorrhagic Escherichia coli serotype
   O157:H7 gastroenteritis, 1466
  in inflammatory bowel disease, 2616
  in intussusception, 2610
  in Plesiomonas shigelloides gastroenteritis,
   1468
Straddle fracture, pelvic, 725, 726f
Straddle injuries, 975
Straight leg raise
 in back pain, 264
 in lumbar radiculopathy, 704
Strain, 567
 gastrocnemius, 804
 in hip trauma, 761-762
 plantaris, 804
Strangulation, 450-451
 penile, 532, 533f
Strangulation obstruction of small bowel,
  1440
Stratified randomization, 3049
Stratum corneum, 842, 914

Stratum germinativum, 842
Street gangs, violence by, 1017-1018, 1020-1022
Streptococcal infection
 in cellulitis, 2198
 in impetigo, 1842, 2202
 in infective endocarditis, 1301
 in rheumatic fever, 1303
 in toxic shock syndrome, 2028, 2028b, 2029,
  2029t, 2200-2201, 2201b
Streptococcal pharyngitis, 274-275, 1109, 1110,
  1111, 1112-1113, 1114
 adult epiglottitis vs., 1115
 in rheumatic fever, 1303, 1304
Streptococcus bovis, 1301
Streptococcus pneumoniae, 1129, 1132, 2016-
  2020, 2020b. See also Pneumococcal disease.
Streptokinase
 in myocardial infarction, 1189
 in pulmonary embolism, 1378t
Streptomycin
 for tuberculosis, 2163t, 2164
 for tularemia, 2131
Stress disorder
 acute, 1746b
 posttraumatic. See Posttraumatic stress
  disorder.
Stress echocardiography, in acute coronary
  syndromes, 1179
Stress fracture, 553
 femoral neck, 755-756
 foot, 837-838
 lower leg, 803-804
 pelvic, 725
 tibial shaft, 800
Stress management, disaster, 3018
Stress polycythemia, 1884-1885
Stress radiographs, in fracture, 557
Stress response
 in anxiety disorders, 1744
 in hemorrhagic shock, 46
 in mood disorders, 1735
 in shock, 43, 44f
Stress test
 ankle, 816-817
 collateral ligament, 774
 elevated arm, 1359
Stress ulcer, in burn injured patient, 924
Stressors, in emergency medicine, 3174-3175
Striae gravidarum, 2723, 2728
Stricture
 esophageal, from caustic ingestion, 2383
 in gastroesophageal reflux, 1389
Stridor
 anaphylaxis vs., 1829
 biphasic, 2520
 causes of, 2521t
 in airway foreign body aspiration, 865, 866
 in anaphylaxis, 2549
 in bacterial tracheitis, 2528
 in epiglottitis, 2523
 in laryngomalacia, 2524
 in laryngotracheal stenosis, 2525
 in neck masses, 1076
 in pediatric upper airway obstruction, 2519-
  2520, 2521t
 in retropharyngeal abscess, 2522
 in subglottic hemangioma, 2525
 in viral croup, 2525
 in vocal cord paralysis, 2524
String of beads sign, in small bowel obstruction,
  1443
Stroke, 1606-1617. See also Intracerebral
  hemorrhage; Subarachnoid hemorrhage.
 acute drug therapy for, 1615-1616, 1615t
 alcohol consumption and, 2869-2870
 anatomy and physiology in, 1607
 antihypertensive drug therapy for, 1614, 1614t,
  1616
 anxiety in, 1748
 cardioembolic, 1608
 clinical features of, 1609-1611, 1610t, 1611f
 diagnosis of, 1612-1613, 1612f
 differential diagnosis in, 1611-1612
 disposition in, 1616-1617
 epidemiology of, 1607-1609, 1607t, 1608b
 fibrinolytic therapy for, 1615, 1615t
 in central retinal artery occlusion, 1057
 in myocardial infarction, 1161
 in systemic lupus erythematosus, 1807

Stroke (Continued)
　management of, 1613-1616, 1613t, 1614t, 1615b
　oropharyngeal dysphagia in, 1396-1397
　pathophysiology of, 1606-1607
　previous, fibrinolytic therapy eligibility and, 1191
　seizure in, 1624
　thrombotic, 1607-1608
　time goals in, 1613t
　vs. high-altitude cerebral edema, 2306
Stroke in evolution, 1609
Stroke syndromes, hypertension in, 1315-1316
Stroke volume
　in heart failure, 1260, 1260f, 1262
　in infants and children, decreased, causes of, 2569, 2569b
Strongyloides stercoralis, 2102t
　dysenteric colitis in, 230t
　gastroenteritis in, 1477t
　in cancer patient with impaired cell-mediated immunity, 2840
　in organ transplant patient, 2849
　neurologic disorders in, 2107
　skin disorders in, 2109
Struvite kidney stones, 1587
Strychnine poisoning, tetanus vs., 2010
Student's t test, 3052, 3052t, 3053
Stun gun, injuries from, 2274
Stupor, 156, 2482
Subacromial bursitis, 1803
Subacromial dislocation, 691
Subacromial syndromes, 693-696, 694t, 695f
Subacute sclerosing panencephalitis, 2054
Subarachnoid hemorrhage, 1635-1637, 1636t, 1637f
　diagnosis of, 1636-1637, 1637f
　dysrhythmia after, 371
　headache in, 174t, 1637, 2677
　Hunt and Hess scale for, 1636, 1636t
　in pregnancy, 2732
　risk factors for, 171b
　spinal, 1682
　traumatic, 377
　treatment of, 1637
Subcalcaneal heel pain, 836-837
Subclavian artery
　aneurysm of, 1354
　compression of, thoracic outlet syndrome from, 1358
　injury to, 544-545
Subclavian steal syndrome, 147t
Subclavian vein
　compression of, thoracic outlet syndrome from, 1358
　injury to, 544-545
　thrombosis of, 1363
Subclavian-axillary artery aneurysm, 1354
Subclavicular dislocation, 697, 698f
Subconjunctival hemorrhage, 285, 296t, 1048, 1048f
Subcoracoid dislocation, 697, 698f
Subcutaneous drug abuse, skin lesions associated with, 1864-1865, 1865f
Subcutaneous emphysema
　chest wall trauma and, 459-460
　in esophageal perforation, 484
　in scuba diving–related disorders, 2286
　tracheobronchial injury and, 466, 466f
Subcutaneous nodules
　in acute rheumatic fever, 2596
　in rheumatic fever, 1304
Subcutaneous tissue, 915
Subdiaphragmatic thrusts, for airway foreign body, 2530
Subdural empyema, in otitis media, 1068
Subdural hematoma, 375-377, 376f
　headache in, 2678
　in children, 335
Subdural hygroma, 377
Subfascial web space infection, 617, 617f, 618
Subglenoid dislocation, 691, 697, 698f
Subglottic hemangioma, 2525
Subglottic stenosis, 2525
Subglottic tracheal disease, 2525-2527
Sublingual capnography, 39
Sublingual glands, 385-386
Subluxation, 564-566
　biceps tendon, 698
　cervical spine, 401, 404, 404f-405f, 427, 428f

Subluxation (Continued)
　glenohumeral joint, 690, 691f
　lens, 1049
　radial head, 666, 666f, 2697-2698, 2697f
　tooth, 1037, 1038f
Subluxation provocation test, in knee trauma, 774
Submandibular gland, stones of, 1075
Submandibular space, 1117
Submersion injuries, 2311-2315
Subperiosteal abscess
　in mastoiditis, 1072
　in osteomyelitis, 2175
Subscapular nerve, 672
Subscapularis muscle, 672, 673f
Subspinous dislocation, 691
Substance abuse, 2882-2896. See also Poisoning/overdose.
　alcohol. See Alcohol intoxication; Alcoholism.
　amphetamines and amphetamine-like drugs in, 2893-2896, 2894t, 2895b
　ancillary studies in, 2885-2886
　anxiety from, 1746b
　by emergency physicians, 3176
　by sexual assault victim, 979
　cocaine in, 2386-2392
　complications of, 2885
　differential diagnosis in, 2885
　epidemiology of, 2882-2883, 2884f
　GHB in, 2489
　hallucinogens in, 2406-2416
　history in, 2883-2884
　in intimate partner violence and abuse, 998
　in pregnancy, 2736, 2790-2794, 2791b, 2883
　ketamine in, 2893
　management of, 2886
　marijuana in, 2411-2412
　mood disorders from, 1739-1740, 1740b, 1740f
　opioids in, 2327t, 2328, 2451-2456
　phencyclidine in, 2413, 2414-2415, 2414t, 2415t, 2416, 2882b, 2891-2893
　physical examination in, 2884-2885
　plant and mushroom poisoning associated with, 2471, 2477
　psychosis from, 1727b, 1728-1729
　referral in, 2886
　reporting requirements for, 3173
　solvents/hydrocarbons in, 2428-2432, 2430f, 2886-2889, 2887t, 2888f, 2889b
　suicide and, 1769
　youth violence and, 1018
Substance dependence, alcohol, 2858
Substituted judgment, 3134
Substituted phenol poisoning, 2463-2464, 2463b
Subtalar joint
　anatomy of, 808, 809f, 820, 820f
　dislocation of, 825-826, 825f
Subtrochanteric fracture, 753-755, 754f
Subungual hematoma, nail bed trauma and, 594, 610-611
Succimer
　for arsenic poisoning, 2424
　for lead poisoning, 2422
　for mercury poisoning, 2426
Succinylcholine
　for emergency intubation, 13-14, 17, 18
　for scleral rupture, 1050
　for tetanus, 2011
　hyperkalemia from, 14, 14t, 1940
　refrigeration of, 14
Sucking chest wound, 462
Sucralfate
　for gastroesophageal reflux, 1390
　for upper gastrointestinal disorders, 1399
Sudden asphyxic asthma, 1084
Sudden death
　epidemiology of, 77
　in heart failure, 1259
　in hydrocarbon poisoning, 2429
　in hypertrophic cardiomyopathy, 1295, 1296
　in mitral valve prolapse, 1305
　in myocardial disease, 1298
　of infant. See Sudden infant death syndrome.
　of young athletes, 2597-2599, 2597b
　trajectory of dying in, 3140, 3140f
Sudden infant death syndrome, 2713-2717
　apparent life-threatening event and, 2718
　caffeine/theophylline and, 2719-2720

Sudden infant death syndrome (Continued)
　definition of, 2714
　diagnosis of, 2716
　epidemiology of, 2713-2714
　etiology and pathophysiology of, 2716, 2716f
　future directions in, 2720
　home monitoring for, 2720
　management of, 2716-2717
　prehospital care in, 2717
　prehospital end-of-life issues related to, 3145-3146
　psychosocial considerations in, 2717, 2717b
　risk factors for, 2714-2716, 2715b
SUDS (single-use diagnostic system) assay for HIV, 2074
Sufentanil, 2922t, 2923
Sugar-tong splint, in humeral shaft fracture, 654, 654f
Suicide, 1766-1774
　by hanging and strangulation, 450
　clinical features of, 1769-1771
　definitions in, 1767
　depression and, 1737, 1768, 1769
　diagnostic strategies in, 1771
　disposition in, 1773-1774, 1773b
　documentation in, 1774
　epidemiology of, 1767, 1767b
　etiology and pathophysiology of, 1767-1769
　history in, 1770-1771, 1770t
　hospitalization indications in, 1773
　in adolescence, 1769
　in elderly person, 1767, 1769-1770
　in terminal illness, 1770
　management of, 1771-1773
　methods used in, 1768-1769
　physical examination in, 1771, 1771t
　prehospital care end-of-life issues related to, 3145
　prevention of, 1774
　psychiatric disorders and, 1768, 1769
　risk determination in, 1772-1773
　risk factors for, 1767, 1767b
　safety precautions in, 1772
　substance abuse and, 1769
Sulfadiazine, for Toxoplasma gondii infection, 2082
Sulfasalazine
　for Behçet's disease, 1815
　for inflammatory bowel disease, 1502
　for rheumatoid arthritis, 1791
Sulfhemoglobin toxicity, cyanosis in, 272-273
Sulfites, allergy to, 1827
Sulfonamides, during pregnancy and lactation, 2784
Sulfonylurea drugs, 1972
　antidotes to, 2329t
　during pregnancy and lactation, 2790
Sulfur mustard exposure, 938-939, 3031
Sulindac, for premature labor, 2807
Sumatriptan
　for cluster headache, 1635
　for migraine, 1633t, 1634, 2680
Sundown syndrome, 2827
Sunflower oil, for tar removal, 927
Super glue, ocular trauma from, 1046
Superficial fascia
　anatomy of, 842
　neck, 442
Superficial femoral vein, 1368
Superficial partial-thickness burn, 918, 919f
Superficial peroneal nerve, 797
Superficial punctate keratitis, 1054
Superfund Amendments and Reauthorization Act of 1986, 930
Superinfection
　in pertussis, 2006
　in tuberculosis, 2151, 2151f
Superior gluteal artery, 717-718
Superior mesenteric artery, 1445
　acute mesenteric ischemia and, 1445-1446, 1446b
　aneurysm of, 1355-1356
　in spinal cord injury, 2907
Superior orbital fracture, 393
Superior peroneal retinaculum, injury to, 818-819, 819f
Superior vena cava syndrome
　in cancer patient, 1909-1911, 1910f
　pacemaker lead–induced, 1250

Supination, of hand, 577f
Supine hypotensive syndrome, in pregnancy, 316, 2725
Suppositories, for constipation, 241t, 242
Suppurative gastritis, 1390, 1391
Supracondylar fracture, 2693-2697, 2694f-2696f, 2694t
    extension, 655-658, 656f-658f
    flexion, 657f, 658-659
Supracondylar process, 648, 648f
Supradiaphragmatic volvulus, 1394
Supraglottic airway disease, 2522-2524
Supralevator abscess, 1513t, 1514
Suprapatellar bursitis, 795-796
Suprascapular nerve, 672
Supraspinatus muscle, 672, 673f
Supraventricular tachycardia, 1226
    in infants and children, 2585-2589, 2586t, 2587f, 2587t, 2588f
    in pediatric cardiac arrest, 109-110, 109t
    paroxysmal, 1233-1235, 1233f, 1234f
    with abnormal conduction, vs. ventricular tachycardia, 1237-1239, 1238t, 1239f, 1240f
Sural nerve, 797
Surface tension of hydrocarbons, 2428
Surgery, recent, fibrinolytic therapy eligibility and, 1191-1192
Surgical mask, for tuberculosis exposure prophylaxis, 2170
Surrogate decision-makers, 3134-3135
Surrogate lists, 3134-3135
Sutural diastasis, 373
Suture
    corner stitch, 851
    half-buried horizontal mattress, 851
    horizontal mattress, 850
    in laceration of extensor mechanism over distal interphalangeal joint, 607, 607f
    interrupted, 849-850
    intradermal (buried), 850
    removal of, 856
    running, 849
    simple, 850
    subcutaneous, for reducing wound tension, 849
    vertical mattress, 850
Suturing
    materials for, 851-853, 852t
    of animal bites, 886-887, 887t
    techniques in, 849-851
Swallowing
    disturbances of. See Dysphagia.
    physiology of, 1395
Swallowing study, in dysphagia, 1397
Swan neck deformity, 607, 607f
SWAT units, tactical emergency medical support in, 3000-3005
Sweat glands, 915
Sweating
    heat loss through, 2255
    in anticholinergic poisoning, 2348
Swimmer's itch, 2109
Swimming pool cleaner, ingestion of, 2381t
Sympathectomy
    for frostbite, 2233
    for peripheral arteriovascular disease, 1350
Sympathetic blockage, for complex regional pain syndrome, 563
Sympathetic nervous system, hyperactivity of, in organophosphate poisoning, 2459
Sympathetic response, to laryngoscopy, 16-17
Sympathomimetic syndrome, in overdosed/poisoned patient, 2327-2328, 2327t
Sympathomimetics. See also specific agents, e.g., Cocaine.
    overdose of, 2386-2393
Synchronized intermittent mechanical ventilation (SIMV), 27
Syncope, 193-198
    anaphylaxis vs., 1830
    ancillary studies in, 195-196, 196t
    chest pain associated with, 185, 186t
    diagnostic approach to, 193-196, 194b, 195b, 195t, 196t
    differential diagnosis in, 194b, 196, 196t, 197t, 198f
    disposition in, 198
    drug-induced, 195, 195b

Syncope (Continued)
    empiric management of, 196, 198, 199f
    epidemiology of, 193
    heat, 2259
    in abdominal aortic aneurysm rupture, 1333
    in aortic dissection, 1325
    in aortic stenosis, 1306
    in children, 2685-2686
    in hypertrophic cardiomyopathy, 1295
    observation in, 3066-3067, 3066b
    pathophysiology of, 193
    physical examination in, 195, 195t
    reflex, 2685
    seizure vs., 165-166, 1626, 2667-2668
Syndesmotic ligaments, anatomy of, 808, 809f
Syndrome of inappropriate antidiuretic hormone (SIADH), 1934, 1934b
Syndromic surveillance, public health reporting and, 3105
Synergistic necrotizing cellulitis, 2209
Synovial fluid analysis
    in acute septic arthritis, 2705, 2706t
    in rheumatic diseases, 1781-1782, 1781t
    in septic arthritis, 1785
Synovial joint, 1777, 1777f
Synovial membrane, glenohumeral, 672, 673f
Synovial spaces, in hand, 585, 586f
Synovitis
    toxic, pediatric limp from, 764
    transient, in children, 2703-2704
Syphilis, 1518t, 1519, 1557t, 1559-1562, 1559t, 1560f, 1561f
    congenital, 2701, 2775
    fracture in, 2701
    in HIV/AIDS, 2087
    in pregnancy, 2764t, 2775
    skin lesions in, 1855-1856, 1855f
    vertigo in, 2683
Syphilitic pharyngitis, 1111, 1112, 1113
Syringomyelia, spinal cord lesions in, 1682-1683
Syrinx, posttraumatic, 435, 436f, 2909
Systemic disease
    diarrhea in, 231b
    in tuberculosis, 2149
    oral manifestations of, 1035, 1035f
    skin lesions associated with, 1860, 1861f, 1862f, 1863f
Systemic infection
    delirium in, 1649
    in animal bite, 885
    in pregnancy, 2773-2775
Systemic inflammatory response, in burn injury, 917-918
Systemic inflammatory response syndrome (SIRS), 49, 49b, 2211, 2212b
Systemic lupus erythematosus, 1805-1812
    clinical features of, 1806-1808, 1806b
    diagnosis of, 1808
    disposition in, 1811-1812
    epidemiology of, 1805
    immune thrombocytopenia in, 1896-1897
    in pregnancy, 1810, 2775-2776
    management of, 1808-1810
    myocarditis in, 1297
    oral manifestations of, 1035, 1035f
    panniculitis in, 1817
    pathophysiology of, 1806
    pericarditis in, 1284
    skin lesions in, 1862t, 1863f
Systemic mastocytosis, 1835
Systemic vascular resistance, in heart failure, 1262
Systolic dysfunction, in heart failure, 1267

T cells
    development of, 1820, 1820f
    in asthma, 1080, 1080f, 2533
    in cell-mediated immunity, 2833
    monoclonal antibody to, for organ transplant patient, 2850-2851
    types of, 1820, 2833
t test, 3052, 3052t, 3053
T wave, 1203
    hyperacute, in myocardial infarction, 1161, 1162f
    in premature ventricular contractions, 1224-1225

T wave (Continued)
    inverted
        differential diagnosis in, 1164
        in acute coronary syndromes, 1163-1164, 1164f
        in pericarditis, 1282
        in Wellen's syndrome, 1163
    pseudonormalization of, 1164
Tabun, 939, 2461, 3030-3031, 3030b, 3031b
TAC, topical, 846, 2933
Tachycardia
    atrial, 1228-1229, 1228f, 1229f
    in asthma, 1084
    in cardiac tamponade, 473
    in high-altitude pulmonary edema, 2303
    in pericarditis, 2592
    in pulmonary embolism, 1372
    in tension pneumothorax, 462
    in Wolff-Parkinson-White syndrome, 1235, 1237
    junctional, 1233-1235, 1233f, 1234f
    narrow-complex, 1226-1235
        atrial fibrillation as, 1230-1233, 1231f, 1232b, 1232f
        atrial flutter as, 1229-1230, 1230f-1231f
        atrial tachycardia as, 1228-1229, 1228f, 1229f
        in infants and children, 2586-2587, 2588f
        junctional tachycardia as, 1233-1235, 1233f, 1234f
        P wave in, 1234f
        sinus tachycardia as, 1227-1228, 1227f
    pediatric, 109-110, 109t
    pseudotachycardia and, 1226
    sinus, 1227-1228, 1227f
        in hyperthyroidism, 1987
        in myocardial contusion, 468
        in pediatric cardiac arrest, 109-110, 109t
    supraventricular. See Supraventricular tachycardia.
    ventricular, 1240-1243, 1241f-1243f
    wide-complex, 1237-1244
        adenosine-induced, 2588, 2589f
        differential diagnosis in, 1237-1239, 1238t, 1239f, 1240f
        in cocaine overdose, 2390
        in infants and children, 2586, 2587f
        torsades de pointes as, 1243-1244, 1243f, 1244b
        treatment of, 1239-1240
        ventricular tachycardia as, 1240-1243, 1241-1243f
Tachycardia-bradycardia syndrome, 1231
Tachydysrhythmia
    in heatstroke, 2264
    in infants and children, 2585-2590
Tachypnea, 175
    in asthma, 1084
    in high-altitude pulmonary edema, 2303
    in pediatric assessment, 2499
    in pneumonia, 2556
Tacrine, for dementia, 1661
Tacrolimus, 2844
    for organ transplant patient, 2851
    toxicity of, 1417
Tactical emergency medical support, 3000-3005
    equipment in, 3003-3004
    forensic science and, 3004
    goals of, 3001, 3001b
    hazardous materials and, 3004
    history of, 3001
    liability in, 3004-3005
    medical threat assessment in, 3004
    phases in, 3002-3003, 3002b
    preventive medicine in, 3004
    remote patient assessment in, 3004
    tactical team structure, training, and integration in, 3001-3003
    training in, 3002, 3002f, 3003
Taenia saginata, 2102t, 2105
Taenia solium, 2102t, 2105, 2109
Takayasu's arteritis, 1813
Talar dome, osteochondral fracture of, 824-825, 825f
Talar neck fracture, 823, 823f
Talar tilt test, 817
Talocalcaneal joint
    anatomy of, 808, 809f, 820, 820f
    dislocation of, 825-826, 825f
Talocrural joint, 808, 809f

Talonavicular dislocation, 825-826, 825f
Talus
    anatomy of, 808, 809f, 810f
    dislocation of, 820, 826
    fracture of, 822-824, 823f, 824f
Tamarind, drug interactions with, 2478t
Tanapox viruses, 2040
Tangential wounds, to head, 369
Tap water irrigation, for wound cleansing, 848
Tape, wound closure, 853
Tape measurement system, in pediatric
    resuscitation, 114, 114f-115f
Tapeworm infection
    anemia in, 2107
    drug therapy for, 2102t
Tar burns, 926-927, 937
Tarasoff v Regents of California, 2967-2968
Tardieu's spots, in near-hanging and
    strangulation, 451
Tardive dyskinesia, antipsychotic-induced, 1732,
    2445, 2447
Tarsal tunnel syndrome, 836-837
Tarsometatarsal joint
    anatomy of, 820, 820f
    fractures and dislocations of, 551t, 828-831,
        829f, 830f
Taser gun injuries, 2274
Taste alterations, in scombroid fish poisoning,
    1472
Tattooing
    in facial trauma, 390
    in intermediate-range handgun wounds, 956-
        957, 956f
Taxus, 2475, 2475f
Teardrop fracture, 551t
    extension, 410-411
    flexion, 401, 403f
Teardrop sign, in orbital wall fracture, 1044,
    1045f
Tears, artificial, 1063b, 1064
Technetium-99m–labeled bone scan, in
    osteomyelitis, 2180-2181, 2180f, 2181f
Teeth. See Tooth (teeth).
Telemedicine, 3105-3106
Telmisartan, 1322t
Temazepam, 2484, 2484t
    for sleep disturbances in demented patient,
        1662
Temperature
    altered perceptions of, in ciguatera fish
        poisoning, 1473
    body. See Body temperature.
    duration of exposure to, burn injury and, 915-
        916, 916f
    of material, burn injury and, 915, 915t
Temporal arteritis, 1813
    headache in, 174t
    risk factors for, 171b
    visual loss in, 1060
Temporal lobe epilepsy, 148t, 1621
Temporomandibular joint
    anatomy of, 1026, 1027f
    dislocation of, 396, 1041-1042, 1041f
    in scuba diving–related disorders, 2283
    trauma to, 395-396
Temporomandibular myofascial pain dysfunction
    syndrome, 1034-1035
Tendinitis/tendinopathy, 567-568, 1794-1801
    Achilles, 1799-1800
    bicipital, 1797
    calcific, 568, 698, 1797-1798
    common sites for, 1796f
    diagnosis of, 1800-1801
    disposition in, 1801
    history in, 1795
    management of, 1801
    of ankle, 818-820, 819f, 1799-1800
    of elbow, 1798-1799
    of foot, 838
    of hand, 604-609, 605f-607f
    of hip, 761-762
    of knee, 794, 795, 1799
    of shoulder, 1796-1798
    of wrist, 1799
    patellar, 1799
    physical examination in, 1795-1796
    rotator cuff, 1796-1797
Tenecteplase, with enoxaparin, in myocardial
    infarction, 1194-1195

Tenesmus
    in inflammatory bowel disease, 1501
    in intestinal amebiasis, 1480
    in radiation proctocolitis, 1505
Tennis elbow. See Epicondylitis.
Tenosynovitis
    bicipital, 697, 697f
    De Quervain's, 1799
    flexor, 616-617
    in gonococcal arthritis, 1788, 2191
    stenosing, in hand, 618
Tensilon test, in myasthenia gravis, 1705
Tension headache, 1635, 2679
Tension pneumomediastinum, 459
Tension pneumopericardium, 1288
Tension pneumothorax, 339, 462, 462f, 463f,
    464
Tenting, in dehydrated infant, 2629
Teratogen, 2779-2780, 2780b
Terazosin, 1321t
Terbinafine, for tinea capitis, 1839
Terbutaline
    for asthma, 1088, 2539t, 2541
    for premature labor, 2806-2807, 2806b
Teres minor muscle, 672, 673f
Terminal illness
    suicide in, 1770
    trajectory of dying in, 3140, 3140f
Terrorism
    role of informatics in, 3105
    weapons used in, 3021-3032. See also
        Weapons of mass destruction.
Terry Thomas sign, in scapholunate dissociation,
    630
Testicular appendage, torsion of, 1597, 2641
Testing requests and requirements, medicolegal
    issues in, 3158-3160
Testis
    anatomy of, 1594, 1594f
    cancer of, 1597
        in children, 2642
        superior vena cava syndrome in, 1909
    physical examination of, 1573, 1594
    torsion of, 1594-1595, 2639-2640, 2640f
    trauma to, 534-535, 535f
    tumor of, 1597
Tetanospasmin neurotoxin, 2009
Tetanus, 2007-2012, 2008f, 2010b, 2012t, 2013t
    cephalic, 2009, 2010
    neonatal, 2009
    prophylaxis against
        in burn injury, 925-926
        in human bites, 891, 891t
        in wound management, 856-857, 857b, 2012,
            2013t
Tetany, hyperventilation, heat cramps vs., 2258
Tetracaine, 846, 2931, 2931t, 2933
Tetracycline
    during pregnancy and lactation, 2784
    for ehrlichiosis, 2138
    for epididymitis, 1597t, 2639
    for Lyme disease–related myocarditis, 1292
    for periodontal abscess, 1033
    for reactive arthritis, 1790
    for relapsing fever, 2129-2130
    for Rocky Mountain spotted fever, 1850
    for syphilis, 1856
Tetrahydrocannabinol (THC), 2411
Tetralogy of Fallot, 2573, 2574f, 2579-2581,
    2579f, 2580f, 2581b
Text teletype writer (TTY), 2905
Thalassemia, 1872-1873, 1872f
Thallium ingestion, radiogardase for, 3023,
    3023t
Thenar mass or eminence, 576, 577f
Thenar muscles, 580, 581f
Thenar space infection, 617, 618
Theophylline
    during pregnancy and lactation, 2789
    for asthma, 1090, 1090t, 2542, 2543t
    for postdural puncture headache, 1641
    serum, in asthma, 1085
    sudden infant death syndrome and, 2719-2720
Thermal burn, 913-928
    airway management and respiratory care in,
        921-923
    anatomy of skin and, 914-915
    burn shock and, 918
    burn wound assessment in, 919-920, 920f

Thermal burn *(Continued)*
    burn wound care in, 924-927, 925f
    catheterization of patient in, 923
    depth of burn injury in, 918-919, 919f
    disposition in, 927, 927b
    epidemiology of, 913-914, 914f
    fluid resuscitation in, 921, 922-923
    gastrointestinal disorders in, 924
    in child abuse, 969-970, 970f, 970t
    in lightning injury, 2273
    in physical assault, 963, 964f
    metabolic response to therapy in, 919
    ocular, 1046
    pain management in, 924
    patient categorization in, 920
    pediatric considerations in, 923
    physiologic changes in, 917-918
    prehospital care in, 921
    thermodynamics of burn injury in, 915-917,
        915t, 916f, 917t
    transportation of patient in, 923-924
    white phosphorus in, 936
    zones of tissue injury in, 917, 917f
Thermal therapy, for fracture, 573-574
Thermogenesis
    decreased, hypothermia and, 2239-2240, 2240b
    increased, heat illness and, 2257
    nonshivering, in burned infant, 923
    physiology of, 2254-2255
    shivering, 2236, 2247
Thermometry
    in heatstroke, 2263
    pediatric, 2508
Thermoregulation
    hypothalamus in, 134
    impaired, hypothermia and, 2240-2241, 2240b
    mechanisms of, 2255-2256
    physiology of
        in cold exposure, 2228, 2236-2237, 2237f
        in heat exposure, 2254-2256
Thermosensors, 2255
Thiamine
    deficiency of
        in alcoholic hepatitis, 1409
        optic neuropathy from, 1060
    for alcohol intoxication, 2860
    for alcohol withdrawal syndrome, 2861, 2863
    for benzodiazepine overdose, 2326
    for toxic alcohol poisoning, 2402
    for Wernicke-Korsakoff syndrome, 2869
Thiazide diuretics
    during pregnancy and lactation, 2788
    hypercalcemia from, 1945
Thiazolidinediones, 1973
Thienopyridines, in acute coronary syndromes,
    1186-1187
Thigh
    compartments of, 737, 737t, 738f
    pain in, atraumatic, 756b
Thioamides, for thyroid storm, 1989
Thiopental
    as induction agent, 15-16
    for procedural sedation and analgesia, in
        children, 2953
Thioridazine, toxicity of, 2445, 2446t
Thiothixene, 2446t
Third stage of labor, 2804-2805
Third trimester
    complications in, 2805-2810
    fetal ultrasonography in, 2802, 2802b, 2802t
Third-degree atrioventricular block, 1220-1221,
    1221f
Third-degree burn, 919, 919f
Third-nerve palsy
    anisocoria in, 1061
    eye movement disorders in, 1062
Thompson test, in Achilles tendon rupture, 818
Thoracentesis, in pleural effusion, 1151-1152
Thoracic aorta
    aneurysm of
        chronic, 482
        superior vena cava syndrome in, 1909
    injury to, in pelvic fracture, 720
    rupture of, 476-482, 477f-479f, 481b
Thoracic duct, injury to, in neck trauma, 450
Thoracic endometriosis syndrome, 1144
Thoracic examination, in multiple trauma, 309
Thoracic lavage, for rewarming in accidental
    hypothermia, 2250

Thoracic outlet syndrome, 1358-1360, 1358f, 1359f, 1693
Thoracic pump model of chest compression, 77, 98
Thoracic spine
    anatomy of, 400f
    fracture-dislocation of, 410f
    vertebral osteomyelitis in, 2184
    vertical body fracture of, 426
Thoracic trauma, 453-486
    cardiovascular injuries in, 467-482
    chest wall injury in, 454-459
    epidemiology of, 453
    esophageal perforation in, 482-485, 482b, 484b, 485f
    in elderly person, 346
    pulmonary injuries in, 459-466
Thoracic vertebrae, 399, 400f
Thoracoabdominal gunshot wounds, 506
Thoracoabdominal stab wounds, 505
Thoracoscopy, in hemothorax, 465
Thoracostomy
    abdominal trauma after, 492
    in children, 339
    in hemothorax, 465
    in pleural effusion, 1151-1152
    in pneumothorax, 463, 464, 464b, 1147-1148
    in tension pneumothorax, 464
Thoracotomy
    in abdominal trauma, 502
    in cardiac tamponade, 475-476, 476t
    in children, 339
    in hemothorax, 465, 465b
    in multiple trauma, 308
    in myocardial rupture, 471
    in tracheobronchial injury, 466
Thought disorders, 1726-1733
    clinical features of, 1726-1728
    diagnosis of, 1728
    differential considerations in, 1727b, 1728-1729, 1728b, 1729t
    disposition in, 1733
    management of, 1730-1733, 1731b
Threat assessment, in tactical emergency medical support, 3004
Three Mile Island nuclear reactor incident, 2317
3-3-2 rule, in direct laryngoscopy, 4, 5f
Thrill, in arteriovenous fistula, 539
Throat culture, in pharyngitis, 1111, 1112
Thrombasthenia, 1899
Thrombectomy
    for arterial thrombosis, 1354
    for peripheral arteriovascular disease, 1349
Thrombin, in bleeding disorders, 1895
Thrombin-sensitive factors, 1892, 1893f
Thromboangiitis obliterans, 1351-1352
Thrombocytopathy, differential diagnosis in, 1896b, 1898-1899
Thrombocytopenia
    cold-induced, 2244
    differential diagnosis in, 1896-1898, 1896b
    dilutional, 1898
    heparin-induced, 1897
    idiopathic, 1897-1898
    immune, 1896-1897
    in alcoholism, 2874
    in systemic lupus erythematosus, 1808
    nonimmune, 1898
    thrombotic, 1467, 1898
Thrombocytopenic purpura
    autoimmune, 1897-1898
    oral manifestations of, 1036
    thrombotic, 1467, 1898
Thrombocytosis, differential diagnosis in, 1896b, 1899
Thromboembolism
    in nephrotic syndrome, 1531
    in pregnancy, 317, 2756-2757
    in prosthetic valve patient, 1308
    in spinal cord injury, 2906-2907
    pathophysiology of, 1343-1344
Thrombolytic therapy
    during pregnancy and lactation, 2766, 2786
    for acute arterial embolism, 1352-1353
    for acute mesenteric ischemia, 1449
    for cerebral venous thrombosis, 1671
    for pacemaker-induced thrombophlebitis, 1250
    for pulmonary embolism, 1377-1378, 1378t, 1379
    for stroke, 1613t, 1615, 1615b

Thrombophlebitis, pacemaker-induced, 1250
Thrombosis
    arterial, 1344, 1347, 1347t, 1353-1354
        embolism vs., 1347t
    in acute coronary syndromes, 1157
    in infective endocarditis, 1301
    in nephrotic syndrome, 2648
    in peripheral vascular injury, 537-538, 538f, 544
    lateral venous sinus, 1068
    of arteriovenous fistula or graft, 1365
    of hemorrhoids, 1510, 1511-1512, 1511f, 1512f
    of saphenous vein, 1370
    pathophysiology of, 1368
    septic, 1123, 1363
    venous, 1368-1371. See also Pulmonary embolism.
        anatomy in, 1368-1369
        cerebral, 1670-1671
        clinical presentation in, 1369
        complications of, 1370-1371
        diagnosis of, 1369-1370, 1369t
        differential diagnosis in, 1369b
        in pregnancy, 2733, 2756-2757
        in spinal cord injury, 2906-2907
        isolated calf, 1370
        mesenteric, 1446, 1446b
        observation in, 3065-3066
        of upper extremity, 1370
        pretest probability of, 1369, 1369t
        proximal vs. distal, 1369
        septic, 1363
        treatment of, 1370
Thrombotic ischemic stroke, 1607-1608
Thrombotic thrombocytopenic purpura, 1467, 1898
Thrombovasculitis, cerebral, in Rocky Mountain spotted fever, 2134
Thromboxane
    as anaphylaxis mediator, 1823, 1823b
    in frostbite, 2229
    in sepsis, 2213
    inhibitors of, in frostbite, 2232
Thrush, oral, 1840-1841
Thumb
    dislocation of
        carpometacarpal joint, 604
        interphalangeal joint, 564, 565f, 603
    metacarpal fractures of, 599-600, 599f
        extra-articular, 599
        intra-articular, 599-600, 599f
        Rolando's, 600
    motions of, 578f
    radial collateral ligament injuries of, 604
    radiography of, 590-591
    ulnar collateral ligament injuries of, 604
Thumb spica cast, in scaphoid fracture, 628, 628f
"Thumbprint sign," in epiglottitis, 2523, 2524f
Thurston Holland's fragment, 551t, 555
Thymectomy, for myasthenia gravis, 1706-1707
Thyroid disorders, 1985-1994
    hypertension in, 1313
    in pregnancy, 2764t, 2772-2773
Thyroid function tests
    in hyperthyroidism, 1987-1988
    in hypothyroidism, 1992-1993
Thyroid gland
    in mood disorders, 1736
    in pregnancy, 2726
Thyroid hormone
    abnormal levels of. See Hyperthyroidism; Hypothyroidism.
    hypercalcemia from, 1945
    replacement of
        for hypothyroidism, 1993-1994
        in pregnancy, 2773
Thyroid storm, 1985-1986, 1986b, 1987
    management of, 1988-1989, 1989t
    vs. heat stroke, 2263
Thyroiditis, 1986, 2773
Thyroid-stimulating hormone
    in hyperthyroidism, 1988
    in hypothyroidism, 1992-1993
Thyrotoxic crisis, 1985
Thyrotoxicosis, 1985-1989
    clinical features of, 1986-1987, 1987b
    diagnosis of, 1987-1988
    differential considerations in, 1988, 1988t

Thyrotoxicosis (Continued)
    etiology of, 1985-1986, 1986b
    management of, 1988, 1989, 1989t
Thyroxine
    in comatose patient, 163
    in hypothermia, 2246-2247
Tibia
    anatomy of, 797
    fracture of
        epiphyseal, 780-781
        proximal
            extra-articular, 797-799
            intra-articular, 777-781
        shaft, 799-801, 801f
        stress, 803-804
        subcondylar, 797-798
        tibial plateau, 777-779, 777f-778f
        tibial spine, 779-780, 780f
        tibial tubercle, 798-799, 798f
    proximal, anatomy of, 770, 771f
Tibial arteries, 797
    anatomy of, 771, 797
    injury to, 547
Tibial condyles
    anatomy of, 770, 771f
    fracture of, 777-779, 777f-778f
Tibial femoral knee dislocation, 787-790, 789f
Tibial nerve, 771, 797
Tibial plateau fracture, 347, 553, 555f
Tibial tubercle apophysitis, 799
Tibialis anterior tendon rupture, 820
Tibialis posterior tendon rupture, 819-820
Tibiofemoral compartments, 770, 771f
Tibiofemoral joint, 770, 771f
Tibiofibular joint
    anatomy of, 797
    fracture at, 799-801, 801f
    proximal, dislocation of, 802-803
Tibiofibular syndesmotic ligaments, distal, injury to, 816, 817
Tibiotalar joint, fracture at, 813, 813f
Tic douloureux, 1664, 1666
    headache in, 1642
    pain in, 1034
Ticarcillin, for mastoiditis, 1072
Tick-borne illness, 2116-2142
    babesiosis as, 2138-2140, 2139f
    Colorado tick fever as, 2140-2141
    ehrlichiosis as, 2137-2138
    identification of ticks in, 2116-2117, 2119f
    Lyme disease as, 2118-2129. See also Lyme disease.
    physiology of, 2117-2118, 2118f
    prophylaxis against, 2142
    Q fever as, 2137
    relapsing fever as, 2129-2130
    Rocky Mountain spotted fever as, 2132-2137. See also Rocky Mountain spotted fever.
    tick paralysis as, 1708, 2141-2142
    tick removal procedure in, 2142, 2142b
    toxin-induced, 908
    tularemia as, 2130-2132
    types of, 2117t
Ticlopidine
    in acute coronary syndromes, 1186-1187
    thrombocytopenia from, 1898
Tics, 2668
Tile's classification of pelvic fractures, 723, 723b
Tillaux fracture, 551t
Tilt table testing, for syncope, 3067
Timolol, 1321t
    for closed-angle glaucoma, 1056
    for increased intraocular pressure, 292
    overdose of, 2373t
Timolol maleate, for central retinal artery occlusion, 1057
Tinea capitis, 1838-1839
Tinea corporis, 1839-1840, 1839f
Tinea pedis, 1840
Tinea unguium, 1840
Tinea versicolor, 1840, 1840f
Tinel's sign
    in carpal tunnel syndrome, 639, 1697
    in thoracic outlet syndrome, 1359
Tinnitus
    in acoustic neuroma, 1668
    vertigo and, 144
Tiotropium, for chronic obstructive pulmonary disease, 1105

Tirofiban, in myocardial infarction, 1186
Tissue
  conductivity of, burn injury and, 916-917
  injury to
    in bone or joint infections, 2176
    zones of, in burn injury, 917, 917f
  ischemia of, in compartment syndrome, 560-
    561, 560b, 561b, 561f
  radiosensitivity of, 2321, 2321f
  resistance of, 2269b
Tissue adhesives, for wound closure, 853-854
Tissue factor, in hemostasis, 1892, 1893f
Tissue plasminogen activator (t-PA)
  during pregnancy and lactation, 2786
  for ischemic stroke, 1615, 1615b
  in myocardial infarction, 1189
    vs. percutaneous coronary intervention,
      1192-1193
  in pulmonary embolism, 1377-1378, 1378t
  mutant forms of, 1189-1190
TMP-SMX. See Trimethoprim-sulfamethoxazole.
Tobacco
  dermal exposure to, 2474
  ingestion of, 2474
  inhalation of. See Smoking.
Tobramycin, for febrile, neutropenic cancer
    patient, 2838t
Tocainide, 1207
Tocolysis
  for placenta previa, 2809
  for premature labor, 2806-2807, 2806b, 2807b
  for PROM, 2808
Toddlers
  developmental milestones in, 2496t, 2497
  fever in
    management of, 2514-2515, 2515f
    pathophysiology of, 2505
  temperature determination in, 2508
Toddler's fracture, 2698, 2698f
Todd's paralysis, 1625
Toe
  decompression of, in burn injury, 925
  fracture of, 834
  interphalangeal dislocation of, 835-836
  metatarsophalangeal dislocation of, 835
  pain in, 837
Toenail, ingrown, 837
Togavirus, 2047-2049
Toilet bowl cleaner, ingestion of, 2381t
Tokaimura, Japan, radiation incident in, 2317
Toluene abuse, 2886-2889
Toluidine blue dye staining technique, in genital
    trauma, 988-989, 988f
Tomography
  computed. See Computed tomography.
  positron emission
    in minor head trauma, 365
    in osteomyelitis, 2181
Tongue
  adult vs. child, 2519, 2520f
  laceration of, 391, 1040
Tonic seizure, 1621
Tonka bean, adverse effects of, 2476t
Tonography, in shock, 50-51
Tonometry, ocular, in red and painful eye, 286-
  287
Tonsillar herniation, 1918
Tonsillectomy, for peritonsillar abscess, 1118
Tonsillitis
  lingual, 1114, 1114f
  recurrent or chronic, treatment of, 1113
Tonsillopharyngitis. See Pharyngitis.
Tooth (teeth), 384. See also Dental entries.
  anatomy of, 1026, 1027f-1029f
  aspiration of, 395, 866
  avulsed, 389-390, 395, 1037-1040, 1038f,
    1039f
  cracked, 1033-1034
  extraction of
    hemorrhage after, 1042
    pain after, 1034
  fracture of, 1036-1037, 1036f
  radiography of, 1030, 1030f
  reimplantation of, 395
  subluxated, 1037-1040, 1038f, 1039f
Tooth sign, in quadriceps rupture, 783
Topical anesthesia, 2933-2934
  allergy to, 846-847
  in wound care, 846

Topiramate
  for seizure, 2675t
  side effects of, 1628t
Torsades de pointes, 1243-1244, 1243f, 1244b
  antipsychotic-induced, 2447, 2449
  in infants and children, 2589-2590
Torsemide, 1321t
Torso examination, in genitourinary trauma, 515
Torus fracture, 554, 556f, 637, 637f, 2690, 2690f
Tossy and Allman classification of
    acromioclavicular joint dislocations, 685-
    686, 686f
Total body surface area assessment, in burn
    injury, 919-920, 920f
Toulene
  abuse of, 2429
  inhalation of, metabolic acidosis from, 1928
Tourniquet injury, of penis, 2638
Toxic alcohol poisoning, 2395-2404
  ethylene glycol in, 2398-2402, 2401t
  isopropyl alcohol in, 2402-2404
  methanol in, 2395-2398
Toxic appearance, as indication for lumbar
    puncture, 2659
Toxic conjunctivitis, 297t
Toxic disaster preparedness, 3017
Toxic encephalopathy, in cancer patient, 1920-
  1921
Toxic epidermal necrolysis
  drug-induced, 1846t
  skin lesions in, 1845-1846, 1846f
Toxic goiter
  diffuse, 1985-1986, 1987
  in pregnancy, 2764t, 2772-2773
  multinodular, 1986
  uninodular, 1986
Toxic megacolon, 1501, 1502f, 2613, 2616
Toxic optic neuropathy, 1060
Toxic shock syndrome, 2027-2031, 2028b, 2029b,
    2029t, 2199-2201, 2200b, 2201b
  pediatric fever in, 2511, 2511b
  skin lesions in, 1846-1847
  streptococcal, 2028, 2028b, 2029, 2029t, 2200-
    2201, 2201b
Toxic syndromes, 1651, 2327-2328, 2327t, 2964t
Toxicologic screen, 2328-2330, 2328b
  drugs, chemicals, and groups not detected by,
    2328b
  for cocaine, 2388
  in abdominal trauma, 495
  in anticholinergic poisoning, 2349
  in comatose patient, 162
  in delirium, 1651
  in hypothermia, 2244
  in substance abuse, 2885-2886
Toxicology. See Poisoning/overdose.
Toxicology laboratory, 2328-2330, 2328b
Toxin(s)
  aplastic anemia from, 1875, 1875t
  botulinum, 2013, 2014
  chronic renal failure from, 1544
  cyanosis from, 269t
  delirium from, 1648
  diarrhea from, 231b
  in bacterial gastroenteritis, 1469-1475, 1480t
  in diphtheria, 2002
  in pertussis, 2005
  in snake venoms, 897-898, 897t
  in toxic shock syndrome, 2029
  inhaled, 2432-2441, 2443t
    carbon monoxide in, 2438-2441
    cyanide and hydrogen sulfide in, 2436-2438,
      2437f
    pulmonary irritants in, 2433t, 2434-2435,
      2434f
    simple asphyxiants in, 2432-2433
    smoke in, 2435-2436
  neuropathy from, 1691b, 1692
  pediatric fever from, 2510-2511
  rhabdomyolysis from, 1979
  seizure from, 1623
  tetanospasmin, 2009
  uremic, 1541
Toxocariasis, 2103t, 2109, 2110
Toxoplasma gondii infection
  in cancer patient with impaired cell-mediated
    immunity, 2840
  in HIV/AIDS, 2081-2082, 2082f

Toxoplasma gondii infection (Continued)
  in organ transplant patient, 2848-2849
  myocarditis in, 1292
  visual disturbances in, 2110
Tracheal disease
  subglottic, 2525-2527
  upper airway obstruction in, 2527-2529, 2529t
Tracheal foreign body, 867, 868f
Tracheal stenosis, 2527
Tracheal tuberculosis, 2151
Tracheitis
  bacterial, 2528-2529, 2529t
  in children, screening for, 2509b
Tracheobronchial injury, 466, 466f
Tracheomalacia, 2527
Tracheostomy
  in neck trauma, 445
  in physically disabled patient, 2907
Tracking systems, computerized, 3101
Traction, in femoral and hip fractures, 746, 748
Traction retinal detachment, 1058
Traction-countertraction reduction method
  for anterior glenohumeral joint dislocation,
    689, 689f
  for hip fracture, 759
  for inferior glenohumeral joint dislocation,
    693, 694f
  for tibial femoral knee dislocation, 789
Tramadol, 1692, 2925
Trandolapril, 1322t
Tranquilization. See also Sedation.
  rapid, 2914b
    for mood disorders, 1741
    for thought disorders, 1730-1731, 1731b
    of combative patient, 2961-2963
Transabdominal ultrasonography, in pregnancy,
    2730, 2730f
Transcondylar fracture, 659, 659f
Transcutaneous blood gas monitoring, 36
Transcutaneous electrical nerve stimulation, 2934
Transection, in peripheral vascular injury, 537
Transesophageal echocardiography
  in aortic dissection, 1327, 1327t
  in aortic rupture, 480, 480f
  in multiple trauma, 313
Transfer. See Patient transfer.
Transferrin, in iron overdose, 2419
Transfusional hemosiderosis, 61
Transfusional therapy, 56-61
  adjuncts in, 58
  clinical features in, 58
  decision making in, 58-59
  hepatitis C infection risk in, 1403
  hypocalcemia after, 1943
  in autoimmune hemolytic anemia, 1883
  in gastrointestinal bleeding, 222
  in hemolytic uremic syndrome, 2655
  in kernicterus prophylaxis, 2603, 2604f
  in multiple trauma, 307-308
  in pelvic fracture, 723, 728, 731
  in peripheral vascular injury, 543
  in placenta previa or abruptio placentae, 2748
  in sickle cell disease, 1880
  in thalassemia, 1872-1873
  massive, 57-58
  outcomes in, 59-61
  pathophysiologic principles in, 57-58, 58t
  refusal of, 3171-3172
  therapeutic modalities in, 59
  thrombocytopenia after, 1897
  viral infection transmission and, 57t, 61
Transfusion-associated graft-versus-host-disease,
    60
Transient ischemic attack (TIA)
  antihypertensive drug therapy for, 1614, 1614t
  anxiety in, 1747
  disposition in, 1617
  epidemiology of, 1607, 1607t, 1608
  previous, fibrinolytic therapy eligibility and,
    1191
Transitional circulation, 118-119, 119t, 2568
Transitions in patient care, as problem area in
    emergency care, 3124
Transplantation, 2846-2856, 3151
  bone marrow
    for aplastic anemia, 1875-1876
    for sickle cell disease, 1881
  complications in, 2847-2851, 2850t, 2851f
  disposition of, 2856

Transplantation (Continued)
  drug toxicity in, 2849-2851, 2850t, 2851f
  heart, 2851-2854, 2852f, 2853f
  immune defects in, 2846-2847
  immunosuppressive therapy for, 2849-2851, 2850t
  infectious complications in, 2847-2849, 2847b
  kidney, 2855
  liver, 2854-2855, 2854f
  lung, 2855-2856
  pancreas, 2856
  rejection in, 2848-2849, 2849f
Transport
  by air, 2994-2999
    administrative structure in, 2995
    aviation physiology and, 2994-2995, 2995t
    clinical concepts and patient care in, 2998-2999
    criteria for, 2998b
    efficacy and cost effectiveness of, 2999
    flight crew in, 2996
    future of, 2999
    medical direction in, 2996
    safety issues in, 2997, 2997b, 2997f, 2998b
    types of missions in, 2995
  interfacility and specialized, 2991-2992, 2991b, 2992b
Transtentorial herniation, after head trauma, 355-356, 355f
Transthoracic echocardiography, in aortic dissection, 1327
Transtracheal jet ventilation, needle cricothyrotomy with, 22, 22f
Transvaginal ultrasonography, in pregnancy, 2730, 2731f
Transverse fracture, 2690, 2691f
Transverse myelitis, 265t, 1682
Transverse spinal cord syndromes, 417, 1677, 1678f
Trapezium
  anatomy of, 622, 623f
  fracture of, 630
Trapezoid
  anatomy of, 622, 623f
  fracture of, 630
Trapezoid ligament, 670-671, 671f
Trauma. See also specific anatomic locations.
  abdominal, 489-512
  air medical transport in, 2998
  alcohol consumption and, 2878
  ankle, 808-820
  birth, postpartum hemorrhage from, 2818
  blunt. See Blunt trauma.
  cardiac, 467-482
  chest wall, 454-459
  dental, 1036-1042
  elbow and humerus, 647-668
  esophageal, 446-447
  facial, 382-396
  femur, 735-768
  foot, 820-839
  forearm, 639-644
  from animal bites, 882-892
  from chemical injuries, 929-939
  from electrical and lightning injuries, 2267-2277
  from motor vehicle crashes. See Motor vehicle crashes; Pedestrian collisions.
  from thermal burns, 913-928
  from venomous animal bites and stings, 894-911
  genitourinary, 514-535
  hand, 592-618
  head, 349-379
  hip, 735-768
  hypothermia and, 2241
  in elderly person, 344-348, 2829
    background of, 344
    clinical features of, 347
    diagnostic strategies in, 347
    disposition in, 348
    epidemiology of, 344-345
    management of, 348
    pathophysiology of, 345
    specific disorders and injuries related to, 345-347
  in pregnancy, 318-326, 2733
    blunt, 318
    diagnostic strategies in, 320-321, 320t, 321t

Trauma (Continued)
    disposition in, 326
    fetal evaluation in, 323-324, 323f, 323t, 324f
    fetal injury in, 319
    fetomaternal hemorrhage and, 321
    management of, 321-326, 322f
    maternal resuscitation in, 322-323
    penetrating, 318-319
    perimortem cesarean section in, 325-326
    placental injury in, 319-320
    prehospital end-of-life issues related to, 3145
    primary survey in, 322-323
    secondary survey in, 323
    uterine injury in, 320
  injury prevention and control in, 940-950. See also Injury prevention and control.
  knee, 770-796
  lower leg, 796-805
  multiple, 300-314
    clinical features in, 309-311, 310f
    diagnostic strategies in, 311-313, 313f
    disposition in, 311
    epidemiology of, 300
    etiology of, 302, 303t
    examination and reassessment in, 305
    in elderly person, 345
    management of, 302-309, 304b
    monitoring in, 305
    prehospital care in, 302-304
    radiologic imaging in, 311-313, 313f
    stabilization in, 305-309
    team approach in, 304
    trauma system and, 300-302, 301f, 302b
  neck, 441-451
  observation in, 3067-3069
  ocular, 1044-1052
  pediatric, 328-342
    abdominal, 340-342
      blunt, 492, 510
      epidemiology of, 489-490
      history in, 493
    cardiothoracic, 338-340
    cervical spine, 336-338, 337f
    child abuse and, 349, 367, 383, 490
    clinical features of, 329-330
    disposition in, 342
    epidemiology of, 328
    facial, 382, 383
    general management principles in, 331-333, 332b, 332t, 333t
    head, 333-336, 334b, 335b, 366-368, 369b
    hip, 763-767, 763f, 765f-767f
    primary survey in, 329-330, 329f, 331t-333t
    renal, 528
    secondary survey in, 330, 330b, 333, 333b, 2501, 2501b, 2502b
    surgical indications in, 332b
  pelvic, 717-734
  penetrating. See Penetrating trauma.
  peripheral vascular, 536-547
  prehospital care in, 2991
  pressure-induced. See Barotrauma.
  pulmonary, 459-466. See also Pulmonary trauma.
  recent, fibrinolytic therapy eligibility and, 1191-1192
  renal, 526-530, 527f, 529f-530f
  rhabdomyolysis in, 1978
  scoring systems for, 300, 301f, 302b
  shoulder, 670-699
  single vs. multisystem, 502, 509
  soft tissue, 566-568. See also Soft tissue injuries.
  spinal, 398-439, 2905-2909
  testicular, 534-535, 535f
  thoracic, 453-486
  urinary tract, 514-535
  vascular. See Vascular injury.
  wound management in, 842-857. See also Wound management.
  wrist, 622-639
Trauma captain, 304
Trauma care system, 948
Trauma series, in child abuse, 973
Trauma system, 300-302, 301f, 302b
Traumatic aneurysm, 1357
Traumatic anxiety, 1746b
Traumatic asphyxia, in chest wall trauma, 459
Traumatic axonal injury, in child abuse, 971

Traumatic brain injury, 349-350. See also Head trauma.
  basilar skull fracture and, 357, 358b
  disseminated intravascular coagulation after, 371
  in children, 366-367
  indirect, 352
  primary, 352
  secondary, 352-353, 353f
  subarachnoid hemorrhage in, 377
Travel restrictions, during pregnancy, 2736
Traveler's diarrhea, 1484-1487, 1486t, 1487b
Trazadone, overdose of, 2361-2362
Treatment
  consent for. See Consent.
  in clinical trials, 3050
  minor category of, medicolegal issues in, 3159
  withholding and withdrawing, bioethical dilemmas in, 3132
Treatment effect, 3051, 3051t
Trematode infections
  drug therapy for, 2098t
  parasites in, 2099t
Trematodicides, 2098t
Tremor
  alcoholic, 2870
  in multiple sclerosis, 1673
  perioral, antipsychotic-induced, 2447
Trench foot, 2228, 2230-2231
Trench mouth, 1033
Treponemal tests, for syphilis, 1562
Triage
  bioethical dilemmas in, 3136
  disaster, 3012-3014, 3013f
    catastrophic casualty, 3013-3014
    routine multiple-casualty, 3012-3013, 3013f
    special categories in, 3014
  failures in emergency care and, 3124
  in electrical and lightning injuries, 2275
  in multiple trauma, 303-304
  in pediatric assessment, 2500, 2500t
  in radiation exposure, 2324, 3023
  marker of death in, 2251
  of private patient, 3157
  scoring systems for, 300, 301f, 302b
Triamcinolone, for asthma, 1089
Triamterene, 1321t
Triangular fibrocartilage complex, 640
Triazolam, 2484, 2484t
Tribec virus, 2047
Trichinella spiralis, 2106
Trichinosis, 1291, 2103t
Trichloroacetic acid, for condylomata acuminata, 1564
Trichlorophenoxyacetic acid, 2465b
Trichobezoar, 873
Trichomoniasis, 1557t, 1567-1568, 1567t, 2103t, 2758
Trichuriasis, 2107
Tricuspid stenosis and regurgitation, 1307
Tricyclic antidepressants
  anticholinergic toxicity of, 2346b
  antidotes to, 2329t
  for anxiety disorders, 1751, 1751t
  for neuropathic pain, 1692
  metabolism of, 2352
  overdose of, 2352-2357, 2353b, 2353f, 2354b, 2355f, 2357t
Trifluoperazine, 2446t
Trifluridine, 2038
Trigeminal nerve, 383-384, 1665t
Trigeminal neuralgia, 1664, 1666
  headache in, 1642
  pain in, 1034
Trigeminovascular theory of headache, 2676
Trigeminy, 1222
Trigger finger, 585, 618
Trihexyphenidyl
  anticholinergic toxicity of, 2345
  for spasticity in cerebral palsy, 2904
Trimalleolar fractures, 813
Trimethadione, during pregnancy and lactation, 2787
Trimethoprim
  for epididymitis, 2639
  for Pneumocystis pneumonia in HIV/AIDS, 2077
Trimethoprim-sulfamethoxazole
  for Aeromonas hydrophila gastroenteritis, 1461t, 1468

Trimethoprim-sulfamethoxazole (Continued)
  for AIDS-related diarrhea, 1484
  for *Cyclospora cayetanensis* gastroenteritis, 1479
  for epididymitis, 1597t
  for *Escherichia coli* food poisoning, 1474
  for granuloma inguinale, 1559t, 1563
  for isosporiasis, 1478
  for otitis media, 1069
  for pertussis, 2006
  for *Plesiomonas shigelloides* gastroenteritis, 1468
  for *Pneumocystis* pneumonia in HIV/AIDS, 2077
  for pneumonia, 2558t
    in HIV-infected patient, 1138-1139
  for prostatitis, 1586
  for *Toxoplasma gondii* infection, 2082
  for urinary tract infection, 1581t, 1582, 1583
  for *Vibrio* fish poisoning, 1472
  hyperkalemia from, 1940
  in HIV/AIDS, side effects of, 2078, 2079t
  prophylactic, in cat bites, 888
Tri-Mix diving, 2280
Tripod fracture, midface, 393, 394f
Tripod position
  in epiglottitis, 2523
  in pediatric assessment, 2498, 2498f
Triptans, for migraine, 1633t, 1634
Triquetral fracture, 629
Triquetrum
  anatomy of, 622, 623f, 625
  dislocation of, 630
Triradiate cartilage, 729
Trismus
  in dental infection, 1032
  in peritonsillitis, 1117
  in temporomandibular joint dislocation, 1041
  in tetanus, 2009
Trisomy 21, 2900t, 2901
Trochanteric bursal calcification, 742, 744f
Trochanteric bursitis, 1803
Trochlea
  anatomy of, 647, 647f
  fracture of, 662
Trochlear nerve, 1665t
Troponin(s), cardiac-specific, in myocardial infarction, 1175-1177, 1175f, 1176t
Troponin-I
  cardiac specificity of, 1177
  in chest pain, 188
  in myocardial contusion, 469
  in pulmonary embolism, predictive value of, 1377, 1378t
Troponin-T
  in chest pain, 188
  in myocardial contusion, 469
  in renal failure, 1177
  mutation of, in hypertrophic cardiomyopathy, 1294-1295
Trousseau's sign, in hypocalcemia, 1943
Truncal mononeuropathy, diabetic, 1971
Trust, failure of, and racial/ethnic disparities in health outcomes, 3110
Truth-telling, as value, 3129
Trypanosomiasis
  African, neurologic disorders in, 2106
  American, 2103t
    fever in, 2105
    myocarditis in, 1291, 2111-2112
  myocarditis in, 1291
Tryptamines, 2406-2408, 2407f
Tryptase, in anaphylaxis, 2548
Tube thoracostomy
  abdominal trauma after, 492
  in children, 339
  in hemothorax, 465
  in pleural effusion, 1151-1152
  in pneumothorax, 463, 464, 464b, 1147-1148
Tuberculin skin test, 2156-2157, 2157b, 2158t
Tuberculoma, 2152, 2161, 2161f
Tuberculosis, 2145-2171
  chest radiography in, 2152-2154, 2152f-2153f, 2159, 2159f
  clinical features of, 2148-2150, 2149t
  complications of, 2150-2151, 2150f
  diagnosis of, 2151-2157, 2152f-2154f
  differential considerations in, 2157
  disposition in, 2169

Tuberculosis (Continued)
  drug-resistant, 2166-2167, 2167b, 2167t
  epidemiology of, 2146
  etiology of, 2147
  extrapulmonary, 2158-2162, 2160f, 2161f, 2167-2168
  history in, 2145-2146
  in alcoholism, 2870
  in bone or joint infections, 2178
  in chronic obstructive pulmonary disease, 1103
  in HIV/AIDS, 1136, 1140-1141, 2078-2079, 2149, 2153-2154, 2166
  in pregnancy, 2764t, 2773-2774
  isolation precautions for, 2147, 2169-2170
  laboratory tests in, 2151-2152
  latent
    testing for, 2158t
    treatment of, 2168-2169, 2168t
  management of, 2162-2169. *See also* Antituberculous agents.
  meningitis in, 2160-2161
    complications of, 1715
    in HIV/AIDS, 2082
    management of, 1722, 2161
    signs and symptoms of, 1714
    spinal, 2161
  microbiology in, 2154-2157, 2154f, 2157b, 2158t
  miliary, 2152, 2159-2160, 2160f
  occupational exposure protocol for, 2170-2171, 2170b
  oral manifestations of, 1035
  pathogenesis of, 2147-2148
  patient history in, 2149, 2149t
  pericarditis in, 1287
  pharyngitis in, 1111, 1112, 1113
  physical examination in, 2150
  postprimary, 2148-2149, 2152-2154, 2153f
  primary, 2152, 2152f
  pulmonary, 2149-2157, 2149t
  renal, urolithiasis vs., 1590-1591
  risk factors for, 2149-2150, 2149b, 2150b
  spinal, 261, 265t, 2159, 2178, 2182, 2182f, 2184-2185
  surgical management of, 2168
  transmission of, 2147
    in emergency department, prevention of, 2169-2171, 2170b
Tuberculostearic acid test, in tuberculosis, 2155
Tuberosity fracture
  in glenohumeral joint dislocation, 698
  ischial, 724, 724f
  navicular, 828
Tubular necrosis, acute, 1534b, 1535-1537, 1536b
  in rhabdomyolysis, 1977, 1977f
  urinary findings in, 1527t
Tubular proteinuria, 1531
Tuft fracture, of distal phalanx, 593-594, 593f
Tularemia, 1131, 2130-2132
Tumor
  atheroembolism from, 1344
  bone, osteomyelitis vs., 2186
  brain
    ataxia in, 2681
    cerebral herniation in, 1918
    headache in, 1637-1638, 2678
    in pregnancy, 2732
  central nervous system, seizure in, 1624
  facial nerve, paralysis from, 1667
  femur or hip, 742, 745f
  malignant. *See* Cancer.
  orbital, red and painful eye in, 294t
  ovarian, 251t
  pancreatic, 1437
  pericardial, 1283-1284
  pregnancy, 1035
  renal, in children, 2646
  spinal cord, 1685
  testicular, 1597
  vertebral body, spinal cord compression in, 1919
Tumor lysis syndrome, acute, 1911-1912, 1911b, 1912b
Tumor necrosis factor, in sepsis, 2213
Tunica adventitia, 1342
Tunica albuginea, 532, 532f
Tunica intima, 1342
Tunica media, 1342
Turf toe, 837

Turner's syndrome, 2901t
Turtle sign, in shoulder dystocia, 2814
Twin gestations
  incidence of, 2722
  labor and delivery in, 2816
Two-dimensional echocardiography, in acute coronary syndromes, 1179
Two-point discrimination test
  for hand, 587
  in nerve injuries, 559
Tympanic membrane
  in otitis media, 1067
  perforation of, in otitis media, 1067
  rupture of, in middle ear barotrauma, 2282
Tympanic membrane thermometer, 2508
Tympanocentesis, in otitis media, 1068
Tympanostomy tubes, for otitis media with effusion, 1070
Type I error
  definition of, 3051t, 3052
  risk of, multiple comparisons and, 3053-3054
Type II error, 3051t, 3052
Typhoidal tularemia, 2131
Tyramine, hypertension and, 1313, 1314b

Uhthoff's phenomenon, in multiple sclerosis, 1672
Ulcer
  atherosclerotic aortic, 1325
  corneal, 289, 289f, 294t, 1052, 1052f, 1054
  decubitus
    in developmentally disabled patient, 2903
    in physically disabled patient, 2907
    in spinal injuries, 438
  foot, in diabetes mellitus, 1351, 1971
  genital, 1557-1564
    in Bartholin cyst and abscess, 1559-1560
    in chancroid, 1557t, 1559t, 1562-1563, 1562f
    in condylomata acuminata, 1559t, 1563-1564, 1564
    in granuloma inguinale, 1559t, 1563
    in herpes simplex virus infection, 1557-1559, 1557t, 1558f, 1559t, 1858
    in lymphogranuloma venereum, 1557t, 1559t, 1562
    in syphilis, 1557t, 1559-1562, 1559t, 1560f, 1561f
  oral, 1036
    in Behçet's disease, 1814
    in HIV/AIDS, 2083
  peptic, 1391-1394, 1391b, 1394b
  stress, in burn-injured patient, 924
  vascular, in diabetes mellitus, 1863f
Ulcerative colitis, 1500-1503, 1502b, 1502f, 1503b
  in children, 2615-2616
  skin lesions in, 1862t
Ulcerative gingivitis, acute necrotic, 1033, 1033f
Ulceroglandular tularemia, 2131
Ulna, 639
Ulnar artery
  anatomy of, 540f, 585-586, 587f, 588f, 622, 625f
  aneurysm of, 1355
  injury to, 546
Ulnar bursa, flexor tendons and, 585, 586f
Ulnar collateral ligament
  anatomy of, 647, 648f
  injury to, 604
Ulnar deviation, of hand, 577f
Ulnar injuries
  fracture in
    Monteggia's, 642, 642f
    pediatric, 644, 644f
    shaft, 641-642
    styloid, 643
  plastic deformation in, 644, 645f
  radioulnar joint disruption in, 636-637
Ulnar nerve
  in elbow, 648-649, 648f
  in hand, 586, 588f, 589f
  in wrist, 622, 625f
  mononeuropathy of, 1695-1696, 1695f, 1696f
  palsy of, 586, 588f
Ulnar slant, of distal radius, 625, 626f
Ulnar styloid, 625
Ulnar surface, of hand, 576, 577f

Ulnar tunnel, 586
Ultrafiltration, for chronic heart failure, 1277
Ultrasonography
  B-mode, 542
  color flow Doppler, 542, 774
  Doppler, 542
    in peripheral arteriovascular disease, 1346, 1348
    in peripheral vascular injury, 541
    in testicular torsion, 1595, 2640
    in testicular trauma, 534, 535f
  duplex, 449, 542
  fetal, in third trimester, 2802, 2802b, 2802t
  in abdominal aortic aneurysm, 1334-1335, 1335f
  in abdominal pain, 216, 216t
  in abdominal trauma, 498-499, 498f
  in acute pancreatitis, 1432-1433
  in acute renal failure, 1538
  in aortic rupture, 480
  in appendicitis, 1454, 1456
  in arthritis, 1780
  in cardiac tamponade, 473-474, 474f
  in cervical vascular injury, 449
  in cholangitis, 1422f
  in cholecystitis, 1419f, 1420
  in cholelithiasis, 1419, 1419f
  in chronic pancreatitis, 1436
  in deep venous thrombosis, 1369
  in diverticular disease, 1494
  in ectopic pregnancy, 2745
  in gastrointestinal foreign body, 874
  in hematuria, 1530
  in jaundice, 244
  in knee trauma, 774
  in multiple trauma, 312-313, 313f
  in ocular foreign body, 860
  in pelvic pain, 250
  in peripheral arteriovascular disease, 1348
  in peripheral vascular injury, 542
  in placenta previa, 2748
  in pneumothorax, 463
  in pregnancy, 2730, 2730f, 2731f
  in pregnant trauma patient, 320
  in renal disorders, 1528
  in renal tumor, 2646
  in septic arthritis, 2188, 2189f, 2190
  in soft tissue foreign body, 878-879
  in tendinopathy, 1801
  in urinary tract infection, 1578
  in urolithiasis, 1589, 1590f, 1591f
  in vaginal bleeding, 256-257, 256t
Ultraviolet keratitis, 1046-1047
Umbilical cord
  clamping and cutting of, 2804
  entanglement of, 2817-2818
  prolapse of, 2817, 2817t
Umbilical cord soufflé, 2728
Umbilical vein cannulation, in neonatal resuscitation, 123
Umbrella tree, 2472
Uncal herniation, 355, 1918
Unconscious sedation, 2914b
Undermining, for reducing wound tension, 849
Undressing, paradoxical, in hypothermia, 2241
Union, in fracture healing, 564
United States, changing demographics in, 3108, 3108t
Univariate models, 3055
Universal donor blood, 57, 58
Universal precautions, noncompliance with, 3081-3082
Universalizability Test, in ethical case analysis, 3132
Unna's boot, for ankle immobilization, 571
Unstable angina
  definition of, 1156
  in differential diagnosis of chest pain, 190t-191t
  management of
    antiplatelet therapy in, 1185-1187
    beta blockers in, 1184-1185
    heparins in, 1187-1188
    morphine in, 1184
  missed diagnosis of, 1160
  ST segment depression in, 1163f
Upper airway obstruction, pediatric, 2519-2530
  evaluation of, 2521, 2521f
  in congenital lesions, 2522, 2524-2525, 2524f, 2527-2528, 2528f

Upper airway obstruction, pediatric (Continued)
  in croup, 2525-2527, 2526f, 2527b
  in epiglottitis, 2523-2524, 2524f
  in foreign body aspiration, 2529-2530
  in laryngeal disease, 2524-2525, 2524f
  in retropharyngeal abscess, 2522-2523, 2523f
  in subglottic tracheal disease, 2525-2527
  in supraglottic disease, 2522-2524
  in tracheal disease, 2527-2529, 2529t
  pathophysiology of, 2519, 2520f
  stridor in, 2519-2520, 2521t
Upper extremity
  aneurysm of, 1354-1355
  deep venous thrombosis of, 1370
  distal, neurologic examination of, 2694t
  escharotomy of, 924-925, 925f
  fracture of, in elderly person, 346
  immobilization of, 569, 569f
  isolated mononeuropathy of, 1693-1697, 1694b
  vascular injury of, 544-546
Upper gastrointestinal bleeding, 220-227
  diagnostic approach to, 220-223, 221b
  differential diagnosis in, 220, 221b, 223
  disposition in, 225-227, 225b, 226t
  management of, 223-225, 223f
  observation in, 3066
Upper respiratory tract infection, 1109-1126
  in adult epiglottitis, 1114-1116, 1115f, 1116f
  in deep space infections of head and neck, 1116-1117, 1116f
  in laryngitis, 1114
  in lingual tonsillitis, 1114, 1114f
  in Ludwig's angina, 1118-1119
  in parapharyngeal abscess, 1121-1123, 1122f
  in peritonsillitis, 1117-1118, 1118f
  in pharyngitis, 1109-1114, 1110f
  in retropharyngeal abscess, 1120-1121, 1120f, 1121f
  in sinusitis, 1123-1126, 1124f, 1125f
  pediatric screening for, 2509b
Upper sulcus, examination of, in red and painful eye, 286
Upper urinary tract trauma
  renal injuries in, 526-530, 527f, 529f-530f
  ureteral injuries in, 530-531, 531f-532f
Upward transtentorial herniation, after head trauma, 356
Uranium, radon exposure from, 2317-2318, 2318f
Urate oxidase, for hyperuricemia, 1914
Urban search and rescue, 3005-3008, 3006b, 3008f, 3019
  crush injury and crush syndrome in, 3007-3008
  medical team operations in, 3006, 3006b
  specific disorders in, 3006-3008, 3008f
  team structure and components in, 3005-3006
Uremia. See also Azotemia.
  clinical manifestations of, 1541-1543, 1542f
  metabolic acidosis in, 1928
  pericarditis in, 1282
Uremic frost, 1542, 1542f
Ureter
  anatomy of, 527, 527f
  obstruction of, in urolithiasis, 1587, 1588f
  trauma to, 530-531, 531f-532f
Ureteral stones, 1586-1593, 1586b, 1589f-1592f, 1593b. See also Urolithiasis.
  abdominal pain in, 210t
  pelvic pain in, 252t
Urethra
  obstruction of, 1538
  prolapse of, 975
  trauma to, 515-519, 516f-520f, 719
Urethral catheterization
  for urinary retention, 1599
  in children, 2643
Urethritis, 1573
  gonococcal, 1565, 1565f
  in urinary tract infection, 1575, 1579-1580, 1579t
  nongonococcal, 1565
Urethrogram, retrograde, in urethral trauma, 517-519, 518f-520f
Urgent care centers, screening requirements related to, 3158
Uric acid crystals, in gouty arthritis, 1785
Uric acid kidney stones, 1587
Uric acid therapy, for gouty arthritis, 1786

Urinalysis, 1525-1527, 1526f, 1527t
  in abdominal pain, 215, 216t
  in acute renal failure, 2649
  in appendicitis, 1454
  in bacterial meningitis, 2662
  in comatose patient, 162
  in diarrhea, 233
  in epididymitis, 2639
  in fever, 137
  in hematuria, 1530, 1602-1603, 2644
  in pediatric urinary tract infections, 2643, 2643t
  in proteinuria, 1532
  in renal stones, 2645
  in rhabdomyolysis, 1980
  in urinary tract infection, 1575-1576
  in urolithiasis, 1588
Urinary alkalinization. See Sodium bicarbonate.
Urinary catheterization
  in children, 2643
  in genitourinary trauma, 515, 517, 518f
  in hypothermia, 2244-2245
  in urinary retention, 1599-1600
Urinary disorders, 1524-1604. See also specific disorders, e.g., Renal failure.
Urinary fluorescence, in ethylene glycol poisoning, 2400
Urinary outlet obstruction
  acute renal failure in, 1533-1534, 1533b, 1538
  in phimosis, 2636
Urinary retention, 1598-1601, 1598b, 1599b, 1600f
  clinical features of, 1599, 1599b
  drug-induced, 1599, 1599b
  in cauda equina syndrome, 706
  in spinal cord injury, 2908-2909
  management of, 1599-1601, 1600f
Urinary sediment, microscopic examination of, 1525-1527, 1526f
Urinary tract. See also Genitourinary entries.
  foreign body in, 877-878
  in pregnancy, 2725-2726
Urinary tract infection, 1573-1586
  bacteriology in, 1574-1575
  complicated, 1573
  definition of, 1573
  diagnosis of, 1575-1578, 1577b
  differential considerations in, 1579-1581, 1579t, 1580f
  epidemiology of, 1573-1574
  in chronic renal failure, 1547
  in diabetes mellitus, 1578
  in elderly person, 2828
  in men, 1573, 1574, 1585-1586
  in patient with indwelling catheters, 1578-1579
  in pregnancy, 1578, 2757-2758
  in sickle cell disease, 1578
  in spinal cord injury, 2909
  in women, 1573, 1574
  lower, 1576, 1581-1582, 1581t
  pathophysiology of, 1574
  pediatric, 1573, 1583-1585, 2510, 2642-2644, 2643b, 2643t
    clinical features of, 1583, 1583t
    diagnosis of, 1583-1584, 1584f
    treatment of, 1584-1585
  pelvic pain in, 251t
  signs and symptoms of, 1575
  terminology related to, 1573
  uncomplicated, 1573
  upper, 1581t, 1582-1583
Urinary tract trauma, 514-535
  bladder injuries in, 519-526, 521f-526f
  clinical features of, 515
  Foley catheter placement in, 515, 517, 518f
  in pelvic fracture, 719
  penile injuries in, 532-534, 532f-534f
  renal injuries in, 526-530, 527f, 529f-530f
  testicular injuries in, 534-535, 535f
  ureteral injuries in, 530-531, 531f-532f
  urethral injuries in, 515-519, 516f-520f
Urine collection methods, 1575
  in children, 1584, 2642-2643
Urine culture
  in epididymitis, 2639
  in pediatric fever, 2509-2510
  in urinary tract infection, 1576-1577, 1577b
Urine dipstick tests, in urinary tract infection, 1575-1576

Urine microscopy, in urinary tract infection, 1576
Urine output, 1525
Urine protein/creatinine ratio, in proteinuria, 2647
Urine test
    for PCP, 2415
    in nausea and vomiting, 203
Urokinase
    for occluded catheters, 1362b
    in frostbite, 2233
    in pulmonary embolism, 1378t
Urolithiasis, 1586-1593
    clinical features of, 1588
    diagnosis of, 1588-1590
    differential considerations in, 1590-1591, 1593b
    epidemiology of, 1586-1587, 1586b
    imaging of, 1589-1590, 1589f-1592f
    laboratory tests in, 1588-1589
    management of, 1591-1593, 1593b
    pathophysiology of, 1587, 1588f
    risk factors for, 1586b, 1587
    types of, 1587
Urologic disorders, 1524-1604. See also specific disorders, e.g., Renal failure.
Urologic examination, 1572-1573, 1573f
Uropathogens, in urinary tract infection, 1574-1575
Urticaria, 1834, 1834f, 1835
    causes of, 1865t
    drug-induced, 1844-1845, 1844f, 1846t-1847t
    in anaphylaxis, 1825t, 2547
    internal malignancy associated with, 1864
    skin lesions in, 1847-1848, 1848f
    transfusion-related, 60
Urticaria pigmentosa, 1835
Uterine activity, measurement of, 2800
Uterine atony
    postpartum hemorrhage from, 2818
    vaginal bleeding in, 258
Uterine contractions, in maternal trauma, 320
Uterine curettage, after miscarriage, 2742
Uterine exploration, and placental removal, for postpartum hemorrhage, 2819
Uterine inversion, 2820
Uterine packing, for postpartum hemorrhage, 2819
Uterine rupture, 2820
    in maternal trauma, 320
    vaginal bleeding in, 257, 257t
Uterine size, gestational age and, 323, 323f, 2728
Uterine soufflé, 2728
Uterus, in pregnancy, 317, 2723
Uveitis, anterior, 287, 287f, 289, 295t
Uvular deviation, in peritonsillitis, 1117, 1118f

Vaccine. See also Immunization.
    anthrax, 3026
    BCG, 2170-2171, 2170b
    diphtheria, 2002, 2004, 2012, 2012t
    Haemophilus influenzae, 1723
    hepatitis A, 2035t
    hepatitis B, 1406, 2035t
    influenza, 2055
    influenza A and B, 2035t
    Japanese encephalitis virus, 1723
    Lyme disease, 2126-2127
    measles, 2035t, 2053
    meningococcal, 1723, 2024
    mumps, 2035t
    pertussis, 2005, 2007
    pneumococcal, 1129, 1723, 2017, 2019-2020, 2020b
    polio, 2035t, 2056-2057
    rabies, 2035t, 2068, 2068b
    rubella, 2035t, 2048-2049
    smallpox, 2035t, 3029
    tetanus, 856-857, 857t, 2008, 2011-2012, 2012t, 2013t
    varicella, 1859, 2035t, 2043
    yellow fever, 2035t
Vaccine Information Statement (VIS), 925-926
Vaccinia virus, 2040
Vacuum device, for anorectal foreign body removal, 876, 876f
Vagal maneuvers, for supraventricular tachycardia, 2588

Vagal nerve stimulation, for seizures in developmentally disabled patient, 2899
Vagina
    foreign body in, 877-878
    in pregnancy, 2723
    tear of, postpartum hemorrhage from, 2818-2819
Vaginal birth after cesarean section, 2820
Vaginal bleeding, 254-259
    ancillary studies in, 256-257, 256t
    diagnostic approach to, 254-257, 255t, 256t
    differential diagnosis in, 255t, 257, 257t-258t
    disposition in, 259
    empiric management of, 257, 259, 259f, 260f
    epidemiology of, 254
    history in, 255-256
    in ectopic pregnancy, 2743
    in pelvic fracture, 720
    in pregnancy, 2727
        differential diagnosis in, 2753t
        during second half, 2747-2748
        epidemiology of, 254
        first-trimester, 2740-2741, 2746f
        pathophysiology of, 254
        third-trimester, 2808-2810
        treatment of, 257, 259
    pathophysiology of, 254
    pelvic pain associated with, 249
    physical examination in, 256, 256t
    rapid assessment and stabilization in, 254-255
Vaginal breech delivery, 2813, 2813b
Vaginal examination
    in genitourinary trauma, 515
    in pelvic fracture, 719
    in sexual assault victim, 987-988, 987b
Vaginitis
    atrophic, 1569
    chemical, 1569
    dysuria in, 1580
    in pregnancy, 2758
Vaginosis, bacterial, 1567t, 1568-1569, 2758
Vagus nerve, 1665t
Valacyclovir
    for genital herpes, 1557t, 1559, 1858
    for herpes simplex esophagitis, 1387
    for herpes simplex virus infection, 2042
    indications for, 2038
    prophylactic, in monkey bites, 888, 889t
Valerian, adverse effects of, 2476t
Valgus displacement of fracture, 552, 553f
Validity of study, 3059, 3059t
Valproic acid
    during pregnancy and lactation, 2786-2787
    for bipolar disorder, 1742
    for seizure, 1627, 1627t, 1628t, 2675, 2675t
    for status epilepticus, 2672t, 2673
    overdose of, antidotes to, 2329t
    side effects of, 1628t
Valsalva maneuver, for dysrhythmias, 1214
Valsartan, 1322t
Values
    religious, 3129-3130, 3130b
    societal and bioethical, 3129, 3129b
Valve replacement
    for aortic regurgitation, 1307
    for aortic stenosis, 1306-1307
Valvular heart disease, 1304-1308. See also specific types, e.g., Aortic stenosis.
    heart failure in, 1265, 1268
    in children, 2517
    in pregnancy, 2763t, 2767
Valvular injuries, traumatic, 472
Vancomycin
    for Clostridium difficile enterocolitis, 1475
    for febrile, neutropenic cancer patient, 2838, 2838t
    for febrile cancer patient, 1909
    for pediatric fever, 2514
    for peritonitis in dialysis patient, 1552, 1553t
    for pneumococcal disease, 2019
Vapor-permeable dressings, in wound management, 855
Varicella, 2042-2043, 2042f
    in children, screening for, 2509b
    skin lesions in, 1858-1859, 1859f
    smallpox vs., 1860, 1860t, 1861f, 3029
Varicella vaccine, 1859, 2035t, 2043
Varicella-zoster virus, 2042-2043, 2042f. See also Herpes zoster.
    drugs for, 2037t

Varicella-zoster virus (Continued)
    in cancer patient with impaired cell-mediated immunity, 2840
    in HIV/AIDS, 2085
    in organ transplant patient, 2848
    in pneumonia, 1130
Varicocele, 2641
Variola virus, 3028
Varus displacement of fracture, 552, 553f
Vasa previa, 257, 257t, 2810
Vascular access
    during cardiopulmonary resuscitation, 91-92
    in adult resuscitation, 91-92
    in hemodialysis, problems related to, 1364-1366, 1549-1550
    in multiple trauma, 307
    in neonatal resuscitation, 123
    in pediatric resuscitation, 99, 99f
    in procedural sedation and analgesia, 2942
    in shock, 50
Vascular dementia, 1656, 1657, 1659
Vascular disorders
    abdominal aortic aneurysm in, 1330-1340
    aortic dissection in, 1324-1329
    cyanosis in, 273
    differential diagnosis in, 1896, 1896b
    hypertension in, 1310-1322
    peripheral, 1342-1366. See also Peripheral arteriovascular disease.
    pulmonary embolism and venous thrombosis in, 1368-1381
Vascular endothelial cells, in hemostasis, 1892, 1893f
Vascular injury
    hard vs. soft findings of, 539
    high-risk, 540, 540f
    in electrical and lightning injuries, 2271, 2273
    in foot trauma, 838
    in hand trauma, 613-614
    in hip trauma, 762
    in spinal injuries, 413, 415f
    in tibial femoral knee dislocation, 787, 788, 789
    major, 544
    minor, 544
    peripheral, 536-547
        clinical features of, 539-541, 540f
        diagnostic strategies in, 541-543
        disposition in, 547
        epidemiology of, 536-537
        of lower extremity, 546-547
        of upper extremity, 544-546
        pathophysiology of, 537-539, 538f
        treatment of, 543-544
    to neck, 448-450
Vascular ring, 2527-2528, 2528f
Vascular shunt, in arterial injury, 544
Vascular steal, in arteriovenous fistula or graft, 1366
Vascular supply. See Blood supply.
Vascular theory of headache, 2676
Vascular ulcer, in diabetes mellitus, 1863f
Vasculitis, 1812-1817
    central nervous system, seizure in, 1624
    classification of, 1812b
    drug-induced, 1844-1845, 1846t
    granulomatous, 1814
    hypersensitivity, 1815-1817
    in Kawasaki disease, 2025
    in systemic lupus erythematosus, 1807, 1808
    large vessel, 1813
    medium vessel, 1813-1815
    mononeuropathy multiplex in, 1699
    pathophysiology of, 1344, 1812-1813
    small vessel, 1815-1817
Vasoconstriction, cold-induced, 2228
Vasodilation
    heat loss through, 2255
    in sepsis, 2213
Vasodilators, 1321t
Vasogenic cerebral edema
    after head trauma, 354
    in high-altitude cerebral edema, 2299-2300, 2306, 2306f
Vaso-occlusive crisis, in sickle cell disease, 1880
Vasopressin. See Antidiuretic hormone.
Vasopressors
    for anaphylaxis, 1833
    for cardiac arrest, 92

Vasopressors (Continued)
for sepsis, 2219-2220, 2219t
for septic shock, 53
for toxic shock syndrome, 2030
for ventricular fibrillation and pulseless
ventricular tachycardia, 84
Vasospasm
cerebral, in traumatic subarachnoid
hemorrhage, 377
coronary, in acute coronary syndromes, 1157
Vasospastic disorders, 1344, 1347, 1357
Vater's ampulla carcinoma, 1423
Vault fracture of skull, 373
VDRL (Venereal Disease Research Laboratory)
test, in syphilis, 1856
Vecuronium
for tetanus, 2011
in intubated, mechanically ventilated patient,
31
in rapid sequence intubation, 14-15, 15t
Vegetation, in infective endocarditis, 1301, 1302
Vegetative state, 156
Vegetative symptoms, in depression, 1737
Vein graft, for peripheral arteriovascular disease,
1350
Velpeau bandage, 569
Vena caval interruption, in pulmonary embolism,
1377
Venereal Disease Research Laboratory test, in
syphilis, 1856
Venlafaxine, overdose of, 2362, 2362t
Venography
in cerebral venous thrombosis, 1670
in deep venous thrombosis, 1369
in pulmonary embolism, 1377
in thoracic outlet syndrome, 1360
Venomous animal injuries, 894-911
arthropods in, 903-908
epidemiology of, 894-895, 895t
hymenoptera in, 903-905
allergy to, 1827, 2547
rhabdomyolysis from, 1979
marine animals in, 908-911
scorpions in, 907-908
snakes and other reptiles in, 895-903, 897f,
897t, 900t
spiders in, 905-907
venom delivery in, 895
Venous access
in adult resuscitation, 91-92
in pediatric resuscitation, 99
Venous admixture, in pulmonary embolism, 1372
Venous air embolism, in neck trauma, 444, 450
Venous catheterization, postresuscitation, 87
Venous hypertension
from arteriovenous fistula or graft, 1366
in superior vena cava syndrome, 1910
Venous injuries, 544
Venous insufficiency, chronic, lower extremity
ulcers in, 1351
Venous pressure, in pregnancy, 2725, 2726f
Venous system
of femur and hip, 737, 737t
of hand, 586
of pubis, 718
Venous thrombosis, 1368-1371. See also
Pulmonary embolism.
anatomy in, 1368-1369
cerebral, 1670-1671
clinical presentation in, 1369
complications of, 1370-1371
diagnosis of, 1369-1370, 1369t
differential diagnosis in, 1369b
in pregnancy, 2733, 2756-2757
in spinal cord injury, 2906-2907
mesenteric, 1446, 1446b
observation in, 3065-3066
of upper extremity, 1370
pretest probability of, 1369, 1369t
proximal vs. distal, 1369
septic, catheter-related, 1363
treatment of, 1370
Venovenous rewarming, 2250t, 2251
VENTIDC mnemonic, in central nervous system
oxygen toxicity, 2283
Ventilation
assisted. See Ventilatory support.
differential lung, in pulmonary contusion,
461

Ventilation (Continued)
failure of, as indication for intubation, 2-3
mechanical. See Mechanical ventilation.
minute
carbon dioxide arterial pressure and, 1923
during acclimatization to high altitude, 2297-
2298
in metabolic acidosis, 1929
transtracheal jet, needle cricothyrotomy with,
22, 22f
Ventilation-perfusion inequality, in pulmonary
embolism, 1372
Ventilation-perfusion scan, in pulmonary
embolism, 1375, 1376t
Ventilatory support, 26-33. See also Airway
management; Intubation
after brain resuscitation, 68
basic approaches to, 26-27
evolving therapies in, 33
in acute respiratory distress syndrome, 1141
in adult resuscitation, 87
in asthma, 1092-1093
in chronic obstructive pulmonary disease,
1103-1105, 1103t-1105t
in flail chest, 458
in multiple trauma, 306
in neonatal resuscitation, 122-123
in pediatric resuscitation, 108-109
in pediatric trauma, 329-330, 332t
in pregnant trauma patient, 322
in shock, 51-52
initial settings and ongoing monitoring in, 29-
30, 29t
invasive, 27-28. See also Mechanical
ventilation.
noninvasive, 28-29, 28f
evolving therapies in, 33
in asthma, 1091-1092
in chronic obstructive pulmonary disease,
1104, 1104t
initial settings and ongoing monitoring in,
29-30, 29t
outcomes in, 32-33
patient management in, 31
patient selection for, 29
outcomes in, 32-33
patient management in, 30-31
special clinical circumstances in, 31-32
Ventricle
penetrating injury to, 472
rupture of, 470-472
Ventricular assist device, for chronic heart
failure, 1277
Ventricular bigemy, 1222, 1222f
Ventricular contractility abnormalities, in dilated
cardiomyopathy, 1294
Ventricular dysrhythmias
in beta blocker overdose, 2375
in chlorinated hydrocarbon poisoning, 2463
in myocardial contusion, 469
Ventricular fibrillation
in hypothermia, 2238, 2246
in infants and children, 112-113, 112f, 2586t,
2590
treatment of, 84, 112-113, 112f
Ventricular paced rhythms, ST segment elevation
in, 1169, 1171f
Ventricular pacemaker, ICDs as, 1255
Ventricular parasystole, 1226, 1226b, 1226f
Ventricular septal defect, in infants and children,
2577
Ventricular tachycardia, 1240-1243, 1241f-1243f
bidirectional (alternating), 1241, 1243f
electrocardiography in, 1238-1239, 1241f-
1243f
in infants and children, 2586t, 2589-2590
monomorphic, 1240-1241, 1242f
polymorphic, 1241, 1243-1244, 1243f
pulseless, in infants and children, 2586t, 2590
sustained vs. nonsustained, 1240
vs. supraventricular tachycardia with abnormal
conduction, 1237-1239, 1238t, 1239f, 1240f
Ventriculoperitoneal shunt, pediatric fever in,
2517
Verapamil, 1210-1211, 1321t
during pregnancy and lactation, 2788
for atrial flutter, 1229
for dysphagia, 1398
for hypertrophic cardiomyopathy, 1295

Verapamil (Continued)
overdose of, 2376, 2377t
side effects of, 1210-1211
Verbal management techniques, for combative
patient, 2958
Vertebrae, 399, 400f
Vertebral artery
dissection of
ataxia in, 2681
headache in, 1638-1639
injury to, 448
occlusion of, spinal cord syndromes from, 420,
420f
stroke involving, 1607, 1609-1610
Vertebral body
compression fracture of, 553, 555f
tumor of, spinal cord compression in, 1919
Vertebral column. See Spinal column.
Vertebral osteomyelitis, 261, 265t, 2159, 2178,
2182, 2182f, 2184-2185
Vertebrobasilar arterial injuries, 448
Vertebrobasilar insufficiency, 146, 147t
Vertebrobasilar migraine, 148t
Vertical body burst fracture, 411-412, 411f-413f,
426, 427f
Vertical compression injuries of spinal cord, 411-
413, 411f-414f
Vertical mattress suture, 850
Vertical shear pelvic fracture, 727, 730f
Vertigo, 142-149
alternobaric, in scuba diving–related disorders,
2286, 2287t
benign paroxysmal positional, 147t, 2683
causes of, 143b
diagnostic approach to, 143-146, 143b, 143t,
145b, 145t, 148f
differential diagnosis in, 143, 143b, 143t, 146,
147t-148t
disposition in, 146, 149
hearing loss and, 144, 2684b, 2684f
management of, 146, 149f
pathophysiology of, 142-143
pediatric, 2682-2685, 2683b, 2684b, 2684f
Very important persons (VIPs), 2978t, 2980
Vesical calculus, 1593
Vesicants, as chemical weapons, 938-939, 3031
Vesicoureteral reflux, 1574
Vesicular lesions, 1839t, 1857-1860
Vesicular stomatitis, 2054
Vestibular apparatus, 142
cold water testing of, in comatose patient, 161,
162f
Vestibular neuronitis, 147t, 2683
Vestibular system, 142-143
Vestibule, 384
Vestibule cardiopulmonary resuscitation, 89
Vestibulocochlear nerve, 1665t
Veterans Affairs, 3018-3019
Vibration stress, during air medical transport,
2995
Vibrio fish poisoning, 1470t, 1471-1472
Vibrio gastroenteritis, 2626
Vibrio parahaemolyticus
dysenteric colitis in, 229t
gastroenteritis in, 1461t, 1462t, 1465-1466
Vicryl suture, 852t
Victim identification, in physical assault, 960
Vidarabine, 2038
Video and rigid fiberoptic laryngoscopy, 21, 22f
Videoesophagram, in dysphagia, 1397
Vigabatrin, for infantile spasms, 2666
Villous adenoma, 1938
Vincent's angina, 1033, 1111-1112, 1113
Violation producing factors, as source of failures
in emergency department, 3121, 3121t
Violence. See also Abuse; Combative patient.
differential considerations in, 2964-2965, 2965b
functional vs. organic etiology of, 2963, 2964t
in PCP intoxication, 2414, 2415-2416, 2891,
2892
intimate partner. See Intimate partner violence
and abuse.
barriers to diagnosis of, 998
clinical features of, 996-998
definitions of, 995, 995t
disposition in, 1004-1005, 1005b
documentation of, 1000-1001, 1003-1004
during pregnancy, 997, 2734-2735, 2734t
epidemiology of, 995-996

Violence (Continued)
  improving emergency department response
    to victims of, 1005-1006
  legal considerations in, 1004-1005
  referral in, 1004
  risk assessment in, 1000, 1002b, 1003b
  risk factors for injury related to, 996
  screening for, 998-999, 999b, 1000f, 1001f,
    1002b
  use of emergency department in, 996
  validation of patient's experience in, 999-
    1000
  media, 1018
  pathogenesis of, 2957
  reporting requirements for, 3172
  sexual. See Sexual abuse; Sexual assault.
  suicide and, 1768
  youth, 1017-1022
    drug abuse and, 1018
    firearms and, 1018-1019
    in schools, 1017-1018
    prevention strategies for, 1019-1020, 1021-
      1022
    street gangs and, 1017-1018, 1020-1022
Viral detecting testing, for HIV, 2074
Viral infection, 2033-2058
  antiviral chemotherapy for, 2035-2039, 2036t-
    2037t
  classification of, 2033, 2034t
  DNA, 2034t, 2039-2046
  exanthems in, 1849
  immunization for, 2033-2034, 2035t
  in acute gastroenteritis, 1475-1476, 2624-2625
  in arthritis, 1788
  in cancer patient with impaired cell-mediated
    immunity, 2840
  in conjunctivitis, 297t
  in COPD exacerbation, 1099
  in croup, 2525-2527, 2526f, 2527b, 2529t
  in diarrhea, 228, 230b
  in encephalitis. See Encephalitis, viral.
  in esophagitis, 1386, 1387
  in febrile cancer patient, 1908
  in hepatitis, 1402-1406, 1403f, 1403t, 1405t,
    1407t, 1408f
  in HIV/AIDS. See HIV/AIDS.
  in laryngotracheobronchitis, 2525-2527, 2526f,
    2527b
  in meningitis. See Meningitis, viral.
  in otitis media, 1066
  in pancreatitis, 1428
  in pharyngitis, 274, 275t, 1109
  in pneumonia, 1129, 1130, 1139, 2555, 2557-
    2560, 2563t
  in sinusitis, 1123
  pediatric hyperpyrexia in, 2506
  risk of, blood transfusions and, 57t, 61
  RNA, 2034t, 2046-2058
  unclassified, 2058
  urticaria in, 1848
Viral vaccines, 2033, 2035t
Visceral aneurysm, 1355-1356
Visceral bias, 3122
Visceral injuries, in pelvic fracture, 719
Visceral larva migrans, 2103t, 2109, 2110
Visceral pain, 209, 211
Viscosity, of hydrocarbons, 2428
Viscus, perforated, abdominal pain in, 215t
Visual acuity assessment, in red and painful eye,
  285-286
Visual agnosia, in ischemic stroke, 1609
Visual Analogue Pain Scale, 2917b
Visual disturbance
  in botulism, 2014
  in ethylene glycol poisoning, 2399
  in hyperviscosity syndrome, 1912
  in methanol poisoning, 2396
  in parasitic infection, 2109-2110
Visual field testing, in red and painful eye, 286
Visual loss. See also Blindness.
  acute, 1056-1061, 1057f-1059f
  chiasmal, 1060
  functional, 1060-1061
  in central retinal artery occlusion, 1057, 1057f
  in central retinal vein occlusion, 1057, 1057f
  in macular disorders, 1059, 1059f
  in methanol poisoning, 2395, 2396
  in multiple sclerosis, 2910
  in posterior vitreous detachment, 1058

Visual loss (Continued)
  in retinal breaks and detachments, 1057-1058
  in vitreous hemorrhage, 1058-1059
  neuroophthalmologic, 1059-1061
  postchiasmal, 1060
  prechiasmal, 1059
Visually impaired patient, 2905
Vital signs
  in abdominal pain, 213
  in asthma, 2534, 2535t
  in back pain, 262-263
  in chest pain, 187t
  in comatose patient, 159, 159t
  in cyanosis, 269
  in dyspnea, 178t
  in gastrointestinal bleeding, 222
  in headache, 172t
  in infants and children, 2495, 2495t, 2571, 2571t
  in nausea and vomiting, 202, 202t
  in newborn, 119t
  in overdosed/poisoned patient, 2326
  in pancreatitis, 1429
  in pelvic pain, 250t
  in pregnancy, 2727-2728
  in seizure, 167
  in syncope, 195t
  in vaginal bleeding, 256t
  in vertigo, 144
  monitoring of
    during procedural sedation and analgesia,
      2943
    in multiple trauma, 304
    toxic syndromes and, 2964t
Vitamin A intoxication, hypercalcemia from,
  1945
Vitamin B deficiency, causes of, 1874b
Vitamin B12 deficiency, megaloblastic anemia
  from, 1873-1875, 1874f, 1874t, 1875t
Vitamin C, for complex regional pain syndrome,
  563
Vitamin D
  deficiency of, hypocalcemia in, 1942
  in calcium homeostasis, 1941-1942
  in phosphate homeostasis, 1950
Vitamin E
  for dementia, 1661
  for Peyronie's disease, 534
Vitamin K, for cholestasis, 1416-1417
Vitamin K-sensitive factors, 1892, 1893f, 1894
Vitamin supplementation, during pregnancy, 2736
Vitrectomy, 1050
Vitreous
  hemorrhage of, 1050, 1058-1059
  posterior detachment of, 1058
Vocal cord paralysis, 2524-2525
Volar compartment of forearm, 640, 640t
Volar extrinsic ligaments of wrist, 622, 624f
Volar intercalated segment instability (VISI), 631-
  632, 633f
Volar surface, of hand, 576, 577f
Volar tilt, of distal radius, 626, 626f
Volatility, of hydrocarbons, 2428
Voltage, electrical injury and, 2269, 2270
Volume
  depletion of. See Hypovolemia.
  excess of. See Hypervolemia.
  repletion of. See Fluid resuscitation.
Volume-cycled ventilation, 27
Volvulus
  cecal, 1497-1498, 1499, 1499f
  colonic, 1497-1499, 1498f, 1499b, 1499f
  gastric, 1394-1395
  midgut, malrotation with, 2606-2608, 2607f,
    2608f
  sigmoid, 1497, 1498, 1498f, 1499
  small bowel, 1441
Vomiting, 200-207
  after pediatric head trauma, 334
  ancillary studies in, 202-203
  chest pain associated with, 185, 186t
  definition of, 200
  differential considerations in, 201-202, 201t,
    203, 204t-206t, 207f
  disposition in, 207, 209
  epidemiology of, 200
  history in, 202
  hypokalemia from, 1938
  in abdominal aortic aneurysm rupture, 1333
  in abdominal trauma, 493

Vomiting (Continued)
  in Aeromonas hydrophila gastroenteritis, 1467
  in appendicitis, 2619
  in asthma, 2536
  in Bacillus anthracis gastroenteritis, 1469
  in Bacillus cereus food poisoning, 1471
  in bacterial meningitis, 2659
  in cholecystitis, 1420
  in cholelithiasis, 1418
  in chronic renal failure, 1542
  in ciguatera fish poisoning, 1473
  in Escherichia coli food poisoning, 1474
  in esophagitis, 1387
  in gastric volvulus, 1394
  in gastritis, 1391
  in gastroesophageal reflux, 2610
  in hemorrhagic Escherichia coli serotype
    O157:H7 gastroenteritis, 1467
  in hypertrophic pyloric stenosis, 2604-2605
  in infants and children, 203, 206, 208t, 2605,
    2606t, 2627t, 2628b
  in intracerebral hemorrhage, 1610
  in intussusception, 2610
  in large bowel obstruction, 1496
  in malrotation with midgut volvulus, 2606
  in necrotizing enterocolitis, 2608
  in opioid overdose, 2453
  in pancreatitis, 1429
  in Plesiomonas shigelloides gastroenteritis,
    1468
  in pneumonia, 2556
  in pregnancy, 204t, 206, 2756
  in salmonellosis, 1463
  in small bowel obstruction, 1442
  in staphylococcal food poisoning, 1470
  in urolithiasis, 1588
  in Vibrio fish poisoning, 1472
  in Vibrio parahaemolyticus gastroenteritis,
    1466
  in viral gastroenteritis, 1476
  management of, 203, 206, 207f, 208b, 208t
  metabolic alkalosis from, 1930
  of blood, 221
  palliative care for, 3153-3154
  parental instruction sheet for, 2628b
  pathophysiology of, 200-201, 201f
  physical examination in, 202, 202t
  rapid assessment and stabilization in, 201t,
    202
  sequelae of, 201-202
Vomiting center, 200, 201f
Vomitus, content of, 202
Von Willebrand's disease, 1898, 1902-1903
Vulvar tears, postpartum hemorrhage from, 2818-
  2819
Vulvovaginal candidiasis, 1567t, 1568
Vulvovaginitis, 1567-1569, 1567t
VX, 2461, 3030-3031, 3030b, 3031b
V-Y wound closure, 851

Waiting times in emergency department, violent
  behavior and, 2966
Waldenstrom's macroglobulinemia,
  hyperviscosity syndrome in, 1912
Waldvogel classification of osteomyelitis, 2174
Wall motion abnormalities, 1179
Wallenberg's syndrome, 147t
War, role of informatics in, 3105
Warfarin
  during pregnancy and lactation, 2785-2786
  for acute mesenteric ischemia, 1449
  for deep venous thrombosis, 1370
Warm ischemia, in peripheral vascular injury,
  537
Warm-reacting antibodies, in autoimmune
  hemolytic anemia, 1883
Warts
  genital, 1518t, 1519-1520, 1563-1564, 1564f,
    2045
  laryngeal, 2045
WASH regimen
  for anal fissures, 1513
  for hemorrhoids, 1511, 1511b
Wasp stings. See Hymenoptera stings.
Water balance, regulation of, 1933
Water brash, in gastroesophageal reflux, 1388
Water deficit, calculation of, 1937

Water depletion heat exhaustion, 2259
Water hemlock, 2472, 2472f
Water moccasins, 896
Water retention, in pregnancy, 2724
"Water-bottle" appearance of heart, 474, 475f
Water-hammer pulse, 1307
Waterhouse-Friderichsen syndrome, 2022
Water-soluble contrast enema
    in diverticular disease, 1494
    in large bowel obstruction, 1496-1497
Weakness, 138-141. See also Palsy; Paralysis.
    acute, emergent, causes of, 1689b
    definitive management of, 141
    diagnostic approach to, 138-139, 139f, 139t,
        140b, 140t
    differential diagnosis in, 138, 139t, 140, 140b
    disposition in, 141
    empiric management of, 140-141, 141b
    epidemiology of, 138
    in botulism, 2014
    in rhabdomyolysis, 1979
    in toluene abuse, 2888
    neuromuscular disorders and, 139, 139t, 140b,
        1702-1709
    neuropathies and, 1687-1701
    pathophysiology of, 138
    shoulder, 674
Weapon searches, in emergency department, 2966
Weapons of mass destruction, 3021-3032
    anthrax and, 3021, 3024-3026, 3025f, 3026b,
        3026f
    biologic, 3023-3029, 3024b
    chemical, 937-939, 938t, 3029-3032, 3030b,
        3031b
    disaster preparedness for, 3017-3018
    likely candidates for use in, 3022b
    nuclear, 2316, 3022
    plague and, 3027-3028, 3027f, 3028b
    planning and response to events involving,
        resources and contact for, 3022b
    radiologic, 3022-3023, 3023t
    smallpox and, 3028-3029, 3028f, 3029f
    threat of, features of, 3022b
Web Bulb Globe Thermometer index, 2257
Wedge fracture, of cervical spine, 401, 402f
Wegener's granulomatosis, 1035, 1814
Weight gain
    during pregnancy, 2724, 2736
    in hypothyroidism, 1991
Weight loss
    in hyperthyroidism, 1986
    in inflammatory bowel disease, 1501
    in intestinal amebiasis, 1480
    in pancreatic carcinoma, 1437
    products for, misidentification of plant used in,
        2476
Wellens criteria, 1237, 1238t
Wellen's syndrome, 1163
Wellness strategies for emergency physician,
    3176-3178, 3176b, 3177b
Wenckebach phenomenon
    in atrioventricular block, 1218-1219, 1218t,
        1219b, 1220f
    in other conduction disorders, 1219
Wernicke-Korsakoff syndrome, 2869
Wernicke's aphasia, 1609
West Nile virus, 2049-2050
West syndrome, 2665-2666
Western blot assay
    for HIV, 2073-2074
    for Lyme disease, 2125
Western medicine, role expectations in, 3115-
    3116
Wharton's ducts, 385-386
Wharton's jelly, 2805
Wheal, 1839t
Wheezing
    in airway foreign body aspiration, 865, 866
    in asthma, 1081, 1083, 1084, 2532-2533, 2537
    in bronchiolitis, 2545
    in pediatric assessment, 2498
    in pneumonia, 2556
Whiplash, 2684-2685
Whipworm infestation, 2107
Whirlpool hydrotherapy, for frostbite, 2234
White blood cell casts, in urinary sediment,
    1526, 1526f
White blood cell count
    agents and conditions that elevate, 1889b

White blood cell count (Continued)
    decreased, 52, 1888-1889, 1889f
    in abdominal trauma, 495
    in alcoholism, 2874
    in asthma, 1085
    in back pain, 707
    in bacterial meningitis, 2661-2662, 2661t
    in diarrhea, 233
    in hypothermia, 2243
    in osteomyelitis, 2179
    in pediatric bacteremia, 2506
    in pediatric fever, 2508-2509, 2513
    in pertussis, 2006
    in pneumonia, 1134, 2560-2561
    in pregnancy, 318
    in septic arthritis, 2189, 2705
    in transient synovitis, 2703
    increased. See Leukocytosis.
    normal values for, 1886t
    peritoneal lavage, 501
    rationale for selection of, 1889
White blood cell differential count
    normal values for, 1886t
    rationale for selection of, 1889
White blood cell disorders, 1886-1889. See also
        specific disorder, e.g., Eosinophilia.
    abnormal values in, 1887
    in alcoholic hepatitis, 1409
    normal values and influences in, 1886-1887,
        1886t
    physiology and pathophysiology of, 1886
White phosphorus, thermal burn from, 936
White-white tears, meniscal, 792
Whole blood
    anaphylactic-type reactions to, 1827
    transfusion of, 58
Whole-body irradiation, acute radiation
        syndrome after, 2317t, 2321-2322, 2321f
Whole-bowel irrigation
    in beta blocker overdose, 2374
    in cocaine body packing/stuffing, 2391
    in iron overdose, 2420
    in lithium toxicity, 2444
    in opioid overdose, 2455
    in overdosed/poisoned patient, 2330
Whooping cough, 2004-2007, 2005f, 2006b, 2559-
        2560
Wide-complex tachycardia, 1237-1244
    adenosine-induced, 2588, 2589f
    differential diagnosis in, 1237-1239, 1238t,
        1239f, 1240f
    in cocaine overdose, 2390
    in infants and children, 2586, 2587f
    torsades de pointes as, 1243-1244, 1243f, 1244b
    treatment of, 1239-1240
    ventricular tachycardia as, 1240-1243, 1241-
        1243f
Wilcoxon rank sum test, 3052, 3052t, 3053
Wilcoxon signed rank test, 3053
Wild animal bite, 885
Will, living, 3133
Winterbottom's sign, in African trypanosomiasis,
    2106
Wire suture, 852t
Withdrawal
    anxiety in, 1748
    from alcohol, 2860-2863
        clinical features of, 2860-2861
        differential considerations in, 2860
        disposition in, 2879
        hypertension in, 1314
        management of, 2861-2863
        pathophysiology of, 2860
        seizure in, 1623, 2863
    from barbiturates, 2482
    from benzodiazepines, 2486, 2486b
    from GHB, 2490
    from opioids, 2451-2456
        clinical features of, 2454
        diagnosis of, 2454
        differential diagnosis in, 2454
        disposition in, 2455
        management of, 2455-2456
        pathophysiology and pharmacology of, 2452
        seizure in, 2670
Withholding and withdrawing treatment,
        bioethical dilemmas in, 3132
Wolff-Parkinson-White syndrome, 1235-1237,
        1235b, 1236f, 1237f, 2589

Wood distillates, toxicity of, 2429t
Woodruff, adverse effects of, 2476t
Wood's corkscrew maneuver, for shoulder
        dystocia, 2815
Wood's lamp, in sexual assault examination, 985,
        985b
Word catheter, for Bartholin abscess, 1560
Word salad, in schizophrenia, 1728
Workers' compensation, 3077-3078
Work-related injuries/illness. See Occupational
        medicine.
Wormwood, adverse effects of, 2476t
Wound
    assessment of, in thermal burns, 919-920, 920f
    cleansing of, 847-848, 848t
    closure of, 849-854
        decision making in, 849
        in animal bites, 886-887, 887t
        materials in, 851-854, 852t
        suture technique in, 849-851
        wound tension considerations in, 849
    contraction of, skin tension lines and, 843,
        843f, 844f
    debridement of, 847
    healing of, phases in, 842-843
    infection of
        in animal bites, 883-884, 885-886, 885t
        risk factors for, 844-845, 844b
    irrigation of, 848
    microscopic examination of, in forensic
        emergency medicine, 960
    radioactive contamination of, 2321
    tetanus-prone, 2008
Wound ballistics, handgun, 954-955
Wound botulism, 2013, 2014, 2015
Wound management, 842-857
    anesthesia in, 845-847
    antibiotic prophylaxis in, 854-855
    biomechanical properties of skin and, 843
    burn, 924-927, 925f
    clinical features and diagnostic strategies in,
        843-845
    disposition in, 855-857, 856b, 857b
    drains, dressings, and immobilization in, 855
    foreign body assessment in, 845, 878
    history taking in, 843
    in animal bites, 886-889, 886b, 887t
    in electrical and lightning injuries, 2276
    in facial trauma, 390-391
    in fingertip amputation, 610
    in human bites, 891-892, 891t
    in rabies, 2068, 2068b
    in radiation exposure, 2323
    in snakebite, 902
    physical examination in, 845
    skin preparation in, 847
    tetanus prophylaxis in, 856-857, 857b, 2012,
        2013t
Wrist
    anatomy of, 622, 623f-625f
    as link mechanism, 632f
    examination of, in arthritis, 1778
    tendinopathy of, 1799
Wrist flexion test, 639, 639f
Wrist splint, 569, 569f
Wrist trauma, 622-639
    carpal injuries in, 627-632, 628f, 630f-633f
    clinical features of, 622, 625
    distal radius and ulna injuries in, 632-639,
        634f-638f
    radiography in, 625-627, 626f-628f, 628t
    soft tissue injuries in, 639, 639f
Wristdrop, 586, 588f
    humeral shaft fracture and, 655
    in radial mononeuropathy, 1695

Xanthochromia, in subarachnoid hemorrhage,
        1636-1637, 1718
Xanthoma diabeticorum, 1972
Xerosis, in HIV/AIDS, 2084-2085

Yarrow, adverse effects of, 2476t
Yellow fever, 2035t, 2049-2050
Yellow jacket stings. See Hymenoptera stings.
Yellow-bellied sea snake envenomation, 901

Yergason's test
    in bicipital tendinopathy, 1797
    in bicipital tenosynovitis, 697, 697f
Yersinia enterocolitica
    in dysenteric colitis, 229t
    in gastroenteritis, 1461t, 1462t, 1465, 2625
Yew trees, 2475, 2475f
Yohimbine
    adverse effects of, 2476t
    drug interactions with, 2478t
Youth violence, 1017-1022

Zafirlukast
    for asthma, 1090
    for chronic asthma, 2542, 2543t

Zalcitabine, in HIV/AIDS, side effects of,
    2079t
Zaleplon, overdose of, 2486-2487
Zanamivir
    for influenza, 2055
    indications for, 2037-2038
Zebra fish envenomation, 910
Zidovudine
    for HIV/AIDS, 2087-2088
    side effects of, 2079t
Zieve's syndrome, 2874
Zileuton, for chronic asthma, 2542, 2543t
Zinc supplement therapy, in infectious diarrhea,
    2628
Ziprasidone
    for agitation in delirious patient, 1654

Ziprasidone *(Continued)*
    for mood disorders, 1741
    for psychosis in demented patient, 1662
    for rapid tranquilization, 2962
    for thought disorders, 1731
    toxicity of, 2446, 2446t
Zolendronate, for hypercalcemic cancer patient,
    1916
Zollinger-Ellison syndrome, peptic ulcer disease
    in, 1391
Zolmitriptan, for migraine, 2680
Zolpidem
    for insomnia in acute mountain sickness, 2302
    overdose of, 2486
Zoonotic infection, in pneumonia, 1131
Zygomatic fracture, 394

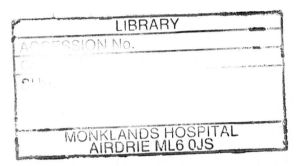